The SURGICAL WORD Book

Claudia Tessier, CAE, RHIA
Executive Director, Mobile Healthcare Alliance (MoHCA)
Co-chair, ASTME31 Continuity of Care Record Initiative
Consultant, Healthcare Documentation, Washington DC

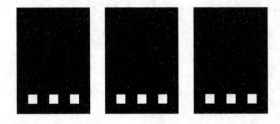

Third Edition

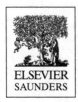

ELSEVIER
SAUNDERS

ELSEVIER
SAUNDERS

11830 Westline Industrial Drive
St. Louis, Missouri 63146

The Surgical Word Book, 3rd edition   0-7216-0020-4

ISBN-13: 978-0-7216-0020-8
ISBN-10: 0-7216-0020-4

Acquisitions Editor: *Susan Cole*
Associate Developmental Editor: *Lisa M. Neumann*
Publishing Services Manager: *Gayle May*
Project Manager: *Joseph Selby*
Designer: *Amy Buxton*

Printed in the United States of America

Last digit is the print number: 9   8   7   6   5   4

Acknowledgements

I am grateful to all who have contributed directly or indirectly to the preparation of this 3rd edition of *The Surgical Word Book*: Janel Heath for designing the database that facilitated its electronic preparation; Marge Parker, who assisted in data entry; Peggy Hughes, whose content knowledge and editorial expertise contributed significantly to proofreading and copyediting the manuscript; Jori Schultz, whose impressive data entry and proofreading talents provided great assistance in preparing this edition; and the Elsevier personnel for their expert assistance and guidance throughout its preparation, including not only those I can name, Susan Cole, Lisa Neumann, Joseph Selby, and Doug Anderson, but also the many others behind the scenes who helped to make this happen.

Notes about This Text

Surgical terminology, as well as my interest in it, continues to grow. This third edition of *The Surgical Word Book* is more than twice the size of the second edition, resulting in over 200,000 entries and close to 3000 categories.

Like previous editions, the 3rd edition of *The Surgical Word Book* (*SWB*) requires no table of contents or index. All entries are in alphabetical order for easy access. Its cross-indexed categories include surgical instruments and materials (for example, bandages, forceps, and retractors), as well as such topics as incisions, operations, and positions.

The cross-indexing feature is of particular value when you are uncertain of a spelling or when an eponym or other modifier is applied to the term in question. For example, you can find the entry "Tessier elevator" in alphabetical order under "T" as well as within the category "elevator." If you thought the spelling to be "Teffier," a quick check through the "T" entries under "elevator" would identify "Tessier" as the correct spelling. If the physician dictated "Tessier retractor," you would not find it under "retractor," but by checking the general alphabetical listings you would find "Tessier dislodger," "Tessier elevator," "Tessier operation," etc., and these other entries would support the use of the eponym with retractor as well. Cross-indexing encourages and helps you to explore alternative spellings and uses.

Category lists include only those entries that do not begin with the category term. Entries that begin with the category term are treated as separate entries and are alphabetized accordingly. Thus:

> roller
>> Devonshire roller
>> Unger adenoid pressure roller
> roller bandage
> roller dressing

Consistent with evolving medical transcription styles and practices, the possessive form with eponyms is used minimally in this text. I encourage you to adopt this usage as much as possible for consistency and clarity. Similarly, accent marks have generally been omitted; thus, Björk is presented as Bjork.

Hyphenation is minimized, but where used, such terms, including eponyms, are alphabetized as if they were one word. Thus,

> salpingolysis
> salpingo-oophorectomy
> salpingo-ovariolysis
> salpingopalatine fold

> *and*

> Sachs retractor
> Sachs vein retractor
> Sachs-Cushing retractor

Other punctuation marks (commas, virgules, periods) are ignored in alphabetizing, as are parenthetical entries.

Abbreviations are placed alphabetically as if the abbreviations themselves were words; meanings are given in parentheses. In addition, some expanded terms are followed by their abbreviations (in parentheses).

Plurals formed by standard English rules are not included. Those formed by Latin or Greek rules are noted in parentheses; many are cross-referenced.

> falces (*sing.* falx)
> falx (*pl.* falces)

An entry preceded by a numeral is placed at the beginning of the letter section the numeral would be in if the numeral were spelled out. Thus, "4-point fixation" is at the beginning of the Fs, along with "4-prong retractor," "4-quadrant biopsy," etc. For the most part I have used numerals rather than writing out numbers; when numbers are written out, they are in their appropriate alphabetical place.

In the interests of saving space in the 3rd edition, terms easily found in other references, such as Latin forms for arteries, muscles, nerves, tendons, and veins (i.e., arteriae, musculi, nervi, tendini, and venae), are omitted. For the same reason, terms such as "Rush clamp" are not included when expanded versions of such terms (e.g., "Rush bone clamp") are included.

I have sought again to make this a compact, easy-to-use, and comprehensive text at an affordable price. Intended primarily for medical transcriptionists, *The Surgical Word Book* will also be useful to teachers, managers, supervisors, students, coders, and other healthcare professionals.

Preparation of a fourth edition begins with the completion of this third edition. Should you identify additions, inaccuracies, or inconsistencies, please send them to me c/o Medical Transcription, Editorial, Elsevier, 11830 Westline Industrial Dr., St. Louis, MO 63146. Your suggestions will be welcomed.

Claudia Tessier, CAE, RHIA
Washington, D.C.
June 2004

abdominal aortic
   aneurysmectomy
abdominal aortic artery
abdominal aortic
   counterpulsation device
abdominal aortic
   endarterectomy
abdominal aortic plexus
abdominal aortogram
abdominal aponeurosis
abdominal approach
abdominal apron
abdominal axial subcutaneous
   pedicle flap
abdominal ballottement
abdominal bandage
abdominal binder
abdominal brace
abdominal brace position
abdominal bruit
abdominal canal
abdominal cardiac reflex
abdominal cavity
abdominal circumference
abdominal colectomy
abdominal colic
abdominal compartment
   syndrome
abdominal complication
abdominal contents
abdominal contouring
abdominal cramp
abdominal dermolipectomy
abdominal distention
abdominal domain
abdominal drainage
abdominal esophagus
abdominal evisceration
abdominal examination
abdominal exploration
abdominal external oblique
   muscle
abdominal fasciocutaneous flap
abdominal fat
abdominal fat pad
abdominal film
abdominal fissure
abdominal fistula
abdominal flaccidity
abdominal fluid collection
abdominal fluid wave
abdominal girth

abdominal guarding
abdominal gunshot wound
abdominal gutter
abdominal heart
abdominal hemorrhage
abdominal hernia
abdominal hydatid disease
abdominal hysterectomy
abdominal hysteropexy
abdominal hysterotomy
abdominal ileitis
abdominal imaging
abdominal impalement
abdominal incision
abdominal incision dehiscence
abdominal incisional hernia
abdominal internal oblique
   muscle
abdominal iron deposition
abdominal irradiation
abdominal kidney
abdominal lap pad
abdominal lavage
abdominal left ventricular assist
   device (ALVAD)
abdominal lipectomy
abdominal lymph node biopsy
abdominal malignancy
abdominal midline incisional
   hernioplasty
abdominal migraine
abdominal muscle deficiency
   syndrome
abdominal myomectomy
abdominal needle
abdominal nephrectomy
abdominal nephrotomy
abdominal ostium
abdominal pad
abdominal panniculus
abdominal pannus
abdominal paracentesis
abdominal patch electrode
abdominal peritoneum
abdominal pool
abdominal pregnancy
abdominal pressure
abdominal pressure technique
abdominal procedure
abdominal proctocolectomy
abdominal pull-through
   operation

abdominal pulse
abdominal rectopexy
abdominal reflex
abdominal reflux
abdominal region
abdominal reservoir
abdominal respiration
abdominal respiratory motion
abdominal retractor
abdominal rigidity
abdominal ring
abdominal ring retractor
abdominal sac
abdominal sacropexy
abdominal salpingo-
    oophorectomy
abdominal salpingotomy
abdominal scissors
abdominal scoop
abdominal sculpturing
abdominal section
abdominal sequela
abdominal situs inversus
abdominal space
abdominal splenectomy
abdominal stoma
abdominal stool
abdominal strain gauge
abdominal structure
abdominal surgery
abdominal surgery instrument set
abdominal tap
abdominal tenderness
Abdominal Trauma Index (ATI)
abdominal trocar
abdominal tumor
abdominal ultrasound
abdominal vagotomy
abdominal vascular accident
abdominal version
abdominal view
abdominal viscera
abdominal viscus
abdominal volume
abdominal wall
abdominal wall insufficiency
abdominal wall lifting
abdominal wall mass
abdominal wall mobility
abdominal wall reconstruction
abdominal wall
    rhabdomyosarcoma

abdominal wall venous pattern
abdominal wall zones (1-4)
abdominal washout
abdominal wound closure
abdominal x-ray (AXR)
abdominal zipper
abdominal zones
abdominal-diaphragmatic
    respiration
abdominalis
  aorta abdominalis
  globus abdominalis
  tunica abdominalis
abdominal-perineal resection
    (APR)
abdominal-sacral
    colpoperineopexy
abdominal-vascular retractor
abdominis
  adipositas abdominis
  aponeurosis of musculus
    transversus abdominis
  diastasis recti abdominis
  hydrops abdominis
  paracentesis abdominis
  regiones abdominis
abdominocardiac reflex
abdominocentesis
abdominohysterectomy
abdominoinguinal incision
abdominoparacentesis
abdominopelvic abscess
abdominopelvic amputation
abdominopelvic cavity
abdominopelvic irradiation
abdominopelvic mass
abdominopelvic splanchnic nerve
abdominopelvic viscus
abdominoperineal excision
abdominoperineal proctectomy
abdominoperineal resection (APR)
abdominoperineal resection of
    colon
abdominoperineal resection of
    rectum
abdominoplasty
  Callia abdominoplasty
  endoscopic abdominoplasty
    (muscle plication)
  endoscopically assisted
    abdominoplasty
  fleur-de-lis abdominoplasty

abdominoplasty (*continued*)
  French-line abdominoplasty
  Grazer abdominoplasty
  high lateral tension
    abdominoplasty
  male abdominoplasty
  mini-tuck abdominoplasty
  Mladick abdominoplasty
  modified abdominoplasty
  modified Weinhold
    abdominoplasty
  muscle-access abdominoplasty
  partial subfascial
    abdominoplasty
  Pitanguy abdominoplasty
  progressive tension suture
    technique in
    abdominoplasty
  Regnault abdominoplasty
  T-excision abdominoplasty
  Victoria's Secret short incision
    abdominoplasty
abdominosacral resection
abdominoscopy
abdominothoracic arch
abdominothoracic flap
abdominothoracic incision
abdominouterotomy
abdominovaginal hysterectomy
Abdopatch
Abdopatch Gel Z Adhesive
  dressing
Abdopatch Gel Z self-adhesive
  scar treatment
abduce
abducens nerve (cranial nerve 6)
abducens nerve sign
abducent nerve
abduction
  arytenoid abduction
  Gilbert stage shoulder
    abduction
  radial abduction
  thumb abduction
abduction contraction of hip
abduction deformity
abduction exercises
abduction pillow
abduction splint
abduction traction technique
abduction-external rotation
  fracture

abducto valgus
abducto varus
abductor
abductor hallucis flap
abductor hallucis muscle
abductor muscle
abductor paralysis
abductorplasty
  flexor pollicis longus
    abductorplasty
  Smith flexor pollicis longus
    abductorplasty
abductor wedge osteotomy
abductus
  hallux abductus
  metatarsus abductus
  pes abductus
Abel-Aesculap-Pratt tenaculum
Abell tenotomy scissors
Abell hysteropexy
Abell operation
Abell uterine suspension
Abell-Gilliam suspension
Abelson adenotome
Abelson cannula
Abelson cricothyrotomy cannula
Abelson cricothyrotomy trocar
Aberdeen knot
Aberhart disposable urinal bag
Aberhart hemostatic bag
Abernaz strut forceps
Abernethy operation
Abernethy sarcoma
aberrant artery
aberrant AV bypass tract
aberrant bile duct
aberrant breast
aberrant breast tissue
aberrant cystic duct
aberrant ganglion
aberrant goiter
aberrant hepatic duct
aberrant mongolian spot
aberrant pancreas
aberrant regeneration
aberrant sebaceous glands of
  anus
aberrant third nerve
  degeneration
aberrant thyroid
aberrant tissue
aberrant vessel

aberration
angle of aberration
chromatic lens aberration
color aberration
coma aberration
curvature aberration
dioptric aberration
distantial aberration
distortion aberration
intraventricular aberration
lateral aberration
lens aberration
longitudinal aberration
meridional aberration
monochromatic aberration
newtonian aberration
oblique aberration
optical aberration
regeneration aberration
sexual aberration
spherical lens aberration
ventricular aberration
zonal aberration
aberrometer
Shack-Hartmann aberrometer
ABG (axiobuccogingival)
ABGs (arterial blood gases)
ABI PRISM Dye Terminator
Cycle Sequencing Ready
Reaction Kit
ability
impaired ability
AbioCor replacement heart
Abiomed BVAD 5000 cardiac
device (biventricular assist
device)
ABL (axiobuccolingual)
Ablaser laser delivery catheter
ablate
ablated skin
ablatio retinae
ablation
accessory conduction ablation
adrenal ablation
androgen ablation
atrioventricular junctional
ablation
carbon dioxide laser plaque
ablation
catheter ablation
celiac alcohol ablation
char-free ablation

ablation (*continued*)
cold forceps ablation
cold snare ablation
Concept ablation
continuous-wave laser
ablation
coronary rotational ablation
cryogenic ablation
cryosurgical ablation
dioiodine ablation
direct-current shock ablation
electrode catheter ablation
endometrial ablation
endoscopic mucosal ablation
ethanol ablation
fast-pathway radiofrequency
ablation
His bundle ablation
homogeneous ablation
inner ear ablation
Kent bundle ablation
laparoscopic uterine nerve
ablation
laser uterosacral nerve
ablation
liver wire TC ablation
marrow ablation
mucosal ablation
Nd:YAG laser ablation
needle ablation
neoadjuvant total androgen
ablation
nerve rootlet ablation
organ ablation
ovarian ablation
panretinal ablation
parathyroid tumor ablation
percutaneous ethanol
ablation
percutaneous radical
cryosurgical ablation
percutaneous radiofrequency
catheter ablation
percutaneous tumor ablation
peripheral panretinal ablation
photothermal laser ablation
pituitary ablation
procerus and corrugator
ablation
pulsed laser ablation
radiofrequency catheter
ablation (RFCA)

ablation (*continued*)
  radiofrequency thermal
    ablation (RFTA)
  radioiodine ablation
  rectoscopic endometrial
    ablation
  renal cyst ablation
  rollerball endometrial ablation
  rotational ablation
  slow-pathway ablation
  stereotactic surgical ablation
  surgical ablation
  surgical estrogen ablation
  ThermaChoice thermal
    balloon ablation
  thermal ablation
  thyroid nodule ablation
  tissue ablation
  toric ablation
  transcatheter ablation
  transurethral needle ablation
  tumor ablation
  valve ablation
  visual laser ablation
ablation catheter
ablation placentae
ablation therapy
ablative cardiac surgery
ablative device
ablative hormonal therapy
ablative instrument
ablative laser angioplasty
ablative laser therapy
ablative procedure
ablative technique
ablator (*spelled also* ablater)
  cautery ablator
  Concept ablator
  endometrial ablator
  radiofrequency ablator
Ablator temperature control
  device
Ablaza aortic wall retractor
Ablaza patent ductus clamp
Ablaza-Blanco cardiac valve
  retractor
Ablaza-Blanco retractor
Ablaza-Morse approximator
Ablaza-Morse rib approximator
abluent
ablution
abnormal bleeding

abnormal frenulum attachment
abnormal frenum attachment
abnormal lobulation
abnormal occlusal relationship
abnormal occlusal wear
abnormal occlusion
abnormal parathyroid gland
abnormality
  anatomic abnormality
  bleeding abnormality
  caliceal abnormality
  clotting abnormality
  congenital abnormality
  cutaneous vascular
    abnormality
  cytologic abnormality
  dislocation contour
    abnormality
  diverticulation abnormality
  DNA ploidy abnormality
  electrical activation
    abnormality
  electrolyte abnormality
  extremity abnormality
  fetal abnormality
  focal abnormality
  genetic abnormality
  ictal abnormality
  inherited abnormality
  intraretinal microvascular
    abnormalities (IRMA)
  joint abnormality
  limb reduction abnormality
  mammographic abnormality
  maxillofacial abnormality
  microvascular abnormalities
  migration abnormality
  mucosal abnormality
  nondermatomal sensory
    abnormality (NDSA)
  nonpalpable mammographic
    abnormality
  oral cavity abnormality
  osseous abnormality
  persistent breast abnormality
  pulmonary vascular
    abnormality
  regional wall motion
    abnormality (RWMA)
  renal abnormality
  reproductive tract
    abnormality

abnormality (*continued*)
  retrosternal abnormality
  rostrocaudal extent signal
    abnormality
  segmental wall motion
    abnormality (SWMA)
  significant abnormality
  skeletal abnormality
  small bowel congenital
    abnormality
  soft tissue abnormality
  structural abnormality
  suspicious abnormality
  tissue texture abnormality
  tympanomastoid abnormality
  urinary tract abnormality
  vascular abnormality
  ventilation/perfusion
    abnormality
  ventricular depolarization
    abnormality
abnormally hyperplastic gland
ABO barrier
Abocath catheter
abocclusion
aborad
aboral
abortion
  cervical abortion
  complete abortion
  Csapo abortion
  drug-induced abortion
  elective abortion (EAB)
  epizootic abortion
  habitual abortion
  imminent abortion
  incomplete abortion
  induced abortion
  inevitable abortion
  late abortion
  late-term abortion
  missed abortion
  septic abortion
  spontaneous abortion (SAB)
  suction abortion
  therapeutic abortion (TAB)
  threatened abortion
  tubal abortion
  vacuum abortion
abortive clonus
abortive pneumonia
à-boule bougie

Aboulker stent
above-elbow amputation
  (AE amputation, AEA)
above-knee amputation
  (AK amputation, AKA)
ABR (anterior band remover)
abrachia
abrachiocephalia
Abradabloc dermabrasion
  instrument
abradant
abrade
abrader (*see also* cartilage
  abrader)
  Dingman otoplasty cartilage
    abrader
  Haverhill dermal abrader
  Howard corneal abrader
abrader bur
abrading instrument
Abraham cannula
Abraham contact lens
Abraham elevator
Abraham enterotome
Abraham iridectomy laser lens
Abraham iridotomy
Abraham knife
Abraham laryngeal cannula
Abraham peripheral button
  iridotomy lens
Abraham rectal curet
Abraham tonsil knife
Abraham tonsillar knife
Abraham YAG laser lens
Abraham-Pankovich tendo
  calcaneus repair
Abramowicz artery
Abrams biopsy needle
Abrams heart reflex
Abrams needle
Abrams pleural biopsy punch
Abrams reflex
Abrams-Lucas flap heart valve
Abramson catheter
Abramson hook
Abramson retractor
Abramson sump drain
Abramson tube
Abramson-Allis breast clamp
Abramson-Dedo
  microlaryngoscope
abrasio corneae

abrasion
  acid abrasion
  arthroplasty abrasion
  betel nut abrasion
  bobby pin abrasion
  cervical abrasion
  contusions and abrasions
  corneal abrasion
  facial abrasions
  occupational abrasion
  pleural abrasion
  superficial abrasion
  truncal abrasions
abrasion of cornea
abrasion resistance
abrasive
  aluminum oxide abrasive
  diatomaceous silicon dioxide
    abrasive
  FF abrasive
  FFF abrasive
  flint abrasive
  garnet abrasive
  iron oxide abrasive
  quartz abrasive
  recrystallized kaolinite
    abrasive
  silicon carbide abrasive
  silicon dioxide abrasive
  sodium-potassium aluminum
    silicate abrasive
  zirconium silicate abrasive
abrasive brush biopsy
abrasive disk
abrasive point
abrasive strip
abrasiveness
abrasor
Abrikosov tumor
abruptio placentae
abscess
  abdominal abscess
  abdominopelvic abscess
  actinomycotic brain abscess
  acute abscess
  alveolar abscess
  amebic hepatic abscess
  anal abscess
  anastomotic abscess
  anorectal abscess
  apical abscess
  aponeurotic abscess

abscess (*continued*)
  appendiceal abscess
  arthrifluent abscess
  axillary abscess
  Bezold abscess
  bicameral abscess
  blind abscess
  bone abscess
  bowel abscess
  brain abscess
  breast abscess
  Brodie metaphysial abscess
  Brodie abscess
  buccal space abscess
  button abscess
  canalicular abscess
  caseocavernous abscess
  caseous abscess
  cerebral abscess
  chronic apical abscess
  chronic subareolar abscess
  circumscribed abscess
  cold abscess
  collar-button abscess
  colonic abscess
  conjunctival abscess
  corneal abscess
  crypt abscess
  cuff abscess
  cutaneous abscess
  deep interloop abscess
  dentoalveolar abscess
  diffuse abscess
  dorsal hand abscess
  Douglas abscess
  drainage of abscess
  drained abscess
  dry abscess
  echinococcal liver abscess
  encapsulated brain abscess
  enteroperitoneal abscess
  epidural abscess
  esophageal abscess
  extradural abscess
  fecal abscess
  first-stage draining of liver
    abscess
  fluctuant abscess
  follicular abscess
  frontal abscess
  gallbladder wall abscess
  gas abscess

abscess (*continued*)

gas-forming liver abscess
glandular abscess
gravitation abscess
growth plate abscess
hepatic abscess
Highmore abscess
horseshoe abscess
hot abscess
hypostatic abscess
incision and drainage of
    abscess
inferior pole peritonsillar
    abscess
infraorbital space abscess
interloop abscess
intermesenteric abscess
interradicular abscess
intersphincteric abscess
intra-abdominal abscess
intradural abscess
intrahepatic abscess
intramammary abscess
intramastoid abscess
intramesenteric abscess
intramural abscess
intramuscular abscess
intramusculature abscess
intraosseous abscess
intraperitoneal abscess
ischiorectal abscess
kidney abscess
lacrimal abscess
lacunar abscess
lateral alveolar abscess
liver abscess
local abscess
localized abscess
loculated abscess
lumbar epidural abscess
lung abscess
mammary abscess
marsupialization of abscess
masseter abscess
mastoid abscess
mesentery abscess
metaphysial abscess
metastatic abscess
midpalmar space abscess
migrating abscess
miliary abscess
milk abscess

abscess (*continued*)

missile track abscess
mixed abscess
Monro abscess
Munro abscess
nasal septal abscess
nasopharyngeal abscess
necrotic abscess
orbital abscess
ovarian abscess
pancreatic abscess
paracolic abscess
paranephric abscess
parapharyngeal space abscess
pararectal abscess
paravaginal abscess
parotid gland abscess
Pautrier abscess
pelvic abscess
perforating abscess
perianal fistula abscess
periapical abscess
periappendiceal abscess
pericecal abscess
pericholecystic abscess
pericolic abscess
pericolonic abscess
pericoronal abscess
periesophageal abscess
perihepatic abscess
perineal abscess
perinephric abscess
periprosthetic breast
    abscess
perirectal abscess
peritoneal cavity abscess
peritonsillar abscess
periumbilical abscess
periureteral abscess
periurethral abscess
perivesical abscess
phlegmonous abscess
pilonidal abscess
point of abscess
postoperative abscess
postpharyngeal abscess
Pott abscess
premammary abscess
premasseteric space abscess
prevertebral space abscess
primary abscess
psoas abscess

abscess (*continued*)
pterygomandibular space
  abscess
pulmonary abscess
pyogenic abscess
radicular abscess
recrudescent abscess
rectal abscess
recurrent cutaneous abscess
residual abscess
retrobulbar abscess
retrocecal abscess
retromammary abscess
retroperitoneal abscess
retroperitoneal-iliopsoas
  abscess
retropharyngeal abscess
retrorectal abscess
ring abscess
run-around abscess
satellite abscess
secondary abscess
soft tissue abscess
space of Retzius abscess
spinal cord abscess
spinal epidural abscess (SEA)
splenic abscess
stellate abscess
stercoral abscess
sterile abscess
stitch abscess
subaponeurotic abscess
subdiaphragmatic abscess
subdural abscess
subepidermal abscess
subgaleal abscess
subhepatic abscess
sublingual space abscess
submammary abscess
submandibular space abscess
submasseteric space abscess
submental space abscess
subperiosteal orbital abscess
  (SPOA)
subperitoneal abscess
subphrenic abscess
subungual abscess
supralevator perirectal abscess
surgical abscess
temporal fossa abscess
testicular abscess
thenar space abscess

abscess (*continued*)
thyroid abscess
tonsillar abscess
Tornwaldt abscess
traumatic abscess
tuberculous abscess
tubo-ovarian abscess
tympanomastoid abscess
vestibular abscess
vitreous abscess
von Bezold abscess
wandering abscess
wound abscess
abscess forceps
abscess formation
abscess knife
abscess lancet
abscess ring
Abscession biliary drainage
  catheter
Abscession catheter
Abscession fluid drainage
  catheter
Abscession needle
abscise
abscission
  corneal abscission
abscission needle
absconsio
Absolok endoscopic clip
  applicator
Absolok forceps
Absolute absorbable screw
absolute bowel sounds
absolute cardiac dullness (ACD)
absolute construction
absolute curative resection
absolute glaucoma
absolute noncurative resection
absolute pocket
absolute quantity
absolute threshold
absorb
absorbable catgut
absorbable dressing
absorbable dusting powder
absorbable film
absorbable gauze
absorbable gelatin film
absorbable gelatin sponge
absorbable plate
absorbable sponge

absorbable stent
absorbable sutures
absorbefacient
absorbent cotton
absorbent gauze
absorbent paper point
absorbent point
absorbent sterile towel
absorbent vessels
absorber
 Hollister wound exudate
  absorber
 hyCURE hydrolyzed protein
  powder and exudate
  absorber
 laser fume absorber
Absorb-its material
absorptiometry
absorption anesthesia
absorption lacuna
Aburel operation
abut
abutment
 Dalla Bona ball and socket
  abutment
 implant abutment
 multiple abutment
 multirooted abutment
AC (acromioclavicular)
AC (axiocervical)
AC joint
AC lens
AC separation
acacia
acalculus
acampsia
acantha
acanthesthesia
acanthion
acantholysis
acanthoma
 basal cell acanthoma
 clear cell acanthoma
acanthomatous ameloblastoma
acanthomatous pattern
acanthosis
acanthotic
ACAT (automated computerized
 axial tomography)
ACAT 1 intraaortic balloon pump
ACBE (air contrast barium
 enema)

acceleration
 angular acceleration
acceleration injury
acceleration/deceleration injury
accelerator
 Becker accelerator
 electron linear accelerator
 serum thrombotic accelerator
Accelerator II aspirator
accelerator tip
accelerometer
Accent-DG balloon
Ac'cents permanent lash liner
AccePressure heel cup
access
 cavity access
 cutdown access
 exit access
 intraoral access
 palatal access
 piriform aperture access
 preparotid access
 random access
 submental access
 translabial access
 venous access
access cavity
access emergency
access flap
access incision
access opening
access peak flowmeter
access preparation
Access-Blocker
accessible lesion
accessiflexor
accessoria, accessoriae
 thyroidea accessoria
 cartilagines nasales accessoriae
accessories
 biopsy accessories
 Bovie accessories
 Bovie Chuck-It accessories
 Chuck-It disposable
  accessories
 Frankfeldt snare accessories
 Storz cleaning accessories
 Storz cystoscopic accessories
accessorius
 lien accessorius
accessory
 Auto Glide walker accessory

accessory bone
accessory adrenal gland
accessory arteriovenous
  connection
accessory auricles
accessory AV connection
accessory blood vessels
accessory bone
accessory cartilage
accessory cephalic vein
accessory collateral ligament
accessory conduction ablation
accessory cuneate nucleus
accessory duct
accessory eye implant
accessory feminizing operation
accessory gland
accessory hemiazygos vein
accessory hepatic duct
accessory instruments
accessory ligament
accessory mammary tissue
accessory maxillary hiatus
accessory maxillary ostium
accessory maxillary sinus ostium
accessory nasal cartilage
accessory navicular bone
accessory nerve (cranial nerve 11)
accessory nerve sign
accessory nerves
accessory node
accessory obturator artery
accessory ostium
accessory ovary
accessory palatine canal
accessory pancreas
accessory pancreatic duct
accessory parotid gland
accessory phrenic nerves
accessory placenta
accessory quadrate cartilage
accessory saphenous vein
accessory sign
accessory sinuses of nose
accessory spleen
accessory structure
accessory suprarenal gland
accessory thyroid gland
accessory trocar
ACCHN (adenoid cystic
  carcinoma of head and
  neck)

accident
  abdominal vascular accident
  cerebrovascular accident
    (CVA)
  cochleovascular accident
  industrial accident
  intracerebrovascular accident
  intraoperative vascular
    accident
  postcerebrovascular accident
accidental hemorrhage
accidental pulp exposure
ACCO cotton roll
ACCO impression material
ACCO orthodontic appliance
Accolade hip prosthesis
Accolade surgical
  instrumentation
accommodation
  binocular accommodation
  light and accommodation
  nerve accommodation
accommodation disorder
accommodation reflex
accommodative asthenopia
accompanying artery of sciatic
  nerve
accompanying vein of
  hypoglossal nerve
accompli
  fait accompli
ACCOR dental matrix
accordion
  subdermal accordion
accordion abdomen
accordion drain
accordion graft
accordion implant
accordion prosthesis
accoucheur's hand
accreta
  placenta accreta
accretio
accretion line
Accu-Beam suction & irrigation
  cannula
Accucap CO_2/O_2 monitor
Accu-Chek Easy glucose monitor
Accu-Chek II Freedom blood
  glucose monitor
Accu-Chek III blood glucose
  meter

Accucom cardiac output
  monitor
Accucore II biopsy needle
accuDEXA bone densitometer
Accu-dyne antiseptic products
Accudynemic adjustable
  damping
Accufilm articulating film
Accufix pacemaker
Accuflex punch
Accu-Flo button
Accu-Flo connector
Accu-Flo CSF reservoir
Accu-Flo dural film
Accu-Flo pressure valve
Accu-Flo spring catheter
Accu-Flo U-channel stripping
  cannula
Accu-Flo ventricular cannula
Accu-Flo ventricular catheter
AccuGel impression material
AccuGel lens
Accugraft
Accuguide syringe
Accuject dental needle
AccuLase excimer laser
Accu-Line chamfer resection
  guide
Accu-Line distal femoral resector
Accu-Line knee instrumentation
Accu-Line patellar instrument
Accu-line Products skin marker
Accu-Line surgical marker
Accu-Line tibial resector
Acculink self-expanding stent
Acculith pacemaker
AccuMark calibrated infant
  feeding tube
AccuMax bed
AccuMax self-adjusting pressure
  management mattress
Accu-Measure personal body fat
  tester
Accu-Measure skinfold calipers
Accu-Mix impression material
accumulation
  focal accumulation
  pus accumulation
accumulative radiation
Accu-Path acetabular cup
AccuPort seal
AccuPressure infusion pump

AccuProbe 600 cryotherapy
  probe
Accura hydrocephalus shunt
accuracy
  diagnostic accuracy
  submillimetric accuracy
Accuracy Neurotron 1000
  machine
accuracy timer
Accurate catheter
accurate débridement
Accurate Surgical and Scientific
  Instruments (ASSI)
Accuratome precurved
  papillotome
Accurette endometrial suction
  curet
AccuroX mask
AccuRx constant flow
  implantable pump
Accusate pulse oximeter
AccuScan CO_2 laser scanner
Accuscanner transducer
Accu-Scope colposcope
Accu-Scope microscope
AccuSharp endoscope
AccuSharp instrument
Accu-Sorb gauze sponge
AccuSpan tissue expander
Accu-Spense cavity liner
Accustaple
Accu-Temp cautery
Accu-Temp hot wire cautery
Accutome low-speed diamond
  saw
Accutorr A1 blood pressure
  monitor
Accutorr bedside monitor
Accutorr monitor
Accutorr oscillometric device
Accutracker blood pressure
  monitor
Accutracker II ambulatory blood
  pressure monitoring
Accuvac smoke evacuation
  attachment
ACD (absolute cardiac dullness)
ACD resuscitator
ACE (autologous-cultured
  epithelium)
Ace adherent bandage
Ace adherent dressing

Ace aerosol cloud enhancer
ACE Autografter bone filter
ACE balloon
Ace bandage
ACE bone screw tack
ACE bone screw tacking kit
Ace brace
Ace cannulated cancellous hip
   screw
Ace cannulated cancellous screw
Ace captured hip screw
Ace Colles technique
Ace cortical bone screw
Ace elastic dressing
ACE Exact Torque disposable
   ratchet
ACE fixed-wire balloon catheter
Ace halo pelvic girdle
Ace halo-cast assembly
Ace hip screw
Ace Kyle prosthesis
Ace longitudinal strips dressing
Ace low-profile MR halo
Ace Mark III halo
ace of spades sign
ACE OsteoGenic distractor
Ace pin
Ace rubber elastic dressing
Ace screw
Ace spica bandage
ACE spline driver
ACE surgical tray
ACE trephine bur
Ace Trippi-Wells tong cervical
   traction
Ace Unifix fixator
Ace Universal tong cervical
   traction
Ace Universal tongs
Ace wire tension assembly
Ace wrap
Ace/Normed osteodistractors
Ace-Colles frame technique
Ace-Colles half ring
Ace-Fischer external fixator
Ace-Fischer frame
Ace-Hershey halo jig
Ace-Hesive dressing
acellular dermis
acellular muscle graft
acentric glide
acentric occlusion

acentric relation
acephalobrachia
acephalopodia
acephalorhachia
acetabula (acetabulum)
acetabular allograft
acetabular angle guide
acetabular augmentation graft
acetabular cavity
acetabular component
acetabular cup arthroplasty
acetabular cup gauge
acetabular cup positioner
acetabular cup template
acetabular cup trial
acetabular endoprosthesis
acetabular extensile approach
acetabular grater
acetabular guide
acetabular index
acetabular knife
acetabular notch
acetabular positioner
acetabular protrusio deformity
acetabular reamer
acetabular reconstruction plate
acetabular rim fracture
acetabular seating hole
acetabular shell guide
acetabular skid
acetabulectomy
acetabuloplasty
acetabulum (*pl* acetabula)
   protrusio acetabulum
   shelf reconstruction of
      acetabulum
   sunken acetabulum
acetate
acetazolamide (Diamox)
acetic acid
acetohydroxamic acid
   irrigation
acetowhite lesion
acetylcholine chloride
   (Miochol)
acetylcholinesterase
acetylsalicylic acid (ASA)
ACF (anterior cervical fusion)
achalasia
   esophageal achalasia
   sphincteral achalasia
achalasia balloon dilation

achalasia dilator
acheiria
acheiropodia
Achiever balloon dilatation
    catheter
Achiever balloon dilator
Achilles
    Thompson squeeze test of
        Achilles
Achilles bursa
Achilles densitometer
Achilles jerk
Achilles reflex
Achilles tendon resurfacing
Achilles tendon rupture
Achillis
    tendo Achillis
achillodynia
achillorrhaphy
achillotenotomy
    plastic achillotenotomy
achillotomy
Achillotrain active Achilles
        tendon support
achlorhydria
achlorhydria apepsia
achondroplasia
achondroplasty
achroacytosis of lacrimal gland
achromatic lens
achromatic mass
achromic patch
acid
    acetic acid
    acetylsalicylic acid (ASA)
    alpha hydroxyl acid (AHA)
    aluminum acetate and acetic
        acid
    aminocaproic acid
    arachidonic acid
    ascorbic acid
    azelaic acid
    bicinchoninic acid (BCA)
    boric acid
    carbolic acid
    caustic acid
    cevitamic acid
    citric acid
    ethacrynic acid
    Gly Derm alpha hydroxy acid
    Gly Derm glycolic acid
    glycolic acid

acid (*continued*)
    hydrochloric acid
    kojic acid
    lactic acid
    nucleic acid
    poly L-lactic acid (PLLA)
    polyglycolic acid
    retinoic acid
    salicylic acid
    stomach acid
    tannic acid
    trichloroacetic acid (TCA)
    trichloroacetic acid (TCA) peel
    uric acid
acid abrasion
acid aspiration
acid burn
acid etch bonding technique
acid gland
acid mucopolysaccharide
acidosteophyte
Acier stainless steel suture
acinar cancer
acinar carcinoma
acinar cell
acinar gland
acinar lumen
acinar pattern
acinar tissue
acinarization of pancreas
acini (*sing.* acinus)
acinic
acinic cell carcinoma
acinic cell tumor
acinous adenoma
acinous cancer
acinous carcinoma
acinous cell carcinoma
acinous gland
acinus (*pl.* acini)
    serous acinus
acircular amputation
Ackerman bar joint
Ackerman clip
Ackerman lingual bar
Ackerman needle
Ackerman-Proffitt classification
        of malocclusion
Ackrad balloon-bearing catheter
Ackrad Bronchitrac L suction
        catheter
Ackrad Cervicet dilator

Ackrad esophageal balloon
  catheter
Ackrad H/S Elliptosphere
  catheter
Ackrad Tampa catheter set
ACL (anterior cruciate ligament)
ACL drill
ACL drill guide
ACL graft knife
ACL guide
ACL reconstruction
ACL repair
Acland clamp
Acland clamp approximator
Acland clasp
Acland clip
Acland double-clamp
  approximator
Acland microvascular clamp
Acland microvascular clamp
  applier
Acland needle
Acland repair
Acland-Banis arteriotomy set
Acland-Buncke counterpressor
aclasia
aclasis
  tarsoepiphyseal aclasis
ACLS (advanced cardiac life
  support)
Acme articulator
ACMI ACN-2 flexible
  cystonephroscope
ACMI Alcock catheter
ACMI antroscope
ACMI bag
ACMI battery cord
ACMI biopsy loop electrode
ACMI bronchoscope
ACMI Bunts catheter
ACMI CAN-2 flexible
  cystonephroscope
ACMI catheter
ACMI cautery
ACMI coated Foley catheter
ACMI cystoscope
ACMI cystoscopic tip
ACMI cystourethroscope
ACMI duodenoscope
ACMI Emmett hemostatic
  catheter
ACMI endoscope

ACMI esophagoscope
ACMI fiberoptic colonoscope
ACMI flexible sigmoidoscope
ACMI forceps
ACMI gastroscope
ACMI hysteroscope
ACMI irrigating valve
ACMI laparoscope
ACMI light source connector
ACMI light-carrying bundle
ACMI Marici bronchoscope
ACMI Martin endoscopic
  forceps
ACMI Martin endoscopy
  forceps
ACMI Martin forceps
ACMI Micro-H hysteroscope
ACMI Micro-Hysteroscope
ACMI microlens
  cystourethroscope
ACMI microlens Foroblique
  telescope
ACMI microlens telescope
ACMI monopolar electrode
ACMI nasopharyngoscope
ACMI operating colonoscope
ACMI operating coloscope
ACMI Owens catheter
ACMI pediatric resectoscope
ACMI Pezzer drain
ACMI positive pressure
  catheter
ACMI proctoscope
ACMI proctosigmoidoscope
ACMI resectoscope
ACMI resistor
ACMI retrograde electrode
ACMI severance catheter
ACMI teaching attachment
ACMI telescope
ACMI Thackston catheter
ACMI Transvaginal Hydro
  laparoscope
ACMI ulcer-measuring device
ACMI ureteral catheter
ACMI urethroscope
ACMI Valentine tube
ACMI valve
ACMI Word Bartholin gland
  catheter
Acmistat catheter
Acmix Foley catheter

acne
  colloid acne
  comedo acne
  comedonal acne
  cystic acne
  miliary acne
  nodulocystic acne
  papular acne
  pustular acne
acne albida
acne artificialis
acne atrophica
acne cachecticorum
acne ciliaris
acne conglobata
acne cosmetica
acne erythematosa
acne fulminans
acne hypertrophica
acne indurata
acne keloidalis
acne keratosa
acne lancet
acne miliaris
acne necrotica
acne papulosa
acne punctata
acne rosacea
acne sebacea
acne simplex
acne tarsi
acne urticata
acne varioliformis
acne vulgaris
acneform (*also* acneiform)
acneform lesion
acnegenic
acneiform
acneiform dermatitis
acneiform eruption
acneiform lesion
Acolysis coronary probe
Acoma scanner
Acorde bur
acorn
  rubber acorn
acorn cannula
acorn carver
Acorn CorCap cardiac support
    device
Acorn II nebulizer
Acorn nebulizer

acorn reamer
acorn-shaped eye implant
acorn-tipped bougie
acorn-tipped catheter
Acosta classification of pelvic
    endometriosis
acoustic duct
acoustic enhancement
acoustic impedance probe
acoustic interface
acoustic macula
acoustic microscope
acoustic myograph
acoustic nerve
acoustic nerve sign
acoustic neuroma
acoustic neurotomy
acoustic otoscope
acoustic rhinometry
acoustic shadow
acoustic window
acousticofacial ganglion
acousticofacial nerve bundle
acousticopalpebral reflex
AC-PC line
ACPS
    (acrocephalopolysyndactyly)
Acquacel Hydrofiber dressing.
acquired anaphylaxis
acquired blepharoptosis
acquired cholesteatoma
acquired cornification disorder
acquired defect
acquired deformity
acquired eccentric jaw relation
acquired harelip
acquired hernia
acquired immunodeficiency
    syndrome (AIDS)
acquired immunoglobulin A
    deficiency
acquired megacolon
acquired myotonia
acquired nasopharyngeal
    stenosis
acquired ventricular septal defect
acquisition
  image acquisition
  multiple gated acquisition
    (MUGA)
acquisition time
Acra-Cut cranial perforator

Acra-Cut Spiral craniotome
  blade
Acrad HS catheter
  (hysterosalpingography
  catheter)
acral anesthesia
acral-lentiginous melanoma
acrania
Acrax prosthesis
Acrel ganglion
acroagnosis
acroangiodermatitis
acrobrachycephaly
acrocephalia
acrocephalopolysyndactyly
  (ACPS)
acrocephalosyndactylia (ACS)
acrocephalosyndactyly
  type I acrocephalosyndactyly
  type II acrocephalosyndactyly
acrocephalosyndactyly (ACS)
acrocephaly
AcroChamber
acrochordon
acrocontracture
acrodermatitis
  papular acrodermatitis
acrodermectasia
acrodont
acrodynia
acrodysplasia
acroedema
acrofacial dysostosis
acrofacial syndrome
acrofacial vitiligo
Acro-Flex artificial disk
acrokeratosis
  paraneoplastic acrokeratosis
acrokeratosis paraneoplastica
acrokeratosis verruciformis of
  Hopf
acrolect
AcroMed Isola Device
acromegalic arthropathy
acromegalic face
acromegalic gigantism
acromegaly
acromial bone
acromial bursa
acromial process
acromioclavicular articulation
acromioclavicular disk

acromioclavicular dislocation
  harness sling
acromioclavicular injury
  classification
acromioclavicular joint
  dislocation
acromioclavicular ligament
acromioclavicular separation
acromioclavicular space
acromiocoracoid ligament
acromiohumeral
acromion
  Neer resection of acromion
acromion process
acromion scapulae
acromionectomy
  Armstrong acromionectomy
acromionizer bur
acromioplasty
  anterior acromioplasty
  McLaughlin acromioplasty
  McShane-Leinberry-Fenlin
    acromioplasty
  Neer acromioplasty
  Smith-Petersen acromioplasty
acromioscapular
acromiothoracic approach
acromiothoracic artery
acromphalus
acromyotonia
acro-osteolysis
acropachy
  thyroid acropachy
acroparalysis
acroparesthesia
acropathy
acrosclerosis
acrospiroma
  eccrine acrospiroma
acrosyndactyly
Acrotorque bur
Acrotorque hand engine
Acry Island border dressing
AcryDerm border island dressing
AcryDerm dressing
AcryDerm hydrogel sheet
AcryDerm Strands absorbent
  wound dressing
acrylic ball eye implant
acrylic bar prosthesis
acrylic bite block
acrylic bone cement

acrylic cap splint
acrylic cement
acrylic conformer eye implant
acrylic ear splint
acrylic eye implant
acrylic graft
acrylic implant
acrylic lens
acrylic mold
acrylic plastic
acrylic prosthesis
acrylic resin dressing
acrylic resin teeth
acrylic splint
acrylic surgical splint
acrylic wafer TMJ splint
acrocyanosis
AcrySof foldable intraocular
    lens
ACS (acrocephalosyndactyly)
ACS Amplatz guidewire
ACS Anchor Exchange device
ACS Angioject
ACS angioplasty catheter
ACS balloon catheter
ACS catheter
ACS Concorde coronary
    dilatation catheter
ACS Concorde OTW catheter
ACS Eclipse
ACS Endura coronary dilation
    catheter
ACS exchange guidewire
ACS exchange guiding catheter
ACS exchange wire
ACS floppy-tip guidewire
ACS floppy-tip guiding catheter
ACS Flowtrack-40 catheter
ACS gold-standard guidewire
ACS gold-standard wire
ACS guidewire
ACS Gyroscan
ACS Hi-Torque Balance
    guidewire
ACS Hi-Torque Balance
    Middleweight catheter
ACS HI-Torque Balance
    Middleweight guidewire
ACS Hi-Torque Floppy II
    exchange wire
ACS Hi-Torque Iron Man
    guidewire

ACS Indeflator 20/30 inflation
    device
ACS JL4 catheter
ACS JL4 French catheter
ACS LIMA guide
ACS LIMA guidewire
ACS microglide wire
ACS Mini catheter
ACS Monorail perfusion balloon
    catheter
ACS Multi-Link Duet coronary
    stent
ACS Multi-Link OTW Duet stent
ACS Multi-Link RX Duet stent
ACS Multi-Link Tristar coronary
    stent
ACS needle
ACS OTW (over-the-wire)
    Lifestream coronary
    dilatation catheter
ACS OTW Comet coronary
    dilation catheter
ACS OTW HP coronary
ACS OTW Lifestream coronary
    dilation catheter
ACS OTW Photon coronary
    dilation catheter
ACS OTW Solaris coronary
    dilation catheter
ACS percutaneous introducer
ACS percutaneous introducer set
ACS RX Comet coronary
    dilatation catheter
ACS RX Comet VP catheter
ACS RX coronary dilatation
    catheter
ACS RX Ellipse angioplasty
    catheter
ACS RX Gemini catheter
ACS RX Lifestream catheter
ACS Rx Multi-Link coronary stent
ACS RX multilink stent
ACS RX Rocket catheter
ACS RX Solaris coronary
    dilatation catheter
ACS RX Streak angioplasty
    catheter
ACS SOF-T guidewire
ACS SULP II balloon
ACS Torquemaster catheter
ACS Tourguide II guiding
    catheter

ACS Tx2000 VP catheter
ACS Viking
ACS Viking catheter
ACST Tx2000 coronary
    dilatation catheter
ACT
Act joint support
ACT Microcoil
ACTH (adrenocorticotropic
    hormone)
Acticoat silver-based burn
    dressing
Acticon neosphincter implant
Actifoam active hemostat
Actifoam collagen sponge
Actifoam hemostat
Actifoam hemostat sponge
actinic
actinic cheilitis
actinic damage
actinic granuloma
actinic keratosis
actinic reticuloid
actinic skin changes
actinomycosis
    cervical actinomycosis
    cervicofacial actinomycosis
actinomycotic brain abscess
actinophytosis
    staphylococcal actinophytosis
actinotherapy
action
    anesthesia action
    bacteriolytic action
    calorigenic action
    capillary action
    centripetal action
    faulty valve action
    heart action
    knee action
    microbial action
    rasping action
    stress action
    tamponade action
Action Eyes and Albany eye
    guards
action line
action of anesthetic
Action OR pad
Action OR table pads
Actipatch Therapy
Actis venous flow controller

Actis venous flow device
Activase
activated balloon expandable
    intravascular stent
activated dermis
activated graft
activated resin
activating adjusting instrument
    (AAI)
activation
activation map-guided surgical
    resection
activator
    Andresen activator
    Andresen-Haupl activator
    Bimler activator
    cutout activator
    Karwetsky U-bow activator
    Klammt elastic open activator
    Metzelder modification
        activator
    palate-free activator
    Pfeiffer-Grobety activator
    Schmuth modification
        activator
    Schwarz bow-type activator
    Wunderer modification
        activator
activator modification
active anaphylaxis
active appliance therapy
active assistive motion therapy
active bowel sounds
Active Cath catheter
active chronic inflammation
active duodenal ulcer
active hemorrhage
active immunity
active length needle
Active Life convex one-piece
        urostomy pouch with
        Durahesive skin barrier
Active Life one-piece drainage
        pouch
Active Life one-piece opaque
        stoma cap
Active Life one-piece precut
        closed-end pouch
active MRI stent (AMRIS)
active phase arrest
active range of motion (AROM)
active source of bleeding

active vasodilation
active-assistive range of motion
actively bleeding varices
Activent antimicrobial
    ventilation tube
Activent ear tube
activities of daily living (ADL)
Activitrax pacemaker
Activitrax single-chamber
    responsive pacemaker
Activitrax variable-rate
    pacemaker
activity
    cerebral paroxysmal activity
    delta activity
    dysrhythmic activity
    ectopic activity
    EEG activity
    electric activity
    fetal cardiac activity
    fetal somatic activity
    functional activity
    identifiable electrical activity
    intrinsic fibroblastic activity
    motor activity
    nerve activity
    peristaltic activity
    phasic activity
    regenerative activity
    renewed tumor activity
    respiratory activity
    rhythmic activity
    secretory activity
    spikey activity
    tertiary peristaltic activity
    vasomotor activity
    voluntary activity
activity-guided pacemaker
activity-sensing pacemaker
actocardiotocograph fetal
    monitor
ACT-one coronary stent
Actros pacemaker
actual cautery
actuation
actuator
    NYU-Hosmer electric elbow
    and prehension actuator
AcuBlade robotic laser
Acu-Brush
Acucare bed
Acucise balloon

Acucise cutting balloon device
Acucise RP retrograde
    endopyelotomy catheter
Acucise ureteral cutting cautery
AcuClip endoscopic multiple-
    clip applier
Acu-Derm IV/TPN dressing
Acu-Derm wound dressing
Acu-Dyne antiseptic
Acufex alignment guide
Acufex arthroscope
Acufex arthroscopic instruments
Acufex basket
Acufex bioabsorbable Suretac
    suture
Acufex bioabsorbable suture
    anchor
Acufex curved basket forceps
Acufex drawknife
Acufex drill guide
Acufex duckbill punch
Acufex Edge
Acufex guide
Acufex handle
Acufex linear grasper
Acufex linear punch
Acufex microsurgical
    instruments
Acufex MosaicPlasty instrument
Acufex power shaver
Acufex rotary basket forceps
Acufex rotary punch
Acufex scissors
Acufex straight basket forceps
Acufex TAG rod
Acufex-Suretac implant
Acuflex impression material
Acuflex intraocular lens implant
acuity visual projector
Acumaster acupuncture needle
AcuMatch L series cemented
    femoral stem
AcuMatch M series modular
    femoral hip prosthesis
AcuMed suture anchor
AcuMed tension band pin
acuminatum (*pl.* acuminata)
    acuminate wart
    condyloma acuminatum
    giant condyloma acuminatum
AcuNav diagnostic ultrasound
    catheter

AcuNav ultrasound catheter
acupoint
acupressure
acupuncture anesthesia
acupuncture instruments
acupuncture laser
acupuncture technique
acupuncture treatment
Acu-Ray x-ray unit
Acurette microcuret
Acuscope microcurrent
   stimulator
AcuSeal cardiovascular patch
acusection
AcuSnare polypectomy device
AcuSnare snare
Acuson 128EP imager
Acuson 128EP scanner
Acuson color Doppler
Acuson computed sonography
Acuson echocardiographic
   equipment
Acuson linear array transducer
Acuson ultrasound scanner
Acuson V5M multiplane TEE
   transducer
Acuson V5M transesophageal
   echocardiographic monitor
Acuspot
   710 Acuspot
   Sharplan Laser 710 Acuspot
Acuspot Sharplan Laser 710 A
acustici
   cartilago meatus acustici
   dentes acustici
acute abscess
acute and chronic inflammation
acute angle
acute aortic dissection
acute atrophic oral candidiasis
acute cardiac event
acute cheilitis
acute coronary syndrome
acute digestive bleeding
acute disconnection syndrome
acute disseminated histiocytosis X
acute fracture
acute frontal sinusitis
acute gastric mucosal lesion
acute graft-versus-host disease
acute hemorrhagic inflammation
acute hepatic rupture

acute hordeolum
acute infective endocarditis (AIE)
acute inflammation
acute intestinal obstruction
acute ionization detector
acute laryngitis
acute mandibular plane angle
acute maxillary sinusitis
acute myocardial infarction (AMI)
acute otitis media (AOM)
acute phase of burn injury
acute physiology and chronic
   health evaluation (APACHE)
acute pyogenic membrane
acute radiation syndrome
acute rejection of liver
   transplant
acute renal failure (ARF)
acute respiratory distress
   syndrome (ARDS)
acute respiratory failure
acute scalp cellulitis
acute subdural hematoma
acute submandibular sialadenitis
acute supraglottic laryngitis
acute surgical abdomen
acute traumatic lesion
acute tubular necrosis
acute ventricular assist device
   (AVAD)
acute warning sign
AcuTect DVT imaging agent
ACUTENS transcutaneous nerve
   stimulator
acute-tipped mammascope
acuti
   dentes acuti
Acutome 2000 Reich-Hasson
   laparoscopic CO_2 laser
   coupler
AcuTouch tissue forceps
AcuTrainer bladder retraining
   device
Acutrak fusion screw
Acutrak Mini screw
Acutrak Plus screw
Acutrak screw
Acuvue bifocal lens
Acuvue disposable contact lens
Acuvue Etafilcon A lens
acyanotic
acyclovir

AD (anterior displacement)
AD (right ear)
ad lib
Ada dissecting scissors
ADAC/Vertex dual-headed
    SPECT camera
adactyly
ADAD gamma camera
Adair adenotome
Adair breast clamp
Adair breast tenaculum
Adair clamp
Adair forceps
Adair hemostat
Adair procedure
Adair screw compressor
Adair tenaculum
Adair uterine forceps
Adair uterine tenaculum
Adair-Allis forceps
Adair-Allis tenaculum
Adair-Veress needle
Adam and Eve rib belt splint
adamantine membrane
adamantinoma
Adamkiewicz
    artery of Adamkiewicz
Adamkiewicz artery
Adamount pocket mounts
Adams advancement of round
    ligaments
Adams ankle arthrodesis
Adam's apple
Adams aspirator
Adams ball
Adams clasp
Adams crushing of nasal septum
Adams ectropion operation
Adams excision of palmar fascia
Adams hip operation
Adams kidney stone filter
Adams modification of Bethune
    tourniquet
Adams operation
Adams operation for ectropion
Adams orthodontic clip
Adams otoplasty
Adams position
Adams retractor
Adams rib contractor
Adams saw
Adams tourniquet

Adams-DeWeese vena caval clip
Adams-Horwitz ankle fusion
Adamson retractor
Adams-Stokes disease
Adams-Stokes syncope
Adante PTCA balloon catheter
adapalene gel
Adaptar contact lens
adaptation
    epithelial adaptation
    marginal adaptation
adaptation disease
adaptational approach
adapted instruments
adapter (see also adaptor)
    Air-Lon adapter
    Alcock catheter adapter
    Alcock conical catheter adapter
    AMSCO Hall adapter
    Bard-Tuohy-Borst adapter
    BD adapter
    Bernaco adapter
    BioLase laser adapter
    Bodai adapter
    Brown-Roberts-Wells ring
        adapter
    butterfly adapter
    cannula tubing adapter
    catheter tubing adapter
    Christmas tree adapter
    chuck adapter
    circuit adapter
    C-mount adapter
    coil machine adapter
    collet screwdriver adapter
    Cook plastic Luer-Lok adapter
    Cooper laser adapter
    Cordis-Dow shunt adapter
    Curry hip nail counterbore
        with Lloyd adapter
    cystoscope-urethroscope
        adapter
    dual adapter
    ear suction adapter
    E-to-A adapter
    fiberoptic cable adapter
    Foregger-Racine adapter
    Freestyle CAPD catheter adapter
    friction-fit adapter
    Grace plate 4-hole adapter
    Greenberg Maxi-Vise adapter
    halo-ring adapter

adapter (*continued*)
  House suction adapter
  Hudson adapter
  Jacobs chuck adapter
  Kaufman adapter
  King connector adapter
  KleenSpec otoscope adapter
  Lloyd adapter
  Luer suction cannula adapter
  Luer-Lok adapter
  Mayfield skull clamp adapter
  Medi-Jector adapter
  Merrimack laser adapter
  metal adapter
  Morch swivel adapter
  Neuroguide suction-irrigation
    adapter
  Nickell cystoscope adapter
  pediatric Racine adapter
  Peep-Keep II adapter
  peripheral interface adapter
  power adapter
  resectoscope adapter
  Rosenblum rotating adapter
  rotating adapter
  SACH foot adapter
  SafeTrak epidural catheter
    adapter
  Sanders ventilation adapter
  sheath with side-arm adapter
  Sheehy-Urban sliding lens
    adapter
  Shiley pressure-relief adapter
  side-arm adapter
  sleeve adapter
  Storz catheter adapter
  Storz fiberoptic cable adapter
  suction adapter
  swivel adapter
  Telestill photo adapter
  terminal electrode adapter
  Trinkle chuck adapter
  tubing adapter
  Tuohy-Borst adapter
  UAM Osteon bur adapter
  Universal T-adapter
  ventilation adapter
  Venturi ventilation adapter
  Volk retinal scale adapter
  Volk Ultra Field aspherical
    lens adapter
  Volk yellow filter adapter

adapter (*continued*)
  Wullstein chuck adapter
  Xanar laser adapter
  Zeiss cine adapter
adapter band
adapter catheter
Adapteur multifunctional drill
    guide
Adaptic dressing
Adaptic gauze
Adaptic gauze dressing
Adaptic gauze packing
Adaptic II dental restorative
    material
Adaptic needle holder
Adaptic nonadhering dressing
adaptive correction
adaptive immunity
adaptive temporomandibular
    joint remodeling
adaptor (*see also* adapter)
  Toomey adaptor
Adasoy procedure
ADC (axiodistocervical)
ADC Medicut shears
Adcon adhesive control gel
Adcon-L
ADD (angled delivery device)
ADD side-directed probe
Add-a-Cath catheter
Add-a-Clamp
Adden herniorrhaphy
Addison disease
Addison maneuver
Addison plane
Addison point
additive
Addix needle
Addix tier
add-on graft
ADD'Stat laser
adducta
  coxa adducta
adduction
  hip adduction
adduction contracture of hip
adduction deformity
adduction position
adduction traction technique
adduction-internal rotation
    deformity
adductor canal

adductor hiatus
adductor longus muscle
adductor longus muscle rupture
adductor magnus muscle
adductor muscle
adductor paralysis
adductor pollicis
adductor tenotomy
adductor tubercle
adductorius
    canalis adductorius
adductovarus deformity
adductus
    metatarsus adductus
AddVent atrial-ventricular
    pacemaker
Adelmann finger disarticulation
Adelmann operation
adenectomy
adenoadipose flap
adenocarcinoma
    alveolar adenocarcinoma
    ampullary adenocarcinoma
    anaplastic adenocarcinoma
    annular adenocarcinoma
    appendiceal adenocarcinoma
    bile duct adenocarcinoma
    bronchial adenocarcinoma
    bronchioalveolar
        adenocarcinoma
    bronchiolar adenocarcinoma
    bronchogenic
        adenocarcinoma
    cervical adenocarcinoma
    colloid adenocarcinoma
    colonic adenocarcinoma
    colorectal adenocarcinoma
    cystic adenocarcinoma
    duct cell adenocarcinoma
    duodenal adenocarcinoma
    endometrial adenocarcinoma
    esophageal adenocarcinoma
    exophytic adenocarcinoma
    gastric adenocarcinoma
    giant cell adenocarcinoma
    infiltrating duct
        adenocarcinoma
    invasive adenocarcinoma
    kidney adenocarcinoma
    medullary adenocarcinoma
    mesonephric adenocarcinoma
    metastatic adenocarcinoma

adenocarcinoma (*continued*)
    mucinous cell adenocarcinoma
    ovarian clear cell
        adenocarcinoma
    pancreatic adenocarcinoma
    papillary adenocarcinoma
    peritoneal adenocarcinoma
    pleomorphic adenocarcinoma
    primary adenocarcinoma
    prostatic adenocarcinoma
    renal adenocarcinoma
    scirrhous adenocarcinoma
    sebaceous adenocarcinoma
    secretory adenocarcinoma
    serous adenocarcinoma
    signet-ring adenocarcinoma
    spontaneous adenocarcinoma
    stomach adenocarcinoma
    sweat-gland adenocarcinoma
    ulcerating adenocarcinoma
    undifferentiated
        adenocarcinoma
    uterine adenocarcinoma
    vaginal adenocarcinoma
    vulvar adenoid cystic
        adenocarcinoma
adenocarcinoma in Barrett
    esophagus
adenochondroma
adenochondrosarcoma
adenocystic carcinoma
adenofibroma
adenohypophysectomy
adenoid cancer
adenoid curet
adenoid cutter
adenoid cystic carcinoma
adenoid cystic carcinoma of
    head and neck (ACCHN)
adenoid face
adenoid facies
adenoid forceps
adenoid instruments
adenoid punch
adenoid squamous cell
    carcinoma
adenoidectomy
adenoides
    carcinoma epitheliale
        adenoides
adenoids
adenolipoma

adenolipomatosis
adenoma (*pl.* adenomas,
 ademonata)
acinous adenoma
adnexal adenoma
adrenal adenoma
apocrine adenoma
basal cell adenoma
basaloid monomorphic
 adenoma (BMA)
bile duct adenoma
bronchial adenoma
Brunner adenoma
canalicular adenoma
carcinoma ex pleomorphic
 adenoma
colonic adenoma
colorectal adenoma
double adenomas
ductal adenoma
duodenal adenoma
ectopic parathyroid adenoma
fibroid adenoma
follicular adenoma
hepatic adenoma
hepatocellular adenoma
Huerthle adenoma
kidney adenoma
liver cell adenoma
malignant adenoma
malignant pleomorphic
 adenoma
moderately differentiated
 adenoma
monoclonal adenoma
monomorphic adenoma
mucinous adenoma
oncocytic adenoma
papillary cystic adenoma
parathyroid adenoma
pedunculated adenoma
pituitary adenoma
pleomorphic adenoma
polypoid adenoma
prostatic adenoma
recurrent pleomorphic
 adenoma
renal adenoma
salivary gland pleomorphic
 adenoma
sebaceous adenoma
sessile adenoma

adenoma (*continued*)
single adenoma
sporadic pituitary adenoma
sweat-gland adenoma
thyroid adenoma
tracheal adenoma
tubular adenoma
tubulovillous adenoma
upper adenoma
villous adenoma
well-differentiated adenoma
well-localized adenoma
adenoma of breast
adenoma sebaceum
adenoma sudoriparum
adenomammectomy
adenomastectomy
adenomata (*sing.* adenoma)
adenomatosis oris
adenomatosum
 carcinoma adenomatosum
adenomatous goiter
adenomatous hyperplasia
adenomatous polyp
adenomyofibroma
adenomyosarcoma
adenomyosis
adenopapillary carcinoma
adenopathy
axillary adenopathy
cervical adenopathy
gross adenopathy
hilar adenopathy
inguinal adenopathy
lymph node adenopathy
palpable adenopathy
regional adenopathy
retroperitoneal adenopathy
scalene adenopathy
supraclavicular adenopathy
adenopexy
adenosatellite virus
adenosquamous carcinoma
adenotome
Abelson adenotome
Adair adenotome
adenotome blade
Box adenotome
Box-DeJager adenotome
Breitman adenotome
Cullom-Mueller adenotome
Daniels adenotome

adenotome (*continued*)
  direct-vision adenotome
  guillotine adenotome
  Kelly adenotome
  Kelly direct-vision adenotome
  LaForce adenotome
  LaForce-Grieshaber adenotome
  LaForce-Stevenson adenotome
  LaForce-Storz adenotome
  Mueller-LaForce adenotome
  Myles guillotine adenotome
  reverse adenotome
  Shambaugh reverse
    adenotome
  Shulec adenotome
  Sluder adenotome
  St. Clair-Thompson
    adenotome
  Stevenson LaForce
    adenotome
  Storz-LaForce adenotome
  Storz-LaForce-Stevenson
    adenotome
  V. Mueller-LaForce
    adenotome
adenotome blade
adenotomy
adenotonsillectomy
adenovirus
ADEPT (Advanced Elements of
  Pacing Trial)
adequacy
adequate
Aderer alloy
adhere
adherence
  immune adherence
adherence obstruction
adherence syndrome
adherens
  macula adherens
adherent bandage
adherent capsule
adherent cataract
adherent lens
adherent pericardium
adherent placenta
adherent stent
adherent tongue
AD-Hese-Away dressing
adhesiolysis
  abdominal adhesiolysis

adhesion
  amniotic adhesions
  anomalous mesenteric
    adhesion
  attic adhesion
  banjo-string adhesions
  capsular adhesions
  cell-cell adhesion
  cell-extracellular matrix
    adhesion
  cervicovaginal adhesions
  conjunctival adhesions
  cortical adhesions
  dense adhesions
  division of adhesions
  dry adhesions
  fibrinous adhesion
  fibrous adhesion
  fiddle-string adhesions
  filamentous adhesion
  filmy adhesions
  flexor tendon adhesion
  freeing up of adhesions
  hard adhesions
  hepatodiaphragmatic
    adhesions
  intestinal adhesions
  intra-abdominal adhesions
  intraperitoneal adhesions
  laparoscopic lysis of adhesion
  laryngeal adhesion
  lysed adhesions
  lysis of adhesions
  membranous adhesion
  meningeal adhesions
  mesenteric adhesions
  obstructing adhesions
  omental adhesions
  paratubular adhesions
  parauterine adhesions
  pelvic adhesions
  pericholecystic adhesions
  perigastric adhesions
  peritoneal adhesion
  piano-wire adhesion
  pleural adhesion
  postoperative adhesions
  primary adhesion
  Randall lip adhesion
  secondary adhesion
  serologic adhesion
  sublabial adhesion

adhesion (*continued*)
 takedown of adhesions
 tenacious adhesion
 tendon adhesions
 thick adhesions
 thin adhesions
 tight adhesions
 violin-string adhesions
adhesion barrier
adhesion formation
adhesion lysis
adhesiotomy
adhesive
 Adcon adhesive control gel
 ADTRA composite external
   fixator ring adhesive
 Aron Alpha adhesive
 autologous fibrin tissue
   adhesive
 BA bone cement adhesive
 bioactive bone cement
   adhesive
 Biobond tissue adhesive
 Biobrane adhesive
 BioGlue
 biologic fibrogen adhesive
 Bond-Eze bond adhesive
 bone cement adhesive
 Brown sterile adhesive
 Cel Touch adhesive
 Chewrite denture adhesive
 Coe-Pak paste adhesive
 composite external fixator
   ring adhesive
 Coverlet adhesive
 Cover-Roll gauze adhesive
 cyanoacrylate adhesive
 cyanoacrylate tissue adhesive
 denture adhesive
 Dermabond topical skin
   adhesive
 fibrin glue adhesive
 fibrin sealant adhesive
 gelatin-resorcin-formalin tissue
   glue adhesive
 HA adhesive
 Histoacryl glue adhesive
 hydroxyapatite adhesive
 Hy-Tape adhesive
 Implast bone cement adhesive
 Indermil tissue adhesive
 karaya adhesive

adhesive (*continued*)
 Klutch denture adhesive
 ligand adhesive
 LiquiBand topical wound-
   closure adhesive
 Liquiderm liquid adhesive
 LPPS hydroxyapatite adhesive
 Mammopatch gel self adhesive
 MCW cement adhesive
 MDS adhesive
 methyl methacrylate cement
   adhesive
 Nexacryl tissue adhesive
 Nu-Hope adhesive
 Orthomite II adhesive
 Orthoset radiopaque bone
   cement adhesive
 Palacos cement adhesive
 Plastodent dental impression
   adhesive
 Scanpor acrylate adhesive
 Silastic medical adhesive
 silicone adhesive
 Simplex cement adhesive
 stoma cap microporous
   adhesive
 Superglue adhesive
 Sur-Fit adhesive
 surgical appliance adhesive
 Surgical Simplex P radiopaque
   adhesive
 Tisseel biologic fibrogen
   adhesive
 T-Stick adhesive
 Urihesive expandable adhesive
 Uro-Bond II brush-on silicone
   adhesive
 Zimmer low-viscosity adhesive
adhesive absorbent dressing
adhesive aluminum splint
adhesive band
adhesive bandage
adhesive capsulitis
adhesive cement
adhesive colpitis
adhesive disease
adhesive drape
adhesive dressing board
adhesive flange
adhesive gauze
adhesive ileus
adhesive inflammation

adhesive needle holder
adhesive otitis media
adhesive pericarditis
adhesive phlebitis
adhesive plaster
adhesive plastic drape
adhesive pleurisy
adhesive pyelophlebitis
adhesive silicone gel (Cica-Care)
adhesive silicone implant
adhesive syndrome
adhesive tape remover
adhesive tape strips
adhesive tenosynovitis
adhesive vulvitis
adhesiveness
adiadochokinesis
Adie pupil
Adie syndrome
adipectomy
adipo aspirate
adipocele
adipocyte
adipodermal graft
adipofascial axial pattern cross-
    finger flap
adipofascial sural flap
adipofascial turnover flap
adipogenic growth factor-treated
    flaps
adiponecrosis
adiposa
    blepharoptosis adiposa
    capsula adiposa
    hernia adiposa
    seborrhea adiposa
adiposa hernia
adipose
adipose body of cheek
adipose capsule of kidney
adipose fold
adipose fossae
adipose graft
adipose infiltration
adipose layers of anterior
    abdominal wall
adipose ligament
adipose renal capsule
adipose sarcoma
adipose theory
adipose tissue
adipose tissue extract

adiposis dolorosa
adiposis universalis
adipositas abdominis
adipositas ex vacuo
adipositis
adiposity
    localized adiposity
adiposus
    arcus adiposus
    panniculus adiposus
aditus
    laryngeal aditus
adjacent tissue
adjunct therapy
adjunctive balloon angioplasty
adjunctive chemotherapy
adjunctive procedure
adjunctive rhinoplasty
adjunctive screw fixation
adjunctive suppressive medical
    therapy
adjustable advanced
    reciprocating gait orthosis
adjustable anterior guide
adjustable articulator
adjustable axis face-bow
adjustable breast implant
adjustable cross splint
adjustable cup reamer
adjustable external suture
adjustable headrest
adjustable leg and ankle
    repositioning mechanism
    (ALARM)
adjustable nail
adjustable ostomy appliance belt
adjustable pedicle connector
adjustable ring gastroplasty
adjustable saline breast implant
adjustable screw
adjustable skull traction tongs
adjustable splint
adjustable strap arm sling
adjustable thigh antiembolism
    stockings (ATS)
adjustable vaginal stent
adjustable-suture strabismus
    surgery
Adjust-A-Flow colostomy
    irrigation kit
Adjusta-Rak hanger
Adjusta-Wrist splint

adjusted occlusion
adjustment
adjustment occlusion
adjustment of cardiac pacemaker
adjuvant
  anesthesia adjuvant
adjuvant chemoradiation therapy
adjuvant chemotherapy
adjuvant drug therapy
adjuvant irradiation
adjuvant therapy
Adkins spinal arthrodesis
Adkins spinal fusion
Adkins strut
Adkins technique spinal
  arthrodesis
ADL (activities of daily living)
Adler attic ear punch
Adler bone forceps
Adler forceps
Adler lens loupe
Adler operation
Adler punch
Adler punch forceps
Adler tripronged lens error loop
Adler-Kreutz forceps
admaxillary
admaxillary gland
administration
  buccal drug administration
  concomitant administration
  drug administration
  epidural administration
  intramuscular administration
  intraocular administration
  intraperitoneal drug
    administration
  intraspinal administration
  intrathecal administration
  intravenous administration
  IV administration
  oral administration
  oxygen administration
  parenteral administration
  postischemic administration
  preischemic administration
  route of administration
  sequential administration
  transdermal administration
  transnasal administration
  vasodilator administration
admixture lesion

adnata
  alopecia adnata
adnexa
  ocular adnexa
adnexa oculi
adnexa uteri
adnexal adenoma
adnexal area
adnexal carcinoma
adnexal forceps
adnexal hemangioma
adnexal mass
adnexal metastasis
adnexal region
adnexal skin tumor
adnexal structures
ADNR (anterior displacement,
  no reduction)
adolescent cataract
adolescent vaginal speculum
ADR Ultramark 4 ultrasound
ADR Ultramark ultrasound
ADR ultrasound
adrenal ablation
adrenal adenoma
adrenal body
adrenal carcinoma
adrenal cortical hyperfunction
adrenal cortical hypofunction
adrenal feminization syndrome
adrenal gland biopsy
adrenal gland cyst
adrenal hemorrhage
adrenal medulla graft
adrenal medulla transplantation
adrenal medullary implants
adrenal metastasis
adrenal veins
adrenalectomize
adrenalectomy
  bilateral total adrenalectomy
  complete adrenalectomy
  Hugh Young adrenalectomy
  ipsilateral adrenalectomy
  laparoscopic adrenalectomy
  open adrenalectomy
  transperitoneal laparoscopic
    adrenalectomy
adrenalorrhaphy
adrenalotomy
adrenergic
adrenoceptor

adrenocortical carcinoma
adrenocortical extract
adrenocorticotropic hormone
    (ACTH)
Adrian-Flat prosthesis
adromia
Adson aneurysm needle
Adson angular hook
Adson artery forceps
Adson aspirating tube
Adson bayonet dressing forceps
Adson bipolar forceps
Adson blunt hook
Adson blunt knife
Adson bone rongeur
Adson brain clip
Adson brain forceps
Adson brain hook
Adson brain retractor
Adson brain suction tip
Adson brain suction tube
Adson brain-exploring cannula
Adson bur
Adson cannula
Adson cerebellar retractor
Adson chisel
Adson clamp
Adson clip
Adson conductor
Adson cranial rongeur
Adson dissecting hook
Adson dissector
Adson drainage cannula
Adson dressing forceps
Adson drill guide
Adson dura protector
Adson dural hook
Adson dural knife
Adson dural needle holder
Adson dural protector
Adson dural scissors
Adson elevator
Adson enlarging bur
Adson exploring cannula
Adson forceps
Adson ganglion scissors
Adson Gigli saw
Adson headrest
Adson hemostat
Adson hook
Adson hypophyseal forceps
Adson knife

Adson knot tier
Adson laminectomy chisel
Adson maneuver
Adson microbipolar forceps
Adson microdressing forceps
Adson microforceps
Adson microtissue forceps
Adson monopolar forceps
Adson needle
Adson needle holder
Adson neurosurgical suction tube
Adson perforating bur
Adson periosteal elevator
Adson pickup
Adson retractor
Adson rongeur
Adson saw conductor
Adson saw guide
Adson scalp clip
Adson scalp needle
Adson scissors
Adson sharp hook
Adson sharp knife
Adson sign
Adson speculum
Adson spiral drill
Adson splanchnic retractor
Adson straight suction tube
Adson suction tube
Adson suture needle
Adson test
Adson thumb forceps
Adson tissue forceps
Adson tooth forceps
Adson tube
Adson twist drill
Adson Vital tissue forceps
Adson-Beckman retractor
Adson-Biemer forceps
Adson-Brown clamp
Adson-Brown tissue forceps
Adson-Callison tissue forceps
Adson-Coffey scalenectomy
Adson-Love periosteal elevator
Adson-Mixter forceps
Adson-Murphy trocar point
    needle
Adson-Rogers cranial bur
Adson-Rogers perforating drill
Adson-Shaefer dural guide
Adson-Toennis scissors
Adson-Vital tissue forceps

adsorb
adsorbent
adsorption
ADTRA composite external
    fixator ring adhesive
adult acquired micrognathia
adult cardiovascular surgery
adult Chiari malformation
adult familial hyaline membrane
    disease
adult intussusception
adult laryngoscope
adult respiratory distress
    syndrome (ARDS)
adult reverse-bevel laryngoscope
adult scoliosis surgery
adult sigmoidoscope
adult teratoma
AdultPatch
    Trans-Ver-Sal AdultPatch
adult-to-adult living related
    donor living transplant
adult-type well-differentiated
    liposarcoma
Advance EX self-adhesive
    urinary external catheter
Advanced beta 200 otoscope
advanced breast biopsy
    instrumentation (ABBI)
advanced cardiac life support
    (ACLS)
Advanced Collection breast
    pump
advanced local invasion
Advanced NMR Systems scanner
Advanced Surgical suture
    applier
advanced therapeutic
    endoscopy
advanced tumor perforation
advancement
    capsular advancement
    five-flap V-Y advancement
    frontal bone advancement
    fronto-orbital advancement
    galea frontalis advancement
    horizontal maxillary
        advancement
    hyoid advancement
    Johnson pronator
        advancement
    LeFort III facial advancement

advancement (*continued*)
    lip border advancement
    mandibular advancement
    mandibular osteotomy
        advancement
    mandibular osteotomy-
        genioglossus advancement
    maxillofacial skeletal
        advancement
    monobloc advancement
    mucosal advancement
    tendon advancement
    Tessier type of frontal bone
        advancement
    tongue-in-groove
        advancement
    transanal pouch advancement
    transcranial monobloc
        frontofacial advancement
    Verhoeff advancement
    volar flap advancement
    V-Y advancement
    V-Y lip roll mucosal
        advancement
    Wagner advancement
advancement flap graft
advancement forceps
advancement genioplasty
advancement needle
advancement of muscle
advancement of ocular muscle
advancement of rectal flap
advancement of round ligament
advancement of superior
    oblique muscle
advancement of tendon
advancement procedure
advancing
    steadily advancing
Advantage ultrasound
advantageous
AdvanTeq II TENS unit
Advent Flurofocon contact lens
Advent implant
Advent pachymeter
adventitia
    membrana adventitia
    tunica adventitia
adventitial bed
adventitial cells
adventitial sheath
adventitial tissue

adventitious breath sounds
adventitious bursa
adventitious cyst
adventitious membrane
adventitious sounds
adverse event
advisable
adynamic bladder
adynamic ileus
adynamic intestinal obstruction
AE (above-elbow, aryepiglottic)
AE amputation (above-elbow
   amputation)
AE fold (aryepiglottic fold)
AE-7277 Rubenstein LASIK
   cannula
Aebli corneal suction scissors
Aebli scissors
Aebli tenotomy scissors
Aebli-Manson scissors
Aeby muscle
Aeby plane
AEC pacemaker
AED (aerodynamic equivalent
   diameter)
AED automatic external
   defibrillator
AEI button for replacement
   gastrostomy
Aequalis humeral head implant
Aequitron apnea monitor
Aequitron pacemaker
Aequitron ventilator
AER+ automatic endoscope
   reprocessor
aerate
aeration time
aeremia
aerobic bacteria
AeroChamber bronchial inhaler
AeroChamber facemask
AeroChamber metered-dose
   inhaler
AeroChamber pediatric spacer
   device
aerodermectasia
aerodynamic equivalent
   diameter (AED)
AeroEclipse device
aeroembolism
aero-flo tip catheter
aerogram

aerography
aerohydrotherapy
Aero-Kromayer lamp
aeroperitoneum
aeroplane splint
Aeroplast dressing
Aeroplasty
Aerosol Cloud Enhancer
aerosol therapy
aerosol-barrier pipette tip
aerosolize
aerosolized pollutant exposure
AeroSonic personal ultrasonic
   nebulizer
AeroTech II nebulizer
aerotitis media
aerotolerant anaerobe
aerotome
   Hall-Serge aerotome
Aerozoin skin conditioner
AERx electronic inhaler
AES antiembolic stockings
Aescula lead
Aesculap alpha vessel clip
Aesculap argon ophthalmic laser
Aesculap cast-cutting
   instruments
Aesculap drill
Aesculap excimer laser
Aesculap forceps
Aesculap instruments
Aesculap needle holder
Aesculap saw
Aesculap skull perforator
Aesculap traction bow
Aesculap-Meditec excimer laser
Aesculap-Pratt tenaculum
AE-series implantable pronged
   unipolar electrode
Aesop 2000, 3000 endoscopic
   stabilizer robot
aesthesioneuroblastoma
aesthetic (*variant of* esthetic)
aesthetic appearance
aesthetic procedure
aesthetic surgery
Aesthetica C topical vitamin C
   skin care product
aesthetician (*also* esthetician)
AF (antifog, antifogging)
AF agent (antifog agent)
AF solution (antifog solution)

AF tube (antifog tube)
AFB needle guide (aortofemoral
    bypass needle guide)
AFBG (aortofemoral bypass graft)
afferent clot
afferent fibers
afferent jejunostomy
afferent limb
afferent loop
afferent lymphatic
afferent nerve
afferent veins
afferent-efferent pathway
Affinity bed
Affinity pacemaker
affix
affixa
    lamina affixa
afflux
AFH (anterior facial height)
AFI Micros 5 microscope
AFO (ankle-foot orthosis)
AFO brace
AFocus catheter
AFP pacemaker
A-frame orthosis
afterbirth
aftercare
aftercataract bur
aftereffect
after-glide
afterload
afterload applicator
afterload colpostat
afterload reduction
afterloading catheter
afterloading colpostat
afterloading implant
afterloading screw
afterloading tandem (AL tandem)
afterloading technique
afterperception
aftersensation
aftertreatment
afunctional occlusion
AG Bovie electrosurgical unit
AGA (appropriate for gestational
    age)
aganglionic bowel
agar hydrocolloid impression
    material
agar impression material

agar-alginate impression material
Agarloid impression material
Agarose gel electrophoresis
agate burnisher
AGC
    anatomic graduated
        components
AGC dual-pivot resection guide
AGC knee program implant
AGC Modular Tibial II
    component
AGC porous anatomic femoral
    component
AGC unicondylar knee
    component
age
    appropriate for gestational
        age (AGA)
    bone age
    fertilization age
    fetal age
    gestational age
    Greulich-Pyle bone age
    large for gestational age (LGA)
    mental age (MA)
    small for gestational age (SGA)
AGE (angle of greatest extension)
Agee 4-pin fixation device
Agee carpal tunnel release
Agee device
Agee Digit Widget mini-external
    fixator
Agee endoscope
Agee fiberoptic carpal tunnel
    operation
Agee force-couple splint
    reduction
Agee sign
Agee WristJack
agenesis
    corpus callosum agenesis
    gonadal agenesis
    penile agenesis
    tracheal agenesis
    vaginal agenesis
agenetic fracture
agent
    AcuTect DVT imaging agent
    AF agent (antifog agent)
    AGF binding agent
    alcohol anesthetic agent
    alkylating agent

agent (*continued*)

alphaprodine anesthetic agent
Americaine anesthetic agent
amethocaine anesthetic agent
amobarbital anesthetic agent
Amytal anesthetic agent
Anectine anesthetic agent
Anestacon anesthetic agent
anesthetic agent
anesthetic induction agent
anesthetizing agent
Aneuroplast hemostatic agent
anticholinesterase anesthetic
    agent
antifogging agent
antiinflammatory agent
antineoplastic agent
antipruritic agent
antipyrotic agent
application of therapeutic
    agent
Avertin anesthetic agent
basal hypnotic agents
benoxinate hydrochloride
    anesthetic agent
benzocaine anesthetic agent
benzoquinonium chloride
    anesthetic agent
binding agent
Blockaine anesthetic agent
blocking agent
bone wax hemostatic agent
Brevital anesthetic agent
bupivacaine hydrochloride
    anesthetic agent
butacaine anesthetic agent
butethamine hydrochloride
    anesthetic agent
Butyn anesthetic agent
Carbocaine hydrochloride
    anesthetic agent
carbon dioxide anesthetic
    agent
cavity lining agent
Cetacaine anesthetic agent
chemical agent
chemotherapeutic agent
chloramine anesthetic agent
chloroprocaine hydrochloride
    anesthetic agent
cinchocaine anesthetic agent
Citanest anesthetic agent

agent (*continued*)

cocaine anesthetic agent
cocaine hydrochloride
    anesthetic agent
contrast agent
curare anesthetic agent
Cyclaine anesthetic agent
cyclomethycaine sulfate
    anesthetic agent
cyclopentane anesthetic agent
cyclopropane anesthetic
    agent
decamethonium bromide
    anesthetic agent
decamethonium iodide
    anesthetic agent
Demerol anesthetic agent
dibucaine hydrochloride
    anesthetic agent
diethyl oxide anesthetic agent
Dilaudid anesthetic agent
divinyl ether anesthetic agent
Duranest anesthetic agent
Dyclone anesthetic agent
dyclonine hydrochloride
    anesthetic agent
Eaton agent
edrophonium chloride
    anesthetic agent
electronarcosis agent
ether anesthetic agent
ethocaine anesthetic agent
Ethrane anesthetic agent
ethyl chloride anesthetic agent
ethyl ether anesthetic agent
ethyl oxide anesthetic agent
ethyl vinyl ether anesthetic
    agent
ethylene anesthetic agent
etidocaine hydrochloride
    anesthetic agent
Evipal anesthetic agent
Fluothane anesthetic agent
Forane anesthetic agent
gallamine anesthetic agent
ganglionic blocking agent
gaseous agent
halogenated agent
halothane anesthetic agent
helium anesthetic agent
hemostatic agent
hexobarbital anesthetic agent

agent (*continued*)

hexylcaine hydrochloride
  anesthetic agent
Holocaine anesthetic agent
hypnotic agents
hypotensive agents
immunosuppressive agent
inactivating agent
infusion of chemotherapeutic
  agent
inhalation agent
Innovar anesthetic agent
keratolytic agent
ketamine hydrochloride
  anesthetic agent
lidocaine hydrochloride
  anesthetic agent
lignocaine anesthetic agent
lipotropic agent
Lorfan anesthetic agent
Marcaine hydrochloride
  anesthetic agent
meperidine anesthetic agent
mepivacaine hydrochloride
  anesthetic agent
methohexital sodium
  anesthetic agent
methoxyflurane anesthetic
  agent
Metycaine hydrochloride
  anesthetic agent
morphine anesthetic agent
myoneural blocking agent
Myoview injectable
  radioactive diagnostic agent
narcotic agent
Nembutal anesthetic agent
NeoTect imaging agent
Nesacaine-CE anesthetic agent
neuromuscular blocking
  agents
Nisentil anesthetic agent
nitrous oxide anesthetic agent
Novocain anesthetic agent
Nupercaine hydrochloride
  anesthetic agent
Ophthaine anesthetic agent
OptiMARK MRI agent
Optison echocardiography
  agent
oral agent
Oxaine anesthetic agent

agent (*continued*)

oxethazaine anesthetic agent
paralytic agent
Penthrane anesthetic agent
pentobarbital anesthetic agent
Pentothal anesthetic agent
Percaine anesthetic agent
piperocaine hydrochloride
  anesthetic agent
PIPIDA hepatobiliary
  scanning agent
Pontocaine anesthetic agent
pramoxine hydrochloride
  anesthetic agent
prilocaine hydrochloride
  anesthetic agent
procaine hydrochloride
  anesthetic agent
proparacaine hydrochloride
  anesthetic agent
propoxycaine hydrochloride
  anesthetic agent
ProstaScint diagnostic
  imaging agent
sclerosing agent
secobarbital anesthetic agent
Seconal anesthetic agent
sodium pentothal anesthetic
  agent
SON anesthetic agent
succinylcholine anesthetic
  agent
suction hemostatic agent
Surfacaine anesthetic agent
synaptic blocking agents
Tensilon anesthetic agent
tetracaine hydrochloride
  anesthetic agent
thermal agents
thialbarbitone anesthetic
  agent
thiamylal sodium anesthetic
  agent
thiopental sodium anesthetic
  agent
tocolytic agent
topical cocaine anesthetic
  agent
trichloroethylene anesthetic
  agent
Trilene anesthetic agent
Trimar anesthetic agent

agent (*continued*)
Tronothane hydrochloride
anesthetic agent
vasoconstrictive agent
vasodilating agent
vasopressor agent
ventilation agent
vinyl ether anesthetic agent
vinyl ethyl ether anesthetic
agent
virucidal agent
viscoelastic agents
wetting agent
age-related macular
degeneration
AGF (angle of greatest flexion)
AGF (autologous growth factor)
AGF binding agent
AGF gel
Agfa Medical scanner
agger (*pl.* aggares)
agger nasi cells
agger perpendicularis
agglomerated
agglutinant
agglutinate
vasoactive agglutinate
agglutination technique
agglutinative
aggravate
aggregate
mineral trioxide aggregate
(MTA)
aggregate anaphylaxis
aggregate gland
aggregate human IgG (AHuG)
aggregati
folliculi lymphatici aggregati
aggressive infantile fibromatosis
aggressive lesion
aggressive skin care program
(Obagi)
aggressive surgical approach
Aggressor meniscal blade
Aggressor meniscal shaver
agility drill
aging
barnacles of aging
facial aging
vector of aging
agitation
abdominal agitation

aglossia-adactylia syndrome
agminate gland
agminated blue nevus
agnathia
Agnew canaliculus knife
Agnew canthoplasty
Agnew keratome
Agnew knife
Agnew needle
Agnew operation
Agnew splint
Agnew tattooing needle
Agnew traction
Agnew-Hunt reduction
Agnew-Verhoeff incision
agnosia
finger agnosia
agonal clot
agonal respirations
agonal thrombosis
agonal thrombus
agonist
agonistic muscle
agraffe
agraffe clamp
agranulocytic ulceration
agraphia
agria
Agricola (*also* Agrikola)
Agrikola eye speculum
Agrikola lacrimal sac retractor
Agrikola refractor
Agrikola retractor
Agrikola tattooing needle
Agris rasp
Agris-Dingman dissector
Agris-Dingman submammary
dissector
agrius
AgX antimicrobial Foley catheter
AHA (alpha hydroxyl acid)
AHA (alphahydroxy acid)
Ahern knot
AHG (antihemophilic globulin)
AHI (apnea-hypopnea index)
AHJ (artificial hip joint)
Ahlfeld sign
Ahlquist-Durham clip
Ahlquist-Durham embolism
clamp
Ahlquist-Durham vena cava clip
Ahmed glaucoma artificial valve

Ahn thrombectomy catheter
AHO (Albright hereditary
    osteodystrophy)
AHuG (aggregated human IgG)
AI (aortic insufficiency)
AI 5200 diagnostic ultrasound
AI angle
AICA (anterior inferior
    communicating artery)
Aicardi syndrome
AICD (automatic implantable
    cardioverter-defibrillator)
AICD (automatic internal
    cardioverter-defibrillator)
AICD device
AICD pacemaker
AICD plus Tachylog device
AICD-B pacemaker
AICD-BR pacemaker
aid
    bioptic aid
    cryostat frozen sectioning aid
    Servox speech aid (post-
        laryngectomy)
    walking aids
AID (artificial insemination
    donor)
AID (automatic implantable
    defibrillator)
AID-B defibrillator
AID-B pacemaker
AIDS (acquired
        immunodeficiency
        syndrome)
AIDS-related complex (ARC)
AIDS-related cryptococcal
    meningitis
AIE (acute infective
    endocarditis)
AIH (artificial insemination
    husband)
Ailee needle
AIM 7 thermocouple input
    module
AIM CPM (continuous passive
    motion)
Aim retractor
aimer
    Arthrotek femoral aimer
    Paddu tibial aimer
Ainslie acrylic splint
Ainsworth arch

Ainsworth punch
AIO compression plate
air
    ambient air
    complemental air
    escape of air
    free air
    germ-laden air
    inhaled air
    injection of air
    intramural colonic air
    intraperitoneal air
    liquid air
    proctoscopic air
    residual air
    retroperitoneal injection of air
    tidal air
    trapping of air
air aspirator needle
air bag
air bed
air block
air bronchogram sign
air bubble
air cannula
air cell casts
air cells
air chamber
air collection
air compressor
air contrast barium enema
    (ACBE)
air cyst
air cystogram
air dermatome
air dome sign
air drill
air embolism
air embolus
air exchange
air inflatable tube
air inflatable vessel occluder
    clamp
air injection cannula
air insufflation
air myelography
air pillow
air plethysmograph
Air Plus low-air-loss bed
air pressure dressing
air pyelogram
air saccule

air sacs
air saw
air sinus
air space disease
air splint
Air Supply air purifier
air syringe
air trapping
air tube
air velocity index
AIR1517 vacuum-formed static
     air wheelchair cushion
air-bone gap
air-boot
   Jobst postoperative air-boot
airbrasive technique
Aircast Air-Stirrup leg brace
Aircast brace
Aircast Cryo Cuff
Aircast fracture brace
Aircast pneumatic brace
Aircast Swivel-Strap brace
Aircast walking brace
air-core magnet
air-driven
air-driven artificial heart
air-driven saw
Aire-Cuf endotracheal tube
Aire-Cuf tracheostomy tube
air-filled loop
AirFlex carpal tunnel splint
airflow limitation
airflow management
airflow obstruction
airflow resistance
air-fluid exchange
air-fluid level
air-fluid line
air-fluidized bed
airfoam splint
air-gap technique
AirGEL ankle brace
airgun retractor
Airkair seat cushion
AIRLens contact lens
Airlife cannula
Airlife Dual Spray MiniSpacer
Airlife MediSpacer
Airlift balloon retractor
AirLITE support pad
Air-Lon adapter
Air-Lon decannulation plug

Air-Lon inhalation cannula
Air-Lon inhalation catheter
Air-Lon laryngectomy tube
Air-Lon plug
Air-Lon tracheal tube brush
Air-Lon tube
AIR-O-EASE static air flotation
     mattress
Air-O-Pad pad
airplane position
airplane splint
air-powered drill
air-powered nebulizer
Airprene hinged knee prosthesis
Airprene hinged knee support
air-puff tonometer
Air-Shield-Vickers syringe tip
Airsoft dry replacement mattress
air-spaced electrode
airsplint
air-stirrup ankle brace
Airstrip composite dressing
airtight closure
airway
   anatomic airway
   anatomical airway
   Beck mouth tube airway
   Berman disposable airway
   Berman intubating pharyngeal
        airway
   binasal pharyngeal airway
   blocked airway
   clear airways
   Coburg-Connell airway
   Combitube airway
   Concord/Portex airway
   Connell airway
   disposable airway
   double-lumen gastric
        laryngeal mask airway
   esophageal obturator airway
   Foerger airway
   Guedel rubber airway
   large mask airway
   laryngeal mask airway (LMA)
   LMA-Unique disposable
        laryngeal mask airway
   Lumbard airway
   Luomanen oral airway
   major airway
   nasal airway
   nasopharyngeal airway

airway (*continued*)
  obstructed airway
  oral pharyngeal airway
  oropharyngeal airway
  pediatric airway
  pharyngeal airway
  Portex nasopharyngeal airway
  Robertazzi nasopharyngeal
    airway
  rubber airway
  Safar-S airway
  Sarfar-S airway
  suction airway
  upper airway
airway compromise
airway elastance
airway gas monitoring
airway management
airway obstruction
airway occlusion technique
airway pattern
airway pressure release
    ventilation (APRV)
airway protection
airway reactivity
airway resistance
airway responsiveness
airway score
airway shunting
airway smooth muscle (ASM)
airway suction
airway, breathing, circulation
    protocol (ABC protocol)
Airy rings
Aitken epiphysial fracture
    classification
AJ (ankle jerk)
AJCC (American Joint
    Committee on Cancer)
AJCC staging
AJCC TNM tumor classification
Ajmalin liver injury
A-K diamond knife
AK-10 dialysis machine
AKA (above-knee amputation)
Akahoshi Nucleus Sustainer
Akahoshi phaco prechopper
AKC varicose vein operation
Aker lens pusher
Aker pusher
Akerlund deformity
Akerlund diaphragm

Akin bunionectomy
akinesia
  Nadbath akinesia
  O'Brien akinesia
  orbital akinesia
  Van Lint-Atkinson akinesia
  Van Lint-O'Brien akinesia
akinesis
akinetic
Akins valve re-do forceps
Akiyama prosthesis
Akron tilt table
Akros DFD wheelchair wedge
    cushion
Akros extended-care mattress
Akros mattress
AkroTech mattress
Akton pad
Akton positioning roll
Akutsu III total artificial heart
Akutsu artificial heart
AL (axiolingual)
AL II guiding catheter
AL reconstruction
AL tandem (afterloading tandem)
AL-1 catheter
ala (*pl.* alae)
  Burkitt lymphoma of nasal ala
  nasal ala
  sacral ala
  thyroid ala
ALA (axiolabial)
ala auris
ala cerebelli
ala cinerea
ala cristae galli
ala ilii
ala major ossis sphenoidalis
ala minor ossis sphenoidalis
ala nasi
ala of ilium
ala of nose
ala of the ethmoid
ala parva ossis sphenoidalis
ala temporalis ossis sphenoidalis
Alabama needle holder
Alabama University forceps
Alabama-Green needle holder
alacrima
alae protector
ala-facial groove
Alanson amputation

alar area
alar artery of nose
alar base
alar batten cartilage
alar bone
alar branch of external maxillary
     artery
alar cartilage
alar chest
alar cinch
alar collapse
alar crease
alar dome and cartilage
alar facial groove
alar fascia
alar flaring
alar flutter
alar folds
alar groove
alar incision
alar lamina
alar ligament
alar muscle
alar osteotome
alar pinching
alar protector
alar reconstruction
alar retractor
alar rim collapse
alar rim excision
alar scapula
alar screw
alar spine
alar suspension stitch
alar wedge excision
alar-columellar relation
alar-facial junction
ALARM (adjustable leg and
     ankle repositioning
     mechanism)
alarplasty
alba
   linea alba
   lingua alba
   lingua villosa alba
   lochia alba
   materia alba
   stria alba
Albany eye guard
Albarran bridge
Albarran cystoscope
Albarran gland

Albarran laser cystoscope
Albarran lens
Albarran urethroscope
Albarran-Reverdin needle
Albee arthrodesis
Albee bone graft calipers
Albee bone saw
Albee drill
Albee fracture table
Albee fusion
Albee graft
Albee hip operation
Albee hip reconstruction
Albee olive-shaped bur
Albee operation
Albee orthopedic fracture table
Albee osteotome
Albee osteotomy
Albee saw
Albee shelf procedure
Albee spinal fusion
Albee table
Albee technique
Albee-Compere fracture table
Albee-Delbert procedure
Albee-Delbet operation
Albers-Schoenberg disease
Albers-Schoenberg marble
     bones
Albers-Schoenberg chalk bones
Albers-Schoenberg position
Albert bronchoscope
Albert knee operation
Albert operation
Albert position
Albert slotted bronchoscope
Albert sutures
Albert-Andrews laryngoscope
Albert-Chase procedure
Albert-Lembert gastroplasty
Albert-Smith pessary
albicans
   corpus albicans
   stria albicans
albicantia
   corpora albicantia
albida
   acne albida
albidum
   atrophoderma albidum
Albion-Ford stethoscope
Albizzia nail

Albrecht bone
Albright disease
Albright hereditary
    osteodystrophy (AHO)
Albright hip synovectomy
Albright syndrome
Albright-Chase arthroplasty
Albright-Hadorn syndrome
Albright-McCune-Sternberg
    syndrome
albuginea
albugineotomy
albumin-coated vascular graft
albuminized woven Dacron tube
    graft
Alcatel pacemaker
Alcock bag
Alcock bladder syringe
Alcock boots
Alcock canal
Alcock catheter
Alcock conical catheter adapter
Alcock hemostatic bag
Alcock hemostatic catheter
Alcock lithotrite
Alcock obturator
Alcock plug
Alcock return-flow hemostatic
    catheter
Alcock syringe
Alcock-Hendrickson lithotrite
Alcock-Timberlake obturator
alcohol
    polyvinyl alcohol
alcohol anesthetic agent
alcohol fixation
alcohol-fixed gastric biopsy
alcoholic cirrhosis
alcoholic fatty liver
alcoholic varices
alcohol injection
    percutaneous alcohol
        injection
Alcon A-OK crescent knife
Alcon A-OK phacoemulsification
    slit knife
Alcon A-OK ShortCut knife
Alcon aspirator
Alcon cautery
Alcon crescent blade
Alcon cryoextractor
Alcon cryophake

Alcon cryosurgical unit
Alcon CU-15 4-mil needle
Alcon cystitome
Alcon Digital B 2000 ultrasound
Alcon disposable drape
Alcon hand cautery
Alcon I-knife
Alcon indirect ophthalmoscope
Alcon intraocular lens
Alcon irrigating needle
Alcon lens
Alcon microsponge
Alcon Phaco-Emulsifier
Alcon pocket blade
Alcon reverse cutting needle
Alcon spatula needle
Alcon sponge
Alcon surgical instruments
Alcon surgical knife
Alcon sutures
Alcon taper-cut needle
Alcon taper-point needle
Alcon tonometer
Alcon vitrectomy probe
Alcon vitrector
Alcott catheter
aldehyde-tanned bovine carotid
    artery graft
Alden loop gastric bypass
Alden retractor
Alden-Senturia specimen
    collector
Alderkreutz tissue forceps
Alder-Reilly anomaly
aldosterone-producing
    carcinoma
Aldrete needle
Aldridge operation
Aldridge rectus fascia sling
Aldridge sling procedure
Aldridge urethropexy
Aldridge-Studdefort urethral
    suspension
Aleman meniscotomy knife
alveolar fistula
Aleppo button
ALERT catheter
ALERT Companion II defibrillator
Alert-TD catheter
Alesen tube
Alexander antrostomy punch
Alexander approximator

Alexander biopsy punch
Alexander bone lever
Alexander chisel
Alexander costal periosteotome
Alexander dressing forceps
Alexander elevator
Alexander gouge
Alexander incision
Alexander mastoid chisel
Alexander mastoid gouge
Alexander needle
Alexander operation
Alexander osteotome
Alexander otoplasty knife
Alexander periosteotome
Alexander prostatectomy
Alexander punch
Alexander raspatory
Alexander retractor
Alexander rib rasp
Alexander rib stripper
Alexander shortening of round
    ligaments
Alexander syringe
Alexander technique
Alexander tonsil needle
Alexander-Adams hysteropexy
Alexander-Adams operation
Alexander-Adams uterine
    suspension
Alexander-Ballen orbital
    retractor
Alexander-Farabeuf costal
    periosteotome
Alexander-Farabeuf elevator
Alexander-Farabeuf forceps
Alexander-Farabeuf
    periosteotome
Alexander-Farabeuf rib rasp
Alexander-Matson retractor
Alexander-Reiner ear syringe
alexandrite laser
alexandrite long-pulsed laser
Alexian Brothers overhead
    fracture frame
Alexian Hospital retractor
ALEXlazr
    Candela ALEXlazr
ALEXlazr laser
Alezzandrini syndrome
Alfa II electrode
Alfonso eyelid speculum

Alfonso guarded bur
Alfonso speculum
Alfreck retractor
Alfred Becht temporary crown
Alfred M. Large vena cava clamp
Alfred snare
alganesthesia
Algee impression material
algefacient
algeoscopy
Alger brush
algesia
algesimeter
    Björnström algesimeter
algesimetry (*also* algesiometry)
algesthesia
algetic
Al-Ghorab modification
Al-Ghorab procedure
AlgiDERM alginate wound
    dressing
AlgiDERM wound packing
alginate
    Hydro-Jel alginate
alginate impression material
alginate wound dressing
AlgiSite alginate wound dressing
Algisorb wound dressing
Algitec impression material
algogenesia
algogenesis
algogenic
algorithm
    bone algorithm
Algosteril alginate wound
    dressing
Alien WildEyes lens
aligner
    Charnley femoral inlay aligner
    femoral aligner
    Geo-Matt 30-degree body
        aligner
    patellar aligner
    tibial aligner
alignment
    fracture alignment
    orbicular alignment
    overall alignment
alignment catheter
alignment cord
alignment curve
AliMed diabetic night splint

AliMed Freedom arthritis
  support
AliMed QualCraft wrist support
AliMed surgical drape
aliment
alimentary canal
alimentary tract duplication
alimentation
  parenteral alimentation
  total parenteral alimentation
alimentation catheter
A-line (arterial line)
Aliplast custom molded foot
  orthosis
aliquot
alisphenoid area
alisphenoid bone
alisphenoid canal
alisphenoid cartilage
Aliston procedure
Alivium prosthesis cup
Aljan prosthesis
alkali burn
alkali caustic
alkaline battery cautery
Alken approach
Alken set
alkylating agent
Allan bone lengthening
Allan calcaneus procedure
allantoic circulation
allantoic membrane
Allarton operation
Allconox
All-Cord bench engine
All-Cord surgical engine
Alldress multilayer wound
  dressing
Allegist syringe
Allen anastomosis clamp
Allen applicator
Allen arm surgery table
Allen cecostomy trocar
Allen clamp
Allen correction
Allen cyclodialysis
Allen ePTFE ocular implant
Allen eye implant
Allen eye introducer
Allen fetal stethoscope
Allen finger trap
Allen forceps

Allen hand surgery table
Allen implant
Allen laparoscopic stirrups
Allen maneuver
Allen operation
Allen orbital implant
Allen pliers
Allen reduction
Allen retractor
Allen root pliers
Allen saw
Allen screw
Allen sphere introducer
Allen spherical eye introducer
Allen stereo separator
Allen Supramid implant
Allen test
Allen trocar
Allen uterine forceps
Allen well leg holder
Allen wire threader
Allen wrench
Allen-Barkan forceps
Allen-Barkan knife
Allen-Braley intraocular lens
  implant
Allen-Braley forceps
Allen-Brown prosthesis
Allen-Brown shunt
Allen-Brown vascular access
  shunt
Allen-Burian trabeculotome
Allen-Hanbury knife
Allen-headed screwdriver
Allen-Heffernan nasal speculum
Allen-Kocher clamp
Allen-Schiøtz plunger retractor
  tonometer
Allen-Thorpe goniolens
Allen-Thorpe gonioscopic prism
Allen-type hex key
Allerdyce approximator
Allerdyce dissector
Allerdyce elevator
Allergan Medical Optics
Allergan-Humphrey lensometer
Allergan-Humphrey
  photokeratoscope
Allergan-Simcoe C-loop
  intraocular lens
allergen exposure
allergic inflammation

allergic reaction (*type I-IV*)
allergic shock
allergic sialadenitis
allergy
    drug allergy
    dye allergy
Allevyn adhesive hydrocellular
    dressing
Allevyn dressing
Allevyn hydrophilic
    polyurethane dressing
Allevyn Island dressing
Allgower suture technique
Alliance catheter
alligator cable
alligator clip
alligator crimper forceps
alligator forceps
alligator grasping forceps
alligator MacCarty scissors
alligator nasal forceps
alligator pacing cable
alligator scissors
alligator skin
alligator-type grasping forceps
Allingham colotomy
Allingham excision of rectum
Allingham operation
Allingham rectal speculum
Allingham ulcer
All-In-One laparoscopic electrode
all-inside repair
Allis catheter
Allis clamp
Allis delicate tissue forceps
Allis dissector
Allis dry dissector
Allis forceps
Allis hemostat
Allis inhaler
Allis intestinal forceps
Allis lung retractor
Allis maneuver
Allis Micro-Line pediatric
    forceps
Allis periosteal elevator
Allis retractor
Allis thoracic forceps
Allis tissue clamp
Allis tissue forceps
Allis tissue-holding forceps
Allis-Abramson breast biopsy

Allis-Abramson breast biopsy
    forceps
Allis-Adair forceps
Allis-Adair intestinal forceps
Allis-Adair tissue forceps
Allis-Coakley forceps
Allis-Coakley tonsil forceps
Allis-Duval forceps
Allis-Ochsner forceps
Allison clamp
Allison forceps
Allison gastroesophageal reflux
    operation
Allison gastroesophageal reflux
    repair
Allison herniorrhaphy
Allison hiatal hernia repair
Allison lung retractor
Allison lung spatula
Allison sutures
Allison technique
Alliston GE reflux correction
Allis-Willauer forceps
Allman acromioclavicular injury
    classification
Allman ankle reconstruction
Allman classification of AC joint
all-metal ear syringe
AlloAnchor RC
Alloclassic Zweymuller hip
    arthroplasty
AlloDerm acellular dermal graft
AlloDerm cellular dermal graft
AlloDerm onlay graft
AlloDerm preserved human
    dermis
AlloDerm processed tissue graft
Alloderm spacer graft
AlloDerm universal dermal
    tissue graft
allogeneic bone crib
allogeneic graft
allogeneic keratinocyte graft
allogeneic lyophilized bone graft
    implant material
allogeneic material
allogeneic transplantation
allogenic bone graft
allogenic fetal graft
allogenically vascularized
    prefabricated flap
allogenous bone graft

allogotrophia
allograft
  acetabular allograft
  AlloGro freeze-dried bone
    allograft
  bovine allograft
  cancellous freeze-dried
    allograft
  cortical bone allograft
  cortical freeze-dried allograft
  cryopreserved heart-valve
    allograft
  decalcified freeze-dried bone
    allograft (DFDBA)
  demineralized freeze-dried
    bone allograft (DFDBA)
  femoral cortical ring allograft
  freeze-dried bone allograft
  fresh frozen allograft
  functioning allograft
  hepatic allograft
  intercalary allograft
  intestinal allograft
  liver allograft
  MTE allograft
  napkin ring calcar allograft
  organ allograft
  osteoarticular allograft
  osteochondral allograft
  pancreaticoduodenal allograft
  Proplast allograft
  renal allograft
  Silastic allograft
  Tutoplast processed allograft
allograft bone vise
allograft corneal rejection
allograft extraction
allograft joint replacement
allograft reaction
allograft rejection
allograft survival
allograft tissue transplantation
allograft transplantation
allograft wound covering
allograft-host junction
AlloGrip bone vise
AlloGro freeze-dried bone
  allograft
alloimplant
allokeratoplasty
AlloMatrix injectable putty bone
  graft substitute

allometric
allopathic keratoplasty
alloplast
alloplastic AMA
alloplastic augmentation
  genioplasty
alloplastic chin augmentation
alloplastic crib
alloplastic facial implant
alloplastic implants
alloplastic reconstruction
alloplastic transplant
alloplasty
Allo-Pro prosthesis
allotransplantation
  inlet allotransplantation
  liver allotransplantation
allotriodontia
alloy
  Aderer alloy
  amalgam alloy
  Arjalloy alloy
  Ceradelta alloy
  Ceramalloy alloy
  Cerapall alloy
  Cer-Mate alloy
  Cer-On R alloy
  cobalt-chromium alloy
  cobalt-chromium-
    molybdenum alloy
  Co-Cr-Mo alloy
  Co-Cr-W-Ni alloy
  Coltene alloy
  Coronet alloy
  Co-Span alloy
  Degucast alloy
  Degudent alloy
  Densilay alloy
  Dentsply alloy
  E-G alloy
  Eligoy metal alloy
  Everest alloy
  Fulcast alloy
  GFH alloy
  GM alloy
  Hammond alloy
  Imperial alloy
  Leff alloy
  Lumi alloy
  Maxigold alloy
  Midas alloy
  Midigold alloy

alloy (*continued*)
Minigold alloy
Ostalloy 202 alloy
Phase-A-Caps alloy
Phasealloy alloy
Primalloy alloy
Remanium alloy
Safco alloy
Shasta alloy
Sierra alloy
Stabilor alloy
Steldent alloy
Summar alloy
Summit alloy
Thriftcase alloy
Tivanium Ti-6A1-4V alloy
Ultracast alloy
Vera bond alloy
Victory alloy
Vitallium alloy
Wilgnath alloy
Wilkadium alloy
Wilkoro alloy
Wil-Tex alloy
Zimaloy cobalt-chromium-
molybdenum alloy
alloy-forming metal
all-PMMA one-piece C-loop
intraocular lens
Allport cutting bur
Allport eustachian bur
Allport gauze packer
Allport hook
Allport incus hook
Allport mastoid bayonet
retractor
Allport mastoid searcher
Allport mastoid sound
Allport operation
Allport packer
Allport ptosis correction
procedure
Allport retractor
Allport searcher
Allport-Babcock mastoid
searcher
Allport-Babcock retractor
Allport-Babcock searcher
Allport-Babcock sound
Allport-Gifford retractor
All-Pro automatic film developer
all-purpose lamp

all-purpose stretcher
all-purpose transilluminator
Allskin marker
all-trans retinoic acid aqueous
gel
All-Tronics scanner
Allurion foot prosthesis
Alm clip applier
Alm dilator
Alm microsurgery retractor
Alm minor surgery retractor
Alm self-retaining retractor
Almeida forceps
Almoor extrapetrosal drainage
Almoor operation
Alnico magneprobe magnet
aloe stitch scissors
aloe tape dressing
Aloetherm diathermy
Aloka echocardiograph machine
Aloka linear ultrasound
Aloka MP-PN ultrasound probe
Aloka OB/GYN ultrasound
Aloka SSD-720 real-time scanner
Aloka transducer
Aloka ultrasound diagnostic
equipment
Aloka ultrasound linear scanner
Aloka ultrasound sector scanner
Alonso-Lej classification
alopecia
burn alopecia
cicatricial alopecia
marginal alopecia
marginal traumatic alopecia
pressure alopecia
radiation alopecia
scarring alopecia
traumatic alopecia
alopecia adnata
alopecia areata
alopecia capitis totalis
alopecia cicatrisata
alopecia circumscripta
alopecia follicularis
alopecia liminaris frontalis
alopecia marginalis
alopecia orbicularis
alopecia seborrheica
alopecia senilis
Alor 5/500
Alouette amputation

Alouette operation
Alpar intraocular lens implant
Alpern cortex
    aspirator/hydrodissector
Alpha 1 penile implant
Alpha Chymar
alpha cradle
Alpha fiberoptic pocket
    otoscope
alpha hydroxyl acid (AHA)
alpha loop maneuver
alpha sigmoid loop
alpha$_2$-macroglobulin
AlphaCare monitor
alpha-chymotrypsin cannula
alpha-fetoglobulin
alpha-fetoprotein
alpha-hydroxy acid (AHA)
    (*written also* alphahydroxy
    acid)
alphaprodine anesthetic agent
AlphaStar operating room table
Alport syndrome
ALR cystoresectoscope
ALRI (anterolateral rotatory
    instability)
Alsus-Knapp eyelid repair
Alsus-Knapp operation
alta
    patella alta
Alta cancellous screw
Alta CFX reconstruction rod
Alta channel bone plate
Alta condylar buttress plate
Alta cortical screw
Alta cross-locking screw
Alta distal fracture plate
Alta femoral bolt
Alta femoral intramedullary rod
Alta femoral plate
Alta humeral rod
Alta intramedullary rod
Alta reconstruction rod
Alta supracondylar bone plate
Alta supracondylar screw
Alta tibial rod
Alta tibial-humeral rod
Alta transverse screw
Altchek vaginal mold
Altemeier operation
Altemeier rectal prolapse
    procedure

Alter lip retractor
alterative inflammation
altercursive intubation
altering route of administration
alternans
    pulsus alternans
alternate-day therapy
alternating sutures
alternation
alternative approach
alternative communication
    device
alternative surgical approach
alternatives of management
    (AOM)
alternator
    film alternator
Altmann classification of
    congenital aural atresia
Altmann needle
Alton Deal pressure infuser
Altona finger extension device
Alumafoam nasal splint
Alumina cemented total hip
    prosthesis
aluminum acetate and acetic
    acid
aluminum alloy fork
aluminum bridge splint
aluminum cortex retractor
aluminum cranioplasty
aluminum eye shield
aluminum fence splint
aluminum finger cot splint
aluminum foam splint
aluminum mallet
aluminum oxide abrasive
aluminum paste
aluminum splint
aluminum wire sutures
ALVAD (abdominal left
    ventricular assist device)
ALVAD artificial heart
Alvarado orthopedic guide
Alvarado Orthopedic Research
    instruments (AOR
    instruments)
Alvarado surgical knee holder
Alvarez prosthesis
Alvarez valve prosthesis
Alvarez-Rodriguez cardiac
    catheter

Alvegniat pump
alveodental suppuration
Alveoform Biograft
Alveograf binder
Alveograf bone-grafting material
alveolabial groove
alveolabial sulcus
alveolabialis
alveolar abscess
alveolar adenocarcinoma
alveolar angle
alveolar arch derangement
alveolar arch of mandible
alveolar arch of maxilla
alveolar area
alveolar artery
alveolar assimilation
alveolar atrophy
alveolar body
alveolar bone defect
alveolar bone density
alveolar bone graft
alveolar border of mandible
alveolar border of maxilla
alveolar branch of internal
    maxillary artery
alveolar canal of maxilla
alveolar capillary
alveolar cavity
alveolar cell carcinoma
alveolar cleft
alveolar crest
alveolar dead space
alveolar dehiscence
alveolar duct
alveolar ectasia
alveolar extension palatoplasty
alveolar fibers
alveolar fistula
alveolar foramina
alveolar gland
alveolar grafting
alveolar height
alveolar hemorrhage
alveolar index
alveolar limbus of mandible
alveolar limbus of maxilla
alveolar margin
alveolar mucosa
alveolar nerve
alveolar osteitis
alveolar periosteum

alveolar plate fenestration
alveolar point
alveolar point-basion line
alveolar point-meatus plane
alveolar point-nasal point line
alveolar point-nasion line
alveolar process
alveolar profile angle
alveolar ridge
alveolar septum
alveolar sinus
alveolar socket wall fracture
alveolar soft part sarcoma
    (ASPS)
alveolar support
alveolar supporting bone
alveolar surface of mandible
alveolar surface of maxilla
alveolar ventilation
alveolar yokes of mandible
alveolar yokes of maxilla
alveolar-arterial oxygen gradient
alveolar-capillary membrane
alveolate
alveolectomy
    mandibular alveolectomy
    maxillary alveolectomy
    partial alveolectomy
    recontouring alveolectomy
alveoli (*sing.* alveolus)
alveolingual groove
alveolingual sulcus
alveolitis
    extrinsic allergic alveolitis
alveolobasilar line
alveolobuccal groove
alveolobuccal sulcus
alveolocapillary membrane
alveolocapillary partial pressure
    gradient
alveolodental canals
alveolodental membrane
alveolonasal line
alveoloplasty
    interradicular alveoloplasty
    intraseptal alveoloplasty
    maxillary alveoloplasty
alveoloplasty reparative closure
alveolotomy
alveolus (*pl.* alveoli)
    buccal alveolus
    canine alveolus

alveolus (*continued*)
  cleft alveolus
  dental alveolus
  lingual alveolus
  mandibular alveolus
  maxillary alveolus
  maxillary first molar alveolus
  mesiobuccal alveolus
  mucous alveolus
  salivary gland alveolus
  serous alveolus
  supramentale mandibular
    alveolus
alveolus dentalis
alveoplasty
alvine calculus
Alvis curet
Alvis fixation forceps
Alvis forceps
Alvis operation
Alvis ptosis correction procedure
Alvis spud
Alvis-Lancaster sclerotome
Alvogyl surgical dressing
Alwall artificial kidney
Alway groover
always-lower-the-fold-a-specific-
    amount philosophy
Alyea clamp
Alyea vas clamp
Alzate catheter
Alzer Model 2001 osmotic
    minipump
ALZET continuous infusion
    osmotic pump
Alzheimer lamp
AMA (augmentation of the
    mandibular angle)
Amadeus ventilator
AMA-Fab scintigraphy
amalgam
  dental amalgam
  marginal integrity of amalgam
amalgam alloy
amalgam carrier
amalgam condenser
amalgam filling
amalgam matrix
amalgam plugger elevator
amalgam scraper
amalgamator
  crown amalgamator

Amark perimeter
Amato body
amaurosis
  Burn amaurosis
amazon thorax
Amazr catheter
amber latex catheter
Amberg lateral sinus line
AMBI compression hip screw
AMBI reamer
Ambicor inflatable prosthesis
Ambicor penile prosthesis
ambient air
ambient oxygen
ambiguity
ambiguous external genitalia
Ambil Skin Tone
Ambler dilator
amblyopia
Ambrose eye forceps
Ambrose operation
Ambrose suture forceps
Ambrose ureterovesicoplasty
Ambu bag
Ambu CardioPump
Ambu respirator
Ambu resuscitator
Ambu-E valve
ambulant
ambulation
  independent ambulation
  standing ambulation
ambulatory anesthesia
ambulatory electrogram monitor
    (AEM)
ambulatory gynecologic
    laparoscopy
ambulatory hemorrhoidectomy
ambulatory Holter monitor
ambulatory infusion
    management device
ambulatory surgery
ambulatory venous
    hypertension
Ambulift
ambustion
Ambuy infant resuscitator
AMC needle
AMC wrist prosthesis
Amcath catheter
AMD artificial urinary sphincter
Amdur lid forceps

AME bone growth stimulator
AME PinSite shield
amebic cyst
amebic hepatic abscess
amebic perforation
amelia
amelioration
ameloblastic carcinoma
ameloblastic fibroma
ameloblastic fibrosarcoma
ameloblastic hemangioma
ameloblastic sarcoma
ameloblastoma
  acanthomatous
    ameloblastoma
  desmoplastic ameloblastoma
  intraosseous ameloblastoma
  melanotic ameloblastoma
  mural ameloblastoma
  peripheral ameloblastoma
  pigmented ameloblastoma
  unicystic ameloblastoma
Amelogen dental implant
Amenabar capsular forceps
Amenabar capsule forceps
Amenabar counterpressor
Amenabar discission hook
Amenabar iris retractor
Amenabar knife
Amenabar lens
Amenabar retractor
amenable
amenorrhea
Amercal intraocular lens
Amercal-Shepard intraocular
  lens
Americaine anesthetic agent
American artificial larynx
American Association for
  Surgery of Trauma Organ
  Injury Scale classification
American Board of Surgery
  (ABS)
American Catheter Corporation
  biopsy forceps
American circle nephrostomy
  tube
American Dilation System
  dilator
American Endoscopy automatic
  reprocessor
American endoscopy dilator

American endoscopy
  esophageal dilator
American endoscopy
  mechanical lithotriptor
American Hamilton stretcher
American Hanks uterine dilator
American Heart Association
  classification
American Heyer-Schulte brain
  retractor
American Heyer-Schulte chin
  prosthesis
American Heyer-Schulte
  elastomer
American Heyer-Schulte malar
  prosthesis
American Heyer-Schulte
  mammary prosthesis
American Heyer-Schulte
  rhinoplasty prosthesis
American Heyer-Schulte stent
American Heyer-Schulte
  testicular prosthesis
American Heyer-Schulte T-tube
American Heyer-Schulte-
  Hinderer malar prosthesis
American Heyer-Schulte-
  Radovan tissue expander
  prosthesis
American Heyer-Schulte-
  Robertson suprapubic
  trocar
American Hydron instruments
American intraocular lens
American Joint Committee on
  Cancer (AJCC) staging
American Lapidus bed
American laryngectomy
  technique
American Medical Electronics
  PinSite shield
American Medical Optics (AMO)
  Baron lens
American Medical Optics
  intraocular lens
American Medical source
  laparoscope
American Medical Systems
  inflatable penile
  prosthesis
American Medical Systems
  penile prosthesis

American Optic R-inhibited
  pacemaker
American Optical Cardiocare
  pacemaker
American Optical coagulator
American Optical Company
  instruments
American Optical
  ophthalmometer
American Optical oximeter
American Optical
  photocoagulator
American Optical R-inhibited
  pacemaker
American pattern scissors
American pattern umbilical
  scissors
American Shared-CuraCare
  scanner
American silk suture
American Society for
  Gastrointestinal Endoscopy
  (ASGE)
American Society of
  Anesthesiologists
  classification
American Sterilizer operating
  table
American tracheotomy tube
American umbilical scissors
American V. Mueller urological
  instruments
American vascular stapler
American wire gauge
Amersham CDCS A-type needle
Amersham J tube
Amerson bone elevator
Ames reflectance meter
Ames shunt
Ames ventriculoperitoneal shunt
amethocaine anesthetic agent
ametropia
  position ametropia
Amfit orthotics
AMI (acute myocardial
  infarction)
amiantacea
  tinea amiantacea
Amici disk
Amici line
Amici striae
Amico chisel

Amico drill
Amico extractor
Amico osteotome
Amicon arteriovenous blood
  tubing set
Amicon D-20 filter
Amicon diafilter
Amicus blood collection
  separator
amide-type local anesthesia unit
aminocaproic acid
aminophylline
Amko vaginal speculum
AML (anatomic medullary
  locking)
AML orthopedic prosthesis
AML total hip prosthesis
Ammon blepharoplasty
Ammon blue dye
Ammon canthoplasty
Ammon dacryocystotomy
Ammon eyelid repair
Ammon horn
Ammon operation
Ammon scleral prominence
amnesia
  patch amnesia
amnestic effect
amnifocal lens
Amnihook amniotic membrane
  perforator
Amnihook perforator
amniocentesis
  genetic amniocentesis
amniogram
amnion
  human amnion
amnion graft
amnion rupture
amnioscope
  Erosa amnioscope
  Saling amnioscope
amnioscopy
amniotic adhesions
amniotic amputation
amniotic band
amniotic cavity
amniotic cyst
amniotic fluid embolism
amniotic fold
amniotic hernia
amniotic infection syndrome

amniotic membrane
amniotic sac
amniotic trocar
amniotome
  Baylor amniotome
  Beacham amniotome
  Glove-n-Gel amniotome
amniotomy
AMO Advent contact lens
AMO Array foldable intraocular
  lens
AMO HPF 500 pump
AMO intraocular lens
AMO intraocular lens implant
AMO laser
AMO lensometer
AMO phacoemulsification lens-
  folder forceps
AMO photokeratoscope
AMO refractometer
AMO scleral implant
AMO Sensar intraocular lens
AMO vitreous aspiration cutter
AMO YAG 100 laser
amobarbital anesthetic agent
A-mode echocardiogram
A-mode image
Amoena breast form
Amoils cryoextractor
Amoils cryopencil
Amoils cryophake
Amoils cryoprobe
Amoils cryosurgical unit
Amoils iris retractor
Amoils probe
Amoils refractor
Amoils retractor
Amoils-Keeler cryounit
AMO-PhacoFlex lens and
  inserter
amorphous calcification
AMP dialysis
AmpErase electrocautery
ampere
amphiarthrodial joint
amphiarthrosis
amphiarthrotic pubic symphysis
amphibolic fistula
amphibolous fistula
amphicrine carcinoma
amphidiarthrodial joint
amphidiarthrosis

Amplatz angiography needle
Amplatz aortography catheter
Amplatz cardiac catheter
Amplatz catheter
Amplatz Clot Buster
Amplatz coronary catheter
Amplatz dilator
Amplatz femoral catheter
Amplatz goose neck snare
Amplatz guide
Amplatz Hi-Flo torque-control
  catheter
Amplatz II curve
Amplatz injector
Amplatz left I catheter
Amplatz left II catheter
Amplatz microsnare
Amplatz needle
Amplatz retinal snare
Amplatz sheath
Amplatz Super Stiff guidewire
Amplatz technique
Amplatz thrombectomy device
  (Clot Buster)
Amplatz torque wire
Amplatz tube guide
Amplatz ventricular septal
  defect device
Amplatzer septal occluder
Amplex guidewire
Amplicor typing kit
amplification
  light amplification
amplifier
amplitude
  maximum amplitude
amplitude of fusion
amplitude-summation
  interferential current therapy
ampule
ampulla (*pl.* ampullae)
  Henle ampulla
  hepatopancreatic ampulla
  rectal ampulla
  Vater ampulla
ampulla canaliculi lacrimalis
ampulla ductus lacrimalis
ampulla of lacrimal canaliculus
ampulla of Vater
ampullaris
  crista ampullaris
  cupula cristae ampullaris

ampullary adenocarcinoma
ampullary aneurysm
ampullary cancer
ampullary carcinoma
ampullary crest
ampullary nerve
ampullary stenosis
amputated
  ligated and amputated
amputating knife
amputating saw
amputating ulcer
amputation
  abdominopelvic amputation
  above-elbow amputation
    (AE amputation, AEA)
  above-knee amputation
    (AK amputation, AKA)
  acircular amputation
  AE amputation (above-elbow
    amputation)
  AK amputation (above-knee
    amputation)
  Alanson amputation
  Alouette amputation
  amniotic amputation
  amniotic band amputation
  aperiosteal amputation
  aperiosteal supracondylar
    tendoplastic amputation
  avulsion amputation
  Batch-Spittler-McFadden
    amputation
  BE amputation (below-elbow
    amputation)
  Béclard amputation
  below-elbow amputation
    (BE amputation, BEA)
  below-knee amputation
    (BK amputation, BKA)
  Berger interscapular
    amputation
  bilateral amputation
  birth amputation
  BK amputation (below-knee
    amputation)
  bloodless amputation
  Bonney cervical amputation
  border ray amputation
  Boyd amputation
  Boyd ankle amputation
  Bunge amputation

amputation (*continued*)
  Burgess below-knee
    amputation
  Béclard amputation
  Callander amputation
  Carden amputation
  celsian amputation
  central amputation
  central ray amputation
  cervical amputation
  chop amputation
  Chopart amputation
  cinematic amputation
  cineplastic amputation
  circular amputation
  circular open amputation
  closed amputation
  closed flap amputation
  coat-sleeve amputation
  congenital above-elbow
    amputation
  congenital amputation
  congenital below-elbow
    amputation
  consecutive amputation
  corporectomy amputation
  cutaneous amputation
  degloved amputation
  diaclastic amputation
  Dieffenbach amputation
  disarticular amputation
  double-flap amputation
  dry amputation
  Dupuytren amputation
  eccentric amputation
  elliptical amputation
  endoplastic amputation
  extremity amputation
  Farabeuf amputation
  fingertip amputation
  fishmouth amputation
  flap amputation
  flapless amputation
  Forbes amputation
  forearm amputation
  forefoot amputation
  forequarter amputation
  galvanocaustic amputation
  Gordon-Taylor hindquarter
    amputation
  Gritti amputation
  Gritti-Stokes amputation

amputation (*continued*)
  guillotine amputation
  Guyon amputation
  Hancock amputation
  hand amputation
  Hey amputation
  hindfoot amputation
  hindquarter amputation
  Hueston finger amputation
  immediate amputation
  incomplete amputation
  index ray amputation
  interilioabdominal amputation
  interinnominoabdominal
    amputation
  intermediary amputation
  intermediate amputation
  interpelviabdominal
    amputation
  interphalangeal amputation
  interscapular amputation
  interscapulothoracic
    amputation
  interthoracoscapular
    amputation
  intrapyretic amputation
  intrauterine amputation
  Jaboulay amputation
  Kendrick method below-knee
    amputation
  kineplastic amputation
  King-Steelquist hindquarter
    amputation
  Kirk amputation
  Krukenberg amputation
  Kutler amputation
  labiomental amputation
  labiopalatal amputation
  Langenbeck amputation
  Larrey amputation
  LeFort amputation
  linear amputation
  Lisfranc amputation
  Littlewood amputation
  Mackenzie amputation
  Maisonneuve amputation
  major amputation
  Malgaigne amputation
  mediate amputation
  mediotarsal amputation
  Mikulicz-Vladimiroff
    amputation

amputation (*continued*)
  minor amputation
  mixed amputation
  modified Chopart amputation
  multiple amputation
  multiple ray amputation
  musculocutaneous
    amputation
  natural amputation
  nipple-areolar amputation
  oblique amputation
  one-stage amputation
  open amputation
  operative amputation
  osteoplastic amputation
  oval amputation
  partial amputation
  pathologic amputation
  penile amputation
  periosteoplastic amputation
  phalangophalangeal
    amputation
  Pirogoff amputation
  Pollock amputation
  primary amputation
  pulp amputation
  Péan amputation
  quadruple amputation
  racket amputation
  ray amputation
  rectangular amputation
  Ricard amputation
  Roger amputation
  root amputation
  secondary amputation
  shoulder amputation
  Sorondo hindquarter
    amputation
  Sorondo-Ferre hindquarter
    amputation
  spontaneous amputation
  Steelquist amputation
  Stokes amputation
  Stokes-Gritti amputation
  subastragalar amputation
  subperiosteal amputation
  supracervical amputation
  supracondylar amputation
  surgical amputation
  Syme amputation
  Syme ankle disarticulation
    amputation

amputation (*continued*)
  synchronous amputation
  Tansini breast amputation
  tarsal amputation
  tarsometatarsal amputation
  tarsotibial amputation
  Teale amputation
  tendinomyoplastic
    amputation
  tendoplastic amputation
  tertiary amputation
  Terwilliger amputation
  through-knee amputation
  transcarpal amputation
  transiliac amputation
  transmetatarsal amputation
    (TMA)
  transpelvic amputation
  transverse amputation
  traumatic amputation
  Tripier amputation
  triple amputation
  two-stage Syme amputation
  Vasconcelos amputation
  Vermale amputation
  Vladimiroff-Mikulicz
    amputation
  Wagner modification of Syme
    amputation
  Wagner two-stage Syme
    amputation
  Wilms amputation
  Wyeth amputation
amputation by transfixion
amputation in contiguity
amputation in continuity
amputation knife
amputation neuroma
amputation rake
amputation retractor
amputation saw
amputation screw
amputation stump
amputation technique
amputation through surgical
    neck of humerus
amputee
Amreich vaginal extirpation
AMRI (anteromedial rotatory
    instability)
AMS 700CX-series penile
    prosthesis

AMS Ambicore penile prosthesis
AMS artificial urethral sphincter
AMS autoclavable laparoscope
AMS Coaguloop
AMS CX penile prosthesis
    cylinder
AMS disposable trocar
AMS Endoview camera
AMS Hydroflex penile prosthesis
AMS inflatable penile prosthesis
AMS malleable penile prosthesis
AMS M-series malleable penile
    prosthesis
AMS rasp
AMS semirigid penile prosthesis
AMS Sphincter 800 urinary
    prosthesis
AMS Ultrex penile prosthesis
AMS ureteral stent
AMS urethral stent
AMSCO Hall adapter
AMSCO head holder
AMSCO hysteroscope
AMSCO light
AMSCO Orthairtome drill
Amset ALPS
Amset R-F rod
Amset R-F screw
AMSI artificial urinary sphincter
Amsler aqueous transplant
    needle
Amsler chart marker
Amsler corneal graft operation
Amsler grid
Amsler needle
Amsler operation
Amsler scleral marker
Amsoft lens
Amspacher-Messenbaugh
    technique
Amsterdam biliary stent
Amsterdam stent
Amsterdam tube
Amsterdam ventilator
Amsterdam-type prosthesis
Amstrong beveled grommet
    drain tube
Amstrong beveled grommet
    myringotomy tube
Amstrong ventilation tube
Amstutz cemented hip
    prosthesis

Amstutz femoral component
Amstutz total hip replacement
Amstutz-Wilson osteotomy
Amtech-Killeen pacemaker
AM-UP-75WET dialyzer
Amussat incision
Amussat operation
Amussat probe
amygdaloid body
amygdaloid fossa
amygdaloidectomy
amygdalotomy
amylase
amyloid kidney
amyloid macroglossia
amyloid oral cavity disease
amyloid tongue
amyloidosis
   cutaneous amyloidosis
   hereditary neuropathic
     amyloidosis
   lichenoid amyloidosis
   nodular amyloidosis
amyotonia
amyotrophic lateral sclerosis
   (ALS)
amyotrophy
Amytal anesthetic agent
AN69 membrane dialyzer
ANA (antinuclear antibody)
anabiosis
anabiotic
anaclasis
anaclitic therapy
anaerobe
   aerotolerant anaerobe
anaerobic bacteria
anaerobic cellulitis
anaerobic clostridial cellulitis
anaerobic culture
anaerobic streptococcus
anaeroplasty
Anagnostakis operation
anakhre
anal abscess
anal anastomosis
anal atresia
anal bulging
anal canal
anal column
anal crypt
anal dilatation

anal dilator
anal endoscopy
anal fissure
anal fistula
anal fistulectomy
anal fistulotomy
anal foreign body
anal gland
anal ileostomy with preservation
   of sphincter
anal manometry
anal orifice
anal papillae
anal pit
anal plate
anal prolapse
anal protrusion
anal reflex
anal retractor
anal speculum
anal sphincter
anal sphincter reconstruction
anal sphincter tone
anal sphincterotomy
anal squamous intraepithelial
   lesion
anal stenosis
anal stretch operation
anal stricture
anal tags
anal tone
anal verge
anal wink
analgesia
   ceiling analgesia
   conduction analgesia
   dermatomal level of
     analgesia
   fixed-dose patient-controlled
     analgesia (FDPCA)
   infiltration analgesia
   inhalation analgesia
   interpleural analgesia
   intrathecal opioid labor
     analgesia
   local analgesia
   multimodal analgesia
   narcolocal analgesia
   obstetrical analgesia
   opioid analgesia
   parenteral analgesia
   paretic analgesia

analgesia (*continued*)
    patient-controlled analgesia
        (PCA)
    patient-controlled epidural
        analgesia (PCEA, PEA)
    patient-controlled intranasal
        analgesia (PCINA)
    perineal analgesia
    perioperative analgesia
    permeation analgesia
    pinprick analgesia
    postoperative analgesia
    preemptive analgesia
    preoperative analgesia
    rescue analgesia
    spinal analgesia
    supplementary analgesia
    surface analgesia
    thoracic epidural analgesia
    tracheal topical analgesia
analgesia permeation
analgesic
    intranasal analgesic
    intrathecal analgesic
    intravenous analgesic
    narcotic analgesic
    NSAID analgesic
    opioid analgesic
    oral analgesic
    parenteral analgesic
    pediatric analgesic
    postoperative analgesic
    spinal analgesic
    transdermal analgesic
    Zydone analgesic
analgesic abuse headache
analgesic cell therapy
    implantable device
analgesic effect
analgesic index
analgesic infusion
analog
Analog knee orthosis
Analogic Anatom 2000 mobile
    CT scanner
analogous rhythm
analogous tissue
analogue
analysis
    body composition analysis
    Bolton analysis
    cephalometric analysis

analysis (*continued*)
    Cohen analysis
    deformity analysis
    densitometric analysis
    dental analysis
    displacement analysis
    Doppler analysis
    facial analysis
    failure analysis (FA)
    flow-cytometry analysis
    free-body analysis
    gastric analysis
    Histalog gastric analysis
    image analysis
    immunoradiometric analysis
        (IRMA)
    Mantel-Haenszel analysis
    nasofacial analysis
    occlusal analysis
    occlusal cephalometric
        analysis
    occlusion analysis
    proportional facial analysis
    pulsed Doppler spectral
        analysis
    qualitative analysis
    quantitative analysis
    spectral analysis
    Tweed analysis
    Van Slyke analysis
    Z-plane analysis
analysis of variance (ANOVA)
analytic reconstruction
analytical electron microscope
    (AEM)
analyzer
    automated cerebral blood
        flow analyzer
    automatic chemical analyzer
    automatic clinical analyzer
    gas analyzer
    Humphrey lens analyzer
    Humphrey vision analyzer
    laser microprobe mass
        analyzer
    Myograph 2000 neuromuscular
        function analyzer
    ultrasound bone analyzer
Anametric knee prosthesis
Anametric prosthesis
anaphylactic crisis
anaphylactic hypersensitivity

anaphylactic reaction
anaphylactic shock
anaphylactogenesis
anaphylactogenic
anaphylactoid crisis
anaphylactoid reaction
anaphylactoid shock
anaphylaxis
   acquired anaphylaxis
   active anaphylaxis
   aggregate anaphylaxis
   antiserum anaphylaxis
   cutaneous anaphylaxis
   homologous anaphylaxis
   local anaphylaxis
   reverse anaphylaxis
anaplastic adenocarcinoma
anaplastic carcinoma
anaplasty
anapophysis
anarrhexis
anasarca
anasarca trocar
Anastaflo intravascular shunt
Anastaflo stent
Anastasia bougie
anastigmatic aural magnifier
Anastomark flexible coronary
   graft marker
anastomose
anastomosed graft
anastomosis (*pl.* anastomoses)
   2-clamp anastomosis
   2-layer anastomosis
   Abbé intestinal anastomosis
   anal anastomosis
   aneurysm by anastomosis
   antecolic anastomosis
   anterocolic anastomosis
   antiperistaltic anastomosis
   aortic anastomosis
   aorticopulmonary
     anastomosis
   arterial anastomosis
   arteriolovenular
     anastomosis
   arteriovenous anastomosis
   Baffe anastomosis
   Baker anastomosis
   basting stitch anastomosis
   Béclard anastomosis
   beveled anastomosis

anastomosis (*continued*)
   bidirectional cavopulmonary
     anastomosis
   bidirectional superior
     cavopulmonary
     anastomosis
   biliary enteric anastomosis
   biliary intestinal anastomosis
   biliodigestive anastomosis
   Billroth anastomosis
   Billroth I, II gastrointestinal
     anastomosis
   bladder neck-to-urethra
     anastomosis
   Blalock anastomosis
   Blalock-Taussig anastomosis
   bowel anastomosis
   Brackin ureterointestinal
     anastomosis
   Braun anastomosis
   bulboprostatic urethral
     anastomosis
   Béclard anastomosis
   carotid-basilar anastomosis
   carotid-vertebral anastomosis
   cavopulmonary anastomosis
   cervical anastomosis
   choledochocholedochostomy
     side-to-side anastomosis
   circular anastomosis
   Clado anastomosis
   cobra-head anastomosis
   Coffey ureterointestinal
     anastomosis
   coloanal anastomosis
   colocolic anastomosis
   colocolonic anastomosis
   coloendoanal anastomosis
   colon resection and
     anastomosis
   colonic pouch anal
     anastomosis
   colorectal anastomosis
   conjoined anastomosis
   Cooley anastomosis
   Cooley intrapericardial
     anastomosis
   Cooley modification of
     Waterston anastomosis
   cornual anastomosis
   Couvelaire ileourethral
     anastomosis

anastomosis (*continued*)
  cross-facial nerve graft
    anastomosis
  crucial anastomosis
  cruciate anastomosis
  crunch-stick anastomosis
  crushing anastomosis
  curved end-to-end
    anastomosis
  Daines-Hodgson anastomosis
  D-D anastomosis
  DeBakey-Reynolds
    anastomosis
  delayed direct coloanal
    anastomosis
  Dennis anastomosis
  dismembered anastomosis
  distal anastomosis
  dog ear of anastomosis
  duct-to-duct anastomosis
  duct-to-mucosa anastomosis
  elliptical anastomosis
  endoanal anastomosis
  endogenous anastomosis
  end-to-back bowel
    anastomosis
  end-to-end anastomosis (EEA)
  end-to-end splenoadrenal
    anastomosis
  end-to-side anastomosis
  end-weave anastomosis
  enteric anastomosis
  erosive anastomosis
  esophageal anastomosis
  esophageal-jejunal
    anastomosis
  esophagocolic anastomosis
  esophagogastric anastomosis
  esophagojejunal anastomosis
  extended end-to-end
    anastomosis
  extraabdominal anastomosis
  extracorporeal anastomosis
  extrapleural anastomosis
  extravesical anastomosis
  fishmouth anastomosis
  flexor tendon anastomosis
  Fontan atriopulmonary
    anastomosis
  Furniss anastomosis
  Furniss ureterointestinal
    anastomosis

anastomosis (*continued*)
  Galen anastomosis
  Gambee anastomosis
  gastroduodenal anastomosis
  gastroileal anastomosis
  gastrointestinal anastomosis
    (GIA)
  gastrojejunal anastomosis
  genicular anastomosis
  Glenn anastomosis
  graft anastomosis
  Haight anastomosis
  handmade anastomosis
  handsewn anastomosis
  hand-sutured ileoanal
    anastomosis
  heel and toe of anastomosis
  heel-toe anastomosis
  hepatojejunal anastomosis
  heterocladic anastomosis
  Higgins ureterointestinal
    anastomosis
  Hofmeister anastomosis
  Hofmeister-Polya anastomosis
  homocladic anastomosis
  Horsley anastomosis
  Hoyer anastomosis
  H-shaped anal anastomosis
  H-shaped ileal pouch-anal
    anastomosis
  hypoglossal facial nerve
    anastomosis
  Hyrtl anastomosis
  ileal pouch-anal anastomosis
    (IPAA)
  ileal pouch-distal rectal
    anastomosis
  ileal-sigmoid anastomosis
  ileoanal anastomosis
  ileoileal anastomosis
  ileorectal anastomosis (IRA)
  ileosigmoid anastomosis
  ileotransverse colon
    anastomosis
  ileovesical anastomosis
  infrahepatic caval anastomosis
  intact anastomosis
  intercoronary anastomosis
  intermesenteric arterial
    anastomosis
  intestinal anastomosis
  intracorporeal anastomosis

anastomosis (*continued*)
  intragastric anastomosis
  intrathoracic anastomosis
  intravesical anastomosis
  invaginating anastomosis
  isoperistaltic anastomosis
  Jacobson anastomosis
  jejunoileal anastomosis
  jejunojejunal anastomosis
  Joel-Baker anastomosis
  J-shaped anal anastomosis
  J-shaped ileal pouch-anal
    anastomosis
  Kocher anastomosis
  Kugel anastomosis
  laparoscopic bilioenteric
    anastomosis
  LeDuc anastomosis
  leptomeningeal anastomosis
  Lich-Gregoir anastomosis
  longitudinal side-to-side
    anastomosis
  Longmire anastomosis
  lymphaticovenous
    anastomosis
  Martin-Gruber anastomosis
  McCleery-Miller anastomosis
  mechanical anastomosis
  mesocaval anastomosis
  microneurovascular
    anastomosis
  microsurgical tubocornual
    anastomosis
  microvascular anastomosis
  mucosa-to-mucosa anastomosis
  Nakayama anastomosis
  nerve anastomosis
  nondismembered anastomosis
  onlay patch anastomosis
  pancreatic anastomosis
  pancreaticogastric
    anastomosis
  pancreaticogastrointestinal
    anastomosis
  pancreaticogastrostomy
    anastomosis (PGA)
  pancreaticojejunal
    anastomosis
  pancreaticojejunostomy
    anastomosis (PJA)
  Parks ileoanal anastomosis
  Parks transanal anastomosis

anastomosis (*continued*)
  Pemberton sigmoid
    anastomosis
  percutaneous portocaval
    anastomosis
  peristaltic anastomosis
  Politano-Leadbetter
    anastomosis
  Polya anastomosis
  portacaval anastomosis
  portal systemic anastomosis
  portoportal anastomosis
  portopulmonary venous
    anastomosis
  portosystemic anastomosis
  Potts anastomosis
  Potts aortic-pulmonary artery
    anastomosis
  Potts-Smith anastomosis
  Potts-Smith side-to-side
    anastomosis
  precapillary anastomosis
  precostal anastomosis
  primary anastomosis
  primary end-to-end
    anastomosis
  Puestow anatomosis
  pulmonary aortic anastomosis
  pulmonary innominate
    anastomosis
  pulmonary subclavian
    anastomosis
  pyeloileocutaneous
    anastomosis
  rectosigmoid anastomosis
  retrocolic anastomosis
  retroperitoneal anastomosis
  Riche-Cannieu anastomosis
  right-angled end-to-side
    anastomosis
  Riolan anastomosis
  Roux-en-Y anastomosis
  Roux-en-Y hepaticojejunal
    anastomosis
  Schmidel anastomosis
  Schoemaker anastomosis
  Schoemaker-Billroth I, II
    anastomosis
  side-to-end anastomosis
  side-to-side anastomosis
  sigmoid anastomosis
  small vessel anastomosis

anastomosis (*continued*)
    spinal accessory nerve-facial
      nerve anastomosis
    splenoadrenal anastomosis
    splenorenal anastomosis
    S-shaped anal anastomosis
    S-shaped ileal pouch-anal
      anastomosis
    STA-MCA anastomosis
    stapled coloanal anastomosis
    stapled ileoanal anastomosis
    State colorectal anastomosis
    State end-to-end anastomosis
    stenotic esophagogastric
      anastomosis
    stirrup anastomosis
    subclavian aortic anastomosis
    subcutaneous anastomosis
    Sucquet anastomosis
    Sucquet-Hoyer anastomosis
    superior mesenteric-caval
      anastomosis
    supraoptic anastomosis
    surgical anastomosis
    suspension anastomosis
    suture anastomosis
    sutureless bowel anastomosis
    systemic-to-pulmonary artery
      anastomosis
    takedown of anastomosis
    temporal-cerebral arterial
      anastomosis
    tension-free anastomosis
    tensionless anastomosis
    terminoterminal anastomosis
    transanal mucosectomy with
      handsewn anastomosis
    transureteroureteral
      anastomosis
    triple anastomosis
    two-layer anastomosis
    ureterocolonic anastomosis
    ureteroileal anastomosis
    ureteroileobladder anastomosis
    ureteroileocutaneous
      anastomosis
    ureterointestinal anastomosis
    ureterosigmoid anastomosis
    ureterotubal anastomosis
    ureteroureteral anastomosis
    urethrocecal anastomosis
    valved conduit anastomosis

anastomosis (*continued*)
    vascular anastomosis
    venous anastomosis
    venous-to-venous anastomosis
    vesicourethral anastomosis
    von Haberer-Finney
      anastomosis
    Waterston extrapericardial
      anastomosis
    wide elliptical anastomosis
    wide-open anastomosis
    W-shaped anal anastomosis
    W-shaped ileal pouch-anal
      anastomosis
    Z-shaped anastomosis
anastomosis arteriolovenularis
anastomosis arteriovenosa
anastomosis clamp
anastomosis forceps
anastomosis of Riolan
anastomotic abscess
anastomotic branch of artery
anastomotic breakdown
anastomotic button
anastomotic complication
anastomotic dehiscence
anastomotic edge
anastomotic failure
anastomotic fistula
anastomotic foramen
anastomotic leakage
anastomotic operation
anastomotic site
anastomotic stricture rate
anastomotic stump leak
anastomotic ulcer
anastomotic ulceration
anastomotic varix
anastomotic vein
anastomotic vessel
anatomic abnormality
anatomic airway
anatomic barrier
anatomic closure
anatomic dead space
anatomic diagnosis
anatomic event
anatomic fracture
anatomic graduated components
    (AGC)
anatomic imaging
anatomic insertion

anatomic localization
anatomic medullary locking
    (AML)
anatomic neck
anatomic occlusion
anatomic plane
anatomic porous replacement
    (APR)
anatomic position
Anatomic Precoat hip prosthesis
anatomic repair
anatomic ridge
anatomic snuffbox
Anatomic/Intracone reamer
anatomical airway
anatomical dead space
anatomical position
anatomical sphincter
anatomical Tobin malar
    prosthetic implant
anatomically
    incision closed anatomically
anatomique
    tabatière anatomique
Anatomique osteal prosthesis
anatomy
    anomalous anatomy
    biliary anatomy
    Billroth II anatomy
    cervicothoracic pedicle
        anatomy
    cleft-affected anatomy
    congenitally altered anatomy
    coronary vessel anatomy
    dental anatomy
    designed after natural
        anatomy (DANA)
    fetal intracranial anatomy
    general anatomy
    gingival anatomy
    immune system anatomy
    internal anatomy
    intracranial anatomy
    intrahepatic anatomy
    knee anatomy
    Lowsley lobar anatomy
    macroscopic anatomy
    minute anatomy
    native anatomy
    neurovascular anatomy
    normal planar MR anatomy
    oncologic anatomy

anatomy (*continued*)
    pathological anatomy
    pedicle anatomy
    peritoneal anatomy
    plantar compartmental
        anatomy
    radiologic anatomy
    surface anatomy
    surgical anatomy
    systematic anatomy
    vascular anatomy
    zonal anatomy
Ancap braided silk suture
Ancap silk suture
anchor
    Acufex bioabsorbable suture
        anchor
    Acumed suture anchor
    Arthrex FASTak suture
        anchor
    AxyaWeld bone anchor
    Bio-Anchor suture anchor
    Bio-Fastak suture/anchor
    Biologically Quiet suture
        anchor
    Bio-Phase suture anchor
    BioROC EZ suture anchor
    BioSphere suture anchor
    Bio-Statak suture anchor
    Bone Bullet suture anchor
    Catera suture anchor
    Corkscrew suture anchor
    DRG Sherlock threaded
        suture anchor
    endosteal implant anchor
    E-Z ROC anchor
    FASTak suture anchor
    FastIn threaded anchor
    fixation anchor
    Hall sacral anchor
    Harpoon suture anchor
    implant anchor
    Innovasive Devices ROC SX
        suture anchor
    Isola spinal implant system
        anchor
    Kurer anchor
    LactoScrew suture anchor
    Lemoine-Searcy anchor
    Mainstay urologic soft tissue
        anchor
    mini Bio-Phase suture anchor

anchor (*continued*)
  Mitek absorbable bone
    anchor
  Mitek anchor
  Mitek Fastin threaded anchor
  Mitek GII Easy Anchor
  Mitek GII suture anchor
  Mitek GL anchor
  Mitek Knotless anchor
  Mitek Ligament anchor
  Mitek Micro anchor
  Mitek Mini GII anchor
  Mitek Mini GLS anchor
  Mitek Panalok anchor
  Mitek rotator cuff anchor
  Mitek Tacit threaded anchor
  Ogden soft tissue to bone
    anchor
  PaBA anchor
  Panalok absorbable anchor
  Panalok RC QuickAnchor Plus
    suture anchor
  Parachute Corkscrew suture
    anchor
  PeBA anchor
  Radix anchor
  Revo suture anchor
  ROC XS suture anchor
  Searcy fixation anchor
  Sherlock threaded suture
    anchor
  SmartAnchor-D suture anchor
  SmartAnchor-L suture anchor
  Statak suture anchor
  Stryker wedge suture anchor
  suture anchor
  Tacit threaded anchor
  TAG Rod II suture anchor
  TALON fixation anchor
  Therap-Loop door anchor
  Ti-Screw suture anchor
  traction anchor
  UltraFix anchor
  UltraSorb suture anchor
  Zest Anchor Advanced
    Generation (ZAAG) bone
    anchor
  Zest implant anchor
Anchor all-nylon hand brush
anchor band
Anchor brush dispenser
anchor endosteal implant

anchor hook
Anchor needle holder
Anchor needle-sterilizing box
anchor plate
anchor screw
Anchor soft tissue biopsy
  device
anchor splint
Anchor spring-suture needle
  holder
Anchor sterilizer box
Anchor surgical needle
anchor suture
anchor with suture ligature
anchor/fixation
anchor/Snap-Pak
  Mitek Panalot RC
    anchor/Snap-Pak
anchorage
  Baker anchorage
  cervical anchorage
  cranial anchorage
  dynamic anchorage
  major anchorage
  maxillary anchorage
  maxillomandibular anchorage
  multiple anchorage
  occipital anchorage
  reinforced anchorage
  simple anchorage
anchorage bend
anchorage control
anchorage procedure
anchored catheter
anchoring
  fascial anchoring
anchoring fibril
anchoring peg
anchoring point
anchoring screw
anchoring sutures
Anchorlok soft tissue anchor
anchovy arthroplasty
anchovy procedure
anconeal
anconeus muscle
anconeus muscle flap
Ancrofil clasp wire
Ancure stent-graft
Andermann syndrome
Anders disease
Andersch ganglion

Andersen mercury-weighted tube
Andersen triad
Anderson (Abrams modified)
    biopsy punch
Anderson acetabular prosthesis
Anderson ankle fusion
Anderson antrum punch
Anderson biopsy punch
Anderson clamp
Anderson columella prosthesis
Anderson converse iris scissors
Anderson curet
Anderson distractor
Anderson double ball
Anderson double-end knife
Anderson double-end retractor
Anderson elevator
Anderson five-prong bear claw
Anderson flexible suction tube
Anderson modification of
    Berndt-Harty classification
Anderson nasal strut
Anderson operation
Anderson portoenterostomy
Anderson splint
Anderson suction tube
Anderson suture pusher and
    double hook
Anderson tibial lengthening
Anderson traction bow
Anderson tractor
Anderson tube
Anderson-Adson retractor
Anderson-Adson self-retaining
    retractor
Anderson-D'Alonzo odontoid
    fracture classification
Anderson-Fowler osteotomy
Anderson-Hutchins technique
Anderson-Hutchins tibial
    fracture operation
Anderson-Hutchins unstable
    tibial shaft fracture
Anderson-Hynes pyeloplasty
Anderson-Neivert osteotome
Ando aortic clamp
Ando motor-driven probe
Andre hook
Andresen activator
Andresen monoblock appliance
Andresen removable
    orthodontic appliance
Andresen-Haupl activator
Andrews applicator
Andrews bottle operation
Andrews chisel
Andrews comedo extractor
Andrews cotton applicator
Andrews decompressor
Andrews ear applicator
Andrews forceps
Andrews frame
Andrews gouge
Andrews hydrocelectomy
Andrews iliotibial band
    reconstruction
Andrews infant laryngoscope
Andrews inguinal herniorrhaphy
Andrews knee reconstruction
Andrews laryngoscope
Andrews mastoid gouge
Andrews nasal applicator
Andrews operation
Andrews osteotome
Andrews retractor
Andrews rigid chest support
    holder
Andrews six keys to normal
    occlusion
Andrews spinal frame
Andrews spinal surgery table
Andrews suction tip
Andrews technique
Andrews tenodesis
Andrews tongue depressor
Andrews tonsil forceps
Andrews tonsil-seizing forceps
Andrews tracheal retractor
Andrews-Hartmann forceps
Andrews-Hartmann rongeur
Andrews-Pynchon
    decompressor
Andrews-Pynchon tongue
    depressor
Andrews-Pynchon tube
Andrews-Yankauer suction tube
androgen ablation
androgen insensitivity syndrome
androgenous
android pelvis
Andy Gump deformity
Andy Gump facies
AnEber probe
anecdotal procedure

anechoic
Anectine anesthetic agent
Anel dilatation of lacrimal duct
Anel lacrimal duct dilation
Anel lacrimal probe
Anel lacrimal syringe
Anel operation
Anel syringe
anemia of hemodialysis
anemia
    aplastic anemia
    burn wound anemia
    sickle cell anemia
aneroid manometry
aneroid sphygmomanometer
Anestacon anesthetic agent
anesthesia
    absorption anesthesia
    acral anesthesia
    acupuncture anesthesia
    ambulatory anesthesia
    angiospastic anesthesia
    ankle block anesthesia
    axillary anesthesia
    axillary block anesthesia
    balanced anesthesia
    barbiturate burst-suppression
        anesthesia
    basal anesthesia
    Bier anesthesia
    Bier arm block anesthesia
    Bier block anesthesia
    block anesthesia
    bolus intravenous anesthesia
    brachial anesthesia
    bupivacaine anesthesia
    bypass anesthesia
    cardiac anesthesia
    cardiovascular anesthesia
    caudal anesthesia
    centroneuroaxis anesthesia
    cerebral anesthesia
    cervical anesthesia
    cervical plexus anesthesia
    chemical anesthesia
    circle absorption anesthesia
    circular block anesthesia
    closed anesthesia
    closed-circuit anesthesia
    cocaine anesthesia
    coinduction of anesthesia
    colonic anesthesia

anesthesia (*continued*)
    combined epidural-general
        anesthesia
    combined sacral and caudal
        block anesthesia
    combined spinal-epidural
        anesthesia (CSEA)
    compression anesthesia
    computer-assisted anesthesia
    conduction anesthesia
    continuous caudal anesthesia
    continuous epidural
        anesthesia
    continuous lumbar peridural
        anesthesia
    continuous peridural
        anesthesia
    continuous spinal anesthesia
    corneal anesthesia
    Corning anesthesia
    crossed anesthesia
    dental anesthesia
    depth of anesthesia
    diagnostic anesthesia
    differential spinal anesthesia
    digital block anesthesia
    dissociative anesthesia
    drop anesthesia
    Droperidol anesthesia
    ear anesthesia
    electric anesthesia
    electricity-induced anesthesia
    endobronchial anesthesia
    endotracheal anesthesia
    endotracheal insufflation
        anesthesia
    epidural anesthesia (EA)
    ether antheisa
    examination under anesthesia
        (EUA)
    extradural anesthesia
    failed anesthesia
    fast-track cardiac anesthesia
    fentanyl anesthesia
    field block anesthesia
    fitness for general anesthesia
    fractional anesthesia
    frost anesthesia
    gauntlet anesthesia
    general anesthesia (GA)
    general endotracheal
        anesthesia (GET)

anesthesia (*continued*)
- general inhalation anesthesia
- general insufflation anesthesia
- geriatric anesthesia
- GET anesthesia (general endotracheal anesthesia)
- girdle anesthesia
- glove anesthesia
- graded spinal anesthesia
- gustatory anesthesia
- Gwathmey oil-ether anesthesia
- gynecologic anesthesia
- high spinal anesthesia
- high-pressure anesthesia
- Hunstad system for tumescent anesthesia
- hydrate microcrystal theory of anesthesia
- hyperbaric spinal anesthesia
- hyperthermia of anesthesia
- hypnosis anesthesia
- hypobaric spinal anesthesia
- hypotensive anesthesia
- hypothermic anesthesia
- hysterical anesthesia
- induced anesthesia
- induction of anesthesia
- infiltration anesthesia
- infiltrative local anesthesia
- infraorbital anesthesia
- inhalant anesthesia
- inhalation anesthesia
- inhalation mask anesthesia
- inhalational anesthesia
- instillation of anesthesia
- insufflation anesthesia
- intercostal anesthesia
- intracavitary anesthesia
- intraligamentary anesthesia
- intramedullary anesthesia
- intranasal anesthesia
- intraoral anesthesia
- intraorbital anesthesia
- intraosseous anesthesia
- intraperitoneal anesthesia
- intrapleural anesthesia
- intrapulpal anesthesia
- intraspinal anesthesia
- intrathecal anesthesia
- intratracheal anesthesia
- intravenous anesthesia

anesthesia (*continued*)
- intravenous block anesthesia
- intravenous regional anesthesia (IVRA)
- intravenous sedation anesthesia
- intubation anesthesia
- isobaric spinal anesthesia
- IV anesthesia
- Kulenkampff anesthesia
- laryngeal anesthesia
- leg-block anesthesia
- level of anesthesia
- lid block anesthesia
- ligamental anesthesia
- lining anesthesia
- local anesthesia
- local infiltrative anesthesia (LIA)
- Lorfan anesthesia
- low central venous pressure anesthesia
- low spinal anesthesia
- low thoracic level epidural anesthesia
- lumbar epidural anesthesia
- MAC anesthesia
- MacIntosh blade anesthesia
- management of anesthesia
- maternal anesthesia
- Meltzer anesthesia
- mixed anesthesia
- modified Van Lint anesthesia
- monitored anesthesia care
- muscular anesthesia
- nasoendotracheal anesthesia
- nasotracheal intubation anesthesia
- neonatal anesthesia
- nerve block anesthesia
- nerve compression anesthesia
- nerve-blocking anesthesia
- neuroleptanalgesia anesthesia
- neurosurgical anesthesia
- newborn anesthesia
- no-absorption anesthesia
- nonrebreathing anesthesia
- nose anesthesia
- O'Brien anesthesia
- obstetric anesthesia
- obstetrical anesthesia
- olfactory anesthesia

anesthesia (*continued*)
  one-lung anesthesia
  open anesthesia
  open drop anesthesia
  open endotracheal inhalation
    anesthesia
  open inhalation anesthesia
  ophthalmologic anesthesia
  opioid anesthesia
  oral anesthesia
  orbital anesthesia
  oropharyngeal anesthesia
  orthopedic anesthesia
  outpatient anesthesia
  painful anesthesia
  palatine block anesthesia
  paracervical block anesthesia
  paraneural anesthesia
  parasacral anesthesia
  paravertebral anesthesia
  parenteral anesthesia
  partial rebreathing anesthesia
  patient-controlled epidural
    anesthesia
  patient-controlled intravenous
    anesthesia
  Pavulon anesthesia
  pediatric radiotherapy
    anesthesia
  pelvirectal anesthesia
  peribulbar anesthesia
  peridural anesthesia
  perineal anesthesia
  perineural anesthesia
  periodontal anesthesia
  periodontal ligament
    anesthesia
  peripheral nerve block
    anesthesia
  permeation anesthesia
  pharyngeal anesthesia
  pharyngeal insufflation
    anesthesia
  plexus anesthesia
  Ponka technique for local
    anesthesia
  postcesarean anesthesia
  postoperative anesthesia
  preemptive anesthesia
  pregnancy-induced anesthesia
  preperitoneal anesthesia
  presacral anesthesia

anesthesia (*continued*)
  pressure anesthesia
  pudendal anesthesia
  pudendal block anesthesia
  rapid-sequence induction of
    anesthesia
  Raplon anesthesia
  rebreathing anesthesia
  rectal anesthesia
  refrigeration anesthesia
  regional anesthesia (RA)
  regional block anesthesia
  respiration assisted anesthesia
  respiration unassisted
    anesthesia
  retrobulbar anesthesia
  risk management of
    anesthesia
  risk of anesthesia
  SAB anesthesia (subarachnoid
    block anesthesia)
  sacral block anesthesia
  saddle block spinal anesthesia
  satisfactory general anesthesia
  SDC anesthesia
  segmental epidural anesthesia
  selective anesthesia
  semiclosed endotracheal
    anesthesia
  semiopen endotracheal
    inhalation anesthesia
  single injection anesthesia
  single-breath induction of
    anesthesia
  spinal anesthesia (SA)
  splanchnic anesthesia
  stellate ganglion block
    anesthesia
  stocking anesthesia
  stocking-glove anesthesia
  subarachnoid block
    anesthesia (SAB anesthesia)
  Sublimaze anesthesia
  supraclavicular brachial block
    anesthesia
  surface anesthesia
  surgical anesthesia
  Surital anesthesia
  sympathetic block anesthesia
  tactile anesthesia
  therapeutic anesthesia
  thermal anesthesia

anesthesia (*continued*)
  thermic anesthesia
  thoracic anesthesia
  throat anesthesia
  to-and-fro anesthesia
  toe-block anesthesia
  topical anesthesia
  total intravenous anesthesia
    (TIVA)
  total spinal anesthesia
  transdermal anesthesia
  transient anesthesia
  transsacral anesthesia
  transtracheal anesthesia
  traumatic anesthesia
  tumescent anesthesia
  twilight anesthesia
  unilateral anesthesia
  unmonitored local anesthesia
  urologic anesthesia
  Van Lint anesthesia
  variable-dose patient-controlled
    anesthesia (VDPCA)
  Versed anesthesia
  visceral anesthesia
  volatile anesthesia
anesthesia action
anesthesia adjuvant
anesthesia block needle
anesthesia breathing circuit
anesthesia dolorosa
anesthesia record
anesthesia time
anesthesia tube
anesthesiologist
anesthesiology
anesthetic
  action of anesthetic
  cardiac anesthetic
  Cetacaine topical anesthetic
  Chirocaine anesthetic
  EMLA anesthetic
  epidural anesthetic
  eutectic mixture of local
    anesthetics (EMLA)
  flammable anesthetic
  Forane general anesthetic
  gas anesthetic
  general anesthetic
  halogenated volatile
    anesthetic
  Hurricaine local anesthetic

anesthetic (*continued*)
  hyperbaric local anesthetic
  inhaled anesthetic
  injection of local anesthetic
  instillation of anesthetic
  intradermal anesthetic
  intramuscular anesthetic
  intraperitoneal anesthetic
  intrathecal anesthetic
  intravenous anesthetic
  levobupivacaine anesthetic
  local anesthetic
  low-dose anesthetic
  Mesocaine anesthetic
  multiple mechanism inhaled
    anesthetic
  multiple site inhaled
    anesthetic
  Naropin anesthetic
  opioid anesthetic
  oral anesthetic
  paracervical anesthetic
  pediatric anesthetic
  polymer anesthetic
  preoperative anesthetic
  primary anesthetic
  Raplon anesthetic
  rectal anesthetic
  regional anesthetic
  ring block digital anesthetic
  ropivacaine anesthetic
  secondary anesthetic
  Septocaine anesthetic
  single mechanism inhaled
    anesthetic
  single site inhaled anesthetic
  spinal anesthetic
  topical anesthetic
  trace anesthetic
  volatile anesthetic
  walking epidural anesthetic
anesthetic agent
anesthetic and fluid
    management
anesthetic approach
anesthetic block
anesthetic blockade
anesthetic circuit
anesthetic consideration
anesthetic cutoff
anesthetic depth
anesthetic emergence

anesthetic gas
anesthetic hepatitis
anesthetic hepatotoxicity
anesthetic immediate recovery
anesthetic index
anesthetic induction
anesthetic leprosy
anesthetic management
anesthetic monitoring
anesthetic potency
anesthetic record
anesthetic risk
anesthetic shock
anesthetic technique
anesthetic time
anesthetic tolerance
anesthetic tube
anesthetic vapor
anesthetist
anesthetist's stool
anesthetist's table
anesthetize
anesthetizing agent
anetoderma
   Schweninger-Buzzi
     anetoderma
aneuploid cell line
aneuploidy
Aneuroplast acrylic material
Aneuroplast hemostatic agent
aneuroplastic kit
aneuroplasty
AneuRx aortic aneurysm stent-
   graft
aneurysm
   abdominal aneurysm
   abdominal aortic aneurysm
     (AAA, triple A)
   ampullary aneurysm
   anterior circulation aneurysm
   aortic aneurysm
   aortoiliac aneurysm
   arterial aneurysm
   arteriosclerotic aneurysm
   arteriovenous aneurysm
   atherosclerotic aneurysm
   AV aneurysm (arteriovenous
     aneurysm)
   axial aneurysm
   axillary artery aneurysm
   balloon occlusion of
     aneurysm

aneurysm (*continued*)
   basilar artery aneurysm
   basilar bifurcation aneurysm
   basilar tip aneurysm
   Bérard aneurysm
   berry aneurysm
   bifurcation aneurysm
   cardiac aneurysm
   carotid aneurysm
   celiac artery aneurysm
   Charcot-Bouchard aneurysm
   circulation aneurysm
   clavicular fracture aneurysm
   coiled intracranial aneurysm
   complex intracranial
     aneurysm
   compound aneurysm
   congenital cerebral aneurysm
   consecutive aneurysm
   coronary artery aneurysm
   Crisp aneurysm
   cylinder aneurysm
   cylindroid aneurysm
   cystogenic aneurysm
   descending aortic aneurysm
   diffuse aneurysm
   discrete aneurysm
   dissecting aneurysm
   ectatic aneurysm
   embolic aneurysm
   embolomycotic aneurysm
   endogenous aneurysm
   endovascular aneurysm
   exogenous aneurysm
   false aneurysm
   femoral artery aneurysm
   fusiform aneurysm
   hernial aneurysm
   iliac artery aneurysm
   infraclinoid aneurysm
   innominate aneurysm
   intracranial aneurysm
   intramural aneurysm
   isolated iliac artery aneurysm
   leaking aneurysm
   miliary aneurysm
   mitral valve aneurysm
   mural aneurysm
   mycotic aneurysm
   Park aneurysm
   pelvic aneurysm
   peripheral aneurysm

aneurysm (*continued*)
  phantom aneurysm
  popliteal aneurysm
  posterior circulation
    aneurysm
  Pott aneurysm
  pulmonary aneurysm
  pulsating aneurysm
  Rasmussen aneurysm
  resected aneurysm
  Richet aneurysm
  Rodriguez aneurysm
  ruptured aneurysm
  saccular aneurysm
  serpentine aneurysm
  Shekelton aneurysm
  shunt for aortic aneurysm
  spurious aneurysm
  subclavian artery aneurysm
  supraclinoid aneurysm
  suprasellar aneurysm
  thoracic aneurysm
  thoracoabdominal aneurysm
  traction aneurysm
  traumatic false aneurysm
  true aneurysm
  tubular aneurysm
  varicose aneurysm
  venous aneurysm
  ventricular aneurysm
  verminous aneurysm
  wrapping of abdominal aortic
    aneurysm
  wrapping of aneurysm
aneurysm by anastomosis
aneurysm clamp
aneurysm clip
aneurysm forceps
aneurysm in orbit
aneurysm management
aneurysm neck dissector
aneurysm needle
aneurysm repair
aneurysm tissue
aneurysm wrapping
aneurysmal bone cyst (ABC)
aneurysmal clip
aneurysmal coil
aneurysmal dilatation
aneurysmal dilation
aneurysmal disease
aneurysmal hematoma

aneurysmal hemorrhage
aneurysmal rupture
aneurysmal varix
aneurysmectomy
  abdominal aortic
    aneurysmectomy
  aortic aneurysmectomy
  apicoseptal aneurysmectomy
  conventional aortic
    aneurysmectomy
  elective aneurysmectomy
  laparoscopic-assisted
    aneurysmectomy
  Matas aneurysmectomy
aneurysmoid varix
aneurysmoplasty
  Matas aneurysmoplasty
aneurysmorrhaphy
aneurysmotomy
ANF (antinuclear factor)
AngeFlex lead
Angeion 2000 ICD generator
angel hair plane
AngeLase combined mapping-
    laser probe
Angelchik antireflux prosthesis
Angell curet
Angell gauze packer
Angell-James dissector
Angell-James hypophysectomy
    forceps
Angell-James punch forceps
Angell-Shiley bioprosthetic heart
    valve
Angell-Shiley bioprosthetic
    valve
Angell-Shiley xenograft
    prosthetic valve
angel's kiss
Angelucci operation
Angelucci ptosis correction
    procedure
angel-wing deformity
AngelWings device
Ange-Med Sentinel ICD device
Anger camera
Anger scintillation camera
Angestat hemostasis introducer
Angetear tear-away introducer
angiectomy
angiitis
  granulomatous angiitis

angina
  abdominal angina
  crescendo angina
  Prinzmetal angina
  vasospastic angina
  Vincent angina
angina-guided therapy
angioaortic arch study
angiocardiogram
angiocardiography
  intravenous
    angiocardiography
  IV angiocardiography
  venous angiocardiography
Angiocath flexible catheter
Angiocath PRN catheter
angiocatheter
  angiocatheter with looped
    polypropylene suture
  Brockenbrough angiocatheter
  Corlon angiocatheter
  Deseret angiocatheter
  Eppendorf angiocatheter
  Gensini angiocatheter
  Mikro-tip angiocatheter
angiocatheter with looped
    polypropylene suture
angiocentric
    immunoproliferative lesion
angiocentric
    lymphoproliferative lesion
angiochondroma
angioclast
Angiocor prosthetic valve
Angiocor rotational
    thrombolizer
angiodermatitis
angiodynagraphic evaluation
angiodysplasia
angiodysplastic lesion
angioendotheliomatosis
  reactive
    angioendotheliomatosis
angiofibroma
  juvenile angiofibroma
  juvenile nasopharyngeal
    angiofibroma
  nasopharyngeal angiofibroma
Angioflow high-flow catheter
angiofollicular
angiogenesis
  HBO-induced angiogenesis

angiogenesis (*continued*)
  hyperbaric oxygen-induced
    angiogenesis
  therapeutic angiogenesis
angiogenesis factor
angiogenic
angiogram
  1st-pass nuclide rest and
    exercise angiogram
  1st-pass radionuclide
    angiogram
  4-vessel angiogram
  arch angiogram
  biplane orthogonal angiogram
  Brown-Dodge angiogram
  cardiac angiogram
  carotid angiogram
  cerebral angiogram
  contrast angiogram
  coronary angiogram
  digital subtraction angiogram
  ECG-synchronized digital
    subtraction angiogram
  Epistar subtraction angiogram
  equilibrium radionuclide
    angiogram
  fluorescein angiogram
  FluoroPlus angiogram
  gated blood pool angiogram
  gated nuclear angiogram
  gated radionuclide angiogram
  helical computed
    tomographic angiogram
  indocyanine green angiogram
  left coronary angiogram
  levophase of angiogram
  MEDIS off-line quantitative
    coronary angiogram
  on-table angiogram
  postangioplasty angiogram
  pulmonary angiogram
  pulmonary artery wedge
    angiogram
  radionuclide angiogram
  rest and exercise gated
    nuclear angiogram
  serial angiogram
  single-plane angiogram
  sitting-up view angiogram
  splenic system angiogram
  superior mesenteric
    angiogram

angiogram (*continued*)
  Tagarno 3SD cineprojector for angiogram
  transvenous digital subtraction angiogram
  ventricular angiogram
angiographic balloon occlusion catheter
angiographic catheter
angiographic embolization
angiographic evaluation
angiographic guidewire
angiographic intervention
angiographic portacaval shunt
angiographic road-mapping technique
angiographic series
angiographically occult intracranial vascular malformation (AOIVM)
angiography
  abdominal angiography
  arch angiography
  biplane angiography
  biplane cerebral angiography
  carotid angiography
  celiac angiography
  cerebral angiography
  coronary angiography
  digital subtraction angiography (DSA)
  digitized subtraction angiography
  fluorescein angiography
  IDIS angiography (intraoperative digital subtraction angiography)
  intra-arterial digital subtraction angiography
  intraoperative digital subtraction angiography (IDIS angiography)
  magnetic resonance angiography (MRA)
  mesenteric angiography
  pudendal artery angiography
  renal angiography
  selective angiography
  spiral computed tomography angiography
  supra-aortic angiography

angiography (*continued*)
  synchrotron-based transvenous angiography
  vascular angiography
  vertebral angiography
  visceral angiography
angiography catheter
angiography needle
Angioguard catheter device
angioinvasive lesion
AngioJet catheter
AngioJet saline jet-vacuum device catheter
AngioJet thrombectomy catheter
angiokeratoma Mibelli
  angiokeratoma verrucous
  angiokeratoma circumscriptum
angiokeratoma corporis diffusum
angiokeratoma of Fordyce
angiokeratosis
Angio-Kit catheter
angiolaser
  pulsed angiolaser
angioleiomyoma
  laryngeal angioleiomyoma
angiolipoma
  subcutaneous angiolipoma
angiolith
angiolupoid
angiolymphangioma
angiolymphoid hyperplasia with eosinophilia
angioma (*pl.* angiomas, angiomata)
  bleeding angioma
  capillary angioma
  cavernous angioma
  cherry angioma
  congenital tufted angioma
  encephalic angioma
  hereditary hemorrhagic angioma
  hypertrophic angioma
  plexiform angioma
  senile angioma
  simple angioma
  spider angioma
  strawberry angioma
  superficial angioma
  telangiectatic angioma
  tufted angioma

angioma arteriale racemosum
angioma cavernosum
angioma cutis
angioma pigmentosum
   atrophicum
angioma serpiginosum
angioma simplex
angioma venosum racemosum
angiomata
   spider angiomata
angiomatoid fibrous
   histiocytoma (AFH)
angiomatoid myosarcoma
angiomatosis
   cephalotrigeminal
     angiomatosis
   cerebroretinal angiomatosis
   encephalotrigeminal
     angiomatosis
   hemorrhagic familial
     angiomatosis
   retinocerebral angiomatosis
angiomatosis of retina
angiomatous lymphoid
   hamartoma
Angiomedics catheter
angiomegaly
angiomyolipoma
   hemorrhagic angiomyolipoma
angiomyoma cutis
angiomyoneuroma
angiomyosarcoma
angioneoplasm
angioneurectomy
angioneuroma
angioneuromyoma
angioneuropathy
angioneurotic edema of vessels
angioneurotomy
AngioOPTIC microcatheter
angio-osteohypertrophy
   syndrome
angiopancreatitis
angiopathy
   giant cell hyaline angiopathy
angiopathy of retina
angiophakomatosis
angiopigtail catheter
angioplasty
   ablative laser angioplasty
   adjunctive balloon angioplasty
   aortoiliac angioplasty

angioplasty (*continued*)
   Axiom DG balloon
     angioplasty
   balloon coarctation
     angioplasty
   balloon coronary angioplasty
   balloon dilation angioplasty
   balloon laser angioplasty
   bootstrap two-vessel
     angioplasty
   brachiocephalic vessel
     angioplasty
   carotid angioplasty
   complementary balloon
     angioplasty
   coronary balloon angioplasty
   culprit lesion angioplasty
   Dotter-Judkins percutaneous
     transluminal angioplasty
   excimer laser coronary
     angioplasty
   facilitated angioplasty
   Gruentzig balloon catheter
     angioplasty
   Hartzler Micro II balloon for
     coronary angioplasty
   high-risk angioplasty
   Ho:YAG laser angioplasty
   iliac artery angioplasty
   infrapopliteal transluminal
     angioplasty
   Kinsey rotation atherectomy
     extrusion angioplasty
   kissing balloon angioplasty
   laser angioplasty
   laser-assisted balloon
     angioplasty
   LASTAC coronary angioplasty
   low-speed rotational
     angioplasty
   multilesion angioplasty
   one-vessel angioplasty
   Osypka rotational angioplasty
   patch-graft angioplasty
   percutaneous balloon
     angioplasty
   percutaneous transluminal
     angioplasty (PTA, PTLA)
   percutaneous transluminal
     coronary angioplasty (PTCA)
   percutaneous transluminal
     renal angioplasty (PTRA)

angioplasty (*continued*)
  peripheral laser angioplasty
    (PLA)
  postcoronary angioplasty
  renal angioplasty
  rescue angioplasty
  salvage balloon angioplasty
  subclavian vein patch
    angioplasty
  supported angioplasty
  Tactilaze angioplasty
  thermal/perfusion balloon
    angioplasty
  thulium:YAG laser angioplasty
  tibioperoneal trunk angioplasty
  tibioperoneal vessel
    angioplasty
  transluminal balloon
    angioplasty
  transluminal coronary artery
    angioplasty
  vein patch angioplasty
  vibrational angioplasty
angioplasty balloon catheter
angioplasty sheath
angioplasty-related vessel
    occlusion
angiopressure
angioproliferative lesion
angioreticuloendothelioma
angiorrhaphy
  arteriovenous angiorrhaphy
angiosarcoma
angiosclerosis
angioscope
  Baxter angioscope
  Coronary Imagecath
    angioscope
  flexible angioscope
  Imagecath rapid exchange
    angioscope
  Masy angioscope
  Mitsubishi angioscope
  Olympus angioscope
  Optiscope angioscope
angioscopic valvulotome
angioscopy
  fluorescein fundus
    angioscopy
  fundal angioscopy
  percutaneous transluminal
    angioscopy

Angio-Seal catheter
Angio-Seal hemostatic puncture
    closure device
Angioskop-D
angiosomal flap
angiospasm
  labyrinthine angiospasm
angiospastic anesthesia
AngioStent cardiovascular stent
angiostomy
angiostrophe
angiostrophy
angiotomy
angiotribe
  Ferguson angiotribe
  Zweifel angiotribe
angiotribe forceps
angiotripsy
angle
  acute angle
  acute mandibular plane angle
  AI angle
  alveolar angle
  alveolar profile angle
  anomaly angle
  anopouch angle
  anorectal angle
  antegonial angle
  anterior angle
  augmentation of the
    mandibular angle (AMA)
  auriculocephalic angle
  auriculomastoid angle
  auriculo-occipital angle
  axial line angle
  basal mandibular angle
  basilar angle
  Bauman angle
  Bennett angle
  biorbital angle
  blunted costophrenic angle
  blunting of costophrenic
    angle
  Böhler calcaneal angle
  Bohlet angle
  Broca basilar angle
  Broca facial angle
  buccal angle
  bucco-occlusal line angle
  calcaneal inclination angle
  calcaneal-second metatarsal
    angle inclination angle

angle (*continued*)
Camper angle
cardiodiaphragmatic angle
cardiohepatic angle
cardiophrenic angle
carrying angle
caudal septal angle
cavity line angle
cephalic angle
cephalometric angle
cerebellar pontine angle
cerebellopontine angle
cervicoisthmic angle
cervicomental angle
Codman x-ray angle
columellar-labial angle
columellar-lobular angle
conchoscaphoid angle
costal angle
costophrenic angle
costosternal angle
costovertebral angle
craniofacial angle
cricothyroid angle
Daubenton angle
declination angle
deformity angle
distal angle
distobuccal line angle
distobucco-occlusal point
    angle
distolabial line angle
distolabioincisal point angle
distolinguo-occlusal point
    angle
disto-occlusal point angle
duodenojejunal angle
Ebstein angle
elevation angle
epigastric angle
ethmoid angle
external angle
facial plane angle
filtration angle
flip angle
Frankfort mandibular angle
    (FMA)
Frankfort mandibular incisor
    angle (FMIA)
gantry angle
Gissane angle
gonial angle

angle (*continued*)
hepatic-renal angle
hepatorenal angle
Hilgenreiner angle
hypsiloid angle
incisal angle
incisal mandibular plane angle
    (IMPA)
inclination angle
infrasternal angle
intergonial angle
interincisal angle
iridocorneal angle
Jacquart angle
kyphotic angle
labial angle
labioincisal line angle
lateral incisal guide angle
left venous angle
line angle
lingual angle
linguoincisal line angle
linguo-occlusal angle
Louis angle
Ludwig angle
lumbosacral angle
magnetization precession angle
mandibular angle
maxillary angle
medial angle
mesiobuccal line angle
mesiobucco-occlusal point
    angle
mesiolabial line angle
mesiolabioincisal point angle
mesiolingual line angle
mesiolinguo-occlusal point
    angle
mesio-occlusal line angle
metafacial angle
Mikulicz angle
nail-to-nail bed angle
nasofrontal angle
nasolabial angle
neck-shaft angle
obtuse angle
obtuse cervicomandibular
    angle
occipital angle
occlusal plane angle
occlusal rest angle
olfactory angle

angle (*continued*)
  ophryospinal angle
  orifacial angle
  parietal angle
  Pauwels angle
  pelvic-femoral angle
  pelvifemoral angle
  pelvic-vertebral angle
  phrenopericardial angle
  piriform angle
  Pirogoff angle
  point angle
  pontine angle
  prophy angles
  prophylactic angles
  protrusive incisal guide angle
  proximal articular set angle
    (PASA)
  pubic angle
  Quatrefage angle
  radiolunate angle
  Ranke angle
  rest angle
  rib-vertebral angle
  right venous angle
  sacrohorizontal angle
  scaphoconchal angle
  scapholunate angle
  sella-nasion-subspinale angle
    (SNA, S-N-A)
  sella-nasion-supramentale
    angle (SNB, S-N-B)
  Serres angle
  sharp angle
  sinodural angle
  sphenoidal angle
  splenic-renal angle
  splenorenal angle
  sternal angle
  sternoclavicular angle
  subcarinal angle
  subpubic angle
  subscapular angle
  substernal angle
  sulcus angle
  superior angle
  talocalcaneal angle
  tip angle
  Topinard angle
  tracheal bifurcation angle
  Trautmann angle
  urethrovesical angle

angle (*continued*)
  venous angle
  Virchow angle
  Virchow-Holder angle
  visor angle
  Vogt angle
  Weisbach angle
  Welcker angle
  xiphoid angle
  Y angle
  Z angle
angle arch
angle band
angle bisection technique
angle board
Angle classification of
    malocclusion (Class I, II, III,
    IV malocclusion)
angle drain
Angle Eager I microprocessor
angle implants of Taylor
angle knife
Angle malocclusion
    classification
angle of aberration
angle of femoral torsion
angle of greatest extension (AGE)
angle of greatest flexion (AGF)
angle of His
angle of jaw
angle of Louis
angle of Ludwig
angle of mouth
angle of Mulder
angle of orientation
angle of reflection
angle of Sylvius
angle port pump
angle splint
angle sutures
angle vessel hook
Anglebasic E arch appliance
angle-closure glaucoma
angled ball-end electrode
angled balloon catheter
angled biter
angled blade plate fixation
angled cannula
angled capsular forceps
angled clamp
angled clip
angled counterpressor

angled curet
angled DeBakey clamp
angled decompression retractor
angled delivery device (ADD)
angled director
angled discission hook
angled elevator
angled guidewire
angled iris retractor
angled iris spatula
angled left cannula
angled lens loop
angled needle holder
angled nucleus removal loop
angled peripheral vascular
    clamp
angled pigtail catheter
angled pleural tube
angled probe
angled right cannula
angled ring curet
angled scissors
angled stone forceps
angled suction tube
angled telescope
angled vein retractor
Angle-Pezzer drain
angle-tip electrode
angle-tip Glidewire
angle-tip guidewire
angle-tip urethral catheter
angry-looking ulcer
Angstrom II implantable
    cardioverter defibrillator
Angstrom MD implantable
    single-lead cardioverter-
    defibrillator
angular acceleration
angular artery
angular deformity
angular displacement
angular elevator
angular facial vein
angular forceps
angular frequency
angular gyrus
angular incision
angular knife
angular line
angular nasal artery
angular needle holder
angular oval punch

angular position
angular position of the ramus
angular rongeur
angular saw
angular scissors
angular spine
angular stomatitis
angular tract of cervical fascia
angular vein
angular vestibular nucleus
angularis
    blepharitis angularis
    dens angularis
    spina angularis
angular-tip electrode
angulate
angulated catheter
angulated forceps
angulated fracture
angulated iris spatula
angulated lesion
angulated blade electrode
angulated needle holder
angulated vein hemostat
angulation
    vertical angulation
angulation deformity
angulation fracture
angulation of ureter
angulation osteotomy
angulus
Angus-Esterlie recorder
anhaustral colonic gas pattern
anhepatic stage of liver
    transplantation
anhydride
    methacryloxyethyl trimellitic
        anhydride (META)
ani
    prolapsus ani
    sphincter ani
    tendinous arch of levator ani
animal graft
animation
· facial animation
    forehead animation
Anis aspirating cannula
Anis ball reverse-curvature
    capsular polisher
Anis capsulotomy forceps
Anis corneal forceps
Anis corneal scissors

Anis corneoscleral forceps
Anis disk capsular polisher
Anis forceps
Anis intraocular lens forceps
Anis irrigating vectis
Anis microforceps
Anis microsurgical eye
    instruments
Anis microsurgical needle holder
Anis microsurgical tying forceps
Anis needle holder
Anis posterior chamber capsule
    intraocular lens
Anis staple implant cataract lens
Anis staple lens
Anis straight corneal forceps
Anis tying forceps
Anis-Barraquer needle holder
anisocoria
anisodactylous
anisodactyly
anisognathous
anisomastia
anisomelia
anisometropia
Anita-Busch chondrocutaneous
    flap
Ankeney retractor
Ankeney sternal retractor
ankle
    extensor retinaculum of ankle
    Hoke arthrodesis of foot and
        ankle
    Nélaton dislocation of ankle
    Syme amputation at ankle
    tailor's ankle
    Tillaux fracture of ankle
ankle air stirrup
ankle block
ankle bone
ankle fusion
ankle jerk (AJ)
ankle joint
ankle mortise
ankle orthosis (AO)
ankle prosthesis
ankle rehab pump
ankle strategy
ankle weight
ankle-brachial index
ankle-foot orthosis (AFO)
ankyloblepharon

ankylocheilia
ankyloglossia
ankyloglossia superior syndrome
ankyloproctia
ankylosed
ankylosing hyperostosis
ankylosing spondylitis
ankylosis
    artificial ankylosis
    Barton operation for ankylosis
    bony ankylosis
    cricoarytenoid ankylosis
    extracapsular ankylosis
    false ankylosis
    fibro-osseous ankylosis
    fibrous ankylosis
    glossopalatine ankylosis
    intracapsular ankylosis
    joint ankylosis
    juxta-articular ankylosis
    ligamentous ankylosis
    spurious ankylosis
    surgical ankylosis
    temporomandibular joint
        ankylosis
    TMJ ankylosis
    zygomatic-coronoid ankylosis
ankylotic
ankylotomy
Ann Arbor clamp
Ann Arbor classification
Ann Arbor double towel clamp
Ann Arbor Hodgkin lymphoma
    stages I, IE, II, IIE, IIIE, IIIS,
    IIISE, IV
Ann Arbor phrenic retractor
Ann Arbor retractor
Ann Arbor towel clamp
Annandale knee operation
Annandale operation
ANNE anesthesia infuser
anneal
annular adenocarcinoma
annular band
annular cartilage
annular constricting lesion
annular corneal graft operation
annular detector
annular gouge
annular ligament
annular pulley
annular scleritis

annular sphincter
annular stricture
annular-array transducer
annulare
  granuloma annulare
annuli (*sing.* annulus)
AnnuloFlex annuloplasty ring
AnnuloFlex flexible
    annuloplasty ring
annuloplasty
  Carpentier annuloplasty
  DeVega tricuspid valve
    annuloplasty
  Gerbode annuloplasty
  isolated annuloplasty
  mitral annuloplasty
  prosthetic ring annuloplasty
  septal annuloplasty
  tricuspid valve annuloplasty
  Wooler-type annuloplasty
annuloplasty valve
annulorrhaphy
annulus (*pl.* annuli; *see also*
  anulus)
  bony annulus
  superior annulus
  tympanic annulus
  Vieussens annulus
  Zinn annulus
annulus ciliaris
annulus gouge
annulus of Zinn
annulus tendineus communis
annulus tympanicus
ano
  fissure in ano
  fistula in ano
  in ano
anococcygeal body
anococcygeal nerves
anocutaneous line
anode tube
anoderm-preserving
    hemorrhoidectomy
anodontia
  partial anodontia
  total anodontia
anodontia vera
anomalies
  unruptured vascular anomalies
anomalous anatomy
anomalous artery

anomalous fixation
anomalous innominate artery
    compression syndrome
anomalous insertion
anomalous junction of the
    pancreatobiliary duct
    (AJPBD)
anomalous mesenteric adhesion
anomalous position
anomaly
  4th branch anomaly
  Alder-Reilly anomaly
  anorectal anomaly
  arterial anomaly
  atrioventricular junction
    anomaly
  Axenfeld anomaly
  branchial anomaly
  branchial cleft anomaly
  cardiac anomaly
  cervical anomaly
  chest wall anomaly
  Chiari anomaly
  cleft anomaly
  coloboma anomaly
  congenital anomaly
  congenital conotruncal
    anomaly
  conjoined nerve-root anomaly
  conotruncal anomaly
  coronary artery anomaly
  craniofacial anomaly
  Cruveilhier-Baumgarten
    anomaly
  cutaneous vascular anomaly
  dental anomaly
  dentofacial anomaly
  double-inlet ventricle anomaly
  Duane anomaly
  duplication anomaly
  dysgnathic anomaly
  Ebstein cardiac anomaly
  Epstein anomaly
  eugnathic anomaly
  facet anomaly
  fetal cardiac anomaly
  fetal chest anomaly
  fetal gastrointestinal anomaly
  fetal vascular anomaly
  fixation anomaly
  Freund anomaly
  genetic anomaly

anomaly (*continued*)
  genitourinary anomaly
  gestant anomaly
  hand anomaly
  heart anomaly
  Heberden anomaly
  hemifacial microsomia
    anomaly
  intracranial dural vascular
    anomaly
  jugular bulb anomaly
  kidney anomaly
  Kimerle anomaly
  Kleeblattschädel anomaly
  Klippel-Feil anomaly
  lacrimal angle duct anomaly
  laryngeal anomaly
  limb reduction anomaly
  maxillofacial anomaly
  megadolichovertebrobasilar
    anomaly
  Michel anomaly
  Moebius anomaly
  Mondini anomaly
  morning glory optic disk
    anomaly
  müllerian duct anomaly
  nevoid anomaly
  numerary renal anomaly
  occipitoatlantoaxial anomaly
  oculocephalic vascular
    anomaly
  oral anomaly
  orthopedic anomaly
  osseous anomaly
  Pelger-Huët anomaly
  Peters anomaly
  Poland anomaly
  postsurgical anomaly
  pragmatic anomaly
  presacral anomaly
  pulmonary valve anomaly
  renal anomaly
  reticulate pigmented anomaly
  root anomaly
  segmentation anomaly
  Shone anomaly
  Sprengel anomaly
  structural anomaly
  Taussig-Bing anomaly
  temporal bone anomaly
  third branchial anomaly

anomaly (*continued*)
  tracheobronchial anomaly
  Uhl anomaly
  umbilical cord anomaly
  Undritz anomaly
  urinary tract anomaly
  urogenital anomaly
  uterine anomaly
  VACTERL anomaly
  vaginal anomaly
  vascular anomaly
  venous anomaly
  ventricular inflow anomaly
  vertebral, anal,
    tracheoesophageal, radial,
    and renal anomaly
  viscerobronchial
    cardiovascular anomaly
  vitelline duct anomaly
anomaly angle
anomaly of Zahn
anonychia
anoperineal
anophthalmos
anoplasty
  cutback anoplasty
  House advancement anoplasty
  Martin anoplasty
  Y-V anoplasty
anoplasty treatment
anopouch angle
anorchism
anorectal abscess
anorectal angle
anorectal anomaly
anorectal carcinoma
anorectal disorder
anorectal dressing
anorectal fistula
anorectal foreign body
anorectal junction
anorectal line
anorectal malformation
anorectal manometry
anorectal orifice
anorectal outlet obstruction
anorectal ring
anorectal space
anorectal sphincter
anorectal stenosis
anorectal surgery
anorectal variceal bleeding

anorectocolonic
anorectoplasty
  Laird-McMahon anorectoplasty
anorectum
anoscope
  Bacon anoscope
  Bensaude anoscope
  Bodenheimer anoscope
  Boehm anoscope
  Brinkerhoff anoscope
  Buie-Hirschman anoscope
  Burnett anoscope
  Disposo-Scope anoscope
  Fansler anoscope
  Fansler-Ives anoscope
  fiberoptic anoscope
  Goldbacher anoscope
  Hirschman anoscope
  Ives anoscope
  Ives-Fansler anoscope
  KleenSpec disposable
    anoscope
  Muer anoscope
  Munich-Crosstreet anoscope
  Otis anoscope
  Pratt anoscope
  Proscope anoscope
  Pruitt anoscope
  rotating anoscope
  rotating speculum anoscope
  Sims anoscope
  Sklar anoscope
  slotted anoscope
  Smith anoscope
  speculum anoscope
  Welch Allyn anoscope
anoscope speculum
anoscope with obturator
anoscopic examination
anoscopy
anoscopy with biopsy
anoscopy with excision
anosigmoidoscope
anosigmoidoscopy
anosmia
anospinal
anotia
anotus
ANOVA (analysis of variance)
anoxia
  cerebral anoxia
  hypoxia and anoxia

anthropometric evaluation
ANS (anterior nasal spine)
ansa
  Haller ansa
ansa (*pl.* ansae)
ansa cervicalis
ansa galeni
ansa hypoglossi
ansa hypoglossus muscle
ansa subclavia
Ansaldo AU560 ultrasound
anserine bursa
anserinus
  pes anserinus
Anson-McVay hernia repair
Anson-McVay herniorrhaphy
Anson-McVay operation
Anspach 65K drill
Anspach cement eater
Anspach cranial perforator
Anspach craniotome
Anspach diamond dissecting
  cutter
Anspach leg holder
Antagon
antagonist
  barbiturate antagonist
  narcotic antagonist
antagonistic muscle
antalgic gait
antebrachial fascia
antebrachial region
antebrachial vein
antecedent sign
antecolic anastomosis
antecolic gastrectomy
antecolic gastrojejunostomy
antecolic jejunostomy
antecolic long-loop isoperistaltic
  gastrojejunostomy
antecubital approach
antecubital arteriovenous fistula
antecubital fossa
antecubital space
anteflexed uterus
anteflexion
antegonial angle
antegonial notch
antegonial notching
antegrade aortogram
antegrade approach
antegrade biliary drainage

antegrade blood flow
antegrade catheterization
antegrade continence enema
     procedure
antegrade double balloon-double
     wire technique
antegrade flow
antegrade internal stent
antegrade island flap
antegrade pyelography
antegrade ureteral stent
antegrade urography
antegrade valvulotome
antegrade/retrograde
     cardioplegia technique
antegrade/retrograde
     compression nail
antehelical fold
antemortem clot
antenatal dislocation
antenna procedure
Antense anti-tension device
antepartum hemorrhage
antepartum monitor
antephase
anterior abdominal injury
anterior abdominal wall
anterior acromioplasty
anterior active mask
     rhinomanometry
anterior acute-flexion elbow
     splint
anterior alveolar branch of
     maxillary nerve
anterior ampullary nerve
anterior and posterior repair
     (A&P repair)
anterior angle
anterior annular ligament
anterior anodal patch electrode
anterior approach
anterior arch length
anterior aspiration
anterior auricular groove
anterior auricular muscle
anterior auricular nerve
anterior auricular vein
anterior axillary approach
anterior axillary fold
anterior axillary line (AAL)
anterior band
anterior band remover (ABR)

anterior bulbi camera
anterior capsule forceps
anterior capsulolabral
     reconstruction
anterior capsulotomy
anterior cardiac veins
anterior cavernous syndrome
anterior cecal artery
anterior central gyrus
anterior cerebral artery
anterior cerebral vein
anterior cerebrospinal fasciculus
anterior cervical fusion (ACF)
anterior cervical lip
anterior cervical surgery vocal
     cord damage
anterior cervicothoracic
     junction surgery
anterior chamber
anterior chamber hyphema
anterior chamber intraocular
     lens
anterior chamber maintainer
anterior chamber synechia
     scissors
anterior chamber tube shunt
     encircling band
anterior chest wall flap
anterior choroidal artery
anterior ciliary artery
anterior circulation aneurysm
anterior circumflex humeral
     artery
anterior clear space
anterior clinoid process
anterior colon resection
anterior colporrhaphy
anterior column
anterior commissure
anterior commissurotomy
anterior communicating artery
anterior complete dislocation
anterior component
anterior condylar vein
anterior condyloid canal of
     occipital bone
anterior condyloid foramen
anterior conjunctival artery
anterior cord compression
anterior corneal curvature
anterior cornu
anterior corpectomy

anterior correction
anterior cranial fossa
anterior craniectomy
anterior cricoid split
anterior crossbite
anterior cruciate ligament (ACL)
anterior crurotomy nipper
anterior cyst
anterior diskectomy
anterior displacement (AD)
anterior displacement no
    reduction (ADNR)
anterior distraction
anterior divergence
anterior drawer sign
anterior epineurotomy
anterior ethmoid
anterior ethmoidal air cell
anterior ethmoidectomy
anterior extensile approach
anterior external arcuate fibers
anterior facial height (AFH)
anterior facial vein
anterior femoral resection guide
anterior focal point
anterior fontanelle
anterior footplate pick
anterior force
anterior forceps
anterior fracture
anterior fundoplasty
anterior funiculus
anterior fusion operation
anterior gastrectomy
anterior gastrojejunostomy
anterior gastropexy
anterior gastrotomy
anterior gray commissure
anterior ground bundle
anterior hairline incision
anterior heel
anterior helical rim free flap
anterior hip dislocation
anterior iliac obturator hernia
anterior inferior cerebellar
    artery
anterior inferior communicating
    artery (AICA)
anterior inferior iliac spine
anterior inguinal herniorrhaphy
anterior intercostal veins
anterior internal fixation

anterior internal stabilization
anterior interosseous artery
anterior interosseous nerve
anterior interventricular groove
anterior intraoccipital joint
anterior intraoccipital
    synchondrosis
anterior iridodialysis
anterior jejunostomy
anterior jugular vein
anterior labial nerve
anterior labial vein
anterior labrum periosteum
anterior lacrimal crest
anterior ligament
anterior lingual gland
anterior mallear fold
anterior mallear ligament
anterior mandibular posturing
anterior mandibulectomy
anterior median fissure
anterior medullary velum
anterior meningeal artery
anterior metallic fixation
anterior middle meatus
anterior naris
anterior nasal spine (ANS)
anterior nephrectomy
anterior nerve roots
anterior oblique position
anterior occlusion
anterior ostium
anterior palatal bar
anterior palatine groove
anterior palatine sutures
anterior partial laryngectomy
anterior pelvic exenteration
anterior pillar of fauces
anterior plate fixation
anterior polar cataract
anterior Polya operation
anterior Polya procedure
anterior port scalp excision
anterior process
anterior pull skin stretch (APSS)
anterior quadriceps
    musculocutaneous flap
anterior quadrilateral triplane
    frame
anterior rectopexy
anterior rectus fascia
anterior resection clamp

anterior retinal orbital canal
anterior retroperitoneal
    decompression
anterior rhinoscopy
anterior rhizotomy
anterior sagittal pelvic inlet
anterior sandwich patch
    technique
anterior scalene muscle
anterior scaler
anterior screw fixation
anterior scrotal nerves
anterior scrotal veins
anterior segment forceps
anterior septum
anterior serratus muscle
anterior sheath
anterior short-segment
    stabilization
anterior shoulder dislocation
anterior skin flap
anterior skull base
anterior spinal artery
anterior spinal fixation
anterior spinal fusion
anterior splint
anterior stabilization procedure
anterior sternomastoid approach
anterior subperiosteal implant
anterior superficialis muscle
anterior superior alveolar artery
anterior superior iliac spine
anterior surface of maxilla
anterior surgical exposure
anterior suspension of hyoid
    bone
anterior suspensory ligament
anterior symblepharon
anterior synechia
anterior table
anterior talocalcaneal ligament
anterior talofibular ligament
anterior temporal diploic vein
anterior thalamotomy
anterior thoracoplasty
anterior tibial artery
anterior tibial muscle
anterior tibial sign
anterior tibial tendon
anterior tibial vein
anterior transabdominal approach
anterior transhepatic approach

anterior transthoracic approach
anterior tympanic artery
anterior urethropexy
anterior uterus
anterior vagal trunk
anterior vertical canal
anterior view
anterior vitrectomy
anterior wall antral ulcer
anterior white commissure
anterior-chamber irrigator
anterior-inferior dislocation
anterior-posterior compression
anterior-posterior
    cystoresectoscope
anterior-posterior otoplasty
anterior-superior iliac spine
    (ASIS)
anteroapical
anterocolic anastomosis
anterocrural celiac plexus block
anterodistal border
anterograde direction
anterograde transseptal
    technique
anteroinferior aspect
anterolateral approach
anterolateral aspect
anterolateral cordotomy
anterolateral dislocation
anterolateral displacement
anterolateral fontanelle
anterolateral infarction
anterolateral ligament
anterolateral region
anterolateral rotatory instability
    (ALRI)
anterolateral sulcus
anterolateral thigh flap
anterolateral thoracoplasty
anterolateral thoracotomy
    incision
anterolisthesis
anteromedial bundle
anteromedial incision
anteromedial retropharyngeal
    approach
anteromedial rotatory instability
    (AMRI)
anteromedian
antero-oblique position
anteroposterior (AP)

anteroposterior compression
anteroposterior correction
anteroposterior curve
anteroposterior dysplasia
anteroposterior facial dysplasia
anteroposterior x-ray view
anteroseptal infarct
anteroseptal myocardial
    infarction (AMI)
anterosuperior iliac spine (ASIS)
anterosuperior quadrant
anterotransverse diameter
anteroventral
anteversion
anteverted position
antevesical hernia
anthelicis
   crura anthelicis
   crus anthelicis
anthelix
   crura of anthelix
   fossa of anthelix
Anthony aspirating tube
Anthony cast boot
Anthony compressor
Anthony elevator
Anthony enucleation compressor
Anthony gorget
Anthony mastoid tube
Anthony orbital compressor
Anthony pillar retractor
Anthony quadrisected dilator
Anthony retractor
Anthony suction tube
Anthony tube
Anthony-Fisher antrum balloon
Anthony-Fisher balloon
Anthony-Fisher forceps
Anthron heparinized catheter
Anthron II catheter
anthropometric measurement
anthropometric total hip
anthropometry
anthroposcopy
Antia composite flap of helical
    cartilage
antiangiogenic effect
antiantibody formation
antiarrhythmic therapy
antibacterial
antibacterial personal catheter
antibasement membrane

antibiotic
   IV antibiotic
   bactericidal antibiotic
   bacteriostatic antibiotic
   broad-spectrum antibiotic
   infusion of antibiotics
   oral antibiotic
   precannulation antibiotic
antibiotic irrigation
antibiotic prophylaxis
antibiotic removal device
antibiotic-coated stent
antibiotic-loaded acrylic
    cement total joint
    prosthesis
antibiotic-resistant
antibiotic-soaked swabs
antibodies
   anti-silicone surface-associated
    antigen antibodies (anti-
    SSAA(X))
   antinuclear antibody (ANA)
   collagen antibody
   fluorescent antibody
   monoclonal antibody
   myoclonal antibodies
   surface antibody
anticavitation drill
anticholinesterase anesthetic
    agent
anticoagulant
   lupus anticoagulant
   oral anticoagulant
anticoagulant effect
anticoagulant monitoring
anticoagulant therapy
anticoagulated blood
anticoagulation
   oral anticoagulation
   prophylactic anticoagulation
   systemic anticoagulation
anticoagulation therapy
anticus
antiembolic hose
antiembolic position
antiembolism stockings
antiemetic therapy
antiepithelial serum
antifog solution
antifog tube
antifog, antifogging (AF)
antifungal therapy

antigen
  carcinoembryonic antigen
    (CEA)
  epithelial membrane antigen
    (EMA)
  heterogenetic antigen (HLA)
  human lymphocyte antigens
  organ-specific antigen
  tissue-specific antigen
antigen-antibody reaction
antigenic
antigenicity
antiglaucoma peripheral
  iridectomy
antiglomerular basement
  membrane
antihelical fold
antihelix
  superior crus of antihelix
  unfurling of antihelix
antihemophilic globulin (AHG)
antihemorrhagic stent
antihormonal therapy
anti-incontinence penile
  prosthesis
anti-incontinence procedure
anti-infective
anti-inflammatory agent
antilymphocytic serum
antilymphoid therapy
antimesenteric border
antimesenteric enterotomy
antimesenteric fat pad
antimesocolic side of cecum
antimicrobial barrier
antimicrobial catheter
antimicrobial removal device
antimony pH electrode
antineoplastic
antineoplastic agent
antinuclear
antinuclear antibody (ANA)
antinuclear factor (ANF)
antiperistalsis
antiperistaltic
antiperistaltic anastomosis
antiperistaltic gastrojejunostomy
antiperistaltic jejunostomy
antiperistaltic operation
antipruritic agent
antipyretic
antireflux operation

antireflux prosthesis
antireflux therapy
antireflux ureteral implantation
  technique
antirejection drug therapy
antiretroviral therapy
antirotation guide
antiseborrheic
antisepsis
Anti-Sept bactericidal scrub
  solution
antiseptic
  Acu-dyne antiseptic
antiseptic dressing
antiseptic surgery
antiserum
  trivalent botulinum
    antiserum
antiserum anaphylaxis
antishock suit
antisialagogue
antisialic
anti-silicone surface-associated
  antigen antibodies (anti-
  SSAA(X))
antisiphon device
antisiphon valve
antispasmodic
antispastic
antistriated muscle biopsy
antitachycardia pacemaker
antitension line (ATL)
antithrombotic therapy
antithymocyte globulin (ATG)
antitoxin
  botulinum antitoxin
  bovine antitoxin
  gas gangrene antitoxin
  tetanus antitoxin
antitragicus
  musculus antitragicus
antitragicus muscle
antitragohelicina
  fissura antitragohelicina
antitragohelicine fissure
antitragus muscle
anti-Trendelenburg position
antitrismus
antitubular basement membrane
antiviral
antiwaves cannula
Antole-Condale elevator

Antoni classification of
   schwannoma morphology
Antoni-Hook lumbar puncture
   cannula
antonina
   facies antonina
antra (*sing.* antrum)
antral balloon
antral biopsy
antral bur
antral cannula
antral carcinoma
antral chisel
antral curet
antral drain
antral edema
antral exclusion
antral floor
antral folds
antral forceps
antral gouge
antral irrigator
antral knife
antral membrane
antral mucosa
antral mycosis
antral needle
antral perforator
antral punch
antral rasp
antral resection
antral retractor
antral rongeur
antral sarcoma
antral saw
antral sinus cannula
antral stenosis
antral stoma
antral stricture
antral syringe
antral trephine
antral trocar
antral ulcer
antral wash tube
antral window operation
antrectomy
antroaural fistula
antrobuccal
antroduodenectomy
antrodynia
Antron catheter
antronasal

antrosaucerization
antroscope
   ACMI antroscope
   Nagashima right-angle
      antroscope
   Reichert antroscope
antroscopy
antrostomy
   Caldwell-Luc maxillary
      antrostomy
   inferior meatal antrostomy
   intraoral antrostomy
   middle meatal antrostomy
   nasal antrostomy
antrostomy punch
antrotomy
   frontal antrotomy
   mastoid antrotomy
   maxillary antrotomy
antrum (*pl.* antra)
   distal antrum
   ethmoid antrum
   falx of maxillary antrum
   frontal antrum
   Highmore antrum
   mastoid antrum
   maxillary antrum
   pyloric antrum
   tympanic antrum
   Valsalva antrum
   Willis antrum
antrum auris
antrum balloon
antrum ethmoidale
antrum instruments (*see also*
   antral)
antrum mastoideum
antrum of Willis
antrum pyloricum
antrum rasp
antrum-exploring needle
antrum-irrigating tube
anuli (*sing.* anulus; *see also*
   annulus)
anuloplasty
   Gerbode anuloplasty
   Wooler mitral anuloplasty
anulus (*pl.* anuli)
anulus fibrosus
anulus of Zinn
anulus tympanicus
anuria

anus
  aberrant sebaceous glands of
    anus
  artificial anus
  decompression of imperforate
    anus
  ectopic anus
  imperforate anus type I, II, III,
    IV
  preternatural anus
Anustim electronic
  neuromuscular stimulator
anvil
  Bunnell anvil
anxiety
  separation anxiety
any-angle splint
Anzio catheter
AO (ankle orthosis)
AO blade plate
AO brace
AO cancellous screw
AO clamp
AO classification
AO compression plate
AO condylar blade plate
AO contoured T plate
AO cortex screw
AO drill bit
AO dynamic compression plate
  construct
AO external fixation
AO femoral distractor
AO fixateur interne
  instrumentation
AO gouge
AO guidepin
AO hook plate
AO indirect ophthalmoscope
AO internal fixator
AO lag screw
A-O minus cylinder Phoroptor
AO notched instrumentation
A-O osteotome
AO plate bender
A-O plus cylinder Phoroptor
AO procedure
AO reconstruction plate
AO reduction forceps
AO Reichert scientific
  instruments
AO rigid fixation

AO screw
AO semitubular plate
AO slotted medullary nail
AO small fragment plate
AO spinal internal fixation
AO spongiosa screw
AO spoon plate
AO stopped-drill guide
AO tap
AO technique
AO tension band
AO/ASIF orthopedic surgical
  instruments and implants
AOA cervical immobilization
  brace
AOA-CHICK halo traction
AOD (arteriosclerotic occlusive
  disease)
AOI compression plate
AOIVM (angiographically occult
  intracranial vascular
  malformation)
Aolka sector ultrasound
AOM (alternatives of
  management)
AOO pacemaker (atrial
  asynchronous)
AOR (Alvarado Orthopedic
  Research instruments)
AOR check traction device
AOR collateral ligament retractor
AOR guide
AOR instruments
aorta (pl. aortae)
  appendicular aorta
  arch of aorta
  arcuate aorta
  ascending aorta (AA)
  cannulation of aorta
  coarctation of aorta
  crossclamped aorta
  decannulation of aorta
  deep articular aorta
  descending aorta
  dextropositioned aorta
  dissection of aorta
  dynamic aorta
  ectasia of aorta
  eggshell aorta
  elongated aorta
  fusiform widening of
    abdominal aorta

aorta (*continued*)
  infrarenal aorta
  kinked aorta
  Kono patch enlargement of
    ascending aorta
  overriding aorta
  porcelain aorta
  posterior articular aorta
  proximal aorta
  pseudocoarctation of aorta
  pulsating aorta
  recoarctation of aorta
  retroesophageal aorta
  straddling aorta
  terminal aorta
  thoracic aorta
  throbbing aorta
  tortuous aorta
  ventral aorta
  Waldhausen subclavian flap
    repair of coarctation of
    aorta
aorta abdominalis
aorta aneurysm clamp
aorta aneurysm forceps
aorta ascendens
aorta clamp
aorta descendens
aorta forceps
aorta occluder
aorta punch
aorta retractor
aorta thoracica
aorta valve retractor
aorta vent needle
aorta-and-runoff arteriogram
aortae
  arcus aortae
aortic anastomosis
aortic aneurysm
aortic aneurysm clamp
aortic aneurysm forceps
aortic aneurysm graft
aortic aneurysm repair
aortic aneurysm tissue
aortic aneurysmal disease
aortic aneurysmectomy
aortic arch arteriography
aortic arch cannula
aortic arch disease
aortic atheromatous disease
aortic balloon pump

aortic bifurcation
aortic bioprosthetic valve
aortic blood pressure
aortic body
aortic body tumor
aortic cannula
aortic catheter
aortic clamp
aortic clamping
aortic commissure
aortic conduit
aortic crossclamp
aortic crossclamp time
aortic cross-clamping
aortic cuff
aortic curet
aortic cusp
aortic dicrotic notch pressure
aortic dilator
aortic director ellipse cannula
aortic dissection
aortic foramen
aortic forceps
aortic graft placement
aortic hiatus
aortic hypoplasia
aortic incompetence
aortic insufficiency
aortic intramural hematoma
aortic isthmus
aortic knob
aortic knuckle
aortic laceration
aortic lymph node
aortic murmur
aortic neck
aortic nipple
aortic node metastasis
aortic notch
aortic occluder
aortic occlusion clamp
aortic occlusion forceps
aortic occlusive disease (AOD)
aortic opening
aortic orifice
aortic patch
aortic perfusion
aortic plexus
aortic pressure
aortic pullback pressure
aortic pulmonary window
aortic punch

aortic reconstructive surgery
aortic regurgitation
aortic regurgitation murmur
aortic retractor
aortic ring
aortic root perfusion needle
aortic root velocity waveform
aortic runoff
aortic rupture
aortic sac
aortic scissors
aortic 2nd sound (A2)
aortic septal defect
aortic sinotubular junction
aortic sound
aortic stump blow-out
aortic sulcus
aortic sump tube
aortic suprarenal artery
aortic thrill
aortic transection
aortic tube graft
aortic valve
aortic valve area
aortic valve atresia
aortic valve brush
aortic valve disease
aortic valve gradient
aortic valve insufficiency
aortic valve leaflet
aortic valve prosthesis
aortic valve repair
aortic valve replacement
aortic valve resistance
aortic valve restenosis
aortic valve retractor
aortic valve rongeur
aortic valve velocity profile
aortic valvotomy
aortic valvuloplasty
aortic valvulotomy
aortic vent needle
aortic wall
aortic window
aortic-femoral bypass
aortic-left ventricular tunnel
aorticocoronary bypass
aorticopulmonary anastomosis
aorticopulmonary septal
   defect
aorticopulmonary shunt
aorticopulmonary window

aorticopulmonary window
   operation
aorticorenal
aorticorenal ganglion
aortoannular ectasia
aortoarteriography
aortobifemoral bypass
aortobi-iliac bypass
aortocarotid bypass
aortocaval fistula
aortocoronary
aortocoronary bypass
aortocoronary snake graft
aortocoronary vein bypass
aortocoronary-saphenous vein
   bypass
aortoduodenal fistula
aortoenteric fistula
aortoesophageal fistula
aortofemoral
   Gore-Tex aortofemoral (AF)
      fistula
aortofemoral bypass
aortofemoral bypass graft (AFBG)
aortofemoral prosthesis
aortogastric fistula
aortograft duodenal fistula
aortogram
   abdominal aortogram
   antegrade aortogram
   arch aortogram
   contrast aortogram
   digital subtraction
      supravalvular aortogram
   flush aortogram
   Huber needle for translumbar
      aortogram
   lumbar aortogram
   retrograde aortogram
   supravalvular aortogram
   thoracic arch aortogram
   transbrachial arch aortogram
   translumbar aortogram
aortogram catheter
aortogram needle
aortogram with distal runoff
aortographic chronic active
   hepatitis
aortographic suction tip
aortography
   abdominal aortography
   arch aortography

aortography (*continued*)
 Dos Santos needle for
  aortography
 lumbar aortography
 percutaneous translumbar
  aortography
 thoracic aortography
 venous aortography
 visceral aortography
aortography catheter
aortography needle
aortohepatic arterial graft
aortoiliac
aortoiliac aneurysm
aortoiliac angioplasty
aortoiliac bypass
aortoiliac endarterectomy
aortoiliac occlusive disease
aortoiliofemoral bypass
aortoiliofemoral endarterectomy
aortoplasty
 patch aortoplasty
aortopulmonary
aortopulmonary fenestration
aortopulmonary shunt
aortopulmonary tunnel
aortopulmonary window
aortorenal bypass
aortorenal reconstruction
aortorrhaphy
aortosigmoid fistula
aorto-subclavian-carotid-
  axilloaxillary bypass
aortotomy
aortotomy incision
aortovein bypass graft
aortoventriculoplasty
AO-Titanium microplate
AP (anteroposterior)
AP cutting block
AP diameter of chest
AP femoral sizer
AP sizer
APACHE-II point
apart
 eye width apart
apatite calculus
apatite urine tract stones
APC-3, -4 collimator
Apdyne phenol applicator kit
ape hand
ape-hand deformity

apepsia
 achlorhydria apepsia
aperiosteal amputation
aperiosteal supracondylar
  tendoplastic amputation
aperistaltic esophagus
Apert disease
Apert hirsutism
Apert syndrome
Apert-Crouzon disease
apertognathia
 compound apertognathia
 infantile apertognathia
 simple apertognathia
apertognathia repair
apertognathism
apertura (*pl.* aperturae)
apertura externa canaliculi
  cochleae
apertura piriformis
apertura sinus frontalis
apertura sinus sphenoidalis
aperture
 bony anterior nasal aperture
 eye aperture
 frontal sinus aperture
 inferior pelvic aperture
 inferior thoracic aperture
 laryngeal aperture
 lateral aperture
 medial aperture
 multiple apertures
 nasal aperture
 orbital aperture
 pharyngeal aperture
 piriform aperture
 pupillary aperture
 pyriform aperture
 sphenoid sinus aperture
 superior pelvic aperture
 superior thoracic aperture
 upper thorax aperture
aperture of inguinal hernia
aperture of sphenoid sinus
apertures of abdomen
apex (*pl.* apices)
 cardiac apex
 closed apex
 darwinian apex
 flaring apex
 open apex
 orbital apex

apex (*continued*)
  pulmonary apex
  radiographic apex
  retropapillary apex
  true apex (TA)
apex auriculae
apex blunderbuss
apex cardiogram
apex cornea
apex fracture
apex linguae
apex locator
apex nasi
apex of duodenal bulb
apex of external ring
apex of heart
apex of petrous part of
    temporal bone
apex of the brow
apex of tongue
apex partis petrosae ossis
    temporalis
apex pin
apex radicis dentis
apex satyri
Apexo elevator
APF Moore-type femoral stem
Apfelbaum bipolar forceps
Apfelbaum cerebellar retractor
Apfelbaum micromirror
Apgar score
aphagia
aphakia
aphakic correction
aphalangia
aphasia
  infantile aphasia
  motor aphasia
apheresis
aphonic bruit
aphtha (*pl.* aphthae)
aphthae
  Bednar aphthae
  Mikulicz aphthae
aphthae major
aphthae minor
aphthoid ulcer
aphthosis
aphthous stomatitis
aphthous ulcer
aphthous-type lesion
API osteotome

API universal foam chin strap
apical abscess
apical base
apical cyst
apical dental ligament
apical fenestration
apical gland
apical granuloma
apical impulse
apical lordotic x-ray view
apical murmur
apical radiolucency
apical space
apical thoracoplasty
apically repositioned flap in
    mucogingival surgery
apicectomy
apices
  petrous apices
apices (*sing.* apex)
apicitis curet
apicoaortic conduit heart valve
apicoaortic shunt heart valve
apicoectomy
apicolysis
  extrafascial apicolysis
  extrapleural apicolysis
apicolysis retractor
apicoseptal aneurysmectomy
apicostomy
aplasia
  cochlear aplasia
  condylar aplasia
  gonadal aplasia
  labyrinthine aplasia
  müllerian duct aplasia
  salivary gland aplasia
  thymic aplasia
aplasia cutis congenita
aplastic anemia
Apley
  grinding test of Apley
Apley grind test
Apley knee test
Apley maneuver
Apley sign
Apley test
Apley traction
Apligraf (graftskin) graft
Apligraf skin graft material
Apligraf venous ulcer graft
    material

apnea
  Arvee model 2400 infant
    apnea
  deglutition apnea
  induced apnea
  obstructive sleep apnea
  peripheral apnea
  vagal apnea
apnea alarm mattress
apnea monitor
apnea neonatorum
apnea-hypopnea index (AHI)
apneic
apneustic respirations
apocope
apocoptic
apocrine adenoma
apocrine carcinoma
apocrine gland
apocrine metaplasia
apocrine retention cyst
apocrine sweat glands
Apogee ultrasound device
Apollo 3 triple-lumen
  papillotome
Apollo hip prosthesis
Apollo knee prosthesis
APOLT technique
aponeurectomy
aponeurorrhaphy
aponeurosis (*pl.* aponeuroses)
  abdominal aponeurosis
  Denonvilliers aponeurosis
  epicranial aponeurosis
  extensor aponeurosis
  external oblique
    aponeurosis
  fibrovascular aponeurosis
  internal oblique aponeurosis
  levator aponeurosis
  lingual aponeurosis
  musculotendinous
    aponeurosis
  palatal aponeurosis
  palatine aponeurosis
  palmar aponeurosis
  Petit aponeurosis
  rhomboid aponeurosis
  temporal aponeurosis
  thoracolumbar aponeurosis
  transverse bundles of palmar
    aponeurosis

aponeurosis (*continued*)
  transversus abdominis
    aponeurosis
  triangular aponeurosis
  Zinn aponeurosis
aponeurosis epicranialis
aponeurosis linguae
aponeurosis of biceps brachii
aponeurosis of external oblique
  muscle
aponeurosis of insertion
aponeurosis of musculus
  transversus abdominis
aponeurosis of origin
aponeurosis of velum
aponeurosis of Zinn
aponeurosis palatina
aponeurositis
aponeurotic
aponeurotic abscess
aponeurotic blepharoptosis
aponeurotic closure
aponeurotic falx
aponeurotic fascia
aponeurotic fibroma
aponeurotic flap
aponeurotic galea
aponeurotic laxity
aponeurotic layer
aponeurotic musculature
aponeurotica
  galea aponeurotica
  lateral galea aponeurotica
aponeurotica galea
aponeurotome
aponeurotomy
apophysary point
apophysial (*also* apophyseal)
apophysial fracture
apophysial point
apophysis
  cerebral apophysis
  genial apophysis
apoplexy
  uteroplacental apoplexy
APOPPS, transtibial prosthetic
  socket
apoptosis
  resuscitation-induced
    pulmonary apoptosis
  selective lectin-triggered
    apoptosis

A-Port implantable port
A-Port vascular access
apostematosa
　cheilitis glandularis
　　apostematosa
apostematous cheilitis
apotreptic therapy
apparatus lacrimalis
apparatus of Perroncito
apparent death
appearance
　aesthetic appearance
　beaten silver appearance
　bone-within-a-bone appearance
　chamois yellow appearance
　chipmunk cheek appearance
　coiled-spring appearance
　copper wire appearance
　cosmetic appearance
　cotton-wool appearance
　cystlike appearance
　dirty-lung appearance
　esthetic appearance
　flat-face appearance
　gland appearance
　gross appearance
　ground-glass appearance
　honeycomb appearance
　lamina dura-like appearance
　micrognathic appearance
　mottled appearance
　onion peel appearance
　pruned-tree appearance
　slapped cheek appearance
　slapped face appearance
　snarl-tip appearance
　string-of-beads appearance
　sunken-eye appearance
　sunken-face appearances
　worm-eaten appearance
Appel-Bercie sheath
appendage
　auricular appendage
　cecal appendage
　epiploic appendages
　filamentous appendage
　omental appendage
　testicular appendage
　uterine appendage
　vermicular appendage
　vermiform appendage
　vesicular appendages

appendage clamp
appendages of the eye
appendages of the skin
appendalgia
appendectomy
　auricular appendectomy
　colonoscopic appendectomy
　emergency appendectomy
　incidental appendectomy
　interval appendectomy
　inversion appendectomy
　inversion-ligation
　　appendectomy
　laparoscopic appendectomy
　　(LA)
　laser-assisted appendectomy
　McBurney appendectomy
　negative appendectomy
　open appendectomy (OA)
　percutaneous appendectomy
　Weir appendectomy
appendectomy clamp
appendectomy incision
appendectomy retractor
appendectomy sponge
appendectomy spoon
appendiceal abscess
appendiceal adenocarcinoma
appendiceal base
appendiceal cancer
appendiceal fecalith
appendiceal gangrene
appendiceal intussusception
appendiceal mass
appendiceal mesentery
appendiceal perforation
appendiceal retractor
appendiceal stump
appendiceal tissue
appendicealgia
appendicectasis
appendicectomy
appendices (*sing.* appendix)
appendices epiploicae
appendicism
appendicitis
　fulminating appendicitis
　perforating appendicitis
　perforative appendicitis
　stercoral appendicitis
　subperitoneal appendicitis
　suppurative appendicitis

appendicitis by contiguity
appendicitis granulosa
appendicitis larvata
appendicitis obliterans
appendiclausis
appendicocecostomy
appendicocele
appendicocystostomy
  continent cutaneous
    appendicocystostomy
  dismembered reimplanted
    appendicocystostomy
  nonplicated
    appendicocystostomy
  orthotopic
    appendicocystostomy
  plicated appendicocystostomy
  reversed reimplanted
    appendicocystostomy
appendicoenterostomy
appendicolith
appendicolithiasis
appendicolysis
appendicopathia
appendicopathy
appendicosis
appendicostomy
appendicotomy
appendicovesicostomy
  Mitrofanoff
    appendicovesicostomy
appendicular aorta
appendicular artery
appendicular ataxia
appendicular vein
appendiculoradiogram
appendix (*pl.* appendices,
  appendixes)
  auricular appendix
  cecal appendix
  ensiform appendix
  guillotine amputation of
    appendix
  inflamed appendix
  lumen of appendix
  Morgagni appendix
  perforated appendix
  retrocecal appendix
  ruptured appendix
  stump of appendix
  vermiform appendix
  virulent appendix

appendix cerebri
appendix inverter
appendix of epididymis
appendix tapes
appendix vermiform
appendix vermiformis
appendolithiasis
appendoroentgenogram
appendoroentgenography
appendotome
appendotome knife
applanation
applanation tonometer
applanation tonometry
applanator
  Johnston LASIK flap
    applanator
applanometer
apple
  Adam's apple
apple cheek contour
Apple laparoscopic stone
  grabber
Apple Medical bipolar forceps
Apple trocar
apple-core lesion
apple-peel bowel
appliance (*see also* fracture
  appliance)
  stick-and-carrot appliance
  ACCO orthodontic appliance
  Andresen monoblock
    appliance
  Andresen removable
    orthodontic appliance
  Anglebasic E arch appliance
  arch bar facial fracture
    appliance
  Balters appliance
  Begg light wire appliance
  Bimler appliance
  biphasic pin appliance
  Bipro orthodontic appliance
  Bradford fracture appliance
  Buck fracture appliance
  Cameron fracture appliance
  Case appliance
  craniofacial fracture appliance
  Crozat removable orthodontic
    appliance
  Denholtz muscle anchorage
    appliance

appliance (*continued*)

dental arch bar facial fracture appliance

Dewald halo spinal appliance

double-band navel appliance

Erich facial fracture appliance

expansion plate appliance

extraoral fracture appliance

facial fracture appliance

Fairdale orthodontic appliance

fixed appliance

FracSure appliance

fracture appliance

Fraenkel appliance

Gentle Touch colostomy appliance

Gerster fracture appliance

Goldthwait fracture appliance

Graber appliance

Hasund appliance

Hawley appliance

Hibbs fracture appliance

Hyrax appliance

ileostomy appliance

intraoral fracture appliance

Jackson appliance

Janes fracture appliance

Jelenko facial fracture appliance

Jewett fracture appliance

Jobst appliance

Johnson twin-wire appliance

Joseph septal fracture appliance

Karaya adhesive appliance

Karaya adhesive ileostomy appliance

Karaya ring ileostomy appliance

Karaya seal ileostomy appliance

Kesling appliance

Latham appliance

Level Anchorage appliance

light wire appliance

lip habit appliance

mandibular advancement appliance (MAA)

mandibular orthopaedic repositioning appliance

Margolis appliance

appliance (*continued*)

Marlen colostomy appliance

Mayne muscle control appliance

microstomia prevention appliance

Mitek anchor appliance

monobloc appliance

Muhlmann appliance

multiphase appliance

Nord appliance

Nu-Comfort colostomy appliance

obturator appliance

Ormco appliance

orthodontic appliance

ostomy appliance

palatal expansion appliance

palate-splitting appliance

prosthetic appliance

Proxi-Floss cleaning appliance

Remedy colostomy appliance

Remedy ileostomy appliance

removable appliance

ribbon arch appliance

Roger Anderson facial fracture appliance

Roger Anderson pin fixation appliance

SACH orthopaedic appliance

Schacht colostomy appliance

Seep-Pruf ileostomy appliance

soft ankle, cushioned heel orthopaedic appliance

split plate appliance

Stockfisch appliance

surgical appliance

TheraSnore oral appliance

Unitek appliance

Universal appliance

Vasocillator fracture appliance

vinyl palatal appliance

W.W. Walker appliance

Whip appliance

Whitman fracture appliance

Wilson fracture appliance

Winter facial fracture appliance

wire appliance

appliance modification

application
  arch bar application
  Ernst radium application
  Fletcher-Suit application
  intracavitary application
  intranasal application
  intrauterine radium
    application
  Jelenko arch bar application
  laparoscopic clip application
  Lathbury application
  ovoid radium application
  radium application
  Sayre cast application
  topical application
  Trabecular Metal Technology
    for knee, hip, and shoulder
    applications
applicator
  90Sr-loaded eye applicator
  Absolok endoscopic clip
    applicator
  afterload applicator
  Allen applicator
  Andrews cotton applicator
  Andrews ear applicator
  Andrews nasal applicator
  applicator forceps
  aural applicator
  Barth double-end applicator
  beta irradiation applicator
  beta therapy eye applicator
  beta-ray applicator
  Bloedorn applicator
  Brown cotton applicator
  Brown nasal applicator
  Brown-Dean cotton applicator
  Bárány applicator
  Buck ear applicator
  Buck nasal applicator
  Burnett applicator (sizes A, B,
    etc.)
  calcium alginate applicator
  Campbell applicator
  Campbell-type Heyman
    fundus applicator
  cesium applicator
  Chaoul applicator
  Clark applicator
  Cohen suture applicator
  colpostat applicator
  Copalite applicator

applicator (*continued*)
  corneal applicator
  cotton ear applicator
  cotton nasal applicator
  cotton-tipped applicator
  Dean cotton applicator
  Delclos applicator
  Delrin applicator
  ear applicator
  Edslab applicator
  Ernst radium applicator
  eustachian applicator
  Falope-ring applicator
  Farrell nasal applicator
  Farrior suction applicator
  Filshie clip minilaparotomy
    applicator
  Fletcher loading applicator
  Fletcher-Suit afterloading
    applicator
  Garney rubber band
    applicator
  Gass dye applicator
  Gifford applicator
  Gifford corneal applicator
  global force applicator
  Grafco cotton tip applicator
  Henschke seed applicator
  HEX heat applicator
  Holinger applicator
  Hotz ear applicator
  Huzly tampon applicator
  infrared applicator
  intracavitary afterloading
    applicator
  intracavitary gynecologic
    applicator
  iontophoretic applicator
  Ivan laryngeal applicator
  Ivan nasopharyngeal
    applicator
  Jackson laryngeal applicator
  Jobson-Horne cotton
    applicator
  Kevorkian-Younge uterine
    applicator
  Kumar applicator
  Kyle ear applicator
  laryngeal applicator
  Lathbury cotton applicator
  Lejeune cotton applicator
  loading applicator

applicator (*continued*)
  Ludwig middle ear applicator
  Ludwig sinus applicator
  Mayfield clip applicator
  metal applicator
  Mick seed applicator
  Mick TP-200 applicator
  Milex Jel-Jector vaginal
    applicator
  minilaparotomy Falope-ring
    applicator
  MIRALVA applicator
  Monel metal radium
    applicator
  Montrose dressing applicator
  multifire clip applicator
  multiload occlusive clip
    applicator
  nasal applicator
  nasopharyngeal applicator
  NeuroAvitene applicator
  Nucletron applicator
  Playfair uterine caustic
    applicator
  Plummer Vinson radium
    esophageal applicator
  Plummer-Vinson radium
    applicator
  postnasal applicator
  Pynchon applicator
  radioactive applicator
  radioisotope applicator
  radium applicator
  Ralks sinus applicator
  ratchet applicator
  resorbable thread clip
    applicator
  ring applicator
  Roberts applicator
  Sawtell laryngeal applicator
  Sawtell nasal applicator
  sealed applicator
  sonic applicator
  Stille laryngeal applicator
  Storz applicator
  strontium-90 ophthalmic beta
    ray applicator
  Syed radium applicator
  Syed-Puthawala-Hedger
    esophageal applicator
  tampon applicator
  tandem applicator

applicator (*continued*)
  Ter-Pogossian cervical radium
    applicator
  Turnbull applicator
  Uckermann cotton applicator
  Uebe applicator
  University of Iowa cotton
    applicator
  Wang applicator
  Wolf-Yoon applicator
  Wood applicator
  Yoon-ring applicator
applicator forceps
applicator jar
Applied Biosystems 340A
    nucleic acid extractor
Applied Medical mini
    ureteroscope
applier
  Acland microvascular clamp
    applier
  AcuClip endoscopic multiple-
    clip applier
  Advanced Surgical suture
    applier
  Alm clip applier
  aneurysm clip applier
  Autoclip applier
  automatic hemoclip applier
  Auto Suture Clip-A-Matic clip
    applier
  bayonet clip applier
  Biemer vessel clip applier
  clip applier
  cranial aneurysm clip applier
  Crockard transoral clip
    applier
  Endo Clip applier
  Gam-Mer clip applier
  Hamby right-angle clip
    applier
  Heifitz clip applier
  hemoclip applier
  hemostatic clip applier
  Hulka clip applier
  Kaufman clip applier
  Kees clip applier
  Kerr clip applier
  LDS clip applier
  Ligaclip MCA multiple-clip
    applier
  Malis clip applier

applier (*continued*)
- Mayfield miniature clip applier
- Mayfield temporary aneurysm clip applier
- McFadden Vari-Angle clip applier
- microarterial clamp applier
- microclip applier
- mini applier
- Mount-Olivecrona clip applier
- Mt. Clemens Hospital clip applier
- Multifire Endo hernia clip applier
- multiloaded clip applier
- Olivecrona clip applier
- pivot aneurysm clip applier
- pivot microanastomosis clip applier
- Raney scalp clip applier
- Right Clip applier
- Sano clip applier
- Schwartz clip applier
- Scoville clip applier
- Scoville-Drew clip applier
- Spetzler clip applier
- Sugita jaws clip applier
- surgical clip applier
- suture clip applier
- Vari-Angle clip applier
- Vari-Angle McFadden clip applier
- vascular clip applier
- Weck clip applier
- Yasargil clip applier
- Zmurkiewicz clip applier

Appolionio implant cataract lens
Appolito operation
Appolito suture technique
Appose disposable skin stapler
Appose skin stapler
apposition
- compensatory periosteal bone apposition

apposition sutures
approach
- Abbott knee approach
- Abbott-Carpenter posterior approach
- Abbott-Lucas approach
- abdominal approach

approach (*continued*)
- acetabular extensile approach
- acromiothoracic approach
- adaptational approach
- aggressive surgical approach
- Alken approach
- alternative surgical approach
- anesthetic approach
- antecubital approach
- antegrade approach
- anterior acromioplasty approach
- anterior approach
- anterolateral approach
- anteromedial retropharyngeal approach
- Aufranc approach
- Austin Moore southern approach
- Avila approach
- axillary subpectoral approach
- Bailey-Badgley cervical spine approach
- Banks-Laufman approach
- basal subfrontal approach
- Bennett posterior shoulder approach
- Berger-Bookwalter posterior approach
- Berke approach
- bicoronal subperiosteal approach
- bilateral ilioinguinal approach
- bilateral sacroiliac approach
- Blair approach
- Bosworth approach
- Boyd approach
- Boyd-Sisk approach
- brachial artery approach
- Brackett-Osgood posterior approach
- Brewser arthrotomy approach
- Brodsky-Tullos-Gartsman approach
- Broomhead medial approach
- brow-lift approach (modified trichophytic)
- Brown knee approach
- Brown lateral approach
- Bruner approach
- Bruser knee approach
- Bruser lateral approach

approach (*continued*)

Bryan-Morrey elbow approach

Bryan-Morrey extensive posterior approach

buccopharyngeal approach

buttonhole approach

Caldwell-Luc approach

Callahan approach

Campbell posterior shoulder approach

Campbell posterolateral approach

Campbell-Molesworth-Campbell approach

Carnesale acetabular extensile approach

Carnesale hip approach

Case knee approach

case-by-case approach

Cave hip approach

central approach

cerebellopontine angle approach

cervical approach

cervicothoracic approach

Charnley approach

Charnley-Mueller approach

choledochal fiberoscopic approach

classical approach

Cloward cervical disk approach

cochleovestibular approach

Codman saber-cut shoulder approach

Colonna-Ralston ankle approach

Colonna-Ralston approach

Colonna-Ralston medial approach

combined anterior and posterior approach

combined laparoscopic and thoracoscopic approach

combined low cervical and transthoracic approach

combined presigmoid-transtransversarium intradural approach

combined transsylvian and middle fossa approach

approach (*continued*)

conservative approach

consortial approach

Coonse-Adams knee approach

Cozen approach

Cubbins shoulder approach

Cubbins-Callahan-Scuderi approach

curved approach

curved L approach

Darrach-McLaughlin approach

deltoid-splitting shoulder approach

deltopectoral approach

Dickinson approach

distal interphalangeal joint approach

dorsal finger approach

dorsal midline approach

dorsalward approach

dorsolateral approach

dorsomedial approach

dorsoplantar approach

dorsoradial approach

dorsorostral approach

dorsoulnar approach

double-doughnut approach

double-seton modified surgical approach

Duran approach

DuVries approach

endaural approach

Endius approach

endonasal approach

endovascular approach

extended frontal approach

extended iliofemoral approach

extended subfrontal approach

extensile approach

external pharyngotomy approach

extrabursal approach

extralaryngeal approach

extraoral approach

extraperitoneal approach

extrapharyngeal approach

extravesical Lich approach

extreme lateral transcondylar approach

Fahey approach

approach (*continued*)

far lateral inferior suboccipital approach

fascial sling approach

femoral artery approach

Fernandez extensile anterior approach

flank approach

foraminal approach

fornix approach

Fowler-Philip approach

frontal cortical approach

frontotemporal approach

Garceau approach

Gardner shoulder approach

gasless laparoscopic approach

Gatellier-Chastang ankle approach

Gatellier-Chastang posterolateral approach

genetic approach

Gibson approach

Gillies approach

Gillquist approach

Gordon approach

Guleke-Stookey approach

Hardinge lateral approach

Harmon cervical approach

Harmon modified posterolateral approach

Harmon shoulder approach

Harris anterolateral approach

Hay lateral approach

Henderson approach

Henry anterior strap approach

Henry extensile approach

Henry posterior interosseous nerve approach

Henry radial approach

Hibbs approach

Hodgson approach

Hoffmann approach

Hoppenfeld-Deboer approach

Howorth approach

humeral approach

idiographic approach

Iliff approach

iliofemoral approach

ilioinguinal acetabular approach

approach (*continued*)

immunocytochemical approach

inferior extradural approach

inferior transvermian approach

inferior-lateral endonasal transsphenoidal approach

infralabyrinthine approach

inframammary approach

infratemporal fossa approach

infratentorial supracerebellar approach

Inglis-Ranawat-Straub approach

inguinal approach

Insall approach

interfascial approach

interforniceal approach

interhemispheric approach

interscalene approach

intradural approach

intranasal approach

intraoral approach

intratentorial supracerebellar approach

inverted U approach

J approach

Japanese approach

Jones-Brackett approach

Judet approach

Kaye minimal-incision anterior approach

keyhole approach

Kikuchi-MacNap-Moreau approach

Kocher curved L approach

Kocher lateral J approach

Kocher-Gibson posterolateral approach

Kocher-Langenbeck approach

Kocher-McFarland arthroplasty approach

Koenig-Schaefer medial approach

Kraske parasacral approach

Kugel approach

L approach

labioglossomandibular approach

labiomandibular approach

laparoscopic approach

approach (*continued*)

lateral deltoid splitting approach

lateral extracavitary approach

lateral Gatellier-Chastung approach

lateral J approach

lateral Kocher approach

Lazepen-Gamidov anteromedial approach

Leslie-Ryan anterior axillary approach

lesser sac approach

Letournel approach

Letournel-Judet approach

limbal approach

lingual approach

Lortat-Jacob approach

Ludloff medial approach

lumbar approach

mandibular swing approach

Mayo approach

McAfee approach

McConnell extensile approach

McConnell median and ulnar nerve approach

McFarland-Osborne lateral approach

McLaughlin approach

McWhorter posterior shoulder approach

Mears-Rubash approach

medial extradural approach

medial parapatellar capsular approach

middle fossa approach

midlateral approach

midline medial approach

midline spinal approach

minimally invasive approach

Minkoff-Jaffe-Menendez posterior approach

Mize-Bucholz-Grogen approach

modified Risdon approach

Molesworth-Campbell elbow approach

Moore posterior approach

multidisciplinary approach

multiple-stage approach

Murphy approach

approach (*continued*)

neurosurgical approach

nonoperative approach

Norwich approach

Ollier arthrodesis approach

Ollier lateral approach

open laparoscopic approach

operative approach

orbitozygomatic temporopolar approach

oropharyngeal approach

Osborne posterior approach

otomicrosurgical transtemporal approach

palmar approach

paramedian approach

pararectus approach

paraspinal approach

parieto-occipital approach

patella turndown approach

percutaneous transhepatic approach

percutaneous transjugular approach

peroral approach

Perry extensile anterior approach

petrosal approach

Pfannenstiel transverse approach

Phemister medial approach

Planas approach

plantar approach

Pogrund lateral approach

postaural approach

postauricular approach

posterior costotransversectomy approach

posterior inverted-U approach

posterior laparoscopic approach

posterior lumbar approach

posterior midline approach

posterior occipitocervical approach

posterior transolecranon approach

posterolateral approach

posteromedial approach

preperitoneal approach

approach (*continued*)
   presigmoid-
      transtransversarium
      intradural approach
   proprioceptive
      neuromuscular facilitation
      approach
   proximal interphalangeal joint
      approach
   pterional approach
   pulp approach
   Putti posterior approach
   Putti-Abbott approach
   rapid-volume approach
   Redman approach
   regressive reconstructive
      approach
   Reinert acetabular extensile
      approach
   retrograde endoscopic
      approach
   retrograde femoral approach
   retrolabyrinthine presigmoid
      approach
   retroperitoneal approach
   retropharyngeal approach
   retroseptal transconjunctival
      approach
   retrosigmoid approach
   rhinoseptal approach
   Risdon approach
   Roaf approach
   Roberts approach
   Roos transaxillary approach
   Rowe posterior shoulder
      approach
   saber-cut approach
   sacral-foraminal approach
   sacroperineal approach
   screw-plate approach
   sensorimotor stimulation
      approach
   shot-gun approach
   skull-base approach
   Smith-Petersen approach
   Smith-Petersen-Cave-Van
      Gorder anterolateral
      approach
   Smith-Robinson anterior
      approach
   Smith-Robinson cervical disk
      approach

approach (*continued*)
   somatic gene-transfer
      approach
   Somerville anterior approach
   Southwick-Robinson anterior
      cervical approach
   Spetzler anterior transoral
      approach
   split-heel approach
   split-patellar approach
   stabilization approach
   standard open approach
   sternum-splitting approach
   subchoroidal approach
   subciliary approach
   subclavicular approach
   subfrontal approach
   subfrontal-transbasal
      approach
   sublabial midline rhinoseptal
      approach
   sublabial transsphenoidal
      approach
   submental tuck approach
   suboccipital-subtemporal
      approach
   suboccipital-transmeatal
      approach
   subperiosteal approach
   subtemporal-intradural
      approach
   superior-intradural approach
   supine-oblique approach
   supracerebellar approach
   supraclavicular approach
   supraduodenal approach
   supraorbital-pterional
      approach
   supratentorial approach
   surgical approach
   suspended-pedicle approach
   Swedish approach
   sylvian approach
   systematic approach
   Szilagyi approach
   takedown abdominal
      approach
   Taylor approach
   team approach
   therapeutic approach
   Thompson anterolateral
      approach

approach (*continued*)
Thompson anteromedial
approach
Thompson posterior radial
approach
Thompson-Henry approach
thoracic approach
thoracoabdominal
extrapleural approach
thoracolumbar retroperitoneal
approach
thoracoscopic approach
thoracotomy approach
thumb metacarpophalangeal
joint approach
too superficial approach
transabdominal approach
transacromial approach
transanal approach
transantral approach
transaxillary approach
transblepharoplasty
approach
transbrachioradialis approach
transcallosal transventricular
approach
transcanine approach
transcavernous transpetrous
apex approach
transcerebellar hemispheric
approach
transcervical approach
transclavicular approach
transcoccygeal approach
transcochlear approach
transconjunctival approach
transcortical transventricular
approach
transcranial frontal-temporal-
orbital approach
transcubital approach
transcystic approach
transduodenal approach
transdural approach
transfibular approach
transfrontal approach
transgluteal approach
transhepatic approach
transhiatal approach
translabyrinthine and
suboccipital approach
transmandibular approach

approach (*continued*)
transmandibular-
glossopharyngeal approach
transmastoid approach
transmaxillary approach
transmeatal approach
transmural approach
transolecranon approach
transoral approach
transpalatal approach
transpalpebral approach
transpapillary approach
transpedicular approach
transperitoneal approach
transpleural approach
transradial approach
transrectal transphincteric
approach
transseptal approach
transsinus approach
transsphenoidal approach
transsternal approach
transsylvian approach
transtentorial approach
transthoracic approach
transtorcular approach
transtrochanteric approach
transvaginal approach
transvenous approach
transverse approach
transxiphoid approach
trapdoor approach
triradiate acetabular extensile
approach
triradiate transtrochanteric
approach
unilateral sacroiliac approach
vaginal wall approach
Van Gorder approach
vertical midline approach
volar finger approach
volar midline approach
volar radial approach
volar ulnar approach
volarward approach
Wadsworth elbow approach
Wadsworth posterolateral
approach
Wagoner approach
Wagoner posterior approach
Watson-Jones anterior
approach

approach (*continued*)
  Watson-Jones lateral approach
  whole-face injection approach
  Wilson approach
  Wiltberger anterior cervical
    approach
  Wiltse-Spencer paraspinal
    approach
  Yee posterior shoulder
    approach
  Young approach
  zigzag approach
  Z-plasty approach
appropriate for gestational age
  (AGA)
approximate lethal
  concentration
approximated
  cutaneous edges
    approximated
  loosely approximated
  skin edges approximated
  subcutaneous tissues
    approximated
approximation
  direct approximation
  Friedewald approximation
  skin approximation
  successive approximation
  tissue approximation
  vocal fold approximation
  wound approximation
approximation forceps
approximation suture technique
approximation sutures
approximator
  Ablaza-Morse rib
    approximator
  Acland double-clamp
    approximator
  Alexander approximator
  Allerdyce approximator
  Bailey rib approximator
  Ballenger-Hajek approximator
  Biemer approximator
  Bruni-Wayne clamp
    approximator
  Brunswick-Mack approximator
  Bunke-Schulz clamp
    approximator
  Christoudias approximator
  clip approximator

approximator (*continued*)
  Henderson clamp
    approximator
  hook approximator
  Ikuta clamp approximator
  Iwashi clamp approximator
  Kleinert-Kutz clamp
    approximator
  Lalonde tendon approximator
  Leksell sternal approximator
  Lemmon rib approximator
  Lemmon sternal
    approximator
  Link approximator
  microanastomosis clip
    approximator
  Microspike approximator
  nerve approximator
  Neuromeet nerve ending
    approximator
  Neuromeet soft tissue
    approximator
  Nunez sternal approximator
  Pilling Wolvek sternal
    approximator
  pivot microanastomosis
    approximator
  rib approximator
  sternal approximator
  Tamai clamp approximator
  Vari-Angle temporary clip
    approximator
  Wolvek sternal approximator
approximator clamp
appy (appendectomy)
appy tape
APR (abdominoperineal
  resection)
APR (anatomic porous
  replacement)
APR (auropalpebral reflex)
APR acetabular cup
APR cement fixation
apraxia
  innervation apraxia
  neural apraxia
Aprema III device
APRL hooks (Army Prosthetics
  Research Laboratory
  hooks)
A-Probe
  Soft-Touch A-Probe

apron
  abdominal apron
  Aufranc groin apron
  lead apron
  lingual apron
  redundant abdominal apron
apron band
apron flap procedure
apron skin incision
apron U-shaped incision
AP-T image
apudoma
Aqua Glycolic skin care
    Products
Aquacel Ag antimicrobial wound
    dressing
Aquacel Hydrofiber wound
    dressing
Aquaflex contact lenses
Aquaflex ultrasound gel pad
Aquaflo hydrogel wound
    dressing
Aquamatic dressing
Aquamatic K-Calcification
    calibration well
Aquamatic K-Module
Aquamatic K-Pads
Aquamatic K-Thermia
    equipment
AquaMmed hydrotherapy device
AquaNot swim mold
Aquapad heating pad
Aquaphor gauze
Aquaphor gauze dressing
Aquaplast alloplastic material
Aquaplast cast
Aquaplast dressing
Aquaplast mask
Aquaplast mold
Aquaplast nasal splint
Aquaplast rapid setting splint
    material
Aquaplast splint
Aquaplast splinting materials
Aquaplast tie-down dressing
aquapuncture
Aqua-Purator suction device
Aquasight lens
Aquasorb border with
    Covaderm tape
Aquasorb transparent hydrogel
    dressing

Aquatech cast padding
Aquatrek device
Aquavac
aqueduct
  cerebral aqueduct
  fallopian aqueduct
  sylvian aqueduct
  ventricular aqueduct
aqueduct of Cotunnius
aqueduct of midbrain
aqueduct of Sylvius
aqueduct of vestibule vein
aqueductal intubation
aqueous
  aqueous transplant needle
  aqueous tube shunt
aqueous extract
aqueous glutaraldehyde (Cidex)
aqueous humor
aqueous transplant needle
aqueous tube shunt
aqueous Zephiran
Aquilion CT scanner
Aquirre gastrectomy
AR 1000 refractor
AR+ portable heart monitor
AR-1 catheter
AR-2 diagnostic catheter
AR-2 guiding catheter
arachidonic acid
arachnoid Beaver blade
arachnoid cyst
arachnoid granulations
arachnoid hemorrhage
arachnoid knife
arachnoid mater
arachnoid membrane
arachnoid space
arachnoid-shape Beaver blade
arachnophlebectomy needle
Arago argon laser
Araki-Sako technique
araldehyde-tanned bovine
    carotid artery graft
Arani double-loop guiding
    catheter
Arani guide
Arans pulley passer
Arantius body
Arantius duct
arborescens
  lipoma arborescens

arborescent cataract
arborization
   pattern arborization
   pulmonary arborization
arborization heart block
arborization pattern
Arbrook Hemovac
Arbuckle antral knife
Arbuckle antral saw
Arbuckle probe
Arbuckle sinus probe
Arbuckle-Shea trocar
Arbuthnot Lane disease
arc
   auricular arc
   binauricular arc
   Gilula arc
   nasobregmatic arc
   naso-occipital arc
   reflex arc
   Riolan arc
   sensorimotor arc
ARC (AIDS-related complex)
arc of Gilula
arc of rotation of
   fasciocutaneous flap
Arc-22 catheter
arcade
   capillary arcade
   Frohse arcade
   gastroepiploic arcade
   intestinal arterial arcade
   lumbar arcades
   mesenteric arcade
   pancreaticoduodenal arterial
     arcade
   Riolan arcade
   temporal arcade
arcade of Frohse
arcade of Riolan
Arcelin view
arch
   abdominothoracic arch
   Ainsworth arch
   alveolar arch
   angle arch
   anterior palatine arch
   aortic arch
   arterial arch
   atlas arch
   axillary arch
   azygos vein arch

arch (*continued*)
   Bimler arch
   branchial cleft arch
   costal arch
   crural arch
   deep crural arch
   deep palmar arch
   deep plantar arch
   deep volar arch
   dental arch
   dentulous dental arch
   digital venous arch
   double aortic arch
   expansion of the arch
   extramedullary alignment
     arch
   faucial arch
   femoral arch
   FemoStop femoral artery
     compression arch
   glossopalatine arch
   Gothic arch
   hemal arch
   hyoid arch
   hyoid branchial arch
   iliopectineal arch
   inferior dental arch
   inferior palpebral arch
   interrupted aortic arch
   jugular arch
   jugular venous arch
   labial arch
   Langer arch
   Langer axillary arch
   lingual arch
   longitudinal arch
   lower arch
   malar arch
   mandibular arch
   mandibular branchial arch
   mandibular visceral arch
   maxillary arch
   Mershon arch
   nasal arch
   nasal venous arch
   neural arch
   oral arch
   palatal arch
   palatine arch
   palatoglossal arch
   palatomaxillary arch
   palatopharyngeal arch

arch (*continued*)
  palmar arch
  palmar radial arch
  pharyngopalatine arch
  plantar arch
  posterior arch
  posterior palatine arch
  premandibular arch
  prepancreatic arch
  pubic arch
  radiocarpal arch
  red rubber arch
  right aortic arch
  Riolan arch
  rubber arch
  saddle arch
  saddle-shaped arch
  Salus arch
  Shenton arch
  Simon expansion arch
  superciliary arch
  superficial femoral arch
  superficial palmar arch
  superficial plantar arch
  superior palpebral arch
  supraorbital arch
  tarsal arch
  tendinous arch
  transverse aponeurotic arch
  transverse arch
  Treitz arch
  upper arch
  U-shaped arch
  utility arch
  vascular epiploic arch
  vertebral arch
  W arch
  Wilson Bimetric arch
  wire arch
  zygomatic arch
arch and carotid arteriography
arch angiogram
arch angiography
arch aortogram
arch aortography
arch arteriogram
arch arteriography
arch bar (*see also* bar)
arch bar application
arch bar cutter
arch bar facial fracture appliance
arch bar fixation

arch bar frame
arch discrepancy
arch form
arch fracture
arch length
arch length deficiency
arch of abdominal aorta
arch of aorta
arch of larynx
arch rake retractor
arch support
arch wire
arch-and-slouch position
arched palate
Archer forceps
Archer splinter forceps
arches
  alveolar arches
  branchial arches
  labial and lingual arches
  paired vertebral arches
  pharyngeal arches
  postoral arches
arch-expander
  Ormco orthodontic arch-
    expander
Archimedean drill
architecture
  breast architecture
  hepatic architecture
  lesion architecture
archwire
  Jarabak-type archwire
  multiple loop archwire
arciform
arciform vein of kidney
Arco atomic pacemaker
Arco lithium pacemaker
Arco pacemaker
Arcon articulator
Arcon semiadjustable articulator
arcuata
  eminentia arcuata
  zona arcuata
arcuata eminence
arcuate
arcuate aorta
arcuate arteries
arcuate arteries of kidney
arcuate artery of foot
arcuate incision
arcuate ligaments

arcuate line
arcuate nerve fiber bundle
arcuate papillae of tongue
arcuate popliteal ligament
arcuate pubic ligament
arcuate skin stapler
arcuate suture
arcuate suture technique
arcuate transverse keratotomy
arcuate veins
arcuate veins of kidney
arcuatus
   uterus arcuatus
arcus (*pl.* arcus)
arcus adiposus
arcus alveolaris
arcus alveolaris mandibulae
arcus alveolaris maxillae
arcus aortae
arcus cornealis
arcus dentalis inferior
arcus dentalis superior
arcus glossopalatinus
arcus juvenilis
arcus marginalis
arcus palatini
arcus palatoglossus
arcus palatopharyngeus
arcus palpebralis inferior
arcus palpebralis superior
arcus pharyngopalatinus
arcus senilis
arcus superciliaris
arcus tarseus inferior
arcus tarseus superior
arcus tendineus
arcus zygomaticus
ARD bandage
Ardee denture liner
area
   adnexal area
   alar area
   alisphenoid area
   alveolar area
   aortic valve area
   articulation area
   auriculomastoid area
   Bamberger area
   BANS area (back, arm, neck, shoulder area)
   bilabial area
   body surface area (BSA)

area (*continued*)
   cardiac area
   circumscribed area
   conjunctivotarsal area
   contact area
   cortical area
   Cotton cartilage graft to cricolaryngeal area
   crural area
   draped area
   ecchymotic area
   echogenic area
   echo-spared area
   faucial area
   flank area
   flying T pelvic area
   frontoparietal area
   fusion area
   genital area
   glottal area
   gyrous area
   hair-bearing area
   hypothalamic area
   inguinal area
   interplacodal area
   intertriginous area
   Kiesselbach area
   Krönig area
   labiodental area
   Laimer-Haeckerman area
   linguoalveolar area
   linguodental area
   Little area
   lytic area
   malar area
   masseteric area
   mesobranchial area
   midtemporal area
   motor area
   mottled area
   nasal cross-sectional area
   nasopharyngeal area
   olfactory area
   painted area
   palatal area
   parasymphysis area
   parietal area
   parotid-masseteric area
   patchy area
   Patrick trigger area
   periareolar area
   perihilar area

area (*continued*)
  perineal area
  perispinal area
  postauricular area
  posterior palatal seal area
  postpalatal seal area
  preauricular area
  prelacrimal area
  premotor area
  rarefied area
  raw area
  reconstruction of heel and
    plantar area
  reddened area
  saddle area
  sagittal area
  scapular area
  scrotal area
  silent area
  skip areas
  sloughed area
  Soemmering area
  somatosensory area
  sonolucent area
  stress-bearing area
  subcostal area
  subglottic area
  submitral area
  subsegmental area
  supporting area
  supra-areolar area
  supraclavicular area
  supraorbital area
  suprarenal area
  surface area
  surgically denervated area
  suspicious area
  sylvian area
  tailbone area
  temporal area
  tissue-bearing area
  total body surface area (TBSA)
  trigger area
  ulcerated area
  ulcerating area
  velar area
  Warthin area
area (*pl.* areae, areas)
area hypoglossi
area nerve facialis
area of facial nerve
areas of innervation

areata
  alopecia areata
areatus
areflexia
Arem retractor
Arem-Madden retractor
Arenberg dural palpator
    elevator
Arenberg endolymphatic sac
    knife
Arenberg-Denver inner-ear valve
Arenberg-Denver inner-ear valve
    implant
Arenberg-Denver valve
areola (*pl.* areolae)
  Chaussier areola
  coning of areola
  second areola
  umbilical areola
areola mammae
areola of mammary gland
areola of nipple
areola papillaris
areolar
areolar complex
areolar demarcation
areolar gland
areolar grafting
areolar incision
areolar reconstruction
areolar scar
areolar tissue
areolar venous plexus
areola-to-inframammary fold
    distance (A-IMF)
areolomammary complex
ARF (acute renal failure)
ArF excimer laser
Argamaso-Lewis composite flap
Argen dental attachment
Arglaes wound dressing
argon beam coagulation
argon beam coagulator
argon blue laser
argon gas
argon gas anticoagulator
argon green laser
argon guidewire
argon ion laser
argon laser
argon laser iridectomy
argon laser photocoagulator

argon laser photocoagulator
    cautery
argon laser therapy
argon laser-induced scars
argon plasma coagulator
argon pump dye laser
argon tunable dye laser
argon vessel dilator
argon-fluoride laser
argon-krypton laser
argon-pumped tunable dye laser
Argyle anti-reflux valve
Argyle arterial catheter
Argyle catheter
Argyle chest tube
Argyle CPAP nasal cannula
Argyle endotracheal tube
Argyle Medicut R catheter
Argyle oxygen catheter
Argyle Penrose tubing
Argyle Sentinel Seal chest tube
Argyle silicon Salem sump
Argyle trocar
Argyle trocar catheter
Argyle tube
Argyle umbilical vessel catheter
Argyle umbilical wedge catheter
Argyle Dennis-tube
Argyle Salem sump anti-reflux
    valve
Argyle Salem sump pump
Argyle Salem sump tube
Argyll Robertson operation
Argyll Robertson pupil
Argyll Robertson strap operation
    for ectropion of eyelid
Argyll Robertson sutures
Argyll Robertson suture
    technique
argyria
argyrophilic
argyrophilic collagen fiber
argyrophilic fibril
argyrosis
arhinia (*variant of* arrhinia)
Aria CABG
Aria coronary bypass
Aria graft
Aria prosthetic coronary artery
    bypass graft
Arie reductive mammaplasty
Arie-Pitanguy breast reduction

Arie-Pitanguy mammaplasty
Arie-Pitanguy mammary ptosis
    operation
Arie-Pitanguy operation
A-ring
    esophageal A-ring
Arion implant
Arion operation
Arion rod eye prosthesis
Arion sling operation
Aristocort
Arixtra
Arizona condylar tibial plateau
    prosthesis
Arjalloy alloy
Arkan sharpening-stone needle
ARK-Juno refractor
Arlt epicanthus repair
Arlt eyelid repair
Arlt fenestrated lens scoop
Arlt lens loupe
Arlt lens scoop
Arlt line
Arlt loupe
Arlt operation
Arlt pterygium excision
Arlt recess
Arlt scoop
Arlt sinus
Arlt suture technique
Arlt sutures
Arlt-Jaesche excision
Arlt-Jaesche operation
Arlt-Jaesche recessus
Arlt-Jaesche sinus
Arlt-Jaesche trachoma
arm
    articulated optical arm
    brawny arm
    inferior lateral cutaneous
        nerve of arm
    Krukenberg arm
    superior lateral cutaneous
        nerve of arm
    tackler's arm
    Utah artificial arm
    Y-nailing of arm
ARM (artificial rupture of
    membranes)
arm and shoulder immobilizer
arm extension position
arm flap

arm lift
arm position
arm retractor
arm splint
Armaly-Drance technique
armboard
    double armboard
armed bougie
arm-extension position
Armistead procedure
Armistead technique
Armistead ulnar lengthening
    operation
armored heart
Armour dural knife
Armour endotracheal tube
Armour knife
Armour tube
armpit
armrest
Armsby operation
Arm-Sling shirt
Armstrong acromionectomy
Armstrong beveled grommet
    drain tube
Armstrong beveled grommet
    myringotomy tube
Armstrong CPR mask
Armstrong hand-held pulse
    oximeter
Armstrong repair
Armstrong tube
Armstrong V9 vent tube
Armstrong ventilation tube
Armstrong V-vent tube
Armstrong warmer
Armstrong-Schuknecht stapes
    prosthesis
Army bone gouge
Army chisel
Army osteotome
Army pattern bone gouge
Army pattern chisel
Army pattern osteotome
Army Prosthetics Research
    Laboratory hooks (APRL
    hooks)
Army-Navy retractor
Arndorfer esophageal motility
    probe
Arndorfer pneumocapillary
    infusion pump

Arneth classification
Arnett LeFort implant
Arnoff external fixation device
Arnold
    foramen of Arnold
Arnold body
Arnold brace
Arnold bundle
Arnold canal
Arnold ganglion
Arnold ligament
Arnold nerve
Arnold-Bruening intracordal
    injection set
Arnold-Bruening syringe
Arnold-Chiari deformity
Arnold-Chiari malformation
Arnold-Chiari syndrome
Arnott bed
Arnott dilator
Arnott one-piece all-PMMA
    intraocular lens
Arnoux sign
AromaScan aroma analysis
    device
Aron Alpha adhesive
Aron Alpha glue
Aronson esophageal retractor
Aronson lateral sternomastoid
    retractor
Aronson medial esophageal
    retractor
Aronson-Fletcher antrum
    cannula
Aronson-Prager technique
AROSupercut scissors
around-the-clock oral
    maintenance
    bronchodilator therapy
aroused
    fully aroused
arrangement
    lesion arrangement
    tongue-in-groove arrangement
Array foldable intraocular lens
Array multifocal intraocular
    lens
array processor
Array ultrasound transducer
arrector muscles of hair
Arrequi KPL laparoscopic knot
    pusher

Arrequi laparoscopic knot
  pusher ligator
arrest
  active phase arrest
  cardiac arrest
  cardiopulmonary arrest
  cardiorespiratory arrest
  epiphyseal arrest
  growth arrest
  respiratory arrest
  sinus arrest
arrest of labor
arrester-heart revascularization
  technique
Arrhigi
  pont of Arrhigi
arrhinia (*spelled also* arhinia)
arrhinia malformation
arrhythmia
  junctional arrhythmia
  nodal arrhythmia
  perpetual arrhythmia
arrhythmia control device
  (ACD)
Arrhythmia Net arrhythmia
  monitor
Arrhythmia Net monitor
Arrhythmia Research 1200 EPX
  electrocardiograph
arrhythmogenesis
arrow
Arrow articulation paper
  forceps
Arrow AutoCAT intraaortic
  balloon pump
Arrow balloon wedge catheter
Arrow Berman angiographic
  balloon
arrow blade
Arrow Blue FlexTip
arrow clasp
Arrow Flex intraaortic balloon
  catheter
Arrow FlexTip Plus catheter
Arrow Hi-flow infusion set
Arrow Multi-Lumen Access
  Catheter (MAC)
Arrow multilumen catheter
Arrow PICC
Arrow pneumothorax kit
Arrow pullback atherectomy
  catheter

Arrow pulmonary artery
  catheter
Arrow QuadPolar electrode
  catheter
Arrow QuickFlash arterial
  catheter
Arrow Raulerson introducer
  syringe
Arrow sheath
Arrow TheraCath epidural
  catheter
Arrow TransAct intraaortic
  balloon pump
Arrow true torque wire guide
Arrow tube
Arrow Twin Cath catheter
Arrow TwinCath multilumen
  peripheral catheter
Arrow two-lumen hemodialysis
  catheter
Arrow-Berman angiographic
  balloon
Arrow-Berman balloon
  angioplasty catheter
Arrow-Berman balloon catheter
Arrow-Clarke thoracentesis
  device
Arrow-Fischell EVAN needle
ArrowFlex intra-aortic balloon
  catheter
ArrowFlex intra-aortic balloon
  catheter
ArrowFlex sheath
ArrowGard Blue antiseptic-
  coated catheter
ArrowGard Blue central venous
  catheter
ArrowGard Blue Line catheter
ArrowGard central venous
  catheter
Arrowhead canthoplasty
Arrowhead operation
Arrow-Howes multilumen
  catheter
Arrow-Howes quad-lumen
  catheter
arrow-pin clasp
Arrowsmith corneal marker
Arrowsmith electrode
Arrowsmith fixation forceps
Arrowsmith-Clerf pin-closing
  forceps

Arrow-Trerotola percutaneous
    thrombolytic device
Arrow-Trerotola PTD catheter
Arrow-Trerotola rotator drive
    unit
arrow-tube
    middle ear arrow-tube
Arroyo cataract extraction
Arroyo dacryostomy
Arroyo expressor
Arroyo forceps
Arroyo implant
Arroyo keratoplasty
Arroyo operation
Arroyo protector
Arroyo trephine
Arruga capsule forceps
Arruga cataract extraction
Arruga curved capsular forceps
Arruga dacryocystostomy
Arruga dacryostomy
Arruga encircling suture
Arruga expressor
Arruga extraction hook
Arruga eye expressor
Arruga eye holder
Arruga eye implant
Arruga eye retractor
Arruga eye speculum
Arruga eye trephine
Arruga forceps
Arruga globe retractor
Arruga globe speculum
Arruga implant
Arruga keratoplasty
Arruga lacrimal trephine
Arruga lens
Arruga lens expressor
Arruga movable eye implant
Arruga needle holder
Arruga operation
Arruga operation for retinal
    detachment
Arruga protector
Arruga retractor
Arruga saw
Arruga speculum
Arruga surface electrode
Arruga tenotomy
Arruga tip forceps
Arruga trephine
Arruga-Berens operation

Arruga-Gill forceps
Arruga-McCool capsular forceps
Arruga-McCool capsule forceps
Arruga-McCool forceps
Arruga-Moura-Brazil orbital
    implant
Arslan fenestration of inner ear
Arslan operation
ART transducer
ArtAssist arterial assist device
ArtAssist compression dressing
ArtAssist dressing
ArtAssist wrap
Artec balloon catheter
Artecoll injectable microimplant
artefact (*see* artifact)
Artegraft collagen vascular graft
arteria
    sphenopalatina, arteria
arteriae
    conjunctivales anteriores,
        arteriae
    conjunctivales posteriores,
        arteriae
arterial anastomosis
arterial aneurysm
arterial anomaly
arterial arch
arterial bleeding
arterial blood collection
arterial blood gases (ABGs)
arterial blood needle
arterial cannula
arterial cannulation anesthetic
    technique
arterial catheter
arterial catheterization
arterial circle of Willis
arterial circulation
arterial clamp
arterial cutdown
arterial decortication
arterial disorder
arterial embolectomy
arterial embolectomy catheter
arterial embolization
arterial filter
arterial flap
arterial forceps
arterial graft
arterial graft prosthesis
arterial groove

arterial hemorrhage
arterial hypoxemia
arterial injury
arterial insufficiency of lower
    extremities
arterial irrigation catheter
arterial line (A-line)
arterial line pressure bag
arterial line transducer
arterial loop
arterial mean line
arterial needle
arterial occlusion
arterial occlusive disease
arterial oscillator
    endarterectomy
    instrument
arterial oxygen saturation (SaO$_2$)
arterial plexus
arterial pressure
arterial prosthesis
arterial puncture
arterial reconstructive
    procedure
arterial reconstructive surgery
arterial runoff
arterial scissors
arterial sheath
arterial silk suture
arterial silk sutures
arterial spider
arterial switch
arterial switch operation
arterial switch procedure
arterial thrombosis
arterial transfusion of blood
arterial ulcer
arterial wall dissection
arterial-arterial fistula
arterial-enteric fistula
arterialization
arterialized flap
arterial-portal fistula
arteriectasis
arteriectomy
arteries
    abdominal aortic artery
    aberrant artery
    Abramowicz artery
    accessory obturator artery
    acromiothoracic artery
    Adamkiewicz artery

arteries (*continued*)
    alar branch of external
        maxillary artery
    alveolar artery
    alveolar branch of internal
        maxillary artery
    anastomosis of ascending
        aorta to pulmonary artery
    anastomosis of internal
        mammary artery to
        coronary artery
    anastomosis of mesenteric
        arteries
    anastomosis of right atrium to
        pulmonary artery
    anastomosis of right
        subclavian artery to
        pulmonary artery
    anastomosis of superior vena
        cava to distal right
        pulmonary artery
    anastomosis of superior vena
        cava to pulmonary artery
    anastomotic branch of artery
    aneurysm of pancreatic artery
    aneurysm of splenic artery
    angular artery
    angular nasal artery
    anomalous artery
    anterior cecal artery
    anterior cerebral artery
    anterior choroidal artery
    anterior ciliary artery
    anterior circumflex humeral
        artery
    anterior communicating
        artery
    anterior conjunctival artery
    anterior ethmoidal artery
    anterior ethmoidal branch of
        ophthalmic artery
    anterior inferior cerebellar
        artery
    anterior inferior
        communicating artery
        (AICA)
    anterior interosseous artery
    anterior meningeal artery
    anterior spinal artery
    anterior superior alveolar
        artery
    anterior tibial artery

arteries (*continued*)

anterior tibial recurrent artery
anterior tympanic artery
aortic suprarenal artery
appendicular artery
arcuate arteries
arcuate artery
ascending cervical artery
ascending palatine artery
ascending pharyngeal artery
auditory artery
auricular artery
auriculotemporal artery
axillary artery
balloon-like dilation of artery
banding of pulmonary artery
basilar artery
beading of arteries
bilateral internal mammary
　artery (BIMA)
bilateral internal mammary
　artery (BIMA)
　reconstruction
brachial artery
brachiocephalic artery
bronchopulmonary segmental
　artery (BPSA)
buccal artery
buccinator artery
callosomarginal artery
caroticotympanic artery
carotid artery
caudal artery
celiac artery
cerebellar artery
cerebral artery
cervical artery
choroid artery
choroidal artery
ciliary arteries
cilioretinal artery
circumflex artery
circumflex coronary artery
circumflex femoral artery
circumflex humeral artery
circumflex iliac artery
circumflex scapular artery
clogged artery
closed disruption of digital
　artery
coarctation of pulmonary
　arteries

arteries (*continued*)

coccygeal artery
colic artery
collateral artery
collateral digital artery
common carotid artery
common carotid artery (CCA)
common iliac artery
common interosseous artery
common palmar digital
　arteries
common plantar digital
　arteries
communicating artery
compression of carotid artery
conjunctival arteries
convolutional artery
copper wire arteries
corkscrew arteries
coronary arteries
cremasteric artery
cricothyroid artery
cubital artery
cystic artery
deep auricular artery
deep brachial artery
deep cervical artery
deep circumflex iliac artery
deep external pudendal artery
deep femoral artery
deep inferior epigastric artery
deep lingual artery
deep middle cerebral artery
deep temporal artery
deferential artery
dental artery
descending genicular artery
descending palatine artery
diaphragmatic artery
digital artery
digital collateral artery
dolichoectatic artery
dorsal artery
dorsal digital arteries
dorsal lingual artery
dorsal metacarpal arteries
dorsal metatarsal arteries
dorsal nasal branch of
　ophthalmic artery
dorsalis pedis artery
duodenal artery
ectatic carotid artery

arteries (*continued*)
  ectatic vertebral artery
  efferent artery
  end artery
  epicardial coronary artery
  epigastric artery
  episcleral artery
  esophageal artery
  ethmoidal artery
  external carotid artery
  external iliac artery
  external mammary artery
  external maxillary artery
  external pudendal artery
  external spermatic artery
  facial artery
  facioscapulohumeral artery
  fallopian artery
  femoral artery
  fibular artery
  first dorsal metatarsal artery
  flushing of artery
  frontal artery
  funicular artery
  gastric arteries
  gastroduodenal artery
  gastroepiploic artery
  genicular artery
  gluteal artery
  great anterior radicular
    artery
  greater palatine artery
  Gruentzig dilatation of renal
    arteries
  hardening of arteries
  Heiss artery
  helicine artery
  hemorrhoidal arteries
  hepatic artery
  Heubner artery
  highest intercostal artery
  hyaloid artery
  hypogastric arteries
  ileal arteries
  ileocolic artery
  iliac artery
  ilioinguinal artery
  iliolumbar artery
  inferior alveolar artery
  inferior artery
  inferior cerebellar arteries
  inferior epigastric artery

arteries (*continued*)
  inferior gluteal artery
  inferior labial artery
  inferior laryngeal artery
  inferior mesenteric artery
    (IMA)
  inferior pancreaticoduodenal
    arteries
  inferior phrenic arteries
  inferior rectal artery
  inferior suprarenal artery
  inferior thyroid artery
  inferior tympanic artery
  inferior ulnar artery
  inferior vesical artery
  infrahyoid artery
  infraorbital artery
  infraorbital branch of interior
    maxillary artery
  inguinal artery
  innominate artery
  intercostal arteries
  intercostal artery
  interior maxillary branch of
    external carotid artery
  interlobar arteries
  interlobular arteries
  internal auditory artery
  internal carotid artery
  internal iliac artery
  internal mammary artery
    (IMA)
  internal maxillary artery
  internal pudendal artery
  internal rectal artery
  internal spermatic artery
  internal thoracic artery
  interosseous artery
  interradicular artery
  interventricular artery
  intestinal arteries
  intramural artery
  ipsilateral common carotid
    artery
  jejunal arteries
  Kugel artery
  labial arteries
  labial artery
  labyrinthine arteries
  labyrinthine artery
  lacrimal artery
  laryngeal artery

arteries (*continued*)

lateral circumflex femoral artery

lateral inferior genicular artery

lateral nasal artery

lateral palpebral arteries

lateral plantar artery

lateral posterior nasal arteries

lateral sacral arteries

lateral striate arteries

lateral superior genicular artery

lateral tarsal arteries

lateral tarsal artery

lateral thoracic artery

left anterior descending artery (LAD)

left colic artery

left coronary artery

left gastric artery

left gastroepiploic artery

left pulmonary artery

lesser palantine arteries

lesser palatine artery

levotransposition of great arteries (L-transposition of great arteries)

lienal artery

ligation of artery

lingual artery

long ciliary arteries

long posterior ciliary artery

lowest thyroid artery

L-transposition of great arteries (levotransposition of great arteries)

lumbar arteries

lumen of artery

lumen of bronchial artery

main pulmonary artery

major palatine artery

malleolar artery

mammary artery

mandibular artery

marginal artery

masseteric artery

maxillary artery

medial anterior malleolus artery

medial circumflex femoral artery

arteries (*continued*)

medial inferior genicular artery

medial palpebral arteries

medial plantar artery

medial superior genicular artery

medial tarsal arteries

medial tarsal artery

median artery

median sacral artery

medullary artery

meningeal arteries

meningeal artery

mental artery

mesenteric artery

mesenteric inferior artery

mesenteric superior artery

metacarpal arteries

metatarsal arteries

metatarsal artery

middle cerebral artery (MCA)

middle colic artery

middle collateral artery

middle genicular artery

middle meningeal artery

middle rectal artery

middle suprarenal artery

middle temporal artery

middle vesical artery

musculocutaneous artery

musculophrenic artery

Mustard transposition of great arteries

nasal accessory artery

nasal arteries

nasal artery

Neubauer artery

nutrient artery

obturator artery

occipital artery

ophthalmic artery

ovarian artery

palatine artery

palmar digital arteries

palmar interosseous arteries

palmar metacarpal arteries

palpebral arteries

palpebral artery

pancreaticoduodenal arteries

perforating alveolar artery

perforating arteries

arteries (*continued*)

- perfusion of coronary artery
- pericallosal artery
- pericardiacophrenic artery
- perineal artery
- peroneal artery
- petrosal artery
- pharyngeal artery
- pharyngeal branch of internal maxillary artery
- phrenic arteries
- pipestem artery
- plantar artery
- plantar digital arteries
- plantar metatarsal arteries
- popliteal artery
- postauricular artery
- posterior alveolar artery
- posterior auricular artery
- posterior auricular branch of external carotid artery
- posterior cecal artery
- posterior cerebral artery
- posterior circumflex humeral artery
- posterior communicating artery
- posterior conjunctival arteries
- posterior descending artery (PDA)
- posterior ethmoidal artery
- posterior ethmoidal branch of ophthalmic artery
- posterior inferior cerebellar artery (PICA)
- posterior inferior communicating artery (PICA)
- posterior intercostal arteries
- posterior interosseous artery
- posterior labial artery
- posterior lateral nasal arteries
- posterior meningeal artery
- posterior palatine artery
- posterior septal artery
- posterior spinal artery
- posterior superior alveolar artery
- posterior tibial artery
- posterior tibial recurrent artery
- posterior tympanic artery

arteries (*continued*)

- posterolateral nasal artery
- preventricular artery
- profunda femoris artery
- proper hepatic artery
- proper palmar digital arteries
- proper palmar digital artery
- proper plantar digital arteries
- proper plantar digital artery
- pudendal artery
- pulmonary artery (PA)
- radial artery
- radial collateral artery
- radial index artery
- radial recurrent artery
- radicular artery
- ranine artery
- recanalization of artery
- rectal artery
- recurrent artery
- recurrent interosseous artery
- renal artery
- retinal artery
- retroauricular artery
- right colic artery
- right coronary artery
- right gastric artery
- right gastroepiploic artery
- right pulmonary artery
- sacral arteries
- saphenous artery
- scapular artery
- sciatic artery
- segmental arteries
- septal artery
- septal posterior nasal arteries
- septal posterior nasal artery
- short ciliary arteries
- short gastric arteries
- short gastric branch of lienal artery
- short posterior ciliary artery
- sigmoid arteries
- sigmoidal branch of inferior mesenteric artery
- silver-wire appearance of retinal arteries
- silver-wiring of retinal arteries
- single internal mammary artery (SIMA) reconstruction
- small arteries

arteries (*continued*)

spermatic artery
sphenopalatine artery
sphenopalatine branch of
    internal maxillary artery
spinal artery
spinal artery
spinoneural artery
splayed arteries
splenic artery
stapedial artery
stenotic femoral artery
sternocleidomastoid artery
stylomandibular artery
stylomastoid artery
subclavian artery
subcostal artery
sublingual artery
submental artery
subscapular artery
sulcus of subclavian artery
superficial brachial artery
superficial circumflex iliac
    artery
superficial epigastric artery
superficial palmar artery
superficial palmar branch of
    radial artery
superficial perineal artery
superficial petrosal artery
superficial temporal artery
superficial temporal branch of
    external carotid artery
superior alveolar artery
superior auricular artery
superior cerebellar artery
superior epigastric artery
superior gluteal artery
superior hemorrhoidal artery
superior hemorrhoidal branch
    of inferior mesenteric
    artery
superior labial artery
superior laryngeal artery
superior mesenteric artery
superior pancreaticoduodenal
    artery
superior pharyngeal artery
superior rectal artery
superior superficial epigastric
    artery
superior suprarenal artery

arteries (*continued*)

superior thyroid artery
superior tympanic artery
superior ulnar collateral
    artery
superior vesical artery
supraorbital artery
suprarenal arteries
suprascapular artery
supratrochlear artery
sural arteries
sylvian artery
tarsal arteries
temporal arteries
temporal artery
terminal artery
testicular artery
thoracic artery
thoracoacromial artery
thoracodorsal artery
thyroid artery
thyroid ima artery
tibial artery
tonsillar artery
transection of artery
transnasal ligation of internal
    maxillary artery
transposition of great arteries
    (TGA)
transverse cervical artery
transverse facial artery
triangle of lingual artery
trigeminal artery
tympanic artery
ulnar artery
ulnar recurrent artery
umbilical artery
urethral artery
uterine artery
vaginal artery
vertebral artery
vesical artery
vestibulocochlear artery
vidian artery
volar artery
Zinn artery
zygomatico-orbital artery
arteriocapillary
arteriococcygeal gland
arteriogenesis
arteriogram
    aorta-and-runoff arteriogram

arteriogram (*continued*)
  aortic arch arteriogram
  arch arteriogram
  biplane pelvic arteriogram
  biplane quantitative coronary
    arteriogram
  brachial arteriogram
  carotid arteriogram
  cerebral arteriogram
  coronary arteriogram
  femoral arteriogram
  four-vessel arteriogram
  Judkins technique for
    coronary arteriogram
  longitudinal arteriogram
  percutaneous arteriogram
  percutaneous femoral
    arteriogram
  pruned-tree arteriogram
  pulmonary artery arteriogram
  renal arteriogram
  retrograde arteriogram
  selective coronary
    arteriogram
  Sones selective coronary
    arteriogram
  subclavian arteriogram
  vertebral arteriogram
  wedge arteriogram
arteriogram needle
arteriography
  aortic arch arteriography
  arch and carotid arteriography
  arch arteriography
  brachial arteriography
  carotid arteriography
  catheter arteriography
  celiac arteriography
  cerebral arteriography
  coronary arteriography
  femoral arteriography
  infrahepatic arteriography
  Judkins selective coronary
    arteriography
  percutaneous arteriography
  percutaneous carotid
    arteriography (PCA)
  percutaneous transfemoral
    arteriography
  pudendal arteriography
  pulmonary arteriography
  renal arteriography

arteriography (*continued*)
  Sones arteriography
  Sones coronary
    arteriography
  vertebral arteriography
  visceral arteriography
arteriography needle
arteriola (*pl.* arteriolae)
arteriolar attenuation
arteriolar narrowing
arteriole
  capillary arteriole
  efferent glomerular arteriole
  glomerular arteriole
  Isaacs-Ludwig arteriole
  main arteriole (MA)
  postglomerular arteriole
  preglomerular arteriole
  pulmonary arteriole
  spiral arterioles
arterioles of kidney
arteriolith
arteriolovenular anastomosis
arteriolovenularis
  anastomosis
    arteriolovenularis
arteriomegaly
arteriopathy
  hypertensive arteriopathy
arterioplasty
arterioportal fistula
arterioportobiliary fistula
arteriorrhaphy
arteriorrhexis
arteriosclerosis
  decrescent arteriosclerosis
  hypertensive arteriosclerosis
  intimal arteriosclerosis
  Mönckeberg arteriosclerosis
arteriosclerotic
arteriosclerotic aneurysm
arteriosclerotic cardiovascular
    disease (ASCVD)
arteriosclerotic gangrene
arteriosclerotic kidney
arteriosclerotic occlusive
    disease (AOD)
arteriosclerotic peripheral
    vascular disease (ASPVD)
arteriosinusoidal penile fistula
arteriospasm
arteriostrepsis

arteriosus
 ductus arteriosus
 patent ductus arteriosus (PDA)
 truncus arteriosus
arteriotomy
 brachial arteriotomy
 distal arteriotomy
 end-to-side arteriotomy
 femoral arteriotomy
 transverse arteriotomy
arteriotomy incision
arteriotomy scissors
arteriotrepsis
arteriovenosa
 anastomosis arteriovenosa
arteriovenostomy
arteriovenous (AV)
arteriovenous anastomosis
arteriovenous aneurysm
arteriovenous angiorrhaphy
arteriovenous catheter
arteriovenous fistula (AVF)
arteriovenous Gore-Tex fistula
 (AV Gore-Tex fistula)
arteriovenous Gore-Tex graft (AV
 Gore-Tex graft)
arteriovenous hemangioma
arteriovenous malformation
 (AVM)
arteriovenous oxygen difference
 (AVDO$_2$)
arteriovenous shunt
arteriovenous shunt site
arteriovenous subclavian fistula
arteritis
 cranial arteritis
 giant cell arteritis
 Horton arteritis
 inflammatory arteritis
 temporal arteritis
 temporal giant cell arteritis
arteritis nodosa
artery ectasia
artery forceps
artery island flap
artery ligation
artery occlusion
artery of Adamkiewicz
artery of bulb of penis
artery of Drummond
artery of pterygoid canal
artery reconstruction

ArthoPlastics ankle
 instrumentation
Arthopor acetabular cup
arthralgia
 temporomandibular arthralgia
arthrectomy
Arthrex arthroscope
Arthrex Bio-Corkscrew suture
 anchor
Arthrex Bio-FASTak suture
 anchor
Arthrex Bio-Transfix cross pin
 fixation
Arthrex Bird-Beak
Arthrex coring reamer
Arthrex drill guide
Arthrex FASTak suture anchor
Arthrex FiberWire suture
Arthrex meniscal dart
Arthrex meniscal dart gun
Arthrex OATS bone plug
Arthrex Penetrator
Arthrex sheathed interference
 screw
Arthrex tibial tunnel guide
Arthrex TissueTak II
 bioabsorbable implant
Arthrex Transfix II cross pin
 fixation
Arthrex zebra pin
arthrifluent abscess
arthritides (*sing.* arthritis)
arthritis (*pl.* arthritides)
 Bekhterev arthritis (*also*
  Bechterev)
 Charcot arthritis
 gouty arthritis
 joint rheumatoid arthritis
 navicular arthritis
 rheumatoid arthritis (RA)
 sarcoid arthritis
 septic arthritis
 viral arthritis
 Yersinia arthritis
Arthro Force basket cutting
 forceps
Arthro Force hook scissors
ArthroCare Rubo-Vac device
ArthroCare thermal wand
arthrocentesis
arthrochalasis
arthrochondritis

arthroclasia
arthrodentosteodysplasia
arthrodesia
arthrodesis
  Abbott arthrodesis
  Adams ankle arthrodesis
  Adkins spinal arthrodesis
  Adkins technique spinal
    arthrodesis
  Albee arthrodesis
  atlantoaxial arthrodesis
  Baciu-Filibiu ankle arthrodesis
  Badgley arthrodesis
  Badgley hip arthrodesis
  Bailey-Badgley arthrodesis
  Batchelor-Brown
    extraarticular subtalar
    arthrodesis
  beak modification with triple
    arthrodesis
  Blair arthrodesis
  Bost arthrodesis
  Brittain arthrodesis
  Brittain knee arthrodesis
  Brittain shoulder arthrodesis
  Brittain-Dunn arthrodesis
  Brockman-Nissen arthrodesis
  Brockman-Nissen wrist
    arthrodesis
  Campbell arthrodesis
  Carceau-Brahms ankle
    arthrodesis
  Carroll arthrodesis
  Chandler arthrodesis
  Charnley arthrodesis
  Charnley compression
    arthrodesis
  Chuinard-Petersen arthrodesis
  Coltart arthrodesis
  compression arthrodesis
  cone arthrodesis
  cricoarytenoid arthrodesis
  Davis hip arthrodesis
  Dennyson-Fulford arthrodesis
  Dunn-Brittain foot arthrodesis
  Dunn-Brittain triple
    arthrodesis
  excisional arthrodesis
  extension injury posterior
    atlantoaxial arthrodesis
  extra-articular arthrodesis
  Fischer arthrodesis

arthrodesis (*continued*)
  Gant arthrodesis
  Gill shoulder arthrodesis
  Gill-Stein radiocarpal
    arthrodesis
  Guttmann arthrodesis
  Guttmann subtalar arthrodesis
  Haddad-Riordan wrist
    arthrodesis
  Henderson arthrodesis
  Henderson hip arthrodesis
  Hibbs arthrodesis
  Hibbs hip arthrodesis
  hip arthrodesis
  Hoke triple talus arthrodesis
  Horwitz-Adams ankle
    arthrodesis
  Houston shoulder arthrodesis
  intra-articular arthrodesis
  ischiofemoral arthrodesis
  joint arthrodesis
  Key knee arthrodesis
  Kirkaldy-Willis hip arthrodesis
  Lambrinudi triple arthrodesis
  Liebolt arthrodesis
  Lucas-Murray knee arthrodesis
  McKeever arthrodesis
  Menelaus triple arthrodesis
  Mich compression arthrodesis
  Millender-Nalebuff wrist
    arthrodesis
  Moberg arthrodesis
  Nalebuff wrist arthrodesis
  Potenza finger arthrodesis
  Potter knee arthrodesis
  Putti arthrodesis
  Putti knee arthrodesis
  Putti shoulder arthrodesis
  radiolunate arthrodesis
  resection arthrodesis
  reverse Cole arthrodesis
  Robinson-Riley cervical
    arthrodesis
  Ryerson triple arthrodesis
  scaphoid-capitate
    arthrodesis
  Schneider arthrodesis
  Seddon arthrodesis
  Seddon wrist arthrodesis
  shoulder arthrodesis
  small joint arthrodesis
  Smith-Petersen arthrodesis

arthrodesis (*continued*)
  Smith-Petersen wrist
    arthrodesis
  Stamm arthrodesis
  Staples elbow arthrodesis
  Steindler arthrodesis
  Stone hip arthrodesis
  subtalar arthrodesis
  tarsometatarsal truncated-
    wedge arthrodesis
  Thompson-Compere hip
    arthrodesis
  tibiocalcaneal arthrodesis
  tibiotalocalcaneal arthrodesis
  transfibular arthrodesis
  triplane arthrodesis
  triple arthrodesis
  Trumble arthrodesis
  Trumble hip arthrodesis
  truncated tarsometatarsal
    wedge arthrodesis
  truncated-wedge arthrodesis
  Uematsu shoulder arthrodesis
  Van Gorder arthrodesis
  Watson-Jones arthrodesis
  Wickstrom arthrodesis
  Wickstrom wrist arthrodesis
  Wilson arthrodesis
  wrist arthrodesis
arthrodesis screw
arthrodial articulation
arthrodial cartilage
arthrodial joint
ArthroDistractor
ArthroDistractor distractor
arthroendoscopy
arthroereisis
Arthrofile orthopaedic rasp
arthrogram
  Judet arthrogram
arthrographic capsular
    distention and rupture
    technique
arthrography
  opaque arthrography
arthrogryposis
  congential multiple
    arthrogryposis
arthrogryposis multiplex
    congenita
ArthroGuide carbon dioxide
    laser

arthrokatadysis
arthrolith
Arthro-Lok knife
Arthro-Lok system of Beaver
    blades
arthrolysis
arthrometer
  Robinson pocket
    arthrometer
  Stryker knee arthrometer
arthrometry
ArthroPasser
arthropathy
  acromegalic arthropathy
  Charcot arthropathy
  chondrocalcific arthropathy
  cuff tear arthropathy
  hemophilic arthropathy
  hydroxyapatite arthropathy
  inflammatory arthropathy
  osteopulmonary arthropathy
  rotator cuff arthropathy
arthrophyte
arthroplastic
arthroplastic implant
arthroplasty
  abrasion arthroplasty
  acetabular cup arthroplasty
  Albright-Chase arthroplasty
  Alloclassic Zweymuller hip
    arthroplasty
  anchovy arthroplasty
  Ashworth arthroplasty
  Ashworth hand arthroplasty
  Ashworth implant
    arthroplasty
  Aufranc cup arthroplasty
  Aufranc mold for cup
    arthroplasty
  Aufranc-Turner arthroplasty
  Austin Moore arthroplasty
  Austin Moore endoprosthetic
    arthroplasty
  Austin Moore hip arthroplasty
  autogenous interpositional
    shoulder arthroplasty
  Bahler elbow arthroplasty
  Bechtol arthroplasty
  bipolar hip arthroplasty
  Bosworth shoulder
    arthroplasty
  Bryan arthroplasty

arthroplasty (*continued*)
- Campbell interpositional arthroplasty
- Campbell resection arthroplasty
- capitellocondylar total elbow arthroplasty
- capsular interposition arthroplasty
- carpometacarpal arthroplasty
- Carroll arthroplasty
- Carroll-Taber arthroplasty
- cartilaginous arthroplasty
- cartilaginous cup arthroplasty
- cemented arthroplasty
- cemented total hip arthroplasty
- cementless total hip arthroplasty
- Charnley arthroplasty
- Charnley total hip arthroplasty
- Charnley-Mueller arthroplasty
- Clayton forefoot arthroplasty
- Colonna arthroplasty
- Colonna trochanteric arthroplasty
- condylar implant arthroplasty
- constrained ankle arthroplasty
- constrained shoulder arthroplasty
- convex condylar implant arthroplasty
- Coonrad total elbow arthroplasty
- Coonrad-Morrey total elbow arthroplasty
- Coventry arthroplasty
- Cracchiolo forefoot arthroplasty
- Crawford-Adams arthroplasty
- Crawford-Adams cup arthroplasty
- Crawford-Adams hip arthroplasty
- Cubbins arthroplasty
- Cubbins shoulder arthroplasty
- cuff tear arthroplasty
- cup arthroplasty
- Curtis arthroplasty
- Darrach wrist arthroplasty
- DePuy arthroplasty

arthroplasty (*continued*)
- Dewar-Barrington arthroplasty
- distraction arthroplasty
- duToit-Roux arthroplasty
- Eaton plate arthroplasty
- Eaton implant arthroplasty
- Eaton volar plate arthroplasty
- Eden-Hybbinette arthroplasty
- Eden-Hybbinette shoulder arthroplasty
- elbow arthroplasty
- ELP stem for hip arthroplasty
- endoprosthetic arthroplasty
- Ewald capitellocondylar total elbow arthroplasty
- Ewald elbow arthroplasty
- Ewald-Walker kinematic knee arthroplasty
- excision arthroplasty
- fascial arthroplasty
- finger joint arthroplasty
- forefoot arthroplasty
- gap arthroplasty
- Geomedic arthroplasty
- Girdlestone resection arthroplasty
- Gristina-Webb total shoulder arthroplasty
- Gunston arthroplasty
- Harrington total hip arthroplasty
- Head hip arthroplasty
- Helal flap arthroplasty
- hemiresection interposition arthroplasty
- hip arthroplasty
- Hungerford-Krackow-Kenna knee arthroplasty
- ICLH arthroplasty
- ICLH double-cup arthroplasty
- implant arthroplasty
- Inglis triaxial total elbow arthroplasty
- Insall-Burstein arthroplasty
- Insall-Burstein-Freeman knee arthroplasty
- interposition arthroplasty
- interpositional arthroplasty
- interpositional elbow arthroplasty
- interpositional gap arthroplasty

arthroplasty (*continued*)

interpositional shoulder arthroplasty

intracapsular temporomandibular joint arthroplasty

joint arthroplasty

Jones resection arthroplasty

Judet arthroplasty

Kates forefoot arthroplasty

Keller arthroplasty

Keller resection arthroplasty

knee arthroplasty

Kocher-McFarland hip arthroplasty

Kocher-Osborn hip arthroplasty

Kutes arthroplasty

Larmon forefoot arthroplasty

low-friction arthroplasty (LFA)

MacAusland elbow arthroplasty

Magnuson arthroplasty

Magnuson-Stack arthroplasty

Magnuson-Stack shoulder arthoplasty

Mann-DuVries arthroplasty

Matchett-Brown hip arthroplasty

Mayo modified total elbow arthroplasty

Mayo resection arthroplasty

McAtee-Tharias-Blazina arthroplasty

McKee-Farrar total hip arthroplasty

Memford-Gurd arthroplasty

Meuli arthroplasty

Millender arthroplasty

Miller-Galante knee arthroplasty

modified mold and surface replacement arthroplasty

mold acetabular arthroplasty

mold arthroplasty

monospherical total shoulder arthroplasty

Morrey-Bryan total elbow arthroplasty

Mould arthroplasty

MP joint arthroplasty

Mueller hip arthroplasty

arthroplasty (*continued*)

Mumford-Gurd arthroplasty

NEB hip arthroplasty

Neer unconstrained shoulder arthroplasty

New England Baptist arthroplasty

Nicola shoulder arthroplasty

Niebauer trapeziometacarpal arthroplasty

noncemented total hip arthroplasty

Ollier-Murphy approach in hip arthroplasty

perichondral arthroplasty

Post total shoulder arthroplasty

Pritchard arthroplasty

prosthetic arthroplasty

prosthetic replacement arthroplasty

Putti-Platt arthroplasty

resection arthroplasty

revision hip arthroplasty

rotator cuff tear arthroplasty

Schlein arthroplasty

Schlein elbow arthroplasty

semiconstrained total elbow arthroplasty

shoulder arthroplasty

Silastic lunate arthroplasty

silicone elastomer arthroplasty

silicone implant arthroplasty

silicone rubber arthroplasty

silicone wrist arthroplasty

small joint arthroplasty

Smith-Petersen cup arthroplasty

Speed arthroplasty

Stanmore shoulder arthroplasty

Steffee thumb arthroplasty

Suave-Kapandji arthroplasty

surface replacement hip arthroplasty

Swanson arthroplasty

Swanson Convex condylar arthroplasty

Swanson radial head implant arthroplasty

arthroplasty (*continued*)
    Swanson silicone wrist arthroplasty
    tendon interposition arthroplasty
    Tharies hip arthroplasty
    total ankle arthroplasty
    total articular replacement arthroplasty (TARA)
    total articular resurfacing arthroplasty
    total elbow arthroplasty
    total hip arthroplasty
    total joint arthroplasty
    total knee arthroplasty
    total patellofemoral joint arthroplasty
    total shoulder arthroplasty
    total wrist arthroplasty
    triaxial total elbow arthroplasty
    Tupper arthroplasty
    ulnar hemiresection interposition arthroplasty
    unconstrained shoulder arthroplasty
    unicompartmental knee arthroplasty
    Vainio arthroplasty
    Vainio MP arthroplasty
    volar plate arthroplasty
    volar shelf arthroplasty
    Volz arthroplasty
    Walldius knee arthroplasty
    Whitman arthoplasty
    Wilson-McKeever arthroplasty
arthroplasty gouge
ArthroProbe laser
arthrorisis
ArthroRivet soft tissue tack
arthroscope
    4M 30-degree arthroscope
    Acufex arthroscope
    Arthrex arthroscope
    Baxter angled arthroscope
    Circon arthroscope
    Citscope arthroscope
    Codman arthroscope
    Concept Intravision arthroscope
    Direct-Coupler arthroscope
    Downs arthroscope

arthroscope (*continued*)
    Dyonics arthroscope
    Dyonics needle scope arthroscope
    Dyonics rod lens arthroscope
    Eagle arthroscope
    Eagle straight-ahead arthroscope
    examining arthroscope
    fiberoptic arthroscope
    Flexiscope arthroscope
    Hopkins arthroscope
    Lumina rod lens arthroscope
    Medical Dynamics 5990 needle arthroscope
    O'Connor operating arthroscope
    Panoview arthroscope
    Richard Wolf arthroscope
    Sapphire View arthroscope
    spinal arthroscope
    standard arthroscope
    Stork arthroscope
    Storz arthroscope
    Storz examining arthroscope
    Stryker arthroscope
    Takagi arthroscope
    Watanabe arthroscope
    Wolf arthroscope
    Zimmer arthroscope
arthroscopic abrasion chondroplasty
arthroscopic ankle holder
arthroscopic anterior cruciate ligament reconstruction (AACLR)
arthroscopic augmentation
arthroscopic banana blade
arthroscopic cannula
arthroscopic entry portal
arthroscopic examination
arthroscopic instruments
arthroscopic knife
arthroscopic laser surgery
arthroscopic leg holder
arthroscopic meniscectomy
arthroscopic microdiskectomy
arthroscopic osteotome
arthroscopic probe
arthroscopic punch
arthroscopic scissors

Arthroscopic Screw Installation (ASI)
arthroscopic shaver
arthroscopic sheath
arthroscopic surgery
arthroscopic synovectomy
arthroscopic synovector
arthroscopy
   diagnostic and operative arthroscopy
   Gillquist arthroscopy
   laser arthroscopy
   midcarpal arthroscopy
   Mumford arthroscopy
   needle arthroscopy
   operative arthroscopy
   radiocarpal arthroscopy
   Ringer arthroscopy
   total knee arthroscopy (TKA)
   Watanabe arthroscopy
arthroscopy knife
Arthroscrew arthroscopic suturing device
Arthrosew arthroscopic suturing device
arthrosis
   Charcot arthrosis
   temporomandibular arthrosis
arthrosis deformans
arthrostomy
Arthrotek calibrated cylinder
Arthrotek Ellipticut hand instruments
Arthrotek femoral aimer
Arthrotek tibial fixation device
arthrotome
   Hall arthrotome
arthrotomy
   eye drill in arthrotomy
   Magnuson-Stack shoulder arthrotomy
   operative arthrotomy
   parapatellar arthrotomy
arthrotomy with drainage
arthrotomy with exploration
arthrotomy with removal
ArthroWand
   CAPS arthroWand
arthroxesis
Arthur splinter forceps
Arthur Ward planisphere
Arthus reaction

articular
articular capsule
articular cartilage
articular cartilage lesion
articular cavity
articular crest
articular disk
articular eminence
articular eminence of temporal bone
articular facet
articular fossa of mandible
articular fossa of temporal bone
articular fracture
articular fragment
articular insert
articular mass separation fracture
articular muscle
articular osteotome
articular pillar fracture
articular surface
articular surface of mandibular fossa
articular tubercle
articular tubercle of temporal bone
articulare
Articu-Lase laser
Articu-Lase laser mirror
articulate
articulated
articulated chin implant
articulated chin prosthesis
articulated external fixator
articulated optical arm
articulating paper forceps
articulatio (*pl.* articulationes)
articulation
   acromioclavicular articulation
   arthrodial articulation
   articulator articulation
   atlantoaxial articulation
   atlantooccipital articulation
   balanced articulation
   bicondylar articulation
   brachiocarpal articulation
   brachioulnar articulation
   calcaneoastragaloid articulation
   calcaneocuboid articulation
   capitolunate articulation

articulation (*continued*)
capitular articulation
carpal articulation
carpometacarpal articulation
chondrosternal articulation
Chopart articulation
condylar articulation
coracoclavicular articulation
costocentral articulation
costosternal articulation
costotransverse articulation
costovertebral articulation
coxofemoral articulation
cranial coronal ring
    articulation
craniovertebral articulation
cricoarytenoid articulation
cricothyroid articulation
Deep Test of Articulation
dental articulation
deviant articulation
ellipsoidal articulation
external ligament of
    mandibular articulation
external ligament of
    temporomandibular
    articulation
glenohumeral articulation
hinged articulation
humeral articulation
humeroradial articulation
humeroulnar articulation
iliosacral articulation
incudomalleolar articulation
incudostapedial articulation
infantile articulation
intercarpal articulation
interchondral articulation
intercostal articulation
intermetacarpal articulation
intermetatarsal articulation
interphalangeal articulation
intertarsal articulation
lateral ligament of
    temporomandibular
    articulation
Lisfranc articulation
mandibular articulation
maxillary articulation
mediocarpal articulation
metacarpocarpal
    articulations

articulation (*continued*)
metacarpophalangeal
    articulation
metatarsocuneiform
    articulation
metatarsophalangeal
    articulations
occipitoatlantal articulation
patellofemoral articulation
peg-and-socket articulation
phalangeal articulation
place of articulation
proximal radioulnar
    articulation
radiocapitellar articulation
radiocarpal articulation
radioulnar articulation
sacrococcygeal articulation
sacroiliac articulation
scaphocapitate articulations
scapholunate articulation
scapuloclavicular articulation
secondary articulation
spheroid articulation
sternoclavicular articulation
sternocostal articulation
subtalar articulation
superior tibial articulation
talocalcaneal articulation
talocalcaneonavicular
    articulation
talonavicular articulation
tarsometatarsal articulations
temporomandibular
    articulation
temporomandibular joint
    articulation
temporomaxillary articulation
tibiofemoral articulation
tibiofibular articulation
tibiotarsal articulation
transverse tarsal articulation
triquetropisiform articulation
trochoid articulation
trochoidal articulation
Vermont spinal fixator
    articulation
vomerosphenoidal
    articulation
articulation area
articulation curve
articulation disorder

articulation index
articulation of pisiform bone
articulation osteotome
articulation test
articulations of fingers
articulations of foot
articulations of hand
articulator
  Acme articulator
  adjustable articulator
  Arcon articulator
  Arcon semiadjustable
    articulator
  Balkwell articulator
  Bergström articulator
  Bonwill articulator
  Christensen articulator
  Denar articulator
  Denar-Witzig articulator
  Dentatus articulator
  Evans articulator
  Galetti articulator
  Gariot articulator
  Granger articulator
  Gysi articulator
  Hanau articulator
  Handy II articulator
  hinge articulator
  hinged articulator
  KSK articulator
  Ney articulator
  non-Arcon articulator
  Oliair articulator
  Olyco articulator
  Olympia articulator
  plain-line articulator
  quick-mount face-bow
    articulator
  semi-adjustable articulator
  Steele articulator
  Stuart articulator
  Walker articulator
  Whip-Mix articulator
articulator articulation
articulatory procedure
Articul-eze hip ball
artifact
  beam hardening artifact
  eye movement artifact
  interfering artifact
  lead artifact
  muscular artifact

artifact (*continued*)
  posterior ghosting artifacts
  skin lesion artifact
  trigeminal nerve artifact
artificial saliva
artificial
artificial ankylosis
artificial anus
artificial blood
artificial classification cavity
artificial ear
artificial endocrine pancreas
artificial erection test
artificial eye
artificial fat pad
artificial fistulation
artificial gut
artificial heart
artificial hip joint (AHJ)
artificial insemination
artificial insemination donor
    (AID)
artificial insemination husband
    (AIH)
artificial intravaginal
    insemination
artificial joint implant
artificial kidney
artificial larynx
artificial leech
artificial lung
artificial mastoid
artificial nose
artificial pacemaker
artificial palate
artificial respiration
artificial rupture of membranes
    (ARM)
artificial sphincter
artificial stoma
artificial valve
artificial velum
artificial ventilation
artificial vertebral body
artificialis
  acne artificialis
Arti-holder tweezers
Artilk forceps
artiodactylous
Artisan phakic intraocular lens
Artisan wide-angle vaginal
    speculum

Artmann chisel
Artmann disarticulation chisel
Artmann elevator
Artmann raspatory
Artoscan MRI scanner
Artus cutting tip
ARUM Colles fixation pin
Arvee model 2400 infant apnea
arycorniculata
   synchondrosis arycorniculata
aryepiglottic (AE)
aryepiglottic fascia
aryepiglottic fold (AE fold)
aryepiglottic fold of Collier
aryepiglottic muscle
arytenoid
arytenoid abduction
arytenoid cartilage
arytenoid glands
arytenoid muscle
arytenoid perichondritis
arytenoid process
arytenoidea, arytenoidea
   cartilago arytenoidea
   basis cartilaginis arytenoideae
   facies articularis cartilaginis
      arytenoideae
   facies medialis cartilaginis
      arytenoideae
   facies posterior cartilaginis
      arytenoideae
arytenoidectomy
arytenoidopexy
arytenoids
Arzbacher pill electrode
Arzco electrode
Arzco model 7 cardiac
   stimulator
Arzco pacemaker
Arzco Tapsul pill electrode
AS (Auto Suture)
asacroliticus
Asahi blood plasma pump
Asahi hollow fiber dialyzer
Asahi Plasmaflo plasma
   separator
Asahi pressure controller
Asai operation
ASAP channel-cut automated
   biopsy needle
ASAP channel-cut automated
   biopsy needle

ASAP PinPoint guiding
   introducer needle
ASAP prostate biopsy needle
ASC Monorel catheter
ASCAD (atherosclerotic
   coronary artery disease)
A-scan
A-scan scanner
A-scan ultrasound
ascendens
   aorta ascendens
   colon ascendens
ascending aorta (AA)
ascending aorta-to-pulmonary
   artery shunt
ascending cervical artery
ascending colon
ascending lumbar vein
ascending palatine artery
ascending pharyngeal artery
ascending pyelogram
ascending pyelography
ascending ramus
ascending ramus of the
   mandible
ascending technique
ascending urogram
ascending urography
Ascension PyroCarbon MCP
   implant
Ascent catheter
Ascent guiding catheter
Asch clamp
Asch forceps
Asch nasal clamp
Asch nasal splint
Asch nasal-straightening forceps
Asch operation
Asch septal forceps
Asch septal straightener
Asch septal-straightening
   forceps
Asch septum-straightening
   forceps
Asch splint
Asch straightener
Asch uterine secretion scoop
Ascher syndrome
Aschner reflex
Aschoff body
Aschoff cell
Aschoff node

Aschoff nodule
Aschoff-Tawara node
ascites
    bile ascites
    blood-tinged ascites
    bloody ascites
    chylous ascites
    cloudy ascites
    Crosby-Cooney operation for
        ascites
    dialysis-related ascites
    drainage of ascites
    exudative ascites
    fatty ascites
    hemorrhagic ascites
    hydremic ascites
    massive ascites
    milky ascites
    nephrogenic ascites
    pancreatic ascites
    pseudochylous ascites
    refractory ascites
    straw-colored ascites
    tense ascites
    transudative ascites
ascites drainage tube
ascites shunt
ascites suction tube
ascitic fluid
Ascon instruments
ascorbic acid
ascribe
ASCVD (arteriosclerotic
    cardiovascular disease)
ASD (atrioseptal defect)
ASDOS umbrella occluder
ASE bandage (axilla, shoulder,
    and elbow bandage)
Aselli pancreas
asepsis
    integral asepsis
    isolation and asepsis
aseptic
aseptic felon
aseptic fever
aseptic necrosis
aseptic saw
aseptic surgery
aseptic technique
aseptic wound
aseptic-antiseptic
asepticism

Asepto aspirating syringe
Asepto bulb syringe
Asepto irrigation syringe
Asepto suction tube
Asepto syringe
ASH (asymmetric septal
    hypertrophy)
Ash catheter
Ash dental forceps
Ash septum-straightening
    forceps
Ash Split Cath dual-lumen
    catheter
Ashbell hook
Ashby fluoroscopic foreign
    body forceps
Ashby forceps
Asher high-pull face-bow
Asherman chest seal
Ashford mammilliplasty
Ashford mammaplasty
Ashford retracted nipple
    operation
Ashhurst splint
Ashhurst-Bromer ankle fracture
    classification
ash-leaf patch
Ashley breast prosthesis
Ashley cleft palate elevator
Ashley elevator
Ashley repair
Ashley retractor
Ashman phenomenon
Ashworth arthroplasty
Ashworth Dow Corning
    prosthesis
Ashworth hand arthroplasty
Ashworth implant arthroplasty
Ashworth-Blatt implant
ASI (Arthroscopic Screw
    Installation)
ASI uroplasty TCU dilatation
    catheter
ASICO multi-angled diamond
    knife
ASID Bonz PP infusion pump
ASIF broad dynamic
    compression bone plate
ASIF plate
ASIF screw
ASIF screw and washer
ASIF screw fixation technique

ASIF screw pin
ASIF T plate
ASIF twist drill
ASIS (anterior-superior iliac spine)
ASIS femoral head locator
askew
Ask-Upmark kidney
Aslan 2-mm minilaparoscope
Aslan endoscopic scissors
Aslan needle holder
Asner screw
Asnis 2 guided screw
Asnis 3 guided screw
Asnis cannulated screw
Asnis guided screw
Asnis III cannulated screw
Asnis pin
Asnis pinning
Asnis screw
Asnis technique
aspect
    anteroinferior aspect
    anterolateral aspect
    buccal aspect
    caudal aspect
    cellulite aspect
    cephalad aspect
    contralateral aspect
    distal aspect
    dorsal aspect
    dumpling aspect (orange skin phenomenon)
    inferolateral aspect
    inferomedial aspect
    inner aspect
    ipsilateral aspect
    laminar cortex posterior aspect
    lateral aspect
    medial aspect
    median aspect
    medicolegal aspect
    outer aspect
    paraspinous aspect
    perichondrium on the cranial aspect
    physiologic aspect
    plantar aspect
    posterior aspect
    posteroinferior aspect
    posterolateral aspect

aspect (continued)
    posteromedial aspect
    puriform aspect
    radial aspect
    rostral aspect
    spinous aspect
    superior aspect
    superolateral aspect
    turgescent aspect
    ulnar aspect
    ventral aspect
    volar aspect
Aspen cervical thoracic orthosis
Aspen digital ultrasound
Aspen electrocautery
Aspen laparoscopic electrode
Aspen ultrasound platform
aspera
    linea aspera
aspergilloma formation
aspermia
aspheric cataract lens
Aspheric lens implant
aspheric viewing lens
aspherical ophthalmoscopic lens
asphyxiating thoracic dysplasia
Aspiradeps dissector
Aspiradeps lipodissector
aspirate
    adipo aspirate
    nasogastric aspirate
    NG aspirate
aspirated foreign body
aspirating cannula
aspirating curet
aspirating dissector
aspirating needle
aspirating syringe
aspirating tip
aspirating trocar
aspirating tube
aspiration
    acid aspiration
    Alcon aspiration
    anterior aspiration
    bone marrow aspiration
    breast cyst aspiration
    bronchoscopy with aspiration
    cataract aspiration
    cervical aspiration
    cold knife cone aspiration

aspiration (*continued*)
  corporeal aspiration
  CT scan-guided needle
    aspiration
  CT-directed needle aspiration
  CT-guided fine-needle
    aspiration
  cyst aspiration
  dilatation and aspiration
    (D&A)
  endoscopic transesophageal
    fine-needle aspiration
  epididymal sperm aspiration
  EUS-guided fine-needle
    aspiration
  fine-needle aspiration (FNA)
  fluid aspiration
  foreign body aspiration
  full-thickness rectal aspiration
  gastric fluid aspiration
  guided fine-needle aspiration
  hematoma aspiration
  iliac crest bone aspiration
  image-guided pancreatic core
    aspiration
  irrigation and aspiration
    (I&A)
  joint aspiration
  lateral aspiration
  lipoma aspiration
  Mammotest Plus breast
    aspiration
  meconium aspiration
  medial aspiration
  menstrual aspiration
  Michele vertebral aspiration
  microscopic epididymal
    sperm aspiration
  microsurgical epididymal
    sperm aspiration
  mineral oil aspiration
  mucosal needle aspiration
  myringotomy with aspiration
  needle aspiration
  negative aspiration
  percutaneous aspiration
  percutaneous balloon
    aspiration
  percutaneous CT-guided
    aspiration
  percutaneous epididymal
    sperm aspiration

aspiration (*continued*)
  percutaneous fine-needle
    aspiration
  peritoneal aspiration
  permucosal needle aspiration
  pleural fluid aspiration
  preoperative percutaneous
    aspiration
  pulmonary aspiration
  real-time endoscopic
    ultrasound-guided fine-
    needle aspiration
  recurrent aspiration
  Scheie cataract aspiration
  seminal vesicle aspiration
  silent aspiration
  sonography guided aspiration
  sperm aspiration
  stereotactic aspiration
  sternal puncture by aspiration
  suction aspiration
  suprapubic aspiration
  suprapubic needle aspiration
  tracheal aspiration
  transbronchial needle
    aspiration
  transthoracic needle
    aspiration
  transtracheal aspiration
  ultrasonic aspiration
  ultrasound guided fine-needle
    aspiration
  uterine aspiration
  vacuum aspiration
  vitreous aspiration
aspiration biopsy
aspiration biopsy cytology
    (ABC)
aspiration biopsy needle
aspiration cannula
aspiration curettage
aspiration needle
aspiration needle biopsy
aspiration of bronchus
aspiration of cortex
aspiration of lung
aspiration of sinuses
aspiration of vitreous
aspiration pneumonia
aspiration pneumonitis
aspiration portal
aspiration prophylaxis

aspiration syringe
aspiration tulip device
aspirator
   Accelerator II aspirator
   Adams aspirator
   Alcon aspirator
   Aspirette endocervical
     aspirator
   blue-tip aspirator
   Bovie ultrasound aspirator
   bronchoscopic aspirator
   Broyles aspirator
   Carabelli aspirator
   Care-e-Vac portable aspirator
   Carmody aspirator
   Carmody electric aspirator
   Castroviejo orbital aspirator
   cataract aspirator
   Cavi-Pulse cavitation
     ultrasound surgical
     aspirator
   Cavitron aspirator
   Cavitron ultrasonic aspirator
     (CUSA)
   Cavitron Ultrasonic Surgical
     aspirator (CUSA)
   Clerf aspirator
   Cogsell tip aspirator
   Cook County aspirator
   Cook County Hospital
     aspirator
   Cooper aspirator
   CUSA aspirator
   CUSA Excel ultrasonic
     aspirator
   DeLee meconium trap
     aspirator
   DeLee trap aspirator
   DeLee trap meconium
     aspirator
   DeVilbiss Vacu-Aide aspirator
   Dia pump aspirator
   Dieulafoy aspirator
   Egnell uterine aspirator
   electric aspirator
   Endo-Assist sponge aspirator
   endocervical aspirator
   endometrial aspirator
   faucet aspirator
   Fibra Sonics phaco aspirator
   Fink cataract aspirator
   Flex-O-Jet aspirator

aspirator (*continued*)
   Fluvog aspirator
   Frazier suction tip aspirator
   Fritz aspirator
   Frye aspirator
   Frye portable aspirator
   gallbladder aspirator
   Gesco aspirator
   Gomco aspirator
   Gomco portable suction
     aspirator
   Gomco suction aspirator
   Gomco uterine aspirator
   Gottschalk aspirator
   Gottschalk middle ear
     aspirator
   Gradwohl sternal bone
     marrow aspirator
   GynoSampler endometrial
     aspirator
   Hahnenkratt aspirator
   Hu-Friedy suction tip aspirator
   Huzly aspirator
   Hydrojette aspirator
   Junior Tompkins portable
     aspirator
   Kelman aspirator
   Leasure aspirator
   Legacy Series 2000
     Cavitron/Kelman phaco-
     emulsifier aspirator
   Lukens aspirator
   LySonix 250 aspirator
   meconium aspirator
   middle ear aspirator
   Monoject bone marrow
     aspirator
   nasal aspirator
   Nugent aspirator
   Nugent soft cataract
     aspirator
   Penberthy double-action
     aspirator
   Pilling-Negus clamp-on
     aspirator
   portable aspirator
   portable suction aspirator
   Potain aspirator
   Printz aspirator
   red-tip aspirator
   Selector ultrasonic aspirator
   Senoran aspirator

aspirator (*continued*)
    Sharplan Ultra ultrasonic
       aspirator
    Sklar-Junior Tompkins
       aspirator
    soft cataract aspirator
    Sonocut ultrasonic aspirator
    Sonop ultrasonic aspirator
    Sorensen aspirator
    Stat aspirator
    Stedman aspirator
    Stedman suction pump
       aspirator
    suction aspirator
    suction pump aspirator
    surgical aspirator
    Taylor aspirator
    Thorek aspirator
    Thorek gallbladder aspirator
    Tompkins aspirator
    Ultra ultrasonic aspirator
    ultrasonic surgical aspirator
    Universal aspirator
    uterine aspirator
    Vabra aspirator
    Vabra cervical aspirator
    vacuum aspirator
    Vent-O-Vac aspirator
    Walker aspirator
    yellow-tip aspirator
aspirator cannula
aspirator/hydrodissector
    Alpern cortex
       aspirator/hydrodissector
Aspirette endocervical aspirator
aspirin
    methocarbamol and aspirin
Aspir-Vac probe
Aspisafe nasogastric tube
asplenia
asplenic
A-splint dental splint
ASPS (alveolar soft part
    sarcoma)
ASPVD (arteriosclerotic
    peripheral vascular disease)
ASR blade
ASR scalpel
Assal-Javid cerebrospinal shunt
assay
    coagulation factor assay
    estrogen assay

assay (*continued*)
    intraoperative iPTH assay
    Maximal Static Response
       Assay (MSRA)
assay technique
assembly
    Ace halo-cast assembly
    Ace wire tension assembly
    Brown-Roberts-Wells arc ring
       assembly
    dilating catheter gastrostomy
       tube assembly
    Dosick bellows assembly
    emergency oxygen mask
       assembly
    Geild retractable blade assembly
    infant nasal cannula assembly
    Kellman nose cone assembly
    Kellman transducer assembly
    KLI dual control assembly
    Konigsberg 5-channel solid-
       state catheter assembly
    linear array-hydrophone
       assembly
    malleostapedial assembly
    malleus footplate assembly
    malleus stapes assembly
    Massie nail assembly
    Vabra assembly
Assess esophageal testing kit
Assess peak flow meter
assessment
    awake neurological assessment
    cytological assessment
    echocardiographic assessment
    endoscopic color Doppler
       assessment
    extrapyramidal function
       assessment
    histologic assessment
    histological assessment
    intraoperative assessment
    jugular bulb catheter
       placement assessment
    neurological assessment
    noninvasive assessment
    nutritional assessment
    overall assessment
    peritoneal cytological
       assessment
    weight estimation and
       assessment

Assézat triangle
ASSI (Accurate Surgical and
    Scientific Instruments)
ASSI bipolar coagulating forceps
ASSI breast dissector
ASSI breast dissector angulated
ASSI breast dissector spatulated
ASSI cannula
ASSI cranial blades
ASSI disposable cranio blade
ASSI dual-ended surgical
    instruments
ASSI forceps
ASSI METE-5168 Microspike
    approximator clamp
ASSI METS-3668 Microspike
    approximator clamp
ASSI Microspike approximator
    clamp
ASSI MKCV-2040 Microspike
    approximator clamp
ASSI MSPK-3678 Microspike
    approximator clamp
ASSI nasal and sinus instruments
ASSI Polar-Mate bipolar
    coagulator
ASSI S&T microsurgical
    instrument
ASSI Super-Cut scissors
ASSI wire pass drill
assimilation
    alveolar assimilation
    labial assimilation
    velar assimilation
assimilation pelvis
assist
    circulatory assist
    standby assist
assistance
    laparoscopic assistance
    minimal assistance
    respiratory assistance
    standby assistance
    ventilatory assistance
assistant
    surgical assistant
    suture assistant
Assistant Free calibrated
    femoral-tibial spreader
Assistant Free retractor
Assistant Free Stulberg leg
    positioner

Assistant Free suture
assist-control mode ventilation
assisted
    suction assisted
assisted breech delivery
assisted circulation
assisted reproductive technique
assisted respiration
assisted ventilation
associated injury
associated myofascial trigger
    point
Association for the Study of
    Internal Fixation (ASIF)
    plate
Asta ligature scissors
Asta-Cath device
Astech peak flow meter
asterion
asternal rib
asternia
asteroid body
Astham Check peak flowmeter
asthenia
    neurocirculatory asthenia
asthenopia
    accommodative asthenopia
    muscular asthenopia
    tarsal asthenopia
asthma
    extrinsic asthma
asthmatic
    cardiac asthmatic
astigmatic keratotomy
astigmatic marker
astigmatism
    corneal astigmatism
    oblique astigmatism
astigmatism correction
Astler-Coller A, B1, B2, C1, C2
    classification
Astler-Coller classification of
    Dukes C carcinoma
Astler-Coller modification of
    Dukes classification
astomia
Aston face-lift scissors
Aston nasal retractor
Aston submental retractor
Astra pacemaker
astragalectomy
    Whitman astragalectomy

astragalonavicular joint
astragalus
  aviator's astragalus
AstrinGYN solution
astrocytoma
Astron investment material
Astropulse cuff
Astro-Trace Universal adapter clip
Asuka PTCA catheter
ASVIP pacemaker
asymmetric, asymmetrical
asymmetric bilateral cleft
asymmetric chin
asymmetric distribution
asymmetric folds of eyes
asymmetric hyperplasia
asymmetric maxillomandibular
  growth
asymmetric reflexes
asymmetric septal hypertrophy
  (ASH)
asymmetric surgery
asymmetric unit membrane
asymmetry
  Blount procedure for bone
    growth asymmetry
  domal asymmetry
  facial asymmetry
  forehead asymmetry
  tumofactive asymmetry
  vertical nipple asymmetry
asymptomatic
asymptomatic gallstone
asynchronous bilateral breast
  cancer
asynchronous mode pacemaker
asynchronous pacemaker
asynchronous ventricular VOO
  pacemaker
asynclitic position
Atad cervical ripening device
Atad Ripener device
ataractic
ataraxia
Atasoy palmar flap
Atasoy triangular advancement
  flap
Atasoy volar V-Y flap
Atasoy V-Y technique
Atasoy-Kleinert flap
Atasoy-Kleinert volar V-Y
  advancement flap

Atasoy-type repair
ataxia
  appendicular ataxia
  cerebellar ataxia
  equilibratory ataxia
  Friedreich ataxia
  hereditary ataxia
  locomotor ataxia
ataxia-telangiectasia
ataxic gait
ataxis
  cerebellar ataxis
atelectasis
  bibasilar atelectasis
  focus of atelectasis
  lobar atelectasis
  lobular patches of atelectasis
  phenomenon of compression
    atelectasis
  resorption atelectasis
  segmental atelectasis
atelectatic band
atelectatic rales
Aten olecranon screw
ATG (antithymocyte globulin)
athelia
Athens forceps
Athens suture spreader
atherectomy
  Auth atherectomy
  coronary angioplasty versus
    excisional atherectomy
  coronary rotational
    atherectomy
  directional coronary
    atherectomy
  high-speed rotational
    atherectomy
  Kinsey atherectomy
  percutaneous coronary
    rotational atherectomy
  percutaneous transluminal
    atherectomy
  retrograde atherectomy
  rotational coronary
    atherectomy
  Simpson atherectomy
  transluminal extraction
    atherectomy
  atherectomy catheter
atherectomy cutter
atherectomy device

atherectomy index
atheroablation laser
AtheroCath
    DVI Simpson AtheroCath
    Simpson coronary AtheroCath
    Simpson peripheral
        AtheroCath
AtheroCath Bantam coronary
    atherectomy catheter
AtheroCath catheter
AtheroCath GTO coronary
    atherectomy catheter
AtheroCath spinning blade
    catheter
atheroma
    embolized atheroma
atheroma embolism
atheromatosis
atheromatosis cutis
atheromatous
atheromatous plaque
atherosclerosis
atherosclerotic aneurysm
atherosclerotic cardiovascular
    disease (ASCVD)
atherosclerotic carotid artery
    lesion
atherosclerotic coronary artery
    disease (ASCAD)
atherosclerotic heart disease
Athlete coronary guidewire
athlete's heart
Athos laser
athyreosis
ATI (abdominal trauma index)
Atkin epiphysial fracture
Atkins esophagoscopic telescope
Atkins knife
Atkins nasal splint
Atkins tonsil knife
Atkins tonsillar knife
Atkins-Cannard tracheotomy
    tube
Atkins-Cannard tube
Atkinson 25-G short curved
    cystotome
Atkinson corneal scissors
Atkinson endoprosthesis
Atkinson eye knife
Atkinson introducer
Atkinson keratome
Atkinson lid block

Atkinson needle
Atkinson prosthesis
Atkinson retrobulbar needle
Atkinson sclerotome
Atkinson sclerotomy
Atkinson silicone rubber tube
Atkinson single-bevel blunt-tip
    needle
Atkinson technique
Atkinson tip peribulbar needle
Atkinson tube stent
Atkinson-Walker scissors
Atkins-Tucker laryngoscope
Atkins-Tucker shadow-free
    laryngoscope
Atkins-Tucker surgical shield
ATL (antitension line)
ATL duplex scanner
ATL high definition imaging
    systems
ATL Mark 600 real-time scanner
ATL real-time NeurosectOR
    scanner
ATL real-time ultrasound
ATL Ultramark-series ultrasound
ATL/ADR Ultramark 4/9 HDI
    ultrasound
Atlanta hip brace
atlantal fracture
Atlanta-Scottish Rite brace
Atlanta-Scottish Rite hip brace
Atlantic O-Dor-Less Pouches
Atlantic ileostomy catheter
Atlantis SR coronary
    intravascular ultrasound
    catheter
atlantoaxial arthrodesis
atlantoaxial articulation
atlantoaxial dislocation
atlantoaxial fracture-dislocation
atlantoaxial fusion
atlantoaxial instability
atlantoaxial joint
atlantoaxial lesion
atlantoaxial rotatory fixation
atlantoaxial stabilization
atlanto-occipital fusion
atlanto-occipital membrane
atlanto-occipital articulation
atlanto-occipital extension
atlanto-occipital joint
atlanto-occipital joint dislocation

atlanto-occipital stabilization
atlas
    Greulich-Pyle atlas
atlas arch
Atlas balloon dilatation catheter
Atlas LP PTCA balloon dilatation
    catheter
Atlas orthogonal percussion
    instrument
Atlas ULP PTCA balloon
    dilatation catheter
atlas-axis combination fracture
Atlas-Storz eye magnet
Atlee bronchus clamp
Atlee clamp
Atlee dilator
Atlee uterine dilator
Atmolit suction unit
atomizer
    cocaine atomizer
    Dench atomizer
    DeVilbiss atomizer
    Jackson atomizer
    Jackson laryngeal atomizer
    Kidde atomizer
    laryngeal atomizer
    Proetz atomizer
    Storz atomizer
atonia
atonic
atonic bladder
atonic labor
atonic ulcer
atonicity
atony
    gastric atony
    intestinal atony
    sphincter atony
    uterine atony
atony of uterus
atopic dermatitis
atopic dermatitis rash
atopic line
Atosoy procedure
ATP hydrolysis
Atrac multipurpose balloon
    catheter
Atrac-II double-balloon catheter
Atra-Grip clamp
Atra-Grip forceps
Atraloc needle
Atraloc surgical needle

Atraloc sutures
Atraloc-Ethilon sutures
Atrauclip grip clamp
Atrauclip hemostatic clip
Atraum with Clotstop drain
atraumatic bowel clamp
atraumatic braided silk
    sutures
atraumatic chromic sutures
atraumatic clamp
atraumatic curved grasper
atraumatic distending
    obturator
atraumatic forceps
atraumatic intestinal clamp
atraumatic needle
atraumatic suture needle
atraumatic suture technique
atraumatic sutures
atraumatic tenaculum
atraumatic tissue forceps
atraumatic visceral forceps
Atraumax peripheral vascular
    clamp
atresia
    Altmann classification of
        congential aural atresia
    anal atresia
    aortic valve atresia
    aural atresia
    biliary atresia
    bony atresia
    celiac atresia
    choana atresia
    choanal atresia
    Coleman classification of
        congenital aural atresia
    de la Cruz classification of
        congenital aural atresia
    duodenal atresia
    enteroinsular atresia
    esophageal atresia
    extrahepatic biliary atresia
    Fontan tricuspid atresia
    intestinal atresia
    intrahepatic atresia
    Kasai procedure for biliary
        atresia
    laryngeal atresia
    meatal atresia
    oral atresia
    prepyloric atresia

atresia (*continued*)
  Pulec and Freedman
    classification of congenital
    aural atresia
  Schuknecht classification of
    congenital aural atresia
  tracheal atresia
  tricuspid atresia
atresia plate
atretic
atretoblepharia
atretolemia
atretorrhinia
atria (*sing.* atrium)
atrial and ventricular
    implantable cardioverter
    defibrillator
atrial baffle
atrial baffle operation
atrial balloon septostomy
atrial cannula
atrial clamp
atrial cuff
atrial demand-inhibited
    pacemaker
atrial demand-triggered
    pacemaker
atrial electrode
atrial fibrillation
atrial flutter
atrial instruments
atrial kick
atrial lead
atrial ostium primum defect
atrial pacemaker
atrial pacemaker lead
atrial pacing wire
atrial retractor
atrial septal defect
atrial septal defect single disk
    closure device
atrial septal resection
atrial septal retractor
atrial synchronous ventricular-
    inhibited pacemaker
atrial tachycardia
atrial tracking pacemaker
atrial triggered ventricular-
    inhibited pacemaker
Atrial View Ventak implantable
    cardioverter-defibrillator
atrial-femoral artery bypass

atrial-well technique
Atricor Cordis pacemaker
Atricor pacemaker
atriocommissuropexy
atriofascicular bypass tract
atrio-His pathway
atrio-His tract
atrio-Hisian bypass tract
atrionodal bypass tract
atrioplasty
atriopressor reflex
atrioseptal defect (ASD)
atrioseptopexy
atrioseptoplasty
atrioseptostomy
atrioseptostomy catheter
atriotomy
atrioventricular (AV)
atrioventricular block (AV block)
atrioventricular bundle
    (AV bundle)
atrioventricular canal
atrioventricular canal defect
atrioventricular conduction defect
    (AV conduction defect)
atrioventricular connection
    anomaly
atrioventricular dissociation
atrioventricular groove
atrioventricular junction
atrioventricular junction anomaly
atrioventricular junctional
    ablation
atrioventricular junctional
    pacemaker (AV junctional
    pacemaker)
atrioventricular malformation
    (AVM)
atrioventricular node
atrioventricular orifice
atrioventricular ring
atrioventricular septal defect
atrioventricular sequential
    demand pacemaker
    (AV sequential demand
    pacemaker)
atrioventricular sequential
    pacemaker (AV sequential
    pacemaker)
atrioventricular synchronous
    pacemaker (AV synchronous
    pacemaker)

atrioventricular valve
atrioventricular valve
   replacement
atrioventriculostomy
Atri-pace I bipolar flared pacing
   catheter
atrium
   common atrium
   filling of right atrium
   left atrium
atrium (*pl.* atria)
atrium (wrapped) Advanta graft
Atrium hemodialysis graft
atrophia
atrophia cutis
atrophia cutis senilis
atrophia maculosa varioliformis
   cutis
atrophia striata et maculosa
atrophic
atrophic acne scar
atrophic catarrh
atrophic excavation
atrophic facial acne scar
atrophic fenestration
atrophic fracture
atrophic gastritis
atrophic glossitis
atrophic inflammation
atrophic kidney
atrophic lichen planus
atrophic papulosis
atrophic pharyngitis
atrophic rhinitis
atrophic scar
atrophic white scar
atrophica
   acne atrophica
   hyperkeratosis figurata
      centrifuga atrophica
   stria atrophica
atrophicum
   angioma pigmentosum
      atrophicum
atrophie blanche
atrophied
atrophied papilla
atrophoderma
   progressive idiopathic
      atrophoderma
   senile atrophoderma
atrophoderma albidum

atrophoderma biotripticum
atrophoderma diffusum
atrophoderma maculatum
atrophoderma neuriticum
atrophoderma of Pasini and
   Pierini
atrophoderma pigmentosum
atrophoderma senilis
atrophoderma striatum
atrophodermatosis
atrophy
   alveolar atrophy
   blue atrophy
   Buchwald atrophy
   Charcot-Marie-Tooth atrophy
   choroid atrophy
   choroidal atrophy
   compensatory atrophy
   concentric atrophy
   cortical atrophy
   Cruveilhier atrophy
   Dejerine-Sottas atrophy
   denervated muscle atrophy
   dermal atrophy
   diffuse alveolar atrophy
   diffuse atrophy
   disuse atrophy
   eccentric atrophy
   epidermal atrophy
   fat atrophy
   fatty atrophy
   focal atrophy
   gastric atrophy
   glandular atrophy
   graft atrophy
   hemifacial atrophy
   hemilingual atrophy
   horizontal atrophy
   Hunt atrophy
   inflammatory atrophy
   interstitial atrophy
   iris atrophy
   ishemic muscular atrophy
   linear atrophy
   lobar atrophy
   macular atrophy
   muscle atrophy
   muscular atrophy
   myelopathic muscular atrophy
   myofiber atrophy
   neural atrophy
   neurotropic atrophy

atrophy (*continued*)
  olivopontocerebellar atrophy
  pathologic atrophy
  physiologic atrophy
  pigmentary atrophy
  pressure atrophy
  progressive hemifacial
    atrophy
  quadriceps atrophy
  Romberg hemifacial atrophy
  senile atrophy
  skin atrophy
  testicular atrophy
  thenar atrophy
  unilateral facial atrophy
  vaginal atrophy
  Wucher atrophy
atrophy of fat
atropine
atropine methyl nitrate
ATS Open Pivot Bileaflet heart
  valve
attached cranial section
attached craniotomy
attached gingiva extension
attached island
attachment
  abnormal frenulum
    attachment
  abnormal frenum attachment
  Accuvac smoke evacuation
    attachment
  ACMI teaching attachment
  Albarran cystoscope
    attachment
  Argen dental attachment
  B-1 craniotome attachment
    (*also* B-2, etc.)
  bar clip attachment
  bar sleeve attachment
  Bivona tracheostomy tube
    with talk attachment
  camera attachment
  cerebellar attachment
  clip-on attachment
  closed chain exercise
    attachment
  condom catheter attachment
  Dalbo extracoronal
    attachment
  Dalbo stud attachment
  Dalla Bona attachment

attachment (*continued*)
  Distaflex dental attachment
  epithelial attachment
  eustachian attachment
  extracoronal attachment
  eyepiece attachment
  Gottlieb epithelial attachment
  Hader dental attachment
  high frenum attachment
  Hudson cerebellar
    attachment
  implant superstructure
    attachment
  lingual attachment
  Mayfield-Kees table
    attachment
  McCollum attachment
  mesenteric attachments
  MP video endoscopic lens
    attachment
  multiphase attachment
  muscular attachment
  O-ring attachments
  pacemaker lead attachment
  pathometer attachment
  peritoneal attachments
  photo-kerato attachment
  Pierson attachment
  Planarm Haag Streit
    attachment
  PRAFO KAFO attachment
  Preci-Slot dental attachment
  Roach ball precision
    attachment
  slit-lamp camera attachment
  specular attachment
  Stern dental attachment
  Storz attachment
  Storz eyepiece attachment
  Storz teaching attachment
  Strauss dental attachment
  Tach-EZ dental attachment
  Tasserit shoulder attachment
  teaching attachment
  Thomas leg splint with
    Pearson attachment
  Thomas splint with Pearson
    attachment
attachment epithelium
attachment of pacemaker
  electrodes
attachment of prosthesis

attack
  fatal heart attack
  heart attack
  massive heart attack
  silent attack
  vasovagal attack
Attain steroid-eluting lead
attained
  hemostasis attained
attempted passage of instrument
Attenborough arthroplasty of knee
Attenborough knee prosthesis
Attenborough total knee
    prosthesis
Attends pad and guard
attenuate
attenuated lower uterine segment
attenuated virus
attenuation
  arteriolar attenuation
  beam attenuation
  broadband attenuation
  digital beam attenuation
  heterogeneous attenuation
  high attenuation
  interaural attenuation
  signal attenuation
  tissue attenuation
  ultrasonic attenuation
attenuation correction
attenuation level
attenuation of tendon
attic adhesion
attic cannula
attic dissector
attic ear punch
attic hook
atticoantral
atticoantrostomy
atticoantrotomy
atticocotomy
atticomastoid
atticotomy
  transmeatal atticotomy
atticus punch
attrition
attrition rupture of extensor
    tendon
attritional occlusion
Atwood bridge remover
Atwood crown remover
Atwood loop

Atwood orthodontic cement
A-type dental implant
atypia
  epithelial atypia
  melanocytic atypia
atypical
atypical carcinoid tumor
atypical cleft
atypical coloboma
atypical dislocation
atypical erythema multiforme
atypical fibroxanthoma
atypical hyperplasia (AH)
atypical junction
atypical lipoma
atypical melanocytic hyperplasia
atypical mole
atypical mycobacterium
atypical nevus
atypical pityriasis rosea
atypism
  cervical atypism
Auchincloss mastectomy
Auchincloss operation
Auclair operation
audiography
audiological evaluation
audiometer
audiometry
Audisil silicone ear mold
    material
auditory artery
auditory brain mapping
auditory canal
auditory closure
auditory nerve
auditory tube
auditory veins
Auenbrugger sign
Auer rod
Auerbach ganglion
Auerbach mesenteric plexus
Aufranc approach
Aufranc arthroplasty gouge
Aufranc awl
Aufranc Cobra retractor
Aufranc cup
Aufranc cup arthroplasty
Aufranc dissector
Aufranc femoral neck retractor
Aufranc finishing ball reamer
Aufranc finishing cup reamer

Aufranc gouge
Aufranc groin apron
Aufranc hip prosthesis
Aufranc hip retractor
Aufranc hook
Aufranc mold for cup
    arthroplasty
Aufranc offset reamer
Aufranc periosteal elevator
Aufranc psoas retractor
Aufranc push retractor
Aufranc reamer
Aufranc retractor
Aufranc trochanteric awl
Aufranc-Turner acetabular cup
Aufranc-Turner arthroplasty
Aufranc-Turner cemented hip
    prosthesis
Aufranc-Turner hip prosthesis
Aufrecht sign
Aufricht elevator
Aufricht fiberoptic light
    retractor
Aufricht glabellar rasp
Aufricht nasal elevator
Aufricht nasal rasp
Aufricht nasal retractor
Aufricht rasp
Aufricht raspatory
Aufricht retractor
Aufricht retractor-speculum
Aufricht scissors
Aufricht septal speculum
Aufricht septum speculum
Aufricht speculum
Aufricht-Britetrac nasal retractor
Aufricht-Lipsett nasal rasp
Aufricht-Lipsett rasp
Aufricht-Lipsett raspatory
auger
    footplate auger
    Hough auger
    Hough footplate auger
    Hough stapedial footplate
        auger
    stapedial footplate auger
auger wire
Augmen bone-grafting material
augmentation
    alloplastic augmentation
    alloplastic chin augmentation
    alveolar ridge augmentation

augmentation (*continued*)
    arthroscopic augmentation
    autologous augmentation
    autologous human collagen
        augmentation
    bladder augmentation
    breast augmentation
    calf augmentation
    camouflage augmentation
    cheek augmentation
    chin augmentation
    connective tissue
        augmentation
    cystoplasty augmentation
    donor-specific bone marrow
        augmentation
    endoscopic breast
        augmentation
    endoscopic transaxillary breast
        augmentation (ETBA)
    extraarticular augmentation
    Farrior graft augmentation
    fat augmentation
    Fomon graft augmentation
    full-spectrum breast
        augmentation
    gastroileac augmentation
    gingival augmentation
    Gore-Tex lip augmentation
    hamstring ligament
        augmentation
    Hogan and Converse graft
        augmentation
    ileocecocystoplasty bladder
        augmentation
    iliotibial band graft
        augmentation
    labor augmentation
    Larson anterior cruciate
        augmentation
    Leach-Schepsis-Paul
        augmentation
    ligament augmentation
    lip augmentation
    Longacre graft augmentation
    Mainz pouch augmentation
    malar alloplastic
        augmentation
    malar facial augmentation
    malar shell augmentation
    mastopexy breast
        augmentation

augmentation (*continued*)
  mentoplasty augmentation
  midface alloplastic
    augmentation
  Millard graft augmentation
  Musgrave and Dupertuis graft
    augmentation
  open transaxillary breast
    augmentation (OTBA)
  permanent lip augmentation
  PermaRidge alveolar ridge
    augmentation
  pharyngeal wall augmentation
  premandible alloplastic
    augmentation
  premandibular augmentation
  preprosthetic augmentation
  reverse augmentation
  ridge augmentation
  silicone lip augmentation
  simultaneous areolar
    mastopexy and breast
    augmentation (SAMBA)
  slotted acetabular
    augmentation
  soft tissue augmentation
  subantral augmentation
  submandibular augmentation
  submucosal urethral
    augmentation
  submuscular breast
    augmentation
  subpectoral augmentation
  synthetic augmentation
  temporary lip augmentation
  thiol augmentation
  transaxillary breast
    augmentation (TBA)
  transaxillary subpectoral
    augmentation
  transumbilical breast
    augmentation (TUBA)
  ureteral bladder augmentation
augmentation cystoplasty
augmentation genioplasty
augmentation graft
augmentation mammaplasty
augmentation of labor
augmentation of the mandibular
    angle (AMA)
augmentation plaque
augmentation procedure

augmentation surgery
augmentation therapy
augmentation with implant
augmentative communication
    device
augnathus
August automatic gauze packer
Augustine boat nail
Augustine nail
Ault clamp
Ault intestinal clamp
Ault intestinal occlusion clamp
Aumence eyelid speculum
Aura desktop laser
aural applicator
aural atresia
aural fistula
aural forceps
aural magnifier
aural microscope
aural myiasis
aural speculum
auricular fissure
Aureomycin gauze
Aureomycin gauze dressing
Aureomycin sutures
auricle
  accessory auricles
  concha of auricle
  innominate fossa of auricle
  supernumerary auricles
auricle clamp
auricula (*pl.* auriculae)
  apex auriculae
  cartilago auriculae
  concha auriculae
  cymba conchae auriculae
  fossa navicularis auriculae
  fossa triangularis auriculae
  ponticulus auriculae
auricula dextra
auricula sinistra
auricular appendage
auricular appendage catheter
auricular appendage clamp
auricular appendage forceps
auricular appendectomy
auricular appendix
auricular arc
auricular artery
auricular artery clamp
auricular branch

auricular cartilage
auricular cartilage graft
auricular composite graft
auricular fibrillation
auricular fissure of temporal
    bone
auricular ganglion
auricular helix
auricular hillock
auricular ligation
auricular muscle
auricular nerve
auricular point
auricular premature contraction
auricular prosthesis
auricular reconstruction
auricular reflex
auricular region
auricular repositioning
auricular rim-based reverse-
    flow-type of flap
auricular standstill
auricular tag
auricular trauma
auricular tubercle
auricular tubercle of Darwin
auricular veins
auriculare
auricularis
auriculectomy
auriculocephalic angle
auriculocephalic sulcus
auriculocranial
auriculoinfraorbital plane
auriculomastoid
auriculomastoid angle
auriculomastoid area
auriculomastoid line
auriculo-occipital angle
auriculopalpebral reflex
auriculotemporal
auriculotemporal artery
auriculotemporal nerve
auriculotemporal nerve
    syndrome
auriculotemporal neuralgia
auriculoventricular
auriculoventricular groove
auriculoventricular interval
auriculoventricular orifice
auriculoventricular valve
auriform

auris
    ala auris
    antrum auris
    hematoma auris
auris (pl. aures)
auris externa
auris interna
auris media
auris sinister
auriscope
    Zeiss-Bruening anastigmatic
        auriscope
auropalpebral reflex (APR)
Aurora diode laser
Aurora dual-chamber pacemaker
Aurora HL laser
Aurora MR breast imaging
    system scanner
Aurora pulse generator
aurotherapy
Aurovest investment material
Ausculscope carotid bruit
    detector
auscultation
    chest clear to percussion and
        auscultation
    clear to auscultation
    inspection, palpation,
        percussion, and
        auscultation (IPAA)
    Korányi auscultation
    lungs clear to percussion and
        auscultation
    percussion and auscultation
        (P&A)
auscultation sites of heart valves
auscultatory findings
auscultatory gap
auscultatory percussion
auscultatory sound
auscultatory triangle
auscultoscope
Aus-Jena-Gullstrand lens loop
Ausman microsurgery
    instrument
Auspitz sign
Austin attic dissector
Austin awl
Austin bunionectomy
Austin chisel
Austin clip
Austin dental knife

Austin dental retractor
Austin dissection knife
Austin dissector
Austin duckbill elevator
Austin elevator
Austin endolymph dispersement
 shunt
Austin excavator
Austin Flint murmur
Austin Flint phenomenon
Austin Flint respiration
Austin footplate elevation
Austin footplate elevator
Austin forceps
Austin gauge
Austin knife
Austin measuring gauge
Austin middle ear instrument
Austin Moore arthroplasty
Austin Moore bone reamer
Austin Moore bone-measuring
 instrument
Austin Moore corkscrew femoral
 head remover
Austin Moore corkscrew
Austin Moore curved
 endoprosthesis
Austin Moore endoprosthetic
 arthroplasty
Austin Moore extractor
Austin Moore head
Austin Moore hip arthroplasty
Austin Moore hip prosthesis
Austin Moore impactor
Austin Moore inside-outside
 calipers
Austin Moore instruments
Austin Moore mortising chisel
Austin Moore outside calipers
Austin Moore pin
Austin Moore prosthesis
Austin Moore prosthesis-sizing
 set
Austin Moore rasp
Austin Moore reamer
Austin Moore southern
 approach
Austin Moore straight-stem
 endoprosthesis
Austin Moore-Murphy bone
 lever
Austin Moore-Murphy bone skid

Austin needle
Austin otological microsurgery
 set
Austin oval curet
Austin pick
Austin piston
Austin retractor
Austin right-angle elevator
Austin sickle knife
Austin sterilizing storage rack
Austin strut calipers
Austin-Moore bone-measuring
 instrument
Austin-Moore prosthesis rasps
Austin-Shea tympanoplasty
Australian orthodontic wire
Australian Special Plus wire
Auth atherectomy
Auth atherectomy catheter
Auth knife
Autima II dual chamber
 pacemaker
Autima II dual-chamber cardiac
 pacemaker
Autima II pacemaker
Auto Glide walker accessory
auto injector
Auto Ref keratometer
 instrument
Auto Suture (AS)
Auto Suture clip
Auto Suture Clip-A-Matic clip
 applier
Auto Suture curet
Auto Suture device
Auto Suture endoscopic suction-
 irrigation device
Auto Suture forceps
Auto Suture Mini-CABG
 occlusion clamp
Auto Suture Multifire Endo GIA
 30 stapler
Auto Suture One-Shot
 anastomotic device
Auto Suture Premium CEEA
 stapler
Auto Suture Soft Thoracoport
Auto Suture surgical mesh
Auto Suture surgical stapler
Auto Suture SurgiStitch
autoallergic
autoamputation

autoanaphylaxis
autoantibody
autoanticomplement
autoantigen
autoaugmentation
    bladder autoaugmentation
Auto-Band Steri-Drape
Auto-Band Steri-Drape drape
Autoblock safety syringe
AutoCat intra-aortic balloon
    pump
autocaval fistula
autochthonous graft
autochthonous stone
autoclasia
autoclasis
autoclavable
autoclave
Autoclip
    Totco Autoclip
Autoclip applier
Autoclip remover
Autoclix fingerstick lancer
    device
Autocon electrosurgical unit
autocystoplasty
autodermic
autodermic graft
autodigestion of pancreatic
    tissue
autodrainage
autoepidermic graft
autoerotic rectal trauma
Autoflex II continuous passive
    motion units (CPM units)
autofunduscope
autogenetic graft
autogenic graft
autogenous graft
autogenous transplant
autogenous bone graft
autogenous bone grafting
autogenous cartilage graft
autogenous composite tissue
autogenous corticocancellous
    graft
autogenous fascia lata sling
    procedure
autogenous fascial heterograft
autogenous fat graft
autogenous graft
autogenous grafting

autogenous interpositional
    shoulder arthroplasty
autogenous keratoplasty
autogenous nerve graft
autogenous reconstruction
autogenous strip
autogenous tooth
    transplantation
autogenous transplant
autogenous vein
autogenous vein bypass
autogenous vein graft
autograft
    bone autograft
    cranial autografts
    cultured autograft
    cultured epithelial autograft
    cultured epithelium autograft
        (CEA)
    free-revascularized autograft
    iliac autograft
    parathyroid autograft
    pulmonary autograft (PA)
    Russell fibular head autograft
autograft extender
autograft fusion
autograft harvesting
autograft material
Autografter
    ACE Autografter
autografting
    cultured epithelial
        autografting
autographism
autohemotherapy
autoimmune
autoimmune connective tissue
    disorder
autoimmune demyelination
autoimmune disorder
autoimmune hemolysis
autoimmune phenomenon
autoimmune reaction
autoimmune response
autoimmunity
autoinfection
Autolet fingerstick device
autologous augmentation
autologous blood
autologous blood stem cell
    transplantation
autologous bone

autologous bone marrow transplant
autologous bone marrow transplantation (ABMT)
autologous clot
autologous donor
autologous fat graft
autologous fat transplantation
autologous fat-injection techniques
autologous fat-transplanting techniques
autologous fibrin tissue adhesive
autologous graft
autologous growth factor (AGF)
autologous human collagen
autologous human collagen augmentation
autologous iliac crest bone graft
autologous implant
autologous patient donor
autologous pericardial patch
autologous platelet gel
autologous rib bone graft
autologous stem
autologous tissue flaps
autologous transfusion
autologous vein graft
autologous-cultured epithelium (ACE)
autolysis
autolytic debridement
autolytic debridement cream
autolyzed
automated
automated cerebral blood flow analyzer
automated computerized axial tomography (ACAT)
automated corneal shaper (ACS)
automated endoscope reprocessor
automated endoscopic system for optimal positioning surgical robot
automated external defibrillator pacemaker (AEDP)
automated hemisphere perimeter
automated intravitreal scissors
automated large-core liver biopsy

automated laser fluorescence sequencer
automated percutaneous diskectomy
automated refractor
automated retractor
automated trephine
automatic catheter
automatic chemical analyzer
automatic clinical analyzer
automatic corneal trephine
automatic cranial drill
automatic endoscopic reprocessor
automatic external defibrillator (AED)
automatic finger
automatic gas sequence
automatic Hemoclip applier
automatic implantable cardiovascular defibrillator (AICD)
automatic implantable cardioverter-defibrillator (AICD)
automatic internal cardioverter-defibrillator (AICD)
automatic intracardiac defibrillator
automatic needle driver
automatic ratchet snare
automatic rotating tourniquet
automatic screwdriver
automatic single-needle monitor (ASN monitor)
automatic skin retractor
automatic stapling device
automatic suction device
automatic tourniquet
automatic twin syringe injector
Automator computerized distraction device
autonomic
autonomic blockade
autonomic ganglion block
autonomic nerve block
autonomic neurogenic bladder
auto-ophthalmoscope
auto-ophthalmoscopy
AutoPap automated screening device
AutoPap reader

autoperfusion balloon
autoperfusion balloon catheter
autophagocytosed cellular
   material
Autophor femoral prosthesis
Autophor hip component
Autophor total hip
autoplastic graft
autoplasty
   peritoneal autoplasty
Autoplot
autopsy
   laparoscopic autopsy
autopsy blade
autopsy blade handle
autopsy handle
autoradiographic film
autoradiographic technique
autoradiography
   dip coating autoradiography
   thick-layer autoradiography
autoregulation
autoreinfusion
autorotation
autorrhaphy
autosomal
autosomal dominant
autosomal dominant polycystic
   kidney disease
autosomal recessive
Autostat hemostatic clip
Autostat ligating clip
Auto Suture (AS)
Auto Suture Clip-A-Matic clip
   applier
Auto Suture curet
Auto Suture EEA instrument
Auto Suture forceps
Auto Suture GIA stapler
Auto Suture stapler
Auto Suture surgical stapler
Auto Suture Surgiclip
Auto Suture TA-50 staple gun
Auto Suture technique
Autosyringe insulin pump
Autosyringe pump
autotome drill
Autotrans system for blood
   recovery
autotransfusion
autotransfusor-prepared platelet
   gel

autotransplant
autotransplantation
   colostomy pyloric
      autotransplantation
   pancreatic autotransplantation
posttraumatic
      autotransplantation
   pyloric autotransplantation
   renal autotransplantation
autotrophic fixation
Autraugrip forceps
Autraugrip tissue forceps
Auvard Britetrac speculum
Auvard clamp
Auvard cranioclast
Auvard speculum
Auvard weighted vaginal retractor
Auvard weighted vaginal
      speculum
Auvard-Remine speculum
Auvard-Remine vaginal speculum
Auvard-Remine weighted
      speculum
Auvard-Zweifel basiotribe
Auvard-Zweifel forceps
Auvray incision
auxiliary lens
auxiliary partial orthotopic liver
      transplantation (APOLT)
auxiliary transplant
AV (aortic valve, atriovenous,
      atrioventricular)
AV aneurysm (arteriovenous
      aneurysm)
AV block (atrioventricular block)
AV bundle (atrioventricular
      bundle)
AV conduction defect
      (atrioventricular
      conduction defect)
AV DeClot catheter
AV fistula (arteriovenous fistula)
AV fistula needle
AV Gore-Tex fistula
      (arteriovenous Gore-Tex
      fistula)
AV Gore-Tex graft (arteriovenous
      Gore-Tex graft)
AV Impulse foot pump
AV junctional pacemaker
      (atrioventricular junctional
      pacemaker)

A-V malformation
AV Miniclinic (atrioventricular
    Miniclinic)
AV nodal modification
AV node (atrioventricular node)
AV repair (aortic valve repair)
AV sequential demand
    pacemaker (atrioventricular
    sequential demand
    pacemaker)
AV sequential pacemaker
    (atrioventricular sequential
    pacemaker)
AV shunt (arteriovenous shunt)
AV synchronous pacemaker
    (atrioventricular
    synchronous pacemaker)
AVA (arteriovenous anastomosis)
AVA 3Xi venous access device
available arch length
Avalox skin clip
Avance hearing enhancer
Avant Gauze nonwoven gauze
Avanta soft skeletal implant
Avanti introducer
avascular
avascular fragment
avascular graft
avascular necrosis
avascular space
avascular tissue
avascularization
AVCO aortic balloon
AVDO$_2$ (arteriovenous oxygen
    difference)
AVE GFX coronary stent
AVE Micro stent
Aveline Gutierrez
    parotidectomy
Avellis syndrome
Avenida dilator
Avenida-Torres dilator
average flow rate
Averett total hip
    endoprosthesis
Avertin anesthetic agent
AVF (arteriovenous fistula)
aviator's astragalus
aviator's ear
aviator's fracture
avidin-biotin-peroxidase
    complex (ABC)

Avila approach
Avila operation
Avila technique
Avina female urethral plug
Avionics two-channel Holter
    recorder
avis
    calcar avis
Avitene fibrillar collagen
Avitene hemostatic material
Avitene microfibrillar collage
    hemostat
Avitene microfibrillar collagen
    hemostat
Avitene sandwich
Avitene Ultrafoam collagen
    hemostat
Avius sequential pacemaker
Avius sequential pacemaker
    avivement
avivement
    Avius sequential pacemaker
    avivement
AVM (arteriovenous
    malformation)
AVM (atrioventricular
    malformation)
AVN (avascular necrosis)
AvocetPT rapid prothrombin
    time meter
Avodart
avoidance maneuver
AV-Paceport thermodilution
    catheter
Avtifoam active hemostat
avulsed fragment
avulsed laceration
avulsed wound
avulsion
    cortex avulsion
    mechanical avulsion
    nerve avulsion
    phrenic avulsion
    traumatic avulsion
avulsion amputation
avulsion chip fracture
avulsion flap injury
avulsion fracture
avulsion injury
avulsion of caruncula lacrimalis
avulsion of epiphysis
avulsion of eyeball

avulsion of finger
avulsion of nerve
avulsion of optic nerve
avulsion stress fraction
avulsion technique
awake craniotomy
awake neurological assessment
awaken
  failure to awaken
awareness
  body awareness
  level of awareness
awl
  Aufranc awl
  Aufranc trochanteric awl
  Austin awl
  bone awl
  Carroll awl
  Carter-Rowe awl
  curved awl
  DePuy awl
  Ferran awl
  Kelsey-Fry bone awl
  Kirklin sternal awl
  lacrimal awl
  Mark II kodros radiolucent
    awl
  Mustarde awl
  Obwegeser awl
  pointed awl
  reamer awl
  reaming awl
  rectangular awl
  rib brad awl
  Rochester awl
  Rush pin reamer awl
  starter awl
  Stedman awl
  sternal perforating awl
  sternum perforating awl
  Swanson scaphoid awl
  T-handle bone awl
  T-handled awl
  trochanteric awl
  Uniflex distal targeting awl
  Wangensteen awl
  Wilson awl
  Wilson right-angled awl
  wire-passing awl
  Zelicof orthopaedic awl
  Zuelzer awl
Axenfeld anomaly

Axenfeld loop
Axenfeld nerve loop
Axenfeld suture technique
Axenfeld sutures
Axer operation
Axer technique
Axer tendon transfer into talus
Axer-Clark procedure
axes (*sing.* axis)
Axhausen cleft lip repair
Axhausen needle holder
axial advancement flap
axial anchor screw
axial aneurysm
axial cataract
axial compression
axial compression injury
axial computed tomography
  scan
axial dorsal flap
axial fixation
axial flag flap
axial flap
axial frontonasal flap
axial fusiform cataract
axial gradiometer
axial hiatal hernia
axial lesion
axial line angle
axial loading fracture
axial myopia
axial pattern scalp flap
axial pattern vascularized skin
  flap
axial plane
axial point
axial projection
axial resolution
axial rotation joint
axial skeleton
axial spin-echo image
axial surface cavity
axial temporoparietal facial flap
axial tractor
axial-based flap
axilla (*pl.* axillae)
axilla, shoulder, and elbow
  bandage (ASE bandage)
axillary
axillary abscess
axillary adenopathy
axillary anesthesia

axillary approach
axillary arch
axillary artery
axillary artery aneurysm
axillary artery catheterization
axillary block
axillary block anesthesia
axillary block anesthetic
    technique
axillary breast tissue
axillary bypass
axillary catheter
axillary contracture
axillary endoscopic reduction
axillary fascia
axillary flap
axillary fold
axillary foramen
axillary fossa
axillary gland
axillary hematoma
axillary hidradenitis
axillary incision
axillary insertion
axillary line
axillary lymphadenectomy
axillary lymph node dissection
    (ALND)
axillary lymphadenopathy
axillary nerve
axillary node
axillary node dissection
axillary node metastasis
axillary perivascular technique
axillary region
axillary skin lesion
axillary space
axillary subpectoral approach
axillary sweat gland
axillary tail of Spence
axillary technique of brachial
    plexus block
axillary vascular injury
axillary vein
axilloaxillary bypass
axillobifemoral
axillobifemoral bypass
axillobifemoral bypass graft
axillofemoral
axillofemoral bypass
axillounifemoral bypass
axiobuccal

axiobuccocervical (ABC)
axiobuccogingival (ABG)
axiobuccolingual (ABL)
axiobuccolingual plane
axiocervical (AC)
axiodistal
axiodistocervical
axiodistogingival
axiodistoincisal
axiodisto-occlusal
axioincisal
axiolabial
axiolabiogingival
axiolabiolingual
axiolabiolingual plane
axiolingual
axiolingual (AL) reconstruction
axiolinguocervical
axiolinguogingival
axiolinguo-occlusal
Axiom DG balloon angioplasty
Axiom DG balloon angioplasty
    catheter
Axiom double sump pump
Axiom drain
Axiom knee component
Axiom thoracic trocar
axiomesial
axiomesiocervical
axiomesiodistal
axiomesiodistal plane
axiomesiogingival
axiomesioincisal
axiomesio-occlusal
axio-occlusal
axiopulpal
Axios pacemaker
axis
    basibregmatic axis
    basicranial axis
    basifacial axis
    binauricular axis
    bowel axis
    celiac axis
    cephalocaudal axis
    cerebrospinal axis
    ciliary axis
    condylar axis
    conjugate axis
    craniofacial axis
    cylinder axis
    deutan axis

axis (*continued*)
 facial axis
 flexion-extension axis
 hinge axis
 hypothalamic-hypophysial-
  ovarian-endometrial axis
 hypothalamic-pituitary-adrenal
  axis
 hypothalamic-pituitary-ovarian
  axis
 hypothalamic-pituitary-
  testicular axis
 long axis
 long posterior ciliary axis
 longitudinal axis
 mandibular axis
 mechanical axis
 mesentericoportal axis
 midpapillary short axis
 opening axis
 optic axis
 orbital axis
 pelvic axis
 protan axis
 radial-ulnar deviation axis
 sagittal axis
 short axis
 short posterior ciliary axis
 supraoptico-hypophyseal axis
 Tessier cleft axis
 thoracic axis
 thyroid axis
 transverse axis
 transverse horizontal axis
 vertical axis
 Y axis
axis (*pl.* axes)
axis corpuscle
axis deviation
axis fixation
axis fracture
axis ligament
axis of rotation
axis pelvis
axis traction
axis-atlas fracture
axis-atlas joint
Axisonic II ultrasound
axis traction forceps
axometer
axon
 dendrites and axons

axon (*continued*)
 injured axon
 motor axon
 myelinated axon
axonal
axonal continuity
axonal damage
axonal demyelination
axonal growth
axonal injury
axonal regeneration
axonotmesis
axonometic injury
Axostim nerve stimulator
Axxcess ureteral catheter
Axxess spinal cord stimulator
Axya bone anchor system and
  kit (BAK)
AxyaWeld bone anchor
AxyaWeld instrument
Ayers cardiovascular needle
  holder
Ayers chalazion forceps
Ayers forceps
Ayers needle holder
Ayers spatula
Ayers sphygmomanometer
Ayers T-piece
Ayerst instruments
Ayerst knife
Aylesbury cervical spatula
Aylett operation
Ayre brush
Ayre cervical spatula
Ayre cone knife
Ayre knife
Ayre spatula-Zelsmyr Cytobrush
  technique
Ayre tube
Ayre-Scott cervical cone knife
Ayre-Scott knife
Azar corneal scissors
Azar cystitome
Azar flexible-loop anterior
  chamber intraocular lens
Azar forceps
Azar intraocular forceps
Azar iris retractor
Azar lens forceps
Azar lens hook
Azar lid speculum
Azar Mark II intraocular lens

Azar needle holder
Azar Tripod eye implant
Azar Tripod implant cataract
   lens
Azar Tripod lens
Azar tying forceps
Azar utility forceps
azelaic acid
Aztec ear
Aztec type
azygoesophageal line

azygogram
azygography
azygoportal interruption
azygos
   vena azygos
azygos arch
azygos fissure
azygos lobe
azygos vein
azygos vein arch
azygous

B

B
  mucopolysaccharidosis type III
    Sanfilippo B (MPS-IIIB)
  point B
B cell line
B phenotypic lymphocyte
B point
B&D needle
B&L pinch gauge
B&S gauge sutures (Brown-
  Sharp)
BE glass abdominal retractor
BH Moore procedure
BIP (Breast Implant Protector)
BIP biopsy instrument
BUS Endotron-Lipectron
  ultrasonic scalpel
B-1 craniotome attachment
  (*also* B-2, etc.)
B-12 dental curet
BA bone cement
BA bone cement adhesive
Babbitt metal
Babcock clamp
Babcock empyema trocar
Babcock Endo Grasp
Babcock forceps
Babcock inguinal herniorrhaphy
Babcock intestinal forceps
Babcock jointed vein stripper
Babcock lung-grasping forceps
Babcock needle
Babcock operation
Babcock plate
Babcock raspatory
Babcock retractor
Babcock stainless steel suture
  wire
Babcock suture wire
Babcock thoracic tissue-holding
  forceps
Babcock tissue clamp
Babcock tissue forceps

Babcock trocar
Babcock tube
Babcock vein stripper
Babcock Vital atraumatic forceps
Babcock Vital intestinal forceps
Babcock Vital tissue forceps
Babcock wire sutures
Babcock wire-cutting scissors
Babcock-Beasley forceps
Babinski percussion hammer
Babinski reflex
Babinski sign
baby Adson brain retractor
baby Adson forceps
baby Allis forceps
baby Balfour retractor
baby Barraquer needle holder
baby Bishop clamp
baby Collin abdominal retractor
baby costal periosteotome
baby Crile forceps
baby Crile needle holder
baby Crile-Wood needle holder
Baby Dopplex 3000 antepartum
  fetal monitor
baby dressing forceps
baby hemostatic forceps
baby Inge bone spreader
baby Inge laminar spreader
baby intestinal tissue forceps
baby Kocher clamp
baby Lane bone-holding forceps
baby Metzenbaum scissors
baby Mikulicz forceps
baby Miller blade
baby Miller laryngoscope
baby Mixter forceps
baby mosquito forceps
baby needle holder
baby Overholt forceps
baby pylorus clamp
baby retractor
baby rib contractor

baby Roux retractor
baby Satinsky clamp
baby scope
baby Senn-Miller retractor
baby spur crusher
baby Tischler biopsy punch
baby tissue forceps
baby Weitlaner self-retaining
    retractor
BabyBeat ultrasound instrument
BABYbird II respirator
BABYbird II ventilator
BABYbird respirator
Babyflex ventilator
babygram
Babytherm IC gel mattress
Bachmann bundle
bacitracin dressing
bacitracin irrigation
bacitracin ointment
bacitracin solution
bacitracin strips
Baciu-Filibiu ankle arthrodesis
back
    drawn back
    low back
    lower back
    rolled back
    V-Y push back
back brace
Back Bubble gravity traction unit
Back Bull lumbar support
    cushion
back manipulation
back pressure
back range-of-motion device
Back Specialist electric table
back table
back vest
back, leg and chest
    dynamometer
backache
back-and-forth suture technique
back-and-forth vibrating
    cannulas
backbar device
backbiter
    MicroFrance pediatric
        backbiter
BackBiter instrument
backbiting bone punch
backbiting forceps

backbiting rongeur
backbleeding
backbone
backcut incision
backcutting knife
BackCycler continuous passive
    motion device
Back-Ease aromatherapy
    hot/cold pack
backfire fracture
backflow
    pyelovenous backflow
backflow bleeding
backflush
Backhaus cervical knife
Backhaus clip
Backhaus dilator
Backhaus towel clamp
Backhaus towel clip
Backhaus towel forceps
Backhaus-Jones towel clamp
Backhaus-Kocher towel clamp
Backhaus-Roeder forceps
Back-Huggar lumbar support
    cushion
back-knee deformity
Backlund stereotactic
    instrument
Backmann thyroid retractor
BackMaster device
back-stop laser probe
back-stopped laser instruments
backstroke injury
BackThing lumbar support
back-up position
backward autorotation of the
    mandible
backward masking
backward position
backward-biting ostrum punch
backward-cutting knife
backward-cutting scissors
Bacon anoscope
Bacon bone rongeur
Bacon cranial forceps
Bacon cranial retractor
Bacon cranial rongeur
Bacon forceps
Bacon periosteal raspatory
Bacon proctoscope
Bacon raspatory
Bacon retractor

Bacon rib shears
Bacon rongeur
Bacon rongeur forceps
Bacon shears
Bacon thoracic shears
Bacon-Babcock operation
Bacstop check valve
bacteremia
  gram-negative bacteremia
  gram-positive bacteremia
bacteria
  aerobic bacteria
  anaerobic bacteria
  vegetative bacteria
bacterial barrier
bacterial complication
bacterial contamination
bacterial endocarditis
bacterial filter
bacterial infection
bacterial keratoconjunctivitis
bacterial meningitis (BM)
bacterial mucosal infiltration
bacterial septicemia
bacterial sialadenitis
bacterial virus
bactericidal antibiotic
bactericidal concentration
bacteriolytic
bacteriolytic action
bacteriostatic
bacteriostatic antibiotic
bacteriostatic barrier
Badal operation
Baden Silastic rod
Badenoch urethroplasty
badger's triangle
Badgley arthrodesis
Badgley combination procedure
Badgley hip arthrodesis
Badgley iliac wing resection
Badgley laminectomy retractor
Badgley nail
Badgley operation
Badgley plate
Badgley retractor
Badgley technique
Bado classification
Baehr-Lohlein lesion
Baek musculocutaneous pedicle
    technique
Baelz disease

Baer bone rongeur
Baer bone-cutting forceps
Baer forceps
Baer rib shears
Baer vesicle
Baerveldt glaucoma implant
    tube
Baerveldt seton implant
Baerveldt shunt tube
Baffe anastomosis
baffle
  atrial baffle
  fabric baffle
  Gore-Tex baffle
  intra-atrial baffle
  pericardial baffle
baffle anastomosis
baffle fenestration
baffle operation
baffle transplant
bag
  2-way hemostatic bag
  3M limb isolation bag
  3-point spreader bag
  Aberhart disposable urinal
      bag
  Aberhart hemostatic bag
  ACMI bag
  air bag
  Alcock hemostatic bag
  Ambu bag
  arterial line pressure bag
  Bard bag
  Bard Dispoz-A-Bag leg bag
  Bardex hemostatic bag
  Barnes bag
  bile bag
  Biohazard bag
  Bogota bag
  Bomgart stomal bag
  bowel bag
  Brake hemostatic bag
  breathing bag
  Brodney hemostatic bag
  Bunyan bag
  Cardiff resuscitation bag
  Champetier de Ribes
      obstetrical bag
  cheek bag
  CLO cool Bag
  Coloplast bag
  Coloplast colostomy bag

bag (*continued*)
Coloplast urine leg bag
colostomy bag
Conveen bedside drainage bag
Conveen deluxe contoured leg bag
coudé hemostatic bag
Curity leg bag
Davol bag
Deluxe Button Bag
DeRoyal Surgical grab bag
dialysate bag
Diamed leg bag
Douglas bag
drainage bag
Duval bag
Dynacor leg bag
Emmet hemostatic bag
Endobag specimen bag
EndoMate grab bag
Endopouch Pro specimen-retrieval bag
Endosac specimen bag
Endo Sock retrieval bag
exudate disposal bag
Foley hemostatic bag
Foley Alcock bag
Foley Alcock hemostatic bag
four-point spreader bag
Freedom T-tap leg bag
Frenta enteral feeding bag
Gambro freezing bag
gauze tissue bag
GEM nonlatex medical bag
Grafco colostomy bag
Grafco ileostomy bag
Greck ileostomy bag
Hagner hemostatic bag
Hagner urethral bag
Hemofreeze blood bag
hemostatic bag
Hendrickson hemostatic bag
Heyer-Schulte disposal bag
Heyer-Schulte Pour-Safe exudate bag
Higgins hemostatic bag
Hofmeister drainage bag
Hollister colostomy bag
Hollister drainage bag
Hollister urostomy bag
Hope resuscitation bag

bag (*continued*)
hydrostatic bag
ice bag
ileostomy bag
Incono bag
infusible pressure infusion bag
Infu-Surg pressure infuser bag
intestinal bag
intracervical bag
isolation bag
Karaya seal ileostomy stomal bag
Kern bag
Lahey bag
Lapides collecting bag
Lapides ileostomy bag
latex bag
Le Bag
Lifesaver disposable resuscitator bag
Lyster water bag
Mac-Lee enema bag
malar bag
manual resuscitation bag
Marlen ileostomy bag
Marlen leg bag
Marlen weightless bag
Melmed blood freezing bag
micturition bag
millinery bag
Mosher bag
Nesbit hemostatic bag
night drainage bag
ostomy bag
Owen hemostatic bag
Paul condom bag
Paul hemostatic bag
Pearman transurethral hemostatic bag
pear-shaped fluted bag
Peel Pak bag
Pennine leg bag
Perry ileostomy bag
Petersen rectal bag
Pilcher hemostatic bag
Pilcher hemostatic suprapubic bag
Pilcher suprapubic hemostatic bag
Plummer bag
pneumatic bag
Politzer air bag

bag (*continued*)
Politzer bag
Ponsky Endo-Sock specimen
    retrieval bag
prostatectomy bag
rebreathing bag
replacement collection bag
Robinson bag
Rusch leg bag
Rutzen ileostomy bag
severance transurethral bag
Shea-Anthony bag
short-tip bag
short-tip hemostatic bag
sleeve bag
Soft Guard XL fecal
    incontinence bag
Sones hemostatic bag
sterile isolation bag
stomal bag
suprapubic bag
suprapubic hemostatic bag
SureGrip breathing bag
Sur-Fit colostomy bag
Sur-Fit urinary drainage bag
Surgi-Flo leg bag
Swenko bag
Tassett vaginal cup bag
Tedlar bag
Teflo-Kapton freezing bag
Thackston retropubic bag
trauma induced saddle bag
Travenol heart bag
Uri-Drain leg bag
urinary leg bag
Urocare latex reusable leg bag
Uro-Safe vinyl disposable leg
    bag
vaginal bag
Van Hove bag
Versi-Splint carry bag
Vi-Drape bowel bag
Voorhees bag
VPI urinary leg bag
Whitmore bag
Wolf hemostatic bag
bag and mask
Bag Bath
bag catheter
bag extraction
bag of waters
bag-and-mask ventilation

Bagby compression plate
Bagby plate
BagEasy disposable manual
    resuscitator
bag-fixated intraocular lens
bagged
bagged mask ventilation
bag-gel implant
bagginess of eyes
bagging
Baggish hysteroscope
Baghdad boil
Baghdad button
Bagley helical basket
Bagley-Wilmer expressor
Bagley-Wilmer lens expressor
bag-of-bones technique
Bagolini lens
bagpipe vertebral outgrowth
bag-valve resuscitator
bag-valve mask-assisted
    ventilation
Bahama suture scissors
Bahler elbow arthroplasty
Bahn spud
Bahnson aortic aneurysm clamp
Bahnson aortic cannula
Bahnson aortic clamp
Bahnson cannula
Bahnson clamp
Bahnson retractor
Bahnson sternal retractor
Bahnson-Brown forceps
Baikoff lens
Bailey aortic clamp
Bailey aortic valve rongeur
Bailey aortic valve-cutting
    forceps
Bailey baby rib contractor
Bailey bur
Bailey cannula
Bailey catheter
Bailey chalazion forceps
Bailey conductor
Bailey contractor
Bailey dilator
Bailey drill
Bailey duckbill clamp
Bailey forceps
Bailey foreign body remover
Bailey Gigli-saw guide
Bailey lacrimal cannula

Bailey leukotome
Bailey operation
Bailey pliers
Bailey punch
Bailey rib approximator
Bailey rib contractor
Bailey rib elevator
Bailey rib spreader
Bailey rod
Bailey rongeur
Bailey round knife
Bailey saw conductor
Bailey shooter
Bailey skull bur
Bailey spreader
Bailey transthoracic catheter
Bailey wire saw
Bailey-Badgley anterior cervical
    approach
Bailey-Badgley arthrodesis
Bailey-Badgley cervical spine
    approach
Bailey-Badgley cervical spine
    fusion
Bailey-Badgley technique
Bailey-Cowley clamp
Bailey-Dubow femoral shaft
    procedure
Bailey-Dubow technique
Bailey-Gibbon contractor
Bailey-Gibbon rib contractor
Bailey-Glover-O'Neill
    commissurotomy knife
Bailey-Glover-O'Neill knife
Bailey-Glover-O'Neill
    valvulotome
Bailey-Morse clamp
Bailey-Morse knife
Bailey-Morse mitral knife
Bailey-Williamson forceps
Bailey-Williamson obstetrical
    forceps
Bailliart goniometer
Bailliart
    ophthalmodynamometer
Bailliart ophthalmoscope
Bailliart tonometer
bail-lock brace
bail-lock splint
bailout autoperfusion balloon
    catheter
bailout catheter

bailout stent
bailout valvuloplasty
Baim catheter
Baim pacing catheter
Baim-Turi cardiac device
Baim-Turi monitoring/pacing
    catheter
Baim-Turi pacing
Bainbridge anastomosis clamp
Bainbridge hemostatic forceps
Bainbridge intestinal clamp
Bainbridge intestinal forceps
Bainbridge reflex
Bainbridge resection forceps
Bainbridge thyroid forceps
Bainbridge vessel clamp
Bair Hugger fluid warming
    device
Bair Hugger infant warming
    device
Bair Hugger patient heating unit
Bair Hugger patient warming
    blanket
Baird chalazion forceps
Baird Electric System 5000 Power
    Plus electrosurgical unit
Baird forceps
Bairnsdale ulcer
Baiter modification of Shirodkar
    procedure
baja
    patella baja
BAK cage
BAK laparoscopic procedure
BAK/C cervical interbody fusion
    implant
BAK/Proximity interbody fusion
    implant
Bakamjian flap
Bakamjian pedicle flap
Bakamjian tubed flap
Bakelite cystoscopy sheath
Bakelite dental chisel
Bakelite hammer
Bakelite mallet
Bakelite resectoscope sheath
Bakelite retractor
Bakelite spatula
Bakelite-handled osteotome
Baker anastomosis
Baker anchorage
Baker capsular contracture

Baker classification of capsular
    contracture (*grades 1-4*)
Baker composite graft
Baker continuous flow capillary
    drain
Baker cyst
Baker forceps
Baker grade
Baker contracture (*grades 1-4*)
Baker intestinal decompression
    tube
Baker jejunostomy tube
Baker patellar advancement
    operation
Baker patellar tendon procedure
Baker procedure
Baker punch
Baker pyridine extraction
Baker self-sumping tube
Baker syndrome
Baker technique
Baker tissue forceps
Baker translocation operation
Baker velum
Baker-Gordon peel
Baker-Hill osteotomy
Baker-Lima-Baker mask (BLB mask)
Bakes bile duct dilator
Bakes common duct dilator
Bakes probe
Bakes-Pearce dilator
Bakst cardiac scissors
Bakst scissors
Bakst valvulotome
BAL (bronchoalveolar lavage)
Balacescu technique
Balacescu-Golden technique
Baladi Inverter
balance
    delicate balance
    occlusal balance
    occlusion balance
balance bridge
Balance hip prosthesis
balance pad
balance padding orthosis
balanced anesthetic technique
balanced articulation
balanced contact between the
    cusps
balanced force instrumentation
    technique

balanced general anesthesia
balanced salt solution (BSS)
balanced suspension
balanced traction device
balanic hypospadias
balanitis
    Follmann balanitis
balanoplasty
Balbiani body
bald gastric fundus
bald tongue
baldness
    Juri II, III degree of male
        pattern baldness
    male pattern baldness
Baldwin butterfly ventilation
    tube
Baldwin operation
Baldy operation
Baldy-Webster hysteropexy
Baldy-Webster operation
Baldy-Webster operation for
    retrodisplacement of uterus
Baldy-Webster procedure
Baldy-Webster uterine
    suspension
Balectrode pacing catheter
Balectrode pacing probe
BALF (bronchoalveolar lavage
    fluid)
Balfour 4th blade extension
Balfour abdominal retractor
Balfour bladder blade
Balfour center blade
Balfour center-blade abdominal
    retractor
Balfour clamp
Balfour gastrectomy
Balfour gastric resection
Balfour gastroenterostomy
Balfour lateral blade
Balfour pediatric abdominal
    retractor
Balfour pediatric retractor
Balfour retractor
Balfour retractor with
    fenestrated blade
Balfour retractor with
    fenestrated blades
Balfour self-retaining retractor
Balkan femoral splint
Balkan fracture frame

Balkin Up & Over introducer
Balkwell articulator
ball
  Adams ball
  Anderson double ball
  Articul-eze hip ball
  birthing ball
  Body Ball
  Cajal axonal retraction ball
  cauterizing ball
  cold-weld femoral ball
  cotton balls
  Finger Fitness Spring Ball
  fungus ball
  Gertie ball
  Gripp squeeze ball
  gym ball
  Gymnastik ball
  Gymnic ball
  hair ball
  hand exercise ball
  HeavyMed ball
  ice ball
  Jurgan pin ball
  KBM cotton ball
  Ledraplastic exercise ball
  PhysioGymnic exercise ball
  Physio-Roll VisuaLiser exercise
    ball
  Pinky ball
  plastic ball
  polyethylene ball
  Silastic ball
  Slo-Mo ball
  Spondex sponge ball
  squeeze ball
  Stycar graded ball
  Super Pinky ball
  Swiss ball
  Thera-Band exercise ball
  Theragym ball
  therapy ball
  Wooden Wobble balance ball
ball burnisher
ball coagulator
ball dissector
ball electrode
ball electrode desiccation
ball extractor
ball fastener
ball forceps
ball heart valve

ball joint block
ball nerve hook
ball poppet
ball reamer
ball reusable electrode
ball tipped scissors
ball valve prosthesis
ball wedge
Ballade needle
Ballance mastoid spoon
Ballance sign
ball-and-cage prosthesis
ball-and-cage prosthetic valve
ball-and-cage valve prosthesis
ball-and-socket ankle prosthesis
ball-and-socket joint
ball-and-socket osteotomy
Ballantine clamp
Ballantine hemilaminectomy
    retractor
Ballantine hysterectomy forceps
Ballantine uterine curet
Ballantine-Drew coagulator
Ballantine-Peterson forceps
Ballantine-Peterson
    hysterectomy forceps
Ballard examination
ball-cage prosthesis
ball-cage valve
Ballen eye repair
Ballen-Alexander forceps
Ballen-Alexander orbital
    retractor
Ballen-Alexander retractor
ball-end elevator
ball-end hook
Ballenger bur
Ballenger cartilage knife
Ballenger chisel
Ballenger elevator
Ballenger ethmoid curet
Ballenger follicle electrode
Ballenger gouge
Ballenger hysterectomy forceps
Ballenger mastoid bur
Ballenger mucosa knife
Ballenger mucosal knife
Ballenger nasal knife
Ballenger nose knife
Ballenger periosteotome
Ballenger raspatory
Ballenger septal elevator

Ballenger septal knife
Ballenger sponge forceps
Ballenger sponge-holding
    forceps
Ballenger swivel knife
Ballenger tonsil forceps
Ballenger tonsillar forceps
Ballenger tonsil-seizing forceps
Ballenger urethroscope
Ballenger-Foerster forceps
Ballenger-Hajek approximator
Ballenger-Hajek chisel
Ballenger-Hajek elevator
Ballenger-Lillie bur
Ballenger-Lillie mastoid bur
Ballenger-Sluder guillotine
Ballenger-Sluder tonometer
Ballenger-Sluder tonsillectome
Baller-Gerold syndrome
ballet sign
Ball-Hoffman operation
ballistic energy generator
ballistic movement
ballistics
    wound ballistics
ballistocardiogram
ballistocardiography
Ballobes gastric balloon
ball-occluder valve
balloon
    Accent-DG balloon
    ACE balloon
    ACS SULP II balloon
    Acucise balloon
    angioplasty balloon
    Anthony-Fisher antral balloon
    Anthony-Fisher antrum
        balloon
    Anthony-Fisher balloon
    antral balloon
    antrum balloon
    Arrow-Berman angiographic
        balloon
    autoperfusion balloon
    AVCO aortic balloon
    Ballobes gastric balloon
    banana-shaped balloon
    Bandit low-profile over-the-
        wire balloon
    Bardex balloon
    barium enema retention
        balloon

balloon (*continued*)
    barostat balloon
    Baxter Intrepid balloon
    Baylor balloon
    Baylor cervical balloon
    bifoil balloon
    Bilisystem stone-removal
        balloon
    Blue Max high-pressure
        balloon
    Brandt cytology balloon
    Brighton balloon
    Brighton epistaxis balloon
    catheter balloon
    centering balloon
    compliant balloon
    Cook balloon
    counterpulsation balloon
    Cribier-Letac aortic
        valvuloplasty balloon
    cutting balloon
    cylindrical balloon
    Datascope balloon
    delivery balloon
    detachable balloon
    Distaflex balloon
    doughnut-shaped balloon
    electrode balloon
    electro-detachable balloon
    Eliminator dilatation balloon
    endocapsular balloon
    Epistat double balloon
    epistaxis balloon
    esophageal balloon
    Express balloon
    extraction balloon
    Extractor XL triple-lumen
        retrieval balloon
    fixed-wire balloon
    Fogarty balloon
    Foley balloon
    Force balloon
    Fox balloon
    Fox postnasal balloon
    French Swan-Ganz balloon
    Garren-Edwards balloon
    Garren-Edwards gastric
        balloon
    gastric balloon
    Gau gastric balloon
    Giesy ureteral dilatation
        balloon

balloon (*continued*)
  Gruentzig balloon
  Gruentizig balloon
  Guidant balloon
  Hadow balloon
  Hartzler angioplasty balloon
  Hartzler Micro II angioplasty
    balloon
  helix balloon
  Helmstein balloon
  high-compliance latex
    balloon
  Honan balloon
  Hunter balloon
  Hunter-Sessions balloon
  hydrostatic balloon
  inflated balloon
  Inoue self-guiding balloon
  Integra II balloon
  intra-aortic balloon
  intra-aortic counterpulsation
    balloon
  intragastric balloon
  intraocular balloon
  Katzin-Long balloon
  Kaye tamponade balloon
  kissing balloon
  Kontron balloon
  Kontron intra-aortic balloon
  laser balloon
  latex balloon
  Lo-Profile balloon
  low-compliance balloon
  low-profile angioplasty
    balloon
  LPS balloon
  Mansfield balloon
  mercury-containing balloon
  metrizamide-filled balloon
  Micross SL balloon
  Microvasic Rigiflex balloon
  Microvasive retrieval balloon
  Microvasive Rigiflex through-
    the-scope balloon
  Microvasive Rigiflex TTS
    balloon
  Monorail Speedy balloon
  nasomaxillary balloon
  NC Cobra balloon
  noncompliant balloon
  nondetachable endovascular
    balloon

balloon (*continued*)
  nondetachable occlusive
    balloon
  NoProfile balloon
  NuMED single balloon
  occlusion balloon
  occlusive balloon
  Olbert balloon
  Omega-NV balloon
  Omni SST balloon
  Omniflex balloon
  Origin balloon
  Origin PDB 1000 balloon
  Orion balloon
  Owen balloon
  Passage exchange balloon
  PDB preperitoneal distention
    balloon
  Percival gastric balloon
  Percor-Stat intra-aortic balloon
  PET balloon
  Piccolino balloon
  pillow-shaped balloon
  Pivot balloon
  POC balloon
  polyethylene terephthalate
    balloon
  polyolefin copolymer balloon
  polyvinyl chloride balloon
  positron emission
    tomography balloon (PET
    balloon)
  postnasal balloon
  preperitoneal distention
    balloon
  Prime balloon
  ProCross Rely balloon
  Provocative sensitivity balloon
  pulmonary balloon
  Quantum TTC biliary balloon
  QuickFurl balloon
  QuickFurl double-lumen
    balloon
  QuickFurl single-lumen
    balloon
  Rashkind balloon
  rectal balloon
  RediFurl balloon
  RediFurl double-lumen
    balloon
  RediFurl single-lumen balloon
  retrieval balloon

balloon (*continued*)

Riepe-Bard gastric balloon
Rigiflex achalasia balloon
Rigiflex balloon
Rigiflex TTS balloon
Rushkin balloon
Schneider-Shiley balloon
Schwarten Microglide LP balloon
Sci-Med Express Monorail balloon
scintigraphic balloon
Seloris balloon
Sengstaken balloon
Sengstaken-Blakemore balloon
Sengstaken-Blakemore esophageal balloon
Shadow balloon
Shea-Anthony balloon
Short Speedy balloon
Simpson epistaxis balloon
sinus balloon
sizing balloon
Slinky balloon
Soft-Wand atraumatic tissue manipulator balloon
Soto USCI balloon
Spacemaker II balloon
Spears USCI laser balloon
Stack autoperfusion balloon
Stealth catheter balloon
stone-retrieval balloon
Stretch balloon
Taylor gastric balloon
TEGwire balloon
Ten balloon
ThermaChoice uterine balloon
thigh balloon
through-the-scope balloon
Thruflex balloon
transluminal balloon
trefoil Schneider balloon
Triad PET balloon
Tri-Ex radiopaque triple-lumen extraction balloon
Tru-Trac high-pressure PTA balloon
Tyshak balloon
ultrasmall-shafted balloon
Ultra-Thin balloon
USCI PET balloon

balloon (*continued*)

Wilson-Cook dilating balloon
Wilson-Cook gastric balloon
windowed balloon
windowed esophageal balloon
wire-guided hydrostatic balloon
Xomed dual-chamber balloon
balloon angioplasty
balloon angioplasty catheter
balloon aortic valvuloplasty
balloon atrial septotomy
balloon biliary catheter
balloon catheter angioplasty
balloon catheter sealing device
balloon catheter technique
balloon cell formation
balloon cell nevus
balloon cholangiogram
balloon coarctation angioplasty
balloon coronary angioplasty
balloon counterpulsation
balloon decompression
balloon dilatation catheter
balloon dilating catheter
balloon dilation angioplasty
balloon dissection
balloon dissector
balloon embolectomy
balloon embolectomy catheter
balloon esophagoplasty
balloon expandable intravascular stent
balloon expandable stent
balloon expansion
balloon fenestration procedure
balloon flotation catheter
balloon inflation
balloon laser angioplasty
balloon mitral commissurotomy
balloon mitral valvuloplasty
balloon nasostat
balloon occlusion of aneurysm
balloon photodynamic therapy
balloon pulmonary valvuloplasty
balloon pump
balloon reflex manometry
balloon rupture
balloon septostomy
balloon shunt
balloon sickness

balloon tamponade
balloon tamponade technique
balloon tuboplasty
balloon valvotomy
balloon valvuloplasty
balloon valvuloplasty catheter
balloon wedge pressure catheter
balloon-catheter and basket-
    retrieval technique
balloon-centered argon laser
balloon-expandable flexible coil
    stent
balloon-expandable metallic stent
balloon-flotation pacing catheter
balloon-imaging catheter
ballooning esophagoscope
balloon-like dilation of artery
balloon-occluded retrograde
    transvenous obliteration
    (B-RTO)
Balloon-on-a-Wire cardiac device
balloon-tipped angiographic
    catheter
balloon-tipped flow-directed
    catheter
ballotable
ballotable patella
ballottement
    abdominal ballottement
    indirect ballottement
    ocular ballottement
    renal ballottement
ballottement test
ball-peen splint
ballpoint scissors
Ball's operation
ball-tip coagulating electrode
ball-tip nerve hook
ball-tip reamer
ball-tipped scissors
ball-type prosthesis
ball-type retractor
ball-type valve
ball-valve obstruction
ball-valve prosthesis
ball-valve thrombus
ball-valved
ball-wedge catheter
balm
    Lipikar balm
    post laser balm
    protective recovery balm

Balmer tongue depressor
Balnetar graft materials
Balnetar implant
Balnetar prosthesis
Baloser hysteroscope
balsa wood block
Balser hook plate
Balshi packer
Balters appliance
Baltherm thermal dilution
    catheter
Baltimore nasal scissors
Baltimore Therapeutic
    Equipment work stimulator
Bamberger area
Bamberger sign
bamboo spine
Bamby clamp
Bamp collar
Ba-N (basion-nasion)
Ba-N plane (basion-nasion plane)
Banaji cannula
Banaji spatula
banana
    Beaver blade banana
banana Beaver blade
banana blade
banana catheter
banana finger extension splint
banana fracture
banana knife
banana peel sheath
banana plug dipolar generator
banana-shaped balloon
Bancroft-Plenk gastrectomy
Bancroft-Plenk operation
band
    adapter band
    adhesive band
    amniotic band
    anchor band
    angle band
    annular band
    anterior band
    anterior chamber tube shunt
        encircling band
    apron band
    atelectatic band
    BB band
    belly band
    broad adhesive band
    broad band

band (*continued*)
  Can-Do Exercise band
  coffer band
  copper band
  Cosgrove-Edwards
    annuloplasty band
  Dentaform band
  elastic band
  elastic rubber band
  encircling band
  ExerBand therapy band
  exercise band
  Falope-ring tubal occlusion
    band
  fibrous band
  Fit-Lastic therapy band
  Flexi-Ty vessel band
  fracture band
  GelBand arm band
  Harris band
  Hehnenkratt matrix band
  His band
  hymenal band
  iliotibial band (ITB)
  Impala rubber band
  Jobst air band
  Johnson dental band
  Ladd band
  Lane band
  lateral band
  latex band
  latex O band
  lip furrow band
  Lukens orthodontic band
  Magill band
  Magill orthodontic band
  Marlex band
  Matas band
  Matas vessel band
  matrix band
  MB band
  Meckel band
  mentalis band
  Mersilene band
  mesocolic band
  metal band
  MM band
  Muehrcke band
  oligoclonal band
  omental adhesive band
  omental band
  Ormco preformed band

band (*continued*)
  Orthoband traction band
  orthodontic band
  palatoglossal band
  Parham band
  Parham-Martin band
  Parma band
  patellar band
  PD copper band
  PD SS matrix band
  periosteal band
  peritoneal band
  placental band
  platysmal band
  Ray-Tec band
  Remak band
  REP Bands exercise band
  scultetus binder band
  Silastic band
  silicone elastomer band
  Simonart band
  snap gauge band
  Storz band
  T band
  table band
  Thera-Band Max band
  Thera-Band therapy band
  tissue band
  Tofflemire matrix band
  tooth band
  tourniquet band
  True Blue exercise band
  T-type matrix band
  ventricular band
  vessel band
  Vistnes rubber band
  Watzke band
  Xercise band
  Zipper Medical
    hypoallergenic
    tracheostomy tube neck
    band
band keratitis
band keratopathy
band ligation
band placement
bandage (*see also* dressing)
  3M Clean Seals waterproof
    bandage
  4-layer bandage
  4-tailed bandage
  abdominal bandage

bandage (*continued*)
    Ace adherent bandage
    Ace spica bandage
    adherent bandage
    adhesive bandage
    ARD bandage
    ASE bandage (axilla, shoulder,
        and elbow bandage)
    axilla, shoulder, and elbow
        bandage (ASE bandage)
    Band-Aid bandage
    barrel bandage
    Barton bandage
    Baynton bandage
    Bennell bandage
    binocle bandage
    binocular bandage
    Borsch bandage
    Bulkee II gauze bandage
    Buller bandage
    butterfly bandage
    capeline bandage
    Cellamin resin plaster-of-Paris
        bandage
    Cellona resin plaster-of-Paris
        bandage
    Champ elastic bandage
    circular bandage
    ClearSite bandage
    Coban bandage
    Coflex bandage
    cohesive bandage
    collodion-treated self-adhesive
        bandage
    Comperm tubular bandage
    Comperm tubular elastic
        bandage
    compression bandage
    Comprilan bandage
    Conco elastic bandage
    Conform stretch bandage
    cotton elastic bandage
    cotton-wool bandage
    Cover-Roll stretch bandage
    cravat bandage
    crepe bandage
    crucial bandage
    Curad plastic bandage
    demigauntlet bandage
    Desault bandage
    Desault wrist bandage
    Dressinet netting bandage

bandage (*continued*)
    DuoDERM SCB sustained
        compression bandage
    DuraCast plaster bandage
    Dyna-Flex elastic bandage
    Dyna-Flex Layer Three
        bandage
    Dyna-Flex Layer Two bandage
    E-cotton bandage
    elastic adhesive bandage
    elastic bandage
    elastic foam bandage
    Elastikon bandage
    Elastomull bandage
    Elastomull elastic gauze
        bandage
    Elastoplast bandage
    Esmarch bandage
    eye bandage
    Fabco gauze bandage
    fiberglass bandage
    figure-of-eight bandage
    fixation bandage
    flat eye bandage
    flexible bandage
    Flexicon gauze bandage
    Flexilite conforming elastic
        bandage
    Flexilite gauze bandage
    FoaMTrac traction bandage
    Fractura Flex bandage
    Fractura Flex elastic bandage
    Fricke bandage
    Galen bandage
    Garretson bandage
    gauntlet bandage
    gauze bandage (*see also*
        gauze, gauze dressing)
    Gauztape bandage
    Gauztex bandage
    Genga bandage
    Gibney bandage
    Gibney fixation bandage
    Gibson bandage
    Guibor Expo flat eye bandage
    Haftelast self-adhering
        bandage
    Hamilton bandage
    hammock bandage
    Heliodorus bandage
    Hermitex bandage
    Hippocrates bandage

bandage (*continued*)
Hollister medial adhesive bandage
Hueter bandage
Hydron burn bandage
Hypertie bandage
immobilizing bandage
immovable bandage
Kerlix bandage
Kerlix gauze bandage
Kiwisch bandage
Kling bandage
Kling gauze bandage
Kold Wrap cold compression bandage
Larrey bandage
Liquiderm liquid healing bandage
Lister bandage
long-stretch bandage
Maisonneuve bandage
many-tailed bandage
Marlex bandage
Martin bandage
Medi-Band bandage
moleskin bandage
monocular bandage
Morton bandage
MPM bandage
oblique bandage
Orthoflex elastic plaster bandage
Ortho-Trac adhesive skin traction bandage
Ortho-Vent bandage
Pearlcast polymer plaster bandage
perineal bandage
plaster bandage
plaster-of-Paris bandage (POP bandage)
Plast-O-Fit thermoplastic bandage
polyurethane bandage
POP bandage (plaster-of-Paris bandage)
pressure bandage
Priessnitz bandage
Profore 4-layer bandage
protective bandage
REB rubber-reinforced bandage

bandage (*continued*)
recurrent bandage
reverse bandage
reversed bandage
Ribble bandage
Richet bandage
Robert Jones bandage
roller bandage
rubber-reinforced bandage
Sayre bandage
scarf bandage
scultetus bandage
Setopress high-compression bandage
Seutin bandage
short-stretch bandage
Shur-Band self-closure elastic bandage
Silesian bandage
sling-and-swathe bandage
Sof-Band bulky bandage
Sof-Kling conforming bandage
Spandage bandage
spica bandage
spiral bandage
spiral reverse bandage
spray bandage
starch bandage
Stepty-P hemostasis bandage
Steri-Band bandage
Steri-Strips bandage
stockinette amputation bandage
stockinette bandage
SurePress high-compression bandage
Sureseal cellulose sponge bandage
Sureseal pressure bandage
Surgiflex bandage
suspensory bandage
Telfa 4 x 4 bandage
Theden bandage
Thera-Boot bandage
Thermophore bandage
Thillaye bandage
thumb Spica bandage
triangular bandage
Tricodur compression support bandage

bandage (*continued*)
  Tricodur Epi (elbow)
    compression support
    bandage
  Tricodur Omos (shoulder)
    compression support
    bandage
  Tricodur Omos compression
    support bandage
  Tricodur Talus (ankle)
    compression support
    bandage
  Tru-Support EW bandage
  Tru-Support SA bandage
  T-spica bandage
  Tubegauz seamless tubular
    knitted cotton bandage
  TubiFast bandage
  Tubigrip elastic support
    bandage
  Tubigrip elastic support
    bandages
  Tubipad bandage
  Tubiton tubular bandage
  Tuffnell bandage
  Unna boot bandage
  Unna-Flex paste bandage
  Velpeau bandage
  Webril bandage
  wet bandage
  woven elastic bandage
  zinc oxide bandage
bandage plaster shears
bandage scissors (*see* scissors)
bandage shears (*see* scissors)
bandage soft contact lens
BandageGuard half-leg guard
BandageGuard half-leg protector
Band-Aid brand surgical dressing
Band-Aid operation
bandaletta
bandeau
  supraorbital bandeau
bandeau defect
banded gastroplasty
Bandi procedure
Bandi technique
banding
  hemorrhoidal banding
  Kuzmak gastric banding
  laparoscopic adjustable
    silicone gastric banding

banding (*continued*)
  laparoscopic gastric banding
  Mueller-Dammann pulmonary
    artery banding
  open adjustable silicone
    gastric banding
  PA banding (pulmonary artery
    banding)
  pulmonary artery banding
  Uchida tubal banding
banding of pulmonary artery
Bandit catheter
Bandit low-profile over-the-wire
    balloon
Bandl obstetric ring
band-ligator device
bandpass filter
bane bone rongeur
Bane hook
Bane mastoid rongeur
Bane rongeur forceps
Bane-Hartmann bone rongeur
Banff classification
Bangerter angled iris spatula
Bangerter forceps
Bangerter muscle forceps
Bangerter operation
Bangerter pterygium operation
Bangerter spatula
Bangs bougie
banjo cast
banjo curet
banjo traction splint
banjo tractor
banjo-string adhesions
bank
  bone bank
  donor bank
  organ bank
  temporal bone bank
  tissue bank
Bankart fracture
Bankart lesion
Bankart operation for shoulder
    dislocation
Bankart procedure
Bankart rasp
Bankart reconstruction
Bankart rectal retractor
Bankart repair
Bankart retractor
Bankart shoulder dislocation

Bankart shoulder lesion
Bankart shoulder prosthesis
Bankart shoulder repair
Bankart shoulder repair set
Bankart shoulder retractor
Bankart tack
Bankart-Magnuson shoulder
    repair
Bankart-Putti-Platt operation
banked freeze-dried bone
banking
    cryopreserved tissue
        banking
Banks bone graft
Banks graft
Banks-Laufman incision
Banks-Laufman technique
Banks-Michel herniorrhaphy
Bannayan-Riley-Ruvalcaba
    syndrome
Banner enucleation knife
Banner enucleation snare
Banner flap
Banner forceps
Banner snare
Banner snare enucleator
Banno catheter
Bannon-Klein implant
BANS area (back, arm, neck,
    shoulder area)
Bansal LASIK forceps
Bantam Bovie coagulator
Bantam Bovie unit
Bantam coagulator
Bantam irrigation set
Bantam wire cutter
Bantam wire scissors
Bantam wire-cutting scissors
bar (see also arch bar,
    crossbar)
    Ackerman lingual bar
    acrylic bar
    anterior palatal bar
    arch bar
    Bendick dental arch bar
    Berens prism bar
    Bill bar
    Bookwalter horizontal bar
    Bose bar
    Brookdale bar
    buccal bar
    Buck extension bar

bar (*continued*)
    Burns prism bar
    calcaneonavicular bar
    clasp bar
    connector bar
    Denis Browne bar
    dental arch bar
    distraction bar
    double lingual bar
    Dynamic Mesh
        craniomaxillofacial pre-
        angled connecting bar
    Erich arch bar
    Erich arch malleable bar
    Erich dental arch bar
    Erich-Winter arch bar
    Essig arch bar
    facial fracture appliance
        dental arch bar
    Fillauer bar
    fixed arch bar
    fracture bar
    Gerster traction bar
    Goldman bar
    Goldthwait bar
    Goshgarian transpalatal bar
    grab bar
    Greenberg bar
    Hader implant bar
    Hahnenkratt lingual bar
    hex bar
    intramedullary bar
    Jelenko arch bar
    Jelenko bar
    Jewett bar
    Joseph septal bar
    Kangoo Thera-P bar
    Kazanjian bar
    Kennedy bar
    labial bar
    Leyla self-retaining tractor bar
    lingual bar
    Livingston bar
    Livingston intramedullary
        bar
    Lockjaw arch bar
    longitudinal spinal bar
    lumbrical bar
    major connector bar
    mandibular arch bar
    maxillary arch bar
    mesostructure bar

bar (*continued*)
   mesostructure conjunction
      bar
   minor connector bar
   Niro arch bars
   occlusal rest bar
   palatal bar
   Passavant bar
   posterior thigh bar
   retainer arch bar
   retention bar
   Roger Anderson fixation bar
   screw alignment bar
   Simonart bar
   skiascopy bar
   spondylitic bar
   spreader bar
   stabilizing bar
   stall bars
   strut bar
   supraorbital bar
   T bar
   tapered fissure bar
   tarsal bar
   Thera-P exercise bar
   Tommy hip bar
   Tommy trapeze bar
   traction bar
   transpalatal bar
   trapeze bar
   unilateral bar
   unsegmented bar
   valgus bar
   Vistnes applier bar
   Winter arch bar
   Zielke derotator bar
bar bolt fixation
bar clip attachment
bar drill
Bar incision
bar joint
bar prism
bar resection
bar T-tube
bar-and-shoe orthosis
Bárány applicator
Bárány box
Bárány chair
Bárány sign
Bárány speculum
barb staple
Barbara needle

Barbara pelvimeter
barbed broach
barbed epicardial pacing lead
barbed myringotome
barbed Richards staple
barbed snare
barbed stapler
barber chair position
barber pole sign
barber's pilonidal sinus
barbiturate
   short-acting barbiturate
barbiturate antagonist
barbiturate burst-suppression
   anesthesia
barbotage
barb-tip lead
barbula hirci
Barcat technique
Barcelona colon anastomosis
   modification
Bard absorption drape
Bard absorption dressing
Bard adhesive and barrier film
   remover
Bard AlgiDerm dressing
Bard alligator cup
Bard ambulatory PCA device
Bard arterial cannula
Bard automatic reprocessor
Bard bag
Bard balloon-directed pacing
   catheter
Bard bioptic gun
Bard Biopty cut needle
Bard Biopty gun
Bard biopsy needle
Bard BladderScan bladder
   volume instrument
Bard button
Bard cardiopulmonary support
   pump
Bard catheter
Bard cervical cannula
Bard clamp
Bard clamshell septal
   occluder
Bard closed-end adhesive
   pouch
Bard coil stent
Bard Commander PTCA
   guidewire

Bard Companion papillotome
Bard Composix Kugel patch
Bard Composix mesh graft
Bard constant contact cord
Bard Cunningham incontinence
    clamp
Bard cystoscope tip
Bard dilator
Bard disposable male external
    catheter
Bard Dispoz-A-Bag leg bag
Bard drainage adhesive pouch
Bard electrode
Bard electrophysiology
    catheter
Bard evacuator
Bard Extra Ileo B pouch
Bard Federal containment
    device
Bard forceps
Bard gastrostomy catheter
Bard gastrostomy feeding tube
Bard graft
Bard guiding catheter
Bard helical catheter
Bard implant
Bard Infus-OR syringe-type
    infusion pump
Bard irrigation sleeve
Bard leg bag holder
Bard male external catheter
Bard Memotherm colorectal
    stent
Bard mesh PerFix hernia plug
Bard Neurostim peripheral
    nerve stimulator
Bard nonsteerable bipolar
    electrode
Bard ostomy pouch
Bard oval cup
Bard PCA pump
Bard PDA umbrella
Bard PEG tube
Bard pouch
Bard probe
Bard prosthesis
Bard protective barrier film
Bard PTFE graft
Bard resectoscope
Bard security pouch
Bard self-adhesive fecal
    containment device

Bard Sequence II Plus
    incontinent skin care kit
Bard soft double-pigtail stent
Bard Sperma-Tex preshaped
    mesh graft
Bard sterile infection control
    tray
Bard sterile red rubber
    catheter
Bard Stinger S ablation catheter
Bard tip
Bard Touchless intermittent
    catheter
Bard TransAct intraaortic balloon
    pump
Bard TransAct intra-aortic
    balloon pump
Bard tube
Bard universal Foley catheter
    sterile insertion tray
Bard urethral catheter sterile
    tray
Bard urethral dilator
Bard Visilex mesh graft
Bard x-ray ureteral catheter
Bard XT coronary stent
Bardach cleft rhinoplasty
Bardach modification of
    Obwegeser mandibular
    osteotomy
Bardam catheter
Bardam red rubber catheter
Bard-Apter valve
Bardco catheter
Bardeen pad
Bardeen primitive disk
Bardeleben bone-holding
    forceps
Bardeleben rasp
Bardelli operation
Bardenheuer extension
Bardenheuer incision
Bardenheuer ligation
Bardet-Biedl syndrome
Bardex all silicone sterile Foley
    catheter
Bardex balloon
Bardex drain
Bardex Foley catheter
Bardex hemostat
Bardex hemostatic bag
Bardex IC sterile Foley catheter

Bardex Lubricath Foley catheter
Bardex Lubricath sterile Foley
    tray
Bardex silicone Foley catheter
Bardex stent
Bardex-Bellini drain
Bardex-Foley balloon catheter
Bardex-Foley return-flow
    retention catheter
Bard-Hamm fulgurating
    electrode
Bardic cannula
Bardic catheter
Bardic curet
Bardic cutdown catheter
Bardic translucent catheter
Bardic tube
Bardic Uro Sheath reusable male
    external catheter
Bardic vein catheter
Bardic-Deseret Intracath
    catheter
Bard-Marlex mesh
Bard-Parker autopsy blade
Bard-Parker blade
Bard-Parker dermatome
Bard-Parker disposable scalpel
Bard-Parker handle
Bard-Parker humidifier
Bard-Parker instrument sterilizer
Bard-Parker keratome
Bard-Parker knife
Bard-Parker razor
Bard-Parker scalpel
Bard-Parker scissors
Bard-Parker sterilizer
Bard-Parker transfer forceps
Bard-Parker trephine
BardPort implanted port
Bard-Steigmann-Goff variceal
    ligation kit
Bard-Tuohy-Borst adapter
Bard-U-Cath self-adhering male
    external catheter
bare scleral technique
Bareskin knee positioner
bariatric operation
bariatric surgery
barium
    evacuation of barium
    fleck of barium
    ingestion of barium

barium (*continued*)
    reflux of barium
    residual barium
    retained barium
    Sol-O-Pake barium
barium column
barium enema retention balloon
barium esophagogram
barium esophagram
barium examination
barium ingestion
barium meal
barium sediment
barium suspension
barium swallow
barium-impregnated poppet
Barkan bident retractor
Barkan cyclodialysis
Barkan double cyclodialysis
    operation
Barkan forceps
Barkan goniolens
Barkan gonioscope
Barkan gonioscopic lens
Barkan goniotomy
Barkan goniotomy knife
Barkan goniotomy lens
Barkan goniotomy operation
Barkan illuminator
Barkan implant
Barkan infant lens
Barkan infant lens implant
Barkan iris forceps
Barkan knife
Barkan light
Barkan membrane
Barkan operating lens
Barkan operation
Barkan scissors
Barkan technique
Barkan-Cordes linear cataract
    operation
Barker bunionectomy
Barker calipers
Barker needle
Barker operation
Barker point
Barker Vacu-tome dermatome
Barker Vacu-tome suction knife
Barkman reflex
Barlow disease
Barlow forceps

Barlow maneuver
Barlow syndrome
barnacles of aging
Barnard mitral valve prosthesis
Barnard operation
Barnes bag
Barnes cervical dilator
Barnes common duct dilator
Barnes compressor
Barnes dilator
Barnes internal decompression
 trocar
Barnes nasal suction tube
Barnes scissors
Barnes speculum
Barnes suction tube
Barnes trocar
Barnes vessel scissors
Barnes-Crile hemostatic forceps
Barnes-Dormia stone basket
Barnes-Hill forceps
Barnes-Hind lens
Barnes-Hind ophthalmic
 dressing
Barnes-Simpson forceps
Barnes-Simpson obstetrical
 forceps
Barnhill adenoid curet
Barnhill adenoid knife
Barnhill-Jones curet
Baron ear knife
Baron ear tube
Baron forceps
Baron intraocular lens
Baron lens
Baron palate elevator
Baron retractor
Baron suction tube
Baron suction tube-cleaning
 wire
Baron-Frazier suction tube
barostat balloon
barotitis media
Barouk button
Barouk cannulated bone screw
Barouk microscrew
Barouk microstaple
Baroux button
Barr anal speculum
Barr body
Barr bolt
Barr crypt hook

Barr fistula hook
Barr fistula probe
Barr nail
Barr open reduction and
 internal fixation
Barr operation
Barr pin
Barr procedure
Barr rectal fistular hook
Barr rectal probe
Barr rectal retractor
Barr rectal speculum
Barr self-retaining rectal
 retractor
Barr self-retaining retractor
Barr speculum
Barr tendon transfer operation
Barr tibial fracture fixation
Barracuda flexible cystoscopic
 hot biopsy forceps
barrage cryopexy
Barraquer applanation
 tonometer
Barraquer baby needle holder
Barraquer brush
Barraquer cannula
Barraquer cilia forceps
Barraquer ciliary forceps
Barraquer Colibri forceps
Barraquer conjunctiva forceps
Barraquer conjunctival forceps
Barraquer corneal dissector
Barraquer corneal forceps
Barraquer corneal knife
Barraquer corneal section
 scissors
Barraquer corneal trephine
Barraquer corneoscleral scissors
Barraquer curved holder
Barraquer cyclodialysis spatula
Barraquer enzymatic zonulolysis
 operation
Barraquer erysiphake
Barraquer eye needle holder
Barraquer eye shield
Barraquer eye speculum
Barraquer fixation forceps
Barraquer hemostatic mosquito
 forceps
Barraquer implant
Barraquer iris scissors
Barraquer iris spatula

Barraquer irrigator
Barraquer irrigator spatula
Barraquer J-loop intraocular lens
Barraquer keratomileusis
Barraquer keratoplasty knife
Barraquer knife
Barraquer lid retractor
Barraquer microkeratome
Barraquer microneedle holder
Barraquer mosquito forceps
Barraquer needle carrier
Barraquer needle holder
Barraquer needle holder clamp
Barraquer operating room
    tonometer
Barraquer operation
Barraquer razor bladebreaker
Barraquer scissors
Barraquer section scissors
Barraquer silk sutures
Barraquer solid speculum
Barraquer spatula
Barraquer speculum
Barraquer suture forceps
Barraquer suture technique
Barraquer tonometer
Barraquer trephine
Barraquer vitreous strand
    scissors
Barraquer wire guide
Barraquer wire lid speculum
Barraquer zonulolysis
Barraquer-Carriazo
    microkeratome
Barraquer-Colibri eye speculum
Barraquer-DeWecker iris scissors
Barraquer-Douvas eye speculum
Barraquer-Floyd speculum
Barraquer-Karakashian scissors
Barraquer-Katzin forceps
Barraquer-Kratz speculum
Barraquer-Krumeich-Swinger
    refractive set
Barraquer-Krumeich-Swinger
    refractor
Barraquer-Krumeich-Swinger
    retractor
Barraquer-Troutman corneal
    forceps
Barraquer-Troutman needle
    holder
Barraquer-Vogt needle

Barraquer-von Mandach capsule
    forceps
Barraquer-von Mandach clot
    forceps
Barraquer-Zeiss microscope
Barraya forceps
Barraya tissue forceps
Barré pyramidal sign
Barré sign
barred teeth
barrel bandage
barrel cervix
barrel chest
barrel cutting bur
barrel dressing
barrel guide
barrel knot suture
barrel-hooping compression
barreling distortion
barrel-shaped chest
barrel-shaped lesion
barrel-shaped thorax
barrel-type chest
Barrett appendix inverter
Barrett epithelium
Barrett esophagus
Barrett flange lens manipulator
Barrett forceps
Barrett hebosteotomy needle
Barrett hydrodelineation
    cannula
Barrett hydrogel intraocular
    lens
Barrett intestinal forceps
Barrett inverter
Barrett irrigating lens
    manipulator
Barrett knife
Barrett lens forceps
Barrett needle
Barrett placenta forceps
Barrett syndrome
Barrett tenaculum forceps
Barrett ulcer
Barrett uterine knife
Barrett uterine tenaculum
    forceps
Barrett-Adson cerebellum
    retractor
Barrett-Adson retractor
Barrett-Allen placental forceps
Barrett-Allen uterine forceps

Barrett-Allen uterine-elevating
    forceps
Barrett-Murphy intestinal
    forceps
Barrie-Jones angled crocodile
    forceps
Barrie-Jones
    canaliculodacryorhinostomy
    operation
Barrie-Jones forceps
Barrie-Jones operation
barrier
    ABO barrier
    adhesion barrier
    anatomic barrier
    antimicrobial barrier
    bacterial barrier
    bacteriostatic barrier
    blood-air barrier
    blood-brain barrier (BB)
    blood-cerebral barrier
    blood-cerebrospinal fluid
        barrier
    blood-liquor barrier
    blood-ocular barrier
    blood-optic nerve barrier
    blood-thymus barrier
    blood-urine barrier
    Capset bone graft barrier
    cerebrospinal fluid-brain
        barrier
    Durahesive skin barrier
    elastic barrier
    endothelial barrier
    epithelial barrier
    fenestrated sterile field barrier
    gastric mucosal barrier
    gel barrier
    integumentary barrier
    Interceed absorbable
        adhesion barrier
    Marlen SkinShield adhesive
        skin barrier
    motion barrier
    mucosal barrier
    Nu-Hope adhesive waterproof
        skin barrier
    ocular barrier
    Oxiplex adhesive barrier
    pathologic barrier
    physical barrier
    physiologic barrier

barrier (*continued*)
    placental barrier
    posterior capsular zonular
        barrier
    side-bending barrier
    skin barrier
    sterile field barrier
    Vitacuff tissue-interface
        barrier
barrier breach
Barrier fenestrated sterile field
barrier function
Barrier laparoscopy drape
Barrier laparoscopy LAVH pack
barrier layer
barrier membrane
Barrier phaco extracapsular
    pack
barrier protection
barrier sheet
barrier technique
barrier zone
arron alligator forceps
Barron disposable trephine
Barron donor corneal punch
Barron epikeratophakia
    trephine
Barron hemorrhoid ligation
Barron hemorrhoidal banding
    technique
Barron hemorrhoidal ligator
Barron ligation
Barron pump
Barron radial vacuum trephine
Barron retractor
Barron-Hessburg corneal
    trephine
Barr-Record clubfoot surgery
Barr-Record operation for talipes
    equinovarus
Barr-Shuford rectal speculum
Barr-Shuford speculum
Barsky alar cartilage relocation
Barsky cleft closure
Barsky cleft lip repair
Barsky cleft palate raspatory
Barsky elevator
Barsky forceps
Barsky hook
Barsky macrodactyly reduction
Barsky nasal osteotome
Barsky nasal rasp

Barsky nasal retractor
Barsky nasal scissors
Barsky operation
Barsky osteotome
Barsky pharyngoplasty
Barsky procedure
Barsky rasp
Barsky raspatory
Barsky retractor
Barsky scissors
Barsky technique
bar-sleeve attachment
Barstow stapler
Bart abdominoperipheral
    angiography unit
Barth applicator
Barth double-end applicator
Barth hernia
Barth mastoid curet
Barth mastoid knife
Bartholdson-Stenstrom rasp
Bartholin cystectomy
Bartholin duct
Bartholin gland catheter
Bartholin glands
Bartholin, Skene, and urethral
    glands (BSU glands)
bartholinitis
Bartkiewicz two-sided drain
Bartlett fascia stripper
Bartlett nail-fold excision
Bartlett procedure
Bartlett stripper
Bartlett-Edwards profilometer
Bartley anastomosis clamp
Bartley partial-occlusion clamp
bar-to-bar clamp
Barton bandage
Barton blade
Barton double hook
Barton dressing
Barton forceps
Barton fracture
Barton hook
Barton maneuver
Barton obstetrical forceps
Barton operation
Barton operation for ankylosis
Barton suction
Barton tongs wrench
Barton traction device
Barton traction handle

Barton-Cone tongs
Barton-Smith fracture
Baruch circumcision scissors
Baruch scissors
Barwell operation
BAS-300 transurethral
    thermotherapy device
basal anesthesia
basal bone
basal cell acanthoma
basal cell adenoma
basal cell carcinoma
basal cell epithelioma (BCE)
basal cell hyperplasia
basal cell membrane
basal cell nevus syndrome
basal cell papilloma
basal cephalocele
basal ganglia guide
basal ganglia hematoma
basal ganglionic lesion
basal hypnotic agents
basal infolding
basal iridectomy
basal joint reflex
basal lamina of choroid
basal lamina of ciliary body
basal layer
basal line
basal mandibular angle
basal neck fracture
basal ophthalmoplegia
basal rales
basal skull fracture
basal squamous cell
    carcinoma
basal subfrontal approach
basal vein
basale
    stratum basale
basalioma
basalis
    decidua basalis
basaloid carcinoma
basaloid cell
basaloid monomorphic
    adenoma (BMA)
basaloid tumor
basaloma
Baschui pigtail catheter
Bascom procedure for repair
    of pilonidal sinus

base
  alar base
  anterior skull base
  apical base
  appendiceal base
  cartridge base
  cavity preparation base
  cilia base
  CM-Band silicone rubber base
  columellar base
  conductive base
  extension base
  fixation base
  hemoclip cartridge base
  lung base
  mandibular base
  metal base
  occult malformation of the
    skull base
  record base
  skull base
  temporary base
  vitreous base
  Weir resection of the alar base
base material
base of arytenoid cartilage
base of bladder
base of flap
base of prostate
base of skull
base of stapes
base of tongue (BOT)
base plane
base plate
baseball elbow
baseball finger
baseball finger fracture
baseball finger splint
baseball splint
baseball stitch
baseball suture technique
basedoid
Basedow disease
Basedow paralysis
basedowian
basedownian disease
basedownian symptom
base-down prism
baseline
  Reid baseline
baseline capacity evaluation
Baseline dynamometer

baseline parameters
baseline procedure
baseline study
baseline view
basement membrane zone
basement membrane zone
  injury
basement tissue
basement tissue zone
baseplate
  stabilized baseplate
baseplate material
bas-fond
bas-fond formation
basialveolar length
basibregmatic axis
basic fibroblastic growth factor
  (bFGF)
basic instrument set
basic technique
basicervical fracture
basicranial axis
basicranial flexure
basicranial sagittal growth
basifacial axis
basihyal bone
basilar angle
basilar artery aneurysm
basilar artery migraine
basilar bifurcation
basilar bifurcation aneurysm
basilar bone
basilar cartilage
basilar femoral neck fracture
basilar fracture
basilar groove of occipital bone
basilar groove of sphenoid bone
basilar invagination
basilar kyphosis
basilar lamina
basilar membrane
basilar plexus
basilar process
basilar prognathism
basilar projection
basilar region
basilar segment
basilar sinus
basilar skull fracture
basilar spine
basilar suture technique
basilar tip aneurysm

Basile hip screw
Basile screw
basilemma
basilic hiatus
basilic vein
basiloma
basiloma terebrans
basin
   ear basin
   emesis basin
   Goldnamer ear basin
   pus basin
   solution basin
   sponge basin
basinasal line
basiocciptal
basioglossus
basion-nasion (Ba-N) plane
basio-occipital bone
basiotribe
   Auvard-Zweifel basiotribe
basiotripsy
   fetal basiotripsy
basipharyngeal canal
Basis breast pump
basis cartilaginis arytenoideae
basis cranii externa
basis cranii interna
basis mandibulae
basis nasi
basis pontis
basisphenoid
basisphenoid bone
basivertebral veins
Basix pacemaker
basket (*see also* stone basket)
   6-wire spiral-tip Segura
     basket
   Acufex basket
   Bagley helical basket
   Barnes-Dormia stone basket
   biliary stone basket
   Browne stone basket
   Councill stone basket
   disposable stone basket
   Dormia biliary stone basket
   Dormia gallstone basket
   Dormia stone basket
   Dormia ureteral basket
   Dormia ureteral stone
     basket
   Duette basket

basket (*continued*)
   Eliminator stone extraction
     basket
   Ellik kidney stone basket
   Ellik stone basket
   endotriptor stone-crushing
     basket
   Ferguson stone basket
   gallstone basket
   Gemini paired helical wire
     basket
   Glassman basket
   Hobbs stone basket
   Howard basket
   Howard stone basket
   instrument basket
   Johns Hopkins stone basket
   Johnson stone basket
   Johnson ureteral basket
   Johnson ureteral stone basket
   laser lithotriptor basket
   Levant stone dislodger basket
   Medi-Tech multipurpose
     basket
   Medi-Tech stone basket
   Mill-Rose spiral stone basket
   Mitchell stone basket
   Moss-Harms basket
   Olympus stone retrieval basket
   parrot-beak basket
   Pfister stone basket
   Pfister-Schwartz stone basket
   Positrap mini-retrieval basket
   Pursuer CBD helical basket
   Robinson stone basket
   rotary basket
   Rutner stone basket
   Schutte shovel-nose basket
   Segura CBD basket
   Segura stone basket
   Segura-Dretler stone basket
   sphincterotomy basket
   sterilizing basket
   stone basket
   stone-holding basket
   stone-retrieval basket
   Sur-Catch paired-wire basket
   ultrasonic cleaner basket
   ureteral stone basket
   Vantec stone basket
   VPI stone basket
   Wilson-Cook stone basket

basket cart
basket chisel
basket extraction technique
basket forceps
basket fragmentation technique
basket impaction
basket retriever
basketball heels
basket-cutting forceps
basketing technique
basket-punch forceps
basket-style scleral supporter
   speculum
basket-type crushing forceps
basocellulare
   carcinoma basocellulare
basolateral membrane
basosquamous carcinoma (BSC)
basosquamous cell carcinoma
basovertical projection
Bass technique
Basset operation
Bassett electrical stimulation
   device
Bassini herniorrhaphy
Bassini inguinal hernia repair
Bassini inguinal herniorrhaphy
Bassini method
Bassini operation
Bassini repair
Bassini technique
Bassini-Stetten hernia repair
basswood splint
bastard sutures
Basterra operation
basting stitch anastomosis
basting suture
Bastow laminectomy raspatory
BAT (bilateral advancement
   transposition)
bat ear
bat ear surgery
Batch knee disarticulation
Batchelor osteotomy of hip
Batchelor plate
Batchelor technique
Batchelor-Brown extra-articular
   subtalar arthrodesis
Batchelor-Girdlestone
   disarticulation
Batch-Spittler-McFadden
   amputation

Batch-Spittler-McFadden knee
   disarticulation
Batch-Spittler-McFaddin
   technique
Bateman bipolar cup hip
   prosthesis
Bateman denervation of knee or
   elbow
Bateman finger joint prosthesis
Bateman hemiarthroplasty
Bateman modification of Mayer
   transfer operation
Bateman operation
Bateman prosthesis
Bateman tendon transfer
Bateman Universal proximal
   femur prosthesis (UPF
   prosthesis)
Bateman UPF II bipolar
   endoprosthesis
Bateman UPF II shoulder
   prosthesis
Bateman UPF prosthesis
   (Universal proximal femur
   prosthesis)
Bates decision
Bates gastrostomy
Bates operation for urethral
   stricture
bath
   Bag Bath
   blitz bath
   Downing hot air bath
   Greville hot air bath
   Nauheim carbonated bath
   Russian bath
   Sandor foam bath
   Schott bath
bath for the nerve
bath respirator
bathrocephaly
bathtub deformity of facial fat
Batista procedure
Batista procedure for left
   ventricular reduction
Baton laser pointer
batrachian position
Batson plexus
Batson vein complex
Batson-Carmody elevator
Batt tip
batten graft

battery-assisted heart assist device
battery-powered endoscope
batting
   Dacron batting
Battle incision
Battle operation
Battle sign
battledore incision
battledore placenta
Battle-Jalaguier-Kammerer incision
bat-wing catheter
bat-wing configuration
batwing dissector
Batzdorf cervical wire passer
Baudelocque diameter
Baudelocque operation
Baudelocque operation for extrauterine pregnancy
Baudelocque pelvimeter
Baudet-Fontan operation
Bauer air valve
Bauer dissecting forceps
Bauer kidney pedicle clamp
Bauer retractor
Bauer sponge forceps
Bauer technique
Bauer Temno biopsy needle
Bauer-Black sutures
Bauerfeind ankle brace
Bauerfeind Comprifix knee brace
Bauerfeind MalleoLoc ankle orthosis
Bauerfeind silicone heel pad
Bauer-Jackson classification
Bauer-Tondra-Trusler cleft lip repair
Bauer-Tondra-Trusler operation for syndactylism
Bauer-Tondra-Trusler technique
Bauer-Trusler-Tondra cleft lip repair
Bauhin
   valve of Bauhin
Bauhin glands
Bauhin valve
Baum bumps
Baum needle holder
Baum operation
Baum scissors

Baum tonsil needle holder
Bauman angle
Baumanometer sphygmomanometer
Baumberger forceps
Baume classification
Baumgard and Schwartz technique
Baumgard-Schwartz tennis elbow technique
Baumgarten gland
Baumgarten Vital wire twister
Baumgartner forceps
Baumgartner holder
Baumgartner needle holder
Baumgartner punch
Baumgartner Vital needle holder
Baum-Hecht forceps
Baum-Hecht tarsorrhaphy forceps
Baum-Metzenbaum sternal needle holder
Baumrucker clamp irrigator
Baumrucker electrode
Baumrucker incontinence clamp
Baumrucker irrigator
Baumrucker post-TUR irrigation clamp
Baumrucker resectoscope
Baumrucker urinary incontinence clamp
Baumrucker-DeBakey clamp
Bausch & Lomb Duoloupe lens loupe
Bausch & Lomb manual keratometer
Bausch & Lomb Optima lens
Bausch & Lomb Surgical L161U lens
Bausch articulation paper forceps
Bausch-Lomb instruments
Bausch-Lomb lens
Bausch-Lomb loupe
Bausch & Lomb-Thorpe slit lamp
Bavarian splint
Bavrona tube
Baxa oral dispenser
Baxter angioplasty catheter
Baxter angioscope
Baxter angled arthroscope

Baxter CA-210 filter
Baxter dilatation catheter
Baxter disposable blade
Baxter fiberoptic
    spectrophotometry
    catheter
Baxter Flo-Gard 8200 volumetric
    infusion pump
Baxter Intrepid balloon
Baxter mechanical valve
    prosthesis
Baxter personal Von-Loc ice
    pack
Baxter PSN dialyzer
Baxter V. Mueller laparoscopic
    instrumentation
Baxter-D'Astous procedure
Baxter V. Mueller catheter
Bay external fixator
Bayer/Technicon H1 automated
    flow cytometer
Bayless neurosurgical head
    holder
Bayley infant scale
Baylor adjustable cross splint
Baylor amniotic perforator
Baylor amniotome
Baylor balloon
Baylor cervical balloon
Baylor hammer
Baylor intracardiac sump tube
Baylor metatarsal splint
Baylor splint
Baylor stump
Baylor sump tube
Baylor total artificial heart
Bayne-Klug centralization
Baynton bandage
Baynton dressing
Baynton operation
bayonet
    Lucae bayonet
bayonet aneurysm clip
bayonet bipolar electrosurgical
    forceps
bayonet clip applier
bayonet curet
bayonet dislocation
bayonet fracture position
bayonet handle
bayonet incision
bayonet knife

bayonet microscissors
bayonet molar forceps
bayonet monopolar forceps
bayonet needle holder
bayonet osteotome
bayonet rongeur
bayonet root tip forceps
bayonet saw
bayonet scissors
bayonet separator
bayonet transsphenoidal mirror
bayonet-point wire
bayonet-tip electrode
bayonet-type forceps
bayonet-type incision
Bazex syndrome
Bazin disease
BB band
B-B graft
BB shot forceps
BCA (bicinchoninic acid)
BCC (basal cell carcinoma)
BCD Plus cardioplegic unit
BCE (basal cell epithelioma)
B-chain cystometrogram
BCI (blunt carotid injury)
BCI 3301 hand-held pulse
    oximeter
BCLP (bilateral cleft lip palate)
B-craniotome
B-curve
BD adapter
BD adapter
BD bone marrow biopsy needle
BD butterfly swab dressing
BD Fleischer spinal
    sphygmomanometer
BD gun
BD Insyte Autoguard shielded
    intravenous catheter
BD irrigating tip
BD Luer syringe
BD Luer-Lok syringe
BD Multifit control syringe
BD needle
BD Potain thoracic trocar
BD Safety-Gard needle
BD SafetyGlide shielding
    hypodermic needle
BD spinal needle
BD stopcock
BD Yale syringe

BDH hip prosthesis
BDP pad
BE amputation (below-elbow amputation)
beach chair position
beach chair positioner
Beacham amniotome
Bead ethmoid forceps
Bead ethmoidal forceps
beaded cerclage wire
beaded filaments
beaded guidewire
beaded hepatic duct
beaded hip pin
beaded-tip scissors
beaded-wires traction bow
beading of arteries
beading of myelin
beading sign
beads
   rachitic beads
beak
   cutaneous polly beak
   fibrous polly beak
   parrot beak
   polly beak
beak fracture
beak modification with triple arthrodesis
beaked cowhorn forceps
beaked pelvis
beaked sheath
beak-like protrusion of nose
Beale intraocular implant lens
Beale lens
Beall bulldog clamp
Beall circumflex artery scissors
Beall disk heart valve
Beall disk valve prosthesis
Beall heart valve
Beall mitral obturator
Beall mitral valve prosthesis
Beall prosthetic valve
Beall valve
Beall-Feldman-Cooley sump tube
Beall-Morris ascending aortic clamp
Beall-Surgitool ball-cage prosthetic valve
Beall-Surgitool disk prosthetic valve
Beall-Surgitool prosthetic valve

Beall-Webel-Bailey technique
beam
   defocused beam
   dose and beams
   electron beam
   fluoroscopy beam
   focused beam
   laser beam
   tangential beam
   x-ray beam
BEAM (brain electrical activity mapping)
beam attenuation
beam hardening artifact
beam splitter
Beamer stent
bean forceps
Bear 1, 2, adult-volume ventilator
Bear 5 respirator
bear claw ulcer
Bear Cub infant ventilator
Bear NUM-1 tidal volume monitor
Bear respirator
Bear ventilator
Beard cataract knife
Beard cystoscope
Beard cystotome
Beard eye speculum
Beard knife
Beard lid knife
Beard operation
Beard speculum
Beard-Cutler operation
bearded distribution
Beardsley aortic dilator
Beardsley cecostomy trocar
Beardsley clamp
Beardsley dilator
Beardsley empyema tube
Beardsley esophageal retractor
Beardsley forceps
Beardsley intestinal clamp
Beardsley trocar
Beardsley tube
bearing
   Steinmann pin with ball bearing
bearing-seating forceps
bear-track pigmentation
Beasley-Babcock tissue forceps
BeasyTrans transfer device

beat
  capture beats
  dropped beat
  ectopic beat
  escape beats
  forced beat
  isolated premature beats
  nodal beat
  premature beat
  skipped beat
  synchronous with heart beat
beaten silver appearance
Beath guidewire
Beath needle
Beath operation
Beath pin
beating-heart bypass surgery
Beatson operation
Beatson ovariotomy
beat-to-beat variation of fetal
    heart rate
Beatty aluminum finger splint
Beatty decompressor
Beatty pillar retractor
Beatty tongue depressor
beat-up osteotome
beat-up periosteal elevator
Beau line
Beaufort setting orthosis
Beaulieu camera
Beaupre cilia forceps
Beaupre epilation forceps
beauty mark
Beaver Arthro-Lok blade
Beaver bent blade
Beaver blade
Beaver blade cataract knife
Beaver blade chuck handle
Beaver blade discission knife
Beaver blade handle
Beaver blade keratome
Beaver blade rosette
Beaver cataract blade
Beaver cataract cryoextractor
Beaver cataract knife
Beaver cataract knife blade
Beaver chondroplasty blade
Beaver chuck handle
Beaver cryoextractor
Beaver curet
Beaver cutter
Beaver DeBakey blade

Beaver discission blade
Beaver discission knife blade
Beaver dissector
Beaver ear knife
Beaver electrode
Beaver eye surgery blade
Beaver finger ring saw
Beaver goniotomy needle knife
Beaver handle
Beaver keratome
Beaver knife
Beaver lamellar blade
Beaver limbus blade
Beaver microblade
Beaver Microsharp blade
Beaver miniblade
Beaver Mini-Blade
Beaver myringotomy blade
Beaver Ocu-1 curved cystotome
Beaver Optimum blade
Beaver phacokeratome blade
Beaver retractor
Beaver rhinoplasty blade
Beaver ring cutter
Beaver saw
Beaver scleral Lundsgaard blade
Beaver surgical blade
Beaver surgical blade handle
Beaver tail-tip electrode
Beaver tonsillar knife
Beaver tonsillectomy blade
Beaver Xstar knife
Beaver-Lundsgaard blade
Beaver-Okamura blade
beaver-tail retractor
Beaver-Ziegler blade
Bebax orthosis
Bebax plaster cast
Beccaria sign
Bechert capsular polisher
Bechert forceps
Bechert intraocular lens cannula
Bechert intraocular lens implant
Bechert intraocular scissors
Bechert irrigating spatula
Bechert lens-holding forceps
Bechert microsurgery
    instruments
Bechert nucleus rotator
Bechert one-piece all-PMMA
    intraocular lens
Bechert spatula

Bechert-Hoffer nucleus rotator
Bechert-Kratz cannulated
    nucleus retractor
Bechert-McPherson tying
    forceps
Bechert-Sinskey needle holder
Bechterew (*variant of*
    Bekhterev)
Bechtol arthroplasty
Bechtol cemented hip
    prosthesis
Bechtol glenohumeral joint
    prosthesis
Bechtol hip prosthesis
Bechtol implant
Bechtol prosthesis
Bechtol screw
Beck I, II operation
Beck abdominal scoop
Beck aortic clamp
Beck bull's eye lamp
Beck cardiopericardiopexy
Beck clamp
Beck forceps
Beck gastrostomy
Beck gastrostomy scoop
Beck knife
Beck loop
Beck miniature aortic clamp
Beck mouth tube airway
Beck operation
Beck pericardial raspatory
Beck pliers
Beck poudrage
Beck rasp
Beck raspatory
Beck scoop
Beck shunt
Beckterev
    line of Beckhterev
Beck tonsillar knife
Beck tonsillectome
Beck triad
Beck twisted wire snare loop
Beck vascular clamp
Beck vessel clamp
Beckenbaugh correction
Beckenbaugh technique
Becker accelerator
Becker accelerator cannula
Becker brace
Becker breast prosthesis

Becker corneal section
    spatulated scissors
Becker corneal suture scissors
Becker dissector cannula
Becker dissector tip
Becker flap
Becker flat dissector tip
Becker goniogram
Becker gonioscopic prism
Becker Grater dissecting
    cannula
Becker hair hamartoma
Becker hand prosthesis
Becker implant
Becker mammary prosthesis
Becker nevus
Becker operation
Becker orthopedic spinal system
    orthotic device
Becker probe
Becker retractor
Becker round tip dissector
Becker scissors
Becker screwdriver
Becker septal scissors
Becker septum scissors
Becker skull trephine
Becker spatulated corneal
    section scissors
Becker technique
Becker tendon repair
Becker tip
Becker tissue expander
Becker tissue expander
    prosthesis
Becker trephine
Becker twist dissector tip
Becker-Joseph saw
Becker-Park eye speculum
Becker-Park speculum
Becker-Parkin pliers
Beckerscope binocular
    microscope
Beck-Jianu gastrostomy
Beck-Jianu operation
Beckman adenoid curet
Beckman distractor
Beckman goiter retractor
Beckman J5.0 elutriation rotor
Beckman JE-10X elutriation
    rotor
Beckman laminectomy retractor

Beckman nasal scissors
Beckman nasal speculum
Beckman probe
Beckman retractor
Beckman self-retaining retractor
Beckman Silastic bulb
Beckman speculum
Beckman stomach electrode
Beckman thyroid retractor
Beckman-Adson laminectomy
    blade
Beckman-Adson laminectomy
    retractor
Beckman-Adson retractor
Beckman-Colver nasal speculum
Beckman-Eaton laminectomy
    blade
Beckman-Eaton laminectomy
    retractor
Beckman-Eaton retractor
Beckman-Weitlaner laminectomy
    retractor
Beckman-Weitlaner retractor
Beck-Mueller tonsillectome
Beck-Potts aorta and pulmonic
    clamp
Beck-Potts aortic clamp
Beck-Potts clamp
Beck-Potts pulmonic clamp
Beck-Satinsky clamp
Beck-Schenck tonsil knife
Beck-Schenck tonsil snare
Beck-Schenck tonsillectome
Beck-Stefee total ankle
    prosthesis
Beck-Storz tonsil snare
Beckwith syndrome
Beckwith-Wiedemann
    syndrome
Béclard amputation
Béclard anastomosis
Béclard hernia
Béclard sign
Béclard suture technique
Béclard triangle
becquerel (Bq)
Becton open reduction
Becton technique
Becton-Dickinson guidewire
Becton-Dickinson Teflon-
    sheathed needle
bedewing of cornea

Bedfont carbon monoxide
    monitor
Bedge antireflux mattress
Bedge pillow
Bednar aphthae
Bednar tumor
bedrest
bedroom fracture
Bedrossian eye speculum
bedside air chair
bedside laparoscopy
bedside suction tube
bedsore
Beebe binocular loupe
Beebe collar scissors
Beebe forceps
Beebe hemostatic forceps
Beebe lens
Beebe lens loupe
Beebe scissors
Beebe wire-cutting forceps
Beebe wire-cutting scissors
beefy red mucosa
beefy tongue
Beehler pupil dilator
Beekhuis-Supramid mentoplasty
    augmentation implant
Beer blade
Beer canaliculus knife
Beer cataract flap operation
Beer cataract knife
Beer cilia forceps
Beer ciliary forceps
beer heart
Beer operation
beer-can capsulotomy
Beeson cast spreader
Beeson plaster spreader
Beeth needle
Beevor phenomenon
Beevor sign
Begg appliance
Begg light wire differential force
    technique
Behavior Assessment System for
    Children monitor
behavior modification
behavioral technique
Behen ear forceps
behind-sternum column
    esophagoplasty
behind-the-ear listening device

Behnken unit
Behrend cystic duct forceps
Behrend periosteal elevator
Beimer-Clip aneurysm clip
Beir local anesthesia
Beird eye catheter
Bekhterev arthritis (*also*
    Bechterew)
Bekhterev sign
Bekhterev spondylitis
Bekhterev symptom
Bekhterev test
Bekhterev-Mendel reflex
Bel-Air orthopedic stockinette
Belcher clamp
Belfield operation
Belfield vasotomy
Belin needle holder
Bell
    Gomco bell
    long nerve of Bell
Bell clamp
Bell erysiphake
bell flap nipple reconstruction
Bell fracture table
Bell operation
Bell palsy
Bell phenomenon
Bell scissors
Bell spasm
Bell sutures
Bell tonometer
bell-clapper deformity
bell-clapper deformity of testis
Bell-Dally cervical dislocation
Bell-Dally dislocation of first
    cervical vertebra
Bellevue surgical wadding
Bellevue anesthesia unit
Bellfield wire retractor
bellied bougie
Bellini drain
Bellini tube
Bellini tubules
Bellman retractor
Bellocq cannula
Bellocq sound
Bellocq tube
bellows
    chest bellows
Bellows cryoextractor
Bellows extractor

Bellows cryophake
Bellows murmur
Bellows pack
Bellows sound
bellows suction
bellows traction
Bell-Tawse open reduction
    technique
Bell-Tawse procedure
Bell-Tawse technique
Bellucci alligator scissors
Bellucci cannula
Bellucci curet
Bellucci ear forceps
Bellucci ear scissors
Bellucci elevator
Bellucci forceps
Bellucci hook
Bellucci knife
Bellucci lancet knife
Bellucci nasal suction tube
Bellucci otolaryngology
    scissors
Bellucci pick
Bellucci suction tube
Bellucci tube
Bellucci-Paparella scissors
Bellucci-Wullstein retractor
belly
    drum belly
    muscle belly
    posterior belly
    prune belly
belly band
belly bath intraperitoneal
    chemotherapy
belly bath therapy
belly of the muscle
belly tap
Belmas operation
Belmont collar
Bel-O-Pak suction tube
Belos compression pin
below-elbow amputation
    (BE amputation, BEA)
below-knee amputation
    (BK amputation, BKA)
below-knee prosthesis
below-knee walking cast
Belscope blade
Belscope laryngoscope
Belsey Mark II fundoplication

Belsey IV fundoplasty
Belsey Mark IV 240-degree
    fundoplication
Belsey Mark IV antireflux
    operation
Belsey Mark IV fundoplication
Belsey Mark IV gastropexy
Belsey Mark IV operation
Belsey Mark IV repair
Belsey antireflux operation
Belsey esophagoplasty
Belsey fundoplication procedure
Belsey fundoplication technique
Belsey herniorrhaphy
Belsey hiatal hernia repair
Belsey operation
Belsey partial fundoplication
Belsey perfusor
Belsey repair
Belsey two-thirds wrap
    fundoplication
belt
    adjustable ostomy appliance
        belt
    control belt
    heavy twill belt
    Hollister belt
    Lapides elastic belt
    lumbosacral belt
    Marlen belt
    Marsan belt
    Mayo sacroiliac belt
    Posey belt
    restraint belt
    rib belt
    Robinson belt
    sacroiliac belt
    safety belt
    seat belt
    Silesian belt
    traction belt
    Velcro belt
Belt hypospadias repair
belt loop gastropexy
Belt prostatectomy
Belt technique
belt-approach incision
Belt-Fugua hypospadias repair
Belz lacrimal sac rongeur
Belz rongeur
Belzer machine
Bemis suction canister

Benaron forceps
Benaron scalp-rotating forceps
Bence Jones body
bench
    dissection bench
bench back test
bench examination
bench knot pusher-tier
bench surgery
bench surgical technique
Benchekroun ileal valve
bend
    anchorage bend
    cautery bend
    knee bend
Bend-A-Boot foot splint
bender
    Bunnell knuckle bender
    French rod bender
    Gratloch wire bender
    plate bender
    rod bender
    Rush pin bender
    Tessier bone bender
    Tuffier bone bender
Bendick dental arch bar
bending
    forward bending
    left lateral bending
bending fracture
bending pliers
Bendixen-Kirschner traction
    bow
Benedict gastroscope
Benedict operating gastroscope
Benedict operation
Benedict retractor
benediction hand
Benedict-Roth spirometer
Benelli mastopexy
Beneventi retractor
Beneventi self-retaining retractor
Beneys tonsil compressor
Bengash needle
Benger probe
Bengolea arterial forceps
Bengolea artery forceps
Bengolea forceps
benign adenomatous polyp
benign biliary stricture
benign bone lesion
benign cellular blue nevus

benign cephalic histiocytosis
benign chondroma
benign cystic teratoma
benign duodenocolic fistula
benign dyskeratosis
benign dysphagia
benign epidermal pigmented
　lesion
benign epithelial neoplasm
benign esophageal disorder
benign familial chronic
　pemphigus
benign fibrous histiocytoma
benign hemangiopericytoma
benign hyperplasia
benign inflammatory disease
benign intraepithelial
　dyskeratosis
benign juvenile melanoma
benign lipoblastoma
benign liver cyst
benign lymphadenosis
benign lymphocytoma cutis
benign lymphoepithelial lesion
　(BLL)
benign lymphoproliferative
　lesion
benign mesenchymal neoplasm
benign mesenchymal tumor
benign migratory glossitis
benign mixed tumor
benign mucous membrane
　pemphigoid
benign necrotizing otitis externa
　(BNOE)
benign neoplasm
benign nevus
benign papillary stenosis
benign papular acantholytic
　dermatitis
benign papular acantholytic
　dermatosis
benign pemphigus
benign pneumatic colonoscopy
　complication
benign prostatic hyperplasia
　(BPH)
benign prostatic hypertrophy
benign subcutaneous cyst
benign symmetric lipomatosis
benign systemic mastocytosis
benign tumor

benign ulcer
benign vascular lesion
benign-acting renal cell
　carcinoma
benignity
Benique catheter guide
Benique dilator
Benique sound
Benjamin binocular slimline
　laryngoscope
Benjamin pediatric operating
　laryngoscope
Benjamin syndrome
Benjamin tube
Benjamin-Havas fiberoptic light
　clip
Benjamin-Lindholm
　microsuspension
　laryngoscope
Ben-Jet tube
Benke everter
Bennell bandage
Bennell elevator
Bennell forceps
Bennell fracture
Bennett angle
Bennett approach
Bennett bone elevator
Bennett bone lever
Bennett bone retractor
Bennett cilia forceps
Bennett classification
Bennett comminuted fracture
Bennett common duct dilator
Bennett dislocation
Bennett elevator
Bennett epilation forceps
Bennett foreign body spud
Bennett fracture-dislocation
Bennett lesion
Bennett monitoring
　spirometer
Bennett movement
Bennett nail biopsy
Bennett operation
Bennett posterior shoulder
　approach
Bennett pressure-cycled
　ventilator
Bennett raspatory
Bennett respirator
Bennett retractor

Bennett self-retaining retractor
  blade
Bennett spud
Bennett tibia retractor
Bennett valve
Bennett ventilator
Benoist scale
benoxinate hydrochloride
  anesthetic agent
Bensaude anoscope
Benson baby pyloric separator
Benson pyloric clamp
Benson pylorus separator
Benson pylorus spreader
Benson separator
bent blade
bent blade plate
bent blunt blade
bent blunt needle
bent fracture
bent hook
bent malleable retractor
bent needle
Bent operation
Bent shoulder excision
Bentall cardiovascular prosthesis
Bentall composite graft
  technique
Bentall inclusion technique
Bentall procedure
Bentley button
Bentley filter
Bentley oxygenator
Bentley transducer
bent-nail syndrome
Bentson exchange straight
  guidewire
Bentson floppy-tip guidewire
Bentson Glidewire guidewire
Bentson guidewire
Bentson wire
Bentson-Hanafee-Wilson
  catheter
Bentson-type Glidewire
  guidewire
Benzac AC Gel
benzocaine anesthetic agent
benzoin
  tincture of benzoin
benzoquinonium chloride
  anesthetic agent
Berard aneurysm

Beraud valve
Berbecker needle
Berbecker pliers
Berbecker wire cutter
Berbridge scissors
Berchtold cautery
Berci-Shore choledochoscopy
Berci-Shore nephroscope
Berci-Ward
  laryngonasopharyngoscope
Berci-Ward
  laryngopharyngoscope
Bercovici wire lid speculum
Berens bident electrode
Berens blade
Berens capsular forceps
Berens capsule forceps
Berens cataract knife
Berens clamp
Berens compressor
Berens conical eye implant
Berens corneal dissector
Berens corneal knife
Berens corneal transplant
  forceps
Berens corneal transplant
  scissors
Berens corneoscleral punch
Berens corneoscleral transplant
Berens dilator
Berens enucleation compressor
Berens esophageal retractor
Berens everter
Berens expressor
Berens eye implant
Berens eye retractor
Berens eye speculum
Berens forceps
Berens glaucoma knife
Berens graft
Berens hook
Berens implant
Berens iridocapsulotomy
  scissors
Berens iris knife
Berens keratome
Berens keratoplasty knife
Berens lens expressor
Berens lens loupe
Berens lens scoop
Berens lid elevator
Berens lid everter

Berens lid retractor
Berens loupe
Berens marking calipers
Berens mastectomy retractor
Berens mastectomy skin flap
    retractor
Berens muscle clamp
Berens muscle forceps
Berens muscle recession forceps
Berens needle holder
Berens operation
Berens orbital compressor
Berens orbital implant
Berens partial keratome
Berens plastic spatula
Berens prism bar
Berens prosthesis
Berens pterygium transplant
Berens pterygium transplant
    operation
Berens ptosis forceps
Berens ptosis knife
Berens punch
Berens punctum dilator
Berens pyramidal eye implant
Berens recession forceps
Berens retractor
Berens scissors
Berens scleral hook
Berens sclerectomy
Berens sclerectomy operation
Berens sclerotomy knife
Berens scoop
Berens skin flap retractor
Berens spatula
Berens speculum
Berens sphere eye implant
Berens suturing forceps
Berens thyroid retractor
Berens tonometer
Berens-Rosa eye implant
Berens-Rosa scleral implant
Berens-Smith operation
Berenstein guiding catheter
Berenstein occlusion balloon
    catheter
Bereyea transurethral bladder
    suspension
Bergen retractor
Bergenhem implantation of
    ureter into rectum
Bergenhem procedure

Berger biopsy forceps
Berger crusher
Berger disease
Berger forceps
Berger interscapular amputation
Berger loop
Berger operation
Berger sign
Berger space
Berger spur crusher
Berger symptom
Berger-Bookwalter posterior
    approach
Bergeret-Reverdin needle
Bergeron pillar forceps
Berges-Reverdin needle
Berget lens loupe
Bergey classification
Bergh ciliary forceps
Berghmann-Foerster sponge
    forceps
Bergland-Warshawksi phaco/
    cortex kit
Bergman bandage scissors
Bergman forceps
Bergman mallet
Bergman plaster saw
Bergman plaster scissors
Bergman scalpel
Bergman tissue forceps
Bergman tracheal retractor
Bergman wound retractor
Bergmann hernia
Bergmann hydrocele repair
Bergmann incision
Bergmann layer
Bergmann Optical laser scanner
Bergmann-Israel incision
Berke approach
Berke cilia forceps
Berke clamp
Berke double-end lid everter
Berke forceps
Berke operation
Berke ptosis clamp
Berke ptosis correction
Berke ptosis forceps
Berkefeld filter
Berke-Jaeger lid plate
Berke-Leahy technique
Berkeley Bioengineering bipolar
    cautery

Berkeley Bioengineering brass
 scleral plug
Berkeley Bioengineering
 infusion terminal port
Berkeley Bioengineering
 mechanized scissors
Berkeley Bioengineering
 ocutome
Berkeley Bioengineering ptosis
 forceps
Berkeley cannula
Berkeley clamp
Berkeley forceps
Berkeley retractor
Berkeley suction cup
Berkeley suction machine
Berkeley suction unit
Berkeley Vacurette machine
Berkeley-Bonney self-retaining
 abdominal retractor
Berkeley-Bonney vaginal clamp
Berke-Motais operation
Berke-Motais ptosis correction
Berkovits-Castellanos hexapolar
 electrode
Berkowitz-Bellis herniorrhaphy
Berlin curet
Berlin edema
Berlin tulip flap
Berlind-Auvard retractor
Berlind-Auvard vaginal speculum
Berliner neurosurgical hammer
Berliner percussion hammer
berlock dermatitis
Berman airway
Berman angiographic catheter
Berman aortic clamp
Berman balloon flotation
 catheter
Berman cardiac catheter
Berman disposable airway
Berman eye director
Berman foreign body locator
Berman intubating pharyngeal
 airway
Berman localizer
Berman locator device
Berman magnet
Berman metal locator
Berman vascular clamp
Berman-Gartland procedure
Berman-Moorhead metal locator

Berman-Werner probe
Bermuda Triangle
Berna infant abdominal retractor
Berna retractor
Bernaco adapter
Bernard duct
Bernard flap
Bernard lip reconstruction
 procedure
Bernard operation
Bernard uterine forceps
Bernard-Burow cheiloplasty
Bernard-Burow operation
Bernard-Burow technique
Bernay gauze packer
Bernay hydrocele trocar
Bernay retractor
Bernay sponge
Bernay tracheal retractor
Bernay uterine gauze packer
Berndorfer syndrome
Berndt hip ruler
Berndt-Harty classification
Berne clips hemostat
Berne nasal forceps
Berne nasal rasp
Berne nasal raspatory
Bernell grid
Bernhard clamp
Bernhard towel forceps
Bernheimer fibers
Bernoulli effect
Bernstein catheter
Bernstein gastroscope
Bernstein light
Bernstein modification
 gastroscope
Bernstein nasal retractor
Bernstein retractor
Bernstein test
Berridge gauze scissors
berry aneurysm
Berry circle
Berry clamp
Berry forceps
Berry ligament
Berry operation
Berry pile clamp
Berry raspatory
Berry rib raspatory
Berry rotating inlet
Berry rotating sheath

Berry sternal needle holder
Berry uterine-elevating
    forceps
Berry-Lambert elevator
Bertel position
Bertel x-ray position
Bertillon calipers
Bertin bone
Bertin hip retractor
Bertin ligament
Bertrandi suture technique
Bertrandi sutures
Berwick dye
Besnier rheumatism
Besnier-Boeck-Schaumann
    disease
Best bite block
Best colon clamp
Best common duct stone
    forceps
Best direct forward-vision
    telescope
Best forceps
Best gallstone forceps
Best intestinal clamp
Best operation
Best right-angle colon clamp
Best telescope
beStent 2 coronary stent
beStent 2 laser-cut stent
beStent balloon-expandable
    stent
beStent coronary stent
beta
    transforming growth factor
    beta (TGF-β)
beta finger-grip catheter
    connector
beta irradiation applicator
beta ray microscope
beta therapy eye applicator
beta-adrenergic blockade
Betabed bed
Beta-Cap II catheter closure
Beta-Cap closure system for
    catheters
Beta-Cath
Beta-Cath catheter
Betacel-Biotronik pacemaker
Betaclassic surgical table
Betadine Helafoam solution
Betadine scrub

Betadine soap
Betadine solution
beta-lactose pack
Beta-Rail catheter
beta-ray applicator
beta-scintillation counter
betatron irradiation
betel carcinoma
betel nut abrasion
Bethea sheet holder
Bethea sign
Bethesda System for Pap smear
    classification
Bethke iridectomy
Bethke operation
Bethune bone cutter
Bethune clamp
Bethune elevator
Bethune hook
Bethune lobectomy tourniquet
Bethune lung tourniquet
Bethune nerve hook
Bethune periosteal elevator
Bethune phrenic retractor
Bethune retractor
Bethune rib rongeur
Bethune rib shears
Bethune tourniquet
Bethune-Coryllos rib shears
Bettman empyema tube
Bettman gauze
Bettman-Forash thermopore
Bettman-Forash thoracotome
Bettman-Noyes fixation
    forceps
Bettman-Noyes forceps
Beurrier connector
Bevan abdominal incision
Bevan gallbladder forceps
Bevan hemostatic forceps
Bevan incision
Bevan operation
Bevan-Rochet operation
beveled, bevelled
beveled anastomosis
beveled chisel
beveled septal cartilage
beveled speculum
beveled thin-walled needle
beveled vein
bevel-point Rush pin
Beverly referential valve

Beverly-Douglas lip-tongue
adhesion technique
BeWo choriocarcinoma cell line
Beyea operation
Beyer atticus punch
Beyer bone rongeur
Beyer endaural rongeur
Beyer forceps
Beyer laminectomy rongeur
Beyer needle
Beyer paracentesis needle
Beyer pigtail probe
Beyer punch
Beyer rongeur forceps
Beyer-Lempert rongeur
Beyer-Stille bone rongeur
bezoar
Bezold abscess
Bezold ganglion
Bezold mastoiditis
Bezold perforation
Bezold reflex
Bezold sign
Bezold symptom
Bezold triad
Bezold-Edelman tuning fork
Bezold-Jarisch reflex
BF large-core bronchoscope
bFGF (basic fibroblastic growth
factor)
BFO Kit
BFO orthosis
BGC Matrix dressing
B-H anterior chamber irrigator
B-H (Bishop-Harman) forceps
B-H irrigating cannula
BHTU microscope
biactive coagulation set cautery
Biad camera
Bianchi valve
biangled hook
Bi-Angular shoulder prosthesis
biarticulate
Bias hip prosthesis
Bias porous metal hip prosthesis
BIAS prosthesis
bias stockinette
bias-cut stockinette dressing
Biatin foam dressing
biatrial hypertrophy
biatriatum
cor triloculare biatriatum

biauricular
biaxial joint
BIB (biliointestinal bypass)
bibasally
bibasilar atelectasis
bibasilar rales
bibeveled cutting instrument
bibulous
bicameral abscess
bicanalicular silicone tube
BICAP bipolar hemostatic probe
BICAP bipolar laparoscopic
probe
BICAP cautery
BICAP II cautery
BICAP monopolar electrode
BICAP probe
BICAP silver ACE
BICAP unit
bicapsular
Bicarbon Sorin valve
bicarotid trunk
bicaval
Bicek retractor
Bicek vaginal retractor
Bi-Centric endoprosthesis
bicephalic trims
biceps bipolar coagulator
biceps brachii flap
biceps interval lesion
biceps jerk
biceps muscle
biceps reflex
biceps tendon sheath
Bicer-val mitral heart valve
Bicer-val prosthetic valve
Bichat
fatty ball of Bichat
Bichat deep cheek pads
Bichat fat pad
Bichat fossa
Bichat membrane
Bichat protuberance
bicinchoninic acid (BCA)
bicipital groove
bicipital rib
bicipital tendinitis
Bick ectropion repair
Bick procedure
Bickel intramedullary nail
Bickel intramedullary rod
Bickel ring

Bickel-Moe procedure
Bickle microsurgical knife
BiCoag bipolar laparoscopic
    forceps
Bicol collagen sponge
bicollis uterus
Bicomatic bipolar cable
Bicon dental implant
biconcave contact lens
biconcave lens
bicondylar ankle prosthesis
bicondylar articulation
bicondylar joint
bicondylar T-shaped fracture
bicondylar Y-shaped fracture
Bicon-Plus cup
biconvex intraocular lens
biconvex lens
Bicor catheter
Bicoral implant
bicornis uterus
bicornuate uterus
bicoronal approach
bicoronal forehead lift
bicoronal incision
bicoronal ridge
bicoronal scalp flap
bicoronal subperiosteal
    approach
bicoronal synostosis
bicortical iliac bone block
bicortical screw fixation
bicortical superior border screw
bicoudate catheter
bicoudé catheter
bicurved needle
bicuspid
    mandibular bicuspid
    maxillary bicuspid
bicuspid aortic valve
bicuspid teeth
bicuspid valvotomy
bicuspid valvulotomy
bicuspidate
bicuspides
    dentes bicuspides
bicuspidization
bicuspis
    dens bicuspis
bicycle dynamometer
bicycle ergonometer
bicycle spoke fracture

bicylindrical lens
bidactylous
bidactyly
bident retractor
Bidet toilet insert
bidirectional
bidirectional cavopulmonary
    anastomosis
bidirectional four-pole
    Butterworth high-pass
    digital filter
bidirectional ligation
bidirectional rhytidectomy
bidirectional shunt
bidirectional superior
    cavopulmonary
    anastomosis
bidiscoidal placenta
Biebl loop
BIEF (bilateral inferior epigastric
    artery flap)
Biegelseisen needle
Bielawski heart clamp
Bielschowsky head tilt test
Bielschowsky maneuver
Bielschowsky operation
Bielschowsky-Jansky disease
Biemer approximator
Biemer vessel clip
Biemer vessel clip applier
biepicondylar line
Bier amputation
Bier amputation saw
Bier anesthesia
Bier arm block anesthesia
Bier block anesthesia
Bier combined treatment
Bier lumbar puncture needle
Bier operation
Bier passive hyperemia
Bier treatment
Bierer ovum forceps
Bierer tenaculum
Bierer vacuum
Bierhoff crutch
Bierman needle
Biermer sign
Biesenberger mammaplasty
Biesenberger operation
Biesenberger reduction
    mammaplasty
Biesiadecki fossa

Biestek thyroid retractor
Biethium ostomy rod
Bietti eye implant
Bietti implant cataract lens
Bietti lens
bifascicular block
bifascicular heart block
biferious pulse
bifid clitoris
bifid cranium
bifid epiglottis
bifid gallbladder retractor
bifid hook
bifid nose
bifid pelvis
bifid pinna
bifid retractor
bifid thumb
bifid thumb deformity
bifid tongue
bifid uvula
bifida
   occult spina bifida
   spina bifida
bifidity
   tip bifidity
bifidity of the columella
bifidum
   cranium bifidum
bifixation
bifocal demand DVI pacemaker
bifocal demand pacemaker
bifocal eye implant
bifocal fixation
bifocal glasses
bifocal intracorneal lens
bifocal lens
bifocal multiplane rectal
   transducer
bifocal pacer
bifoil balloon catheter
bifoveal fixation
bifrontal craniotomy
bifrontal incision
bifurcated aortofemoral
   prosthesis
bifurcated bladeplate
bifurcated drain extension
bifurcated J-shaped tined atrial
   pacing and defibrillation
   lead
bifurcated ligament

bifurcated retractor
bifurcated seamless prosthesis
bifurcated vascular graft
bifurcation
   aortic bifurcation
   basilar bifurcation
   carotid artery bifurcation
   carotid bifurcation
   coronary bifurcation
   iliac bifurcation
   portal bifurcation
   venous bifurcation
bifurcation aneurysm
bifurcation graft
bifurcation involvement
bifurcation lesion
bifurcation of gallbladder
bifurcation of renal pelvis
bifurcation of root
bifurcation of trachea
bifurcation of ureter
bifurcation of vessels
bifurcation osteotomy
bifurcation point
bifurcation prosthesis
bifurcational lesion
Bigelow calvarium clamp
Bigelow clamp
Bigelow dislocation
Bigelow evacuator
Bigelow forceps
Bigelow ligament
Bigelow litholapaxy
Bigelow lithotrite
Bigelow maneuver
Bigelow operation
Bigelow sutures
bigeminal pregnancy
bigeminal pulse
bigeminal rhythm
bigeminy
   nodal bigeminy
   ventricular bigeminy
Bihrle dorsal clamp
Bihrle dorsal clamp-T-C needle
   holder
bijaw osteotomy
bijaw segmental dentoalveolar
   setback osteotomy
bike brace
bikini
   disposable bikini

bikini incision
bikini skin incision
bikini wax
bilabe
bilabial
bilaminar
bilaminar membrane
BiLAP bipolar cautery
BiLAP bipolar cautery unit
BiLAP bipolar needle electrode
bilateral abductor paralysis
bilateral adductor paralysis
bilateral adrenal hemorrhage
bilateral advancement
    transposition (BAT)
bilateral amputation
bilateral approach
bilateral balanced occlusion
bilateral bundle branch block
bilateral canthopexy
bilateral cleft
bilateral cleft lip and palate
    (BCLP)
bilateral cleft lip-associated
    nose
bilateral cleft palate
bilateral condylar fracture
bilateral coronal suture
bilateral coronal synostosis
bilateral coronal synostosis
    reoperation
bilateral coronoidectomies
bilateral facial paralysis
bilateral flexion deformity
bilateral forehead remodeling
bilateral fronto-orbital
    remodeling
bilateral gingivoperiosteoplasty
bilateral gluteus maximus
    transposition
bilateral hermaphroditism
bilateral hypesthesia
bilateral ilioinguinal approach
bilateral inferior epigastric
    artery flap (BIEF)
bilateral inguinal hernia (BIH)
bilateral inguinal hernia repair
bilateral inguinal hernia repair
    procedure
bilateral inguinal hernia repair
    technique
bilateral interfacetal dislocation

bilateral internal mammary
    artery (BIMA)
bilateral internal mammary
    artery (BIMA)
    reconstruction
bilateral lithotomy
bilateral lymphadenectomy
bilateral malposition
bilateral mandibular sagittal split
    osteotomy
bilateral masseteric hypertrophy
bilateral McKissock reduction
    mammaplasty
bilateral mesiocclusion
bilateral myocutaneous graft
bilateral neck dissection
bilateral neck exploration
bilateral pectoralis major muscle
    flap
bilateral procedures
bilateral resection
bilateral rotational flap
bilateral sacroiliac approach
bilateral sagittal split
    advancement osteotomy
bilateral sagittal split osteotomy
    (BSSO)
bilateral subcostal incision
bilateral total adrenalectomy
bilateral transabdominal incision
bilateral ventricular assist device
    (BIVAD)
bilateral vestibular
    deafferentation
bilateral V-Y Kutler flap
bilaterally
    downgoing Babinski
    bilaterally
    equal and active bilaterally
    equal bilaterally
    incision extended bilaterally
bilayer patch hernia repair
Bilboa-Dotter nasogastric tube
bile
    interlobular bile
    viscous bile
bile acid circulation
bile ascites
bile bag
bile canaliculi
bile concretion
bile duct

bile duct adenocarcinoma
bile duct adenoma
bile duct calculus
bile duct cannulation
bile duct carcinoma
bile duct catheterization
bile duct dilatation
bile duct exploration
bile duct injury
bile duct ligation
bile duct lumen
bile duct manipulation
bile duct proliferation
bile duct stone
bile duct stricture
bile fluid examination
bile leak
bile leakage
bile plug
bile salts
bile stasis
bile tract drainage
bileaflet heart valve
bileaflet prosthesis
bileaflet tilting-disk prosthetic
    valve
bile-plug syndrome
bile-stained fluid
bile-tinged fluid
bilevel chisel
bilharzial carcinoma
Bilhaut-Cloquet procedure
Bilhaut-Cloquet wedge resection
bili light
Bili-Mask
Bili-Mask eye shield
biliary anatomy
biliary atresia
biliary balloon catheter
biliary balloon probe
biliary calculus
biliary cannulation
biliary carcinoma
biliary catheter
biliary dilatation
biliary dilation
biliary drainage
biliary duct balloon dilator
biliary duct prosthesis
biliary dyskinesia
biliary endoprosthesis
biliary endoprosthesis insertion

biliary endoscopy
biliary enteric anastomosis
biliary enteric bypass
biliary fistula
biliary intestinal anastomosis
biliary leakage
biliary lithotripsy
biliary manometry
biliary obstruction
biliary plexus
biliary procedure
biliary radicle
biliary reconstruction
biliary retractor
biliary sphincter
biliary sphincterotomy and stent
    placement
biliary stent
biliary stone basket
biliary tract cancer
biliary tract disease
biliary tract obstruction
biliary tract stone
biliary tract tray
biliary tree
biliary-bronchial fistula
biliary-cutaneous fistula
biliary-duodenal fistula
biliary-duodenal pressure
    gradient
biliary-enteric anastomosis
    operation
biliary-enteric fistula
Bili-Dosimeter
BiliLight
biliocystic fistula
biliodigestive anastomosis
bilioduodenal prosthesis
bilioenteric fistula
biliointestinal bypass (BIB)
biliopancreatic bypass (BPB)
biliopancreatic shunt
biliopleural fistula
bilious
biliptysis
bilirubin
    postexchange bilirubin
bilirubin concentration
bilirubin pigment gallstone
bilirubinate stone
Bilisystem ERCP cannula
Bilisystem stone-removal balloon

Bilisystem wire-guided
    papillotome
Bili-Timer
Bill axis traction handle
Bill bar
Bill maneuver
Bill traction handle forceps
Billeau curet
Billeau ear curet
Billeau ear hook
Billeau ear knife
Billeau ear loop
Billeau ear wax curet
Billeau loop
Billeau Teflon-coated loop
Billeau-House ear loop
billet
Billingham-Bookwalter rectal
    fenestrated blade
billowing mitral valve syndrome
Billroth anastomosis
Billroth curet
Billroth forceps
Billroth gastrectomy
Billroth gastroduodenoscopy
Billroth gastroenterostomy
Billroth gastrojejunostomy
Billroth gastrostomy
Billroth hypertrophy
Billroth I anastomosis
Billroth I gastroduodenostomy
Billroth I gastroenterostomy
Billroth I gastrointestinal
    anastomosis
Billroth I gastrostomy
Billroth I operation
Billroth I partial gastrectomy
Billroth I procedure
Billroth I technique
Billroth I gastrectomy
Billroth II gastrectomy
Billroth I, II reconstruction
Billroth II anastomosis
Billroth II anatomy
Billroth II gastrectomy
Billroth II gastroenterostomy
Billroth II gastrointestinal
    anastomosis
Billroth II gastrojejunostomy
Billroth II gastrostomy
Billroth II operation
Billroth II procedure

Billroth II technique
Billroth operation
Billroth ovarian retractor
Billroth ovarian trocar
Billroth retractor
Billroth tongue excision
Billroth tube
Billroth tumor forceps
Billroth uterine tumor forceps
Billroth-Stille retractor
bilobar disease
bilobar liver metastasis
bilobar resection
bilobate placenta
bilobed fasciocutaneous flap
bilobed gallbladder
bilobed placenta
bilobed polypoid lesion
bilobed skin flap technique
bilobed transposition flap
bilocular femoral hernia
bilocular joint
biloculare
    cor biloculare
bilocularis uterus
Bilos pin extractor
Bilson fixable-removable cross
    arch bar splint
Biltzer laryngeal blade
bilumen implant
bilumen mammary implant
BIMA (bilateral internal
    mammary artery)
BIMA reconstruction
bimalleolar ankle fracture
bimalleolar fracture
bimanual examination
bimanual pelvic examination
bimanual percussion
bimanual version
bimastoid line
bimaxillary dentoalveolar
    protrusion
bimaxillary prognathism
bimaxillary protrusion
bimaxillary protrusive
    occlusion
bimaxillary relationship
bimeter gnathodynamometer
Bi-Metric hip prosthesis
Bi-Metric Interlok femoral
    prosthesis

Bi-Metric porous primary
    femoral prosthesis
Bimler activator
Bimler appliance
Bimler arch
Bimler elastic plate
bimucosa
    fistula bimucosa
binangle
binangled chisel
binary fission
binasal cannula
binasal pharyngeal airway
binaural fusion
binaural stethoscope
binauricular arc
binauricular axis
binder
    abdominal binder
    Alveograf binder
    breast binder
    compression binder
    Dale abdominal binder
    Dale surgical binder
    HK binder
    obstetrical binder
    Orthomatrix binder
    Osteograf binder
    Scultetus binder
    Texal-Muller chest binder
    Velcro binder
Binder implant
Binder submalar implant
Binder syndrome
binding agent
Binet scale
Binet system of classification
Bing syringe
Bing stylet
Bingham knee prosthesis
Bing-Siebenmann
    malformation
Bing-Taussig heart procedure
Binkhorst collar stud intraocular
    lens
Binkhorst collar stud lens
    implant
Binkhorst equation
Binkhorst eye implant
Binkhorst 4-loop iris-fixated
    implant
Binkhorst hooked cannula

Binkhorst intraocular lens
    implant
Binkhorst irrigating cannula
Binkhorst lens forceps
Binkhorst lens implant
Binkhorst mustache lens
    intraocular lens
Binkhorst tip
Binkhorst 2-loop modified
    J loop intraocular lens
Binkhorst 2-loop intraocular
    lens implant
Binkhorst 2-loop lens
Binkhorst-Fyodorov lens
Binne operation
Binner diaphoscope
Binner head lamp
Binnie operation
binocle bandage
binocular accommodation
binocular bandage
binocular eye dressing
binocular fixation forceps
binocular fusion
binocular indirect
    ophthalmoscope with SPF
binocular instrument
binocular loupe
binocular microscope
binocular microscopy
binocular ophthalmoscope
binocular prism
binocular prism loupe
binocular shield
binocular slit lamp
binocular surgical loupe
binocular tube
binotic
Bio Core therapeutic mattress
Bio Foam Eggcrate
Bio Gard critical care flotation
    unit
bioabsorbable double-spiral
    stent
bioabsorbable interference
    screw
Bio-Absorbable staple
bioabsorbable closure device
bioacrylic interface
bioactive bone cement adhesive
Bio-Anchor suture anchor
bioartificial liver support device

bioavailability
Biobond tissue adhesive
Biobrane adhesive
Biobrane dressing
Biobrane experimental skin
    substitute
Biobrane glove dressing
Biobrane glove graft
Biobrane graft material
Biobrane sheet
Biobrane skin substitute
Biobrane wound covering
Biobrane wound dressing
Biobrane/HF graft material
Biobrane/HF substitute skin
    graft
Biobrane/HF wound dressing
BioCare implant
Biocell anatomical
    reconstructive mammary
    implant
Biocell RTV breast implant
Biocell RTV implant
Biocell RTV saline-filled breast
    implant
Biocell smooth surface implant
Biocell textured implant
Biocell textured shell surface
    implant
Biocell textured silicone
Biocell textured surface implant
Biocell wrap
Bioceram 2-stage series II
    endosteal dental implant
bioceramic implant material
bioceramics
biochemical metastasis
Bio-Chromatic hand prosthesis
biocidal
Bioclad with pegs reinforced
    acetabular prosthesis
Bioclusive drape
Bioclusive dressing
Bioclusive MVP Select
    transparent dressing
Bioclusive transparent dressing
Biocol temporary dressing
biocompatibility
    implant biocompatibility
biocompatible bone graft
    substitute material
biocompatible spacing material

biocompression pneumatic
    sleeve
Biocon impedance
    plethysmography cardiac
    output monitor
Biocor heart valve
Biocor porcine stented aortic
    valve
Biocor porcine stented mitral
    valve
Biocor stentless porcine aortic
    valve
Biocoral graft
Biocoral implant
BioCore collagen dressing
BioCuff screw
BioCuff washer
BioCurve saline-filled breast
    implant
biodegradable plate fixation
biodegradable polymer scaffold
biodegradable stent
biodegradable surgical tack
biodegradation
    implant biodegradation
Biodel implant
Biodex isokinetic dynamometer
Biodex isokinetic testing machine
Biodex machine
Biodex test
Biodex XYZ imaging table
BioDimensional saline-filled
    implant
BioDimensional tissue expander
BiodivYsio AS (added support)
    stent
BiodivYsio OC (open cell) stent
BiodivYsio SV (small vessel)
    stent
Biodrape dressing
Biodynamic acetabular
    component
biodynamics
BioDyne II kinetic therapy low-
    air-loss bed
bioequivalent
Bio-eye hydroxyapatite ocular
    implant
Bio-eye implant
Bio-Fastak suture/anchor
biofeedback
    laryngeal image biofeedback

biofeedback
  electroencephalograph
biofeedback galvanic skin
  response device
biofeedback instrumentation
biofilm
  glycocalyx-enclosed biofilm
  THINSite with BioFilm
  Biofix absorbable rod
Biofix absorbable screw
Biofix arrow gun
Biofix biodegradable implant
Biofix fixation rod
Biofix system pin
BIOflex Magnet Back Support
BIOflex magnetic brace
BIOflex penile orthotic
Biofoot orthotic
biofragmentable anastomotic
  ring
Biogel Diagnostic surgical gloves
Biogel M surgical gloves
Biogel Neotech surgical gloves
Biogel orthopaedic surgical
  gloves
Biogel Reveal/Indicator surgical
  gloves
Biogel Sensor surgical gloves
Biogel Super-Sensitive surgical
  gloves
BioGen nonporous barrier
  membrane
Bio-Gide dental implant
Bio-Gide resorbable barrier
  membrane
Bio-Gide resorbable bilayer
  barrier membrane
Bioglass bone substitute
  material
Bioglass bone graft substitute
  material
Bioglass bone substitute
  material
Bioglass prosthesis
BioGlide catheter
BioGlue surgical patch
bioglycolic lightening gel
biograft
  Alveoform biograft
  Dardik biograft
  Meadox Dardik biograft
Biograft bovine heterograft

Biograft bovine heterograft
  material
biograft umbilical prosthesis
BioGran resorbable synthetic
  bone graft
BioGran synthetic graft
Bio-Groove acetabular
  prosthesis
Bio-Groove hip
Bio-Groove Macrobond HA
  femoral prosthesis
Bio-Groove total hip prosthesis
Bio-Guard spectrum
  antimicrobial bonded
  catheter
biohazard bag
biohazard container
biohazard operating technique
biohazard specimen
BioHorizon implant
bioimpedance
  electrocardiograph
bioimplant
bioingrowth
biointerference screw
Bioject jet injector
Bio-kinetics reader
BioKleen
BioKnit garment electrode
BioLase laser adapter
Biolex cleansers
Biolex impregnated dressing
Biolex wound glue
Biolite ventilation tube
biologic creep of skin
biologic fibrogen adhesive
biologic fixation
biologic response modifier
biological effect
biological tissue valve
Biologically Quiet interference
  screw
Biologically Quiet
  reconstruction screw
Biologically Quiet suture
  anchor
Biologics Airlift bed
Biolox ball head prosthesis
Biolox ceramic ball head for hip
  replacement
Biolox ceramic femoral head
biomagnetic therapy

biomaterial
  Gore-Tex DualMesh
    biomaterial
  Gore-Tex MycroMesh
    biomaterial
Biomatrix ocular implant
biomechanics
Bio-Med MVP-10 pediatric
  ventilator
BioMed TENS unit
BioMedic MicroEncapsulated
  retinol cream
Bio-Medicus arterial catheter
Bio-Medicus centrifugal pump
Bio-Medicus percutaneous
  cannula set
Bio-Medicus pump
biomembrane
BioMend collagen membrane
BioMend membrane
BioMend periodontal material
Biomer microsuturing
  instrument
Biomet AGC knee component
Biomet AGC knee prosthesis
Biomet AGC primary and
  posterior stabilized
  component
Biomet ankle arthrodesis nail
Biomet bed
Biomet Bi-Polar component
Biomet button
Biomet cement removal hand
  chisel
Biomet custom implant
Biomet femoral component
Biomet fracture brace
Biomet hip
Biomet hip prosthesis
Biomet impactor
Biomet instruments
Biomet MARS acetabular
  component
Biomet plug
Biomet Repicci II
  unicompartment knee
  component
Biomet revision acetabular
  component
Biomet shoulder component
Biomet total knee instruments
Biomet total toe prosthesis

Biomet Ultra-Drive cement
  remover
Biomet Velcro wrist support
biometric profile
biometric prosthesis
biometry probe
biomicroscope
biomicroscopic indirect lens
biomicroscopy
Bio-Modular humeral rasp
Bio-Modular shoulder
Bio-Moore II instrumentation
Bio-Moore II stem impactor
Bio-Moore endoprosthesis
Bio-Moore rasp
biomort
bion
Bionic ear prosthesis
Bionicare stimulator
Bionit II vascular prosthesis
Bionit vascular graft
Bionit vascular prosthesis
Bionix disposable nasal
  speculum
Bionix self-reinforced PLLA
  smart screw
Bionix SmartNail bioresorbable
  implant
bio-oncotic gel
Bio-Optics camera
Bio-Optics specular microscope
Bio-Oss
Bio-Oss bone filler graft
Bio-Oss collagen
Bio-Oss corticalis bone graft
  material
Bio-Oss freeze-dried
  demineralized bone
Bio-Oss maxillofacial bone filler
Bio-Oss spongiosa block
Bio-Oss spongiosa bone graft
  material
Bio-Oss synthetic bone
Biopatch antimicrobial dressing
Biopatch antimicrobial foam
  wound dressing
Biopatch foam wound dressing
Bio-Pen biometric ruler
Bio-Phase suture anchor
biophotometer
biophylaxis
Biophysic Medical YAG laser

Biophysic Ophthascan S
instrument
biophysical profile (BPP)
biophysics
dental biophysics
Bioplant hard tissue
replacement synthetic bone
Bioplant HTR synthetic bone
Bioplastique augmentation
material
Bioplastique injectable
microimplant
Bioplastique polymer
Bio-Plug
Bio-Plug canal plug
Bioplus dispersive electrode
BioPolyMeric femoropopliteal
bypass graft
BioPolyMeric graft
BioPolyMeric vascular graft
Biopore membrane
biopotential skin electrode
Biopro implant for the proximal
phalanx
bioprogressive technique
bioprosthesis
Carpentier-Edwards
bioprosthesis
bioprosthetic heart valve
biopsy
4-quadrant biopsy
4-quadrant cervical punch
biopsy
4-point biopsy
abdominal lymph node
biopsy
abrasive brush biopsy
adrenal gland biopsy
alcohol-fixed gastric biopsy
Allis-Abramson breast biopsy
anoscopy with biopsy
antistriated muscle biopsy
antral biopsy
aspiration biopsy
aspiration needle biopsy
automated large-core liver
biopsy
Bennett nail biopsy
bioptic biopsy
bisection biopsy
bite biopsy
bladder biopsy

biopsy (*continued*)
blind percutaneous liver
biopsy
bone marrow aspiration and
biopsy
bone marrow biopsy
bougienage biopsy
brain biopsy
breast biopsy
bronchial biopsy
bronchial brush biopsy
bronchoscopic needle biopsy
bronchoscopy with biopsy
bronchotomy with biopsy
brush biopsy
Campylobacter-like organism
biopsy
catheter-guided biopsy
cervical biopsy
cervical cone biopsy
cervical punch biopsy
channel and core biopsy
chorionic villi biopsy (CVB)
chorionic villus biopsy
CLO biopsy
coin biopsy
cold biopsy
cold blade biopsy
cold cone biopsy
cold cup biopsy
colonoscopic biopsy
colorectal biopsy
colposcopic-directed punch
biopsy
computer tomography-guided
biopsy
cone biopsy
conization biopsy
core needle biopsy
corporeal biopsy
cortical biopsy
Crosby-Kugler capsule for
biopsy
CT-guided liver biopsy
CT-guided needle aspiration
biopsy
cutting needle biopsy
cystoscopic biopsy
cytobrush biopsy
cytologic biopsy
cytological biopsy
deep-wedge biopsy

biopsy (*continued*)
    diagnostic biopsy
    diagnostic excisional biopsy
    diathermic loop biopsy
    digitally-guided biopsy
    directed biopsy
    directed fine-needle aspiration
        biopsy
    direct-vision liver biopsy
    Dunn biopsy
    elliptical biopsy
    embryo biopsy
    endocervical biopsy
    endometrial biopsy
    endomyocardial biopsy (EMB)
    endoscopic biopsy
    endoscopic small bowel
        biopsy
    endoscopic sphenoidal biopsy
    ERCP-guided biopsy
    esophageal biopsy
    excision and biopsy
    excision and wedge biopsy
    excision biopsy
    excisional biopsy
    exploratory biopsy
    fetal liver biopsy
    fetal skin biopsy
    fine-needle aspiration biopsy
        (FNAB)
    fine-needle biopsy
    FNA biopsy
    forage core biopsy
    Fosnaugh nail biopsy
    fractional biopsy
    gastrointestinal biopsy
    guided transcutaneous biopsy
    guillotine needle biopsy
    hilar biopsy
    hot biopsy
    ileal biopsy
    iliac crest biopsy
    image-guided breast biopsy
        (GBB)
    image-guided fine-needle
        aspiration biopsy
    image-guided stereotactic
        brain biopsy
    incisional biopsy
    internal mammary node
        biopsy
    intestinal biopsy

biopsy (*continued*)
    intramedullary tumor biopsy
    intraocular foreign biopsy
    intraoperative biopsy
    Jako biopsy
    Jamshidi muscle needle
        biopsy
    jejunal biopsy
    jumbo biopsy
    Kevorkian punch biopsy
    Keyes punch biopsy
    kidney biopsy
    Kuschner-Tandatnick
        endometrial biopsy
    laparoscopic liver biopsy
    large-core needle aspiration
        biopsy
    large-particle biopsy
    lift-and-cut biopsy
    liquid biopsy
    liver biopsy
    lumbar spine biopsy
    lung biopsy
    lymph node biopsy
    mammary node biopsy
    mediastinal lymph node
        biopsy
    mediastinal node biopsy
    Menghini percutaneous liver
        biopsy
    Menghini technique for
        percutaneous liver biopsy
    minimally invasive biopsy
    mirror-image breast biopsy
    mucosal biopsy
    multiple core biopsy
    muscle biopsy
    nasopharyngeal biopsy
    native renal biopsy
    needle aspiration biopsy
    needle core biopsy
    needle localization breast
        biopsy
    needle-localized open biopsy
        (NLOB)
    negative biopsy
    negative breast biopsy
    nerve biopsy
    node biopsy
    onion-bulb changes on biopsy
    open biopsy
    optical biopsy

biopsy (*continued*)
  out-of-phase endometrial
    biopsy
  outpatient biopsy
  pancreatic biopsy
  paracollicular biopsy
  parathyroid biopsy
  pelvic aspiration biopsy
  percutaneous excisional
    breast biopsy (PEBB)
  percutaneous fine-needle
    aspiration biopsy
  percutaneous fine-needle
    pancreatic biopsy
  percutaneous liver biopsy
  percutaneous native renal
    biopsy
  percutaneous needle liver
    biopsy
  percutaneous pancreas biopsy
  pericardial biopsy
  perineal biopsy
  perineal needle biopsy
  peritoneal biopsy
  peroral intestinal biopsy
  PET-guided biopsy
  pinch biopsy
  pipelle biopsy
  pleural biopsy
  point-in-space stereotactic
    biopsy
  positron emission
    tomography-guided biopsy
  pouch biopsy
  preoperative biopsy
  pseudotumor
    cerebromeningeal biopsy
  punch biopsy
  random bladder biopsy
  rectal suction biopsy
  renal biopsy
  saucerized biopsy
  scalene biopsy
  scalene fat pad biopsy
  scalene node biopsy (SNB)
  scan-directed biopsy
  Scher nail biopsy
  secondary diagnostic biopsy
  second-look biopsy
  sentinel node biopsy (SNB)
  serial percutaneous liver
    biopsy

biopsy (*continued*)
  shave biopsy
  shave excision biopsy
  single biopsy
  skeletal biopsy
  skin biopsy
  skinny-needle biopsy
  SLN biopsy
  small incisional biopsy
  snap-frozen biopsy
  snare excision biopsy
  snare loop biopsy
  sonoguided biopsy
  spinal infection biopsy
  sponge biopsy
  StereoGuide stereotactic
    needle core biopsy
  stereotactic aspiration
    biopsy
  stereotactic brain biopsy
  stereotactic core breast
    biopsy
  stereotactic needle core
    biopsy
  stereotactic percutaneous
    needle biopsy
  stereotactic-guided biopsy
  sternal biopsy
  strip biopsy
  submitted for biopsy
  suction biopsy
  supraclavicular lymph node
    biopsy
  sural nerve biopsy
  surface biopsy
  surgical biopsy
  surgical excision biopsy
  synovial biopsy
  systematic sextant biopsy
  tangential biopsy
  targeted brain biopsy
  temporal artery biopsy
  testicular biopsy
  thin-needle biopsy
  thoracic spine biopsy
  thyroid needle biopsy
  tissue biopsy
  total biopsy
  tracheal biopsy
  transbronchial lung biopsy
  transcutaneous biopsy
  transfemoral liver biopsy

biopsy (*continued*)

transgastric fine-needle aspiration biopsy
transitional zone biopsy
transjugular hepatic biopsy
transjugular liver biopsy
transnasal biopsy
transpapillary biopsy
transrectal perineal needle biopsy
transrectal ultrasound-guided sextant biopsy
transthoracic biopsy
transthoracic needle aspiration biopsy
transthoracic percutaneous fine-needle aspiration biopsy
transurethral biopsy
transurethral perineal biopsy
transvenous liver biopsy
trephine needle biopsy
trophectoderm biopsy
Tru-Cut needle biopsy (TCNB, TNB)
ultrasonography-guided fine-needle aspiration biopsy
ultrasound-guided anterior subcostal liver biopsy
ultrasound-guided automated large-core breast biopsy
ultrasound-guided biopsy
ultrasound-guided core breast biopsy
ultrasound-guided core-needle biopsy (US-CNB)
ultrasound-guided echo biopsy
ultrasound-guided fine-needle aspiration biopsy (US-FNAB)
ultrasound-guided stereotactic biopsy
ureteral biopsy
Vabra endometrial biopsy
vaginal cone biopsy
Valls needle biopsy
Valls-Ottolenghim-Schajowicz needle biopsy
ventricular endomyocardial biopsy
Verman needle biopsy

biopsy (*continued*)

Vertical lip biopsy
video-assisted excisional biopsy
Vim-Silverman technique for liver biopsy
vulvar biopsy
Watson capsule biopsy
wedge excisional biopsy
wedge hepatic biopsy
wedge liver biopsy
wide resection biopsy
wire-guided breast biopsy
wound biopsy
Zaias nail biopsy
biopsy accessories
biopsy after radiation
biopsy by curettage
biopsy cannula
biopsy cavity
biopsy curet
biopsy forceps
biopsy gun
biopsy instruments
biopsy loop electrode
biopsy needle
biopsy probe
biopsy punch
biopsy punch forceps
biopsy sample
biopsy set
biopsy site
biopsy specimen
biopsy specimen forceps
biopsy suction curet
biopsy technique
biopsy telescope
biopsy thorascope
biopsy tongs
biopsy volume
biopsy-proven metastasis
Biopsys
bioptic aid
bioptic biopsy
bioptic telescope
bioptome
Bycep PC Jr bioptome
Caves bioptome
Caves-Schultz bioptome
Cordis bioptome
King cardiac bioptome
Mansfield bioptome

bioptome (*continued*)
    Scholten endomyocardial
        bioptome
    Stanford bioptome
    Stanford-Caves bioptome
Biopty cut biopsy needle
Biopty cut needle
Biopty gun
Bio-Pump for bypass surgery
Bio-Pump pump
Biorate pacemaker
biorbital angle
BioRCI bioabsorbable screw
bioresorbable
bioresorbable guided tissue
    membrane
bioresorbable implant
biorhythm
BioROC EZ suture anchor
Bio-R-Sorb resorbable poly-
    L-lactic acid ministaple
Biosearch anal biofeedback
    device
Biosearch female intermittent
    urinary catheter
Biosearch jejunostomy kit
Biosearch male intermittent
    urinary catheter
Biosearch needle
Bio-SET needleless device
BioSkin support
BioSorb endoscopic browlift
    screw
BioSorb resorbable urology stent
BioSorb suture
Biosound 2000 II ultrasound
    unit
Biosound Surgiscan
    echocardiograph
Biosound wide-angle monoplane
    ultrasound scanner
Biospal filter
Biospan anatomical tissue
    expander
BioSpan breast tissue expander
BioSpec MR imaging system
    scanner
BioSphere suture anchor
Bio-Statak suture anchor
Biostil blood transfusion set
BioStinger bioabsorbable
    meniscal implant

BioStinger fixation device
BioStinger-V bioabsorbable
    meniscal repair device
Biostop G cement restrictor
Biosyn suture
biosynthetic wound covering
Biosystems feeding tube
Biot breathing
Biot sign
BioTac biopsy cannula
BioTac ECG electrode
biotesting
Biothotic foot orthosis
Biothotic orthotic mold
biotome
Biotrack coagulation monitor
BioTrainer exercise meter
biotripticum
    atrophoderma biotripticum
Biotronic demand pacemaker
Biotronik lead
Bio-Vascular prosthetic valve
Bio-Vent implant
Biovert ceramic implant
Biovert implant material
Biovue catheter
Biox III ear oximeter
BiPAP unit
BiPAP (bilevel positive airway
    pressure)
bilevel positive airway pressure
    (inBiPAP)
biparietal
biparietal craniotomy
biparietal diameter (BPD)
biparietal hump
biparietal suture
biparietal suture technique
bipartita
    placenta bipartita
bipartite patella
bipartite placenta
bipartition
    transcranial facial bipartition
bipartitus uterus
bipedal
bipedicle delay flap
bipedicle digital visor flap
bipedicle dorsal flap
bipedicle flap
bipedicle mucoperiosteal flap
bipedicle TRAM flap

bipedicled
bipedicled delay flap
bipennate muscle
bipenniform structure
biphalangeal thumb
biphase external pin fixation
biphase pin fixation
biphasic
bi-Phasic exfoliator
biphasic growth cycle
biphasic pin
biphasic pin appliance
biphasic response
bipivotal hinge knee brace
biplanar fixator
biplanar fluoroscopy
biplanar forehead lift
biplane angiography
biplane cerebral angiography
biplane cineangiogram
biplane fluoroscopy
biplane intracavitary plane
biplane orthogonal angiogram
biplane pelvic arteriogram
biplane projection
biplane quantitative coronary
    arteriogram
biplane sector probe
biplane view
biplaner II control
bipolar
    E-series bipolar
bipolar affective disorder (BAD)
bipolar bayonet forceps
bipolar catheter
bipolar catheter electrode
bipolar cautery scissors
bipolar circumactive probe (BIC
    inAP)
bipolar coagulating forceps
bipolar coagulation-suction
    forceps
bipolar coaptation forceps
bipolar connecting cord
bipolar cup hip prosthesis
bipolar cutting forceps
bipolar depth electrode
bipolar diathermy adapter clip
bipolar diathermy forceps tip
bipolar disorder
bipolar electrocautery
bipolar electrocautery forceps

bipolar electrocoagulation
bipolar electrode
bipolar electrosurgery
bipolar electrosurgical unit
bipolar endostasis probe
bipolar eye forceps
bipolar glass electrode
bipolar hemostasis probe
bipolar hip arthroplasty
bipolar irrigating forceps
bipolar irrigating stylet
bipolar laparoscopic forceps
bipolar lead
bipolar limb leads
bipolar long-shaft forceps
bipolar Medtronic pacemaker
bipolar microforceps
bipolar myocardial electrode
bipolar needle
bipolar pacemaker leads
bipolar pacing catheter
bipolar pacing electrode
    catheter
bipolar placement of
    electrodes
bipolar probe
bipolar prosthesis
bipolar radiofrequency
    resurfacing
bipolar suction forceps
bipolar temporary pacemaker
    catheter
bipolar total hip
bipolar transsphenoidal
    forceps
bipolar urological loop
bipolar version
BiPort hemostasis introducer
    sheath kit
BIPP ribbon gauze
biprism applanation tonometer
biprong muscle marker
Biopulse stimulator
Birbeck granule
Birch trocar
Bircher bone-holding clamp
Bircher cartilage clamp
Bircher meniscus knife
Bircher operation
Bircher-Ganske meniscal
    cartilage forceps
Bircher-Weber technique

Birch-Hirschfeld entropion
    operation
Birch-Hirschfeld lamp
Bird 8400STi ventilator
Bird machine
Bird Mark 8 respirator
Bird micronebulizer
Bird neonatal CPAP generator
Bird cup
Bird pressure-cycled ventilator
Bird respirator
Bird table
Bird vacuum extractor
bird-beak deformity
bird-beak jaw
birdcage head coil
birdcage resonator
birdcage splint
bird-face
bird-face retrognathism
bird-headed dwarf
bird's beak distal esophagus
bird's eye view
bird's nest IVC filter
bird's nest lesion
bird's-eye catheter
bi-refringence
bi-refringent
Bireks dissecting forceps
Birkett hemostatic forceps
Birkett hernia
Birks Mark II Colibri forceps
Birks Mark II grooved forceps
Birks Mark II hook
Birks Mark II micro cross-action
    holder
Birks Mark II micro push/pull
    spatula
Birks Mark II microneedle-
    holder forceps
Birks Mark II needle-holder
    forceps
Birks Mark II straight forceps
Birks Mark II suture-tying
    forceps
Birks Mark II toothed forceps
Birks Mark II trabeculectomy
    scissors
Birnbaum procedure for vaginal
    prolapse
Birnberg bow intrauterine
    device

Birnberg traction bow
Biro dermal nevus scissors
Birtcher cautery
Birtcher coagulator
Birtcher defibrillator
Birtcher electrocautery probe
Birtcher electrode
Birtcher electrosurgery unit
Birtcher electrosurgical
    generator
Birtcher electrosurgical needle
Birtcher endoscopic forceps
Birtcher hyfrecator cautery
    guidewire
Birtcher hyfrecator
    electrosurgical unit
Birtcher Hyfrecutter
Birtcher laparoscopic coagulator
Birtcher proctological electrode
    set
Birtcher proctology set
Birtcher proctosigmoid
    desiccation set
birth
    breech birth
    cesarean birth
    complicated birth
    instrument birth
    live birth
    multiple births
    post-term birth
    premature birth
    uncomplicated birth
    vaginal birth
birth amputation
birth canal laceration
birth cushion
birth defect
birth fracture
birth injury
birth trauma
birthing ball
birthing chair
birthing position
birthing room
birthmark
    café au lait birthmark
    hemangioma birthmark
    macular vascular birthmark
    port-wine stain birthmark
    strawberry birthmark
    telangiectatic birthmark

birthmark (*continued*)
  vascular birthmark
  vascular malformation
    birthmark
Birt-Hogg-Dubé syndrome
Bischoff corona
Bischoff crown
Bischoff myelotomy
Bischoff operation
bisect
bisected
bisected mass
bisected minigraft dilator
bisecting angle cone position
bisecting angle technique
bisection biopsy
bisector line
Biset catheter
bisected angle radiograph
bis-GMA (bisphenol A-glycidyl
    methacrylate)
Bishop antrum perforator
Bishop antrum trocar
Bishop bone clamp
Bishop chisel
Bishop classification
bishop collar deformity
Bishop gouge
Bishop mastoid chisel
Bishop mastoid gouge
Bishop oscillatory electric bone
    saw
Bishop perforator
Bishop retractor
Bishop saw
Bishop sphygmoscope
Bishop tendon tucker
Bishop tissue forceps
Bishop-Black tendon tucker
Bishop-Black tucker
Bishop-Coop enterostomy
Bishop-DeWitt tendon tucker
Bishop-Harman anterior
    chamber cannula
Bishop-Harman anterior
    chamber irrigating cannula
Bishop-Harman anterior
    chamber irrigator
Bishop-Harman bladebreaker
Bishop-Harman dressing forceps
Bishop-Harman foreign body
    forceps

Bishop-Harman iris forceps
Bishop-Harman irrigating
    cannula
Bishop-Harman knife
Bishop-Harman mules
Bishop-Harman tip
Bishop-Harman tissue forceps
Bishop-Koop ileostomy
Bishop-Peter tendon tucker
bi-iliac diameter
Biskra button
bismuth benign bile duct
    stricture classification
bismuth bile duct stricture type
    I-V classification
bismuth line
bismuth pigmentation
BiSNARE bipolar polypectomy
    snare
Bi-Soft contact lens
Bi-Soft lens
bisphenol A-glycidyl
    methacrylate (bis-GMA)
bispherical lens
Bisping electrode
bispinous diameter
bisque-baked prosthesis
bissac
  en bissac
  hernia en bissac
Bissell operation
bistable imaging
bistoury
  Brophy bistoury
  Converse bistoury
  Converse button-end bistoury
  ear bistoury
  Jackson bistoury
  Jackson tracheotomic
    bistoury
  nasal bistoury
  tracheal bistoury
  tracheotomic bistoury
bistoury blade
bistoury knife
bisubcostal incision
Biswas Silastic vaginal pessary
bit
  drill guide with drill bit
  Zimalate twist drill bit
bite
  deep bite

bite (*continued*)
   mature bite
   open bite
   skeletal open bite
   stork bite
   stork's bite
   underhung bite
bite biopsy
bite biopsy forceps
bite block
bite force
bite force transducer
bite line
bite plane therapy
bite protector
bite splint
bite-block
   lollipop bite-block
Bi-tec forceps
bitemporal
bitemporal craniotomy
bitemporal diameter
biteplane
biter
   parrot-beak basket biter
   suction biter
biterminal electrode
bitewing technique
biting
   cheek biting
   lip biting
   tongue biting
biting forceps
biting punch
biting rongeur
Bitome bipolar sphincterotome
Bitome catheter
Bitoric lens
Bitpad digitizer
Bitumi monobjective
   microscope
BIVAD (bilateral left and right
   ventricular assist device)
bivalve nasal splint implant
bivalve, bivalved
bivalved anal speculum
bivalved cannula
bivalved cast
bivalved ear speculum
bivalved elliptical incision
bivalved incision
bivalved plaster cast

bivalved retractor
bivalved speculum
bivalved tube
biventricular assist device
   (BVAD)
Bivona cuff maintenance
   device
Bivona duckbill voice prosthesis
Bivona epistaxis catheter
Bivona Fome-Cuf tube
Bivona low-resistance voice
   prosthesis
Bivona customized
   tracheostomy tube
Bivona sleep apnea
   tracheostomy tube
Bivona tracheostomy tube
Bivona tracheostomy tube with
   talk attachment
Bivona TTS tracheostomy tube
Bivona Ultra Low voice
   prosthesis
Bivona voice prosthesis
Bivona-Colorado button
Bivona-Colorado dummy
   prosthesis
Bivona-Colorado sizing device
Bivona-Colorado voice
   prosthesis
bizygomatic breadth
Bizzarri-Guiffrida kinfe
Bizzarri-Guiffrida laryngoscope
Bjerrum scotoma
Bjerrum scotometer
Bjerrum screen
Bjerrum sign
Björk diathermy forceps
Björk drill
Björk flap tracheostomy
Björk method of Fontan
   procedure
Björk operation
Björk prosthesis
Björk rib drill
Björk-Shiley aortic valve
   prosthesis
Björk-Shiley convexoconcave
   60-degree valve prosthesis
Björk-Shiley floating disk
   prosthesis
Björk-Shiley graft
Björk-Shiley mitral valve

Björk-Shiley mitral valve
   prosthesis
Björk-Shiley Monostrut valve
Björk-Shiley prosthetic aortic
   valve
Björk-Shiley prosthetic mitral
   valve
Björk-Shiley valve prosthesis
Björk-Stille diathermy forceps
Björnström algesimeter
BK amputation (below-knee
   amputation)
B-K dysplastic nevi
B-K moles
BK prosthesis, (below-knee
   prosthesis)
BL (buccolingual)
black blood clot
Black bone and skin rasp
black box of upper GI tract
black braided nylon sutures
black braided silk sutures
black cancer
Black clamp
Black classification
black currant rash
black eschar
black faceted stone
black light lamp
black line
Black Max midsize knee
Black meatus clamp
black mole cancer
black patch syndrome
black pigment gallstone
Black rasp
Black repair
Black retractor
black silk sutures
Black technique
black twisted sutures
black/white occluder
BlackBeauty ureteral stent
Black-Brostrom staple technique
Blackburn skull traction tractor
Blackburn technique
Blackburn trephine
Black Decker needle
black-dot heel
blackened hemostat
blackened laser instruments
blackened speculum

Blackett-Healy position
Blackmon needle
Blackstone anterior cervical
   plate
Blackwood meniscal repair
Blackwood suture instrument
Black-Wylie dilator
Black-Wylie obstetric dilator
bladder
   adynamic bladder
   atonic bladder
   autonomic neurogenic
      bladder
   base of bladder
   catheterization of bladder
   complete emptying of
      bladder
   contracted urinary bladder
   cord bladder
   denervated bladder
   dome of bladder
   double bladder
   dyssynergic bladder
   ectopic bladder
   exstrophy of bladder
   fasciculated bladder
   filling of bladder
   hourglass bladder
   hyperreflexic bladder
   hypertonic bladder
   hyporeflexic bladder
   hypotonic bladder
   ileal bladder
   ileocecal bladder
   infundibulum of urinary
      bladder
   irrigated bladder
   irrigation of bladder
   irritable bladder
   kidneys, ureters, bladder
      (KUB)
   neurogenic bladder
   neuropathic bladder
   orthotopic bladder
   poorly compliant bladder
   pseudoneurogenic bladder
   reflex neurogenic bladder
   ruptured bladder
   sigmoid bladder
   stammering bladder
   string bladder
   trabeculated bladder

bladder (*continued*)
  uninhibited neurogenic
    bladder
  unstable bladder
  urachal sinus of bladder
  urinary bladder
  valve bladder
bladder augmentation
bladder autoaugmentation
bladder biopsy
bladder blade
bladder bubble
bladder calculus
bladder carcinoma classification
bladder catheterization
bladder chimney procedure
bladder dilator
bladder distention
bladder diverticulectomy
bladder dome
bladder drainage
bladder ectopia
bladder evacuator
bladder fistula
bladder flap hematoma
bladder flap tube
bladder forceps
bladder hemorrhage
bladder hernia
bladder irrigating valve
bladder irrigation control clamp
bladder laceration
bladder mucosa
bladder neck contracture
bladder neck elevator test
bladder neck preserving
  technique
bladder neck ridge
bladder neck spreader
bladder neck support pessary
bladder neck suspension
bladder neck-to-urethra
  anastomosis
bladder outlet reconstruction
bladder pacemaker
bladder perforation
bladder pillars
bladder pressure
bladder reflection
bladder replacement urinary
  pouch
bladder retractor

bladder sound
bladder specimen forceps
bladder stimulation
bladder stone
bladder suspension
bladder syringe
bladder temperature
bladder trocar
bladder tube
bladder wall
BladderManager portable
  ultrasonic device
BladderManager portable
  ultrasound scanner
BladderManager ultrasound
bladder-neck support prosthesis
bladder-prostate model
BladderScan BVI2500 scanner
BladderScan monitor
BladderScan ultrasound
blade
  3-pronged rake blade
  5-prong rake blade
  Acra-Cut Spiral craniotome
    blade
  adenotome blade
  Aggressor meniscal blade
  Alcon crescent blade
  Alcon pocket blade
  anterior commissure
    laryngoscope blade
  arachnoid Beaver blade
  arachnoid-shape Beaver blade
  arachnoid-shape blade
  arrow blade
  Arthro-Lok system of Beaver
    blades
  arthroscopic banana blade
  ASR blade
  ASSI cranial blades
  ASSI disposable cranio blade
  autopsy blade
  baby Miller blade
  Balfour bladder blade
  Balfour blade
  Balfour center blade
  Balfour lateral blade
  Balfour retractor with
    fenestrated blades
  banana Beaver blade
  banana blade
  Bard-Parker autopsy blade

blade (*continued*)
Bard-Parker blade
Barton blade
Baxter disposable blade
Beaver Arthro-Lok blade
Beaver bent blade
Beaver blade
Beaver cataract blade
Beaver cataract knife blade
Beaver chondroplasty blade
Beaver DeBakey blade
Beaver discission blade
Beaver discission knife blade
Beaver eye surgery blade
Beaver keratome blade
Beaver lamellar blade
Beaver limbus blade
Beaver Microsharp blade
Beaver myringotomy blade
Beaver Optimum blade
Beaver phacokeratome
    blade
Beaver rhinoplasty blade
Beaver surgical blade
Beaver tonsillectomy blade
Beaver-Lundsgaard blade
Beaver-Lundsgaard scleral
    blade
Beaver-Okamura blade
Beaver-Ziegler blade
Beckman-Adson laminectomy
    blade
Beckman-Eaton laminectomy
    blade
Beer blade
Belscope blade
Bennett self-retaining
    retractor blade
bent blade
bent blunt blade
Berens blade
Billingham-Bookwalter rectal
    fenestrated blade
Biltzer laryngeal blade
bistoury blade
bladder blade
Blount bent blade
bone saw blade
Bookwalter malleable
    retractor blade
Bookwalter rectal blade
Bookwalter retractor blade

blade (*continued*)
Bookwalter vaginal Deaver
    blade
Bookwalter-Cook anal rectal
    blade
Bookwalter-Gelpi point
    retractor blade
Bookwalter-Kelly retractor
    blade
Bookwalter-Mayo blade
Bookwalter-Parks anal
    sphincter blade
Bovie blade
Bowen BAS-30 blade
breakable blade
Brown dermatome blade
capsulotomy blade
carbolized knife blade
carbon steel blade
carving blade
Caspar blade
cast blade
Castroviejo blade
Castroviejo razor blade
cataract blade
center blade
cervical biopsy blade
cervical blade
chisel blade
chondroplastic Beaver blade
chondroplastic blade
chondroplasty Beaver blade
circular blade
CLM articulating
    laryngoscope blade
Cloward blade
Cloward single-tooth retractor
    blade
Collin radiopaque sternal blade
conization instrument blade
Converse retractor blade
Cooley-Pontius sternal blade
CooperVision Surgeon-Plus
    Ultrathin blade
copper blade
Cottle blade
Cottle nasal knife blade
crescent blade
crescentic blade
Crile blade
Crockard small-tongue
    retractor blade

blade (*continued*)
- Curdy blade
- Curdy-Hebra blade
- curved meniscotome blade
- David blade
- David-Crowe tongue blade
- Davidoff blade
- Davis-Crowe tongue blade
- Dean blade
- Deaver blade
- DeBakey Beaver blade
- DeBakey blade
- deep spreader blade
- Denis Browne abdominal retractor blade
- Denis Browne malleable copper retractor blade
- Denis Browne mastoid pediatric retractor blade
- Denis Browne pediatric abdominal retractor blade
- Denis Browne-Hendren pediatric retractor blade
- dermatome blade
- diamond blade
- Dingman mouthgag tongue depressor blade
- discission blade
- Dixon center blade
- double-angled blade
- double-vector blade
- Duotrak blade
- Dyonics arthroscopic blade
- Dyonics disposable arthroscope blade
- ear surgery Beaver blade
- ear surgery blade
- Edge blade
- Edge coated blade
- electrodermatome sterile blade
- E-Mac laryngoscope blade
- Emir razor blade
- Endo-Assist blade
- Endo-Assist retractable blade
- English MacIntosh fiberoptic laryngoscope blade
- Epstein hemilaminectomy blade
- expandable blade
- eye blade
- eye knife blade

blade (*continued*)
- eye surgery blade
- Feather carbon breakable blade
- Field blade
- Flagg stainless steel laryngoscope blade
- folding blade
- Franceschetti-type freeblade
- Fugo blade
- Genesis diamond blade
- Gigli-saw blade
- Gill blade
- Gillette Blue Blade
- Gill-Hess blade
- Gott-Balfour blade
- Gott-Harrington blade
- Gott-Seeram blade
- Goulian blade
- Grieshaber blade
- Guedel blade
- Guedel laryngoscope blade
- Hammond blade
- Hammond winged retractor blade
- Hebra blade
- hemilaminectomy blade
- Hemostatix scalpel blade
- Hendren blade
- Hendren pediatric retractor blade
- Hendren retractor blade
- Henley retractor blade
- Hibbs blade
- Hibbs retractor blade
- Hibbs spinal retractor blade
- Hopp anterior commissure laryngoscope blade
- Hopp blade
- Hopp laryngoscope blade
- Horgan blade
- Horgan center blade
- Hoskins razor fragment blade
- House blade
- House detachable blade
- House knife blade
- House ophthalmic blade
- incisor arthroscopic blade
- infant urethrotome blade
- jigsaw blade
- Katena double-edged sapphire blade

blade (*continued*)
K-blade
K-blade microsurgical blade
Keeler retractable blade
Kellan sutureless incision
blade
keratome blade
Knapp blade
knife blade
LaForce adenotome blade
LaForce blade
lamellar blade
laminectomy blade
laminectomy retractor blade
lancet blade
Lange blade
laryngoscope blade
laryngoscope folding blade
LaserSonics EndoBlade
Leivers blade
Lemmon blade
Lieberman wire aspirating
speculum with V-shape
blades
Lite blade
Lundsgaard blade
MacIntosh blade
MacIntosh fiberoptic
laryngoscope blade
Magrina-Bookwalter vaginal
Deaver blade
Mako shaver blade
malleable blade
Martin blade
Martinez corneal trephine
blade
Mastel trifaceted diamond
blade
McPherson-Wheeler blade
meniscectomy blade
Merlin arthroscopy blade
Merlin bendable blade
Meyerding laminectomy
blade
Meyerding retractor blade
Micro-Sharp blade
microvitreoretinal blade
(MVR)
Miller fiberoptic laryngoscope
blade
miniature blade
mini-meniscus blade

blade (*continued*)
Morse blade
mouthgag tongue depressor
blade
Mueller tongue blade
Mullins blade
Murphy-Balfour center
blade
MVR blade
Myocure blade
myringotomy knife blade
nasal knife blade
nasal saw blade
New Skimmer blade
notchplasty blade
Nounton blade
ocutome vitreous blade
ophthalmic blade
Optimum blade
Orandi blade
Orbit blade
Orca surgical blade
Organdi blade
Otocap myringotomy blade
Oxiport blade
Padgett blade
Padgett dermatome blade
Park blade
Parker-Bard blade
Paufique blade
pediatric Hendren retractor
blade
pediatric mastoid retractor
blade
Personna Plus MicroCoat
surgeon's blade
Personna prep blades
Personna surgical blade
PowerCut drill blade
RAD Airway laryngeal blade
RAD40 sinus blade
RADenoid adenoidectomy
blade
ramus blade
razor blade
rectangular blade
Reese dermatome blade
replaceable blade
retractor blade
retrograde Beaver blade
retrograde meniscal blade
Rew-Wyly blade

blade (*continued*)

Rhein 3-D trapezoid diamond blade
ribbon blade
ring tongue blade
rosette blade
Rubin blade
Rusch laryngoscope blade
Satterlee bone saw blade
scalpel blade
ScalpelTec keratome slit blade
ScalpelTec wound-enlargement blade
scapular blade
Schanz Scheie blade
Scheie blade
scimitar blade
scleral blade
sclerotome blade
Scoville retractor blade
self-retaining retractor blade
semilunar-tip blade
serrated blade
Sharpoint blade
Sharpoint crescent blade
Sharpoint spoon blade
Sharpoint V-lance blade
Sharptome crescent blade
shoulder blade
sickle blade
sickle-shape blade
sickle-shaped Beaver blade
sickle-shaped blade
side blade
side-cutting blade
Skimmer blade
slimcut blade
slit blade
Sofield retractor blade
spear blade
spinal retractor blade
Sputnik Russian razor blade
stainless steel blade
sterile electrodermatome blade
sternal blade
sternal retractor blade
Storz disposable blade
straight blade
Stryker blade
Superblade
Super-Cut blade

blade (*continued*)

surgical blade
surgical saw blade
Surgistar ophthalmic blade
Swann-Morton blade
Swann-Morton surgical blade
Swiss blade
Synovator arthroscopic blade
synovectomy blade
tapered blade
Taylor laminectomy blade
Taylor spinal retractor blade
Temperlite saw blade
Thornton arcuate blade
Thornton tri-square blade
throw-away manual dermatome blade
Tiger blade
tongue blade
tongue retractor blade
Tooke blade
Torpin vectis blade
trephine blade
Tricut blade
tri-radial resector blade
Troutman blade
tubular blade
Tucker-Luikart blade
Turner-Warwick blade
Typhoon cutter blade
Typhoon microdebrider blade
UltraEdge keratome blade
ultra-thin surgical blade
Universal nasal saw blade
urethrotome blade
V. Mueller myringotomy blade
Vascutech circular blade
vectis blade
V-lance blade
Weck-Prep blade
Weinberg blade
Welch Allyn laryngoscope blade
Wheeler blade
winged retractor blade
wire side blade
Wisconsin laryngoscope blade
Wood tongue blade
X-Acto blade
Yu-Holtgrewe malleable blade
Zalkind-Balfour blade
Ziegler blade
Zimmer Gigli-saw blade

blade and balloon atrial
   septostomy
blade electrode
blade endosteal implant
blade handle
blade holder
blade knife
bladeplate
bladeplate fixation
bladeplate fixation device
blade retractor
blade scalpel
blade septostomy catheter
bladebreaker
   Barraquer razor bladebreaker
   Bishop-Harman bladebreaker
   Castroviejo bladebreaker
   Castroviejo razor
      bladebreaker
   I-tech-Castroviejo
      bladebreaker
   Jarit bladebreaker
   minirazor bladebreaker
   razor bladebreaker
   Troutman bladebreaker
   Vari bladebreaker
bladebreaker holder
bladebreaker knife
blade-form device
blade-form implant
bladeplate
   bifurcated bladeplate
   fixed-angle AO bladeplate
Blade-Wilde ear forceps
Blainville ears
Blair 4-prong retractor
Blair approach
Blair arthrodesis
Blair chisel
Blair cleft palate clamp
Blair cleft palate elevator
Blair cleft palate knife
Blair elevator
Blair epicanthus repair
Blair fusion
Blair Gigli-saw guide
Blair head drape
Blair hook
Blair incision
Blair knife
Blair modification of Gellhorn
   pessary

Blair nasal chisel
Blair operation
Blair palate hook
Blair ptosis correction operation
Blair retractor
Blair saw guide
Blair serrefine
Blair silicone drain
Blair talar body fusion blade
   plate
Blair technique
Blair tibiotalar arthrodesis blade
   plate
Blair-Brown graft
Blair-Brown implant
Blair-Brown knife
Blair-Brown needle
Blair-Brown needle holder
Blair-Brown operation
Blair-Brown procedure
Blair-Brown prosthesis
Blair-Brown retractor
Blair-Brown skin graft
Blair-Brown skin graft knife
Blair-Brown vacuum retractor
Blair-Brown-McDowell operation
Blair-Byars hypospadias
   technique
Blair-Byars operation
Blair-Ivy loop
Blair-Morris technique
Blair-Omer technique
Blair-Wehrbein operation
Blaisdell skin pencil
Blake curet
Blake drain
Blake dressing forceps
Blake ear forceps
Blake embolus forceps
Blake esophageal tube
Blake forceps
Blake gallstone forceps
Blake gingivectomy knife
Blake knife
Blake rake
Blake silicone drain
Blake uterine curet
Blakemore esophageal tube
Blakemore nasogastric tube
Blakemore tube
Blakemore-Sengstaken tube
Blakesley decompressor

Blakesley ethmoid forceps
Blakesley forceps
Blakesley grasper
Blakesley lacrimal trephine
Blakesley laminectomy rongeur
Blakesley retractor
Blakesley septal bone forceps
Blakesley septal compression
    forceps
Blakesley septal forceps
Blakesley tongue depressor
Blakesley trephine
Blakesley uvula retractor
Blakesley uvular retractor
Blakesley-Weil upturned
    ethmoid forceps
Blakesley-Wilde ear forceps
Blakesley-Wilde ethmoid forceps
Blakesley-Wilde nasal forceps
Blalock anastomosis
Blalock clamp
Blalock forceps
Blalock operation
Blalock procedure
Blalock pulmonary artery clamp
Blalock pulmonic stenosis clamp
Blalock shunt
Blalock suture
Blalock sutures
Blalock-Hanlon atrial septectomy
Blalock-Hanlon operation
Blalock-Hanlon procedure
Blalock-Kleinert forceps
Blalock-Niedner pulmonic
    stenosis clamp
Blalock-Taussig anastomosis
Blalock-Taussig operation
Blalock-Taussig procedure
Blalock-Taussig shunt ligation
blanch
blanchable red lesion
Blanchard clamp
Blanchard cryptotome
Blanchard hemorrhoid forceps
Blanchard pile clamp
Blanchard traction device
Blanchard traction device blade
    plate
blanche
    atrophie blanche
blanched cutaneous elevation
blanched skin

blanching of hand
blanching of sclera
blanching of trabecular
    meshwork
blanching reaction
Blanco retractor
Blanco scissors
Blanco valve spreader
Bland cervical traction forceps
Bland cervical traction
    vulsellum
Bland perineal retractor
bland thrombosis
Bland vulsellum forceps
Blandin and Nuhn glands
Blandin ganglion
Blandin glands
Blandin-Nuhn cyst
Blandy urethroplasty
blank
    implant blank
blanket
    Bair Hugger patient warming
        blanket
    continuous blanket
    cooling blanket
    hypothermia blanket
    K-Thermia blanket
    mucociliary blanket
    mucous blanket
    Therm-O-Rite blanket
blanket suture technique
Blaschko line
Blasius duct
Blasius lid flap operation
Blasius lid operation
Blasius operation
Blaskovics canthoplasty
    operation
Blaskovics dacryostomy
    operation
Blaskovics eyelid shortening
    technique
Blaskovics flap
Blaskovics lid operation
Blaskovics operation
Blaskovics ptosis correction
blast injury
blastic lesion
blastic metastasis
blastoma
blastomycetic dermatitis

blastomycosis
cutaneous blastomycosis
keloidal blastomycosis
laryngeal blastomycosis
blastomycosis-like pyoderma
Blasucci catheter
Blasucci clamp
Blasucci curved-tip ureteral
catheter
Blasucci pigtail ureteral catheter
Blasucci tip
Blasucci ureteral catheter
Blatt operation
Blatt procedure
Blatt-Ashworth procedure
Blauth hypoplastic thumb
(Types I, II, IIA, IIIB, IV, V)
Blauth knee prosthesis
Blaydes angled lens forceps
Blaydes corneal forceps
Blaydes lens-holding forceps
Blazina patellofemoral repair
Blazina procedure
Blazina prosthesis
BLB mask (Boothby, Lovelace,
Bulbulian mask)
bleaching cream
bleb
pleural bleb
bleb resection
Bleck iliopsoas recession
Bleck recession technique
bled
Bledsoe adjustable post-up brace
Bledsoe cast brace
Bledsoe knee brace
Bledsoe leg brace
Bledsoe passive motion exerciser
bleed
esophageal variceal bleed
gap bleed
gastrointestinal bleed
gel bleeds
GI bleed
intracerebral bleed
maternal bleed
postgastrectomy bleed
postpolypectomy bleed
sentinel bleed
silicone gel bleed
trocar wound bleed
variceal bleed

bleed of tattoo pigment
bleeder
episcleral bleeder
ligation of bleeders
preperitoneal bleeder
subcutaneous bleeders
superficial bleeders
bleeding
abnormal bleeding
active source of bleeding
acute digestive bleeding
anorectal variceal bleeding
arterial bleeding
backflow bleeding
chronic digestive bleeding
colorectal bleeding
concomitant bleeding
copious bleeding
digestive bleeding
distal bleeding
dysfunctional uterine
bleeding
esophageal variceal bleeding
esophagogastric variceal
bleeding
excessive bleeding
external bleeding
fresh bleeding
gastric variceal bleeding
gastrointestinal bleeding
implantation bleeding
intermenstrual bleeding
intestinal bleeding
intraabdominal bleeding
intracranial bleeding
intraoperative bleeding
intrathoracic bleeding
irregular bleeding
massive bleeding
massive lower GI bleeding
midtrimester bleeding
minimal bleeding
occult bleeding
painless rectal bleeding
pinpoint gastric mucosal
defect bleeding
placentation bleeding
portal hypertensive bleeding
postcoital bleeding
postextraction bleeding
postmenopausal bleeding
postnasal bleeding

bleeding (*continued*)
  postoperative bleeding
  profuse bleeding
  rectal bleeding
  recurrent vaginal bleeding
  retroperitoneal bleeding
  subarachnoid bleeding
  uncontrollable bleeding
  upper gastrointestinal
    bleeding
  uterine bleeding
  vaginal bleeding
  venous bleeding
bleeding abnormality
bleeding angioma
bleeding complication
bleeding controlled with direct
  pressure
bleeding controlled with
  electrocautery
bleeding episode
bleeding esophageal varices
bleeding lesion
bleeding needle
bleeding point
bleeding risk
bleeding site ligation
bleeding site localization
bleeding time coagulation panel
bleeding tumor
bleeding vessel
Bleier clip for tubal sterilization
Blenderm patch technique
Blenderm surgical tape dressing
Blenderm tape
blennorrhagia
blennorrhagic
blennorrhagic inflammation
blennorrhagica
  keratoderma blennorrhagica
  keratosis blennorrhagica
blennorrhea
  Stoerk blennorrhea
blepharal
blepharectomy
blepharedema
blepharelosis
blepharism
blepharitis
  seborrheic blepharitis
blepharitis angularis
blepharitis ciliaris

blepharitis oleosa
blepharitis rosacea
blepharoadenoma
blepharoatheroma
blepharochalasia
blepharochalasis
  Kreiker blepharochalasis
blepharochalasis forceps
blepharochalasis repair
blepharoclonus
blepharocoloboma
blepharodermatochalasis
blepharodiastasis
blepharokeratoconjunctivitis
blepharomelasma
blepharopachynsis
blepharophimosis
blepharophyma
blepharopigmentation
blepharoplasty
  Ammon blepharoplasty
  Bossalino blepharoplasty
  Budinger blepharoplasty
  Burow blepharoplasty
  Castanares bilateral
    blepharoplasty
  CO_2 laser blepharoplasty
  combined upper
    blepharoplasty
  combined upper lid
    blepharoplasty
  cosmetic blepharoplasty
  Denonvilliers blepharoplasty
  Dupuy-Dutemps
    blepharoplasty
  Fox blepharoplasty
  functional blepharoplasty
  laser incisional blepharoplasty
  laser lower lid
    transconjunctival
    blepharoplasty
  lid-fracturing blepharoplasty
  long-skin flap blepharoplasty
  lower blepharoplasty
  modified Loeb and de la Plaza
    technique blepharoplasty
  Morel-Fatio blepharoplasty
  skin-muscle flap
    blepharoplasty
  skin-muscle blepharoplasty
  transconjunctival
    blepharoplasty (TCB)

blepharoplasty (*continued*)
  transconjunctival lower lid
    blepharoplasty
  upper blepharoplasty
blepharoplasty clip
blepharoplasty incision
blepharoplegia
blepharoptosis
  acquired blepharoptosis
  aponeurotic blepharoptosis
  cicatricial blepharoptosis
  congenital blepharoptosis
  dysmyogenic blepharoptosis
  external levator resection to
    repair blepharoptosis
  false blepharoptosis
  involutional blepharoptosis
  mechanical blepharoptosis
  myogenic blepharoptosis
  neurogenic blepharoptosis
  senile blepharoptosis
  structural blepharoptosis
  traumatic blepharoptosis
blepharoptosis adiposa
blepharoptosis repair
blepharoptosis-related blindness
blepharorrhaphy
  Elschnig blepharorrhaphy
blepharospasm
blepharosphincterectomy
blepharostat
  Goldman-McNeill blepharostat
  McNeill-Goldmann
    blepharostat
  Schachar blepharostat
blepharostat clamp
blepharostat ring
blepharostenosis
blepharosynechia
blepharotomy
Blessig cyst
Blessig groove
Blessig-Iwanoff cyst
bleuâtres
  taches bleuâtres
blighted ovum
blind abscess
blind clamping
blind dilatation
blind end
blind endosonography probe
blind fistula

blind foramen
blind foramen of frontal bone
blind gut
blind insertion
blind limb
blind lithotripsy
blind loop syndrome
blind medullary nail
blind nailing
blind nasal intubation anesthetic
  technique
blind nasotracheal intubation
  anesthetic technique
blind osteotomy
blind percutaneous liver biopsy
blind pouch syndrome
blind rectal pouch
blind Rush nailing
blind stump
blind upper esophageal pouch
blindness
  blepharoptosis-related
    blindness
  cortical blindness
  functional blindness
blind-spot projection technique
B-Line utility cart
blink
  poor blink
blink reflex
Bliskunov implantable femoral
  distractor
blister
  blood blister
  fracture blister
BlisterFilm transparent dressing
BlisterFilm transparent wound
  dressing
BLL (benign lymphoepithelial
  lesion)
bloc (*see also* block)
  en bloc
Bloch-Paul-Mikulicz operation
Bloch-Sulzberger disease
Bloch-Sulzberger syndrome
block (*see also* bloc)
  d-tubocurarine block
  3-in-one block
  2-point nerve block
  4-in-1 cutting block
  acrylic bite block
  air block

block (*continued*)
  anesthetic block
  ankle block
  anterior-posterior cutting
    block
  anterocrural celiac plexus
    block
  A-P cutting block
  arborization block
  arborization heart block
  Atkinson lid block
  atrioventricular block
    (AV block)
  autonomic ganglion block
  autonomic nerve block
  AV block (atrioventricular
    block)
  axillary block
  axillary technique of brachial
    plexus block
  ball joint block
  balsa wood block
  Best bite block
  bicortical iliac bone block
  Bier block
  bifascicular block
  bifascicular heart block
  bilateral bundle branch
    block
  Bio-Oss spongiosa block
  bite block
  bone block
  brachial plexus block (BPB)
  Brightbill corneal cutting
    block
  Brightbill cutting block
  bundle branch block
  Bunnell block
  calipers block
  Campbell bone block
  carotid artery block
  catheter technique for
    brachial plexus block
  caudal block
  cecal block
  celiac plexus block
  central block
  Cerrobend trim block
  cervical plexus block
  cervical plexus nerve block
  ciliovitrectomy block
  complete heart block

block (*continued*)
  complete left bundle branch
    block (CLBBB)
  cord block
  corneal block
  cryogenic block
  cutting block
  cutting Delrin block
  cutting Teflon block
  Dembone demineralized
    cortical dental block
  depolarization block
  depolarizing block
  differential nerve block
  differential spinal block
  digital block
  digital nerve block
  direct obturator nerve block
  disposable Styrofoam block
  dorsal penile nerve block
    (DPNB)
  dynamic block
  ear block
  ENT bite block
  epidural block
  ESI bite block
  Ethox bite block
  exit block
  external nasal nerve block
  extradural block
  fascicular heart block
  femoral nerve block
  field block
  Fine folding block
  ganglion block
  ganglion impar block
  gasserian ganglion block
  GeneraBloc bite block
  glossopharyngeal nerve block
  greater occipital nerve block
  Greco cutting block
  Guilford-Wright cutting block
  hand block
  Hara infiltration block
  heart block
  hepatic outflow block
  His bundle heart block
  House block
  House cutting block
  House Teflon cutting block
  House Delrin cutting block
  iliohypogastric nerve block

block (*continued*)
  ilioinguinal nerve block
  ilioinguinal-iliohypogastric
    nerve block (INB)
  incomplete left bundle
    branch block
  incomplete right bundle
    branch block
  indirect obturator nerve block
  inferior alveolar nerve block
  infiltration block
  infraorbital block
  infraorbital nerve block
  inguinal field block
  inguinal perivascular block
  intercostal fossa block
  intercostal nerve block
  interpleural block
  Interpore block
  Interpore porous
    hydroxyapatite block
  interscalene block
  interscalene brachial plexus
    block
  interventricular heart block
  intrahepatic block
  intranasal block
  intrapleural block
  intraspinal block
  Jackson bite block
  laparoscopic celiac plexus
    pain block
  laryngeal block
  lead block
  left bundle branch block
  Lell bite block
  lingual block
  local field block
  local nerve block
  loge de Guyon ulnar nerve
    block
  lower extremity nerve block
  lumbar nerve block
  lumbar plexus block
  lumbar sympathetic block
  mandibular nerve block
  mantle block
  MaxBloc bite block
  maxillary nerve block
  mechanical block
  median nerve block
  mental nerve block

block (*continued*)
  metal and rubber block
  methyl methacrylate block
  midfemoral block
  Mikhail bone block
  Mobitz heart block
  Mobitz I AV, II AV heart block
  Mobitz I, II block
  motor point block
  nasopalatine nerve block
  nerve block
  Neumann calipers block
  neuraxial neurolytic block
  neurolytic celiac plexus block
    (NCPB)
  neuromuscular block
  New Orleans corneal cutting
    block
  nondepolarizing block
  O'Brien block
  obturator nerve block
  Omni Bloc bite blocks
  Ora-Gard disposable intraoral
    bite block
  orbicularis block
  Oxyguard mouth block
  paracervical block
  paraffin block
  paraneural block
  parasacral block
  paravertebral block
  paravertebral lumbar
    sympathetic block
  pelvic block
  penile block
  peri-infarction block
  perineural block
  peripheral nerve block
  phase I, II block
  phrenic nerve block
  Plexiglas tissue equivalency
    block
  portal block
  posterior bone block
  preganglionic sympathetic
    block
  presacral block
  prognostic block
  psoas sheath block
  pudendal block
  punch block
  pupillary block

block (*continued*)
  push-up block
  radial nerve block
  regional block
  retrobulbar nerve block
  retrocrural celiac plexus
    block
  right bundle-branch block
  ring block
  sciatic nerve block
  sensory block
  Shepard calipers block
  Shepard-Kramer calipers
    block
  shielding block
  shock block
  silicone block
  sinoatrial exit block
  sinus block
  sinus exit block
  skull block
  Southern Eye Bank corneal
    cutting block
  Spaeth facial nerve block
  Speed-E-Rim denture bite
    block
  spinal block
  spinal subarachnoid block
  splanchnic block
  Stahl calipers block
  Steinberg infiltration block
  stellate ganglion block
  subarachnoid block
  subclavian perivascular block
  subdural block
  supraclavicular block
  supraorbital nerve block
  supratrochlear nerve block
  sympathetic block
  sympathetic nerve block
  Tanne corneal cutting block
  Teflon block
  Teflon strut-cutting block
  Teflon-Delrin cutting block
  therapeutic nerve block
  thoracic nerve block
  thoracolumbar nerve block
  tibial augmentation block
  tibial cutting block
  tracheal block
  transsacral block
  tubal block

block (*continued*)
  ulnar nerve block
  Ultima Bloc bite block
  upper extremity nerve
    block
  uterosacral block
  Van Lint lid block
  Van Lint-Atkinson lid akinetic
    block
  ventricular block
  Wenckebach block
  Wright-Guildford cutting
    block
  wrist block
  yoke block
block anesthesia
block anesthesia needle
Block cardiac device
block dissection
Block entropion repair
Block gastric hemostat
block injection
block needle
block osteotomy
Block right coronary guiding
    catheter
block technique
blockade
  anesthetic blockade
  autonomic blockade
  beta-adrenergic blockade
  cholinergic blockade
  epidural blockade
  epidural neural blockade
  flickering blockade
  ganglionic blockade
  gasserian ganglion blockade
  interscalene blockade
  lytic blockade
  myoneural blockade
  neuromuscular blockade
    (NMB)
  nondepolarizing blockade
  onset of blockade
  preganglionic cardiac
    sympathetic blockade
  pulmonary sympathetic
    blockade
  sensory blockade
  stellate ganglion blockade
  sympathetic blockade
  temporary nerve blockade

blockage
  bypass blockage
  complete blockage
  ganglion blockage
  tendon blockage
  urinary blockage
Blockaine anesthetic agent
blocked airway
blocked breathing passage
blocked nasal passage
blocker
  ganglion blocker
  hook blocker
Blocker operation
blocking agent
blocking procedure
Block-Paul-Mixter operation
Block-Potts intestinal forceps
Bloedorn applicator
Blohmka tonsil forceps
Blohmka tonsil hemostat
Blohmka tonsillar forceps
Blohmka tonsillar hemostat
Blohmka vesicostomy
Blom-Singer esophagoscope
Blom-Singer indwelling low-
    pressure voice prosthesis
Blom-Singer postlaryngectomy
    valve
Blom-Singer tracheoesophageal
    fistula
Blom-Singer tracheoesophageal
    prosthesis
Blom-Singer vocal
    reconstruction
blood
  anticoagulated blood
  arterial transfusion of blood
  artificial blood
  autologous blood
  blood-retinal blood
  Cell Saver blood
  cleansing blood
  cord blood
  deoxygenated blood
  extravasation of blood
  flow of blood
  Fluosol artificial blood
  inflow of arterial blood
  occult blood
  osmolarity of blood
  oxygenated blood

blood (*continued*)
  passage of blood
  peripheral blood
  refusion of blood
  sludged blood
  streaked with blood
  whole blood
blood agar plate
blood alcohol concentration
blood blister
blood calculus
blood cell separator
blood channels
blood clot
blood coagulation
blood coagulation disorder
blood coagulation factor
blood count
blood expander
blood flow imaging
blood flow rate
blood patch
blood patch injection
blood perfusion
blood perfusion monitor
blood pressure
blood pressure cuff
blood pressure monitoring
blood pressure recorder
blood product
blood pump
blood sampling instrument
blood staining
blood supply
blood transfusion
blood vessel bridges
blood vessel formation
blood vessel invasion (BVI)
blood vessel supporter
blood warmer cuffs
blood-air barrier
blood-borne macrophage
blood-borne pathogen
blood-brain barrier (BB)
blood-cerebral barrier
blood-cerebrospinal fluid barrier
blood-contacting catheter
blood-flow probe
blood-fluid warmer
blood-gas exchange
Bloodgood inguinal
    herniorrhaphy

Bloodgood operation
Bloodgood syndrome
bloodless amputation
bloodless circumcision clamp
bloodless decerebration
bloodless field
bloodless operation
bloodless phlebotomy
bloodless zone of necrosis
blood-liquor barrier
blood-ocular barrier
blood-optic nerve barrier
blood-retinal blood
Bloodshot WildEyes lens
blood-thymus barrier
blood-tinged
blood-tinged ascites
blood-urine barrier
Bloodwell forceps
Bloodwell tissue forceps
Bloodwell vascular forceps
Bloodwell vascular tissue
    forceps
Bloodwell-Brown forceps
bloody ascites
bloody peritoneal fluid
bloody stool
bloody tap
Bloom programmable stimulator
Bloom syndrome
Bloomberg lens forceps
Bloomberg SuperNumb
    anesthetic ring
Bloomberg trabeculotome set
Bloom-Raney modification of
    Smith-Robinson technique
blot hemorrhage
Blot perforator
Blot scissors
blot-and-dot hemorrhage
blotchy
blot hemostat
Blount bent blade
Blount blade plate
Blount bone retractor
Blount bone spreader
Blount brace
Blount disease
Blount displacement osteotomy
Blount double-prong retractor
Blount epiphyseal staple
Blount fracture staple

Blount hip retractor
Blount knee retractor
Blount knee staple
Blount knife
Blount laminar spreader
Blount nylon mallet
Blount operation
Blount osteotome
Blount osteotomy
Blount plate
Blount procedure for bone
    growth asymmetry
Blount retractor
Blount scoliosis osteotome
Blount single-prong retractor
Blount splint
Blount staple
Blount tracing technique
Blount V-blade
Blount-Schmidt-Milwaukee
    brace
blow
    sharp blow
blow-by oxygen
blow-by ventilator
blower
    DeVilbiss powder blower
    powder blower
blowhole decompressing
    colostomy
blow-hole ileostomy
blow-in fracture
blowing wound
blown pupil
blow-out
    aortic stump blow-out
blow-out fracture
blow-out fracture of orbital floor
blow-out lesion
blow-out view projection
blow-up gloves
blue
    Bonney blue
    methylene blue
    toluidine blue
blue atrophy
blue Cook sheath
blue cotton sutures
blue dome breast cyst
blue dome cyst
Blue FlexTip catheter
blue line

Blue Line cuffed endotracheal
tube
Blue Line orthotic
blue mantle
Blue Max balloon catheter
Blue Max cannula
Blue Max high-pressure balloon
Blue Max triple-lumen catheter
blue nevus
Blue Peel chemical peel
blue rectal suction tip
blue ring pessary
blue rubber bleb nevus
syndrome
blue sclera
blue Shepard grommet tube
blue sponge dressing
blue spot
blue toe syndrome
blue twisted cotton sutures
blue-black monofilament sutures
blue-gray lesion
Bluemle pump
blue-tip aspirator
Blum arterial scissors
Blum forceps
Blumberg sign
Blumensaat line
Blumenthal anterior chamber
maintainer
Blumenthal bone rongeur
Blumenthal irrigating cystotome
Blumenthal lesion
Blumenthal rongeur
Blumenthal uterine dressing
forceps
Blumer rectal shelf
Blumer shelf
Blundell-Jones operation
Blundell-Jones osteotomy
Blundell-Jones technique
blunderbuss
apex blunderbuss
blunt abdominal trauma
blunt and sharp dissection
blunt bullet-tip cannula
blunt carotid injury (BCI)
blunt dissecting hook
blunt dissection and snare
technique
blunt dissector
blunt elevator

blunt eversion carotid
endarterectomy
blunt forceps
blunt hook
blunt hook dissector
blunt injury
blunt iris hook
blunt lacrimal probe
blunt lipoplasty by tunnelization
blunt liver injury
blunt needle
blunt nerve hook
blunt obturator
blunt periosteal elevator
blunt probe
blunt rake retractor
blunt retractor
blunt scissors
blunt suction lipectomy
blunt suction tube
blunt suction-assisted lipoplasty
blunt torso injury
blunt trocar
blunted costophrenic angle
blunt-end sialogram needle
blunting
sulcus blunting
blunting of calyces
blunting of costophrenic angle
blunting of nerve
blunting of sulcus
blunting of valve
blunt-nose hemostat
Bluntport disposable trocar
blunt-ring curet
blunt-suction-assisted lipoplasty
blunt-tip probe
blunt-tipped cannula
blunt-tipped extraction cannula
blunt-tipped obturator
blur point
blush
tumor blush
BM (bacterial meningitis)
BM (buccomesial)
BMA (basaloid monomorphic
adenoma)
BMD (bone mineral density)
BMI (body mass index)
B-mode imaging
B-mode scanning
B-mode ultrasound

BMP (bone morphogenic protein)
BMP-2 (bone morphogenic protein-2)
BMSI 5000 electroencephalograph
BMT (bone marrow transplant)
Bülau trocar
BNOE (benign necrotizing otitis externa)
Bürker chamber
BO (bucco-occlusal)
board
  adhesive dressing board
  angle board
  cartilage cutting board
  cutting board
  Fisher tape board
  Flexisplint flexed-arm board
  graft board
  grid maze board
  nasal cartilage-cutting board
  powder board
  rocker board
  spine board
  tape board
board splint
boardlike retractor
Boari bladder flap
Boari bladder flap procedure
Boari button
Boari flap
Boari operation
Boari ureteral flap repair
Boari-Küss flap
Boari-Ockerblad flap reimplantation
Boariplasty
Boas point
Boas sign
boat hook
boat nail
boatlike abdomen
boat-shaped abdomen
boat-shaped heart
Bobath sling
Bobb cholelithotomy
Bobb operation
bobbin
  Reuter stainless steel bobbin
bobbin myringotomy tube

bobbin-type laryngectomy button
bobby pin abrasion
Bobechko rod
Bobechko sliding barrel hook
Bobechko spreader
Boberg lens
Boberg-Ans intraocular lens
Boberg-Ans lens implant
Bocca neck dissection
Bochadalek foramen
Bochdalek
  foramen of Bochdalek
Bochdalek ganglion
Bochdalek hernia
Bochdalek muscle
Bochdalek valve
Bock foot
Bock ganglion
Bock knee prosthesis
Bock knife
Bock nerve
Bodai adapter
Bodansky unit
Bodenham dermabrasion cylinder
Bodenham saw
Bodenham-Blair skin graft knife
Bodenham-Humby skin graft knife
Bodenheimer anoscope
Bodenheimer proctoscope
Bodenheimer rectal speculum
Bodenstab tourniquet
BODI Dynamic orthosis
BODI knee extension orthosis
Bodian discission knife
Bodian lacrimal pigtail probe
Bodian minilacrimal probe
Bodian scissors
bodies (see body)
bodily movement
bodkin
Bodkin thread holder
Bodnar knee retractor
body
  adipose body
  adrenal body
  alveolar body
  Amato body
  amygdaloid body
  anal foreign body

body (*continued*)

anococcygeal body
anorectal foreign body
aortic body
Arantius body
Arnold body
artificial vertebral body
Aschoff body
aspirated foreign body
asteroid body
Balbiani body
Barr body
basal lamina of ciliary body
Bence Jones body
body righting reflex rigid
    body
Bracht-Wachter body
brassy body
Cabot ring body
calcified free body
cancer body
carotid body
cartilaginous loose body
caudate body
cavernous body
central fibrous body
chromaffin body
chromatinic body
ciliary body
coccidian body
coccygeal body
colloid body
colonic foreign body
compressed body
compressible cavernous body
corneal foreign body
Creola body
crescent body
cystoid body
cytoid body
dense body
detached loose body
donated body
duodenal foreign body
Dutcher body
Ehrlich inner body
Elschnig body
esophageal foreign body
esophageal Lewy body
external geniculate body
fat body
fibrin bodies

body (*continued*)

fibrous loose body
foreign body
foreign body (FB)
free body
Gamma-Gandy body
gastric foreign body
gelatin compression body
geniculate body
glomus body
Goldmann-Larson foreign
    body
Gordon elementary body
Hamazaki-Wesenberg body
Harting body
Hassall body
Heinz body
Heinz-Ehrlich body
hematoxylin body
Henle body
Hensen body
Highmore body
Hirano body
Howell-Jolly body
hyaline body
hyaloid body
hypoplastic mandibular body
impacted foreign body
infrapatellar fat body
ingested foreign body
intervertebral body
intraarticular loose body
intraluminal foreign body
intraorbital foreign body
intrauterine foreign body
intravascular foreign body
iris ciliary body
irregularly shaped body
Jaworski body
juxtaglomerular body
juxtarestiform body
Kelvin body
ketone bodies
Lallemand body
Lallemand-Trousseau body
Landolt body
lateral geniculate body
Lewy bodies
Lieutaud body
lifeless body
loose body
loose intraarticular body

body (*continued*)
- lower GI tract foreign body
- Luys body
- lyssa body
- malpighian body
- mamillary body
- mammary body
- mammillary body
- Maragiliano body
- Maxwell body
- May-Hegglin body
- melon seed body
- metallic foreign body
- metallic foreign body (MFB)
- mineral oil foreign body
- Mueller duct body
- Mott body
- multilamellar body
- multivesicular body
- Neill-Mooser body
- nerve cell body
- newtonian body
- olivary body
- osteocartilagnious loose body
- osteochondral loose body
- owl eye inclusion body
- pampiniform body
- pancreatic body
- paranephric body
- paranephric fat body
- paraterminal body
- parotid body
- pectinate body
- pedunculated loose body
- perineal body
- pineal body
- pituitary body
- Prowazek-Greef body
- psammoma body
- pubic body
- pyknotic body
- radiopaque foreign body
- rectal foreign body
- refractile body
- rice bodies
- Reilly body
- relaxed perineal body
- removal of foreign body
- residual body
- restiform body
- retained foreign body
- rice body

body (*continued*)
- Rosenmueller body
- Ross body
- round body
- Rucker body
- sand body
- Sandström body
- Savage perineal body
- Schaumann body
- Schiller-Duvall body
- Schmorl body
- sclerotomy with removal of foreign body
- Seidelin body
- spongy body
- S-shaped body
- striate body
- suprarenal body
- swaying of body
- Symington anococcygeal body
- thoracic vertebral body
- thrombogenic foreign body
- thyroid body
- Todd bodies
- total body
- tracheobronchial foreign body
- trapezoid body
- ultimobranchial body
- upper GI tract foreign body
- vagal body
- vaginal foreign body
- vermiform body
- Verocay bodies
- vertebral body
- vitreous body
- vitreous foreign body
- wall of body
- Wesenberg-Hamazaki body
- Winkler body
- wolffian body
- X body
- Y body
- yellow body

Body Armor walker cast
body awareness
body cast syndrome
body cavity
body cell mass
body coil
body composition analysis
body contouring
body dysmorphic disorder

body fat
body fluid
Body Gard neoprene support
body habitus
body hematocrit-venous
    hematocrit ratio
body image
body image disorder
body image dissatisfaction
body jacket
body mass index (BMI)
body of fornix
body of gallbladder
body of Luys
body of mandible
body of maxilla
body of sphenoid bone
body of hamate
body of tongue
body position
body positron
Body prop positioning splint
body righting reflex
body righting reflex rigid body
body scanning technique
body schema
body sculpting
body section radiography
body side integration
body stalk
body surface area (BSA)
body surface burned
body surface Laplacian mapping
body temperature
body tumor
body weight
Body Wrap foam positioner
BodyBilt chair
body-contour surgery
BodyCushion positioner
body-fluid exchange
BodyIce cold pack
BodyIce wrap
Body-Solid exercise equipment
body-to-ramus transition
Boebinger tongue depressor
Boeck sarcoid
Boeck sarcoid disease
Boehler (also Böhler)
Boehler angle of calcaneus
Boehler bone rongeur
Boehler clamp

Boehler fracture frame
Boehler pin
Boehler reducing frame
Boehler splint
Boehler tongs
Boehler traction bow
Boehler tractor
Boehler wire splint
Boehler-Braun frame
Boehler-Braun splint
Boehm anoscope
Boehm cord
Boehm current controller
Boehm drop syringe
Boehm proctoscope
Boehm sigmoidoscope
Boehringer kit
Boer craniotomy forceps
Boerema anterior gastropexy
Boerema hernia repair
Boerema-Crile operation
Boerhaave gland
Boerhaave syndrome
Boerhaave tear
Boerma obstetrical forceps
Boettcher antral trocar
Boettcher artery forceps
Boettcher hemostat
Boettcher hook
Boettcher pulmonary artery
    clamp
Boettcher pulmonary artery
    forceps
Boettcher scissors
Boettcher tonsil artery forceps
Boettcher tonsil hook
Boettcher tonsil scissors
Boettcher trocar
Boettcher-Fralow snare
Boettcher-Jennings mouth gag
Boettcher-Schmidt antrum trocar
Boettcher-Schmidt forceps
Boettcher space
boggy prostate
boggy swelling
boggy uterus
Bogle rongeur
Bogorad syndrome
Bogota bag
Bograb Universal offset ossicular
    prosthesis
Bogros space

Bogue operation
Boehm operation
Böhler (*see* Boehler)
Boehler-Braun fracture frame
Boehler calcaneal angle
Boehler guideline
Boehler hip nail
Boehler-Knowles hip pin
Boehler os calcis clamp
Boehler plaster cast breaker
Boehler reducing fracture frame
Boehler rongeur
Bohlet angle
Bohlman cervical fusion technique
Bohlman pin
Bohlman triple-wire technique
Bohlman vertebrectomy
Bohn nodules
Bohr effect
Boies cutting forceps
Boies forceps
Boies nasal fracture elevator
Boies plastic surgery elevator
Boiler septal trephine
Boiler trephine
Boilo head mirror
Boilo laryngeal mirror
Boilo retinoscope
Boitzy open reduction
BOLD (blood oxygen level
    dependent)
Bolder hemostat
Boldrey brace
Bolex cine-camera
Bolex gastrocamera
Boley dental gouge
Boley gauge
Boley gouge
Boley retractor
Boll cells
Bollinger knee brace
bolster
    cotton bolster
    Hollister bridge suture bolster
    knee bolster
    muscular bolster
    retention suture bolster
    roll control bolster
    rubber bolster
    Teflon felt bolster
    Telfa bolster
    tie-over bolster

bolster buddy
bolster finger
bolster operation
bolster suture technique
bolt
    Alta femoral bolt
    Barr bolt
    Camino microventricular bolt
    Camino ventricular bolt
    cannulated bolt
    DePuy bolt
    Fenton tibial bolt
    Herzenberg bolt
    hexhead bolt
    Hubbard bolt
    Hubbard-Nylok bolt
    I bolt
    ICP Camino bolt
    Norman tibial bolt
    Nylok bolt
    Philly bolt
    Richmond bolt
    solid hex bolt
    tibial bolt
    transfixion bolt
    trochanteric bolt
    Webb stove bolt
    Wilson bolt
    wire fixation bolt
    Zimmer tibial bolt
bolt fixation
Bolt sign
Bolton analysis
Bolton forceps
Bolton nasion plane
Bolton point
Bolton-Broadbent plane
Boltzmann distribution
Boltzmann factor
bolus (*pl.* boluses)
    intravenous bolus
bolus chase technique
bolus dressing
bolus injection
bolus intravenous anesthesia
bolus intravenous anesthetic
    technique
bolus ties over graft
bolused
bombé
    iris bombé
Bomgart stomal bag

Bonaccolto capsule fragment
    forceps
Bonaccolto cup jaws forceps
Bonaccolto eye implant
Bonaccolto fragment forceps
Bonaccolto jeweler's forceps
Bonaccolto jeweler's-type
    forceps
Bonaccolto magnet tip forceps
Bonaccolto monoplex orbital
    implant material
Bonaccolto orbital implant
Bonaccolto scleral ring
Bonaccolto trephine
Bonaccolto utility forceps
Bonaccolto utility pickup
    forceps
Bonaccolto-Flieringa operation
Bonaccolto-Flieringa scleral
    ring
Bonaccolto-Flieringa vitreous
    operation
Bonanno catheter
Bonchek-Shiley cardiac jacket
Bond arm splint
Bond forceps
Bond placenta forceps
Bond splint
Bondek absorbable suture
Bond-Eze bond adhesive
Bondy mastoidectomy
    (type I, II, III)
Bondy operation
bone
    accessory bone
    accessory navicular bone
    acromial bone
    alar bone
    Albers-Schoenberg marble
        bones
    Albers-Schoenberg chalk
        bones
    Albrecht bone
    alisphenoid bone
    allogeneic bone
    alveolar bone
    alveolar supporting bone
    ankle bone
    anterior condyloid canal of
        occipital bone
    anterior suspension of hyoid
        bone

bone (*continued*)
    apex of petrous part of
        temporal bone
    articular eminence of
        temporal bone
    articular fossa of temporal
        bone
    articular tubercle of temporal
        bone
    articulation of pisiform bone
    auricular fissure of temporal
        bone
    autologous bone
    banked freeze-dried bone
    basal bone
    basihyal bone
    basilar bone
    basilar groove of occipital
        bone
    basilar groove of sphenoid
        bone
    basio-occipital bone
    basisphenoid bone
    Bertin bone
    Bio-Oss freeze-dried
        demineralized bone
    Bio-Oss synthetic bone
    Bioplant hard tissue
        replacement synthetic bone
    Bioplant HTR synthetic bone
    blind foramen of frontal bone
    body of sphenoid bone
    boss of bone
    breakdown of bone
    breast bone
    bregmatic bone
    brittle bone
    bucket-handle view of facial
        bones
    bundle bone
    calcaneal bone
    Calcibon synthetic bone
    calvarial bone
    cancellated bone
    cancellous bone
    cancellous cellular bone
    capitate bone
    caries of bone
    carpal bones
    carpal row bones
    cavernous groove of sphenoid
        bone

bone (*continued*)
cecal foramen of frontal bone
cerclage of fractured bone
cerebral crests of cranial bone
chalk bones
chalky bones
cheek bone
clavicle bone
coccygeal bone
coccyx bone
collar bone
compact bone
conchal crest of palatine bone
condyle bone
contour of nasal bones
cortical bone
corticocancellous bone
costal bone
crest of palatine bone
cuboid bone
cuneiform bone
curetted bone
cut end of bone
decalcified freeze-dried bone
decalcified freeze-dried
    cortical bone (DFDCB)
Dembone demineralized
    human bone
Dembone freeze-dried bone
demineralization of bone
demineralized bone (DMB)
demineralized freeze-dried
    bone (DFBD)
dermal bone
diastasis of cranial bone
dislocation of bone
drainage of bone
ear bone
eburnated bone
ectethmoid bones
ectocuneiform bone
ectopic bone
endochondral bone
entocuneiform bone
epactal bones
epihyal bone
epipteric bone
ethmoid bone
ethmoidal bone
ethmoidal sulcus of nasal
    bone
exoccipital bone

bone (*continued*)
exposed bone
facial bones
femoral bone
fibular bone
flank bone
Flower bone
foot bones
fracture of bone
fractured bone
fragment of bone
freeze-dried bone
freeze-dried demineralized
    bone (FDDB)
frontal angle of parietal bone
frontal bone
fusion of bone
gladiolus bone
glandular fossa of frontal bone
glenoid fossa of temporal
    bone
great wing of sphenoid bone
greater horn of hyoid bone
greater multangular bone
greater palatine sulcus of
    palatine bone
greater wing of sphenoid
    bone
groove of lacrimal bone
guttering of bone
hamate bone
hamulus of ethmoid bone
hamulus of hamate bone
haunch bone
haversian bone
heel bone
hemiseptum of interalveolar
    bone
hip bone
horizontal plate of palatine
    bone
humeral bone
hyoid bone
iliac bone
ilium bone
immature bone
incus bone
inferior angle of parietal bone
inferior maxillary bone
inferior turbinal crest of
    palatine bone
inferior turbinate bone

bone (*continued*)

inner table frontal bone
innominate bone
intermaxillary bone
interparietal bone
interproximal bone
intrachondrial bone
intrajugular process of
  temporal bone
invasive fungal infection of
  temporal bone
ischial bone
ivory bones
jugal bone
jugular crest of great wing of
  sphenoid bone
Kidner removal of accessory
  navicular bone
knee bone
lacrimal bone
lacrimal sulcus of lacrimal
  bone
Lambone demineralized
  laminar bone
Lambone freeze-dried bone
lamellar bone
lamellated bone
laminar bone
lateral condyle bone
lateral horn of hyoid bone
lateral mastoid bone
lateral surface of zygomatic
  bone
lateral wall of sphenoid
  bone
lengthening of bone
lenticular bone
lesser horn of hyoid bone
lesser multangular bone
lingual bone
long bone
lunate bone
malar bone
malar crest of great wing of
  sphenoid bone
malar surface of zygomatic
  bone
malleus bone
mandibular bone
marble bones
marginal process of malar
  bone

bone (*continued*)

marginal tubercle of
  zygomatic bone
masticatory bone
mastoid angle of parietal bone
mastoid bone
mature bone
maxillary bone
maxillary process of
  zygomatic bone
maxillary surface of
  perpendicular plate of
  palatine bone
medial turbinate bone
meniscal bone
mesocuneiform bone
metacarpal bones
metatarsal bone
midshaft of bone
monocortical bone
multangular bone
mylohyoid groove of inferior
  maxillary bone
nailing of bone
nasal bone
nasal crest of palatine bone
nasal spine of frontal bone
nasal spine of palatine bone
navicular bone
nutrient canal of bone
occipital angle of parietal
  bone
occipital bone
orbital bone
orbital border of sphenoid
  bone
orbitosphenoidal bone
Osteomin freeze-dried bone
osteonic bone
outer table of frontal bone
Paget disease of bone
palatal bone
palate bone
palatine bones
palatine groove of palatine
  bone
palatomaxillary groove of
  palatine bone
parietal angle of the sphenoid
  bone
parietal bone
patella bone

bone (*continued*)
    pelvic bone
    percussion of bone
    periosteal bone
    petrous bone
    phalangeal bone
    Pirie bone
    pisiform bone
    porous bones
    posterior border of petrous
        portion of temporal bone
    postsphenoid bone
    prefrontal bone
    pterygoid bone
    pterygoid ridge of sphenoid
        bone
    pubic bone
    pyramidal tuberosity of
        palatine bone
    radial bone
    ramus bone
    refracture of bone
    refractured bone
    regenerated bone
    replacement bone
    resorption of bone
    rider's bone
    ring of bone
    Riolan bones
    rudimentary bone
    sacral bone
    scaphoid bone
    scroll bones
    semilunar bone
    septal bones
    sesamatic bone
    sesamoid bones
    shaft of bone
    shin bone
    shortening of bone
    sieve bone
    sphenoid bone
    sphenoidal turbinate bones
    sphenopalatine notch of
        palatine bone
    spine of sphenoid bone
    spongy bone
    squamous bone
    stapes bone
    stirrup bone
    styloid bone
    subchondral bone

bone (*continued*)
    subperiosteal bone
    superior border of petrous
        portion of temporal bone
    superior maxillary bone
    superior surface of horizontal
        plate of palatine bone
    superior turbinal crest of
        palatine bone
    superior turbinate bone
    supernumerary bone
    supporting bone
    supraorbital arch of frontal
        bone
    supraorbital rim of frontal
        bone
    supreme turbinate bone
    sutural bones
    synthetic bone
    tarsal bone
    temporal bone
    temporal process of
        zygomatic bone
    temporal surface of frontal
        bone
    temporal surface of zygomatic
        bone
    thickened bone
    thigh bone
    toe bones
    trabecular bone
    trapezium bone
    trapezoid bone
    triangular bone
    triquetral bone
    tuft of bone
    turbinate bone
    tympanic bone
    ulnar styloid bone
    unciform bone
    uncinate bone
    upper jaw bone
    vaginal process of sphenoid
        bone
    vascular bundle implantation
        into bone
    vesalian bone
    Vesalius bone
    vomer bone
    wormian bone
    woven bone
    wrist bone

bone (*continued*)
  xanthomatosis of bone
  xenogeneic bone
  yoke bone
  zygomatic bone
  zygomatic crest of great wing
    of sphenoid bone
  zygomatic process of frontal
    bone
  zygomatic process of
    temporal bone
bone abduction instrument
bone abscess
bone age
bone algorithm
bone attenuation coefficient
bone autogenous graft
bone autograft
bone awl
bone bank
bone biopsy instruments
bone block
bone block procedure
Bone Bullet suture anchor
bone bur
bone calipers
bone callus
bone cement
bone cement adhesive
bone chip
bone chip graft
bone chisel
bone clamp
bone collector
bone crater
bone crib
bone crusher
bone curet
bone cutter
bone cyst
bone cyst excision
bone decay
bone defect
bone densitometer
bone density
bone deposition
bone destruction
bone disease
bone dissection
bone dowel
bone drill
bone duction

bone elevator
bone exposure
bone extension clamp
bone femoral plug
bone file
bone fixation device
bone fixation wire
bone flap
bone flap fixation plate
bone forceps
bone formation
bone fragment
bone gouge
bone graft decompression
bone graft extrusion
bone graft harvesting technique
bone graft holder
bone graft material
bone graft peg
bone graft placement
bone graft repair
bone graft substitute
bone graft substitute graft
Bone grafter instrument
bone grafting instrument
bone growth chambers
bone growth stimulation
bone growth stimulator (*see*
    stimulator)
bone guide
bone hand drill
bone harvest
bone hole punch
bone hook
bone hump
bone impactor
bone implant
bone implant material
bone infarct
bone ingrowth
bone injection gun
bone island
bone landmarks
bone lesion
bone lever
bone liquefaction
bone mallet
bone margin
bone marrow aspiration
bone marrow aspiration and
    biopsy
bone marrow biopsy

bone marrow biopsy needle
bone marrow dysfunction
bone marrow embolism
bone marrow examination
bone marrow failure
bone marrow graft
bone marrow infiltration
bone marrow lesion
bone marrow needle
bone marrow pressure
bone marrow tap
bone marrow transplant
bone marrow transplantation
bone matrix
bone metastasis
bone mineral density (BMD)
bone morphogenic protein
bone morphogenic protein-2
    (BMP-2)
bone mulch screw
bone pain
bone peg graft
bone plate
bone plug
bone powder
bone prosthesis
bone punch forceps
bone punch rongeur
bone rasp
bone recession
bone reconstruction
bone remodeling
bone resection
bone resorption
bone retractor
bone rongeur
bone salts
bone saw
bone saw blade
bone scalpel
bone scan
bone screw
bone screw depth gauge
bone sequestrum
bone shears
bone skid
bone spicule
bone spur
bone step-off at ZF suture
bone step-off at
    zygomaticofrontal suture
bone stock

bone substitute material
bone technique
bone threshold
bone trabecula
bone wax (see wax)
bone wax dressing
bone wax hemostatic agent
bone wax sutures
bone whorl
bone window
bone windowing
bone-anchored prosthesis
bone-biting forceps
bone-biting rongeur
bone-cement interface
BoneCollector device
bone-cutting double-action
    forceps
bone-cutting forceps
bone-cutting rongeur
bone-holding clamp
bone-holding forceps
bone-implant interface
bone-inductive protein
bone-ingrowth fixation
bonelet
bone-ligament dissection
Boneloc cement
bone-measuring calipers
BonePlast bone void filler
BonePlast graft
bone-reduction forceps
bone-retinaculum-bone autograft
    graft
BoneSource HA cement
BoneSource hydroxyapatite
    cement
BoneSource implant
bone-splitting forceps
bone-tendon-bone graft
bone-to-bone graft
bone-within-a-bone
    appearance
Bonferroni correction
Bonferroni-Holm procedure
Bonfiglio bone graft
Bonfiglio modification
Bonfiglio modification of
    Phemister technique
Bongort Lifestyles Closed-End
    pouches
Bongort Max-E-Pouch

Bongort one-piece drainable pouch
Bongort one-piece ostomy pouch
Bongort urinary diversion pouch
Bonina-Jacobson tube
Bonn European suturing forceps
Bonn iris forceps
Bonn iris hook
Bonn iris scissors
Bonn microhook
Bonn microiris hook
Bonn miniature iris scissors
Bonn peripheral iridectomy forceps
Bonn suturing forceps
Bonnano catheter
Bonnano tube
Bonner position
Bonnet enucleation of eyeball
Bonnet enucleation operation
Bonnet operation
Bonnet sign
Bonney abdominal hysterectomy
Bonney blue ink
Bonney blue stress incontinence test
Bonney cervical amputation
Bonney cervical dilator
Bonney clamp
Bonney clip
Bonney forceps
Bonney hysterectomy
Bonney inflator
Bonney insufflator
Bonney needle
Bonney operation
Bonney retrograde inflator
Bonney suture needle
Bonney sutures
Bonney tissue forceps
Bonney uterine tube
Bonnie balloon catheter
Bonola technique
Bonta mastectomy knife
Bonwill articulator
Bonwill triangle
bony ankylosis
bony annulus
bony anterior nasal aperture
bony atresia

bony atretic plate
bony bridge resection
bony bridging
bony caval opening
bony cavity of nose
bony chin button
bony choanae
bony cleft
bony crater
bony deformity
bony demineralization
bony destruction
bony discontinuity
bony dissection
bony element destruction
bony erosion
bony excess
bony excrescence
bony exposure
bony forehead
bony fragment
bony frontal sinus
bony hard palate
bony heart
bony impaction
bony ingrowth
bony island
bony kyphos
bony labyrinth
bony landmarks
bony lesion
bony maxillary sinus
bony metastasis
bony mobilization
bony nasal septum
bony necrosis and destruction
bony orbit of eye
bony overhand
bony palate
bony pathologic change
bony plate
bony pogonion
bony procedure
bony projection
bony prominence
bony protuberance
bony pyramid
bony rasping
bony reconstruction
bony regeneration
bony repositioning
bony retrusion

bony ridge
bony rongeur
bony septation
bony septum
bony sphenoethmoidal recess
bony sphenoidal sinus
bony spicules
bony spur
bony sutures
bony table
bony tarsus
bony union
bony vault
bony vault collapse
bony volume
Bonzel iridodialysis
Bonzel operation
Boo-Chai craniofacial cleft
Boo-Chai scissors
book
   cast book
   Ishihara test chart book
Book syndrome
Bookler swivel-ball laparoscopic
   instrument holder
Bookwalter horizontal bar
Bookwalter malleable retractor
   blade
Bookwalter rectal blade
Bookwalter retractor blade
Bookwalter retractor ring
Bookwalter ring retractor
Bookwalter segmented ring
Bookwalter vaginal Deaver blade
Bookwalter vaginal retractor
   ring
Bookwalter-Balfour retractor
Bookwalter-Cook anal rectal
   blade
Bookwalter-Gelpi point retractor
   blade
Bookwalter-Goulet retractor
Bookwalter-Harrington retractor
Bookwalter-Hill-Ferguson rectal
   retractor
Bookwalter-Kelly retractor blade
Bookwalter-Magrina vaginal
   retractor
Bookwalter-Mayo blade
Bookwalter-Parks anal sphincter
   blade
Bookwalter-ring retractor

Bookwalter-St. Mark deep pelvic
   retractor
boomerang bladder needle
boomerang needle holder
boomerang-shaped lesion
boomerang-shaped rectus
   abdominis
      musculocutaneous free flap
boomerang-shaped skin paddle
boost technique
Booster clip
boot
   Alcock boot
   Bunny boot
   Calamary cast boot
   Cam walker boot
   Chukka boot
   compression boot
   Dome paste boot
   gelatin compression boot
   gelatinous compression boot
   Gelocast Unna boot
   Gibney boot
   Jobst boot
   Junod boot
   Mollo boot
   moon boot
   plaster boot
   rocker boot
   Spenco boot
   TED pneumatic compression
      boot
   UltraGait 2 walker boot
   Unna boot
   Unna paste boot
   Venodyne boot
   walking boot
   Wilke boot
boot brace
Boothby-Lovelace-Bulbulian
   mask (BLB mask)
bootie cast
boot-shaped heart
bootstrap 2-vessel angioplasty
bootstrap dilation
boot-top fracture
Boplant graft
Bora centralization
Bora operation
Bora procedure
Bora technique
borazone blade cutting machine

borborygmus
Borchard bone wire guide
Borchard Gigli-saw guide
Borchard wire threader
Borchardt olive-shaped bur
Borden-Spencer-Herndon
    osteotomy
border
    alveolar border
    anterodistal border
    antimesenteric border
    cardiac border
    caudal border
    demarcated border
    frontal border
    heart border
    indurated border
    interosseous border
    irregular border
    lateral border
    lateral upper lip vermilion
        border
    mandibular border
    medial border
    mesenteric border
    mucocutaneous border
    nasal border
    occipital border
    outer border
    parietal border
    pupillary border
    raised border
    shifting border
    sphenoidal border
    squamous border
    sternal border
    superior border
    tragal border
    vermilion border
    white roll border
    white roll-flare vermilion
        border
border involvement
border molding
border of cardiac dullness
border of ramus
border ray amputation
border tissue movement
border tissue of Jacoby
borderline malignant
    hemangiopericytoma
bore trocar

Boren-Mayo table
Bores U-shaped forceps
Bores corneal fixation forceps
Bores incision spreader
Bores radial marker
Bores twist fixation ring
Bores U-shaped forceps
Borge bile duct clamp
Borge catheter
Borggreve operation
Borggreve-Hall technique
boric acid
boring cancer
boron counter
boron neutron-capture therapy
Boros esophagoscope
Borrmann gastric cancer typing
    systems (types I-IV)
    classification
Borsch bandage
Borsch dressing
Borst side-arm introducer set
Borst-Jadassohn type
    intraepidermal epithelioma
Borthen operation
Bortone shears
Bortz clamp
Boruchoff forceps
Bosch yaws
Bose bar
Bose hook
Bose nail fold removal
Bose nail fold excision
Bose operation
Bose retractor
Bose tracheal hook
Bose tracheostomy hook
Bosher commissurotomy knife
Bosher knife
Bosker TMI surgery
Bosker transmandibular
    implant
Bosniak classification
boss of bone
Bossalino blepharoplasty
Bossalino blepharoplasty
    operation
Bossalino operation
bosselated surface
bosselated uterus
bosselation
Bossi cervical dilator

bossing
  excessive supraorbital bossing
    (fullness)
  frontal bossing
  tip bossing
Bost arthrodesis
Bost operation for talipes
  equinovarus
Bostick staple
Boston bivalve brace
Boston bivalve cast
Boston Children's frame
Boston Envision lens
Boston gauze sponge
Boston Lying-In cervical forceps
Boston Lying-In cervical-
  grasping forceps
Boston model trephine
Boston overlap brace
Boston post-op hip orthosis
Boston Scientific Sonicath
  imaging catheter
Boston scoliosis brace
Boston soft body jacket
Boston soft corset
Boston trephine
Bosworth approach
Bosworth coracoclavicular
  screw
Bosworth crown drill
Bosworth decompressor
Bosworth femoroischial
  transplantation
Bosworth fracture
Bosworth fusion
Bosworth headband
Bosworth nasal saw
Bosworth nasal snare
Bosworth nasal speculum
Bosworth nasal wire speculum
Bosworth nerve root retractor
Bosworth operation
Bosworth plate
Bosworth procedure
Bosworth retractor
Bosworth saw
Bosworth screw
Bosworth shoulder arthroplasty
Bosworth snare
Bosworth speculum
Bosworth spinal fusion
Bosworth spline plate

Bosworth temporary crown
Bosworth tendo calcaneus
  repair
Bosworth tongue depressor
Bosworth-Joseph nasal saw
Bosworth-Shawler incision
BOT (base of tongue)
Botallo duct
Botallo foramen
both-bone fracture
both-column fracture
Botox
botryomycosis
Böttcher (see Bottcher)
Bottcher (also Böttcher)
Bottini operation
bottle
  DeVilbiss bottle
  dropper bottle
  eye dropper bottle
  glass bottle
  Imperatori antral wash bottle
  sealed vacuum bottle
  sinus wash bottle
  spray bottle
  trap bottle
  Van Osdel antral wash bottle
  water-seal drainage bottle
  Ziegler wash bottle
bottle hernia operation
bottle operation
bottle repair
bottlemaker's cataract
bottom
  weaver's bottom
bottom out
bottom-shaped nose
botulinum antitoxin
botulinum toxin serotype A
  (BTX-A)
botulinus antitoxin
botulism
  wound botulism
botulism antitoxin
Botvin iris forceps
Botvin vulsellum forceps
Botvin-Bradford eye enucleator
Bouchard nodes
Bouchard nodules
bouche de tapir
Boucheron speculum
Bouchut laryngeal tube

bougie (*see also* searcher, sound)
- á-boule bougie
- acorn-tipped bougie
- Anastasia bougie
- armed bougie
- Bangs bougie
- bellied bougie
- bronchoscopic bougie
- Buerger bougie
- Buerger dilating bougie
- bulbous bougie
- caustic bougie
- Celestin bougie
- Celestin dilator bougie
- Chevalier Jackson bougie
- common duct bougie
- conic bougie
- conical bougie
- Cooper bougie
- coudé bougie
- cylindrical bougie
- dilatable bougie
- dilating bougie
- Dittel dilating urethral bougie
- Dourmashkin bougie
- Dourmashkin tunneled bougie
- ear bougie
- elastic bougie
- elbowed bougie
- EndoLumina illuminated bougie
- esophageal mercury-filled bougie
- eustachian bougie
- exploratory bougie
- filiform Jackson bougie
- Fort urethral bougie
- French bougie
- Friedman-Otis bougie
- frontal sinus bougie
- fusiform bougie
- Gabriel Tucker bougie
- Garceau bougie
- Gruber medicated bougie
- Guyon dilating bougie
- Guyon exploratory bougie
- Harold Hayes eustachian bougie
- Hegar bougie
- Hertel bougie

bougie (*continued*)
- Holinger infant bougie
- Holinger-Hurst bougie
- Hurst esophageal bougie
- Hurst mercury bougie
- Hurst mercury-filled bougie
- Hurst mercury-filled esophageal bougie
- infant bougie
- Jackson esophageal bougie
- Jackson radiopaque bougie
- Jackson steel-stem woven filiform bougie
- Jackson tracheal bougie
- Klebanoff bougie
- Klebanoff common duct bougie
- large-diameter bougie
- LeFort filiform bougie
- Maloney mercury bougie
- Maloney tapered mercury filled esophageal bougie
- Maloney-type bougie
- medicated bougie
- mercury-filled esophageal bougie
- mercury-weighted bougie
- mercury-weighted rubber bougie
- Miller bougie
- olive-tipped bougie
- Otis urological bougie
- Phillips urethral whip bougie
- Plummer bougie
- Plummer modified bougie
- polyvinyl bougie
- radiopaque bougie
- Ravich bougie
- rectal bougie
- retrograde bougie
- Ritter bougie
- rosary bougie
- Rusch bougie
- Ruschelit urethral bougie
- Savary bougie
- Savary-Gilliard Silastic flexible bougie
- Savary-Gilliard wire-guided bougie
- soluble bougie
- sounds and bougies
- spiral-tipped bougie

bougie (*continued*)
    Szuler eustachian bougie
    tapered rubber bougie
    through-the-scope bougie
    tracheal bougie
    Trousseau esophageal bougie
    Tucker retrograde bougie
    tunneled bougie
    Urbantschitsch eustachian
      bougie
    ureteral bougie
    urethral whip bougie
    Wales bougie
    Wales rectal bougie
    Waltham-Street bougie
    wax bougie
    wax-tipped bougie
    whalebone eustachian bougie
    whalebone filiform bougie
    whip bougie
    whistle bougie
    Whistler bougie
    wire-guided polyvinyl bougie
    woven bougie
    yellow-eyed dilating bougie
bougie à boule
bougie dilator
bougie guide
bougie urethrotome
bougienage
    esophageal bougienage
    urethral bougienage
bougienage biopsy
bougienage technique
bougie-urethrotome
    Hertel bougie-urethrotome
    Storz bougie-urethrotome
Bouillaud sign
Bouilly operation
bounce point
bound
    upper bound
bounding pulse
bounding pupil
bouquet
    Riolan bouquet
Bourassa catheter
Bourdon tube pressure gauge
Bourns electronic adult
    respirator
Bourns humidifier
Bourns infant respirator

Bourns infant ventilator
Bourns LS104-150 infant
    ventilator
Bourns-Bear I ventilator
Bourns-Bear ventilator
boutonniere deformity
boutonniere hand dislocation
boutonniere incision
boutonniere repair
boutonniere splint
Bovero muscle
Bovie
    clinic Bovie
    coagulating current Bovie
    green Bovie
    liquid conductor Bovie
    Ritter Bovie
    underwater Bovie
Bovie accessories
Bovie blade
Bovie cautery
Bovie Chuck-It accessories
Bovie chuck-type handle
Bovie coagulating current
Bovie coagulating forceps
Bovie coagulating-current
    hemostat
Bovie coagulation
Bovie coagulation cautery
Bovie coagulation tip
Bovie coagulator
Bovie conization electrode
Bovie CSV coagulator
Bovie cutting current
Bovie cutting-current hemostat
Bovie electrocautery device
Bovie electrocautery unit
Bovie electrocoagulation unit
Bovie electrode
Bovie electrosurgical unit
Bovie endoscopic connecting
    cord
Bovie grounding pad
Bovie holder
Bovie knife
Bovie liquid conductor
Bovie needle
Bovie retinal detachment unit
Bovie suction device
Bovie ultrasound aspirator
Bovie unit
Bovie wet-field cautery

bovied
Bovin vaginal speculum
bovine allograft
bovine antitoxin
bovine cartilage
bovine collagen implant
bovine collagen material
    prosthesis
bovine collagen plug device
bovine face
bovine graft material
bovine heart valve
bovine heterograft
bovine implant
bovine pericardial valve
bovine pericardial heart valve
    xenograft
bovine pericardial prosthesis
bovine pericardium dural graft
bovine prosthesis
bovine-derived bone filler
Bovino scleral-spreading forceps
bow
    Anderson traction bow
    beaded-wires traction bow
    Bendixen-Kirschner traction
        bow
    Birnberg traction bow
    Boehler traction bow
    Crutchfield traction bow
    cupid's bow
    extension bow
    Framer finger extension bow
    high point of cupid's bow
    IUD bow
    Kirschner bow
    Kirschner wire traction bow
    lip traction bow
    Logan lip traction bow
    Pease-Thomson traction bow
    Steinmann traction bow
    traction bow
bow intrauterine device (bow
    IUD)
bowel
    aganglionic bowel
    apple-peel bowel
    dead bowel
    evacuation of bowel
    infarcted bowel
    intussuscepted bowel
    ischemic bowel

bowel (*continued*)
    knuckle of bowel
    Ladd procedure for
        malrotation of bowel
    large bowel
    lazy bowel
    loop of bowel
    lumen of bowel
    plication of bowel
    small bowel
    strangulated bowel
bowel abscess
bowel anastomosis
bowel axis
bowel bag
bowel bypass
bowel contents
bowel dilatation
bowel dilation
bowel forceps
bowel grasper
bowel injury
bowel intussusception
bowel lavage
bowel loop
bowel lumen
bowel obstruction
bowel pattern
bowel perforation
bowel prep regimen
bowel refashioning procedure
bowel resection
bowel retractor
bowel sounds
bowel stoma
bowel tones
bowel wall
bowel wall hematoma
Bowen AMS rasp
Bowen BAS-30 blade
Bowen chisel
Bowen disease
Bowen double-bladed scalpel
Bowen gooseneck chisel
Bowen gouge
Bowen osteotome
Bowen PEG tube
Bowen periosteal elevator
Bowen precancerous dermatosis
Bowen rasp
Bowen suction loose body
    forceps

Bowen suture drill
Bowen wire tightener
Bowen-Grover meniscotome
bowenoid carcinoma of vulva
bowenoid cells
bowenoid papulosis
Bower PEG tube
Bowers cannula
Bowers technique
bowing
    fracture bowing
bowing deformity
bowing fracture
bowing of fracture
bowing of nail
bowing of vocal cords
bowl
    conchal bowl
    ear bowl
    mastoid bowl
    solution bowl
bowl curet
bowl fistula
bowl of ear
Bowlby arm splint
Bowlby splint
bowleg
bowleg brace
bowleg deformity
bowler hat sign
bowler's thumb
Bowles stethoscope
Bowles technique
bowling-pin incision
Bowman capsule
Bowman cataract needle
Bowman ciliary muscle
Bowman dilator
Bowman disks
Bowman eye knife
Bowman eye speculum
Bowman glands
Bowman iris needle
Bowman iris scissors
Bowman lacrimal dilator
Bowman lacrimal probe
Bowman lamina
Bowman layer
Bowman membrane
Bowman muscle
Bowman needle
Bowman operation

Bowman probe
Bowman scissors
Bowman slitting of canaliculus
Bowman space
Bowman stop needle
Bowman strabismus scissors
Bowman tube
bowstring
bowstring sign
bow-tie knot
bow-tie stitch
box
    Anchor needle-sterilizing box
    Bárány box
    bronchoscopic battery box
    eye knife box
    eye knife plastic box
    House sterilizing box
    Logan box
    ointment box
    Panje voice box
    plastic eye knife box
    voice box
Box adenotome
Box curet
Box osteotome
Box technique
box-top technique of nipple
        reconstruction
boxcarring
Box-DeJager adenotome
boxer's ear
boxer's elbow
boxer's fracture
boxing of nipple
box-joint forceps
Boxwood hammer
Boxwood mallet
boxy tip deformity
Boyce needle holder
Boyce position
Boyce sign
Boyce tube
Boyce-Vest procedure
Boyd table
Boyd ankle amputation
Boyd approach
Boyd bone graft
Boyd classification
Boyd disarticulation
Boyd dissecting scissors
Boyd graft

Boyd hip disarticulation
Boyd implant
Boyd incision
Boyd intraocular implant lens
Boyd lens
Boyd operation
Boyd orbital implant
Boyd perforator
Boyd point
Boyd posterior bone block elbow
Boyd posterior incision
Boyd retractor
Boyd table
Boyd tonsillar scissors
Boyd-Anderson biceps tendon repair
Boyd-Anderson technique
Boyd-Bosworth procedure
Boyden chamber assay device
Boyden chamber technique
Boyden sphincter
Boyd-Griffin trochanteric fracture classification
Boyd-McLeod tennis elbow procedure
Boyd-McLeod tennis elbow technique
Boyd-Sisk approach
Boyd-Sisk posterior capsulorrhaphy
Boyd-Sisk shoulder procedure
Boyd-Stille tonsillar scissors
Boyer bursa
Boyer cyst
Boyes brachioradialis transfer technique
Boyes muscle clamp
Boyes operation
Boyes technique
Boyes-Goodfellow hook retractor
Boyle uterine elevator
Boyle-Davis mouth gag
Boyle-Rosin clip
Boyne dental prosthesis
Boynton needle holder
Boys-Allis tissue forceps
Boys-Allis tissue-holding forceps
Boys-Smith laser lens
Boytchev procedure
Bozeman catheter

Bozeman clamp
Bozeman curet
Bozeman dilator
Bozeman dressing forceps
Bozeman hook
Bozeman LR dressing forceps
Bozeman LR packing forceps
Bozeman LR uterine-dressing forceps
Bozeman needle holder
Bozeman operation
Bozeman position
Bozeman scissors
Bozeman speculum
Bozeman suture technique
Bozeman uterine-dressing forceps
Bozeman uterine-packing forceps
Bozeman-Douglas dressing forceps
Bozeman-Douglas uterine-dressing forceps
Bozeman-Finochietto needle holder
Bozeman-Fritsch catheter
Bozeman-Wertheim needle holder
Bozzi foramen
Bozzolo sign
BP Cuff pressure infuser
BP fistula
BP surgical handle
BP transfer forceps
BPB (biliopancreatic bypass)
BPD (biparietal diameter)
BPH (benign prostatic hypertrophy)
BPP (biophysical profile)
BPS spinal angiographic catheter
BPSA (bronchopulmonary segmental artery)
Bq (becquerel)
bra
   compression bra
   E-Z-ON surgical bra
   Jobst bra
   lead bra
Braasch bladder specimen forceps
Braasch bulb catheter
Braasch bulb technique

Braasch bulb ureteral catheter
Braasch catheter
Braasch cystoscope
Braasch direct catheterization cystoscope
Braasch direct cystoscope
Braasch forceps
Braasch ureteral catheter
Braasch ureteral dilator
Braasch-Bumpus prostatic punch
Braasch-Kaplan direct-vision cystoscope
Braastad costal arch retractor
brace with burs
bracelet test
brachial anesthesia
brachial arteriogram
brachial arteriography
brachial arteriotomy
brachial artery
brachial artery approach
brachial bypass
brachial cleft cyst
brachial coronary catheter
brachial dance
brachial dermolipectomy
brachial fascia
brachial gland
brachial muscle
brachial plexus
brachial plexus block (BPB)
brachial plexus block anesthetic technique
brachial plexus infiltration
brachial plexus nerve
brachial plexus repair
brachial plexus traction injury
brachial veins
brachialis muscle
brachioaxillary bridge graft fistula
brachiocarpal articulation
brachiocephalic artery
brachiocephalic trunk
brachiocephalic veins
brachiocephalic vessel angioplasty
brachiocrural
brachiocubital
brachiocyrtosis
brachiogram

brachioradial ligament
brachioradial muscle
brachioradial reflex
brachioradialis flap
brachioradialis muscle
brachiosubclavian bridge graft fistula
brachiotomy
brachioulnar articulation
Bracht maneuver
Bracht-Wachter lesion
brachybasia
brachybasophalangia
brachycephalic
brachycephalism
brachycephalofrontonasal dysplasia
brachycephalous
brachycephaly
   frontal brachycephaly
   occipital brachycephaly
brachycheilia
brachycnemic
brachycranic
brachydactylic
brachydactyly
   Haws type brachydactyly
brachydactyly type C
brachyesophagus
brachyfacial
brachyglossal
brachygnathia
brachygnathous
brachykerkic
brachyknemic
brachymelia
brachymesophalangia
brachymetacarpalia
brachymetapody
brachymetatarsia
brachymorphic
brachyphalangia
brachyprosopic
brachyrhinia
brachyrhyncus
brachyskelous
brachystaphyline
brachystasis
brachysyndactyly
brachytelephalangia
brachytherapy
brachyturricephaly

brachytypical
brachyuranic
bracing
   fracture bracing
   Hosmer Dorrance fracture
     bracing
Bracken anterior chamber
   cannula
Bracken fixation forceps
Bracken iris forceps
Bracken irrigating cannula
Bracken scleral fixation forceps
Bracken tissue-grasping forceps
Bracken-Forkas corneal forceps
bracket
   ligatureless bracket
   metal bracket
   multiphase bracket
   wall bracket
bracket modification
bracketed splint
Brackett dental probe
Brackett hip osteotomy
Brackett operation
Brackett probe
Brackett technique
Brackett-Osgood knee
   procedure
Brackett-Osgood posterior
   approach
Brackett-Osgood-Putti-Abbott
   technique
Brackin incision
Brackin technique
Brackin ureterointestinal
   anastomosis
Brackmann facial nerve monitor
Brackmann grade
Brackmann TORP
Braden flushing reservoir
Braden-CSF flushing reservoir
Bradford enucleation neurotome
Bradford forceps
Bradford fracture appliance
Bradford fracture frame
Bradford fusion
Bradford snare enucleator
Bradford thyroid forceps
Bradford thyroid traction
   vulsellum forceps
Bradford-Young Y-V plasty
Bradshaw-O'Neill aorta clamp

Brady suspension splint
bradyarrhythmia
Brady-Jewett technique
bradykinesia
brady-tachy syndrome
Bragard sign
Bragg peak proton-beam
   therapy
Bragg-Paul pulsator
Bragg-Paul respirator
Brahms mallet toe procedure
Brahms procedure
braid
   polypropylene braid
Braid strabismus
braided diagnostic catheter
braided Ethibond sutures
braided Mersilene sutures
braided Nurolon sutures
braided nylon sutures
braided occlusion device
braided polyamide sutures
braided polyester fiber
braided polyester sutures
braided silk sutures
braided Spectra UHMWPE
   surgical cable
braided titanium cable
braided Vicryl sutures
braided wire sutures
braid-like lesion
brain
   Broca motor speech area of
     brain
   compression of brain
   convexes of brain
   hemisphere of brain
   herniation of brain
   labyrinth of brain
   lobe of brain
   lobotomy of brain
   membrane of brain
   sulci in brain
   third ventricle of brain
   Wernicke area of brain
brain abscess
brain biopsy cannula
brain biopsy needle
brain clip
brain clip carrier
brain clip forceps
brain concussion

brain contusion
brain death
brain depressor
brain dressing forceps
brain edema
brain electrical activity
    map/mapping (BEAM)
brain elevator
brain forceps
brain herniation
brain hook
brain injury
brain knife
brain laceration
brain mapping
brain metastasis
brain probe
brain retractor
brain scan
brain scissors
brain silicone-coated retractor
brain spatula
brain spatula forceps
brain spatula spoon
brain spatula with insulation
brain speculum
brain spoon
brain stem
brain suction tip
brain suction tube
brain tissue forceps
brain transplantation
brain trocar
brain tumor forceps
brain-exploring cannula
brain-exploring trocar
brainstem compression
brainstem hemorrhage
brainstem lesion
Braithwaite clip remover
Braithwaite forceps
Braithwaite nasal chisel
Braithwaite skin graft knife
Brake hemostatic bag
Braley operation
Braley stretching of
    supratrochlear nerve
Bralon suture
Bran opponensplasty
branch
    auricular branch
    buccal branch

branch (*continued*)
    caudal branch
    circumflexed branch
    cochlear branch
    conus branch
    esophageal branch
    facial nerve branches
    frontal branch
    ganglionic branches
    gastroepiploic branch
    genicular branch
    internal branch
    joint branch
    labial branches
    lingual branch
    mammary branches
    marginal mandibular branch
    mental branches
    nasal branches
    nerve branch
    orbital branches
    perforating branches
    secondary branch
    septal branch
    stylohyoid branch
    zygomatic branch
    zygomaticofacial branch
    zygomaticotemporal branch
branch lesion
branch vein occlusion
branched calculus
branched vascular graft
branchial anomaly
branchial arches
branchial cartilage
branchial cleft anomaly
branchial cleft arch
branchial cleft cyst
branchial cleft sinus
branchial cleft sinusectomy
branchial cyst
branchial fistula
branchial pouch
branching tubule formation
branchiogenic carcinoma
branchiogenic cyst
branchiogenous cyst
branchioma
Brand opponensplasty
Brand passing forceps
Brand shunt-introducing forceps
Brand tendon passer

Brand tendon repair
Brand tendon stripper
Brand tendon transfer
Brand tendon transfer technique
Brand tendon-holding forceps
Brand tendon-passing forceps
Brand tendon-tunneling forceps
Brandt brassiere
Brandt cytology balloon
Brandt treatment
Brandt-Andrews maneuver
brandy nose
Brandy scalp stretcher I, rear
    closure
Brandy scalp stretcher II, front
    closure
Branemark endosteal implant
Branemark implant
Branemark osseointegration
    implant
Brannon-Wickstrom technique
branny desquamation
Bransford-Lewis ureteral dilator
Brant aluminum splint
Brantigan interbody fusion cage
Brantigan procedure
Brantigan-Voshell procedure
Brantley-Turner retractor
Brantley-Turner vaginal retractor
Branula cannula
brash
Brasivol soap
brass mallet
brass scleral plug
brass wire
brassiere
    Brandt brassiere
    Foerster surgical support
        brassiere
    skin brassiere
brassiere-type dressing
brassy body
Brauer cardiolysis
Brauer chisel
Brauer operation
Braun anastomosis
Braun cranioclast
Braun decapitation hook
Braun depressor
Braun episiotomy scissors
Braun forceps
Braun frame

Braun graft
Braun implant
Braun ligature carrier
Braun needle
Braun obstetrical hook
Braun operation
Braun pinch graft technique
Braun prosthesis
Braun shoulder procedure
Braun skin graft
Braun speculum
Braun stent
Braun technique
Braun uterine depressor
Braun uterine tenaculum
Braun uterine tenaculum
    forceps
Braun-Fernwald sign
Braun-Jaboulay gastrectomy
Braun-Jaboulay
    gastroenterostomy
Braun-Jardine-DeLee hook
Braun-Schroeder single-tooth
    tenaculum
Braun-Stadler bandage scissors
Braun-Stadler episiotomy
    scissors
Braun-Stadler sternal shears
Braunstein fixed calipers
Braunwald heart valve
Braunwald prosthesis
Braunwald valve
Braunwald-Cutter ball prosthetic
    valve
Braunwald-Cutter ball-valve
    prosthesis
Braunwald-Cutter caged-ball
    heart valve
Braunwald-Cutter prosthesis
Braunwald-Cutter prosthetic
    valve
Braun-Wangensteen graft
Braun-Wangensteen operation
Braun-Wangensteen prosthesis
Braun-Yasargil right-angle clip
Brawley antrum rasp
Brawley antrum raspatory
Brawley frontal sinus rasp
Brawley nasal suction tip
Brawley nasal suction tube
Brawley rasp
Brawley refractor

Brawley scleral wound retractor
Brawley sinus rasp
Brawley suction tip
Brawley tube
Brawner orbital implant
brawny arm
brawny edema
brawny induration
brawny trachoma
Braxton Hicks contraction
Braxton Hicks sign
Braxton Hicks version
Brazelton neonatal assessment
   scale
Brazilian leishmaniasis
bread-and-butter pericardium
bread-knife valvulotome
bread-loaf fashion
breadth
   bizygomatic breadth
   maxilloalveolar breadth
   midfacial breadth
   zygomatic breadth
breadth of mandible
breadth of mandibular ramus
breadth of palate
break point
break shock
breakable blade
BreakAway absorptive wound
   dressing
breakaway lap cushion
breakaway pin
breakdown
   anastomotic breakdown
   epithelial breakdown
   muscle breakdown
   sepsis-induced muscle
     breakdown
   skin breakdown
breakdown of bone
breaker
   Boehler plaster cast breaker
   cast breaker
   Jarit-Mason cast breaker
   Swiss blade breaker
   Woelfe-Boehler cast breaker
Breakstone lithotripter
breast
   aberrant breast
   caked breast
   constricted breast

breast (*continued*)
   contralateral breast
   cystic breast
   Haagensen triple biopsy of
     breast
   hypoplastic tuberous breast
   Kajava classification of
     supernumerary nipples and
     breasts
   lactating breast
   paraumbilical perforator
     adiposal flap reconstruction
     of breast
   pendulous breasts
   pole of the breast
   postmenopausal breasts
   ptotic breast
   shaping of breast
   shotty breast
   Snoopy breast
   striae of breasts
   tail of breast
   tubular breasts
breast abscess
breast architecture
breast augmentation
breast binder
breast biopsy
breast bone
breast bridge
breast calipers
breast cancer
breast carcinoma
breast cone
breast conservation therapy
   (BCT)
breast contour
breast cyst aspiration
breast folds
breast hypertrophy
breast hypoplasia
breast implant
breast implant capsular
   contracture
breast implant protection
   (B.I.P.)
breast implant valve
breast incision
breast irradiation
breast lift
breast localization needle
breast metastasis

breast mobility
breast mound
breast mound reconstruction
breast parenchyma
breast pinch test
breast plate
breast prosthesis
breast ptosis (grades I-IV)
breast pump
breast reconstruction
breast reduction
breast resection
breast shadow
breast sizer
breast strap
breast surgery
breast symmetry
breast tenaculum
breast tenaculum forceps
breast tissue
breast tissue is coned
Breast Vest Exu-Dry one-piece
    wound dressing
breast volume
BreastAlert DTS screening
    device
breast conserving procedure
breast conserving surgery
breast conserving technique
breast conserving therapy
breast mound form
breast preservation therapy
breaststroke injury
breaststroker's knee
breath
    short of breath (SOB)
    shortness of breath (SOB)
Breathe-Easy nasal splint
breathing
    Biot breathing
    continuous positive pressure
        breathing (CPPB)
    decelerated breathing
    frog breathing
    glossopharyngeal breathing
    intermittent positive pressure
        breathing (IPPB)
    Kussmaul breathing
    labored breathing
    mouth breathing
    rhythmic breathing
    shallow breathing

breathing (*continued*)
    sign mechanism for ventilator
        breathing
breathing bag
breathing pacemaker
breathing tube
breath-operated inhaler
Brecher new methylene blue
    technique
Brecher-Cronkite technique
Brecht feeder
Breck pin
Breck pin cutter
Breckenmacher tract
Breda disease
Bredall amalgam plugger
breech
    footling breech
    frank breech
breech birth
breech delivery
breech extraction
breech presentation
breeder reactor
Breen retractor
Breeze infant ventilator
Breeze respirator
bregmamastoid suture
bregma-menton radiograph
bregmatic bone
bregmatic fontanelle
bregmatic space
bregmatomastoid suture
    technique
bregmocardiac reflex
Breinin suction cup
Breisky Navritrol retractor
Breisky pelvimeter
Breisky vaginal retractor
Breisky vaginal speculum
Breisky-Navratil straight
    retractor
Breisky-Navratil vaginal speculum
Breisky-Stille speculum
Breitman adenotome
Bremer halo cervical traction
Bremer halo crown traction
Bremer halo crown traction set
Bremmer halo traction
Bremmer-Breeze splint
Brems astigmatism marker
Brenman camera

Brennen biosynthetic surgical mesh
Brenner carotid bypass shunt
Brenner forceps
Brenner gastrojejunostomy technique
Brenner inguinal herniorrhaphy
Brenner operation
Brenner rectal probe
Brent eyebrow reconstruction
Brent pressure earring
Brent pressure earrings for keloid surgery
brephoplastic graft
Breschet canal
Breschet hiatus
Breschet sinus
Breschet veins
Brescia fistula
Brescia-Cimino AV fistula
Brescia-Cimino graft
Brescia-Cimino shunt
Brescio-Breisky-Navratil speculum
Brescio-Cimino arteriovenous fistula
Bresgen cannula
Bresgen catheter
Bresgen frontal sinus probe
Bresgen sinus probe
Breslow classification for malignant melanoma
Breslow measurements
Breslow microstaging system for malignant melanoma
Breslow staging
Breslow thickness
Brett bone graft
Brett operation
Brett osteotomy
Brett technique
Brett-Campbell tibial osteotomy
Breuer-Hering inflation reflex
Breuerton x-ray view
brevicollis
Brevi-Kath epidural catheter
Brevital anesthetic agent
Brewer infarcts
Brewer kidney
Brewer operation
Brewer speculum
Brewer vaginal speculum

Brewerton view radiograph
Brewster arthrotomy approach
Brewster phrenic retractor
Brewster retractor
Brewster sinus punch
Bricker ileal conduit
Bricker ileoureterostomy
Bricker loop
Bricker operation
Bricker ureteroileostomy
Brickner position
Brickner sign
bridge
    3-way bridge
    Albarran bridge
    balance bridge
    blood vessel bridges
    breast bridge
    broad nasal bridge
    Burns converting bridge
    catheter deflecting bridge
    ceramometal implant bridge
    colostomy bridge
    combination sleeve bridge
    cystourethroscope bridge
    dental bridge
    double bridge
    extension bridge
    fixed bridge
    intercellular bridges
    loop ostomy bridge
    Maryland bridge
    membrane bridge
    nasal bridge
    one-horn bridge
    palmar skin bridge
    pediatric bridge
    retention suture bridge
    Rochette bridge
    Short bridge
    stationary bridge
    telescope adapting bridge
    telescope bridge
    three-way bridge
    Trestle prostatic bridge
    Wappler bridge
Bridge clamp
Bridge deep-surgery forceps
bridge flap
bridge graft
Bridge hemostatic forceps
Bridge intestinal forceps

bridge of nose
Bridge operation
bridge organ transplantation
bridge pedicle flap
bridge pedicle flap operation
bridge plate fixation
bridge prosthesis
bridge splint
Bridge telescope
bridged loop-gap resonator
bridgeless mask
bridge-like lesion
Bridgemaster nasal splint
bridging osteophytes
Bridle procedure
bridle stricture
bridle sutures
Briggs laryngoscope
Briggs operation
Briggs retractor
Briggs strabismus operation
Briggs transilluminator
Brigham brain tumor forceps
Brigham dressing forceps
Brigham forceps
Brigham thumb tissue forceps
Brigham total knee prosthesis
Bright disease
Brightbill corneal cutting block
Brighton epistaxis balloon
Bright-Ring keratoscope
Brill-Symmers disease
brim of pelvis
Brimfield cannulated grasping
    hook
Brimfield magnetic retriever
Brimms Quik-Fix denture repair
    kit
brimstone liver
Brinell hardness indenter point
B-ring
    esophageal B-ring
Brink PeriPyriform implant
Brinker hygienic tissue retractor
Brinkerhoff anoscope
Brinkerhoff proctoscope
Brinkerhoff rectal speculum
Brinton disease
brisement forcé
brisement therapy
brisk hemorrhage
brisk reflexes

Brisman-Nova carotid
    endarterectomy shunt
Brissaud-Marie syndrome
Bristow lever
Bristow operation
Bristow periosteal elevator
Bristow rasp
Bristow screw
Bristow zygomatic elevator
Bristow-Bankart humeral
    retractor
Bristow-Bankart soft tissue
    retractor
Bristow-Helfet procedure
Bristow-Latarjet procedure
Bristow-May procedure
Brite Lite III light
Britetrac fiberoptic instrument
Britetrac illuminator
Britetrac speculum
British test
Britt argon laser
Britt argon pulsed laser
Britt BL-12 laser
Britt krypton laser
Britt pulsed argon laser
Brittain arthrodesis
Brittain chisel
Brittain fusion
Brittain knee arthrodesis
Brittain operation
Brittain shoulder arthrodesis
Brittain-Dunn arthrodesis
brittle bone disease
brittle failure
brittle material
brittle nail syndrome
BRK transseptal needle
BRK-series transseptal needle
broach
    barbed broach
    Charnley femoral broach
    crescent broach
    DuaLock broach
    ELP broach
    endodontic broach
    femoral broach
    femoral prosthetic broach
    Firtel broach
    Fred Thompson broach
    glenoid fin broach
    Harris broach

broach (*continued*)
   intramedullary broach
   Koenig metatarsal broach
   metacarpal broach
   metatarsal stem broach
   Mittlemeir broach
   Monaco broach
   orthopedic broach
   phalangeal broach
   root canal broach
   series II femoral broach
   smooth broach
   square-hole broach
   starter broach
   Swanson intramedullary
     broach
   Swanson metatarsal broach
   tibial broach
broach extractor
broaching
broad adhesive band
broad AO dynamic compression
   plate
broad band
broad forehead
broad ligament hernia
broad ligament of uterus
broad nasal bridge
broad, boxy or ball tips (3 Bs of
   tip surgery)
broadband attenuation
broad-based polyp
broad-based type B Cormack-
   Lamberty pedicled
   fasciocutaneous flap
Broadbent inverted sign
Broadbent operation
Broadbent registration point
Broadbent sign
broadbill hemostat with push
   fork
broad-blade forceps
broad-spectrum antibiotic
Broca basilar angle
Broca facial angle
Broca motor speech area of
   brain
Broca pouch
Broca region
Broca space
Broca visual plane
Brock auricle clamp

Brock auricular clamp
Brock biopsy forceps
Brock cardiac dilator
Brock cardiac dilator rongeur
Brock commissurotomy knife
Brock incision
Brock infundibular punch
Brock infundibulectomy
Brock mitral valve knife
Brock operation
Brock probe
Brock pulmonary valve knife
Brock punch
Brock syndrome
Brock valvotomy
Brock valvulotome
Brockenbrough angiocatheter
Brockenbrough cardiac device
Brockenbrough catheter
Brockenbrough
   commissurotomy
Brockenbrough curved needle
Brockenbrough curved-tip
   occluder
Brockenbrough mapping
   catheter
Brockenbrough modified
   bipolar catheter
Brockenbrough needle
Brockenbrough sign
Brockenbrough technique
Brockenbrough transseptal
   catheter
Brockenbrough transseptal
   commissurotomy
Brockenbrough transseptal
   needle
Brockhurst technique
Brockington pile clamp
Brockman clubfoot procedure
Brockman incision
Brockman operation
Brockman technique
Brockman-Nissen arthrodesis
Brockman-Nissen wrist
   arthrodesis
Brödel bloodless line
Broders tumor classification
   (grades 1-4)
Brodhead uterine gauze packing
Brodie metaphysial abscess
Brodie director

Brodie disease
Brodie finger
Brodie fistula probe
Brodie joint
Brodie knee
Brodie ligament
Brodmerkel colon
    decompression set
Brodney catheter
Brodney hemostatic bag
Brodney urethrographic cannula
Brodney urethrographic clamp
Brodsky-Tullos-Gartsman
    approach
Broesike fossa
Broggi-Kelman dipstick gauge
Brom repair
Brombach perimeter
Bromley foreign body operation
Bromley operation
Bromley uterine curet
Brompton cocktail
Brompton Hospital retractor
Brompton mixture
Brompton solution
Bron implant cataract lens
Bron suction tube
bronchi (*sing.* bronchus)
bronchial adenocarcinoma
bronchial adenoma
bronchial biopsy forceps
bronchial breath sounds
bronchial brush biopsy
bronchial brushings
bronchial bud
bronchial carcinoma
bronchial catheter
bronchial check-valve
bronchial dilator
bronchial drainage
bronchial forceps
bronchial fracture
bronchial glands
bronchial inflammation
bronchial lavage
bronchial lumen
bronchial obstruction
bronchial sleeve resection
bronchial stump
bronchial sutures
bronchial tree
bronchial tube

bronchial veins
bronchial washings
bronchial grasping forceps
bronchiectasis
    capillary bronchiectasis
    saccular bronchiectasis
bronchioalveolar
    adenocarcinoma
bronchiolar adenocarcinoma
bronchiole
bronchioloalveolar carcinoma
bronchitis
    fibrinous bronchitis
    putrid bronchitis
bronchitis suction tube
Bronchitrac L catheter
Bronchitrac L flexible suction
    catheter
bronchoalveolar carcinoma
bronchoalveolar lavage (BAL)
bronchoalveolar lavage fluid
    (BALF)
bronchobiliary fistula
Broncho-Cath double-lumen
    endotracheal tube
bronchocele sound raspatory
bronchocentric granulomatosis
bronchocutaneous fistula
bronchodilation
bronchodilator (*see also* dilator)
    Marax bronchodilator
bronchoesophageal fistula
bronchoesophageal muscle
bronchofiberscope
bronchogenic adenocarcinoma
bronchogram
    tantalum bronchogram
bronchography
    Cope bronchography
    percutaneous transtracheal
        bronchography
broncholithiasis
bronchomediastinal
bronchophony
bronchoplasty repair
bronchopleural fistula
bronchopleurocutaneous fistula
    (BPCF)
bronchopneumonia
bronchopulmonary dysplasia
    (BPD)
bronchopulmonary fistula

bronchopulmonary foregut
   malformation
bronchopulmonary segmental
   artery (BPSA)
bronchopulmonary segments
bronchorrhaphy
bronchoscope
   ACMI bronchoscope
   ACMI Marici bronchoscope
   Albert slotted bronchoscope
   BF large-core bronchoscope
   Broyles bronchoscope
   Broyles-Negus bronchoscope
   Bruening bronchoscope
   Chevalier Jackson
      bronchoscope
   coagulation bronchoscope
   costophrenic bronchoscope
   Davis bronchoscope
   Doesel-Huzly bronchoscope
   double-channel irrigating
      bronchoscope
   Dumon laser bronchoscope
   Dumon-Harrell bronchoscope
   emergency ventilation
      bronchoscope
   Emerson bronchoscope
   flexible fiberoptic
      bronchoscope
   folding emergency ventilation
      bronchoscope
   Foregger bronchoscope
   Foroblique bronchoscope
   Fujinon bronchoscope
   Fujinon flexible
      bronchoscope
   Haslinger bronchoscope
   Holinger infant
      bronchoscope
   Holinger ventilating fiberoptic
      bronchoscope
   Holinger-Jackson
      bronchoscope
   hook-on bronchoscope
   infant bronchoscope
   irrigating bronchoscope
   Jackson costophrenic
      bronchoscope
   Jackson full-lumen
      bronchoscope
   Jackson full-lumen standard
      bronchoscope

bronchoscope (*continued*)
   Jackson standard
      bronchoscope
   Jackson staple bronchoscope
   Jesberg bronchoscope
   Jesberg infant bronchoscope
   Kernan-Jackson bronchoscope
   Kernan-Jackson coagulating
      bronchoscope
   Killian bronchoscope
   Life Imaging System and
      White Light bronchoscope
   Machida bronchoscope
   Marici bronchoscope
   Michelson bronchoscope
   Michelson infant
      bronchoscope
   Moersch bronchoscope
   Negus bronchoscope
   Negus-Broyles bronchoscope
   Olympus fiberoptic
      bronchoscope
   open-tube rigid bronchoscope
   pediatric bronchoscope
   Pentax bronchoscope
   Pilling bronchoscope
   respiration bronchoscope
   Riecker bronchoscope
   Riecker respiration
      bronchoscope
   Safar ventilation
      bronchoscope
   Savary bronchoscope
   SFB-I right-angled
      bronchoscope
   Shapshay laser bronchoscope
   single-channel fiberoptic
      bronchoscope
   slotted bronchoscope
   standard bronchoscope
   Storz emergency ventilation
      bronchoscope
   Storz folding emergency
      ventilation bronchoscope
   Storz infant bronchoscope
   Tucker bronchoscope
   ventilation bronchoscope
   Waterman folding
      bronchoscope
   Xanar laser bronchoscope
   Yankauer bronchoscope
bronchoscope-guided intubation

bronchoscopic aspirating tube
bronchoscopic aspirator
bronchoscopic battery box
bronchoscopic biopsy forceps
bronchoscopic bougie
bronchoscopic brush
bronchoscopic cleaner
bronchoscopic cleaning tool
bronchoscopic face shield
bronchoscopic forceps handle
bronchoscopic guide
bronchoscopic instrument guide
bronchoscopic magnet
bronchoscopic needle biopsy
bronchoscopic photodynamic
    therapy
bronchoscopic probe
bronchoscopic rotation forceps
bronchoscopic rule
bronchoscopic ruler
bronchoscopic specimen
    collector
bronchoscopic sponge carrier
bronchoscopic suction tube
bronchoscopic telescope
bronchoscopy
    fiberoptic bronchoscopy
        (FOB)
    nonfiberoptic bronchoscopy
bronchoscopy anesthetic
    technique
bronchoscopy disposable
    suction tube
bronchoscopy sponge
bronchoscopy with aspiration
bronchoscopy with biopsy
bronchoscopy with dilatation
bronchoscopy with drainage
bronchoscopy with insertion
bronchoscopy with irrigation
bronchoscopy with removal
bronchospasm
    induced bronchospasm
bronchospirometric catheter
bronchospirometry
bronchostomy
bronchotome
bronchotomy
bronchotomy with biopsy
bronchotomy with exploration
bronchotomy with removal
bronchovesicular markings

bronchovesicular respiration
bronchus (*pl.* bronchi)
    aspiration of bronchus
    cardiac bronchus
    ectatic bronchus
    eparterial bronchus
    hyparterial bronchus
    left main bronchus
    left upper lobe bronchus
    lingular bronchus
    main bronchus
    mainstem bronchus
    middle lobe bronchus
    right bronchus
    segmental bronchus
    stump of bronchus
    tracheal bronchus
bronchus clamp
bronchus forceps
bronchus-grasping forceps
Bronkhorst High Tec controller
Bronner clamp
Bronson foreign body removal
    operation
Bronson magnet
Bronson operation
Bronson speculum
Bronson-Magnion eye magnet
Bronson-Magnion forceps
Bronson-Park speculum
Bronson-Ray
    Hardy bayonet modification of
        Bronson-Ray
Bronson-Ray curet
Bronson-Ray pituitary curet
Bronson-Turner foreign body
    locator
Bronson-Turtz iris retractor
Bronson-Turtz refractor
Bronson-Turtz speculum
bronze mallet
bronze sutures
bronze wire sutures
bronzinum
    chloasma bronzinum
Brook wire-stitch scissors
Brookdale bar
Brooke Army Hospital splint
Brooke disease
Brooke epithelioma
Brooke fashion
Brooke ileostomy

Brooke tumor
Brooker double-locking
    unreamed tibial nail
Brooker wire
Brooker-Wills interlocking nail
Brooker-Wills nail
Brooks adenoid punch
Brooks gallbladder scissors
Brooks punch
Brooks scissors
Brooks technique
Brooks-Jenkins atlantoaxial
    fusion technique
Brooks-Jenkins fusion
Brooks-Seddon transfer
Brooks-Seddon transfer
    technique
Brooks-type fusion
Broomhead ankle surgery
Broomhead approach
Broomhead medial approach
broomstick cast
Brophy bistoury
Brophy bistoury knife
Brophy cleft palate knife
Brophy cleft palate operation
Brophy dressing forceps
Brophy elevator
Brophy forceps
Brophy gag
Brophy knife
Brophy mouth gag
Brophy needle
Brophy operation
Brophy periosteal elevator
Brophy periosteotome
Brophy plastic surgery scissors
Brophy plate
Brophy scissors
Brophy tenaculum
Brophy tenaculum retractor
Brophy tissue forceps
Brophy tooth elevator
Brophy-Deschamps needle
Broselow tape
Brostrom injection technique
Brostrom procedure
Brostrom-Gould foot procedure
Broviac atrial catheter
Broviac catheter
Broviac hyperalimentation
    catheter

brow
    apex of the brow
    contour of the brow
    hairline of brow
    ptotic brow
    surprise look caused by
        overcorrection of central
        brow
brow fixation
brow lift
brow lift suspension screw
brow position
brow presentation
brow ptosis
brow tape
brow-anterior position
brow-down position
brow-forehead lift
brow-lift approach (modified
    trichophytic)
Brown and Sharpe suture gauge
    (B&S suture gauge)
brown adipose tissue
Brown air dermatome
Brown and McDowell alar
    cartilage relocation
Brown & Sharp digital
    electronic calipers
Brown applicator
Brown bone elevator
Brown cannula
Brown chisel
Brown clamp
Brown cleft palate knife
Brown cleft palate needle
Brown cotton applicator
Brown dermatome
Brown dermatome blade
Brown dermatotome
Brown dissecting scissors
Brown ear speculum
Brown electric dermatome
Brown electrodermatome
Brown elevator
brown fat
Brown forceps
Brown hook
Brown knee approach
Brown knee joint reconstruction
Brown knife
Brown lateral approach
Brown lip clamp

Brown mallet
Brown nasal applicator
Brown nasal splint
Brown needle
Brown needle holder
Brown operation
Brown periosteotome
brown pigment gallstone
Brown push-back palatoplasty
Brown rasp
Brown raspatory
Brown retractor
Brown saw
Brown scissors
Brown side-grasping forceps
Brown snare
Brown sphenoid cannula
Brown staphylorrhaphy needle
Brown sterile adhesive
Brown suture hook
Brown syndrome
Brown technique
Brown tendon sheath syndrome
Brown thoracic forceps
Brown tissue forceps
Brown tissue hook
Brown tonsil snare
Brown tonsillar snare
Brown tonsillectome
Brown tooth elevator
brown tumor
Brown uvula retractor
Brown uvular retractor
brown/black pigmentation
Brown-Adson forceps
Brown-Adson side-grasping
    forceps
Brown-Adson tissue forceps
Brown-Bahnson bayonet forceps
Brown-Bahnson forceps
Brown-Beard technique
brown-black lesion
Brown-Blair dermatome
Brown-Blair operation
Brown-Blair skin graft knife
Brown-Bovari machine
Brown-Brenn stain
Brown-Brenn technique
Brown-Buerger cystoscope
Brown-Buerger dilator
Brown-Buerger forceps
Brown-Buerger hemostat

Brown-Burr modified Gillies
    retractor
Brown-Cushing forceps
Brown-Davis gag
Brown-Davis mouth gag
Brown-Dean cotton applicator
Brown-Dodge angiogram
Brown-Dohlman corneal implant
Brown-Dohlman eye implant
Brown-Dohlman implant
Brown-Dohlman Silastic corneal
    implant
Browne basket
Browne hypospadias repair
Browne orthosis
Browne retractor set
Browne splint
Browne stone basket
Browne urethral reconstruction
brownian motion
brownian movement
Browning vein
Brown-Joseph saw
Brown-McDowell procedure
Brown-McHardy air-filled
    pneumatic dilator
Brown-McHardy dilator
Brown-McHardy pneumatic
    dilator
Brown-McHardy pneumatic
    mercury bougie dilation
Brown-Mueller T-bar fastener
Brown-Mueller T-fastener set
Brown-Pusey corneal trephine
Brown-Pusey trephine
Brown-Roberts-Wells arc ring
    assembly
Brown-Roberts-Wells base ring
Brown-Roberts-Wells CT
    stereotaxic guide
Brown-Roberts-Wells head frame
Brown-Roberts-Wells head ring
    halo
Brown-Roberts-Wells headrest
Brown-Roberts-Wells ring
    adapter
Brown-Sanders fascial needle
Brown-Sequard injection
Brown-Sequard lesion
Brown-Sequard paralysis
Brown-Sequard syndrome
Brown-Swan forceps

brown-tail rash
Brown-Whitehead mouth gag
Brown-Wickham technique
browpexy
    endoscopy browpexy
brow-posterior position
brow-tail region
brow-up position
brow-up presentation
brow-upper lid complex
Broyle ligament
Broyles anterior commissure
    laryngoscope
Broyles aspirator
Broyles bronchoscope
Broyles dilator
Broyles esophageal dilator
Broyles esophagoscope
Broyles forceps
Broyles laryngoscope
Broyles laryngoscopy
Broyles nasopharyngoscope
Broyles optical forceps
Broyles optical laryngoscope
Broyles retrograde cystoscope
Broyles telescope
Broyles tube
Broyles wasp-waist
    laryngoscope
Broyles-Negus bronchoscope
Bruce bundle
Bruce protocol
brucellosis
Bruch gland
Bruch mastoid retractor
Bruch membrane
Bruck protocol
Bruecke fibers
Bruecke lens
Bruecke muscle
Bruecke tube
Bruel & Kjaer axial transducer
Bruel & Kjaer ultrasound
Bruel & Kjaer transvaginal
    ultrasound probe
Bruel & Kjaer ultrasound
    scanner
Bruening biting tip
Bruening bronchoscope
Bruening cannula
Bruening chisel
Bruening cutting-tip forceps

Bruening ear snare
Bruening electroscope
Bruening esophagoscope
Bruening esophagoscopy
    forceps handle
Bruening ethmoid exenteration
    forceps
Bruening forceps
Bruening forceps stylet
Bruening intracordal injection
    set
Bruening Japanese anastigmatic
    aural magnifier
Bruening nasal snare
Bruening nasal-cutting septal
    forceps
Bruening nasal-cutting septum
    forceps
Bruening otoscope
Bruening otoscope set
Bruening pneumatic otoscope
Bruening pressure syringe
Bruening punch
Bruening retractor
Bruening septal forceps
Bruening septum forceps
Bruening snare
Bruening speculum
Bruening syringe
Bruening tongue depressor
Bruening tonsillar snare
Bruening-Arnold intracordal
    injection set
Bruening-Citelli forceps
Bruening-Citelli rongeur
Bruening-Storz anastigmatic
    aural magnifier
Bruening-Storz diagnostic head
Bruening-Work diagnostic
    head
Bruggeman needle
Bruhat laser fimbrioplasty
Bruhat maneuver
Bruhat technique
bruised tissue
bruise-like macules
bruit
    abdominal bruit
    aphonic bruit
    carotid bruit
    false bruit
    intracranial bruit

bruit (*continued*)
  placental bruit
  supraclavicular bruit
  thyroid bruit
bruit de clapotement
Bruker scanner
Brun bone curet
Brun bone knife
Brun chisel
Brun curet
Brun ear curet
Brun guarded chisel
Brun mastoid curet
Brun plaster shears
Brun plastic shears
Brun plastic surgery scissors
Brun scissors
Bruner approach
Bruner vaginal speculum
brunescent
brunescent cataract
Brunetti chisel
Bruni counterpressor
Bruni-Wayne clamp
  approximator
Brunn cyst
Brunn membrane
Brunner adenoma
Brunner chisel
Brunner colon clamp
Brunner dissector
Brunner forceps
Brunner glands
Brunner goiter dissector
Brunner incision
Brunner intestinal clamp
Brunner intestinal forceps
Brunner ligature needle
Brunner modified incision
Brunner palmar incision
Brunner probe
Brunner raspatory
Brunner retractor
Brunner rib shears
Brunner sigmoid anastomosis
  forceps
Brunner tissue forceps
Bruns bone curet
Brunschwig arterial forceps
Brunschwig artery forceps
Brunschwig forceps
Brunschwig operation

Brunschwig
  pancreatoduodenectomy
Brunschwig retractor
Brunschwig total pelvic
  exenteration
Brunschwig viscera forceps
Brunschwig visceral forceps
Brunschwig visceral retractor
Brun-Stadler episiotomy scissors
Brunswick total hip
Brunswick-Mack approximator
Brunswick-Mack bur
Brunswick-Mack chisel
Brunswick-Mack rotating drill
Brunton otoscope
Bruser approach
Bruser incision
Bruser knee approach
Bruser lateral approach
Bruser lateral incision
Bruser skin incision
Bruser technique
brush
  Air-Lon tracheal tube brush
  Anchor all-nylon hand brush
  aortic valve brush
  Ayre brush
  Barraquer brush
  bronchoscopic brush
  bur brush
  cleaning brush
  contour instrument cleaning
    brush
  cytological brush
  denture brush
  endotracheal tube brush
  Geenan cytology brush
  Gill biopsy brush
  Glassman brush
  Haidinger brush
  hand nylon scrub brush
  hand scrub brush
  Kurten wire brush
  Mill-Rose cytology brush
  nylon hand scrub brush
  nylon scrub brush
  ophthalmic sable brush
  polishing brush
  protected bronchoscopic
    brush
  sable brush
  stomach brush

brush (*continued*)
    Storz cleaning brush
    tracheal tube brush
    Wagner laryngeal brush
brush biopsy
brush biopsy kit
brush burn
brush cytology
brush dispenser
Brushfield spots
brushings
    bronchial brushings
    lung brushings
brusque dilatation of esophagus
BRW (Brown-Roberts-Wells)
BRW CT stereotaxic guide
Bryan arthroplasty
Bryan procedure
Bryan technique
Bryan-Morrey approach
Bryan-Morrey elbow approach
Bryan-Morrey extensive
    posterior approach
Bryan-Morrey technique
Bryant lumbar colotomy
Bryant mitral hook
Bryant nasal forceps
Bryant operation
Bryant sign
Bryant traction
Bryant tractor
Bryant's traction
Brymill cryosurgical probe
Brymiss cryoprobe
BSC (basosquamous carcinoma)
BSC (burn scar contracture)
B-scan
B-scan reflectivity
B-scan ultrasound
B-scan ultrasound machine
BSS (balanced salt solution)
BSSO (bilateral sagittal split
    osteotomy)
BSU (Bartholin, Skene, and
    urethral glands)
BTE listening device
BTR (buccal triangular ridge)
bubble
    air bubble
    bladder bubble
    eye bubble
    Garren gastric bubble

bubble (*continued*)
    Garren-Edwards gastric
        bubble
    gastric air bubble
    gastric bubble
    Guibor Expo eye bubble
    intragastric bubble
    Riepe gastric bubble
    stomach bubble
bubble chamber equipment
bubble formation
bubble oxygenator
bubble trap oxygenator pump
bubble ventriculography
bubbly bone lesion
bubo
bubonulus
bubonocele
buccal
buccal alveolar plate
buccal alveolus
buccal angle
buccal artery
buccal aspect
buccal bar
buccal branch
buccal cavity
buccal cervical ridge
buccal contour
buccal cortical plate
buccal crossbite
buccal curve
buccal cyst
buccal defect
buccal drug administration
buccal embrasure
buccal envelope flap
buccal epithelium
buccal fat
buccal fat extractor
buccal fat extractor tip
buccal fat pad
buccal glands
buccal lymph node
buccal mucosa
buccal mucosa graft
buccal mucosa graft for urethra
    reconstruction
buccal mucosal defect
buccal mucosal flap
buccal mucosal graft
buccal muscle

buccal musculomucosal flap
buccal nerve
buccal neuralgia
buccal occlusion
buccal osteotomy
buccal pedicle-flap operation
buccal region
buccal ridge
buccal shelf
buccal space
buccal space abscess
buccal sulcus
buccal tablet
buccal triangular ridge (BTR)
buccal tube
buccal vestibule
buccal view
buccalis
    leukoplakia buccalis
    linea alba buccalis
    regio buccalis
buccinator
buccinator artery
buccinator crest
buccinator fascia
buccinator muscle
buccinator myomucosal flap
buccinator nerve
buccinator plication
buccinator space
buccoaxiogingival
buccocervical
buccodistal
buccogingival
buccolabial
buccolingual (BL)
buccolingual curvature
buccolingual diameter
buccolingual plane
buccolingual relation
buccomandibular zone
buccomaxillary
buccomesial (BM)
bucconeural duct
bucco-occlusal (BO)
bucco-occlusal line angle
buccopalatal
buccopalatal height
buccopharyngeal
buccopharyngeal approach
buccopharyngeal fascia
buccopharyngeal space

buccoversion
buccula
Buchbinder catheter
Buchbinder Omniflex catheter
Buchbinder Thruflex Over-the-
    Wire catheter
Buch-Gramcko gouge
Buchholz acetabular cup
Buchholz hip prosthesis
Buchholz knee prosthesis
Buchholz prosthesis
Buchholz total hip prosthesis
Buchwald atrophy
Buchwald tongue depressor
Buchwalter retractor
Buck applicator
Buck bone curet
Buck convoluted traction device
Buck curet
Buck dissecting knife
Buck ear applicator
Buck ear curet
Buck ear knife
Buck ear probe
Buck extension
Buck extension bar
Buck extension frame
Buck extension splint
Buck extension traction
Buck fascia
Buck femoral cement restrictor
Buck femoral cement restrictor
    inserter
Buck foreign body forceps
Buck fracture appliance
Buck hook
Buck knee brace
Buck knife
Buck mastoid curet
Buck myringotome
Buck myringotome knife
Buck myringotomy knife
Buck nasal applicator
Buck neurological hammer
Buck operation
Buck osteotome
Buck percussion hammer
Buck periosteal elevator
Buck plug
Buck probe
Buck restrictor
Buck splint

Buck traction
Buck traction splint
Buck tractor
Buck Universal convoluted
    traction unit
Buck wax curet
bucket
    Denis Browne bucket
    hospital bucket
    kick bucket
    Lenox bucket
bucket-handle fracture
bucket-handle incision
bucket-handle tear
bucket-handle tear of meniscus
bucket-handle view of facial
    bones
Buck-Gramcko bone lever
Buck-Gramcko incision
Buck-Gramcko pollicization
Buck-Gramcko technique
Buck-House curet
Buckingham drill
Buckingham mirror
buckle
    encircling operation for
        scleral buckle
    segmental buckle
buckle fracture
buckle fracture of phalanx
Buckley chisel
buckling
    cortical buckling
    midsystolic buckling
    scleral buckling
buckling fracture of the phalanx
buckling of cortex
buckling of knee
buckling of sclera
buckling operation
Bucknall procedure
Bucknall urethral reconstruction
Buck's traction
Buckstein colonic insufflator
Buckstein insufflator
Buckston suture
Bucky diaphragm
Bucky digital x-ray device
Bucky film
Bucky grid
Bucky hand drill
Bucky high-contrast imaging

Bucky rays
Bucky studies
Bucky technique
Bucky view tray
bucrylate
Bucy cordotomy knife
Bucy knife
Bucy laminectomy rongeur
Bucy retractor
Bucy spinal cord retractor
Bucy suction tube
Bucy tube
Bucy-Frazier cannula
Bucy-Frazier coagulating-suction
    cannula
Bucy-Frazier coagulation
    cannula
Bucy-Frazier suction cannula
Bucy-Frazier suction tube
bud
    bronchial bud
    limb bud
    taste bud
    tooth bud
Bud bur
Budd-Chiari syndrome
Budd-Chiari syndrome with
    Behçet disease
Budd-Chiari syndrome without
    Behçet disease
Budde halo neurosurgical
    retractor
Budde halo ring
Budde halo ring retractor
Budde-Greenberg-Sugita
    stereotactic head frame
buddy splint
buddy strap
buddy tape
buddy wire
Budin hammertoe splint
Budin joint
Budin toe splint
Budinger blepharoplasty
Budinger blepharoplasty
    operation
Budinger operation
Buechel-Pappas total ankle
    prosthesis
Buedding squeegee cortex
    extractor and polisher
Bueleau empyema trocar

Buerger bougie
Buerger dilating bougie
Buerger disease
Buerger exercises
Buerger needle
Buerger prostatic needle
Buerger punch
Buerger snare
Buerger-McCarthy bladder
    forceps
Buerger-McCarthy forceps
Buerger-McCarthy scissors
Buerger-Oliver dilator
Buerhenne catheter
Buerhenne technique
Buettner-Parel cutter
Buettner-Parel vitreous cutter
Buffalo dental cement
buffalo hump
buffer
buffing sponge
Bugbee electrocautery
Bugbee electrode
Bugbee fulgurating electrode
Bugg-Boyd procedure
Bugg-Boyd technique
Buie biopsy forceps
Buie cannula
Buie clamp
Buie electrode
Buie fistula probe
Buie forceps
Buie fulgurating electrode
Buie fulguration electrode
Buie hemorrhoidectomy
Buie irrigator
Buie operating scissors
Buie operation
Buie pile clamp
Buie position
Buie probe
Buie rectal forceps
Buie rectal irrigator
Buie rectal scissors
Buie rectal suction tip
Buie rectal suction tube
Buie retractor
Buie scissors
Buie sigmoidoscope
Buie specimen forceps
Buie suction tube
Buie technique

Buie tube
Buie-Hirschman anoscope
Buie-Hirschman clamp
Buie-Hirschman pile clamp
Buie-Hirschman proctoscope
Buie-Hirschman speculum
Buie-Smith anal retractor
Buie-Smith rectal speculum
Buie-Smith retractor
Buie-Smith speculum
buildup eye implant
Buelau trocar
bulb
    apex of duodenal bulb
    Beckman Silastic bulb
    Braasch bulb
    dilating bulb
    duodenal bulb
    hair bulb
    inflation of bulb
    jugular bulb
    nystagmus bulb
    olfactory bulb
    saphenous bulb
    self-inflating bulb
    Selrodo bulb
    sigmoidoscope inflation bulb
    suction bulb
    Westlake bull's eye bulb
bulb and thumb screw valve
bulb catheter
bulb deformity
bulb dynamometer
bulb grenade
bulb of inferior jugular vein
bulb of occipital horn of lateral
    ventricle
bulb of penis
bulb of vestibule
bulb retractor
bulb suction
bulb suture
bulb syringe
bulb ureteral catheter
bulbar peptic ulcer
bulbi
    fascia bulbi
    vagina bulbi
bulbiform
bulbocavernosus fat flap
bulbocavernosus reflex
bulbocavernous glands

bulbocavernous muscle
bulbocavernous reflex
bulbomembranous
bulbomimic reflex
bulb-operated nebulizer
bulboprostatic urethral
    anastomosis
bulbosity of nasal tip
bulbourethral
bulbourethral glands
bulbous bougie
bulbous catheter
bulbous cervix
bulbous dilatation
bulbous nasal tip
bulbous tip of nose
bulbous turbinates
bulbous urethra
bulbous-tip ear syringe
bulboventricular fold
bulbus
bulbus urethrae
bulge
    periocular bulge
    reduction of lower palpebral
        bulge
bulging
    anal bulging
bulging disk
bulk
    muscle bulk
bulk pack technique
Bulkee II gauze bandage
Bulkee super fluff sponge
bulky compressive dressing
bulky dressing
bulky hand dressing
bulky pressure dressing
bulla (*pl.* bullae)
    ethmoid bulla
    ethmoidal bulla
    hemorrhagic bulla
    intraepidermal bulla
    superficial bullae
bulla ethmoidalis
bulla ethmoidalis cava nasi
bulla ethmoidalis ossis
    ethmoidalis
Bullard intubating laryngoscope
bulldog
    vascular bulldog
bulldog clamp

bulldog clamp-applier forceps
bulldog clamp-applying forceps
bulldog forceps
bulldog head
bulldog hemostat
bulldog microclamp
bulldog nasal scissors
bulldog scissors
Buller bandage
Buller eye shield
bullet forceps
bullet probe
bullet tenaculum
bullet tip catheter
bullet-shaped cannula
bullosa
    concha bullosa
    epidermolysis bullosa
    generalized atrophic benign
        epidermolysis bullosa
        (GABEB)
    myringitis bullosa
bullous
bullous edema
bullous erythema multiforme
bullous granulomatous
    inflammation
bullous hemorrhagic pyoderma
    gangrenosum
bullous lesion
bullous lichen planus
bullous myringitis
bullous pemphigoid
bullous skin lesion
bullous-like edema
bull's eye lamp
bull's eye lesion
bull's eye macular lesion
Bullseye femoral guide
Bulnes-Sanchez retractor
Bumgardner dental holder
Bumke pupil
Bumm curet
Bumm placental curet
Bumm uterine curet
bump
    Baum bumps
    pump bump
bumped up
bumper fracture
bumper-fender fracture
Bumpus forceps

Bumpus resectoscope
Bumpus specimen forceps
bunching
bunching maneuver
bunching suture technique
bunching sutures
Buncke quartz needle
Buncke technique
bundle
    ACMI light-carrying bundle
    acousticofacial nerve bundle
    anterior ground bundle
    anteromedial bundle
    arcuate nerve fiber bundle
    Arnold bundle
    atrioventricular bundle
      (AV bundle)
    AV bundle (atrioventricular
      bundle)
    Bachmann bundle
    Bruce bundle
    cingulum bundle
    clip-on light bundles
    coherent bundle
    commissural bundle
    Drualt bundle
    extracostal bundle
    extravelar muscle bundle
    fiber bundle
    fiberoptic bundle
    fiberoptic light bundle
    forebrain bundle
    Gierke respiratory bundle
    Held bundle
    Helweg bundle
    high-intensity light bundle
    His bundle
    His-Tawara bundle
    Hoche bundle
    IG bundle
    image guide bundle
    inferior arcuate bundle
    inferior alveolar neurovascular
      bundle
    intercostal bundle
    intermediate bundle
    interwoven bundle
    James bundle
    Keith bundle
    Kent bundle
    Kent-His bundle
    Killian bundle

bundle (*continued*)
    Krause respiratory bundle
    lateral ground bundle
    LG bundle
    light guide bundle
    Lissauer bundle
    Loewenthal bundle
    longitudinal bundle
    longitudinal medial bundle
    maculopapillary bundle
    maculopapular bundle
    Mahaim bundle
    main bundle
    master IG bundle
    Meynert retroflex bundle
    Meynert bundle
    microfilament bundle
    Monakow bundle
    muscle bundle
    neovascular bundle
    nerve bundle
    nerve fiber bundle
    neurovascular bundle
    olfactory bundle
    olivocochlear bundle
    orbital neurovascular bundle
    papillomacular nerve fiber
      bundle
    paracentral nerve fiber
      bundle
    Pick bundle
    posterior longitudinal bundle
    posterolateral bundle
    precommissural bundle
    predorsal bundle
    principal fiber bundle
    Rathke bundle
    Schütz bundle
    sensory nerve fiber bundle
    sinospiral muscle bundle
    solitary bundle
    Stanley-Kent bundle
    superior arcuate bundle
    superior gluteal neurovascular
      bundle
    thalamomammillary bundle
    Thorel bundle
    Türck bundle
    vascular bundle
    Vicq d'Azyr bundle
bundle bone
bundle branch block

bundle fiber
bundle of His
bundle of Kent
bundle of Stanley Kent
bundle-branch block
Bundt cross-legged clip
Bunge amputation
Bunge curet
Bunge exenteration spoon
Bunge meatotome
Bunge scissors
Bunge spoon
Bunge ureteral meatotome
Bunim forceps
Bunim urethral forceps
bunion
    dorsal bunion
    tailor's bunion
bunion deformity
bunion dissector
bunion formation
bunion operation
bunion osteotomy
bunion shield
bunionectomy
    Akin bunionectomy
    Austin bunionectomy
    Barker bunionectomy
    cap bunionectomy
    chevron bunionectomy
    closing ABD wedge
        bunionectomy
    crescentic bunionectomy
    Drato bunionectomy
    DuVries-Mann modified
        bunionectomy
    Hammond bunionectomy
    Hauser bunionectomy
    Hiss bunionectomy
    Hohmann bunionectomy
    Jones bunionectomy
    Joplin bunionectomy
    Keller bunionectomy
    Kreuscher bunionectomy
    Lapidus bunionectomy
    Logracino bunionectomy
    Ludloff bunionectomy
    Mayo bunionectomy
    Mayo-Heuter bunionectomy
    McBride bunionectomy
    McKeever bunionectomy
    Mitchell bunionectomy

bunionectomy (*continued*)
    offset reverse dome
        bunionectomy (ORD
        bunionectomy)
    opening ABD wedge
        bunionectomy
    ORD bunionectomy (offset
        reverse dome
        bunionectomy)
    Peabody bunionectomy
    Peabody-Mitchell
        bunionectomy
    Reverdin bunionectomy
    Reverdin-Laird bunionectomy
    Reverdin-McBride
        bunionectomy
    Silver bunionectomy
    Silver-Skin bunionectomy
    Stamm bunionectomy
    Stone bunionectomy
    tailor bunionectomy
    tricorrectional bunionectomy
    Wilson bunionectomy
bunionette
bunk-bed fracture
Bunke clamp
Bunker forceps
Bunker implant
Bunker intraocular implant lens
Bunker lens
Bunker modification of Jackson
    laryngeal forceps
Bunke-Schulz clamp
    approximator
Bunnnel tendon transfer
Bunnell active hand splint
Bunnell anvil
Bunnell atraumatic technique
Bunnell bipedicle digital visor
    flap
Bunnell bipedicle flap
Bunnell block
Bunnell bone drill
Bunnell digital exertion
    measurer
Bunnell dissecting probe
Bunnell dressing
Bunnell drill
Bunnell finger extension splint
Bunnell finger loop
Bunnell finger splint
Bunnell flap

Bunnell forwarding probe
Bunnell gutter splint
Bunnell hand and finger
   splints
Bunnell hand drill
Bunnell knuckle bender
Bunnell knuckle bender splint
Bunnell knuckle bender with
   outrigger
Bunnell ligament repair
Bunnell modification of
   Steindler flexorplasty
Bunnell modified safety-pin
   splint
Bunnell needle
Bunnell operation
Bunnell outrigger splint
Bunnell probe
Bunnell procedure
Bunnell pull-out wire
Bunnell reverse knuckle-bender
   splint
Bunnell safety pin splint
Bunnell sign
Bunnell splint
Bunnell stitch
Bunnell suture technique
Bunnell sutures
Bunnell tendon needle
Bunnell tendon passer
Bunnell tendon repair
Bunnell tendon stripper
Bunnell tendon transfer
Bunnell tendon transfer
   technique
Bunnell test
Bunnell wire pull-out suture
Bunnell-Howard arthrodesis
   clamp
Bunnell-Littler dressing
Bunnell-Williams procedure
Bunny boot
Bunny Boot foot splint
bunny scrunch lines
Bunt catheter
Bunt forceps holder
Bunt instrument holder
Bunt tendon stripper
Bunyan bag
bupivacaine anesthesia
bupivacaine hydrochloride
   anesthetic agent

buprenorphine narcotic
   analgesic therapy
bur
   abrader bur
   Acorde bur
   acromionizer bur
   Acrotorque bur
   Adson bur
   Adson enlarging bur
   Adson perforating bur
   Adson-Rogers cranial bur
   aftercataract bur
   Alfonso guarded bur
   Allport bur
   Allport eustachian bur
   antral bur
   Bailey bur
   Bailey skull bur
   Ballenger bur
   Ballenger mastoid bur
   Ballenger-Lillie bur
   Ballenger-Lillie mastoid bur
   barrel cutting bur
   bone bur
   Borchardt olive-shaped bur
   brace with burs
   Brunswick-Mack bur
   Bud bur
   Burwell bur
   Burwell corneal bur
   Caparosa bur
   Caparosa cutting bur
   carbide bur
   carbide finishing bur
   carbide mastoid bur
   cataract bur
   Cavanaugh bur
   Cavanaugh sphenoid bur
   Cavanaugh-Israel bur
   choanal bur
   coarse carbide cone bur
   coarse-olive bur
   Cone bur
   conical bur
   corneal bur
   corneal foreign body bur
   countersink bur
   cranial bur
   Cross corneal bur
   crosscut bur
   crosscut fissure bur
   crosscut straight fissure bur

bur (*continued*)
- curetting bur
- Cushing bur
- Cushing cranial bur
- cutting bur
- cylinder bur
- Davidson bur
- decortication bur
- Densco bur
- dental bur
- dentate bur
- denture vulcanite bur
- dermabrasion bur
- D'Errico bur
- D'Errico enlarging bur
- D'Errico perforating bur
- Dialom bur
- diamond barrel bur
- diamond bur
- diamond finishing bur
- diamond-coated bur
- diamond-dust bur
- Doyen bur
- Doyen cylindrical bur
- Doyen spherical bur
- Dyonics arthroplasty bur
- Dyonics bur
- electric bur
- electrically driven bur
- end-cutting fissure bur
- endodontic bur
- enlarging bur
- eustachian bur
- excavating bur
- Farrior bur
- Feldman bur
- fenestration bur
- Ferris Smith-Halle bur
- Ferris Smith-Halle sinus bur
- FG diamond bur
- fine olive bur
- finish bur
- finishing bur
- Fisch cutting bur
- fissure bur
- flame bur
- flame-tip bur
- fluted finishing bur
- foreign body bur
- Frey-Freer bur
- Gam-Mer bur
- Gates-Glidden bur

bur (*continued*)
- gold bur
- Guilford-Wright bur
- Hall bone bur
- Hall bur
- Hall mastoid bur
- Hannahan bur
- high-speed bur
- high-speed diamond 3-tiered depth cutting bur
- high-speed diamond wheel bur
- high-speed steel bur
- high-speed tungsten carbide bur
- high-speed 2-grit bur
- high-torque bur
- Hough-Wullstein crurotomy saw bur
- House bur
- House-Wullstein perforating bur
- Hudson brace bur
- Hudson brace with bur
- Hudson bur
- Hudson conical bur
- Hudson cranial bur
- Hu-Friedy dental bur
- inverted cone bur
- Jordan bur
- Jordan perforating bur
- Jordan-Day bur
- Jordan-Day cutting bur
- Jordan-Day fenestration bur
- Jordan-Day polishing bur
- Kopetzky sinus bur
- lacrimal sac bur
- large nail spicule bur
- Le Blonde R diamond dental bur
- Lee diamond bur
- Lempert bur
- Lempert diamond-dust polishing bur
- Lempert fenestration bur
- Light-Veley bur
- Lindermann bur
- long coarse bur
- low-speed Christmas tree diamond bur
- low-speed tapered carbide bur
- Marin bur

bur (*continued*)
- Martin bur
- Masseran trepan bur
- mastoid bone bur
- mastoid bur
- McKenzie bur
- McKenzie enlarging bur
- Micro-Aire bur
- M-series bur (M-1, M-2, etc.)
- MTM 2 bur
- Mueller bur
- neurosurgical bur
- new happy bur
- old smoothie bur
- orthopedic bur
- Osteon bur
- oval cutting bur
- Parapost bur
- paronychia bur
- Patton bur
- pear-shaped bur
- perforating bur
- pilot bur
- pineapple bur
- pineapple contouring bur
- plug-finishing bur
- pointed cone bur
- polishing bur
- primary trimming bur
- Red Witch bur
- Redi Bur
- rhinoplasty diamond bur
- rosehead bur
- Rosen bur
- Rotablator rotating bur
- rotary bur
- round bur
- round cutting bur
- round diamond bur
- Sachs bur
- Sachs skull bur
- Scheer-Wullstein cutting bur
- Shannon bur
- Shea bur
- short coarse bur
- short fine bur
- side-cutting Swanson bur
- sinus bur
- skull bur
- slotting bur
- small nail spicule bur
- Smoothie Junior bur

bur (*continued*)
- Somerset bur
- sphenoidal bur
- spherical bur
- spiral fluted tungsten carbide bur
- Starlite Omni-AT bur
- Stille bur
- Storz corneal bur
- straight fissure bur
- straight shank bur
- Stryker bur
- Stumer perforating bur
- Super-Cut diamond bur
- Surgair bur
- surgical bur
- Surgitome bur
- Thomas bur
- tungsten carbide bur
- Turbo-Jet dental bur
- vulcanite bur
- Wachsberger bur
- wheel bur
- Wilkerson bur
- Wilkerson choanal bur
- Willstein diamond bur
- wire pass bur
- wire-passing bur
- Worst corneal bur
- Wullstein bur
- Wullstein high-speed bur
- Yazujian bur
- Yazujian cataract bur
- Zimmer bur

bur brush
bur cells
bur drill
bur hole
bur hole cover
bur hole transducer
bur neck
bur saw
Buratto flap forceps
Buratto flap protector
Buratto irrigating cannula
Buratto LASIK forceps
Buratto ophthalmic forceps
Buratto technique
bur-bearing catheter
Burch biopsy forceps
Burch bladder suspension procedure

Burch bladder suspension
    technique
Burch bladder suspension
Burch calipers
Burch colposuspension
Burch colpourethropexy
Burch evisceration
Burch eye calipers
Burch eye evisceration
    operation
Burch fixation pick
Burch forceps
Burch hook
Burch iliopectineal ligament
    urethrovesical suspension
Burch modification
Burch operation
Burch ophthalmic pick
Burch pick
Burch procedure
Burch retropubic urethropexy
Burch technique
Burch urethropexy
Burch-Greenwood tendon
    tucker
Burch-Greenwood tucker
Burckhardt operation
Burdach tract
Burdick cautery
Burdick Eclipse ECG machine
Burdick electrosurgical unit
Burdick microtherm diathermy
    unit
Burdick microwave diathermy
    electrosurgical unit
Burdick muscle stimulator
    generator
Burdick Zoalite
Burdizzo clamp vasectomy
Burdizzo vasectomy
Buretrol device
Burford clamp
Burford coarctation forceps
Burford forceps
Burford retractor
Burford rib retractor
Burford rib spreader
Burford spreader
Burford-Finochietto infant rib
    spreader
Burford-Finochietto retractor
Burford-Finochietto rib retractor

Burford-Finochietto rib spreader
Burford-Finochietto spreader
Burford-Lebsche knife
Burford-Lebsche sternal knife
Burger technique for
    scapulothoracic
    disarticulation
Burger triangle
Burgess below-knee amputation
Burgess nail
Burgess operation
Burgess table
Burgess technique
Burget nasal splint
Burhenne biliary duct stone
    extraction
Burhenne steerable catheter
bur-hole button
bur-hole cover
bur-hole incision
bur-hole placement
Burian-Allen contact lens
Burian-Allen contact lens
    electrode
buried
buried cortex
buried de-epithelialized local
    flap
buried dermal flap
buried flap
buried free forearm flap transfer
buried mass far-and-near suture
    technique
buried penis
buried sutures
buried tonsil
Burke bariatric treatment system
    powered bariatric bed
Burke plus low-air-loss bed
Burkhalter modification of Stiles-
    Bunnell technique
Burkhalter procedure
Burkhalter technique
Burkhalter transfer technique
Burkhalter-Reyes method of
    phalangeal fracture
Burkitt lymphoma
Burkitt lymphoma of nasal ala
Burlar process
Burlar tubercle
Burlisher clamp
Burman technique

burn
 1st-degree burn
 2nd-degree burn
 3rd-degree burn
 4th-degree burn
 acid burn
 alkali burn
 brush burn
 cement burn
 chemical burn
 concrete burn
 contact burn
 corneal alkali burn
 corneal burn
 electric burn
 electrical burn
 flash burn
 friction burn
 full-thickness burn
 irrigation burn
 laryngeal burn
 partial-thickness burn
 plaster cast application burn
 powder burn
 radiation burn
 road burn
 slag burn
 superficial burn
 thermal burn
 tissue burn
 x-ray burn
burn alopecia
Burn amaurosis
burn boutonnière deformity
burn classification
burn classification (1st to 4th
 degree)
burn claw
burn debridement
burn eschar
burn injury
Burn Jel dressing
burn process
burn reconstruction
burn scar carcinoma
burn scar contracture (BSC)
burn scar treatment
burn shock
burn wound
burn wound anemia
burn wound management
burn wound regimen

burned
 body surface burned
 rule of nines formula for
  percentage of body surface
  burned
burned out mucosa
burner syndrome
Burnett anoscope
Burnett applicator (sizes A, B,
 etc.)
Burnett cylinder
Burnett mouth positioning
 device
Burnett Pap smear kit
Burnett Sani-Spec disposable
 speculum
Burnett syndrome
Burnham bandage scissors
Burnham biopsy forceps
Burnham finger bandage
 scissors
Burnham forceps
Burnham scissors
burning feet syndrome
burning pain
burnisher
 ball burnisher
burnishing
burn-out procedure
Burns bone forceps
Burns bridge telescope
Burns chisel
Burns converting bridge
Burns forceps
Burns guarded chisel
Burns plate
Burns prism bar
Burns space
Burns telescope
Burns-Haney incision
Burow blepharoplasty
Burow cheiloplasty
Burow flap
Burow flap operation
Burow operation
Burow solution
Burow technique
Burow triangle
Burow triangle deformity
Burow vein
BURP maneuver
Burr butterfly needle

Burr corneal ring
Burr silicone button
burred Wright reamer
Burrows technique
bursa (*pl.* bursae)
  Achilles bursa
  acromial bursa
  adventitious bursa
  anserine bursa
  Boyer bursa
  calcaneal bursa
  Fleischmann bursa
  hyoid bursa
  iliopectineal bursa
  iliopsoas bursa
  incision and drainage of bursa
  injection of bursa
  Luschka bursa
  Monro bursa
  nasopharyngeal bursa
  olecranon bursa
  omental bursa
  pharyngeal bursa
  prepatellar bursa
  radial bursa
  retrohyoid bursa
  retromammary bursa
  scapulothoracic bursa
  splenic recess of omental
    bursa
  subacromial bursa
  subdeltoid bursa
  subscapular bursa
  subtendinous bursa
  Tornwaldt bursa
  ulnar bursa
  Voshell bursa
bursal cyst
bursal flap
bursata
  exostosis bursata
bursectomy
bursitis
  Duplay bursitis
bursocentesis
bursolith
bursopathy
bursotomy
burst
  short bursts
  tone burst
burst fracture

burst pacemaker
bursting dislocation
bursting fracture
burst-type laceration
Burton black light
Burton Fresnel floor light
Burton laryngoscope
Burton line
Burton osteotome
Burton sign
Buruli lesion
Buruli ulcer
Burwell bur
Burwell corneal bur
Burwell-Scott modification of
    Watson-Jones incision
burying of appendiceal stump
burying of fimbriae in uterine
    wall
Busacca nodules
Busch scissors
Busch umbilical cord scissors
Busch umbilical scissors
Buschke-Ollendorf sign
Buselmeier shunt
Busenkell posterior hip retractor
Bush intervertebral curet
Bush stabilized cutting loop
Bush ureteral illuminator
Bushey compression clamp
bushing
  reamer bushing
but
  Allport cutting but
butacaine anesthetic agent
Butchart staging classification
Butcher saw
butethamine hydrochloride
    anesthetic agent
Butler bayonet forceps
Butler dental retractor
Butler fifth toe operation
Butler pillar retractor
Butler retractor
Butler stimulator
Butler technique
Butler tonsil suction tube
Butler tonsillar suction tube
butt
butt joint
Butte dissector
Butterfield cystoscope

butterfly
butterfly adapter
butterfly bandage
butterfly catheter
butterfly clip
Butterfly cushion
butterfly drain
butterfly dressing
butterfly flap
butterfly fracture
butterfly fracture fragment
butterfly fragment
butterfly heart valve
butterfly IV needle
butterfly needle
butterfly needle infusion port
butterfly patch
butterfly pattern of perihilar
    edema
butterfly-shaped monoblock
    vertebral plate
Butterworth bidirectional four-
    pole high-pass digital filter
buttock
    Merkel cell carcinoma of
        buttock
buttocks lift
button
    Accu-Flo button
    Aleppo button
    anastomotic button
    Baghdad button
    Bard button
    Baroux button
    Bentley button
    Biomet button
    Biskra button
    Bivona-Colorado button
    Boari button
    bobbin-type laryngectomy
        button
    bony chin button
    bur-hole button
    Burr silicone button
    Charnley suture button
    Chlumsky button
    collar button (*see also*
        button)
    Converse fracture-wiring
        button
    coronary artery button
    Davy surgical button

button (*continued*)
    DiaTAP vascular access button
    Drummond button
    Emesay suture button
    Endo button
    fixation button
    gastrostomy button
    Graether collar button
    Groningen button
    Helsper laryngectomy button
    Husen button
    implant button
    Jaboulay button
    Kazanjian button
    Kazanjian tooth button
    Kistner button
    Kistner tracheal button
    Lardennois button
    Lee lingual button
    ligament button
    lingual button
    Microvaise One Step Button
    Moore button
    Moore tracheostomy buttons
    Murphy button
    Murphy-Johnson anastomosis
        button
    myringotomy with insertion
        of polyethylene collar
        buttons
    Norris button
    oriental button
    Panje voice button
    patellar button
    peritoneal button
    Perspex button
    polyethylene collar button
    polypropylene button
    pull-out button
    Reuter bobbin collar button
    Reuter button
    Sheehy button
    Sheehy collar button
    Silastic suture button
    silicone button
    Smithwick buttonhook button
    Spitzy button
    stoma button
    Surgitek button
    suture button
    Teflon button
    Teflon collar button

button (*continued*)
    Todd bur hole button
    Todd button
    tracheal button
    tracheostomy button
    Villard button
    voice button
button (*see also* collar button,
    buttonhook)
button abscess
button cautery
button drainage
button electrode
button farcy
Button gastrostomy device
button hook
button infuser
button knife
button lip lens manipulator
button one-step gastrostomy
Button One-Step gastrostomy
    device
button spacer
button suture technique
button sutures
button technique
buttoned device
button-end knife
buttonhole
buttonhole approach
buttonhole deformity
buttonhole fracture
buttonhole incision
buttonhole iridectomy
buttonhole mitral stenosis
buttonhole opening
buttonhole operation
buttonhole puncture technique
    for hemodialysis needle
    insertion
buttonhole skin incision
buttonhole suture technique
buttonholing of skin
buttonhook
    Graether buttonhook
    Graether collar buttonhook
    Smithwick buttonhook
    Smithwick silk buttonhook
buttonhook (*see also* hook)
buttonhook nerve retractor
buttonhook retractor
button-nosed knife

Button-One Step gastrostomy
    device
button-tip manipulator
buttress
    fragmatic buttress
    maxillary buttress
    nasomaxillary buttress
    Omni pretibial buttress
    pterygomaxillary buttress
    Teflon pledget suture buttress
    zygomatic buttress
    zygomaticomaxillary buttress
buttress grafts
buttress pad
buttress plate
buttress thread screw
buttressed hook
buttressing
buttress-type plate
butyl cyanoacrylate glue
butyl methacrylate
Butyn anesthetic agent
Buxton bolus suture technique
Buxton clamp
Buxton uterine clamp
Buyes air-vent suction tube
Buzard-Thornton fixation ring
Buzzard maneuver
Buzzi operation
BV-2 needle
BVAD (biventricular assist
    device)
BVS pump
B-W graft
Bx Velocity coronary artery
    stent
Bx Velocity sirolimus-coated
    stent
by
    precipitated by
by mouth (per os, p.o., po, PO)
Byars mandibular prosthesis
Bycep biopsy forceps
Bycep PC Jr bioptome
Bycroft-Brunswick thyroid
    retractor
Byers flap
Byers prosthesis
Byers repair
Byford retractor
bypasss
    cross femoral-femoral bypasss

bypass (*continued*)
  Alden loop gastric bypass
  aorta to first obtuse marginal
    branch bypass
  aorta to marginal branch
    bypass
  aorta to posterior descending
    coronary artery bypass
  aortic-femoral bypass
  aorticocoronary bypass
  aortobifemoral bypass
  aortobi-iliac bypass
  aortocarotid bypass
  aortocoronary bypass
  aortocoronary vein bypass
  aortocoronary-saphenous vein
    bypass
  aortofemoral bypass
  aortoiliac bypass
  aortoiliofemoral bypass
  aortorenal bypass
  aorto-subclavian-carotid-
    axilloaxillary bypass
  Aria coronary bypass
  atrial-femoral artery bypass
  autogenous vein bypass
  axillary bypass
  axilloaxillary bypass
  axillobifemoral bypass
  axillofemoral bypass
  axillounifemoral bypass
  axilobifemoral bypass
  biliary enteric bypass
  biliointestinal bypass (BIB)
  biliopancreatic bypass
    (BPB)
  bowel bypass
  brachial bypass
  cardiac bypass (CBP)
  cardiopulmonary bypass
    (CPB)
  carotid artery bypass
  carotid-axillary bypass
  carotid-carotid bypass
  carotid-subclavian artery
    bypass
  carotid-subclavian bypass
  cervical-to-MCA bypass
  CFA-SFA bypass
  coronary artery bypass
    (CAB)
  coronary bypass

bypass (*continued*)
  crossover bypass
  DTAF-F bypass (descending
    thoracic aortofemoral-
    femoral bypass)
  duodenoileal bypass (DIB)
  ECIC bypass (extracranial-
    intracranial bypass)
  endovascular
    cardiopulmonary bypass
  end-to-end jejunoileal bypass
  end-to-side jejunoileal bypass
  end-to-side vein bypass
  exclusion bypass
  EXS femoropopliteal bypass
  extra-anatomic bypass
  extracorporeal bypass
  extracorporeal venous bypass
  extracranial-intracranial
    bypass
  extracranial-intracranial
    bypass (ECIC bypass)
  fem-fem bypass (femoral-
    femoral bypass)
  femoral bypass
  femoral crossover bypass
  femoral vein-femoral artery
    bypass
  femoral-femoral bypass
    (fem-fem bypass)
  femoral-popliteal artery
    bypass
  femoral-popliteal bypass
    (fem-pop bypass)
  femoral-tibial bypass (fem-tib
    bypass)
  femoral-tibial-peroneal bypass
  femoroaxillary bypass
  femorodistal bypass
  femorofemoral bypass
  femorofemoral crossover
    bypass
  femoropopliteal bypass
  femoropopliteal saphenous
    vein bypass
  femorotibial bypass
  fem-pop bypass (femoral-
    popliteal bypass)
  fem-tib bypass (femoral-tibial
    bypass)
  fibrillator subclavian-
    subclavian bypass

bypass (*continued*)
  gastric bypass
  gastric bypass (GBP)
  gastric loop bypass
  gastric loop-type bypass
  Greenville gastric bypass
  Gregory instruments for in
    situ saphenous vein bypass
  Griffen Roux-en-Y bypass
  Hallberg biliointestinal bypass
  hand-assisted laparoscopic
    gastric bypass
  heart bypass
  heart-lung bypass
  hepatorenal bypass
  ileojejunal bypass
  iliopopliteal bypass
  in situ bypass
  infracubital bypass
  infrainguinal bypass
  infrapopliteal bypass
  internal mammary artery
    bypass (IMAB)
  intestinal bypass
  ipsilateral nonreversed
    greater saphenous vein
    bypass
  jejunal bypass
  jejunoileal bypass (JIB)
  laparoscopic gastric bypass
  left atrium to distal arterial
    aortic bypass
  left atrium-to-femoral artery
    circulatory bypass
  left heart bypass
  Litwak aortic bypass
  Litwak left atrial-aortic
    bypass
  long limb gastric bypass
  long-limb gastric artery
    bypass
  loop gastric bypass
  lower extremity bypass
  lymphaticovenous bypass
  minimally invasive direct
    coronary artery bypass
    (MIDCAB)
  natural bypass
  nonanatomic renal bypass
  obturator bypass
  off-pump coronary artery
    bypass

bypass (*continued*)
  off-pump coronary artery
    bypass (OPCAB)
  operative biliary bypass
  palliative bypass
  pancreatic bypass
  pancreatoduodenectomy
    bypass
  partial bypass
  partial ileal bypass
  Payne-DeWind jejunoileal
    bypass
  percutaneous femoral-femoral
    cardiopulmonary bypass
  percutaneous subclavian-
    subclavian bypass
  peripheral artery bypass
  petrous-to-supraclinoid bypass
  popliteal bypass
  primary antecubital jump
    bypass (PAJB)
  pulmonary bypass
  pulsatile cardiopulmonary
    bypass
  renal artery-reverse
    saphenous vein bypass
  reversed bypass
  right heart bypass
  Roux-en-Y biliary bypass
  Roux-en-Y gastric bypass
  saphenous ICA bypass
  saphenous vein bypass
  Scopinaro pancreaticobiliary
    bypass
  Scopinary pancreaticobiliary
    bypass
  Scott jejunoileal bypass
  side-to-vein bypass
  Silastic ring vertical-banded
    gastric bypass (SRVGB)
  simple bypass
  subclavian-carotid bypass
  subclavian-subclavian bypass
  superficial temporal artery-to-
    MCA bypass
  temporary aortic shunt
    subclavian-subclavian
    bypass
  total cardiopulmonary bypass
  transected vertical gastric
    bypass
  venovenous bypass

bypass (*continued*)
  venovenous bypass (VVB)
  venovenous extracorporeal
    bypass
  vertical gastric bypass
  weaned off bypass
bypass anesthesia
bypass blockage
bypass failure
bypass graft
bypass graft catheter
bypass graft catheterization
bypass machine
bypass occluded segment
bypass operation
bypass procedure
bypass prosthesis
bypass Speedy balloon catheter
bypass surgery
bypass technique
bypass tract
bypass tube

bypass vein graft
bypassable
BYR-300 imaging and
    illumination platform
Byrd EndoPlastic retractor
Byrel pacemaker
Byrel SX pacemaker
Byrel SX/Versatrax pacemaker
Byrne expulsive hemorrhage
    lens
Byrom Smith operation
Byron intraocular implant lens
Byron lens
Byron Smith correction of
    ectropion
Byron Smith ectropion
    operation
Byron Smith lazy-T correction
Byron Smith lazy-T procedure
Byron Smith operation
Bywaters lesion
Byzantine arch palate

C sliding osteotomy
C&S (culture and sensitivity)
C. L. Jackson head-holding
    forceps
C. Ti. brace
C.L. Jackson head-holding
    forceps
C.R. Bard catheter
C.R. Bard Urolase fiber
C-2 OsteoCap hip prosthesis
CA (carcinoma)
CA (cervicoaxial)
CA membrane hollow-fiber
    dialyzer
CA monitor (cardiac-apnea
    monitor)
CA-5000 drill-guide isometer
caseous inflammation
CAB (coronary artery bypass)
CABG (coronary artery bypass
    graft)
CABG'd (slang for coronary
    artery bypass grafted)
cabinet respirator
cable
    alligator cable
    alligator pacing cable
    Bicomatic bipolar cable
    braided Spectra UHMWPE
        surgical cable
    braided titanium cable
    cautery cable
    chrome-cobalt cable
    coaxial cable
    control cable
    Dall-Miles cable
    Dwyer cable
    ESI Lite-Pipe fiberoptic cable
    European/German bipolar
        cable
    fiberoptic cable
    fiberoptic light cable
    fiberoptic Lite-Piper cable

cable (*continued*)
    FlexStrand cable
    Gallie fusion-using cable
    internal fiberoptic cable
    interspinous cable
    Oklahoma City cable
    Old Martin bipolar cable
    OxyLead interconnect cable
    resectoscope cable
    SecureStrand cable
    Songer cable
    Storz cable
    Storz fiberoptic light cable
    Storz resectoscope cable
    Sullivan variable stiffness
        cable
    titanium cable
    world standard Olsen bipolar
        cable
cable graft
cable tie
cable twister orthosis
cable wire suture technique
cable wire sutures
cable-operated hand
        prosthesis
Cabot cannula
Cabot leg splint
Cabot Medical Corporation
        diagnostic laparoscope
Cabot Medical Corporation
        operating laparoscope
Cabot ring body
Cabot splint
Cabot trocar
Cabral coronary
        reconstruction
CABS (coronary artery bypass
        surgery)
cachecticorum
    acne cachecticorum
cachexia
    cancer cachexia

cacogenesis
cacomelia
cacomorphosis
CAD (computerized assisted
   design; coronary artery
   disease)
CAD hip prosthesis
CAD prosthesis
CAD reamer
CAD/CAM (computer-assisted
   design/computer-assisted
   manufacturing)
cadaver
   donor cadaver
   homograft cadaver
cadaver donor (CAD)
cadaver-derived fascia lata
cadaveric donor
cadaveric donor hepatectomy
cadaveric donor transplantation
cadaveric graft
cadaveric hand transplant
cadaveric homograft
cadaveric knee
cadaveric organ
cadaveric organ donation
cadaveric reaction
cadaveric transplant
cadaveric whole organ
   transplant
CADD-Plus intravenous infusion
   pump
CADD-TPN pump
Cadence defibrillator
Cadence TVL nonthoracotomy
   lead
Cadet defibrillator
Cadlow shoulder stabilizer
cadmium iodide detector
cadmium selenide Vidicon video
   camera
Cadwell 5200A somatosensory
   evoked potential unit
   device
Caffey disease
Caffey syndrome
Caffey-Silverman disease
Caffiniere prosthesis
cage catheter device
cage-back brace
caged-ball heart valve
caged-ball valve prosthesis

caged-disk heart valve
Cagot ear
CAHD (coronary arteriosclerotic/
   atherosclerotic heart
   disease)
Cairns clamp
Cairns forceps
Cairns maneuver
Cairns operation
Cairns retractor
Cairns rongeur
Cairns-Dandy hemostasis
   forceps
Cajal axonal retraction ball
caked breast
caked kidney
Cal-20 central dialysate
   preparation unit
Calamary cast boot
Calamary cast shoe
calamus scriptorius
Calandriello open hip reduction
Calandriello procedure
Calandruccio clamp
Calandruccio compression
   device
Calandruccio external fixator
Calandruccio frame
Calandruccio nail
calcaneal apophysis occult
   compression injury
calcaneal avulsion fracture
calcaneal bone
calcaneal bursa
calcaneal facet
calcaneal fracture reduction
calcaneal gait
calcaneal inclination angle
calcaneal region
calcaneal spur
calcaneal spur cookie orthosis
calcaneal stance position
calcaneal sulcus
calcaneal tendon
calcaneal tuberosity
calcaneal-2nd metatarsal angle
   inclination angle
calcaneoapophysitis
calcaneoastragaloid
calcaneocavovarus deformity
calcaneocavus deformity
calcaneocuboid articulation

calcaneodynia
calcaneofibular ligament
calcaneonavicular bar
calcaneonavicular ligament
calcaneoplantar
calcaneotibial
calcaneovalgocavus
calcaneovalgus
   talipes calcaneovalgus
calcaneovalgus deformity
calcaneovarus
   talipes calcaneovarus
calcaneovarus deformity
calcaneus
   Boehler angle of calcaneus
   talipes calcaneus
   tendon calcaneus
calcar
calcar avis
calcar femorale
calcar pedis
calcar reamer
calcar replacement femoral
   prosthesis
calcareous cataract
calcareous deposit
calcareous infiltration
calcareous metastasis
calcareous pancreatitis
calcarine fissure
calcarine sulcus
Calcibon synthetic bone
calciferous canals
calcific change
calcific degeneration
calcific density
calcific deposit
calcific metamorphosis
calcific shadow
calcific tendinitis
calcification
   amorphous calcification
   capsular calcification
   cerebral calcification
   curvilinear calcification
   diffuse calcification
   dystopic calcification
   dystrophic calcification
   eggshell calcification
   intracranial calcification
   irregular calcification
   ligamentous calcification

calcification (*continued*)
   mottled calcification
   periarticular calcification
   pineal calcification
   soft tissue calcification
   spiculated calcification
   subcutaneous calcification
   submitral calcification
   subperiosteal calcification
   tooth-like calcification
   tracheal calcification
calcification line
calcification of breast implant
calcification zone
calcified cartilage
calcified cephalhematoma
calcified density
calcified focus
calcified free body
calcified gallbladder
calcified granulomatous
   inflammation
calcified lesion
calcified liver metastasis
calcified lymph node
calcified mass
calcified node
calcified nodule
calcified organ
calcified tissue
calcified tissue scissors
calciform papilla
calcifying cyst
calcifying epithelioma of
   Malherbe
calcifying metastasis
calcinosis
calcinosis circumscripta
calciotraumatic line
calcipenia
calciphylaxis
Calcipulpe cavity liner
Calcitek drill
Calcitek implant
Calcitek retaining screw
Calcitek spline
Calcitite alloplastic bone
   replacement material
Calcitite bone graft
Calcitite hydroxyapatite
calcitonin
calcium alginate applicator

calcium alginate gel
calcium bilirubinate stone
calcium chloride
calcium concretion
calcium phosphate ceramic
    implant
calcium pump
calcium pyrophosphate
    deposition disease
calcium sodium alginate wound
    dressing
calciuria
calcospherite mineralization
Calculair spirometer
calculated date of confinement
calculated dose
calculation
    computer dose calculation
    dose calculation
calculi (*sing.* calculus)
    lucent calculi
    renal calculi
calculus formation
calculous gallbladder
calculus (*pl.* calculi)
    alvine calculus
    apatite calculus
    bile duct calculus
    biliary calculus
    bladder calculus
    blood calculus
    branched calculus
    caliceal diverticular calculus
    cat's eye calculus
    cerebral calculus
    cholesterol calculus
    combination calculus
    common duct calculus
    coral calculus
    crushing of calculus
    cystine calculus
    decubitus calculus
    dendritic calculus
    ductal calculus
    encysted calculus
    extraction of calculus
    fibrin calculus
    gallbladder calculus
    gastric calculus
    hard calculus
    hemic calculus
    hepatic calculus

calculus (*continued*)
    hepatic duct calculus
    impacted calculus
    incision and removal of
        calculus
    infection calculus
    intestinal calculus
    lacrimal calculus
    lung calculus
    mammary calculus
    matrix calculus
    metabolic calculus
    mulberry calculus
    nasal calculus
    nephritic calculus
    opaque calculus
    ovarian calculus
    oxalate calculus
    pancreatic calculus
    pharyngeal calculus
    pleural calculus
    pocketed calculus
    preputial calculus
    primary renal calculus
    prostatic calculus
    radiolucent calculus
    removal of calculus
    renal calculus
    salivary calculus
    secondary renal calculus
    spermatic calculus
    staghorn calculus
    stomach calculus
    struvite calculus
    tonsillar calculus
    urethral calculus
    urinary calculus
    vesical calculus
    vesicoprostatic calculus
    weddellite calculus
    whewellite calculus
calculus extraction
calculus migration
Calcusplit pneumatic
    lithotriptor
Calcutript electrohydraulic
    lithotriptor
Calcutript lithotripter
Caldani ligament
Caldwell cannula
Caldwell guide
Caldwell hanging cast

Caldwell needle
Caldwell operation
Caldwell projection
Caldwell x-ray view
Caldwell-Coleman flatfoot
　technique
Caldwell-Coleman technique
Caldwell-Durham procedure
Caldwell-Luc maxillary
　antrostomy
Caldwell-Luc operation
Caldwell-Luc window operation
Caldwell-Moloy classification
calf (*pl.* calves)
calf augmentation
calf compression unit
calf reduction
Calgiswab dressing
Calhoun needle
Calhoun-Hagler lens extraction
　operation
Calhoun-Hagler lens needle
Calhoun-Merz needle
caliber
　small caliber
calibrated clubfoot splint
calibrated depth gauge
calibrated grasping tube
calibrated guide pin
calibrated pin
calibrated position
calibrated probe
calibrated triangle of septal
　cartilage
calibrated V-Lok cuff
calibrated-tip threaded guide pin
calibration
calibration gauge
calibration tonometer
calibration well
calibrator
　Fogarty calibrator
　isotope calibrator
　screw depth calibrator
Calibri forceps
caliceal abnormality
caliceal cups
caliceal cyst
caliceal dilatation
caliceal diverticulum
caliceal extension
caliceal fistula

caliceal pattern
caliceal stone
calicectasis
calicectomy
calices (*sing.* calix)
caliculus ophthalmicus
caliectasis
caliectomy
Caligamed ankle orthosis
Caligamed brace
calipers
　Accu-Measure skinfold
　　calipers
　Albee bone graft calipers
　Austin Moore inside-outside
　　calipers
　Austin Moore outside calipers
　Austin strut calipers
　Barker calipers
　Berens marking calipers
　Bertillon calipers
　bone calipers
　Braunstein fixed calipers
　breast calipers
　Brown and Sharp digital
　　electronic calipers
　Burch calipers
　Castroviejo calipers
　Castroviejo-Schacher angled
　　calipers
　Cone ice-tong calipers
　Cottle calipers
　digital calipers
　EKG calipers
　electric calipers
　eye calipers
　Fat-O-Meter skinfold calipers
　FatTrack Digital body fat
　　calipers
　FatTrack skinfold calipers
　Green eye calipers
　Harpenden skinfold calipers
　House strut calipers
　ice-tong calipers
　Jameson calipers
　Jameson eye calipers
　John Green calipers
　Kapp Surgical Instrument
　　total hip calipers
　Ladd calipers
　Lafayette skinfold calipers
　Lang/Jamar skinfold calipers

calipers (*continued*)
Lange skin-fold calipers
Machemer calipers
McGaw skinfold calipers
Mendez degree calipers
middle ear calipers
Mipron digital computer calipers
Mitutoyo Digimatic calipers
ophthalmic calipers
Osher internal calipers
Paparella rasp calipers
Ruddy stapes calipers
ruler calipers
Sentalloy digital calipers
skinfold calipers
Storz calipers
Stahl calipers
strut calipers
Tenzel calipers
Tesa S.A. hand-held electronic digital calipers
Thomas calipers
Thorpe calipers
Thorpe-Castroviejo calipers
tibial calipers
tonsillar calipers
Townley femur calipers
Townley inside-outside femur calipers
V. Mueller ruler calipers
Vernier calipers
walking calipers
x-ray calipers
calipers block
calipers strut
Cali-Press graft press
calix (*pl.* calices)
effacement of calix
superior pole of calix
calix tube
Callaghan sutures
Callahan approach
Callahan extension of cervical injury
Callahan fixation forceps
Callahan flange
Callahan forceps
Callahan fusion technique
Callahan lacrimal rongeur
Callahan lens loupe
Callahan modification speculum

Callahan operation
Callahan retractor
Callahan rongeur
Callahan scleral fixation forceps
Callahan zonule lens stripper
Callander amputation
Callaway formula
Callender brace
Callender cell-type classification
Callender clip
Callender derotational brace
Callender technique hip prosthesis
Callia abdominoplasty
Callia floating umbilicus procedure
Callisen operation
Callison-Adson tissue forceps
callosal disconnection syndrome
callosi
corporis callosi
genu corporis callosi
callosomarginal artery
callus
bone callus
central callus
definitive callus
ensheathing callus
fracture callus
inner callus
intermediate callus
internal callus
medullary callus
myelogenous callus
permanent callus
temporary callus
callus distraction
callus formation
calcaneal bursa
CALM (café au lait macule)
Calman carotid clamp
Calman ring clamp
Calnan-Nicolle synthetic joint prosthesis
calomel electrode
caloric irrigation
caloric nystagmus
caloric requirements for burn patients
calorie-to-nitrogen ratio
calorigenic action
Calot jacket

Calot node
Calot operation
Calot triangle
Caltagirone chisel
Caltagirone knife
Caltagirone skin graft knife
Caluso PEG (percutaneous
    endoscopic gastrostomy
    tube)
calvarectomy
calvaria (*pl.* calvariae)
calvarial bone
calvarial clamp
calvarial defect
calvarial deformity
calvarial hook
calvarial lesion
calvarial repair
calvarium
calvarium clamp
calvarium flap
clavate papilla
Calve cannula
calvities
calyceal (*see* caliceal)
calycectasis (*see* calicectasis)
calycectomy (*see* calicectomy)
calyces renales majores
calyces renales minores
Calypso Rely catheter
calyx (*pl.* calyces) (*see* calix)
CAM (cell adhesion molecule)
CAM (controlled ankle
    motion)
CAM Lock knee joint
CAM procedure (Coblation-
    Assisted Microdisc)
CAM stimulator
CAM tent
CAM Walker boot
CAM Walker walking brace
Camber axis hinge
cambium
Cambridge classification
Cambridge defibrillator
Cambridge electrocardiograph
Cambridge jelly electrode
Cameco syringe pistol aspiration
    device
Camel tube
camelback sign
Camel-Lindbergh pump

camera
  3-head camera
  4-head camera
  Anger camera
  anterior bulbi camera
  binocular camera
  cardiac camera
  cataract camera
  cine camera
  chip camera
  closed-circuit camera
  digital camera
  endoscopic camera
  field-of-view camera
  fundus camera
  fundus-retinal camera
  gamma camera
  gamma scintillation camera
  gantry-free gamma camera
  hand camera
  hand-held fundus camera
  high-resolution digital camera
  immersible video camera
  instant camera
  intraoral camera
  microprocessor-controlled
    camera
  miniature camera
  mirror reflex lens camera
  monochromic camera
  multicrystal gamma camera
  multiwire camera
  ophthalmoscope camera
  photon emission camera
  pinhole camera
  positron scintillation camera
  radiosotope camera
  reflex camera
  retinal camera
  retroillumination camera
  rotating gamma camera
  scintillation camera
  single-crystal gamma camera
  single-headed camera
  single-head rotating gamma
    camera
  slip-ring camera
  spinal camera
  variable angle gamma camera
  video camera
  video display camera
  zoom lens camera

camera attachment
camera equipment
cameral fistula
Cameron cautery
Cameron electrosurgical unit
Cameron elevator
Cameron femoral component
    removal
Cameron fracture appliance
Cameron fracture device
Cameron gastroscope
Cameron lesion
Cameron omni-angle
    gastroscope
Cameron ulcer
Cameron-Haight elevator
Cameron-Lorenz cautery
Cameron-Miller
    electrocoagulation unit
Cameron-Miller electrode
Cameron-Miller type monopolar
    forceps
Camey enterocystoplasty
Camey enterocystoplasty
    urinary diversion
Camey I operation
Camey II operation
Camey ileocystoplasty
Camey procedure
Camey reservoir
cam-guided trephine
Camille Bernard lip repair
Camino catheter
Camino fiberoptic monitor
Camino intracranial catheter
Camino intracranial pressure
    monitoring device
Camino intraparenchymal
    fiberoptic device
Camino micromanometer
    catheter
Camino microventricular bolt
Camino microventricular bolt
    catheter
Camino OLM intracranial
    pressure monitoring kit
Camino postcraniotomy
    subdural pressure
    monitoring kit
Camino subdural screw
Camino transducer catheter
Camino ventricular bolt

Camitz opponensplasty
Camitz technique
Cammann stethoscope
Camo disposable dental splint
camouflage
    cosmetic camouflage
    long-term tip graft camouflage
camouflage augmentation
camouflage make-up
camouflage prosthesis
Camp brace
Camp collar
Camp corset
Camp grid cassette
Campbell applicator
Campbell approach
Campbell arthrodesis
Campbell bone block
Campbell catheter
Campbell De Morgan spots
Campbell elevator
Campbell forceps
Campbell gouge
Campbell graft
Campbell interpositional
    arthroplasty
Campbell lacrimal sac retractor
Campbell ligament
Campbell ligature-carrier
    forceps
Campbell miniature sound
Campbell needle
Campbell bone graft
Campbell operation
Campbell osteotome
Campbell refractor
Campbell resection
    arthroplasty
Campbell rest strap
Campbell retractor
Campbell rongeur
Campbell slit lamp
Campbell sound
Campbell splint
Campbell technique
Campbell trocar
Campbell-Boyd tourniquet
Campbell-French sound
Campbell-Goldthwait patella
    dislocation operation
Campbell-Molesworth-Campbell
    approach

Campbell-type Heyman fundus
applicator
Campbell-Young incontinence
repair
Camp-Coventry position
Camper angle
Camper chiasm
Camper fascia
Camper line
Camper plane
Camp-Lewin collar
Campodonico operation
campotomy
Camp-Sigraris stockings
camptocormia
camptodactylia
camptodactylism
camptodactyly
camptomelia
camptomelic syndrome
camptospasm
Campylobacter-like organism
biopsy
campylodactyly
campylognathia
Canad meniscal knife
Canadian Cardiovascular Society
classification
Canadian chest retractor
Canadian crutches
Canadian hip disarticulation
prosthesis
Canadian knee orthosis
Canakis beaded hip pin
canal
abdominal canal
accessory palatine canal
adductor canal
Alcock canal
alimentary canal
alisphenoid canal
alveolar canal
alveolodental canals
anal canal
anterior ethmoid canal
anterior retinal orbital canal
anterior vertical canal
Arnold canal
artery of pterygoid canal
atrioventricular canal
auditory canal
basipharyngeal canal

canal (*continued*)
birth canal
Breschet canal
calciferous canals
carotid canal
carpal canal
cartilage canal
central canal
cervical canal
ciliary canals
Cloquet canal
cochlear canal
common canal
condylar canal
Corit canal
craniopharyngeal canal
crural canal
dehiscence of mandibular
canal
dehiscent mandibular canal
diploic canals
Dorello canal
ear canal
endocervical canal
ethmoid canal
eustachian canal
external auditory canal (EAC)
external canal
external ear canal
facial canal
fallopian canal
femoral canal
fenestration of semicircular
canal
Ferrein canal
fibro-osseous flexor tendon
canal
filling of pulp canal
flexor canal
galactophorous canals
geniculum of facial canal
genu of facial canal
greater palatine canal
Guidi canal
Guyon canal
Hannover canal
haversian canal
Hering canal
hernial canal
hiatus of facial canal
hiatus of fallopian canal
His canal

canal (*continued*)
  horizontal canal
  Hovius canal
  Hunter canal
  Huschke canal
  hyaloid canal
  hypoglossal canal
  incisive canal
  infraorbital canal
  inguinal canal
  interfacial canals
  internal auditory canal
  intramedullary canal
  irruption canal
  Kürsteiner canals
  lacrimal canal
  lateral canal
  lesser palatine canal
  mandibular canal
  mandibular neurovascular
    canal
  maxillary canal
  medullary canal
  membranous canal
  mental canal
  mesiobuccal canal
  nasal canal
  nasolacrimal canal
  nasopalatine canal
  nerve of pterygoid canal
  neural canal
  Nuck canal
  optic canal
  orbital canal
  palatine canal
  palatomaxillary canal
  palatovaginal canal
  pelvic canal
  Petit canal
  pharyngeal canal
  pleuroperitoneal canal
  posterior internal orbital
    canal
  pterygoid canal
  pterygopalatine canal
  pudendal canal
  pulp canal
  rectal canal
  recurrent canal
  Reissner canal
  Rivinus canals
  root canal

canal (*continued*)
  ruffed canal
  sacral canal
  Santorini canal
  Schlemm canal
  scleral canal
  scleroticochoroidal canal
  semicircular canals
  serous canal
  Sondermann canal
  sphenopalatine canal
  sphenopharyngeal canal
  spinal canal
  spurious aperture of facial
    canal
  Stensen canal
  Sucquet canals
  Sucquet-Hoyer canals
  supraciliary canal
  supraoptic canal
  supraorbital canal
  tarsal canal
  temporal canal
  tortuous root canal
  Tourtual canal
  uterine canal
  vertebral canal
  vestibular canal
  vidian canal
  Volkmann canal
  vomerine canal
  vomerobasilar canal
  vomerorostral canal
  vomerovaginal canal
  Walther canal
  zygomaticofacial canal
  zygomaticotemporal canal
canal chisel
canal curvature
canal irrigation
canal knife
Canal Master drill
canal of Cloquet
canal of Corti
canal of Guidi
canal of Nuck
canal of Petit
canal of Schlemm
canal rays
canal reamer
canal wall-down mastoidectomy
canal wall-up mastoidectomy

canal wall-up technique
Canale technique
canalicular
canalicular abscess
canalicular adenoma
canalicular duct
canalicular laceration
canalicular scissors
canaliculi (*sing.* canaliculus)
canaliculitis
canaliculodacryocystostomy
canaliculodacryorhinostomy
canaliculoplasty
canaliculorhinostomy
canaliculus (*pl.* canaliculi)
   bile canaliculi
   Bowman slitting of
     canaliculus
   intercellular canaliculus
   lacrimal canaliculus
   mastoid canaliculi
   secretory canaliculus
canaliculus chordae tympani
canaliculus cochleae
canaliculus dilator
canaliculus innominatus
canaliculus knife
canaliculus lacrimalis
canaliculus mastoideus
canaliculus of chorda tympani
canaliculus of cochlea
canaliculus probe
canaliculus punch
canaliculus tympanicus
canaliculus vein
canalis
canalis adductorius
canalith repositioning
   procedure
canalization
canaloplasty
canals and drums
canals for lesser palatine nerves
canals of cartilage
canals of Recklinghausen
canals of Scarpa
Canals-N root canal filling
   material
Can-Am brace
Cancell therapy
cancellated bone
cancelli (*sing.* cancellus)

cancellous and cortical bone
   graft
cancellous bone
cancellous cellular bone
cancellous formation
cancellous freeze-dried allograft
cancellous graft
cancellous insert graft
cancellous pin
cancellous screw
cancellous tissue
cancellus (*pl.* cancelli)
cancer
   acinar cancer
   acinous cancer
   adenoid cancer
   American Joint Committee on
     Cancer (AJCC) staging
   ampullary cancer
   appendiceal cancer
   asynchronous bilateral breast
     cancer
   biliary tract cancer
   black cancer
   black mole cancer
   boring cancer
   breast cancer
   cervical cancer
   claypipe cancer
   clinically node-negative breast
     cancer
   colloid cancer
   colon cancer
   colorectal cancer
   cystic cancer
   dermoid cancer
   digestive glandular cancer
   duct cancer
   ductal cancer
   early gastric cancer
   endobronchial cancer
   endometrial cancer
   endothelial cancer
   epidermal cancer
   epidermoid cancer
   epiesophageal cancer
   epithelial cancer
   esophageal cancer
   esophagogastric cancer
   European Organization for
     Research and Treatment of
     Cancer (EORTC)

cancer (*continued*)
  extrahepatic bile duct cancer
  extrathoracic spread of
    cancer
  familial breast cancer
  familial colon cancer (FCC)
  gallbladder cancer
  gastric cancer
  genitourinary cancer
  glandular cancer
  Gleason staging of prostate
    cancer
  Haagensen staging of breast
    cancer (A, B, etc.)
  hard cancer
  hard palate cancer
  hematogenous spread of
    cancer
  hepatocellular cancer
  hereditary breast cancer
  hereditary nonpolyposis
    colon cancer (HNPCC)
  high-risk papillary cancer
  inoperable cancer
  intraductal cancer
  intraoral cancer
  invasive breast cancer
  invasive ductal cancer
  islet cell cancer
  laryngeal cancer
  latent cancer
  life-threatening cancer
  localized cancer
  localized prostate cancer
  low rectal cancer
  low-risk papillary cancer
  lung cancer
  Markel cell cancer
  melanotic cancer
  metastatic cancer
  metastatic colorectal cancer
  mule spinners cancer
  nasal cavity cancer
  neuroendocrine cancer
  node-positive breast cancer
  nonpalpable invasive breast
    cancer
  obstructing colorectal
    cancer
  obstructive esophagogastric
    cancer
  occult cancer

cancer (*continued*)
  operable cancer
  oral cancer
  oral cavity cancer
  ovarian cancer
  pancreas cancer
  pancreatic head cancer
  papillary cancer
  penile cancer
  perforated cancer
  periampullary cancer
  peritoneal cancer
  pitch workers cancer
  postgastrectomy cancer
  primary cancer
  prostate cancer
  prostatic cancer
  proximal gastric cancer
  QUART procedure for breast
    cancer
  rectal cancer
  rectum cancer
  resectable periampullary
    cancer
  Robson staging of renal
    cancer (I-IV)
  scirrhous cancer
  skin cancer
  smokers' cancer
  soft-palate cancer
  spindle cell cancer
  stomach cancer
  suture line cancer
  synchronous bilateral breast
    cancer
  systemic cancer
  tar cancer
  telangiectatic cancer
  terminal cancer
  testicular cancer
  thyroid cancer
  tubular cancer
  Union Internationale Contre
    Le Cancer (UICC)
  unresectable periampullary
    cancer
  urologic system cancer
  villous duct cancer
  virulent cancer
  Whitmore-Jewett classification
    for staging of prostate
    cancer

cancer (*continued*)
  W-J classification for staging
    of prostate cancer
  young onset cancer
cancer body
cancer cachexia
cancer cell collector
cancer genetics
Cancer Genetics Network
cancer in situ
cancer invasion
cancer juice
cancer lesion
cancer pain
cancer status
Cancer Surveillance Program
cancer susceptibility syndrome
cancerous
cancerous growth
cancerous mass
cancerous region
cancerous tissue
cancra (*sing.* cancrum)
cancriform
cancrum (*pl.* cancra)
cancrum nasi
cancrum oris
candy cane cannula style II
Candela laser
Candela laser lithotriptor
Candela lithotripsy
Candela miniscope
Candela pulsed dye laser
candidal
candidal angular cheilitis
candidal infection
candidiasis
  acute atrophic oral candidiasis
  chronic hyperplastic candidiasis
  cutaneous candidiasis
  esophageal candidiasis
  localized mucocutaneous
    candidiasis
  mucocutaneous candidiasis
  oral candidiasis
  oropharyngeal candidiasis
  vaginal candidiasis
candidiasis in facelift skin flap
candle
  cesium candle
  urethral candle
  vaginal candle

candle vaginal cesium implant
candy cane cannula
cane
  Double Duty cane
  Duke pistol-grip cane
  English cane
  tripod cane
Cane bone-holding forceps
Cane forceps
Canfield facial plastics garment
Canfield operation
Canfield tonsil knife
Canfield tonsillar knife
canine alveolus
canine eminence
canine fossa
canine muscle
canine prominence
canine smile
canine teeth
canine transmissible tumor
canine-to-canine lingual splint
canister
  Bemis suction canister
  Lipovacutainer canister
  Sorensen reusable canister
canker sore
Cann-Ease moisturizing nasal gel
Cannon Bio-Flek nasal splint
Cannon endarterectomy loop
Cannon point
Cannon ring
Cannon stripper
Cannon vein stripper
cannon waves
cannonball metastasis
cannonball pulse
Cannon-Rochester elevator
Cannon-Rochester lamina
    elevator
Cannon-type stripper
Cannu-Flex guidewire
cannula (*pl.* cannulas, cannulae)
  7277 Rubenstein LASIK
    cannula
  2-stage Sarns cannula
  2-way cataract-aspirating
    cannula
  3-hole aspiration cannula
  4-pronged liposuction cannula
  Abelson cricothyrotomy
    cannula

cannula (*continued*)
Abraham laryngeal cannula
Accu-Beam suction &
    irrigation cannula
Accu-Flo U-channel stripping
    cannula
Accu-Flo ventricular
    cannula
acorn cannula
Adson brain-exploring
    cannula
Adson drainage cannula
Adson exploring cannula
air cannula
air injection cannula
Airlife cannula
Air-Lon inhalation cannula
alpha-chymotrypsin cannula
angled cannula
angled left cannula
angled right cannula
Anis aspirating cannula
anterior chamber cannula
anterior chamber irrigating
    cannula
Antoni-Hook lumbar puncture
    cannula
antral cannula
antral sinus cannula
aortic arch cannula
aortic direct ellipse cannula
aortic perfusion cannula
Argyle CPAP nasal cannula
Aronson-Fletcher antrum
    cannula
arterial cannula
aspirating cannula
aspiration cannula
aspirator cannula
atrial cannula
attic cannula
back-and-forth vibrating
    cannulas
Bahnson aortic cannula
Bahnson cannula
Bailey cannula
Bailey lacrimal cannula
Banaji cannula
Bard arterial cannula
Bard cervical cannula
Bardic cannula
Barraquer cannula

cannula (*continued*)
Barrett hydrodelineation
    cannula
Bechert intraocular lens
    cannula
Becker accelerator cannula
Becker dissector cannula
Becker Greater dissecting
    cannula
Becker Greater Grater
    dissecting cannula
Bellocq cannula
Bellucci cannula
Bergström-Stille muscle
    cannula
Berkeley cannula
B-H irrigating cannula
Bilisystem ERCP cannula
binasal cannula
Binkhorst hooked cannula
Binkhorst irrigating cannula
biopsy cannula
BioTac biopsy cannula
Bishop-Harman anterior
    chamber cannula
Bishop-Harman anterior
    chamber irrigating cannula
Bishop-Harman irrigating
    cannula
bivalved cannula
Blue Max cannula
blunt bullet-tip cannula
blunt-tipped extraction
    cannula
Bowers cannula
Bracken anterior chamber
    cannula
Bracken irrigating cannula
brain biopsy cannula
brain cannula
brain-exploring cannula
Branula cannula
Bresgen cannula
Brodney urethrographic
    cannula
Brown sphenoid cannula
Bruening cannula
Bucy-Frazier coagulating-
    suction cannula
Bucy-Frazier coagulation
    cannula
Bucy-Frazier suction cannula

cannula (*continued*)
- Buie cannula
- bullet-shaped cannula
- Buratto irrigating cannula
- Cabot cannula
- Caldwell cannula
- Calve cannula
- Campbell suprapubic cannula
- candy cane cannula
- Cantlie cannula
- Carabelli mirror cannula
- cardiovascular cannula
- Casselberry sphenoid cannula
- Castaneda cannula
- Castroviejo cyclodialysis cannula
- cataract-aspirating cannula
- caval cannula
- CellFriendly cannula
- cerebral cannula
- cervical cannula
- Charlton cannula
- Chilcott venoclysis cannula
- Christmas-tree cannula
- Churchill cardiac suction cannula
- Cimochowski cardiac cannula
- Circon ACMI cannula
- Clagett cannula
- clysis cannula
- coagulating-suction cannula
- Coakley frontal sinus cannula
- coaxial cannula
- Cobe small vessel cannula
- Cobra cannula
- Cobra K cannula
- Cobra K+ cannula
- Cobra+ cannula
- Codman cannula
- Cohen intrauterine cannula
- Cohen tubal insufflation cannula
- Cohen uterine cannula
- Cohen-Eder cannula
- Cohen-Eder uterine cannula
- Coleman aspiration cannula
- Coleman V-dissector infiltration cannula
- Colt cannula
- Concept cannula
- Concorde disposable suction cannula

cannula (*continued*)
- Concorde suction cannula
- cone biopsy cannula
- Cone cerebral cannula
- Cone-Bucy cannula
- Continental cannula
- Contour ERCP cannula
- Cooper cannula
- Cooper chemopallidectomy cannula
- Cooper double-lumen cannula
- Cope needle introducer cannula
- Core Dynamics disposable cannula
- coronary artery cannula
- coronary perfusion cannula
- cortex-aspirating cannula
- cortical cleaving hydrodissector cannula
- Corydon hydroexpression cannula
- Cosmetech cannula
- cricothyrotomy cannula
- curved cannula
- curved cricothyrotomy cannula
- cyclodialysis cannula
- dacryocystorhinostomy cannula
- Day attic cannula
- De La Vega vitreous-aspirating cannula
- Delima ethmoid cannula
- DeRoyal cannula
- Devonshire-Mack cannula
- DeWecker syringe cannula
- Dexide disposable cannula
- Digiflex cannula
- DirectFlow arterial cannula
- disposable cystotome cannula
- DLP aortic root cannula
- Dohrmann-Rubin cannula
- Dorsey ventricular cannula
- double irrigating-aspirating cannula
- double-lumen cannula
- double-lumen irrigation cannula
- Dougherty anterior chamber cannula
- Douglas cannula

cannula (*continued*)
Dow Corning cannula
Drews irrigating cannula
Duke cannula
Dulaney antral cannula
duodenoscope cannula
Dupuis cannula
ear cannula
egress cannula
Eichen irrigating cannula
Elecath ECMO cannula
Elsberg brain-exploring
cannula
Elsberg ventricular cannula
Embol-X arterial cannula
EndoForehead cannula
endometrial cannula
Endo-Pool suction cannula
Endotrac cannula
Entree II cannula
Entree Plus cannula
ERCP cannula
Eriksson muscle biopsy
cannula
esophagoscopic cannula
Ethicon disposable cannula
Everett fallopian cannula
exploring cannula
extractor-injector cannula
eye and ear cannula
fallopian cannula
Fasanella lacrimal cannula
Fazio-Montgomery cannula
Feaster hydrodissecting
cannula
Fein cannula
Fem-Flex II femoral
cannulae
femoral artery cannula
femoral perfusion cannula
Fink cul-de-sac cannula
Fish infusion cannula
Fisher ventricular cannula
flap cannula
flap dissector cannula
flattened irrigating cannula
Fletcher-Pierce cannula
Flexicath silicone subclavian
cannula
Floyd loop cannula
Fluoro Tip ERCP cannula
flute cannula

cannula (*continued*)
Ford Hospital ventricular
cannula
Franklin-Silverman biopsy
cannula
Frazier brain-exploring
cannula
Frazier cannula
Frazier ventricular cannula
Freeman Blue-Max cannula
Freeman positioning cannula
frontal sinus cannula
Fujita suction cannula
Futch antral cannula
gallbladder cannula
Galt aspirating cannula
Gans cyclodialysis cannula
Gans eye cannula
Gass cataract-aspirating
cannula
Gass retinal detachment
cannula
Gass vitreous-aspirating
cannula
G-bevel cannula
Genitor mini-intrauterine
insemination cannula
Gesco cannula
Ghormley double cannula
Gill double I&A cannula
Gill double Luer-Lok
cannula
Gill sinus cannula
Gill-Welsh irrigating cannula
Gill-Welsh aspirating cannula
Gill-Welsh double cannula
Gill-Welsh olive-tip cannula
Gimbel fountain cannula
Girard irrigating cannula
Goddio disposable cannula
Goldstein anterior chamber
cannula
Goldstein anterior chamber-
irrigating cannula
Goldstein irrigating cannula
Goldstein lacrimal cannula
golf tee hollow titanium
cannula
golf tee UAL cannula
goniotomy knife cannula
Gonzalez specialized
dissecting cannula

cannula (*continued*)
- Goodfellow frontal sinus cannula
- Gott cannula
- Grafco cannula
- Gram cannula
- gravity infusion cannula
- Gregg cannula
- Grinfeld cannula
- Grizzard subretinal cannula
- Gromley-Russell cannula
- Gruentzig femoral stiffening cannula
- guiding cannula
- Gulani triple function LASIK cannula
- Gundry cannula
- Hahn cannula
- Hajek cannula
- Harvard cannula
- Hasson open-laparoscopy cannula
- Hasson stable access cannula
- Hasson-Eder laparoscope cannula
- Hasson-Eder laparoscopy cannula
- Hassoon balloon uterine elevator cannula
- Haverfield brain cannula
- Havlicek spiral cannula
- Haynes brain cannula
- Healon injection cannula
- Heartport Endovenous drainage cannula
- HeartPort Endoclamp balloon cannula
- Hendon venoclysis cannula
- Hepacon cannula
- Heyer-Schulte-Fischer ventricular cannula
- Heyner double cannula
- high-flow coaxial cannula
- Hilton sutureless infusion cannula
- Hilton self-retaining infusion cannula
- Hirschman hooked cannula
- Hoen ventricular cannula
- Hoffer forward-cutting knife cannula
- Holinger cannula

cannula (*continued*)
- hollow cannula
- Holman-Mathieu cannula
- Holman-Mathieu salpingography cannula
- Hudgins salpingography cannula
- Hudson all-clear nasal cannula
- Hulka uterine cannula
- Hulten-Stille cannula
- HUMI cannula
- Hunt-Reich secondary cannula
- Huse cannula
- Hyde frog irrigating cannula
- I&A coaxial cannula
- iliac-femoral cannula
- Illouz suction cannula
- infiltration cannula
- inflow cannula
- infusion cannula
- infusion/infiltration cannula
- Ingals flexible silver cannula
- Ingals rectal injection cannula
- ingress-egress cannula
- inhalation cannula
- injection cannula
- inlet cannula
- insertion of cannula
- Interlink threaded lock cannula
- intra-arterial cannula
- intracardiac cannula
- Intraducer peritoneal cannula
- intragastric cannula
- intraocular cannula
- intraocular lens cannula
- intrauterine balloon cannula
- intrauterine balloon-type cannula
- intrauterine cannula
- intrauterine insemination cannula
- IPAS flexible cannula
- iris hook cannula
- irrigating cannula
- irrigating-aspirating cannula
- I-tech cannula
- IUI disposable cannula
- Jarcho self-retaining uterine cannula
- Jarit air injection cannula

cannula (*continued*)
Jarit disposable cannula
Jarit lacrimal cannula
Jensen-Thomas I&A cannula
Jetco spray cannula
Johnson double cannula
J-shaped I&A cannula
Judd cannula
Kahn trigger cannula
Kahn uterine cannula
Kahn uterine trigger cannula
Kanavel brain-exploring cannula
Kanavel exploring cannula
Kara cataract-aspirating cannula
Karickhoff double cannula
Karman cannula
Katena cannula
Katzenstein rectal cannula
Keeler-Keislar lacrimal cannula
Keisler lacrimal cannula
Kellan hydrodissection cannula
Kelman cyclodialysis cannula
Kesilar cannula
Keyes-Ultzmann-Luer cannula
Khouri hydrodissection cannula
Kidde uterine cannula
Killian antral cannula
Killian antrum cannula
Killian nasal cannula
Killian-Eicken cannula
Kleegman cannula
Klein curved cannula
Knolle anterior chamber irrigating cannula
Knolle-Pearce cannula
Kos attic cannula
Kos cannula
Kraff cortex cannula
Krause nasal snare cannula
Kreutzmann cannula
lacrimal cannula
lacrimal irrigating cannula
Lamb cannula
Landolt cannula
laparoscopy cannula
large antral cannula
large-bore cannula

cannula (*continued*)
laryngeal cannula
laser-assisted intrastromal keratomileusis cannula
lens cannula
Leon cannula
Leon cobra cannula
Lewicky threaded infusion cannula
Lichtwicz antral cannula
Lifemed cannula
ligature cannula
Lillie attic cannula
Lindeman self-retaining uterine vacuum cannula
Linvatec cannula
liposuction cannula
liquid vitreous-aspirating cannula
Littell cannula
Litwak cannula
Look coaxial flexible disposable cannula
Look I&A coaxial cannula
Luebke uterine vacuum cannula
Luer tracheal cannula
Lukens cannula
lumen cannula
Luongo sphenoid irrigating cannula
LV apex cannula (left ventricular apex cannula)
Makler cannula
Malette-Spencer coronary cannula
Malström-Westman cannula
Mandelbaum cannula
Marlow disposable cannula
Maumenee goniotomy cannula
maxillary sinus cannula
Mayo coronary perfusion cannula
Mayo-Ochsner suction trocar cannula
McCain TMJ cannula
McCaskey sphenoid cannula
McGoon cannula
McIntyre anterior chamber cannula
McIntyre coaxial cannula

cannula (*continued*)
McIntyre lacrimal cannula
McIntyre-Binkhorst irrigating cannula
mediastinal cannula
Medicut cannula
Medi-Tech flexible stiffening cannula
Menghini cannula
Mercedes tip cannula
metal cannula
metal-ball tip cannula
metallic-tip cannula
metal-tipped cannula
microaire cannulas
middle ear suction cannula
mirror cannula
Mladick concave cannula
Mladick convex cannula
Moehle cannula
Moncrieff anterior chamber irrigating cannula
monitoring cannula
Montgomery tracheal cannula
Morris cannula
Morwel cannula
motorized cannula
Mueller coronary perfusion cannula
MultAport cannula
MVS cannula
Myerson-Moncrieff cannula
Myles sinus antral cannula
Myles sinus cannula
nasal cannula
Neal fallopian cannula
Neubauer lancet cannula
New York Eye and Ear cannula
Nichamin hydrodissection cannula
nucleus delivery cannula
Oaks double straight cannula
O'Gawa cataract-aspirating cannula
O'Gawa irrigating cannula
O'Gawa 2-way I&A cannula
olive-tipped cannula
Olympus disposable cannula
Olympus monopolar cannula
O'Malley-Heintz infusion cannula

cannula (*continued*)
oscillating cannula
Osher air-bubble removal cannula
Osher lens-vacuuming cannula
outflow cannula
outlet cannula
Pacifico cannula
Packo pars plana cannula
Padgett shark-mouth cannula
Padgett-Concorde suction cannula
Park irrigating cannula
Paterson laryngeal cannula
Patton cannula
Pautler infusion cannula
Peacekeeper cannula
Pearce coaxial I&A cannula
Peczon I&A cannula
Pemco cannula
Pereyra ligature cannula
perfusion cannula
Pierce attic cannula
Pierce coaxial I&A cannula
Pinto superficial dissection cannula
plastic cannula
polyethylene cannula
Polystan perfusion cannula
portal cannula
Portex nylon cannula
Portnoy ventricular cannula
Post trocar and washing cannula
Post washing cannula
Power cannula
Pritchard cannula
ProForma cannula
Pye cannula
Pynchon cannula
pyramid cannula
Rabinov cannula
Ramirez Silastic cannula
Randolph cyclodialysis cannula
Ranfac cannula
reciprocating cannula
rectal injection cannula
Reddick-Saye cannula
reel aspiration cannula
Reipen cannula

cannula (*continued*)

Research Medical straight multiple-holed aortic cannula
return-flow cannula
Rica tracheostomy cannula
Rigg cannula
Riordan flexible silver cannula
Robb antral cannula
Robles cutting point cannula
Rockey mediastinal cannula
Rockey trachea cannula
Rohrschneider cannula
Rolf-Jackson cannula
Roper alpha-chymotrypsin cannula
Rosenberg dissecting cannula
Rowsey cannula
Rowsey fixation cannula
Rubin fallopian tube cannula
Rycroft cannula
Sachs brain-exploring cannula
saphenous vein cannula
Sarns aortic arch cannula
Sarns soft-flow aortic cannula
Sarns 2-stage cannula
Sarns venous drainage cannula
Schanz cannula
Scheie anterior chamber cannula
Scheie cataract-aspirating cannula
Scott attic cannula
Scott rubber ventricular cannula
Scott ventricular cannula
Sedan cannula
Seletz ventricular cannula
self-retaining infusion cannula
self-retaining irrigating cannula
self-sealing cannula
Semm uterine vacuum cannula
Sewall antral cannula
Shahinian lacrimal cannula
shark-mouth cannula
Shark-tip cannula
Sheets cannula
Sheets irrigating vectis cannula

cannula (*continued*)

Shepard incision irrigating cannula
Shepard radial keratotomy irrigating cannula
side-cutting cannula
side-port cannula
sidewall infusion cannula
Silastic coronary artery cannula
silicone cannula
Silver cannula
Silverman-Boeker cannula
Simcoe cortex cannula
Simcoe double-barreled cannula
Simcoe II PC double cannula
Simcoe nucleus delivery cannula
Simcoe reverse I&A cannula
Simcoe reverse-aperture cannula
Sims cannula
single-holed suction cannula
single-lumen cannula
sinus antral cannula
sinus cannula
sinuscopy cannula
sinus-irrigating cannula
Skillern sphenoid cannula
Slade cannula
Sluijter-Mehta cannula
small-bore cannula
SMI cannula
smooth cannula
soft tissue shaving cannula
soft-tipped cannula
Solos disposable cannula
Soresi cannula
Southey cannula
SpaceSEAL balloon tip cannula
spatula cannula
spatula tip cannula
Spencer cannula
sphenoidal cannula
Spielberg sinus cannula
Spizziri-Simcoe cannula
stable access cannula
standard single port cannula
Stangel fallopian tube cannula
step-down cannula

cannula (*continued*)

- Steriseal disposable cannula
- Storz disposable cannula
- Storz needle cannula
- straight lacrimal cannula
- Strauss cannula
- stress on cannula
- subclavian cannula
- subretinal fluid cannula
- sub-Tenon anesthesia cannula
- suction cannula
- suprapubic cannula
- surgical cannula
- Swets goniotomy cannula
- Sylva irrigating cannula
- TAC2 atrial caval cannula
- Tandem XL triple-lumen ERCP cannula
- Teflon ERCP cannula
- Tenner eye cannula
- Tenner lacrimal cannula
- Texas cannula
- thin disposable cannula
- Thomas I&A cannula
- Thurmond nucleus-irrigating cannula
- Tibbs arterial cannula
- Toledo V-dissector cannula
- Toomey angled cannula
- Toomey G-bevel cannula
- Toomey standard cannula
- Topper cannula
- Torchia nucleus-aspirating cannula
- tracheal cannula
- tracheostomy cannula
- tracheotomy cannula
- transseptal cannula
- Tremble sphenoid cannula
- Trendelenburg cannula
- Trevisani cannula
- TriEye cannula
- trigeminus cannula
- trigger cannula
- Tri-Port sub-Tenon anesthesia cannula
- Trocan disposable CO_2 trocar and cannula
- Troutman alpha-chymotrypsin cannula
- trumpet cannula
- TruPro lacrimal cannula

cannula (*continued*)

- tubal insufflation cannula
- Tulevech lacrimal cannula
- Tulip cannula
- tumescent infiltrator cannula
- Turnbull cannula
- Ulanday double cannula
- Uldall subclavian hemodialysis cannula
- Ultra-Sil cannula
- ultrasonic cannula
- Unitech Toomey cannula
- Unitri cannula
- Universal cannula
- urethral instillation cannula
- urethrographic cannula
- USCI cannula
- U-shaped cannula
- uterine self-retaining cannula
- uterine trigger cannula
- uterine vacuum cannula
- Vabra cannula
- vacuum intrauterine cannula
- vacuum uterine cannula
- Van Alyea antral cannula
- Van Alyea frontal sinus cannula
- Van Alyea sphenoid cannula
- Van Osdel irrigating cannula
- Vancaillie uterine cannula
- Vance prostatic aspiration cannula
- VC2 atrial caval cannula
- vein graft cannula
- Veirs cannula
- vena caval cannula
- Venflon cannula
- venoclysis cannula
- venous cannula
- ventricular cannula
- Veress laparoscopic cannula
- Veress peritoneum cannula
- Vidaurri cannula
- Viking cannula
- Viscoflow angled cannula
- Visitec anterior chamber cannula
- Visitec I&A cannula
- Vitalcor cardioplegia infusion cannula
- vitreous-aspirating cannula
- Von Eichen antral cannula

cannula (*continued*)
Wallace Flexihub central
venous pressure cannula
washout cannula
Webb cannula
Webster infusion cannula
Weck disposable cannula
Weil lacrimal cannula
Weiner cannula
Weisman cannula
Wells cannula
Wells Johnson cannula
Welsh cortex-stripper cannula
Welsh flat olive-tipped double
cannula
Wergeland double cannula
West lacrimal cannula
wire-wound cannula
Wisap disposable cannula
Wolf disposable cannula
Wolf drainage cannula
Wolf return-flow cannula
Ximed disposable cannula
Yankauer middle meatus
cannula
Zinn endoillumination
infusion cannula
Zylik cannula
cannula clamp
cannula guard
cannula scissors
cannula tubing adapter
cannula with locking dilator
cannulate
cannulated
cannulated bolt
cannulated bronchoscopic
forceps
cannulated cancellous lag screw
cannulated cortical step drill
cannulated drill
cannulated forceps
cannulated four-flute reamer
cannulated nail
cannulated obturator
cannulated reamer
cannulated wire threader
cannulation
bile duct cannulation
biliary cannulation
duct cannulation
ductal cannulation

cannulation (*continued*)
endoscopic retrograde
cannulation
endoscopic transpapillary
cannulation
ERCP cannulation
ex vivo cannulation
femoral vein cannulation
intravenous cannulation
percutaneous arterial
cannulation
peripheral venous
cannulation
postsphincterotomy ERCP
cannulation
retrograde cannulation
selective cannulation
selective ductal cannulation
transpapillary cannulation
unilateral pedicle cannulation
vascular cannulation
venous cannulation
cannulation catheter
cannulation of aorta
cannulization (*see* cannulation)
Canon auto refraction
keratometer
Canon automatic keratometer
Canon perimeter
Canon refractor
Canon scanner
can-opener capsulotomy
Can-Opt stand-alone dual lumen
ERCP catheter
cant
occlusal cant
occlusive cant
cant of mandible
cant of upper lip
canted finger hook
Cantelli sign
cantering rhythm
canthal drift
canthal hypertelorism
canthal lift
canthectomy
canthi (*sing.* canthus)
canthitis
cantholysis
inferior cantholysis
lateral cantholysis
superior cantholysis

canthomeatal flap
canthomeatal line
canthopexy
  bilateral canthopexy
  lateral canthopexy
canthoplasty
  Agnew canthoplasty
  Ammon canthoplasty
  Arrowhead canthoplasty
  Imre canthoplasty
  Imre lateral canthoplasty
  inferior retinacular lateral
    canthoplasty
  lateral canthoplasty
  medial canthoplasty
  provisional canthoplasty
  tarsal strip canthoplasty
canthorrhaphy
  Elschnig canthorrhaphy
canthotomy
  external canthotomy
  lateral canthotomy
canthus (*pl.* canthi)
  external canthus
  inner canthus
  internal canthus
  lateral canthus
  medial canthus
  nasal canthus
  outer canthus
  temporal canthus
cantilever
cantilever effect
cantilever graft
cantilevered bone graft
Cantlie cannula
Cantlie line
Cantor intestinal tube
Cantor tube
Cantwell-Ransley epispadias
  repair
canvas brace
Canyon auto refractometer
Canyons irrigation syringe
cap
  chin cap
  Gelfilm cap
  hypothermia cap
  ice cap
  knee cap
  Luer tip cap
  phrygian cap

cap (*continued*)
  pyloric cap
  root cap
  skull cap
  stockinette cap
  syringe cap
  Vitallium cap
  Zimmer tibial nail cap
  Zinn cap
cap bunionectomy
cap grafts
cap splint
cap technique
capacitive radiofrequency
capacity
  cranial capacity
  electric capacity
  flow capacity
  knot holding capacity (KHC)
  maximum breathing capacity
  stomach capacity
  ventilatory capacity
  vital capacity
CAPARES (Coronary Angioplasty
    Amlodipine in Restenosis
    Study)
Caparosa bur
Caparosa cutting bur
Caparosa wire crimper
CAPD (continuous ambulatory
    peritoneal dialysis)
CAPDH probe
Cape Town technique
capeline
capeline bandage
Capello slim-line abduction
    pillow
Capello technique
Capener brace
Capener coil splint
Capener finger splint
Capener nail
Capener nail plate
Capener technique
Capes clamp
Capetown aortic prosthetic valve
Capetown prosthesis
cap-fitted endoscope
cap-fitted panendoscope
caphalotrigonal technique
capillaroscopy
  nail-fold capillaroscopy

capillary
   alveolar capillary
   lymph capillary
   lymphatic capillary
capillary action
capillary angioma
capillary arcade
capillary arteriole
capillary bed
capillary bed shunt
capillary bronchiectasis
capillary dilation
capillary drainage
capillary embolism
capillary flames
capillary flow dialyzer
capillary fracture
capillary fragility test
capillary hemangioma
capillary hemorrhage
capillary hyperfiltration
capillary loop
capillary lymphangioma
capillary malformation
capillary microscope
capillary muscle
capillary nevus
capillary plexus
capillary points of ooze
capillary pressure
capillary refill
capillary refill time
capillary resistance test
capillary stenosis
capillary tube
capillary vascular malformation
capillary vessel
capillary wedge pressure
Capintec instant gamma counter
Capintec nuclear VEST monitor
Capio CL transvaginal suture-
    capturing device
Capiox hollow flow oxygenator
Capiox II oxygenator
Capiox-E bypass system
    oxygenator
CAPIS compression plate
CAPIS reconstruction plate
capital epiphysis
capital fragment
capital operation
capitate bone

capitate dislocation
capitate fracture
capitate papillae
capitellar fracture
capitellocondylar
capitellocondylar total elbow
    arthroplasty
capitellum
   Kocher fracture of capitellum
capitis
   lateral rectus capitis
   paracentesis capitis
   regio frontalis capitis
   seborrhea capitis
   vitiligo capitis
capitolunate articulation
capitolunate joint
capitolunate ligament
capitonnage
capitonnage suture technique
capitular articulation
capitular joint
capitular process
capitulum humerae
capitulum mandibulae
capitulum of humerus
capitulum of stapes
capitulum processus
    condyloidei
Caplan angular scissors
Caplan dorsal scissors
Caplan double-action scissors
Caplan nasal bone scissors
Caplan nasal scissors
Capner boutonniere splint
Capner gouge
Capner splint
Capnocheck capnometer
Capnogard capnograph monitor
Capnomac Ultima monitor
capnometer
   Capnocheck capnometer
   Cardiocap capnometer
   MicroSpan capnometer
Capp point
capped elbow
capped knee
capped lead
capping
capping technique
Cappio suture passer
Caprolactam suture

CAPS arthroWand
Capset bone graft barrier
Capsitome cystotome
CAPSO (cautery-assisted palatal
    stiffening operation)
capsotomy (see capsulotomy)
capstan knot
Capsuel CPAP manometer
capsula adiposa
capsula articularis articulationis
    temporomandibularis
capsula articularis mandibulae
capsular adhesions
capsular advancement
capsular calcification
capsular cataract
capsular contracture
capsular decidua
capsular dissection
capsular exfoliation syndrome
capsular fixation
capsular flap pyeloplasty
capsular forceps
capsular hemiplegia
capsular imbrication
capsular incision
capsular interposition
    arthroplasty
capsular invasion
capsular joint
capsular knife
capsular ligament
capsular mineralization
capsular occlusion
capsular opacities
capsular polisher
capsular reefing
capsular shift procedure
capsular space
capsular-style lens
capsule
    adherent capsule
    adipose capsule
    adipose renal capsule
    articular capsule
    Bowman capsule
    Carey capsule
    Castroviejo transplant-grafting
        capsule
    contracture of joint capsule
    Crosby capsule
    Crosby-Kugler capsule

capsule (continued)
    drug release capsule
    Ernst radium capsule
    exposed capsule
    external capsule
    fibrous capsule
    fibrous renal capsule
    gelatinous capsule
    Gerota capsule
    Glisson capsule
    glomerular capsule
    Heyman capsule
    internal capsule
    joint capsule
    lateral capsule
    lens capsule
    M2A capsule
    malpighian capsule
    medial capsule
    midcarpal capsule
    nasal capsule
    parotid capsule
    pelvioprostatic capsule
    perinephric capsule
    periprosthetic fibrous capsule
    platinum iridium capsule
    posterior capsule
    prostatic capsule
    radiocarpal joint capsule
    radium capsule
    reefing of joint capsule
    salivary gland capsule
    Schweigger capsule
    splenic capsule
    stripping of kidney capsule
    suprarenal capsule
    synovial capsule
    tear of capsule
    temporomandibular joint
        capsule
    Tenon capsule
    thyroid capsule
    traumatic capsule
    tumor capsule
capsule flap technique
capsule forceps
capsule forceps technique
capsule fragment forceps
capsule fragment spatula
capsule of corpora
capsule of glomerulus
capsule of kidney

capsule of knee
capsule of spleen
capsule of temporomandibular
    joint
capsule of Tenon
capsule polisher
capsule tumor
capsulectomy
    pituitary capsulectomy
    renal capsulectomy
    total capsulectomy
capsule-grasping forceps
Capsulform lens
capsulitis
    adhesive capsulitis
capsulodesis
    Zancolli capsulodesis
capsuloganglionic hemorrhage
capsulolenticular
capsulolenticular cataract
capsulopalpebral fascia
capsuloplasty
    Zancolli capsuloplasty
capsulorrhexis forceps
capsulorrhaphy
    Boyd-Sisk posterior
        capsulorrhaphy
    duToit-Roux capsulorrhaphy
    duToit-Roux staple
        capsulorrhaphy
    medial capsulorrhaphy
    pants-over-vest
        capsulorrhaphy
    posterior capsulorrhaphy
    Rockwood posterior
        capsulorrhaphy
    Roux-DuToit staple
        capsulorrhaphy
    staple capsulorrhaphy
    Tibone posterior
        capsulorrhaphy
capsulotome
    Darling capsulotome
capsulotomy
    anterior capsulotomy
    beer-can capsulotomy
    can-opener capsulotomy
    Castroviejo capsulotomy
    closed capsulotomy
    Curtis PIP joint capsulotomy
    Darling capsulotomy
    dorsal transverse capsulotomy

capsulotomy (*continued*)
    dorsolateral and medial
        capsulotomy
    L-type capsulotomy
    open capsulotomy
    posterior capsulotomy
    renal capsulotomy
    triangular capsulotomy
    T-shaped capsulotomy
    Vannas capsulotomy
    Verhoeff-Chandler
        capsulotomy
    YAG capsulotomy
    YAG laser capsulotomy
capsulotomy blade
capsulotomy forceps
capsulotomy scissors
CapSure cardiac pacing lead
CapSure electrode
CapSure tool for soft tissues
Captiflex polypectomy snare
Captivator polypectomy snare
capture beats
Capuron point
caput (*pl.* capita)
caput angulare musculi quadrati
        labii superioris
caput forceps
caput infraorbitale musculi
        quadrati labii superioris
caput malleus
caput mandibulae
caput medusae
caput progeneum
caput quadratum
caput succedaneum
caput ulnae syndrome
caput zygomaticum musculi
        quadrati labii superioris
Carabelli aspirator
Carabelli cancer cell collector
Carabelli cannula
Carabelli collector
Carabelli endobronchial tube
Carabelli irrigator
Carabelli lumen finder
Carabelli mirror cannula
Carabelli tube
Carabelt lower back support
CaraGlass fiberglass casting tape
Carapace disposable face shield
Carapace face shield

Carass ventilator
Carassini spool
Carasyn hydrogel wound
    dressing
Carb-Bite needle holder
Carb-Bite tissue forceps
Carb-Edge scissors
carbide bur
carbide finishing bur
carbide mastoid bur
carbide-jaw forceps
carbide-jaw needle holder
carbide-jaw scissors
Carbocaine hydrochloride
    anesthetic agent
CarboFlex odor-control dressing
carbolic acid
carbolize
carbolized knife blade
CarboMedics Top-Hat supra-
    annular valve
CarboMedics bileaflet prosthetic
    heart valve
CarboMedics cardiac valve
    prosthesis
CarboMedics valve device
carbon
    polymeric carbon
    Pyrolite carbon
    pyrolitic carbon
carbon arc lamp
carbon arc light
Carbon Copy HP foot prosthesis
Carbon Copy II foot prosthesis
Carbon Copy II lightweight
    prosthesis
carbon dioxide (CO_2)
carbon dioxide (CO_2) laser
    scalpel
carbon dioxide anesthetic agent
carbon dioxide cautery
carbon dioxide concentration
carbon dioxide fixation
carbon dioxide insufflation
carbon dioxide laser
carbon dioxide laser plaque
    ablation
carbon dioxide pressure
carbon dioxide therapy
carbon fiber
carbon implant
carbon ion therapy

carbon steel blade
carbonaceous material
carbon-fiber-composite cage
carbon-fiber-reinforced cage
Carboplast II sheet orthotic
    material
Carborundum disk
Carborundum polisher
Carbo-Seal ascending aortic
    prosthesis
Carbo-Seal cardiovascular
    composite graft
Carbo-Seal graft material
Carbo-Zinc skin barrier material
carbuncle
    kidney carbuncle
carbuncular
carbunculoid
Carceau-Brahms ankle
    arthrodesis
carcinectomy
carcinoembryonic antigen (CEA)
carcinogen
carcinogenesis
    radiation-induced
        carcinogenesis
carcinogenic
carcinoid
    laryngeal carcinoid
    oncocytoid carcinoid
carcinoid tumor
carcinoid valve disease
carcinoma (*pl.* carcinomas,
    carcinomata)
    acinar carcinoma
    acinic cell carcinoma
    acinous carcinoma
    acinous cell carcinoma
    adenocystic carcinoma
    adenoid cystic carcinoma
    adenoid squamous cell
        carcinoma
    adenopapillary carcinoma
    adenosquamous carcinoma
    adnexal carcinoma
    adrenal carcinoma
    adrenocortical carcinoma
    aldosterone-producing
        carcinoma
    alveolar cell carcinoma
    ameloblastic carcinoma
    amphicrine carcinoma

carcinoma (*continued*)
  ampullary carcinoma
  anaplastic carcinoma
  anorectal carcinoma
  antral carcinoma
  apocrine carcinoma
  Astler-Coller classification of
    Dukes C carcinoma
  basal cell carcinoma
  basal squamous cell
    carcinoma
  basaloid carcinoma
  basosquamous carcinoma (BSC)
  basosquamous cell carcinoma
  benign-acting renal cell
    carcinoma
  betel carcinoma
  bile duct carcinoma
  bilharzial carcinoma
  biliary carcinoma
  bladder carcinoma
  Borrmann type I-IV carcinoma
  branchiogenic carcinoma
  breast carcinoma
  bronchial carcinoma
  bronchioloalveolar carcinoma
  bronchoalveolar carcinoma
  burn scar carcinoma
  cecal carcinoma
  central mucoepidermoid
    carcinoma
  cerebriform carcinoma
  cervical carcinoma
  chimney sweep's carcinoma
  cholangitis carcinoma
  choroid plexus carcinoma
  clay pipe carcinoma
  clear cell hepatocellular
    carcinoma
  colloid carcinoma
  colon carcinoma
  colonic carcinoma
  colorectal carcinoma
  Columbia staging system for
    breast carcinoma
  columnar cuff carcinoma
  comedo carcinoma
  corpus carcinoma
  cortisol-producing carcinoma
  cribriform carcinoma
  curettage of basal cell
    carcinoma

carcinoma (*continued*)
  cutaneous metastatic breast
    carcinoma
  cylindrical carcinoma
  cystic carcinoma
  dendritic carcinoma
  differentiated carcinoma
  differentiated thyroid
    carcinoma
  disseminated carcinoma
  duct carcinoma
  duct cell carcinoma
  ductal carcinoma
  Dukes classification of
    carcinoma (A, B, C, or D)
  dye workers carcinoma
  eccrine carcinoma
  Edmondson grading system
    for hepatocellular
    carcinoma
  embryonal carcinoma
  embryonal cell carcinoma
  encephaloid gastric
    carcinoma
  endometrial carcinoma
  epibulbar carcinoma
  epidermoid carcinoma
  epithelial carcinoma
  epithelial-myoepithelial
    carcinoma
  esophageal carcinoma
  ethmoid sinus carcinoma
  excavated gastric carcinoma
  exophytic carcinoma
  extrahepatic abdominal
    carcinoma
  FAB staging of carcinoma
    (French, American, British
    staging)
  fallopian tube carcinoma
  false cord carcinoma
  fibroepithelioma basal cell
    carcinoma
  follicular carcinoma
  follicular thyroid carcinoma
  French, American, British
    staging of carcinoma (FAB)
  gallbladder carcinoma
  gastric carcinoma
  gastric stump carcinoma
  gastrointestinal carcinoma
  gelatiniform carcinoma

carcinoma (*continued*)
  gelatinous carcinoma
  genital carcinoma
  giant cell carcinoma
  glandular carcinoma
  glassy cell carcinoma
  Gleason score of prostatic
    carcinoma
  glottic carcinoma
  glottic squamous cell
    carcinoma
  granulosa cell carcinoma
  gynecological carcinoma
  gyriform carcinoma
  hair-matrix carcinoma
  hematoid carcinoma
  hepatic cell carcinoma
  hepatocellular carcinoma
    (HCC)
  hereditary nonpolyposis
    colon carcinoma (HNPCC)
  hilar carcinoma
  hypernephroid carcinoma
  hypopharyngeal carcinoma
  hypopharyngeal squamous
    cell carcinoma
  in situ squamous cell
    carcinoma
  infantile embryonal
    carcinoma
  infiltrated duct cell carcinoma
  infiltrating carcinoma
  infiltrating ductal cell
    carcinoma
  infiltrating lobular carcinoma
  infiltrative basal cell
    carcinoma
  infiltrative carcinoma
  inflammatory breast
    carcinoma
  inflammatory carcinoma
  infraglottic carcinoma
  infraglottic squamous cell
    carcinoma
  inoperable carcinoma
  insular carcinoma
  intermediate carcinoma
  intraductal carcinoma
  intraepidermal carcinoma
  intraepithelial carcinoma
  intraepithelial nonkeratinizing
    carcinoma

carcinoma (*continued*)
  intraosseous carcinoma
  invasive breast carcinoma
  invasive carcinoma
  invasive ductal carcinoma
  invasive lobular carcinoma
  Japanese classification for
    gastric carcinoma (JCGC)
  Jewett classification of
    bladder carcinoma
  juvenile carcinoma
  juvenile embryonal carcinoma
  keratinizing squamous cell
    carcinoma
  Kulchitsky cell carcinoma
  large cell carcinoma
  laryngeal carcinoma
  laryngeal neuroendocrine
    carcinoma
  latent carcinoma
  lateral aberrant thyroid
    carcinoma
  lenticular carcinoma
  leptomeningeal carcinoma
  lingual thyroid carcinoma
  lobular carcinoma
  local recurrence of carcinoma
  lung carcinoma
  lymphoepithelial carcinoma
  maxillary sinus carcinoma
  medullary carcinoma
  meibomian gland carcinoma
  melanotic carcinoma
  meningeal carcinoma
  Merkel cell carcinoma
  metaplastic carcinoma
  metastatic basal cell
    carcinoma
  metastatic carcinoma
  metastatic colorectal
    carcinoma
  metastatic prostatic
    carcinoma
  metastatic renal cell
    carcinoma
  metatypical carcinoma
  microcystic adnexal
    carcinoma
  microinvasive carcinoma
  micropapillary carcinoma
  microscopic multifocal
    medullary carcinoma

carcinoma (*continued*)

microtrabecular hepatocellular carcinoma

moderately differentiated neuroendocrine carcinoma

Mohs excision of basal cell carcinoma

morbilliform basal cell carcinoma

morpheaform basal cell carcinoma

mucinous carcinoma

mucoepidermal carcinoma

mucoepidermoid carcinoma (MEC)

mucus-producing adenopapillary carcinoma (MPAPC)

napkin-ring carcinoma

nasopharyngeal carcinoma (NPC)

neuroendocrine carcinoma

neuroendocrine skin carcinoma

nevoid basal cell carcinoma

nodular basal cell carcinoma

nodular ulcerative basal cell carcinoma

noninfiltrating lobular carcinoma

nonkeratinizing carcinoma

oat cell carcinoma

occult carcinoma

oncoplastic carcinoma

oral squamous cell carcinoma (oral SCC)

orofacial carcinoma

oropharyngeal carcinoma

ovarian carcinoma

Paget carcinoma

pancreatic carcinoma

papillary gastric carcinoma

papillary squamous carcinoma

papillary thyroid carcinoma

parathyroid carcinoma

parenchymatous carcinoma

parotid carcinoma

penile carcinoma

periampullary carcinoma

periportal carcinoma

periurethral duct carcinoma

pharyngeal wall carcinoma

carcinoma (*continued*)

pigmented basal cell carcinoma

pilomatrixoma carcinoma

polypoid superficial gastric carcinoma

preinvasive carcinoma

prickle cell carcinoma

primary bile duct carcinoma

primary carcinoma

primary intraosseous carcinoma

prostatic carcinoma

pure insular carcinoma

radiation-induced carcinoma

rectal carcinoma

rectosigmoid carcinoma

recurrent basal cell carcinoma

recurrent squamous cell carcinoma

renal cell carcinoma

renal pelvis carcinoma

resectable carcinoma

reserve cell carcinoma

salivary duct carcinoma (SDC)

salivary gland carcinoma (SGC)

sarcomatoid carcinoma

scar carcinoma

schistosomal bladder carcinoma

Schmincke-Regaud lymphoepithelial carcinoma

schneiderian carcinoma

scirrhous carcinoma

sclerosing basal cell carcinoma

sebaceous carcinoma

secondary carcinoma

secretory carcinoma

sigmoid colon carcinoma

signet-ring carcinoma

signet-ring cell carcinoma

sinonasal carcinoma

small cell lung carcinoma

small cell neuroendocrine carcinoma

small round cell carcinoma

spheroidal cell carcinoma

spindle cell carcinoma

splenic flexure carcinoma

sporadic renal cell carcinoma

carcinoma (*continued*)
  squamous cell carcinoma
    (SCC)
  stage B, C carcinoma
  string carcinoma
  string cell carcinoma
  subglottic squamous cell
    carcinoma
  subungual squamous cell
    carcinoma
  superficial basal cell
    carcinoma
  supraglottic carcinoma
  supraglottic squamous cell
    carcinoma
  swamp carcinoma
  sweat gland carcinoma
  terminal carcinoma
  terminal duct carcinoma
  testicular carcinoma
  thymic carcinoma
  thyroid carcinoma
  trabecular carcinoma
  transglottic squamous cell
    carcinoma
  transitional cell carcinoma
  tuberous carcinoma
  tuberous sclerosis-associated
    renal cell carcinoma
  tubular carcinoma
  undifferentiated carcinoma
  undifferentiated squamous
    cell carcinoma
  unresectable squamous cell
    carcinoma
  urachal carcinoma
  ureteral carcinoma
  urethral carcinoma
  urothelial carcinoma
  uterine papillary serous
    carcinoma
  vaginal carcinoma
  verrucous carcinoma
  Von Brunn nests in bladder
    carcinoma
  vulvar carcinoma
  vulvovaginal carcinoma
  well differentiated carcinoma
  wolffian duct carcinoma
  yolk sac carcinoma
carcinoma adenomatosum
carcinoma basocellulare

carcinoma cutaneum
carcinoma en cuirasse
carcinoma epitheliale adenoides
carcinoma ex pleomorphic
  adenoma
carcinoma in situ (CIS)
carcinoma of nasopharynx
carcinoma of uncertain primary
  site
carcinoma simplex
carcinoma stage irresectable
carcinoma telangiectaticum
carcinomatosis
carcinomatous lesion
carcinosis
  miliary carcinosis
Carcon stent
CARD (cardiac automatic
  resuscitative device)
Cardak percutaneous catheter
  introducer
Cardarelli sign
cardboard splint
Carden amputation
Carden bronchoscopy tube
Carden disarticulation
Carden double-lumen
  endotracheal tube
Carden jetting device
Carden laryngoscopy tube
cardia
  crescent of cardia
  gastric cardia
cardia of stomach
cardiac anesthesia
cardiac aneurysm
cardiac angiogram
cardiac anomaly
cardiac apex
cardiac apnea monitor
cardiac area
cardiac arrest
Cardiac Assist intra-aortic
  balloon catheter
cardiac asthmatic
cardiac automatic resuscitative
  device (CARD)
cardiac balloon pump
cardiac border
cardiac bronchus
cardiac bypass (CBP)
cardiac care unit (CCU)

cardiac catheter
cardiac catheter microphone
cardiac catheterization
cardiac chamber
cardiac compensation
cardiac compression
cardiac contractility
cardiac decompression
cardiac defect
cardiac defibrillator
cardiac depressant
cardiac dilatation
cardiac dilation
cardiac dilator
cardiac disease
cardiac Doppler examination
cardiac dullness
cardiac effusion
cardiac event
cardiac examination
cardiac failure (CF)
cardiac fibrillation
cardiac fluoroscopy
cardiac function
cardiac ganglion
cardiac glands of esophagus
cardiac herniation
cardiac hypertrophy
cardiac impairment
cardiac impression
cardiac impulse
cardiac infant catheter
cardiac infarction
cardiac instability
cardiac intervention
cardiac irradiation
cardiac irregularity
cardiac massage
cardiac metastasis
cardiac monitor
cardiac monitor strip
cardiac monitoring
cardiac mucosa
cardiac murmur
cardiac muscle
cardiac nerves
cardiac notch
cardiac notch of lung
cardiac orifice
cardiac output
cardiac output recorder
cardiac pacemaker

cardiac pacing
cardiac patch
cardiac perforation
cardiac perfusion
cardiac plexus
cardiac position
cardiac probe
cardiac profile
cardiac puncture
cardiac rate
cardiac resuscitation
cardiac retraction clip
cardiac revascularization
cardiac rhythm
cardiac rupture
cardiac scissors
cardiac series
cardiac shadow
cardiac shock
cardiac shunt
cardiac shunt detection
cardiac silhouette
cardiac size
cardiac souffle
cardiac sounds
cardiac sphincter
cardiac status
cardiac stimulant
cardiac study
cardiac stump
cardiac surgery
cardiac syncope
cardiac tamponade
cardiac transplant
cardiac transplantation
cardiac tumor
cardiac tumor plop
cardiac ultrasound
cardiac valve dilator
cardiac valve leaflets
cardiac valvular malformation
cardiac veins
cardiac ventriculography
cardiac workup
cardiectomy
Cardiff resuscitation bag
Cardillo retractor
Cardima Pathfinder
    microcatheter
cardinal ligaments
cardinal point
cardinal position

cardinal signs of inflammation
cardinal suture
cardinal symptom
cardinal vein
cardinal vessel
Cardio Tactilaze peripheral
  angioplasty laser catheter
cardioangiogram
CardioBeeper CM-12L monitor
Cardiocap 5-patient monitor
Cardiocap capnometer
cardiocentesis
CardioCoil coronary stent
CardioCoil self-expanding
  coronary stent
Cardio-Control pacemaker
Cardio-Cool myocardial pouch
Cardio-Cool myocardial
  protection pouch
Cardio-Cuff
  Childs Cardio-Cuff
CardioData MK-3 Holter scanner
cardiodiaphragmatic angle
CardioDiary heart monitor
cardiodilator
  Starck cardiodilator
cardiodiosis
cardioesophageal junction
cardioesophageal junction
  dilator
cardioesophageal sphincter
CardioFix pericardium patch
Cardioflon suture
cardiogenic shock
cardiogram
  apex cardiogram
  esophageal cardiogram
  ultrasound cardiogram
cardiography
  apex cardiography
Cardio-Green dye
Cardio-Grip anastomosis clamp
Cardio-Grip aortic clamp
Cardio-Grip bronchus clamp
Cardio-Grip iliac forceps
Cardio-Grip ligature carrier
Cardio-Grip pediatric clamp
Cardio-Grip renal artery clamp
Cardio-Grip tangential occlusion
  clamp
Cardio-Grip tissue forceps
Cardio-Grip vascular clamp

Cardioguide 4000
  electrocardiographic
  monitor
cardiohepatic angle
cardiohepatic sulcus
cardiohepatic triangle
cardiokymograph
cardiokymographic test
cardiologic magnification
cardiolysis
  Brauer cardiolysis
Cardiomarker catheter
CardioMatic electrocardiograph
Cardiomed Bodysoft epidural
  catheter
Cardiomed endotracheal
  ventilation catheter
Cardiomed thermodilution
  catheter
cardiomegaly
Cardiomemo device
cardiometer
Cardiometrics cardiotomy
  reservoir
Cardiometrics Flow-wire
  guidewire
cardiometry
cardiomyopathy
  hypertrophic cardiomyopathy
  (HCM)
cardiomyopexy
cardiomyoplasty
  dynamic cardiomyoplasty
cardiomyotomy
  Heller cardiomyotomy
  laparoscopic cardiomyotomy
  stomach cardiomyotomy
  videolaparoscopic
  cardiomyotomy
Cardionyl suture
cardio-omentopexy
Cardio-Pace Medical Durapulse
  pacemaker
Cardiopass graft
cardiopathy
  fatty cardiopathy
  nephropathic cardiopathy
cardiopericardiopexy
  Beck cardiopericardiopexy
cardiophrenic angle
cardioplasty
cardioplegia

cardioplegic needle
cardioplegic solution
cardioplegic technique
cardiopneumonopexy
Cardiopoint cardiac surgery
    needle
Cardiopoint needle
cardiopressor reflex
cardioprotective effect
cardiopulmonary arrest
cardiopulmonary bypass
cardiopulmonary bypass (CPB)
cardiopulmonary circulation
cardiopulmonary complication
cardiopulmonary murmur
cardiopulmonary resuscitation
cardiopulmonary resuscitator
cardiopulmonary support
cardiopuncture
cardiorespiratory arrest
cardiorespiratory complication
cardiorespiratory failure
cardiorespiratory murmur
cardiorespiratory sign
cardiorrhaphy
cardioschisis
Cardioscint nuclear detector
cardioscope
    Carlens cardioscope
CardioSeal septal occluder
Cardioserv defibrillator
cardiospasm
cardiospasm dilator
cardiosplenopexy
Cardiotach fetal monitor
cardiothoracic ratio
cardiothoracic surgery
cardiothymic silhouette
cardiotomy
cardiotomy reservoir
cardiotomy reservoir chest
    drainage
cardiotoxic effect
cardiovalvulotome
cardiovalvulotomy
cardiovascular
cardiovascular adverse effect
cardiovascular anastomotic clamp
cardiovascular anesthesia
cardiovascular bulldog clamp
cardiovascular cannula
cardiovascular circulation

cardiovascular clamp
cardiovascular collapse
cardiovascular complication
cardiovascular disease
cardiovascular disturbance
cardiovascular finger-to-nose
cardiovascular forceps
cardiovascular function
cardiovascular imaging
    technique
cardiovascular implant
cardiovascular malformation
cardiovascular monitor
cardiovascular needle holder
cardiovascular patch graft
cardiovascular physiology
cardiovascular Prolene suture
cardiovascular response
cardiovascular retractor
cardiovascular scissors
cardiovascular shunt
cardiovascular silhouette
cardiovascular silk suture
cardiovascular structures
cardiovascular stylet
cardiovascular support
cardiovascular surgery
cardiovascular sutures
cardiovascular thoracic needle
    holder
cardiovascular tissue forceps
cardiovascular tourniquet
cardioversion
    chemical cardioversion
    defibrillation and electrical
        cardioversion
    electric cardioversion
cardioversion paddles
cardioverted
cardioverter
    Lown cardioverter
cardioverter-defibrillator
    automatic implantable
        cardioverter-defibrillator
    automatic internal
        cardioverter-defibrillator
        (AICD)
Cardiovit AT-10 monitor
carditis
Cardix EZ cardiac pacing lead
Cardona corneal prosthesis
    forceps

Cardona corneal prosthesis
    trephine
Cardona eye prosthesis
Cardona fiberoptic diagnostic
    lens
Cardona focalizing fundus lens
    implant
Cardona focalizing goniolens
Cardona forceps
Cardona goniofocalizing implant
Cardona keratoprosthesis
Cardona laser
Cardona lens
Cardona threading lens forceps
CARE electrode
C-area in nose
Care-e-Vac portable aspirator
Carey capsule
Carey Ranvier technique
Carey-Coombs murmur
Carey-Coons biliary
    endoprosthesis kit
Carey-Coons soft stent
Cargile membrane
Cargile sutures
Carhart notch
caries
    dental caries
caries classification
caries of bone
carina
    tertiary carina
carina fornicis
carina of trachea
carina urethralis vaginae
carinate abdomen
carinatum
    pectus carinatum
carious lesion
carious pulp exposure
carious restoration margin
carious teeth
Carl P. Jones traction splint
Carl Zeiss instruments
Carl Zeiss lens
Carl Zeiss lensometer
Carl Zeiss myringotomy tube
Carl Zeiss tonometer
Carl Zeiss YAG laser
Carlens bronchospirometric
    catheter
Carlens cardioscope

Carlens catheter
Carlens curet
Carlens double-lumen
    endotracheal tube
Carlens fiberoptic
    mediastinoscope
Carlens forceps
Carlens mediastinoscope
Carlens needle
Carlens retractor
Carlens tracheotomy retractor
Carlens tube
Carlens-Stille tracheal retractor
Carlo Traverso maneuver
C-arm fluoroscope
C-arm fluoroscopy
C-arm fluoroscopy unit
C-arm image intensifier
C-arm portable x-ray unit
Carmack curet
Carmack ear curet
Carmalt arterial forceps
Carmalt artery forceps
Carmalt clamp
Carmalt forceps
Carmalt hemostat
Carmalt hemostatic forceps
Carmalt hysterectomy forceps
Carmalt splinter forceps
Carmalt thoracic forceps
Carmalt tube
Carman rectal tube
Carman tube
Carmault hemostat
Carmel clamp
carmine dye
Carmody aspirator
Carmody drill
Carmody electric aspirator
Carmody forceps
Carmody perforator drill
Carmody pump
Carmody thumb tissue forceps
Carmody tissue forceps
Carmody valvulotome
Carmody-Batson elevator
Carmody-Batson operation
Carmody-Brophy forceps
carmustine wafer
Carnesale acetabular extensile
    approach
Carnesale hip approach

Carnesale technique
Carnesale-Stewart-Barnes hip
    dislocation classification
Carnochan operation
carnosus
    panniculus carnosus
Carol Gerard screw
Caroli syndrome
Carolina Doppler
Carolina rocker
Caroline finger retractor
Caroli-Sarles classification
carotenoderma
carotenemia
caroticoclinoid foramen
caroticotympanic
caroticotympanic artery
caroticotympanic nerves
carotid
carotid ablative procedure
carotid air cell
carotid aneurysm
carotid angiogram
carotid angiogram needle
carotid angiography
carotid angioplasty
carotid arterial beds
carotid arteriogram
carotid arteriography
carotid artery
carotid artery bifurcation
carotid artery block
carotid artery bypass
carotid artery bypass clamp
carotid artery clamp
carotid artery compression
carotid artery disease
carotid artery dissection
carotid artery forceps
carotid artery occlusion
carotid artery stenosis
carotid bifurcation
carotid bifurcation
    endarterectomy
carotid body
carotid body tumor
carotid bruit
carotid bypass shunt
carotid canal
carotid cavernous sinus
carotid circulation
carotid clamp

carotid clamping
carotid compression
carotid endarterectomy (CEA)
carotid endarterectomy shunt
carotid eversion endarterectomy
carotid foramen
carotid ganglion
carotid genu
carotid gland
carotid groove
carotid injury
carotid isolation
carotid massage
carotid nerve
carotid plexus
carotid preservation technique
carotid pulsation
carotid pulse
carotid pulse tracing
carotid puncture
carotid sheath
carotid shunt
carotid sinus
carotid sinus nerve
carotid sinus reflex
carotid sinus sensitivity
carotid sinus stimulation
carotid sinus syncope
carotid sinus syndrome
carotid space
carotid steal syndrome
carotid stent
carotid subclavian
    endarterectomy
carotid sulcus
carotid surgery
carotid syncope
carotid triangle
carotid vein
carotid vessel
carotid-axillary bypass
carotid-basilar anastomosis
carotid-carotid bypass
carotid-cavernous sinus fistula
    (CCSF)
CarotidCoil stent
carotid-dural fistula
carotid-subclavian artery
    bypass
carotid-subclavian bypass
carotid-subclavian transposition
carotid-vertebral anastomosis

carotid-vertebral vein bypass
    graft
carotodynia
carp mouth
carpal
carpal articulation
carpal bone stress fracture
carpal bones
carpal boss
carpal canal
carpal compression test
carpal dislocation
carpal fracture
carpal height measurement
carpal height ratio
carpal instability
Carpal Lock cock-up wrist splint
Carpal Lock wrist brace
carpal lunate implant
carpal prosthesis
carpal row
carpal row bones
carpal scaphoid screw
carpal synchondrosis
carpal tunnel
carpal tunnel decompression
carpal tunnel projection
carpal tunnel release
carpal tunnel release system
    (CTRS)
carpal tunnel release system
    device
carpal tunnel surgery relief kit
carpal tunnel syndrome
carpals
carpectomy
    distal-row carpectomy
    Omer-Capen carpectomy
    proximal row carpectomy
Carpel speculum
Carpenter dissector
Carpenter enucleator
Carpenter knife
Carpenter syndrome (CTS)
Carpenter tonsil kinfe
Carpentier annuloplasty
Carpentier annuloplasty ring
    prosthesis
Carpentier pericardial valve
Carpentier ring
Carpentier ring heart valve
Carpentier stent

Carpentier tricuspid
    valvuloplasty
Carpentier valve
Carpentier-Edwards aortic valve
    prosthesis
Carpentier-Edwards
    bioprosthesis
Carpentier-Edwards
    bioprosthetic valve
Carpentier-Edwards
    glutaraldehyde-preserved
    porcine xenograft
    prosthesis
Carpentier-Edwards mitral
    annuloplasty valve
Carpentier-Edwards pericardial
    valve
Carpentier-Edwards Physio
    annuloplasty ring
Carpentier-Edwards porcine
    prosthetic valve
Carpentier-Edwards porcine
    supra-annular valve
Carpentier-Edwards valve
Carpentier-Edwards valve
    prosthesis
Carpentier-Edwards xenograft
Carpentier-Rhone-Poulenc mitral
    rings prosthesis
carpet lesion
carpocarpal
carpometacarpal (CMC) joint
carpometacarpal arthroplasty
carpometacarpal articulation
carpometacarpal disarticulation
carpometacarpal fracture-
    dislocation
carpometacarpal joint
    dislocation
carpometacarpal joint fracture
carpometacarpal ligament
carpopedal
carpopedal contraction
carpopedal spasm
carpophalangeal
Carpue operation
Carpue rhinoplasty
Carpule needle
Carpule syringe
carpus
    greater arc injury of the carpus
    lesser arc injury of the carpus

carpus curvus
Carr lobectomy tourniquet
Carr tourniquet
Carra Sorb H dressing
Carra Sorb M dressing
CarraFilm transparent dressing
CarraFilm transparent film
    dressing
CarraGauze hydrogel wound
    dressing pad
CarraKleenz cleansers
CarraSmart foam
CarraSmart foam dressing
CarraSorb H calcium alginate
    wound dressing
CarraSorb M freeze-dried gel
    wound dressing
Carrasyn hydrogel
Carrasyn hydrogel dressing
Carrel clamp
Carrel hemostatic forceps
Carrel mosquito forceps
Carrel operation
Carrel patch
Carrel suture technique
Carrel sutures
Carrel treatment
Carrel tube
Carrel-Dakin treatment
Carrel-Girard screw
Carrell fibular substitution
    technique
Carrell resection
Carrel-Lindbergh pump
Carriazo-Barraquer
    microkeratome
Carrie traction
carrier (see also ligature carrier,
    ligature passer, sponge
    carrier, suture carrier, tube
    carrier)
  amalgam carrier
  Barraquer needle carrier
  brain clip carrier
  Braun ligature carrier
  bronchoscopic sponge carrier
  Cardio-Grip ligature carrier
  Cave-Rowe ligature carrier
  clamp carrier
  Converta-Litter carrier
  Cooley ligature carrier
  cotton carrier

carrier (continued)
  DeBakey ligature carrier
  deep ligature carrier
  Deschamps carrier
  Deschamps ligature carrier
  double-headed stereotactic
    carrier
  ear snare wire carrier
  Endo-Assist endoscopic
    ligature carrier
  Endoclose suture carrier
  Favaloro-Semb ligature carrier
  Favaloro ligature carrier
  fiberoptic light carrier
  Finochietto clamp carrier
  Fitzwater ligature carrier
  foil carrier
  Fragen carrier
  gauze pad carrier
  goiter ligature carrier
  Goldwasser suture carrier
  Jackson sponge carrier
  Kilner suture carrier
  Kwapis ligature carrier
  Lahey carrier
  Lahey ligature carrier
  laryngeal sponge carrier
  ligature carrier
  light carrier
  linear in-line ligature carrier
  London College foil carrier
  Macey tendon carrier
  Madden ligature carrier
  Mayo carrier
  Mayo goiter ligature carrier
  miniature carrier
  Miya hook ligament carrier
  Miya hook ligature carrier
  nasal snare wire carrier
  proctologic cotton carrier
  Raz double-prong ligature
    carrier
  Rica cotton carrier
  sigmoidoscope light carrier
  sponge carrier
  Storz cotton carrier
  suture carrier
  Tauber ligature carrier
  tendon carrier
  Thermafil plastic carrier
  tube carrier
  Wangensteen carrier

carrier (*continued*)
  Wangensteen deep ligature
    carrier
  Wangensteen ligature carrier
  Yasargil ligature carrier
  Young ligature carrier
Carrington cleansers
Carrington dermal wound gel
Carrion penile prosthesis
Carrion-Small penile implant
Carrobend cast
Carroll aluminum hammer
Carroll aluminum mallet
Carroll arthrodesis
Carroll arthroplasty
Carroll awl
Carroll bone hook
Carroll bone-holding forceps
Carroll dressing forceps
Carroll elevator
Carroll finger goniometer
Carroll forearm tendon stripper
Carroll hook
Carroll hook curet
Carroll needle
Carroll needle holder
Carroll offset hand retractor
Carroll osteotome
Carroll periosteal elevator
Carroll retractor
Carroll rongeur
Carroll self-retaining spring
    retractor
Carroll skin hook
Carroll technique
Carroll tendon passer
Carroll tendon retriever
Carroll tendon-passing forceps
Carroll tendon-pulling forceps
Carroll tissue forceps
Carroll-Adson dural forceps
Carroll-Adson forceps
Carroll-Bennett finger retractor
Carroll-Bunnell drill
Carroll-Girard screw
Carroll-Legg osteotome
Carroll-Legg periosteal elevator
Carroll-Smith-Petersen
    osteotome
Carroll-Taber arthroplasty
carrying angle
Carson catheter

Carson internal-external
    endopyelotomy stent
Carson model catheter
Carson Zero Tip balloon
    dilatation catheter
Carswell grapes
cart
  basket cart
  B-Line utility cart
  case cart
  crash cart
  Datel endoscopy travel cart
  Harloff cart
  K-Thermia OR cart
  MetroFlex endoscopic cart
  OR cart
Cartella eye shield
Carten mitral valve retractor
Carter clamp
Carter curet
Carter elevator
Carter eye elevator
Carter intranasal splint
Carter introducer sphere
Carter knife
Carter operation
Carter pillow
Carter retractor
Carter septal knife
Carter septal speculum
Carter speculum
Carter sphere introducer
Carter spherical eye introducer
Carter splenectomy
Carter splint
Carter submucous curet
Carter Tubal Assistant surgical
    instrument
Carter-Glassman resection clamp
Carter-Rowe awl
Carter-Rowe view
Carter submucous elevator
Carter-Thomason suture passer
Carticel knee-cartilage
    replacement product
cartilage
  accessory cartilage
  accessory nasal cartilage
  accessory quadrate cartilage
  alar batten cartilage
  alar cartilage
  alar dome and cartilage

cartilage (*continued*)

alisphenoid cartilage
annular cartilage
Antia composite flap of
    helical cartilage
arthrodial cartilage
articular cartilage
arytenoid cartilage
auricular cartilage
base of arytenoid cartilage
basilar cartilage
beveled septal cartilage
bovine cartilage
branchial cartilage
calcified cartilage
calibrated triangle of septal
    cartilage
canals of cartilage
colliculus of arytenoid
    cartilage
conchal cartilage
condylar cartilage
connecting cartilage
corniculate cartilage
cornua of thyroid cartilage
costal cartilage
cricoid cartilage
cuneiform cartilage
Davis composite flap of
    conchal cartilage
diarthrodial cartilage
dislocation of cartilage
domal cartilage
ear cartilage
ensiform cartilage
epactal cartilages
epiglottic cartilage
eustachian cartilage
external semilunar
    cartilage
facet cartilage
falciform cartilage
floating cartilage
foot pods of alar cartilage
fracture of cartilage
gingival cartilage
greater alar cartilage
Huschke cartilage
hyaline articular cartilage
hyaline cartilage
hyoid cartilage
hypsiloid cartilage

cartilage (*continued*)

inferior horn of thyroid
    cartilage
innominate cartilage
interarticular cartilage
interosseous cartilage
interventricular cartilage
intervertebral cartilage
intraarticular cartilage
intrathyroid cartilage
investing cartilage
Jacobson cartilage
joint cartilage
laryngeal cartilage
lateral cartilage
lateral crus of greater alar
    cartilage
lesser alar cartilage
loose cartilage
lower lateral cartilage
Luschka cartilage
Luschka laryngeal cartilage
mandibular cartilage
meatal cartilage
Meckel cartilage
medial crus of lower lateral
    cartilage
Meyer cartilage
Morgagni cartilage
morselized cartilage
nasal cartilage
nasal dome cartilage
oblong fovea of arytenoid
    cartilage
ossifying cartilage
palpebral cartilage
paraseptal cartilage
patellar facet cartilage
permanent cartilage
quadrangular cartilage
quadrilateral cartilage
Reichert cartilage
returning cartilage
rib cartilage
rigid ball-shaped alar
    cartilages
sail of cartilage
Santorini cartilage
Seiler cartilage
semilunar cartilage
septal cartilage
sesamoid cartilages

cartilage (*continued*)
  soft cartilage
  splayed alar cartilage
  sternal cartilage
  sternum cartilage
  supra-arytenoid cartilage
  temporary cartilage
  tendon cartilage
  thyroid cartilage
  tissue-engineered cartilage
  torn cartilage
  torn knee cartilage
  tracheal cartilage
  tragal cartilage
  triangular cartilage
  triquetrous cartilage
  triradiate cartilage
  triticeal cartilage
  tympanomandibular cartilage
  uniting cartilage
  unossified cartilage
  upper lateral nasal cartilage
  ventral cleft of thyroid
    cartilage
  vomerine cartilage
  vomeronasal cartilage
  Weitbrecht cartilage
  Wrisberg cartilage
  xiphoid cartilage
  Y cartilage
  yellow cartilage
cartilage abrader (*see also*
    abrader)
  cartilage abrader
  corneal abrader
  Dingman abrader
  Dingman otoplasty cartilage
    abrader
  Haverhill dermal abrader
  Howard abrader
  Howard corneal abrader
  Iverson dermabrader
  lid dermabrader
  Lieberman abrader
  Montague abrader
  sandpaper dermabrader
  Stryker dermabrader
cartilage canal
cartilage case-grafting technique
cartilage chisel
cartilage clamp
cartilage corpuscle

cartilage crusher
cartilage cutting board
cartilage edge
cartilage elastic pullover
    kneecap splint
cartilage flap
cartilage forceps
cartilage graft
cartilage grafting
cartilage guide
cartilage implant
cartilage inflammation
cartilage island
cartilage knife
cartilage matrix
cartilage of nasal septum
cartilage overgrowth
cartilage prosthesis
cartilage punch
cartilage ring
cartilage scaffolding
cartilage scissors
cartilage scoring
cartilage shaping
cartilage space
cartilage stripper
cartilage tear
cartilage-breaking technique
cartilage-hair hypoplasia
cartilage-holding forceps
cartilage-molding technique
cartilage-weakening
    technique
cartilaginea
  exostosis cartilaginea
cartilagines (*sing.* cartilago)
cartilagines alares minores
cartilagines laryngis
cartilagines nasales
cartilagines nasales accessoriae
cartilagines nasi
cartilagines tracheales
cartilaginous
cartilaginous arthroplasty
cartilaginous autologous thin
    septal graft
cartilaginous collagen
cartilaginous cup arthroplasty
cartilaginous disk
cartilaginous exostosis
cartilaginous graft
cartilaginous growth

cartilaginous growth plate
  disorder
cartilaginous joint
cartilaginous loose body
cartilaginous portion
cartilaginous pyramid
cartilaginous ring
cartilaginous septum
cartilaginous support
cartilaginous tissue
cartilaginous tube
cartilaginous tumor
cartilaginous vault
cartilago (*pl.* cartilagines)
cartilago alaris major
cartilago arytenoidea
cartilago auriculae
cartilago corniculata
cartilago costalis
cartilago cricoidea
cartilago cuneiformis
cartilago epiglottica
cartilago meatus acustici
cartilago sesamoidea laryngis
cartilago thyroidea
cartilago tritcea
cartilago vomeronasalis
Carti-Loid syringe
Cartman lens insertion forceps
Cartmill feeding tube kit
cartridge base
cartwheel fracture
cartwheel motion
Cartwright heart prosthesis
Cartwright implant
Cartwright valve prosthesis
Cartwright vascular prosthesis
caruncle
  lacrimal caruncle
  Stensen duct caruncle
  sublingual caruncle
  submaxillary caruncle
caruncle clamp
caruncle forceps
caruncula (*pl.* carunculae)
caruncula lacrimalis
caruncula salivaris
caruncula sublingualis
carved cartilage graft
carver
  acorn carver
  Vehe carver

carving blade
CAS connector
CAS-200 image cytometer
Casanellas lacrimal operation
Casanellas operation
cascade
  coagulation cascade
  complementary cascade
cascade stomach
Casco heating pad
case
  aneurysm clip case
  clean case
  clean-contaminated case
  contaminated case
  endoscopic sterilizing case
  infected case
  instrument sterilizing case
  operable case
  Storz sterilizing case
Case appliance
case cart
Case enamel cleaver
Case knee approach
caseated tissue
caseating
caseating granuloma
caseating granulomatous
  inflammation
caseation
  tuberculous caseation
caseation necrosis
case-by-case approach
caseocavernous abscess
caseous
caseous abscess
caseous cataract
caseous necrosis
caseous pneumonia
CA-series dialyzer
Casey operation
Casey pelvic clamp
CASH (cruciform anterior spinal
  hyperextension)
CASH brace
CASH orthosis
CaSki cell line
Caslick operation
Caspar alligator forceps
Caspar anterior cervical plate
Caspar anterior instrumentation
Caspar blade

Caspar cervical retractor
Caspar cervical screw
Caspar disk space spreader
Caspar distraction pin
Caspar distractor
Caspar drill
Caspar forceps
Caspar hook
Caspar ring opacity
Caspar rongeur
Caspar speculum
Caspar trapezoidal plate
Caspar vertebral body spreader
Caspari repair
Caspari soft tissue tack
Caspari suture punch
CASS TrueTaper collimator
Cassel operation
Casselberry cannula
Casselberry position
Casselberry sphenoid cannula
Casselberry sphenoid tube
Casselberry sphenoid washing
    tube
Casselberry suture punch
Casselberry tube
Casser fontanelle
Casser muscle
casserian fontanelle
casserian muscle
cassette
    Camp grid cassette
    x-ray cassette
cassette cup collecting device
Cassidy-Brophy dressing forceps
Cassidy-Brophy forceps
cast
    3-finger spica cast
    air cell casts
    application of cast
    Aquaplast cast
    banjo cast
    Bebax plaster cast
    below-knee walking cast
    bivalved cast
    bivalved plaster cast
    Body Armor walker cast
    body cast
    bootie cast
    Boston bivalve cast
    broomstick cast
    Caldwell hanging cast

cast (*continued*)
    Carrobend cast
    Comfort Cast
    Contura cast
    corrective cast
    Cotrel body cast
    Cotton-Loader position cast
    Cutter cast
    cylinder cast
    dermoplasty cast
    diagnostic cast
    EDF cast
    epithelial cast
    Equilizer short leg walking
        cast
    figure-eight cast
    Fractura Flex
    Fractura Flex cast
    Freedom Thumb spica cast
    Frejka cast
    gel cast
    gnathostatic cast
    Gypsona
    Gypsona cast
    half-shell cast
    halo body cast
    halo cast
    hanging arm cast
    hanging cast
    Hexcel cast
    Hexcelite cast
    Hexcelite long-arm cast
    Hexcelite thermoplastic cast
    hinged cast
    hip spica cast
    immobilized in cast
    immobilized in plaster cast
    Kite cast
    Kite corrective cast
    LAE cast
    LBE cast
    leg cast
    Lite hip cast
    localizer cast
    long above-elbow cast
    long arm navicular cast
    long below-elbow cast
    long leg cylinder cast
    long leg plaster cast
    long leg walking cast
    long-arm cast (LAC)
    long-armed cast

cast (*continued*)

   long-leg cast (LLC)
   master cast
   MaxCast
   MBE cast
   medium below-elbow cast
   Minerva cast
   modified cast
   Muenster cast
   Munster cast
   Neufeld cast
   O'Donoghue cotton cast
   Orfizip knee cast
   Ortho-Glass
   Orthoplast slipper cast
   paddy bear cast
   panty cast
   patellar tendon-bearing cast
     (PTB)
   petaling the cast
   Petrie spica cast
   plaster cast
   plaster-of-Paris cast
   pontoon spica cast
   preoperative cast
   PTB cast
   reapplication of cast
   replaced in cast
   Risser cast
   Risser localizer scoliosis cast
   Risser turnbuckle cast
   Risser-Cotrel body cast
   SAE cast
   Sarmiento cast
   SBE cast
   semirigid fiberglass cast
   serial wedged cast
   short above-elbow cast
   short arm cylinder cast
   short arm navicular cast
   short below-elbow cast
   short leg cylinder cast
   short leg nonwalking cast
   short leg nonweightbearing
     cast
   short leg plaster cast
   short-arm cast (SAC)
   short-arm thumb spica cast
   short-leg cast (SLC)
   short-leg walking cast (SLWC)
   slipper cast
   spica cast

cast (*continued*)

   standard above-elbow cast
   sugar-tong cast
   supportive halo cast
   thumb spica cast
   toe spica cast
   total contact cast
   turnbuckle cast
   Univalve cast
   Unna boot cast
   Velpeau cast
   walking cast
   walking heel cast
   Warm N Form cast
   waxy cast
   well-leg cast
cast blade
cast boot
Cast Boot hip abduction brace
cast brace
cast breaker
cast cap splint
cast cells
cast cutter
Cast Gard cast protector
cast immobilization
cast iron struma
cast knife
cast liner
cast lingual splint
cast material
cast padding
cast removal
cast shoe
cast sock
cast spreader
cast syndrome
CastAlert device
Castallo eye speculum
Castallo eyelid retractor
Castallo lid retractor
Castallo refractor
Castallo retractor
Castallo speculum
Castanares bilateral blepharoplasty
Castanares facelift scissors
Castanares scissors
Castaneda anastomosis clamp
Castaneda cannula
Castaneda clamp
Castaneda infant sternal retractor
Castaneda multipurpose clamp

Castaneda partial-occlusion clamp
Castaneda procedure
Castaneda suture tag forceps
Castaneda vascular clamp
Castaneda vascular forceps
Castaneda-Malecot catheter
Castaneda-Mixter clamp
Castaneda-Mixter forceps
Castaneda-Mixter thoracic clamp
Castaway leg brace
Castech extremity support
Castellani paint
Castelli tube
Castelli-Paparella collar button
    tube
Castelli-Paparella myringotomy
    tube
Castens ascites trocar
Castens hydrocele trocar
Castens trocar
Castex rigid dressing
Casteyer prostatic punch
CastGuard
Castillo catheter
casting
    Cotrel casting
    Gumby technique for thumb
        casting
    Hexcelite intermediate phase
        casting
casting bone wax
casting machine
casting model
casting mold
casting tape
Castle laminectomy table
Castle procedure
Castle sterilizer
Castle surgical light
Castleman lymphoma
Castmate plaster bandage
    dressing
cast-molded PMMA intraocular
    lens
Castorit investment material
castration
Castro-Martinez keratome
Castroviejo acrylic eye implant
Castroviejo adjustable retractor
Castroviejo angled keratome
Castroviejo anterior synechia
    scissors

Castroviejo blade
Castroviejo blade holder
Castroviejo bladebreaker
Castroviejo bladebreaker knife
Castroviejo calipers
Castroviejo cannula
Castroviejo capsular forceps
Castroviejo capsule forceps
Castroviejo capsulotomy
Castroviejo clamp
Castroviejo clip-applying forceps
Castroviejo compressor
Castroviejo cornea-holding
    forceps
Castroviejo corneal dissector
Castroviejo corneal
    microscissors
Castroviejo corneal scissors
Castroviejo corneal section
    scissors
Castroviejo corneal transplant
    marker
Castroviejo corneal transplant
    scissors
Castroviejo corneal transplant
    trephine
Castroviejo corneal trephine
Castroviejo corneoscleral
    forceps
Castroviejo corneoscleral punch
Castroviejo corneoscleral suture
    forceps
Castroviejo cross-action capsular
    forceps
Castroviejo cyclodialysis cannula
Castroviejo cyclodialysis spatula
Castroviejo dermatome
Castroviejo dilator
Castroviejo discission knife
Castroviejo dissector
Castroviejo double-end dilator
Castroviejo double-end lacrimal
    dilator
Castroviejo double-end spatula
Castroviejo electrode
Castroviejo electromucotome
Castroviejo enucleation snare
Castroviejo erysiphake
Castroviejo eye calipers
Castroviejo eye speculum
Castroviejo eye suture forceps
Castroviejo fixation forceps

Castroviejo forceps
Castroviejo implant
Castroviejo iridectomy
Castroviejo iridocapsulotomy
    scissors
Castroviejo iris scissors
Castroviejo keratectomy
Castroviejo keratome
Castroviejo keratoplasty scissors
Castroviejo knife
Castroviejo lacrimal dilator
Castroviejo lacrimal sac probe
Castroviejo lens clamp
Castroviejo lens loop
Castroviejo lens loupe
Castroviejo lid forceps
Castroviejo lid retractor
Castroviejo marking calipers
Castroviejo microcorneal
    scissors
Castroviejo microneedle holder
Castroviejo microscissors
Castroviejo mosquito lid clamp
Castroviejo needle
Castroviejo needle holder
Castroviejo needle holder clamp
Castroviejo operation
Castroviejo ophthalmic knife
Castroviejo orbital aspirator
Castroviejo oscillating razor
Castroviejo punch
Castroviejo radial iridotomy
Castroviejo razor
Castroviejo razor blade
Castroviejo razor blade holder
Castroviejo razor bladebreaker
Castroviejo razor holder
Castroviejo refractor
Castroviejo retractor
Castroviejo scissors
Castroviejo scleral fold forceps
Castroviejo scleral marker
Castroviejo scleral shortening
    clip
Castroviejo sclerotome
Castroviejo section scissors
Castroviejo snare
Castroviejo snare enucleator
Castroviejo spatula
Castroviejo speculum
Castroviejo spoon
Castroviejo surface electrode

Castroviejo suture forceps
Castroviejo suturing forceps
Castroviejo synechia scissors
Castroviejo synechia spatula
Castroviejo tenotomy scissors
Castroviejo transplant forceps
Castroviejo transplant trephine
Castroviejo transplant-grafting
    capsule
Castroviejo transplant-grafting
    forceps
Castroviejo trephine
Castroviejo twin knife
Castroviejo tying forceps
Castroviejo Vital needle holder
Castroviejo vitreous-aspirating
    needle
Castroviejo wide grip handle
    forceps
Castroviejo-Arruga capsular
    forceps
Castroviejo-Arruga capsule
    forceps
Castroviejo-Arruga forceps
Castroviejo-Barraquer needle
    holder
Castroviejo-Barraquer speculum
Castroviejo-Colibri corneal
    forceps
Castroviejo-Furniss cornea-
    holding forceps
Castroviejo-Galezowski dilator
Castroviejo-Green needle holder
Castroviejo-Kalt needle holder
Castroviejo-Kalt traction handle
Castroviejo-McPherson
    keratectomy scissors
Castroviejo-Schacher angled
    calipers
Castroviejo-Scheie
    cyclodiathermy
Castroviejo-Simpson forceps
Castroviejo-Steinhauser
    mucotome
Castroviejo-Troutman needle
    holder
Castroviejo-Troutman scissors
Castroviejo-Vannas capsulotomy
    scissors
Castroviejo-Wheeler discission
    knife
cat cry syndrome

cat epithelium
CAT scan (computerized axial tomography scan)
CAT scanner
cat sneer exercise
catabolic condition
catabasial
Catalano capsular forceps
Catalano corneoscleral forceps
Catalano dilator
Catalano intubation set
Catalano muscle hook
Catalano needle holder
Catalano tubing
Catalano tying forceps
Catalyst machine
Catamaran swim plug
cataract
  adherent cataract
  adolescent cataract
  anterior polar cataract
  arborescent cataract
  axial cataract
  axial fusiform cataract
  bottlemakers cataract
  brunescent cataract
  calcareous cataract
  capsular cataract
  capsulolenticular cataract
  caseous cataract
  central cataract
  cerulean cataract
  cheesy cataract
  choroidal cataract
  complicated cataract
  contusion cataract
  coralliform cataract
  coralliformis cataract
  coronary cataract
  cortical cataract
  cryoextraction of cataract
  cupuliform cataract
  cystic cataract
  degenerative cataract
  developmental cataract
  diabetic cataract
  discission of cataract
  extracapsular extraction of cataract
  extraction of cataract
  fibroid cataract
  flap operation cataract

cataract (*continued*)
  floriform cataract
  fusiform cataract
  general cataract
  glassblowers cataract
  glaucomatous cataract
  hard cataract
  hedgers cataract
  heterochromic cataract
  hypermature cataract
  immature cataract
  incipient cataract
  infantile cataract
  intumescent cataract
  irradiation cataract
  Koby cataract
  lacteal cataract
  lamellar cataract
  lenticular cataract
  lightning cataract
  mature cataract
  membranous cataract
  mixed cataract
  morgagnian cataract
  myotonic cataract
  naphthalinic cataract
  needling of cataract
  nuclear cataract
  O'Brien cataract
  overripe cataract
  peripheral cataract
  polar cataract
  posterior subcapsular cataract (PSC)
  puddlers cataract
  punctate cataract
  pyramidal cataract
  ripe cataract
  rosette cataract
  sanguineous cataract
  secondary cataract
  sedimentary cataract
  senile cataract
  snowflake cataract
  snowstorm cataract
  Soemmering ring cataract
  spindle cataract
  spindle-shaped cataract
  stationary cataract
  stellate cataract
  subcapsular cataract
  sunflower cataract

cataract (*continued*)
　　sutural cataract
　　total cataract
　　traumatic cataract
　　unripe cataract
　　Vogt cataract
　　zonular cataract
cataract aspiration
cataract aspirator
cataract blade
cataract bur
cataract extraction
cataract extraction operation
cataract extractor
cataract flap operation
cataract formation
cataract irradiation
cataract knife
cataract knife guard
cataract lamp
cataract lens
cataract mask
cataract mask ring
cataract needle
cataract operation
cataract pencil
cataract probe
cataract procedure
cataract rotoextractor extractor
cataract scissors
cataract spoon
cataract suction unit
cataract surgery
cataract-aspirating cannula
cataract-aspirating needle
catarrh
　　atrophic catarrh
　　hypertrophic catarrh
　　nasal catarrh
　　postnasal catarrh
catarrhal
catarrhal inflammation
catarrhal otitis media
catastrophic brain damage
catastrophic brain injury
catastrophic event
catch-up growth
catenating
Catera suture anchor
caterpillar flap
catgut
　　absorbable catgut

catgut (*continued*)
　　chromic catgut
　　fast-absorbing catgut
　　fine plain catgut
　　formaldehyde catgut
　　iodine catgut
　　iodochromic catgut
　　Rica surgical catgut
　　SMIC surgical catgut
catgut ligature
catgut needle
catgut plain ties
catgut sutures (CGS)
cathartic colon
Cathcart endoprosthesis
Cathcart orthocentric hip
　　prosthesis
Cathelin segregator
cathematic catheter
catheter
　　2-way catheter
　　3-way catheter
　　3-way Foley catheter
　　3-way irrigating catheter
　　4-eye catheter
　　4-lumen polyvinyl
　　　　manometric catheter
　　4-wing catheter
　　4-wing Malecot retention
　　　　catheter
　　5-French angiographic catheter
　　5-French stiff catheter
　　6-eye catheter
　　7F Hydrolyser thrombectomy
　　　　catheter
　　8-lumen catheter
　　8-lumen esophageal
　　　　manometry catheter
　　8-lumen manometry catheter
　　A1 Port multipurpose
　　　　catheter
　　A2 Port multipurpose
　　　　catheter
　　Abbokinase catheter
　　Ablaser laser delivery catheter
　　ablation catheter
　　Abocath catheter
　　Abramson catheter
　　Abscession biliary drainage
　　　　catheter
　　Abscession fluid drainage
　　　　catheter

catheter (*continued*)
abscission catheter
Accu-Flo spring catheter
Accu-Flo ventricular catheter
Accurate catheter
ACE fixed-wire balloon catheter
Achiever balloon dilatation catheter
Ackrad balloon-bearing catheter
Ackrad Bronchitrac L suction catheter
Ackrad esophageal balloon catheter
Ackrad H/S Elliptosphere catheter
ACMI Alcock catheter
ACMI Bunts catheter
ACMI catheter
ACMI coated Foley catheter
ACMI Emmett hemostatic catheter
ACMI Owens catheter
ACMI positive pressure catheter
ACMI severance catheter
ACMI Thackston catheter
ACMI ureteral catheter
ACMI Word Bartholin gland catheter
Acmistat catheter
Acmix Foley catheter
acorn-tipped catheter
Acrad HS catheter (hysterosalpingography catheter)
ACS angioplasty catheter
ACS balloon catheter
ACS catheter
ACS Concorde coronary dilatation catheter
ACS Concorde dilatation catheter
ACS Concorde OTW catheter
ACS Endura coronary dilatation catheter
ACS Endura coronary dilation catheter
ACS exchange guiding catheter

catheter (*continued*)
ACS floppy-tip guiding catheter
ACS guiding catheter
ACS Hi-Torque Balance Middleweight catheter
ACS JL4 catheter
ACS JL4 French catheter
ACS Mini catheter
ACS Monorail perfusion balloon catheter
ACS OTW coronary dilatation catheter
ACS RX catheter
ACS RX coronary dilatation catheter
ACS Torquemaster catheter
Active Cath catheter
Acucise RP retrograde endopyelotomy catheter
AcuNav diagnostic ultrasound catheter
AcuNav ultrasound catheter
Adante PTCA balloon catheter
adapter catheter
Add-a-Cath catheter
Advance EX self-adhesive urinary external catheter
aero-flo tip catheter
AFocus catheter
afterloading catheter
AgX antimicrobial Foley catheter
Ahn thrombectomy catheter
Air-Lon inhalation catheter
AL-2 guiding catheter
AL-1 catheter
Alcock catheter
Alcock hemostatic catheter
Alcock return-flow hemostatic catheter
Alcott catheter
Alert-TD catheter
α demeure catheter
alignment catheter
alimentation catheter
Alliance catheter
Allis catheter
Alvarez-Rodriguez cardiac catheter
Alzate catheter
Amazr catheter

catheter (*continued*)

amber latex catheter
Amcath catheter
Amplatz aortography catheter
Amplatz cardiac catheter
Amplatz catheter
Amplatz coronary catheter
Amplatz femoral catheter
Amplatz Hi-Flo torque-control catheter
anchored catheter
Angiocath flexible catheter
Angiocath PRN catheter
Angioflow high-flow catheter
angiographic balloon occlusion catheter
angiographic catheter
angiography catheter
AngioJet thrombectomy catheter
Angio-Kit catheter
Angiomedics catheter
angiopigtail catheter
angioplasty balloon catheter
angioplasty guiding catheter
Angio-Seal catheter
angled balloon catheter
angled pigtail catheter
angle-tip urethral catheter
angulated catheter
Anthron heparinized catheter
Antibacterial personal catheter
antimicrobial catheter
Antron catheter
Anzio catheter
aortic catheter
aortogram catheter
aortography catheter
AR-1 catheter
AR-2 diagnostic catheter
AR-2 guiding catheter
Arani catheter
Arani double-loop guiding catheter
Arc-22 catheter
Argyle arterial catheter
Argyle catheter
Argyle Medicut R catheter
Argyle oxygen catheter
Argyle trocar catheter

catheter (*continued*)

Argyle umbilical wedge catheter
Arrow FlexTip Plus catheter
Arrow multilumen catheter
Arrow pulmonary artery catheter
Arrow QuadPolar electrode catheter
Arrow QuickFlash arterial catheter
Arrow TheraCath epidural catheter
Arrow TwinCath catheter
Arrow TwinCath multilumen peripheral catheter
Arrow 2-lumen hemodialysis catheter
Arrow-Berman balloon angioplasty catheter
Arrow-Berman balloon catheter
ArrowFlex intra-aortic balloon catheter
ArrowGard Blue antiseptic-coated catheter
ArrowGard Blue central venous catheter
ArrowGard Blue line catheter
ArrowGard central venous catheter
Arrow-Howes multilumen catheter
Arrow-Howes quad-lumen catheter
Arrow-Trerotola PTD catheter
arterial catheter
arterial embolectomy catheter
arterial irrigation catheter
arteriovenous catheter
ASC Monorel catheter
Ascent catheter
Ascent guiding catheter
Ash catheter
Ash Split Cath dual-lumen catheter
ASI uroplasty TCU dilatation catheter
Asuka PTCA catheter
atherectomy catheter
AtheroCath Bantam coronary atherectomy catheter

catheter (*continued*)

AtheroCath catheter
AtheroCath GTO coronary atherectomy catheter
AtheroCath spinning blade catheter
Atlantic ileostomy catheter
Atlantis SR coronary intravascular ultrasound catheter
Atlas balloon dilatation catheter
Atlas LP PTCA balloon dilatation catheter
Atlas ULP PTCA balloon dilatation catheter
Atrac multipurpose balloon catheter
Atrac-II double-balloon catheter
Atri-pace I bipolar flared pacing catheter
auricular appendage catheter
Auth atherectomy catheter
automatic catheter
autoperfusion balloon catheter
AV DeClot catheter
AV-Paceport thermodilution catheter
axillary catheter
Axiom DG balloon angioplasty catheter
Axxcess ureteral catheter
bag catheter
Bailey catheter
Bailey transthoracic catheter
bailout autoperfusion balloon catheter
bailout catheter
Baim catheter
Baim pacing catheter
Baim-Turi monitoring-pacing catheter
Balectrode pacing catheter
balloon angioplasty catheter
balloon biliary catheter
balloon catheter
balloon dilatation catheter
balloon dilating catheter
balloon embolectomy catheter

catheter (*continued*)

balloon flotation catheter
balloon valvuloplasty catheter
balloon wedge pressure catheter
balloon-flotation pacing catheter
balloon-imaging catheter
balloon-tipped angiographic catheter
balloon-tipped flow-directed catheter
ball-wedge catheter
Baltherm thermal dilution catheter
banana catheter
Bandit catheter
Banno catheter
Bard balloon-directed pacing catheter
Bard catheter
Bard disposable male external catheter
Bard electrophysiology catheter
Bard gastrostomy catheter
Bard guiding catheter
Bard helical catheter
Bard male external catheter
Bard sterile red rubber catheter
Bard Stinger S ablation catheter
Bard Touchless intermittent catheter
Bard x-ray ureteral catheter
Bardam catheter
Bardam red rubber catheter
Bardco catheter
Bardex all silicone sterile Foley catheter
Bardex catheter
Bardex Foley catheter
Bardex I.C. sterile Foley catheter
Bardex Lubricath Foley catheter
Bardex silicone Foley catheter
Bardex-Foley balloon catheter
Bardex-Foley return-flow retention catheter
Bardic catheter

catheter (*continued*)
Bardic cutdown catheter
Bardic translucent catheter
Bardic Uro Sheath reusable male external catheter
Bardic vein catheter
Bardic-Deseret Intracath catheter
Bard-U-Cath self-adhering male external catheter
Bartholin gland catheter
Baschui pigtail catheter
bat-wing catheter
Baxter angioplasty catheter
Baxter dilatation catheter
Baxter fiberoptic spectrophotometry catheter
Baxter V. Mueller catheter
BD Insyte Autoguard shielded intravenous catheter
Beird eye catheter
Benique catheter
Béniqué catheter
Béniqué catheter guide
Bentson-Hanafee-Wilson catheter
Berenstein guiding catheter
Berenstein occlusion balloon catheter
Berman angiographic catheter
Berman balloon flotation catheter
Berman cardiac catheter
Berman catheter
Bernstein catheter
Beta-Cap closure system for catheters
Beta-Cath catheter
Beta-Rail catheter
Bicor catheter
bicoudate catheter
bicoudé catheter
bifoil balloon catheter
biliary balloon catheter
biliary catheter
BioGlide catheter
Bio-Guard spectrum antimicrobial bonded catheter
Bio-Medicus arterial catheter
Biosearch female intermittent urinary catheter

catheter (*continued*)
Biosearch male intermittent urinary catheter
Biovue catheter
bipolar catheter
bipolar pacing catheter
bipolar pacing electrode catheter
bipolar temporary pacemaker catheter
bird's-eye catheter
Bi-Set catheter
Bitome catheter
Bivona epistaxis catheter
bladder catheter
blade septostomy catheter
Blasucci catheter
Blasucci curved-tip ureteral catheter
Blasucci pigtail ureteral catheter
Blasucci ureteral catheter
Block right coronary guiding catheter
blood-contacting catheter
Blue FlexTip catheter
Blue Max balloon catheter
Blue Max triple-lumen catheter
Bonnano catheter
Bonnie balloon catheter
Borge catheter
Boston Scientific Sonicath imaging catheter
Bourassa catheter
Bozeman catheter
Bozeman-Fritsch catheter
BPS spinal angiographic catheter
Braasch bulb catheter
Braasch bulb ureteral catheter
Braasch catheter
Braasch ureteral catheter
brachial coronary catheter
braided diagnostic catheter
Bresgen catheter
Brevis-Kaith epidural catheter
Brockenbrough catheter
Brockenbrough mapping catheter
Brockenbrough modified bipolar catheter

catheter (*continued*)

Brockenbrough transseptal catheter
Brodney catheter
bronchial catheter
Bronchitrac L catheter
Bronchitrac L flexible suction catheter
bronchospirometric catheter
Broviac atrial catheter
Broviac catheter
Broviac hyperalimentation catheter
Buchbinder catheter
Buchbinder Omniflex catheter
Buchbinder Thruflex OTW catheter
BUD drainage catheter
Buerhenne catheter
bulb catheter
bulb ureteral catheter
bulbous catheter
bullet tip catheter
Bunt catheter
bur-bearing catheter
Burhenne steerable catheter
butterfly catheter
bypass graft catheter
bypass Speedy balloon catheter
C.R. Bard catheter
Calypso Rely catheter
cam blade-tipped catheter
Camino catheter
Camino intracranial catheter
Camino micromanometer catheter
Camino microventricular bolt catheter
Camino transducer catheter
Campbell catheter
Campbell infant catheter
Campbell ureteral catheter
Campbell urethral catheter
cannulation catheter
Can-Opt stand-alone dual lumen ERCP catheter
Cardiac Assist intra-aortic balloon catheter
cardiac catheter
cardiac infant catheter

catheter (*continued*)

Cardio Tactilaze peripheral angioplasty laser catheter
Cardiomarker catheter
Cardiomed Bodysoft epidural catheter
Cardiomed endotracheal ventilation catheter
Cardiomed thermodilution catheter
Carlens bronchospirometric catheter
Carlens catheter
Carson catheter
Carson model catheter
Carson Zero Tip balloon dilatation catheter
Castaneda-Malecot catheter
Castillo catheter
cathematic catheter
Cath-Finder catheter
Cath-Guide closed suction catheter
CathLink 20 catheter
Cathlon IV catheter
Cathmark suction catheter
Caud-a-Kaith epidural catheter
caval catheter
Cayote OTW balloon catheter
Combo catheter
cecostomy catheter
central catheter
central venous catheter
central venous pressure catheter
cephalad catheter
Cereblate catheter
cerebral catheter
C-Flex catheter
Chaffin catheter
Chaffin tube catheter
Cheetah angioplasty catheter
Chemo-Port catheter
Chilli cooled ablation catheter
cholangiocath catheter
cholangiographic catheter
cholangiography catheter
Cholangiolapcath catheter
chorionic villus sampling catheter
Chubby balloon catheter
Cisco covered needle catheter

catheter (*continued*)

cisterna magna catheter
Clark expanding mesh catheter
Clark helix catheter
Clark rotating cutter catheter
Clay Adams PE-series catheter
Clear Advantage latex free
  catheter
Clear Advantage silicone male
  catheter
CliniCath catheter
CliniCath peripherally
  inserted catheter
cloverleaf catheter
cloverleaf EP catheter
coaxial catheter
Cobe-Tenckhoff peritoneal
  dialysis catheter
cobra catheter
cobra OTW balloon catheter
cobra-shaped catheter
Codman ventricular silicone
  catheter
Codman-Holter catheter
coil catheter
Coil-Cath catheter
coil-tipped catheter
colon motility catheter
combination biliary brush
  catheter
Comfort Cath I, II catheter
Conceptus Soft Seal cervical
  catheter
Conceptus Soft torque uterine
  catheter
Conceptus VS catheter
condom catheter
conductance catheter
cone tip catheter
conformation of right heart
  catheter
conical catheter
conical-tip catheter
Constantine catheter
Constantine flexible metal
  catheter
ConstaVac catheter
Constellation mapping
  catheter
continuous irrigation catheter
Contour balloon dilatation
  catheter

catheter (*continued*)

Conveen curved-tapered
  intermittent catheter
Conveen female intermittent
  catheter
Conveen Security self-sealing
  male external catheter
Cook arterial catheter
Cook Cardiovascular infusion
  catheter
Cook catheter
Cook pigtail catheter
Cook Spectrum catheter
Cook TPN catheter
Cook yellow pigtail catheter
Cool Tip catheter
Cooled ThermoCath catheter
Cope loop nephrostomy
  catheter
Cordis BriteTip guiding
  catheter
Cordis catheter
Cordis Ducor I, II, III coronary
  catheter
Cordis Ducor pigtail catheter
Cordis guiding catheter
Cordis Lumelec catheter
Cordis pigtail catheter
Cordis Predator balloon
  catheter
Cordis Predator PTCA balloon
  catheter
Cordis Son-II catheter
Cordis Titan balloon dilatation
  catheter
Cordis Trakstar PTCA balloon
  catheter
Cordis TransTaper tip catheter
Cordis Webster diagnostic-
  ablation deflectable tip
  catheter
Cordis Webster mapping
  catheter
Corlon catheter
coronary angiographic
  catheter
coronary catheter
coronary dilatation catheter
coronary guiding catheter
coronary seeking catheter
coronary sinus
  thermodilution catheter

catheter (*continued*)

corset balloon catheter

Cotton graduated dilation catheter

coudé catheter

coudé assist catheter

coudé catheter

coudé suction catheter

coudé urethral catheter

coudé-tip catheter

coudé-tip demeure catheter

Councill catheter

Councill retention catheter

Cournand catheter

Cournand quadpolar catheter

Coxeter catheter

Coxeter prostatic catheter

CPV catheter

Cribier-Letac catheter

CritiCath PA catheter

CritiCath thermodilution catheter

Critikon balloon temporary pacing catheter

Critikon balloon thermodilution catheter

Critikon balloon wedge pressure catheter

Critikon balloon-tipped endhole catheter

Critikon catheter

Critikon-Berman angiographic balloon catheter

CrossSail coronary dilatation catheter

CrossSail coronary dilation catheter

cryoablation catheter

CryoCath catheter

CUI catheter

Cummings catheter

Cummings 4-wing catheter

Cummings 4-wing Malecot retention catheter

Cummings nephrostomy catheter

Cummings-Pezzer catheter

cup catheter

Curl Cath catheter

curved catheter

cutdown catheter

catheter (*continued*)

CVIS intravascular US imaging catheter

CVP catheter

CVS catheter

Cynosar catheter

Cystocath catheter

Dacron catheter

Dakin catheter

Damato curved catheter

Datascope catheter

Datascope percutaneous translucent balloon catheter

Datascope intra-aortic balloon pump catheter

Datascope true sheathless catheter

Davis catheter

Davol catheter

Davol rubber catheter

Davol sterile red rubber catheter

de Pezzer catheter

de Pezzer mushroom-tipped catheter

de Pezzer self-retaining catheter

Dearor model catheter

decapolar electrode catheter

decapolar pacing catheter

decompression catheter

decompression-feeding catheter

decompressive enteroclysis catheter

deflectable quadripolar catheter

DeKock 2-way bronchial catheter

Delcath double-balloon catheter

DeLee catheter

DeLee infant catheter

DeLee tracheal catheter

demeare catheter

Dent sleeve catheter

DeOrio intrauterine insemination catheter

Derek-Harwood-Nash catheter

Desai VectorCath catheter

Deseret flow-directed thermodilution catheter

catheter (*continued*)

Desert catheter
Desilets catheter
Desilets-Hoffman catheter
Devonshire catheter
Devonshire-Mack catheter
DeWeese caval catheter
Diaflex ureteral dilatation catheter
diagnostic catheter
diagnostic ultrasound imaging catheter
Dialy-Nate catheter
dialysis catheter
Diasonics catheter
Digiflex high-flow catheter
dilatation balloon catheter
dilating catheter
dilating pressure balloon catheter
dilation catheter
dilator catheter
Dispatch infusion catheter
disposable catheter
distal catheter
DLP cardioplegic catheter
DLP infant ventricular catheter
DLP left atrial pressure monitoring catheter
Dobbhoff catheter
dog-leg catheter
Doppler coronary catheter
Dormia stone basket catheter
Dorros brachial internal mammary guiding catheter
Dorros infusion and probing catheter
Dorros infusion-probing catheter
Dorros probing catheter
Dotter caged-balloon catheter
Dotter coaxial catheter
double-chip micromanometer catheter
double-current catheter
double-J indwelling catheter
double-J ureteral catheter
double-lumen balloon stone extractor catheter
double-lumen Broviac catheter

catheter (*continued*)

double-lumen catheter
double-lumen Hickman catheter
double-lumen Hickman-Broviac catheter
double-lumen Silastic catheter
double-lumen subclavian catheter
double-lumen Swan-Ganz catheter
double-thermistor coronary sinus catheter
Dover silicone Foley catheter
Dover catheter
Dover Premium Teflon-coated latex Foley catheter
Dover Teflon-coated latex Foley catheter
Dover Texas Catheter Disposable Male Catheter
Dow Corning catheter
Dow Corning ileal pouch catheter
Dowd II prostatic balloon dilatation catheter
drainage catheter
Drew-Smythe catheter
drill-tip catheter
Du Pen catheter
dual-lumen catheter
dual-sensor micromanometric high-fidelity catheter
Dualtherm dual-thermistor thermodilution catheter
Ducor angiographic catheter
Ducor balloon catheter
Ducor cardiac catheter
Ducor HF catheter
Ducor-Cordis pigtail catheter
duo-decapolar catheter
Duo-Flow catheter
DURAglide stone balloon catheter
DURAglide stone removal balloon catheter
DVI Simpson AtheroCath catheter
Dynacor Foley catheter
Dynacor suction catheter
EAC catheter
Easy catheter

catheter (*continued*)

Easy Rider neurovascular catheter
E-cath catheter
echo catheter
echo transponder electrode catheter
EchoMark angiographic catheter
EchoMark catheter
EchoMark salpingography catheter
Edge dilatation catheter
EDM infusion catheter
Edslab catheter
Edslab cholangiography catheter
Edwards catheter
Edwards diagnostic catheter
Ehrlich catheter
Eichelter-Schenk vena cava catheter
EID percutaneous central venous large-bore catheter
El Gamal coronary bypass catheter
El Gamal guiding catheter
elbowed catheter
Elecath catheter
Elecath electrophysiologic stimulation catheter
Elecath thermodilution catheter
electrode catheter
electrohemostasis catheter
Elite guide catheter
embolectomy catheter
en chemise catheter
Encapsulon epidural catheter
Endeavor nondetachable silicone balloon catheter
end-hole balloon-tipped catheter
end-hole catheter
end-hole fluid-filled catheter
end-hole French catheter
end-hole pigtail catheter
end-hole ureteral catheter
EndoCPB catheter
endoscopic retrograde cholangiopancreatography catheter

catheter (*continued*)

EndoSonics balloon dilatation catheter
EndoSound endoscopic ultrasound catheter
Endotak C lead catheter
Endotak Catheter lead catheter
endotracheal catheter
Endura dilatation catheter
Enhanced Torque 8F guiding catheter
Enhanced Torque guiding catheter
EnSite cardiac catheter
Entact dilation and occlusion catheter
Envy catheter
Eppendorfer cardiac catheter
Eppendorfer catheter
EPTFE ventricular shunt catheter
ERCP catheter
ERCPeel Away catheter
Erythroflex catheter
Erythroflex hydromer-coated central venous catheter
esophageal balloon catheter
esophageal manometry catheter
esophageal perfusion catheter
esophagoscopic catheter
eustachian catheter
Everyday self-adhering urinary external catheter
Everett eustachian catheter
Everett fallopian catheter
Evermed catheter
Evert-O-Cath
Evert-O-Cath drug delivery catheter
exdwelling ureteral occlusion balloon catheter
expandable access catheter
Explorer pre-curved diagnostic EP catheter
Express OTW balloon catheter
Express PTCA catheter
Extended Wear self-adhering urinary external catheter
external ureteral catheter

catheter (*continued*)

Extractor 3-lumen retrieval balloon catheter
ExtraSafe catheter
Extreme laser catheter
extrusion balloon catheter
E-Z Cath catheter
FACT catheter
FACT coronary balloon angioplasty catheter
FACT-22 catheter
Falcon coronary catheter
Falcon single-operator exchange balloon catheter
fallopian catheter
FAST balloon catheter (flow-assisted, short-term balloon catheter)
FAST balloon flotation catheter
FAST right heart cardiovascular catheter
FasTracker-18 infusion catheter
faucial catheter
faucial eustachian catheter
female catheter
femoral cerebral catheter
femoral guiding catheter
femoral hemodialysis catheter
fenestrated catheter
Feth-R-Cath epidural catheter
Feth-R-Kath epidural catheter
fiberoptic oximeter catheter
fiberoptic pressure catheter
filiform catheter
filiform-tipped catheter
fine-bore catheter
Finesse guiding catheter
Finesse large-lumen guiding catheter
flat-blade-tipped catheter
Flex-Cath double-lumen intra-aortic balloon catheter
Flexguard tip catheter
flexible catheter
flexible metal catheter
Flexi-Cath double-lumen intra-aortic balloon catheter
Flexitip catheter
Flexxicon Blue catheter

catheter (*continued*)

Flexxicon Blue dialysis catheter
Flexxicon catheter
Flexxicon II PC internal jugular catheter
floating catheter
flotation catheter
Flow Rider flow-directed catheter
Flow Rider neurovascular catheter
flow-assisted short-term balloon catheter
flow-directed balloon cardiovascular catheter
flow-directed balloon-tipped catheter
flow-directed catheter
FloWire Doppler catheter
flow-oximetry catheter
fluid-filled balloon-tipped flow-directed catheter
fluid-filled catheter
Focus -PV balloon catheter
Fogarty adherent clot catheter
Fogarty arterial embolectomy catheter
Fogarty anterior irrigation catheter
Fogarty balloon biliary catheter
Fogarty balloon catheter
Fogarty catheter
Fogarty dilation catheter
Fogarty embolus catheter
Fogarty gallstone catheter
Fogarty graft thrombectomy catheter
Fogarty irrigation catheter
Fogarty occlusion catheter
Fogarty Thru-Lumen catheter
Fogarty venous irrigation catheter
Fogarty venous thrombectomy catheter
Fogarty-Chin catheter
Fogarty-Chin extrusion balloon catheter
Fogarty-Chin peripheral dilatation catheter
Folatex catheter

catheter (*continued*)

Foley acorn-bulb catheter
Foley balloon catheter
Foley catheter
Foley cone-tip catheter
Foley 3-way catheter
Foley-Alcock bag catheter
Foley-Alcock catheter
Foltz catheter
Foltz-Overton cardiac catheter
Force balloon dilatation
    catheter
ForeRunner coronary sinus
    guiding catheter
Formex barium catheter
Fountain infusion catheter
Franz monophasic action
    potential catheter
Freedom external catheter
Freedom Pak Seven catheter
Freeway PTCA catheter
French angiographic catheter
French catheter
French Cope loop
    nephrostomy catheter
French curve out-of-plane
    catheter
French double-lumen catheter
French Foley catheter
French Gesco catheter
French in-plane guiding
    catheter
French JR4 Schneider catheter
French MBIH catheter
French mushroom-tipped
    catheter
French pigtail nephrostomy
    catheter
French red-rubber Robinson
    catheter
French Robinson catheter
French SAL catheter
French shaft catheter
French Silastic Foley catheter
French sizing of catheter
French Teflon pyeloureteral
    catheter
French tripolar His catheter
Friend catheter
Friend-Hebert catheter
Fritsch catheter
Frydman catheter

catheter (*continued*)

FullFlow catheter
FullFlow perfusion dilation
    catheter
Furniss catheter
Furniss female catheter
fused-tip catheter
Gambro catheter
Ganz-Edwards coronary
    infusion catheter
Garceau catheter
Garceau ureteral catheter
gastroenterostomy catheter
Gauder Silicon PEG catheter
Gauderer-Ponsky catheter
Gazelle balloon dilatation
    catheter
Geenan graduated dilation
    catheter
Gensini catheter
Gensini coronary
    arteriography catheter
Gensini Teflon catheter
Gentle-Flo suction catheter
Gesco catheter
Gibbon catheter
Gibbon urethral catheter
Gilbert balloon catheter
Gilbert catheter
Gilbert pediatric balloon
    catheter
Gilbert pediatric catheter
Gilbert plug-sealing catheter
Gilbert-type Bardex Foley
    catheter
Gizmo catheter
Glidecath hydrophilic coated
    catheter
Glidewire catheter
Glidex coated Percuflex
    catheter
Glo-Tip ERCP catheter
Goeltec catheter
Gold Probe bipolar
    hemostasis catheter
Gold Probe electrohemostasis
    catheter
Goodale-Lubin cardiac
    catheter
Goodale-Lubin catheter
Gore-Tex catheter
Gore-Tex peritoneal catheter

catheter (*continued*)
Gorlin catheter
Gorlin pacing catheter
Gould PentaCath 5-lumen
  thermodilution catheter
Gould PentaCath
  thermodilution catheter
Gouley catheter
Gouley whalebone filiform
  catheter
Goutz catheter
graduated catheter
graduated-sized catheter
Graft ACE fixed-wire balloon
  catheter
graft-seeker catheter
graft-seeking catheter
Graham catheter
Greenfield caval catheter
Grigor fiberoptic guiding
  catheter
Grollman catheter
Grollman pigtail catheter
Grollman pulmonary artery-
  seeking catheter
Groshong catheter
Groshong double-lumen
  catheter
Gruentzig 20-30 dilating
  catheter
Gruentzig arterial balloon
  catheter
Gruentzig balloon
  angiography catheter
Gruentzig balloon catheter
Gruentzig catheter
Gruentzig D dilating catheter
Gruentzig D-G dilating
  catheter
Gruentzig Dilaca catheter
Gruentzig G dilating catheter
Gruentzig S dilating catheter
Gruentzig steerable catheter
Gruentzig balloon catheter
Guardian catheter
guide catheter
Guidefather catheter
guiding catheter
Guyon ureteral catheter
GyneSys Dx diagnostic
  catheter
H-1 catheter

catheter (*continued*)
Hagner bag catheter
Hagner catheter
Hakim catheter
Hakko Dwellcath catheter
Halo catheter
Halo XP catheter
Halocath catheter
Hamilton-Steward catheter
Hanafee catheter
Hancock embolectomy
  catheter
Hancock fiberoptic catheter
Hancock hydrogen detection
  catheter
Hancock luminal
  electrophysiologic
  recording catheter
Hancock thermodilution
  catheter
Hancock wedge-pressure
  catheter
Harris catheter
Harris uterine injector
  catheter
Hartmann catheter
Hartmann eustachian catheter
Hartzler ACS coronary dilation
  catheter
Hartzler ACX II catheter
Hartzler balloon catheter
Hartzler catheter
Hartzler dilatation catheter
Hartzler Excel catheter
Hartzler LPS dilatation
  catheter
Hartzler Micro catheter
Hartzler Micro II catheter
Hartzler Micro XT catheter
Hartzler Micro-600 catheter
Hartzler RX-14 balloon
  catheter
Hartzler Ultra Lo-Profile
  catheter
Hassan catheter
Hatch catheter
headhunter catheter
headhunter visceral
  angiography catheter
HealthShield antimicrobial
  mediastinal wound drainage
  catheter

catheter (*continued*)
   HealthShield catheter
   Heartport Endocoronary Sinus
      catheter
   helical catheter
   helical PTCA dilatation
      catheter
   helical-tip Halo catheter
   helium-filled balloon catheter
   Helix PTCA dilatation
      catheter
   Hemo-Cath catheter
   hemodialysis catheter
   Hemoject injection catheter
   hemostatic catheter
   Hepacon catheter
   heparin-coated catheter
   hexapolar catheter
   Heyer-Schulte catheter
   Heyer-Schulte-Pudenz cardiac
      catheter
   H-H open-end alimentation
      catheter
   Hi5 Torq Flow catheter
   Hickman catheter
   Hickman indwelling catheter
   Hickman indwelling right
      atrial catheter
   Hickman tunneled catheter
   Hickman-Broviac catheter
   Hidalgo catheter
   Hieshima coaxial catheter
   Higgins catheter
   high-fidelity catheter
   high-fidelity micromanometric
      catheter
   high-flow catheter
   high-speed rotation dynamic
      angioplasty catheter
   Hilal modified headhunter
      catheter
   His bundle catheter
   His catheter
   Hi-Torque floppy guide
      catheter
   Hobbs dilatation balloon
      catheter
   hockey-stick catheter
   Hohn catheter
   Hohn central venous catheter
   Hollister catheter
   Hollister external catheter

catheter (*continued*)
   Hollister self-adhesive
      catheter
   Holt self-retaining catheter
   Holter distal atrial catheter
   Holter distal peritoneal
      catheter
   Holter lumboperitoneal
      catheter
   Holter ventricular catheter
   Holter-Hausner catheter
   hooked catheter
   Hopkins Percuflex drainage
      catheter
   hot-tipped catheter
   Hryntschak catheter
   HUI catheter
   Huibregtse-Katon ERCP
      catheter
   Hunter-Sessions vena cava-
      occluding balloon catheter
   Hurwitt catheter
   Hurwitz dialysis catheter
   Hyams catheter
   HydraCross TLC PTCA
      catheter
   HydroCath central venous
      catheter
   Hydrogel-coated PTCA
      balloon catheter
   Hydromer grafted catheter
   hydrostatic balloon catheter
   Hymes double-lumen catheter
   hyperalimentation catheter
   hysterosalpingography
      catheter
   IAB catheter (intra-aortic
      balloon catheter)
   ICP catheter
   ICP-T fiberoptic ICP
      monitoring catheter
   Illumen-8 guiding catheter
   Illumen-9 guiding catheter
   ILUS catheter
   Imager Torque selective
      catheter
   imaging-angioplasty balloon
      catheter
   Impersol catheter
   implantable cardioverter-
      defibrillator catheter
   Impra peritoneal catheter

catheter (*continued*)

InDura catheter
indwelling catheter
indwelling Foley catheter
indwelling silicone catheter
indwelling subclavian
    catheter
indwelling venous catheter
infant catheter
infant female catheter
infant male catheter
inferior vena cava catheter
Infiniti catheter
inflatable catheter
inflatable Foley bag catheter
Infusaid catheter
InfusaSleeve II catheter
Infuse-a-Port catheter
infusion catheter
Ingram catheter
injection electrode catheter
Inmed whistle tip urethral
    catheter
Innervision ventricular
    catheter
Inoue balloon catheter
insertion of catheter
inside-the-needle catheter (INC)
inside-the-needle infusion
    catheter
Insuflon catheter
Insure-A-Cath catheter
Insyte AutoGuard catheter
Intact catheter
Integra catheter
Intellicath pulmonary artery
    catheter
intercostal catheter
internal mammary artery
    catheter
Interpret ultrasound catheter
interventional catheter
Intimax biliary catheter
Intimax cholangiography
    catheter
Intimax occlusion catheter
Intimax vascular catheter
intra-aortic balloon catheter
intra-arterial chemotherapy
    catheter
intracardiac catheter
Intracath catheter

catheter (*continued*)

intracoronary guiding catheter
intracoronary perfusion
    catheter
intracranial pressure catheter
Intraducer peritoneal catheter
intraductal imaging catheter
intramedullary catheter
Intran disposable intrauterine
    pressure measurement
    catheter
Intran intrauterine pressure
    measurement catheter
intrapleural catheter
Intrasil catheter
intraurethral prostatic bridge
    catheter
intrauterine catheter
intrauterine insemination
    catheter
intrauterine pressure catheter
intravascular ultrasound
    catheter
intravenous catheter
intravenous pacing catheter
intravenous ultrasound
    catheter
intraventricular pressure
    monitoring catheter
Intrepid balloon catheter
Intrepid percutaneous
    transluminal coronary
    angioplasty catheter
Intrepid PTCA catheter
introducer catheter
irrigating catheter
irrigation catheter
Itard catheter
Itard eustachian catheter
ITC radiopaque balloon
    catheter
IUI catheter
IV catheter
IVUS catheter
Jackman coronary sinus
    electrode catheter
Jackson orthogonal catheter
Jackson-Pratt catheter
Jacques catheter
Jaeger-Whiteley catheter
James lumbar peritoneal
    catheter

catheter (*continued*)

Javid catheter
JB catheter
JB-1 catheter
Jehle coronary perfusion
  catheter
Jelco catheter
Jelco intravenous catheter
Jelm catheter
Jelm two-way catheter
Jinotti dual-purpose catheter
JL catheter
JL-4 catheter (Judkins left,
  4 cm)
JL-5 catheter (Judkins left,
  5 cm)
Jocath Maestro coronary
  balloon catheter
Jography angiographic
  catheter
Joguide coronary guiding
  catheter
Jo-Kath catheter
Josephson catheter
Josephson quadripolar
  catheter
Jostra catheter
JR catheter
JR-4 catheter (Judkins right,
  4 cm)
JR-5 catheter (Judkins right,
  5 cm)
Judkins catheter
Judkins coronary catheter
  (left/right)
Judkins curve LAD catheter
Judkins curve LCX catheter
Judkins curve STD catheter
Judkins guiding catheter
Judkins left coronary catheter
Judkins right coronary
  catheter
Judkins torque-control
  catheter
Judkins USCI catheter
jugular venous catheter
J-Vac catheter
Kaminsky catheter
Karmen catheter
Katon catheter
Katzen long balloon dilatation
  catheter

catheter (*continued*)

Kaufman catheter
Kearns bag catheter
Kensey atherectomy catheter
kidney internal splint catheter
  (KISS catheter)
kidney internal stent catheter
  (KISS catheter)
kidney internal stent catheter
Kifa catheter
Kifia catheter
Kimball catheter
Kimny catheter
King catheter
King guiding catheter
King multipurpose catheter
King multipurpose coronary
  graft catheter
kink-resistant catheter
kink-resistant peritoneal
  catheter
Kinsey atherectomy catheter
Kish urethral catheter
KISS catheter (kidney internal
  splint/stent catheter)
Koala intrauterine pressure
  catheter
Konigsberg catheter
Kontron catheter
Kontron balloon catheter
Kumpe catheter
Lacricath lacrimal duct
  catheter
lacrimal balloon catheter
Lahey catheter
Landmark midline catheter
Lane catheter
Lane rectal catheter
laparoscopic
  cholangiographic catheter
Lapides catheter
Lapras catheter
large-bore catheter
large-lumen catheter
laser catheter
laser delivery catheter
latex catheter
Latis catheter
Latis dual-lumen graft-cleaning
  catheter
Latson multipurpose catheter
lavaging catheter

catheter (*continued*)

L-Cath peripherally inserted neonatal catheter
Ledor pigtail catheter
LeFort catheter
LeFort male catheter
LeFort urethral catheter
left coronary catheter
left heart catheter
left Judkins catheter
left ventricular clamp catheter
left ventricular sump catheter
Lehman aortographic catheter
Lehman catheter
Lehman pancreatic manometry catheter
Lehman ventriculography catheter
LeMaitre biliary catheter
lensed fiber-tip laser delivery catheter
Leonard catheter
Leroy catheter
LeRoy ventricular catheter
LeVeen catheter
Levin tube catheter
Leycom volume conductance catheter
Lifecath catheter
LifeJet high-flow chronic dialysis catheter
Lifemed catheter
Lifestream coronary dilatation catheter
Lifestream coronary dilation catheter
Lillehei-Warden catheter
Lincoff design of Storz scleral buckling balloon catheter
Lionheart catheter
Livewire Duo-Decapolar catheter
Livewire TC Compass ablation catheter
Lloyd bronchial catheter
Lloyd catheter
Lloyd double catheter
Lloyd esophagoscopic catheter
lobster-tail catheter
Lofric disposable urethral catheter

catheter (*continued*)

long ACE fixed-wire balloon catheter
Long Brite Tip guiding catheter
Long Skinny OTW balloon catheter
Longdwel catheter
Longdwel Teflon catheter
long-term internal jugular catheter
Lo-Profile balloon catheter
Lo-Profile II balloon catheter
Lo-Profile steerable dilatation catheter
low-profile balloon-positioning catheter
low-speed rotation angioplasty catheter
LPS catheter
Lucae eustachian catheter
Lumaguide infusion catheter
lumbar peritoneal catheter
lumbar subarachnoid catheter
Lumelec catheter
Lumelec pacing catheter
Lunderquist catheter
Lynx OTW catheter
Lynx OTW balloon catheter
Magill endotracheal catheter
Maglinte catheter
magnet-tipped flexible catheter
Mahurkar catheter
Mahurkar curved extension catheter
Mahurkar dual-lumen catheter
Mahurkar dual-lumen dialysis catheter
Mahurkar dual-lumen femoral catheter
Mahurkar dual-lumen femoral dialysis catheter
male catheter
Malecot 2-wing catheter
Malecot 4-wing catheter
Malecot catheter
Malecot nephrostomy catheter
Malecot reentry catheter
Malecot self-retaining urethral catheter

catheter (*continued*)

Malecot Silastic catheter
Malecot suprapubic cystostomy catheter
Malecot urethral catheter
Mallinckrodt angiographic catheter
Mallinckrodt catheter
Mallinckrodt vertebral catheter
Maloney catheter
Manashil sialography catheter
Mandelbaum catheter
Manhurkar catheter
Mani catheter
Mani cerebral catheter
manometer-tipped catheter
manometric catheter
Mansfield Atri-Pace 1 catheter
Mansfield balloon catheter
Mansfield balloon dilatation catheter
Mansfield dilatation balloon catheter
Mansfield orthogonal electrode catheter
Mansfield Scientific dilatation balloon catheter
Mansfield-Webster catheter
Mansfield-Webster deflectable curve catheter
mapping catheter
mapping-ablation catheter
Marathon guiding catheter
Marinr catheter
Mark IV Moss decompression-feeding catheter
marker catheter
Marlin thoracic catheter
Marrs intrauterine catheter
Maryfield introducer catheter
mastoid catheter
Maverick balloon dilatation catheter
Max Force balloon dilatation catheter
Max Force catheter
Max Force TTS biliary balloon dilatation catheter
Maxxum balloon catheter
McCarthy catheter
McCaskey antral catheter

catheter (*continued*)

McCaskey catheter
McGoon coronary perfusion catheter
McIntosh double-lumen catheter
McIntosh double-lumen hemodialysis catheter
McIver catheter
McIver nephrostomy catheter
Meadox Surgimed catheter
measuring-mounting catheter
Med-Co flexible catheter
Medcomp catheter
Medena continent ileostomy catheter
mediastinal catheter
Medicut catheter
Medina catheter
Medina ileostomy catheter
MediPort-DL double-lumen catheter
Meditech arterial dilatation catheter
Meditech balloon catheter
Meditech catheter
Meditech Mansfield dilating catheter
Medi-tech occlusion balloon catheter
Meditech steerable catheter
Medrad catheter
Medtronic balloon catheter
Medtronic Transvene electrode catheter
MegaSonics PTCA catheter
Memokath catheter
memory catheter
Menlo Care catheter
Mentor coudé catheter
Mentor Foley catheter
Mentor Self-Cath soft catheter
Mentor straight catheter
Mentor Tele-Cath ileal conduit sampling catheter
Mentor-Urosan external catheter
Mercator catheter
Mercier catheter
metal ball-tip catheter
metal catheter
metallic-tip catheter

catheter (*continued*)

Metaport catheter
Metras bronchial catheter
Metras catheter
metro catheter
Mewissen infusion catheter
Micro catheter
Micro-Guide catheter
microinvasive catheter
micromanometer catheter
micromanometer-tip catheter
MicroMewi multiple sidehole
    infusion catheter
MicroMewi multi-sidehole
    infusion catheter
Micro-Soft Stream sidehole
    infusion catheter
Microsoftrac catheter
MicroTip catheter
Micro-Transducer catheter
MicroVac catheter
Microvasive Rigiflex balloon
    catheter
MicroView sheath-based
    catheter
microendoscopic optical
    catheter
midstream aortogram catheter
Mikaelsson catheter
Mikro-Tip micromanometer-
    tipped catheter
Millar catheter
Millar Doppler catheter
Millar micromanometer
    catheter
Millar pigtail angiographic
    catheter
Millar urodynamic catheter
Millenia balloon catheter
Miller septostomy catheter
Miller-Abbott catheter
Mills operative peripheral
    angioplasty catheter
MiniBard catheter
Mini-Profile dilatation catheter
Minispace catheter
Mirage OTW balloon catheter
Missouri catheter
Mitsubishi angioscopic
    catheter
Mixter catheter
Molina needle catheter

catheter (*continued*)

MoniTorr CIP lumbar catheter
monofoil catheter
Monorail angioplasty catheter
Monorail catheter
Monorail imaging catheter
Monorail Piccolino catheter
Morris catheter
Morris thoracic catheter
Moss decompression feeding
    catheter
Moss Suction Buster catheter
MP-A-1 catheter
MP-A-2 catheter
MPF catheter
MPR drain catheter
MS Classique balloon
    dilatation catheter
MTC Ventcontrol ventricular
    catheter
Mueller catheter
Mullins transseptal catheter
multi-access catheter
multielectrode basket
    catheter
multielectrode impedance
    catheter
multiflanged Portnoy catheter
Multiflex catheter
multilayer design catheter
multilumen catheter
multilumen manometric
    catheter
Multi-Med triple-lumen
    catheter
Multi-Med triple-lumen
    infusion catheter
multiplex catheter
multipolar electrode catheter
multipolar impedance
    catheter
multipurpose catheter
multisensor catheter
Multistim electrode catheter
mushroom catheter
Mylar catheter
Mystic balloon catheter
Namic catheter
NarrowFlex intra-aortic
    balloon catheter
nasal catheter
nasobiliary catheter

catheter (*continued*)

nasocystic catheter
nasopancreatic catheter
nasotracheal catheter
nasovesicular catheter
NavAblator catheter
Naviport hollow-lumen
  guiding catheter
NBIH catheter
NC Bandit catheter
NC Big Ranger OTW balloon
  catheter
NDSB occlusion balloon
  catheter
Neal catheter
needle tip catheter
Neonatal Y TrachCare catheter
Neoplex catheter
Neo-Sert umbilical vessel
  catheter
Neostar Pheres-Flow triple-
  lumen catheter
nephrostomy catheter
Nestor guiding catheter
NeuroEdge neurovascular
  catheter
Neuroguide Visicath viewing
  catheter
Nexus 2 linear ablation
  catheter
Niagara temporary dialysis
  catheter
Nichols-Jehle coronary
  multihead catheter
NIH cardiomarker catheter
NIH catheter
NIH Image catheter
NIH left ventriculography
  catheter
NIH marking catheter
nondetachable silicone
  balloon catheter
nonflotation catheter
nonflow-directed catheter
nontraumatizing catheter
NoProfile balloon catheter
Norfolk intrauterine
  aspiration catheter
Norton flow-directed Swan-
  Ganz thermodilution
  catheter
Nova thermodilution catheter

catheter (*continued*)

NovaCath multilumen
  infusion catheter
Novoste catheter
Numed intracoronary
  Doppler catheter
Nutricath catheter
Nutricath silicone elastomer
  catheter
Nycore angiography catheter
Nycore angiography pigtail
  catheter
Nycore catheter
Nélaton catheter
Nélaton urethral catheter
occlusion catheter
octapolar catheter
Odman-Ledin catheter
Olbert balloon catheter
Olbert balloon dilatation
  catheter
Olbert NoProfile balloon
  dilatation catheter
olivary catheter
olive-tipped catheter
Olympus II PTCA dilatation
  catheter
Olympus wash catheter
Omni catheter
OmniCath atherectomy
  catheter
Omniflex balloon catheter
On-Command catheter
one-hold angiographic
  catheter
Onik-Cohen percutaneous
  access catheter
Opaca-Garcea ureteral
  catheter
open-ended ureteral catheter
OpenSail balloon catheter
Opta 5 catheter
Optical catheter
Opticath oximeter catheter
Opticon catheter
Opti-Flow permanent dialysis
  catheter
Opti-Plast XT balloon catheter
OptiQue sensing catheter
Optiscope catheter
Optiva catheter
Oracle Focus PTCA catheter

catheter (*continued*)

Oracle Focus ultrasound imaging catheter

Oracle intravascular ultrasound catheter

Oracle Megasonics catheter

Oracle MegaSonics coronary balloon/imaging catheter

Oracle Micro intravascular ultrasound catheter

Oracle Micro Plus PTCA catheter

Oral-Cath catheter

Oreopoulos-Zellerman catheter

OTN catheter (over-the-needle catheter)

OTW catheter (over-the-wire)

over-the-needle (OTN) infusion catheter

over-the-wire (OTW balloon catheter)

Owatusi double catheter

Owen catheter

Owen Lo-Profile dilation catheter

oximetric catheter

oximetry catheter

PA Watch position-monitoring catheter

Pacel bipolar pacing catheter

pacemaker catheter

Paceport catheter

Pacewedge dual-pressure bipolar pacing catheter

Pacifico catheter

pacing catheter

Panther catheter

Paparella catheter

Parahisian EP catheter

ParCA catheter

Park blade septostomy catheter

Parodi catheter

partially-implantable catheter

Passage balloon dilation catheter

Passage catheter

passage of catheter

Passport Balloon-on-a-Wire dilatation catheter

Pathfinder catheter

catheter (*continued*)

PBN hysterosalpingography catheter

PDT guiding catheter

PE Plus II balloon dilatation catheter

PE Plus II peripheral balloon catheter

pectoral catheter

pediatric balloon catheter

pediatric catheter

pediatric Foley catheter

pediatric pigtail catheter

Pedicath catheter

peel-away banana catheter

peel-away catheter

peel-off catheter

pennate suction catheter

Pennine Nélaton catheter

PENSIL catheter (Penn State Intravascular Lung catheter)

PentaCath catheter

Pentalumen catheter

PentaPace QRS catheter

Per-C-Cath catheter

Percor dual-lumen intra-aortic balloon catheter

Percor intra-aortic balloon catheter

Percor-DL catheter (dual-lumen catheter)

Percor-Stat DL catheter (dual-lumen catheter)

Percuflex nephrostomy catheter

percutaneous catheter

percutaneous central venous catheter

percutaneous drainage catheter

percutaneous nephrostomy Malecot catheter

percutaneous rotational thrombectomy catheter

percutaneous transhepatic biliary drainage catheter

percutaneous transhepatic pigtail catheter

percutaneous transluminal coronary angioplasty catheter

perfusion catheter

catheter (*continued*)

Periflow peripheral balloon angioplasty-infusion catheter
Periflow peripheral balloon catheter
peripheral atherectomy catheter
peripheral long-line catheter
peripherally inserted central catheter (PICC)
peripherally inserted central catheter (PICC) line
peripherally inserted central venous catheter (PICVC)
peritoneal catheter
peritoneal dialysis catheter
peritoneal reflux control catheter
Perma-Cath catheter
permanent silicone catheter
PermCath dual-lumen catheter
Per-Q-Cath
Per-Q-Cath CVP catheter
Perry pediatric Foley latex catheter
Perry-Foley catheter
Personal Catheter silicone intermittent catheter
pervenous catheter
Pezzer catheter
Pezzer mushroom-tipped catheter
Pezzer self-retaining urethral catheter
Pezzer suprapubic cystostomy catheter
Pfeifer catheter
Phantom V Plus balloon dilatation catheter
Phantom V Plus catheter
Pharmaseal catheter
Pharmex disposable catheter
Phillips catheter
Phillips urethral catheter
Phillips urologic catheter
Phoenix Anti-Blok ventricular catheter
Piccolino Monorail catheter
Pico-ST II low-profile balloon catheter
Pico-T II PTCA balloon catheter

catheter (*continued*)

pigtail catheter
Pilcher bag catheter
Pilcher catheter
Pilotip catheter
Pinkerton balloon catheter
Pipelle endometrial suction catheter
Pivot fixed-wire balloon catheter
plastic catheter
plastic Tiemann catheter
Pleurovac chest catheter
Pleurx catheter
Pleurx pleural catheter
pneumatic balloon catheter
POC Bandit catheter
Polaris LE catheter
Polaris steerable diagnostic catheter
Pollack ureteral catheter
Pollock catheter
POLY balloon catheter
Poly-Cath catheter
polyethylene catheter
polyethylene intravenous catheter
PolyFlo peripherally inserted central catheter
Polysil-Foley catheter
Polystan catheter
Polystan venous return catheter
PolyTech nonlatex self-adhering urinary external catheter
polyurethane nasoenteric catheter
polyvinyl catheter
pop-on self-adhering male external catheter
Port-A-Cath implantable catheter
portal catheter
Porterfield catheter
Portex chorionic villus sampling catheter
Portex-Gibbon catheter
Portnoy catheter
Portnoy multiflanged catheter
Portnoy ventricular catheter
Porto-vac catheter
position-sensing catheter

catheter (*continued*)
Positrol catheter
Positrol II Bernstein catheter
Positrol USCI catheter
Pousson pigtail catheter
Powerflex balloon catheter
Predator balloon catheter
preformed catheter
preformed Cordis catheter
preshaped catheter
Priestly catheter
Prima Laser catheter
Pro-Bal protected balloon-tipped catheter
probe balloon catheter
probe catheter
probing catheter
probing sheath exchange catheter
Procath electrophysiology catheter
ProCross Rely OTW balloon catheter
Profile Plus balloon dilatation catheter
Profile Plus catheter
Profile Plus dilatation catheter
Proflex dilatation catheter
Pro-Flo XT catheter
Prostaprobe catheter
prostatic bridge catheter
prostatic catheter
ProSys silicone sterile 2-way, 3-way Foley catheter
Pruitt irrigation catheter
Pruitt occlusion catheter
Pruitt-Inahara balloon-tipped perfusion catheter
PTBD catheter (percutaneous transhepatic biliary drainage catheter)
PTCA catheter
Pudenz barium cardiac catheter
Pudenz infant cardiac catheter
Pudenz peritoneal catheter
Pudenz ventricular catheter
Pudenz-Heyer vascular catheter
pulmonary arterial catheter
pulmonary artery catheter
pulmonary flotation catheter

catheter (*continued*)
pulmonary triple-lumen catheter
pulse spray catheter
Pursuit catheter
pusher catheter
push-pull catheter
Putnam evacuator catheter
pyeloureteral catheter
Q-cath catheter
Quadra-Flo infusion catheter
quadripolar 6-French diagnostic electrophysiology catheter
quadripolar catheter
quadripolar electrode catheter
quadripolar pacing catheter
quadripolar steerable electrode catheter
quadripolar steerable mapping/ablation catheter
Quanticor catheter
Quantum Ranger OTW balloon catheter
quick catheter
QuickFlash arterial catheter
Quinton biopsy catheter
Quinton catheter
Quinton central venous catheter
Quinton dual-lumen catheter
Quinton Mahurkar double-lumen catheter
Quinton Mahurkar dual lumen catheter
Quinton Mahurkar dual-lumen peritoneal catheter
Quinton peritoneal catheter
Quinton PermCath catheter
Quinton Q-Port catheter
R1 Rapid Exchange balloon catheter
Raaf Cath vascular catheter
Raaf catheter
Raaf double-lumen catheter
Raaf dual-lumen catheter
Racz catheter
Racz epidural catheter
radial artery catheter
Radiofocus Glidewire angiography catheter

catheter (*continued*)

radiofrequency-generated thermal balloon catheter
radiopaque calibrated catheter
radiopaque catheter
radiopaque ERCP catheter
radiopaque Silastic catheter
railway catheter
Raimondi catheter
Raimondi peritoneal catheter
Raimondi spring peritoneal catheter
Raimondi ventricular catheter
Ramirez winged catheter
Ranfac cholangiographic catheter
Ranger OTW balloon catheter
rapid exchange balloon catheter
rapid exchange Flowtrack catheter
Raptorail catheter
Rashkind balloon catheter
Rashkind catheter
Rashkind septostomy balloon catheter
rat-tail catheter
RC1, RC2 catheter
Rebar microvascular catheter
recessed balloon septostomy catheter
rectal catheter
red Robinson catheter
red rubber catheter
Reddick cystic duct cholangiogram catheter
Reddick-Saye screw catheter
RediFurl catheter
Redifurl Taperseal catheter
RediFurl TaperSeal IAB catheter
RediGuard catheter
RediGuard IAB catheter
reference catheter
Ref-Star EP catheter
Reif catheter
Release-NF catheter
Reliance urinary control insert catheter
Rentrop catheter
Rentrop infusion catheter

catheter (*continued*)

reperfusion catheter
Replogle catheter
retention catheter
retrograde femoral catheter
retrograde occlusion balloon catheter
retroperfusion catheter
return-flow catheter
return-flow hemostatic catheter
return-flow retention catheter
Revivac catheter
Reynolds infusion catheter
RF Ablatr ablation catheter
RF balloon catheter
RF Marinr catheter
RF Performer catheter
rheolytic catheter
Rhyder diagnostic catheter
Rica eustachian catheter
right coronary catheter
right Judkins catheter
right-angle chest catheter
Rigiflex ABD balloon dilatation catheter
Rigiflex biliary balloon dilatation catheter
Rigiflex OTW balloon dilatation catheter
Rigiflex TTS balloon dilatation catheter
RIJ catheter
Ring biliary drainage catheter
Ring catheter
Ring-McLean catheter
RITA ablation catheter
Ritchie catheter
Rivas vascular catheter
Robinson catheter
Robinson urethral catheter
Rochester Medical silicone Foley catheter
Rochester Medical self-adhering male external catheter
Rockey-Thompson catheter
Rodriguez catheter
Rodriguez-Alvarez catheter
Rolnel catheter
Rosch catheter
Ross catheter

catheter (*continued*)

Rotacs motorized catheter
Rothene catheter
round-tip catheter
rove magnetic catheter
Royal Flush angiographic flush catheter
Rusch-Uchida transjugular liver access needle-catheter
rubber catheter
rubber-shod catheter
Rumel catheter
Rusch bronchial catheter
Rusch catheter
Rusch coudé catheter
Rusch external catheter
Ruschelit catheter
Rusch-Foley catheter
Rutner catheter
Rutner nephrostomy balloon catheter
Rutner wedge catheter
RX perfusion catheter
RX Streak balloon catheter
Sable balloon catheter
Sable PTCA balloon catheter
Sacks QuickStick catheter
Sacks Single-Step catheter
Safe-Dwel Plus catheter
Safe-T-Coat heparin-coated thermodilution catheter
Saf Touch catheter
Salmon catheter
Salvage catheter
Saratoga sump catheter
Sarns wire-reinforced catheter
Schneider catheter
Schneider-Shiley catheter
Schneider-Shiley dilatation catheter
Schoonmaker catheter
Schoonmaker femoral catheter
Schoonmaker multipurpose catheter
Schrötter catheter
Schwarten balloon dilatation catheter
Science-Med balloon catheter
Sci-Med angioplasty catheter
Sci-Med guiding catheter
Sci-Med skinny catheter

catheter (*continued*)

Sci-Med SSC Skinny catheter
scleral buckling catheter
Scoop 1, 2 catheter
Scoop transtracheal catheter
Scrotter catheter
Security+ self-sealing Urisheath external catheter
Seidel catheter
Seldinger cardiac catheter
Seldinger catheter
Selecon coronary angiography catheter
Selective-HI catheter
Seletz catheter
Self-Cath coudé tipped catheter
Self-Cath soft catheter
Self-Cath straight tipped female catheter
Self-Cath straight tipped pediatric catheter
Self-Cath straight tipped soft catheter
self-guiding catheter
self-retaining catheter
Sellheim uterine catheter
semirigid catheter
Semm uterine catheter
Semm uterine vacuum catheter
Sensation intra-aortic balloon catheter
sensing catheter
Sentron pigtail angiographic micromanometer catheter
Sentron pigtail microtip-manometer catheter
septostomy balloon catheter
Seroma-Cath wound drainage catheter
SET three-lumen thrombectomy catheter
S-G catheter
Shadow OTW balloon catheter
Shadow-Stripe catheter
Shaldon catheter
shaver catheter
Shaw catheter
Sheldon catheter
shellac-covered catheter

catheter (*continued*)

Shepherd hook catheter
shepherd's hook catheter
Sherpa guiding catheter
Shiley catheter
Shiley guiding catheter
Shiley irrigation catheter
Shiley JL-4 guiding catheter
Shiley JR-4 guiding catheter
Shiley MultiPro catheter
Shiley soft-tip guiding
    catheter
Shiley-Ionescu catheter
SHJR4s catheter (side-hold
    Judkins right, curve 4, short
    catheter)
Shone catheter
short-arm Grollman catheter
ShortCutter catheter
Shulitz catheter
sialographic catheter
side-hole catheter
side-hole pigtail catheter
sidewinder catheter
sidewinder percutaneous
    intra-aortic balloon catheter
Siegel-Cohen dilating catheter
Silastic Brand sterile Foley
    catheter
Silastic catheter
Silastic elastomer infusion
    catheter
Silastic ileal reservoir catheter
Silastic mushroom catheter
Silcath subclavian catheter
silicone elastomer catheter
silicone elastomer infusion
    catheter
silicone epistaxis catheter
silicone Robinson catheter
silicone rubber Dacron-cuffed
    catheter
Silicore catheter
Silitek catheter
silk-and-wax catheter
Sil-Med catheter
silver catheter
Simmons 1, 2, 3 catheter
Simmons catheter
Simmons II, III catheter
Simmons sidewinder catheter
Simplastic catheter

catheter (*continued*)

Simplus catheter
Simplus dilatation catheter
Simpson atherectomy
    catheter
Simpson AtheroCath catheter
Simpson coronary AtheroCath
    catheter
Simpson suction catheter
Simpson Ultra Lo-Profile II
    balloon catheter
Simpson-Robert ACS dilatation
    catheter
Simpson-Robert catheter
single need catheter
single-lumen balloon stone
    extractor catheter
single-lumen infusion catheter
single-stage catheter
Skene catheter
Skinny balloon catheter
Skinny dilatation catheter
Skinny OTW balloon catheter
Sleek catheter
Slider catheter
sliding-rail catheter
Slinky balloon catheter
Slinky catheter
Slinky PTCA catheter
Slip-Sheen catheter
Smart position-sensing
    catheter
SMIC eustachian catheter
snare catheter
Soaker catheter
Soehendra dilating catheter
Soehendra Universal catheter
soft catheter
SOF-T guiding catheter
Soft Seal cervical catheter
Soft Torque uterine catheter
Soft-Cell permanent dual-
    lumen catheter
Softip arteriography catheter
Softip catheter
Softip diagnostic catheter
Softouch Cobra 1, 2 catheter
Softouch guiding catheter
Softouch Headhunter 1
    catheter
Softouch Multipurpose B2
    catheter

catheter (*continued*)
Softouch Simmons 1, 2
catheter
Softouch spinal angiography
catheter
Softouch cardiac pigtail
catheter
Softrac-PTA catheter
Soft-Vu angiographic catheter
Soft-Vu Omni flush catheter
Solera thrombectomy catheter
solid-state esophageal
manometry catheter
solid-tip catheter
Solo catheter
SoloPass catheter
Sones Cardio-Marker catheter
Sones catheter
Sones coronary catheter
Sones Hi-Flow catheter
Sones Positrol catheter
Sones vent catheter
Sones female Dacron catheter
Sonicath endoluminal
ultrasound catheter
Sonicath imaging catheter
Sonicath intravascular
ultrasound catheter
Sorenson thermodilution
catheter
SOS Omni catheter
Soules intrauterine
insemination catheter
Spectra-Cath STP catheter
Spectranetics support
catheter
Spectraprobe-PLS laser
angioplasty catheter
Spectrum silicone Foley
catheter
Speedy balloon catheter
Spetzler catheter
Spetzler subarachnoid
catheter
SPI-Argent II peritoneal
dialysis catheter
spinal catheter
SpineCATH catheter
SpineCATH intradiscal
catheter
spiral-tipped catheter
split-sheath catheter

catheter (*continued*)
Spring catheter
Sprint catheter
Spyglass angiography catheter
Squibb catheter
Squire catheter
St. Bartholomew barium
catheter
Stack perfusion coronary
dilatation catheter
Stamey catheter
Stamey Malecot catheter
Stamey open-tip ureteral
catheter
Stamey ureteral catheter
Stamey-Malecot catheter
standard 6-lumen perfused
catheter
Standard Care sterile urethral
catheter
standard ERCP catheter
standard Lehman catheter
Stanford end-hole pigtail
catheter
Stargate falloposcopy catheter
StatLock-Foley catheter
Stealth angioplasty balloon
catheter
steerable catheter
steerable decapolar electrode
catheter
steerable guidewire catheter
steering catheter
Steerocath catheter
stenting catheter
Steri-Cath catheter
Stertzer brachial guiding
catheter
Stertzer catheter
Stillette catheter
stimulating catheter
Stitt catheter
Storz bronchial catheter
Storz scleral buckling balloon
catheter
Storz-DeKock 2-way bronchial
catheter
straight catheter
straight flush percutaneous
catheter
straight-tipped catheter
Streamline peripheral catheter

catheter (*continued*)

Stress Cath catheter
Stretzer bent-tip USCI catheter
Stringer tracheal catheter
Stripseal catheter
styletted catheter
styletted tracheobronchial catheter
Sub-4 small-vessel balloon dilatation catheter
subclavian apheresis catheter
subclavian catheter
subclavian dialysis catheter
subclavian hemodialysis catheter
subclavian vein access catheter
submicroinfusion catheter
Suction Buster catheter
suction catheter
Suggs catheter
Sugita catheter
SULP II balloon catheter
SULP II catheter
sump catheter
sump pump catheter
Super Torque Plus catheter
Super-9 guiding catheter
Supercath intravenous catheter
Superflow guiding catheter
Superior suction catheter
Supra-Foley catheter
suprapubic catheter
Supreme electrophysiology catheter
Sure Seal Golden Drain catheter
SureCath port access catheter
Sureflow catheter
Surflo IV catheter
surgically implanted hemodialysis catheter
Surgimedics cholangiography catheter
Surgitek catheter
Surgitek double-J ureteral catheter
Surpass catheter
Swan-Ganz balloon flotation catheter

catheter (*continued*)

Swan-Ganz bipolar pacing catheter
Swan-Ganz catheter
Swan-Ganz flow-directed catheter
Swan-Ganz guidewire catheter
Swan-Ganz Pacing catheter
Swan-Ganz pulmonary artery catheter
Swan-Ganz thermodilution catheter
swan-neck Missouri catheter
swan-neck pediatric Coil-Cath catheter
Switzerland dilatation catheter
Syntel latex-free embolectomy catheter
TAC atherectomy catheter
Tactilaze angioplasty laser catheter
Takumi PTCA catheter
Talon balloon dilatation catheter
Tandem thin-shaft transureteroscopic balloon dilatation catheter
tapered catheter
tapered-tip hydrophilic-coated push catheter
Tauber catheter
Tauber male urethrographic catheter
Taut cholangiographic catheter
Taut cystic duct catheter
Taut M55, M56, M57 catheter
TEC extraction catheter
Tefcat intrauterine insemination catheter
Teflon catheter
Teflon ERCP catheter
Teflon guiding catheter
Teflon injection catheter
Teflon needle catheter
Teflon-tipped catheter
TEGwire balloon dilatation catheter
Telescope catheter
telescoping plugged catheter
temporary pacing catheter

catheter (*continued*)

Ten system balloon catheter
Tenckhoff 2-cuff catheter
Tenckhoff catheter
Tenckhoff peritoneal catheter
Tenckhoff peritoneal dialysis catheter
Tenckhoff renal dialysis catheter
Tennis Racquet angiographic catheter
Tennis Racquet catheter
Terumo SP coaxial catheter
Terumo Surflo intravenous catheter
Tesio catheter
tetrapolar esophageal catheter
Texas catheter
Texax condom catheter
ThermaChoice catheter
thermistor catheter
thermistor thermodilution catheter
thermodilution balloon catheter
thermodilution catheter
thermodilution pacing catheter
thermodilution Swan-Ganz catheter
thin-wall introducer catheter
Thompson bronchial catheter
Thompson catheter
ThoraCath catheter
thoracic catheter
thrombectomy catheter
thrombosuction catheter
Thruflex PTCA balloon catheter
Tiemann catheter
Tiemann coudé catheter
Tiemann Foley catheter
Tiemann Neoflex catheter
Timberlake catheter
tip-deflecting catheter
Tis-U-Trap endometrial suction catheter
Tital balloon catheter
Titan Mega PTCA dilatation catheter
Titan Mega XL PtCA dilatation catheter

catheter (*continued*)

Titan-Mega catheter
TLC Baxter balloon catheter
Tolantins bone marrow infusion catheter
Tomac catheter
Tomac-Nelaton catheter
toposcopic catheter
Torcon angiographic catheter
Torcon catheter
Torcon NB selective angiographic catheter
Torktherm torque control catheter
Toronto-Western catheter
torque-control balloon catheter
totally implantable catheter
Tourguide guiding catheter
TPN catheter
Trabucco double balloon catheter
Trac Plus catheter
Tracer catheter
Tracer OTW intravascular mapping catheter
TrachCare multi-access catheter
tracheal catheter
Tracker infusion catheter
Tracker Soft Stream side-hole microinfusion catheter
Tracker-18 Unibody catheter
Trakstar balloon catheter
transcervical tubal access catheter
transcutaneous extraction catheter
transducer-tipped catheter
transfemoral endoaortic occlusion catheter
translumbar inferior vena cava catheter
transluminal angioplasty catheter
transluminal endarterectomy catheter
transluminal extraction catheter
transluminal extraction catheter (TEC)

catheter (*continued*)

   transnasal intraduodenal
      feeding catheter
   transoral catheter
   Transport catheter
   transseptal catheter
   transthoracic catheter
   transtracheal oxygen catheter
   transurethral catheter
   transvenous pacemaker
      catheter
   Trattner catheter
   Trattner urethrographic
      catheter
   trefoil balloon catheter
   Triguide catheter
   Trilogy low-profile balloon
      dilatation catheter
   triple thermistor coronary
      sinus catheter
   triple-lumen Arrow catheter
   triple-lumen balloon flotation
      thermistor catheter
   triple-lumen biliary
      manometry catheter
   triple-lumen catheter
   triple-lumen central catheter
   triple-lumen central venous
      catheter
   triple-lumen manometric
      catheter
   triple-lumen manometry
      catheter
   tripolar catheter
   tripolar Damato curve
      catheter
   tripolar electrode catheter
   tripolar with Damato curve
      catheter
   Trocath peritoneal dialysis
      catheter
   Troeltsch eustachian catheter
   True Sheathless catheter
   T-TAC catheter
   TTS (through the scope)
      catheter
   T-tube catheter
   TUN-L-KATH epidural
      catheter
   tunnelable ventricular ICP
      catheter
   Tuohy catheter

catheter (*continued*)

   twist drill catheter
   Tygon catheter
   Tyshak balloon valvuloplasty
      catheter
   UAC catheter (umbilical artery
      catheter)
   UCAC diagnostic catheter
   Uldall subclavian hemodialysis
      catheter
   Ultraflex self-adhering male
      external catheter
   UltraFuse catheter
   Ultramer catheter
   umbilical artery catheter (UAC)
   umbilical catheter
   umbilical vein catheter
   umbilical venous catheter
   UMI catheter
   UNI shunt catheter
   Unicath all-purpose catheter
   Universal drainage catheter
   Uniweave catheter
   Ureflex ureteral catheter
   Uresil biliary catheter
   Uresil embolectomy
      thrombectomy catheter
   Uresil irrigation catheter
   Uresil occlusion balloon
      catheter
   ureteral catheter
   ureteral dilatation catheter
   ureteral occlusion catheter
   urethral catheter
   urethrographic catheter
   Uridome catheter
   Uridrop catheter
   urinary catheter
   Urocare Foley catheter
   Uro-Cath molded latex male
      external catheter
   Uro-Con Texas style male
      external catheter
   urodynamic catheter
   Urofoam-1, -2 adhesive foam
      strip for male external
      catheter
   urologic catheter
   urological catheter
   UroMax II catheter
   UroMax II high-pressure
      balloon catheter

catheter (*continued*)

Uro-San Plus external catheter
USCI Bard catheter
USCI catheter
USCI Finesse guiding catheter
USCI guiding catheter
USCI Mini-Profile balloon dilatation catheter
USCI Positrol coronary catheter
uterine cornual access catheter
uterine ostial access catheter
V. Mueller embolectomy catheter
Vabra catheter
Vacurette catheter
vacuum aspiration catheter
valve-ended catheter
valvuloplasty balloon catheter
Van Aman pigtail catheter
Van Buren catheter
van Sonnenberg gallbladder catheter
van Sonnenberg catheter
van Sonnenberg sump catheter
van Sonnenberg-Wittich catheter
Van Tassel angled pigtail catheter
Van Tassel pigtail catheter
Vance percutaneous Malecot nephrostomy catheter
Vance-Kish urethral illuminated catheter
Vantec occlusion balloon catheter
Vantec ureteral balloon dilatation catheter
Variflex catheter
Vas-Cath catheter
Vas-Cath Opti-Plast peripheral angioplasty catheter
vascular access catheter
vascular catheter
Vascu-Sheath catheter
Vaso-Cath peritoneal dialysis catheter
Vaxcel catheter
Vector large-lumen catheter
Vector large-lumen guiding catheter

catheter (*continued*)

VectoX large-lumen guiding catheter
Venaport catheter
venous catheter
venous irrigation catheter
venous thrombectomy catheter
venting catheter
Ventra catheter
Ventric True Tech ICP catheter
ventricular catheter
ventriculography catheter
Ventureyra ventricular catheter
Verbatim balloon catheter
Veripath peripheral guiding catheter
Versaflex steerable catheter
vertebrated catheter
vessel-sizing catheter
Viper PTA catheter
Virden catheter
Virden rectal catheter
Visicath viewing catheter
Vision PTCA catheter
Visi-Tube catheter
Vitalcor catheter
Vitalcor venous catheter
Vitalcor venous return catheter
Vitatron E catheter
Vitax female catheter
Vitesse catheter
Vitesse Cos laser catheter
Vitesse E-II coronary catheter
Vivonex jejunostomy catheter
VNUS Closure catheter
VNUS Restore catheter
Voda catheter
Von Andel biliary dilation catheter
Von Andel catheter
Von Andel dilation catheter
VPI nonadhesive condom catheter
Vueport balloon-occlusion catheter
Vygon Nutricath S catheter
Walrus Advancit catheter
Walther catheter
Walther female catheter

catheter (*continued*)
  wash catheter
  washing catheter
  Watanabe catheter
  water-infusion esophageal
    manometry catheter
  water-perfused catheter
  wave guide catheter
  Weber catheter
  Weber rectal catheter
  Weber winged catheter
  Webster coronary sinus
    catheter
  Webster orthogonal electrode
    catheter
  wedge catheter
  wedge Cook catheter
  wedge pressure balloon
    catheter
  Western external urinary
    catheter
  Wexler catheter
  whalebone filiform catheter
  whistle-tip catheter
  whistle-tip Foley catheter
  whistle-tip ureteral catheter
  Wholey balloon occlusion
    catheter
  Wholey-Edwards catheter
  Wick catheter
  Wideband urinary catheter
  Williams L-R guiding catheter
  Wilson-Cook catheter
  Wilson-Cook fine-needle-
    aspiration catheter
  Wilton-Webster coronary
    sinus catheter
  Wilton-Webster coronary
    sinus thermodilution
    catheter
  Wilton-Webster
    thermodilution flow and
    pacing catheter
  Winer catheter
  winged catheter
  Winston SD catheter
  wire stylet catheter
  Wiseguide catheter
  Wishard catheter
  Wishard tip catheter
  Wishard ureteral catheter
  Witzel enterostomy catheter

catheter (*continued*)
  Wolf catheter
  Wolf nephrostomy catheter
  Wolf nephrostomy bag
    catheter
  Woodruff catheter
  Woodruff
    ureteropyelographic
    catheter
  Word Bartholin gland catheter
  Word catheter
  Workhorse percutaneous
    transluminal angioplasty
    balloon catheter
  woven catheter
  woven Dacron catheter
  woven-silk catheter
  Xemex pulmonary artery
    catheter
  Xpeedior 100 catheter
  Xpeedior catheter
  X-Sizer catheter
  X-Trode electrode catheter
  XXL balloon dilatation
    catheter
  Yankauer catheter
  Yankauer eustachian catheter
  Y-trough catheter
  Zavod bronchospirometry
    catheter
  Zavod catheter
  Zimmon catheter
  Z-Med balloon catheter
  Z-Med catheter
  Zucker cardiac catheter
  Zucker catheter
  Zucker multipurpose bipolar
    catheter
  Zuma coronary guiding
    catheter
  Zuma guiding catheter
  Zurich dilatation catheter
catheter ablation
catheter ablation of bundle of
    His
catheter adapter
catheter arteriography
catheter balloon
catheter balloon valvuloplasty
    (CBV)
catheter care kit
catheter clamp

catheter connector
catheter coudé
catheter deflecting bridge
catheter deflecting mechanism
catheter dilatation
catheter dilation
catheter drainage
catheter embolectomy
catheter embolism
catheter entrapment
catheter exchange
catheter fin
catheter fixation
catheter forceps
catheter forming wires
catheter fragment
catheter gauge
catheter guide
catheter guide holder
catheter guidewire
catheter in place
catheter insertion
catheter introducer
catheter leg strap
catheter leg tube holder
catheter manipulation
catheter mapping
catheter needle
catheter obstruction
catheter placement
catheter plug
catheter position
catheter positioned
catheter probe ultrasound
catheter sepsis
catheter sheath
catheter site
catheter stylet
catheter technique for brachial
    plexus block
catheter tip
catheter tip occluder
catheter tip placement
catheter tray
catheter tubing adapter
catheter ultrasound probe
catheter vitrector
catheter waist tube holder
catheter was parked
catheter wick
catheter wire stylet
catheter-based ultrasound probe

catheter-borne sector transducer
catheter-dilator
    female catheter-dilator
catheter-directed fenestration
catheter-directed interventional
    procedure
catheter-guided biopsy
catheter-guided endoscopic
    intubation
catheter-induced pulmonary
    artery hemorrhage
catheter-introducing forceps
catheterization
    antegrade catheterization
    arterial catheterization
    axillary artery catheterization
    bile duct catheterization
    bladder catheterization
    bypass graft catheterization
    cardiac catheterization
    central venous catheterization
    chronic catheterization
    clean intermittent
        catheterization
    combined heart catheterization
    coronary catheterization
    coronary sinus catheterization
    cystic duct catheterization
    diagnostic cardiac
        catheterization
    dip and plateau at cardiac
        catheterization
    heart catheterization
    hepatic vein catheterization
    in-and-out catheterization
    intermittent catheterization
    interventional cardiac
        catheterization
    Judkins-Sones technique of
        cardiac catheterization
    left cardiac catheterization
    left heart catheterization
    long-term epidural
        catheterization
    male catheterization
    percutaneous catheterization
    percutaneous transhepatic
        cardiac catheterization
    portal vein catheterization
    probe catheterization
    pulmonary artery
        catheterization

catheterization (*continued*)
   retrograde catheterization
   retrourethral catheterization
   right heart catheterization
   Seldinger cardiac
      catheterization
   Seldinger cystic duct
      catheterization
   selective catheterization
   Sones cardiac catheterization
   subclavian vein
      catheterization
   Swan-Ganz catheterization
   Swan-Ganz pulmonary
      catheterization
   thoracic epidural
      catheterization
   tracheal catheterization
   transfemoral venous
      catheterization
   transhepatic catheterization
   transnasal bile duct
      catheterization
   transpapillary catheterization
   transseptal left heart
      catheterization
   transvaginal fallopian tube
      catheterization
   transvaginal tubal
      catheterization
   umbilical artery
      catheterization
   umbilical vein catheterization
   ureteral catheterization
   urethral catheterization
   urinary catheterization
catheterization of bladder
catheterization of duct
catheterization of eustachian
   tube
catheterization of heart
catheterization of lacrimonasal
   duct
catheterization technique
catheterize
catheterized specimen
catheterizing Foroblique
   telescope
Catheter-Secure tape
catheter-securing technique
catheter-tip syringe
catheter-tipped manometer

Cath-Finder catheter
Cath-Guide Closed Suction
   catheter
CathLink 20 catheter
CathLink 20 implanted port
CathLink implantable vascular
   access device
Cath-Lok catheter locking device
Cathlon IV catheter
Cathmark suction catheter
cathode
cathode ray oscilloscope
cathode ray tube (CRT)
cathotomy
   lateral cathotomy
Cath-Secure catheter holder
Cath-Secure Dual Tab holder
Cath-Secure hypoallergenic
Cath-Secure tape
Cath-Strip catheter fastener
cation exchange
catlin
catlin amputating knife
catlin amputation knife
catling (*see* catlin)
Catrix dressing
cat's ear
cat's eye calculus
cat's paw retractor
Cattell forked-type T-tube
Cattell gallbladder tube
Cattell herniorrhaphy
Cattell operation
Cattell T-tube
Cattell tube
Catterall classification
Catterall classification of Perthes
   disease (I-IV)
Catterall prosthesis
cauda equina
cauda equina compression
cauda equina syndrome
cauda helicis
caudad
Caud-a-Kaith epidural catheter
caudal
caudal anesthesia
caudal artery
caudal aspect
caudal block
caudal border
caudal branch

caudal condensation of the
transverse fascial tissues
caudal direction
caudal displacement
caudal elevator
caudal epidural anesthetic
technique
caudal flexure
caudal fragment
caudal helix
caudal hook
caudal lamina resection
caudal ligament
caudal needle
caudal pancreaticojejunostomy
caudal pole
caudal rotation
caudal sac
caudal septal angle
caudal septal reduction
caudal septum
caudal transtentorial herniation
caudal transverse fissure
caudalward
caudate
caudate body
caudate lobe
caudate lobe of liver
caudate nucleus
caudate process
caudocephalad
caudocranial hemiaxial view
caudocranial view
cauliflower ear
cauliflower excrescence
caulking gun
Cault punch
cause
    fundamental cause
    precipitating cause
    predisposing cause
    proximate cause
    secondary cause
    undetermined cause
Causse piston
Causse-Shea prosthesis
Causse-Shea tube
caustic
    alkali caustic
caustic acid
caustic bougie
caustic pencil

cauterization
    cervical cauterization
    destruction of lesion by
        cauterization
    electrosurgical cauterization
    scleral cauterization
    Ziegler cauterization
cauterization of cervix
cauterization of lesion
cauterization of nose
cauterize
cauterizing ball
cautery
    Aaron cautery
    Accu-Temp cautery
    Accu-Temp hot wire cautery
    ACMI cautery
    actual cautery
    Acucise ureteral cutting
        cautery
    Alcon cautery
    Alcon hand cautery
    alkaline battery cautery
    argon laser photocoagulator
        cautery
    Berchtold cautery
    Berkeley Bioengineering
        bipolar cautery
    biactive coagulation set
        cautery
    bicap cautery
    BiLap bipolar cautery
    bipolar cautery
    Birtcher cautery
    Birtcher hyfrecator cautery
    Bovie cautery
    Bovie coagulation cautery
    Bovie wet-field cautery
    Burdick cautery
    button cautery
    Cameron cautery
    Cameron-Lorenz cautery
    Cameron-Miller cautery
    carbon dioxide cautery
    chemical cautery
    coagulation cautery
    Codman Mentor Wet-Field
        cautery
    cold cautery
    Colorado tip cautery
    Concept cautery
    Concept disposable cautery

cautery (*continued*)

- Concept eye cautery
- Concept handheld cautery
- Corrigan cautery
- Currentrol cautery
- cutting cautery
- Davis Bovie cautery
- Denis bipolar cautery
- disposable cautery
- Disposolette cautery
- Downes cautery
- electric cautery
- electrocautery cautery
- Endocut cautery device
- endoscopic laser cautery
- Eraser cautery
- Eraser-tip cautery
- excision and cautery
- eye cautery
- fine cautery
- Fine micropoint cautery
- galvanic cautery
- gas cautery
- Geiger cautery
- Geiger-Downes cautery
- Gonin cautery
- Goodhill cautery
- Graefe cautery
- hand cautery
- hand-control cautery
- Hawkins cervix conization cautery
- heat cautery
- Hildreth cautery
- Hildreth ocular cautery
- hook cautery
- Hotsy high-temperature cautery
- insulated cautery
- Ishihara I-Temp cautery
- I-Stat cautery
- I-Temp cautery
- Khosia cautery
- linear cautery
- looped cautery
- L-shaped cautery
- Magielski cautery
- Magielski coagulation cautery
- MegaDyne cautery
- Mentor cautery
- Mentor Wet-Field cautery
- micropoint cautery

cautery (*continued*)

- Mills cautery
- Mira cautery
- Mira tip eye cautery
- monopolar cautery
- Mueller alkaline battery cautery
- Mueller cautery
- Mueller Currentrol cautery
- National cautery
- needlepoint cautery
- NeoKnife cautery
- Neo-Med cautery
- ocular cautery
- ophthalmic cautery
- Op-Temp cautery
- Oxycel cautery
- Paquelin cautery
- Parker-Heath cautery
- pencil cautery
- pencil-tip cautery
- penlight cautery
- Percy cautery
- phacoemulsification cautery
- potential cautery
- Prince cautery
- Prince eye cautery
- pure cutting cautery
- retinal puncture cautery
- right-angle bipolar cautery
- Rommel cautery
- Rommel-Hildreth cautery
- Schanz cautery
- Scheie cautery
- Scheie ophthalmic cautery
- Schepens eye cautery
- silver nitrate cautery
- snare cautery
- solar cautery
- Souttar cautery
- spot cautery
- Statham cautery
- steam cautery
- stepped-down cautery
- straight cautery
- suction cautery
- sun cautery
- Todd cautery
- unipolar cautery
- Valley Lab cautery
- virtual cautery
- von Graefe cautery

cautery (*continued*)
  Wadsworth-Todd eye cautery
  Walker cautery
  Wappler cautery
  Wappler cold cautery
  Wepsic fiberoptic cautery
  wet-field cautery
  wet-field eraser cautery
  Wills Hospital eye cautery
  wound cautery
  xenon arc photocoagulation
    cautery
  Ziegler cautery
cautery ablator
cautery bend
cautery cable
cautery clamp
cautery conization
cautery electrode
cautery for retinal detachment
cautery handle
cautery hook
cautery incision
cautery knife
cautery knife electrode
cautery operation
cautery pencil
cautery snare
cautery transformer
cautery unit
cava (*pl.* cavae)
  cannulation of vena cava
  decannulation of vena cava
  foramen venae cavae
  Greenfield titanium inferior
    vena cava (IVC) filter
  inferior vena cava
  Simon nitinol inferior vena
    cava (IVC) filter
  superior vena cava
  thoracic inferior vena cava
  vena cava
cavagram
caval cannula
caval catheter
caval drainage
caval filter
caval fold
caval insertion
caval nodes
caval occlusion clamp
caval snare

caval tourniquet
caval valve
cavamesenteric shunt
Cavanaugh bur
Cavanaugh sphenoid bur
Cavanaugh-Israel bur
Cavanaugh-Wells tonsil forceps
Cavanaugh-Wells tonsillar
  forceps
cavascope
Cave cartilage knife
Cave gouge
Cave hip approach
Cave incision
Cave knee retractor
Cave knife
Cave operation
Cave retractor
Cave scaphoid gouge
Cave scaphoid spatula
Cave spatula
caved-in chest
CaverMap surgical device
cavernoma
cavernomatous changes
cavernosal alpha blockade
  technique
cavernoscope
cavernoscopy
cavernosography
cavernosometry
cavernospongiosum shunt
cavernosum
  angioma cavernosum
  corpus cavernosum
  fibroma cavernosum
cavernotome
cavernotomy
cavernous
cavernous angioma
cavernous body
cavernous groove
cavernous groove of sphenoid
  bone
cavernous hemangioma
cavernous
  lymphangiohemangioma
cavernous lymphangioma
cavernous malformation
cavernous nerves of clitoris
cavernous nerves of penis
cavernous portion of urethra

cavernous sinus
cavernous sinus fistula
cavernous sinus syndrome
cavernous urethra
cavernous veins of penis
Cave-Rowe ligature carrier
Cave-Rowe operation
Cave-Rowe patellar procedure
Cave-Rowe shoulder dislocation
    technique
Caves bioptome
Caves-Schultz bioptome
CAVH (continuous
    arteriovenous
    hemofiltration)
caviar lesion
Cavi-Jet dental prophylaxis
    device
Cavilon barrier ointment
Cavin osteotome
Cavin shunt
Cavi-Pulse cavitation ultrasound
    surgical aspirator
cavitary disease
cavitary lesion
cavitary lung lesion
cavitary mass
cavitary small-bowel lesion
cavitas (*pl.* cavitates)
cavitas dentis
cavitating inflammation
cavitation of lobe
cavitation phenomenon
Cavitec cavity liner
Cavitron aspirator
Cavitron cataract extraction
    unit
Cavitron cautery unit
Cavitron dental unit
Cavitron dissection
Cavitron dissector
Cavitron laser
Cavitron machine
Cavitron phacoemulsification
    unit
Cavitron Phaco-Emulsifier
Cavitron scalpel
Cavitron ultrasonic aspirator
    (CUSA)
Cavitron Ultrasonic Surgical
    aspirator (CUSA)
Cavitron-Kelman cataract unit

Cavitron-Kelman
    phacoemulsification
Cavitron-Kelman
    phacoemulsification
    machine
Cavitron-Kelman surgical unit
cavity
    abdominal cavity
    abdominopelvic cavity
    access cavity
    acetabular cavity
    alveolar cavity
    amniotic cavity
    articular cavity
    artificial classification cavity
    axial surface cavity
    biopsy cavity
    body cavity
    buccal cavity
    chest cavity
    chorionic cavity
    complex cavity
    compound cavity
    cotyloid cavity
    cranial cavity
    cystic cavity
    dental cavity
    distal cavity
    DO cavity
    ear cavity
    endodontic cavity
    endolymphatic cavity
    endometrial cavity
    epidural cavity
    exocelomic cavity
    faucial cavity
    fenestration cavity
    fissure cavity
    frontal sinus cavity
    gingival cavity
    glenoid cavity
    greater peritoneal cavity
    idiopathic bone cavity
    incisal cavity
    inferior laryngeal cavity
    inflammatory cavity
    infraglottic cavity
    insufflated peritoneal cavity
    intermediate laryngeal cavity
    intracranial cavity
    intraperitoneal cavity
    joint cavity

cavity (*continued*)
  junctional cavity
  labial cavity
  laryngeal cavity
  laryngopharyngeal cavity
  laser cavity
  lesser peritoneal cavity
  lingual cavity
  lung cavity
  marrow cavity
  mastoid cavity
  maxillary sinus cavity
  Meckel cavity
  mediastinal cavity
  medullary cavity
  miniature uterine cavity
  nasal cavity
  neovaginal cavity
  nephrotomic cavity
  nonseptate cavity
  open cavity
  optic papilla cavity
  optical cavity
  oral cavity
  orbital cavity
  pelvic cavity
  pelvic peritoneal cavity
  pericardial cavity
  perilymphatic cavity
  peritoneal cavity
  pharyngeal cavity
  pharyngonasal cavity
  pit and fissure cavity
  pleural cavity
  postexcision cavity
  prepared cavity
  prostatic cavity
  proximal cavity
  pulmonary cavity
  pulp cavity
  residual cystic cavity
  retroperitoneal cavity
  Retzius cavity
  Rosenmueller cavity
  saclike cavity
  seroma cavity
  sinonasal cavity
  sinus cavity
  smooth surface cavity
  Stafne idiopathic bone cavity
  subarachnoid cavity
  subdural cavity

cavity (*continued*)
  subglottic cavity
  superior laryngeal cavity
  synovial cavity
  syringohydromyelic cavity
  thoracic cavity
  trigeminal cavity
  tympanic cavity
  tympanomastoid cavity
  uterine cavity
  vitreous cavity
  wound cavity
cavity access
cavity classification
cavity debridement
cavity line angle
cavity liner
cavity lining
cavity lining agent
cavity margin
cavity of concha
cavity preparation
cavity preparation base
cavity primer
cavity seal
cavity test
cavity toilet
cavity wall
cavity
cavogram
cavography
  superior vena cavography
cavohepatic junction
Cavoline cavity liner
cavopulmonary anastomosis
cavosurface margin
cavovalgus
  talipes cavovalgus
cavovarus
cavovarus deformity
CAVU (continuous
    arteriovenous
    ultrafiltration)
cavum (*pl.* cava)
cavum concha
cavum conchae
cavum conchal cartilage graft
cavum dentis
cavum epidurale
cavum nasi
cavum septi pellucidi
cavum subarachnoideale

cavum subdurale
cavum trigeminale
cavum tympani
cavum uteri
cavum vergae
cavus
  pes cavus
  talipes cavus
cavus deformity
Cawood nasal splint
Cawthorne destruction
Cawthorne operation
Cawthorne-Day procedure
cayenne pepper spot
Caylor scissors
Cayo saw
Cayote OTW balloon catheter
Cazenave vitiligo
C-bar web-spacer
CB laser
CBD (common bile duct)
CBD choledochoscope
CBD stone
CBI stereotactic head holder
CBI stereotactic ring
CBV (catheter balloon
  valvuloplasty)
C-C (convexo-concave)
CCA (common carotid artery)
C-Casting tape
CCB (cancellous cellular bone)
CCG (costochondral graft)
CCH (circumscribed choroidal
  hemangioma)
CCK femoral stem provisional
  guide
CCL orthotic
C-clamp
  Fukushima C-clamp
CCMS (cerebrocostomandibular
  syndrome)
CCOmbo catheter
CCRN (congenital cartilaginous
  rest of the neck)
CCS (composite cultured skin)
CCS endocardial pacing lead
CCSF (carotid-cavernous sinus
  fistula)
CCT (computerized cranial
  tomography)
CCU (coronary care unit;
  cardiac care unit)

CD (conjugate diameter)
C-D hook
C-D instrumentation device
C-D screw modification
CD-5 needle
C-DAK artificial kidney
C-DAK dialyzer
CDH (congenital dislocated hip)
CDH (congenital dysplasia of hip)
CDH Precoat Plus hip prosthesis
CDH stapler
CDI 2000 blood gas monitor
cDNA probe
CDO brace
CDR (cup-disk ratio)
CE angle of Wiberg
CE-2 cryostat
CE-24 needle
CEA (carcinoembryonic antigen)
CEA (carotid endarterectomy)
CEAP classification of venous
  disorders
cebocephaly
Cebotome drill
cecal
cecal appendage
cecal appendix
cecal block
cecal carcinoma
cecal colonoscopy
cecal cystoplasty
cecal deformity
cecal distention
cecal fold
cecal foramen
cecal foramen of frontal bone
cecal foramen of tongue
cecal hernia
cecal imbrication procedure
cecal intussusception
cecal mesocolic lymph nodes
cecal vault
cecal volvulus
Cecar electrode
cecectomy
Cecil cotton
Cecil dressing
Cecil hypospadias repair
Cecil operation
Cecil procedure
Cecil transurethral resection of
  prostate

Cecil TURP
Cecil urethral stricture
　operation
Cecil-Culp hypospadias repair
Cecil-Culp operation
Cecil-Culp urethroplasty
cecocele
cecocolic
cecocolic intussusception
cecocolon
cecocolopexy
cecocoloplicopexy
cecocolostome
cecocolostomy
cecocystoplasty
cecofixation
cecoileostomy
cecopexy
cecoplication
cecoptosis
cecorectal
cecorrhaphy
cecosigmoidostomy
cecostomy
　percutaneous catheter
　　cecostomy
　tube cecostomy
cecostomy catheter
cecostomy retractor
cecostomy trocar
cecotomy
cecum
　antimesocolic side of cecum
　hepatic cecum
　mobile cecum
　mobilized cecum
　nondescent of cecum
cecum mobile
Cedar anesthesia face rest
Cedars-Sinai classification
CEEA stapler (curved end-to-end
　anastomosis stapler)
CeeOn heparinized intraocular
　lens
cefadroxil
cefamandole
cefazolin sodium
ceiling analgesia
Cel Touch adhesive
Cel Touch white indicator
　powder
Celay InCeram crown

Celay milling unit
celectome
Celestin bougie
Celestin dilator bougie
Celestin endoesophageal
　prosthesis
Celestin endoesophageal tube
Celestin endoprosthesis
Celestin esophageal tube
Celestin graduated dilator
Celestin graft material
Celestin implant
Celestin latex rubber tube
Celestin procedure
Celestin prosthesis
Celestin tube
celiac
celiac alcohol ablation
celiac angiography
celiac arteriography
celiac artery
celiac artery aneurysm
celiac artery compression
　syndrome (CCS)
celiac atresia
celiac axis
celiac band syndrome
celiac clamp
celiac dimple
celiac ganglion
celiac glands
celiac lymph node metastasis
celiac lymph nodes
celiac nerves
celiac nodal involvement
celiac plexus
celiac plexus block
celiac plexus block anesthetic
　technique
celiac plexus reflex
celiac trunk
celiacography
celiectomy
celiocentesis
celioenterotomy
celiogastrotomy
celiohysterectomy
celiomyomectomy
celiomyomotomy
celioparacentesis
celiopyosis
celiorrhaphy

celioscope
celioscopy
celiotomy
   exploratory celiotomy
   vaginal celiotomy
   ventral celiotomy
celiotomy incision
Celita Elite knife
Celita Sapphire knife
cell
   acinar cells
   adventitial cells
   agger nasi cells
   air cells
   anterior ethmoidal air cells
   Aschoff cells
   basaloid cells
   Boll cells
   bowenoid cells
   bur cells
   carotid air cells
   cast cells
   cochlear cells
   collagen-producing cells
   columnar cells
   cone cells
   connective tissue cells
   cultured periosteal cells
   dendritic cells
   desquamated cells
   desquamated epithelial cells
   endothelial cells
   episquamous cells
   epithelial cells
   epithelioid cells
   ethmoid air cells
   ethmoid cells
   ethmoidal air cells
   ethmoidal cells
   ethmoidal labyrinth cells
   fat cells
   fiber cells
   floor cells
   foreign body giant cells
   Golgi cells
   Huerthle cells
   horn cells
   immunocompetent cells
   inflammation cells
   inflammatory cells
   infralabyrinthine air cells
   infundibular cells

cell (*continued*)
   interdigitating dendritic cells
     (IDC)
   irradiated cells
   K cells
   keratinized cells
   Langerhans cells
   Langerhans-type giant cells
   lutein cells
   lymph cells
   lymphocyte cells
   macular hair cells
   malpighian cells
   Markel cells
   Martinotti cells
   mast cells
   mastoid air cells
   mastoid tip cells
   matrix cells
   mature cells
   media wall of agger nasi cells
   medullary cells
   melanin-pigmented cells
   meningothelial cells
   Merkel cells
   mesenchymal cells
   mesothelial cells
   microvillar cells
   migratory cells
   Mikulicz cells
   monocytoid cells
   mother cells
   mucoserous cells
   mucous cells
   mucus-secreting cells
   mulberry cells
   multinucleated dentinoblastic
     cells
   multinucleated giant cells
   myeloid cells
   myoepithelial cells
   myofibroblast cells
   myoid cells
   nerve cells
   Neumann cells
   neural crest cells
   neuroepithelial cells
   neurosensory cells
   nevus cells
   oncocytic epithelial cells
   packed red blood cells
   Paget cells

cell (*continued*)
  pavement cells
  pediculated cells
  peg cells
  pericapillary cells
  perivascular cells
  petrous pyramid air cells
  pillar cells
  plasmid-carrying cells
  polymorphonuclear cells
  precornified cells
  prefollicle cells
  preganglionic cells
  pulpar cells
  Purkinje cells
  pus cells
  reserve cells
  reticular cells
  reticuloendothelial cells
  reticulum cells
  round cells
  sarcogenic cells
  satellite cells
  scavenger cells
  Schultze cells
  Schwann cells
  sedimented red cells
  sentinel cells
  Sertoli cells
  sheets of nevus cells
  spermatogenic cells
  spider cells
  spindle cells
  stipple cells
  supporting cells
  supraorbital air cells
  syncytial cells
  target cells
  taste cells
  tegmental cells
  theca lutein cells
  thecal cells
  transplanted fat cells
  Virchow cells
  whorled cells
cell adhesion molecule (CAM)
cell and flare
cell collection
cell line
cell membrane
Cell Saver 4 cardiopulmonary
    bypass blood centrifuge
    and washing equip

Cell Saver 4 cardiopulmonary
    bypass blood centrifuge
    and washing equipment
Cell Saver 5
Cell Saver blood
Cell Saver Haemolite
cell separation technique
Cellamin bandage
Cellamin resin plaster-of-Paris
    bandage
cell-cell adhesion
cell-extracellular matrix
    adhesion
cell-free zone
CellFriendly cannula
cell-mediated
cell-mediated immune response
cell-mediated immunity
Cellolite
Cellolite material
Cellolite patty
Cellona bandage
Cellona resin plaster-of-Paris
    bandage
cellophane
cellophane dressing
cell-poor zone
cell-rich zone
cells
cell-seeded stent
CellSpray
cell-to-extracellular matrix
    crosstalk
celltrifuge device
cellular
cellular blue nevus
cellular damage
cellular debris
cellular infiltration
cellular pleomorphism
cellular wrinkle filler
cellularity
  high cellularity
cellules
cellulite
  Chesterfield sofa cellulite
  phenomenon of cellulite
cellulite aspect
cellulite phenomenon
cellulitic defect
cellulitis
  acute scalp cellulitis
  anaerobic cellulitis

cellulitis (*continued*)
    anaerobic clostridial cellulitis
    demarcated cellulitis
    orbital cellulitis
    periorbital cellulitis
    peritonsillar cellulitis
    preseptal cellulitis
    submaxillary cellulitis
    synergistic necrotizing
      cellulitis
cellulocutaneous
cellulocutaneous flap
celluloid
celluloid graft material
celluloid implant
celluloid implant material
celluloid linen sutures
celluloid matrix
celluloid prosthesis
celluloid sutures
celluloid thread
cellulose
cellulose acetate device dialyzer
cellulose gauze
cellulose surgical sponge
cellulose-based membrane
Celluron dental roll
Cell-VU disposable semen
    analysis chamber
celoscope
celoscopy
celotomy
celsian amputation
celsian lithotomy
celsian operation
Celsite brachial port
Celsite implanted port
Celsite pediatric port
Celsus lithotomy
Celsus operation
Celsus spasmodic entropion
    operation
Celsus-Hotz operation
CEM handswitching nosecone
Cemax PACS platform
Cemax/Icon scanner
cement
    acrylic bone cement
    acrylic cement
    adhesive cement
    antibiotic-loaded acrylic
      cement
    Atwood orthodontic cement

cement (*continued*)
    BA bone cement
    bone cement
    Boneloc cement
    BoneSource HA cement
    BoneSource hydroxyapatite
      cement
    Buffalo dental cement
    Ceramasave dental cement
    Ceramco dental cement
    Ceramlin dental cement
    CMW bone cement
    Coe-pak cement
    Compacement dental cement
    composite dental cement
    Conclude dental cement
    copper phosphate cement
    dental cement
    DePuy I bone cement
    dermatome cement
    Diaket root canal cement
    Duall cement
    Duo adhesive cement
    Durelon dental cement
    Eastman dental cement
    Endurance bone cement
    Epoxylite CBA dental resin
      cement
    Freegenol cement
    Fuji dental cement
    Gembase dental cement
    Gemcem dental cement
    Gemcore dental cement
    glass ionomer cement
    Howmedica Simplex P
      cement
    Implast bone cement
    IMProv cement
    inorganic dental cement
    Ketac Fil cement
    Ketac Silver cement
    Kirkland cement
    low viscosity cement (LVC)
    low viscosity bone cement
    LVC cement (low viscosity
      cement)
    master cement
    methyl methacrylate bone
      cement
    methyl methacrylate cement
    modified zinc oxide-eugenol
      cement
    My-Bond Carbo cement

cement (*continued*)

Mynol endodontic cement
Neutrocim dental cement
Nobetec dental cement
Nogenol dental cement
Norian SRS cement
organic dental cement
Orthocomp cement
orthodontic cement
Orthoset cement
Osteobond copolymer bone
cement
Palacos bone cement
Palacos cement
Palacos radiopaque bone
cement
Petralit dental cement
PMMA bone cement
polycarboxylate cement
polyethylene cement
polymethyl methacrylate
bone cement
Pronto cement
prosthetic antibiotic-loaded
acrylic cement
radiopaque bone cement
resin cement
Roth dental cement
Selfast dental cement
Shofu dental cement
Simplex cement
Simplex P cement
Simplex P premixed bone
cement
Simplex P&C cement
Simplex P bone cement
silicate cement
Skin-Bond skin cement
SRS injectable cement
Sulfix-6 cement
Super-Dent orthodontic
cement
SuperEBA cement
Surgical Simplex cement
Surgical Simplex P radiopaque
bone cement
Tempbond dental cement
Temrex dental cement
Terlux cement
tooth cement
Torbot cement
VersaBond cement

cement (*continued*)

Wacker Sil-Gel 504 silicone
cement
Zimmer bone cement
Zimmer low viscosity cement
cement burn
cement centralizer
cement disease
cement eater
cement eater drill
cement gun
cement interface
cement line
cement mantle
cement removal
cement restrictor
cement restrictor inserter
cement spacer inserter
cement spatula
cement technique
cemental lesion
cemental line
cemental repair
cement-bone interface
cemented arthroplasty
cemented gingiva
cemented total hip arthroplasty
cementifying fibroma
cementing line
cementless
Cementless Sportorno hip
arthroplasty stem device
cementless technique
cementless total hip
arthroplasty
cementoma
cementophyte
cement-removal hand chisel
cementum fracture
cementum hyperplasia
Cencit facial scanner
Cencit surface scanner
Centaur trial cup
Centec Propoint knee brace
center
ciliospinal center
ejaculation center
ganglionic center
genitospinal center
metacarpal epiphyseal centers
motor center
nerve center

center (*continued*)
    optic center
    ossification centers
    rectovesical center
    semioval center
    sudorific centers
    swallowing center
    tendinous center
    vasomotor center
    vesicospinal center
center blade
center of ridge
center of rotation
center of rotation of wrist
center-action forceps
centering balloon
centering collar
centering drill
centering genioplasty
centering ring
Centermark vascular access
    device
CenterPointLock 2-piece ostomy
    system closed mini-pouch
Centers for Disease Control HIV
    infection classification
centesis
centigray (cGy)
centimeter (cm)
centimeter subtraction ruler
Centimist nebulizer
Centra-Flex lens
central amputation
central anesthetic technique
central anticholinergic
    syndrome
central approach
central artery of retina
central block
central blunt-tipped
    mammascope
central callus
central canal
central cataract
central catheter
central cerebral sulcus
central chemoreflex loop
central chondrosarcoma
central compartment
central cone technique
    reduction
central cord syndrome

central core disease (CCD)
central core wire
central dislocation
central duplication
central facial paralysis
central fat
central fibroma
central fibromatosis
central fibrous body
central fixation
central fossa
central fracture
central fusion
central giant cell granuloma
central giant cell tumor
central heel pad syndrome
central hemangioma
central hepatectomy
central herniation
central iridectomy
central lesion
central masking
central mentum (CM)
central mucoepidermoid
    carcinoma
central nervous system (CNS)
central nervous system disease
central nervous system
    malformation
central nervous system shunt
central occlusion
central ossifying fibroma
central palmar space
central ray amputation
central Recklinghausen disease,
    type II
central resorption
central retinal lens
central slip sparing technique
central stellate laceration
central sutures incised
central tendon
central tendon of diaphragm
central tendon of perineum
central terminal electrode
central vein of retina
central vein of suprarenal gland
central veins of liver
central venous cannulation
    anesthetic technique
central venous catheter
central venous catheterization

central venous line
central venous pressure (CVP)
central venous pressure catheter
central venous pressure line
central venous pressure
    monitoring
central vermilion
central vision
central yellow point
central zone inflammation
central-bearing point
Centralign Precoat hip
    prosthesis
centralization
   Bayne-Klug centralization
   Bora centralization
   Manske-McCarroll-Swanson
     centralization
   tendon centralization
centralizer
   cement centralizer
centrally balanced occlusion
Centrax bipolar endoprosthesis
centric
   Myo-monitor centric
   point centric
   retruded centric
centric checkbite
centric contact
centric fusion
centric interocclusal record
centric jaw relation
centric maxillomandibular
    record
centric occluding relation
centric occlusion
centric position
centric relation
centric relation occlusion
centrically balanced occlusion
centriciput
Centricon-10 filter
centrifugal pump
centrifuge microscope
centrilobular lesion
centripetal action
centripetal extrusion
centripetal nerve
centripetal venous pulse
Centrix PDQ ligator
Centrix syringe
centrocecal scotoma

centrofacial
centrofacial hyperpigmentation
centroneuroaxis anesthesia
centroparietal regions
Centry bicarbonate dialysis
    control unit
Centry dialysis unit
Centry II dialysis machine
Centurion needleless catheter
    extensions
Centurion SorbaView window
    dressing
Century birthing chair
Century urodynamics chair
cephalad
cephalad aspect
cephalad catheter
cephalad direction
cephalad fragment
cephalalgia
cephalgia
cephalhematocele
cephalhematoma
cephalhematoma deformans
cephalic
cephalic angle
cephalic blade forceps
cephalic flexure
cephalic ganglion
cephalic index
cephalic presentation
cephalic reflexes
cephalic skeleton
cephalic triangle
cephalic trim cap graft
cephalic trim cartilage remnants
cephalic vein
cephalic vein graft
cephalic version
cephalocaudad
cephalocaudad diameter
cephalocaudal
cephalocaudal axis
cephalocele
   basal cephalocele
   frontal cephalocele
   frontoethmoidal cephalocele
   occipital cephalocele
   oral cephalocele
   parietal cephalocele
   sincipital cephalocele
cephalocentesis

cephalodactyly
  Vogt cephalodactyly
cephalogram
  lateral cephalogram
cephalography
cephalomedullary nail fracture
cephalomegaly
cephalomelus
cephalometer
  radiographic cephalometer
cephalometric
cephalometric analysis
cephalometric angle
cephalometric correction
cephalometric laminagraphy
cephalometric landmark
cephalometric plane
cephalometric radiograph
cephalometric radiography
cephalometric relationship
cephalometric roentgenogram
cephalometric standards
cephalometric tracing
cephalometrics
cephalometry
cephalonia
cephalo-oculocutaneous
    telangiectasia
cephalopagus
cephalopalpebral reflex
cephalopelvic disproportion
    (CPD)
cephalopolysyndactyly
    syndrome
cephalostat
  portable cephalostat
  Porta-Stat cephalostat
cephalothoracopagus
cephalothoracopagus
    disymmetros
cephalothoracopagus
    monosymmetros
cephalotomy
cephalotrigeminal angiomatosis
ceraceous
Ceradelta alloy
Ceramalloy alloy
Ceramasave dental cement
Ceramco dental cement
Ceramco porcelain kit
CeraMed bone grafting material
ceramic

ceramic endosteal implant
ceramic hip prosthesis
ceramic ossicular prosthesis
ceramic total hip
Ceramion prosthesis
Ceramlin dental cement
ceramometal implant bridge
ceramometal margin
CeraOne abutment implant
Cerapall alloy
CeraSPECT camera
ceratocricoid muscle
ceratopharyngeal muscle
Ceravital incus replacement
    prosthesis
cerclage
  cervical cerclage
  McDonald cerclage
  McDonald cervical cerclage
  Shirodkar cerclage
  Shirodkar-Barter cervical
    cerclage
  Shirodkar-Page cerclage
  Thiersch cerclage
cerclage for retinal
    detachment
cerclage of cervix
cerclage of fractured bone
cerclage operation
cerclage wire
cerclage wire fixation
cerebellar artery
cerebellar ataxia
cerebellar attachment
cerebellar cortex
cerebellar degeneration
cerebellar ectopia
cerebellar electrodes
cerebellar gait
cerebellar gliosis
cerebellar hematoma
cerebellar hemisphere
cerebellar hemorrhage
cerebellar notch
cerebellar peduncle
cerebellar pontine angle
cerebellar retractor
cerebellar rigidity
cerebellar sclerosis
cerebellar stimulation
cerebellar tonsil
cerebellar veins

cerebelli
  ala cerebelli
  corpus cerebelli
  crura cerebelli
  falx cerebelli
  pons cerebelli
  tentorium cerebelli
cerebellomedullary cistern
cerebellomedullary
    malformation syndrome
cerebellopontile angle
cerebellopontine
cerebellopontine angle
cerebellopontine angle
    approach
cerebellopontine angle cistern
cerebellopontine angle
    syndrome
cerebellopontine angle tumor
cerebellum
  quadrangular lobule of
    cerebellum
  tentorium of cerebellum
  vermis of cerebellum
cerebellum retractor
Cereblate catheter
cerebral
cerebral abscess
cerebral air embolism
cerebral anesthesia
cerebral angiogram
cerebral angiography
cerebral angiography needle
cerebral anoxia
cerebral apophysis
cerebral aqueduct
cerebral aqueduct compression
cerebral arteriogram
cerebral arteriography
cerebral arteriovenous
    malformation
cerebral artery
cerebral blood flow
cerebral calcification
cerebral calculus
cerebral cannula
cerebral catheter
cerebral circulation
cerebral compression
cerebral concussion
cerebral contusion
cerebral cortex

cerebral cranium
cerebral crests of cranial bone
cerebral death
cerebral decompression
cerebral decortication
cerebral edema
cerebral embolism
cerebral epidural space
cerebral event
cerebral finger-to-nose
cerebral fissure
cerebral fornix
cerebral fossa
cerebral function
cerebral function monitor
cerebral gigantism
cerebral hemicorticectomy
cerebral hemiplegia
cerebral hemisphere
cerebral hemorrhage
cerebral hernia
cerebral herniation
cerebral infarction
cerebral injury
cerebral lateralization
cerebral lesion
cerebral metabolic rate (CMR)
cerebral metastasis
cerebral nerves
cerebral origin
cerebral palsy
cerebral palsy pathological
    fracture
cerebral paraplegia
cerebral paresis
cerebral paroxysmal activity
cerebral peduncle
cerebral perfusion
cerebral protective therapy
cerebral reference line
cerebral retractor
cerebral seizure
cerebral sinusography
cerebral spasm
cerebral spinal fluid drainage
cerebral thrombosis
cerebral trauma
cerebral tumor
cerebral vascular
    malformation
cerebral vasoconstriction
cerebral vein

cerebral venous sinus thrombosis (CVST)
cerebral ventricles
cerebral ventriculography
cerebral yokes of bone of cranium
cerebral-sacral loop
cerebration
cerebri
  appendix cerebri
  crura cerebri
  crus cerebri
  falx cerebri
  fornix cerebri
  gyri cerebri
  gyri profundi cerebri
  gyri transitivi cerebri
  pseudomotor cerebri
  pseudotumor cerebri
  velamenta cerebri
cerebriform carcinoma
cerebriform tongue
cerebroangiophotoscintigram
cerebrocostomandibular syndrome (CCMS)
cerebromedullary tube
cerebro-ocular
cerebroretinal angiomatosis
cerebrospinal
cerebrospinal axis
cerebrospinal endarteritis
cerebrospinal fasciculus
cerebrospinal fluid (CSF)
cerebrospinal fluid fistula
cerebrospinal fluid leak
cerebrospinal fluid otorrhea
cerebrospinal fluid rhinorrhea
cerebrospinal fluid shunt
cerebrospinal fluid-brain barrier
cerebrospinal pressure
cerebrospinal rhinorrhea
cerebrostomy
cerebrovascular
cerebrovascular accident (CVA)
cerebrovascular blood circulation
cerebrovascular complication
cerebrovascular disease
cerebrovascular event
cerebrovascular insufficiency
cerebrovascular malformation

cerebrovascular obstructive disease
cerebrovascular occlusion
cerebrovascular resistance
cerebrum
  convolutions of cerebrum
  gyri of cerebrum
  longitudinal fissure of cerebrum
Cer-Mate alloy
Cer-On R alloy
Cerrobend radiation cut-outs
Cerrobend trim block
cerulean cataract
cerumen
  impacted cerumen
  inspissated cerumen
cerumen inspissatum
ceruminal impaction
ceruminoma
ceruminous gland
ceruminous gland tumor
Cerva Crane halter
Cervex-Brush cervical cell collector
cervical abortion
cervical abrasion
cervical acceleration-deceleration syndrome
cervical actinomycosis
cervical adenocarcinoma
cervical adenopathy
cervical amputation
cervical anastomosis
cervical anchorage
cervical anesthesia
cervical anomaly
cervical AOA halo traction
cervical approach
cervical artery
cervical aspiration
cervical atypism
cervical biopsy
cervical biopsy blade
cervical biopsy curet
cervical biopsy forceps
cervical biopsy punch forceps
cervical blade
cervical block kit
cervical brace
cervical branch of facial nerve
cervical canal

cervical cancer
cervical cannula
cervical carcinoma
cervical cauterization
cervical cerclage
cervical cesarean section
cervical chain
cervical cheek
cervical clamp
cervical collar
cervical collar brace
cervical compression syndrome
cervical cone biopsy
cervical cone knife
cervical conization
cervical conization electrode
cervical cord injury
cervical cordotomy
cervical cordotomy knife
cervical corpectomy
cervical culture
cervical curet
cervical curettage
cervical curvature
cervical curve
cervical cyst
cervical decompression surgery
cervical dilation
cervical dilator
cervical discharge
cervical disk
cervical disk excision
cervical disk instruments
cervical disk retractor
cervical disk surgery
cervical diskectomy
cervical drill
cervical drill guard
cervical dysplasia
cervical dystocia
cervical ectopy
cervical erosion
cervical esophagogastrostomy
cervical esophagoplasty
cervical esophagostomy
cervical esophagus
cervical fascia
cervical fistula
cervical flap
cervical flexure
cervical foraminal punch
cervical forceps

cervical fusion
cervical fusion syndrome
cervical ganglion
cervical glands
cervical grasping forceps
cervical heart
cervical hemostatic forceps
cervical humeral flap
cervical hydrocele
cervical hygroma
cervical hyperesthesia
cervical immobilization
cervical immobilization device
cervical incision
cervical incompetence
cervical inflammation
cervical insemination
cervical insertion of radium
cervical interbody fusion
cervical intraepithelial neoplasia
　(CIN)
cervical knife
cervical laceration
cervical laminectomy punch
cervical leakage
cervical lesion
cervical line (CL)
cervical loop
cervical lymph node
cervical mallet
cervical manipulation
cervical margin
cervical mediastinoscopy
cervical metastasis
cervical midline disk herniation
cervical midline pterygium
cervical mobilization
cervical muscle contraction
cervical musculature
cervical needle
cervical neoplasia
cervical nerve root injection
cervical nerves
cervical neural canal
cervical node
cervical node dissection
cervical orthosis (CO)
cervical os
cervical Pap smear
cervical patagium
cervical plate
cervical platysma

cervical pleura
cervical plexus
cervical plexus anesthesia
cervical plexus block
cervical plexus block anesthetic
    technique
cervical plexus nerve block
cervical polyp
cervical position
cervical pregnancy
cervical punch
cervical punch biopsy
cervical punch forceps
cervical radium insertion
cervical range-of-motion device
cervical range-of-motion
    instrument
cervical region
cervical retractor
cervical rib
cervical rib syndrome
cervical roll
cervical rongeur
cervical rotational flap
cervical screw insertion
    technique
cervical sleep pillow
cervical smear
cervical spine
cervical spine fracture
cervical spine internal fixation
cervical spine kyphotic
    deformity
cervical spine laminectomy
cervical spine posterior fusion
cervical spine screw-plate
    fixation
cervical spine stabilization
cervical spine stabilization
    procedure
cervical spondylolysis
cervical spondylotic myelopathy
    fusion technique
cervical sprain
cervical stenosis
cervical stump
cervical support
cervical suture needle
cervical sutures
cervical swab
cervical sympathectomy
cervical sympathetic nerve

cervical tenaculum
cervical thoracic orthosis
cervical traction
cervical traction forceps
cervical traction tongs
cervical tube flap
cervical vein
cervical vertebrae
cervical vessel compression
cervical visor flap
cervical-lumbar hammer
cervicales
    vertebrae cervicales
cervicalis
    ansa cervicalis
    inferior root of ansa cervicalis
    lamina superficialis fasciae
        cervicalis
    linea alba cervicalis
    superior root ansa cervicalis
cervical-to-MCA bypass
cervicectomy
cervicoaxial (CA)
cervicobrachial
cervicobrachialgia
cervicobregmatic diameter
cervicodynia
cervicofacial
cervicofacial actinomycosis
cervicofacial contour
cervicofacial face lift
cervicofacial fat
cervicofacial flaccidity
cervicofacial flap
cervicofacial hemangioma
cervicofacial liposurgery
cervicofacial rhytidectomy
cervicofacial rhytidectomy
    procedure
cervicofacial sling
cervicoisthmic angle
cervicomandibular angle
    correction through
    Guyuron procedure
cervicomedullary deformity
cervicomedullary junction
    compression
cervicomental angle
cervico-occipital
cervicoplasty
cervicothoracic
cervicothoracic approach

cervicothoracic ganglion
cervicothoracic jacket
cervicothoracic junction
   stabilization
cervicothoracic junction
   surgery
cervicothoracic orthosis
cervicothoracic pedicle anatomy
cervicotrochanteric
cervicotrochanteric displaced
   fracture
cervicouterine ganglion
cervicovaginal adhesions
cervicovaginal fistula
Cer-View lateral vaginal
   retractor
CerviSoft cytology collection
   device
Cervital partial ossicular
   replacement prosthesis
   (PORP)
Cervital PORP (partial ossicular
   replacement prosthesis)
Cervital TORP (total ossicular
   replacement prosthesis)
Cervital total ossicular
   replacement prosthesis
   (TORP)
cervitome
Cervitrak device
cervix
  A&P repair of cervix
  anterior and posterior repair
    of cervix (A&P repair)
  barrel cervix
  bulbous cervix
  cauterization of cervix
  cerclage of cervix
  clean cervix
  cold conization of cervix
  conization of cervix
  conization of uterine cervix
  dilatation of cervix
  dilation of cervix
  discission of cervix
  effaced cervix
  effacement of cervix
  electroconization of cervix
  erosion of cervix
  fish-mouth cervix
  Fleming conization of cervix
  friable cervix

cervix (*continued*)
  guillotine amputation of
    cervix
  implant cervix
  incompetent cervix
  irregular cervix
  lip of cervix
  mosaicism of cervix
  parous cervix
  ripe cervix
  strawberry cervix
  Sturmdorf amputation of
    cervix
  TFT cervix (tight fingertip
    dilated)
  Universal joint cervix
  uterine cervix
  vaginal cervix
cervix dentis
cervix forceps
cervix suture needle
cervix uteri
cervix-holding forceps
cesarean birth
cesarean delivery
cesarean forceps
cesarean hysterectomy
cesarean operation
cesarean resection
cesarean section
cesarean section incision
cesium applicator
cesium candle
cesium cylinder
cesium fluoride scintillation
   detector
cesium insertion
cesium irradiation
cesium mold
cesium needle
cesium radiation
cesium sources
cesium therapy
cesium tube
cesium tube radiation
cesium-137 wire
cessation
Cetacaine anesthetic agent
Cetacaine topical anesthetic
cevitamic acid
CF (cardiac failure)
CF-200Z Olympus colonoscope

CFA-SFA bypass
CFC pheresis (continuous-flow
    centrifugation pheresis)
CFE Taperloc hip prosthesis
C-fiber
C-flap
C-Flex Amsterdam stent
C-Flex catheter
C-Flex supine cervical traction
C-Flex ureteral stent
C-form osteotomy
CFS hip prosthesis
CFS rhinorrhea
CFS total hip (contoured
    femoral stem total hip)
CF-UM3 echocolonoscope
CFV (continuous-flow
    ventilation)
CFV wrist
CGI-1 contact lens
C-graft
CGS (catgut suture)
cGy (centigray)
Chadwick scissors
Chadwick-Bentley classification
Chaffin catheter
Chaffin suction tube
Chaffin sump tube
Chaffin tube
Chaffin tube catheter
Chaffin-Pratt concept unit
Chaffin-Pratt drain
Chaffin-Pratt percolator hanger
    holder
Chaffin-Pratt suction tube
Chaffin-Pratt suction unit
Chaffin-Pratt tube
Chagas disease
chagoma
chain
    cervical chain
    ganglionated chain
    iliac chain
    lymphatic chain
    ossicular chain
    periaortic chain
    spinal sympathetic chain
    superior cervical chain
    superior ossicular chain
    sympathetic chain
chain ligatures
chain saw

chain suture technique
chain sutures
chain-of-lakes configuration
chain-of-lakes deformity
chain-of-lakes filling defect
chain-of-lakes sign
chair lift
chair pad
chair shower
chair-back brace
chair-table
    hydraulic chair-table
Chajchir dissector
Chakirgil technique
chalazion
chalazion clamp
chalazion curet
chalazion excision
chalazion forceps
chalazion knife
chalazion punch
chalazion retractor
chalazion trephine
chalazodermia
chalinoplasty
chalk bones
chalky bones
Challenger digital applanation
    tonometer
chamaecephalic
chamaecephalous
chamaecephaly
chamaeprosopic
chamaeprosopy
chamber
    Abbé-Zeiss counting chamber
    air chamber
    anterior chamber
    Buerker chamber
    bone growth chambers
    Boyden chamber
    cardiac chamber
    Cell-VU disposable semen
      analysis chamber
    drill chamber
    drip chamber
    Finn chamber
    Fisher-Paykel water-feed
      chamber
    flush chamber
    heart chamber
    high-pressure chamber

chamber (*continued*)
  hyperbaric chamber
  Hyper-Oxy portable
    hyperbaric chamber
  Makler reusable semen
    analysis chamber
  Microcell chamber
  moisture chamber
  MR 290 humidification chamber
  multiwire proportional
    chamber
  nasal chamber
  parallel-plate flow chamber
  plasma clot diffusion chamber
  pocket chamber
  portable topical hyperbaric
    oxygen extremity chamber
  posterior chamber
  Pudenz flushing chamber
  pulp chamber
  reentrant well chamber
  reformation of chamber
  Sechrist hyperbaric chamber
  Sechrist monoplace
    hyperbaric chamber
  shallow chamber
  Shandon cytospin chamber
  Storn Von Leeuwen chamber
  Ussing chamber
  vitreous chamber
  Wilson chamber
chamber doughnut pessary
chamber irrigation
chamber of eye
chamber rupture
chamber size
Chamberlain decompressor
Chamberlain incision
Chamberlain line
Chamberlain mediastinoscopy
Chamberlain mediastinotomy
Chamberlain procedure
Chamberlain tongue depressor
Chamberlain-Fries atraumatic
  retractor
Chamberlen forceps
Chamberlen obstetrical forceps
Chambers diaphragm
Chambers doughnut pessary
Chambers intrauterine cup
Chambers intrauterine pessary
Chambers pessary

Chambers procedure
Chambers technique
chamfer
chamfer cut
chamfer guide
chamfer jig
chamfer reamer
chamfer saw
chamfered
chamois yellow appearance
Champ cardiac device
Champ elastic bandage
champagne cork deformity
Champetier de Ribes obstetrical
  bag
Champion stent
Champion sutures
Championniere bone drill
Championniere forceps
Champy bone plate
Champy miniplate
Chan wrist rest
Chance fracture
Chance lumbar spine fracture
Chance vertebral fracture
chancre
chancriform
chancroid
  serpiginous chancroid
Chandler arthrodesis
Chandler bone elevator
Chandler elevator
Chandler felt collar splint
Chandler forceps
Chandler hammer
Chandler hip fusion
Chandler iridectomy
Chandler iris forceps
Chandler knee retractor
Chandler laminectomy retractor
Chandler mallet
Chandler retractor
Chandler spinal perforating
  forceps
Chandler spinal-perforating
  forceps
Chandler splint
Chandler table
Chandler technique
Chandler unreamed interlocking
  tibial nail
Chandler vitreous operation

Chandler V-pacing probe
Chandler-Verhoeff lens
　　extraction
Chandler-Verhoeff operation
Chang bone-cutting forceps
Chang Quick Chop combo
　　ophthalmic instrument
change
　　actinic skin changes
　　bony pathologic change
　　calcific change
　　cavernomatous changes
　　cystic change
　　degenerative bone changes
　　degenerative change
　　edematous change
　　erythematous change
　　fibrocystic change
　　fibrotic changes
　　fractional area change (FAC)
　　functional change
　　gown change
　　hetching changes
　　induced change
　　inflammatory change
　　involutional ovarian changes
　　macular change
　　no appreciable change
　　no significant change
　　nonspecific change
　　oncocytoid change
　　osteoarthritic changes
　　parenchymatous change
　　pathologic change
　　pigmentary changes
　　postoperative change
　　postpeel pigmentary changes
　　postural changes
　　pressure changes
　　pseudopolypoid changes
　　pupillary change
　　senescent changes
　　SLAC pattern of degenerative
　　　　change
　　stasis changes
　　structural change
　　subjective change
change point
changer
　　film changer
　　tube changer
Chang-Miltner incision

channel
　　blood channels
　　EEG channel
　　engorged collateral venous
　　　　channels
　　lymph channel
　　lymphatic channel
　　perineural channels
　　vascular channel
channel and core biopsy
channel dissector
channel retractor
channel shoulder pin technique
channel ulcer
Chaoul applicator
Chaoul tube
Chaoul voltage x-ray tube
Chapchal technique
Chapman-Dintenfass perforator
Chaput anal operation
Chaput forceps
Chaput fracture
Chaput operation
Chaput tissue forceps
charcoal filter
Charcot arthritis
Charcot arthropathy
Charcot arthrosis
Charcot foot
Charcot joint
Charcot operation
Charcot prosthesis
Charcot sign
Charcot triad
Charcot-Bottcher filament
Charcot-Bouchard aneurysm
Charcot-Leyden crystals
Charcot-Marie-Tooth atrophy
Charcot-Marie-Tooth disease
Chardack-Greatbatch
　　　　implantable cardiac pulse
　　　　generator
Chardack Medtronic pacemaker
Chardack pacemaker
Chardack-Greatbatch
　　　　implantable cardiac pulse
　　　　generator
Chardack-Greatbatch
　　　　pacemaker
Charest head frame
char-free ablation
char-free carbon-dioxide laser

charge
  electric charge
  positive charge
CHARGE (coloboma, heart
    anomaly, choanal atresia,
    retardation, and genital and
    ear anomalies)
charge-coupled device
charge-coupled device
    monochrome camera
charge-coupled device scanner
charge-coupled device video
    camera
charged particle beam therapy
charged particles
charged-particle irradiation
charger
Charles anterior segment sleeve
Charles contact lens
Charles flute needle
Charles infusion sleeve
Charles intraocular lens
Charles irrigating lens
Charles lens
Charles needle
Charles operation
Charles procedure
Charles vacuuming needle
Charles vitrector with sleeve
Charleston nighttime bending
    brace
Charleston scoliosis brace
Charlin syndrome
Charlton antral needle
Charlton antral trocar
Charlton antrum needle
Charlton cannula
Charlton needle
Charlton trocar
Charnley acetabular cup
Charnley acetabular cup
    prosthesis
Charnley approach
Charnley arthrodesis
Charnley arthrodesis clamp
Charnley arthroplasty
Charnley bone clamp
Charnley bone clasp
Charnley brace handle
Charnley cement restrictor
Charnley cemented hip
    prosthesis

Charnley centering drill
Charnley centering ring
Charnley clamp
Charnley compression
Charnley compression
    arthrodesis
Charnley compression fusion
Charnley compression-type
    knee fusion
Charnley compressor
Charnley cup
Charnley cup-trimming scissors
Charnley deepening reamer
Charnley device
Charnley double-ended bone
    curet
Charnley drain tube
Charnley drill
Charnley expanding reamer
Charnley external fixation clamp
Charnley femoral broach
Charnley femoral condyle radius
    gauge
Charnley femoral condyle drill
Charnley femoral inlay aligner
Charnley femoral inlay guillotine
Charnley femoral lever
Charnley femoral prosthesis
    neck punch
Charnley femoral prosthesis
    pusher
Charnley flat-back femoral
    component
Charnley foam suture pad
Charnley forceps
Charnley gouge
Charnley hip prosthesis
Charnley horizontal retractor
Charnley implant
Charnley incision
Charnley initial incision
    retractor
Charnley knee prosthesis
Charnley knee retractor
Charnley narrow stem
    component
Charnley offset-bore cup
Charnley pilot drill
Charnley pin
Charnley pin clamp
Charnley pin retractor
Charnley prosthesis

Charnley rasp
Charnley reamer
Charnley retractor
Charnley saw
Charnley self-retaining retractor
Charnley socket gauge
Charnley standard stem retractor
Charnley starting drill
Charnley suction drain
Charnley suture button
Charnley suture forceps
Charnley taper reamer
Charnley tibial onlay jig
Charnley total hip arthroplasty
Charnley total hip prosthesis
Charnley trochanter file
Charnley trochanter holder
Charnley trochanter reamer
Charnley trochanter wire
Charnley wire passer
Charnley wire-holding forceps
Charnley-Barnes hemostat
Charnley-cobra total hip
    prosthesis
Charnley-Ferreira trochanter
    reattachment
Charnley-Hastings prosthesis
Charnley-Moore hip prosthesis
Charnley-Mueller approach
Charnley-Mueller arthroplasty
Charnley-Mueller cemented hip
    prosthesis
Charnley-Mueller hip prosthesis
Charnley-Mueller rasp
Charnley-Riches arterial forceps
Charnow notched ruler
Charretera flap
Charriere amputation saw
Charriere aseptic metacarpal saw
Charriere bone saw
Charriere saw
Charriere scale
chart
    cystometer chart
    Jaeger reading chart
    kymograph chart
    Lund-Browder burn chart
    Snellen eye chart
Charters technique
char-zone depth
Chassaignac axillary muscle
Chassaignac space

Chassaignac tubercle
Chassar Moir sling procedure
Chassar Moir-Sims procedure
Chassard-Lapiné maneuver
Chassin tube
Chaston eye pad
Chatfield-Girdlestone splint
Chatzidakis implant
Chauffard point
chauffeur's fracture
Chauffin-Pratt tube
Chausse view
Chaussier areola
Chaussier line
Chaussier tube
Chavasse squint hook
Chavasse strabismus hook
Chaves procedure
Chaves scapula surgery
Chaves-Rapp muscle transfer
    technique
Chaves-Rapp scapula surgery
Chayet corneal marker
CHD (congenital heart defect)
CHD (congenital hip dislocation)
CHD (congestive heart disease)
CHD (coronary heart disease)
Cheanvechai-Favaloro retractor
Cheatle forceps
Cheatle slit
Cheatle slit for colostomy
    takedown
Cheatle sterilizer forceps
Cheatle sterilizing forceps
Cheatle syndrome
Cheatle-Henry hernia
Cheatle-Henry incision
Cheatle-Henry operation
check ligament
checkbite
    centric checkbite
Check-Flo introducer
checkrein deformity
checkrein procedure
checkup
check-valve
    bronchial check-valve
check-valve obstruction
check-valve sheath
cheek
    adipose body of cheek
    cervical cheek

cheek (*continued*)
  cleft cheek
  collapsed cheek
  drapery swag of cheek
  fat body of cheek
  laxity of cheeks
  postmaxillectomy collapsed
    cheek
  rosy apple cheeks
  vestibule of cheek
cheek advancement flap
cheek and tongue retractor
cheek augmentation
cheek bag
cheek biting
cheek bone
cheek compression
cheek flap
cheek glands
cheek hollows
cheek implant
cheek mucous-muscle flap
cheek muscle
cheek pad
cheek pouch
cheek retractor
cheek rotation flap
cheek tone
cheek tooth
cheek-lip flap
cheesy cataract
Cheetah angioplasty catheter
Cheever tonsillectomy
Cheft leg holder
cheilalgia
cheilectomy
  Garceau cheilectomy
  Mann-Coughlin-DuVries
    cheilectomy
  Sage-Clark cheilectomy
cheilectropion
cheilion
cheilitis
  actinic cheilitis
  acute cheilitis
  angular cheilitis
  apostematous cheilitis
  candidal angular cheilitis
  commissural cheilitis
  contact cheilitis
  granulomatosa cheilitis
  granulomatous cheilitis

cheilitis (*continued*)
  impetiginous cheilitis
  solar cheilitis
  Volkmann cheilitis
cheilitis exfoliativa
cheilitis glandularis
cheilitis glandularis
    apostematosa
cheilitis granulomatosa
cheilitis venenata
cheilitis-glossitis-gingivitis
    syndrome
cheiloalveoloschisis
cheiloangioscopy
cheilocarcinoma
cheilognathopalatoschisis
cheilognathoprosoposchisis
cheilognathoschisis
cheilognathouranoschisis
cheiloncus
cheilophagia
cheiloplasty
  Abbe stage I cheiloplasty
  Abbe stage II cheiloplasty
  Abbe-Estlander cheiloplasty
  Bernard-Burow cheiloplasty
  Burow cheiloplasty
  Chopart cheiloplasty
  Cronin cheiloplasty
  Estlander cheiloplasty
  Estlander flap cheiloplasty
  Hagedorn cheiloplasty
  Millard cheiloplasty
  Simon cheiloplasty
  Stein cheiloplasty
  Tennison cheiloplasty
  Webster cheiloplasty
  Webster modification of
    Bernard-Burow
    cheiloplasty
  Wolfe cheiloplasty
cheilorrhaphy
cheiloschisis
cheilosis
cheilostomatoplasty
cheilotomy
  Garceau cheilotomy
cheirology
cheiromegaly
cheiroplasty
cheiropodalgia
cheirospasm

cheloidalis
  folliculitis cheloidalis
Chelsea-Eaton anal speculum
Chelsea-Eaton speculum
chemabrasion
chemexfoliation
chemical agent
chemical anesthesia
chemical burn
chemical capnography
chemical cardioversion
chemical cautery
chemical decortication
chemical dermatitis
chemical exchange
chemical exposure
chemical face peeling
chemical hemostasis
chemical hysterectomy
chemical labyrinthectomy
chemical pallidectomy
chemical peel
chemical peel of skin
chemical peeling
chemical shift
chemical sympathectomy
chemicocautery
chemocauterization
chemocautery
chemocoagulation
chemodectoma
chemodectomy
chemofoliation
chemolysis
chemoneurolysis
chemonucleolysis
  double-needle
    chemonucleolysis
chemonucleolysis table
chemopallidectomy
chemopallidectomy scissors
chemopallidothalamectomy
chemopeel
Chemo-Port catheter
Chemo-Port perivena catheter
  system device
chemoprophylaxis
chemoradiotherapy effect
chemosis
chemosurgery
  Mohs micrographic
    chemosurgery

chemosurgical gingivectomy
chemosurgical superficial
  dermatologic peel
chemotactic factor
chemotactic factor for
  macrophage (CFM)
chemotaxis
chemothalamectomy
chemotherapeutic agent
chemotherapy
  adjunctive chemotherapy
  adjuvant chemotherapy
  belly bath intraperitoneal
    chemotherapy
  combination chemotherapy
  concurrent chemotherapy
  dose of chemotherapy
  fractionation with
    chemotherapy
  fractionation without
    chemotherapy
  high-dose chemotherapy
  induction chemotherapy
  infusion chemotherapy
  infusional chemotherapy
  initial systemic chemotherapy
  intraarterial chemotherapy
    (IAC)
  intraperitoneal chemotherapy
  intraperitoneal hyperthermic
    chemotherapy (IPHC)
  intrapleural chemotherapy
  intravesical chemotherapy
  irradiation and chemotherapy
  maintenance chemotherapy
  Mohs chemotherapy
  postoperative chemotherapy
  postoperative systemic
    chemotherapy
  preoperative induction
    chemotherapy
  preoperative systemic
    chemotherapy
  radiation and chemotherapy
  second-line chemotherapy
  systemic chemotherapy
chemotherapy protocol
Chermel bone chisel
Chermel bone gouge
Chermel osteotome
Cherney abdominal incision
Cherney incision

Cherney lower transverse
    abdominal incision
Cherney suture technique
Cherney sutures
Cherney thyroid nodule
Cherney-Winklesnit abdominal
    incision
Chernez incision
Chernov hook
Chernov notched ruler
Chernov tracheostomy hook
Cheron forceps
Cheron uterine dressing forceps
cherry angioma
Cherry brain probe
Cherry drill
Cherry extractor
Cherry forceps
cherry hemangioma
Cherry laminectomy self-
    retaining retractor
Cherry osteotome
Cherry probe
Cherry retractor
Cherry scissors
Cherry screw extractor
Cherry Secto dissector
cherry sponge
cherry spot
Cherry S-shaped brain
    retractor
Cherry S-shaped scissors
Cherry tongs
Cherry traction tongs
Cherry-Adson forceps
Cherry-Austin drill
Cherry-Crandall procedure
Cherry-Kerrison forceps
Cherry-Kerrison laminectomy
    rongeur
Cherry-Kerrison rongeur
    forceps
cherry-picking procedure
cherubic facies
cherubism
Cheshire electrosurgical pencil
Cheshire-Poole-Yankauer suction
    instrument
chessboard graft
chessboard implant
chessboard prosthesis
chessboard skin graft

chest
    alar chest
    AP diameter of chest
    barrel chest
    barrel-shaped chest
    barrel-type chest
    caved-in chest
    crushing sensation in chest
    drainage of chest
    expansion of chest
    flail chest
    flat chest
    foveated chest
    funnel chest
    hourglass chest
    hyperaerated chest
    keeled chest
    pigeon chest
    silent chest
chest bellows
chest cardiac massage
chest cavity
chest clear to percussion and
    auscultation
chest compression
chest congestion
chest cuirass
chest diameter
chest drainage
chest dressing
chest examination
chest film
chest flap
chest lesion
chest mediastinum
chest muscles
chest nodules
chest pain
chest percussion
chest physical therapy
chest port
chest position
chest spreader
chest thump
chest tightness
chest tube
chest tube drainage (CTD)
chest tube stripper
chest wall
chest wall anomaly
chest wall defect
chest wall fixation

chest wall invasion
chest wall reconstruction
chest wall stabilization
chest x-ray
Chester forceps
Chester sponge forceps
Chesterfield canape aspect
Chesterfield sofa cellulite
Chester-Winter procedure
Chevalier Jackson bougie
Chevalier Jackson
    bronchoesophagoscopy
    forceps
Chevalier Jackson bronchoscope
Chevalier Jackson
    esophagoscope
Chevalier Jackson forceps
Chevalier Jackson gastroscope
Chevalier Jackson laryngeal
    speculum
Chevalier Jackson laryngectomy
Chevalier Jackson laryngoscope
Chevalier Jackson operation
Chevalier Jackson scissors
Chevalier Jackson speculum
Chevalier Jackson tracheal
    tube
Chevalier Jackson tube
chevron
chevron bunionectomy
chevron hallux valgus
    correction
chevron incision
chevron laceration
chevron marking technique
chevron osteotomy
chevron technique
chevron-shaped incision
chew-in technique
Chewrite denture adhesive
Cheyne dissector
Cheyne dry dissector
Cheyne operation
Cheyne periosteal elevator
Cheyne retractor
Cheyne-Stokes sign
CHF (congestive heart failure)
CHI (closed head injury)
Chiari anomaly
Chiari II syndrome
Chiari malformation
    (types I, II, III, IV)

Chiari operation for congenital
    hip dislocation
Chiari osteotomy
Chiari technique
Chiari-Arnold syndrome
chiasm
    Camper chiasm
    optic chiasm
    tendinous chiasm
chiasm of Camper
chiasm of digits of hand
chiasm of digitus of hand
chiasm of flexor sublimis
chiasm of musculus flexor
    digitorum
chiasm opticum
chiasma
chiasma formation
chiasmal compression
chiasmal lesion
chiasmal metastasis
chiasmatic cistern
chiasmatic groove
Chiazzi operation
Chiba biopsy needle
Chiba eye needle
Chiba needle
Chiba percutaneous
    cholangiogram
Chiba transhepatic
    cholangiography needle
Chicago classification
Chicco breast pump
Chick CLT operating frame
Chick CLT operating table
Chick fracture table
Chick operating table
Chick patient transfer device
Chick sterile dressings
Chick surgical light
Chick surgical table
chicken fat clot
chicken-bill rongeur
chicken-bill rongeur forceps
Chick-Foster orthopedic bed
Chick-Hyde fracture table
Chick-Langren table
chief artery of thumb
Chiene incision
Chiene operation
Chiene test for femoral neck
    fracture

Chiesi powder inhaler
Chilaiditi syndrome
chilblain
Chilcott cannula
Chilcott venoclysis cannula
Child classification of liver
    disease
Child clip-applying forceps
Child esophageal varix
child esophagoscope
Child forceps
Child hepatic dysfunction
    classification
Child hepatic risk criteria
    classification
Child intestinal forceps
Child liver disease classification
Child operation
Child operative risk grading
    system (A, B, C)
Child pancreatectomy
Child pancreaticoduodenostomy
child rectal dilator
childhood thyroid irradiation
Child-Phillips forceps
Child-Pugh classification
Children's Hospital dressing
    forceps
Children's Hospital brain spatula
Children's Hospital clip
Children's Hospital dressing
    forceps
Children's Hospital forceps
Children's Hospital hand drill
Children's Hospital intestinal
    forceps
Children's Hospital mallet
Children's Hospital pediatric
    retractor
Children's Hospital screwdriver
Children's Hospital spatula
Childress ankle fixation
    technique
Childress operation
child-restraint device
Childs Cardio-Cuff
child's rib spreader
child-size eye speculum
Childs-Phillips bowel plication
Childs-Phillips forceps
Childs-Phillips intestinal
    plication needle

Childs-Phillips needle
Childs-Phillips plication needle
Child-Turcotte classification of
    liver reserve
Child-Turcotte hepatic surgery
    classification
Chilli cooled ablation catheter
Chimani pharyngeal forceps
chimney sweeps carcinoma
chin
    asymmetric chin
    double chin
    extended anatomical chin
    galouche chin
    microlipofilling of the cheeks
        and chin
    ptosis of the chin
    senile chin
    weak chin
    witch's chin
chin augmentation
chin cap
chin deformity
chin elevation
chin implant
chin lift
chin muscle
chin notch
chin point
chin position
chin prosthesis
chin protuberance
chin reflex
chin retraction sign
chin strap
chin support
chin tuck
chin-contouring procedure
Chinese fingerstraps traction
    device
Chinese fingertrap suture
Chinese flap
Chinese twisted silk sutures
chink
    glottal chink
    glottic chink
chin-nose view
ChinUpps cervicofacial support
chip
    bone chip
    Dembone demineralized
        cancellous chips

chip (*continued*)
  Dembone demineralized
    cortical chips
  Dembone demineralized
    corticocancellous chips
  fracture chip
  ice chips
chip fracture
chip graft
chip syringe
chipmunk cheek appearance
Chirocaine anesthetic
Chiroflex lens
Chiron microkeratome
chiroplasty
chiropractic adjusting
    instrument
chiropractic treatment of
    fracture
Chiroslide measuring device
chisel
  Adson chisel
  Adson laminectomy chisel
  Alexander bone chisel
  Alexander chisel
  Alexander mastoid chisel
  Amico chisel
  Andrews chisel
  antral chisel
  Army chisel
  Army pattern chisel
  Artmann chisel
  Artmann disarticulation chisel
  Austin chisel
  Austin Moore mortising chisel
  Bakelite dental chisel
  Ballenger chisel
  Ballenger-Hajek chisel
  Basket chisel
  beveled chisel
  bilevel chisel
  binangled chisel
  Biomet cement removal hand
    chisel
  Bishop chisel
  Bishop mastoid chisel
  Blair chisel
  Blair nasal chisel
  bone chisel
  Bowen chisel
  Bowen gooseneck chisel
  Braithwaite nasal chisel

chisel (*continued*)
  Brauer chisel
  Brittain chisel
  Brown chisel
  Bruening chisel
  Brun chisel
  Brun guarded chisel
  Brunetti chisel
  Brunner chisel
  Brunswick-Mack chisel
  Buckley chisel
  Burns chisel
  Burns guarded chisel
  Caltagirone chisel
  canal chisel
  cartilage chisel
  cement-removal hand chisel
  Chermel bone chisel
  Cinelli chisel
  Cinelli-McIndoe chisel
  Clawicz chisel
  Clevedent-Gardner chisel
  Clevedent-Wakefield chisel
  Cloward chisel
  Cloward puka chisel
  Cloward spinal fusion chisel
  Cloward-Harman chisel
  Cobb chisel
  Compere bone chisel
  Compere chisel
  contra-angle chisel
  Converse chisel
  Converse guarded chisel
  Converse guarded nasal chisel
  Converse nasal chisel
  Cooley chisel
  cornea chisel
  corneal chisel
  costotome chisel
  Cottle antral chisel
  Cottle chisel
  Cottle crossbar chisel
  Cottle crossbar fishtail chisel
  Cottle curved chisel
  Cottle fishtail chisel
  Councilman chisel
  Crane bone chisel
  Crane chisel
  crossbar chisel
  crossbar fishtail chisel
  crurotomy chisel
  curved chisel

chisel (*continued*)
Dautrey chisel
Derlacki chisel
Derlacki-Shambaugh chisel
D'Errico chisel
D'Errico laminectomy chisel
disarticulation chisel
dissecting chisel
double safe-sided chisel
double-guarded chisel
Duray-Read chisel
Duray-Wood chisel
Dworacek-Farrior canal chisel
Ecker-Roopenian chisel
Eicher chisel
Eicher tri-fin chisel
endaural surgery chisel
ethmoidal chisel
Farrior-Derlacki chisel
Farrior-Dworacek canal chisel
Faulkner antral chisel
Faulkner antrum chisel
Faulkner chisel
Faulkner trocar chisel
Faulkner-Browne chisel
fishtail chisel
Fomon chisel
Fomon nasal chisel
footplate chisel
fracture chisel
Freer bone chisel
Freer chisel
Freer lacrimal chisel
Freer nasal chisel
Freer submucous chisel
French chisel
frontal sinus chisel
Gardner bone chisel
Gardner chisel
Goldman chisel
Goldman guarded chisel
gold-paneled chisel
gooseneck chisel
guarded chisel
Hajek chisel
Hajek septal chisel
Halle chisel
Harmon chisel
Hatch chisel
Heermann chisel
Henderson chisel
Hibbs bone chisel

chisel (*continued*)
Hibbs chisel
hollow chisel
Holmes chisel
Hough chisel
House chisel
House footplate chisel
House-Derlacki chisel
J.E. Sheehan chisel
Jenkins chisel
Jordan-Hermann chisel
Joseph chisel
Katsch chisel
Keyes bone-splitting chisel
Keyes chisel
Kezerian chisel
Killian chisel
Killian frontal sinus chisel
Killian-Claus chisel
Killian-Reinhard chisel
Kilner chisel
Kos chisel
Kreischer bone chisel
Kreischer chisel
lacrimal chisel
lacrimal sac chisel
Lambert-Lowman chisel
Lambotte bone chisel
Lambotte chisel
Lambotte splitting chisel
laminectomy chisel
Lebsche chisel
Lebsche sternal chisel
Lexer chisel
Lorenz chisel
Lowman chisel
Lowman-Hoglund chisel
Lucas chisel
MacAusland chisel
Magielski chisel
Magielski stapes chisel
Magnum chisel
Mannerfelt chisel
Martin cartilage chisel
mastoid chisel
McIndoe chisel
McIndoe nasal chisel
Metzenbaum chisel
Meyerding chisel
middle ear chisel
Miles bone chisel
Moberg chisel

chisel (*continued*)
  monoangle chisel
  Moore chisel
  Moore hollow chisel
  Moore prosthesis mortising
    chisel
  mortising chisel
  Murphy chisel
  nasal chisel
  Neivert chisel
  Nordent bone chisel
  Nordent-Oschsenbein
    periodontic chisel
  Obwegeser splitting chisel
  Oratek chisel
  orthopedic chisel
  Partsch bone chisel
  Partsch chisel
  Passow chisel
  peapod chisel
  Peck chisel
  pick chisel
  pterygoid chisel
  puka chisel
  Read chisel
  Rica mastoid chisel
  Richards chisel
  Richards-Hibbs chisel
  Rish chisel
  Roberts chisel
  Roberts hip dissecting chisel
  Rollet chisel
  Rubin nasal chisel
  Schuknecht chisel
  Schwartze chisel
  septal chisel
  Sewall chisel
  Sewall ethmoidal chisel
  Shambaugh-Derlacki chisel
  Sheehan chisel
  Sheehan nasal chisel
  Sheehy-House chisel
  Silver chisel
  Simmons chisel
  single safe-sided chisel
  sinus chisel
  Skoog nasal chisel
  small bone chisel
  SMIC bone chisel
  SMIC mastoid chisel
  SMIC sternal chisel
  Smillie cartilage chisel

chisel (*continued*)
  Smillie chisel
  Smillie meniscectomy chisel
  Smith-Peterson chisel
  Smith-Peterson chisel
  spinal fusion chisel
  splitting chisel
  stapes chisel
  Stille bone chisel
  Stille chisel
  Stille-pattern bone chisel
  submucous chisel
  Swedish-pattern chisel
  Swiderski nasal chisel
  tri-fin chisel
  Troutman chisel
  Troutman mastoid chisel
  twin-pattern chisel
  U.S. Army bone chisel
  U.S. Army chisel
  unibevel chisel
  Virchow chisel
  vulcanite chisel
  Walsh chisel
  Walsh footplate chisel
  Ward nasal chisel
  Wedelstaedt chisel
  West bone chisel
  West chisel
  West lacrimal chisel
  West nasal chisel
  White bone chisel
  White chisel
  Wilmer chisel
  Wilmer wedge chisel
  Worth chisel
chisel blade
chisel elevator
chisel fracture
chisel fracture of radius
chisel guard
chisel knife
chisel-osteotome
  crossbar chisel-osteotome
  nasal chisel-osteotome
chi-square test
Chitten-Hill retractor
chloasma
  melanoderma chloasma
chloasma bronzinum
chloasma gravidarum
chloramine

chloramine anesthetic agent
chloramine catgut suture
chloramine catgut sutures
chloramine-T technique
chloramphenicol
chloroma
Chloromycetin
chloromyeloma
chloroprocaine hydrochloride
    anesthetic agent
Chlumsky button
CHM (hypertrophic
    cardiomyopathy)
Cho anterior cruciate ligament
    reconstruction
Cho technique
Cho tendon technique
Cho 2-portal Dyonics endoscope
Cho-Dionics 2-portal endoscope
choana (*pl.* choanae)
    primary choana
    secondary choana
    bony choanae
choana atresia
choana narium
choanae osseae
choanal
choanal atresia
choanal bur
choanal opening
choanal plug
choanal polyp
choanal stenosis
chocolate cyst
Choice PT guidewire
choke vessel
choked disk
cholangiectasis
cholangioadenoma
Cholangiocath catheter
cholangiocholangiostomy
cholangiocholecystocholedoche-
    ctomy
cholangioenterostomy
cholangiogastrostomy
cholangiogram
    balloon cholangiogram
    Chiba percutaneous
        cholangiogram
    common duct cholangiogram
    contrast selective
        cholangiogram

cholangiogram (*continued*)
    cystic duct cholangiogram
    endoscopic cholangiogram
    endoscopic retrograde
        cholangiogram (ERC)
    false-negative cholangiogram
    fine-needle percutaneous
        cholangiogram
    fine-needle transhepatic
        cholangiogram
    intraoperative cholangiogram
    intravenous cholangiogram
        (IVC)
    nasobiliary catheter
        cholangiogram
    percutaneous cholangiogram
    percutaneous transhepatic
        cholangiogram
    preoperative retrograde
        cholangiogram
    retrograde cholangiogram
    serial cholangiograms
    thin-needle percutaneous
        cholangiogram
    transhepatic cholangiogram
        (THC)
    T-tube cholangiogram (TTC)
cholangiographic catheter
cholangiographic technique
cholangiography
    completion cholangiography
    delayed operative
        cholangiography
    drip-infusion cholangiography
    endoscopic retrograde
        cholangiography
    infusion cholangiography
    intraoperative dynamic
        cholangiography
    intravenous cholangiography
        (IVC)
    IV cholangiography
    magnetic resonance imaging
        cholangiography
    MRI cholangiography
    operative cholangiography (OC)
    percutaneous
        cholangiography
    percutaneous hepatobiliary
        cholangiography
    percutaneous transhepatic
        cholangiography (PTC)

cholangiography (*continued*)
  skinny needle
    cholangiography
  transabdominal
    cholangiography
  transhepatic
    cholangiography
  T-tube cholangiography
cholangiography catheter
cholangiography clamp
cholangiography tube
cholangiohepatoma
cholangiojejunostomy
  intrahepatic
    cholangiojejunostomy
Cholangiolapcath catheter
cholangiopancreatogram
  endoscopic retrograde
    cholangiopancreatogram
    (ERCP)
cholangiopancreatography
  endoscopic
    cholangiopancreatography
  endoscopic retrograde
    cholangiopancreatography
    (ERCP)
  magnetic resonance
    cholangiopancreatography
cholangiopancreatoscopy
  peroral
    cholangiopancreatoscopy
cholangioscope
  adaptable baby
    cholangioscope
  Olympus cholangioscope
  prototype cholangioscope
cholangioscopy
  intraductal cholangioscopy
  percutaneous transhepatic
    cholangioscopy
  peroral cholangioscopy
cholangiostomy
cholangiotomy
cholangitis carcinoma
cholefistula
cholecyst
cholecystalgia
cholecystatony
cholecystectasia
cholecystectomy
  2-trocar laparoscopic
    cholecystectomy

cholecystectomy (*continued*)
  3-trocar technique
    cholecystectomy
  combined laparoscopic
    splenectomy and
    cholecystectomy
  laparoscopic cholecystectomy
    (LC)
  laparoscopic laser
    cholecystectomy (LLC)
  laser laparoscopic
    cholecystectomy (LLC)
  microlaparoscopic
    cholecystectomy
  minilaparoscopic
    cholecystectomy
  needlescopic laparoscopic
    cholecystectomy
  open cholecystectomy
  percutaneous
    cholecystectomy
  prophylactic cholecystectomy
  retrograde cholecystectomy
  surgical cholecystectomy
  transcylindrical
    cholecystectomy
cholecystectomy treatment
cholecystelectrocoagulectomy
cholecystendysis
cholecystenteric
cholecystenteric fistula
cholecystenteroanastomosis
cholecystenterorrhaphy
cholecystenterostomy
cholecystgastric fistula
cholecystgastrostomy
cholecystic
cholecystitis
cholecystitis with lithiasis
cholecystnephrostomy
cholecystocecostomy
cholecystocholangiogram
cholecystocholangiography
cholecystocholedochal fistula
cholecystocolic fistula
cholecystocolonic
cholecystocolonic fistula
cholecystocolostomy
cholecystocolotomy
cholecystoduodenal fistula
cholecystoduodenal ligament
cholecystoduodenocolic fistula

cholecystoduodenocolic fold
cholecystoduodenostomy
  Jenckel
    cholecystoduodenostomy
cholecystoelectrocoagulectomy
cholecystoendoprosthesis
cholecystoenterostomy
cholecystogastric
cholecystogastric fistula
cholecystogastrostomy
cholecystogram
cholecystography
cholecystoileostomy
cholecystointestinal fistula
cholecystojejunostomy
cholecystokinetic
cholecystolithiasis
cholecystolithotomy
cholecystolithotripsy
cholecystonephrostomy
cholecystopancreatostomy
cholecystopathy
cholecystopexy
cholecystoptosis
cholecystopyelostomy
cholecystorrhaphy
cholecystoscopy
cholecystostomy
  laparoscopy-guided
    subhepatic
    cholecystostomy
  percutaneous cholecystostomy
  surgical cholecystostomy
cholecystotomy
  laparoscopic cholecystotomy
  transpapillary endoscopic
    cholecystotomy
choledocha
choledochal
choledochal cyst
choledochal cyst disease
choledochal fiberoscopic
  approach
choledochal sphincter
choledochal sphincterotomy
choledochectomy
choledochendysis
choledochitis
choledochocholedochorrhaphy
choledochocholedochostomy
choledochocholedochostomy
  side-to-side anastomosis

choledochocolonic fistula
choledochoduodenal fistula
choledochoduodenal
  fistulotomy
choledochoduodenal junction
choledochoduodenal junctional
  stenosis
choledochoduodenostomy
choledochoenteric fistula
choledochoenterostomy
choledochofiberoscopy
choledochofiberscope
choledochogastrostomy
choledochogram study
choledochography
choledochohepatostomy
choledochoileostomy
choledochojejunostomy
  loop choledochojejunostomy
  retrocolic
    choledochojejunostomy
choledocholith
choledocholithiasis
choledocholithotomy
choledocholithotripsy
choledochopancreatic ductal
  junction
choledochopancreatostomy
choledochoplasty
choledochorrhaphy
choledochoscope
  Berci-Shore choledochoscope
  fiberoptic choledochoscope
  Fujinon flexible
    choledochoscope
  Olympus choledochoscope
  Storz choledochoscope
choledochoscope-nephroscope
choledochoscopy
  Berci-Shore choledochoscopy
  cystic duct choledochoscopy
  jejunostomy tract
    choledochoscopy
  operative choledochoscopy
  postoperative
    choledochoscopy
  T-tube tract choledochoscopy
choledochosphincterotomy
choledochostomy
choledochotomy
choledochotomy incision
choledochus

choledochus cyst
choledogram
cholelithiasis
cholelithotomy
cholelithotripsy
cholelithotrity
cholemia
cholepathia
choleperitoneum
cholescintigraphy
cholesteatoma
    acquired cholesteatoma
    congenital cholesteatoma
    iatrogenic cholesteatoma
cholesterol
cholesterol calculus
cholesterol cleft
cholesterol gallstone
cholesterol granuloma cyst
cholesterol stone
cholinergic blockade
chondral
chondral edge
chondral fracture
chondral fragment
chondrectomy
chondrification
chondritis
chondroblast
chondroblastic sarcoma
chondroblastoma
chondrocalcific arthropathy
chondrocalcinosis
chondrocarcinoma
chondrocranium
chondrocutaneous flap
chondrocyte
chondrodermatitis
chondrodermatitis helicis
    nodularis
chondrodermatitis nodularis
    chronica helicis
chondrodynia
chondrodysplasia
chondrodystrophia
chondrodystrophia calcificans
    congenita
chondrodystrophia congenita
    punctata
chondrodystrophia fetalis
chondrodystrophia fetalis
    calcificans

chondrodystrophy
    familial chondrodystrophy
    hyperplastic
        chondrodystrophy
    hypoplastic
        chondrodystrophy
chondroectodermal dysplasia
chondroendothelioma
chondroethmoidal junction
chondrofasciocutaneous
chondrofibroma
chondrogenesis
chondrogenic sarcoma
chondroglossus muscle
chondroid
chondrolipoma
chondrolysis
chondroma
    benign chondroma
    condylar chondroma
    extraskeletal chondroma
    juxtacortical chondroma
    laryngeal chondroma
    malignant chondroma
    nasal chondroma
    synovial chondroma
chondromalacia
    generalized chondromalacia
    patellar chondromalacia
    systemic chondromalacia
chondromalacia fetalis
chondromalacia of larynx
chondromatosis
    Reichel chondromatosis
chondromatous
chondromatous growth
chondrometaplasia
chondromucoid
chondromucosal graft
chondromyxofibroma
chondromyxoma
chondronecrosis
chondro-osseous
chondro-osteodystrophy
chondropathology
chondropharyngeal muscle
chondroplasia
chondroplastic
chondroplastic Beaver blade
chondroplastic blade
chondroplasty
chondroplasty Beaver blade

chondroporosis
chondroradionecrosis
chondrosarcoma
  central chondrosarcoma
  extraosseous chondrosarcoma
  extraskeletal chondrosarcoma
  mesenchymal
    chondrosarcoma (MC)
chondrosarcomatosis
chondrosis
chondroskeleton
chondrosternal
chondrosternal articulation
chondrosternal depression
chondrosternoplasty
chondrotome
  Dyonics chondrotome
  Stryker chondrotome
chondrotomy
chop amputation
Chopart amputation
Chopart ankle dislocation
Chopart articulation
Chopart brace
Chopart cheiloplasty
Chopart dislocation
Chopart fracture
Chopart joint
Chopart operation
Chopart partial foot prosthesis
choppy sea sign
chord incision
chorda (*pl.* chordae)
chorda dorsalis
chorda gubernaculum
chorda saliva
chorda spermatica
chorda tendineae chordis
chorda tympani nerve
chorda tympani pusher
chordae tendineae rupture
chordal rupture
chordal tissue
chordate
chordectomy
chordee
chordee release
chordis
chorditis
chorditis cantorum
chorditis fibrinosa
chorditis nodosa

chorditis tuberosa
chorditis vocalis
chorditis vocalis inferior
chordoma (*pl.* chordomas)
  craniocervical chordoma
  dedifferentiated chordoma
  skull base chordoma
chordotomy
chorea
  Huntington chorea
  laryngeal chorea
choreiform movements
choreoathetosis
chorioallantoic membrane
choriocarcinoma
choriomeningitis
chorion
chorion membranes
chorionic
chorionic cavity
chorionic cyst
chorionic plaque
chorionic tissue
chorionic vesicle
chorionic villi
chorionic villi biopsy (CVB)
chorionic villi sampling
chorionic villus biopsy
chorionic villus sampling
    catheter
chorioretinal
chorioretinitis
choriovitelline placenta
choristoma
choroid
  basal lamina of choroid
  crescent choroid
  Haller layer of choroid
  knuckle of choroid
choroid artery
choroid atrophy
choroid detachment
choroid plexus
choroid plexus carcinoma
choroid point
choroid vein
choroidal artery
choroidal atrophy
choroidal cataract
choroidal hemangioma
choroidal hemorrhage
choroidal infiltration

choroidal lesion
choroidal metastasis
choroidal neovascular
    membrane
choroidal rupture
choroidal vessels
choroidectomy
choroiditis
Chorus pacemaker
Chow technique
Choyce anterior chamber lens
Choyce eye implant
Choyce implant
Choyce implant cataract lens
Choyce intraocular lens forceps
Choyce lens
Choyce lens forceps
Choyce lens-inserting forceps
Choyce Mark eye implant
Choyce Mark intraocular lens
Choyce Mark VII eye implant
Choyce MK II keratoprosthesis
Choyce-Tennant lens
Choyce Mark VIII lens
Chrisman-Snook ankle
    procedure
Chrisman-Snook ankle
    technique
Chrisman-Snook procedure
Chrisman-Snook reconstruction
Christensen articulator
Christiansen total hip
Christie gallbladder retractor
Christmas tree adapter
Christmas tree cannula
Christmas tree rasp
Christopher-Stille forceps
Christopher-Williams overtube
Christopher-Williams tube
Christoudias approximator
Christoudias fascial closure device
Christoudias fascial wound
    closure device
chromaffin body
Chromaser dermatology laser
chromated catgut sutures
chromatic lens aberration
chromatinic body
chromatography
    gas chromatography
    gas-liquid chromatography
    gas-solid chromatography

chromic
chromic blue dyed sutures
chromic catgut mattress sutures
chromic catgut sutures
chromic collagen sutures
chromic gut sutures
chromic ligatures
chromic sutures
chromicized catgut sutures
chromium-cobalt alloy implant
chromocystoscopy
chromohydrotubation
chromomycosis
chromopertubation
chromosomal mosaicism
chromotubation
chromoureteroscopy
chronaximeter
chronic opioid analgesic therapy
    (COAT)
chronic daily headache (CDH)
chronic paroxysmal hemicrania
    (CPH)
chronic renal failure (CRF)
chronic suppurative otitis media
    (CSOM)
Chronicure wound dressing
Chronocor IV external
    pacemaker
Chronos pacemaker
chronotropic effect
Chrys surgical CO_2 laser
CHS (compression hip screw)
CHS supracondylar bone plate
Chu foldable lens cutter
Chubb tonsil forceps
Chubb tonsillar forceps
Chubby balloon catheter
chuck
    3-point chuck
    Gam-Mer chuck
    gold-handled chuck
    hand chuck
    Jacobs chuck
    Jacobs snap-lock chuck
    Jacobs T-handled chuck
    key chuck
    pin chuck
    press-button chuck
    Steinmann pin chuck
    T-handle Jacob chuck
    T-handle Zimmer chuck

chuck (*continued*)
  Trinkle chuck
  Wozniak Sur-Lok chuck
chuck adapter
chuck cutter
chuck drill
chuck handle
chuck handle holster
chuck key
Chuck-It disposable accessories
Chuinard femoral osteotomy
Chuinard-Petersen arthrodesis
Chuinard-Peterson ankle fusion
Chukka boot
Chun-gun transillumination
Church cardiovascular scissors
Church deep surgery scissors
Church pediatric scissors
Church scissors
Churchill cardiac suction
  cannula
Churg-Strauss vasculitis
Chuter endovascular device
Chux incontinent dressing
Chvostek sign
Chvostek-Trousseau sign
Chvostek-Weiss sign
chyle
chyle cyst
chyle fat
chyle fistula
chylectasis
chyli
  cisterna chyli
chylous
chylous ascites
chylous fluid
chylous leak
chylous leakage
Chymodiactin
chymonucleolysis
chymopapain
Ciaccio glands
Ciaglia percutaneous
  tracheostomy introducer
Ciba Soft lens
Ciba Thin lens
Cibathin lens
Cibis electrode
Cibis liquid silicone procedure
Cibis operation
Cibis procedure

Cibis ski needle
Cibis-Vaiser muscle retractor
Cica-Care silicone gel sheet
  dressing
Cica-Care silicone gel sheeting
Cica-Care topical gel sheet
  dressing
cicatrectomy
cicatrices (*sing.* cicatrix)
cicatricial
cicatricial alopecia
cicatricial blepharoptosis
cicatricial contraction
cicatricial depression
cicatricial entropion
cicatricial horn
cicatricial kidney
cicatricial stenosis
cicatricial stricture
cicatricial tissue
cicatricotomy
cicatrisata
cicatrix (*pl.* cicatrices)
  filtering cicatrix
  hypertrophic cicatrix
  trophic cicatrix
  vicious cicatrix
cicatrizant
cicatrization
  epithelial cicatrization
  exuberant cicatrization
cicatrize
cicatrizing enteritis
Cicherelli bone rongeur
Cicherelli forceps
Cicherelli rongeur
Cicherelli rongeur forceps
cidal level
Cidex solution
Cierny-Mader technique
CIF needle
CIF-4 needle
cigar handle basket punch
cigarette drain
cigarette-paper scarring
cigarette-paper scars
Cikloid dressing
Cilacalcin double-chambered
  syringe
cilastatin
Cilastin tube
Cilco argon laser

Cilco extractor
Cilco Frigitronics laser
Cilco Hoffer Laseridge laser
Cilco intraocular lens
Cilco krypton laser
Cilco laser
Cilco Lasertek argon laser
Cilco lens
Cilco lens forceps
Cilco MonoFlex lens
Cilco ophthalmic endoscope
Cilco Optiflex intraocular lens
Cilco perimeter
Cilco posterior chamber
    intraocular lens
Cilco ultrasound unit
Cilco vitrector
Cilco YAG laser
Cilco-Simcoe II lens
Cilco-Sonometrics lens
cilectomy
cilia
cilia base
cilia forceps
cilia suture forceps
ciliaris
    acne ciliaris
    annulus ciliaris
    blepharitis ciliaris
    corona ciliaris
    corpus ciliaris
    radix longa ganglii ciliaris
    zonula ciliaris
ciliarotomy
ciliary
ciliary arteries
ciliary axis
ciliary body
ciliary canals
ciliary disk
ciliary flush
ciliary folds
ciliary ganglion
ciliary glands
ciliary immobility
ciliary injection
ciliary ligament
ciliary margins
ciliary motion
ciliary muscle
ciliary nerves
ciliary procedure

ciliary processes
ciliary reflex
ciliary region
ciliary veins
ciliary vessels
ciliary zonule
ciliectomy
ciliodestructive surgery
ciliogenesis
cilioretinal artery
cilioretinal vein
ciliospinal center
ciliotomy
ciliovitrectomy block
cilium (*pl.* cilia)
cilium pacemaker
Cimino arteriovenous fistula
Cimino arteriovenous shunt
Cimino AV fistula
Cimino dialysis shunt
Cimino fistula
Cimino-Brescia arteriovenous
    fistula
Cimochowski cardiac cannula
CIN (cervical intraepithelial
    neoplasia)
cinch operation
cinch suture
cinching
cinching operation
cinchocaine anesthetic agent
Cincinnati ACL brace
Cincinnati incision
Cincinnati technique
cinctured
cine camera
cine CT
cine CT scanner
cine gastrocamera
cine magnetic resonance
    imaging (cine MRI)
cine microscope
cineangiocardiogram
cineangiocardiography
cineangiogram
    biplane cineangiogram
    coronary cineangiogram
    left ventricular
      cineangiogram
    radionuclide cineangiogram
    selective coronary
      cineangiogram

cineangiography
cinearteriogram
cinebronchogram
cine-camera
cinefluorography
Cinelli chisel
Cinelli elevator
Cinelli guarded osteotome
Cinelli osteotome
Cinelli periosteal elevator
Cinelli scissors
Cinelli-Fomon scissors
Cinelli-McIndoe chisel
cine-magnetic resonance
    imaging
cinematic amputation
cinematization
cinephonation study
cineplastic amputation
cineplastic procedure
cineplastic surgery
cineplastics
cineplasty
    Spittle biceps muscle
        cineplasty
    Vanghetti cineplasty
cineradiogram
cineradiographic examination
cineradiography
cines and plain films
cingulate gyrus
cingulate herniation
cingulate sulcus
cingulectomy
cinguli gyrus
cingulotomy
cingulum bundle
cingulum dentis
cingulum modification
cingulumotomy
Cintor knee prosthesis
cionectomy
cionorrhaphy
cionotome
cionotomy
Cipro cystitis pack
Circadia dual-chamber rate-
    adaptive pacemaker
circadian event recorder
CircAid elastic stockings
circinate
circinate exudate

circle
    Berry circle
    Haller circle
    Hovius circle
    Minsky circle
    Willis circle
    Zinn circle
circle absorption anesthesia
circle knife
circle loop biliary drainage
circle nephrostomy tube
circle of Willis
circlet
Circline magnifier
circling silicone tape
CircOlectric bed
CircOlectric sling
Circon ACMI cannula
Circon ACMI diagnostic
        laparoscope
Circon ACMI hysteroscope
Circon ACMI trocar
Circon arthroscope
Circon camera
Circon leg holder
Circon Tripolar forceps
Circon video camera
Circon videohydrothoracoscope
Circon-ACMI electrohydraulic
        lithotriptor probe
Circon-ACMI endoscope
Circon-ACMI lithotriptor
CircPlus compression dressing
CircPlus wrap
circuit
    anesthesia breathing circuit
    anesthetic circuit
    neuronal circuit
    ventilation circuit
circuit adapter
circular amputation
circular anastomosis
circular bandage
circular blade
circular block anesthesia
circular cherry-red lesion
circular cup bronchoscopic
        biopsy forceps
circular dental ligament
circular enterorrhaphy
circular external fixator
circular fibers

circular fibers of ciliary muscle
circular flap
circular fold
circular griseotomy
circular guillotine incision
circular incision
circular intraluminal stapler
circular lesion
circular mechanical stapler
circular muscle
circular myotomy
circular open amputation
circular punch
circular rasp
circular saw
circular stapler
circular stapling device
circular subcutaneous island
   flap
circular suture technique
circular sutures
circular tape
circular twin saw
circular with Passavant ridge
   pattern of closure
circulating blood volume
circulation
   airway, breathing, and
     circulation (ABC)
   allantoic circulation
   arterial circulation
   assisted circulation
   bile acid circulation
   cardiopulmonary circulation
   cardiovascular circulation
   carotid circulation
   cerebral circulation
   cerebrovascular blood
     circulation
   collateral abdominal
     circulation
   collateral arterial circulation
   collateral circulation
   collateral mesenteric
     circulation
   compensatory circulation
   conjunctival circulation
   coronary circulation
   coronary collateral circulation
   cross circulation
   cutaneous collateral
     circulation

circulation (*continued*)
   derivative circulation
   ductal-dependent pulmonary
     circulation
   enterohepatic circulation
   episcleral circulation
   extracorporeal circulation
   extracranial carotid
     circulation
   femoral circulation
   fetal circulation
   fetoplacental circulation
   greater circulation
   hepatic circulation
   hyperdynamic circulation
   hypophyseal portal
     circulation
   hypothalamic-hypophysial
     portal circulation
   intervillous circulation
   intracranial circulation
   left dominant coronary
     circulation
   lymph circulation
   mesenteric circulation
   perichondral circulation
   peripheral circulation
   persistent fetal circulation
   placental circulation
   portal circulation
   portal-collateral circulation
   portal-hypophysial circulation
   portosystemic collateral
     circulation
   posterior fossa circulation
   pulmonary circulation
   retinal circulation
   sinusoidal circulation
   sludging of circulation
   spinal cord circulation
   splanchnic circulation
   systemic circulation
   systemic venous circulation
   thalamic circulation
   thebesian circulation
   umbilical circulation
   uteroplacental circulation
   venous circulation
   vitelline circulation
circulation aneurysm
circulation rate
circulation time

circulation volume
circulator
circulator fold
circulatory
circulatory arrest anesthetic
    technique
circulatory arrest procedure
circulatory assist
circulatory collapse
circulatory compromise
circulatory control
circulatory decompensation
circulatory embarrassment
circulatory overload
circulatory system function
Circulon dressing
Circulon wrap
circumalveolar fixation
circumanal glands
circumareolar
circumareolar incision
circumareolar scar
circumcaval ureter
circumcise
circumcision
    Kantor circumcision
    Plastibell circumcision
    ritual circumcision
    sleeve-resection
        circumcision
circumcision clamp
circumcision suture technique
circumcisional clamp
circumcisional incision
circumcisional scissors
circumcisional shield
circumcisional sutures
circumcorneal incision
circumcorneal injection
circumcoronal wire
circumcostal gastropexy
circumdential wire
circumduction
circumduction maneuver
circumductor table
circumference
    abdominal circumference
    head circumference
    occipitofrontal circumference
circumference of the chest at
    the inframammary crease
    (C-IMC)

circumference of the chest at
    the nipple (C-N)
circumferential
circumferential bipolar montage
circumferential dressing
circumferential esophageal
    reconstruction
circumferential
    esophagomyotomy
circumferential extremity coil
circumferential fibrocartilage
circumferential fracture
circumferential implantation
circumferential incision
circumferential lesion
circumferential mesorectal
    excision
circumferential mobilization
circumferential mucosal
    dissection
circumferential para-axillary
    superficial tumescent
    (CAST) liposuction
circumferential strip
circumferential tearing of skin
circumferential venolysis
circumferential wire-loop
    fixation
circumferential wiring
circumferentially
circumferentiating skin incision
circumflex
circumflex artery
circumflex artery of scapula
circumflex artery scissors
circumflex coronary artery
circumflex femoral artery
circumflex femoral veins
circumflex humeral artery
circumflex iliac artery
circumflex iliac superficial fascia
circumflex iliac vein
circumflex nerve
circumflex scapular artery
circumflex scapular flap
circumflex scapular pedicle
circumflex scissors
circumflex vessel
circumflexed branch
circumlental space
circumlimbal incision
circumlinear incision

circummandibular
circummandibular fixation
circummandibular wiring
circumocular
circumoral
circumoral incision
circumorbital
Circumpress chin strap
Circumpress facelift dressing
circumscribed
circumscribed abscess
circumscribed area
circumscribed choroidal
    hemangioma (CCH)
circumscribed gangrene
circumscribed inflammation
circumscribed labyrinthitis
circumscribed lesion
circumscribed precancerous
    melanosis
circumscribed scleroderma
circumscribed vitiligo
circumscribing incision
circumscripta
    alopecia circumscripta
    calcinosis circumscripta
    osteoporosis circumscripta
circumscriptum
    angiokeratoma
      circumscriptum
    lymphangioma
      circumscriptum
Circumstraint restraint
circumtractor
circum-umbilical incision
circumvallate papilla
circumvent
circumzygomatic
circumzygomatic fixation
circumzygomatic wiring
cirrhosis
    alcoholic cirrhosis
    coarse nodular cirrhosis
    Laennec cirrhosis
    perioportal cirrhosis
    periportal cirrhosis
cirrhotic
cirrhotic gastritis
cirrhotic liver
Cirrus composite prosthetic foot
Cirrus foot prosthesis
cirsectomy

cirsenchysis
cirsodesis
cirsotome
cirsotome knife
cirsotomy
CIS (carcinoma in situ)
Cisco covered needle catheter
cistern
    cerebellomedullary cistern
    cerebellopontine angle
      cistern
    chiasmatic cistern
    great cistern
    interpeduncular cistern
    subarachnoidal cisterns
cisterna
    subarachnoid cisterna
    suprasellar cisterna
cisterna chyli
cisterna magna
cisterna magna catheter
cisternal herniation
cisternal puncture
cisternal tap
cisternogram
    metrizamide cisternogram
cisternography
    oxygen cisternography
    RISA cisternography
Citanest anesthetic agent
Citelli forceps
Citelli laminectomy punch
Citelli punch
Citelli punch forceps
Citelli rongeur
Citelli sphenoid rongeur
Citelli-Bruening ear forceps
Citelli-Meltzer atticus punch
Citelli-Meltzer punch
citrate
citric acid
Citscope arthroscope
Civiale forceps
Civiale lithotrity
Civiale operation
Civinni spine
CL (cervical line)
CL (cleft lip)
CLA (cleft lip alveolus)
Clado anastomosis
Clado point
Claes scleral depressor

Clagett Barrett
  esophagogastrostomy
Clagett cannula
Clagett closure
Clagett needle
Clagett operation
Clagett S-cannula
Clairborne clamp
clam enterocystoplasty
clam ileocystoplasty
clamp
  3-bladed clamp
  Abadie clamp
  Abadie enterostomy clamp
  Ablaza clamp
  Ablaza patent ductus clamp
  Abramson-Allis breast clamp
  Acland clamp
  Acland microvascular clamp
  Adair breast clamp
  Adair clamp
  Adson clamp
  Adson-Brown clamp
  agraffe clamp
  Ahlquist-Durham embolism
    clamp
  air inflatable vessel occluder
    clamp
  Alfred M. Large clamp
  Alfred M. Large vena cava
    clamp
  Allen anastomosis clamp
  Allen clamp
  Allen intestinal clamp
  Allen-Kocher clamp
  Allis clamp
  Allis tissue clamp
  Allison clamp
  Alyea clamp
  Alyea vas clamp
  anastomosis clamp
  Ando aortic clamp
  aneurysm clamp
  angled clamp
  angled DeBakey clamp
  angled peripheral vascular
    clamp
  Ann Arbor clamp
  Ann Arbor double towel
    clamp
  Ann Arbor towel clamp
  anterior resection clamp

clamp (*continued*)
  AO clamp
  aorta aneurysm clamp
  aorta clamp
  aortic aneurysm clamp
  aortic cannula clamp
  aortic clamp
  aortic occlusion clamp
  appendage clamp
  approximator clamp
  arterial clamp
  Asch clamp
  Atlee bronchus clamp
  Atlee clamp
  Atra-grip clamp
  atraumatic bowel clamp
  atraumatic clamp
  atraumatic intestinal clamp
  Atraumax peripheral vascular
    clamp
  atrial clamp
  Ault clamp
  Ault intestinal clamp
  Ault intestinal occlusion
    clamp
  auricle clamp
  auricular appendage clamp
  auricular artery clamp
  Auvard clamp
  Babcock clamp
  Babcock tissue clamp
  baby Bishop clamp
  baby Kocher clamp
  baby pylorus clamp
  baby Satinsky clamp
  Backhaus clamp
  Backhaus towel clamp
  Backhaus-Jones towel clamp
  Backhaus-Kocher towel clamp
  Bahnson aortic aneurysm
    clamp
  Bahnson aortic clamp
  Bahnson appendage clamp
  Bahnson clamp
  Bailey aortic clamp
  Bailey clamp
  Bailey duckbill clamp
  Bailey-Cowley clamp
  Bailey-Morse clamp
  Bainbridge anastomosis clamp
  Bainbridge clamp
  Bainbridge intestinal clamp

clamp (*continued*)
  Bainbridge vessel clamp
  Balfour clamp
  Ballantine clamp
  Bamby clamp
  Bard clamp
  Bard Cunningham
    incontinence clamp
  Barraquer needle holder
    clamp
  Bartley anastomosis clamp
  Bartley partial-occlusion
    clamp
  bar-to-bar clamp
  Bauer kidney pedicle clamp
  Baumrucker incontinence
    clamp
  Baumrucker post-TUR
    irrigation clamp
  Baumrucker urinary
    incontinence clamp
  Baumrucker-DeBakey clamp
  Beall bulldog clamp
  Beall-Morris ascending aortic
    clamp
  Beardsley clamp
  Beardsley intestinal clamp
  Beck aortic clamp
  Beck clamp
  Beck miniature aortic clamp
  Beck vascular clamp
  Beck vessel clamp
  Beck-Potts aorta and
    pulmonic clamp
  Beck-Potts aortic clamp
  Beck-Potts clamp
  Beck-Potts pulmonic clamp
  Beck-Satinsky clamp
  Belcher clamp
  Bell clamp
  Benson pyloric clamp
  Berens clamp
  Berens muscle clamp
  Berke clamp
  Berke ptosis clamp
  Berkeley clamp
  Berkeley-Bonney vaginal
    clamp
  Berman aortic clamp
  Berman clamp
  Berman vascular clamp
  Bernhard clamp

clamp (*continued*)
  Berry clamp
  Berry pile clamp
  Best clamp
  Best colon clamp
  Best intestinal clamp
  Best right-angle colon clamp
  Bethune clamp
  Bielawski heart clamp
  Bigelow calvaria clamp
  Bigelow calvarium clamp
  Bigelow clamp
  Bihrle dorsal clamp
  Bircher bone-holding clamp
  Bircher cartilage clamp
  Bishop bone clamp
  Black clamp
  Black meatal clamp
  Black meatus clamp
  bladder irrigation control
    clamp
  Blair cleft palate clamp
  Blalock clamp
  Blalock pulmonary artery
    clamp
  Blalock pulmonary clamp
  Blalock pulmonic stenosis
    clamp
  Blalock-Niedner clamp
  Blalock-Niedner pulmonic
    clamp
  Blalock-Niedner pulmonic
    stenosis clamp
  Blanchard clamp
  Blanchard pile clamp
  Blasucci clamp
  blepharostat clamp
  bloodless circumcision clamp
  Boehler clamp
  Boehler os calcis clamp
  Boettcher pulmonary artery
    clamp
  bone clamp
  bone extension clamp
  bone-holding clamp
  Bonney clamp
  Borge bile duct clamp
  Borge clamp
  Bortz clamp
  Boyes clamp
  Boyes muscle clamp
  Bozeman clamp

clamp (*continued*)

Bradshaw-O'Neill aorta clamp
Bradshaw-O'Neill aortic clamp
Bradshaw-O'Neill clamp
Bridge clamp
Brock auricle clamp
Brock auricular clamp
Brock clamp
Brockington pile clamp
Brodney clamp
Brodney urethrographic clamp
bronchus clamp
Brown clamp
Brown lip clamp
Brunner colon clamp
Brunner intestinal clamp
Buie clamp
Buie pile clamp
Buie-Hirschman clamp
Buie-Hirschman pile clamp
bulldog clamp
Bunke clamp
Bunnell-Howard arthrodesis clamp
Burford clamp
Burlisher clamp
Bushey compression clamp
Buxton clamp
Buxton uterine clamp
Cairns clamp
Calandruccio clamp
Calman carotid clamp
Calman ring clamp
calvarial clamp
calvarium clamp
cannula clamp
Capes clamp
Cardio-Grip anastomosis clamp
Cardio-Grip aortic clamp
Cardio-Grip bronchus clamp
Cardio-Grip pediatric clamp
Cardio-Grip renal artery clamp
Cardio-Grip tangential occlusion clamp
Cardio-Grip vascular clamp
cardiovascular anastomotic clamp
cardiovascular bulldog clamp
cardiovascular clamp

clamp (*continued*)

Carmalt clamp
carotid artery bypass clamp
carotid artery clamp
carotid clamp
Carrel clamp
Carter clamp
Carter-Glassman resection clamp
cartilage clamp
caruncle clamp
Casey pelvic clamp
Castaneda 1MM vascular clamp
Castaneda anastomosis clamp
Castaneda clamp
Castaneda vascular clamp
Castaneda multipurpose clamp
Castaneda partial-occlusion clamp
Castaneda vascular clamp
Castaneda-Mixter clamp
Castaneda-Mixter thoracic clamp
Castroviejo clamp
Castroviejo lens clamp
Castroviejo mosquito lid clamp
Castroviejo needle holder clamp
catheter clamp
cautery clamp
caval occlusion clamp
C-clamp
celiac clamp
cervical clamp
chalazion clamp
Charnley arthrodesis clamp
Charnley bone clamp
Charnley clamp
Charnley external fixation clamp
Charnley pin clamp
cholangiography clamp
circumcision clamp
circumcisional clamp
Clairborne clamp
Clevis clamp
cloth-shod clamp
coarctation clamp
Codman cartilage clamp

clamp (*continued*)
- Codman clamp
- Codman towel clamp
- Collier thoracic clamp
- Collin clamp
- Collin umbilical clamp
- colon clamp
- colostomy clamp
- columella clamp
- columellar clamp
- Conger perineal urethrostomy clamp
- contour block clamp
- Cooley acutely-curved clamp
- Cooley anastomosis clamp
- Cooley aortic aneurysm clamp
- Cooley aortic cannula clamp
- Cooley aortic clamp
- Cooley bronchial clamp
- Cooley bronchus clamp
- Cooley bulldog clamp
- Cooley carotid clamp
- Cooley caval occlusion clamp
- Cooley clamp
- Cooley coarctation clamp
- Cooley cross-action bulldog clamp
- Cooley curved cardiovascular clamp
- Cooley double-angled clamp
- Cooley graft clamp
- Cooley iliac clamp
- Cooley multipurpose clamp
- Cooley neonatal vascular clamp
- Cooley partial occlusion clamp
- Cooley patent ductus clamp
- Cooley pediatric clamp
- Cooley pediatric vascular clamp
- Cooley peripheral vascular clamp
- Cooley renal artery clamp
- Cooley renal clamp
- Cooley subclavian clamp
- Cooley tangential pediatric clamp
- Cooley vascular clamp
- Cooley vena cava clamp
- Cooley vena caval catheter clamp

clamp (*continued*)
- Cooley vena caval clamp
- Cooley-Baumgarten aortic clamp
- Cooley-Beck clamp
- Cooley-Beck vessel clamp
- Cooley-Derra anastomosis clamp
- Cooley-Derra clamp
- Cooley-Satinsky clamp
- Cooley-Satinsky multipurpose clamp
- Cope clamp
- Cope crushing clamp
- Cope modification of Martel intestinal clamp
- Cope-DeMartel clamp
- cordotomy clamp
- Cottle clamp
- Cottle columella clamp
- Cottle columellar clamp
- cotton-roll rubber-dam clamp
- Crafoord aortic clamp
- Crafoord auricular clamp
- Crafoord clamp
- Crafoord coarctation clamp
- Crafoord-Sellors auricular clamp
- Crawford auricle clamp
- Crenshaw caruncle clamp
- Crile appendiceal clamp
- Crile clamp
- Crile crushing clamp
- Crile hemostatic clamp
- Crile-Crutchfield clamp
- Cross clamp
- cross-action bulldog clamp
- cross-action clamp
- cross-action towel clamp
- Cruickshank clamp
- Cruickshank entropion clamp
- crushing clamp
- Crutchfield carotid artery clamp
- Crutchfield clamp
- Cunningham clamp
- Cunningham incontinence clamp
- Cunningham urinary incontinence clamp
- curved cardiovascular clamp
- curved clamp

clamp (*continued*)
  curved Mayo clamp
  curved mosquito clamp
  curved-8 clamp
  Cushing clamp
  cystic duct catheter clamp
  Dacron graft clamp
  Daems bronchial clamp
  Daems clamp
  D'Allesandro clamp
  Dandy clamp
  Daniel clamp
  Daniel colostomy clamp
  Dardik clamp
  D'Assumpcao clamp
  David-Baker clamp
  David-Baker lip clamp
  Davidson clamp
  Davidson muscle clamp
  Davidson pulmonary vessel
    clamp
  Davidson vessel clamp
  Davila atrial clamp
  Davis aneurysm clamp
  Davis aortic aneurysm clamp
  Davis clamp
  Dean MacDonald clamp
  Dean MacDonald gastric
    resection clamp
  Deaver clamp
  DeBakey aortic aneurysm
    clamp
  DeBakey aortic clamp
  DeBakey aortic exclusion
    clamp
  DeBakey arterial clamp
  DeBakey bulldog clamp
  DeBakey clamp
  DeBakey coarctation clamp
  DeBakey cross-action bulldog
    clamp
  DeBakey curved peripheral
    vascular clamp
  DeBakey miniature
    multipurpose clamp
  DeBakey multipurpose clamp
  DeBakey patent ductus clamp
  DeBakey pediatric clamp
  DeBakey peripheral vascular
    clamp
  DeBakey right-angled
    multipurpose clamp

clamp (*continued*)
  DeBakey ring-handled bulldog
    clamp
  DeBakey S-shaped peripheral
    vascular clamp
  DeBakey tangential clamp
  DeBakey tangential occlusion
    clamp
  DeBakey vascular clamp
  DeBakey-Bahnson clamp
  DeBakey-Bahnson vascular
    clamp
  DeBakey-Bainbridge clamp
  DeBakey-Bainbridge vascular
    clamp
  DeBakey-Beck clamp
  DeBakey-Craafoord vascular
    clamp
  DeBakey-Derra anastomosis
    clamp
  DeBakey-Harken auricle
    clamp
  DeBakey-Harken auricular
    clamp
  DeBakey-Harken clamp
  DeBakey-Howard aortic
    aneurysm clamp
  DeBakey-Howard aortic
    aneurysmal clamp
  DeBakey-Howard clamp
  DeBakey-Kay aortic clamp
  DeBakey-Kay clamp
  DeBakey-McQuigg-Mixter
    bronchial clamp
  DeBakey-Satinsky vena cava
    clamp
  DeBakey-Satinsky vena caval
    clamp
  DeBakey-Semb clamp
  DeBakey-Semb ligature-carrier
    clamp
  DeCourcy clamp
  DeCourcy goiter clamp
  DeMartel clamp
  DeMartel vascular clamp
  DeMartel-Wolfson
    anastomosis clamp
  DeMartel-Wolfson
    anastomotic clamp
  DeMartel-Wolfson clamp
  DeMartel-Wolfson colon
    clamp

clamp (*continued*)
- DeMartel-Wolfson intestinal anastomotic clamp
- DeMartel-Wolfson intestinal clamp
- Demel wire clamp
- Demos tibial artery clamp
- Dennis anastomotic clamp
- Dennis clamp
- Dennis intestinal clamp
- Derra anastomosis clamp
- Derra aortic clamp
- Derra clamp
- Derra vena cava clamp
- Derra vestibular clamp
- Desmarres clamp
- Desmarres lid clamp
- Devonshire-Mack clamp
- DeWeese clamp
- DeWeese vena cava clamp
- Dick bronchus clamp
- Dick pressure clamp
- Dieffenbach bulldog clamp
- Dieffenbach clamp
- Diethrich aortic clamp
- Diethrich clamp
- Diethrich graft clamp
- Diethrich microcoronary bulldog clamp
- Diethrich shunt clamp
- Dingman cartilage clamp
- Dingman clamp
- disposable muscle biopsy clamp
- dissecting clamp
- distraction clamp
- Dixon-Thomas-Smith clamp
- Dixon-Thomas-Smith colonic clamp
- Dixon-Thomas-Smith intestinal clamp
- Dobbie-Trout bulldog clamp
- Dobbie-Trout clamp
- Doctor Collins clamp
- Doctor Collins fracture clamp
- Doctor Long clamp
- Dogliotti-Gugliel mini clamp
- Dolphin cord clamp
- Donald clamp
- double Softjaw clamp
- double towel clamp
- double-angled clamp

clamp (*continued*)
- Downing clamp
- Doyen clamp
- Doyen intestinal clamp
- Doyen towel clamp
- drape clamp
- dreamer clamp
- duckbill clamp
- ductus clamp
- duodenal clamp
- Duval lung clamp
- Earle clamp
- Earle hemorrhoidal clamp
- Eastman clamp
- Eastman intestinal clamp
- Edebohls clamp
- Edebohls kidney clamp
- Edna towel clamp
- Edwards clamp
- Edwards double Softjaw clamp
- Edwards handleless clamp
- Edwards single Softjaw clamp
- Edwards spring clamp
- Eisenstein clamp
- endoaortic clamp
- English clamp
- enterostomy clamp
- entropion clamp
- Erhardt clamp
- Erhardt lid clamp
- Ewald-Hudson clamp
- Ewing lid clamp
- exclusion clamp
- extension bone clamp
- extension clamp
- extracutaneous vas fixation clamp
- Falk clamp
- Falk vaginal cuff clamp
- Farabeuf bone clamp
- Farabeuf-Lambotte bone-holding clamp
- Farabeuf-Lambotte clamp
- Fauer peritoneal clamp
- Favaloro proximal anastomosis clamp
- Favorite clamp
- feather clamp
- Fehland clamp
- Fehland intestinal clamp
- Fehland right-angled colon clamp

clamp (*continued*)
   femoral clamp
   Ferguson bone clamp
   Ferrier gingival clamp
   ferrule clamp
   fetal cord clamp
   fine-toothed clamp
   Finochietto arterial clamp
   Finochietto artery clamp
   Finochietto bronchial clamp
   Finochietto clamp
   Fitzgerald aortic aneurysm
      clamp
   flexible aortic clamp
   flexible retractor pressure
      clamp
   flexible retractor sliding
      clamp
   flexible vascular clamp
   flow-regulator clamp
   Fogarty clamp
   Fogarty Hydragrip clamp
   Fogarty vascular clamp
   Fogarty-Chin clamp
   Ford clamp
   Forrester clamp
   Foss anterior resection clamp
   Foss cardiovascular clamp
   Foss clamp
   Foss intestinal clamp
   Frahur cartilage clamp
   Frahur clamp
   Frazier-Adson clamp
   Frazier-Adson osteoplastic
      clamp
   Frazier-Adson osteoplastic
      flap clamp
   Frazier-Sachs clamp
   Freeman clamp
   Friedrich clamp
   Friedrich-Petz clamp
   Fukushima C-clamp clamp
   full-curved clamp
   Furness anastomosis clamp
   Furness-McClure-Hinton
      clamp
   Furniss anastomotic clamp
   Furniss clamp
   Furniss-Clute anastomosis
      clamp
   Furniss-Clute clamp
   Furniss-Clute duodenal clamp

clamp (*continued*)
   Furniss-McClure-Hinton clamp
   gallbladder ring clamp
   Gam-Mer aneurysm clamp
   Gam-Mer occlusion clamp
   Gandy clamp
   Gant clamp
   Garcia aorta clamp
   Garcia aortic clamp
   Gardner skull clamp
   Garland clamp
   Garland hysterectomy clamp
   Gaskell clamp
   gastric clamp
   gastroenterostomy clamp
   gastrointestinal clamp
   gate clamp
   Gavin-Miller clamp
   Gemini clamp
   Gerald clamp
   Gerbode patent ductus clamp
   Gerster bone clamp
   GI clamp
   gingival clamp
   Gladstone-Putterman
      transmarginal rotation
      entropion clamp
   Glass liver-holding clamp
   Glassman anterior resection
      clamp
   Glassman bowel atraumatic
      clamp
   Glassman clamp
   Glassman gastroenterostomy
      clamp
   Glassman gastrointestinal
      clamp
   Glassman intestinal clamp
   Glassman liver-holding clamp
   Glassman noncrushing
      gastroenterostomy clamp
   Glassman noncrushing
      gastrointestinal clamp
   Glassman-Allis clamp
   Glover auricular clamp
   Glover auricular-appendage
      clamp
   Glover bulldog clamp
   Glover clamp
   Glover coarctation clamp
   Glover curved clamp
   Glover patent ductus clamp

clamp (*continued*)

Glover spoon anastomosis clamp
Glover spoon-shaped anastomosis clamp
Glover vascular clamp
Glover-DeBakey clamp
Glover-Stille clamp
goiter clamp
Goldblatt clamp
Goldstein Microspike approximator clamp
Goldvasser clamp
Gomco bell clamp
Gomco bloodless circumcision clamp
Gomco circumcision clamp
Gomco clamp
Gomco umbilical cord clamp
Gomco-Bell clamp
Goodhill tonsillar hemostatic clamp
Goodwin bone clamp
Goodwin clamp
Grafco incontinence clamp
Grafco umbilical cord clamp
graft clamp
Grant abdominal aortic aneurysmal clamp
Grant aneurysmal clamp
Grant aortic aneurysm clamp
Grant clamp
grasping clamp
Gray clamp
Green bulldog clamp
Green clamp
Green lid clamp
Green suction tube-holding clamp
Greenberg clamp
Gregory baby profunda clamp
Gregory bulldog clamp
Gregory carotid bulldog clamp
Gregory clamp
Gregory external clamp
Gregory stay suture clamp
Gregory vascular miniature clamp
Gross clamp
Gross coarctation clamp
Gross coarctation occlusion clamp

clamp (*continued*)

Grover Atra-grip clamp
Grover auricular appendage clamp
Grover clamp
Gusberg hysterectomy clamp
Gussenbauer clamp
gut and colon clamp
gut clamp
Gutgeman auricular appendage clamp
Gutgeman clamp
Guyon clamp
Guyon kidney clamp
Guyon vessel clamp
Guyon-Péan clamp
Guyon-Péan vessel clamp
Haberer intestinal clamp
half-curved clamp
Halifax interlaminar clamp
Halsted clamp
Halsted straight mosquito clamp
handleless clamp
Haney clamp
Harken auricular clamp
Harken clamp
Harrah lung clamp
Harrington clamp
Harrington hook clamp
Harrington-Carmalt clamp
Harrington-Mixter clamp
Harrington-Mixter thoracic clamp
Hartmann clamp
Harvey Stone clamp
Hatch clamp
Hausmann vascular clamp
Haverhill clamp
Haverhill-Mack clamp
Hayes anterior resection clamp
Hayes clamp
Hayes colon clamp
Hayes intestinal clamp
Heaney clamp
Heartport endoaortic clamp
Heifitz cerebral aneurysm clamp
Heifitz clamp
Heitz-Boyer clamp
hemoclip clamp
hemorrhoidal clamp

clamp (*continued*)

hemostatic clamp
hemostatic thoracic clamp
Hendren cardiovascular clamp
Hendren clamp
Hendren ductus clamp
Hendren megaureter clamp
Hendren ureteral clamp
Henley subclavian artery
   clamp
Henley vascular clamp
Herbert Adams clamp
Herbert Adams coarctation
   clamp
Herff clamp
Herrick clamp
Herrick kidney clamp
Herrick kidney pedicle clamp
Herrick pedicle clamp
Hesseltine clamp
Hesseltine umbilical cord
   clamp
Hex-Fix Universal swivel
   clamp
Heyer-Schulte biopsy clamp
Heyer-Schulte clamp
Heyer-Schulte muscle biopsy
   clamp
Hibbs clamp
hilar clamp
Hirsch mucosal clamp
Hirschman clamp
Hirschman pile clamp
Hoff towel clamp
Hoffmann clamp
Hoffmann ligament clamp
Hohmann clamp
Hollister clamp
Holter pump clamp
Hopener clamp
Hopkins aortic clamp
Hopkins aortic occlusion
   clamp
Hopkins clamp
Hopkins hysterectomy clamp
Howard-DeBakey aortic
   aneurysm clamp
Hudson clamp
Hufnagel aortic clamp
Hufnagel ascending aortic
   clamp
Hufnagel clamp

clamp (*continued*)

Hufnagel valve-holding clamp
Hugh Young pedicle clamp
Hume aortic clamp
Hume clamp
Humphries aortic aneurysm
   clamp
Humphries aortic clamp
Humphries clamp
Humphries reverse-curve
   aortic clamp
Hunt clamp
Hunt colostomy clamp
Hunter-Satinsky clamp
Hurson flexible pressure
   clamp
Hurson flexible pressure
   clamp
Hurson flexible sliding clamp
Hurwitz clamp
Hurwitz esophageal clamp
Hurwitz intestinal clamp
Hyams clamp
Hyams meatus clamp
hydraclip clamp
Hydragrip clamp
Hymes meatal clamp
hysterectomy clamp
iliac clamp
Iliff clamp
incontinence clamp
infant vascular clamp
interlaminar clamp
intestinal anastomosis clamp
intestinal clamp
intestinal occlusion clamp
intestinal resection clamp
intestinal ring clamp
isoelastic rip clamp
Ivory rubber dam clamp
Jackson bone clamp
Jackson bone-extension clamp
Jackson bone-holding clamp
Jackson clamp
Jacobs clamp
Jacobson bulldog clamp
Jacobson clamp
Jacobson microbulldog clamp
Jacobson modified vessel
   clamp
Jacobson vessel clamp
Jacobson-Potts clamp

clamp (*continued*)

Jacobson-Potts vessel clamp
Jahnke anastomosis clamp
Jahnke-Cook-Seeley clamp
Jako clamp
Jameson muscle clamp
Janko clamp
Jansen clamp
Jarit anterior resection clamp
Jarit cartilage clamp
Jarit intestinal clamp
Jarit meniscal clamp
Jarvis clamp
Jarvis pile clamp
Javid bypass clamp
Javid carotid artery bypass
  clamp
Javid carotid artery clamp
Javid carotid clamp
Javid clamp
Jesberg clamp
Jesberg laryngectomy clamp
Johns Hopkins bulldog clamp
Johns Hopkins clamp
Johns Hopkins coarctation
  clamp
Johns Hopkins modified Potts
  clamp
Johnston clamp
Jones clamp
Jones thoracic clamp
Jones towel clamp
Joseph clamp
Joseph septal clamp
Judd clamp
Judd-Allis clamp
Juevenelle clamp
Julian-Damian clamp
Julian-Fildes clamp
Kalt needle holder clamp
Kane clamp
Kane obstetrical clamp
Kane umbilical clamp
Kane umbilical cord clamp
Kantor circumcision clamp
Kantor clamp
Kantrowitz clamp
Kantrowitz hemostatic clamp
Kantrowitz thoracic clamp
Kapp clamp
Kapp microarterial clamp
Kapp-Beck bronchial clamp

clamp (*continued*)

Kapp-Beck clamp
Kapp-Beck coarctation clamp
Kapp-Beck colon clamp
Kapp-Beck-Thomson clamp
Karamar-Mailatt tarsorrhaphy
  clamp
Kartchner carotid artery
  clamp
Kartchner carotid clamp
Kaufman clamp
Kaufman kidney clamp
Kay aortic anastomosis clamp
Kay aortic clamp
Kay clamp
Kay-Lambert clamp
Kelly clamp
Kelsey clamp
Kelsey pile clamp
Kern bone clamp
Kern bone-holding clamp
Kern clamp
Kersting colostomy clamp
K-Gar clamp
K-Gar umbilical clamp
Khan-Jaeger clamp
Khodadad clamp
kidney clamp
kidney pedicle clamp
Kiefer clamp
Kindt arterial clamp
Kindt artery clamp
Kindt carotid artery clamp
Kindt carotid clamp
Kindt clamp
King clamp
Kinsella-Buie clamp
Kinsella-Buie lung clamp
Kitner clamp
Kleinert-Kutz clamp
Kleinschmidt appendectomy
  clamp
Klevas clamp
Klinikum-Berlin tubing clamp
Klintmalm clamp
Klute clamp
Knutsson penile clamp
Knutsson urethrography
  clamp
Kocher clamp
Kocher intestinal clamp
Kolodny clamp

clamp (*continued*)

Krosnick vesicourethral
suspension clamp
Kutzmann clamp
Ladd clamp
Ladd lid clamp
Lahey bronchial clamp
Lahey clamp
Lahey thoracic clamp
Lalonde bone clamp
Lambert aortic clamp
Lambert-Kay aorta clamp
Lambert-Kay clamp
Lambert-Kay vascular clamp
Lambert-Lowman bone clamp
Lambert-Lowman clamp
Lambotte bone-holding clamp
Lambotte clamp
Lamis patella clamp
Lamis patellar clamp
Lane bone-holding clamp
Lane clamp
Lane gastroenterostomy
clamp
Lane intestinal clamp
Lane towel clamp
laparoscopic Allis clamp
Large clamp
Large vena cava clamp (Alfred
M. Large)
Large vena caval clamp
laryngectomy clamp
LCC lung compression clamp
Leahey clamp
Lees clamp
Lees vascular clamp
Lees wedge resection clamp
Leland-Jones clamp
Leland-Jones peripheral
vascular clamp
Leland-Jones vascular clamp
Lem-Blay circumcision clamp
Lem-Blay clamp
Lewin bone clamp
Lewin bone-holding clamp
Lewin clamp
lid clamp
Liddle aorta clamp
Liddle aortic clamp
Life-Lok clamp
ligament clamp
Lillie rectus tendon clamp

clamp (*continued*)

Lin clamp
Lindner anastomosis clamp
Linnartz clamp
Linnartz intestinal clamp
Linnartz stomach clamp
Linton clamp
Linton tourniquet clamp
lion-head clamp
lion-jaw clamp
lip clamp
Litwak clamp
liver-holding clamp
Lloyd-Davis clamp
lobster-type clamp
Locke bone clamp
locking clamp
Lockwood clamp
Longmire-Storm clamp
Lorna nonperforating towel
clamp
Lowman bone clamp
Lowman bone-holding clamp
Lowman clamp
Lowman-Gerster bone clamp
Lowman-Hoglund clamp
Lulu clamp
lung clamp
lung exclusion clamp
MacDonald clamp
Madden clamp
Madden intestinal clamp
Maingot clamp
Malgaigne clamp
Malis hinge clamp
Marcuse tube clamp
marginal clamp
Marlen clamp
Martel clamp
Martel intestinal clamp
Martin cartilage clamp
Martin clamp
Martin muscle clamp
Mason clamp
Mason vascular clamp
Masters intestinal clamp
Masterson clamp
Masterson pelvic clamp
Masters-Schwartz intestinal
clamp
Masters-Schwartz liver clamp
Mastin clamp

clamp (*continued*)
  Mastin muscle clamp
  Matthew cross-leg clamp
  Mattox aortic clamp
  May kidney clamp
  Mayfield aneurysm clamp
  Mayfield head clamp
  Mayfield skull clamp
  Mayfield 3-pin skull clamp
  Mayo clamp
  Mayo kidney clamp
  Mayo vessel clamp
  Mayo-Guyon clamp
  Mayo-Guyon kidney clamp
  Mayo-Guyon vessel clamp
  Mayo-Lovelace clamp
  Mayo-Lovelace spur crushing
    clamp
  Mayo-Robson intestinal
    clamp
  McCleery-Miller clamp
  McCleery-Miller intestinal
    anastomosis clamp
  McCleery-Miller intestinal
    clamp
  McCullough hysterectomy
    clamp
  McDonald clamp
  McDonald gastric clamp
  McDougal prostatectomy
    clamp
  McDougal prostatectomy
    clamps
  McGuire clamp
  McKenzie clamp
  McLean clamp
  McNealey-Glassman clamp
  McNealey-Glassman-Mixter
    clamp
  McQuigg clamp
  meatal clamp
  meatus clamp
  Meeker gallstone clamp
  Meeker right-angle clamp
  megaureter clamp
  meniscal clamp
  metal clamp
  metallic clamp
  Michel aortic clamp
  Michel clamp
  microarterial clamp
  microbulldog clamp

clamp (*continued*)
  Microspike approximator
    clamp
  microvascular clamp
  Mikulicz clamp
  Mikulicz peritoneal clamp
  Mikulicz-Radecki clamp
  Miles clamp
  Miles rectal clamp
  Millard clamp
  Millin clamp
  miniature bulldog clamp
  mini-Ullrich bone clamp
  Mitchel aortotomy clamp
  Mitchel-Adam clamp
  Mitchel-Adam multipurpose
    clamp
  Mixter clamp
  Mixter ligature-carrier clamp
  Mixter right-angle clamp
  Mixter thoracic clamp
  Mogen circumcision clamp
  Mohr clamp
  Mohr pinchcock clamp
  Moorehead clamp
  Moorehead lid clamp
  Moorehead lip clamp
  Moreno clamp
  Moreno gastroenterostomy
    clamp
  Moria-France
    dacryocystorhinostomy
    clamp
  Morris aortic clamp
  mosquito clamp
  mosquito hemostatic clamp
  mosquito lid clamp
  mouse-tooth clamp
  Moynihan clamp
  Moynihan towel clamp
  Mueller aortic clamp
  Mueller bronchial clamp
  Mueller clamp
  Mueller pediatric clamp
  Mueller vena cava clamp
  Mueller vena caval clamp
  Muir cautery clamp
  Muir clamp
  Muir rectal cautery clamp
  Mulligan anastomosis clamp
  multipurpose clamp
  muscle biopsy clamp

clamp (*continued*)

muscle clamp
mush clamp
Myles clamp
Myles hemorrhoidal clamp
myocardial clamp
Nakayama clamp
Naraghi-DeCoster reduction
   clamp
needle holder clamp
neonatal vascular clamp
nephrostomy clamp
nerve-approximating clamp
Nichols aortic clamp
Nicola clamp
Nicola tendon clamp
Niedner anastomosis clamp
Niedner clamp
Niedner pulmonic clamp
noncrushing anterior
   resection clamp
noncrushing bowel clamp
noncrushing clamp
noncrushing
   gastroenterostomy clamp
noncrushing gastrointestinal
   clamp
noncrushing intestinal clamp
noncrushing liver-holding
   clamp
noncrushing vascular clamp
nonperforating towel clamp
Noon AV fistula clamp
Noon AV fistular clamp
Nunez aortic clamp
Nunez auricular clamp
Nunez clamp
Nussbaum clamp
Nussbaum intestinal clamp
occluding clamp
occlusion clamp
occlusion multipurpose clamp
Ochsner aortic clamp
Ochsner arterial clamp
Ochsner artery clamp
Ochsner clamp
Ochsner thoracic clamp
Ockerblad clamp
Ockerblad kidney clamp
Ockerblad vessel clamp
O'Connor clamp
O'Connor lid clamp

clamp (*continued*)

O'Hanlon gastrointestinal
   clamp
O'Hanlon intestinal clamp
Olivecrona aneurysm clamp
Olsen cholangiogram clamp
O'Neill cardiac clamp
O'Neill clamp
O'Shaughnessy clamp
ossicle-holding clamp
osteoplastic flap clamp
padded clamp
parametrium clamp
Parham-Martin bone clamp
Parham-Martin bone-holding
   clamp
Parham-Martin clamp
Parker clamp
Parker-Kerr clamp
Parker-Kerr intestinal clamp
Parsonnet aortic clamp
partial occlusion clamp
partially occluding clamp
Partipilo clamp
patellar cement clamp
patellar clamp
patent ductus clamp
Payr clamp
Payr gastrointestinal clamp
Payr pylorus clamp
Payr resection clamp
Payr stomach clamp
Péan clamp
Péan hemostatic clamp
Péan hysterectomy clamp
Péan intestinal clamp
Péan vessel clamp
pediatric bulldog clamp
pediatric vascular clamp
pedicle clamp
Peers towel clamp
pelvic clamp
Pemberton clamp
Pemberton sigmoid clamp
Pemberton spur-crushing
   clamp
penile clamp
penis clamp
Pennington clamp
Percy clamp
pericortical clamp
peripheral vascular clamp

clamp (*continued*)
- peritoneal clamp
- Petz clamp
- phalangeal clamp
- Phaneuf clamp
- phantom clamp
- Phillips clamp
- Phillips rectal clamp
- pile clamp
- Pilling clamp
- Pilling microanastomosis clamp
- Pilling pediatric clamp
- pinchcock clamp
- pin-to-bar clamp
- Pitanguy clamp
- placenta clamp
- placental clamp
- placing of clamp
- Plastibell circumcision clamp
- Plastibell clamp
- plate-holding clamp
- point-of-reduction clamp
- Pomeranz aortic clamp
- Poppen aortic clamp
- Poppen clamp
- Poppen-Blalock carotid artery clamp
- Poppen-Blalock clamp
- Poppen-Blalock-Salibi carotid clamp
- Poppen-Blalock-Salibi clamp
- post-TUR clamp
- post-TUR irrigation clamp
- post-TUR irrigation control clamp
- Potts aortic clamp
- Potts cardiovascular clamp
- Potts clamp
- Potts coarctation clamp
- Potts divisional clamp
- Potts ductus clamp
- Potts patent ductus clamp
- Potts pulmonic clamp
- Potts-DeBakey clamp
- Potts-Niedner aorta clamp
- Potts-Niedner aortic clamp
- Potts-Niedner clamp
- Potts-Satinsky clamp
- Potts-Smith aortic clamp
- Potts-Smith aortic occlusion clamp

clamp (*continued*)
- Potts-Smith pulmonic clamp
- Poutasse clamp
- Poutasse renal artery clamp
- Presbyterian Hospital clamp
- Presbyterian Hospital occluding clamp
- Presbyterian Hospital T-clamp
- Presbyterian Hospital tubing clamp
- Preshaw clamp
- Price muscle biopsy clamp
- Price muscle clamp
- Price-Thomas bronchial clamp
- Price-Thomas clamp
- Prince clamp
- Prince muscle clamp
- Pringle clamp
- Providence Hospital clamp
- ptosis clamp
- Pudenz-Heyer clamp
- pulmonary arterial clamp
- pulmonary artery clamp
- pulmonary clamp
- pulmonary embolism clamp
- pulmonary nodulectomy clamp
- pulmonary vessel clamp
- pulmonic clamp
- pulmonic stenosis clamp
- Putterman levator resection clamp
- Putterman ptosis clamp
- pylorus clamp
- Quick Bend flex clamp
- Ralks clamp
- Ralks thoracic clamp
- Ramstedt clamp
- Ranieri clamp
- Rankin anastomosis clamp
- Rankin clamp
- Rankin intestinal clamp
- Rankin stomach clamp
- Ranzewski clamp
- Ranzewski intestinal clamp
- ratchet clamp
- Ravich clamp
- Rayport muscle clamp
- reamer clamp
- rectal clamp
- Redo intestinal clamp
- Reich-Nechtow arterial clamp

clamp (*continued*)

Reich-Nechtow clamp
Reinhoff swan neck clamp
renal artery clamp
renal clamp
renal pedicle clamp
resection clamp
reverse-curve clamp
Reynolds clamp
Reynolds dissecting clamp
Reynolds resection clamp
Reynolds vascular clamp
Rhinelander clamp
Rica arterial clamp
Rica microarterial clamp
Rica stem clamp
Rica vessel clamp
Richards bone clamp
Richards clamp
Rienhoff arterial clamp
Rienhoff clamp
right-angle clamp
right-angle colon clamp
ring clamp
ring-handled bulldog clamp
ring-jawed holding clamp
R-N clamp
Robin chalazion clamp
Rochester clamp
Rochester hook clamp
Rochester sigmoid clamp
Rochester-Kocher clamp
Rochester-Péan clamp
Rockey clamp
Rockey vascular clamp
Roe aortic clamp
Roe aortic tourniquet clamp
Roeder clamp
Roeder towel clamp
Roosen clamp
Roosevelt clamp
Roosevelt gastroenterostomy
    clamp
Roosevelt gastrointestinal
    clamp
root rubber dam clamp
rubber-dam clamp
rubber-shod clamp
Rubin bronchial clamp
Rubin bronchus clamp
Rubin clamp
Rubio wire-holding clamp

clamp (*continued*)

Rubovits clamp
Ruel aorta clamp
Rumel clamp
Rumel myocardial clamp
Rumel rubber clamp
Rumel thoracic clamp
Rush bone clamp
Rush clamp
S.S. White clamp
Salibi carotid artery clamp
Salibi carotid clamp
Salibi clamp
Santulli clamp
Sarnoff aortic clamp
Sarnoff clamp
Sarot arterial clamp
Sarot artery clamp
Sarot bronchial clamp
Sarot bronchus clamp
Sarot clamp
Satinsky anastomosis clamp
Satinsky aortic clamp
Satinsky clamp
Satinsky pediatric clamp
Satinsky vascular clamp
Satinsky vena cava clamp
Schaedel cross-action towel
    clamp
Schlein clamp
Schlesinger clamp
Schnidt clamp
Schoemaker intestinal
    clamp
Schumacher aorta clamp
Schumacher aortic clamp
Schutz clamp
Schwartz arterial aneurysm
    clamp
Schwartz bulldog clamp
Schwartz clamp
Schwartz intracranial clamp
Schwartz vascular clamp
Scoville-Lewis clamp
screw occlusive clamp
Scudder clamp
Scudder intestinal clamp
Scudder stomach clamp
Sehrt clamp
Seidel bone-holding clamp
Sellor clamp
Selman clamp

clamp (*continued*)
- Selverstone carotid artery clamp
- Selverstone carotid clamp
- Selverstone clamp
- Semb bone-holding clamp
- Semb bronchus clamp
- Senning bulldog clamp
- Senning clamp
- Senning featherweight bulldog clamp
- Senning-Stille clamp
- septal clamp
- serrefine clamp
- shape memory clamp
- Sheehy ossicle-holding clamp
- Sheldon clamp
- Shoemaker intestinal clamp
- shutoff clamp
- side-biting clamp
- sidewinder aortic clamp
- Siegler-Hellman clamp
- sigmoid anastomosis clamp
- sigmoid clamp
- Silber microvascular clamp
- Silber vasovasostomy clamp
- Sims-Maier clamp
- Singley clamp
- Singley intestinal clamp
- Siniscal eyelid clamp
- skull clamp
- Slim Fit flex clamp
- Slocum meniscal clamp
- slotted nerve clamp
- SMIC intestinal clamp
- Smith bone clamp
- Smith clamp
- Smith cordotomy clamp
- Smith marginal clamp
- Smithwick anastomotic clamp
- Smithwick clamp
- Softjaw clamp
- Softjaw handless clamp
- Somers clamp
- Somers uterine clamp
- Southwick clamp
- speed lock clamp
- sponge clamp
- spoon anastomosis clamp
- spoon clamp
- spur-crushing clamp
- S-shaped peripheral vascular clamp

clamp (*continued*)
- St. Mark clamp
- St. Vincent tube clamp
- stainless steel clamp
- Stallard head clamp
- Stanton cautery clamp
- Stanton cautery with mousetrap clamp
- Stanton clamp
- Stayce adjustable clamp
- Stay-Rite clamp
- Steinhauser bone clamp
- Stemp clamp
- stenosis clamp
- Stepita clamp
- Stepita meatal clamp
- Stepita meatus clamp
- Stetten intestinal clamp
- Stevenson clamp
- Stille clamp
- Stille kidney clamp
- Stille vessel clamp
- Stille-Crawford clamp
- Stille-Crawford coarctation clamp
- Stimson pedicle clamp
- Stiwer towel clamp
- Stockman clamp
- Stockman meatal clamp
- Stockman penile clamp
- Stockman penis clamp
- stomach clamp
- Stone clamp
- Stone intestinal clamp
- Stone stomach clamp
- Stone-Holcombe anastomosis clamp
- Stone-Holcombe clamp
- Stone-Holcombe intestinal clamp
- Stony splenorenal shunt clamp
- Storey clamp
- Storz meatal clamp
- Storz meatus clamp
- straight clamp
- straight Crile clamp
- straight mosquito clamp
- Stratte clamp
- Stratte kidney clamp
- Strauss clamp
- Strauss meatal clamp
- Strauss meatus clamp

clamp (*continued*)

Strauss metal clamp
Strauss penile clamp
Strauss-Valentine penile clamp
Strelinger colon clamp
Strelinger right-angle colon
    clamp
Subramanian aortic clamp
Subramanian clamp
Subramanian classic miniature
    aortic clamp
Subramanian miniature aortic
    clamp
Subramanian sidewinder
    aortic clamp
Sugarbaker retrocolic clamp
Sugita head clamp
Sumner clamp
Surgimed clamp
Swan aortic clamp
Swan clamp
swan-neck clamp
Swenson ring-jawed holding
    clamp
Swiss bulldog clamp
Sztehlo clamp
Sztehlo umbilical clamp
T-clamp
tangential clamp
tangential occlusion clamp
tangential pediatric clamp
Tatum clamp
Tatum meatal clamp
Taufic cholangiography clamp
Tehl clamp
temporalis transfer clamp
tension clamp
Textor vasectomy clamp
Thoma clamp
Thompson carotid artery
    clamp
Thompson carotid vascular
    clamp
Thompson clamp
Thomson lung clamp
thoracic clamp
Thorlakson lower occlusive
    clamp
Thorlakson upper occlusive
    clamp
Thumb-Saver introducer
    clamp

clamp (*continued*)

tissue occlusion clamp
tonsil clamp
tonsillar clamp
towel clamp
Trendelenburg-Crafoord
    clamp
Trendelenburg-Crafoord
    coarctation clamp
Treves intestinal clamp
trochanter-holding clamp
truncus clamp
Trusler clamp
Trusler infant vascular clamp
tube-occluding clamp
tubing clamp
Tucker appendix clamp
turkey-claw clamp
Tydings tonsil clamp
Tydings tonsillar clamp
Tyrrell clamp
Ullrich tubing clamp
Ulrich bone-holding clamp
umbilical clamp
umbilical cord clamp
Umbilicutter clamp
Universal wire clamp
upper occlusive clamp
ureteral clamp
urethrographic cannula clamp
urethrographic clamp
urinary incontinence clamp
uterine clamp
V. Mueller aortic clamp
V. Mueller auricular
    appendage clamp
V. Mueller bulldog clamp
V. Mueller cross-action bulldog
    clamp
V. Mueller vena cava clamp
vaginal cuff clamp
Valdoni clamp
Vanderbilt clamp
Vanderbilt University vessel
    clamp
Vanderbilt vessel clamp
Varco dissecting clamp
Varco gallbladder clamp
vas clamp
Vasconcelos-Barretto clamp
VascuClamp minibulldog
    vessel clamp

clamp (*continued*)

VascuClamp vascular clamp
vascular clamp
vascular graft clamp
vasovasostomy clamp
Veidenheimer clamp
Veidenheimer resection
    clamp
vena cava clamp
vena caval clamp
Verbrugge bone clamp
Verbrugge bone-holding
    clamp
Verbrugge clamp
Verse-Webster clamp
vessel clamp
vessel peripheral clamp
vessel-occluding clamp
vestibular clamp
Virtus splinter clamp
voltage clamp
von Petz clamp
von Petz intestinal clamp
von Petz stomach clamp
Vorse occluding clamp
Vorse tube-occluding clamp
Vorse-Webster clamp
Vorse-Webster tube-occluding
    clamp
vulsellum clamp
Wadsworth lid clamp
Walther clamp
Walther kidney pedicle clamp
Walther pedicle clamp
Walther-Crenshaw clamp
Walther-Crenshaw meatal
    clamp
Walther-Crenshaw meatus
    clamp
Walton clamp
Walton meniscal clamp
Walton meniscus clamp
Wangensteen anastomosis
    clamp
Wangensteen clamp
Wangensteen gastric-crushing
    anastomotic clamp
Wangensteen patent ductus
    clamp
Warthen clamp
Warthen spur-crushing clamp
Watts clamp

clamp (*continued*)

Watts locking clamp
Weaver chalazion clamp
Weaver clamp
Weber aortic clamp
Weck clamp
Weck-Edna nonperforating
    towel clamp
wedge resection clamp
Weldon miniature bulldog
    clamp
Wells clamp
Wells pedicle clamp
Wertheim clamp
Wertheim kidney pedicle
    clamp
Wertheim-Cullen clamp
Wertheim-Cullen kidney
    pedicle clamp
Wertheim-Cullen pedicle
    clamp
Wertheim-Reverdin clamp
Wertheim-Reverdin pedicle
    clamp
West Shur cartilage clamp
Wester clamp
Wester meniscal clamp
White clamp
Whitver clamp
Whitver penile clamp
Wikstroem gallbladder clamp
Wikstroem-Stilgust clamp
Willett clamp
Williams clamp
Wilman clamp
Wilson clamp
Winkelmann circumcision
    clamp
Winston cervical clamp
wire-tightening clamp
Wirthlin splenorenal clamp
Wirthlin splenorenal shunt
    clamp
Wister clamp
Wister vascular clamp
Wolfson clamp
Wolfson intestinal clamp
Wolfson spur-crushing clamp
Wood bulldog clamp
Wylie J clamp
Wylie carotid artery clamp
Wylie clamp

clamp (*continued*)
    Wylie hypogastric clamp
    Wylie lumbar bulldog clamp
    X-clamp
    Yasargil carotid clamp
    Yasargil clamp
    Yellen circumcision clamp
    Yellen clamp
    Young clamp
    Young renal pedicle clamp
    Zachary-Cope clamp
    Zachary-Cope-DeMartel clamp
    Zachary-Cope-DeMartel colon
        clamp
    Zachary-Cope-DeMartel triple-
        colon clamp
    Z-clamp
    Zeppelin clamp
    Ziegler-Furniss clamp
    Zimmer cartilage clamp
    Zimmer clamp
    Zinnanti clamp
    Zipser clamp
    Zipser meatal clamp
    Zipser penile clamp
    Zipser penis clamp
    Zutt clamp
    Zweifel appendectomy clamp
    Zweifel pressure clamp
clamp carrier
clamp clip
Clamp Ease device
clamp forceps
clamp holder
clamp insert
clamp lamp
clamp-and-sew technique
clamp-carrier forceps
clamped
    doubly clamped
    serially clamped
clamped, cut, and ligated
clamped, cut, and tied
clamping
    aortic clamping
    blind clamping
    carotid clamping
    portal triad clamping
    selective vascular clamping
        (SVC)
clamping and tying
clamp-on telescope

clamshell brace
clamshell closure
clamshell device
clamshell incision
clamshell prosthesis
clamshell technique
Clancy cruciate ligament
    reconstruction
Clancy ligament technique
Clancy patellar tendon graft
Clancy whipstitch
Clancy-Zoellner procedure
clapotement
Clapton line
Clar head light
ClariFlex intraocular lens
Clarion cochlear implant
Clark applicator
Clark capsule fragment forceps
Clark classification of malignant
    melanoma (levels I-IV)
Clark common duct dilator
Clark dilator
Clark expanding mesh catheter
Clark eye speculum
Clark forceps
Clark helix catheter
Clark ligator scissor forceps
Clark nevi
Clark operation
Clark oxygen electrode
Clark perineorrhaphy
Clark rotating cutter catheter
Clark speculum
Clark technique
Clark transfer technique
Clark vein stripper
Clark-Axer technique
Clarke stereotactic instrument
Clarke-Fournier glossitis
Clark-Elder classification of
    malignant melanoma
Clarke-Reich ligator
Clark-Guyton forceps
Clark-McGovern classification of
    malignant melanoma
Clark-Reich knot pusher
Clark-Southwick-Ogden
    modification
Clark-Verhoeff capsule forceps
Clark-Verhoeff forceps
Clarus peristaltic pump

Clarus spinescope
Clas von Eichen needle
clasp
  Acland clasp
  Adams clasp
  arrow clasp
  arrow-pin clasp
  Charnley bone clasp
  Crozat clasp
  Damon clasp
  Duyzings clasp
  embrasure clasp
  EPI Sport epicondylitis clasp
  extended clasp
  eyelet clasp
  Hahnenkraft dental clasp
  infrabulge clasp
  lingual clasp
  mesiodistal clasp
  movable-arm clasp
  multiple clasp
  preformed clasp
  Roach clasp
clasp bar
clasp knife
CLASP procedure
clasped thumb
clasped thumb deformity
clasp-knife reflex
clasp-knife rigidity
clasp-knife spasticity
Classen-Demling papillotome
classic abdominal Semm
    hysterectomy
classic DSRS technique
classic multiple organ failure
    syndrome
classic, classical
classical approach
classical cesarean section
classical incision
classical Judd-Mayo overlap
    midline incisional
    hernioplasty
classical sign of rejection
classical subtotal resection
classical technique
classical transverse incision
classification
  Ackerman-Proffitt
    classification
  Acosta classification

classification (*continued*)
  acromioclavicular injury
    classification
  Aitken epiphysial fracture
    classification
  AJCC TNM tumor
    classification
  Allman acromioclavicular
    injury classification
  Alonso-Lej classification
  American Heart Association
    classification
  American Society of
    Anesthesiologists
    classification
  Anderson modification of
    Berndt-Harty classification
  Anderson-D'Alonzo odontoid
    fracture classification
  Angle malocclusion
    classification
  Ann Arbor classification
  AO classification
  Arneth classification
  Ashhurst-Bromer ankle
    fracture classification
  Astler-Coller A, B1, B2, C1, C2
    classification
  Astler-Coller modification of
    Dukes classification
  Bado classification
  Bailyn classification
  Banff classification
  Bauer-Jackson classification
  Baume classification
  Bennett classification
  Bergey classification
  Berndt-Harty classification
  Bethesda System for Pap
    smear classification
  Binet system of classification
  BIRADS classification
  Bishop classification
  bismuth bile duct stricture
    type I-V classification
  Black classification
  bladder carcinoma
    classification
  Borrmann gastric cancer
    classification
  Bosniak classification
  Boyd classification

classification (*continued*)
 Boyd-Griffin trochanteric
  fracture classification
 Breslow classification
 Breslow melanoma
  classification
 Broders tumor classification
  (grades 1-4)
 burn classification (1st to 4th
  degree)
 Butchart staging classification
 Caldwell-Moloy classification
 Callender cell-type
  classification
 Cambridge classification
 Canadian Cardiovascular
  Society classification
 caries classification
 Carnesale-Stewart-Barnes hip
  dislocation classification
 Caroli-Sarles classification
 Casten classification
 Catterall classification
 cavity classification
 CEAP classification
 Cedars-Sinai classification
 Centers for Disease Control
  HIV infection classification
 Chadwick-Bentley
  classification
 Chicago classification
 Child hepatic dysfunction
  classification
 Child hepatic risk criteria
  classification
 Child liver disease
  classification
 Child-Pugh classification
 Child-Turcotte hepatic
  surgery classification
 clean operative wound
  classification
 clean-contaminated operative
  wound classification
 cleft palate classification
 clinical pathologic
  classification
 Codman classification
 Cohen-Rentrop classification
 Colonna hip fracture
  classification
 Colton classification

classification (*continued*)
 contaminated operative
  wound classification
 Cori classification
 Correa classification
 Couinaud classification
 Coventry-Johnson
  classification
 Croften classification
 Crowe classification
 Cummer classification
 Dagradi esophageal variceal
  classification
 Danis-Weber ankle fracture
  classification (types A, B, C)
 Danis-Weber ankle injury
  classification
 de Groot classification
 DeBakey classification
 Delbet hip classification
 DeLee classification
 Denis Browne spinal fracture
  classification
 denture classification
 Denver classification
 Dexter-Grossman
  classification
 Diamond classification
 Dias-Tachdijian physical injury
  classification
 dichotomous classification
 Dickhaut-DeLee discoid
  meniscus classification
 dirty operative wound
  classification
 Dripps classification
 Duane classification
 Dubin-Amelar varicocele
  classification
 Dukes classification
 Dyck-Lambert classification
 Eckert-Davis classification
 Edmondson-Steiner
  classification
 Efron jackknife classification
 Egawa classification
 El-Ahwany humeral
  supracondylar fracture
  classification
 Ellis classification
 Enna classification
 Enneking classification

classification (*continued*)
  Epstein hip dislocation
    classification
  Epstein-Thomas classification
  Essex-Lopresti calcaneal
    fracture classification
  Essex-Lopresti classification
  Evans intertrochanteric
    fracture classification
  FAB classification
  Federation of Gynecology and
    Obstetrics classification
  Fielding classification
  Fielding femoral fracture
    classification
  Fielding-Magliato
    subtrochanteric fracture
    classification
  Flatt classification
  Foucher epiphysial injury
    classification
  fracture classification
  Franz-O'Rahilly classification
  Fredrickson
    hyperlipoproteinemia
    classification
  Fredrickson-Levy-Lees
    classification
  Freeman calcaneal fracture
    classification
  French-American-British
    classification
  Frykman radial fracture
    classification
  Fraenkel neurologic deficit
    classification
  functional capacity
    classification
  Garden femoral neck fracture
    classification
  Gartland humeral
    supracondylar fracture
    classification
  Gartland Universal radial
    fracture classification
  gastric mucosal pattern
    classification
  Gell and Coombs
    classification
  Goldman classification
  Grantham femur fracture
    classification

classification (*continued*)
  Greenfield spinocerebellar
    ataxia classification
  Guhl classification
  Gustilo puncture wound
    classification
  Gustilo-Anderson open
    fracture classification
  Haggitt classification
  Halverson classification
  Halverson-McVay hernia
    classification
  Hannover classification
  Hansen fracture classification
  Hara gallbladder inflammation
    classification
  Hardcastle tarsometatarsal
    joint injury classification
  Hawkins talar fracture
    classification
  Henderson classification
  Hepatitis Activity Index
    classification
  Hinchey diverticulitis grade
    classification
  HIV classification
  Hoaglund-States classification
  Hohl tibial condylar fracture
    classification
  Hohl-Luck tibial plateau
    fracture classification
  Hohl-Moore classification
  Holdsworth spinal fracture
    classification
  House-Brackmann
    classification
  Hughston classification
  Hunt-Hess neurological
    classification
  Ideberg glenoid fracture
    classification
  immunologic classification
  Ingram-Bachynski hip fracture
    classification
  Insall patellar injury
    classification
  international cancer of cervix
    classification
  international stage
    classification
  Isaacson classification (IC)
  Jansky classification

classification (*continued*)
  Japanese cancer classification
  Jeffrey radial fracture
    classification
  Jensen classification
  Jewett and Whitmore
    classification
  Johner-Wruhs tibial fracture
    classification
  Jones-Barnes-Lloyd-Roberts
    classification
  Kajava classification
  Kalamchi classification
  Karnofsky rating scale
    classification
  Kasugai classification
  Kauffman-White classification
  Kazangia and Converse facial
    fracture classification
  Kazangia and Converse
    mandibular fracture
    classification
  Keil tumor cell classification
  Keith-Wagener hypertensive
    retinopathy classification
    (I-IV)
  Keith-Wagener-Barker
    classification
  Kelami classification
  Kellam-Waddel classification
  Kennedy classification
  Kernohan system of glioma
    classification
  KESS constipation scoring
    system classification
  Key-Conwell pelvic fracture
    classification
  Kiel classification
  Kilfoyle humeral medial
    condylar fracture
    classification
  Killip-Kimball heart failure
    classification
  Kocher classification
  KWB classification
  Kyle-Gustilo classification
  Kyle-Gustilo-Premer
    classification
  Lagrange humeral
    supracondylar fracture
    classification
  Lancefield classification

classification (*continued*)
  Lanza scale for drug-induced
    mucosal damage
    classification
  Lauge-Hansen ankle fracture
    classification
  Lauren gastric carcinoma
    classification
  Le Fort classification
  Leishman classification
  Lennert classification
  Letournel-Judet acetabular
    fracture classification
  Leung thumb loss classification
  Levine-Harvey classification
  Lindell classification
  Linell-Ljungberg classification
  Lloyd-Roberts-Catteral-
    Salamon classification
  Loesche classification
  Lown classification
  Lukes and Butler Hodgkin
    disease classification
  Lukes-Collins classification
  lymph node classification
  MacCallan classification
  Macewen classification
  MacNichol-Voutsinas
    classification
  Mallampati oropharyngeal
    classification
  Mallampati pharyngeal
    visibility classification
  Marseille pancreatitis
    classification
  Mason radial head fracture
    classification
  Mast-Spieghel-Pappas
    classification
  Masuka modified thymic
    carcinoma classification
  Mathews olecranon fracture
    classification
  Mayo carpal instability
    classification
  Mayo rheumatoid elbow
    classification
  McNeer classification
  Melone distal radius fracture
    classification
  Meyers-McKeever avulsion
    fracture classification

classification (*continued*)
  Meyers-McKeever tibial
    fracture classification
  microinvasive carcinoma
    classification
  Milch condylar fracture
    classification
  Milch elbow fracture
    classification
  Milch humeral fracture
    classification
  Ming gastric carcinoma
    classification
  Minnesota EKG classification
  Moore tibial plateau fracture
    classification
  morphologic classification
  Moss classification
  Mueller femoral
    supracondylar fracture
    classification
  Mueller tibial fracture
    classification
  multiaxial classification
  Munro-Parker laparoscopic
    hysterectomy classification
  Nalebuff classification
  Neer femur fracture
    classification
  Neer shoulder fracture
    classification
  Neer-Horowitz humeral
    fracture classification
  New York Heart Association
    heart disease classification
  Newman radial neck and head
    fracture classification
  Nicoll classification
  Niemeier classification
  Nyhus classification
  Ogden epiphysial fracture
    classification
  Ogden knee dislocation
    classification
  O'Rahilly diabetes classification
  ordinal classification
  Orthopaedic Trauma
    Association classification
  Outerbridge classification
  Paley classification
  Papavasiliou olecranon
    fracture classification

classification (*continued*)
  Paris classification
  pathologic classification
  Pauwels femoral neck fracture
    classification
  Pell-Gregory classification
  Pennal classification
  Pipkin femoral fracture
    classification
  Pipkin posterior hip
    dislocation classification
  Pipkin subclassification of
    Epstein-Thomas
    classification
  Poland epiphysial fracture
    classification
  Poland physical injury
    classification
  Potter classification
  Pugh classification
  Pulec-Freedman classification
  Quinby pelvic fracture
    classification
  Quénu-Küss tarsometatarsal
    injury classification
  Rai classification
  Ranawat classification
  Ranson acute pancreatitis
    classification
  Rappaport classification
  Rentrop classification
  Riseborough-Radin
    intercondylar fracture
    classification
  Ruetter classification
  Rockwood acromioclavicular
    injury classification
  Rockwood clavicular fracture
    classification
  Rosenthal nail injury
    classification
  round-robin classification
  Rowe calcaneal fracture
    classification
  Rowe-Lowell hip dislocation
    classification
  Rowe-Lowell system for
    fracture-dislocation
    classification
  Ruedi-Allgower classification
  Runyon classification
  Russe classification

classification (*continued*)
  Russell-Taylor classification
  Rutkow-Robbins-Gilbert
    classification
  Rutledge extended
    hysterectomy classification
  Rye Hodgkin disease
    classification
  Sage-Salvatore
    acromioclavicular joint
    injury classification
  Saha shoulder muscle
    classification
  Sakellarides calcaneal fracture
    classification
  Salter epiphysial fracture
    classification
  Salter-Harris epiphysial
    fracture classification
  Santiani-Stone classification
  Sassouni classification
  Savary-Mille grading scale
    classification
  scalar classification
  Schatzker tibial plateau
    fracture classification
  Scheie classification
  Schuknecht classification
  Schwarz classification
  Seattle classification
  Seddon classification
  Seinsheimer femoral fracture
    classification
  Severin classification
  Shaffer-Weiss classification
  Shaher-Puddu classification
  Shelton femoral fracture
    classification
  Shimada classification
  Singh osteoporosis
    classification
  Siurala classification
  Skinner classification
  Snyder classification
  Solcia classification
  Sonnenberg classification
  Sorbie calcaneal fracture
    classification
  Spaulding classification
  Speed radial head fracture
    classification
  Spetzler-Martin classification

classification (*continued*)
  Stark classification
  Steinbrocker classification
  Suda type I, II, III papilla
    classification
  Sunderland nerve injury
    classification
  surgical wound classification
  Swanson classification
  Sydney system gastritis
    classification
  Tachdjian classification
  Tessier classification
  Thomas classification
  Thompson-Epstein femoral
    fracture classification
  Three Color Concept of
    wound classification
  thrombolysis in myocardial
    infarction classification
  Tile classification
  TIMI classification
  TNM carcinoma classification
  tongue thrust classification
  Torg classification
  Torode-Zieg classification
  Toronto pelvic fracture
    classification
  Tronzo intertrochanteric
    fracture classification
  Tscherne classification
  Tscherne-Gotzen tibial
    fracture classification
  tumor, node, metastasis
    carcinoma classification
  UICC tumor classification
  Vaughan Williams
    antiarrhythmic drug
    classification
  Veau classification
  Venn-Watson classification
  Visick dysphagia classification
  Vostal radial fracture
    classification
  Wagener-Clay-Gipner retinal
    lesion classification
  Wagner diabetic foot
    classification
  Walter Reed classification
  Warren-Marshall classification
  Wassel thumb duplication
    classification

classification (*continued*)
Watanabe discoid meniscus
classification
Watson-Jones tibial fracture
classification
Watson-Jones tibial tubercle
avulsion fracture
classification
Weber physical injury
classification
Weber-Danis ankle injury
classification
Weiland classification
Weissman classification
White classification
Whitehead classification
WHO gastric carcinoma
classification
Wiberg patellar classification
Wiley-Galey classification
Wilkins radial fracture
classification
Winquist femoral fracture
classification
Winquist-Hansen femoral
fracture classification
Winter classification
Wolfe breast carcinoma
classification
World Health Organization
classification
Yacoub and Radley-Smith
classification
Young pelvic fracture
classification
Zickel classification
Zlotsky-Ballard
acromioclavicular injury
classification
Zollinger classification
Classix pacemaker
Classon deep surgery scissors
Classon pediatric scissors
Classon scissors
Claude hyperkinesis sign
claudicant
claudication
intermittent claudication
venous claudication
Claudius fossa
claustrum
clavate clove-hitch sutures

clavate sutures
clavicle
clavicle bone
clavicle excision
clavicle splint
clavicle strap sling
clavicopectoral
clavicotomy
clavicular
clavicular birth fracture
clavicular cross splint
clavicular facet
clavicular fracture aneurysm
clavicular fracture fragment
clavicular incision
clavicular incisure of sternum
clavicular notch
clavicular notch of sternum
clavicular region
clavipectoral
clavipectoral fascia
clavipectoral triangle
clavus (*pl.* clavi)
clavus durum
clavus mollum
claw
Anderson 5-prong bear claw
burn claw
devil's claw
claw deformity
claw forceps
claw hand
claw hand deformity
claw retractor
claw toe
clawfoot
clawfoot deformity
clawhand
Clawicz chisel
clawing deformity
clawing of ring and little fingers
clawtoe deformity
clawtoe position
Clay Adams catheter
clay pipe carcinoma
Clayman corneal forceps
Clayman forceps
Clayman intraocular guide
Clayman intraocular implant
lens
Clayman intraocular lens
Clayman iris hook

Clayman lens
Clayman lens forceps
Clayman lens implant
Clayman lens-holding forceps
Clayman lens-inserting
  forceps
Clayman lid retractor
Clayman spatula
Clayman suturing forceps
Clayman-Kelman intraocular lens
  forceps
Clayman-Kelman lens
Clayman-Knolle irrigating lens
  loop
Clayman-Knolle lens loop
Clayman-McPherson tying
  forceps
Clayman-Troutman corneal
  scissors
Clayman-Vannas scissors
Clayman-Westcott scissors
claypipe cancer
clay-shoveler's fracture
Clayton forefoot arthroplasty
Clayton laminectomy shears
Clayton operation
Clayton osteotome
Clayton procedure with
  panmetatarsal head
  resection
Clayton shears
Clayton splint
Clayton-Fowler technique
CLBBB (complete left bundle
  branch block)
clean acrylic template splint
clean and dry incision
clean case
clean cervix
clean closure
clean contaminated surgery
clean intermittent
  catheterization
clean operation
clean operative wound
  classification
clean wound
clean-contaminated
clean-contaminated case
clean-contaminated operation
clean-contaminated operative
  wound classification

cleaner
  bronchoscopic cleaner
  Mill-Rose instrument cleaner
  ultrasonic cleaner
cleaning brush
cleaning pistol
cleaning tool
Cleanlet lancet
cleansers
  Biolex cleansers
  CarraKleenz cleansers
  Carrington cleansers
  Clinswound cleansers
  Dey-Wash skin wound cleansers
  DiabKlenz wound cleansers
  Hibiclens cleansers
  Hibistat cleansers
  Hibitane cleansers
  Hibiclens skin cleanser
  quaternary ammonium
    chloride skin cleanser
  SAF-Clens chronic wound
    cleanser
  Sea-Clens wound cleanser
  Shur-Clens wound cleanser
  SilqueClenz skin cleanser
  Sorenson sinus cleanser
  Techni-Care wound cleanser
  Septicare cleansers
  Sklar cleansers
  UltraKlenz wound cleansers
cleansing blood
cleansing emulsion
cleansing enema
cleanup
Clear Advantage latex free
  catheter
Clear Advantage silicone male
  catheter
clear airways
clear cell acanthoma
clear cell hepatocellular
  carcinoma
clear cell hidradenoma
clear cell sarcoma
clear lung fields
clear to auscultation
clear to percussion
clear urine
clearance
  interocclusal clearance
  occlusal clearance

clearance technique
ClearCut 2 instrument
Clearfix meniscal dart
Clearfix meniscal screw
ClearSite bandage
ClearSite borderless dressing
ClearSite Hydro Gauze dressing
ClearSite hydrogel absorptive
    borderline wound
    dressing
ClearSite wound dressing
ClearView CO_2 laser
ClearView uterine manipulator
Cleasby iridectomy
Cleasby iridectomy operation
Cleasby iris spatula
Cleasby spatulated needle
cleavage fracture
cleavage lesion
cleavage line
cleavage plane
cleaver
    Case enamel cleaver
    fiber cleaver
    Haefliger cleaver
    Orton enamel cleaver
Cleaves position
Cleeman sign
cleft
    alveolar cleft
    asymmetric bilateral cleft
    atypical cleft
    bilateral cleft
    bony cleft
    Boo-Chai craniofacial cleft
    branchial cleft
    cholesterol cleft
    complete bilateral cleft
    congenital earlobe cleft
    craniofacial cleft
    facial cleft
    Facial Impairment Scales for
      clefts
    fascial cleft
    gluteal cleft
    Hahn cleft
    hyomandibular cleft
    incomplete cleft
    intergluteal cleft
    isolated naso-ocular cleft
    labial cleft
    laryngeal cleft

cleft (*continued*)
    laryngotracheoesophageal
      cleft
    lateral facial cleft
    laterofacial cleft
    median facial cleft
    median maxillary anterior
      alveolar cleft
    mesenchymal cleft
    middle ear cleft
    naso-ocular cleft
    natal cleft
    nose cleft
    oblique facial cleft
    oculofacial cleft
    olfactory cleft
    operated cleft
    oral cleft
    oronaso-ocular cleft
    oro-ocular cleft
    osseous cleft
    palatal cleft
    palatomaxillary cleft
    pharyngeal cleft
    prealveolar cleft
    prepalatal cleft
    primary cleft
    secondary cleft
    soft palate cleft
    Sondergaard cleft
    stenotic cleft
    sternal cleft
    Stillman cleft
    subaponeurotic fascial cleft
    submucous cleft
    symmetrical bilateral cleft
    Tessier classification of
      craniofacial clefts (Tessier
      numbers 0-14)
    thenar cleft
    transverse facial cleft
    type II earlobe cleft
    unilateral cleft
    unoperated cleft
cleft alveolus
cleft anomaly
cleft cheek
cleft closure
cleft earlobe
cleft face
cleft foot
cleft hand

cleft hand deformity
cleft high points
cleft jaw
cleft lip (CL)
cleft lip and palate (CLP)
cleft lip deformity
cleft lip nasal reconstruction
cleft lip nose
cleft lip repair
cleft lip-alveolus (CLA)
cleft margin flap
cleft maxillary segment
cleft mitral valve
cleft muscle of Veau
cleft nose
cleft of lateral aspect of nose
cleft of primary palate
cleft palate
cleft palate and lateral synechia
    syndrome (CPLS)
cleft palate classification
cleft palate elevator
cleft palate forceps
cleft palate impression
cleft palate knife
cleft palate needle
cleft palate operation
cleft palate prosthesis
cleft palate raspatory
cleft palate repair
cleft palate sharp hook
cleft palate tenaculum
cleft rhinoplasty
cleft spine
cleft tongue
cleft uvula
cleft-affected anatomy
clefting
    facial clefting
    midline cranio-orbital clefting
    orofacial clefting
    suprabasal clefting
cleidocranial
cleidocranial dysostosis
cleidocranial dysplasia
cleidocranial dystrophia
cleidotomy
cleidotripsy
Cleland cutaneous ligament
Cleland ligament
Clemetson uterine forceps
clenched fist deformity

clenched fist sign
Clerf aspirating tip
Clerf aspirator
Clerf cancer cell collector
Clerf dilator
Clerf forceps
Clerf laryngeal saw
Clerf laryngectomy tube
Clerf laryngoscope
Clerf needle holder
Clerf saw
Clerf tube
Clerf-Arrowsmith pin closer
Clerf-Arrowsmith safety pin
    closure
Clerk laryngectomy tube
Clerk needle holder
Clevedent crossbar elevator
Clevedent forceps
Clevedent retractor
Clevedent-Gardner chisel
Clevedent-Lucas curet
Clevedent-Miller elevator
Clevedent-Wakefield chisel
Cleveland bone rongeur
Cleveland bone-cutting forceps
Cleveland IMA retractor
Cleveland procedure
Cleveland-Bosworth-Thompson
    operation
Clevis clamp
Clevis dressing
click
    ejection click
    Gallvardin systolic click
    Hamman click
    joint click
    Ortolani click
    rarefaction click
    temporomandibular joint
        click
clicking rales
clicking sensation
clicking sound
click-murmur syndrome
clinch
clinch knot
clincher nail
C-line bipolar coagulator
clinic Bovie
clinic exolever elevator
clinic spasm

clinical defect
clinical diagnosis
clinical electromagnetic
    flowmeter
clinical encephalopathy
clinical evaluation
clinical examination
clinical intestinal transplantation
clinical pathologic classification
clinical signs and symptoms
clinical surgery
clinical syndrome
CliniCath catheter
CliniCath peripherally inserted
    catheter
Clinidine
clinocephaly
clinodactyly
clinoid process
Clinswound cleansers
clip (*see also* clip applier)
    2-way towel clip
    Ackerman clip
    Acland clip
    Adams orthodontic clip
    Adams-DeWeese vena caval
        clip
    Adams-DeWeese vena caval
        serrated clip
    Adson brain clip
    Adson clip
    Adson scalp clip
    Adson scalp hemostasis clips
    Ahlquist-Durham clip
    Ahlquist-Durham vena cava
        clip
    alligator clip
    aneurysm clip
    aneurysmal clip
    angled clip
    Astro-Trace Universal adapter
        clip
    Atrauclip hemostatic clip
    Austin clip
    Auto Suture clip
    Autostat hemostatic clip
    Autostat ligating clip
    Avalox skin clip
    Backhaus clip
    Backhaus towel clip
    bayonet aneurysm clip
    Beimer-Clip aneurysm clip

clip (*continued*)
    Benjamin-Havas fiberoptic
        light clip
    Biemer vessel clip
    bipolar diathermy adapter clip
    Bleier clip
    blepharoplasty clip
    Bonney clip
    Booster clip
    Boyle-Rosin clip
    brain clip
    Braun-Yasargil right-angle clip
    Bundt cross-legged clip
    butterfly clip
    Callender clip
    cardiac retraction clip
    Castroviejo scleral shortening
        clip
    Children's Hospital clip
    clamp clip
    Codman clip
    Colotzmark clip
    cranial aneurysm clip
    crankshaft clip
    cross-legged clip
    curved clip
    Cushing clip
    Cushing-McKenzie clip
    Dandy clip
    Delrin plastic scalp clip
    DeWeese-Hunter clip
    Drake aneurysm clip
    Drake clip
    Drake fenestrated clip
    Drake-Kees clip
    Drew clip
    ear clip
    Edslab jaw spring clip
    Edwards clip
    Edwards parallel-jaw spring
        clip
    Elgiloy clip
    Elgiloy-Heifitz aneurysm clip
    encircling clip
    Endo GIA surgical clip
    Ethicon clip
    Feldstein blepharoplasty clip
    fenestrated aneurysm clip
    fenestrated Drake clip
    ferromagnetic intracerebral
        aneurysm clip
    Filshie clip

clip (*continued*)

   Filshie female sterilization clip
   Flexi-Seal fecal collector & tail
      clip
   Friedman clip
   Friedman tantalum clip
   gate clip
   Guilford-Wright clip
   Hader bar clip
   Halberg clip
   Heath clip
   Hegenbarth clip
   Hegenbarth-Adams clip
   Heifitz aneurysm clip
   Heifitz clip
   Heifitz-Weck clip
   Hemoclip clip
   Hem-o-lok clip
   Hem-o-lok polymer ligating
      clip
   hemostasis clip
   hemostasis scalp clip
   hemostasis silver clip
   hemostatic clip
   Herff clip
   Hesseltine Umbili clip
   holding clip
   Horizon surgical ligating and
      marking clip
   House neurovascular clip
   Housepian aneurysm clip
   Hoxworth clip
   Hulka clip
   Hulka-Clemens clip
   Hylinks clip
   inferior vena cava clip
   Ingraham-Fowler cranium clip
   Ingraham-Fowler tantalum
      clip
   Iwabuchi clip
   Janelli clip
   jaw spring clip
   Kapp clip
   Keer aneurysm clip
   Kerr clip
   Khodadad clip
   Kifa clip
   Koln clip
   laparoscopic tie clip
   Lapro-Clip ligating clip
   LDS clip
   lens clip

clip (*continued*)

   LeRoy clip
   LeRoy disposable scalp clip
   LeRoy infant scalp clip
   LeRoy-Raney scalp clip
   Liga surgical clip
   Ligaclip surgical clip
   L-shaped aneurysm clip
   magazine clip
   Mayfield aneurysm clip
   Mayfield clip
   Mayfield-Kees clip
   McDermott clip
   McFadden aneurysm clip
   McFadden clip
   McFadden cross-legged clip
   McFadden Vari-Angle
      aneurysm clip
   McFadden-Kees clip
   McKenzie clip
   McKenzie hemostasis clip
   McKenzie silver brain clip
   metal clip
   metallic clip
   Michel clip
   Michel scalp clip
   Michel suture clip
   Michel wound clip
   Michel-Wachtenfeldt clip
   microanastomosis clip
   microbulldog clip
   microclamp clip
   MicroMark clip
   microvascular clip
   Miles clip
   Miles skin clip
   Miles Teflon clip
   Miles vena cava clip
   mini-Sugita clip
   Moren-Moretz vena caval clip
   Moretz clip
   Morse towel clip
   Mortson V-shaped clip
   Moynihan clip
   nonferromagnetic clip
   nose clip
   Olivecrona aneurysm clip
   Olivecrona clip
   Olivecrona silver clip
   palmar clip
   parallel jaw clip
   parallel-jaw spring clip

clip (*continued*)

   partial-occlusion inferior vena cava clip
   Paterson long-shank brain clip
   Penfield clip
   Penfield silver clip
   Perneczky aneurysm clip
   Petz clip
   Phynox clip
   Phynox cobalt alloy clip
   pivot aneurysm clip
   plastic scalp clip
   Poly Surgiclip absorbable clip
   Pool Pfeiffer self-locking clip
   primary clip
   Raney clip
   Raney scalp clip
   Raney spring steel clip
   Raney stainless steel scalp clip
   retractor clip
   Rica cross-action towel clip
   Rica silver clip
   Rica suture clip
   right-angle booster clip
   ring clip
   scalp clip
   scalp hemostasis clip
   Scanlan aneurysm clip
   Schaedel clip
   Schepens clip
   Schepens tantalum clip
   Schulec silver clip
   Schutz clip
   Schwartz clip
   Schwasser brain clip
   Schwasser microclip clip
   scleral shortening clip
   Scoville clip
   Scoville-Lewis aneurysm clip
   Scoville-Lewis clip
   Secu clip
   Selman clip
   Seraphim clip
   Serature clip
   Serature spur clip
   silver clip
   skin clip
   Slimline clip
   Smith aneurysm clip
   Smith aneurysmal clip
   Smith clip

clip (*continued*)

   Smithwick clip
   Smithwick silver clip
   Sofield retractor clip
   Spetzler titanium aneurysm clip
   spring clip
   sternal clip
   Stichs wound clip
   straight aneurysm clip
   suction tube clip
   Sugar aneurysm clip
   Sugar clip
   Sugita aneurysm clip
   Sugita clip
   Sugita cross-legged clip
   Sugita side-curved bayonet clip
   Sugita temporary straight clip
   Sugita-Ikakogyo clip
   Sundt booster clip
   Sundt clip
   Sundt encircling clip
   Sundt straddling clip
   Sundt-Kees aneurysm clip
   Sundt-Kees aneurysmal clip
   Sundt-Kees booster clip
   Sundt-Kees clip
   Sundt-Kees encircling patch clip
   Sundt-Kees graft clip
   Sundt-Kees Slimline clip
   surgical clip
   Surgidev iris clip
   suture clip
   Takaro clip
   tantalum clip
   tantalum hemostasis clip
   Teflon clip
   temporary clip
   temporary vascular clip
   temporary vessel clip
   titanium aneurysm clip
   Tomac clip
   Tonnis clip
   Totco clip
   towel clip
   triangular encompassing clip
   umbilical clip
   Uni-Shunt abdominal slip clip
   Uni-Shunt cranial anchoring clip

clip (*continued*)
  Uni-Shunt right-angle clip
  Vari-Angle clip
  vascular clip
  vena cava clip
  vena caval clip
  vessel clip
  Vitallium clip
  von Petz clip
  Wachtenfeldt butterfly clip
  Wachtenfeldt clip
  Wachtenfeldt suture clip
  Wachtenfeldt wound clip
  Weck clip
  window clip
  wing clip
  wound clip
  Yasargil aneurysmal clip
  Yasargil clip
  Yasargil cross-legged clip
  Yasargil-Aesculap spring clip
  Zimmer clip
  Zmurkiewicz brain clip
clip applier
  Sundt aneurysm clip-applier
  Yasargil aneurysm clip-applier
clip applier (*see also* clip)
clip approximator
clip force meter
clip forceps
clip graft
clip occlusion
clip placement
clip remover
clip technique
clip
clip-applying aneurysm forceps
clip-applying forceps
clip-bending forceps
clip-cutting forceps
clip-introducing forceps
clip-on attachment
Clip-on headlight
clip-on light bundles
clip-on/tie-on occluder
clippers
  electric hair clippers
  electric surgical clippers
  hair clippers
  preoperative hair clippers
clip-removing forceps
clip-removing scissors

Clisco covered needle catheter
clitoral incision
clitoral therapy device
clitoridauxe
clitoridectomy
clitoridis
  corpus cavernosum
    clitoridis
  corpus clitoridis
  crus clitoridis
  crus glandis clitoridis
  glans clitoridis
clitoridotomy
clitorimegaly
clitoris
  bifid clitoris
  cavernous nerves of clitoris
  crura of clitoris
  crus of clitoris
  deep artery of clitoris
  deep veins of clitoris
  dorsal artery of clitoris
  dorsal nerve of clitoris
  dorsal veins of clitoris
  frenulum of clitoris
  horn of clitoris
clitoroplasty
clitorotomy
clival
clival lesion
clivogram
clivography
clivus
clivus canal line
clivus metastasis
clivus syndrome
CLM articulating laryngoscope
    blade
CLO biopsy
cloaca (*pl.* cloacae)
cloacal formation
cloacal malformation
cloacal membrane
clockwise direction
clockwise rotation of heart
clogged artery
clomiphene fetal malformation
clonal expansion
clonic contraction
clonic convulsion
clonic seizure
clonic spasm

clonus
  abortive clonus
  drawn ankle clonus
C-loop of duodenum
C-loop posterior chamber lens
Cloquet canal
Cloquet fascia
Cloquet ganglion
Cloquet hernia
Cloquet needle
Cloquet node
close margin
close monitoring
closed
  loosely closed
  skin closed
  wound closed
closed amputation
closed anesthesia
closed apex
closed brachial plexus injury
closed capsulotomy
closed chain exercise
    attachment
closed chest cardiac massage
closed chest commissurotomy
closed chest drainage
closed commissurotomy
closed Cotrel-Dubousset hook
closed degloving injury
closed diaphyseal fracture
closed dislocation
closed disruption of digital
    artery
closed drain
closed drainage
closed drainage tube
closed flap amputation
closed fracture
closed head injury (CHI)
closed heart surgery
closed hemorrhoidectomy
closed in a routine manner
closed in anatomic layers
closed in layers
closed injury
closed iris forceps
closed irrigation
closed Küntscher nail
closed laparoscopy
closed loop
closed manipulative maneuver

closed mini-pouch
closed mitral commissurotomy
closed osteotomy
closed pneumothorax
closed reduction
closed reduction and internal
    fixation
closed reduction and
    percutaneous fixation (CRPF)
closed reduction of dislocation
closed reduction of fracture
closed reduction of fracture-
    dislocation
closed rhinoplasty
closed skull fracture
closed soft tissue injury
closed subcondylar osteotomy
closed suction drain
closed suction drainage
closed suction drainage tube
closed suction tube
closed surgery
closed technique
closed thoracostomy
closed transventricular mitral
    commissurotomy
closed tube drainage
closed tubule fixation technique
closed valvotomy
closed vitrectomy
closed water-seal drainage
closed water-seal suction tube
closed wedge osteotomy
closed-angle glaucoma
closed-bite malocclusion
closed-box suction
closed-break fracture
closed-circuit anesthesia
closed-circuit anesthetic
    technique
closed-end ostomy pouch
closed-gloving technique
closed-loop device
closed-loop intestinal
    obstruction
closed-loop intraocular lens
closed-suction tube
closely spaced electrodes
closer
  Clerf-Arrowsmith pin closer
  safety pin closer
closer forceps

closer water-seal drainage
closer wire
closing ABD wedge
　bunionectomy
closing base wedge
closing base wedge osteotomy
closing forceps
closing pressure
closing ring of Winkler-Waldeyer
Clostridium perfringens
Clostridium tetani
closure (*see also* sutures)
　2nd intention wound closure
　2-layer latex closure
　3rd intention wound closure
　abdominal wall closure
　abdominal wound closure
　airtight closure
　alveoloplasty reparative
　　closure
　anatomic closure
　aponeurotic closure
　auditory closure
　Barsky cleft closure
　Beta-Cap II catheter closure
　Brandy scalp stretcher I, rear
　　closure
　Brandy scalp stretcher II, front
　　closure
　circular with Passavant ridge
　　pattern of closure
　Clagett closure
　clamshell closure
　clean closure
　cleft closure
　Clerf-Arrowsmith safety pin
　　closure
　colostomy closure
　complete closure
　compression skull cap closure
　crowfoot closure
　crural closure
　deep closure
　delayed primary closure
　Dieffenbach plastic closure
　direct closure
　Dorrance closure
　double-umbrella closure
　DuoLock curved tail closure
　early hard palate closure
　epiphysial closure
　esophageal fistula closure

closure (*continued*)
　exit disposable puncture
　　closure
　exstrophy closure
　facial compression finger
　　closure
　facial compression skull cap
　　closure
　fascial closure
　final closure
　first intention wound closure
　fistular closure
　flask closure
　floor-of-mouth closure
　Fontan fenestration closure
　forced-eye closure
　Furlow closure
　general closure (GC)
　geometric broken line closure
　　(GBLC)
　glottic closure
　Gore-Tex closure
　Graham closure
　hand-sutured closure
　Harrington overlapping
　　closure
　Hartmann closure
　ileostomy closure
　imperfect closure
　incision closure
　inconsistent velopharyngeal
　　closure
　Jones closure
　Kleiger closure
　latex closure
　Latzko closure
　layered closure
　Lowsley retractor with hand-
　　sutured closure
　Marlex closure
　Marlex mesh closure
　mastectomy closure
　maxillary antrum closure
　midline aponeurotic closure
　mucosa-to-mucosa closure
　multisided Z-plasty closure
　muscularis tunnel closure
　nonoperative closure
　nonprosthetic closure
　overlapping closure
　palatal closure
　palatopharyngeal closure

closure (*continued*)

   pancreatic slump closure
   percutaneous patent ductus
     arteriosus closure
   peritoneal closure
   plastic closure
   Pratt-Sims closure
   premature airway closure
   premature ductus arteriosus
     closure
   primary closure
   primary wound closure
   prompt surgical closure
   Proxi-Strip wound closures
   pulmonic closure
   pursestring cervical closure
   reparative closure
   retainer closure
   revision and closure
   sandwich patch closure
   scalloped closure
   scalp closure
   secondary closure
   secondary wound closure
   shoelace fasciotomy closure
   single-layer continuous
     closure
   sinus closure
   skin closure
   skull closure
   Smead closure
   Smead-Jones closure
   Steri-Strip skin closure
   Steritapes closure
   stoma closure
   supraglottic closure
   Sure-Closure closure
   Sur-Fit irrigation sleeve tail
     closure
   surgical closure
   suture closure
   sutureless colostomy closure
   SutureStrip Plus wound
     closure
   tension-free closure
   tertiary wound closure
   Tom Jones closure
   Tom Jones hysterectomy
     closure
   tracheoesophageal fistula
     closure
   transcatheter closure

closure (*continued*)

   transmural closure
   umbrella closure
   vacuum assisted closure (VAC)
   Veau straight-line closure
   velopharyngeal closure
   ventricular septal defect
     closure
   visual closure
   von Langenbeck palate
     closure
   V-to-Y closure
   V-to-Y fashion closure
   V-Y closure
   watertight closure
   watertight skin closure
   wound closure
   Y configuration closure
   Z-plasty closure

closure of colostomy
closure of defect
closure of fistula
closure of ostomy
closure of wound
closure pressure
closure principle

clot

   afferent clot
   agonal clot
   antemortem clot
   autologous clot
   black blood clot
   blood clot
   chicken fat clot
   currant jelly clot
   dissolving blood clot
   distal clot
   evacuating clot
   evacuation of blood clots
   evacuation of clots
   exogenous fibrin clot
   external clot
   fresh blood clot
   friable clot
   heart clot
   inhibit blood clots
   internal clot
   laminated clot
   marantic clot
   organized clot
   passage of clots
   passive clot

clot (*continued*)
   plastic clot
   postmortem clot
   proximal clot
   retraction of clot
   Schede clot
   sentinel blood clot
   sleeve clot
   spider-web clot
   stratified clot
   washed clot
clot colic
clot evacuator
clot extension
clot forceps
clot formation
clot propagation
clot regression
clot retraction coagulation panel
clot size
clot stripper
cloth disk
cloth scissors
clothesline drain
clothesline evulsion of maxilla
clothesline injury
clothespin graft
clothespin H spinal fusion
cloth-shod clamp
clot-induced urinary tract
    obstruction
clotting
   graft clotting
   intrauterine clotting
clotting abnormality
clotting factor
cloudy ascites
cloudy fluid
cloudy iris
cloudy urine
Cloutier knee prosthesis
Cloutier operation
Cloutier unconstrained knee
    prosthesis
clove hitch
clove-hitch knot
clove-hitch sutures
cloverleaf catheter
cloverleaf condylar-plate fixation
cloverleaf counterbore
cloverleaf deformity
Cloverleaf EP catheter

cloverleaf excision
cloverleaf nail
cloverleaf pin
cloverleaf pin extractor
cloverleaf plate
cloverleaf rod
cloverleaf skull
cloverleaf skull deformity
cloverleaf skull syndrome
cloverleaf-type deformity
Cloward anterior fusion kit
Cloward anterior spinal fusion
Cloward back fusion
Cloward blade
Cloward blade retractor
Cloward bone graft impactor
Cloward bone punch
Cloward brain retractor
Cloward cautery hook
Cloward cervical disk approach
Cloward cervical dislocation
    reducer
Cloward cervical drill
Cloward cervical drill guard
Cloward cervical retractor
Cloward cervical retractor set
Cloward chisel
Cloward cross-bar handle
Cloward curet
Cloward depth gauge
Cloward double-hinge cervical
    retractor handle
Cloward dowel cutter
Cloward dowel handle
Cloward dowel impactor
Cloward drill
Cloward drill guide
Cloward dural hook
Cloward dural retractor
Cloward elevator
Cloward fusion diskectomy
Cloward guide
Cloward hammer
Cloward hook
Cloward instrument
Cloward intervertebral disk
    rongeur
Cloward intervertebral punch
Cloward laminectomy
    instrument
Cloward laminectomy rongeur
Cloward L-W gauge

Cloward nerve root retractor
Cloward operation
Cloward osteophyte elevator
Cloward osteotome
Cloward periosteal elevator
Cloward pituitary rongeur
Cloward procedure
Cloward puka chisel
Cloward punch
Cloward retractor
Cloward rongeur
Cloward self-retaining retractor
Cloward single-tooth retractor blade
Cloward spanner gauge
Cloward spinal fusion chisel
Cloward spinal fusion osteotome
Cloward spreader
Cloward square punch
Cloward stitch suture
Cloward technique
Cloward tissue retractor
Cloward trephine
Cloward vertebral spreader
Cloward-Cone ring curet
Cloward-Cushing vein retractor
Cloward-Dowel cutter
Cloward-Dowel punch
Cloward-English laminectomy rongeur
Cloward-English punch
Cloward-English rongeur
Cloward-Harman chisel
Cloward-Harper cervical punch
Cloward-Harper laminectomy rongeur
Cloward-Harper punch
Cloward-Hoen laminectomy retractor
Cloward-Hoen retractor
CLP (cleft lip and palate)
CLS total hip
clubbed finger
clubbed penis
clubbing
clubbing of distal phalanges
clubbing of extremities
clubbing of fingers
clubfoot
    Heyman-Herndon tarsometatarsal release for clubfoot

clubfoot (*continued*)
    Hiram Kite three-part cast for clubfoot
clubfoot deformity
clubfoot splint
clubhand
clump kidney
clunial nerves
cluster operation
cluster reduction
cluster tic syndrome
Clute incision
Clutton joint
Clyburn Colles fixator
Clyburn Colles fracture fixator
Clyburn dynamic Colles fixator
Clyman endometrial curet
clysis
clysis cannula
clyster
clysterize
CMC (carpometacarpal) joint
CMD (craniomandibular dysfunction)
CMG (cystometrogram)
C-mount adapter
CMV (continuous mandatory ventilation)
CMV-positive donor
CMW bone cement
CNS (central nervous system)
Contour ERCP cannula
CO_2 (carbon dioxide)
CO_2 cartridge
CO_2 cylinder
CO_2 FeatherTouch SilkLaser
CO_2 generator
CO_2 Heart Laser 2
CO_2 laser
CO_2 laser blepharoplasty
CO_2 laser probe
CO_2 muscle prosthesis
CO_2 Sharplan laser
CO_2 SilkLaser
co-abrasion
coagulate
coagulated bleeders
coagulated bleeding points
coagulating current
coagulating current Bovie
coagulating diathermy
coagulating electrode

coagulating forceps
coagulating knife
coagulating suction cannula
   obturator
coagulating-suction cannula
coagulating-suction forceps
coagulation
  argon beam coagulation
  bipolar coagulation
  blood coagulation
  Bovie coagulation
  cold coagulation
  cutaneous protein
    coagulation
  diffuse intravascular
    coagulation
  disseminated intravascular
    coagulation (DIC)
  electric coagulation
  Elmed coagulation
  endoscopic microwave
    coagulation
  endovascular coagulation
  exogenous anticoagulant
    coagulation
  fibrinolysin coagulation
  free-beam coagulation
  heater-probe coagulation
  infrared coagulation
  intravascular coagulation
  laser coagulation
  light coagulation
  low-current monopolar
    coagulation
  Meyer-Schwickerath light
    coagulation
  microwave coagulation
  monopolar coagulation
  multipolar coagulation
  plasmin coagulation
  sepsis-induced disseminated
    intravascular coagulation
  tissue coagulation
coagulation bronchoscope
coagulation cascade
coagulation cautery
coagulation defect
coagulation disorder
coagulation electrode
coagulation factor
coagulation factor assay
coagulation factor transfusion

coagulation forceps
coagulation meshwork
coagulation necrosis
coagulation pathway
coagulation probe
coagulation profile
coagulation screen
coagulation suction tube
coagulation-aspiration tube
coagulation-aspirator tube
coagulative laser therapy
coagulator (*see also*
    photocoagulator)
  American Optical coagulator
  argon beam coagulator
  argon plasma coagulator
  ASSI Polar-Mate bipolar
    coagulator
  Ball coagulator
  Ballantine-Drew coagulator
  Bantam Bovie coagulator
  Bantam coagulator
  Biceps bipolar coagulator
  bipolar coagulator
  Birtcher coagulator
  Birtcher Hyfrecator
    coagulator
  Birtcher laparoscopic
    coagulator
  Bovie coagulator
  Bovie CSV coagulator
  C-line bipolar coagulator
  Codman-Mentor wet-field
    coagulator
  cold coagulator
  Concept bipolar coagulator
  Cut-Blot coagulator
  electricator coagulator
  Elektrotom BiCut II
    coagulator
  Elmed digital bipolar
    coagulator
  Erbe Unit argon plasma
    coagulator
  Evergreen Lasertek coagulator
  Fabry coagulator
  Fukushima monopolar
    malleable coagulator
  Gram-Mer bipolar coagulator
  Grieshaber microbipolar
    coagulator
  Hildreth coagulator

coagulator (*continued*)
    infrared coagulator
    Jarit bipolar coagulator
    Karl Storz coagulator
    Kirwan bipolar coagulator
    Magielski coagulator
    Makar coagulator
    Malis bipolar coagulator
    Malis coagulator
    Malis solid state coagulator
    Mentor wet-field coagulator
    Mentor wet-field cordless
        coagulator
    Meyer-Schwickerath
        coagulator
    National coagulator
    Polar-Mate bipolar coagulator
    Poppen coagulator
    Poppen electrosurgical
        coagulator
    Redfield inframed coagulator
    Resnick Button bipolar
        coagulator
    Riddle coagulator
    Ritter coagulator
    Ritter-Bantam Bovie
        coagulator
    Scanlan bipolar coagulator
    solid-state coagulator
    Storz microsurgical bipolar
        coagulator
    Tekno coagulator
    Ultroid coagulator
    Walker coagulator
    wet-field coagulator
    xenon arc coagulator
    Zeiss coagulator
Coaguloop resection electrode
coagulopathic disorder
coagulopathy
coagulum
coagulum formation
coagulum pyelolithotomy
Coakley antral curet
Coakley antral trocar
Coakley antrum curet
Coakley cannula
Coakley curet
Coakley ethmoid curet
Coakley forceps
Coakley frontal sinus cannula
Coakley hemostat

Coakley nasal curet
Coakley nasal probe
Coakley nasal speculum
Coakley probe
Coakley sinus curet
Coakley sinus operation
Coakley speculum
Coakley suture technique
Coakley sutures
Coakley tenaculum
Coakley tonsil hemostat
Coakley tonsillar forceps
Coakley trocar
Coakley tube
Coakley wash tube
Coakley-Allis forceps
Coakley-Allis tonsillar forceps
coalescence
coalescent mastoiditis
coapt
coaptation
    end-to-side nerve coaptation
    nerve coaptation
    urethral coaptation
coaptation bipolar forceps
coaptation plate
coaptation site
coaptation splint
coaptation suture technique
coaptation sutures
coarctate retina
coarctation
coarctation clamp
coarctation forceps
coarctation hook
coarctation of aorta
coarctation of pulmonary
        arteries
coarctation of thoracic aorta
coarctation repair
coarctation syndrome
coarctectomy
coarctotomy
coarse
coarse breath sounds
coarse carbide cone bur
coarse crepitation
coarse facial features
coarse folds
coarse nodular cirrhosis
coarse rales
coarse trabeculation

coarse tremor
coarsened mucosal fold pattern
coarse-olive bur
coated biopsy forceps
coated carbon fiber
coated polyester sutures
coated sutures
coated tongue
coated Vicryl sutures
coating
   Calcitite hydroxyapatite
     coating
   Porocoat coating
   porous coating
   Pro/Pel coating
   Solo catheter with Pro/Pel
     coating
   Spring catheter with Pro/Pel
     coating
   Teflon coating
coating material
Coats ring
coat-sleeve amputation
coaxial cable
coaxial cannula
coaxial catheter
coaxial headlight
coaxial nylon connector
coaxial micropuncture
   introducer set
coaxial sheath cut-biopsy needle
coaxial snare
Coballoy twist drill
cobalt blue light
cobalt therapy
cobalt-60 irradiation
cobalt-60 therapy
cobalt-chrome
cobalt-chromium alloy
cobalt-chromium alloy
   prosthesis
cobalt-chromium head
cobalt-chromium implant
cobalt-chromium-molybdenum
   alloy metal implant
cobalt-chromium-molybdenum
   alloy
Coban bandage
Coban dressing
Coban elastic dressing
Coban wrap
Coban wrapping

Cobaugh eye forceps
Cobb bone curet
Cobb chisel
Cobb curet
Cobb elevator
Cobb gouge
Cobb osteotome
Cobb periosteal elevator
Cobb retractor
Cobb scoliosis measuring
   technique
Cobb spinal curet
Cobb spinal elevator
Cobb spinal gouge
Cobb spinal instrument
Cobb spine curet
Cobb syndrome
Cobb technique
Cobbett knife
Cobbett skin graft knife
cobblers suture technique
cobblers sutures
cobblestone degeneration
cobblestone lesion
cobblestone mucosa
cobblestone tongue
cobblestone-like plaques
cobblestoning
cobblestoning of mucosa
cobblestoning sign
cobbling
Cobb-Ragde bladder neck
   suspension
Cobb-Ragde needle
Cobe AV fistular needle
Cobe AV shunt
Cobe blood cell separator
Cobe cardiotomy reservoir
Cobe oxygenator
Cobe dialyzer
Cobe double blood pump
Cobe gun stapler
Cobe Optima hollow-fiber
   membrane oxygenator
Cobe small vessel cannula
Cobe staple gun
Cobe stapler
Cobelli glands
Cobe-Stockert heart-lung
   machine
Cobe-Tenckhoff peritoneal
   dialysis catheter

coblation-based disposable
arthroscopic
Cobra cannula
Cobra cannula tip
Cobra catheter
Cobra K cannula
Cobra K tip
Cobra K+ cannula
Cobra K+ cannula tip
Cobra OTW balloon catheter
cobra plate
cobra retractor
Cobra+ cannula
Cobra+ cannula tip
cobra-head anastomosis
cobra-head drill
cobra-head plate
cobra-head retractor
cobra-hood technique for
transecting graft
cobra-shaped catheter
Coburg-Connell airway
Coburn anterior chamber
intraocular lens implant
Coburn camera
Coburn equiconvex lens
Coburn intraocular lens
Coburn lens
Coburn lensometer
Coburn Mark IX eye implant
Coburn refractor
Coburn tonometer
Coburn-Rodenstock slit lamp
Coburn-Storz intraocular lens
cocaine anesthesia
cocaine anesthetic agent
cocaine atomizer
cocaine hydrochloride
cocaine hydrochloride
anesthetic agent
cocaine-induced respiratory
failure
cocainization
cocainize
coccidian body
coccidioidomycosis
cutaneous
coccidioidomycosis
coccidioidomycosis
tenosynovitis
coccydynia
coccygeal artery

coccygeal body
coccygeal bone
coccygeal fistula
coccygeal ganglion
coccygeal glands
coccygeal joint
coccygeal muscle
coccygeal nerve
coccygeal plexus
coccygeal vertebrae
coccygectomy
coccygeopubic diameter
coccygodynia
coccygotomy
coccyx
coccyx bone
coccyx fracture
cochlea (*pl.* cochleae)
canaliculus of cochlea
coiled cochlea
cupula of cochlea
external aperture of
canaliculus of cochlea
cochleae
apertura externa canaliculi
cochleae
canaliculus cochleae
fenestra cochleae
cochlear aplasia
cochlear branch
cochlear canal
cochlear cells
cochlear degeneration
cochlear duct
cochlear electrical stimulation
cochlear ganglion
cochlear implant
cochlear joint
cochlear lesion
cochlear microphonic
cochlear nerve
cochlear nucleus
cochlear prosthesis
cochlear recess of vestibule
cochleariform process
cochleate uterus
cochleo-orbicular reflex
cochleopalpebral reflex
cochleopapillary reflex
cochleostapedial reflex
cochleovascular accident
cochleovestibular approach

Cock urethrotomy
Cocke large flap retractor
cocked hat procedure
cocked-half flap
Cockett procedure
cockleshell ear
cocktail
    Brompton cocktail
    IV cocktail
    lytic cocktail
    Philadelphia cocktail
cock-up arm splint
cock-up deformity
cock-up hand splint
cock-up wrist support
cocoon dressing
cocoon thread susures
Co-Cr-Mo alloy
Co-Cr-Mo pin
Co-Cr-Mo prosthesis
Co-Cr-W-Ni alloy
Co-Cr-W-Ni alloy prosthesis
cod liver oil-soaked strips
    dressing
Codere orbital floor implant
codfish appearance of vertebrae
codfish deformity
Codivilla bone graft
Codivilla extension
Codivilla graft
Codivilla operation
Codivilla operation for
    pseudarthrosis
Codivilla tendon lengthening
    technique
Codman Accu-Flow shunt
Codman angle
Codman approach
Codman arthroscope
Codman bone gouge
Codman cannula
Codman cartilage clamp
Codman cervical rongeur
Codman clamp
Codman classification
Codman clip
Codman cranioblade
Codman cranioclast
Codman cranioplastic material
Codman disposable ICP lock
Codman disposable perforator
Codman drill

Codman exercises
Codman external drainage
    ventricular set
Codman fallopian tube forceps
Codman frame
Codman guide
Codman Hakim programmable
    valve
Codman ICP monitor
Codman ICP monitoring line
Codman IMA kit
Codman incision
Codman intracranial pressure
    monitor
Codman laminectomy rongeur
Codman lumbar external drain
Codman magnifying loupe
Codman marker
Codman Mentor Wet-Field
    cautery
Codman microimpactor
Codman osteotome
Codman ovary forceps
Codman patty
Codman Rhoton dissector
Codman saber-cut shoulder
    approach
Codman scissors
Codman shunt
Codman sign
Codman skull perforator guard
Codman sponge
Codman sternal saw
Codman towel clamp
Codman triangle
Codman vein stripper
Codman ventricular silicone
    catheter
Codman wire cutter
Codman wire-passing drill
Codman x-ray angle
Codman-Holter catheter
Codman-Kerrison laminectomy
    rongeur
Codman-Leksell laminectomy
    rongeur
Codman-Mentor erasure
Codman-Mentor microscope
Codman-Mentor wet-field
    coagulator
Codman-Schlesinger cervical
    laminectomy rongeur

Codman-Schlesinger cervical rongeur
Codman-Shurtleff cranial drill
Codman-Shurtleff neo-coagulator
Cody magnetic probe
Cody sacculotomy tack
Cody tack
Cody tack inserter
Cody tack procedure
Coe impression material
Coe investment material
coefficient of joint friction
Coe-Pak cement
Coe-Pak paste adhesive
Coe-Pak periodontal dressing
Coe-Soft dressing
coffer band
cofferdam
Coffey incision
Coffey operation
Coffey suspension
Coffey technique (I, II, III)
Coffey ureterointestinal anastomosis
Coffey uterine suspension
Coffey-Witzel jejunostomy technique
Coffin plate
Coffin split plate
Coffin spring
Coffin transpalatal wire
Coffin-Lowry syndrome
Coffin-Siris syndrome
Coffin-type transpalatal wire
Cofield technique
Coflex bandage
Coflex wrap
Cogan syndrome
Cogan-Boberg-Ans lens
Cogan-Boberg-Ans lens implant
Cogent light
Cogent XL illuminator
cognitive mapping
cognitive-behavioral therapy
Cogsell tip aspirator
cog-tooth of malleus
cogwheel
cogwheel motion
cogwheel respiration
cogwheel rigidity
cogwheel sign

Cohan corneal utility forceps
Cohan microscope
Cohan needle holder
Cohan-Barraquer microscope
Cohan-Vannas iris scissors
Cohan-Vannas scissors
Cohan-Westcott scissors
Cohen analysis
Cohen antireflux procedure
Cohen cannula
Cohen corneal forceps
Cohen cross-trigonal technique
Cohen elevator
Cohen intrauterine cannula
Cohen nasal-dressing forceps
Cohen operation
Cohen periosteal elevator
Cohen rasp
Cohen reimplantation
Cohen retractor
Cohen rongeur
Cohen sinus rasp
Cohen sinus raspatory
Cohen suture applicator
Cohen tubal insufflation cannula
Cohen urethroplasty
Cohen uterine cannula
Cohen uterine incision
Cohen-Eder cannula
Cohen-Eder tongs
Cohen-Eder uterine cannula
Cohen-Rentrop classification
Coherent laser
Coherent argon laser
Coherent argon laser photocoagulator
coherent bundle
Coherent CO_2 laser
Coherent CO_2 surgical laser
Coherent EPIC laser
Coherent Novus Omni multiwavelength laser
cohesive anatomic silicone gel breast implants
cohesive bandage
cohesive dressing
cohesive site density
Cohn cardiac stabilizer
Cohort bone screw
Cohort spinal impactor
coil canister
coil catheter

coil dialyzer
coil electrode
coil gland
coil hemodialyzer
coil intrauterine device (coil IUD)
coil machine adapter
coil vascular stent
Coil-Cath catheter
coiled bony structure
coiled cochlea
coiled intracranial aneurysm
coiled position
coiled spiral pusher wire
coiled upon itself
coiled-spring appearance
coil-tipped catheter
coin biopsy
coin lesion
coincidence correction
coinduction of anesthesia
Colanis maneuver
Colapinto needle
Colapinto sheath
Colapinto transjugular biopsy
    set
Colapinto transjugular needle
Colclough laminectomy rongeur
Colclough rongeur
Colcough-Love-Kerrison
    laminectomy rongeur
cold (carbon dioxide) cautery
cold abscess
cold beam laser
cold biopsy
cold biopsy forceps
cold blade biopsy
cold bone scan
cold cardioplegic solution
cold cautery
cold coagulation
cold coagulator
Cold Compress mask
cold cone biopsy
cold coning knife
cold conization
cold conization of cervix
cold cup biopsy
cold cup biopsy forceps
cold cup forceps
cold defect
cold dissection
cold exposure

cold forceps ablation
cold gangrene
cold infusion
cold injury
cold intolerance after fingertip
    injury
cold knife
cold knife cone aspiration
cold knife hook
cold lesion
cold light fountain
cold nodule
cold pack
cold pad
cold pressor test
cold pressor testing maneuver
cold resurfacing technique
cold rolled rod
cold saline-induced paresthesia
    technique
cold scissors
cold snare
cold snare ablation
cold snare excision
cold to the opposite, warm to
    the same (COWS)
cold ulcer
cold urticaria
cold-cone knife
cold-cup resection
Coldhot pack
cold-knife conization
cold-knife dissection
Coldlite speculum
Coldlite transilluminator
Coldlite vaginal speculum
Coldlite-Graves vaginal
    speculum
coldness of extremity
cold-punch resectoscope
cold-weld femoral ball
Cole duodenal retractor
Cole endotracheal tube
Cole fracture frame
Cole hyperextension fracture
    frame
Cole intubation procedure
Cole operation
Cole orotracheal tube
Cole osteotomy
Cole pediatric tube
Cole polyethylene vein stripper

Cole procedure
Cole pull-out wire
Cole retractor
Cole sign
Cole technique
Cole tendon fixation
Cole tube
Cole uncuffed endotracheal tube
Cole vein stripper
colectomy
   abdominal colectomy
   hand-assisted laparoscopic
     colectomy
   ileostomy without colectomy
   laparoscopic colectomy
   laparoscopic-assisted
     colectomy
   laparoscopy-assisted
     colectomy
   left colectomy
   left segmental colectomy
   one-stage left colectomy
   open colectomy
   partial colectomy
   prophylactic colectomy
   restorative colectomy
   subtotal colectomy
   total abdominal colectomy
     (TAC)
   total colectomy (TC)
   transverse colectomy
Coleman aspiration cannula
Coleman classification of
   congenital aural atresia
Coleman design
Coleman flatfoot technique
Coleman operation for talipes
   valgus
Coleman retractor
Coleman technique
Coleman V-dissector infiltration
   cannula
Coleman-Noonan technique
Coleman-Stelling-Jarrett technique
Coleman-Taylor IOL forceps
coli
   haustra coli
   polyposis coli
   tenia libera coli
   tunica muscularis coli
   tunica serosa coli
Colibri corneal forceps

Colibri corneal utility forceps
Colibri eye forceps
Colibri forceps
Colibri microforceps
Colibri mules
Colibri speculum
Colibri-Pierse forceps
Colibri-Storz corneal forceps
Colibri-Storz forceps
colic
   abdominal colic
   clot colic
   esophageal colic
   gallbladder colic
   gallstone colic
   renal colic
colic artery
colic flexure
colic impression
colic omentum
colic patch
colic patch esophagoplasty
colic surface of spleen
colic valve
colic vein
coliplication
colipuncture
colitis perineal complication
CollaCote wound dressing
collagen
   autologous human collagen
   Avitene fibrillar collagen
   Bio-Oss collagen
   bovine collagen
   cartilaginous collagen
   Dermalogen human collagen
   Fibrel collagen
   human collagen
   injectable collagen
   Isolagen human collagen
   microfibrillar collagen
   purified bovine collagen
   remodeling of collagen
   sterilized fibrillar bovine
     collagen
   subepidermal collagen
   Zyderm I collagen
   Zyderm II collagen
   Zyplast collagen
   Zyplast injectable collagen
collagen absorbable suture
collagen antibody

collagen deposition
collagen dressing
collagen fibers
collagen fibrils
collagen graft
collagen hemostatic material
collagen hemostatic material for
    wounds
collagen implant
collagen injection
collagen meniscus implant
collagen molecule
collagen plug
collagen prosthesis
collagen septum
collagen shield
collagen skin test
collagen sponge
collagen sutures
collagen synthesis
collagen tape prosthesis
collagen type
collagen vascular disease
collagen vascular serologic test
collagenase
collagenation
collagenesis
collagenolysis
collagenous
collagenous colitis
collagenous fibers
collagen-producing cells
Collagraft bone graft matrix
Collamer intraocular lens
Collamer one-piece lens
CollaPlug dressing
CollaPlug wound dressing
collapse
    alar collapse
    alar rim collapse
    bony vault collapse
    cardiovascular collapse
    circulatory collapse
    hemodynamic collapse
    massive collapse
    nasal valve collapse
    respiratory collapse
    scapholunate advanced
        collapse (SLAC)
    vascular collapse
collapse of lung
collapsed cheek

collapsed jugular vein
collapsed lung
collapsible tissue retractor
collar
    2+2 Rehab collar
    Bamp collar
    Belmont collar
    Camp collar
    Camp-Lewin collar
    centering collar
    cervical collar
    Colpacs collar
    cone collar
    Cowboy collar
    Dwyer collar
    Exo-Static cervical collar
    foam collar
    Forrester collar
    Headmaster collar
    heated tracheostomy collar
    high-humidity tracheostomy
        collar
    Houston halo traction collar
    implant collar
    MAC cervical collar
    Marlin cervical collar
    Miami Acute Care cervical
        collar
    Miami J cervical collar
    Minerva collar
    Minerva plaster collar
    mucosal collar
    myocervical collar
    Nec Loc cervical collar
    Newport collar
    Peterson cervical collar
    Philadelphia cervical collar
    Philadelphia collar
    plastic collar
    Plastizote cervical collar
    Plastizote collar
    Plastizote neck collar
    Pneu-trac cervical collar
    Queen Anne collar
    Schanz collar
    Stifneck immobilizing collar
    Thomas collar
    thyroid collar
    traction halter collar
collar bone
collar brace
collar button (*see also* button)

collar button-like ulcer
collar dressing
collar incision
collar prosthesis
collar scissors
collar-button abscess
collar-button iris retractor
collar-button tube
collar-button ulceration
collarette
Collastat OBP microfibrillar
    collagen hemostat
CollaTape
CollaTape tape
CollaTape wound dressing
collateral
collateral abdominal circulation
collateral arterial circulation
collateral artery
collateral circulation
collateral digital artery
collateral eminence
collateral ligament rupture
collateral ligaments
collateral mesenteric circulation
collateral vessel
collateralization
collecting duct
collecting structures
collecting tube
collecting tubule
collection
    abdominal air collection
    abdominal fluid collection
    air collection
    arterial blood collection
    cell collection
    duodenal fluid collection
    encysted intraabdominal
        collection
    expired air collection
    extra-axial fluid collection
    extracerebral fluid collection
    fluid collection
    gas collection
    globular collection
    gravitational particle
        collection
    infected collection
    intraglandular fluid collection
    isokinetic collection
    pancreatic fluid collection

collection (*continued*)
    periarticular fluid collection
    pericholecystic fluid
        collection
    perinephric fluid collection
    pleural fluid collection
    posttraumatic subcapsular
        hepatic fluid collection
    pus collection
    quantitative stool collection
    saccular collection
    sputum collection
    subphrenic collection
    urine specimen collection
collection tube
collector
    Alden-Senturia specimen
        collector
    bone collector
    bronchoscopic specimen
        collector
    cancer cell collector
    Carabelli cancer cell collector
    Carabelli collector
    Clerf cancer cell collector
    Conveen drip collector
    Cuputi sputum collector
    Cytobrush Plus cell collector
    Cytopick endocervical and
        uterovaginal cell collector
    Davidson collector
    drainable fecal collector
    Endocell endometrial cell
        collector
    Flexi-Seal fecal collector
    fetal incontinence collector
    Grass force displacement fluid
        collector
    Herchenson esophageal
        cytology collector
    Leukotrap red cell collector
    Lukens collector
    Medscand Cytobrush Plus cell
        collector
    Misstique female external
        urinary collector
    Moffat-Robinson bone pate
        collector
    Papette cervical collector
    Pilling collector
    Senturia-Alden specimen
        collector

collector (*continued*)
 Sheehy Pate Collector
 stool collector
 Storz bronchoscopic
  specimen collector
 Uterobrush endometrial
  sample collector
 Wallach-Papette disposable
  cervical cell collector
 Ware cancer cell collector
 wound drainage collector
 Xomed sinus-secretion
  collector
College forceps
College Park TruStep foot
 prosthesis
College pliers
Collen-Pozzi tenaculum
Coller arterial forceps
Coller artery forceps
Coller forceps
Coller hemostatic forceps
Colles external fixation frame
Colles fascia
Colles fracture
Colles ligament
Colles needle holder
Colles operation
Colles sling
Colles snare
Colles space
Colles splint
collet
collet screwdriver adapter
Colley tissue forceps
Colley traction forceps
colliculus (*pl.* colliculi)
 fascial colliculus
 inferior colliculus
 superior colliculus
colliculus of arytenoid cartilage
Collier
 aryepiglottic fold of Collier
Collier eye needle holder
Collier forceps
Collier hemostatic forceps
Collier needle holder
Collier thoracic clamp
Collier-Crile hemostatic forceps
Collier-DeBakey hemostat
Collier-DeBakey hemostatic
 forceps

Collier-Martin hook
collimation
collimator
 511-keV collimator
 APC-3, -4 collimator
 CASS TrueTaper collimator
 converging collimator
 diverging collimator
 Eureka collimator
 external collimator
 fan-beam collimator
 high-resolution multileaf
  collimator
 high-sensitivity collimator
 Leur-par collimator
 long-bore collimator
 low-energy collimator
 Machlett collimator
 medium-energy collimator
 Micro-Cast collimator
 multileaf collimator
 multirod collimator
 parallel-hole medium
  sensitivity collimator
 pinhole collimator
 slant hole collimator
 Sophy high-resolution
  collimator
 StereoGuide collimator
 Summit LoDose collimator
collimator helmet
Collimator plugging pattern
Collin abdominal retractor
Collin amputating knife
Collin amputation knife
Collin clamp
Collin dissector
Collin dressing forceps
Collin forceps
Collin intestinal forceps
Collin lung-grasping forceps
Collin mesher
Collin mucous forceps
Collin osteoclast
Collin ovarian forceps
Collin pelvimeter
Collin pleural dissector
Collin radiopaque sternal blade
Collin raspatory
Collin rib shears
Collin sound
Collin speculum

Collin sternal self-retaining retractor
Collin tissue forceps
Collin tongue forceps
Collin tongue-seizing forceps
Collin tube
Collin umbilical clamp
Collin uterine curet
Collin uterine-elevating forceps
Collin vaginal speculum
Collin-Beard operation
Collin-Beard procedure
Collin-Duval intestinal forceps
Collin-Duval-Crile intestinal forceps
Collin-Duvall intestinal forceps
Collings electrode
Collings electrosurgery knife
Collings fulguration electrode
Collings knife
Collings knife electrode
Collin-Hartman retractor
Collin-Hartmann retractor
Collin-Pozzi uterine forceps
Collins dynamometer
Collins leg holder
Collins solution
Collins-Mayo mastoid retractor
Collins-Mayo retractor
colliquative degeneration
colliquative necrosis
Collis anterior cervical retractor
Collis antireflux operation
Collis broken femoral stem technique
Collis Eagle I spirometry unit
Collis forceps
Collis gastroplasty
Collis gastroplasty procedure
Collis microforceps
Collis microscissors
Collis microutility forceps
Collis mouth gag
Collis posterior lumbar retractor
Collis repair
Collis scissors
Collis spirometer
Collis technique
Collis Universal laminectomy set
Collis-Belsey repair
Collis-Dubrul femoral stem removal

Collis-Maumenee corneal forceps
Collis-Nissen esophageal lengthening procedure
Collis-Nissen fundoplication
Collis-Nissen gastroplasty
Collis-Nissen operation
Collison body drill
Collison cannulated hand drill
Collison drill
Collison plate
Collison screw
Collison screwdriver
Collison tap drill
Collis-Taylor retractor
collodion
collodion dressing
collodion gauze
collodion membrane
collodion solution
collodion strip
collodion-treated self-adhesive bandage
colloid
colloid acne
colloid adenocarcinoma
colloid bodies
colloid cancer
colloid carcinoma
colloid cyst
colloid formation
colloid goiter
colloid impression material
colloid infusion
colloid milium
Collostat hemostatic sponge
Collostat sponge
collum (pl. colla)
collum dentis
collum mandibulae
Collyer pelvimeter
coloanal anastomosis
coloanal resection
coloboma (pl. colobomas, colobomata)
    atypical coloboma
    typical coloboma
coloboma anomaly
coloboma lentis
coloboma lobuli
coloboma palpebrae

coloboma, heart anomaly, choanal atresia, retardation, and genital and ear anomalies (CHARGE)
colobronchial fistula
colocecostomy
colocentesis
colocholecystostomy
coloclyster
colocolic anastomosis
colocolic intussusception
colocolonic anastomosis
colocolostomy
colocutaneous
colocutaneous fistula
colocystoplasty
coloendoanal anastomosis
colofixation
cologastrocutaneous fistula
cologastrostomy
colohepatopexy
coloileal
coloileal fistula
coloileotomy
cololysis
colon
   abdominoperineal resection of colon
   anterior band of colon
   ascending colon
   cathartic colon
   descending colon
   dilatation of colon
   distal colon
   Duhamel pull-through procedure of colon
   flexure of colon
   fold of colon
   free band of colon
   hypotonic colon
   iliac colon
   iliac flexure of colon
   infarcted transverse colon
   interposition of colon
   irritable colon
   knuckle of colon
   lead-pipe colon
   left colon
   loops of redundant colon
   midsigmoid colon
   midtransverse colon
   pelvic colon

colon (*continued*)
   proximal colon
   resection of colon
   right colon
   rotation of colon
   saccular colon
   sigmoid colon
   splenic flexure of colon
   transposition of colon
   transverse colon
   Waldeyer colon
colon and rectal surgery
colon ascendens
colon cancer
colon carcinoma
colon clamp
colon cut-off sign
colon descendens
colon interposition vaginoplasty
colon motility catheter
colon obstruction
colon perforation
colon procedure
colon resection
colon resection and anastomosis
colon sigmoideum
colon transversum
Colonial retractor
colonic abscess
colonic adenocarcinoma
colonic adenoma
colonic anesthesia
colonic carcinoma
colonic dilation
colonic distention
colonic diverticular hemorrhage
colonic diverticulum
colonic esophagoplasty
colonic fistula
colonic foreign body
colonic inertia
colonic infiltration
colonic insufflator
colonic interposition
colonic intussusception
colonic lavage
colonic loop
colonic metastasis
colonic mucosal line
colonic myenteric plexus
colonic obstruction
colonic patch

colonic perforation
colonic pit
colonic polyp
colonic pouch anal anastomosis
colonic resection
colonic varices
colonic vascular lesion
colonic volvulus
Colonlite bowel prep
Colonna arthroplasty
Colonna hip fracture
    classification
Colonna operation
Colonna reconstruction
Colonna trochanteric
    arthroplasty
Colonna-Ralston ankle approach
Colonna-Ralston approach
Colonna-Ralston incision
Colonna-Ralston medial
    approach
Colonna-Ralston operation
colonofiberoptic scope
colonofiberscope
    Olympus CF-series
        colonofiberscope
    Olympus CG-P-series
        colonofiberscope
    Pentax colonofiberscope
colonorrhagia
colonorrhea
colonoscope
    ACMI fiberoptic colonoscope
    ACMI operating colonoscope
    Fujinon colonoscope
    magnifying colonoscope
    OES colonoscope
    Olympus colonoscope
    Pentax colonoscope
    short bundle colonoscope
    standard colonoscope
    Toshiba colonoscope
    video image colonoscope
    Welch Allyn video
        colonoscope
    ZM-1 colonoscope
colonoscope syringe
colonoscopic
colonoscopic appendectomy
colonoscopic biopsy
colonoscopic evaluation
colonoscopic examination

colonoscopic polypectomy
colonoscopic removal
colonoscopy
    cecal colonoscopy
    complete colonoscopy
    diagnostic colonoscopy
    emergency colonoscopy
    high-magnification
        colonoscopy
    incomplete colonoscopy
    pediatric colonoscopy
    real-time colonoscopy
    splenic flexure colonoscopy
    stomal colonoscopy
    tandem colonoscopy
    therapeutic colonoscopy
    total colonoscopy
    transabdominal colonoscopy
    upper endoscopy and
        colonoscopy
    virtual colonoscopy
colonoscopy complication
colonoscopy complication
colonoscopy per rectum
colonoscopy per stoma
colonoscopy screening
colony formation
colony-stimulating factor (CSF)
colopexia
colopexostomy
colopexotomy
colopexy
Coloplast bag
Coloplast colostomy bag
Coloplast colostomy pouch
Coloplast deluxe irrigation kit
Coloplast dressing
Coloplast economy irrigation set
Coloplast flange
Coloplast flange pouch
Coloplast pouch
Coloplast urine leg bag
coloplasty
coloplasty pouch
coloplasty procedure
coloplication
coloproctectomy
coloproctostomy
coloptosis
colopuncture
color aberration
color Dopplar ultrasound

color flow Doppler scanner
color fusion
color imaging
Colorado electrocautery device
Colorado electrocautery tip
Colorado microdissection
  needle
Colorado MicroNeedle needle
  electrode
Colorado tip cautery
color-coding tape
colorectal adenocarcinoma
colorectal adenoma
colorectal anastomosis
colorectal biopsy
colorectal bleeding
colorectal cancer
colorectal cancer endoscopy
colorectal cancer resection
colorectal carcinoma
colorectal disease
colorectal disorder
colorectal fistula
colorectal hemorrhage
colorectal metastasis
colorectal mucosa
colorectal operation
colorectal polyp
colorectal surgery
colorectosigmoidostomy
colorectostomy
colored tape
color-flow Doppler
color-flow Doppler
  echocardiogram
colorrhaphy
colorvascular Doppler
  ultrasound
coloscopy
Coloset ostomy pouch
colosigmoid resection
colosigmoidostomy
colostomy
  blowhole decompressing
    colostomy
  closure of colostomy
  continent colostomy
  decompression colostomy
  decompressive colostomy
  descending loop colostomy
  Devine colostomy
  diverting colostomy

colostomy (*continued*)
  diverting loop colostomy
  diverting proximal colostomy
  divided colostomy
  divided-stoma colostomy
  double-barreled colostomy
  double-barreled loop
    colostomy
  dry colostomy
  end colostomy
  end-loop colostomy
  end-sigmoid colostomy
  end-to-side colostomy
  end-to-side ileotransverse
    colostomy
  exteriorization colostomy
  fecal diversion colostomy
  Hartmann colostomy
  ileal colostomy
  ileal transverse colostomy
  ileoascending colostomy
  ileosigmoid colostomy
  ileotransverse colostomy
  initial colostomy
  juxta-anal colostomy
  Lazaro da Silva technique
    colostomy
  loop colostomy
  loop transverse colostomy
  Maydl colostomy
  Mikulicz colostomy
  permanent colostomy
  permanent end colostomy
  primary colostomy
  resective colostomy
  sigmoid colostomy
  sigmoid loop colostomy
  sigmoid-end colostomy
  sigmoid loop rod colostomy
  temporary diverting
    colostomy
  temporary end colostomy
  terminal colostomy
  terminal sigmoid colostomy
  transverse colostomy
  transverse-loop rod colostomy
  Turnbull colostomy
  Wangensteen colostomy
  wet colostomy
colostomy bag
colostomy bridge
colostomy clamp

colostomy closure
colostomy loop
colostomy pouch
colostomy pyloric
   autotransplantation
colostomy rod
colostomy site
colostomy soiling
colostomy takedown
colostomy tube
colostrum
colotomy
  Allingham colotomy
  Bryant lumbar colotomy
  ileotransverse colotomy
  lumbar colotomy
Colotzmark clip
colovaginal fistula
colovesical fistula
Coloviras-Rumel thoracic
   forceps
Colpacs
Colpacs collar
Colpacs pack
colpectomy
Colp-Hofmeister operation
colpitis
colpocele
colpoceliocentesis
colpoceliotomy
colpocentesis
colpocleisis
  Latzko colpocleisis
  Latzko partial colpocleisis
  LeFort colpocleisis
  LeFort partial colpocleisis
  McIndoe colpocleisis
  Simon colpocleisis
colpocystotomy
colpocystoureterocystotomy
colpocystourethropexy
colpohysterectomy
colpohysterotomy
colpomyomectomy
colpoperineopexy
  abdominal-sacral
   colpoperineopexy
colpoperineoplasty
colpoperineorrhaphy
colpopexy
colpoplasty
colpopoiesis

colporectopexy
colporrhaphy
  A&P colporrhaphy
  anterior and posterior
   colporrhaphy (A&P repair)
  anterior colporrhaphy
  Goffe colporrhaphy
  Manchester colporrhaphy
  posterior colporrhaphy
  Sturmdorf colporrhaphy
colposcope
  Accu-Scope colposcope
  CooperSurgical overhead
   colposcope
  Cryomedics colposcope
  Frigitronics colposcope
  Jena colposcope
  Leisegang colposcope
  OpMi colposcope
  Wallach colposcope
  Wallach ZoomStar colposcope
colposcopic diagnosis
colposcopic examination
colposcopic-directed punch
  biopsy
colposcopy
  digital imaging colposcopy
  estrogen-assisted colposcopy
Colpostar-V6 colpostat
colpostat
  afterload colpostat
  afterloading colpostat
  Colpostar-V6 colpostat
  dome colpostat
  Fletcher afterloading colpostat
  FSD colpostat
  Henchke colpostat
  Homiak radium colpostat
  Landon colpostat
  Regaud radium colpostat
colpostat applicator
colposuspension
  Burch colposuspension
  laparoscopic needle
   colposuspension
  laparoscopic retropubic
   colposuspension
colpotomy
colpotomy incision
colpoureterocystotomy
colpoureterotomy
colpourethrocystopexy

colpourethropexy
Colson vaporizer
Colt cannula
Coltart arthrodesis
Coltart calcaneotibial fusion
Coltart fracture technique
Coltart talus fracture operation
Coltene alloy
Coltene impression material
Coltex impression material
Colton classification
Colton empyema tube
Colts cutting needle
Columbia staging system for
    breast carcinoma
Columbus McKinnon Hugger
    device
columella (*pl.* columellae)
    bifidity of the columella
    hanging columella
    midline of the columella
    retracted columella
    retrusion of the base of the
        columella
columella breakpoint
columella clamp
columella implant
columella nasi
columellar base
columellar clamp
columellar crease
columellar deformity
columellar flap
columellar implant
columellar jut of nose
columellar reconstruction
columellar repair
columellar stabilization
columellar strut
columellar subluxation
    stabilization
columellar type II
    tympanoplasty
columellar-infratip ratio
columellar-labial angle
columellar-lobular angle
column
    anal column
    anterior column
    barium column
    dimple and columns
    dorsal column

column (*continued*)
    lateral column
    Morgagni column
    philtral column
    posterior column
    radial column
    rectal column
    ventral column
    vertebral column
columnar carpus theory
columnar cells
columnar cuff carcinoma
columnar mucosa
columnar-lined esophagus
Colver dissector
Colver examining hook
Colver examining retractor hook
Colver forceps
Colver hook
Colver knife
Colver needle
Colver retractor
Colver retractor hook
Colver tonsil forceps
Colver tonsil hemostat
Colver tonsil needle
Colver tonsil retractor
Colver tonsillar dissector
Colver tonsillar knife
Colver tonsillar needle
Colver tonsillar pillar-grasping
    forceps
Colver tonsillar retractor
Colver tonsil-seizing forceps
Colver-Coakley forceps
Colver-Coakley tonsil forceps
Colver-Coakley tonsillar forceps
Colver-Dawson decompressor
Colver-Dawson tongue
    depressor
coma
    deep coma
    hyperosmolar coma
    irreversible coma
    prehepatic coma
coma aberration
comatose
Comberg contact lens
Comberg foreign body
    operation
Comberg operation
Combi-40 cochlear implant

CombiDerm absorbent cover
 dressing
CombiDerm dressing
combination biliary brush catheter
combination calculus
combination chemotherapy
combination cone/tube irrigator
 kit
combination cone/tube stoma
 irrigator drain
combination forceps/needle
 holder
combination gel and inflatable
 mammary prosthesis
combination mallet
combination needle electrode
combination of isotonics
 technique
combination skin
combination sleeve bridge
combination stethoscope
combination surgery
combined anterior and posterior
 approach
combined cavus deformity
combined chemoradiation
 therapy
combined contour procedure
combined defect
combined epidural-general
 anesthesia
combined femoral-inguinal
 herniorrhaphy
combined flexion-distraction
 injury and burst fracture
combined frontal-ethmoid-
 sphenoid sinusotomy
combined gastrointestinal
 resection
combined heart catheterization
combined hemorrhoids
combined hiatal hernia
combined injuries
combined internal and external
 version
combined laparoscopic and
 thoracoscopic approach
combined laparoscopic
 splenectomy and
 cholecystectomy
combined low cervical and
 transthoracic approach

combined needle holder and
 scissors
combined operation
combined organ resection
combined penetrating and
 lamellar corneal graft
combined presigmoid-
 transtransversarium
 intradural approach
combined radial-ulnar-humeral
 fracture
combined sacral and caudal
 block anesthesia
combined spinal-epidural
 anesthesia (CSEA)
combined spinal-epidural
 anesthetic technique
combined system disease
combined transsylvian and
 middle fossa approach
combined upper blepharoplasty
combined upper lid
 blepharoplasty
combined version
combined wire guide bone
 elevator
combined-flow lesion
Combisit surgeon's chair
Combitrans transducer
Combitube airway
Combitube endotracheal tube
comblike redness sign
Comby sign
comedo (pl. comedones)
comedo acne
comedo carcinoma
comedo extraction
comedo extractor
comedocarcinoma
comedomastitis
comedonal acne
comedones (sing. comedo)
comedones epidermal nevus
Comfeel contour dressing
Comfeel hydrocolloid dressing
Comfeel Plus pressure relief
 dressing
Comfeel powder
Comfeel Purilon dressing
Comfeel Ulcus occlusive
 dressing
Comfit endotracheal tube

Comfit endotracheal tube holder
Comfort Cath, I, II catheter
Comfort wrist immobilizer
ComfortCuff blood pressure cuff
ComfortWalk2 prosthetic foot
Comfy Elbow orthosis
Comfy elbow splint
Comfy Knee orthosis
completion cholangiography
Comlex dressing
complex regional pain
   syndrome I, II
Command PS pacemaker
Commander angioplasty
   guidewire
Commander PTCA wire
commando glossectomy
commando operation
commando procedure
commando radical glossectomy
commando resection
comma-shaped vertebral outgrowth
comminuted fracture
comminuted intraarticular
   fracture
comminuted orbital fracture
comminuted skull fracture
comminution
   mandibular symphysis
      comminution
commissural
commissural bundle
commissural cheilitis
commissural fusion
commissural myelotomy
commissural pit
commissural pulmonary valve
commissure
   anterior commissure
   anterior gray commissure
   aortic commissure
   Forel commissure
   fused commissures
   great transverse commissure
   Gudden commissure
   habenular commissure
   interthalamic commissure
   labial commissure
   laryngeal commissure
   lateral oral commissure
   lateral palpebral commissure

commissure (*continued*)
   medial palpebral commissure
   Meynet commissure
   optic commissure
   palpebral commissure
   posterior commissure
   superior commissure
   supraoptic commissure
   transverse commissure
commissure laryngoscope
commissure of fornix
commissure of Gudden
commissure of lips of mouth
commissure repair
commissuroplasty
commissurorrhaphy
commissurotomy
   anterior commissurotomy
   balloon mitral
      commissurotomy
   Brockenbrough
      commissurotomy
   Brockenbrough transseptal
      commissurotomy
   closed chest commissurotomy
   closed commissurotomy
   closed mitral
      commissurotomy
   closed transventricular mitral
      commissurotomy
   mitral balloon
      commissurotomy
   mitral commissurotomy
   mitral valve commissurotomy
   open mitral commissurotomy
   percutaneous catheter
      commissurotomy
   percutaneous mitral balloon
      commissurotomy
   percutaneous transatrial
      mitral commissurotomy
   percutaneous transvenous
      mitral commissurotomy
   transventricular mitral valve
      commissurotomy
   tricuspid commissurotomy
commissurotomy knife
committed mode pacemaker
common anterior facial vein
common atrium
common bile duct (CBD)
common bile duct dilator

common bile duct exploration
common bile duct ligation
common bile duct obstruction
common bile duct stone
common blue nevus
common canal
common carotid artery (CCA)
common carotid plexus
common component
common craniosynostosis
common digital vein of foot
common duct
common duct bougie
common duct calculus
common duct cholangiogram
common duct dilator
common duct exploration
common duct obstruction
common duct probe
common duct scoop
common duct sound
common duct stone
common duct stone forceps
common duct tumor
common duct-holding forceps
common extensor muscle of
    digits
common extensors
common facial vein
common fibular nerve
common hepatic duct
common iliac artery
common iliac lymph nodes
common iliac vein
common interosseous artery
common McPherson forceps
common nevus
common palmar digital arteries
common palmar digital nerves
common peroneal nerve
common peroneal nerve
    syndrome
common pH electrode
common plantar digital arteries
common plantar digital nerves
common tendinous ring
common tendon
common wart
communicating artery
communicating fistula
communicating hematoma
communis tendon

Compacement dental cement
compact bone
compact tissue
compactor
    McSpadden compactor
    Micro-Flow compactor (MFC)
Compafill MH dental restorative
    material
Compalay dental restorative
    material
Compamolar dental restorative
    material
Companion 2 blood glucose
    monitor
Companion 2 self-blood glucose
    monitoring device
Companion feeding pump
comparative radiographic
    examination
comparison eyepiece
comparison film
comparison microscope
comparison operation
comparison views
compartment
    central compartment
    decompressed compartment
    extraconal fat compartment
    intraconal fat compartment
    lateral compartment
    medial compartment
    released compartment
    scrotal compartment
    thenar compartment
    tibial compartment
    tissue compartments
compartment compression
    syndrome
compartment of knee
compartment pressure
compartment procedure
compartment syndrome
compartmental
    radioimmunoglobulin
    therapy
compartmental total knee
    prosthesis
Compass hinge
Compass stereotactic frame
Compat enteral feeding pump
Compat surgical feeding tube
compatible findings

Compeed Skinprotector
    dressing
compensated cardiac status
compensating curve
compensating eyepiece
compensation
    cardiac compensation
    depth-gain compensation
compensation technique
compensational frontal
    plagiocephaly
compensatory
compensatory antiinflammatory
    response syndrome (CARS)
compensatory atrophy
compensatory bone resorption
compensatory circulation
compensatory curvature of
    spine
compensatory curve
compensatory deformity
compensatory hypertrophy
compensatory movement
compensatory periosteal bone
    apposition
compensatory synostosis
Compere bone chisel
Compere chisel
Compere femoral lengthening
    procedure
Compere fixation wire
Compere gouge
Compere operation
Compere osteotome
Compere pin
Compere threaded pin
Comperm tubular bandage
Comperm tubular elastic
    bandage
competence
    immunological competence
    velopharyngeal competence
        (VPC)
    venous valvular competence
competency
    lip competency
    velopharyngeal competency
competent ileocecal valve
competent valve
compilation autogenous vein
    graft
complement

complement fixation
complemental air
complementary balloon
    angioplasty
complementary cascade
complementary hypertrophy
complementary induction
complementary therapy
complement-induced lung injury
complete abortion
complete adrenalectomy
complete anterior dislocation
complete atrioventricular
    dissociation
complete A-V dissociation
complete axillary dissection
complete bilateral cleft
complete bilateral deformity
complete blockage
complete circumferential
    mesorectal excision
complete cleft lip
complete cleft palate
complete closure
complete colonoscopy
complete common peroneal
    nerve lesion
complete cutaneous syndactyly
    of all four limbs
complete dislocation
complete duplication
complete emptying of bladder
complete excision
complete facial rejuvenation
complete filling
complete fistula
complete fracture
complete heart block
complete hemostasis
complete hernia
complete implant
complete inferior dislocation
complete integration
complete internal
    hemipelvectomy
complete iridectomy
complete laparoscopic distal
    pancreatectomy (C-LDP)
complete lateral
    hemilaminectomy
complete left bundle branch
    block (CLBBB)

complete mesh excision
complete motor paraplegia
complete obstruction
complete posterior dislocation
complete procedure
complete pulpectomy
complete pulpotomy
complete remission
complete resection
complete right bundle branch
  block (CRBBB)
complete rupture
complete skin-sparing
  mastectomy
complete sphincter relaxation
complete subperiosteal implant
complete superior dislocation
complete surgical exploration
complete syndactyly
complete thymectomy
complete thyroidectomy
complete weightbearing
complete wrap Nissen
  operation
complete-arch blade endosteal
  implant
complex
  AIDS-related complex (ARC)
  areolar complex
  areolomammary complex
  avidin-biotin-peroxidase
    complex (ABC)
  Batson vein complex
  brow-upper lid complex
  craniofacial complex
  DAE complex
  dentofacial complex
  Eisenmenger complex
  epispadias-exstrophy complex
  exstrophy-epispadias complex
  fibrocystic complex
  forehead-brow complex
  fusion complex
  Ghon complex
  Golgi complex
  growth plate complex
  HLA complex
  immune complex
  internal hemorrhoidal
    complex
  junctional complex
  juxtaglomerular complex

complex (*continued*)
  levator complex
  limb-body wall complex
  lip-nose complex
  major histocompatibility
    complex (MHC)
  malar ligament complex
  maxillozygomatic complex
  midface-malar zygomatic
    cheek-bone complex
  modified junctional complex
  ostiomeatal complex
  peripheral triangular
    fibrocartilage complex
  plasmin-inhibitor complex
    (PIC)
  Ranke complex
  short QRS complex
  sling-ring complex
  spike-and-dome complex
  teardrop-shaped nipple-areola
    complex
  triangular fibrocartilage
    complex (TFCC)
  triangular fibrocartilage
    complex (TFCC)
    débridement
  triangular fibrocartilage
    complex (TFCC) meniscus
    tear
  triangular fibrocartilage
    complex (TFCC) tear
  tuberous sclerosis complex
  vertebral subluxation
    complex
  Xase complex
  zygomatic malar complex
    (ZMC)
  zygomatic maxillary complex
    (ZMC)
  zygomaticomaxillary complex
complex adrenal endocrine
  disorder
complex anorectal fistula
complex aortic disease
complex cavity
complex chest mass
complex dissection
complex fracture
complex gonadal endocrine
  disorder
complex hepatojejunostomy

complex intracranial aneurysm
complex left ventricular outflow
    tract obstruction
complex pituitary endocrine
    disorder
complex polysyndactyly
complex regional pain
    syndrome I, II
complex regional pain
    syndromes (CRPS)
complex signal transduction
complex simple fracture
complex superficial
    musculoaponeurotic system
    rhytidectomy
complex thyroid endocrine
    disorder
compliant balloon
Compliant pre-stress bone
    implant
complicated birth
complicated cataract
complicated delivery
complicated dislocation
complicated diverticular disease
complicated fracture
complicated labor
complicated postoperative
    course
complicated recovery
complicated syndactyly
complication
    abdominal complication
    anastomotic complication
    bacterial complication
    benign pneumatic
        colonoscopy complication
    bleeding complication
    cardiopulmonary
        complication
    cardiorespiratory
        complication
    cardiovascular complication
    cerebrovascular complication
    colitis perineal complication
    colonoscopy complication
    concomitant obesity
        complication
    deep abdominal complication
        (DAC)
    delayed complication
    diabetic complication

complication (*continued*)
    disease-related complication
    endoscopy complication
    extraabdominal infective
        complication
    extraintestinal complication
    fatal complications
    feeding complication
    gastroduodenal
        complication
    gastrointestinal complication
    gonadal complication
    hematologic complication
    hemorrhagic complication
    hepatic complication
    immunologic complication
    implant-related complications
        (IRC)
    infection complications
    infectious complication
    infective extraabdominal
        complication
    intraoperative complication
    late complication
    life-threatening complication
    metabolic complication
    neurologic complication
    neurological complication
    neurovascular complication
    nonfatal complication
    nonimmunologic
        complication
    noninfective extraabdominal
        complication
    obstetrical complication
    operative site complication
    opportunistic complication
    oral complication
    pancreatic complication
    perioperative complication
    postbiopsy vascular
        complication
    postoperative complication
    postoperative respiratory
        complication
    postsplenectomy
        complication
    pregnancy complication
    procedures, alternatives,
        indications, complications
        (PAIC)
    pulmonary complication

complication (*continued*)
    recurrent thromboembolic
        complication
    renal complication
    respiratory complication
    sclerotherapy complication
    septic complication
    stomal complication
    surgery complication
    surgical complications
    thromboembolic
        complication
    thrombotic complication
    trocar wound site
        complication
    urologic complication
    vascular complication
    venous-related complication
    wound complication
complication rate
ComPly panty shield
component
    acetabular component
    AGC Modular Tibial II
        component
    AGC porous anatomic femoral
        component
    AGC unicondylar knee
        component
    anatomic graduated
        components (AGC)
    anterior component
    Autophor hip component
    Axiom knee component
    Biodynamic acetabular
        component
    Biomet AGC knee
        component
    Biomet AGC primary and
        posterior stabilized
        component
    Biomet Bi-Polar component
    Biomet femoral component
    Biomet MARS acetabular
        component
    Biomet unicompartment knee
        component
    Biomet revision acetabular
        component
    Biomet shoulder component
    Charnley flat-back femoral
        component

component (*continued*)
    Charnley narrow stem
        component
    cobalt chrome modular head
        component
    common component
    coronary perfusion
        components
    Deyerle component
    direct component
    Dunn-Hess femoral component
    Duramer polyethylene
        component
    electronic component
    femoral component
    filamentous component
    Freeman femoral component
    Harris-Galante hip
        replacement acetabular
        component
    Harris-Galante porous
        acetabular component
    Harris-Galante porous-coated
        femoral component
    Healey revision acetabular
        component
    Hoffmann compact external
        fixation component
    homogeneous component
    hybrid fixation of hip
        replacement component
    individual components
    Interlok primary femoral
        component
    Ionguard titanium modular
        head component
    Iowa hip component
    Isola spinal implant system
        component
    Judet impactor for acetabular
        component
    Kirschner Universal self-
        centering captive-head
        bipolar component
    Kudo elbow component
    Lubinus acetabular
        component
    Madreporic femoral
        component
    Mallory-Head hip component
    Mallory-Head Interlok primary
        femoral component

component (*continued*)
  MARS revision acetabular
    component
  Meridian femoral implant
    component
  Metasul hip joint component
  monoblock femoral
    component
  Morse tape lock of modular
    hip implant component
  NexGen knee component
  noncemented component
  Ogee acetabular component
  Oh femoral component
  Omnifit HA femoral
    component
  Opti-Fix acetabular component
  Opti-Fix femoral component
  Osteolock femoral
    component
  Osteolock acetabular
    component
  Osteonics femoral component
  PCA hip component
  PFC component (Press-Fit
    condylar component)
  polyethylene linear implant
    component
  Precision Osteolock femoral
    component
  Press-Fit condylar component
    (PFC component)
  Press-Fit femoral component
  Profix porous femoral
    component
  Pugh barrel component
  Reliance CM femoral
    component
  roof-reinforcement ring hip
    arthroplasty component
  Rotalok cup cementless
    acetabular component
  Rothman Institute porous
    femoral component
  Smith & Nephew reflection
    acetabular cup implant
    component
  Sofomor-Danek component
  Spectron femoral component
  Springlite foot component
  straight stem femoral
    component

component (*continued*)
  supracondylar barrel-plate
    component
  talar component
  Taperloc femoral component
  Tharies femoral resurfacing
    component
  Tharies hip component
  Ti-BAC acetabular component
  Tilastan femoral components
  Titan femoral component
  trial component
  Tri-Con component
  Ultima C femoral component
  Universal radial component
  Vitallium mesh component
  Vitalock cluster acetabular
    component
  Vitalock solid-back acetabular
    component
  Vitalock talon acetabular
    component
  wandering of disarticulated
    components
  Zimmer Ti-BAC acetabular
    components
component pusher
component ribs
component thin-walled veins
composite addition technique
composite auricular graft
composite bilateral
    infrastructure maxillectomy
composite biodegradable skin graft
composite chondrocutaneous
    flap
Composite Cultured Skin (CCS)
composite dental cement
composite dressing
composite external fixator ring
    adhesive
composite face-lift
composite flap
composite fracture
composite free tissue transfer
composite graft
composite inlay
composite inlay antral and nasal
    bone graft
composite joint
composite mandibular
    reconstruction

composite materials
composite odontoma
composite onlay
composite operation
composite osteomyocutaneous
  preformed flap
composite pelvic resection
composite pelvic resection
  procedure
composite pelvic resection
  technique
composite polymer stent
composite radiograph
composite resection
composite resin restoration
composite rhytidectomy
composite rib graft
composite skin graft
composite spring elastic splint
composite tissue transplantation
composite valve graft
composite wiring fixation
composition
Composix mesh
compound
  Dermatex compound
  Microfil silicone-rubber
    injection compound
  modeling compound
  phenolized gelatin compound
  Stemp compound
  triangular fibrocartilage
    compound
compound aneurysm
compound apertognathia
compound cavity
compound comminuted fracture
compound curved rasp
compound cyst
compound dislocation
compound dressing
compound flap
compound fracture
compound ganglion
compound gland
compound graft
compound joint
compound melanocytoma
compound microscope
compound muscle action
  potential (CMAP)
compound nevus

compound presentation
compound restoration
compound scanner
compound skin flap
compound skull fracture
compound suture technique
compound sutures
compress
  cool compress
  cribriform compress
  dry compress
  fenestrated compress
  graduated compress
  hot compress
  moist compress
  Priessnitz compress
  saline compress
  wet compress
compressed body
compressed fracture
compressed Ivalon patch graft
compressed nerves
compresses
  hot moist compresses
compressible acrylic intraocular
    lens
compressible cavernous body
compression
  anterior cord compression
  anterior-posterior
    compression
  anteroposterior compression
  axial compression
  barrel-hooping compression
  brainstem compression
  cardiac compression
  carotid artery compression
  carotid compression
  cauda equina compression
  cerebral aqueduct
    compression
  cerebral compression
  cervical vessel compression
  cervicomedullary junction
    compression
  Charnley compression
  cheek compression
  chest compression
  chiasmal compression
  chronic nerve compression
  continuous compression
  cord compression

compression (*continued*)
digital compression
direct compression
disk compression
downward compression
duodenal compression
duplex-guided compression
dynamic compression
early supraclavicular
    compression
elastic compression
esophageal compression
external chest compression
external compression
external pneumatic calf
    compression
extradural compression
extradural cord compression
extrinsic bladder compression
extrinsic compression
gastric compression
gentle compression
head compression
image compression
instrumental compression
interfragmentary compression
intermittent pneumatic
    compression
intrinsic compression
ischemic compression
lag screw technique of
    interfragmentary
    compression
lateral compression
limbal compression
lower plexus compression
mechanical variceal
    compression
median nerve compression
napkin-ring compression
nerve compression
nerve root compression
neurovascular cross
    compression (NVCC)
optic chiasm compression
optic tract compression
patella compression
pneumatic compression
prechiasmal compression
progressive compression
radial sensory compression
root compression

compression (*continued*)
spinal cord compression
spot compression
static compression
supraclavicular compression
suprascapular nerve
    compression
thecal sac compression
thoracic outlet compression
tissue compression
tracheal compression
trigeminal nerve compression
uterine compression
variable-release compression
vascular compression
venous compression
vertebral compression
vertical compression
compression anesthesia
compression arthrodesis
compression bandage
compression binder
compression bone conduction
compression boot
compression bra
compression button
    gastrojejunostomy
compression cough
compression cyanosis
compression deformity
compression device
compression dressing
compression earring
compression extension
compression forceps
compression fracture
compression garment
compression girdle
compression hip screw (CHS)
compression hook
compression injury
compression instrumentation
    posterior construct
compression instruments for
    bone plating
compression molding
compression of brain
compression of carotid artery
compression of spinal cord
compression overload
compression paddle
compression paralysis

compression plate
compression plate fixation
compression plating
compression pump
compression reflex
compression rod
compression rod treatment
compression screw
compression screw plate
compression skull cap closure
compression sleeve shin splint
compression splint
compression stockings
compression strain
compression switch
compression syndrome
compression tape
compression technique
compression test
compression testing
compression U-rod
    instrumentation
compression wiring
compression wrench
compression-molded intraocular
    lens
compression-type deformity
compressive internal fixating
    device
compressive plastic splint
compressive strength
compressor
    Adair screw compressor
    air compressor
    Anthony compressor
    Anthony enucleation
        compressor
    Anthony orbital compressor
    Anthony orbital enucleation
        compressor
    Barnes compressor
    Berens compressor
    Berens enucleation
        compressor
    Berens orbital compressor
    Castroviejo compressor
    Charnley compressor
    Conn aortic compressor
    continuous air compressor
    Deschamps compressor
    DeVilbiss air compressor
    DeVilbiss compressor

compressor (*continued*)
    enucleation compressor
    external inflatable
        compressor
    orbital enucleation
        compressor
    Pulmo-Mist compressor
    Riahl coronary compressor
    screw compressor
    Sehrt compressor
    shot compressor
    tonsillar compressor
    tubing compressor
compressor muscle of naris
Comprifix active ankle support
Comprifix ankle splint
Comprilan bandage
Comprol dressing
compromise
    airway compromise
    circulatory compromise
    FAT compromise
    neurovascular compromise
    vascular compromise
CompuCam digital intraoral
    camera
computerized pattern generator
Compu-Neb ultrasonic nebulizer
Compuscan-P pachymeter
computed axial tomography
    (CAT)
computed tomography (CT)
computed tomography laser
    mammography
computed tomography-guided
    selective drainage
computer dose calculation
computer tomography
computer tomography-guided
    biopsy
computer-assisted anesthesia
computer-assisted continuous
        infusion anesthetic
        technique
computer-assisted controlled
        infusion (CACO)
computer-assisted neurosurgical
        navigational system
        (CANS)
computer-assisted operation
computer-assisted stereotactic
        surgery

computer-controlled drug
   administration anesthetic
   technique
computer-controlled infusion
   anesthetic technique
computer-controlled infusion
   pump
computerized assisted design
   (CAD)
computerized assisted design
   prosthesis
computerized axial tomography
   (CAT)
computerized cranial
   tomography (CCT)
computerized electronic
   endoscopy
computerized isokinetic
   dynamometer
computerized muscle-joint
   evaluation
computerized pattern generator
computerized tomography (CT)
Computon microtonometer
Comyns-Berkeley retractor
concave abdomen
concave anterior surface
concave gouge
concave lens
concave loading socket
concave obturator
concave philtral dimple
concave posterior surface
concave sheath
concave sheath and obturator
concavity
   macroscopic concavity
concavity and depression
concavity of spine
concavoconcave
concavoconcave lens
concavoconvex
concavoconvex lens
concealed hemorrhage
concealed graft
concealed hernia
concealer graft
concentration
   1-minimum alveolar
     concentration (1-MAC)
   ambient oxygen
     concentration

concentration (*continued*)
   approximate lethal
     concentration
   bactericidal concentration
   bilirubin concentration
   blood alcohol concentration
   carbon dioxide concentration
   end-tidal nitrogen
     concentration
   hazardous concentration
   inspiratory vapor
     concentration
   intense concentration
   lethal concentration
   mass concentration
   maximal drug concentration
   maximum permissible
     concentration
   minimal alveolar
     concentration
   minimal anesthetic
     concentration (MAC)
   minimal bactericidal
     concentration
   minimum alveolar anesthetic
     concentration (MAC)
   minimum alveolar
     concentration (MAC)
   minimum bactericidal
     concentration
   minimum detectable
     concentration
   minimum effective analgesic
     concentration
   minimum effective
     concentration (MEC)
   minimum lethal concentration
   minimum local analgesic
     concentration (MLAC)
   peak lidocaine concentration
   plasma concentration
   plasma endotoxin
     concentration
   plasma gastrin concentration
   plasma iron concentration
   plasma norepinephrine
     concentration
   plasma renin concentration
   plasma urea concentration
   predialysis plasma phosphate
     concentration
   prick-test concentration

concentration (*continued*)
  radioactive concentration
  renal vein renin concentration
  serum bactericidal
    concentration
  serum bilirubin concentration
  serum calcium concentration
  serum lithium concentration
  steroid concentration
  subanesthetic concentration
  substance concentration
  target plasma concentration
    (TPC)
  thyroid hormone serum
    concentration
  time of maximum
    concentration
  total protein concentration
concentration performance test
concentration procedure
concentration times time
concentrator
  Keystone Plus oxygenator
    concentrator
  Millennium oxygen
    concentrator
  NewLife oxygen concentrator
  SolAiris III oxygen
    concentrator
  stem cell concentrator
concentric atrophy
concentric constriction
concentric hernia
concentric hypertrophy
concentric lesion
concentric needle
concentric needle electrode
concentric pantomography
concentric reduction
concentric swabbing
concentric-needle electrode
Concept 2-pin passer
Concept ablation
Concept ablator
Concept graft passer
Concept arthroscopy rasp
Concept arthroscopic knife
Concept bipolar coagulator
Concept bone tunnel plug
Concept cannula
Concept cautery
Concept curet

Concept dermatome
Concept disposable cautery
Concept eye cautery
Concept handheld cautery
Concept Intra-Arc drive
Concept Intravision arthroscope
Concept mesh grafter
  dermatome
Concept Multi-Liner lining
  needle
Concept nerve stimulator
Concept Ophtho-Bur
Concept screw
Concept suturing needle
Concept tibial guide
Conceptus Robust guidewire
Conceptus Soft Seal cervical
  catheter
Conceptus Soft Torque uterine
  catheter
Conceptus VS (variable softness)
  catheter
concha (*pl.* conchae)
  cavity of concha
  cavum concha
  highest concha
  inferior concha
  inferior ethmoidal concha
  inferior nasal concha
  inferior turbinate concha
  medial nasal concha
  middle nasal concha
  Morgagni concha
  nasal concha
  nasoturbinal concha
  Santorini concha
  sphenoidal concha
  superior nasal concha
  supreme nasal concha
  cavum conchae
  cymba conchae
  sphenoidal nasal conchae
concha auriculae
concha bullosa
concha nasalis
concha nasoturbinal
concha of auricle
concha of cranium
concha of ear
concha Santorini
concha sphenoidalis
conchal

conchal bowl
conchal cartilage
conchal cartilage graft
conchal cartilage-ethmoid bone
    graft
conchal contraction
conchal crest
conchal crest of maxilla
conchal crest of palatine bone
conchal flap
conchal fossa
conchal mastoid angle
conchal mucosa
conchal reduction
conchal retrodisplacement
conchal show
conchal surgery
conchal tip graft
concha-mastoid sutures
conchectomy
conchomastoidal sutures
conchoscaphal sutures
conchoscaphoid angle
conchotome
    Hartmann nasal conchotome
    Henke-Stille conchotome
    Olivecrona conchotome
    Stille conchotome
    Struyken conchotome
    Watson-Williams conchotome
    Weil-Blakesley conchotome
conchotomy
Concise compression hip screw
Concise side plate
Conclude dental cement
Conco elastic bandage
Conco tractor
concomitant administration
concomitant antireflux surgery
concomitant bleeding
concomitant hepatectomy
concomitant obesity
    complication
concomitant spinal cord injury
concomitant symptom
concomitant therapy
Concord line draw syringe
Concord Portex airway
Concorde disposable skin
    stapler
Concorde disposable suction
    cannula

Concorde suction cannula
concrement
concrescence
concrete burn
concrete seborrhea
concretion
    bile concretion
    calcium concretion
concurrent chemotherapy
concurrent findings
concurrent hepatic laceration
concurrent medical condition
concussion (grades 1-3)
    brain concussion
    cerebral concussion
    mild concussion
condenser
    Abbe condenser
    amalgam condenser
    McShirley electromallet
        condenser
    mechanical condenser
    Nordent amalgam condenser
    Universal condenser
condenser point
condensing lens
condition
    catabolic condition
    concurrent medical condition
    congenital condition
    corrected condition
    deteriorated condition
    diffuse condition
    diseased condition
    drug-induced condition
    fibrocystic condition
    functional condition
    gastrointestinal condition
    genetic condition
    hemorrhagic condition
    improved condition
    inactive condition
    infantile condition
    inflammatory condition
    inoperable condition
    irreversible condition
    life-threatening condition
    locally advanced condition
    long-standing condition
    medical systemic condition
    mixed condition
    normal condition

condition (*continued*)
  pathologic condition
  postoperative condition
  predisposing condition
  progressive condition
  secondary condition
  stabilized condition
  stable condition
  stress-induced condition
  stress-related condition
  subacute condition
  systemic condition
  terminal condition
  tumor-like bone condition
conditioning therapy
condom catheter
condom catheter attachment
Condon antibiotic prep
conductance catheter
conducting cord
conduction
  compression bone
    conduction
  delayed conduction
  His-Purkinje conduction
conduction analgesia
conduction anesthesia
conduction defect
conduction disturbance
conduction nerve study
conduction system of heart
conduction time
conduction velocity
conductive base
conductive device
conductive Hydrogel wound
  dressing
conductive V-Lok cuff
conductivity
conductor
  Adson conductor
  Adson saw conductor
  Bailey conductor
  Bailey saw conductor
  Bovie liquid conductor
  Davis conductor
  Davis saw conductor
  esophageal conductor
  flexible esophageal conductor
  Gigli-saw conductor
  Kanavel conductor
  Martel conductor

conductor (*continued*)
  Souttar esophageal conductor
  Storz conductor
  Storz esophageal conductor
  Storz flexible esophageal
    conductor
  Xomed Audiant bone
    conductor
conduit
  aortic conduit
  Bricker ileal conduit
  ileal conduit
  intestinal diversion conduit
conduitogram
conduitography
condylar aplasia
condylar articulation
condylar axis
condylar blade plate
condylar canal
condylar cartilage
condylar chondroma
condylar deformation
condylar displacement
condylar dysplasia
condylar emissary vein
condylar femoral fracture
condylar fossa
condylar fracture
condylar fragment
condylar growth
condylar guide
condylar guide inclination
condylar head
condylar hinge position
condylar hyperplasia
condylar hypoplasia
condylar implant
condylar implant arthroplasty
condylar lag screw plate
condylar neck
condylar neck retractor
condylar path
condylar process fracture
condylar process fracture axial
  anchor screw fixation
condylar prosthesis
condylar screw fixation
condyle
  displaced condyle
  femoral condyle
  lateral condyle

condyle (*continued*)
  mandibular condyle
  medial condyle
  neck of condyle
  occipital condyle
  protrusive condyle
  tibial condyle
condyle bone
condyle dissection
condyle head
condyle of mandible
condyle resection
condyle rod
condylectomy
  Duverney plantar
    condylectomy
  DuVries condylectomy
  mandibular condylectomy
  plantar condylectomy
condylion
condylocephalic nail
condyloid fossa
condyloid joint
condyloid process
condyloma (*pl.* condylomata,
    condylomas)
condyloma acuminatum
condylomata
  vulvar condylomata
condylomata (*sing.* condyloma)
condyloplasty
condylotomy
condylus
cone
  breast cone
  copper sulphate cone
  hot cone
  intraoral cone
  master cone
  narrow cone
  retinal cones
  rods and cones
  transvaginal cone
  truncated cone
cone arthrodesis
cone biopsy
cone biopsy cannula
cone biopsy knife
cone biopsy needle
cone biopsy punch
cone bone punch
cone bur

cone calipers
cone cannula
cone cells
cone cerebral cannula
cone collar
cone curet
cone forceps
cone ice-tong calipers
cone knife
cone laminectomy retractor
cone nasal curet
cone needle
cone projection
cone punch
cone retractor
cone ring curet
cone scalp retractor
cone self-retaining retractor
cone skull punch
cone specimen
cone splint
cone suction biopsy curet
cone suction tube
cone tip catheter
cone tube
cone ventricular needle
cone wire twister
cone wire-twisting forceps
coned AP projection
coned heparin tip
cone-down x-ray view
cone-down projection
cone-down view
cone-shaped amputation
    stump
Confide HIV test kit
confidence ring
configuration
  bat-wing configuration
  chain-of-lakes configuration
  plane configuration
  pulse-wave configurations
  standard configuration
  uterine configuration
configuration and size
confinement
  calculated date of
    confinement
  expected date of confinement
    (EDC)
confirmation
  intraoperative confirmation

confirmation (*continued*)
  intraoperative spatial
    confirmation
confirmatory axillary dissection
confirmatory incision
confluence of sinuses
confluent and reticulated
  papillomatosis
confluent inflammation
confluent rash
confluent shadows
confocal laser scanning
confocal microscope
confocal scanning laser
  ophthalmoscope
confocal scanning laser
  polarimeter
Conform stretch bandage
Conformant dressing
Conformant wound dressing
conformation of right heart
  catheter
conformer
  acrylic conformer
  eye conformer
  eye implant conformer
  Fox conformer
  Fox eye conformer
  implant conformer
  plastic conformer
  Universal conformer
conformer for eye
confrontation fields
confrontation of visual fields
congenerous muscles
congenita
  aplasia cutis congenita
  arthrogryposis multiplex
    congenita
  chondrodystrophia calcificans
    congenita
  cutis marmorata
    telangiectatica congenita
  dyskeratosis congenita
  fistula auris congenita
  hyperkeratosis congenita
  melanosis diffusa congenita
  myopathic arthrogryposis
    multiplex congenita
  neuropathic arthrogryposis
    multiplex congenita
  pachyonychia congenita

congenital abnormality
congenital above-elbow
  amputation
congenital absence of (organ,
  organ part, tissue)
congenital adrenal hyperplasia
congenital alveolar synechia
  syndrome
congenital amputation
congenital anomaly
congenital below-elbow
  amputation
congenital birth defect
congenital blepharoptosis
congenital brain malformation
congenital camptodactyly
congenital carpal synchondrosis
congenital central
  hypoventilation syndrome
congenital cerebral aneurysm
congenital choledochal cyst
congenital cholesteatoma
congenital circumscribed
  hypomelanosis
congenital condition
congenital cystic adenomatoid
  malformation
congenital cystic dilatation
congenital defect
congenital deformity
congenital diaphragmatic hernia
  (CDH)
congenital disease
congenital dislocated hip (CDH)
congenital dislocation
congenital disorder
congenital duplication
congenital dysplasia of hip
  (CDH)
congenital earlobe cleft
congenital ectodermal dysplasia
congenital entropion
congenital epicanthus
congenital facial diplegia
congenital failure
congenital fibromatosis
congenital fracture
congenital generalized
  lipodystrophy
congenital goiter
congenital hand anomaly
congenital hand duplication

congenital heart defect (CHD)
congenital heart malformation
congenital hemangioma
congenital hemangiopericytoma
congenital hernia
congenital hip dislocation
   (CHD)
congenital laryngeal stridor
congenital lens dislocation
congenital lesion
congenital luetic labyrinthitis
congenital malformation
congenital mass
congenital megacolon
congenital myotonia
congenital nevus
congenital postural deformity
congenital pulmonary
   arteriovenous fistula
congenital pyloric membrane
congenital ring syndrome
congenital scapular elevation
congenital sebaceous
   hyperplasia
congenital subglottic
   hemangioma
congenital synchondrosis
congenital telangiectatic erythema
congenital thumb duplication
congenital tufted angioma
congenital tympanic dehiscence
congenital urethroperineal fistula
congenital vascular
   malformation
congenitally altered anatomy
congenital multiple
   arthrogryposis
Conger perineal urethrostomy
   clamp
congested kidney
congested vascular structures
congestion
   chest congestion
   flap congestion
   functional congestion
   nasal congestion
   pleuropulmonary congestion
   pulmonary venous congestion
   vascular congestion
   venocapillary congestion
   venous congestion
congestive cardiac failure

congestive failure
congestive glaucoma
congestive heart disease (CHD)
congestive heart failure (CHF)
congestive splenomegaly
conglobate gland
conglutinant
conglutination
Congo red dye
conic bougie
conic papillae
conic, conical
conical bougie
conical bur
conical catheter
conical centrifuge tube
conical cornea
conical eye implant
conical flap
conical implant
conical inserter tip
conical probe
conical stump
conical trocar
conical-tip catheter
conical-tip electrode
coning of areola
coniotomy
conization
   cautery conization
   cervical conization
   cold conization
   cold-knife conization
   excisional conization
   hot conization
   hot-knife conization
   Hyam conization
   knife conization
   laser cervical conization
   laser conization
   LEEP conization
   loop diathermy cervical
     conization
   loop electrosurgical excision
     procedure conization
   postlaser conization
conization biopsy
conization electrode
conization instrument
conization instrument blade
conization knife
conization of cervix

conization of uterine cervix
conization technique
conjoined anastomosis
conjoined nerve root
conjoined nerve-root anomaly
conjoined organs
conjoined tendon
conjoined twins
conjoint extensor digitorum
 brevis muscle and dorsalis
 pedis osteocutaneous
conjoint extensor digitorum
 brevis muscle and dorsalis
 pedis osteocutaneous isla
conjoint extensor digitorum
 brevis muscle and dorsalis
 pedis osteocutaneous island
 flap
conjugate axis
conjugate deviation
conjugate diameter (CD)
conjugate eye movement
conjugate foramen
conjugate gaze
conjugate measurements
conjugate movement
conjugate paralysis
conjugate point
conjunctiva (*pl.* conjunctivae)
 flap of conjunctiva
 flapping of conjunctiva
 fornix conjunctivae
 fornix of superior conjunctiva
 grattage of conjunctiva
 rolling of conjunctiva
 sclerae and conjunctivae
  (S&C)
 tunica conjunctiva
conjunctival abscess
conjunctival adhesions
conjunctival arteries
conjunctival circulation
conjunctival cul-de-sac
conjunctival cul-de-sac
 reconstruction
conjunctival exudate
conjunctival fixation forceps
conjunctival flap
conjunctival fold
conjunctival forceps
conjunctival fornix
conjunctival hemorrhage

conjunctival incision
conjunctival injection
conjunctival laceration
conjunctival lipoma
conjunctival melanotic lesion
conjunctival membrane
conjunctival patch graft
conjunctival scissors
conjunctival spreader
conjunctival tumor
conjunctival veins
conjunctivales anteriores, ateriae
conjunctivales posteriores,
 ateriae
conjunctiva-Mueller muscle
 excision
conjunctivocystorhinostomy
conjunctivodacryocystorhinos-
 tomy
conjunctivodacryocystostomy
conjunctivoplasty
conjunctivorhinostomy
conjunctivotarsal area
conjunctivotarsal surface
conjunctivo-Tenon flap
Conley incision
Conley mandibular prosthesis
Conley neck incision
Conley pin
Conley prosthesis
Conley radical neck incision
Conley tracheal stent
Conn aortic compressor
Conn operation
Conn pneumatic tourniquet
Conn technique
Conn tourniquet
Conn Universal tourniquet
connate teeth
connecting cartilage
connecting cord
connecting neurons
connecting nipple
connecting plate
connection
 accessory arteriovenous
  connection
 accessory AV connection
 fasciculoventricular
  connection
 Luer-Lok catheter connection
connection cord

connective tissue
connective tissue augmentation
connective tissue cells
connective tissue disease (CTD)
connective tissue disorder
connective tissue graft
connective tissue membrane
connective tissue neoplasm
connective tissue nevus
connective tissue sheath
connective tissue stalk
connector
　Accu-Flo connector
　ACMI light source connector
　adjustable pedicle connector
　beta finger-grip catheter
　　connector
　Beurrier connector
　CAS connector
　catheter connector
　coaxial I&A nylon connector
　Denver connector
　domino spinal
　　instrumentation connector
　drain-to-wall suction
　　connector
　dual bypass connector
　extension tubing with
　　connector
　Holter connector
　Hud-Vent elbow connector
　implant superstructure
　　connector
　intrinsic transverse connector
　Karl Storz light source
　　connector
　linguoplate major connector
　Luer connector
　Luer-Lok jet ventilator
　　connector
　Machida light source
　　connector
　major connector
　McIntyre nylon cannula
　　connector
　mediastinal sump connector
　metal connector
　metal suction connector
　minor connector
　neurosurgical connector
　Olympus light source
　　connector

connector (*continued*)
　palatal connector
　pedicle connector
　Pentax light source connector
　plastic connector
　Prolene Hernia system
　　connector
　Pudenz connector
　quick connector
　Saf-T-Flo T-tube connector
　SidePort AutoControl airway
　　connector
　Storz catheter connector
　straight connector
　suction connector
　tandem connector
　Touhy-Borst connector
　transverse connector
　Tunstal connector
　T-vent connector
　Uni-Gard piggyback
　　connector
　Universal connector
　venous Y connector
　Y-port connector
connector bar
connector forceps
connector tubing
connector with lock washer
Connell airway
Connell breathing tube
Connell cystoscope
Connell ether vapor tube
Connell gastrectomy
Connell incision
Connell inverting suture
Connell operation
Connell stitch
Connell suture technique
Connell sutures
Connolly procedure
Connolly technique
conoid lens
conoid ligament
conoid papillae of tongue
conoid process
conotruncal anomaly
ConQuest male continence
　system leg bag kit
Conrad operation
Conrad orbital blowout fracture
　operation

Conrad-Crosby biopsy needle
Conrad-Crosby bone marrow
   biopsy needle
Conrad-Crosby needle
Conradi line
consanguineous donor
consciousness
   level of consciousness
   regained consciousness
   state of consciousness
consecutive amputation
consecutive aneurysm
consecutive dislocation
consensual reflex
consent
   implied consent
   informed consent
   presumed consent
   waiver and consent
conservation surgery
conservative approach
conservative resection
conservative subtraction-
   addition rhinoplasty (CSAR)
conservative surgery
conservative surgical treatment
conservative therapy
conservative treatment
consistency
   doughy consistency
   fish-flesh consistency
   lesion consistency
consistent findings
consolidant
consolidation of lungs
consonant position
consonating rales
consortial approach
conspicuous
constant current stimulator
constant flow insufflation
constant passive-motion
   machine (CPMM)
Constantine catheter
Constantine flexible metal
   catheter
ConstaVac catheter
Constellation mapping catheter
constrained ankle arthroplasty
constrained hinged knee
   prosthesis
constrained knee prosthesis

constrained nonhinged knee
   prosthesis
constrained reconstruction
constrained shoulder
   arthroplasty
constrained total knee
   prosthesis
constricted blood vessels
constricted breast
constricted ear
constricted web space
constricting eschar
constricting esophageal lesion
constricting lesion
constricting pain
constriction
   concentric constriction
   duodenal constriction
   duodenopyloric constriction
   esophageal constriction
   nares constriction
   naris constriction
   pyloric constriction
   secondary constriction
constriction of pupil
constriction ring
constriction ring syndrome
constrictive edema
constrictive hyperemia
constrictive ring
constrictor
   inferior pharyngeal
     constrictor
   middle pharyngeal constrictor
   superior pharyngeal
     constrictor
constrictor muscle
constrictor muscle of pharynx
constrictor naris
construction
   Abbe vaginal construction
   absolute construction
   costochondral graft mandibular
     ramus construction
   exocentric construction
   ileal reservoir construction
   ileocecal bladder construction
   ileostomy construction
   loop ileostomy construction
   McIndoe-Hayes construction
   pelvic ileal reservoir
     construction

construction (*continued*)
    plastic construction
    single denture construction
    sphincteric construction
    stent construction
    tandem construction
    Thiersch-Duplay urethral
        construction
    U-pouch construction
    vaginal construction
contact
    centric contact
    deflective occlusal contact
    faulty contact
    initial occlusive contact
    interceptive occlusal contact
    linguopalatal contact
    occlusal contact
    perinuclear contact
    point of proximal contact
    premature contact
    retruded contact
contact area
contact area point
contact bandage lens
contact burn
contact cheilitis
contact compressive forceps
contact dermatitis
contact dissolution therapy
contact hysteroscope
Contact Laser bullet probe
Contact Laser chisel probe
Contact Laser conical probe
Contact Laser convex probe
Contact Laser flat probe
Contact Laser interstitial probe
Contact Laser round probe
Contact Laser scalpel
contact lens
contact lens training mirror
contact low-vacuum lens
contact manipulation
contact metastasis
contact ring
contact shell implant
contact shield
contact splint
contact-layer wound dressings
container
    biohazard container
    Dick combination container

container (*continued*)
    instrument retrieval container
    specimen container
contaminated case
contaminated field
contaminated operative wound
        classification
contaminated wound
contamination
    bacterial contamination
    cross contamination
    direct fecal contamination
    environmental contamination
    foreign body contamination
    graft contamination
    hematogenous contamination
    intraoperative contamination
    radon contamination
contents
    abdominal contents
    bowel contents
    cyst content
    escape of gastroduodenal
        contents
    evisceration of orbital
        contents
    exenteration of orbital
        contents
    fecal contents
    gastric contents
    gastroduodenal contents
    intestinal contents
    intra-abdominal contents
    intraocular contents
    oral contents
    orbital contents
    reflux of gastric contents
    retained contents
    stomach contents
Contigen Bard cochlear implant
Contigen Bard collagen implant
Contigen glutaraldehyde
Contigen implant
Contigen tube
contiguity
    amputation in contiguity
    appendicitis by contiguity
contiguous loop
contiguous rib
contiguous spinal fluid reservoir
contiguous ventricular septal
    defect

continence
continent colostomy
continent cutaneous
    appendicocystostomy
continent ileal pouch
continent ileal reservoir
continent ileostomy
Continent operation
Continental cannula
Continental needle
contingency management
continuity
    amputation in continuity
    axonal continuity
    gastrointestinal continuity
continuous air compressor
continuous ambulatory
    peritoneal dialysis (CAPD)
continuous arteriovenous
    hemofiltration (CAVH)
continuous arteriovenous
    ultrafiltration (CAVU)
continuous atrial fibrillation
continuous bar retainer
continuous bladder irrigation
continuous blanket
continuous catgut sutures
continuous catheter drainage
continuous caudal anesthesia
continuous circular inverting
    sutures
continuous clip forceps
continuous compression
continuous cuticular sutures
continuous distending airway
    pressure
continuous endothelium
continuous epidural anesthesia
continuous gum technique
continuous hemostatic sutures
continuous Holter monitor
continuous hyperthermic
    peritoneal perfusion
continuous infusion anesthetic
    technique
continuous insulin delivery
    system (CIDS)
continuous interlocking sutures
continuous intramucosal PCO_2
    measurement
continuous inverting sutures
continuous irrigation

continuous irrigation catheter
continuous irrigation-suction
    resectoscope
continuous key pattern sutures
continuous Lembert sutures
continuous locked sutures
continuous loop wire
continuous loop wiring
continuous lumbar peridural
    anesthesia
continuous mandatory
    ventilation (CMV)
continuous mattress sutures
continuous medical treatment
continuous microinfusion
    device
continuous nasogastric suction
continuous negative airway
    pressure
continuous NG suction
continuous on-line recording
continuous over-and-over
    sutures
continuous passive motion
    device
continuous pericardial lavage
continuous peridural anesthesia
continuous positive airway
    pressure (CPAP)
continuous positive pressure
    breathing (CPPB)
continuous positive pressure
    ventilation (CPPV)
continuous postoperative closed
    lavage
continuous pull-through
    technique
continuous renal replacement
    therapy
continuous rotation-
    advancement
continuous running locked
    sutures
continuous running sutures
continuous sanguineous
    perfusion
continuous silk sutures
continuous spinal anesthesia
continuous spinal anesthetic
    technique
continuous subcutaneous
    insulin infusion pump

continuous subcutaneous
    insulin injection
continuous suction
continuous suction drainage
continuous suction pump
continuous suction tube
continuous suture technique
continuous sutures
continuous tension
continuous U-shaped sutures
continuous venovenous
    hemodialysis (CVVHD)
continuous venovenous
    hemofiltration
continuous wave
continuous wave CO_2 laser
continuous wave laser
continuous-flow nebulizer
continuous-flow resectoscope
continuous-flow ventilation (CFV)
continuous-locking manner
continuously perfused probe
continuous-wave argon laser
continuous-wave arthroscopy
    pump
continuous-wave diode laser
continuous-wave Doppler
    imaging
continuous-wave laser ablation
continuous-wave technique
continuous-wave UAL devices
continuous-wave ultrasound
Continuum knee system implant
contour
    apple cheek contour
    breast contour
    buccal contour
    cervicofacial contour
    lobulated contour
    mandibular contour
    nasal contour
    symmetrical in contour
    uneven contour
    waisting of nerve contour
Contour balloon dilatation
    catheter
contour block clamp
contour defect
contour defect molding kit
contour deformity
Contour Emboli artificial
    embolization device

contour instrument cleaning brush
contour irregularities
Contour laser
contour line
Contour defibrillator
contour of heart
contour of nasal bones
contour of the brow
Contour Profile defibrillator
Contour Profile saline breast
    implant
Contour Profile silicone breast
    implant
contour retractor
contour scalp retractor
contoured anterior spinal plate
contoured anterior spinal plate
    drill guide
contoured anterior spinal plate
    technique
contoured Dow Corning Silastic
    prosthesis
contoured pretragal incision
contour-facilitating instrument
contouring
    abdominal contouring
    body contouring
    facial contouring
    implant contouring
    occlusal contouring
contra-angle chisel
contra-angle head
contra-aperture
contraception
contraceptive
contraceptive technique
contracted abdomen
contracted heart
contracted heel cord
contracted kidney
contracted pelvis
contracted shoulder
contracted toe
contracted urinary bladder
contracted uterus
contractile ring dysphagia
contractile stricture
contractility
    cardiac contractility
    idiomuscular contractility
contracting and relaxing of
    muscles

contracting scar
contraction
  auricular premature
    contraction
  Braxton Hicks contraction
  carpopedal contraction
  cervical muscle contraction
  cicatricial contraction
  clonic contraction
  conchal contraction
  escaped ventricular
    contraction
  expulsion contraction
  fibrillary contractions
  gallbladder contraction
  galvanotonic contractions
  Hicks contraction
  idiomuscular contraction
  involuntary contraction
  ipsilateral contraction
  irregular contractions
  moderate contractions
  multifocal contractions
  muscle contraction
  muscular contraction
  myofibroblast contraction
  myotatic contraction
  palmar contraction
  paradoxical contraction
  premature atrial contraction
    (PAC)
  premature contraction
  premature ventricular
    contraction (PVC)
  premonitory contraction
  propagated contractions
  regular contractions
  rested state contraction
  tertiary contractions
  timed contractions
  tone contraction
  tonic contraction
  ventricular contraction
  wound contraction
  wound matrix contraction
contraction of muscles
contraction of pupil
contraction of uterus
contraction on ventriculogram
contraction pattern
contraction reflex
contraction time

contraction-relaxation cycle
contractor (*see also* rib
    contractor)
  Adams rib contractor
  baby rib contractor
  Bailey baby rib contractor
  Bailey contractor
  Bailey rib contractor
  Bailey-Gibbon contractor
  Bailey-Gibbon rib contractor
  Cooley rib contractor
  Crafoord contractor
  Effenberger contractor
  Finochietto infant rib
    contractor
  Finochietto-Burford rib
    contractor
  Graham rib contractor
  isovolumic contractor
  Lemmon contractor
  Lemmon rib contractor
  Medicon contractor
  rib contractor
  Rienhoff-Finochietto rib
    contractor
  Scanlan-Crafoord contractor
  Sellor contractor
  Sellor rib contractor
  Stille-Bailey-Senning rib
    contractor
  surgical contractor
  Waterman rib contractor
contract-relax technique
contracture
  axillary contracture
  Baker capsular contracture
  Baker classification of
    capsular contracture
    (grades 1-4)
  bladder neck contracture
  breast implant capsular
    contracture
  burn scar contracture (BSC)
  capsular contracture
  Dupuytren contracture
  elbow flexion contracture
  false Dupuytren contracture
  fibrous capsular contracture
  finger contracture
  flexion contracture
  hip flexion contracture
  iris contracture

contracture (*continued*)
  ischemic contracture
  joint contracture
  McCash procedure for
    Dupuytren contracture
  midlamellar contracture
  postpoliomyelitic contracture
  Sakellarides technique for
    forearm contracture
  scar contracture
  Skoog procedure for
    Dupuytren contracture
  Skoog release of Dupuytren
    contracture
  soft tissue contracture
  spherical contracture
  subglandular capsular
    contracture
  thumb-index contracture
  tight contracture
  Volkmann contracture
  Volkmann ischemic
    contracture
contracture of hip
contracture of interosseous
  muscles
contracture of joint capsule
contracture of knee
contracture of ligament
contraflexion brace
contraincision
contraindication to surgery
contralateral aspect
contralateral axillary metastasis
contralateral breast
contralateral carotid artery
  occlusion
contralateral ear
contralateral face
contralateral groin exploration
contralateral movement
contralateral musculature
contralateral organ
contralateral parathyroid gland
contralateral radiation
contralateral sign
contrast
  maximal contrast
contrast agent
contrast angiogram
contrast aortogram
contrast CT scan

contrast echocardiography
contrast enema
contrast enhancement
contrast examination
contrast injection
contrast material
contrast material instillation
contrast medium
contrast selective cholangiogram
contrast-enhanced scan
Contraves microscope
contrecoup contusion
contrecoup fracture
contrecoup injury
Contreet antimicrobial dressings
contributing factor
control
  anchorage control
  biplaner II control
  circulatory control
  endoscopic control
  exsanguination tourniquet
    control
  external tachyarrhythmia
    control
  extrahepatic control
  fluoroscopic control
  gate control
  hemorrhage control
  Hosmer voluntary control 4-
    bar knee orthosis
  infection control
  inflow control
  intrahepatic control
  monitored anesthesia control
  muscle control
  muscular control
  musculoaponeurotic control
  neuromuscular control
  outflow control
  Pringle vascular control
  pronation control
  proximal vascular control
  tourniquet control
  transcriptional control
  vascular control
  voluntary control
  x-ray control
control belt
control cable
control of ventilation
Control Release pop-off needle

control syringe
control wire
controlled bone regeneration
controlled drain
controlled expansion
controlled fistula
controlled mechanical
   ventilation (CMV)
controlled procedure
controlled release anesthetic
   technique
controlled respiration
controlled ventilation
controlled water-added
   technique
controller
   Actis venous flow controller
   Asahi pressure controller
   Boehm current controller
   Bronkhorst High Tec
     controller
   current controller
   galvanic eye current
     controller
   IMED Gemini volumetric
     controller
   IVAC drip controller
   Magneedle controller
   mass flow controller
   shoulder controller
   voice intensity controller
control-mode ventilation
Control-Release needle
Control-Release pop-off needle
ControlWire guidewire
Contura cast
Contura medicated dressing
contused wound
contusion
   brain contusion
   cerebral contusion
   contrecoup contusion
   corneal contusion
   myocardial contusion
   scalp contusion
contusion cataract
contusions and abrasions
conus
   lateral conus
   oblique conus
conus branch
conus elasticus

conus elasticus laryngis
conus medullaris
convalescence
convalescent
convalescing patient
ConvaTec ostomy pouch
ConvaTec urostomy pouch
Conve back support
Conveen bag hanger
Conveen bedside drainage bag
Conveen curved-tapered
   intermittent catheter
Conveen deluxe contoured leg
   bag
Conveen drip collector
Conveen female intermittent
   catheter
convenience occlusion
convenience point
conventional aortic
   aneurysmectomy
conventional concentric
   electromyography
conventional distal
   pancreatectomy
conventional endarterectomy
conventional needle
conventional operation
conventional
   pancreatoduodenectomy
conventional parameter
conventional procedure
conventional reform eye implant
conventional reform implant
conventional shell-type eye
   implant
conventional shunt
conventional silicone elastomer
conventional SMAS (superficial
   musculoaponeurotic
   system) face-lift
conventional static scanner
conventional stent
conventional surgery
conventional suturing
conventional technique
conventional thoracoplasty
conventional transmission
   electron microscope
conventional treatment
convergence of eyes
convergence point

convergence position
convergent beam irradiation
convergent ray
convergent squint
convergent strabismus
converging collimator
converging lens
converging triangular flap
Converse alar elevator
Converse alar retractor
Converse bistoury
Converse blade retractor
Converse button-end bistoury
Converse chisel
Converse curet
Converse double-end curet
Converse double-ended alar
    retractor
Converse double-ended
    retractor
Converse flap
Converse fracture-wiring button
Converse guarded chisel
Converse guarded nasal chisel
Converse guarded osteotome
Converse hinged skin hook
Converse hook
Converse knife
Converse nasal chisel
Converse nasal knife
Converse nasal retractor
Converse nasal rongeur
Converse nasal root rongeur
Converse nasal saw
Converse nasal speculum
Converse nasal tip scissors
Converse needle holder
Converse operation
Converse osteotome
Converse periosteal elevator
Converse plastic surgery
    scissors
Converse rasp
Converse raspatory
Converse retractor
Converse retractor blade
Converse rongeur
Converse saw
Converse scalping flap
Converse scissors
Converse skin hook
Converse skin lines

Converse speculum
Converse splint
Converse sweeper curet
Converse technique
Converse-Gillies needle holder
Converse-Lange rongeur
Converse-MacKenty elevator
Converse-MacKenty periosteal
    elevator
Converse-Wilmer conjunctival
    scissors
conversion of position
conversion table
Converta-Litter carrier
converted rhythm
convertible cystoscope
convertible fin
convertible telescope
convertible telescope and fin
Convertors surgical drapes
convex cartilage graft
convex condylar implant
    arthroplasty
convex forehead
convex fusion
convex lens
convex obturator
convex probe
convex rasp
convex sheath
convex sheath and obturator
convexes of brain
convexity
    forehead convexity
    lateral crural convexity (LAC)
    outer convexity
convexity of lens
convexity of spine
convexoconcave disk prosthetic
    valve
convexoconcave heart valve
convexoconcave lens
convexoconcave valve
    prosthesis
convoluted foam mattress
convoluted seminiferous tubules
convolution mask
convolutional artery
convolutional markings
convolutions of cerebrum
convolutions of Gratiolet
convulsive disorder

convulsive therapy
Conway eye retractor
Conway lid retractor
Conway lid speculum
Conway operation
Conway technique
Conyers technique
Conzett goniometer
Cook arterial catheter
Cook balloon
Cook biopsy gun
Cook cardiovascular infusion
   catheter
Cook catheter
Cook continence cuff
Cook continence ring
Cook County aspirator
Cook County Hospital aspirator
Cook County Hospital tracheal
   suction tube
Cook County suction tube
Cook County tracheal suction
   tube
Cook drainage pouch set
Cook endomyocardial needle
Cook endoscopic curved needle
   driver
Cook eye speculum
Cook filter
Cook flexible biopsy forceps
Cook FlexStent stent
Cook helical stone dislodger
Cook intracoronary stent
Cook introducer
Cook locking stylet
Cook Longdwel needle
Cook micropuncture introducer
Cook osteotome
Cook pacemaker
Cook Peel-Away introducer
Cook percutaneous entry
   needle
Cook pigtail catheter
Cook plastic Luer-Lok adapter
Cook rectal retractor
Cook rectal speculum
Cook retractor
Cook retrievable embolization
   coil
Cook shingle
Cook Spectrum catheter
Cook speculum

Cook stent positioner
Cook stereotaxic guide
Cook straight guidewire
Cook tissue morcellator
Cook transseptal sheath
Cook ureteral stent
Cook urological trocar
Cook Urosoft stent
Cook walking brace
Cook yellow pigtail catheter
Cook-Amplatz dilator
cookie cutter areolar marker
cookie-cutter-type areola marker
Cool Comfort cold pack
Cool Tip catheter
Cool Touch laser
Cooled ThermoCath catheter
Cooley acutely-curved clamp
Cooley anastomosis
Cooley anastomosis clamp
Cooley anastomosis forceps
Cooley aorta retractor
Cooley aortic aneurysm clamp
Cooley aortic cannula clamp
Cooley aortic clamp
Cooley aortic forceps
Cooley aortic retractor
Cooley aortic sump tube
Cooley aortic vent needle
Cooley arterial occlusion
   forceps
Cooley arteriotomy scissors
Cooley atrial retractor
Cooley atrial valve retractor
Cooley auricular appendage
   forceps
Cooley bronchial clamp
Cooley bronchus clamp
Cooley bulldog clamp
Cooley cardiac tucker
Cooley cardiovascular forceps
Cooley cardiovascular scissors
Cooley cardiovascular suction
Cooley cardiovascular suction
   tube
Cooley carotid clamp
Cooley carotid retractor
Cooley caval occlusion clamp
Cooley chisel
Cooley clamp
Cooley coarctation clamp
Cooley coarctation forceps

Cooley coronary dilator
Cooley cross-action bulldog
    clamp
Cooley curved cardiovascular
    clamp
Cooley curved forceps
Cooley Dacron prosthesis
Cooley dilator
Cooley double-angled clamp
Cooley double-angled jaw
    forceps
Cooley femoral retractor
Cooley first-rib shears
Cooley forceps
Cooley graft clamp
Cooley graft forceps
Cooley graft suction tube
Cooley iliac clamp
Cooley iliac forceps
Cooley intracardiac suction tube
Cooley intrapericardial
    anastomosis
Cooley ligature carrier
Cooley microvascular needle
    holder
Cooley mitral valve retractor
Cooley modification of
    Waterston anastomosis
Cooley cardiovascular retractor
Cooley multipurpose clamp
Cooley multipurpose forceps
Cooley needle holder
Cooley neonatal instruments
Cooley neonatal retractor
Cooley neonatal sternal
    retractor
Cooley neonatal vascular clamp
Cooley neonatal vascular
    forceps
Cooley operation
Cooley partial occlusion clamp
Cooley patent ductus clamp
Cooley patent ductus forceps
Cooley pediatric aortic forceps
Cooley pediatric clamp
Cooley pediatric dilator
Cooley pediatric vascular clamp
Cooley peripheral vascular
    clamp
Cooley peripheral vascular
    forceps
Cooley pick

Cooley probe-point scissors
Cooley renal artery clamp
Cooley renal clamp
Cooley retractor
Cooley reverse-cut scissors
Cooley rib contractor
Cooley rib retractor
Cooley rib shears
Cooley scissors
Cooley sternotomy retractor
Cooley subclavian clamp
Cooley suction tube
Cooley sump suction tube
Cooley sump tube
Cooley tangential pediatric
    clamp
Cooley tangential pediatric
    forceps
Cooley tissue forceps
Cooley U-sutures
Cooley valve dilator
Cooley vascular clamp
Cooley vascular dilator
Cooley vascular forceps
Cooley vascular suction tube
Cooley vascular tissue forceps
Cooley vena cava clamp
Cooley vena caval catheter
    clamp
Cooley vena caval clamp
Cooley ventricular needle
Cooley Vital microvascular
    needle holder
Cooley woven Dacron graft
Cooley-Anthony suction tube
Cooley-Baumgarten aortic clamp
Cooley-Baumgarten aortic forceps
Cooley-Beck clamp
Cooley-Beck vessel clamp
Cooley-Bloodwell low profile
    valve
Cooley-Bloodwell mitral valve
    prosthesis
Cooley-Bloodwell-Cutter
    prosthesis
Cooley-Bloodwell-Cutter valve
Cooley-Cutter disk prosthetic
    valve
Cooley-Cutter prosthesis
Cooley-Derra anastomosis clamp
Cooley-Derra anastomosis
    forceps

Cooley-Derra clamp
Cooley-Merz sternal retractor
Cooley-Merz sternum retractor
Cooley-Pontius blade
Cooley-Pontius shears
Cooley-Pontius sternal blade
Cooley-Pontius sternal shears
Cooley-Pontius sternum shears
Cooley-Satinsky clamp
Cooley-Satinsky multipurpose
    clamp
CoolGlide laser
Coolidge tube
cooling blanket
cooling machine
CoolSorb absorbent cold
    transfer dressing
cool-tip laser
CoolTouch Nd:YAG laser
Coombs cord
Coonrad prosthesis
Coonrad total elbow
    arthroplasty
Coonrad wrist prosthesis
Coonrad-Morrey total elbow
    arthroplasty
Coonrad-Morrey total elbow
    prosthesis
Coons Super Stiff long-tip
    guidewire
Coonse-Adams knee approach
Cooper argon laser
Cooper aspirator
Cooper basal ganglia guide
Cooper bougie
Cooper cannula
Cooper chemopallidectomy
    cannula
Cooper chemopallidectomy
    needle
Cooper cryoprobe
Cooper cryostat
Cooper director
Cooper disk cryostat
Cooper double-lumen cannula
Cooper elevator
Cooper endotracheal stylet
Cooper gouge
Cooper guide
Cooper hernia
Cooper herniotome
Cooper implant

Cooper laser adapter
Cooper LaserSonics laser
Cooper lens
Cooper ligament
Cooper ligament repair
Cooper ligature needle
Cooper mallet
Cooper nasal ganglia guide
Cooper needle
Cooper operation
Cooper pallidectomy needle
Cooper reduction
Cooper scissors
Cooper spinal fusion elevator
Cooper spinal fusion gouge
Cooper syndrome
Coopernail sign
Cooper-Rand intraoral artificial
    larynx
CooperSurgical overhead
    colposcope
CooperVision argon laser
CooperVision camera
CooperVision refractor
CooperVision fragmatome
CooperVision imaging perimeter
CooperVision irrigating needle
CooperVision J-loop intraocular
    lens
CooperVision laser
CooperVision microscope
CooperVision ocutome
CooperVision Flex lens
CooperVision spatulated needle
CooperVision blade
CooperVision ultrasound
CooperVision vitrector
CooperVision YAG laser
CooperVision-Cilco-Kelman
    multiflex intraocular lens
CooperVision-Cilco-Novaflex
    anterior chamber
    intraocular lens
coordinate muscle movement
coordinated reflexes
coordinates
coordination
    equilibratory coordination
    motor power and
      coordination
    muscle coordination
co-ossify

Copalite applicator
Cope biopsy needle
Cope bronchography
Cope clamp
Cope crushing clamp
Cope double-ended retractor
Cope gastrointestinal suture
    anchor set
Cope loop nephrostomy
    catheter
Cope loop nephrostomy tube
Cope lung forceps
Cope mandrel guidewire
Cope modification of Martel
    intestinal clamp
Cope needle
Cope needle introducer cannula
Cope nephrostomy tube
Cope pleural biopsy needle
Cope technique
Cope thoracentesis needle
Cope wire
Cope-DeMartel clamp
Copeland anterior chamber
    intraocular lens
Copeland fetal scalp electrode
Copeland intraocular lens
    implant
Copeland lens
Copeland lens implant
Copeland radial loop intraocular
    lens
Copeland radial panchamber
    lens
Copeland retinoscope
Copeland streak retinoscope
Copeland technique
Copeland-Howard
    scapulothoracic fusion
Cope-Saddekni catheter tip
Cope-Saddekni introducer
copious bleeding
copious drainage
copious irrigation
copious lavage
copious peritoneal lavage
copolymer
    LactoSorb copolymer
    silicone copolymer
copolymer ankle-foot orthosis
copolymer stapler
copper band

copper band-acrylic splint
copper blade
copper bromide laser
copper mallet
copper phosphate cement
copper sulphate cone
copper vapor laser
copper vapor pulsed laser
copper wire appearance
copper wire arteries
copper wire effect
copper wiring
copper-7 intrauterine device
copper-7 IUD
copper-clad steel needle
copper-vapor pulsed laser
copper-wire reflex
Coppridge forceps
Coppridge grasping forceps
Coppridge urethral forceps
copula linguae
copular point
coquille plano lens
cor biloculare
cor pacemaker
cor pulmonale
cor triatriatum
cor triloculare biatriatum
coracoacromial
coracoacromial ligament
coracobrachial muscle
coracoclavicular articulation
coracoclavicular ligament
coracoclavicular screw
coracoclavicular screw fixation
coracoclavicular space
coracoclavicular suture fixation
coracoclavicular technique
coracocostal fascia
coracohumeral ligament
coracoid fracture
coracoid notch
coracoid process
Corail stem hip implant
coral calculus
coralliform cataract
coralliformis cataract
coralline PBHA bone graft
coralline porous block
    hydroxyapatite bone graft
Coratomic implantable pulse
    generator

Coratomic pacemaker
Coratomic prosthetic valve
Coratomic R-wave inhibited
    pacemaker
Coratomic R-wave inhibited
    pulse generator
Corb biopsy trocar
Corbett bone rongeur
Corbett bone-cutting forceps
Corbett bone-cutting rongeur
Corbett forceps
Corbett foreign body spud
Corbett spud
Corbin technique
Corbin-Farnsworth defibrillator
Corboy hemostat
Corboy needle holder
cord bladder
cord block
cord blood
cord compression
cord handle
cord injury
cord length
cord lengthening
cord stripping
cord traction syndrome
cord tumor
cordate
cordectomy
    vocal cordectomy
Cordes circular punch
Cordes esophagoscopy forceps
Cordes ethmoidal punch
Cordes forceps
Cordes punch
Cordes punch forceps tip
Cordes semicircular punch
Cordes sphenoid punch
Cordes sphenoidal punch
Cordes square punch
Cordes-New elevator
Cordes-New forceps
Cordes-New laryngeal punch
Cordes-New laryngeal punch
    elevator
Cordes-New laryngeal punch
    forceps
Cordes-New punch
cordiform tendon of
    diaphragm
cordiformis uterus

cordis
    diastasis cordis
    myomalacia cordis
    paracentesis cordis
    theca cordis
Cordis Ancar pacing lead
Cordis Atricor pacemaker
Cordis balloon catheter
Cordis bioptome
Cordis Bioptone sheath
Cordis BriteTip guiding catheter
Cordis catheter
Cordis Chronocor pacemaker
Cordis Crossflex stent
Cordis dilator
Cordis Ducor I, II, III coronary
    catheter
Cordis Ducor pigtail catheter
Cordis Ectocor pacemaker
Cordis fixed-rate pacemaker
Cordis Gemini cardiac
    pacemaker
Cordis Gemini pacemaker
Cordis guiding catheter
Cordis Hakim pump
Cordis Hakim shunt
Cordis implantable drug
    reservoir device
Cordis injector
Cordis lead conversion kit
Cordis Lumelec catheter
Cordis Multicor pacemaker
Cordis multipurpose access port
Cordis Omni Stanicor Theta
    transvenous pacemaker
Cordis Omnicor Stanicor
    pacemaker
Cordis pacemaker
Cordis pigtail catheter
Cordis Powerflex balloon
    catheter
Cordis Predator balloon catheter
Cordis Predator PTCA balloon
    catheter
Cordis radiopaque tantalum
    stent
Cordis SMART stent
Cordis Secor implantable pump
Cordis Sentron transducer
Cordis Sequicor cardiac
    pacemaker
Cordis Sequicor pacemaker

Cordis sheath
Cordis Stabilizer marker wire
Cordis Stanicor unipolar
  ventricular pacemaker
Cordis Titan balloon dilatation
  catheter
Cordis TransTaper tip catheter
Cordis TrapEase permanent vena
  cava filter
Cordis Ventricor pacemaker
Cordis Webster diagnostic-
  ablation deflectable tip
  catheter
Cordis Webster mapping
  catheter
Cordis-Dow shunt adapter
Cordis-Hakin valve
cordless dermatome
cordless monocular indirect
  ophthalmoscope
Cordon Colles fracture splint
Cordonnier ureteroileal loop
cordopexy
cordotomy
  anterolateral cordotomy
  cervical cordotomy
  dorsal cordotomy
  open surgical cordotomy
  percutaneous cordotomy
  posterior column cordotomy
  Rosomoff cordotomy
  Rosomoff percutaneous
    cordotomy
  spinal cordotomy
  spinothalamic cordotomy
  stereotactic cordotomy
  vocal cordotomy
cordotomy clamp
cordotomy hook
cordotomy knife
Cordran tape
cordy pulse
core
  irrigation-aspiration core
  Kellman irrigation-aspiration
    core
  mesodermal core
Core aspiration-injection
  needle
Core CO_2 insufflation needle
core cooling
core drilling procedure

Core Dynamics disposable
  cannula
Core Dynamics disposable
  trocar
core mold stent
core needle biopsy
core reamer
core trocar
core wire guide
corectomy
Core-Flex wire guides
corelysis
Coremetrics fetal apnea monitor
coreometrics
coreoplasty
coretomy
Core-Vent implant
Corex instrument
Corey forceps
Corey ovum forceps
Corey placental forceps
Corey tenaculum
Cor-Flex guide
Cor-Flex guidewire
Cor-Flex wire guide
Corgill bone punch
Corgill punch
Corgill-Hartmann forceps
Corgill-Shapleigh ear curet
Cori classification
Corin total hip
coring biopsy gun
Corinthian stent
Corit canal
cork fashion
cork, leather, and elastic
  orthotic
corkscrew arteries
corkscrew dural hook
corkscrew esophagus
corkscrew femoral head
  remover
corkscrew maneuver
Corkscrew suture anchor
Corlon angiocatheter
Corlon catheter
Cormack-Lamberty
  fasciocutaneous flaps
  (types A-C)
Cormed ambulatory infusion
  pump
Cormed infusion pump

cornea
  abrasion of cornea
  apex cornea
  bedewing of cornea
  conical cornea
  denudation of cornea
  ectasia of cornea
  facet of cornea
  keloid of cornea
  ring ulcer of cornea
  transplantation of cornea
cornea chisel
cornea farinata
cornea globosa
cornea guttata
cornea guttate lesion
cornea opaca
cornea plana
cornea scissors
cornea-holding forceps
corneal abrader
corneal abrasion
corneal abscess
corneal abscission
corneal alkali burn
corneal anesthesia
corneal applicator
corneal astigmatism
corneal block
corneal bur
corneal burn
corneal chisel
corneal contusion
corneal curet
corneal curvature
corneal debrider
corneal degeneration
corneal deposits
corneal dissector
corneal ectasia
corneal edema
corneal erosion
corneal erysiphake
corneal eye implant
corneal facet
corneal fascia lata spatula
corneal fissure
corneal fistula
corneal fixation forceps
corneal flap
corneal forceps
corneal foreign body

corneal foreign body bur
corneal graft
corneal graft operation
corneal graft spatula
corneal hook
corneal implant
corneal incision
corneal infiltrate
corneal inlay
corneal iron line
corneal keloid
corneal knife
corneal knife dissector
corneal laceration
corneal lamellar groove
corneal leakage
corneal light reflex
corneal light shield
corneal loupe
corneal luster
corneal margin
corneal marginal furrow
corneal microscope
corneal monocular loupe
corneal needle
corneal opacification
corneal opacity
corneal pachymeter
corneal perforation
corneal prosthesis forceps
corneal prosthesis trephine
corneal punch
corneal punctate lesion
corneal rasp
corneal reflex
corneal ring
corneal rust ring remover
corneal scarring
corneal scissors
corneal section
corneal section scissors
corneal section spatulated
  scissors
corneal section-enlarging
  scissors
Corneal Shaper microkeratome
corneal space
corneal spatulated scissors
corneal splinter forceps
corneal staining
corneal surface
corneal surgery

corneal suture needle
corneal sutures
corneal swelling
corneal thickness measuring
  equipment
corneal transplant
corneal transplant centering
  ring
corneal transplant forceps
corneal transplant marker
corneal transplant scissors
corneal transplantation
corneal trephination
corneal trephine
corneal tube
corneal ulcer
corneal ulceration
corneal utility forceps
corneal wound
corneal-suturing forceps
cornea-splitting knife
cornea-suturing forceps
corneoblepharon
corneoconjunctivoplasty
corneomandibular reflex
corneomental reflex
corneopterygoid reflex
corneoscleral forceps
corneoscleral incision
corneoscleral junction
corneoscleral laceration
corneoscleral punch
corneoscleral scissors
corneoscleral sutures
corneoscleral suturing forceps
corneoscleral trephination
corneoscleral wound
corneoscleroconjunctival
  sutures
corneoscope
corneous
corner fracture
corner mouth lift
corner retractor
Corner tampon
Cornet forceps
corniculate cartilage
corniculate tubercle
cornification
cornification disorder
cornified cell envelope
cornified epithelium

cornified layer
Corning anesthesia
Corning implant
Corning puncture
Corning silicone
Cornish wool dressing
Cornman dissecting knife
cornoid lamella
cornu (*pl.* cornua)
  anterior cornu
  dorsal cornu
  ethmoid cornu
cornu cutaneum
cornua of thyroid cartilage
cornual anastomosis
cornual implantation
cornual portion of uterus
cornual pregnancy
cornual resection of fallopian
  tube
cornuradicular zone
corollary incision
corolliform papillae of tongue
Corometrics Doppler scanner
Corometrics electrode tip
Corometrics maternal-fetal
  monitor
Corometrics-Aloka
  echocardiograph machine
corona (*pl.* coronae, coronas)
  Bischoff corona
  Zinn corona
  zona corona
corona ciliaris
corona dentis
corona glandis
corona radiata
corona seborrheica
corona vascularis
corona veneris
coronal arc technique
coronal bipolar montage
coronal brow lift
coronal computed tomography
  scan
coronal incision
coronal lift
coronal MRI of wrist
coronal necrosis
coronal orientation
coronal plane correction
coronal plane deformity

coronal reconstruction
coronal split fracture
coronal sulcus
coronal suture
coronal suture lines
coronal synostosis
coronary anastomotic shunt
coronary angiogram
coronary angiographic catheter
coronary angiography
coronary angioplasty
coronary angioplasty versus
    excisional atherectomy
coronary arteries
coronary arteriogram
coronary arteriography
coronary arteriosclerotic heart
    disease (CAHD)
coronary artery aneurysm
coronary artery angioplasty
coronary artery anomaly
coronary artery button
coronary artery bypass (CAB)
coronary artery bypass graft
    (CABG)
coronary artery bypass grafted
    (CABG'd)
coronary artery bypass surgery
    (CABS)
coronary artery cannula
coronary artery disease (CAD)
coronary artery dissection
coronary artery ectasia
coronary artery endarterectomy
coronary artery fistula (CAF)
coronary artery forceps
coronary artery perfusion
coronary artery probe
coronary artery
    revascularization procedure
coronary artery scissors
coronary artery-right ventricular
    fistula
coronary atherosclerotic heart
    disease (CAHD)
coronary balloon angioplasty
coronary bifurcation
coronary blood flow
coronary bypass procedure
coronary bypass surgery
coronary bypass therapy
coronary cannula

coronary care unit (CCU)
coronary cataract
coronary cataract of Vogt
coronary catheter
coronary catheterization
coronary cineangiogram
coronary cineangiography
coronary circulation
coronary collateral circulation
coronary cusps
coronary dilatation catheter
coronary dilator
coronary embolism
coronary endarterectomy
coronary endarterectomy
    spatula
coronary fistula
coronary flow reserve
    technique
coronary guiding catheter
coronary heart disease (CHD)
Coronary Imagecath angioscope
coronary insufficiency
coronary ligaments
coronary occlusion
coronary opacification
coronary perfusion
coronary perfusion cannula
coronary perfusion components
coronary perfusion tip
coronary reflex
coronary rotational ablation
coronary rotational atherectomy
coronary scissors
coronary seeking catheter
coronary sinus
coronary sinus catheterization
coronary sinus suction tube
coronary sinus thermodilution
    catheter
coronary steal phenomenon
coronary sulcus
coronary syndrome
coronary tendon
coronary thrombosis
coronary vasodilator
coronary veins
coronary vessel anatomy
coronary wire
Coronet alloy
Coronet magnet
coronion

coronocanthopexy
coronoid flap
coronoid fossa
coronoid hyperplasia
coronoid line
coronoid process
coronoid process fracture
coronoid process of mandible
coronoidectomy
coronoplasty
coronoradicular stabilization
Corpak feeding tube
Corpak weighted-tip, self-
    lubricating tube
corpectomy
    anterior corpectomy
    cervical corpectomy
    median corpectomy
    vertebral body corpectomy
corpectomy model
corpora (*sing.* corpus)
    capsule of corpora
    erectile corpora
corpora albicantia
corpora cavernosa penis
corpora quadrigemina
corpora santoriana
corporeal aspiration
corporeal biopsy
corporeal cesarean section
corporeal reconstruction
corporeal rotation procedure
corporeal sacrospinous
    suspension
corporectomy amputation
corporis callosi
corporoplasty
    incisional corporoplasty
    modified Essed-Schroeder
        corporoplasty
corpus (*pl.* corpora)
corpus adiposum buccae
corpus adiposum orbitae
corpus albicans
corpus callosum
corpus callosum agenesis
corpus carcinoma
corpus cavernosum
corpus cavernosum clitoridis
corpus cavernosum penis
corpus cavernosum urethrae
corpus cerebelli

corpus ciliaris
corpus clitoridis
corpus costae
corpus linguae
corpus luteal cyst
corpus luteum
corpus luteum cyst
corpus luteum hematoma
corpus mammae
corpus mandibulae
corpus maxillae
corpus of uterus
corpus ossis sphenoidalis
corpus spongiosum penis
corpus spongiosum urethrae
    muliebris
corpus unguis
corpus uteri
corpus vitreum
corpuscle
    axis corpuscle
    cartilage corpuscle
    Golgi corpuscles
    Golgi-Mazzoni corpuscles
    Krause corpuscle
    lingual corpuscle
    Meissner corpuscles
    Meissner tactile corpuscle
    Merkel corpuscles
    Pacini corpuscles
    pacinian corpuscles
    Ruffini corpuscles
    Schwalbe corpuscle
    tactile corpuscles
    tendon corpuscles
    Vater corpuscles
    Vater-Pacini corpuscles
    Virchow corpuscles
    Wagner-Meissner corpuscle
corpuscular volume
Correa classification
corrected condition
corrected cosmetic contact shell
    eye implant
corrected sternal position
correction
    adaptive correction
    Allen correction
    Alliston GE reflux correction
    anterior correction
    anteroposterior correction
    aphakic correction

correction (*continued*)
  astigmatism correction
  attenuation correction
  Beckenbaugh correction
  Berke ptosis correction
  Berke-Motais ptosis correction
  Blaskovics ptosis correction
  Bonferroni correction
  Byron Smith lazy-T correction
  cephalometric correction
  chevron hallux valgus
    correction
  coincidence correction
  coronal plane correction
  cubitus varus correction
  dioptric correction
  elective correction
  epicanthal correction
  frontal plane correction
  hallux varus correction
  hammer toe correction
  heparinase correction
  Higgs spike operation for
    hammer toe correction
  Johnson-Spiegl hallux varus
    correction
  King type IV curve posterior
    correction
  Küstner uterine inversion
    correction
  kyphosis correction
  Mayo hammer toe correction
  notch correction
  occlusal correction
  oligosegmental correction
  one-stage esthetic correction
  operative correction
  optical correction
  phalangeal malunion
    correction
  presurgical orthopedic
    correction (POC)
  presurgical orthopedic
    correction (POC) device
  protamine correction
  ptosis correction
  rhinoplastic correction
  rotational correction
  Ruiz-Mora correction
  scatter correction
  scoliosis correction
  secondary ptosis correction

correction (*continued*)
  skeletal correction
  speech correction
  Steel correction
  strabismus correction
  surgical correction
  talipes correction
  thumb duplication correction
  Tukey post-hoc correction
  Whitlow-Constable alar
    cartilage correction
  Yates correction
corrective cast
corrective operation
corrective orthodontics
corrective procedure
corrective therapy
correlation
Correra line
corresponding point
corridor incision
corridor procedure
Corrigan cautery
Corrigan sign
corroborate
corrugated forehead retractor
corrugator frown
corrugator muscle
corrugator muscle resection
corrugator removal
corrugator supercilii muscle
corset
  Boston soft corset
  Camp corset
  Daw Industries orthopaedic
    corset
  lumbar corset
  lumbosacral corset
  surgical corset
corset balloon catheter
corset platysmaplasty
corset suspension
Corson myoma forceps
Corson needle
Corson needle electrosurgical
    probe
Cortac monitoring electrode
Cortel insertion of steel rods
Cortel technique
cortex (*pl.* cortices)
  aspiration of cortex
  buckling of cortex

cortex (*continued*)
  buried cortex
  cerebellar cortex
  cerebral cortex
  femoral cortex
  impinging on cortex
  mastoid cortex
  rolandic cortex
  sensorimotor cortex
  subcapsular cortex
  windowing of cortex
cortex avulsion
cortex extractor
cortex lentis
cortex of kidney
cortex reflex
cortex retractor
cortex screw
cortex-aspirating cannula
Cortexplorer cerebral blood
    flow monitor
Corti ganglion
Corti rods
cortical
cortical adhesions
cortical anchoring screw
cortical arch of kidney
cortical area
cortical atrophy
cortical biopsy
cortical blindness
cortical bone
cortical bone allograft
cortical bone graft
cortical bone plate
cortical buckling
cortical cataract
cortical cleaving hydrodissector
    cannula
cortical cyst
cortical desmoid
cortical destruction
cortical dysplasia
cortical electrode
cortical electroencephalogram
cortical evoked responses
cortical fracture
cortical fragment
cortical freeze-dried allograft
cortical function
cortical graft
cortical implantation

cortical incision
cortical incision coronary
    dilator
cortical lateralization
cortical lesion
cortical lobules of kidney
cortical mastoidectomy
cortical medullary junction
cortical necrosis
cortical opacification
cortical oral plate
cortical peel
cortical perforation
cortical pin
cortical process
cortical scarring of kidney
cortical screw
cortical spoking
cortical step drill
cortical strut graft
cortical surface
cortical thickening
cortical thickness
cortical thumb
corticectomy
cortices (*sing.* cortex)
corticoadrenal tumor
corticobulbar tract
corticocancellous
corticocancellous block graft
corticocancellous bone
corticocancellous bone graft
corticocancellous graft
corticoid injection
corticomedullary demarcation
corticospinal
corticospinal lesion
corticospinal tract
corticospinal tract lesion
corticosteroid
  intralesional corticosteroid
  oral corticosteroid
  systemic corticosteroid
  topical corticosteroid
corticosteroid rosacea
corticostriatal
corticotomy
cortisol-producing carcinoma
Cortomic pacemaker
Cortoss bone filler
corundum ceramic implant
    material

Corvita endoluminal graft
Corvita endovascular graft
Corvita stent
Corwin forceps
Corwin hemostat
Corwin knife handle
Corwin tonsillar forceps
Corwin tonsillar hemostat
Corwin tonsillar hemostatic
    forceps
Corydon hydroexpression
    cannula
Coryllos periosteal elevator
Coryllos rasp
Coryllos raspatory
Coryllos retractor
Coryllos rib raspatory
Coryllos rib shears
Coryllos thoracoscope
Coryllos-Bethune rib shears
Coryllos-Doyen periosteal
    elevator
Coryllos-Moure rib shears
Coryllos-Shoemaker rib shears
CoSeal fibrin glue
CoSeal premixed surgical
    sealant
CoSeal resorbable synthetic
    sealant
Cosgrove mitral valve
    replacement
Cosgrove mitral valve retractor
Cosgrove-Edwards annuloplasty
    band
Cosman monitor
Cosman telemonitoring
Cosman-Nashold spinal
    stereotaxic guide
Cosman-Roberts-Wells (CRW)
    stereotactic frame
Cosman-Roberts-Wells
    stereotactic ring
cosmesis
Cosmet lens
Cosmetech cannula
cosmetic appearance
cosmetic blepharoplasty
cosmetic camouflage
cosmetic contact shell implant
cosmetic evaluation
cosmetic operation
cosmetic orthodontics

cosmetic outcome
cosmetic problem
cosmetic reconstruction
cosmetic result
cosmetic rhinoplasty
cosmetic score
cosmetic surgery
Cosmolon closure for splint
Cosmos pacemaker
Cosmos pulse-generator
    pacemaker
Co-Span alloy
costa (*pl.* costae)
Costa wire suture scissors
costal angle
costal arch
costal arch retractor
costal bone
costal cartilage
costal cartilage graft
costal chondritis
costal elevator
costal excursion
costal facet
costal groove
costal incisures of sternum
costal margin
costal notch of sternum
costal periosteal elevator
costal periosteotome
costal pleura
CoStasis fibrin glue
costatectomy
costectomy
Costen rongeur
Costen suction tube
Costen syndrome
Costen tube
Costenbader incision spreader
Costenbader retractor
Costen-Kerrison rongeur
costicartilage
costicervical
costispinal
costoaxillary vein
costocentral articulation
costocervical trunk
costochondral graft (CCG)
costochondral graft mandibular
    ramus construction
costochondral graft mandibular
    ramus reconstruction

costochondral graft
    reconstruction
costochondral joint
costochondral junction
costochondral margin
costochondrectomy
costoclavicular ligament
costoclavicular line
costoclavicular maneuver
costoclavicular space
costocolic fold
costodiaphragmatic recess
costoinferior
costomediastinal recess
Coston eye decompressor
Coston iris needle
Coston-Trent cryoretractor
Coston-Trent iris retractor
costophrenic angle
costophrenic bronchoscope
costophrenic septal line
costophrenic sinus
costophrenic sulcus
costoprostatectomy
costosternal angle
costosternal articulation
costosternoplasty
costotome
    Tudor-Edwards costotome
    Vehmehren costotome
costotome chisel
costotomy
costotransverse articulation
costotransverse joint
costotransverse ligament
costotransversectomy
costotransversectomy technique
costoversion thoracoplasty
costovertebral angle
costovertebral articulation
costovertebral joint
cot
    finger cot
    rectal finger cot
Cotrel body cast
Cotrel cast technique
Cotrel casting
Cotrel pedicle screw
Cotrel traction
Cotrel-Dubousset closed hook
Cotrel-Dubousset dynamic
    transverse traction device

Cotrel-Dubousset fixation
Cotrel-Dubousset
    instrumentation (CDI)
Cotrel-Dubousset orthopedic
    brace
Cotrel-Dubousset pediatric rod
Cotrel-Dubousset pedicle screw
    instrumentation
Cotrel-Dubousset pedicular
    instrumentation
Cotrel-Dubousset rod
Cotrel-Dubousset spinal
    instrumentation
Cotrel-Dubousset spinal rod
    fixation
Cotte neurectomy
Cotte operation
Cotting operation
Cotting toenail operation
Cottingham punch
Cottle alar elevator
Cottle alar protector
Cottle alar retractor
Cottle angular scissors
Cottle antral chisel
Cottle biting forceps
Cottle blade
Cottle bone crusher
Cottle bone guide
Cottle bone lever
Cottle bulldog nasal scissors
Cottle bulldog scissors
Cottle calipers
Cottle cartilage guide
Cottle chisel
Cottle chisel osteotome
Cottle clamp
Cottle columella clamp
Cottle columellar clamp
Cottle crossbar chisel
Cottle crossbar chisel osteotome
Cottle crossbar fishtail chisel
Cottle curved chisel
Cottle dorsal scissors
Cottle double hook
Cottle double-edged knife
Cottle double-edged nasal knife
Cottle dressing scissors
Cottle elevator
Cottle elevator-feeler
Cottle fishtail chisel
Cottle forceps

Cottle 4-prong retractor
Cottle graduated elevator
Cottle guide
Cottle heavy septal scissors
Cottle heavy septum scissors
Cottle hook
Cottle hook retractor
Cottle incision
Cottle insertion forceps
Cottle instrument tray and
    spring holder
Cottle knife
Cottle knife guide
Cottle knife guide and retractor
Cottle knife handle
Cottle lower lateral forceps
Cottle mallet
Cottle maneuver
Cottle modified knife handle
Cottle nasal elevator
Cottle nasal hook
Cottle nasal knife
Cottle nasal knife blade
Cottle nasal rasp
Cottle nasal retractor
Cottle nasal saw
Cottle nasal scissors
Cottle nasal speculum
Cottle nasal-biting rongeur
Cottle needle holder
Cottle operation
Cottle osteotome
Cottle periosteal comb
Cottle periosteal elevator
Cottle pillar retractor
Cottle profilometer
Cottle pronged retractor
Cottle protected knife handle
Cottle rasp
Cottle raspatory
Cottle retractor
Cottle rhinoplasty
Cottle saw
Cottle scissors
Cottle septal elevator
Cottle septal speculum
Cottle septum elevator
Cottle septum speculum
Cottle sharp prong retractor
Cottle sharp tenaculum
Cottle sharp-prong retractor
Cottle single-blade retractor

Cottle single-prong tenaculum
Cottle skin elevator
Cottle skin hook
Cottle soft palate retractor
Cottle speculum
Cottle spicule sweeper
Cottle spring scissors
Cottle stent scissors
Cottle suction tube
Cottle sweeper
Cottle tenaculum
Cottle tenaculum hook
Cottle thumb hook retractor
Cottle tissue forceps
Cottle Universal nasal saw
Cottle upper lateral exposing
    retractor
Cottle upper lateral retractor
Cottle Vital dorsal angled
    scissors
Cottle weighted retractor
Cottle-Arruga cartilage forceps
Cottle-Arruga forceps
Cottle-Jansen bone rongeur
Cottle-Jansen forceps
Cottle-Jansen rongeur
Cottle-Jansen rongeur forceps
Cottle-Joseph hook
Cottle-Joseph retractor
Cottle-Joseph saw
Cottle-Kazanjian bone rongeur
Cottle-Kazanjian bone-cutting
    forceps
Cottle-Kazanjian forceps
Cottle-Kazanjian nasal forceps
Cottle-Kazanjian nasal-cutting
    forceps
Cottle-Kazanjian rongeur
Cottle-MacKenty elevator
Cottle-MacKenty elevator rasp
Cottle-MacKenty rasp
Cottle-MacKenty septal elevator
Cottle-Medicon osteotome
Cottle-Neivert retractor
Cottle-Walsham forceps
Cottle-Walsham septal
    straightener
Cottle-Walsham septum
    straightening forceps
Cottle-Walsham septum-
    straightening forceps
Cottle-Walsham straightener

cotton
  absorbent cotton
  Cecil cotton
  Oxycel cotton
  purified cotton
  salicylated cotton
  soaked cotton
  styptic cotton
  sutures tied down over cotton
Cotton ankle fracture
cotton applicator
cotton ball sponge
cotton balls
cotton bolster
cotton bolster dressing
cotton carrier
Cotton cartilage graft
Cotton cartilage graft to
    cricolaryngeal area
cotton Deknatel sutures
cotton ear applicator
cotton elastic bandage
cotton elastic dressing
Cotton fracture
cotton gauze
Cotton graduated dilation
    catheter
cotton nasal applicator
cotton nonabsorbable sutures
Cotton osteotomy
cotton pledget
cotton pledgets dressing
cotton plug
cotton receptacle
Cotton reduction
cotton roll injury
cotton screw
Cotton sphincterotome
cotton sutures
cotton wadding
cotton wool
cotton-ball dressing
cotton-ball hemorrhage of eye
cotton-covered tourniquet
Cotton-Huibregtse biliary stent
    set
Cotton-Huibregtse double pigtail
    stent
Cotton-Leung biliary stent
cottonloader position
cottonoid dissector
cottonoid patty

cottonoid pledget
Cottonoid strips
cotton-roll gingivitis
cotton-roll rubber-dam clamp
cotton-tipped applicator
cotton-wadding dressing
cotton-wool appearance
cotton-wool bandage
cotton-wool exudate
cotton-wool patch
cotton-wool spot
Cottony Dacron hollow suture
Cottony Dacron suture
cotyledon
cotyloid cavity
cotyloid joint
cotyloid ligament
cotyloid notch
Couch-DeRosa-Throop hip
    procedure
couching needle
couch-mounted head frame
coudé
  catheter coudé
  sonde coudé
coudé assist catheter
coudé bag
coudé bougie
coudé catheter
coudé electrode
coudé fulgurating electrode
coudé hemostatic bag
coudé suction catheter
coudé urethral catheter
cough
  compression cough
  deglutitory cough
  nonproductive cough
cough CPR technique
cough fracture
Couinaud classification
Coulevaire uterus
Coulter cell counter
Coulter counter
Coulter cytometer
Coumadin
coumarin pulsed dye laser
coumarin-flashlamp-pumped
    pulsed-dye laser
Coumatrak prothrombin time
    device
Councill basket

Councill catheter
Councill dilator
Councill retention catheter
Councill stone basket
Councill stone dislodger
Councill stone extractor
Councill stone scoop
Councill ureteral dilator
Councill ureteral stone extractor
Councilman chisel
Councilman lesion
Counsellor plug
Counsellor vaginal mold
Counsellor-Davis artificial vagina
  operation
Counsellor-Flor modification of
  McIndoe technique
count
  blood count
  instrument, sponge, and
    needle count
  kick count
  lap count
  needle count
  sponge and lap count
  sponge and needle count
  sponge count
counter
counterbalance
counterbore
  cloverleaf counterbore
  Curry hip nail counterbore
  Lloyd adapter counterbore
  round counterbore
counterclockwise direction
countercurrent extraction
countercurrent heat exchanger
counterextension
CounterForce Plus brace
counterincision
counteropening
counterpressor
  Acland-Buncke counterpressor
  Amenabar counterpressor
  angled counterpressor
  Bruni counterpressor
  Gill counterpressor
counterpressure
counterpulsation
  balloon counterpulsation
  intra-aortic balloon
    counterpulsation

counterpulsation balloon
counterpuncture
counterrotating saw
counterrotational splint
countershock
countersink
countersink bur
countertraction
countertraction splint
Count'R-Force arch brace
coup de sabre
coup de sabre deformity
coup-contrecoup
Coupland elevator
Coupland nasal suction tube
Coupland suction tube
coupled pulse
coupled rhythm
coupler
  Acutome laparoscopic CO_2
    laser coupler
  Ferrier coupler
  Precise anastomotic coupler
coupling head
coupling interval
coupling microscope
Cournand arterial needle
Cournand arteriography needle
Cournand cardiac device
Cournand catheter
Cournand needle
Cournand quadpolar catheter
Cournand-Grino angiography
  needle
Cournand-Grino needle
Cournand-Potts needle
course of dialysis
course of radiation
coursing
Courvoisier gallbladder
Courvoisier gastroenterostomy
Courvoisier incision
Couvelaire ileourethral
  anastomosis
Couvelaire incision
Covaderm composite wound
  dressing
Covaderm Plus tube site
  dressing
Covaderm Plus dressing
cove plane
Coventry arthroplasty

Coventry nail
Coventry osteotomy
Coventry staple
Coventry stapler
Coventry total hip replacement
Coventry wiring
Coventry-Johnson classification
cover screw
coverage flap
covered Gianturco stent
covering
  allograft wound covering
  Biobrane wound covering
  biosynthetic wound covering
  dural covering
  fibroelastic covering
  fibrous covering
  outermost covering
  titanium mini bur hole
    covering
  wound covering
  xenograft wound covering
Coverlet adhesive
Coverlet adhesive dressing
Coverlet adhesive surgical
  dressing
Coverlet Strips wound dressing
Cover-Pad dressing
Cover-Roll adhesive gauze
Cover-Roll dressing
Cover-Roll gauze adhesive
Cover-Roll stretch bandage
Cover-Strip wound closure
  strips
Covertell composite secondary
  dressing
coving
CovRSite dressing
Cowboy collar
Cowden disease
Cowen-Loftus toe-phalanx
  transplantation
cowhorn tooth-extracting
  forceps
Cowper glands
Cowper ligament
Co-Wrap dressing
COWS (cold to the opposite,
  warm to the same)
Cox II ocular laser shield
Cox Maze III procedure
Cox metatarsal spreader

Cox polypectomy snare
Cox regression analysis of
  partially edentulous jaw
Cox skin lines
Cox technique
coxa adducta
coxa flexa
coxa magna
coxa plana
coxa valga
coxa vara
coxa vara luxans
coxarthrosis
Coxeter catheter
Coxeter prostatic catheter
coxofemoral articulation
Cox-Uphoff double-lumen breast
  prosthesis
Cox-Uphoff implant
Cox-Uphoff International tissue
  expander (CUI tissue
  expander)
Cox-Uphoff prosthesis
Cox-Uphoff skin expander
Cozean angled lens forceps
Cozean bipolar forceps
Cozean implantation forceps
Cozean-McPherson angled lens
  forceps
Cozean-McPherson tying forceps
Cozen approach
Cozen-Brockway operation
Cozen-Brockway technique
Cozen-Brockway Z-plasty
C-P (Chaffin-Pratt)
CP (cleft palate)
C-P suction
C-P suction tube
CPAP (continuous positive
  airway pressure)
CPAP ventilator
CPD (cephalopelvic
  disproportion)
CPI Astra pacemaker
CPI automatic implantable
  defibrillator
CPI endocardial defibrillation
  rate-sensing pacing lead
CPI Endotak electrode lead
CPI Endotak transvenous
  electrode
CPI Maxilith pacemaker

CPI Microthin lithium-powered programmable pacemaker
CPI Microthin pacemaker
CPI Minilith pacemaker
CPI pacemaker
CPI porous tined-tip bipolar pacing lead
CPI Sentra endocardial lead
CPI Sweet Tip lead
CPI Ultra II pacemaker
CPI Vigor pacemaker
CPI Vista-T pacemaker
CPI-PRx pulse generator
CPLS (cleft palate and lateral synechia syndrome)
CPM (continuous passive pressure)
AIM CPM
CairTech Knee CPM
CPM device
CPM machine
CPS modular air cranioclast
CPS unitized air cranioclast
CPV catheter
C-R resin syringe
crab hand
crab yaws
Crabtree dissector
Crabtree dissector pick
Cracchiolo forefoot arthroplasty
Cracchiolo procedure
crack fracture
crack growth
crack lung
cracked heel
cracked pot note
cracked-pot resonance
cracked-pot sound
crackles
crackling jaw
cradle arm sling
cradling instrument
Crafon-Oretorp arthroscopy pump
Crafoord aortic clamp
Crafoord arterial forceps
Crafoord auricular clamp
Crafoord bronchial forceps
Crafoord clamp
Crafoord coarctation clamp
Crafoord coarctation forceps
Crafoord contractor

Crafoord forceps
Crafoord hemostat
Crafoord lobectomy scissors
Crafoord lung scissors
Crafoord operation
Crafoord pulmonary forceps
Crafoord retractor
Crafoord scissors
Crafoord thoracic scissors
Crafoord-Cooley tucker
Crafoord-Cooley tunneler
Crafoord-Sellors auricular clamp
Crafoord-Sellors hemostatic forceps
Crafoord-Senning heart-lung machine
Cragg Convertible wire
Cragg endoluminal graft
Cragg wire
Cragg infusion wire
Cragg stent
Cragg thrombolytic brush
Craig abduction splint
Craig angular scissors
Craig biopsy needle
Craig forceps
Craig headrest
Craig headrest holder
Craig nasal-cutting forceps
Craig needle
Craig pin
Craig scissors
Craig septal forceps
Craig septum bone-cutting forceps
Craig septum-cutting forceps
Craig splint
Craig tonsil-seizing forceps
Craig vertebral body biopsy set
Craig-Scott orthosis
Craig-Sheehan retractor
Cramer cleft palate elevator
Cramer splint
Cramer wire splint
cramping abdominal pain
Crampton line
Crampton muscle
Crampton-Tsang percutaneous endoscopic biliary stent set
Crandall syndrome
Crane bone chisel
Crane chisel

Crane dental pick
Crane elevator
Crane flap
Crane gouge
Crane hammer
Crane mallet
Crane osteotome
Crane pick
Craniad cup positioner
cranial anchorage
cranial aneurysm clip
cranial aneurysm clip applier
cranial arteritis
cranial autografts
cranial base defect
cranial base landmark
cranial base neoplasm
cranial base plane
cranial base surgery
cranial bone graft
cranial bone grafting
cranial bone rongeur
cranial bur
cranial capacity
cranial cavity
cranial coronal ring articulation
cranial defect
cranial diameter
cranial drill
cranial duplication
cranial epidural space
cranial extension
cranial flap fixation
cranial fontanelles
cranial forceps
cranial fossa
cranial fossa defect
cranial fracture
cranial growth
cranial halo
cranial insufflation
cranial irradiation
cranial Jacobs hook
cranial nerve dissection
cranial nerve manipulation
cranial nerve sign
cranial nerves (1-12, also I-XII)
cranial neurectomy
cranial operating instruments
cranial perforator
cranial prosthesis
cranial puncture

cranial reflex
cranial retractor
cranial rongeur
cranial rongeur forceps
cranial segment
cranial sinus
cranial suture
cranial suture joint
cranial suture synostosis
cranial synostosis
cranial trauma
cranial trephine
cranial twist drill perforator
cranial vault
cranial vault suture
cranialization
craniamphitomy
craniectomy
    anterior craniectomy
    endoscopic craniectomy
    endoscopic strip craniectomy
    frontal bone advancement
        with strip craniectomy
    keyhole-shaped craniectomy
    linear craniectomy
    partial-thickness craniectomy
    retromastoid suboccipital
        craniectomy
    sagittal craniectomy
    strip craniectomy
    suboccipital craniectomy
cranioaural
cranioblade
    Codman cranioblade
    Kirwan cranioblade
craniobuccal
craniocaudad position
craniocaudad views
craniocaudal views
craniocerebral injury
craniocerebral topography
craniocervical chordoma
craniocervical plate
cranioclasis
cranioclast
    Auvard cranioclast
    Braun cranioclast
    Codman cranioclast
    CPS modular air cranioclast
    CPS unitized air cranioclast
    DeLee-Zweifel cranioclast
    Rica cranioclast

cranioclast (*continued*)
Tarnier cranioclast
Zweifel-DeLee cranioclast
craniodentofacial deformity
craniodiaphyseal dysplasia
craniofacial angle
craniofacial anomaly
craniofacial appliance
craniofacial axis
craniofacial cleft
craniofacial complex
craniofacial deformity
craniofacial disjunction
craniofacial disjunction fracture
craniofacial disorder
craniofacial dysmorphism
craniofacial dysostosis
craniofacial dysplasia
craniofacial fixation
craniofacial fracture appliance
craniofacial hemangioma
craniofacial instrumentation
craniofacial malformation
craniofacial microsomia
craniofacial morphology
craniofacial notch
craniofacial osteogenic sarcoma
craniofacial pathology
craniofacial reconstruction
craniofacial reconstructive
   surgery
craniofacial resection
craniofacial surgery
craniofacial suspension wiring
craniofacial syndromes
craniofaciocervical
craniofenestria
craniolacunia
craniomalacia
craniomandibular dysfunction
   (CMD)
craniomandibular orthopaedic
   repositioning device
craniomaxillofacial
craniomaxillofacial callus
   distraction
craniomaxillofacial mesh
craniomaxillofacial plate
craniomaxillofacial screw
craniomaxillofacial surgery
craniomedial
craniometric diameter

craniometric point
craniometry
cranio-orbital
cranio-orbital neurofibromatosis
cranio-orbital surgery
craniopharyngeal canal
craniopharyngeal duct
craniopharyngeal duct tumor
craniopharyngioma
Cranioplastic acrylic
      cranioplasty material
cranioplastic kit
Cranioplastic material dressing
Cranioplastic powder
cranioplasty
   aluminum cranioplasty
   Curlex cranioplasty
   metallic cranioplasty
   tantalum cranioplasty
craniopuncture
craniorachischisis
craniosacral
craniosacral division
cranioschisis
craniosclerosis
craniosinus fistula
craniospinal irradiation
craniospinal space
craniostenosis
craniostosis
craniosynostectomy
craniosynostosis
      (*pl.* craniosynostoses)
   common craniosynostosis
   Crouzon craniosynostosis
   kleeblattschädel
      craniosynostosis
   metopic craniosynostosis
   Saethre-Chotzen
      craniosynostosis
   secondary craniosynostosis
   single-suture craniosynostosis
   syndromic craniosynostosis
craniotabes
craniotome
   Hall craniotome
   Hall in-and-out craniotome
   Hall neurosurgical craniotome
   Muehr craniotome
   turbo-bit craniotome
   Verbrugge-Souttar craniotome
   Williams craniotome

craniotomy
  attached craniotomy
  awake craniotomy
  bifrontal craniotomy
  biparietal craniotomy
  bitemporal craniotomy
  decompressive craniotomy
  detached craniotomy
  endoscopic frontal
    craniotomy
  fetal craniotomy
  frontal craniotomy
  frontotemporal craniotomy
  left frontal craniotomy (LFC)
  open stereotactic craniotomy
  osteoplastic craniotomy
  posterior fossa craniotomy
  pterional craniotomy
  retromastoid craniotomy
  right temporoparietal
    craniotomy
  stereotactic craniotomy
  supratentorial craniotomy
  Yasargil craniotomy
craniotomy defect
craniotomy flap
craniotomy instrument set
craniotomy scissors
craniotrypesis
craniovac drain
craniovertebral articulation
cranium (*pl.* crania)
  bifid cranium
  cerebral cranium
  cerebral yokes of bone of
    cranium
  concha of cranium
  dysmorphic cranium
  squamous suture of cranium
  synchondroses of cranium
  vertex of bony cranium
  visceral cranium
cranium bifidum
cranium bifidum occultum
cranium clip-applying forceps
crank frame retractor
crank table
crankshaft clip
Cranley-Graff phleborrheogram
Crapeau nasal snare
Crapeau snare
crash cart

crash cesarean section
crash technique
crater
  alveolar process crater
  bone crater
  bony crater
  interalveolar bone crater
crater formation
craterization
crater-shaped erosion
cravat
cravat bandage
Crawford aortic retractor
Crawford auricle clamp
Crawford canaliculus hook
Crawford canaliculus probe
Crawford crutches
Crawford dural elevator
Crawford fascial forceps
Crawford fascial needle
Crawford fascial stripper
Crawford fracture frame
Crawford graft inclusion
    technique
Crawford head frame
Crawford hook
Crawford incision
Crawford lacrimal set
Crawford low-lithotomy
    crutches
Crawford needle
Crawford operation
Crawford retractor
Crawford sling operation
Crawford suture ring
Crawford tube
Crawford-Adams acetabular cup
Crawford-Adams arthroplasty
Crawford-Adams cup
Crawford-Adams cup arthroplasty
Crawford-Adams hip
    arthroplasty
Crawford-Knighton forceps
Crawford-Marxen-Osterfeld
    technique
CRC resection
crease
  alar crease
  circumference of the chest at
    the inframammary crease
    (C-IMC)
  columellar crease

crease (*continued*)
  earlobe crease
  flexion crease
  glabellar crease
  helical crease
  inframammary crease
  labiocolumellar crease
  lateral crease
  lateral neck crease
  midline abdominal crease
  nasolabial crease
  palmar crease
  preauricular crease
  simian crease
  skin crease
  submammary crease
  Sydney crease
  torso crease
  vertical glabellar crease
crease incision
crease line
creation
  kyphosis creation
  lordosis creation
  McIndoe vaginal creation
  Politano-Leadbetter tunnel
    creation
  tunnel creation
Credé maneuver
Credé prophylaxis
Credo operation
Credo razor
Creech aorto-iliac graft
Creech manner
Creech technique
Creed dissection
Creed dissector
creep recovery
creeping infiltrates
creeping thrombosis
creeping vesiculation
Creevy biopsy forceps
Creevy bladder evacuator
Creevy calyx dislodger
Creevy dilator
Creevy evacuator
Creevy irrigator
Creevy operation
Creevy stone dislodger
Creevy urethral dilator
Creevy-Bumpus hemostat
Crego bow traction

Crego closed reduction
Crego elevator
Crego Gigli-saw
Crego operation
Crego osteotomy
Crego periosteal elevator
Crego periosteal retractor
Crego retractor
Crego tendon transfer technique
Crego traction
Crego wire traction
cremaster fascia
cremaster muscle
cremasteric artery
cremasteric fascia
cremasteric layer
cremasteric muscle
cremasteric reflex
Cremer-Ikeda papillotome
Cremer-Ikeda sphincterotome
cremnocele
crenation of tongue
Crenshaw carbuncle forceps
Crenshaw caruncle clamp
Crenshaw caruncle forceps
Crenshaw forceps
crenulated tantalum wire
Creola body
crepe bandage
crepe bandage dressing
crepitant rales
crepitation
  coarse crepitation
crepitation in the lower eyelids
crepitation of mandible on
    manual palpation
crepitus at fracture site
Cresatin dental material
crescendo angina
crescendo murmur
crescendo pattern
crescendo TIAs (crescendo
    transient ischemic attacks)
crescendo-decrescendo murmur
crescent
  Heidenhain crescents
  sublingual crescent
  traumatic crescent
crescent blade
crescent body
crescent broach
crescent choroid

Crescent corneal graft
Crescent graft
crescent incision
crescent of cardia
crescent operation
Crescent plaster knife
crescent snare
crescentic blade
crescentic bunionectomy
crescentic glomerulonephritis
crescentic lobule
crescentic rupture
crescentic-shaped incision
crescentic-shaped skin paddle
Crespo operation
crest
   alveolar crest
   ampullary crest
   anterior lacrimal crest
   articular crest
   buccinator crest
   conchal crest
   deltoid crest
   endoalveolar crest
   ethmoidal crest
   external frontal crest
   external mental crest
   external occipital crest
   falciform crest
   frontal crest
   iliac crest
   ilium crest
   infratemporal crest
   infrazygomatic crest
   inguinal crest
   intermediate sacral crest
   internal occipital crest
   interosseous crest
   intertrochanteric crest
   lacrimal crest
   mandibular crest
   marginal crest
   maxillary crest
   nasal crest
   obturator crest
   occipital crest
   piriform crest
   posterior lacrimal crest
   pubic crest
   sacral crest
   sagittal crest
   sphenoidal crest

crest (*continued*)
   superficial temporal crest
   supinator crest
   supramastoid crest
   supraventricular crest
   terminal crest
   tibial crest
   triangular crest
   trochanteric crest
   urethral crest
   vestibular crest
   vomeropremaxillary crest
   zygomatic crest
crest of alveolar ridge
crest of palatine bone
crest of ridge
crestal bone loss
Crete-Manche implant
cretinism
crevicular epithelium
crevicular incision
cri du chat syndrome
crib
   allogeneic bone crib
   allogeneic crib
   alloplastic crib
   bone crib
   Jackson crib
   lip-sucking habit crib
crib splint
Cribier-Letac aortic valvuloplasty
   balloon
Cribier-Letac catheter
cribriform carcinoma
cribriform compress
cribriform fascia
cribriform hymen
cribriform pattern
cribriform plate
cribriform plate injury
cribriform plate of alveolar
   process
cribriform process
cribriform salivary carcinoma of
   the excretory duct
cribriform sinus
cribriform tissue
cribroethmoid foramen
cribrous lamina
Cricket disposable skin stapler
Cricket pulse oximetry
   monitor

Cricket recording pulse oximeter
Cricket stapling device
cricket thigh
cricoarytenoid ankylosis
cricoarytenoid arthrodesis
cricoarytenoid articulation
cricoarytenoid fixation
cricoarytenoid joint
cricoarytenoid joint ankylosis
cricoarytenoid ligament
cricoarytenoid muscle
cricoesophageal tendon
cricoid cartilage
cricoid pressure anesthetic technique
cricoid ring
cricoid split
cricoidea (*pl.* cricoideae)
  cartilago cricoidea
  facies articularis arytenoidea cricoideae
  facies articularis thyroidea cricoideae
cricoidectomy
cricoidynia
cricopharyngeal dilatation
cricopharyngeal diverticulum
cricopharyngeal muscle
cricopharyngeal myotomy
cricopharyngeal sphincter
cricopharyngeus muscle
cricothyroarytenoid ligament
cricothyroid
cricothyroid angle
cricothyroid artery
cricothyroid articulation
cricothyroid joint
cricothyroid ligament
cricothyroid membrane
cricothyroid muscle
cricothyroid needle puncture
cricothyroid paralysis
cricothyroid trocar
cricothyroidectomy
cricothyroidotomy
cricothyroidotomy and tracheostomy
cricothyrostomy
cricothyrotomy
cricothyrotomy cannula
cricothyrotomy trocar

cricothyrotomy trocar tube
cricotomy
cricotracheal ligament
cricotracheal membrane
cricotracheal resection
cricotracheotomy
cricovocal membrane
Crigler evacuator
Crigler evaluator
Crikelair otoplasty
Crile appendiceal clamp
Crile arterial forceps
Crile blade
Crile clamp
Crile cleft palate knife
Crile crushing clamp
Crile dissector
Crile forceps
Crile gall duct forceps
Crile gall duct hemostat
Crile gall hemostat
Crile gasserian ganglion dissector
Crile gasserian ganglion knife
Crile head traction
Crile hemostat
Crile hemostatic clamp
Crile hemostatic forceps
Crile hook
Crile incision
Crile knife
Crile Micro-Line arterial forceps
Crile Micro-Line artery forceps
Crile needle holder
Crile nerve hook
Crile retractor
Crile single hook
Crile spatula
Crile stripper
Crile thyroid double-ended retractor
Crile vagotomy stripper
Crile wire passer
Crile-Barnes hemostatic forceps
Crile-Crutchfield clamp
Crile-Duval lung-grasping forceps
Crile-Matas operation
Crile-Murray needle holder
Crile-Rankin forceps
Crile-Wood needle holder
Crile-Wood Vital needle holder

crimped Dacron prosthesis
crimped wire
crimped woven prosthesis
crimped-wire prosthesis
crimper (*see also* wire crimper)
   Caparosa wire crimper
   ENT wire crimper
   Farrior wire crimper
   Francis-Gray wire crimper
   Gruppe wire crimper
   Juers crimper
   Juers wire crimper
   McGee crimper
   McGee wire crimper
   McGee-Caparosa wire crimper
   McGee-Priest wire crimper
   pin crimper
   Schuknecht crimper
   Schuknecht Teflon crimper
   Schuknecht wire crimper
   Shiffrin wire crimper
   washer crimper
   wire crimper (*see also* crimper)
crimper closer forceps
crimper forceps
crimper wire
crimping forceps
crinkle
crinkle line
Crinotene dressing
Cripps obturator
Cripps operation
Crisp aneurysm
crisscross fashion
crisscross heart
crisscross suturing
crisscrossing abdominal wall incisions
crista (*pl.* cristae)
crista ampullaris
crista buccinatoria
crista conchalis maxillae
crista conchalis ossis palatini
crista dentalis
crista ethmoidalis maxillae
crista ethmoidalis ossis palatini
crista frontalis
crista galli
crista helicis
crista lacrimalis
crista marginalis

crista nasalis maxillae
crista occipitalis
crista palatina
crista temporalis
Cristobalite investment material
Critchett excision of anterior eyeball
Critchett eye speculum
Critchett operation
Crites laryngeal cotton screw
critical level
critical mass
Criticare monitor
Criticare pulse oximeter
Criticare sensor probe
CritiCath PA catheter
CritiCath thermodilution catheter
Critikon automated blood pressure cuff
Critikon balloon temporary pacing catheter
Critikon balloon thermodilution catheter
Critikon balloon wedge pressure catheter
Critikon balloon-tipped endhole catheter
Critikon catheter
Critikon guidewire
Critikon oximeter
Critikon pressure infuser
Critikon-Berman angiographic balloon catheter
Crobin technique
crochet hook
Crock encircling operation
Crockard hard palate retractor
Crockard ligament grasping forceps
Crockard microdissector
Crockard midfacial osteotomy retractor plate
Crockard odontoid peg-grasping forceps
Crockard pharyngeal retractor
Crockard small-tongue retractor blade
Crockard sublaminar wire guide
Crockard suction tube holder
Crockard transoral clip applier
crocodile biopsy forceps

crocodile forceps
crocodile tears
crocodile tongue
Croften classification
Crohn disease
Cröhnlein procedure
Cronin cheiloplasty
Cronin cleft palate elevator
Cronin implant
Cronin mammary implant
Cronin operation
Cronin palate elevator
Cronin palate knife
Cronin Silastic mammary
    prosthesis
Cronin-Matthews eave flap
Cronkhite-Canada syndrome
crook measuring prosthesis
Crookes lens
Crookes tube
Crookes-Hittorf tube
Crosby capsule
Crosby knife
Crosby reduction
Crosby-Cooney operation for
    ascites
Crosby-Kugler capsule
cross arch fulcrum line
cross circulation
Cross clamp
cross contamination
Cross corneal bur
cross femoral-femoral bypass
cross flap
Cross needle trocar
Cross osteotome
Cross scleral trephine
cross section (noun; *see also*
    cross-section)
cross union
cross-action bulldog clamp
cross-action capsular forceps
cross-action clamp
cross-action forceps
cross-action towel clamp
crossarm flap
crossbar (*see also* bar)
crossbar chisel
crossbar chisel-osteotome
crossbar elevator
crossbar fishtail chisel
crossbar stomach deformity

crossbite
    anterior crossbite
    buccal crossbite
    lingual crossbite
    posterior crossbite
    scissors-bite crossbite
    telescoping crossbite
crossbite occlusion
crossclamp time
crossclamped aorta
crossclamping
crosscut
crosscut bur
crosscut fissure bur
crosscut saw
crosscut straight fissure bur
crossed anesthesia
crossed coil
crossed extensor reflex
crossed fixation
crossed K-wire fixation
crossed reflex
crossed renal ectopia
crossed sword fashion
Crossen puncturing tenaculum
Crossen puncturing tenaculum
    forceps
cross-facial nerve graft
cross-facial nerve graft
    anastomosis
cross-facial technique
cross-finger flap
Crossfire polyethylene material
CrossFlex coronary stent
cross-friction massage
crosshatch
crosshatch incision
crosshatching undermining
cross-head displacement
crossing over
crossing tunnels
Cross-it guidewire
Cross-Jones disk prosthetic valve
Cross-Jones disk valve prosthesis
Cross-Jones mitral valve
Cross-Jones valve prosthesis
cross-leg
cross-leg bypass graft
cross-leg flap
cross-leg graft
cross-leg skin flap
cross-legged clip

cross-lid flap
cross-lip flap
cross-lip pedicle flap
crossmatch
crossover bypass
crossover graft
crossover toe deformity
crossover vasectomy
crosspiece
cross-pin teeth
cross-reactivity
CrossSail coronary dilatation
    catheter
CrossSail coronary dilation
    catheter
cross-section (verb; *see also*
    cross section)
cross-section technique
cross-sectional
cross-sectional anal sphincter
    probe
cross-sectional
    echocardiography
cross-sectional image
cross-sectional plane
cross-sectional projection
cross-sectional view
cross-shaped incision
cross-slot screwdriver
cross-sword technique of Park
cross-table lateral position
cross-talk pacemaker
cross-trigonal repair
cross-tunneling incision
Crosswire guidewire
Crosswire PTCA guidewire
Crotti goiter retractor
Crotti retractor
Crotti thyroid retractor
Crouch corneal protector
Crouzon craniostenotic defect
Crouzon craniosynostosis
Crouzon disease
Crouzon facial deformity
Crouzon syndrome
Crouzon syndromic synostosis
Crowe classification
Crowe pilot point
Crowe pilot point on Steinmann
    pin
Crowe-Davis mouth gag
Crowe-Davis mouth retractor

Crowel-Beard ptosis procedure
Crowe-tip pin
crowfoot closure
crown amalgamator
crown and bridge scissors
Crown biopsy needle
crown debridement
crown drill
crown drill screw
crown fracture
Crown needle
crown saw
crown scissors
crown stent
crown stitch
crown sutures
crown-collar scissors
crown-crimping pliers
crowning of infant's head
crown-of thorns head holder
crown-root fracture
crown-rump length
crown-to-heel
crown-to-rump
crow's feet
crow's foot incision
Crozat appliance
Crozat clasp
Crozat orthodontic wire
Crozat removable orthodontic
    appliance
Crozat therapy
CRT (cardiac resynchronization
    therapy)
crucial anastomosis
crucial bandage
crucial incision
cruciate anastomosis
cruciate eminence
cruciate head bone screw
cruciate head screw
cruciate incision
cruciate ligament guide
cruciate ligament
    reconstruction
cruciate ligament tear
cruciate ligaments
cruciate pulley
cruciate punch
cruciate screw
cruciate-retaining prosthesis
cruciate-sacrificing prosthesis

cruciform anterior spinal
  hyperextension (CASH)
cruciform anterior spinal
  hyperextension orthosis
cruciform eminence
cruciform head bone screw
cruciform screw
cruciform screwdriver
cruciform suture technique
Cruickshank clamp
Cruickshank entropion clamp
Cruiser hip abduction brace
Crump dilator
Crump vessel dilator
Crump-Himmelstein dilator
crumpled aluminum foil
crunch
  Hamman crunch
  Means-Lernan mediastinal
    crunch
crunching sound
crunch-stick anastomosis
crura (*sing.* crus)
crura anthelicis
crura cerebelli
crura cerebri
crura hook
crura of anthelix
crura of clitoris
crural arch
crural area
crural canal
crural closure
crural fascia
crural feet
crural fossa
crural hernia
crural ligament
crural nipper
crural nipper forceps
crural region
crural repair
Cruricast dressing
crurotomy
crurotomy chisel
crurotomy nipper
crurotomy saw
crus (*pl.* crura)
  helical crus
  lateral crus
  medial crus
  posterior crus

crus (*continued*)
  stapedial crus
  superior crus
crus anterius stapedis
crus anthelicis
crus breve incudis
crus cerebri
crus clitoridis
crus commune
crus fornicis
crus glandis clitoridis
crus guide fork
crus helicis
crus laterale
crus mediale
crus of clitoris
crus of diaphragm
crus of fornix
crus of helix
crus of incus
crus of stapes
crus penis
crus posterius stapedis
crush clamp
crush fracture
crush injury
crush kidney
crush syndrome
crush vasectomy technique
crush-border membrane
crushed cartilage graft
crushed chest injury
crushed eggshell fracture
crushed muscle
crusher (*see also* spur crusher)
  baby spur crusher
  Berger crusher
  Berger spur crusher
  bone crusher
  cartilage crusher
  Cottle bone crusher
  DeWitt-Stetten colostomy
    spur crusher
  Garlock spur crusher
  Gross spur crusher
  Hendrickson stone crusher
  Lieberman phaco crusher
  Lowsley stone crusher
  Mayo-Lovelace crusher
  Mayo-Lovelace spur crusher
  Mikulicz crusher
  Mosley stone crusher

crusher (*continued*)
nasal bone crusher
Ochsner-DeBakey crusher
Ochsner-DeBakey spur
crusher
Pemberton spur crusher
Proud fascia crusher
spur crusher
Stetten colostomy crusher
Stetten spur crusher
ultrasonic stone crusher
Warthen crusher
Warthen spur crusher
Wolfson spur crusher
Wurth crusher
Wurth spur crusher
crushing anastomosis
crushing and removal of calculi
crushing chest discomfort
crushing clamp
crushing fracture
crushing injury
crushing of calculus
crushing of nerve
crushing of vas deferens
crushing sensation in chest
crushing technique
crutch and belt femoral closed
nail
crutched stick-type
polyurethane
endoprosthesis
Crutchfield bone drill
Crutchfield carotid artery clamp
Crutchfield clamp
Crutchfield drill
Crutchfield hand drill
Crutchfield operation
Crutchfield reduction technique
Crutchfield skeletal traction
Crutchfield skeletal traction
tongs
Crutchfield skull tongs
Crutchfield skull-tip pin
Crutchfield tongs
Crutchfield tongs prosthesis
Crutchfield tongs traction
Crutchfield traction
Crutchfield traction bow
Crutchfield traction tongs
Crutchfield-Raney drill
Crutchfield-Raney drill point

Crutchfield-Raney tongs
Crutchfield-Raney traction tongs
Cruveilhier atrophy
Cruveilhier fossa
Cruveilhier joint
Cruveilhier nodules
Cruveilhier sign
Cruveilhier tumor
Cruveilhier ulcer
Cruveilhier-Baumgarten anomaly
crux of heart
Cryer dental elevator
Cryer elevator
Cryer root elevator
Cryer Universal forceps
Cryo/Cuff ankle dressing
Cryo/Cuff boot
Cryo/Cuff compression dressing
cryoablation
cryoablation catheter
cryoanalgesia
cryoanesthesia
cryoapplication
cryo-assisted resection
Cryo-Barrages vitreous implant
cryocardioplegia
cryocataract extraction
CryoCath catheter
cryocautery
cryocoagulation
cryoconization
Cryo-Cut microtome
cryodestruction
cryoelectron microscopy
cryoenucleator
Gallie cryoenucleator
cryoextraction of cataract
cryoextraction operation
cryoextractor (*see also*
extractor)
Alcon cryoextractor
Amoils cryoextractor
Beaver cataract cryoextractor
Beaver cryoextractor
Bellows cryoextractor
disposable cryoextractor
Frigitronics cryoextractor
Frigitronics Mark II
cryoextractor
Keeler cryoextractor
Kelman cryoextractor
Krwawicz cryoextractor

cryoextractor (*continued*)
    Rubinstein cryoextractor
    Thomas cryoextractor
cryoextraction operation
cryoflex envelope
cryofrigitronics
cryogenic ablation
cryogenic block
cryogenic cataract extraction
cryogenic eye surgery
cryogenic probe
cryogenic surgery
cryoglue
cryohypophysectomy
cryoleucotomy
Cryolife homograft
Cryolife valvular graft
CryoLife-O'Brien stentless
    porcine heart valve
CryoLife-O'Brien valve
cryolysis
cryomagnet
Cryomedics colposcope
Cryomedics disposable
    electrode
cryo-ophthalmic unit
cryopallidectomy
cryopencil
    Amoils cryopencil
    Mira endovitreal cryopencil
cryopexy
    barrage cryopexy
    double freeze-thaw cryopexy
    retinal cryopexy
cryopexy probe
cryophake
    Alcon cryophake
    Amoils cryophake
    Bellows cryophake
    Frigitronics cryophake
    Keeler cryophake
    Kelman cryophake
    Rubinstein cryophake
cryoprecipitate
cryopreservation
cryopreserved
cryopreserved allograft
cryopreserved aortic homograft
cryopreserved extrapelvic
    ovarian transplantation
cryopreserved heart-valve
    allograft

cryopreserved homograft valve
cryopreserved tissue banking
cryoprobe (*see also* probe)
    Amoils cryoprobe
    Brymiss cryoprobe
    Cooper cryoprobe
    cryoptor cryoprobe
    Frigitronics cryoprobe
    intravitreal cryoprobe
    Kry-Med cryoprobe
    Lee cryoprobe
    Linde cryoprobe
    Rubinstein cryoprobe
    Spembly cryoprobe
    Sudarsky cryoprobe
    Thomas cryoprobe
cryoprostatectomy
cryoprosthesis
cryopter
cryoptor
cryoptor cryoprobe
cryopulvinectomy
cryoretinopexy
cryoretractor
    Coston-Trent cryoretractor
    Harstein iris cryoretractor
    Hartstein iris cryoretractor
cryoscopy
cryostat
    Cooper cryostat
    Cooper disk cryostat
cryostat frozen sectioning aid
cryostat section
cryostat tissue
cryostylet
    disposable cryostylet
    Frigitronics cryostylet
    Kelman cryostylet
cryosurgery
cryosurgical ablation
cryosurgical instrument
cryosurgical interruption of AV
    node
cryosurgical technique
cryosurgical unit
cryosystem
cryothalamectomy
cryothalmotomy
cryotherapy
cryotherapy operation
cryotherapy probe
cryotube

cryounit
crypt
  anal crypt
  Fuchs crypt
  iris crypt
  Lieberkühn crypts
  Luschka crypt
  tonsillar crypts
crypt abscess
crypt hook
crypt knife
cryptectomy
cryptic tonsil
cryptitis
cryptococcal meningitis
cryptodontic brachymetacarpia
cryptogenic septicemia
cryptophthalmia
cryptophthalmos
cryptorchidectomy
cryptorchidism
cryptorchidopexy
cryptoscope
cryptotia
cryptotome
  Blanchard cryptotome
  Pierce cryptotome
cryptotomy
crypts of Lieberkühn
crypts of Luschka
crypts of palatine tonsil
crypts of pharyngeal tonsil
crypts of tonsils
crystalline
crystalline lens
crystallinity
crystallization
crystallized trypsin
crystalloid
crystalloid infusion
Crystar porcelain kit
Csapo abortion
Csapody operation
Csapody orbital repair operation
CSAR (conservative subtraction-
    rhinoplasty)
C-section (cesarean section)
C-section delivery
CSF (cerebrospinal fluid)
CSF (colony-stimulating factor)
CSF flushing reservoir
CSF flushing valve

CSF prosthesis
CSF reservoir
CSF shunt connector forceps
CSF shunt instruments
CSF shunt-introducing forceps
CSF T-tube shunt
C-shaped microplate
C-shaped plate
C-shaped resistive magnet
C-shaped scalp flap
CSII (continuous subcutaneous
    insulin infusion)
C-splint
C-splint immobilizer
C-sponge
CSV Bovie electrosurgical unit
CT (computed tomography,
    computerized
    tomography)
CT densitometer
CT gantry
CT laser mammography
CT scan
CT scan gantry
CT scan-guided needle
    aspiration
CT scanner
CT1 suture
CTD (connective tissue disease)
CT-directed needle aspiration
CT-guided balloon inflation
CT-guided fine-needle
    aspiration
CT-guided liver biopsy
CT-guided needle aspiration
    biopsy
CT-guided selective drainage
CT-guided stereotactic
    evacuation
CTR (carpal tunnel release)
C-Trak hand-held gamma
    detector
C-Trak handheld gamma probe
CTS (carpal tunnel syndrome)
CTS gauge
CTS Gripfit splint
CTT scanner
CTX needle
C-type acupuncture needle
Cu-7 intrauterine device
CU-8 needle
Cubbins approach

Cubbins arthroplasty
Cubbins incision
Cubbins open reduction
Cubbins screw
Cubbins screwdriver
Cubbins shoulder approach
Cubbins shoulder approach
   curved approach
Cubbins shoulder arthroplasty
Cubbins shoulder dislocation
   technique
Cubbins-Callahan-Scuderi
   approach
cube pessary
cubital
cubital artery
cubital fossa
cubital lymph nodes
cubital nerve
cubital region
cubital tunnel
cubital tunnel syndrome
cubital vein
cubitocarpal
cubitoradial
cubitus valgus
cubitus valgus deformity
cubitus varus
cubitus varus correction
cuboid bone
cuboidal epithelium
Cuchica syringe
Cueva cranial nerve electrode
Cueva cranial nerve electrode
   monitoring device
cuff
   aortic cuff
   Astropulse cuff
   atrial cuff
   blood pressure cuff
   blood warmer cuffs
   calibrated V-Lok cuff
   ComfortCuff blood pressure
      cuff
   conductive V-Lok cuff
   Cook continence cuff
   Critikon automated blood
      pressure cuff
   Dacron cuff
   Dinamap blood pressure cuff
   Ducker-Hayes nerve cuff
   elephant cuff

cuff (*continued*)
   endotracheal tube cuff
   epithelial cuff
   Ethoc cuff
   Falk vaginal cuff
   Finapres finger cuff
   finger cuff
   hand cuff
   Honan cuff
   inflatable cuff
   inflatable tourniquet cuff
   inflatable tracheal tube cuff
   joint distraction cuff
   Kendall endotracheal tube
      cuff
   Kidde tourniquet cuff
   mucosal cuff
   musculotendinous cuff
   nerve cuff
   oscillometric blood pressure
      cuff
   Papercuff disposable blood
      pressure cuff
   pneumatic cuff
   Polmedco endotracheal tube
      cuff
   Portex SS endotracheal tube
      cuff
   Portex XL endotracheal tube
      cuff
   pressure cuff
   push cuff
   Push-Ease Quad cuff
   rectal muscle cuff
   reefed vaginal cuff
   right atrial cuff
   rotator cuff
   Rusch endotracheal tube cuff
   Safe-Cuff blood pressure cuff
   Sheridan endotracheal tube cuff
   shoulder cuff
   sphygmomanometer cuffs
   Steri-Cuff disposable
      tourniquet cuff
   suprahepatic caval cuff
   tourniquet cuff
   tracheal tube cuff
   uterine cuff
   vaginal cuff
   V-Lok disposable blood
      pressure cuff
   Watzke cuff

cuff abscess
cuff electrode
Cuff Link orthopedic device
cuff pressure
cuff resection
cuff salpingostomy
cuff sign
cuff suspension
cuff tear arthropathy
cuff tear arthroplasty
cuffed endotracheal tube
cuffed esophageal
   endoprosthesis
cuffed sheet
cuffed tracheostomy tube
cuffed tube
cuffless tube
CuffPatch soft tissue
   reinforcement
cuff-type inactive electrode
CUI artificial breast prosthesis
CUI catheter
CUI chin prosthesis
CUI columellar implant
CUI dorsal implant
CUI eye sphere prosthesis
CUI gel mammary prosthesis
CUI joint
CUI malar implant
CUI myringotomy tube
CUI nasal prosthesis
CUI rhinoplasty implant
CUI saline mammary prosthesis
CUI tendon prosthesis
CUI testicular prosthesis
CUI tissue expander (Cox-Uphoff
   International tissue expander)
CUI urological drain
cuirass jacket
cuirass respirator
cuirass ventilation
cuirass ventilator
Cukier nasal forceps
Culbertson canal knife
Culcher-Sussman pelvic inlet
   measurement
Culcher-Sussman technique
cul-de-sac
   conjunctival cul-de-sac
   Douglas cul-de-sac
   sacral cul-de-sac
   superior cul-de-sac

cul-de-sac irrigating vectis
cul-de-sac irrigation T-tube
cul-de-sac of Douglas
cul-de-sac of vagina
culdocentesis
culdoplasty
   Halban culdoplasty
   Marion-Moschcowitz
     culdoplasty
   McCall culdoplasty
culdoscope
   Decker culdoscope
   fiberoptic culdoscope
culdoscopy
culdotomy
culdotomy incision
Cullen abduction splint
Cullen obstetrical forceps
Cullen sign
Culler eye forceps
Culler fixation forceps
Culler iris spatula
Culler iris speculum
Culler lens spoon
Culler rectus muscle hook
Culler spatula
Culley splint
Culley ulna splint
Cullom septal forceps
Cullom-Mueller adenotome
Culp biopsy needle
Culp pyeloplasty
Culp ureteropelvioplasty
Culp-Calhoon operation
Culpolase laser
culprit coronary lesion
culprit lesion
culprit lesion angioplasty
Culp-Scardino operation
culture
   anaerobic culture
   cervical culture
   endocervical culture
   fractional culture
   Isolator blood culture
   nasal culture
   negative culture
   positive culture
   smear and culture
   smear culture
   sputum culture
   streak culture

culture (*continued*)
tissue culture
urine culture
culture and sensitivity (C&S)
culture tubes
cultured autografts
cultured autologous
keratinocyte
cultured autologous melanocyte
cultured epithelial autograft
cultured epithelial autografting
cultured epithelium autograft
(CEA)
cultured mucosal graft
cultured periosteal cell
culturing technique
Cummer classification
Cummings catheter
Cummings 4-wing catheter
Cummings 4-wing Malecot
retention catheter
Cummings nephrostomy
catheter
Cummings tube
Cummings-Pezzer catheter
cumulative dose
cumulative radiation effect
cumulative toxicity index
cumulative trauma disorder
cuneiform bone
cuneiform cartilage
cuneiform cartilage of Wrisberg
cuneiform joint
cuneiform ligament
cuneiform osteotomy
cuneiform tubercle
cuneocuboid
cuneonavicular ligament
cuneoscaphoid
Cunningham brace
Cunningham clamp
Cunningham incontinence
clamp
Cunningham urinary
incontinence clamp
Cunningham-Cotton sleeve
Cunningham-Cotton sleeve
coaxial dilator
cup
AccePressure heel cup
Accu-Path acetabular cup
acetabular cup

cup (*continued*)
Alivium prosthesis cup
APR acetabular cup
Arthopor acetabular cup
Aufranc cup
Aufranc-Turner acetabular cup
Bard alligator cup
Bard oval cup
Berkeley suction cup
Bicon-Plus cup
Bird OP cup
Breinin suction cup
Buchholz acetabular cup
caliceal cups
Centaur trial cup
Chambers intrauterine cup
Charnley acetabular cup
Charnley cup
Charnley offset-bore cup
Crawford-Adams acetabluar
cup
Crawford-Adams cup
CRM cup
dry cup
Dual Geometry HA cup
Duraloc acetabular cup
ear cup
Galin silicone bleb cup
Gemini cup
Harris-Galante cup
heel cup
HGP II acetabular cup
Integrity acetabular cup
Interseal acetabular cup
iodine cup
Judet impactor for acetabular
cup
Laing concentric hip cup
large physiological cup
Lord cup
magnetic cup
Malström cup
McBride cup
McGoey-Evans acetabular cup
McGoey-Evans cup
McKee-Farrar acetabular cup
McKee-Farrar cup
Mityvac obstetric vacuum
extractor cup
Mityvac Super M cup
MMS low-profile acetabular
cup

cup (*continued*)
  Mueller-type acetabular cup
  multipolar bipolar cup
  nasal suction cup
  Natural-Loc RM acetabular
    cups
  Natural-Lok acetabular cup
  New England Baptist
    acetabular cup
  Newhart-Smith cup
  O'Connor finger cup
  ocular cup
  O'Harris-Petruso cup
  Omnifit acetabular cup
  ophthalmic cup
  optic cup
  Opti-Fix acetabular cup
  Oves cervical cup
  PCA acetabular cup
  Pierce nasal cup
  prosthetic cup
  Reflection I, V, and FSO
    acetabular cup
  Restoration GAP acetabular
    cup
  Rickham cup
  Riecken PQ premium heel
    cup
  Rotalok acetabular cup
  Rotalok cup
  Silastic obstetrical vacuum
    cup
  Silipos silicone wonder cup
  slit-lamp cup
  Smith-Petersen cup
  Soft Touch cup
  Sorbuthane II heel cup
  S-ROM acetabular cup
  stainless steel cup
  Ster-O2-Mist ultrasonic cup
  suction cup
  Super M vacuum extractor
    cup
  Tender Touch vacuum
    birthing cup
  Ti-BAC I, II acetabular cup
  Titan hip cup
  trial acetabular cups
  trial cup
  Tri-Lock acetabular cup
  Trilogy acetabular cup
  Tuli heel cup

cup (*continued*)
  University of California
    Biomechanics Laboratory
    heel cup
  Vitallium cup
  wet cup
cup arthroplasty
cup biopsy forceps
cup catheter
cup curet
cup ear
cup forceps
cup hip prosthesis
cup impactor
cup insemination
cup palm manual percussor
cup pessary
cup positioner
cup pusher shaft
cup/disk ratio (CDR)
cup-and-ball osteotomy
cup-and-spill stomach
cup-biting forceps
cup-biting punch
cup-cement interface
Cupid's bow
Cupid's bow peak
Cupid's peak
cup-patch technique
cupped curet
cupped disk
cupped ear
cupped forceps
Cupper suture technique
Cupper-Faden operation
cupping of disk
cupping of nerve
Cupraphane dialyzer reaction
cuprophane membrane
cup-shaped curet forceps
cup-shaped ear forceps
cup-shaped electrode
cup-shaped forceps
cup-shaped inner ear forceps
cup-shaped middle ear forceps
cupula cristae ampullaris
cupula of cochlea
cupula of pleura
cupula technique
cupular cecum of cochlear duct
cupuliform cataract
Cuputi sputum collector

Curad plastic bandage
Curad plastic dressing
Curad surgical adhesive dressing
Curaderm dressing
Curaderm hydrocolloid dressing
  material
Curafil dressing
Curafil gel wound dressing
Curafil hydrogel dressing
Curafil hydrogel impregnated
  gauze
Curafoam dressing
Curafoam foam wound dressing
Curafoam island dressing
Curafoam wound dressing
Curagel hydrogel dressing
Curagel hydrogel island wound
  dressing
curare anesthetic agent
Curasol sterile wound dressing
Curasorb calcium alginate
  dressing
curative dose
curative procedure
curative radical total
  gastrectomy
curative resection
curative result
curative sphincter-saving
  operation
curative surgery
curative-intent operation
curative-intent procedure
curative-intent surgery
curb tenotomy
Curdy blade
Curdy knife
Curdy sclerotome
Curdy sclerotome knife
Curdy-Hebra blade
curet
  Abraham rectal curet
  Accurette endometrial suction
    curet
  adenoid curet
  Alvis curet
  Alvis foreign body curet
  Alvis foreign body eye curet
  Anderson curet
  Angell curet
  angled curet
  angled ring curet

curet (*continued*)
  antral curet
  aortic curet
  apicitis curet
  aspirating curet
  Austin oval curet
  Auto-Suture curet
  B-12 dental curet
  Ballantine uterine curet
  Ballenger curet
  Ballenger ethmoid curet
  banjo curet
  Bardic curet
  Barnhill adenoid curet
  Barnhill curet
  Barnhill-Jones curet
  Barth curet
  Barth mastoid curet
  bayonet curet
  Beaver curet
  Beckman adenoid curet
  Bellucci curet
  Berlin curet
  Billeau curet
  Billeau ear curet
  Billeau ear wax curet
  Billroth curet
  biopsy curet
  biopsy suction curet
  Blake curet
  Blake uterine curet
  blunt-ring curet
  bone curet
  bowl curet
  box curet
  Bozeman curet
  Bromley uterine curet
  Bronson-Ray curet
  Bronson-Ray pituitary curet
  Brun bone curet
  Brun curet
  Brun ear curet
  Brun mastoid curet
  Bruns bone curet
  Buck bone curet
  Buck curet
  Buck ear curet
  Buck earring curet
  Buck mastoid curet
  Buck wax curet
  Buck-House curet
  Bumm curet

curet (*continued*)

Bumm placental curet
Bumm uterine curet
Bunge curet
Bush intervertebral curet
Carlens curet
Carmack curet
Carmack ear curet
Carroll hook curet
Carter curet
Carter submucous curet
cervical biopsy curet
cervical curet
chalazion curet
Charnley double-ended bone
curet
Clevedent-Lucas curet
Cloward curet
Cloward-Cone ring curet
Clyman endometrial curet
Coakley antral curet
Coakley antrum curet
Coakley curet
Coakley ethmoid curet
Coakley nasal curet
Coakley sinus curet
Cobb bone curet
Cobb curet
Cobb spinal curet
Cobb spine curet
Collin uterine curet
Concept curet
Cone curet
Cone nasal curet
Cone ring curet
Cone suction biopsy curet
Converse curet
Converse double-end curet
Converse sweeper curet
Corgill-Shapleigh ear curet
corneal curet
cup curet
cupped curet
cylindrical uterine curet
Daubenspeck bone curet
Daviel chalazion curet
Dawson-Yuhl curet
Dawson-Yuhl-Cone curet
DeLee curet
Dench ear curet
Dench uterine curet
DePuy bone curet

curet (*continued*)

DePuy curet
Derlacki curet
Derlacki ear curet
dermal curet
diagnostic curet
disk curet
disposable vacuum curet
double-ended bone curet
double-ended curet
double-ended dental curet
double-ended stapes curet
double-lumen curet
down-biting curet
down-biting Epstein curet
Duncan curet
Duncan endometrial biopsy
curet
Duncan endometrial curet
Dunning curet
ear curet
embolectomy curet
endaural curet
endocervical biopsy curet
endocervical curet
endodontic curet
endometrial biopsy curet
endometrial curet
endotracheal curet
Epstein curet
Epstein down-biting curet
Epstein spinal fusion curet
ethmoidal curet
Explora uterine curet
eye curet
Farrior angulated curet
Farrior ear curet
Faulkner antral curet
Faulkner antrum curet
Faulkner curet
Faulkner double-end ring
curet
Faulkner ethmoid curet
Faulkner ethmoidal curet
Faulkner nasal curet
Faullkner ethmoidal curet
fenestration curet
Ferguson bone curet
Ferguson curet
fine curet
fine-angled curet
Fink chalazion curet

curet (*continued*)
  Fink curet
  flat back curet
  foreign body curet
  fossa curet
  Fowler double-end curet
  Fox curet
  Fox dermal curet
  Franklin-Silverman curet
  Freimuth curet
  Freimuth ear curet
  Frenckner curet
  Frenckner-Stille curet
  frontal sinus curet
  Gam-Mer spinal fusion curet
  Garcia-Rock endometrial
    biopsy curet
  Garcia-Rock endometrial
    suction curet
  Genell biopsy curet
  Gifford corneal curet
  Gifford curet
  Gillquist suction curet
  Gill-Welsh curet
  Goldman curet
  Goldstein curet
  Goodhill double-end curet
  Govons curet
  Govons pituitary curet
  Gracey curet
  Green corneal curet
  Green curet
  Greene endocervical curet
  Greene endocervical uterine
    curet
  Greene placental curet
  Greene uterine curet
  Gross curet
  Gross ear curet
  Guilford-Wright curet
  Gusberg cervical biopsy
    curet
  Gusberg cervical cone curet
  Gusberg curet
  Gusberg endocervical biopsy
    curet
  Gusberg endocervical curet
  Halle bone curet
  Halle curet
  Halle ethmoidal curet
  Halle sinus curet
  Hannon curet

curet (*continued*)
  Hannon endometrial biopsy
    curet
  Hannon endometrial curet
  Hardy bayonet curet
  Hardy hypophysial curet
  Hardy modification of
    Bronson-Ray curet
  Harrison curet
  Harrison scarifying curet
  Harrison-Shea curet
  Hartmann adenoidal curet
  Hartmann curet
  Hatfield bone curet
  Hayden curet
  Hayden tonsil curet
  Hayden tonsillar curet
  Heaney curet
  Heaney endometrial biopsy
    curet
  Heaney uterine curet
  Heath chalazion curet
  Heath curet
  Hebra chalazion curet
  Hebra corneal curet
  Helix endocervical curet
  Helix uterine biopsy curet
  Heyner curet
  Hibbs bone curet
  Hibbs curet
  Hibbs spinal curet
  Hibbs-Spratt curet
  Hibbs-Spratt spinal fusion
    curet
  Hofmeister endometrial
    biopsy curet
  Holden curet
  Holden uterine curet
  Holtz curet
  Holtz ear curet
  Holtz endometrial curet
  hook-type dermal curet
  horizontal ring curet
  Hotz curet
  Hotz ear curet
  Hough curet
  House curet
  House ear curet
  House stapes curet
  House tympanoplasty curet
  House-Buck curet
  House-Paparella curet

curet (*continued*)
  House-Paparella stapes curet
  House-Sanders middle ear
    curet
  House-Saunders middle ear
    curet
  House-Sheehy knife curet
  Houtz endometrial curet
  Howard spinal curet
  Hunter curet
  Hunter large uterine curet
  Hunter uterine curet
  hypophysial curet
  Ingersoll adenoid curet
  Ingersoll curet
  Innomed bone curet
  Innomed curet
  intervertebral curet
  irrigating curet
  irrigating uterine curet
  Jacobson curet
  Jansen bone curet
  Jansen curet
  Jarit reverse adenoid curet
  Jones adenoid curet
  Jones curet
  Jordan-Rosen curet
  Juers ear curet
  Kelly curet
  Kelly-Gray curet
  Kelly-Gray uterine curet
  Kerpel bone curet
  Kevorkian curet
  Kevorkian endocervical curet
  Kevorkian endometrial curet
  Kevorkian-Younge biopsy
    curet
  Kevorkian-Younge curet
  Kevorkian-Younge
    endocervical biopsy curet
  Kevorkian-Younge uterine
    curet
  Kezerian curet
  Kirkland curet
  Kos curet
  Kraff capsule polisher curet
  Kuhn-Bolger angled curet
  Kushner-Tandatnick
    endometrial biopsy curet
  labyrinth curet
  large bowel curet
  large uterine curet

curet (*continued*)
  Laufe aspirating curet
  Laufe-Novak diagnostic curet
  Laufe-Novak gynecologic
    curet
  Laufe-Randall curet
  Laufe-Randall gynecologic
    curet
  Lempert bone curet
  Lempert curet
  Lempert endaural curet
  Lempert fine curet
  long-handle curet
  loop curet
  Lounsbury curet
  Lounsbury placenta curet
  Lounsbury placental curet
  Lucas alveolar curet
  Lucas curet
  Luer bone curet
  Luer curet
  Luongo curet
  Lynch curet
  Magielski curet
  Magnum curet
  Majewski nasal curet
  Malis curet
  Marino rotatable
    transsphenoidal curet
  Marino rotatable
    transsphenoidal horizontal-
    ring curet
  Marino rotatable
    transsphenoidal vertical-
    ring curet
  Marino transsphenoidal curet
  Maroon lip curet
  Martin dermal curet
  Martini bone curet
  mastoid curet
  Mayfield curet
  Mayfield spinal curet
  McCain TMJ curet
  McCall curet
  McCaskey antral curet
  McCaskey curet
  McElroy curet
  Meigs curet
  Meigs endometrial curet
  Meigs uterine curet
  meniscal curet
  Meyerding curet

curet (*continued*)

Meyerding saw-toothed curet
Meyhoeffer bone curet
Meyhoeffer chalazion curet
Meyhoeffer curet
Meyhoeffer bone curet
Meyhoeffer chalazion curet
microbone curet
Microsect curet
middle ear curet
middle ear ring curet
Middleton adenoid curet
Middleton curet
Milan uterine curet
Miles antral curet
Miller curet
MiMark disposable
   endocervical curet
Misdome-Frank curet
Moe bone curet
Molt curet
Moorfields curet
Mosher curet
Mosher ethmoid curet
Moult curet
Mueller curet
Munchen endometrial biopsy
   curet
Myles antral curet
Myles curet
nasal curet
Noland-Budd cervical curet
Noland-Budd curet
Nordent bone curet
Novak biopsy curet
Novak curet
Novak uterine curet
Novak uterine suction curet
Novak-Schoeckaert
   endometrial biopsy curet
Novak-Schoeckaert
   endometrial curet
O'Connor double-edged curet
optical aspirating curet
Orban curet
orthopedic curet
oval-window curet
ovum curet
Paparella angled-ring curet
Paparella curet
Paparella mastoid curet
Paparella stapes curet

curet (*continued*)

Paparella-House curet
periapical curet
Piffard curet
Piffard dermal curet
Piffard placental curet
Pipelle endometrial curet
Pipelle endometrial suction
   curet
Pipelle-deCornier endometrial
   curet
pituitary curet
placenta curet
placental curet
plastic curet
polyvinyl curet
Pratt antral curet
Pratt antrum curet
Pratt curet
Pratt ethmoid curet
Pratt nasal curet
Rand bayonet ring curet
Randall biopsy curet
Randall curet
Randall endometrial biopsy
   curet
Randall uterine curet
Raney curet
Raney spinal fusion curet
Raney stirrup-loop curet
Ray curet
Ray pituitary curet
Read facial curet
Read oral curet
Récamier curet
Récamier uterine curet
rectal curet
Reich curet
Reich-Nechtow cervical
   biopsy curet
Reich-Nechtow curet
Reiner curet
resectoscope curet
retrograde curet
reverse-angle skid curet
reverse-curve adenoid curet
Rheinstaedter curet
Rheinstaedter flushing curet
Rheinstaedter uterine curet
Rhoton blunt-ring curet
Rhoton horizontal-ring curet
Rhoton loop curet

curet (*continued*)

Rhoton pituitary curet
Rhoton spoon curet
Rhoton vertical ring curet
Rica ear curet
Rica lipoma curet
Rica mastoid curet
Rica uterine curet
Richards bone curet
Richards curet
Richards ethmoid curet
Richards mastoid curet
Richards mastoid ethmoid
    curet
Ridpath curet
Ridpath ethmoid curet
right-angle curet
rigid curet
ring bayonet Rand curet
ring curet
Rock endometrial suction
    curet
Rosen curet
Rosen knife curet
Rosenmueller curet
rotatable transsphenoidal
    horizontal ring curet
rotatable transsphenoidal
    vertical ring curet
ruptured disk curet
salpingeal curet
saw-toothed curet
scarifying curet
Schaeffer curet
Schaeffer ethmoid curet
Schaeffer mastoid curet
Schede bone curet
Schede curet
Schroeder curet
Schroeder uterine curet
Schuletz antral curet
Schuletz-Simmons ethmoidal
    curet
Schwartz curet
Schwartz endocervical curet
Scoville curet
Scoville ruptured disk curet
Semmes curet
Semmes spinal fusion curet
serrated curet
Shambaugh adenoidal curet
Shapleigh curet

curet (*continued*)

Shapleigh ear curet
Shapleigh ear wax curet
Sharman curet
sharp curet
sharp derma curet
sharp dermal curet
sharp loop curet
Shea curet
Sheehy-House curet
Simon bone curet
Simon cup uterine curet
Simon spinal curet
Simpson antral curet
Simpson curet
Sims curet
Sims irrigating uterine curet
Sims uterine curet
sinus curet
Skeele chalazion curet
Skeele corneal curet
Skeele curet
Skeele eye curet
Skene uterine curet
Skene uterine spoon curet
skid curet
Skillern curet
Skillern sinus curet
SMIC ear curet
SMIC mastoid curet
SMIC pituitary curet
Smith-Petersen curet
soft rubber curet
sonic curet
spinal curet
spinal fusion curet
sponge ear curet
spoon curet
Sprague ear curet
Spratt bone curet
Spratt curet
Spratt ear curet
Spratt mastoid curet
St. Clair-Thompson adenoid
    curet
St. Clair-Thompson adenoidal
    curet
St. Clair-Thompson curet
stapes curet
stirrup-loop curet
Stiwer curet
Storz resectoscope curet

curet (*continued*)
  stout-neck curet
  straight ring curet
  Strully curet
  Strully ruptured disk curet
  Stubbs adenoid curet
  Stubbs adenoidal curet
  Stubbs curet
  submucous curet
  suction curet
  suction tip curet
  surgical curet
  Sweaper curet
  Synthes facial curet
  Tabb curet
  Tabb ear curet
  Tamsco curet
  Taylor curet
  Temens curet
  T-handled cup curet
  Thomas curet
  Thomas uterine curet
  Thompson adenoid curet
  Thompson curet
  Thorpe curet
  tonsillar curet
  Townsend endocervical
    biopsy curet
  toxemia curet
  Toynbee curet
  transsphenoidal curet
  Uffenorde bone curet
  Ulrich wart curet
  Ultra-Cut Cobb curet
  Unimar Pipelle curet
  up-angled curet
  uterine biopsy curet
  uterine curet
  uterine irrigating curet
  uterine suction curet
  uterine vacuum aspirating
    curet
  uterine-irrigating curet
  V. Mueller mastoid curet
  Vabra suction curet
  Vacurette suction curet
  vacuum curet
  Vakutage curet
  vertical ring curet
  Visitec capsule polisher curet
  Vogel adenoid curet
  Vogel curet

curet (*continued*)
  Vogel infant adenoid curet
  Volkmann bone curet
  Volkmann curet
  Volkmann oval curet
  Voller curet
  Walker curet
  Walker ring curet
  Walker ruptured disk curet
  Wallich curet
  Walsh curet
  Walsh dermal curet
  Walsh hook-type dermal curet
  Walton curet
  wax curet
  Weaver chalazion curet
  Weisman curet
  Weisman ear curet
  Weisman infant ear curet
  West-Beck spoon curet
  Whiting mastoid curet
  Whitney single-use plastic
    curet
  Williger bone curet
  Williger ear curet
  Wolff dermal curet
  Wright-Guilford curet
  Wullstein curet
  Wullstein ring curet
  Yankauer curet
  Yankauer ear curet
  Yankauer salpingeal curet
  Yasargil curet
  Younge endometrial curet
  Younge uterine biopsy curet
  Younge uterine curet
  Zielke curet
  Z-Sampler endometrial
    suction curet
curet forceps
curettage
  aspiration curettage
  biopsy by curettage
  cervical curettage
  destruction of lesion by
    curettage
  diagnostic curettage
  diagnostic dilatation and
    curettage
  dilatation and curettage (D&C)
  dilation and curettage (D&C)
  dull curettage

curettage (*continued*)
  electrodesiccation and
    curettage
  endocervical curettage
  fractional curettage
  fractional dilation and
    curettage
  Guyon curettage
  Gynaspir vacuum curettage
  infrabony pocket curettage
  intrauterine curettage
  irrigation and curettage
  Papineau sequestrectomy and
    curettage
  parametrial curettage
  periapical curettage
  soft tissue curettage
  sternal puncture by curettage
  subgingival curettage
  suction curettage
  suction dilatation and curettage
  uterine curettage
  Vabra curettage
  Vabra uterine aspiration
    curettage
  vacuum curettage
curettage and irrigation
curettage of basal cell carcinoma
curette (*see* curet)
curet forceps
curetted
curetted bone
curettement
curetting bur
curetting
  endocervical curetting (ECC)
  uterine curetting
Curity cover sponge
Curity disposable laparotomy
  sponge
Curity dressing
Curity gauze sponge
Curity irrigation tray
Curity leg bag
Curl Cath catheter
curl-back shell eye implant
curled enamel
Curlex cranioplasty
Curling stress ulcer
Curling ulcer
curly toes
Curon dressing

Curran eye knife
Curran knife needle
currant jelly clot
currant jelly thrombus
current
  Bovie coagulating current
  Bovie current
  Bovie cutting current
  coagulating current
  cutting current
  demarcation current
  direct current
  eddy current
  electric current
  faradic current
  galvanic current
  single-phase current
  surgical current
current controller
current transformer
Currentrol cautery
Curry cerebral needle
Curry hip nail
Curry hip nail counterbore
Curry hip nail counterbore with
  Lloyd adapter
Curry needle
Curry splint
Curry walking splint
currycomb instrument
Curschmann trocar
Curtin incision
Curtin operation
Curtin plantar fibromatosis
  excision
Curtin technique
Curtis arthroplasty
Curtis forceps
Curtis operation
Curtis PIP joint capsulotomy
Curtis technique
Curtis tissue forceps
Curtis-Fisher knee technique
curvature
  anterior corneal curvature
  buccolingual curvature
  canal curvature
  cervical curvature
  corneal curvature
  dextroscoliotic curvature
  downward curvature
  greater curvature

curvature (*continued*)
   lesser curvature
   lumbar curvature
   occlusal curvature
   thoracic cage curvature
curvature aberration
curvature site
curve
   alignment curve
   Amplatz II curve
   anteroposterior curve
   articulation curve
   buccal curve
   cervical curve
   compensating curve
   compensatory curve
   displacement curve
   dose-response curve
   expiratory curve
   flat curve
   Frank-Starling curve
   isodose curve
   isoeffect curve
   labial curve
   lordotic curve
   lumbar curve
   lumbar lordotic curve
   lumbosacral curve
   Monson curve
   occlusal curve
   reversal of cervical curve
   reversal of lumbar curve
   saddle curve
   spherical three-dimensional
     curve
   stress-strain curve
   U-shaped curve
   von Spee curve
curve of occlusion
curve of Spee
curve of von Spee
curve of Wilson
curved approach
curved array transducer
curved awl
curved cannula
curved cardiovascular clamp
curved catheter
curved chisel
curved clamp
curved clip
curved conventional microscissors

curved cricothyrotomy cannula
curved dissecting forceps
curved electrode
curved end-to-end anastomosis
curved end-to-end anastomosis
   stapler (CEEA stapler)
curved flank position
curved forceps
curved gouge
curved hemostat
curved hook
curved incision
curved intraluminal stapler
curved iris forceps
curved iris scissors
curved J-exchange wire
curved Kelly hemostat
curved knife
curved knot-tying forceps
curved laryngeal mirror
curved longitudinal incision
curved magnifying mirror
curved Maryland forceps
curved Mayo clamp
curved Mayo scissors
curved meniscotome blade
curved microbipolar forceps
curved micromonopolar forceps
curved micro-needle holder
curved mosquito clamp
curved mosquito hemostat
curved needle
curved needle eye spud
curved needle holder
curved needle spud
curved nerve hook
curved operating scissors
curved osteotome
curved periosteal elevator
curved periscapular incision
curved radiolucent line
curved retinal probe
curved scissors
curved suture needle
curved tenotomy scissors
curved toenails
curved tractor
curved transjugular needle
curved turbinate scissors
curved turbinectomy scissors
curved tying forceps
curved valvulotome

curved zonule separator
curved-8 clamp
curved-downward incision
curved-needle surgeon knot
curved-on-flat scissors
curved-tip jewelers bipolar
　　forceps
curved-tipped spatula
curvilinear calcification
curvilinear chin implant
curvilinear flattening
curvilinear incision
curvilinear skin incision
curving incision
CurvTek bone tunneling device
CurvTek TSR bone drill
CUSA (Cavitron ultrasonic
　　aspirator)
CUSA aspirator
CUSA dissector
CUSA Excel ultrasonic aspirator
CUSA laparoscopic tip
CUSALap device
CUSALap ultrasonic accessory
　　needle
Cusco speculum
Cusco vaginal speculum
Cushieri maneuver
Cushing aluminum retractor
Cushing angled decompression
　　retractor
Cushing angled retractor
Cushing bayonet forceps
Cushing bipolar forceps
Cushing bipolar neurosurgical
　　forceps
Cushing bivalve retractor
Cushing bone rongeur
Cushing brain depressor
Cushing brain forceps
Cushing brain instruments
Cushing brain retractor
Cushing brain spatula
Cushing brain spatula spoon
Cushing bur
Cushing clamp
Cushing clip
Cushing cranial bur
Cushing cranial drill
Cushing cranial perforator
Cushing cranial rongeur forceps
Cushing decompression forceps

Cushing decompression retractor
Cushing disease
Cushing dressing forceps
Cushing drill
Cushing dural hook
Cushing dural hook knife
Cushing dural knife
Cushing elevator
Cushing flat drill
Cushing forceps
Cushing gasserian ganglion hook
Cushing Gigli-saw guide
Cushing hook
Cushing intervertebral disk
　　rongeur
Cushing knife
Cushing laminectomy rongeur
Cushing little joker elevator
Cushing monopolar forceps
Cushing needle
Cushing nerve hook
Cushing nerve retractor
Cushing operation
Cushing perforator
Cushing perforator drill
Cushing periosteal elevator
Cushing pituitary elevator
Cushing pituitary rongeur
Cushing pituitary spoon
Cushing raspatory
Cushing reflex
Cushing retractor
Cushing rongeur
Cushing saw guide
Cushing self-retaining retractor
Cushing spatula
Cushing spatula spoon
Cushing spoon
Cushing S-retractor
Cushing S-shaped brain spatula
Cushing S-shaped retractor
Cushing staphylorrhaphy
　　elevator
Cushing straight retractor
Cushing stress ulcer
Cushing subtemporal retractor
Cushing suture technique
Cushing sutures
Cushing thumb forceps
Cushing tissue forceps
Cushing tumor
Cushing ulcer

Cushing vein retractor
Cushing ventricular needle
Cushing Vital tissue forceps
Cushing-Brown tissue forceps
Cushing-Gutsch dressing forceps
Cushing-Gutsch tissue forceps
Cushing-Hopkins periosteal
   elevator
Cushing-Kocher retractor
Cushing-Landolt transsphenoidal
   speculum
Cushing-McKenzie clip
Cushing-Taylor carbide-jaw forceps
Cushing Vital tissue forceps
cushioned heel shoe
cushioning suture technique
cushioning sutures
Cushman drain
Cusick eye knife
Cusick goniotomy knife
Cusick operation
Cusick-Sarrail ptosis operation
cusp
   aortic cusp
   balanced contact between the
      cusps
   coronary cusps
cusp fenestration
cusp height
cusp plane
cuspid
   deciduous cuspid
   mandibular cuspid
   maxillary cuspid
cuspid teeth
cuspid-molar position
custocolic fold
Custodis implant
Custodis nondraining procedure
Custodis operation
Custodis scleral buckle operation
Custodis sponge
Custodis sutures
custom drill guide
custom matrix
custom pectus excavatum per
   moulage prosthesis
custom tip
custom total alloplastic TMJ
   reconstruction prosthesis
Custom Ultrasonic automatic
   reprocessor

custom-contoured implant
custom-curved coil
custom-healing orthotic
cut
   Chamfer cut
   stapedial tendon cut
   tangential cut
   tomographic cut
   Veenema-Gusberg prostatic
      biopsy cut
cut and ligated
cut biopsy needle
cut edge
cut end
cut point
cut section
cut snare wire
cut surface
cut taper needle
cut, clamped, and ligated
cut-and-sew technique
cutaneobiliary fistula
cutaneomucouveal syndrome
cutaneoperiosteal flap
cutaneous
cutaneous abscess
cutaneous amputation
cutaneous amyloidosis
cutaneous anaphylaxis
cutaneous blastomycosis
cutaneous blue venus
cutaneous burn injury
cutaneous candidiasis
cutaneous capillary formation
cutaneous coccidioidomycosis
cutaneous collateral circulation
cutaneous edges approximated
cutaneous fibrous histiocytoma
cutaneous flap
cutaneous focal mucinosis
cutaneous forearm flap
cutaneous gangrene
cutaneous gland
cutaneous graft-versus-host
   disease
cutaneous hemorrhoid
cutaneous horn
cutaneous hyperpigmentation
cutaneous hypopigmentation
cutaneous ileocystostomy
cutaneous ileostomy
cutaneous innervation

cutaneous lesion
cutaneous ligaments of
    phalanges
cutaneous malformation
cutaneous melanoma
cutaneous meningioma
cutaneous metastasis
cutaneous metastatic breast
    carcinoma
cutaneous muscle
cutaneous nerve
cutaneous nodule
cutaneous paddle
cutaneous papilloma
cutaneous polly beak
cutaneous protein coagulation
cutaneous punch
cutaneous reaction
cutaneous sarcoidosis
cutaneous sebum
cutaneous sinus
cutaneous stimulators
cutaneous striae
cutaneous suture of palate
cutaneous suture technique
cutaneous sutures
cutaneous tag
cutaneous T-cell lymphoma (CTCL)
cutaneous thoracic patch
    electrode
cutaneous ureterostomy
cutaneous vascular abnormality
cutaneous vascular anomaly
cutaneous vascular lesion
cutaneous vasculitis
cutaneous vasostomy
cutaneous vein
cutaneous vesicostomy
cutaneous-subcutaneous nodule
cut-as-you-go technique
cutback anoplasty
Cut-Blot coagulator
cutdown
    arterial cutdown
    venous cutdown
cutdown access
cutdown catheter
cutdown incision
cutdown instruments
cutdown technique
cuticle nipper
cuticle of hair

cuticle scissors
cuticular fold
cuticular membrane
cuticular stitch
cuticular suture technique
cuticular sutures
Cutifilm Plus waterproof wound
    dressing
Cutinova alginate dressing
Cutinova cavity dressing
Cutinova cavity wound filler
Cutinova cavity wound filling
    material
Cutinova dressing
Cutinova foam dressing
Cutinova Hydro dressing
Cutinova hydroactive dressing
Cutiplast sterile wound
    dressing
cutis
    angioma cutis
    angiomyoma cutis
    atheromatosis cutis
    atrophia cutis
    atrophia maculosa
        varioliformis cutis
    benign lymphocytoma cutis
    fibroma cutis
    retinacula cutis
    sarcomatosis cutis
    sulci cutis
cutis elastica
cutis graft
cutis laxa
cutis marmorata telangiectatica
    congenita
cutis neuroma
cutis osteoma
cutis verrucosa
Cutler eye implant
Cutler flap
Cutler forceps
Cutler implant
Cutler operation
Cutler repair
Cutler-Beard bridge flap
Cutler-Beard bridge flap
    procedure
Cutler-Beard flap
Cutler-Beard operation
Cutler-Beard reconstruction
Cutler-Beard technique

cutoff
   anesthetic cutoff
   DeVilbiss cutoffs
cutout activator
cutout patellar brace
cutout table
cutter (*see also* wire cutter)
   adenoid cutter
   AMO vitreous aspiration cutter
   Anspach diamond dissecting
      cutter
   arch bar cutter
   atherectomy cutter
   Bantam wire cutter
   Beaver cutter
   Beaver ring cutter
   Berbecker wire cutter
   Bethune bone cutter
   bone cutter
   Breck pin cutter
   Buettner-Parel cutter
   Buettner-Parel vitreous cutter
   cast cutter
   Chu foldable lens cutter
   chuck cutter
   Cloward dowel cutter
   Codman wire cutter
   cookie cutter
   Dedo-Webb cutter
   diamond wire cutter
   diamond-pin cutter
   Doret graft cutter
   double-action bone cutter
   double-action plate cutter
   Douvas cutter
   Douvas vitreous cutter
   dowel cutter
   Dual Geometry cutter
   Dyonics cutter
   Dyonics meniscal cutter
   electric cutter
   Elmed Bi-Pol cutter
   Endopath endoscopic linear
      cutter
   Endopath endoscopic
      articulating linear cutter
   Endopath endoscopic linear
      cutter
   Endopath linear cutter
   endoscopic linear cutter
   Ethicon endoscopic linear
      cutter

cutter (*continued*)
   Expand-O-Graft cutter
   Expand-O-Graft disposable
      cutter
   fascial cutter
   finger ring cutter
   flat-end cutter
   Gator meniscal cutter
   Guilford-Wright wire cutter
   guillotine-type cutter
   Heath wire cutter
   Heft Bite pin cutter
   hollow cutter
   Horsley bone cutter
   Horsley spine cutter
   Hough Teflon cutter
   Howmedica Microfixation
      System plate cutter
   infusion suction vitreous cutter
   Intra-Articular Surgical System
      cutter
   Jarit pin cutter
   Kalish Duredge wire cutter
   Kirschner wire cutter
   Kleinert-Kutz bone cutter
   Kloti cutter
   Kloti vitreous cutter
   Kuhlman cast cutter
   Leather valve cutter
   Leibinger Micro System plate
      cutter
   Lempert malleus cutter
   lens glide cutter
   ligature cutter
   Lindeman bone cutter
   Luhr Microfixation System
      plate cutter
   Machemer cutter
   Machemer vitreous cutter
   Machemer vitreous infusion
      suction cutter (Machemer
      VISC)
   Maguire-Harvey cutter
   Maguire-Harvey vitreous
      cutter
   malleus cutter
   Martin diamond wire cutter
   Martin wire cutter
   Martini bone cutter
   meniscal cutter
   Microvit cutter
   milling cutter

cutter (*continued*)

M-Pact cast cutter
nail cutter
nasal stent cutter
Northpedic cast cutter
Nu-Hope hole cutter
O'Malley-Heintz vitreous cutter
O'Malley-Heinz cutter
Parel-Crock cutter
Parel-Crock vitreous cutter
Pendula cast cutter
pin cutter
plaster cast cutter
plate cutter
plug cutter
Polaris reusable cutter
Porter-O-Surgical cutter
Premiere vitreous cutter
Proximate linear cutter
rectal cutter
Reflex articulating endoscopic cutter
rib cutter
right-angled bone cutter
ring cutter
Rochester harvest bone cutter
Rochester recipient bone cutter
rod cutter
Rogers wire cutter
Roos rib cutter
rotating-type cutter
round-end cutter
Schuknecht cutter
Sheets lens cutter
side-cut pin cutter
Sklar bone pin cutter
Sklar cutter
Sklar pin cutter
Spartan jaw wire cutter
Speck-Ange cutter
Stengstrom nerve cutter
stent cutter
Stille cast cutter
Storz Microsystems plate cutter
Stryker cast cutter
suction cutter
surgical cutter
suture cutter
Synthes Microsystem plate cutter

cutter (*continued*)

Szulc bone cutter
T-C pin cutter
Tolentino cutter
Tolentino vitreoretinal cutter
Tolentino vitreous cutter
Utrata foldable lens cutter
Verner-Joel cutter
Vernon wire cutter
Vit Commander vitreous cutter
vitreoretinal infusion cutter
vitreous infusion suction cutter (VISC)
wire cutter (*see also* cutter)
Wister wire-and-pin cutter
Woelfe-Boehler cutter
Wright-Guilford wire cutter
Cutter aortic valve prosthesis
Cutter cast
Cutter cast for disk lesion
Cutter cast tape
Cutter implant
Cutter mitral valve
Cutter SCDK prosthesis
Cutter-Smeloff aortic valve prosthesis
Cutter-Smeloff cardiac valve prosthesis
Cutter-Smeloff disk valve
Cutter-Smeloff heart valve
Cutter-Smeloff mitral valve
cutting balloon
cutting balloon device
cutting block
cutting board
cutting Bovie knife
cutting bur
cutting cautery
cutting current
cutting Delrin block
cutting device
cutting disk
cutting edge
cutting forceps
cutting jig
cutting loop
cutting loop electrode
cutting movement
cutting needle
cutting needle biopsy
cutting Teflon block

cuttlefish disk
Cuvier ducts
CVA (cerebrovascular accident)
CVB (chorionic villi biopsy)
CVIS imaging device
CVIS intravascular imaging
    catheter
CVOD (cerebrovascular
    obstructive disease)
CVP (central venous pressure)
CVP catheter
CVP line
CVS catheter
cyanoacrylate adhesive
cyanoacrylate embolization
cyanoacrylate fixed orbital
    silicone sleds implant
    material
cyanoacrylate glue
cyanoacrylate tissue adhesive
cyanographic contrast material
cyanotic
cyanotic induration
Cyberknife
Cyberlith demand pacemaker
Cyberlith multiprogrammable
    pulse generator
Cyberlith pacemaker
Cybertach automatic-burst atrial
    pacemaker
CyberTach pacemaker
Cyberware 3030RGB digitizer
Cybex back rehabilitation
    equipment
Cybex evaluation
Cybex finger-clip pulse meter
Cybex II isokinetic
    dynamometer
Cybex machine
Cyclaine anesthetic agent
cycle
    biphasic growth cycle
    contraction-relaxation cycle
    isohydric cycle
    ovarian cycle
    ovulation cycle
    uterine cycle
cyclectomy
cyclic irregularity
cyclic loading
cyclic therapy
cyclic treatment

cyclicotomy
cyclitic membrane
cycloanemization
cyclocryotherapy
cyclodestructive procedure
cyclodialysis
    Allen cyclodialysis
    Barkan cyclodialysis
    Gans cyclodialysis
    Heine cyclodialysis
    Kelman cyclodialysis
    Sheets cyclodialysis
cyclodialysis cannula
cyclodialysis spatula
cyclodiathermy
    Castroviejo-Scheie
        cyclodiathermy
cyclodiathermy electrode
cyclodiathermy needle
cyclodiathermy operation
cycloelectrolysis
cycloergometer
cyclographic tomogram
cyclolithopexy
cyclomethycaine sulfate
    anesthetic agent
cyclopentane anesthetic agent
cyclophorometer
cyclophotocoagulation
cycloplegia
cyclopropane anesthetic agent
Cyclops procedure
cyclotomy
cyclotron
cyesis
Cyfra 21-1 IRMS kit
Cygnus transdermal fentanyl
    device
cylinder
    AMS CX penile prosthesis
        cylinder
    Bodenham dermabrasion
        cylinder
    Burnett cylinder
    cesium cylinder
    CO_2 cylinder
    Delclos cylinder
    Delclos vaginal cylinder
    dome cylinder
    drill stop cylinder
    Feldenkrais cylinder
    Fletcher-Delclos dome cylinder

cylinder (*continued*)
  gas cylinder
  Mitroflow cylinders
  penile prosthesis cylinders
  suction cylinder
  TPS-coated cylinder
  Ultrec cylinder
  vaginal cylinder
cylinder aneurysm
cylinder axis
cylinder bur
cylinder cast
cylinder penile distendible
    prosthesis
cylinder penile nondistendible
    prosthesis
cylinder process
cylinder-type implant
cylindrical balloon
cylindrical bougie
cylindrical carcinoma
cylindrical diffuser
cylindrical lens
cylindrical reamer
cylindrical sponge
cylindrical uterine curet
cylindrical zonule separator
cylindrical-object forceps
cylindroid aneurysm
cylindromatous lesion
cylindromatous spiradenoma
cymba conchae
cymba conchae auriculae
cymba conchal cartilage graft
cymbiform
Cymed Micro skin pouch
Cymetra tissue replacement
    graft
Cynosar catheter
Cynosure laser
Cypher stent
Cyrano nose
Cyriax technique
cyst
  adrenal gland cyst
  adventitious cyst
  air cyst
  amebic cyst
  amniotic cyst
  aneurysmal bone cyst (ABC)
  anterior cyst
  antral mucosal cyst

cyst (*continued*)
  apical cyst
  apocrine retention cyst
  arachnoid cyst
  Baker cyst
  benign liver cyst
  benign subcutaneous cyst
  Blandin-Nuhn cyst
  Blessig cyst
  Blessig-Iwanoff cyst
  blue dome breast cyst
  blue dome cyst
  bone cyst
  Boyer cyst
  branchial cleft cyst
  branchial cyst
  branchiogenic cyst
  branchiogenous cyst
  breast cyst
  Brunn cyst
  buccal cyst
  bursal cyst
  calcifying and keratinizing
      odontogenic cyst
  calcifying cyst
  calcifying odontogenic cyst
  caliceal cyst
  cervical cyst
  chocolate cyst
  choledochal cyst
  choledochus cyst
  cholesterol granuloma cyst
  chorionic cyst
  chyle cyst
  colloid cyst
  compound cyst
  congenital choledochal cyst
  corpus luteal cyst
  corpus luteum cyst
  cortical cyst
  daughter cyst
  dentigerous cyst
  dentoalveolar cyst
  dermal cyst
  dermoid cyst
  dermoid inclusion cyst
  desmoid cyst
  double unilateral cysts
  drainage of cyst
  ductal cyst
  duplication cyst
  echinococcal liver cyst

cyst (*continued*)

echinococcus cyst
echinococcus liver cyst
embryonal cyst
endodermal cyst
enteric cyst
enterogenous cyst
enucleation of cyst
epidermal cyst
epidermal inclusion cyst
epidermoid cyst
epithelial cyst
eruption cyst
excision of cyst
false cyst
Favre-Racouchot cyst
fissural cyst
follicular cyst
follicular infundibular cyst
follicular isthmus cyst
follicular odontogenic cyst
ganglion cyst
Gartner cyst
gartnerian cyst
gastric duplication cyst
gastroenterogenous cyst
glandular odontogenic cyst
globulomaxillary cyst
Gorlin cyst
graafian cyst
granddaughter cyst
hemorrhagic cyst
hepatic parasitic cyst
hydatid cyst
hydatid liver cyst
hymenal cyst
hyperplastic cyst
implantation cyst
inclusion cyst
inflammatory cyst
intraluminal cyst
intraoral cyst
intraosseous cyst
intraosseous ganglion cyst
involution cyst
keratinizing epithelial
    odontogenic cyst
keratinous cyst
laryngeal cyst
laryngeal saccular cyst
lateral cyst
lingual cyst

cyst (*continued*)

lymphoepithelial cyst
mandibular cyst
mandibular median cyst
marsupialization of cyst
maxillary cyst
maxillary median anterior
    cyst
maxillary sinus cyst
median alveolar cyst
median anterior maxillary
    cyst
median mandibular cyst
median palatal cyst
meibomian cyst
mesenteric cyst
milia cyst
milk-filled cyst
morgagnian cyst
mother cyst
mucinous cyst
mucosal cyst
mucous cyst
mucous retention cyst
multilobular cyst
multilocular cyst
myoid cyst
myxoid cyst
Naboth cysts
nabothian cyst
nasoalveolar cyst
nasolabial cyst
nasopalatine cyst
nasopalatine duct cyst
nasopharyngeal cyst
neurenteric cyst
nonepithelial bone cyst
old posterior cyst
omental cyst
oophoritic cyst
organizing hemorrhagic cyst
ovarian cyst
ovarian dermoid cyst
palatine papilla cyst
pancreatic cyst
papillary cyst
parakeratinized cyst
paraovarian cyst
parasitic cyst
paroophoritic cyst
parotid cyst
parovarian cyst

cyst (*continued*)
  pedicled cyst
  periosteal cyst
  peripelvic cyst
  pilonidal cyst
  popliteal cyst
  porencephalic cyst
  posterior cyst
  preauricular cyst
  primordial cyst
  proliferating pilar cyst
  radicular cyst
  Rathke pouch cyst
  renal cyst
  residual cyst
  rest cyst
  retention cyst
  saccular cyst
  sacrococcygeal cyst
  salivary gland cyst
  salivary gland retention cyst
  salivary duct cyst
  Sampson cyst
  saucerizing a cyst
  sebaceous cyst
  sequestration cyst
  simple bone cyst
  sinus tract cyst
  soft tissue cyst
  solitary bone cyst
  sphenoidal cyst
  spit cyst
  splenic cyst
  Stafne bone cyst
  subchondral cyst
  sublingual cyst
  sudoriferous cyst
  synovial cyst
  Tansini removal of liver cyst
  Tarlov cyst
  tarsal cyst
  tentorium cyst
  theca-lutein cyst
  thymic cyst
  thyroglossal cyst
  Tornwaldt cyst
  tubo-ovarian cyst
  unicameral bone cyst
  unilocular cyst
  urachal cyst
  vestibular cyst
  vitellointestinal cyst

cyst (*continued*)
  vulvovaginal cyst
  wolffian cyst
  young cyst
cyst aspiration
cyst content
cyst fenestration
cyst puncture device
cyst wall
cystadenocarcinoma
cystadenoma
  hyperplastic cystadenoma
  serous cystadenoma
cystadenoma lymphomatosum
cystauchenotomy
cystectasia
cystectasy
cystectomy
  Bartholin cystectomy
  ovarian cystectomy
  partial cystectomy
  pilonidal cystectomy
  radical cystectomy
  salvage cystectomy
  subtotal cystectomy
  thyroglossal duct cystectomy
  total cystectomy
  vulvovaginal cystectomy
cystenterostomy
  direct cystenterostomy
  endoscopic cystenterostomy
  surgical cystogastrostomy
cystic acne
cystic acute inflammation
cystic adenocarcinoma
cystic adenoid epithelioma
cystic adenomatoid
    malformation (CAM)
cystic artery
cystic bone lesion
cystic breast
cystic cancer
cystic carcinoma
cystic cataract
cystic cavity
cystic change
cystic chronic inflammation
cystic dilatation
cystic dilation
cystic disease
cystic duct
cystic duct catheter clamp

cystic duct catheterization
cystic duct cholangiogram
cystic duct choledochoscopy
cystic duct forceps
cystic duct lumen
cystic duct scoop
cystic duct stump leak
cystic duct-infundibulum
    junction
cystic enlargement
cystic fibroma
cystic form
cystic goiter
cystic granulomatous inflammation
cystic hernia
cystic hidradenoma
cystic hook
cystic hygroma
cystic hyperplasia
cystic kidney
cystic kidney disease
cystic lesion
cystic locules
cystic lymphangioma
cystic lymphoepithelial
    AIDS-related lesion
cystic mass
cystic mastitis
cystic membrane
cystic metastasis
cystic oncocytic metaplasia
cystic plexus
cystic structure
cystic teratoma
cystic tumor
cystic vein
cystic-choledochal junction
cysticolithectomy
cysticolithotripsy
cysticorrhaphy
cysticotomy
cystidoceliotomy
cystidolaparotomy
cystidotrachelotomy
cystine calculus
cystine urinary tract stones
cystis fellea
cystitis
cystitome (*see also* cystotome)
    25G short curved cystitome
    Azar cystitome
    eye cystitome

cystitome (*continued*)
    Graefe cystitome
    Knolle cystitome
    Knolle-Kelman cystitome
    Lieppman cystitome
    McIntyre cystitome
    Nevyas cystitome
    Worth cystitome
cystlike appearance
Cysto Flex stent
Cystocath catheter
cystocatheter
cystocele
cystocele repair
cystochromoscopy
cystocolostomy
cystocope
    telescope of cystocope
    Wilhelm cystocope
cystodiaphanoscopy
cystodrain
cystoduodenostomy
    endoscopic cystoduodenostomy
    pancreatic cystoduodenostomy
cystoelytroplasty
cystoenterocele
cystoepiplocele
cystogastric fistula
cystogastrostomy
    endoscopic cystogastrostomy
cystogenic aneurysm
cystogram
    air cystogram
    excretion cystogram
    excretory cystogram
    iced cystogram
    postvoiding cystogram
    retrograde cystogram
    triple voiding cystogram
    voiding cystogram
cystography
    excretion cystography
    gravity cystography
    postvoiding cystography
cystohepatic triangle
cystohydrodistension
cystoid body
cystojejunostomy
cystolithectomy
cystolitholapaxy
    electrohydraulic
        cystolitholapaxy

cystolithotomy
cystometer
  Lewis cystometer
  Lewis recording cystometer
  recording cystometer
  Uroflo cystometer
  water cystometer
cystometer chart
cystometric study
cystometrogram (CMG)
cystometrography
cystometry
cystonephroscope
  ACMI flexible
    cystonephroscope
cystopanendoscope
cystopericystectomy
cystopexy
cystophotography
cystoplasty
  augmentation cystoplasty
  cecal cystoplasty
  Gil-Vernet ileocecal
    cystoplasty
  human lyophilized dura
    cystoplasty
  ileocecal cystoplasty
  nonsecretory sigmoid
    cystoplasty
  sigmoid cystoplasty
cystoplasty augmentation
cystoproctostomy
cystopyelogram
cystopyelography
cystoradium insertion
cystorectostomy
cystoreductive surgery
cystoresectoscope
  ALR cystoresectoscope
  anterior-posterior
    cystoresectoscope
  Damon-Julian
    cystoresectoscope
  Julian cystoresectoscope
cystorrhaphy
cystosarcoma
cystosarcoma phylloides
cystoscope
  ACMI cystoscope
  Albarran cystoscope
  Beard cystoscope
  Braasch cystoscope

cystoscope (*continued*)
  Braasch direct catheterization
    cystoscope
  Braasch direct cystoscope
  Braasch-Kaplan direct-vision
    cystoscope
  Brown-Buerger cystoscope
  Broyles retrograde cystoscope
  Butterfield cystoscope
  Connell cystoscope
  convertible cystoscope
  direct catheterizing
    cystoscope
  direct-vision cystoscope
  Dourmashkin cystoscope
  female cystoscope
  fiberoptic cystoscope
  Foroblique cystoscope
  French Brown-Buerger
    cystoscope
  French cystoscope
  French Wappler cystoscope
  Graefe cystoscope
  Holth cystoscope
  infant cystoscope
  Judd cystoscope
  Kelly cystoscope
  Kidd cystoscope
  Kirwin cystoscope
  Laidley cystoscope
  Laidley double-catheterizing
    cystoscope
  Leiter cystoscope
  Lowsley-Peterson cystoscope
  McCarthy cystoscope
  McCarthy-Campbell
    cystoscope
  McCarthy-Campbell miniature
    cystoscope
  McCarthy Foroblique
    panendoscope cystoscope
  McCarthy-Peterson
    cystoscope
  McCrae cystoscope
  Miller cystoscope
  Morganstern continuous-flow
    operating cystoscope
  National cystoscope
  National general-purpose
    cystoscope
  Nesbit cystoscope
  obturator cystoscope

cystoscope (*continued*)
  Olympus cystoscope
  Olympus fiberoptic
    cystoscope
  Olympus neonatal cystoscope
  Otis bulb cystoscope
  Otis-Brown cystoscope
  Ravich convertible cystoscope
  Ravich cystoscope
  sheath cystoscope
  Storz cystoscope
  Storz direct-vision cystoscope
  Storz suprapubic cystoscope
  suprapubic cystoscope
  Surgitek graduated cystoscope
  Universal cystoscope
  Wappler cystoscope
  Wheeler cystoscope
  Wilder cystoscope
  Young cystoscope
cystoscope cord
cystoscope obturator
cystoscope sheath
cystoscope tip
cystoscope-urethroscope
cystoscope-urethroscope
    adapter
cystoscopic biopsy
cystoscopic connecting nipple
cystoscopic cord
cystoscopic electrocautery
cystoscopic electrode
cystoscopic electrohydraulic
    lithotripsy
cystoscopic examination
cystoscopic findings
cystoscopic forceps
cystoscopic fulgurating
    electrode
cystoscopic fulguration
cystoscopic rongeur
cystoscopic scissors
cystoscopic snare
cystoscopic ulcer
cystoscopic urography
cystoscopy
  ileobladder cystoscopy
  percutaneous fetal cystoscopy
  steerable cystoscopy
  virtual cystoscopy
cystoscopy and dilatation
cystostomy

Spivack cystostomy
suprapubic cystostomy
trocar cystostomy
tubeless cystostomy
cystostomy tube
cystotome (*see also* cystitome)
  Alcon cystotome
  Atkinson 25-G short curved
    cystotome
  Beard cystotome
  Beaver Ocu-1 curved
    cystotome
  Blumenthal irrigating
    cystotome
  Capsitome cystotome
  double-cutting sharp
    cystotome
  Drews cystotome
  formed nonirrigating
    cystotome
  Graefe cystotome
  Graefe flexible cystotome
  guarded irrigating cystotome
  Holth cystotome
  irrigating cystotome
  Kellman cystotome
  Kelman cystotome
  Knapp cystotome
  knife cannula cystotome
  knife cystotome
  Knolle-Kelman cannulated
    cystotome
  Knolle-Kelman sharp
    cystotome
  Kratz cystotome
  Lewicky formed cystotome
  Lieppman sharp cystotome
  Look cystotome
  McIntyre guarded cystotome
  Mendez cystotome
  Mendez ultrasonic cystotome
  Moorfields cystotome
  Neuhann cystotome
  Nevyas double sharp cystotome
  Sharp point-tip cystotome
  side-cutting irrigating cystotome
  Visatec cystotome
  Visitec cystotome
  Visitec double-cutting
    cystotome
  von Graefe cystotome
  Wheeler cystotome

cystotome (*continued*)
   Wilder cystotome
   Zawadzki cystotome
cystotome (*see also* cystitome)
cystotomy
   longitudinal cystotomy
   suprapubic cystotomy
cystotrachelotomy
cystotrocar
cystoureterogram
cystoureterolithotomy
cystourethral suspension
cystourethrogram
   voiding cystourethrogram
      (VCUG)
cystourethrography
cystourethropexy
   In-Fast cystourethropexy
   obturator shelf
      cystourethropexy
   Pereyra-Raz cystourethropexy
   vaginal cystourethropexy
cystourethroplasty
   Kropp cystourethroplasty
   Leadbetter cystourethroplasty
cystourethroscope
   ACMI cystourethroscope
   ACMI microlens
      cystourethroscope
   Foroblique cystourethroscope
   Microlens cystourethroscope
   O'Donoghue
      cystourethroscope
   Wappler microlens
      cystourethroscope
cystourethroscope bridge
cystourethroscope parts
cystourethroscopy
Cytobrush biopsy
Cytobrush Plus
Cytobrush Plus cell collector
Cytobrush Plus endocervical
   cell sampler
Cytobrush spatula
cytocidal
cytokeratin filament
cytokeratin marker
cytologic abnormality
cytologic biopsy
cytologic diagnosis
cytologic evaluation

cytologic examination
cytologic, cytological
cytological assessment
cytological biopsy
cytological brush
cytology
   aspiration biopsy cytology
      (ABC)
   brush cytology
   endoscopic brush cytology
   endoscopic fine-needle
      aspiration cytology
   endoscopic ultrasonography-
      guided cytology
   fine-needle aspiration
      cytology (FNAC)
   gastric cytology
   guided-needle aspiration
      cytology
   intraoperative touch prep
      cytology
cytology examination
cytomegalovirus-positive
   donor
Cytopick endocervical and
   uterovaginal cell collector
cytoplasmic membrane
cytoreductive surgery
cytoscope
   direct cytoscope
   double-catheterizing
      cytoscope
Cytoxan
Czaja-McCaffrey rigid stent
   introducer-endoscope
Czapski microscope
Czermak eye knife
Czermak keratome
Czermak operation
Czermak pterygium operation
Czermak spaces
Czerny herniorrhaphy
Czerny incision
Czerny operation
Czerny rectal speculum
Czerny suture technique
Czerny sutures
Czerny tenaculum forceps
Czerny-Lembert suture
   technique
Czerny-Lembert sutures

D chromosome ring syndrome
D line
D point
D syringe
D&C (dilation and curettage;
    dilatation and curettage)
  diagnostic D&C
  fractional D&C
  suction D&C
  therapeutic D&C
D&E (dilation and evacuation)
D&G sutures
D&N (distant and near)
D.A.D. mattress
D2 dissection
D2 lymphadenectomy
D2 resection
D3 dialyzer
Dacomed Omni Phase penile
    prosthesis
Dacomed Rigidscan
Dacomed Snap-Gauge
Dacron arterial prosthesis
Dacron batting
Dacron bifurcation prosthesis
Dacron bolstered sutures
Dacron catheter
Dacron cuff
Dacron fiber-coating coil
Dacron graft
Dacron graft clamp
Dacron implant
Dacron intracardiac patch
Dacron knitted graft
Dacron mesh
Dacron netting
Dacron onlay patch graft
Dacron patch graft
Dacron pledget
Dacron preclotted graft
Dacron prosthesis
Dacron retraction tape
Dacron Sauvage graft

Dacron Sauvage patch
Dacron shield
Dacron stent
Dacron sutures
Dacron tape
Dacron tightly woven graft
Dacron traction sutures
Dacron tube graft
Dacron tubular graft
Dacron valve prosthesis
Dacron vascular prosthesis
Dacron velour graft
Dacron vessel prosthesis
Dacron Weave Knit graft
Dacron-backed implant
Dacron-covered stent
Dacron-covered stent graft
dacryoadenectomy
dacryoadenotomy
dacryocystectomy
dacryocystography
dacryocystorhinostomy (DCR)
  endonasal
      dacryocystorhinostomy
  endoscopic
      dacryocystorhinostomy
dacryocystorhinostomy cannula
dacryocystorhinostomy needle
dacryocystorhinostomy
    procedure
dacryocystorhinostomy
    retractor
dacryocystorhinostomy
    trephine
dacryocystostomy
  Arruga dacryocystostomy
  Hogan dacryocystostomy
dacryocystosyringotomy
dacryocystotomy
  Ammon dacryocystotomy
dacryolith
dacryorhinocystostomy
dacryostenosis

dacryostomy
   Arroyo dacryostomy
   Arruga dacryostomy
   Dupuy-Dutemps dacryostomy
   Kuhnt dacryostomy
   Rowinski dacryostomy
dacryotrephine
dactyl speech
dactylitis
dactylocostal rhinoplasty
dactylology
dactylolysis
dactylolysis spontanea
Daems bronchial clamp
Dafilon sutures
Dagger dilator
Daggett procedure
Dagnini reflex
Dagradi esophageal variceal
   classification
Dagrofil sutures
Dahlgren iris scissors
Dahlgren rongeur
Dahlgren-Hudson cranial
   forceps
Dahlman diverticulum excision
Daicoff needle-pulling forceps
Daicoff vascular forceps
Daig atrial screw-in lead
Daig pacemaker
Daig screw-in lead
Dailey operation
Daily cataract needle
Daily cataract operation
Daily cooling jacket
Daily eye knife
Daily fixation hook
Daily keratome
Daily sutures
Dainer-Kaupp needle holder
Daines-Hodgson anastomosis
Daisy I&A instrument
Daisy vitrectomy machine
Daiwa dental needle
Dakin catheter
Dakin dressing
Dakin fluid
Dakin solution
Dakin tube
Dakin tubing
Dalbo extracoronal attachment
Dalbo extracoronal unit

Dalbo stud attachment
Dalbo stud unit
Dale abdominal binder
Dale abdominal support
Dale ankle support
Dale femoral-popliteal
   anastomosis forceps
Dale first rib rongeur
Dale Foley catheter holder
Dale Foley catheter legband
   holder
Dale forceps
Dale gastrostomy tube holder
Dale knee support
Dale nasal dressing holder
Dale oxygen cannula support
Dale pelvic support
Dale rib support
Dale secondary wound dressing
   and holder
Dale surgical binder
Dale tapeless wound dressing
   holder
Dale tennis elbow support
Dale thoracic rongeur
Dale tracheostomy tube holder
Dale traction
Dale ventilator tubing support
Dale wrist support
Dalen-Fuchs nodules
Dalgleish operation
Dalkon shield
Dalkon shield intrauterine
   device
Dalla Bona attachment
Dalla Bona ball and socket
   abutment
Dallas lens-inserting forceps
Dallas operation
Dallas retractor
D'Allesandro clamp
D'Allesandro serial suture-
   holding forceps
Dall-Miles cable
Dall-Miles cerclage wire
Dallop-type fascial prosthesis
Dalrymple sign
dam
   nonlatex dental dam
   post dam
   rubber dam
   rubber punch dam

dam drain
damage
  actinic damage
  anterior cervical surgery vocal
    cord damage
  axonal damage
  catastrophic brain damage
  cellular damage
  end-organ damage
  endothelial damage
  epidermal actinic damage
  irradiation damage
  irreversible brain damage
  lethal damage
  liver damage
  myocardial damage
  nerve damage
  nervous damage
  obturator nerve damage
  operative damage
  permanent damage
  postsurgical nervous damage
  projection fiber damage
  radiation damage
  soft-tissue damage
  structural damage
  subretinal damage
  sun and chemical
    combination damage
  tissue damage
Damascus Disk
Damato curved catheter
D'Amato sign
Damian graft procedure
Damian lumen finder
Dammann-Muller operation
Damon clasp
Damon Scan Mate
Damon-Julian cystoresectoscope
Damon-Julian ring remover
damped waveform
Damshek needle
Damshek sternal trephine
Damshek trephine
Damus-Kaye-Stansel operation
Damus-Kaye-Stansel procedure
Damus-Stansel-Kaye procedure
Dan chalazion forceps
Dana operation
Dana rhizotomy
Dana shoulder prosthesis
Danberg forceps

Danberg iris forceps
Dandy arterial forceps
Dandy clamp
Dandy clip
Dandy hemostatic forceps
Dandy hook
Dandy maneuver
Dandy myocutaneous scalp flap
Dandy needle
Dandy nerve hook
Dandy neurosurgical scissors
Dandy operation
Dandy probe
Dandy rhizotomy
Dandy scalp forceps
Dandy scalp hemostat
Dandy scalp hemostatic forceps
Dandy scissors
Dandy suction tube
Dandy trigeminal scissors
Dandy ventricular needle
Dandy ventriculostomy
Dandy-Cairns brain needle
Dandy-Cairns ventricular needle
Dandy-Kolodny hemostatic
    forceps
Dandy-Walker deformity
Dandy-Walker malformation
Dandy-Walker syndrome
Danek cervical fusion plate
Danek rod
Danek self-retaining retractor
Danforth fetal operation
Danforth operation
Dangel slip knot
Dan-Gradle cilial forceps
Dan-Gradle ciliary forceps
Daniel clamp
Daniel colostomy clamp
Daniel double-punch laser
    laparoscope
Daniel iliac bone graft
Daniel operation
Daniels adenotome
Daniels hemostatic
    tonsillectome
Daniels operation
Daniels tonometer
Daniels tonsillectome
Danis retractor
Danis-Weber ankle fracture
    classification (types A, B, C)

Danis-Weber fracture
Danker-Wohlk contact lens
Dann respirator
Dannheim eye implant
Danniflex CPM machine
Dann-Jennings mouth gag
Dansac colostomy irrigation
    set
Dansac ileal pouch
Dansac Karaya seal pouch
Dansac ostomy pouch
Dantec rotating disk flowmeter
Danus-Fontan procedure
Danus-Stanzel repair
Dap II biopsy needle guide
Darby surgical shoe
d'Arcet metal
Darco medical-surgical shoe and
    toe alignment splint
Darco shoe
Darco toe alignment splint
DarcoGel ankle brace
Dardik biograft
Dardik Biograft vein graft
Dardik clamp
Dardik human graft
Dardik umbilical graft
Dardik umbilical prosthesis
Dardik vein substitute
Dardour flap
Dardour lateral flap
Darier disease
Darier sign
Darier-White disease
Darin intraocular implant lens
Darin lens
darkening of nipples
darkfield examination
darkfield microscope
Darling capsulotome
Darling capsulotomy
Darmstruck lymphoma
Darox cutaneous thoracic patch
    electrode
Darrach elevator
Darrach procedure
Darrach resection
Darrach retractor
Darrach technique
Darrach ulnar resection
Darrach wrist arthroplasty
Darrach-McLaughlin approach

Darrach-McLaughlin shoulder
    technique
dart
    Arthrex meniscal dart
    Clearfix meniscal dart
    intranasal darts
Dart coronary stent
Dart pacemaker
Dartigues kidney-elevating
    forceps
Dartigues uterine-elevating
    forceps
darting incision
dartoid tissue
dartos fascia
dartos fasciocutaneous flap
dartos muscle
dartos musculocutaneous flap
dartos pouch
dartos pouch procedure
Darwin tubercle
darwinian apex
darwinian ear
darwinian tubercle
Das Gupta procedure
Das Gupta scapula procedure
Das Gupta scapular excision
Dash pacemaker
Dash single-chamber rate-
    adaptic pacemaker
dashboard dislocation
dashboard fracture
dashboard perineum
Dasher guidewire
DaSilva dermatome
D'Assumpcao clamp
D'Assumpcao rhytidoplasty
    marker
Dastoor erysiphake
Datascope 300 pulse oximeter
Datascope balloon
Datascope catheter
Datascope percutaneous
    translucent balloon
    catheter
Datascope intra-aortic balloon
    pump
Datascope intra-aortic balloon
    pump catheter
Datascope pulse oximeter
Datascope intra-aortic balloon
    pump

Datascope true sheathless
    catheter
Datex infrared CO_2 monitor
Datex model pulse oximeter
Datta procedure
Dattner needle
Daubenspeck bone curet
Daubenton angle
Daubenton line
Daubenton plane
d'Aubigne femoral
    reconstruction
d'Aubigne operator
d'Aubigne prosthesis
d'Aubigne resection
    reconstruction
daughter cyst
Dautrey osteotome
Dautrey chisel
Dautrey osteotome
Dautrey osteotomy
Dautrey retractor
Dautrey-Munro osteotome
Davat operation for varicocele
Davey-Rorabeck-Fowler
    decompression technique
David blade
David drainage
David interlocking sound
David Letterman sign
David pharyngolaryngectomy
    tube
David rectal speculum
David technique
David-Baker clamp
David-Baker eyelid retractor
David-Baker lip clamp
David-Crowe tongue blade
Davidoff blade
Davidoff cordotomy knife
Davidoff knife
Davidoff retractor
Davidoff trigeminal retractor
Davidson bur
Davidson clamp
Davidson collector
Davidson erector spinae retractor
Davidson forceps
Davidson muscle clamp
Davidson periosteal elevator
Davidson pulmonary vessel
    clamp

Davidson pulmonary vessel
    forceps
Davidson retractor
Davidson scapular retractor
Davidson syringe
Davidson thoracic trocar
Davidson trocar
Davidson vessel clamp
Davidson-Mathieu elevator
Davidson-Mathieu raspatory
Davidson-Mathieu-Alexander
    elevator rasp
Davidson-Mathieu-Alexander
    periosteal elevator
Davidson-Sauerbruch elevator
Davidson-Sauerbruch rasp
Davidson-Sauerbruch rib
    raspatory
Davidson-Sauerbruch-Doyen
    elevator
Davidson-Sauerbruch-Doyen
    periosteal elevator
Daviel cataract extraction
Daviel chalazion curet
Daviel chalazion knife
Daviel knife
Daviel lens loupe
Daviel lens spoon
Daviel loupe
Daviel operation
Daviel scoop
Daviel spoon
Davies-Colley operation
Davila atrial clamp
Davis aneurysm clamp
Davis aortic aneurysm clamp
Davis bayonet forceps
Davis bone skid
Davis Bovie cautery
Davis brain retractor
Davis brain spatula
Davis bronchoscope
Davis capsule forceps
Davis catheter
Davis clamp
Davis coagulating forceps
Davis coagulation electrode
Davis composite flap of conchal
    cartilage
Davis conductor
Davis diathermy forceps
Davis dissector

Davis double-ended retractor
Davis drainage technique
Davis electrode
Davis forceps
Davis foreign body spud
Davis fusion
Davis graft
Davis hemostat
Davis hip arthrodesis
Davis hook
Davis hysteropexy
Davis implant
Davis knife
Davis knife needle
Davis lamp
Davis loop stone dislodger
Davis metacarpal splint
Davis modified Finochietto rib
    spreader
Davis monopolar bayonet
    forceps
Davis mouth gag
Davis muscle-pedicle graft
Davis needle
Davis needle holder
Davis nerve separator
Davis operation
Davis periosteal elevator
Davis pillar retractor
Davis pin
Davis prosthesis
Davis raspatory
Davis retractor
Davis rhytidectomy scissors
Davis rib spreader
Davis ring mouth gag
Davis saw conductor
Davis saw guide
Davis scissors
Davis separator
Davis skid
Davis sound
Davis spatula
Davis splint
Davis spud
Davis sterilizing forceps
Davis stone dislodger
Davis thoracic tissue forceps
Davis tonsillar hemostat
Davis tonsillar knife
Davis tonsillar needle
Davis tooth plate

Davis trephine
Davis uterine suspension
Davis-Crowe mouth gag
Davis-Crowe tongue blade
Davis-Geck eye sutures
Davis-Geck incision
Davis-Geck surgical stapler
Davis-Geck sutures
Davis-Kitlowski otoplasty
Davis-Kitlowski procedure
Davis-Rockey incision
Davol bag
Davol canal wall punch
Davol catheter
Davol colon tube
Davol dermatome
Davol drain
Davol forceps
Davol microrongeur
Davol pacemaker introducer
Davol pillows
Davol punch
Davol rongeur
Davol rongeur forceps
Davol rubber catheter
Davol sterile female cath kit
Davol sterile irrigation tray
Davol sterile red rubber catheter
Davol suction drain
Davol suction tube
Davol sump drain
Davol tourniquet
Davol tube
Davol-Simon dermatome
Davy speculum
Davy surgical button
Davydov procedure
DAW (dispense as written)
DAWG procedure
Dawson-Yuhl curet
Dawson-Yuhl impactor
Dawson-Yuhl osteotome
Dawson-Yuhl periosteal
    elevator
Dawson-Yuhl rongeur forceps
Dawson-Yuhl spinal instruments
Dawson-Yuhl suction tube
Dawson-Yuhl-Cone curet
Dawson-Yuhl-Kerrison rongeur
Dawson-Yuhl-Kerrison rongeur
    forceps
Dawson-Yuhl-Leksell rongeur

Dawson-Yuhl-Leksell rongeur
 forceps
Dawson-Yuhl-Key elevator
Day attic cannula
Day cannula
Day earhook
Day hook
Day knife
Day stapler
Day tonsillar knife
DayTimer carpal tunnel support
Daytona cervical orthosis
DCP (dynamic compression
 plate)
DCR (dacryocystorhinostomy)
DCS (dynamic condylar screw)
DCS implant (dorsal column
 stimulator/stimulation
 implant)
D-D anastomosis
DDD (degenerative disk disease)
DDD pacemaker (dual-sensing,
 pacing, -mode)
DDI mode pacemaker
DDR (direct digital radiography)
DDT lock screw inserter
DDV ligator
De Alvarez forceps
de Andrade-MacNab technique
de Grandmont operation
de Groot classification
De Juan forceps
De La Caffiniere
 trapeziometacarpal
 prosthesis
de la Camp sign
de la Cruz classification of
 congenital aural atresia
de la Plaza transconjunctival
 retractor
De La Vega lens pusher
De La Vega vitreous-aspirating
 cannula
de Lapersonne operation
De Morgan spots
de Musset sign
de Mussy point
de novo lesion
de novo needle-knife technique
de novo tumor
De Paco implant
De Paco prosthesis

de Pezzer (*see also* Pezzer)
de Pezzer catheter
de Pezzer drain
de Pezzer mushroom-tipped
 catheter
de Pezzer self-retaining catheter
de Quervain (*see also* Quervain)
de Quervain fracture
de Quervain granulomatous
 thyroiditis
de Quervain incision
de Quervain release
de Quervain syndrome
de Quervain tenolysis
de Quervain tenosynovitis
de Signeux dilator
de Vincentiis operation
dead bowel
dead hand
dead space
deafferentation
 bilateral vestibular
  deafferentation
 total unilateral vestibular
  deafferentation
 vestibular deafferentation
deafferentation pain syndrome
deaffrication
deafness
 Mondini deafness
 nerve deafness
 neural deafness
 sensorineural deafness
de-aired graft
de-airing procedure
Dean antral needle
Dean antral rasp
Dean antral trocar
Dean applicator
Dean blade
Dean bone rongeur
Dean capsulotomy knife
Dean cotton applicator
Dean curved eye knife
Dean ear snare
Dean fluorosis index
Dean forceps
Dean hemostat
Dean iris knife
Dean iris knife needle
Dean iris needle
Dean knife

Dean knife holder
Dean knife needle
Dean MacDonald clamp
Dean MacDonald gastric
 resection clamp
Dean mastoid rongeur
Dean needle
Dean needle knife
Dean periosteal elevator
Dean periosteotome
Dean rasp
Dean raspatory
Dean rongeur
Dean scissors
Dean tonsil hemostat
Dean tonsillar forceps
Dean tonsillar hemostatic
 forceps
Dean tonsillar knife
Dean tonsillar scissors
Dean trocar
Dean wash tube
Deane tube
Deane unconstrained knee
 prosthesis
Dean-Senturia needle
Dean-Shallcross tonsil-seizing
 forceps
Dean-Trusler scissors
Dearor model catheter
dearterialization
Deaver blade
Deaver clamp
Deaver hemostat
Deaver incision
Deaver retractor
Deaver scissors
Deaver skin incision
Deaver T-drain
Deaver T-tube
Deaver tube
DeBakey aortic aneurysm clamp
DeBakey aortic clamp
DeBakey aortic exclusion clamp
DeBakey aortic forceps
DeBakey arterial clamp
DeBakey arterial forceps
DeBakey Autraugrip forceps
DeBakey ball-valve prosthesis
DeBakey Beaver blade
DeBakey blade
DeBakey bulldog clamp

DeBakey cardiovascular needle
 holder
DeBakey chest retractor
DeBakey clamp
DeBakey classification
DeBakey coarctation clamp
DeBakey cross-action bulldog
 clamp
DeBakey curved peripheral
 vascular clamp
DeBakey dissecting forceps
DeBakey endarterectomy
 scissors
DeBakey forceps
DeBakey graft
DeBakey heart pump
 oxygenator
DeBakey heart valve
DeBakey implant
DeBakey infant and child rib
 spreader
DeBakey intraluminal stripper
DeBakey ligature carrier
DeBakey miniature
 multipurpose clamp
DeBakey multipurpose clamp
DeBakey needle
DeBakey needle holder
DeBakey patent ductus clamp
DeBakey pediatric clamp
DeBakey peripheral vascular
 clamp
DeBakey pickup
DeBakey prosthesis
DeBakey prosthetic valve
DeBakey retractor
DeBakey rib spreader
DeBakey right-angled
 multipurpose clamp
DeBakey ring-handled bulldog
 clamp
DeBakey scissors
DeBakey S-shaped peripheral
 vascular clamp
DeBakey stitch scissors
DeBakey stripper
DeBakey suction tube
DeBakey tangential clamp
DeBakey tangential occlusion
 clamp
DeBakey tangential occlusion
 forceps

DeBakey thoracic forceps
DeBakey tissue forceps
DeBakey tucker
DeBakey tunneler
DeBakey valve hook
DeBakey valve prosthesis
DeBakey valve scissors
DeBakey vascular clamp
DeBakey vascular dilator
DeBakey vascular forceps
DeBakey vascular prosthesis
DeBakey vascular scissors
DeBakey vascular tissue forceps
DeBakey Vital needle holder
DeBakey-Adson suction tube
DeBakey-Bahnson clamp
DeBakey-Bahnson forceps
DeBakey-Bahnson vascular
    clamp
DeBakey-Bainbridge clamp
DeBakey-Bainbridge forceps
DeBakey-Bainbridge vascular
    clamp
DeBakey-Bainbridge vascular
    forceps
DeBakey-Balfour retractor
DeBakey-Beck clamp
DeBakey-Beck multipurpose
    forceps
DeBakey-Coloviras-Rumel
    thoracic forceps
DeBakey-Cooley anastomosis
    forceps
DeBakey-Cooley cardiovascular
    forceps
DeBakey-Cooley dilator
DeBakey-Cooley forceps
DeBakey-Cooley retractor
DeBakey-Cooley valve dilator
DeBakey-Cooley-Deaver
    retractor
DeBakey-Crafoord vascular
    clamp
DeBakey-Creech aneurysm repair
DeBakey-Creech manner
DeBakey-Creech procedure
DeBakey-Derra anastomosis
    clamp
DeBakey-Derra anastomosis
    forceps
DeBakey-Diethrich coronary
    artery forceps

DeBakey-Diethrich vascular
    forceps
DeBakey-Harken auricle clamp
DeBakey-Harken auricular clamp
DeBakey-Howard aortic
    aneurysm clamp
DeBakey-Howard aortic
    aneurysmal clamp
DeBakey-Kay aortic clamp
DeBakey-Kelly hemostatic
    forceps
DeBakey-Liddicoat vascular
    forceps
DeBakey-McQuigg-Mixter
    bronchial clamp
DeBakey-Metzenbaum dissecting
    scissors
DeBakey-Mixter thoracic forceps
DeBakey-Péan cardiovascular
    forceps
DeBakey-Potts scissors
DeBakey-Rankin hemostatic
    forceps
DeBakey-Reynolds anastomosis
    forceps
DeBakey-Rumel thoracic forceps
DeBakey-Satinsky vena cava
    clamp
DeBakey-Semb clamp
DeBakey-Semb forceps
DeBakey-Semb ligature-carrier
    clamp
DeBakey-Surgitool prosthetic
    valve
DeBakey-type aortic dissection
debanding
DeBastiani distractor
DeBastiani external fixator
Debeyre rotator cuff operation
Debeyre-Patte-Elmelik rotator
    cuff technique
deblocking
Deboisans drain
debonding pliers (DP)
Debove membrane
Debove tube
debride
debrided bone surface
debrided necrotic tissue
debridement
    crown debridement
    dental debridement

debridement (*continued*)
   enzymatic debridement
   extensive debridement
debridement
   revision and debridement
   surgical debridement
debridement and irrigation
debridement and revision
debridement needle
debridement of bruised tissue
debridement of compound skull
      fracture
debridement of necrotic tissue
debridement of wound
debridement technique
debrider
   corneal debrider
   Nordson debrider
   Sauer debrider
debris
   cellular debris
   desquamating debris
   Malassez debris
   necrotic debris
debris index
Debrisan dressing
debris-retaining acetabular
      reamer
debubbling procedure
debulking
   ovarian carcinoma debulking
   secondary debulking
   surgical debulking
debulking of tumor
debulking operation
debulking procedure
debulking surgery
Debut ear piercing kit
decalcification
decalcified freeze-dried bone
      allograft (DFDBA)
decalcified freeze-dried cortical
      bone (DFDCB)
decalcify
decamethonium bromide
      anesthetic agent
decamethonium iodide
      anesthetic agent
decannulation
   femoral artery decannulation
   femoral vein decannulation
decannulation of aorta

decannulation of femoral artery
      and vein
decannulation of vena cava
decannulation of ventricle
decannulation plug
decapitation
decapitation hook
decapitation scissors
decapolar electrode catheter
decapolar pacing catheter
decapsulation
decapsulation of kidney
Decasone
decayed teeth
decelerated breathing
deceleration
   fetal decelerations
   late decelerations
deceleration injury
deceleration of heart rate
decellularized human dermis
decentered lens
decentration
decentration of lenses
decerebrate posturing
decerebrate rigidity
decerebration
decidua basalis
decidua capsularis
decidua menstrualis
decidua parietalis
decidua reflexa
decidua serotina
decidua vera
decidual endometritis
decidual fragment
decidual membrane
decidual tissue
deciduous (D)
deciduous cuspid
deciduous placenta
deciduous skin
deciduous teeth
deciduous tissue
deciliter
deck plate
Decker culdoscope
Decker culdoscopy
Decker microforceps
Decker microrongeur
Decker microsurgical forceps
Decker microsurgical rongeur

Decker microsurgical scissors
Decker operation
Decker pituitary rongeur
Decker retractor
Decker scissors
declamping
declamping phenomenon
declamping shock
declination angle
declinator
declive
declotting
decompensated liver disease
decompensation
  circulatory decompensation
  hepatic decompensation
  vascular decompensation
decompensation injury
decompressed compartment
decompression
  3-wall orbital decompression
  anterior retroperitoneal
    decompression
  balloon decompression
  bone graft decompression
  cardiac decompression
  carpal tunnel
    decompression
  cerebral decompression
  Dickson-Wright orbit
    decompression
  endolymphatic sac
    decompression
  endoscopic biliary
    decompression
  endoscopic carpal tunnel
    decompression
  endoscopic decompression
  endoscopic orbital
    decompression
  explosive decompression
  extensive posterior
    decompression
  facial nerve decompression
  gaseous decompression
  gastric decompression
  hydrostatic decompression
  internal decompression
  intestinal decompression
  jugular bulb decompression
  microvascular decompression
    (MVD)

decompression (*continued*)
  Naffziger-Poppen-Craig orbital
    decompression
  nerve decompression
  orbital decompression
  paraclavicular thoracic outlet
    decompression
  percutaneous transhepatic
    decompression (PTD)
  pericardial decompression
  portal decompression
  posterior fossa
    decompression
  retroperitoneal
    decompression
  RFAC-assisted microdisc
    decompression
  Rowbatham orbital
    decompression
  sac-vein decompression
  selective portal
    decompression
  spinal decompression
  subfascial carpal tunnel
    decompression
  suboccipital decompression
  subtemporal decompression
  surgical decompression
  surgical portal decompression
  transantral orbital
    decompression
  transconjunctival endoscopic
    orbital decompression
  transduodenal endoscopic
    decompression
  trigeminal decompression
  tube decompression
  variceal decompression
  vein decompression
  vertebral body
    decompression
  Walsh-Ogura orbital
    decompression
  wide decompression
decompression catheter
decompression colostomy
decompression fasciotomy
decompression incision
decompression jejunostomy
decompression laminectomy
decompression of abdomen
decompression of heart

decompression of imperforate
anus
decompression of orbit
decompression of pericardium
decompression of rectum
decompression of spinal cord
decompression operation
decompression rhachotomy
decompression technique
decompression-feeding catheter
decompressive colostomy
decompressive craniotomy
decompressive enteroclysis
catheter
decompressive laminectomy
decompressive retractor
decompressive surgery
decompressive trocar
decompressive tube
decompressor (see also
compressor)
Andrews decompressor
Andrews-Pynchon
decompressor
Balmer decompressor
Beatty decompressor
Blakesley decompressor
Bosworth decompressor
Chamberlain decompressor
Colver-Dawson decompressor
Coston eye decompressor
Dorsey decompressor
Dunn decompressor
Farlow decompressor
Fraser decompressor
Granberry decompressor
Hamilton decompressor
Israel decompressor
Jobson-Pynchon decompressor
Kellogg decompressor
Layman decompressor
Lewis decompressor
Mullins decompressor
Pirquet decompressor
Proetz decompressor
Pynchon decompressor
Savage intestinal
decompressor
Schepens eye decompressor
Sims vaginal decompressor
Titus decompressor
Wieder decompressor

deconditioning
decorative tattoo
decortical position
decorticate posturing
decorticate rigidity
decorticated flap
decortication
arterial decortication
cerebral decortication
chemical decortication
enzymatic decortication
laparoscopic cyst
decortication
renal cyst decortication
renal decortication
reversible decortication
decortication bur
decortication of heart
decortication of kidney
decortication of lung
decortication technique
DeCourcy clamp
DeCourcy goiter clamp
decreased peristalsis
decrescendo early systolic
murmur
decrescendo murmur
decrescent arteriosclerosis
DeCube therapeutic mattress
Decubi-Care pad dressing
decubital gangrene
decubital necrosis
decubitus
decubitus calculus
decubitus cushion
decubitus film
decubitus position
decubitus ulcer
decussation
dorsal tegmental decussation
Forel decussation
fountain decussation
Held decussation
Meynet decussation
motor decussation
oculomotor decussation
optic decussation
pyramidal decussation
rubrospinal decussation
tectospinal decussation
ventral tegmental decussation
Wernekinck decussation

Deddish-Potts intestinal forceps
dedentition
dedicated push enteroscope
dedifferentiated chordoma
Dedo laryngoscope
Dedo laser laryngoscope
Dedo laser retractor
Dedo machine
Dedo-Jako laryngoscope
Dedo-Jako microlaryngoscope
Dedo-Pilling laryngoscope
Dedo-Webb cutter
Dee elbow hinge
Dee elbow prosthesis
deep abdominal complication
    (DAC)
deep abdominal reflexes
deep abdominal retractor
deep abdominal tenderness
deep and regular respirations
deep artery of clitoris
deep artery of penis
deep artery of tongue
deep articular aorta
deep auricular artery
deep bite
deep blunt rake retractor
deep brachial artery
deep brain extension
deep brain lead
deep brain stimulation
deep cervical artery
deep cervical fascia
deep cervical jugulodigastric
    nodes
deep cervical vein
deep chest therapy
deep circumflex iliac artery
deep circumflex iliac artery-iliac
    crest flap
deep circumflex iliac vein
deep closure
deep coma
deep crural arch
deep Deaver retractor
deep destruction
deep dissection
deep dorsal vein
deep epigastric vessels
deep external pudendal artery
deep facial lymph node
deep facial vein

deep fascia
deep femoral artery
deep femoral vein
deep flexor muscle
deep frostbite
deep hemangioma
deep iliac dissection
deep inferior epigastric artery
deep inferior epigastric vein
deep inguinal ring
deep interloop abscess
deep keratitis
deep knife
deep lamina
deep lateral node
deep layer
deep ligature carrier
deep lingual artery
deep lingual vein
deep lobectomy
deep middle cerebral artery
deep muscle
deep muscular aponeurotic
    system (DMAS)
deep nerve
deep overbite
deep palmar arch
deep palpation
deep parotid lobe
deep parotid node
deep penetrating wound
deep perineal fascia
deep perineal space
deep peroneal nerve
deep petrosal nerve
deep plane face lift
deep plantar arch
deep postanal anorectal space
deep rake retractor
deep retractor
deep scaler
deep scaling
deep space
deep spreader blade
deep structure
deep subdermal
deep suspension suture
deep tear troughs
deep temporal artery
deep temporal fascia (DTF)
deep temporal nerve
deep temporal vein

deep tendon reflexes (DTRs)
deep transverse fibers
deep transverse ligament
deep transverse muscle of
    perineum
deep tumor
deep ulceration
deep veins of clitoris
deep veins of penis
deep venous thrombosis (DVT)
deep vertical overlap
deep volar arch
deepened incision
deepened reamer
deepening pocket
de-epicardialization
de-epithelialization
    periareolar de-epithelialization
    vertical rhomboid de-
        epithelialization
de-epithelialized
de-epithelialized dermal wings
de-epithelialized local flap
de-epithelialized rectus
    abdominis muscle flap
de-epithelialized revascularized
    lateral intercostal flap
de-epithelization (*variant of*
    de-epithelialization)
deep-lobe parotid tumor
deeply anesthetized patient
deep-plane face-lift
deep-plane lift
deep-plane rhytidectomy
deep-seated infection
deep-seated lesion
deep-surgery forceps
deep-surgery scissors
deep-vessel forceps
deep-wedge biopsy
Dees holder
Dees needle
Dees operation
Dees renal needle
Dees suture needle
Dees-Young procedure
defatted
defatted skin graft
defatting
defatting of skin
defatting the umbilical stalk
defecating proctogram

defecation
defecogram
defecography
defect
    3-buttress defect
    acquired defect
    acquired ventricular septal
        defect
    alveolar bone defect
    alveolar ridge defect
    aortic septal defect
    aorticopulmonary septal
        defect
    atrial ostium primum defect
    atrial septal defect (ASD)
    atrioseptal defect (ASD)
    atrioventricular canal defect
    atrioventricular conduction
        defect (AV conduction
        defect)
    atrioventricular septal defect
    AV conduction defect
        (atrioventricular
        conduction defect)
    bandeau defect
    birth defect
    bone defect
    buccal defect
    buccal mucosal defect
    calvarial defect
    cardiac defect
    cellulitic defect
    chain-of-lakes filling defect
    chest wall defect
    clinical defect
    closure of defect
    coagulation defect
    cold defect
    combined defect
    conduction defect
    congenital birth defect
    congenital defect
    congenital heart defect (CHD)
    contiguous ventricular septal
        defect
    contour defect
    cranial base defect
    cranial defect
    cranial fossa defect
    craniotomy defect
    Crouzon craniostenotic defect
    cushion defects

defect (*continued*)
   dentinoenamel defect
   diaphragmatic defect
   direct defect
   dural defect
   endocardial cushion defect
   extirpative defect
   extradural defect
   extraoral defect
   extrinsic defect
   familial defect
   fascial defect
   filling defect
   fixed perfusion defect
   focal defect
   frondlike filling defect
   full-thickness defect
   fusion defect
   genetic defect
   Hanna classification of head
      and neck defects
      (classes A, B, C)
   heart defect
   heminasal defect
   hernia defect
   hot defect
   iatrogenic hernia defect
   indirect defect
   inferoapical defect
   infundibular ventricular septal
      defect
   inherited genetic defect
   interatrial septal defect
   intercalated defect
   interradicular osseous defect
   interventricular conduction
      defect
   interventricular septal defect
      (IVSD)
   intra-atrial conduction defect
   intrabony defect
   intraluminal filling defect
   intraoral mucosal defect
   intrinsic defect
   irradiated surgical defects
   irregular defects
   linear defect
   localized defect
   lucent defect
   luminal defect
   lytic defect
   mandibular defect

defect (*continued*)
   mass defect
   membranous ventricular
      septal defect
   Mohs defect
   motor defect
   muscular defect
   muscular ventricular septal
      defect
   myocardial conduction defect
   napkin-ring defect
   neural arch defect
   neural tube defect
   neurological defect
   obstructive airway defect
   obstructive defect
   one-buttress defect
   orbitomaxillary defect
   orbitonasomaxillary defect
   oromandibular defect
   oropharyngeal defect
   osteoarticular defect
   osteochondral defect
   osteoporotic marrow defect
   parietal defect
   pars defect
   pars flaccida defect
   patch closure of defect
   perfusion defect
   peri-infarction conduction
      defect
   perineal defect
   periodontal bony defect
   periodontal defect
   periodontal intrabony defect
   peritoneal defect
   pharyngoesophageal defect
   pinpoint gastric mucosal
      defect
   pitting defect
   plantar foot defect
   postablation defect
   postinfarction
      ventriculoseptal defect
   postinjury immunologic defect
   postresection defect
   Rastelli type A, B, C
      classification of
      atrioventricular septal defect
   reconstruction of
      maxillectomy and midfacial
      defects

defect (*continued*)
  repair of alveolar ridge defect
  repair of defect
  resorptive defect
  restrictive airway defect
  resulting defect
  reversible ischemic defect
  reversible ischemic
    neurological defect (RIND)
  reversible perfusion defect
  sacrococcygeal defect
  saddle defect
  saddle nose defect
  scintigraphic perfusion defect
  secundum atrial septal defect
  segmental bone defect
  segmental continuity defect
  septal defect
  sinus defect
  slitlike defect
  speech defect
  suboccipital dural defect
  surgical defect
  through-and-through defect
  transcatheter closure of atrial
    septal defect
  triangular defect
  tubular defect
  tumor defect
  two-buttress defect
  valvular defect
  ventilation defect
  ventilation-perfusion defect
  ventral septal defect
  ventricular defect
  ventricular septal defect (VSD)
  ventricular septal wound
    defect
  ventriculoseptal defect
  vertebral arch fusion defect
  V-Y repair of cheek defect
defect closed with sutures
deferent duct
deferentectomy
deferential artery
deferred fracture
deferred shock
defervesce
defervescence
defibrillated heart
defibrillating patient
defibrillation

defibrillation and electrical
  cardioversion
defibrillation paddle
defibrillation patch
defibrillation technique
defibrillator
  AED automatic external
    defibrillator
  AID-B defibrillator
  Angstrom II implantable
    cardioverter defibrillator
  Angstrom MD implantable
    cardioverter defibrillator
  atrial and ventricular
    implantable cardioverter
    defibrillator
  automatic external
    defibrillator (AED)
  automatic implantable
    cardiovascular defibrillator
    (AICD)
  automatic intracardiac
    defibrillator
  Birtcher defibrillator
  Cadence defibrillator
  Cadet defibrillator
  Cambridge defibrillator
  cardiac defibrillator
  Cardioserv defibrillator
  Contour LTV-135D
    defibrillator
  Contour MD defibrillator
  Contour MD implantable
    single-lead cardioverter
    defibrillator
  Contour Profile defibrillator
  Contour V-145D defibrillator
  Corbin-Farnsworth
    defibrillator
  CPI automatic implantable
    defibrillator
  Electrodyne defibrillator
  Endotak defibrillator
  FirstSave automated external
    defibrillator
  Forerunner defibrillator
  Foster defibrillator
  Gem defibrillator
  Gem implantable defibrillator
  Guidant defibrillator
  Hewlett-Packard defibrillator
  implantable atrial defibrillator

defibrillator (*continued*)
  implantable defibrillator
  Intec implantable defibrillator
  IPCO-Partridge defibrillator
  Jewel AF implantable
    defibrillator
  Lifepak defibrillator
  Marquette Responder
    1500 multifunctional
    defibrillator
  Medtronic defibrillator
  Medtronic implantable
    cardioverter defibrillator
  Medtronic defibrillator
  Mini II, II+ automatic
    implantable cardioverter
    defibrillator
  Morris defibrillator
  ODAM defibrillator
  pacer-cardioverter
    defibrillator (PCD)
  PD 2000 defibrillator
  Photon micro implantable
    cardioverter defibrillator
  Phylax implantable
    cardioverter defibrillator
  Porta Pulse 3 defibrillator
  Porta Pulse 3 portable
    defibrillator
  Prizm defibrillator
  Ventak Mini III implantable
    defibrillator
  Ventak Prizm implantable
    defibrillator
  Zoll defibrillator
  Zoll external defibrillator
defibrillator implant
defibrillator paddle
deficit
  nerve deficit
  neurological deficit
  sensory deficit
defined frequency
defined sterilization
definite mass
definitive callus
definitive diagnosis
definitive irradiation
definitive local therapy
definitive prosthesis
definitive resection
definitive stabilization

definitive surgery
definitive therapy
definitive treatment
deflated tourniquet
deflation
deflectable quadripolar catheter
deflected skin flap
deflecting obturator
deflection
  intrinsicoid deflection
  peak-to-peak deflection
  vesicouterine deflection
deflective malocclusion
deflective occlusal
deflective occlusal contact
Deflux system implant
defocused beam
deformation
  condylar deformation
  dentinoblastic deformation
  elastic deformation
  permanent deformation
  viscoelastic deformation
deformation sequence
deformational frontal
    plagiocephaly
deformities
  pelvic deformities
deformity
  2-plance deformity
  3-plane deformity
  abduction deformity
  acetabular protrusio
    deformity
  acquired deformity
  adduction deformity
  adduction-internal rotation
    deformity
  adductovarus deformity
  Akerlund deformity
  Andy Gump deformity
  angel-wing deformity
  angular deformity
  angulation deformity
  ape-hand deformity
  Arnold-Chiari deformity
  back-knee deformity
  bell-clapper deformity
  bifid thumb deformity
  bilateral flexion deformity
  bird-beak deformity
  bishop collar deformity

deformity (*continued*)
- bony deformity
- boutonniere deformity
- bowing deformity
- bowleg deformity
- boxy tip deformity
- bulb deformity
- bunion deformity
- burn boutonniere deformity
- Burow triangle deformity
- buttonhole deformity
- calcaneocavovarus deformity
- calcaneocavus deformity
- calcaneovalgus deformity
- calcaneovarus deformity
- calvarial deformity
- cavovarus deformity
- cavus deformity
- cecal deformity
- cervical spine kyphotic deformity
- cervicomedullary deformity
- chain-of-lakes deformity
- champagne cork deformity
- checkrein deformity
- chin deformity
- clasped thumb deformity
- claw deformity
- claw hand deformity
- clawfoot deformity
- clawing deformity
- clawtoe deformity
- cleft hand deformity
- cleft lip deformity
- clenched fist deformity
- cloverleaf skull deformity
- cloverleaf-type deformity
- clubfoot deformity
- cock-up deformity
- codfish deformity
- columellar deformity
- combined cavus deformity
- compensatory deformity
- complete bilateral deformity
- compression deformity
- compression-type deformity
- congenital deformity
- congenital postural deformity
- contour deformity
- coronal plane deformity
- coup de sabre deformity
- craniodentofacial deformity

deformity (*continued*)
- craniofacial deformity
- crossbar stomach deformity
- crossover toe deformity
- Crouzon facial deformity
- cubitus valgus deformity
- Dandy-Walker deformity
- dentofacial deformity
- dinner fork deformity
- dish-face deformity
- double-bubble breast deformity
- drooping-chin deformity
- duodenal bulb deformity
- duodenal deformity
- ectopic antihelical folding deformity
- edge scalloping deformity
- elevatus deformity
- equinovalgus deformity
- equinus deformity
- Erlenmeyer flask deformity
- eversion-external rotation deformity
- extension deformity
- extrinsic colon deformity
- facial contour deformity
- facial deformity
- finger deformity
- fishtail deformity
- fixed deformity
- flat back deformity
- flexion deformity
- flexion-internal rotational deformity
- foot deformity
- Fowler procedure for boutonniere deformity
- funnel chest deformity
- funnel deformity
- fusiform deformity
- garden spade deformity
- genu valgum deformity
- genu varum deformity
- gibbus deformity
- gingival deformity
- gooseneck deformity
- gross deformity
- Haglund deformity
- hallux valgus deformity
- halo deformity
- hammertoe deformity

deformity (*continued*)

hand deformity
harlequin deformity
hatchet head deformity
Hill-Sachs deformity
hindbrain deformity
hindfoot deformity
hip deformity
hockey-stick deformity
hook-nail deformity
Houghland deformity
hourglass deformity
hourglass nasal deformity
humpback deformity
hyperextension deformity
iatrogenic deformity
internal rotation deformity
intrinsic minus deformity
intrinsic plus deformity
inversion deformity
inverted teardrop areola
  deformity
ipsilateral hand deformity
joint deformity
J-sella deformity
keyhole deformity
Kirner deformity
kleeblattschadel deformity
Klippel-Feil deformity
knock-knee deformity
kyphotic deformity
lambdoid synostosis deformity
lanceolate deformity
lateral facial cleft deformity
Launois-Cléret deformity
limb deformity
lobster hand deformity
lobster claw deformity
lop-ear deformity
lumbar spine kyphotic
  deformity
Madelung deformity
mallet finger deformity
mallet toe deformity
maxillary deformity
Michel deformity
middle vault deformity
Mondini deformity
nasal deformity
nasal tip deformity
one-plane deformity
opera-glass deformity

deformity (*continued*)

parachute deformity
parrot beak deformity
pectus carinatum deformity
pectus deformity
pectus excavatum deformity
pencil-in-cup deformity
penile deformity
pes planus deformity
phrygian cap deformity
pigeon breast deformity
ping-pong ball deformity
Pinocchio tip deformity
planovalgus deformity
plantar flexion-inversion
  deformity
polly beak deformity
polly beak nasal deformity
postmaxillectomy deformity
posttraumatic spinal
  deformity
postural deformity
protrusio deformity
pseudo-boutonniere deformity
pseudomallet deformity
rat-tail deformity
recurvatum angulation
  deformity
residual deformity
riding-pants deformity
ripple deformity
Romberg facial deformity
rotational deformity
round back deformity
round shoulder deformity
sabre-shin deformity
saddle deformity
saddle nose deformity
sagittal deformity
scaphocephalic deformity
septal deformity
shepherd's crook deformity
silver-fork deformity
skeletal deformity
slight deformity
snoopy deformity
soft tissue deformity
spastic thumb-in-palm
  deformity
spinal coronal plane
  deformity
spine deformity

deformity (*continued*)
  spinning-top deformity
  splayfoot deformity
  splenic vein deformity
  split-hand deformity
  split-nail deformity
  spondylitic deformity
  Sprengel deformity
  S-shaped deformity
  SST deformity
  stairstep deformity
  step deformity
  subcondylar deformity
  supination deformity
  Suppan procedure for nail
    deformity
  supratip deformity
  swan-neck deformity
  swan-neck finger deformity
  swayback deformity
  talipes cavus deformity
  talus foot deformity
  thoracic spine kyphotic
    deformity
  thoracic spine scoliotic
    deformity
  thumb deformity
  thumb-in-palm deformity
  Treacher Collins deformity
  trefoil deformity
  triphalangeal thumb
    deformity
  turned-up pulp deformity
  ulnar deviation deformity
  ulnar drift deformity
  unesthetic contour deformity
  unilateral cleft-lip/nose
    deformity
  uni-tip deformity
  valgus deformity
  varus hindfoot deformity
  Velpeau deformity
  volar angulation deformity
  Volkmann claw hand
    deformity
  waterfall deformity
  whistling deformity
  Whitehead deformity
  windblown deformity
  windsock deformity
  windswept deformity
  witch's chin deformity

deformity (*continued*)
  wrist deformity
  Zancolli clawhand deformity
  Zancolli procedure for
    clawhand deformity
  zig-zag compensatory
    deformity
  Z-type deformity
deformity analysis
deformity angle
deformity of earlobe
Defourmental bone rongeur
Defourmental forceps
Defourmental nasal rongeur
Defourmental rongeur
Defourmental rongeur forceps
defunctionalized
defunctioning loop ileostomy
degassing
degenerated tissue
degenerating decidual tissue
degeneration
  aberrant third nerve
    degeneration
  age-related macular
    degeneration
  calcific degeneration
  cerebellar degeneration
  cobblestone degeneration
  cochlear degeneration
  colliquative degeneration
  corneal degeneration
  fatty degeneration
  granular degeneration
  hepaticolenticular
    degeneration
  hyaline degeneration
  lattice degeneration
  lattice retinal degeneration
  lenticular degeneration
  macula degeneration
  macular degeneration
  malignant degeneration
  Monckeberg degeneration
  myxomatous degeneration
  paving-stone degeneration
  Terrien degeneration
  trabecular degeneration
  traction spur from disk
    degeneration
  wallerian degeneration
degeneration of adrenal gland

degenerative bone changes
degenerative cataract
degenerative change
degenerative discogenic endplate disease
degenerative disease
degenerative disk disease (DDD)
degenerative disorder
degenerative encephalopathy
degenerative heart disease
degenerative inflammation
degenerative joint disease (DJD)
degenerative joint disease of
wrist
degenerative mitral valve
insufficiency
degenerative spurring
degenerative status
degenerative tear
degenerative zone
deglove
degloved amputation
degloving
degloving injury
degloving procedure
degloving technique
deglutition
deglutition apnea
deglutition maneuver
deglutition mechanism
deglutition reflex
deglutitory cough
deglutitory disturbance
deglycerated
Degnon sutures
degradable polyglycolide rod
degradation
degrease the skin
Degucast alloy
Degudent alloy
dehiscence
abdominal incision
dehiscence
alveolar dehiscence
anastomotic dehiscence
congenital tympanic
dehiscence
intimal dehiscence
iris dehiscence
Killian dehiscence
levator dehiscence
root dehiscence

dehiscence (*continued*)
Roux limb stump dehiscence
scar dehiscence
soft tissue dehiscence
staple line dehiscence
sternotomy dehiscence
stump dehiscence
suture-line dehiscence
tertiary dehiscence
total dehiscence
wound dehiscence
Zuckerkandl dehiscence
dehiscence of iris
dehiscence of mandibular canal
dehiscence of uterus
dehiscence of wound
dehiscent mandibular canal
dehydration of gingivae
dehydrosterone
deionized water
Deiters nucleus
DeJager elevator
Dejerine percussion hammer
Dejerine sign
Dejerine syndrome
Dejerine-Davis percussion
hammer
Dejerine-Landouzy dystrophy
Dejerine-Roussy syndrome
Dejerine-Sottas atrophy
dekalon sutures
DeKlair operation
Deklene polypropylene sutures
Deklene sutures
Deknatel K-needle
Deknatel needle
Deknatel silk sutures
Deknatel Snowden Pencer
Deknatel sutures
Deknatel tape
Deknatel wound closure tape
DeKock 2-way bronchial
catheter
Del Mar Avionics scanner
Del Mar Avionics 3-channel
recorder
Del Toro operation
Delaborde dilator
Delaborde tracheal dilator
Delaborde-Trousseau tracheal
dilator
DeLaginiere abdominal retractor

Delaire palatoplasty
Delaney phrenic retractor
Delaney retractor
Delarnette scanner
DeLaura knee prosthesis
DeLaura-Verner knee prosthesis
delay line
delay maneuver
delay of muscle flap
delay musculocutaneous flap
delayed closure of wound
delayed complication
delayed conduction
delayed dentition
delayed direct coloanal
    anastomosis
delayed distally based total
    sartorius flap
delayed echolalia
delayed emptying
delayed expansion
delayed flap
delayed graft
delayed healing
delayed hypersensitivity
delayed open reduction
delayed operative
    cholangiography
delayed primary closure
delayed primary repair
delayed primary suture
    technique
delayed reaction
delayed reflex
delayed skin flap
delayed skin flap technique
delayed sutures
delayed transfer flap
delayed union
delayed wound healing
Delbert-Reverdin needle
Delbet hip classification
Delbet splint
Delbet splint for heel fracture
Delcath double-balloon catheter
Delclos applicator
Delclos cylinder
Delclos dilator
Delclos ovoid
Delclos vaginal cylinder
Delcom filling instrument
DeLee catheter

DeLee cervical forceps
DeLee cervix-holding forceps
DeLee classification
DeLee corner retractor
DeLee curet
DeLee dressing forceps
DeLee forceps
DeLee infant catheter
DeLee knife
DeLee laparotrachelotomy knife
DeLee maneuver
DeLee meconium trap aspirator
DeLee obstetrical forceps
DeLee operation
DeLee ovum forceps
DeLee pelvimeter
DeLee retractor
DeLee shuttle forceps
DeLee speculum
DeLee spoon tissue forceps
DeLee suction
DeLee tenaculum
DeLee tracheal catheter
DeLee tracheal trap
DeLee trap aspirator
DeLee trap meconium aspirator
DeLee tube
DeLee Universal retractor
DeLee uterine forceps
DeLee uterine packing forceps
DeLee vaginal retractor
DeLee vesical retractor
DeLee-Breisky pelvimeter
DeLee-Hillis obstetrical head
    stethoscope
DeLee-Hillis obstetrical
    stethoscope
DeLee-Hillis stethoscope
DeLee-Pierce membrane
    perforator
DeLee-Pierce perforator
DeLee-Simpson forceps
DeLee-Zweifel cranioclast
Delerm and Elbaz technique
Delgado electrode
deliberate hypotension
    anesthetic technique
delicate balance
delicate intervertebral disk
    rongeur
delicate needle holder
delicate operating scissors

delicate scissors
delicate skin hook
delicate structure
delicate thumb-dressing forceps
Delima ethmoid cannula
delimiting keratotomy
Delitala T-nail
Delitala T-pins
delivery
   assisted breech delivery
   breech delivery
   cesarean delivery
   complicated delivery
   C-section delivery
   difficult vaginal delivery
   double-footling delivery
   failed forceps delivery
   footling delivery
   forceps delivery
   full-term delivery
   high-forceps delivery
   induced delivery
   instant delivery
   intravitreal delivery
   low-forceps delivery
   midforceps delivery
   Mityvac vacuum extraction
     delivery
   monomanual delivery
   obstetrical delivery
   operative delivery
   outlet forceps delivery
   partial breech delivery
   premature delivery
   prep for delivery
   prior to delivery
   rotation operative delivery
   spontaneous breech delivery
   spontaneous delivery
   spontaneous vaginal delivery
   term delivery
   threatened premature
     delivery
   total breech delivery
   unassisted delivery
   uncomplicated delivery
   vacuum vaginal delivery
   vaginal delivery
   vaginal vertex delivery
delivery assistance sleeve
delivery balloon
delivery guidewire

delivery hose
delivery wire
Dell astigmatism marker
Della Badia laparoscopic
   suturing device
Dellepiane hysterectomy
Deller modification
Dellon generator
Dellon ulnar nerve transposition
Delmege sign
Delorme operation
Delorme rectal prolapse
   operation
Delorme table
Delorme-Fowler operation
Delphian lymph node
Delphian node
Delrin applicator
Delrin biomaterial joint
   replacement prosthesis
Delrin disk heart valve
Delrin frame of valve prosthesis
Delrin heart valve
Delrin joint
Delrin locking-handle forceps
Delrin plastic scalp clip
Delrin push rod
Delrin-handle bone saw
delta activity
Delta dermatoscope
Delta external fixation frame
Delta pacemaker
delta phalanx
Delta Recon proximal drill
   guide
Delta Reconnail
Delta rod
Delta TACT (tuned aperture
   computed tomography)
Delta TRS pacemaker
Delta valve
Delta-FormCast reinforcing resin
Delta-lite casting tape
Delta-lite S-casting tape
Delta-Net stockinette
Delta-Rol cast padding
DeltaTrac II metabolic monitor
Deltec portable external
   infusion device
Deltec-Pharmacia CADD pump
deltoid crest
deltoid eminence

deltoid fascia
deltoid flap
deltoid ligament
deltoid muscle
deltoid region
deltoid-splitting approach
deltoid-splitting incision
deltoid-splitting shoulder
    approach
deltopectoral approach
deltopectoral flap
deltopectoral groove
deltopectoral incision
deltoscapular flap
Deltran disposable transducer
deluxe FIN extractor
deluxe FIN pin
deluxe FIN pin inserter
deluxe head halter
demand cardiac pacemaker
demand flow machine
demand pacemaker
demand-adapted administration
    anesthetic technique
demarcate
demarcated
    sharply demarcated
demarcated border
demarcated cellulitis
demarcated lesion
demarcated margin
demarcation
    areolar demarcation
    corticomedullary demarcation
    line of demarcation
    no line of demarcation
demarcation current
demarcation line
demarcation potential
demarcator
    flap demarcator
    Pitanguy demarcator
    Pitanguy flap demarcator
Demarest forceps
Demarest septal forceps
Demarquay sign
DeMartel appendix forceps
DeMartel clamp
DeMartel conductor saw
DeMartel forceps
DeMartel neurosurgical scissors
DeMartel retractor

DeMartel scalp flap forceps
DeMartel scalp forceps
DeMartel scissors
DeMartel self-retaining brain
    retractor
DeMartel sutures
DeMartel trephine
DeMartel T-wire saw
DeMartel vascular clamp
DeMartel vascular scissors
DeMartel-Wolfson anastomosis
    clamp
DeMartel-Wolfson anastomotic
    clamp
DeMartel-Wolfson clamp
DeMartel-Wolfson clamp holder
DeMartel-Wolfson closing
    forceps
DeMartel-Wolfson colon clamp
DeMartel-Wolfson forceps
DeMartel-Wolfson intestinal
    anastomotic clamp
DeMartel-Wolfson intestinal
    clamp
DeMartel-Wolfson intestinal-
    holding forceps
DeMayo suture passer
DeMayo 2-point discrimination
    device
Dembone demineralized
    cancellous chips
Dembone demineralized cortical
    chips
Dembone demineralized cortical
    dental block
Dembone demineralized cortical
    powder
Dembone demineralized
    corticocancellous chips
Dembone demineralized human
    bone
Dembone freeze-dried bone
Dembone graft
Demel forceps
Demel wire clamp
Demel wire-tightening forceps
Demel wire-twisting forceps
Demel-Ruttin operation
Demerol anesthetic agent
demeure catheter
demifacet
demigauntlet bandage

demigauntlet dressing
demineralization
demineralization of bone
demineralized bone (DMB)
demineralized bone graft
demineralized bone matrix
demineralized bony structure
demineralized cortical bone
    powder
demineralized flexible laminar
    bone strip
demineralized freeze-dried bone
    (DFDB)
demineralized freeze-dried bone
    allograft (DFDBA)
Deming nephropexy
Demling-Classen
    sphincterotome
demonstrable evidence
demonstration eyepiece
Demos tibial arterial clamp
Demos tibial artery clamp
Demours membrane
demucosation
Demuth hip screw
demyelinate
demyelinating disease
demyelinating lesion
demyelination
    autoimmune demyelination
    axonal demyelination
    intramedullary demyelination
    segmental demyelination
demyelinization
DeMyer system of cerebral
    malformation
Denans operation
Denar articulator
Denar-Witzig articulator
denatured homograft
Dench atomizer
Dench ear
Dench ear curet
Dench ear forceps
Dench ear knife
Dench forceps
Dench insufflator
Dench knife
Dench nebulizer
Dench rongeur
Dench uterine curet
Dench vaporizer

Denck esophagoscope
dendrites and axons
dendritic calculus
dendritic carcinoma
dendritic cell
dendritic lesion
dendritic ulcer
denervate
denervated bladder
denervated heart
denervated muscle
denervated muscle atrophy
denervation
    extrinsic denervation
    Krause denervation
    law of denervation
    preganglionic sympathetic
        denervation
    sinoaortic denervation
denervation disease
denervation hypersensitivity
denervation potential
Denham external fixation
Denham external fixation device
Denham pin
Denham skeletal fixation
Denhardt mouth gag
Denhardt-Dingman mouth gag
Denholtz appliance
Denholtz muscle anchorage
    appliance
Denis bipolar cautery
Denis Browne abdominal
    retractor blade
Denis Browne adult retractor set
Denis Browne bar
Denis Browne bucket
Denis Browne cleft palate
    needle
Denis Browne clubfoot splint
Denis Browne forceps
Denis Browne hip splint
Denis Browne malleable copper
    retractor blade
Denis Browne mastoid pediatric
    retractor blade
Denis Browne needle
Denis Browne operation
Denis Browne pediatric
    abdominal retractor blade
Denis Browne pediatric
    retractor

Denis Browne pediatric
    retractor set
Denis Browne procedure
Denis Browne retractor oval
    sprocket frame
Denis Browne ring retractor
Denis Browne spinal fracture
    classification
Denis Browne splint
Denis Browne talipes hobble
    splint
Denis Browne tonsillar forceps
Denis Browne tray
Denis Browne Universal
    retractor set
Denis Browne urethroplasty
    technique
Denis Browne-Hendren
    pediatric retractor blade
Denis Browne pouch
Denker operation
Denker sinus operation
Denker trocar
Denker tube
Denlan magnifying loupe
DenLite illuminated handheld
    mirror
Denman spontaneous version
Dennen forceps
Dennie infraorbital fold
Dennie lines
Dennie-Morgan infraorbital folds
Dennie-Morgan line
Dennis anastomosis
Dennis anastomotic clamp
Dennis clamp
Dennis forceps
Dennis intestinal clamp
Dennis intestinal forceps
Dennis intestinal tube
Dennis operation
Dennis technique
Dennis tube
Dennis-Brooke ileostomy
Denniston dilator
Dennis-Varco
    pancreaticoduodenostomy
Dennyson-Fulford arthrodesis
Denonvilliers aponeurosis
Denonvilliers blepharoplasty
Denonvilliers fascia
Denonvilliers operation

Denonvilliers space
Denpac porcelain powder
dens (*pl.* dentes)
dens angularis
dens anterior screw fixation
dens bicuspis
dens caninus
dens cuspidatus
dens deciduus
dens fracture
dens in dente
dens incisivus
dens invaginatus
dens invaginatus gestant
    odontoma
dens molaris
dens permanens
dens premolaris
dens sapientiae
dens serotinus
dens succedaneus
Dens view of cervical spine
Densco bur
Densco dental handpiece
dense adhesions
dense body
dense bony structure
densification
Densilay alloy
Densite
densitometer
densitometric
densitometric analysis
densitometry
density
    alveolar bone density
    bone density
    bone mineral density (BMD)
    calcific density
    calcified density
    cohesive site density
    linear density
    microvessel density (MVD)
    nodular density
    optical density
    parenchymal density
    radiographic density
    radiolucent density
    radiopaque density
    shadow density
density radiograph
density-dependent repair

Dent sleeve
Dent sleeve catheter
Dent sleeve device
Dentaflex wire
Dentaform band
dental alveoli
dental alveolus
dental amalgam
dental amalgam packer
dental analysis
dental anatomy
dental anesthesia
dental anomaly
dental appliance
dental arch
dental arch bar
dental arch bar facial fracture
    appliance
dental arch bar frame
dental arch expansion
dental artery
dental articulation
dental biophysics
dental bridge
dental bur
dental caries
dental cavity
dental cement
dental crown
dental debridement
dental disease
dental dressing forceps
dental drill
dental dysfunction
dental elevator
dental excavator
dental exostosis
dental extraction
dental fenestration
dental fistula
dental flange
dental forceps
dental handpiece
dental impaction
dental implant
dental implant cover screw
dental impression
dental knife
dental lisp
dental lymph
dental material
dental mold

dental nerve
dental occlusion
dental operculum
dental pick
dental plaque
dental plate
dental pliers
Dental Pro II camera
dental procedure
dental prosthesis
dental pulp
dental pulp extirpation
dental repair
dental restorative surgery
dental retractor
dental rongeur
dental shelf
dental shield
dental splint
dental surgery
dental syringe
dental tool
dental tophus
dentate bur
dentate fascia
dentate fissure
dentate fracture
dentate gyrus
dentate ligament
dentate line
dentate margin
dentate nucleus
dentate sutures
Dentatus articulator
Dentatus reamer
Dentatus screw
dente (*pl. of* dens)
Dentemp filling material
dentes (*pl. of* dens)
dentes acustici
dentes acuti
dentes bicuspides
dentes canini
dentes cuspidati
dentes decidui
dentes incisivi
dentes molares
dentes permanentes
dentes premolares
denticular hymen
denticulate ligament
Dentifix denture repair kit

dentigerous cyst
dentilabial
dentilingual
dentin
dentin (D)
dentin matrix
dentinal lymph
dentinal matrix
dentinoblastic deformation
dentinoblastic injury
dentinocemental junction
dentinoenamel defect
dentinoenamel membrane
dentinogenesis
dentinogenesis hypoplastica
   hereditaria
dentinogenesis imperfecta
dentinogenic
dentinogenic fiber
dentinoid
dentinoid formation
dentinoma
dentinosteoid
dentinum
dentiparous
dentis (genitive of dens)
dentitio difficilis
dentition
   delayed dentition
   mandibular dentition
   maxillary dentition
   mixed dentition
dentitional odontectomy
Dentloid impression material
dentoalveolar
dentoalveolar abscess
dentoalveolar cyst
dentoalveolar dysplasia
dentoalveolar fracture
dentoalveolar joint
dentoalveolar ligament
dentoalveolitis
dentoaural
dentoepithelial
dentoepithelial junction
dentofacial anomaly
dentofacial complex
dentofacial deformity
dentofacial dysplasia
dentofacial esthetics
dentofacial orthopedics
dentofacial surgery

dentofacial zone
dentoform
dentogenic movement
dentogingival fiber
dentogingival junction
dentogingival lamina
dentography
dentolabial dysplasia
dentonomy
dentoperiosteal fiber
dentopulmonary syndrome
dentoskeletal
Dento-Spray oral irrigator
dentosurgical
dentotropic
Dentsply alloy
Dentsply MVS evacuator
dentulism
dentulous
dentulous dental arch
dentulous esthetics
dentulous sore mouth
denture adhesive
denture brush
denture classification
denture impression
denture sore mouth
denture space
denture splint
denture vulcanite bur
dentures
Dentus x-ray film
denudation
   endothelial denudation
   interdental denudation
denudation of cornea
denuded and buried skin
   submental flap
denuded finger
denuded furca
denuded furcation
denuded tissue
Denuse operation
Denver ascites shunt
Denver classification
Denver connector
Denver hydrocephalus shunt
Denver nasal splint
Denver shunt
Denver percutaneous access kit
Denver peritoneovenous shunt
Denver peritoneal-venous shunt

Denver pleuroperitoneal shunt
Denver reservoir
Denver splint
Denver valve
Denver valve shunt
Denver-Krupin valve
Denver-Wells atrial retractor
Denver-Wells sternal retractor
Deon hip
Deon hip prosthesis
DeOrio intrauterine
   insemination catheter
deossification
deoxygenated blood
Depage incision
Depage position
Depage-Janeway gastrostomy
depalatalization
DePalma hip prosthesis
DePalma knife
DePalma modified patellar
   technique
DePalma staple
Depaul tube
dependency skin lines
dependent drainage
depigmentation
depigmented lesion
depigmenting skin
depilation
depilatory dermal forceps
depolarization block
depolarizing block
depolarizing electrode
deposit
   calcareous deposit
   calcific deposit
   corneal deposits
   endochondral bone deposit
   fat deposits
   fatty deposits
   fibrin deposit
deposition
   abdominal iron deposition
   bone deposition
   collagen deposition
   silicone deposition
depot
   fat depot
depot intramuscular injection
depressant
depressed chest wall

depressed fracture
depressed fracture of zygoma
depressed lesion
depressed skull fracture
depressed systolic pressure
depression (*see also* tongue
   depressor)
   chondrosternal depression
   cicatricial depression
   concavity and depression
   inspiratory rib cage depression
   linear depression
   lingual salivary gland
     depression
   marrow depression
   otic depression
   prejowl depression
   radial depression
   respiratory depression
   sternal depression
   superimposed depression
   supratrochlear depression
   trochanteric depression
   twitch depression
   ventilatory depression
   xiphoumbilical depression
depression fracture
depressor (*see also* tongue
   depressor)
   Balmer depressor
   brain depressor
   Braun depressor
   Braun uterine depressor
   Claes scleral depressor
   Cushing brain depressor
   Dunn depressor
   Flynn scleral depressor
   Fraser depressor
   Israel depressor
   Kocher depressor
   O'Connor depressor
   O'Connor scleral depressor
   orbital depressor
   Schepens depressor
   Schepens scleral depressor
   Schocket depressor
   Schocket scleral depressor
   scleral depressor
   Sims uterine depressor
   Spaide depressor
   Urrets-Zavalia depressor
   Wilder scleral depressor

depressor anguli oris muscle
depressor epiglottidis
depressor labii inferioris muscle
depressor labii oris muscle
depressor muscle
depressor muscle of angle of
    mouth
depressor nerve
depressor reflex
depressor septi
depressor septi muscle
depressor septi release
depth
    anesthetic depth
    char-zone depth
    gap depth
    mandibular depth
    maxillary depth
    oral vestibular depth
    pocket depth
    probing depth (PD)
    vestibular depth
depth check drill
depth electrode
depth gauge
depth of anesthesia
depth of anesthesia monitoring
depth of insertion (DOI)
depth plate
depth pulse technique
Depthalon monitoring electrode
depth-gain compensation
DePuy acetabular liner
DePuy arthroplasty
DePuy awl
DePuy bolt
DePuy bone cement
DePuy bone curet
DePuy bone mill
DePuy cannulated reamer
DePuy curet
DePuy drill
DePuy dual-lock hip prosthesis
DePuy extractor
DePuy fracture brace
DePuy fracture frame
DePuy fracture-reducing frame
DePuy head halter
DePuy hip prosthesis with
    Scuderi head
DePuy hook
DePuy I bone cement

DePuy interference screw
DePuy Keystone graft
    instruments
DePuy Lumbar Cage
DePuy nail
DePuy nerve hook
DePuy open-thimble splint
DePuy orthopedic implant
DePuy anterior compression
    plate
DePuy pin
DePuy plate
DePuy Porocoat
    hemiarthroplasty
DePuy prosthesis
DePuy reamer
DePuy retractor
DePuy rocking leg splint
DePuy rolled Colles splint
DePuy rongeur
DePuy screwdriver
DePuy small-joint arthroscopy
    instrument set
DePuy splint
DePuy rod
DePuy support
DePuy Vertigraft bone wedge
DePuy-Potts splint
DePuy-Weiss tonsillar needle
derangement
    alveolar arch derangement
    Hey internal derangement
    internal derangement (ID)
derangement of joint
derangement of knee
derangement of vasomotor
    nerves
derby hat fracture
Derby nail
Derby operation
Derch vaporizer
Derek-Harwood-Nash catheter
Derf ear knife
Derf eye needle holder
Derf forceps
Derf holder
Derf needle holder
Derf scissors
Derf Vital needle holder
derivative circulation
Derlacki capsular knife
Derlacki capsule knife

Derlacki chisel
Derlacki curet
Derlacki duckbill elevator
Derlacki ear curet
Derlacki ear mobilizer
Derlacki elevator
Derlacki gouge
Derlacki knife
Derlacki mobilizer
Derlacki operation
Derlacki ossicle holder
Derlacki punch
Derlacki-Hough mobilizer
Derlacki-Juers head holder
Derlacki-Shambaugh chisel
Derlacki-Shambaugh microscope
Derma laser
Derma Care dressing
Derma K combination laser
Derma K laser
Dermabond topical skin
    adhesive
Dermabond wound closure
    device
dermabrader (*see also* abrader)
    diamond dermabrader
    high-speed dermabrader
    Iverson dermabrader
    lid dermabrader
    sandpaper dermabrader
    Schumann-Schreus
        dermabrader
    Stryker dermabrader
dermabrasion
    spot dermabrasion
    therapeutic dermabrasion
dermabrasion (*also*
    dermoabrasion)
dermabrasion bur
DermaCare electrosurgical
    forceps
dermacarrier
    Tanner mesh graft
        dermacarrier
Dermacea alginate dressing
Dermacea alginate wound
    dressing
Dermacerator handpiece
Dermaclip
DermaCol hydrocolloid wound
    dressing
DermaFilm dressing

Dermaflex Gel
DermaGard prism
Dermagraft graft
Dermagran hydrophilic wound
    dressing
Dermagran zinc-saline hydrogel
    wound dressing
Dermagran-B hydrophilic wound
    dressing
dermal analogue tumor
dermal atrophy
dermal bone
dermal brassiere technique
dermal curet
dermal cyst
dermal elevator
dermal fat free flap
dermal fat free tissue transfer
dermal fat graft
dermal fat pedicle flap
dermal graft
dermal grafting
dermal injection
dermal instrument
dermal lesion
dermal lymphatics
dermal melanosis
dermal network
dermal orbicular pennant
    technique
dermal overgrafting
dermal papillae
dermal pedicle
dermal pedicle technique
dermal pouch
dermal pouch reconstruction
dermal punch
dermal pyramidal flap
dermal route of injection
dermal sinus
dermal suture technique
dermal sutures
dermal tension nonabsorbing
    sutures
dermal tissue
dermal vascular plexus
dermal vascularized pedicle
DermaLase laser
Dermalene polyethylene sutures
Dermalene sutures
Dermalogen human collagen
Dermalogen material

Dermalon cuticular sutures
Dermalon sutures
DermaMend foam
DermaMend foam wound
    dressing
DermaMend hydrogel dressing
Dermamesh graft expander
DermaNet contact-layer wound
    dressing
DermaNet wound contact layer
dermaplaning
Dermapor glove
Dermascrub
Derma-Sil impression material
DermaSite transparent film
    dressing
Dermasoft mattress
DermAssist gel gauze dressing
DermAssist glycerin hydrogel
    dressing
DermAssist hydrocolloid
    dressing
DermAssist transparent site
    dressing
DermAssist wound filling
    material
DermaStat calcium alginate
    wound dressing
Dermastat dermatology
    handpiece
Dermatape
Derma-Tattoo surgical tattoo
Dermatell hydrocolloid
    dressing
Dermatell hydrocolloid dressing
    material
Dermatex compound
dermatitis herpetiformis (DH)
dermatitis medicamentosa
dermatitis venenata
dermatoalloplasty
dermatoautoplasty
dermatocele
dermatochalasis
dermatofibroma protuberans
dermatofibrosarcoma
    protuberans
dermatoheteroplasty
dermatohomoplasty
dermatologic disorder
dermatologic ultraviolet light
dermatomal level of analgesia

dermatomal superficial
    telangiectasia
dermatome (*see* dermatotome)
    air dermatome
    Bard-Parker dermatome
    Barker Vacu-tome dermatome
    Brown air dermatome
    Brown dermatome
    Brown electric dermatome
    Brown-Blair dermatome
    Castroviejo dermatome
    Concept dermatome
    Concept mesh grafter
        dermatome
    cordless dermatome
    DaSilva dermatome
    Davol dermatome
    Davol-Simon dermatome
    DeSilva dermatome
    Down hand dermatome
    drum dermatome
    Duval dermatome
    Duval disposable dermatome
    Duval-Simon portable
        dermatome
    electric dermatome
    Goulian dermatome
    Hall dermatome
    Hood dermatome
    Hood manual dermatome
    Jordan-Day dermatome
    manual dermatome
    Meek-Wall dermatome
    Padgett dermatome
    Padgett manual dermatome
    Padgett-Hood dermatome
    Pitkin dermatome
    Rees dermatome
    Reese dermatome
    Reese-Drum dermatome
    Reuse Expanda-graft
        dermatome
    Rica dermatome
    Schink dermatome
    sick dermatome
    Simon dermatome
    single-use dermatome
    SMIC dermatome
    Strempel dermatome
    Stryker dermatome
    Tanner-Vandeput mesh
        dermatome

dermatome (*continued*)
  Weck dermatome
  Zimmer dermatome
dermatome blade
dermatome cement
dermatomic
dermatomyositis
dermatopathologist
dermatoplastic
dermatoplasty
dermatoscope
dermatosis (*pl.* dermatoses)
  benign papular acantholytic
    dermatosis
  Bowen precancerous
    dermatosis
  papulosa nigra dermatosis
  radiation dermatosis
  Schamberg progressive
    pigmented purpuric
    dermatosis
  temperature-dependent
    dermatosis
dermatosis papulosa nigra
dermatotome
  Brown dermatotome
  drum dermatotome
  electric dermatotome
  Reuse Expanda-graft
    dermatotome
dermatoxenoplasty
Dermex wrap
Dermgran hydrogel wound
  dressing
dermic graft
Dermicare hypoallergenic paper
  tape
Dermicel dressing
Dermicel hypoallergenic cloth
  tape
Dermicel hypoallergenic knitted
  tape
Dermicel tape
Dermiclear tape
Dermiform hypoallergenic
  knitted tape
Dermilite tape
dermis fascia
dermis patch graft
dermis-fat grafting
dermis-fat grafts
dermis-fat passer

Dermiview hypoallergenic
  transparent tape
dermoabrasion (*variant of*
  dermabrasion)
dermoadipose
dermoadipose flap
dermoadipose tissue
dermodesis
dermoepidermal Gillies stitch
dermoepidermal junction
dermofasciectomy
dermofat
dermofat flap
dermofat graft
dermofat technique
dermoid cancer
dermoid cyst
dermoid inclusion cyst
dermoid tumor
Dermo-Jet high pressure injector
Dermo-Jet injector
dermolipectomy
  abdominal dermolipectomy
  brachial dermolipectomy
  U-M dermolipectomy
Dermophase dressing
Dermoplast spray
Dermoplast-Plastazote orthosis
dermoplasty cast
dermoplasty procedure
Dermostat eye implant material
Dermostat implant
Dermostat orbital implant
Dermot-Pierse ball-tipped knife
DeRoaldes nasal speculum
DeRoaldes speculum
derotation brace
derotation osteotomy
derotational pin
DeRoyal cannula
DeRoyal catheter tube holder
DeRoyal HyperControl elbow
  brace
DeRoyal laparotomy sponge
DeRoyal Surgical grab bag
DeRoyal/LMB finger splint
Derra anastomosis clamp
Derra aortic clamp
Derra cardiac valve dilator
Derra cardiovascular forceps
Derra clamp
Derra commissurotomy knife

Derra dilator
Derra forceps
Derra guillotine
Derra guillotine knife
Derra knife
Derra urethral forceps
Derra valve dilator
Derra valvulotome
Derra vena cava clamp
Derra vestibular clamp
Derra-Cooley forceps
D'Errico bayonet pituitary
    forceps
D'Errico brain spatula
D'Errico bur
D'Errico chisel
D'Errico dressing forceps
D'Errico drill
D'Errico enlarging bur
D'Errico forceps
D'Errico hypophyseal forceps
D'Errico knife
D'Errico laminar knife
D'Errico laminectomy chisel
D'Errico nerve elevator
D'Errico nerve retractor
D'Errico nerve root retractor
D'Errico perforating bur
D'Errico perforating drill
D'Errico perforator
D'Errico periosteal elevator
D'Errico retractor
D'Errico skull trephine
D'Errico spatula
D'Errico tissue forceps
D'Errico trephine
D'Errico ventricular needle
D'Errico-Adson retractor
Desai VectorCath catheter
Desault bandage
Desault dislocation
Desault dressing
Desault fracture
Desault hip sign
Desault ligation
Desault ligature
Desault sign
Desault wrist bandage
Desault wrist dislocation
Descemet membrane
Descemet membrane
    detachment

Descemet membrane punch
Descemet operation
descemetocele
descended diaphragm
descended testicle
descending aorta
descending aortic aneurysm
descending brain stem
descending colon
descending duodenum
descending genicular artery
descending loop colostomy
descending necrotizing
    mediastinitis (DNM)
descending palatine artery
descending technique
descending thoracic aorta to
    pulmonary artery shunt
descending urogram
descending urography
descensus uteri
descensus ventriculi
descent of the cheek fat
Deschamps carrier
Deschamps compressor
Deschamps ligature carrier
Deschamps ligature needle
Deschamps needle
Deschamps-Navratil ligature
    needle
Deschamps-Navratil needle
Descot fracture
desensitization
desensitize
Deseret angiocatheter
Deseret flow-directed
    thermodilution catheter
Deseret sump drain
desiccate
desiccated lesion
desiccated thyroid
desiccation
    ball electrode desiccation
    electrosurgical desiccation
    mucous desiccation
desiccation needle
desiccation-fulguration needle
designated donor
designated recipient
designed after natural anatomy
    (DANA)
DesignLine orthotic

designs for vision frame
designs for vision side shield
Desilets catheter
Desilets introducer
Desilets-Hoffman catheter
Desilets-Hoffman catheter
  introducer
Desilets-Hoffman introducer
Desilets-Hoffman introducer set
Desilets-Hoffman micropuncture
  introducer
Desilets-Hoffman pacemaker
  introducer
Desilets-Hoffman sheath
DeSilva dermatome
desired breast width (DBW)
Desjardins dilator
Desjardins forceps
Desjardins gall duct scoop
Desjardins gallbladder scoop
Desjardins gallstone forceps
Desjardins gallstone probe
Desjardins gallstone scoop
Desjardins kidney pedicle
  forceps
Desjardins point
Desjardins probe
Desjardins scoop
Desmarres cardiovascular
  retractor
Desmarres chalazion forceps
Desmarres clamp
Desmarres corneal dissection
Desmarres corneal dissector
Desmarres dissector
Desmarres elevator
Desmarres eye dissector
Desmarres eye speculum
Desmarres fixation pick
Desmarres forceps
Desmarres iris knife
Desmarres knife
Desmarres lid clamp
Desmarres lid elevator
Desmarres lid forceps
Desmarres lid retractor
Desmarres lid speculum
Desmarres marker
Desmarres needle
Desmarres operation
Desmarres paracentesis knife
Desmarres paracentesis needle

Desmarres refractor
Desmarres retractor
Desmarres scarifier
Desmarres valve retractor
Desmarres vein retractor
desmoid cyst
desmoid lesion
desmology
desmolysis
desmolytic
desmolytic stage
desmoplasia
desmoplastic ameloblastoma
desmoplastic fibroma
desmoplastic melanoma
desmosome
desmotomy
desquamate
desquamated cells
desquamated epithelial cell
desquamating debris
desquamating epithelium
desquamation
  branny desquamation
  erosion desquamation
  periungual desquamation
desquamative gingivitis
desquamative nephritis
desquamative pneumonia
Desting prostatic dilatation
  technique
destruction
  bone destruction
  bony destruction
  bony element destruction
  bony necrosis and destruction
  Cawthorne destruction
  cortical destruction
  deep destruction
  moth-eaten bone destruction
  mucosal destruction
  progressive parenchymal
    destruction
  superficial destruction
destruction of lesion
destruction of lesion by
  cauterization
destruction of lesion by
  curettage
destruction of lesion by
  fulguration
destructive bone lesion

destructive injury
destructive interference
    technique
destructive obstetrical hook
destructive process
desultory labor
desultory pain
detachable balloon
detachable coil
detachable stretcher frame
detached cranial section
detached craniotomy
detached loose body
detached retina
detachment
    Arruga operation for retinal
        detachment
    cautery for retinal
        detachment
    cerclage for retinal
        detachment
    choroid detachment
    Descemet membrane
        detachment
    encircling procedure for
        retinal detachment
    exudative retinal
        detachment
    light coagulation for retinal
        detachment
    macula-off retinal detachment
    retinal detachment (RD)
    rhegmatogenous retinal
        detachment
    ruby laser operation for
        retinal detachment
    scleral buckle procedure for
        retinal detachment
    traction detachment
    trapdoor technique for retinal
        detachment
    vitreous detachment
    Zeiss light coagulation for
        retinal detachment
detachment of ligament
detachment of retina
DeTakats-McKenzie brain
    clip-applying forceps
DeTakats-McKenzie
    clip-applying forceps
DeTakats-McKenzie forceps
deteriorated condition

deteriorating neurological
    disorder
deteriorating patient
deterioration
determinant
detorsed
detorsion
detrusor function
detrusor pattern
detrusor response
detrusor sphincter dyssynergia
detrusor urinae
detubation
Deucher abdominal retractor
Deune knee prosthesis
deuterium-tritium generator
Deutschman cataract knife
Deutschman knife
devascularization
devascularize
devascularized material
DeVega annuloplasty
DeVega prosthesis
DeVega tricuspid valve
    annuloplasty
developed flap
development
    mosaic development
    motor development
    prenatal development
    transitional development
developmental cataract
developmental coordination
    disorder
developmental line
Deventer diameter
Deventer pelvis
Deverle fixation
Devers gallbladder tube
Devex mesh
deviant articulation
deviated nasal septum
deviated septum
deviation
    axis deviation
    conjugate deviation
    left axis deviation
    left deviation
    mandibular deviation
    manifest deviation
    medial deviation
    nasoseptal deviation

deviation (*continued*)
  radial deviation
  septal deviation
  tracheal deviation
  ulnar deviation
  wrist radial deviation
  wrist ulnar deviation
device for transverse traction
device therapy
Devices Ltd Pacemaker
DeVilbiss air compressor
DeVilbiss atomizer
DeVilbiss bottle
DeVilbiss compressor
DeVilbiss CPAP manometer
DeVilbiss cranial forceps
DeVilbiss cranial rongeur
DeVilbiss cranial trephine
DeVilbiss cutoffs
DeVilbiss eye irrigator
DeVilbiss forceps
DeVilbiss I&A unit
DeVilbiss irrigating syringe
DeVilbiss irrigator
DeVilbiss Mini-Dop fetal monitor
DeVilbiss nebulizer
DeVilbiss OB-Dop fetal monitor
DeVilbiss powder blower
DeVilbiss Pulmo-Aide nebulizer
DeVilbiss rack
DeVilbiss rongeur
DeVilbiss rongeur forceps
DeVilbiss skull trephine
DeVilbiss speculum
DeVilbiss spirometer
DeVilbiss suction pump
DeVilbiss suction tube
DeVilbiss syringe
DeVilbiss trephine
DeVilbiss Vacu-Aide aspirator
DeVilbiss vaginal speculum
DeVilbiss vaporizer
DeVilbiss-Stacey speculum
devil's claw
devil's incision mammaplasty
Devine antral exclusion
Devine colostomy
Devine hypospadias repair
Devine operation
Devine pyloroplasty
Devine tube
Devine-Devine procedure

Devine-Millard-Aufricht retractor
Devine-Millard-Frazier fiberoptic
  suction tube
Devine-Millard-Frazier suction
  tube
devisceration
devitalization
devitalize
devitalized
devitalized bone graft
devitalized skin
devitalized soft tissue
devitalized tissue
devolvulization
Devon-Pura stent
Devonshire catheter
Devonshire knife
Devonshire needle
Devonshire operation for talipes
  valgus
Devonshire roller
Devonshire technique
Devonshire-Mack cannula
Devonshire-Mack catheter
Devonshire-Mack clamp
Dewald halo spinal appliance
DeWall bubbler-type pump
Dewar elevator
Dewar flask
Dewar posterior cervical
  fixation procedure
Dewar posterior cervical fusion
Dewar procedure
Dewar-Barrington arthroplasty
Dewar-Barrington clavicular
  dislocation technique
Dewar-Barrington procedure
Dewar-Harris operation
Dewar-Harris shoulder
  technique
dewebbing
DeWecker anterior sclerotomy
DeWecker cannula
DeWecker eye implant
DeWecker eye scissors
DeWecker forceps
DeWecker iridectomy scissors
DeWecker iris scissors
DeWecker iris spatula
DeWecker operation
DeWecker scissors
DeWecker sclerotomy

DeWecker syringe cannula
DeWecker-Pritikin iris scissors
DeWecker-Pritikin scissors
DeWeerd ureteropelvioplasty
DeWeese axis traction forceps
DeWeese axis traction
    obstetrical forceps
DeWeese caval catheter
DeWeese clamp
DeWeese vena cava clamp
DeWeese-Hunter clip
Dewey forceps
Dewey obstetrical forceps
DeWitt-Stetten colostomy spur
    crusher
DEXA densitometer
Dexide disposable cannula
Dexide laparoscopic trocar
Dexon absorbable synthetic
    polyglycolic acid sutures
Dexon II sutures
Dexon mesh
Dexon Plus sutures
Dexon polyglycolic acid mesh
Dexon subcuticular sutures
Dexon surgical table
Dexon surgically knitted mesh
Dexon sutures
Dexter-Grossman classification
Dexterity Pneumo Sleeve
Dextran-70 barrier material
dextranomer
dextrocardia
dextroduction of eye
dextroposition
dextropositioned aorta
dextrorotatory scoliosis
dextrorotoscoliosis
dextroscoliotic curvature
dextroversion
Deyerle bone graft plate
Deyerle component
Deyerle drill
Deyerle femoral fracture
    technique
Deyerle fixation device
Deyerle hip fracture reduction
Deyerle nail
Deyerle pin
Deyerle plate
Deyerle procedure
Deyerle punch

Deyerle screw
Deyo device
Dey-Wash skin wound cleansers
DF (distal fossa)
DFDB (demineralized freeze-
    dried bone)
DFDBA (decalcified freeze-dried
    bone allograft)
DFDBA (demineralized freeze-
    dried bone allograft)
DFDCB (decalcified freeze-dried
    cortical bone)
DG Softgut sutures
DG Softgut sutures
DG-L image
DG-T image
Dia pump
Dia pump aspirator
Dia suction
Diab-A-Thotics orthotic
diabetes mellitus
diabetic cataract
diabetic complication
Diabetic D-Sole foot orthosis
diabetic foot
diabetic foot ulcer
diabetic gangrene
diabetic orthosis kit
diabetic puncture
Diabeticorum dressing
DiabGel hydrogel dressing
DiabKlenz wound cleansers
diaclasis
diaclastic amputation
diacondylar fracture
diafiltrate
diafiltration
Diaflex dilator
Diaflex grasping forceps
Diaflex nephrostomy
Diaflex retrieval loop
Diaflex ureteral dilatation
    catheter
diagnosis (pl. diagnoses)
    anatomic diagnosis
    clinical diagnosis
    colposcopic diagnosis
    cytologic diagnosis
    definitive diagnosis
    differential diagnosis
    equivocal diagnosis
    final diagnosis

diagnosis (*continued*)
    final pathological diagnosis
    frozen section diagnosis
    genetic diagnosis
    histologic diagnosis
    histological diagnosis
    histopathologic diagnosis
    initial diagnosis
    microscopic diagnosis
    noninvasive diagnosis
    nonoperative diagnosis
    operative diagnosis
    pathologic diagnosis
    possible diagnosis
    postoperative diagnosis
    prenatal diagnosis
    preoperative diagnosis
    presumptive diagnosis
    radiologic diagnosis
    surgical diagnosis
    unequivocal diagnosis
    working diagnosis
diagnostic accuracy
diagnostic and operative
    arthroscopy
diagnostic anesthesia
diagnostic arthroscopy and
    debridement
diagnostic arthroscopy,
    operative arthroscopy, and
    possible operative
    arthrotomy
diagnostic articulation test
diagnostic biopsy
diagnostic cardiac
    catheterization
diagnostic cast
diagnostic catheter
diagnostic colonoscopy
diagnostic curet
diagnostic curettage
diagnostic D&C
diagnostic dilatation and
    curettage
diagnostic dilemma
diagnostic duodenoscope
diagnostic ear tube
diagnostic excisional biopsy
diagnostic fiberoptic lens
diagnostic fiberoptic
    stomatoscopy
diagnostic finding

diagnostic hysteroscope
diagnostic imaging evaluation
diagnostic investigation
diagnostic laparoscopy
Diagnostic Medical Instruments
    (DMI)
diagnostic mirror
diagnostic modality
diagnostic otoscope
diagnostic peritoneal lavage
    (DPL)
diagnostic procedure
diagnostic program
diagnostic radiation
diagnostic set
diagnostic small bowel series
diagnostic spinal tap
diagnostic step
diagnostic study
diagnostic surgery
diagnostic surgical therapy
diagnostic technique
diagnostic therapy
diagnostic tube
diagnostic ultrasound
diagnostic ultrasound imaging
    catheter
diagnostic value
diagnostic workup
diagnostic x-ray
Diaket root canal cement
dial lock
dial osteotomy
Dialix dialyzer
dial-lock orthosis
Dialock access port
Dialog pacemaker
Dialom bur
dialtor
Dialyflex dialysis fluid
Dialy-Nate catheter
dialysate bag
dialysis
    Abderhalden dialysis
    AMP dialysis
    continuous ambulatory
      peritoneal dialysis (CAPD)
    course of dialysis
    iris dialysis
    lymph dialysis
    maintenance dialysis
    peritoneal dialysis

dialysis access surgery
dialysis catheter
dialysis disequilibrium syndrome
dialysis encephalopathy
   syndrome
dialysis fistula
dialysis fluid
dialysis procedure
dialysis shunt
dialysis therapy
dialysis unit
dialysis-related ascites
dialyzation unit
dialyzed patient
dialyzer membrane
diamagnetic
Diamatrix trapezoidal diamond
   knife
Diamed leg bag
diameter
   aerodynamic equivalent
      diameter (AED)
   anterotransverse diameter
   Baudelocque diameter
   biparietal diameter (BPD)
   bisiliac diameter
   bispinous diameter
   bitemporal diameter
   buccolingual diameter
   cephalocaudad diameter
   cervicobregmatic diameter
   chest diameter
   coccygeopubic diameter
   conjugate diameter (CD)
   cranial diameter
   craniometric diameter
   Deventer diameter
   disk diameter
   extracanthic diameter
   fetal cranial diameters
   frontomental diameter
   fronto-occipital diameter
   inside diameter
   intercanthic diameter
   intertuberal diameter
   Loehlein diameter
   longitudinal diameter
   mento-occipital diameter
   mentoparietal diameter
   midpelvic anteroposterior
      diameter
   midpelvic diameter

diameter (*continued*)
   oblique diameter
   occipitofrontal diameter
   occipitomental diameter
   outside diameter
   parietal diameter
   pelvic diameter
   posterotransverse diameter
   pubosacral diameter
   pubotuberous diameter
   sacropubic diameter
   sagittal diameter
   suboccipitobregmatic
      diameter
   temporal diameter
   transthoracic diameter
   transverse diameter
   vertebromammary diameter
diametric pelvic fracture
diamond barrel bur
diamond blade
diamond blade knife
diamond bur
Diamond classification
diamond dermabrader
diamond disk
diamond drill
diamond electrode
diamond finishing bur
diamond fraise
diamond green marker
diamond grip needle holder
diamond high-speed aid drill
Diamond pacemaker
diamond inlay bone graft
diamond instrument
diamond knife
diamond micrometer
diamond nail
diamond nasal rasp
diamond needle holder
diamond phaco knife
diamond rasp
diamond saw
Diamond SharpPoint needle
Diamond tube
Diamond valve
diamond wafering saw
diamond wire cutter
diamond-coated bur
diamond-dust bur
diamond-dusted knife

diamond-dusted tip
Diamond-Edge Supercut
  scissors
diamond-edged scissors
Diamond-Flex trocar
Diamond-Gould syndactyly
  operation
Diamond-Gould technique
Diamond-Jaw needle holder
Diamond-Lite cardiovascular
  instrument
Diamond-Lite titanium
  instrument
diamond-pin cutter
diamond-point suture needle
diamond-shaped incision
diamond-shaped murmur
Diamontek knife
Dianoux operation
Dianoux trichiasis operation
diaphanography
diaphanoscope
diaphanoscopy
DiaPhine corneal trephination
  device
DiaPhine trephine
DiaPhone corneal trephination
  device
diaphoscope
diaphragm
  Akerlund diaphragm
  Bucky diaphragm
  central tendon of diaphragm
  Chambers diaphragm
  cordiform tendon of
    diaphragm
  crus of diaphragm
  descended diaphragm
  dome of diaphragm
  elevated diaphragm
  elevation of diaphragm
  intermediate tendon of
    diaphragm
  left diaphragm
  oral diaphragm
  Ortho All-Flex diaphragm
  pelvic diaphragm
  pillar of diaphragm
  Potter-Bucky diaphragm
  Ramses diaphragm
  ruptured diaphragm
  styloid diaphragm

diaphragm (*continued*)
  superior fascia of urogenital
    diaphragm
  tenting of diaphragm
  urogenital diaphragm
  wide-seal diaphragm
diaphragm eventration
diaphragm injury
diaphragm inserter
diaphragm laceration
diaphragm of mouth
diaphragm perforation
diaphragm pessary
diaphragm stethoscope
diaphragmatic artery
diaphragmatic crural repair
diaphragmatic defect
diaphragmatic elevation
diaphragmatic eventration
diaphragmatic excursions
diaphragmatic hernia
diaphragmatic hernia repair
diaphragmatic herniation
diaphragmatic herniorrhaphy
diaphragmatic hiatus
diaphragmatic injury
diaphragmatic laceration
diaphragmatic muscle
diaphragmatic nerve
diaphragmatic node
diaphragmatic pleura
diaphragmatic pulmonary infarct
diaphragmatic reflection
diaphragmatic respiration
diaphragmatic rupture
diaphragmatic silhouette
diaphragmatic surface
diaphragmatic surface of heart
diaphragmatocele
diaphyseal-epiphyseal fusion
diaphysectomy
diaphysis
diarthrodial cartilage
diarthrodial joint
diascopic examination
diascopy
Dias-Giegerich fracture
  technique
Dias-Giegerich open reduction
Dias-Giegerich technique
Diasonics Cardiovue Sector
  scanner

Diasonics catheter
Diasonics ultrasound unit
Diasonics Therasonic lithotriptor
Diasonics transducer
Diasonics ultrasound
Dias-Tachdijian physical injury
    classification
diastalsis
diastasis
    ankle mortise diastasis
    iris diastasis
    palpable rib diastasis
    pubic diastasis
    rectus diastasis
    sutural diastasis
    tibiofibular diastasis
diastasis cordis
diastasis fibula
diastasis of cranial bone
diastasis of muscle
diastasis recti
diastasis recti abdominis
Diastat vascular access graft
diastatic fracture
diastatic skull fracture
diastema (pl. diastemata)
diastole
diastolic blood pressure
diastolic fluttering aortic valve
diastolic murmur
diastolic pressure
diastolic rumble
DIASYS Novacor cardiac
    device
DiaTAP vascular access button
    for dialysis patients
diathermal needle
diathermal snare
diathermia knife
diathermic electrode
diathermic eye electrode
diathermic fistulotomy
diathermic forceps
diathermic loop
diathermic loop biopsy
diathermic needle
diathermic precut needle
diathermic resection
diathermic retinal electrode
diathermic scissors
diathermic snare
diathermic therapy

diathermy
    Aloetherm diathermy
    coagulating diathermy
    electrocoagulation diathermy
    medical diathermy
    microwave diathermy
    Mira diathermy
    short-wave diathermy
    surgical diathermy
    ultrasonic diathermy
    underwater diathermy
diathermy and massage
diathermy cord
diathermy dissection
diathermy electrode
diathermy forceps
diathermy hemorrhoidectomy
diathermy knife
diathermy operation
diathermy palatoplasty
diathermy puncture
diathermy scissors
diathermy tip
diathermy unit
diathermy wire
diathesis
DIB (duodenoileal bypass)
Dibbell cleft lip-nasal
    reconstruction
Dibbell cleft lip-nasal revision
dibucaine hydrochloride
    anesthetic agent
DIC (diffuse intravascular
    coagulopathy)
DIC (disseminated intravascular
    coagulation)
DIC tracheostomy tube
diced cartilage graft
dichorionic placenta
dichotomous classification
dichromate dosimeter
dichromography
Dick bronchus clamp
Dick cardiac valve dilator
Dick combination container
Dick dilator
Dick operation
Dick pressure clamp
Dick treatment stand
Dick valve dilator
Dickerson intraocular implant
    lens

Dickerson lens
Dickey operation
Dickey ptosis repair
Dickey-Fox operation
Dickhaut-DeLee discoid
    meniscus classification
Dickinson approach
Dickinson calcaneal bursitis
    technique
Dickinson flow cytometer
Dickson operation
Dickson osteotomy
Dickson shelf operation
Dickson technique
Dickson transplant technique
Dickson-Diveley operation
Dickson-Diveley procedure
Dickson-Willien technique
Dickson-Wright operation
Dickson-Wright orbit
    decompression
dicondylar fracture
dicrotic notch
dicrotic pulse
didactylism
didelphic uterus
didelphys
    uterine didelphys
    uterus didelphys
die
    metal-plated die
    pin-deburring die
    Schuknecht-Paparella wire-
        bending die
    wire-bending die
die punch fracture
Dieckmann intraosseous
    needle
Diederich empyema trocar
Dieffenbach amputation
Dieffenbach bulldog clamp
Dieffenbach clamp
Dieffenbach forceps
Dieffenbach knife
Dieffenbach operation
Dieffenbach otoplasty
Dieffenbach plastic closure
Dieffenbach scalpel
Dieffenbach serrefine
Dieffenbach-Duplay hypospadias
    technique
Dieffenbach-Duplay operation

Dieffenbach-Szymanowski-Kuhnt
    operation
Dieffenbach-Warren operation
Dieffenbach-Webster operation
Dienco flowmeter
Diener forceps
dieresis
Diertz shears
Dieter forceps
Dieter malleus forceps
Dieter nipper
Dieter-House nipper
Diethrich aortic clamp
Diethrich circumflex artery
    scissors
Diethrich clamp
Diethrich coronary artery
    bypass kit
Diethrich coronary artery set
Diethrich coronary scissors
Diethrich graft clamp
Diethrich microcoronary
    bulldog clamp
Diethrich right-angled
    hemostatic forceps
Diethrich scissors
Diethrich shunt clamp
Diethrich valve scissors
Diethrich-Hegemann scissors
diethyl oxide anesthetic agent
Dieulafoy aspirator
Dieulafoy erosion
Dieulafoy lesion
Dieulafoy triad
Dieulafoy ulcer
Dieulafoy vascular malformation
Dieulafoy-like lesion
differential diagnosis
differential force technique
differential nerve block
differential spinal anesthesia
differential spinal block
differential spinal block
    anesthetic technique
differentiated carcinoma
differentiated thyroid carcinoma
differentiation failure
Differin Gel
difficult vaginal delivery
difficult ventilation
diffraction pattern
diffuse abscess

diffuse acute inflammation
diffuse air space disease
diffuse alveolar atrophy
diffuse aneurysm
diffuse atrophy
diffuse breast involvement
diffuse calcification
diffuse chronic inflammation
diffuse colloid goiter
diffuse condition
diffuse enlargement
diffuse esophageal spasm
diffuse fatty infiltration
diffuse fusiform dilatation
diffuse ganglion
diffuse idiopathic sclerosing
    hyperostosis (DISH)
diffuse idiopathic skeletal
    hyperostosis
diffuse intravascular coagulation
diffuse large cell lymphoma
diffuse metastasis
diffuse multimodular goiter
diffuse plane
diffuse pulmonary alveolar
    hemorrhage
diffuse scleritis
diffuse scleroderma
diffuse serous labyrinthitis
diffuse suppurative labyrinthitis
diffuse swelling
diffuse systemic sclerosis
diffuse toxic non-nodular goiter
diffuse ulcerative lesion
diffusely tender abdomen
diffusion-weighted MR imaging
digastric fossa
digastric groove
digastric line
digastric muscle
digastric muscle flap
digastric nerve
digastric ridge
digastric space
digastric triangle
DiGeorge syndrome
digestive bleeding
digestive glandular cancer
digestive system vascular disease
digestive tract
digestive tube
Digi Sleeve stockinette dressing

Digi-Dyne cardiopulmonary
    bypass oxygenator
Digi-Dyne dialyzer
Digiflator digital inflation device
Digiflex cannula
Digiflex high-flow catheter
Digikit finger tourniquet
Digilab perimeter
Digilab pneumatonography
Digilab pneumatonometer
Digirad gamma camera
DigiScope camera
DIGISleeve
digit
    common extensor muscle of
        digits
    extra digit
    replantation of amputated
        digit
    sausage digit
    severed digit
    supernumerary digits
    trigger digit
Digit Aid splint
digit splint
digit tube
digit wrap
Digital Add-On Bucky x-ray
    device
digital artery
digital beam attenuation
digital biometric rule
digital block
digital block anesthesia
digital calipers
Digital Care kit
digital collateral artery
digital compression
digital dilation
digital examination
digital fibromatosis
digital flap
digital furrow
digital goniometer
digital image score
digital imaging colposcopy
digital manipulation
digital nerve
digital nerve block
digital nerve reconstruction
digital readout
digital rectal evacuation

digital rectal examination
digital replantation
digital runoff
digital slide scanner
digital subtraction angiogram
digital subtraction angiography
    (DSA)
digital subtraction supravalvular
    aortogram
digital subtraction technique
digital tonometry
digital vein
digital venous arch
digital x-ray detector
digitalate pulse
digitales dorsales pedis, nevae
digitalization of heart
digitalize
digitally guided biopsy
digital-to-analog converted
digitate impression
Digitate microsurgical
    instrument
digitation
Digitimer pattern reversal
    stimulator
digitized instrument
digitized subtraction
    angiography
digitizing pad
digitoxin
Digitrapper ECG recorder
Digitrapper Mark III sleep
    monitor
Dilamezinsert device
Dilamezinsert dilator
Dilamezinsert penile prosthesis
Dilamezinsert urologic
    instrument
Dilapan hygroscopic cervical
    dilator
Dilapan laminaria
Dilaprobe dilator
dilatable bougie
dilatable lesion
dilatation (*see also* dilation)
    anal dilatation
    Anel lacrimal dilatation
    aneurysmal dilatation
    balloon dilatation
    bile duct dilatation
    biliary dilatation

dilatation (*continued*)
    blind dilatation
    bowel dilatation
    bronchoscopy with dilatation
    bulbous dilatation
    caliceal dilatation
    cardiac dilatation
    catheter dilatation
    congenital cystic dilatation
    cricopharyngeal dilatation
    cystic dilatation
    cystoscopy and dilatation
    diffuse fusiform dilatation
    ductal dilatation
    effacement and dilatation
    endoscopic retrograde
        balloon dilatation
    esophageal dilatation
    ex vacuo dilatation
    fusiform dilatation
    gaseous dilatation
    gastric dilatation
    homatropine dilatation
    junctional dilatation
    pancreatic duct dilatation
    percutaneous stricture
        dilatation (PSD)
    percutaneous transluminal
        balloon dilatation (PTBD)
    periodic dilatation
    periportal sinusoidal
        dilatation
    pneumatic bag esophageal
        dilatation
    pneumatic dilatation
    poststenotic dilatation
    pouch dilatation
    prestenotic dilatation
    pupillary dilatation
    Pusto dilatation
    secondary arrest of dilatation
    segmental dilatation
    transurethral balloon
        dilatation
    urethral dilatation
    uterine dilatation
    Virchow-Robin space
        dilatation
dilatation and aspiration (D&A)
dilatation and curettage (D&C)
dilatation and evacuation (D&E)
dilatation balloon catheter

dilatation of cervix
dilatation of colon
dilatation of common bile duct
dilatation of esophagus
dilatation of organ
dilatation of urethra
dilated gallbladder
dilated organ
dilated pupil
dilated stricture
dilated vessel
dilating bougie
dilating bulb
dilating catheter
dilating catheter-gastrostomy
　　tube assembly
dilating forceps
dilating pressure balloon
　　catheter
dilating probe
dilation (*see also* dilatation)
　achalasia balloon dilation
　anal dilation
　Anel lacrimal duct dilation
　aneurysmal dilation
　balloon dilation
　biliary dilation
　bootstrap dilation
　bowel dilation
　Brown-McHardy pneumatic
　　mercury bougie dilation
　capillary dilation
　cardiac dilation
　catheter dilation
　cervical dilation
　colonic dilation
　cystic dilation
　digital dilation
　ductal dilation
　ectatic dilation
　Eder-Puestow dilation
　endoscopic dilation
　endoscopic papillary balloon
　　dilation
　episcleral vascular dilation
　esophageal dilation
　extrahepatic biliary cystic
　　dilation
　finger dilation
　Frank technique of dilation
　gastric dilation
　Gruentzig balloon dilation

dilation (*continued*)
　hepatic web dilation
　hydrostatic balloon dilation
　idiopathic dilation
　inadequate dilation
　instrumental dilation
　intrahepatic biliary cystic
　　dilation
　intrahepatic ductal dilation
　junctional dilation
　lag dilation
　mechanical ureteral dilation
　medical dilation
　mucosal vascular dilation
　percutaneous balloon
　　dilation
　periportal sinusoidal dilation
　peroral esophageal dilation
　pneumatic bag esophageal
　　dilation
　pneumatic balloon catheter
　　dilation
　pneumostatic dilation
　postoperative ductal dilation
　poststenotic dilation
　progressive dilation
　pupil dilation
　pyloric dilation
　reactive dilation
　rectal dilation
　serial dilation
　submucosal vascular dilation
　through-the-scope balloon
　　dilation (TTT)
　tract dilation
　transurethral balloon
　　dilation
　TTS balloon dilation (through
　　the scope)
　ureteral dilation
　urethral dilation
　Uromat dilation
　ventricular dilation
　Wirsung dilation
dilation and curettage (D&C)
dilation and evacuation (D&E)
dilation catheter
dilation instrument
dilation lag
dilation of cervix
dilation therapy
dilation with metal sound

dilator
  2-bladed dilator
  achalasia dilator
  Achiever balloon dilator
  Alm dilator
  Ambler dilator
  American Dilation System
    dilator
  American endoscopy dilator
  American endoscopy
    esophageal dilator
  American Hanks uterine
    dilator
  Amplatz dilator
  Amplatz facial dilator
  anal dilator
  Anthony quadrisected dilator
  Anthony quadrisected
    minigraft dilator
  aortic dilator
  argon vessel dilator
  Arnott dilator
  Atlee dilator
  Atlee uterine dilator
  Avenida dilator
  Avenida-Torres dilator
  Backhaus dilator
  Bailey dilator
  Bakes bile duct dilator
  Bakes common duct dilator
  Bakes dilator
  Bakes-Pearce dilator
  balloon dilator
  Bard dilator
  Bard urethral dilator
  Barnes cervical dilator
  Barnes common duct dilator
  Barnes dilator
  Beardsley aortic dilator
  Beardsley dilator
  Beehler pupil dilator
  Benique dilator
  Bennett common duct dilator
  Berens dilator
  Berens punctum dilator
  biliary duct balloon dilator
  biliary duct dilator
  bisected minigraft dilator
  Black-Wylie dilator
  Black-Wylie obstetric dilator
  bladder dilator
  Bonney cervical dilator

dilator (*continued*)
  Bossi cervical dilator
  Bossi dilator
  bougie dilator
  Bowman dilator
  Bowman lacrimal dilator
  Bozeman dilator
  Braasch ureteral dilator
  Bransford-Lewis dilator
  Bransford-Lewis ureteral
    dilator
  Brock cardiac dilator
  Brock dilator
  bronchial dilator
  Brown-Buerger dilator
  Brown-McHardy air-filled
    pneumatic dilator
  Brown-McHardy dilator
  Brown-McHardy pneumatic
    dilator
  Broyles dilator
  Broyles esophageal dilator
  Buerger-Oliver dilator
  Béniqué dilator
  canaliculus dilator
  cannula with locking dilator
  cardiac dilator
  cardiac valve dilator
  cardioesophageal junction
    dilator
  cardiospasm dilator
  Castroviejo dilator
  Castroviejo double-end dilator
  Castroviejo double-end
    lacrimal dilator
  Castroviejo lacrimal dilator
  Castroviejo-Galezowski dilator
  Catalano dilator
  Celestin graduated dilator
  cervical dilator
  child rectal dilator
  Clark common duct dilator
  Clark dilator
  Clerf dilator
  common bile duct dilator
  common duct dilator
  Cook-Amplatz dilator
  Cooley coronary dilator
  Cooley dilator
  Cooley pediatric dilator
  Cooley valve dilator
  Cooley vascular dilator

dilator (*continued*)
Cordis dilator
coronary dilator
cortical incision coronary
   dilator
Councill dilator
Councill ureteral dilator
Creevy dilator
Creevy urethral dilator
Crump dilator
Crump vessel dilator
Crump-Himmelstein dilator
Cunningham-Cotton sleeve
   coaxial dilator
Dagger dilator
de Signeux dilator
DeBakey vascular dilator
DeBakey-Cooley dilator
DeBakey-Cooley valve dilator
Delaborde dilator
Delaborde tracheal dilator
Delaborde-Trousseau tracheal
   dilator
Delclos dilator
Denniston dilator
Derra cardiac valve dilator
Derra dilator
Derra valve dilator
Desjardins dilator
Diaflex dilator
Dick cardiac valve dilator
Dick dilator
Dick valve dilator
Dilamezinsert dilator
Dilapan hygroscopic cervical
   dilator
Dilaprobe dilator
disposable cervical dilator
Dittel uterine dilator
Dittman dilator
Dittsburg dilator
Dotter dilator
double-ended dilator
Dourmashkin dilator
duct dilator
Eder-Puestow dilator
Eder-Puestow esophageal
   dilator
Einhorn dilator
Einhorn esophageal dilator
Eliminator PET biliary balloon
   dilator

dilator (*continued*)
Encapsulon vessel dilator
ERCP dilator
esophageal balloon dilator
esophageal dilator
esophagospasm dilator
expandable cervical dilator
expansile dilator
Falope-ring dilator
Feldbausch dilator
Fenton dilator
Fenton uterine dilator
Ferris biliary duct dilator
Ferris dilator
Ferris filiform dilator
fixed cervical dilator
fluoroscopy-guided balloon
   dilator
French dilator
French lacrimal dilator
French-Hanks uterine dilator
French-McRea dilator
Frommer dilator
frontal sinus dilator
Galezowski dilator
Galezowski lacrimal dilator
gall duct dilator
gallstone dilator
Garrett dilator
Garrett vascular dilator
Gerbode dilator
Gerbode mitral dilator
Gerbode mitral valvulotomy
   dilator
Gerbode valve dilator
Gillquist-Oretorp-Stille dilator
Glover dilator
Glover modification of Brock
   aortic dilator
Godelo dilator
Gohrbrand cardiac dilator
Gohrbrand dilator
Goodell dilator
Goodell uterine dilator
Gouley dilator
graduated Garrett dilator
grooved director dilator
Gruentzig balloon dilator
Guyon dilator
Hank uterine dilator
Hank-Bradley uterine dilator
Hanks uterine dilator

dilator (*continued*)

Hanks-Bradley uterine dilator
Hayman dilator
Hearst dilator
Heath dilator
Heath punctum dilator
Hegar dilator
Hegar rectal dilator
Hegar uterine dilator
Hegar-Goodell dilator
Henley dilator
Henning cardiac dilator
Henning dilator
Heyner dilator
Hiebert vascular dilator
high-diameter dilator
Hohn vessel dilator
Hopkins dilator
Hosford dilator
Hosford double-ended
    lacrimal dilator
Hosford eye dilator
Hosford lacrimal dilator
House lacrimal dilator
Hurst bullet-tip dilator
Hurst bullet-tip esophageal
    dilator
Hurst dilator
Hurst esophageal dilator
Hurst esophagus dilator
Hurst mercury dilator
Hurst mercury-filled dilator
Hurst-Maloney dilator
Hurst-Tucker pneumatic
    dilator
Hurtig dilator
hydrophilic dilator
hydrostatic dilator
Iglesias dilator
implant site dilator
incision dilator
infant dilator
Ivinsco cervical dilator
Jackson bronchial dilator
Jackson dilator
Jackson esophageal dilator
Jackson tracheal dilator
Jackson triangular brass
    dilator
Jackson-Mosher cardiospasm
    dilator
Jackson-Mosher dilator

dilator (*continued*)

Jackson-Plummer dilator
Jackson-Trousseau dilator
Jewett uterine dilator
Johnston dilator
Johnston infant dilator
Jolly dilator
Jolly uterine dilator
Jones canaliculus dilator
Jones dilator
Jones lacrimal canaliculus
    dilator
Jones punctum dilator
Jordan dilator
Jordan wire loop dilator
Kahn dilator
Kahn uterine dilator
Kearns bladder dilator
Kearns dilator
Kelly dilator
Kelly orifice dilator
Kelly sphincter dilator
Kelly uterine dilator
Keuch pupil dilator
Keymed dilator
Kleegman dilator
Kohlman dilator
Kohlman urethral dilator
K-Pratt dilator
Krol esophageal dilator
Krol-Koski tracheal dilator
Kron bile duct dilator
Kron dilator
Kron gall duct dilator
Laborde dilator
Laborde tracheal dilator
lacrimal canaliculus dilator
lacrimal dilator
laminaria seaweed obstetrical
    cervical dilator
laminaria seaweed obstetrical
    dilator
Landau dilator
laryngeal dilator
Laufe cervical dilator
Leader-Kohlman dilator
LeFort dilator
LeMaitre-Bookwalter dilator
Luchese mitral valve dilator
Mahoney dilator
Mahorner dilator
Maloney dilator

dilator (*continued*)

Maloney esophageal dilator
Maloney mercury-filled dilator
Maloney mercury-filled
  esophageal dilator
Maloney tapered-tip dilator
Maloney-Hurst dilator
mandrin dilator
Mantz dilator
Mantz rectal dilator
Marritt dilator
McCrae dilator
meatal dilator
Medi-Tech fascial dilator
mercury-filled dilator
mercury-weighted dilator
metal-olive dilator
micrograft dilator
Microvasive controlled radial
  expansion esophageal
  dilator
Microvasive Rigiflex balloon
  dilator
Miller dilator
minigraft dilator
mitral dilator
mitral valve dilator
Mixter common duct
  irrigating Dilaprobe dilator
Mixter dilator
Moersch cardiospasm dilator
Mosher dilator
Muldoon dilator
Muldoon lacrimal dilator
Murphy common duct dilator
Murphy dilator
myocardial dilator
nasal dilator
Nettleship canaliculus dilator
Nettleship dilator
Nettleship-Wilder dilator
Nettleship-Wilder lacrimal
  dilator
Nottingham One-Step tapered
  dilator
Nottingham ureteral dilator
Olbert balloon dilator
olivary dilator
olive dilator
olive-tipped dilator
Optilume prostate balloon
  dilator

dilator (*continued*)

Otis bougie á boule dilator
Ottenheimer common duct
  dilator
Ottenheimer dilator
Outerbridge uterine dilator
over-the-endoscope Witzel
  dilator
over-the-guidewire esophageal
  dilator
Palmer dilator
Palmer uterine dilator
Parsonnet dilator
Patton dilator
Patton esophageal dilator
pediatric rectal dilator
Percor dilator
Pharmaseal disposable
  cervical dilator
Phillips dilator
Pilling dilator
Plummer dilator
Plummer esophageal dilator
Plummer water-filled
  pneumatic esophageal
  dilator
Plummer-Vinson dilator
Plummer-Vinson esophageal
  dilator
pneumatic balloon dilator
pneumatic dilator
pneumostatic dilator
polyvinyl dilator
Porges Neoflex dilator
Potts dilator
Potts expansile dilator
Potts-Riker dilator
Pratt dilator
Pratt rectal dilator
Pratt uterine dilator
probe dilator
progressive dilators
Puestow dilator
punctal dilator
punctum dilator
pupil dilator
pyloric stenosis dilator
quadrisected graft dilator
quadrisected minigraft dilator
Quantum TTC biliary balloon
  dilator
Ramstedt dilator

dilator (*continued*)

Ramstedt pyloric stenosis dilator
Ravich dilator
Ravich ureteral dilator
rectal dilator
Reich-Nechtow dilator
Richards-Moeller pneumatic air-filled dilator
Rider-Moeller cardiac dilator
Rider-Moeller pneumatic dilator
Rigiflex achalasia balloon dilator
Rigiflex balloon dilator
Rigiflex dilator
Rigiflex TTS balloon dilator
Ritter dilator
Ritter meatal dilator
Rockert dilator
Roland dilator
Rolf dilator
Rolf punctum dilator
Royal Hospital dilator
Rubbs aortic dilator
Ruedemann lacrimal dilator
Russell dilator
Russell hydrostatic dilator
Russell peel-away sheath dilator
Saint Mark dilator
Savary dilator
Savary esophageal dilator
Savary tapered thermoplastic dilator
Savary-Gilliard dilator
Savary-Gilliard esophageal dilator
Savary-Gilliard over-the-wire dilator
Scanlan vessel dilator
Simpson lacrimal dilator
Simpson uterine dilator
Sims dilator
Sims uterine dilator
Sinexon dilator
sinus dilator
Sippy dilator
Sippy esophageal dilator
Smedberg dilator
Soehendra catheter dilator
sphincter dilator

dilator (*continued*)

Spielberg dilator
stapes dilator
Starck dilator
Starlinger uterine dilator
Steele bronchial dilator
Steele dilator
Stille uterine dilator
Stucker bile duct dilator
synthetic hygroscopic cervical dilator
Szulc vascular dilator
Taylor pulmonary dilator
Theobald lacrimal dilator
through-the-scope dilator (TTS dilator)
tracheal dilator
tracheoesophageal dilator
tracheoesophageal puncture dilator
transventricular dilator
Trousseau dilator
Trousseau tracheal dilator
Trousseau-Jackson dilator
Trousseau-Jackson esophageal dilator
Trousseau-Jackson tracheal dilator
TTS dilator (through-the-scope dilator)
Tubbs aortic dilator
Tubbs dilator
Tubbs mitral valve dilator
Tubbs 2-bladed dilator
Tucker cardiospasm dilator
Tucker dilator
Turner dilator
ureteral dilator
ureteral stone dilator
urethral dilator
urethral female dilator
urethral male dilator
urethral meatus dilator
uterine dilator
vaginal dilator
valve dilator
van Buren dilator
Vantec dilator
vascular dilator
vein dilator
vessel dilator
Wales dilator

dilator (*continued*)
  Wales rectal dilator
  Walther dilator
  Walther urethral dilator
  Weiss gold dilator
  Wilder dilator
  Wilder lacrimal dilator
  Williams dilator
  Williams lacrimal dilator
  wire loop dilator
  wire loop stapes dilator
  wire-guided oval intracostal
    dilator
  Wise dilator
  Wylie dilator
  Wylie uterine dilator
  Young dilator
  Young pediatric rectal dilator
  Young rectal dilator
  Young vaginal dilator
  Ziegler dilator
  Ziegler lacrimal dilator
  Zipser meatal dilator
dilator catheter
dilator muscle of nose
dilator muscle of pupil
dilator naris
dilator naris muscle
dilator placement
dilator placement failure
dilator probe
dilator-and-sheath technique
dilator-sheath
Dilaudid anesthetic agent
Dileant osteotome
Dillwyn Evans procedure
Dillwyn Evans resection
Dilner-Doughty mouth gag
diluting fluid
dilution-filtration technique
Di-Main retractor
Dimension hip prosthesis
Dimension-C femoral stem
    prosthesis
dimethyl methacrylate
dimethylpolysiloxane
diminished bowel sounds
diminished breath sounds
diminished function
diminished reflexes
diminution
Dimitry chalazion trephine

Dimitry dacryocystorhinostomy
    trephine
Dimitry erysiphake
Dimitry trephine
Dimitry-Bell erysiphake
Dimitry-Thomas erysiphake
Dimon-Hughston fracture
    fixation
Dimon-Hughston technique
dimple and columns
dimple sign
dimpling of breast skin
dimpling of eyeball
dimpling of skin
Dinamap blood pressure cuff
Dinamap blood pressure monitor
Dinamap monitor
Dinamap ultrasound blood
    pressure manometer
Dingman abrader
Dingman bone-holding forceps
Dingman breast dissection
Dingman breast dissector
Dingman cartilage clamp
Dingman clamp
Dingman elevator
Dingman flexible retractor
Dingman Flexsteel retractor
Dingman forceps
Dingman malleable passing
    needle
Dingman mouth gag
Dingman mouth gag frame
Dingman mouth gag tongue
    depressor blade
Dingman needle
Dingman ostectomy
Dingman osteotome
Dingman otoplasty cartilage
    abrader
Dingman passing needle
Dingman periosteal elevator
Dingman retractor
Dingman wire passer
Dingman zygoma elevator
Dingman zygoma hook
Dingman zygoma hook retractor
Dingman zygomatic hook
Dingman-Denhardt mouth gag
Dingman-Millard mouth gag
Dingman-Senn retractor
dinner fork deformity

Dintenfass ear knife
Dintenfass-Chapman ear knife
Dintenfass-Chapman knife
diopter lens
diopter prism
dioptric aberration
dioptric correction
DIP (distal interphalangeal)
dip and plateau at cardiac
    catheterization
dip coating autoradiography
DIP fusion
DIP joint
diphasic wave
diphtheritic membrane
diploic canals
diploic vein
diplopia
Diplos pacemaker
Diprivan technique
dipstick
    anterior chamber dipstick
    Fyodorov dipstick
    Kelman dipstick
    Knolle dipstick
dipyridamole-thallium imaging
    (DTI)
direct approximation
direct catheterizing cystoscope
direct closure
direct component
direct compression
direct crease excision
direct current
direct current
    electrocoagulation
direct current generator
direct cystenterostomy
direct cytoscope
direct defect
direct digital radiography (DDR)
direct drainage
direct electrical nerve stimulator
direct embolectomy
direct fecal contamination
direct field
direct flap
direct forward-vision telescope
direct fracture
direct gonioscopic lens
direct hernia
direct immunofluorescence

direct inguinal hernia
direct insertion technique
direct inspection
direct intraperitoneal
    insemination
direct laryngeal operating
    instruments
direct laryngoscope
direct laryngoscopy
direct ligation
direct manipulation
direct metastasis
direct method for making inlays
direct microlaryngoscopy
direct muscle lysis
direct obturator nerve block
direct ophthalmoscope
direct ophthalmoscopy
direct porcelain matrix
direct radial sutures
direct retainer
direct supraciliary excision
direct transfer flap
direct transverse traction (DTT)
direct visualization
direct/indirect technique
Direct-Coupler arthroscope
direct-current bone growth
    stimulator
direct-current shock ablation
directed biopsy
directed fine-needle aspiration
    biopsy
DirectFlow arterial cannula
direct-focus headlight
direction
    anterograde direction
    caudal direction
    cephalad direction
    clockwise direction
    counterclockwise direction
    flow direction
    line of direction
    pelvic direction
    phase-encoding direction
    principal visual direction
    retrograde direction
    visual direction
    Z direction
directional atherectomy device
directional coronary
    atherectomy

director
  angled director
  Berman eye director
  Brodie director
  Cooper director
  Doyen director
  Durnin angled director
  grooved director
  Kocher goiter director
  Kocher grooved director
  Koenig grooved director
  Larry director
  Larry grooved director
  Larry rectal director
  laser fiber director
  Leksell director
  Leksell grooved director
  ligature director
  Ormco ligature director
  Payr grooved director
  plain-end grooved director
  Pratt director
  Pratt rectal director
  probe-ended grooved
      director
  Putti-Platt director
  Quickert grooved director
  rectal director
  Stiwer grooved director
  Teale director
  Toennis director
  ultrasonic flow director
  Wylie uterine director
DirectRay direct-to-digital x-ray
    capture device
direct-vision adenotome
direct-vision cystoscope
direct-vision internal
    urethrotomy (DVIU)
direct-vision liver biopsy
direct-vision telescope
Direx Tripter X-1
    lithotriptor
dirty operative wound
    classification
dirty surgery
dirty wound
dirty-lung appearance
DISA S-flex coronary stent
disappearing mandible
disarticular amputation
disarticulated

disarticulation
  Adelmann finger
      disarticulation
  Batch knee disarticulation
  Batchelor-Girdlestone
      disarticulation
  Batch-Spittler-McFadden knee
      disarticulation
  Boyd disarticulation
  Boyd hip disarticulation
  Burger technique for
      scapulothoracic
      disarticulation
  Carden disarticulation
  carpometacarpal
      disarticulation
  elbow disarticulation
  hip disarticulation
  joint disarticulation
  Lisfranc disarticulation
  Mazet disarticulation
  Mazet knee disarticulation
  metatarsophalangeal joint
      disarticulation
  radiocarpal disarticulation
  sacroiliac disarticulation
  shoulder disarticulation
  wrist disarticulation
disarticulation chisel
disc (see disk)
DISC nucleoplasty
discectomy (see diskectomy)
discharge
  cervical discharge
  malodorous discharge
  meconium discharge
  mucoid discharge
  mucopurulent discharge
  mucous discharge
  myotonic discharges
  nasal discharge
  neural discharge
  nipple discharge
  penile discharge
  postnasal discharge
  prior to discharge
  purulent discharge
  seropurulent discharge
  spike discharges
  watery discharge
  wound discharge
discharge tube

Dischler rectoscopic suction
   insert
discission blade
discission hook
discission knife
discission needle
discission of cataract
discission of cervix
discission of cervix uteri
discission of lens
discission of pleura
discogenic disease
discoid skin lesion
discoid valve prosthesis
discoidectomy
disconjugate gaze (*also*
   dysconjugate)
disconnection syndrome
discontinuous dissection
discontinuous neck dissection
discopathy
discorraphy
Disc-O-Sit Jr. cushion
Discover Cryo-Therapy unit
Discovery DDDR pacemaker
Discrene breast form
discrepancy
   anterior-posterior discrepancy
   arch discrepancy
   envelope of discrepancy
   leg-length discrepancy
   posterior occlusal
      discrepancy
   transverse discrepancy
   Wagner procedure to correct
      leg length discrepancy
discrete aneurysm
discrete lesion
discrete mass
discrete nodule
discriminator
disease recurrence rate
disease stage
diseased condition
diseased fascia
diseased organ
diseased tissue
disease-related complication
disembowelment
disengagement mechanism
Disetronic infuser syringe pump
dish face

dished-in face
dish-face deformity
dishpan face
dishpan fracture
DISI (dorsal intercalated
   segmental instability)
DISI deformity
DISIDA scan
disimpaction
disimpaction forceps
disinfectant
disinfecting fluid
disinfection
disinsertion
   levator disinsertion
disintegrating stones
disintegration
   endoscopic stone
      disintegration
disintegration rate
disjoint
disjunction
disjunctive nystagmus
disk (*also* disc)
   abrasive disk
   Acro-Flex artificial disk
   acromioclavicular disk
   Amici disk
   articular disk
   Bardeen primitive disk
   Bowman disks
   bulging disk
   Carborundum disk
   cartilaginous disk
   cervical disk
   choked disk
   ciliary disk
   cloth disk
   cupped disk
   cupping of disk
   cutting disk
   cuttlefish disk
   Damascus Disk
   diamond disk
   Double-hesive adhesive disk
   Eigon disk
   emery disk
   Engelmann disk
   extruded disk
   fibrocartilaginous disk
   floppy disk
   free fragment disk

disk (*continued*)
  gelatinous disk
  HCH disk
  herniated disk
  herniation of disk
  Horico disk
  interarticular disk
  intercalated disk
  interpubic disk
  interventricular disk
  intervertebral disk
  isotropic disk
  IV disk (intravertebral disk)
  Krupin eye disk
  Krupin valve with disk
  Lillehei-Kaster pivoting disk
  mandibular disk
  Merkel disk
  Molnar disk
  Moore disk
  Moran-Karaya disk
  Newton disk
  optic disk
  ortho disk
  Placido da Costa disk
  Placido disk
  planoconvex-shaped disk
  polishing disk
  protruded disk
  Ranvier tactile disk
  roof disk
  ruptured disk
  sacrococcygeal disk
  safety-sterility disk
  sandpaper disk
  sharp disk
  slipped disk
  soft disk
  stenopeic disk
  sternoclavicular disk
  Storz safety-sterility disk
  tactile disk
  temporomandibular articular
    disk
  thin disk
  Tracho-Foam adhesive disk
  transverse disk
  vertebral disk
disk compression
disk cupping
disk curet
disk diameter

disk disease
disk drusen hemorrhage
disk electrode
disk elevation
disk endoscope
disk excision
disk explorer
disk extrusion
disk forceps
disk fragment
disk grabber
disk herniation
disk lens intraocular lens
disk lesion
disk mandrel
disk neovascularization
disk oxygenation
disk oxygenator
disk oxygenator pump
disk plication
disk poppet
disk pressure
disk protrusion
disk rongeur
disk space
disk space infection
disk space narrowing
disk space saline acceptance test
disk valve
disk valve prosthesis
disk, disc
Diskard head halter
Disk-Criminator instrument
Disk-Criminator nerve
    stimulation measuring
    device
diskectomy (*also* discectomy)
  anterior diskectomy
  automated percutaneous
    diskectomy
  cervical diskectomy
  Cloward fusion diskectomy
  laminotomy and diskectomy
  lumbar diskectomy
  microlumbar diskectomy
  microsurgical diskectomy
  partial diskectomy
  percutaneous automated
    diskectomy (PAD)
  percutaneous diskectomy
  percutaneous lumbar
    diskectomy

diskectomy (*continued*)
  Robinson anterior cervical
    diskectomy
  Smith-Robinson anterior
    cervical diskectomy
  thoracic diskectomy
  thoracoscopic diskectomy
  transthoracic diskectomy
  Williams diskectomy
diskectomy forceps
diskectomy with Cloward fusion
diskiform process
diskogram
diskogram needle
diskographic needle
diskography
dislocated joint
dislocation
  antenatal dislocation
  anterior complete dislocation
  anterior hip dislocation
  anterior shoulder dislocation
  anterior-inferior dislocation
  anterolateral dislocation
  atlantoaxial dislocation
  atlantooccipital joint
    dislocation
  atypical dislocation
  Bankart dislocation
  Bankart operation for
    shoulder dislocation
  Bankart shoulder dislocation
  bayonet dislocation
  Bell-Dally cervical dislocation
  Bennett dislocation
  Bigelow dislocation
  bilateral interfacetal
    dislocation
  boutonniere hand dislocation
  bursting dislocation
  capitate dislocation
  carpal dislocation
  carpometacarpal joint
    dislocation
  central dislocation
  Chiari operation for
    congenital hip dislocation
  Chopart ankle dislocation
  Chopart dislocation
  closed dislocation
  closed reduction of
    dislocation

dislocation (*continued*)
  complete anterior dislocation
  complete dislocation
  complete inferior dislocation
  complete posterior
    dislocation
  complete superior dislocation
  complicated dislocation
  compound dislocation
  congenital dislocation
  congenital hip dislocation
    (CHD)
  congenital lens dislocation
  consecutive dislocation
  dashboard dislocation
  Desault dislocation
  Desault wrist dislocation
  divergent dislocation
  divergent elbow dislocation
  dorsal perilunate dislocation
  dorsal transscaphoid perilunar
    dislocation
  dysplasia dislocation
  Eden-Hybbinette operation for
    shoulder dislocation
  elbow dislocation
  facet dislocation
  femoral dislocation
  fracture dislocation
  frank dislocation
  gamekeeper's thumb
    dislocation
  glenohumeral joint
    dislocation
  habitual dislocation
  Hill-Sachs shoulder dislocation
  hip dislocation
  incomplete dislocation
  inferior complete closed
    dislocation
  inferior complete compound
    dislocation
  interphalangeal joint
    dislocation
  intraocular lens dislocation
  isolated dislocation
  joint dislocation
  Kienböck dislocation
  knee dislocation
  lens dislocation
  Lisfranc ankle dislocation
  Lisfranc dislocation

dislocation (*continued*)
lumbosacral dislocation
lunate dislocation
luxatio erecta shoulder
    dislocation
mandibular dislocation
manual reduction of
    dislocation
metatarsophalangeal joint
    dislocation
midcarpal dislocation
milkmaid's elbow dislocation
Monteggia dislocation
Nicola operation for shoulder
    dislocation
Nelaton ankle dislocation
Nelaton dislocation
occipitoatlantal dislocation
Omer sternoclavicular
    dislocation
open dislocation
open reduction of dislocation
Otto pelvis dislocation
Palmer transscaphoid
    perilunar dislocation
panclavicular dislocation
parachute jumper's
    dislocation
paralunate dislocation
partial dislocation
patella dislocation
patellar intraarticular
    dislocation
pathologic dislocation
perilunar transscaphoid
    dislocation
perilunate carpal dislocation
perilunate dislocation
peroneal dislocation
phalangeal dislocation
posterior hip dislocation
posterior shoulder dislocation
posteromedial dislocation
prenatal dislocation
primitive dislocation
prosthetic dislocation
proximal tibiofibular joint
    dislocation
radial head dislocation
radiocarpal dislocation
recent dislocation
recurrent dislocation

dislocation (*continued*)
recurrent patellar dislocation
retrosternal dislocation
Ridlon hip dislocation
rotational dislocation
sacroiliac dislocation
scapholunate dislocation
shoulder dislocation
simple dislocation
Smith dislocation
spontaneous hyperemic
    dislocation
sternoclavicular joint
    dislocation
subastragalar dislocation
subcoracoid dislocation
subcoracoid shoulder
    dislocation
subglenoid dislocation
subglenoid shoulder
    dislocation
subspinous dislocation
subtalar dislocation
superior dislocation
swivel dislocation
talar dislocation
tarsal dislocation
tarsometatarsal dislocation
temporomandibular joint
    dislocation
tendon dislocation
teratologic dislocation
Thompson-Epstein
    classification of hip
    dislocations
tibialis posterior dislocation
tibiofibular joint dislocation
transscaphoid perilunate
    dislocation
traumatic atlantooccipital
    dislocation
traumatic dislocation
triquetrolunate dislocation
unilateral interfacetal
    dislocation
unilateral intrafacetal
    dislocation
unreduced dislocation
volar semilunar wrist dislocation
von Rosen view for
    determining hip dislocation
wrist dislocation

dislocation contour abnormality
dislocation fracture
dislocation of bone
dislocation of cartilage
dislocation of joint
dislocation procedure
dislocator
   Kirby lens dislocator
dislodger (*see also* stone
   dislodger)
dismembered anastomosis
dismembered pyeloplasty
dismembered reimplanted
   appendicocystostomy
dismemberment
disorder of cornification
disorganized globe
disparate point
Dispatch infusion catheter
dispense as written (DAW)
dispensing tablet
dispersing electrode
dispersing lens
displaced condyle
displaced fracture
displaced malar fracture
displaced sideburn
displaced zygomatic fracture
displacement analysis
displacement curve
displacement implantation
displacement of fracture
displacement osteotomy
displacement sensing device
displacement syringe
displacement threshold
display technique
disposable acupuncture needle
disposable airway
disposable aortic rotating punch
disposable aspiration needle
disposable bikini
disposable biopsy needle
disposable cannula tip
disposable catheter
disposable cautery
disposable cervical dilator
disposable cord
disposable cryoextractor
disposable cryostylet
disposable cystotome cannula
disposable ear tip

disposable electrode
disposable electrode pad
disposable electrosurgical cord
disposable electrosurgical
   electrode
disposable electrosurgical pencil
disposable endoscopic
   conducting cord
disposable endoscopic
   electrosurgical cord
disposable forceps
disposable ground plate
disposable head halter
disposable injection needle
disposable instrument
disposable intraluminal stapler
disposable iris retractor
disposable laryngoscope
disposable measuring guide
disposable microclamp
disposable muscle biopsy clamp
disposable ocutome
disposable otoscopic ear tips
disposable probe
disposable retractor
disposable scalpel
disposable sigmoidoscope
disposable specimen trap
disposable speculum
disposable sterile scalpel
disposable stone basket
disposable stripper
disposable Styrofoam block
disposable surfaces EMG
   electrode
disposable surgical electrode
disposable suturing needle
disposable syringe
disposable trephine
disposable TUR drape
disposable vacuum curet
disposable vaginal speculum
disposable Yankauer aspirating
   tube
disposable Yankauer suction
   tube
disposable-sheath flexible
   gastroscope
Disposatrode disposable
   electrode
Dispos-A-Ture single-use surgical
   needle

Disposiquet disposable
    tourniquet
Disposolette cautery
Disposo-Scope anoscope
Disposo-Spec disposable
    speculum
disproportion
    cephalopelvic disproportion
        (CPD)
    fetal pelvic disproportion
    fetopelvic disproportion
    skeletal disproportion
disrupted operative wound
disruption
disruption of operative wound
disruption sequence
Disse space
dissecting aneurysm
dissecting cellulitis of scalp
dissecting chisel
dissecting clamp
dissecting forceps
dissecting hook
dissecting intramural
    hematoma
dissecting probe
dissecting scissors
dissecting tonsillar scissors
dissecting vital scissors
dissection
    2-field dissection
    2-team dissection
    3-field dissection
    acute aortic dissection
    aortic dissection
    arterial wall dissection
    axillary lymph node
        dissection (ALND)
    axillary node dissection
    balloon dissection
    bilateral neck dissection
    block dissection
    blunt and sharp dissection
    blunt dissection
    Bocca neck dissection
    bone dissection
    bone-ligament dissection
    bony dissection
    capsular dissection
    carotid artery dissection
    Cavitron dissection
    cervical node dissection

dissection (*continued*)
    circumferential mucosal
        dissection
    cold dissection
    cold-knife dissection
    complete axillary dissection
    complex dissection
    condyle dissection
    confirmatory axillary
        dissection
    coronary artery dissection
    cranial nerve dissection
    Creed dissection
    DeBakey-type aortic
        dissection
    deep dissection
    deep iliac dissection
    Desmarres corneal
        dissection
    diathermy dissection
    Dingman breast dissection
    discontinuous dissection
    discontinuous neck dissection
    elective lymph node
        dissection (ELND)
    elective neck dissection (END)
    electrosurgical dissection
    en bloc dissection
    endoscopic dissection
    epiphenomena of dissection
    esophageal dissection
    ESP dissection
    extensive lymph node
        dissection
    extracapsular dissection
    extrahepatic dissection
    extraperitoneal endoscopic
        pelvic lymph node
        dissection
    facial nerve dissection
    Falcao suction dissection
    field of dissection
    finger dissection
    finger fracture dissection
    fingertip dissection
    flank dissection
    freed by blunt dissection
    freed by sharp dissection
    Freer dissection
    full axillary dissection
    functional lymph node
        dissection

dissection (*continued*)
  functional neck dissection
  gauze dissection
  Gil-Vernet dissection
  groin dissection
  hard palate dissection
  hydraulic dissection
  in situ dissection
  incisural dissection
  inguinal canal dissection
  inguinal node dissection
  inguinal-femoral node
    dissection
  intracapsular dissection
  intradural dissection
  intramural air dissection
  intraparenchymal digital
    dissection
  jugular vein dissection
  Kitner dissection
  knife and scissors dissection
  Kuttner blunt dissection
  laparoscopic pelvic lymph
    node dissection
  lateral cervical node
    dissection
  lateroaortic lymph node
    dissection
  left radical groin dissection
  limited obturator node
    dissection
  lymph node dissection
  lymphatic dissection
  medial dissection
  mediastinal dissection
  mediastinal lymph node
    dissection
  mesoesophageal dissection
  Milligan double-ended
    dissection
  modified neck dissection
    (MND)
  modified radical neck
    dissection
  muscle dissection
  nasal dissection
  neck dissection
  Neivert dissection
  nerve dissection
  nerve-sparing dissection
  Nezhat-Dorsey hydrodissector
  node dissection

dissection (*continued*)
  Pack-Ehrlich deep iliac
    dissection
  para-aortic lymph node
    dissection
  parenchymal dissection
  parotid dissection
  partial zonal dissection
  Patey axillary node dissection
  Pearce nucleus hydrodissector
  pelvic lymph node dissection
    (PLND)
  pelvic node dissection
  periesophageal lymph node
    dissection
  perineal dissection
  peripheral mesh dissection
  perirectal pelvic dissection
  philtral tunnel dissection
  plane of dissection
  postradical neck dissection
  preadventitial dissection
  precise dissection
  radical axillary dissection
  radical lymph node dissection
  radical mediastinal dissection
  radical neck dissection
  retrograde dissection
  retroperitoneal pelvic lymph
    node dissection (RPLND)
  Rhoton dissection
  scissors dissection
  selective inguinal node
    dissection
  selective neck dissection
    (SND)
  sharp and blunt dissection
  sharp dissection
  skin-flap dissection
  soft-tissue dissection
  spiral dissection
  sponge dissection
  spontaneous coronary artery
    dissection
  spud dissection
  standard radical neck
    dissection
  Stanford type A, B aortic
    dissection
  Stanford-type aortic dissection
  stripping and dissection
  subgaleal dissection

dissection (*continued*)
  subligamentous dissection
  submucosal dissection
  submucous dissection
  subperichondrial dissection
  subperiosteal dissection
  subtemporal dissection
  suction dissection
  suprahyoid neck dissection
  supraomohyoid neck
    dissection
  supraperichondrial dissection
  sylvian dissection
  symptomatic traumatic
    dissection
  systemic dissection
  Taussig-Morton node
    dissection
  therapeutic dissection
  therapeutic lymph node
    dissection (TLND)
  thoracic aortic dissection
  tissue dissection
  tongue-jaw-neck dissection
  total laryngectomy with
    radical neck dissection
  transthoracic dissection
  traumatic internal carotid
    artery dissection
  ultrasonic dissection
  vertebral dissection
  water dissection
  Wookey radical neck
    dissection
dissection and snare
dissection and stripping
dissection bench
dissection forceps
dissection hook
dissection knife
dissection margin
dissection of aorta
dissection probe
dissection scissors
dissection snare
dissection tubercle
dissector
  ASSI breast dissector
  attic dissector
  Aufranc dissector
  Austin attic dissector
  Austin dissector

dissector (*continued*)
  Ball dissector
  balloon dissector
  Barraquer corneal dissector
  batwing dissector
  Beaver dissector
  Becker round tip dissector
  Berens corneal dissector
  blunt dissector
  blunt hook dissector
  Brunner dissector
  Brunner goiter dissector
  bunion dissector
  Butte dissector
  Carpenter dissector
  Castroviejo corneal dissector
  Castroviejo dissector
  Cavitron dissector
  Chajchir dissector
  channel dissector
  Cherry Secto dissector
  Cheyne dissector
  Cheyne dry dissector
  Codman Rhoton dissector
  Collin dissector
  Collin pleural dissector
  Colver dissector
  Colver tonsillar dissector
  corneal dissector
  corneal knife dissector
  Cottonoid dissector
  Crabtree dissector
  Creed dissector
  Crile dissector
  Crile gasserian ganglion
    dissector
  CUSA dissector
  Davis dissector
  Desmarres corneal dissector
  Desmarres dissector
  Desmarres eye dissector
  Dingman breast dissector
  dolphin nose dissector
  dolphin-nose monopolar
    electrosurgical dissector
  double-ended dissector
  Doyen rib dissector
  ear dissector
  Effler double-ended
    dissector
  Effler-Groves dissector
  elevator and dissector

dissector (*continued*)

Emory endoplastic electrosurgical dissector
endarterectomy dissector
Endo Dissect dissector
Endo-Assist cutting dissector
endoscopic dissector
facial nerve dissector
Fager pituitary dissector
Falcao dissector
Falcao suction dissector
Field suction dissector
Fisher tonsil dissector
flap knife dissector
Freer dissector
Freer dural dissector
Freer-Sachs dissector
Fukushima dissector
Gannetta dissector
goiter dissector
Gorney dissector
Green corneal dissector
Green dissector
Green eye dissector
Haines arachnoid dissector
Hajek-Ballenger dissector
Hajek-Ballenger septal dissector
Hamrick suction dissector
Hardy dissector
Hardy pituitary dissector
Harris dissector
Hartmann tonsillar dissector
Heath dissector
Heath trephine flap dissector
Henke tonsillar dissector
Herczel dissector
Hitselberger-McElveen neural dissector
Holinger dissector
Holinger endarterectomy dissector
Holinger laryngeal dissector
Hood dissector
House dissector
House-Crabtree dissector
House-Urban dissector
House-Urban rotary dissector
House-Urban vacuum rotary dissector
Hunt arachnoid dissector
Hunt dissector

dissector (*continued*)

Hurd dissector
Hurd tonsil dissector
Hurd tonsillar dissector
Hurd-Morrison dissector
Hurd-Weder tonsil dissector
Hurd-Weder tonsillar dissector
hydrostatic dissector
Inaba-Ezaki dissector
Israel dissector
Israel tonsillar dissector
Jackson-Pratt dissector
Jannetta aneurysm neck dissector
Jannetta dissector
Jazbi dissector
Jazbi suction tonsillar dissector
Jazbi tonsil dissector
Jazbi tonsillar dissector
Jimmy dissector
joker dissector
Judet dissector
Kennerdell-Maroon dissector
Killian dissector
King-Hurd dissector
King-Hurd tonsil dissector
King-Hurd tonsillar dissector
Kistner dissector
Kitner blunt dissector
Kitner dissector
Kleinert-Kutz dissector
knife dissector
Kocher dissector
Kocher goiter dissector
Kocher periosteal dissector
Kurze dissector
lamina dissector
laminar dissector
Lane dissector
Lang dissector
laryngeal dissector
Lemmon intimal dissector
Lewin bunion dissector
Lewin dissector
Lewin sesamoidectomy dissector
Logan dissector
Lopez-Reinke tonsillar dissector
Lothrop dissector
Lynch blunt dissector

dissector (*continued*)
Lynch dissector
Lynch laryngeal dissector
Lynch tonsillar dissector
MacAusland dissector
MacDonald dissector
Madden dissector
Manhattan Eye and Ear
    corneal dissector
Marino rotatable
    transsphenoidal round
    dissector
Marino rotatable
    transsphenoidal spatula
    dissector
Martinez double-ended
    corneal dissector
Maryland dissector
Maryland monopolar
    electrosurgical dissector
McCabe facial nerve dissector
McCabe flap knife dissector
McDonald dissector
McWhinnie dissector
McWhinnie tonsillar dissector
Meeker monopolar
    electrosurgical dissector
microsurgery dissector
microsurgical dissector
Milette-Tyding dissector
Miller tonsillar dissector
Milligan double-ended
    dissector
Mixter dissector
Molt dissector
Moorehead dissector
Morrison-Hurd dissector
Morrison-Hurd tonsillar
    dissector
Mulligan dissector
nasal dissector
needle dissector
Neivert dissector
nerve root laminectomy
    dissector
neural dissector
neurosurgical dissector
Oldberg dissector
Olivecrona dissector
Olivecrona double-ended
    dissector
Olivecrona-Stille dissector

dissector (*continued*)
Olive-tipped monopolar
    electrosurgical dissector
Paton corneal dissector
peanut dissector
Penfield dissector
Pennington septal dissector
Pierce dissector
Pierce submucous dissector
pillar and dissector
pleural dissector
Polaris reusable dissector
Potts dissector
prostatic dissector
Raney dissector
Rayport dural dissector
Reinhoff dissector
Resposable surgical balloon
    dissector
Rhode Island dissector
Rhoton ball dissector
Rhoton round dissector
Rhoton spatula dissector
Rienhoff dissector
Rochester dissector
Rochester laminar dissector
Roger dissector
Roger submucous dissector
Rosen dissector
rotary dissector
rotatable transsphenoidal
    round dissector
rotatable transsphenoidal
    spatula dissector
round dissector
Ruddy dissector
Sachs-Freer dissector
SaphFinder balloon dissector
SaphFinder surgical balloon
    dissector
SaphTrak balloon dissector
Secto dissector
Sens dissector
septal dissector
sesamoidectomy dissector
Sheldon-Pudenz dissector
Silverstein arachnoid dissector
Silverstein auditory canal
    dissector
Sloan dissector
Sloan goiter flap dissector
Smith dissector

dissector (*continued*)
Smith tonsillar dissector
Smithwick dissector
Smithwick nerve dissector
Spacemaker hernia balloon
   dissector
spatula dissector
Spetzler dissector
sponge dissector
spud dissector
square-tipped arterial
   dissector
square-tipped artery dissector
Stallard blunt dissector
Stallard dissector
Stiwer tendon dissector
Stolte dissector
Stolte tonsillar dissector
straight monopolar
   electrosurgical dissector
submammary dissector
submucous dissector
suction dissector
suction tonsillar dissector
synovial dissector
teardrop dissector
tissue plane dissector
Toennis dissector
Toennis-Adson dissector
Toledo dissector
tonsil dissector
tonsil suction dissector
tonsillar dissector
Touma dissector
transsphenoidal dissector
triangle dissector
Troutman corneal dissector
Troutman eye dissector
Troutman nonincisional
   lamellar dissector
Troutman wave-edge corneal
   dissector
ultrasonic dissector
umbrella dissector
vascular dissector
Walker dissector
Walker suction tonsillar
   dissector
Walker tonsil dissector
Walker tonsil suction
   dissector
Wangensteen dissector

dissector (*continued*)
Watson-Cheyne dissector
Watson-Cheyne dry dissector
Weder dissector
West blunt dissector
West hand dissector
West plastic dissector
Wieder dissector
Wieder tonsillar dissector
Woodson double-ended
   dissector
Wynne-Evans tonsil dissector
Wynne-Evans tonsillar
   dissector
Yasargil dissector
Yoshida dissector
Yoshida tonsil dissector
Yoshida tonsillar dissector
Young dissector
Young urological dissector
dissector and pillar
dissector hook
dissector knife
disseminate
disseminated asymptomatic
   unilateral
   neovascularization
disseminated carcinoma
disseminated CMV infection
disseminated disease
disseminated form Albright
   syndrome
disseminated gangrene
disseminated gonococcal
   infection
disseminated herpes simplex
disseminated inflammation
disseminated intravascular
   coagulation (DIC)
disseminated pagetoid
   reticulosis
dissemination
dissemination of disease
dissipate
dissociated anesthesia
dissociated position
dissociation
dissociative anesthesia
dissolution of stone
dissolvable
dissolving blood clot
dissolving gallstone

dissolving kidney stone
Distaflex balloon
Distaflex dental attachment
Distaflo bypass graft
distal anastomosis
distal angle
distal antrum
distal aortic perfusion
distal arteriotomy
distal aspect
distal biceps brachii tendon
    rupture
distal bile duct
distal bleeding
distal catheter
distal cavity
distal clavicular excision
distal clot
distal colon
distal duodenum
distal ectasia
distal end
distal endarterectomy
distal esophageal ring
distal esophagectomy
distal esophagus
distal femoral cutting guide
distal femoral epiphysial fracture
distal femoral resector
distal femoral tensor
distal femoropopliteal bypass
    graft
distal fibula
distal flap
distal force (DF)
distal fossa
distal fragment
distal gastrectomy
distal humeral fracture
distal hypospadias
distal ileitis
distal ileum
distal interphalangeal (DIP)
distal interphalangeal (DIP) joint
distal interphalangeal fusion
distal interphalangeal joint
    approach
distal ischemia
distal ligation
distal locking screw
distal metastasis
distal movement

distal nail matrix
distal nerve graft
distal oblique groove (DOG)
distal occlusion
distal pancreatectomy
distal pancreaticojejunostomy
distal pedicle flap
distal pedicle flap technique
distal phalanx
distal portion of organ
distal procedure
distal radial fracture
distal radioulnar joint prosthesis
    (DRUJ prosthesis)
distal radioulnar joint
    stabilization
distal Roux-en-Y gastric
    operation
distal runoff
distal splenorenal shunt
distal stimulation generator
distal surface
distal targeting device
distal tibiofibular fusion
distal triangular fossa (DTF)
distal tunnel technique
distal ulna
distal vertebral artery
    reconstruction
distal visceral perfusion
distal with excision of ulcer
    gastrectomy
distal-based flap
distal-based island flap
distally based fasciocutaneous
    flap (DBFF)
distal-occlusal
distal-row carpectomy
distance
distant flap
distant metastasis
distant metastatic disease
distant nodal disease
distant skin flap
distantial aberration
distended abdomen
distended afferent loop
distended gallbladder
distending obturator
distention
distoangular position
distobuccal line angle

distobucco-occlusal point angle
distolabial line angle
distolabioincisal point angle
distolinguo-occlusal point angle
disto-occlusal point angle
distortion aberration
distraction
  callus distraction
  craniomaxillofacial callus
    distraction
  forward mandibular
    distraction
  mandibular distraction
  muscle distraction
  palatal distraction
  rigid external distraction
    (RED)
  simple mandibular distraction
  skeletal distraction
distraction arthroplasty
distraction bar
distraction clamp
distraction device
distraction hook
distraction instrumentation
distraction lengthening
distraction of fracture
distraction osteogenesis (DO)
distraction osteosynthesis
distraction pin
distraction rod
distraction screw
distraction technique
distractive extension
distractor
  ACE OsteoGenic distractor
  ArthroDistractor distractor
  Beckman distractor
  Bliskunov implantable femoral
    distractor
  Caspar distractor
  DeBastiani distractor
  femoral distractor
  hook distractor
  Ilizarov distractor
  Kaneda distractor
  Kessler metacarpal distractor
  mandibular distractor
  Mark II distal femur distractor
  Molina mandibular distractor
  Monticelli-Spinelli distractor
  multidirectional distractor

distractor (*continued*)
  Multiguide mandibular
    distractor
  multiplanar mandibular
    distractor
  Orthofix M-100 distractor
  Pinto distractor
  turnbuckle distractor
distractor pin
distribution
distribution of hair
disturbance
disuse atrophy
Dittel dilating urethral bougie
Dittel operation
Dittel sound
Dittel urethral sound
Dittel uterine dilator
Dittel uterine sound
Dittman dilator
Dittrich plug
Dittsburg dilator
diuresed patient
diuresis
diuretic therapy
Diva laparoscopic morcellator
Diva laparoscopic morcellator
    device
divergence
divergent dislocation
divergent elbow dislocation
divergent outlet forceps
divergent strabismus
diverging collimator
diversion
  Camey enterocystoplasty
    urinary diversion
  Duke pouch cutaneous
    urinary diversion
  fecal diversion
  Gil-Vernet ileocecal cystoplasty
    urinary diversion
  ileal conduit urinary diversion
  ileocolonic pouch urinary
    diversion
  Indiana continent reservoir
    urinary diversion
  Khafagy modified ileocecal
    cystoplasty urinary
    diversion
  Koch pouch cutaneous
    urinary diversion

diversion (*continued*)
  Laparostat with fiber
    diversion
  laryngeal diversion
  laryngotracheal diversion
  Mainz pouch cutaneous
    urinary diversion
  orthotopic urinary diversion
  simple diversion
  Studer reservoir urinary
    diversion
  temporary fecal diversion
  urinary diversion
diversion of blood flow
diversion stent
diversionary ileostomy
diverticula (*sing.* diverticulum)
diverticular disease
diverticular hemorrhage
diverticular hernia
diverticulation abnormality
diverticulectomy
  bladder diverticulectomy
  endocavitary bladder
    diverticulectomy
  esophageal diverticulectomy
  Harrington esophageal
    diverticulectomy
  Meckel diverticulectomy
  open diverticulectomy
  pharyngoesophageal
    diverticulectomy
  urethral diverticulectomy
  vesical diverticulectomy
diverticulectomy of
    hypopharynx
diverticulectomy with myotomy
diverticulitis
diverticulogram
diverticulography
diverticulopexy
diverticulosis
diverticulum (*pl.* diverticula)
  caliceal diverticulum
  colonic diverticulum
  cricopharyngeal diverticulum
  epiphrenic diverticulum
  esophageal diverticulum
  false diverticulum
  Ganser diverticulum
  Graser diverticulum
  Heister diverticulum

diverticulum (*continued*)
  hepatic diverticulum
  Hutch bladder diverticulum
  Hutch diverticulum
  hypopharyngeal
    diverticulum
  inflamed diverticulum
  intestinal diverticulum
  intraluminal duodenal
    diverticulum (IDD)
  intramural diverticulum
  jejunal diverticulum
  juxtapapillary diverticulum
  Kirchner diverticulum
  Kommerell diverticulum
  Meckel diverticulum
  midesophageal diverticulum
  Nuck diverticulum
  perforated diverticulum
  periampullary diverticulum
  pharyngoesophageal
    diverticulum
  prostatic diverticulum
  Rokitansky diverticulum
  supradiaphragmatic
    diverticulum
  traction diverticulum
  Zenker diverticulum
diverting bacteremic donor
diverting colostomy
diverting loop colostomy
diverting loop ileostomy
diverting proximal colostomy
diverting stoma
divided and separated
divided and tied
divided colostomy
divided respiration
divided tendon
divided-stoma colostomy
divinyl ether anesthetic agent
Diviplast impression material
division
  craniosacral division
  maxillary division
  reduction division
  thoracicolumbar division
  thoracolumbar division
division I-IV lesion
division line
division of adhesions
division skin lines

divot
  liposuction divot
divulse
divulsion
divulsor
Dix double-ended instrument
Dix foreign body spud
Dix gouge
Dix needle
Dix spud
Dix spud probe
Dixey spatula
Dix-Hallpike maneuver
Dix-Hallpike position
Dix-Hallpike test
Dixon blade
Dixon center blade
Dixon center-blade retractor
Dixon collar scissors
Dixon flamingo forceps
Dixon technique
Dixon-Lovelace hemostatic
  forceps
Dixon-Thomas-Smith clamp
Dixon-Thomas-Smith colonic
  clamp
Dixon-Thomas-Smith intestinal
  clamp
Dixon-Thorpe vitreous foreign
  body forceps
DKS operation
DKS procedure
DLP aortic root cannula
DLP cardioplegic catheter
DLP cardioplegic needle
DLP infant ventricular
  catheter
DLP left atrial pressure
  monitoring catheter
DMB (demineralized bone)
DMI (Diagnostic Medical
  Instruments)
DMI ambulatory surgery table
DMV II contact lens remover
DN acupuncture needle
DNA ploidy abnormality
DNE digital scanner
DNM (descending necrotizing
  mediastinitis)
DNE (do not resuscitate)
DO (distraction osteogenesis)
DO cavity

do not resuscitate (DNR)
Doane knee retractor
Dobbhoff
  Dobbhoff biliary stent
  Dobbhoff gastrectomy feeding
    tube
  Dobbhoff PEG tube
Dobbhoff bipolar coagulation
  probe
Dobbhoff catheter
Dobbhoff feeding tube
Dobbhoff gastrectomy feeding
  tube
Dobbhoff gastric decompression
  tube
Dobbhoff nasogastric feeding
  tube
Dobbhoff PEG tube
Dobbie-Trout bulldog clamp
Dobbie-Trout clamp
DOC guidewire extension
dock wire
Dockhorn retractor
docking needle
docking wire
Docktor forceps
Docktor needle
Docktor suture
Docktor tissue forceps
Doctor Collins clamp
Doctor Collins fracture clamp
Doctor Long clamp
documentation sheath
Dodd perforator
Doderlein operation
Doderlein roll-flap operation
Doderlein-Kronig operation
Dodick lens-holding forceps
Dodick nucleus cracker forceps
Dodick photolysis probe
Dodrill forceps
Doesel-Huzly bronchoscope
Doesel-Huzly bronchoscopic
  tube
DOG (distal oblique groove)
dog chain retractor
dog ear of anastomosis
dog-ear repair
dog-ear sign
dog-earing
dog-leg catheter
dog-leg fracture

dog-legged filiforms
Dogliotti valvulotome
Dogliotti-Gugliel mini clamp
Doherty eye implant
Doherty eye sphere
Doherty graft
Doherty implant
Doherty prosthesis
Doherty spherical eye implant
Dohlman endoscope
Dohlman esophagoscope
Dohlman hook
Dohlman incus hook
Dohlman operation
Dohlman plug
Dohn-Carton brain retractor
Dohrmann-Rubin cannula
Dolan extractor
Dolenc technique
Doleris operation
Doleris uterine suspension
Dolfin extensor tenotomy
dolichocephaly
dolichoectatic artery
dolichopellic pelvis
Doll trochanteric reattachment
    technique
Dolley raspatory
doll's eye maneuver
doll's eye reflex
doll's eye sign
doll's head maneuver
Dolphin cord clamp
Dolphin device
dolphin dissecting forceps
dolphin grasping forceps
Dolphin instrument
dolphin nose dissector
dolphin-billed grasping forceps
dolphin-nose monopolar
    electrosurgical dissector
dolphin-type atraumatic forceps
domal asymmetry
domal cartilage
domal creation sutures
domal divergence
D'Ombrain operation
dome
    bladder dome
    nasal dome
    patellar dome
    surgical dome

dome colpostat
dome cylinder
dome excursion
dome fracture
dome hole plug
dome of bladder
dome of diaphragm
dome paste boot
dome-binding sutures
domed angle-tipped electrode
dominant gland
dominant hemisphere
dominant pattern
dominant pedicle
dominant skin lines
doming of mitral valve leaflet
doming of valve
Dominici tube
domino procedure
domino reflex
domino spinal instrumentation
    connector
domino transplant
Donaghy angled suture needle
    holder
Donahoo marker
Donald clamp
Donald operation
Donald procedure
Donald vulsellum
Donald-Fothergill operation
Donaldson drain tube
Donaldson eustachian tube
Donaldson eye patch
Donaldson fundus camera
Donaldson myringotomy tube
Donaldson Silastic ear tube
Donaldson Teflon tube
Donaldson tube
Donaldson ventilation tube
donated body
donated organ
Donberg iris forceps
Donders line
Donders procedure
DonJoy 4-point Super Sport
    knee brace
DonJoy ALP brace
DonJoy Goldpoint knee brace
DonJoy knee brace
DonJoy knee splint
DonJoy Legend ACL knee brace

Donnati sutures
Donnell Dermedex
Donnez endometrial ablation
    device
Donnheim implant
Donnheim lens
Donoghue knee procedure
donor
    artificial insemination donor
        (AID)
    autologous donor
    autologous patient donor
    cadaver donor (CAD)
    cadaveric donor
    CMV-positive donor
    consanguineous donor
    cytomegalovirus-positive
        donor
    designated donor
    diverting bacteremic donor
    extended criteria donor
        (ECD)
    heart donor
    living relative donor
    living-related donor
    matching donor
    non-heart-beating donor
        (NHBD)
    organ donor
    subhuman primary donor
donor bank
donor bone marrow
    engraftment
donor button forceps
donor cadaver
donor iliac Y graft
donor incision
donor island harvesting
donor kidney
donor nipple
donor organs and tissues
donor pancreatectomy
donor radius fracture
donor recipient
donor screening
donor site
donor site dressing
donor size
donor tissue
donor transfusion
donor transplant
donor typing
donor-specific bone marrow
    augmentation
donor-specific transfusion (DST)
Dontrix gauge
Dooley nail
Dopcord recorder
Doplette Doppler blood flow
    detector
Doplette monitor
Doppler
    2D Doppler
    Acuson color Doppler
    Carolina color spectrum
        Doppler
    color-flow Doppler
    Convergent color Doppler
    Dopplette Doppler
    echo Doppler
    endoscopic color Doppler
    Fetal Pulse Plus fetal Doppler
    Hadeco mini Doppler
    Hadeco intraoperative
        Doppler
    Hadeco Minidop Doppler
    Haemoson ultrasound
        Doppler
    Imex Pocket-Dop OB Doppler
    Imexdop CT Doppler
    IntraDop intraoperative
        Doppler
    MD2 Doppler
    Medasonics transcranial
        Doppler
    Minidop Pocket Doppler
    Mizuho surgical Doppler
    Multi Dopplex II Doppler
    Neuroguard transcranial
        Doppler
    Nicolet Elite obstetrical
        Doppler
    pencil-probe Doppler
    penile Doppler
    power Doppler
    pulse wave Doppler
    pulsed Doppler
    Siemens Quantum Doppler
    Smartdop Doppler
    spectral Doppler
    transcranial Doppler
    Ultrascope obstetrical
        Doppler
Doppler analysis

Doppler auto-correlation
technique
Doppler blood flow detector
Doppler blood flow monitor
Doppler color flow
Doppler color flow Doppler
scanner
Doppler color flow imaging
Doppler color jet
Doppler coronary catheter
Doppler device
Doppler duplex ultrasonography
Doppler echocardiogram
Doppler echocardiography
Doppler effect
Doppler fetal stethoscope
Doppler flow detector
Doppler flow
echocardiographic probe
Doppler flow probe
Doppler flow probe
examination
Doppler FloWire
Doppler flowmeter
Doppler four-beam laser probe
Doppler guidewire
Doppler interrogation
Doppler IntraDop
Doppler laser velocimeter
Doppler monitor
Doppler operation
Doppler pressure gradient
Doppler probe
Doppler pulse evaluation
Doppler pulsed ultrasound
Doppler scope
Doppler signal
Doppler sound device
Doppler stethoscope
Doppler study
Doppler ultrasonic blood flow
detector
Doppler ultrasonic fetal heart
monitor
Doppler ultrasonic flowmeter
Doppler ultrasonic probe
Doppler ultrasonography
Doppler ultrasound
Doppler ultrasound flowmeter
Doppler ultrasound monitor
Doppler ultrasound segmental
blood pressure testing

Doppler ultrasound stethoscope
Doppler-Cavin monitor
dopplergram
dopplergraphy
Doppler-guided artery ligation
hemorrhoidectomy
Doppler-tipped angioplasty
guidewire
Dopplette Doppler
Doptone fetal monitor
Doptone fetal pulse detector
Doptone fetal stethoscope
Doptone monitor
Doptone monitoring
Dor anterior fundoplication
Dor fundoplication procedure
Dor fundoplication technique
Doran pattern stimulator
ophthalmoscope
DORC backflush instrument
DORC handle
DORC microforceps
DORC microforceps and
microscissors
DORC subretinal instrument set
DORC surgical instrument
DORC vitreous shaver
Dorello canal
Dorendorf sign
Doret graft cutter
Dorian rib stripper
Doriot handpiece
Dormed cranial electrotherapy
stimulator
Dormia basket
Dormia biliary stone basket
Dormia dislodger
Dormia gallstone basket
Dormia gallstone lithotripter
Dormia stone basket
Dormia stone basket catheter
Dormia stone dislodger
Dormia ureteral basket
Dormia ureteral stone basket
Dormia ureteral stone dislodger
Dorner gallstone lithotriptor
Dornier compact lithotriptor
Dornier Epos Ultra lithotripter
Dornier extracorporeal
shockwave lithotriptor
Dornier gallstone lithotriptor
Dornier HM-series lithotriptor

Dornier lithotriptor
Dornier Medilas H holmium:
    YAG endourology laser
Dornier scanner
Dornier Urotract cysto table
Dornier waterbath lithotriptor
Dorrance closure
Dorrance operation
Dorrance palatal pushback
Dorrance procedure
Dorros brachial internal
    mammary guiding catheter
Dorros infusion/probing
    catheter
Dorros probing catheter
dorsa (*sing.* dorsum)
dorsal antebrachial cutaneous
    nerve
dorsal aponeurotic fascia
dorsal artery
dorsal artery of clitoris
dorsal artery of foot
dorsal artery of nose
dorsal artery of penis
dorsal aspect
dorsal back roll
dorsal branch of nerve
dorsal bunion
dorsal calcaneocuboid ligament
dorsal carpal ligament
dorsal columella implant
dorsal column
dorsal column stimulation
dorsal column stimulator
    implant (DCS implant)
dorsal condylar surface
dorsal cordotomy
dorsal cornu
dorsal cross-finger flap
dorsal decubitus position
dorsal digital arteries
dorsal digital nerves
dorsal digital veins
dorsal elevated position
dorsal enteric fistula
dorsal excision
dorsal expansion
dorsal fascia
dorsal finger approach
dorsal fissure
dorsal flap
dorsal flexure

dorsal hand abscess
dorsal hood
dorsal hump
dorsal induction
dorsal inertia position
dorsal intercalated segmental
    instability (DISI) deformity
dorsal intercarpal ligament
dorsal interosseous fascia
dorsal interosseous muscles
dorsal ligament
dorsal linear incision
dorsal lingual artery
dorsal lingual mucosa
dorsal lingual veins
dorsal lithotomy
dorsal lithotomy position
dorsal longitudinal incision
dorsal lumbotomy incision
dorsal metacarpal arteries
dorsal metacarpal veins
dorsal metatarsal arteries
dorsal metatarsal veins
dorsal midline approach
dorsal muscle
dorsal mutilation
dorsal nasal branch of
    ophthalmic artery
dorsal nerve
dorsal nerve of clitoris
dorsal nerve of penis
dorsal nerve root
dorsal onlay graft
dorsal pedicle TRAM flap
dorsal penile nerve block
    (DPNB)
dorsal perilunate dislocation
dorsal plaster spine
dorsal plate
dorsal plate and lag screw
    fixation
dorsal point
dorsal position
dorsal radiocarpal ligament
dorsal radioulnar ligament
dorsal recumbent position
dorsal reduction
dorsal reflex
dorsal region
dorsal retinaculum
dorsal rhizotomy
dorsal rigid position

dorsal root entry zone lesion
   (DREZ lesion)
dorsal root entry zone
   procedure
dorsal root ganglion
dorsal root ganglionectomy
dorsal rotation flap
dorsal sacrococcygeal muscle
dorsal scapular nerve
dorsal scissors
dorsal sclerosis
dorsal sensory branch of ulnar
   nerve
dorsal slit of prepuce
dorsal spine
dorsal strut
dorsal subaponeurotic space
dorsal supine incision
dorsal supine position
dorsal surface
dorsal talonavicular ligament
dorsal tegmental decussation
dorsal thoracic fascia
dorsal thoracic fascia free flap
dorsal transposition flap
dorsal transscaphoid perilunar
   dislocation
dorsal transverse capsulotomy
dorsal transverse incision
dorsal vein
dorsal vein patch graft
dorsal veins of clitoris
dorsal veins of penis
dorsal veins of tongue
dorsal venous arch of foot
dorsal vertebrae
dorsal view
dorsal wire-loop fixation
dorsal wrist splint with
   outrigger
dorsal wrist syndrome (DWS)
dorsal-angled scissors
dorsales linguae, venae
dorsalis pedis artery
dorsalis pedis flap
dorsalis pedis pulse
dorsalward approach
Dorsey bayonet forceps
Dorsey cannula
Dorsey cervical foraminal punch
Dorsey decompressor
Dorsey dural separator

Dorsey forceps
Dorsey leukotome
Dorsey needle
Dorsey nerve root retractor
Dorsey punch
Dorsey retractor
Dorsey screwdriver
Dorsey separator
Dorsey spatula
Dorsey tongue depressor
Dorsey transorbital leukotome
Dorsey ventricular cannula
dorsiflexion sign
dorsiflexor
dorsiflexor wedge osteotomy
dorsispinal vein
Dorsiwedge night splint
dorsoanterior
dorsocuboidal reflex
dorsodecubitus position
dorsolateral and medial
   capsulotomy
dorsolateral approach
dorsolateral incision
dorsolateral surface
dorsomedial approach
dorsomedial incision
dorsomedial thalamotomy
dorsomedian
dorsonasal
dorsoplantar approach
dorsoplantar projection
dorsoposterior
dorsoradial approach
dorsorecumbent position
dorsorostral approach
dorsosacral position
dorsoscapular
dorsosupine position
dorsoulnar approach
dorsoventral
dorsum (pl. dorsa)
dorsum linguae
dorsum nasi
dorsum of nose
dorsum of tongue
dorsum pedis reflex
dorsum rotundum
dorsum sellae
Dorton self-retaining retractor
Dos Santos aortography
   needle

Dos Santos lumbar aortography
    needle
Dos Santos needle for
    aortography
dosage adjustment
dosage boost
dosage of medication
dosage range
dose
    calculated dose
    cumulative dose
    curative dose
    identical plane dose
    initial dose
    integral dose
    intravenous dose
    loading dose
    maintenance dose
    massive dose
    maximum accumulated dose
        (MAD)
    maximum permissible dose
        (MPD)
    optimal dose
    oral dose
    radiation absorbed dose (rad)
    rectovaginal dose
    roentgen absorbed dose
        (rad)
    thermal dose
dose and beams
dose calculation
dose fractionation
dose of chemotherapy
dose of medication
dose of radiation
dose profile
dose response
dose-related effect
dose-response curve
Dosick bellows assembly
dosimeter
    dichromate dosimeter
    Gardray dosimeter
    LiF thermoluminescence
        dosimeter
    pencil dosimeter
    Rosenthal-French nebulization
        dosimeter
    silicone diode dosimeter
    single-channel in vivo light
        dosimeter

dosimeter (*continued*)
    thermoluminescent dosimeter
    Victoreen dosimeter
dosimetrist radiation beam
        monitor
dosimetry
    film dosimetry
    rotational x-ray beam
        dosimetry
Doss automatic percolator
        irrigator
dot hemorrhage
dot-and-blot hemorrhage
dot-blot procedure
dot-blot technique
dot-plotted probe
Dott mouth gag
Dott operation
Dott retractor
dotted line
Dotter caged-balloon catheter
Dotter coaxial catheter
Dotter dilator
Dotter operation
dotter technique
Dotter-Judkins percutaneous
        transluminal angioplasty
Dotter-Judkins technique
Dott-Kilner mouth gag
Doubilet sphincterotome
Doubilet sphincterotomy
double adenomas
double aortic arch
double armboard
double balloon device
double Becker ankle brace
double bladder
double breast coil
double bridge
double bubble flushing reservoir
double chin
double club elevator
double concave
double contrast technique
double convex
double cross-lip flap
double decidual sac sign
double dome effect
double dynamic graciloplasty
double elevator
double enterostomy
double exposure

double eyelid operation
double eyelidplasty
double fracture
double freeze-stalk cryopexy
double freeze-thaw cryopexy
double gloving
double graft
double harelip
double hip spica
double hook
double incision
double injection
double irrigating/aspirating
    cannula
double jaw surgery
double J-shaped reservoir
double keyhole loop wire
double kidney
double knot
double lingual bar
double lip
double loop tourniquet
double lumen implant
double opposing Z-plasty
double papilla graft
double papilla pedicle graft
double pedicle flap
double pedicle technique
double pendulum flap
double protrusion
double pyloroplasty
double rectus harvest
double right-angle suture
double safe-sided chisel
double setup endotracheal tube
double simultaneous stimulation
    (DSS)
double skin paddle fibular flap
double Softjaw clamp
double spatula
double spring ball valve
double stapling technique (DST)
double stockinette
double syndactyly
double toe transplantation
double towel clamp
double tunnel
double unilateral cysts
double ureter
double urethra
double uterus
double vagina

double V-Y flap
double V-Y plasty with paired
    inverted Burow triangle
    excisions
double Zielke instrumentation
double-action ankle joint
double-action bone cutter
double-action bone-cutting
    forceps
double-action hump forceps
double-action plate cutter
double-action rongeur
double-action rongeur forceps
double-angled blade
double-angled blade plate
double-angled clamp
double-angled retractor
double-angled valve
double-armed mattress sutures
double-armed retention sutures
double-armed suture technique
double-armed sutures
double-articulated
    bronchoscopic forceps
double-articulated forceps tip
double-articulated laryngeal
    forceps tip
double-ball separator
double-balloon technique
double-balloon valvotomy
double-balloon valvuloplasty
double-band navel appliance
double-barreled colostomy
double-barreled fibular bone
    graft
double-barreled ileostomy
double-barreled loop colostomy
double-barreled needle
double-barreled reservoir
double-bent Hohmann
    acetabular retractor
double-biting rongeur
double-blind procedure
double-bubble breast deformity
double-bubble flushing reservoir
double-bubble isolette
double-bubble sign
double-burst
double-burst stimulation
double-burst transmission
double-button suture technique
double-button sutures

double-camelback sign
double-cannula tracheostomy
  tube
double-cataract mask
double-catheterizing
double-catheterizing cytoscope
double-catheterizing fin
double-catheterizing sheath and
  obturator
double-catheterizing telescope
double-channel endoscope
double-channel irrigating
  bronchoscope
double-channel operating sheath
double-channel sphincterotome
double-channel videoendoscope
double-chip micromanometer
  catheter
double-cobra retractor
double-compartment knee
  replacement
double-concave forceps
double-concave rat-tooth
  forceps
double-concave rotating saw
double-contrast barium enema
  examination
double-contrast barium meal
double-contrast enema
double-contrast study
double-contrast visualization
double-crank retractor
double-cross-plasty
double-crush syndrome
double-cuff urinary sphincter
double-cuffed tube
double-cupped forceps
double-current catheter
double-cutting sharp cystotome
doubled black silk sutures
doubled chromic catgut sutures
doubled pursestring sutures
doubled sutures
double-disk ASD closure device
double-dome reservoir
double-doughnut approach
double-dummy technique
double-edged knife
double-edged sickle knife
double-emulsion-solvent-
  extraction technique
double-end graft

double-end, double-ended
double-ended bone curet
double-ended breast retractors
double-ended chrome probe
double-ended curet
double-ended dental curet
double-ended dilator
double-ended dissector
double-ended elevator
double-ended flap
double-ended flap knife
double-ended graft
double-ended nail
double-ended needle forceps
double-ended nickelene probe
double-ended periosteal
  elevator
double-ended probe
double-ended retractor
double-ended root tip dental
  pick
double-ended silver probe
double-ended spatula
double-ended stapes curet
double-ended suture forceps
double-ended tissue forceps
double-exposed rib
double-eyelid plasty
double-fishhook retractor
double-fixation forceps
double-fixation hook
double-flanged valve sewing
  ring
double-flap amputation
double-flap operation
double-focus tube
double-fold line in double
  eyelidplasty
double-folded cup-patch
  technique
double-footling delivery
double-freeze technique
double-guarded chisel
double-H plate
double-headed P190 stapler
double-headed P190 stapling
  device
double-headed stereotactic
  carrier
Double-hesive adhesive disk
double-hook skin tenaculum
double-hub emulsifying needle

double-immunofluorescence
 microscopy
double-incision fasciotomy
double-inlet ventricle anomaly
double-J dangle stent
double-J indwelling catheter
double-J indwelling catheter
 stent
double-J silicone internal
 ureteral catheter stent
double-J silicone splint
double-J stent catheter stent
double-J ureteral catheter
double-J ureteral stent
double-L spinal rod
double-loop hernia
double-loop pouch
double-looped semitendinosus
 technique
double-lumen (DL)
double-lumen balloon stone
 extractor catheter
double-lumen breast implant
double-lumen breast implant
 material
double-lumen Broviac catheter
double-lumen cannula
double-lumen catheter
double-lumen curet
double-lumen endobronchial
 tube
double-lumen endoprosthesis
double-lumen gastric laryngeal
 mask airway
double-lumen Hickman catheter
double-lumen Hickman-Broviac
 catheter
double-lumen intubation
double-lumen irrigation cannula
double-lumen needle
double-lumen Silastic catheter
double-lumen subclavian
 catheter
double-lumen suction irrigation
 tube
double-lumen Swan-Ganz
 catheter
double-lumen tapered-tip
 papillotome
double-lumen tube
double-needle cataract
 operation

double-needle chemonucleolysis
double-occlusal splint
double-outlet right ventricle
double-paddle flap
double-paddle island flap
double-paddle peroneal tissue
 transfer
double-paddle peroneal tissue
 transfer reconstruction
double-pedicle skin flap
double-pedicle transverse rectus
 abdominis
 musculocutaneous flap
double-pigtail endoprosthesis
double-pigtail prosthesis
double-pigtail stent
double-plate Molteno implant
double-point threshold
double-pronged
double-pronged Cottle hook
double-pronged Fomon hook
double-pronged forceps
double-pronged fork
double-pronged hook
double-puncture laparoscopy
double-reverse alpha sigmoid
 loop
double-ring frame
double-rod
double-rod construct
double-rod penile prosthesis
double-rod technique
double-running penetrating
 keratoplasty suture
double-sealant technique
double-seton modified surgical
 approach
double-skin mastopexy
double-spoon
double-spoon biopsy forceps
double-spoon forceps
double-staple technique
double-stapled ileoanal reservoir
 procedure
double-stapled ileoanal reservoir
 technique
double-stapled technique
double-stem implant
DoubleStent biliary
 endoprosthesis
double-stick technique
double-stop sutures

double-tenaculum hook
double-thermistor coronary
    sinus catheter
double-thickness Sheen graft
double-threaded Herbert
    screw
double-tipped center-threading
    needle
double-tooth tenaculum
double-tube technique
double-umbrella closure
double-umbrella device
double-vector
double-vector blade
double-vector brain spatula
double-velour graft
double-velour knitted graft
double-volume exchange
    transfusion
double-walled incubator
double-webbed needle
double-wire technique
double-woven wire
double-wrap graciloplasty
double-Y incision
doubling time for tumor
doubly armed sutures
doubly clamped and divided
doubly clamped and ligated
doubly ligated
doubly ligated suture
Doubra lens
douche
    Fritsch uterine douche
    jet douche
    nasal douche
    Scotch douche
    Weber douche
    Weber nasal douche
Dougherty anterior chamber
    cannula
Dougherty eye irrigator
Dougherty irrigator
doughnut headrest
doughnut kidney
doughnut lesion
doughnut magnet
doughnut pessary
doughnut sign
doughnut tip suction tube
Doughty tongue plate
doughy abdomen

doughy consistency
Douglas abscess
Douglas antral trocar
Douglas bag
Douglas bag technique
Douglas cannula
Douglas cilia forceps
Douglas ciliary forceps
Douglas cul-de-sac
Douglas eye forceps
Douglas fold
Douglas forceps
Douglas graft
Douglas knife
Douglas line
Douglas measuring plate
    pelvimeter
Douglas mesh skin graft
Douglas mucosal snare
Douglas mucosal speculum
Douglas nasal scissors
Douglas nasal snare
Douglas nasal trocar
Douglas operation
Douglas pelvimeter
Douglas pouch
Douglas procedure
Douglas rectal snare
Douglas skin graft
Douglas snare
Douglas speculum
Douglas suture needle
Douglas sutures
Douglas tonsillar knife
Douglas tonsillar snare
Douglas trocar
douglascele
Douglas-Roberts snare
Dourmashkin bougie
Dourmashkin cystoscope
Dourmashkin dilator
Dourmashkin operation
Dourmashkin tunneled bougie
Douvas roto-extractor
Douvas vitreous cutter
Douvas-Barraquer speculum
Dover silicone Foley catheter
Dover catheter
Dover midstream urine
    collection kit
Dover Premium Teflon-coated
    latex Foley catheter

Dover Teflon-coated latex Foley
    catheter
Dover Texas Catheter disposable
    male catheter
DoveTail geometry
Dow Corning antifoam agent
    dressing
Dow Corning cannula
Dow Corning catheter
Dow Corning contoured Silastic
    prosthesis
Dow Corning cystocatheter
Dow Corning external breast
    form
Dow Corning ileal pouch
    catheter
Dow Corning implant
Dow Corning mammary
    prosthesis
Dow Corning shunt
Dow Corning Silastic prosthesis
Dow Corning Silastic prosthetic
    sizer
Dow Corning silicone
Dow Cystocath
Dow hollow-fiber artificial
    kidney dialyzer
Dow hollow-fiber dialyzer
Dow hollow-fiber hemodialyzer
dowager hump
Dowd, prostatic balloon
    dilatation catheter
dowel bone graft
dowel cutter
dowel grip
dowel spinal fusion
dowel technique
doweling spondylolisthesis
    technique
Dowell hernia repair
Dowell operation
Dower bone plugger
Down epiphyseal knife
Down flow generator
Down hand dermatome
down-angle hook
down-biting curet
down-biting Epstein curet
down-curved rasp
down-cutting rongeur
Downes cautery
Downes nasal speculum

Downey-McGlamery procedure
down-fracture
downgoing Babinski bilaterally
downgoing toes
downgrafting
downhill course
downhill esophageal varices
Downing cartilage knife
Downing cartilage scalpel
Downing clamp
Downing hot air bath
Downing laminectomy retractor
Downing knife
Downing retractor
Downing stapler
Downs arthroscope
downsized circular laminar
    hook
downward compression
downward curvature
downward displacement
downward drainage
downward movement
downward tilting
Doyen abdominal retractor
Doyen abdominal scissors
Doyen bone mallet
Doyen bur
Doyen child abdominal retractor
Doyen clamp
Doyen costal elevator
Doyen costal rasp
Doyen cylindrical bur
Doyen cylindrical drill
Doyen director
Doyen dissecting scissors
Doyen electrode
Doyen elevator
Doyen forceps
Doyen gallbladder forceps
Doyen hysterectomy
Doyen intestinal clamp
Doyen intestinal forceps
Doyen mouth gag
Doyen myoma screw
Doyen needle
Doyen needle holder
Doyen operation
Doyen periosteal elevator
Doyen raspatory
Doyen retractor
Doyen rib dissector

Doyen rib elevator
Doyen rib hook
Doyen rib rasp
Doyen rib raspatory
Doyen rib shears
Doyen rib spreader
Doyen rib stripper
Doyen scissors
Doyen screw
Doyen spatula
Doyen speculum
Doyen spherical bur
Doyen towel clamp
Doyen towel forceps
Doyen trocar
Doyen tumor screw
Doyen uterine forceps
Doyen vaginal hysterectomy
Doyen vaginal retractor
Doyen vaginal speculum
Doyen vulsellum forceps
Doyen-Ferguson scissors
Doyen-Jansen mouth gag
Doyle bi-valved airway splint
Doyle Combo nasal airway splint
Doyle ear dressing
Doyle silicone stent
Doyle intranasal airway splint
Doyle nasal splint
Doyle nasal tampon
Doyle operation
Doyle Shark nasal splint
Doyle splints
Doyle vein stripper
Dozier radiolucent Bennett
    retractor
DP (debonding pliers)
DPA (dual photoabsorptiometry)
DPAP Stealth positive airway
    pressure device
DPM (dual-pedicle
    dermoparenchymal
    mastopexy)
DPNB (dorsal penile nerve block)
DPX-IQ densitometer
Draeger forceps
Draeger high-vacuum erysiphake
Draeger modified keratome
Draeger tonometer
Drager (*also* Dräger, Draeger)
Dräger (*see* Drager)
Draeger (*see* Drager)

Drager MTC transducer
Drager respirometer
Drager thermal gel mattress
Drager ventilator
Drager Volumeter
dragonhead needle
Dragstedt feeding gastrostomy
Dragstedt gastrostomy
Dragstedt graft
Dragstedt implant
Dragstedt operation
Dragstedt prosthesis
Dragstedt skin graft
Dragstedt vagotomy and
    gastrojejunostomy
Dragstedt-Tanner operation
drain
    2-wing drain
    2-wing Malecot drain
    4-wing drain
    4-wing Malecot drain
    Abramson sump drain
    accordion drain
    ACMI Pezzer drain
    angle drain
    Angle-Pezzer drain
    antral drain
    Atraum with Clotstop drain
    Axiom drain
    Baker continuous flow
        capillary drain
    Bardex drain
    Bardex-Bellini drain
    Bartkiewicz 2-sided drain
    Bellini drain
    Blair silicone drain
    Blake drain
    Blake silicone drain
    butterfly drain
    CenterPointLock 2-piece
        ostomy system: stoma
        irrigator drain
    Chaffin-Pratt drain
    Charnley suction drain
    cigarette drain
    closed drain
    closed suction drain
    Clot Stop drain
    clothesline drain
    Codman lumbar external drain
    combination cone/tube stoma
        irrigator drain

drain (*continued*)

- controlled drain
- craniovac drain
- CUI urological drain
- Cushman drain
- dam drain
- Davol drain
- Davol suction drain
- Davol sump drain
- de Pezzer drain
- Deboisans drain
- Deseret sump drain
- dual-sump silicone drain
- DuoDerm drain
- ERCP nasobiliary drain
- extraventricular drain
- filtered dual-sump drain
- filtered mediastinal sump drain
- fluted J-Vac drain
- flute-ended right-angle drain
- Foley straight drain
- Freyer drain
- Freyer suprapubic drain
- Glove drain
- Gomco drain
- Guardian 2-piece ostomy system: stoma irrigator drain
- Guibor lacrimal drain
- Hemaduct wound drain
- Hemovac drain
- Hemovac Hydrocoat drain
- Hendrickson drain
- Hendrickson suprapubic drain
- Heyer-Robertson suprapubic drain
- Heyer-Schulte wound drain
- high-capacity drain
- high-capacity silicone drain
- Hollister irrigator drain
- Hysterovac drain
- Hysto-vac drain
- incise and drain
- intercostal drain
- Jackson-Pratt drain
- Jackson-Pratt Gold wound drain
- Jackson-Pratt Hemaduct drain
- Jackson-Pratt round PVC drain
- Jackson-Pratt silicone flat drain

drain (*continued*)

- Jackson-Pratt silicone round drain
- Jackson-Pratt suction drain
- Jackson-Pratt T-tube drain
- J-Vac closed wound drain
- J-Vac
- Keith drain
- Lahey drain
- large-volume round silicone drain
- latex drain
- Leydig drain
- Malecot 2-wing drain
- Malecot 4-wing drain
- Mantisol drain
- Marion drain
- mediastinal drain
- mesonephric drain
- Mikulicz drain
- Mikulicz-Radecki drain
- Miller-vac drain
- mini-ophthalmic drain
- MMG Golden drain
- Molteno implant drain
- Monaldi drain
- Morris drain
- Morris Silastic thoracic drain
- Mosher drain
- nasocystic drain
- Nelaton rubber tube drain
- papilla drain
- pencil drain
- Penrose drain
- Penrose sump drain
- Perma-Cath drain
- Pezzer drain
- Pharmaseal closed drain
- Pharmaseal drain
- pigtail nephrostomy drain
- polyethylene drain
- polyvinyl drain
- PVC drain
- Quad-Lumen drain
- quarantine drain
- Ragnell drain
- Redivac drain
- Redivac suction drain
- Redon drain
- Reliavac drain
- removal of drain
- Ritter drain

drain (*continued*)

Ritter suprapubic suction drain
Robertson suprapubic drain
rubber drain
rubber-dam drain
Sacks biliary drain
Salem sump drain
seton drain
Shirley sump wound drain
Shirley wound drain
Silastic drain
Silastic thoracic drain
Silastic thyroid drain
silicone drain
silicone hubless flat drain
silicone round drain
silicone sump drain
silicone thoracic drain
Snyder Hemovac drain
Snyder Hemovac silicone sump drain
Snyder mini-Hemovac drain
soft rubber drain
Sof-Wick drain
Solcotrans closed vacuum drain
Sonnenberg sump drain
Sovally suprapubic suction cup drain
spaghetti drain
stab drain
stab-wound drain
Sterivac drain
stoma irrigator drain
Stryker drain
subgaleal drain
suction drain
sump drain
sump Penrose drain
suprapubic drain
suprapubic suction drain
surgical drain
Surgilav drain
Surgivac drain
Taut capillary drain
Teflon nasobiliary drain
thoracic drain
Thora-Drain 3-bottle chest drain
Thora-Klex chest drain
thyroid drain

drain (*continued*)

tissue drain
TLS drain
TLS suction drain
TLS surgical drain
transnasal drain
transnasal pancreaticobiliary drain
transpapillary drain
triple-lumen sump drain
T-tube drain
umbilical tape drain
Uni-sump drain
U-tube drain
Vacutainer drain
vacuum drain
van Sonnenberg sump drain
Varidyne drain
Vigilon drain
Wangensteen drain
Waterman sump drain
water-seal drain
water-trap drain
whistle-tip drain
Wolff drain
wolffian drain
wound drain
Wylie drain
Yeates drain
Younken double-lumen drain
drain site
drain site evisceration
drain tube
drainable fecal collector
drainable ostomy pouch
drainage
2-bottle drainage
3-bottle drainage
abdominal drainage
Almoor extrapetrosal drainage
antegrade biliary drainage
arthrotomy with drainage
bile tract drainage
biliary drainage
bladder drainage
bronchial drainage
bronchoscopy with drainage
button drainage
capillary drainage
cardiotomy reservoir chest drainage
catheter drainage

drainage (*continued*)
  caval drainage
  cerebral spinal fluid drainage
  chest drainage
  chest tube drainage (CTD)
  circle loop biliary drainage
  closed chest drainage
  closed drainage
  closed suction drainage
  closed tube drainage
  closed water-seal drainage
  computed tomography-guided
    selective drainage
  continuous catheter drainage
  continuous suction drainage
  copious drainage
  CT-guided selective drainage
  David drainage
  dependent drainage
  direct drainage
  downward drainage
  DuVal pancreatic drainage
  endoscopic biliary drainage
  endoscopic nasobiliary
    catheter drainage
  endoscopic pancreatic
    drainage
  endoscopic transpapillary cyst
    drainage
  endosonography-guided
    drainage
  external bile drainage
  external bile tract drainage
  external biliary drainage
  external ventricular drainage
  extrapetrosal drainage
  fluid drainage
  gravity drainage
  Greer EZ Access drainage
  hematoma drainage
  incision and drainage (I&D)
  internal drainage
  J-Vac closed wound drainage
  lumbar drainage
  lymphatic drainage
  lymphocele drainage
  Molteno drainage
  nasal drainage
  nasobiliary drainage
  nasogastric drainage
  nasopancreatic drainage
  nephrostomy drainage

drainage (*continued*)
  open drainage
  operative drainage
  orthostatic drainage
  pattern of drainage
  pelvic drainage
  percutaneous abscess and
    fluid drainage (PAFD)
  percutaneous abscess
    drainage (PAD)
  percutaneous antegrade
    biliary drainage
  percutaneous catheter
    drainage
  percutaneous external
    drainage (PED)
  percutaneous transhepatic
    biliary drainage (PTBD)
  percutaneous transhepatic
    drainage (PTD)
  peripancreatic abdominal
    drainage
  perirectal incision and
    drainage
  peritoneal drainage
  portal drainage
  postoperative irrigation-
    suction drainage
  postural drainage
  pseudocyst drainage
  purulent drainage
  Redivac drainage
  retrograde venous drainage
  Rodney Smith drainage
  sanguineous drainage
  sclerotomy with drainage
  serosanguineous drainage
  shunt-site drainage
  simple external drainage
  sinus drainage
  Snyder Surgivac drainage
  spinal fluid drainage
  stereotactic catheter drainage
  strike-through drainage
  suction drainage
  sump drainage
  Surgivac drainage
  thoracic duct drainage (TDD)
  Thoracoseal drainage
  Thora-Drain chest drainage
  thorascopic drainage
  through drainage

drainage (*continued*)
   tidal drainage
   transcystic drainage
   T-tube drainage
   underwater drainage
   underwater-seal drainage
   urinary drainage
   vacuum drainage
   venous drainage
   video thoracoscopic drainage
   Wangensteen drainage
   water-seal drainage
   wound drainage
drainage bag
drainage catheter
drainage from wound
drainage gastroscopy
drainage gastrostomy
drainage of abscess
drainage of ascites
drainage of bone
drainage of chest
drainage of cyst
drainage of gland
drainage of muscle
drainage of organ
drainage of sinus
drainage of tissues
drainage of wound
drainage pattern
drainage pump
drainage to gravity
drainage tube
drainage with myringotomy
drained abscess
draining abscess
draining incisional site
draining lesion
draining wound
drain-to-wall suction connector
drain-to-wall suction tube
Drake aneurysm clip
Drake clip
Drake fenestrated clip
Drake machine
Drake tandem clipping
   technique
Drake tourniquet
Drake uroflometer
Drake-Kees clip
Drake-Willard hemodialysis
   machine

Drake-Willock dialysis machine
Drake-Willock dialyzer
Drapanas mesocaval shunt
Drapanas shunt
drape
   3M drape
   3M small aperture Steri-Drape
     drape
   Abandia drapes
   adhesive drape
   adhesive plastic drape
   Alcon disposable drape
   AliMed surgical drape
   Bard absorption drape
   Barrier laparoscopy drape
   Bioclusive drape
   Blair head drape
   Convertors surgical drapes
   disposable TUR drape
   eye drape
   Eye-Pak drape
   fenestrated drape
   fenestrated sterile drape
   foot drape
   Gator drape
   head drape
   Hough drape
   incise drape
   Ioban antimicrobial incise
     drape
   Ioban drape
   J&J Band-Aid sterile drape
   Johnson & Johnson Band-Aid
     sterile drape
   Lingeman 3-in-1 procedure
     drape
   Lingeman TUR drape
   MB&J hip drape
   MMM drape (3M drape)
   NeuroDrape surgical drape
   O'Connor drape
   operation drape
   operation microscope drape
   OpMi microscopic drape
   Opraflex drape
   Opraflex incise drape
   OpSite drape
   paper drape
   plastic drape
   prep and drape
   procedure drape
   Pro-Ophtha drape

drape (*continued*)

Qualtex surgical drape
Richards drape
Rusch perineal drape
sewn-in waterproof drape
small aperture Steri-Drape
  drape
split drape
sterile drape
surgical drapes
Surgikos disposable drape
Surgi-Site Incise drape
Thompson drape
towel drape
Transelast surgical drape
transparent drape
V. Mueller TUR drape
Viadrape drape
Vi-Drape drape
Visi-Drape Elite ophthalmic
  drape
Visi-Drape Mini Aperture
  drape
Visi-Drape Mini Incise drape
Visiflex drape
Zeiss OpMi drape
drape clamp
draped area
draped free
draped in a routine fashion
draped in a routine manner
draped operative field
draped out of the field
drapery swag of cheek
Drapier needle
draping of field
draping of surgical patient
Drato bunionectomy
drawn ankle clonus
drawn back
dreamer clamp
Dreiling tube
Dreisse meatotome
Dremel rotary tool
dressed tube
dressed wound
DressFlex orthotic
Dressinet netting bandage
dressing (*see also* bandage,
  gauze bandage, gauze
  dressing)
  3M dressing

dressing (*continued*)

3M Microdon dressing
3M SoftCloth adhesive wound
  dressing
3M Tegaderm transparent
  dressing
3M Tegasorb hydrocolloid
  dressing
4-tailed dressing
ABD dressing
Abdopatch Gel Z Adhesive
  dressing
absorbable dressing
Ace adherent dressing
Ace elastic dressing
Ace longitudinal strips
  dressing
Ace rubber elastic dressing
Ace-Hesive dressing
Acry Island border dressing
AcryDerm border island
  dressing
AcryDerm dressing
AcryDerm Strands absorbent
  wound dressing
acrylic resin dressing
Acticoat silver-based burn
  dressing
Acu-Derm IV/TPN dressing
Acu-Derm wound dressing
Adaptic dressing
Adaptic gauze dressing
Adaptic nonadhering dressing
AD-Hese-Away dressing
adhesive absorbent dressing
adhesive dressing
Aeroplast dressing
air pressure dressing
Airstrip composite dressing
AlgiDerm alginate wound
  dressing
AlgiDerm wound dressing
alginate wound dressing
AlgiSite alginate wound
  dressing
Algisorb wound dressing
Algosteril alginate dressing
Algosteril alginate wound
  dressing
Alldress dressing
Alldress multilayer wound
  dressing

dressing (*continued*)

Alldress multilayered wound dressing
Allevyn adhesive hydrocellular dressing
Allevyn cavity dressing
Allevyn dressing
Allevyn foam dressing
Allevyn hydrophilic polyurethane dressing
Allevyn Island dressing
Allevyn tracheostomy dressing
aloe tape dressing
Alvogyl surgical dressing
amniotic membrane dressing
anorectal dressing
antiseptic dressing
Aquacel Ag antimicrobial wound dressing
Aquacel Hydrofiber dressing
Aquacel Hydrofiber wound dressing
Aquaflo dressing
Aquaflo hydrogel wound dressing
Aquamatic dressing
Aquaphor gauze dressing
Aquaplast dressing
Aquaplast tie-down dressing
Aquasorb transparent hydrogel dressing
Arglaes wound dressing
ArtAssist compression dressing
ArtAssist dressing
Aureomycin gauze dressing
bacitracin dressing
Band-Aid brand surgical dressing
Band-Aid dressing
Bard absorption dressing
Bard AlgiDerm dressing
Barnes-Hind ophthalmic dressing
barrel dressing
Barton dressing
Baynton dressing
B-D butterfly swab dressing
BGC Matrix dressing
bias-cut stockinette dressing
Biatin foam dressing

dressing (*continued*)

binocular dressing
binocular eye dressing
Biobrane dressing
Biobrane glove dressing
Biobrane wound dressing
Bioclusive dressing
Bioclusive transparent dressing
Biocol dressing
Biocol temporary dressing
BioCore collagen dressing
Biodrape dressing
Biolex impregnated dressing
Biopatch antimicrobial dressing
Biopatch antimicrobial foam wound dressing
Biopatch foam wound dressing
Bio-occlusive dressing
Bishop-Harman dressing
Blenderm surgical tape dressing
BlisterFilm transparent dressing
BlisterFilm transparent wound dressing
blue sponge dressing
bolus dressing
bone wax dressing
Borsch dressing
brassiere-type dressing
BreakAway absorptive wound dressing
Breast Vest Exu-Dry one-piece wound dressing
bulky compressive dressing
bulky dressing
bulky hand dressing
bulky pressure dressing
Bunnell dressing
Bunnell-Littler dressing
Burn Jel dressing
butterfly dressing
calcium sodium alginate wound dressing
Calgiswab dressing
Carasyn hydrogel wound dressing
CarboFlex odor-control dressing

dressing (*continued*)

CarraFilm transparent dressing

CarraFilm transparent film dressing

CarraSmart foam dressing

CarraSorb H calcium alginate wound dressing

CarraSorb M freeze-dried gel wound dressing

Carrasyn Hydrogel dressing

Carrasyn viscous hydrogel wound dressing

Castex rigid dressing

Castmate plaster bandage dressing

Catrix dressing

Cecil dressing

cellophane dressing

Centurion SorbaView window dressing

chest dressing

Chick sterile dressings

Chronicure wound dressing

Chux incontinent dressing

Cica-Care silicone gel sheet dressing

CicaCare topical gel sheet dressing

Cikloid dressing

CircPlus compression dressing

Circulon dressing

circumferential dressing

Circumpress facelift dressing

ClearSite borderless dressing

ClearSite Hydro Gauze dressing

ClearSite hydrogel absorptive borderline wound dressing

ClearSite wound dressing

Clevis dressing

Coban dressing

Coban elastic dressing

cocoon dressing

cod liver oil-soaked strips dressing

Coe-Pak periodontal dressing

Coe-Soft dressing

cohesive dressing

CollaCote collagen wound dressing

dressing (*continued*)

CollaCote wound dressing

collagen dressing

CollaPlug dressing

CollaPlug wound dressing

collar dressing

CollaTape wound dressing

collodion dressing

Coloplast dressing

CombiDerm absorbent cover dressing

CombiDerm dressing

Comfeel contour dressing

Comfeel hydrocolloid dressing

Comfeel Plus pressure relief dressing

Comfeel Purilon dressing

Comfeel UIcus occlusive dressing

Complex Cu3 dressing

Compeed Skinprotector dressing

Composite Cultured Skin

composite dressing

compound dressing

compression dressing

Comprol dressing

conductive Hydrogel wound dressing

Conformant wound dressing

contact-layer wound dressings

Contreet antimicrobial dressings

Contura medicated dressing

CoolSorb absorbent cold transfer dressing

Cornish wool dressing

cotton bolster dressing

cotton elastic dressing

cotton pledgets dressing

cotton-ball dressing

cotton-wadding dressing

Covaderm composite wound dressing

Covaderm Plus tube site dressing

Covaderm Plus dressing

Coverlet adhesive dressing

Coverlet OR adhesive surgical dressing

dressing (*continued*)

Coverlet Strips wound dressing
Cover-Pad dressing
Cover-Roll dressing
Covertell composite secondary dressing
CovRSite dressing
Co-Wrap dressing
Cranioplastic material dressing
crepe bandage dressing
Crinotene dressing
Cruricast dressing
Cryo/Cuff ankle dressing
Cryo/Cuff compression dressing
Curad plastic dressing
Curad surgical adhesive dressing
Curaderm dressing
Curafil dressing
Curafil gel wound dressing
Curafil hydrogel dressing
Curafoam dressing
Curafoam foam wound dressing
Curafoam island dressing
Curafoam wound dressing
Curagel hydrogel dressing
Curagel hydrogel island wound dressing
Curasol sterile wound dressing
Curasorb calcium alginate dressing
Curity dressing
Curon dressing
Cutifilm Plus waterproof wound dressing
Cutinova alginate dressing
Cutinova cavity dressing
Cutinova dressing
Cutinova foam dressing
Cutinova Hydro dressing
Cutinova hydroactive dressing
Cutiplast sterile wound dressing
Dakin dressing
Debrisan dressing
Decubi-Care pad dressing
demigauntlet dressing

dressing (*continued*)

Derma Care dressing
Dermacea alginate dressing
Dermacea alginate wound dressing
DermaCol hydrocolloid wound dressing
DermaFilm dressing
Dermagran hydrophilic wound dressing
Dermagran zinc-saline hydrogel wound dressing
Dermagran-B hydrophilic wound dressing
DermaMend foam wound dressing
DermaMend hydrogel dressing
DermaNet contact-layer wound dressing
DermaSite transparent film dressing
DermaSORB hydrocolloid/alginate wound dressing
DermAssist gel/gauze dressing
DermAssist glycerin hydrogel dressing
DermAssist hydrocolloid dressing
DermAssist transparent site dressing
DermaStat calcium alginate wound dressing
Dermatell hydrocolloid dressing
Dermgran hydrogel wound dressing
Dermicel dressing
Dermophase dressing
Desault dressing
Diabeticorum dressing
DiabGel hydrogel dressing
Digi Sleeve stockinette dressing
donor site dressing
Dow Corning antifoam agent dressing
Doyle ear dressing
Drilac surgical dressing
Dri-Site dressing
dry dressing

dressing (*continued*)
dry pressure dressing
dry sterile dressing (DSD)
dry textile dressing
dry-and-occlusive dressing
DuoDERM CGF gel dressing
DuoDerm compression
    dressing
DuoDerm dressing
DuoDerm hydrocolloid
    dressing
DuoDerm porous dressing
Dyna-Flex compression
    dressing
Dyna-Flex dressing
Eakin cohesive seal dressing
elastic foam pressure dressing
Elastikon dressing
Elastikon elastic tape dressing
Elastikon wristlet dressing
Elasto dressing
Elasto-Gel hydrogel dressing
Elasto-Gel hydrogel wound
    dressing
Elastomull dressing
Elastoplast dressing
Elastoplast pressure dressing
Elastopore dressing
Elta Dermal hydrogel dressing
Enviclusive semi-occlusive
    adhesive film dressing
Envinet gauze dressing
EpiFilm otologic lamina
    dressing
Epigard dressing
Epilock dressing
Epilock polyurethane foam
    wound dressing
Episeal wound dressing
Esmarch roll dressing
ethylene oxide dressing
Expo Bubble dressing
Expo eye dressing
ExuDerm hydrocolloid
    dressing
ExuDerm RCD hydrocolloid
    dressing
ExuDry absorptive dressing
ExuDry dressing
eye dressing
eye pad dressing
EZ-Derm dressing

dressing (*continued*)
EZ-Derm porcine biosynthetic
    wound dressing
Fabco gauze dressing
Fastrak traction strip dressing
felt dressing
Ferris polyostomy wound
    dressing
Fibracol collagen-alginate
    wound dressing
Fibracol collagen-alginate
    dressing
figure-eight dressing
figure-of-eight dressing
filiform dressing
film wound dressing
fine-mesh dressing
finger-cot dressing
Firbracol collagen-alginate
    dressing
fixed dressing
flats of dressing
Flex foam dressing
Flex-Aid knuckle dressing
FlexDerm wound dressing
Flexfilm wound dressing
FlexiGel gel sheet dressing
Flexigrid dressing
Flexinet dressing
Flexzan dressing
Flexzan Extra dressing
Flexzan foam wound dressing
Flexzan topical wound
    dressing
fluff dressing
fluffed gauze dressing
fluffy compression dressing
foam rubber dressing
foam wound dressing
Foille dressing
FortaDerm dressing
Fowler dressing
Fricke dressing
Fricke scrotal dressing
Fuller rectal dressing
Fuller shield dressing
Fuller shield rectal dressing
Furacin dressing
Furacin gauze dressing
FyBron alginate dressing
FyBron calcium alginate
    dressing

dressing (*continued*)
Galen dressing
Gamgee dressing
Garretson dressing
gauze dressing
gauze stent dressing
Gauztex dressing
gel wound dressing
Gelfilm dressing
Gelfoam dressing
Gelocast dressing
Gel-Syte wound dressing
Gentell alginate wound dressing
Gentell foam wound dressing
Gentell hydrogel dressing
Gentell isotonic saline wet dressing
Gibney dressing
Gibson dressing
Glasscock dressing
Glasscock ear dressing
GraftCyte dressing
GraftCyte gauze wound dressing
GraftCyte moist dressing
GraftCyte moist wound dressing
Griffin bandage lens dressing
GU irrigant dressing
Gypsona plaster dressing
hammock dressing
hand dressing
Harman eye dressing
Harrison interlocked mesh dressing
Hexcel cast dressing
hip spica dressing
hour-glass dressing
Hueter perineal dressing
HyCare G hydrogel dressing
hyCure collagen hemostatic wound dressing
Hydragran absorption dressing
Hydrasorb foam wound dressing
hydroactive dressing
Hydrocol dressing
Hydrocol sacral wound dressing
hydrocolloid dressing

dressing (*continued*)
hydrocolloid occlusive dressing
HydroDerm transparent dressing
hydrofiber dressing
hydrogel dressing
hydrophilic polymer dressing
hydrophilic polyurethane foam dressing
hydrophilic semipermeable absorbent polyurethane foam dressing
HyFil hydrogel dressing
Hypergel dressing
Hypergel hydrogel wound dressing
Hypergel wound dressing
Iamin gel wound dressing
Iamin hydrating gel wound dressing
immobilizing dressing
impermeable dressing
impregnated dressing
Inerpan dressing
Inerpan flexible burn dressing
InteguDerm dressing
Intelligent dressing
IntraSite gel dressing
IntraSite gel wound dressing
Iodoflex absorptive dressing
Iodosorb absorptive dressing
IPOP cast dressing (immediate postoperative prosthesis cast dressing)
Ivalon dressing
J&J dressing
jacket-type chest dressing
jelly dressing
Jelonet dressing
Jobst dressing
Jobst mammary support dressing
Jobst UlcerCare dressing
Johnson & Johnson dressing
Jones dressing
Kalginate alginate wound dressing
Kalginate calcium alginate wound dressing
Kaltostat Fortex dressing
Kaltostat wound dressing

dressing (*continued*)

Kaltostat wound packing dressing
Karaya dressing
Kelikian foot dressing
Kerlix conforming bandage dressing
Kerlix dressing
Kirkland cement dressing
Kling adhesive dressing
Kling conform dressing
Kling dressing
Kling gauze dressing
Koagamin dressing
Koch-Mason dressing
Kollagen dressing
Koylon foam rubber dressing
Larrey dressing
LaserSite wound dressing
Lipisorb dressing
Liquiderm dressing
Lister dressing
Lubafax dressing
Lukens bone wax dressing
LyoFoam A water resistant dressing
LyoFoam C dressing
LyoFoam dressing
LyoFoam T dressing
LyoFoam wound dressing
mammary support dressing
Mammopatch gel self-adhesive dressing
Manchu cotton dressing
many-tailed dressing
Martin rubber dressing
mastoid dressing
Maxorb alginate wound dressing
mechanic's waste dressing
Medical Resources hydrophilic wounddressing
Medici aerosol adhesive tape remover dressing
Medifill collagen hemostatic wound dressing
Medipatch Gel Z adhesive dressing
Medipore Dress-it dressing
Medi-Rip dressing
Mediskin porcine biological wound dressing

dressing (*continued*)

Medline Derma-Gel dressing
Mefilm dressing
Melgisorb calcium alginate dressing
Mepiform dressing
Mepiform self-adherent silicone dressing
Mepilex dressing
Mepilex foam dressing
Mepitel contact-layer wound dressing
Mepitel dressing
Mepitel nonadherent silicone dressing
Mepore absorptive dressing
Merogel dressing
Merogel nasal dressing and sinus stent
Mersilene dressing
Mersilene mesh dressing
Merthiolate dressing
Mesalt sodium chloride impregnated dressing
Metaline dressing
Microdon dressing
Microfoam dressing
Micropore dressing
Micropore surgical tape dressing
Mills dressing
Minnesota Mining and Manufacturing Company dressing (3M dressing)
Mitraflex dressing
Mitraflex foam dressing
Mitraflex sterile spyrosorbent multilayer wound dressing
Mitrathane wound dressing
MMM dressing (3M dressing)
modified Robert Jones dressing
moist dressing
moist interactive dressing
moistened fine mesh gauze dressing
moisture-retentive dressing
moleskin traction hitch dressing
monocular dressing
monocular eye dressing
Montgomery strap dressing

dressing (*continued*)
  Mother Jones dressing
  moustache dressing
  MPM conductive hydrogel
    dressing
  MPM GelPad dressing
  MPM hydrogel dressing
  MPM multilayer dressing
  Multidex maltodextrin wound
    dressing
  MultiPad absorptive dressing
  muslin dressing
  mustache dressing
  nasal-tip dressing
  NDM adhesive wound
    dressing
  NeoDerm dressing
  neoprene dressing
  nonadhering dressing
  nonadhesive dressing
  nonocclusive dressing
  Normigel hydrogel dressing
  Normigel protective wound
    dressing
  N-Terface contact-layer
    wound dressing
  N-Terface graft dressing
  Nu Gauze dressing
  Nu-Derm foam island dressing
  Nu-Gel clear hydrogel wound
    dressing
  NutraCol hydrocolloid wound
    dressing
  NutraDress zinc-saline
    dressing
  NutraFil hydrophilic B
    dressing
  NutraGauze hydrophilic
    wound dressing
  NutraStat calcium alginate
    wound dressing
  NutraVue hydrogel dressing
  Nu-wrap rolls dressing
  Oasis wound dressing
  occlusive collodion dressing
  occlusive dressing
  occlusive moisture-retentive
    dressing
  occlusive semipermeable
    dressing
  O'Donoghue dressing
  odor absorbent dressing

dressing (*continued*)
  oiled silk dressing
  Omiderm transparent
    adhesive film dressing
  open dressing
  Opraflex dressing
  OpSite dressing
  OpSite Flexifix transparent
    film dressing
  OpSite Flexigrid dressing
  OpSite Flexigrid transparent
    adhesive film dressing
  OpSite occlusive dressing
  OpSite Plus dressing
  OpSite wound dressing
  Orthoflex dressing
  Orthoplast dressing
  OsmoCyte island wound care
    dressing
  OsmoCyte PCA pillow wound
    dressing
  OsmoCyte pillow dressing
  Ostic plaster dressing
  Owen cloth dressing
  Owen gauze dressing
  Owen nonadherent surgical
    dressing
  Oxiplex
  Oxycel dressing
  oxyquinoline dressing
  PanoGauze dressing
  PanoGauze hydrogel-
    impregnated gauze dressing
  PanoPlex hydrogel dressing
  PanoPlex hydrogel wound
    dressing
  Paracine dressing
  paraffin dressing
  patch dressing
  peacock dressing
  Peries medicated hygienic
    wire dressing
  petrolatum dressing
  petrolatum gauze dressing
  Piedmont all-cotton elastic
    dressing
  Pillo Pro dressing
  pink dressing
  plaster dressing
  plaster pants dressing
  plaster-of-Paris dressing
  plastic dressing

dressing (*continued*)

pledget dressing
Polyderm foam wound dressing
PolyFlex traction dressing
PolyMem adhesive surgical wound dressing
PolyMem foam wound dressing
PolyMem wound care dressing
Polyskin II dressing
PolyTrach dressing
polyurethane foam dressing
PolyWic dressing
Pope halo dressing
postauricular ear dressing
postnasal dressing
Preptic dressing
Presso-Elastic dressing
Pressoplast compression dressing
Presso-Superior dressing
pressure dressing
pressure patch dressing
Priessnitz dressing
Primaderm dressing
Primaderm foam dressing
Primapore absorptive wound dressing
Primapore tape and gauze wound dressing
Primer compression dressing
Proclude transparent adhesive film dressing
ProCyte transparent adhesive film dressing
Proflavine wool dressing
Profore 4-layer bandage
Profore 4-layer wound dressing
Pro-Ophtha dressing
propylene dressing
protective dressing
pulped muscle dressing
PuraPly wound dressing
Quadro dressing
Queen Anne dressing
Qwik-Clean dressing
Ray-Tec dressing
Red Cross adhesive dressing
Release nonadhering dressing

dressing (*continued*)

removal of dressing
RepliCare hydrocolloid dressing
RepliCare Thin hydrocolloid dressing
Repliderm dressing
Reston dressing
Reston foam dressing
Reston foam wound dressing
Reston hydrocolloid dressing
Restore alginate wound dressing
Restore CalciCare dressing
Restore extra-thin dressing
Restore hydrocolloid dressing
Restore hydrogel dressing
Restore Plus wound care dressing
Rezifilm dressing
Reziplast spray-on dressing
Ribble dressing
ribbon gauze dressing
Richet dressing
Robert Jones bulky soft compressive dressing
Robert Jones compressive dressing
Robert Jones dressing
Rochester dressing
roller dressing
Rondic sponge dressing
Rose bed dressing
Royl-Derm wound hydrogel nonadherent dressing
rubber scan spray dressing
Saf-Gel hydrogel dressing
saline dressing
saline-saturated wool dressing
Sayre dressing
Scan spray dressing
scarlet red gauze dressing
scrotal dressing
scultetus binder dressing
scultetus dressing
SeaSorb alginate wound dressing
Sellotape tie-over dressing
Selofix dressing
Selopor dressing
semicompressive dressing
semiocclusive dressing

dressing (*continued*)

- semiocclusive moisture-retentive dressing
- semiopen dressing
- semipermeable dressing
- semipermeable membrane dressing
- semipressure dressing
- Septisol soap dressing
- Septopack periodontal dressing
- Setopress dressing
- Shah aural dressing
- Shantz dressing
- sheepskin dressing
- sheer spot Band-Aid dressing
- sheet-wadding dressing
- Signadress hydrocolloid dressing
- Silastic dressing
- Silastic foam dressing
- Silastic gel dressing
- silicone dressing
- Silon wound dressing
- Silon-TSR wound dressing
- Siloskin dressing
- Silverlon wound packing strips
- Silverstein dressing
- SIS wound dressing
- SiteGuard transparent adhesive film dressing
- SiteGuard transparent dressing
- Skin-Prep protective dressing
- SkinTegrity hydrogel dressing
- SkinTemp biosynthetic collagen dressing
- sling dressing
- Snugs dressing
- Sof-Foam dressing
- Sof-Rol dressing
- SofSorb absorptive dressing
- SoftCloth absorptive dressing
- Sof-Wick dressing
- SoloSite hydrogel dressing
- Sommers compression dressing
- SorbaView composite wound dressing
- Sorbex Thin hydrocolloid dressing

dressing (*continued*)

- Sorb-It dressing
- Sorbsan alginate dressing
- Sorbsan dressing
- Sorbsan gel block topical wound dressing
- Sorbsan topical wound dressing
- spica dressing
- Spray Band dressing
- Spyrogel hydrogel wound dressing
- squares of dressing
- starch-based copolymer dressing
- Sta-Tite gauze dressing
- stent dressing
- Stericare copolymer absorbent dressing
- Stericare hydrogel gauze dressing
- sterile adhesive bubble dressing
- sterile compression dressing
- sterile dressing
- sterile dry dressing
- Steri-pads dressing
- Stimson dressing
- stockinette dressing
- StrataSorb composite wound dressing
- Stretch Net wound dressing
- Styrofoam dressing
- subclavian Tegaderm dressing
- super-absorptive polymer dressing
- Superflex elastic dressing
- SuperSkin thin film dressing
- Super-Trac adhesive traction dressing
- SurePress compression dressing
- SureSite transparent adhesive film dressing
- Surfasoft dressing
- surgical dressing
- Surgicel dressing
- Surgicel gauze dressing
- Surgicel Nu-Knit dressing
- Surgifix dressing
- Surgiflex dressing
- Surgilast tubular elastic dressing

dressing (*continued*)

Surgi-Pad combined dressing
Surgitube dressing
suspensory dressing
Sween-A-Peel wound dressing
Synthaderm dressing
Synthaderm occlusive wound dressing
synthetic barrier dressing
tap water wet dressing
T-bandage dressing
T-binder pressure dressing
Tegaderm dressing
Tegaderm occlusive dressing
Tegaderm semipermeable dressing
Tegaderm semipermeable occlusive dressing
Tegaderm transparent dressing
Tegagel hydrogel dressing
Tegagen alginate wound dressing
Tegapore contact-layer wound dressing
Tegasorb occlusive dressing
Tegasorb ulcer dressing
Telfa Clear nonadherent wound dressing
Telfa dressing
Telfa gauze dressing
Telfa island dressing
Telfa plastic film dressing
Telfa Plus barrier island dressing
Telfa Xtra absorbent island dressing
Telfamax ultra absorbent dressing
Tensoplast elastic adhesive dressing
Tensor elastic dressing
Tes Tape dressing
Thera-Boot compression dressing
TheraSkin wound dressing
Thillaye dressing
thin film dressing
ThinSite dressing
ThinSite topical wound dressing

dressing (*continued*)

ThinSite with Biofilm hydrogel topical wound dressing
Tielle absorptive dressing
Tielle hydropolymer dressing
tie-over dressing
tie-over Sellotape dressing
Tomac foam rubber traction dressing
Tomac knitted rubber elastic dressing
Transeal transparent adhesive film dressing
Transeal transparent wound dressing
TransiGel woven gauze dressing
Transorb wound dressing
Transorbent topical wound dressing
transparent adhesive film dressing
transparent dressing
Transpore surgical tape dressing
Triad hydrophilic wound dressing
triangular dressing
tube dressing
Tube-Lok tracheotomy dressing
Tubex gauze dressing
TubiGrip dressing
tubular dressing
tulle gras dressing
twill dressing
ulcer dressing
Ultec hydrocolloid dressing
Ultec Pro alginate hydrocolloid dressing
Ultex Thin extra thin hydrocolloid dressing
Ultrafera wound dressing
Uniflex dressing
Unna boot dressing
Unna-Flex compression dressing
Unna-Flex Plus dressing
Unna-Pak compression dressing
upper body dressing

dressing (*continued*)

Usher Marlex mesh dressing
vacuum assisted closure dressing
vapor-permeable dressing
Vari/Moist wound dressing
Varick elastic dressing
Vaseline dressing
Vaseline gauze dressing
Vaseline petrolatum gauze dressing
Vaseline wick dressing
Veingard dressing
Velcro dressing
Velcro fastener dressing
Velpeau dressing
Velpeau stockinette dressing
Velroc dressing
Veni-Gard stabilization dressing
Ventex dressing
Ventifoam traction dressing
Viasorb dressing
Viasorb occlusive film dressing
Victorian collar dressing
Victorian collar-type dressing
Vi-Drape dressing
VigiFoam dressing
Vigilon dressing
Vigilon gel dressing
Vigilon primary wound dressing
Vigilon semipermeable nonocclusive dressing
Vigilon synthetic occlusive dressing
Vioform dressing
Vioform gauze dressing
Viscopaste gauze dressing
VitaCuff dressing
Wangensteen dressing
water dressing
Watson-Jones dressing
Webril dressing
Weck-cel dressing
wet dressing
wet-to-dry dressing
whisk-packets dressing
wick dressing
wood roll dressing
wool roll dressing

dressing (*continued*)

wound dressing
Woun'Dres hydrogel dressing
Woun'Dres natural collagen hydrogel wound dressing
Wound-Span Bridge dressing
wraparound dressing
Xeroflo dressing
Xeroform dressing
Y-bandage dressing
Yield nonadherent gauze dressing
Zephyr rubber elastic dressing
Zim-Flux dressing
Zimocel dressing
Zipzoc stocking compression dressing
Zobec sponge dressing
Zonas porous adhesive tape dressing
Zoroc resin plaster dressing
dressing forceps
dressing jar
dressing scissors
dressing stick
dressing therapy
Drew clip
Drews cannula
Drews capsular polisher
Drews cataract needle
Drews cilia forceps
Drews ciliary forceps
Drews cystotome
Drews forceps
Drews hook
Drews inclined prism
Drews intraocular forceps
Drews intraocular implant lens
Drews intraocular lens forceps
Drews iris retractor
Drews irrigating cannula
Drews lavage needle
Drews lens
Drews pick
Drews polisher
Drews sutures
Drews suture pickup spatula
Drew-Smythe catheter
Drews-Rosenbaum iris retractor
Drews-Rosenbaum retractor
Drews-Sato capsular fragment spatula

Drews-Sato suture-pickup hook
Drews-Sato suture-pickup
  spatula
Drews-Sato tying forceps
Dreyfus prosthesis forceps
DREZ (dorsal route entry zone)
DREZ lesion
DREZ modification of Eriksson
  technique
DREZ procedure
DREZ surgery
DRG Sherlock threaded suture
  anchor
Driessen hinged plate
Drilac surgical dressing
drill
  ACL drill
  Acufex drill
  Adson drill
  Adson spiral drill
  Adson twist drill
  Adson-Rogers perforating drill
  Aesculap drill
  agility drill
  air drill
  air-powered drill
  Albee drill
  Amico drill
  Amsco Orthairtome drill
  Anspach drill
  anticavitation drill
  Archimedean drill
  ASIF twist drill
  ASSI wire pass drill
  automatic cranial drill
  autotome drill
  Bailey drill
  bar drill
  Björk drill
  Björk rib drill
  bone drill
  bone hand drill
  Bosworth crown drill
  Bosworth drill
  Bowen suture drill
  Brunswick-Mack rotating drill
  Buckingham drill
  Bucky hand drill
  Bunnell bone drill
  Bunnell drill
  Bunnell hand drill
  bur drill

drill (*continued*)
  Calcitek drill
  Canal Master drill
  cannulated cortical step drill
  cannulated drill
  Carmody drill
  Carmody perforator drill
  Carroll-Bunnell drill
  Caspar drill
  Cebotome drill
  cement eater drill
  centering drill
  cervical drill
  Championnière bone drill
  Charnley centering drill
  Charnley drill
  Charnley femoral condyle
    drill
  Charnley pilot drill
  Charnley starting drill
  Cherry drill
  Cherry-Austin drill
  Children's Hospital hand drill
  chuck drill
  Cloward cervical drill
  Cloward drill
  Coballoy twist drill
  cobra-head drill
  Codman drill
  Codman wire-passing drill
  Codman-Shurtleff cranial drill
  Collison body drill
  Collison cannulated hand drill
  Collison drill
  Collison tap drill
  cortical step drill
  cranial drill
  crown drill
  Crutchfield bone drill
  Crutchfield drill
  Crutchfield hand drill
  Crutchfield-Raney drill
  CurvTek TSR bone drill
  Cushing cranial drill
  Cushing drill
  Cushing flat drill
  Cushing perforator drill
  dental drill
  depth check drill
  DePuy drill
  D'Errico perforating drill
  Deyerle drill

drill (*continued*)
 diamond drill
 diamond high-speed aid drill
 Doyen cylindrical drill
 driver nail drill
 Elan drill
 Elan-E power drill
 electric drill
 extractor nail drill
 fingernail drill
 Fisch drill
 flat drill
 Galt drill
 Gates-Glidden drill
 glenoid drill
 Gray bone drill
 Gray drill
 Grosse-Kempf bone drill
 Hall air drill
 Hall drill
 Hall Micro-Aire drill
 Hall Neurairtome drill
 Hall Orthairtome drill
 Hall power drill
 Hall step-down drill
 Hall Surgairtome II drill
 Hall surgical drill
 Hall Versipower drill
 Hall-Dundar drill
 Hamby twist drill
 hand drill
 Harold Crowe drill
 Harris-Smith anterior
   interbody drill
 Hewson drill
 high-speed drill
 Hudson cerebellar attachment
   drill
 Hudson cranial drill
 Hudson drill
 initiator drill
 intramedullary drill
 Jacobs chuck drill
 Jordan-Day drill
 Kerr drill
 Kerr electro-torque drill
 Kerr hand drill
 Kirschner bone drill
 Kirschner wire drill
 Küntscher drill
 Kodex drill
 Lentulo drill

drill (*continued*)
 Lentulo spiral drill
 Light-Veley cranial drill
 Light-Veley drill
 Loth-Kirschner drill
 Luck bone drill
 Luck drill
 Lusskin bone drill
 Lusskin drill
 Macewen drill
 Magnuson twist drill
 Mathews drill
 Mathews hand drill
 Mathews load drill
 McKenzie bone drill
 McKenzie cranial drill
 McKenzie drill
 McKenzie perforating twist
   drill
 McKenzie perforator drill
 Michelson-Sequoia air drill
 Micro-Aire drill
 MicroMax Speed drill
 Midas Rex drill
 Mini Stryker power drill
 Minos air drill
 Mira drill
 Modny drill
 Moore bone drill
 Moore drill
 nail drill
 Neil-Moore perforator drill
 Neurain drill
 Neurairtome drill
 nipper nail drill
 Orthairtome II drill
 orthopedic drill
 orthopedic Universal drill
 OsseoCare drill
 Osseodent surgical drill
 osteone air drill
 ototome drill
 ototome otological drill
 Patrick drill
 Pease bone drill
 pencil-tip drill
 penetrating drill
 Penn drill
 Penn finger drill
 perforating drill
 perforating twist drill
 perforator drill

drill (*continued*)
  pilot drill
  pistol-grip hand drill
  Portmann drill
  Posi-Stop drill
  power drill
  Powerforma surgical drill
  pronator drill
  Rainbow drill
  Ralks bone drill
  Ralks drill
  Ralks fingernail drill
  Raney bone drill
  Raney cranial drill
  Raney drill
  Raney perforator drill
  retention drill
  rib drill
  Rica bone drill
  Richards pistol-grip drill
  Richards-Lovejoy bone drill
  Richmond subarachnoid twist drill
  Richter bone drill
  right-angle drill
  Romano curved surgical drill
  root canal drill
  scissors nail drill
  Shea drill
  Shea ear drill
  Sherman-Stille drill
  Skeeter otologic drill
  Sklar bone drill
  skull traction drill
  Smedberg drill
  Smedberg hand drill
  Smedberg twist drill
  SMIC sternal drill
  Smith drill
  spiral drill
  Spirec drill
  step drill
  step-down drill
  Stille bone drill
  Stille cranial drill
  Stille drill
  Stille hand drill
  Stille-pattern bone drill
  Stille-Sherman bone drill
  Stiwer hand drill
  Stryker drill
  Suretac drill

drill (*continued*)
  Surgairtome air drill
  surgical-orthopaedic drill
  suture hole drill
  Synthes drill
  Synthes facial drill
  tap drill
  Thornwald antral drill
  Thornwald drill
  Toti trephine drill
  Treace drill
  Treace stapes drill
  trephine drill
  Trinkle bone drill
  Trinkle power drill
  Trinkle Super-Cut twist drill
  Trowbridge triple-speed drill
  Trowbridge-Campau bone drill
  twist drill
  Uniflex calibrated step drill
  union broach retention drill
  Universal drill
  Universal two-speed hand drill
  Vitallium drill
  Warren-Mack drill
  Warren-Mack rotating drill
  wire drill
  Wolferman drill
  Wullstein drill
  Xoman drill
  Zimalate drill
  Zimalate twist drill
  Zimmer drill
  Zimmer hand drill
  Zimmer Universal drill
  Zimmer-Kirschner hand drill
drill chamber
drill guard
drill guide
drill guide forceps
drill guide with drill bit
drill hole
drill point
drill reamer
drill stop cylinder
drilled bur hole
drilling technique
drill-tip catheter
drill-tipped guidewire
Drinker respirator

Drinker tank respirator
drip chamber
drip infusion
drip phleboclysis
drip pyelogram
drip pyelography
drip-infusion cholangiography
Dripps classification
drip-tube feeding
Dri-Site dressing
drive
   Concept Intra-Arc drive
   exploratory drive
driven equilibrium Fourier
   transform technique
driver (*see also* screwdriver)
   automatic needle driver
   Cook endoscopic curved
     needle driver
   Eby band driver
   femoral head driver
   Flatt driver
   graft driver
   Hall driver
   Haney needle driver
   Harrington hook driver
   Jewett driver
   K wire driver
   Ken driver
   Küntscher driver
   Küntscher nail driver
   laparoscopic needle driver
   Laurus needle driver
   Linvatec driver
   Lloyd nail driver
   Massie driver
   McNutt driver
   McReynolds driver
   Micro Series wire driver
   Milewski driver
   Moore driver
   Moore-Blount driver
   needle driver
   Neufeld driver
   Nystroem nail driver
   Nystroem-Stille driver
   orthodontic band driver
   ParaMax angled driver
   Pereyra needle driver
   polyethylene-faced driver
   prostatic driver
   Pugh driver

driver (*continued*)
   Put-In driver
   Rush driver
   Schneider nail driver
   Sharbaro driver
   surgical pin driver
   Sven Johansson driver
   Szabo-Berci needle driver
   Teflon-coated driver
   tibial driver
   trial driver
   UAM universal fixation driver
   wire driver
   Zimmer driver
   Zimmer Orthair ream driver
driver nail drill
driver-extractor (*see* extractor)
drive-through sign
dromedary hump
Dromos pacemaker
drooping
drooping-chin deformity
droopy nasal tip
drop anesthesia
drop finger
drop foot
drop hand
drop metastasis
drop shoulder
drop-back procedure
drop-entry (closed-body) hook
Droperidol anesthesia
drop-foot brace
drop-foot procedure
drop-foot splint
drop-lock knee brace
drop-lock ring
dropped beat
DropTainer dispenser
Druault bundle
Druck-Schrauben screw
drug administration
drug allergy
drug dosage
drug fever
drug infusion
drug infusion pump
drug infusion sleeve
drug interaction
drug intolerance
drug intoxication
drug reaction

drug regimen
drug release capsule
drug sensitivity
drug therapy
drug use
drug withdrawal
drug-coated stent
drug-eluting stent
drug-induced abortion
drug-induced condition
drug-induced hypothermia
drug-induced
    immunosuppression
drug-infusion pump
drug-resistant
DRUJ prosthesis (distal radial-
    ulnar joint)
drum belly
drum dermatome
drum dermatotome
drum elevator
drum elevator knife
drum membrane
drum probe
drum scraper
drumhead
drumhead elevator
Drummond button
Drummond hook
Drummond hook holder
Drummond spinous wiring
    technique
Drummond wire
Drummond wire technique
Drummond-Morison operation
drums of skin graft
drumstick finger
dry abscess
dry adhesions
dry amputation
dry colostomy
dry compress
dry cup
dry dressing
dry eye syndrome
dry field
dry field technique
Dry Flotation wheelchair
    cushion
dry gangrene
dry hernia
dry incision

dry labor
dry lithotripsy
dry mouth
dry mucous membrane
dry needle holder
dry pack
dry packing
dry pressure dressing
dry socket
dry sterile dressing (DSD)
dry sterile gauze
dry swallows
dry textile dressing
dry textile gauze
dry vermilion
dry-and-occlusive dressing
Dryden-Quickert tube
dry-powder inhaler
DS-9 needle
DSA (digital subtraction
    angiography)
DSD (dry sterile dressing)
D-shaped implant
DSP Micro Diamond-Point
    microsurgery instrument
DSS (double-simultaneous
    stimulation)
DST (donor-specific
    transfusion)
D-Tach needle
D-Tach removable needle
DTAF-F bypass (descending
    thoracic aortofemoral-
    femoral bypass)
DTF (deep temporal fossa)
DTF (distal triangular fossa)
DTRs (deep tendon reflexes)
DTT (direct transverse traction)
Du Pen catheter
Du Pen pump
Dua antireflux valve
Dua stent
dual adapter
dual bypass connector
dual coil transvenous lead
dual distal-lighted laryngoscope
Dual Geometry cutter
Dual Geometry HA cup
dual impression technique
dual nerve root suction retractor
dual octapolar lead
dual onlay cortical bone graft

dual percutaneous endoscopic
    gastrostomy
dual photoabsorptiometry
    (DPA)
dual quadrapolar lead
dual square-ended Harrington
    rod
dual therapy
dual-beam fiberoptic light
    source
dual-chamber AV sequential
    pacemaker
dual-chamber flushing valve
dual-chamber Medtronic
    pacemaker
dual-chamber pacemaker
dual-chambered
dual-chambered implant
dual-chambered prosthesis
dual-compartment gel-inflatable
    mammary implant
dual-contract study
dual-energy x-ray
    absorptiometry
    densitometer
dual-head gamma camera
Dualine digital hearing
    instrument
dual-inlay bone graft
Duall #88 cement
dual-lead electrode
dual-lock Depuy hip prosthesis
dual-lock hip prosthesis
dual-lock prosthesis
dual-lock total hip prosthesis
dual-lumen catheter
dual-lumen papillotome
dual-lumen sump nasogastric
    tube
DualMesh biomaterial
DualMesh biomaterial graft
DualMesh hernia mesh
DualMesh material
DualMesh mesh
DuaLock broach
DuaLock total hip
dual-onlay bone graft
dual-onlay graft
Dualoupe
dual-pass pacemaker
dual-pedicle dermoparenchymal
    mastopexy (DPM)

dual-photon densitometer
dual-photon electrospinal
    orthosis
dual-plane techniques
dual-sensor micromanometric
    high-fidelity catheter
DualStim TENS unit
dual-sump silicone drain
Dualtherm dual-thermistor
    thermodilution catheter
Duane anomaly
Duane classification
Duane retractor
Duane U-clip
DUB (dysfunctional uterine
    bleeding)
Dubecq-Princeteau angulating
    needle holder
Duberstein intraluminal tube
    wick
Dubin-Amelar varicocele
    classification
Dubinet prosthesis
Dubois decapitation scissors
Dubois scissors
Dubois shears
Dubowitz evaluation
Dubowitz examination
Dubowitz syndrome
Dubroff radial loop intraocular
    lens
Duchenne disease
Duchenne trocar
Duchenne-Erb paralysis
Duchenne-Landouzy dystrophy
duckbill clamp
duckbill elevator
duckbill forceps
duckbill rongeur
duckbill speculum
duckbill voice prosthesis
duckbilled anodized spatula
Ducker-Hayes nerve cuff
Duckett procedure
Duckett procedure for
    hypospadias repair
Duckworth-Smith technique
Ducor angiographic catheter
Ducor balloon catheter
Ducor cardiac catheter
Ducor HF catheter
Ducor tip

Ducor-Cordis pigtail catheter
duct
- aberrant bile duct
- aberrant cystic duct
- aberrant hepatic duct
- accessory duct
- accessory hepatic duct
- accessory pancreatic duct
- acoustic duct
- alveolar duct
- Anel dilatation of lacrimal duct
- anomalous junction of the pancreatobiliary duct (AJPBD)
- Arantius duct
- Bartholin duct
- beaded hepatic duct
- Bernard duct
- bile duct
- biliary duct
- Blasius duct
- Botallo duct
- bucconeural duct
- canalicular duct
- catheterization of duct
- catheterization of lacrimonasal duct
- cochlear duct
- collecting duct
- common bile duct (CBD)
- common duct
- common hepatic duct
- Coschwitz duct
- craniopharyngeal duct
- cribriform salivary carcinoma of the excretory duct
- cupular cecum of cochlear duct
- Cuvier ducts
- cystic duct
- deferent duct
- dilatation of common bile duct
- distal bile duct
- eccrine duct
- efferent duct
- ejaculatory duct
- endolymphatic duct
- excision of duct
- excretory duct
- extrahepatic bile duct
- fold of cystic duct

duct (*continued*)
- frontonasal duct
- fusiform widening of duct
- galactophorous duct
- gall duct
- Gartner duct
- genital duct
- guttural duct
- hemithoracic duct
- Hensen duct
- hepatic duct
- hepatocystic duct
- Hering duct
- Hoffmann duct
- hypophyseal duct
- incisive duct
- inferior lacrimal duct
- InSurg common bile duct (CBD) basket
- intercalated duct
- interlobular duct
- intrahepatic bile duct
- intrahepatic biliary duct
- intralobular duct
- jugular duct
- kinking of duct
- lacrimal duct
- lacrimonasal duct
- lactiferous duct
- left hepatic duct
- lingual duct
- lymphatic duct
- main pancreatic duct (MPD)
- mamillary duct
- mammary duct
- mesonephric duct
- metanephric duct
- middle extrahepatic bile duct
- milk ducts
- minor sublingual duct
- muellerian duct
- Mueller duct
- narrowed duct
- nasal duct
- nasofrontal duct
- nasolacrimal duct
- nasopalatine duct
- normal caliber duct
- occluded duct
- omphalomesenteric duct
- ovarian duct
- pancreatic duct

duct (*continued*)
- papillary duct
- paramesonephric duct
- paraurethral duct
- parotid duct
- patent duct
- Pecquet duct
- perilobular duct
- perilymphatic duct
- periotic duct
- pharyngoinfraglottic duct
- preampullary portion of bile duct
- prepapillary bile duct
- probing of lacrimonasal duct
- pronephric duct
- prostatic duct
- Reichel cloacal duct
- reuniens duct
- right hepatic duct
- right lymphatic duct
- Rivinus duct
- saccular duct
- sacculoutricular duct
- salivary duct
- Santorini duct
- Schueller duct
- secretory duct
- segmental duct
- semicircular ducts
- seminal ducts
- Skene duct
- spermatic duct
- Stensen duct
- striated duct
- subclavian duct
- sublingual ducts
- submandibular duct
- submaxillary duct
- subvesical duct
- sudoriferous duct
- superior lacrimal duct
- sweat duct
- tear duct
- Terblanche decompression of common bile duct
- terminal bile duct
- testicular duct
- thoracic duct
- thymic duct
- thyroglossal duct
- thyrolingual duct

duct (*continued*)
- uniting duct
- utricular duct
- utriculosaccular duct
- vestibulo-infraglottic duct
- vitelline duct
- Walther duct
- Wharton duct
- Wirsung duct
- Wirsung pancreatic duct
- wolffian duct

duct cancer
duct cannulation
duct carcinoma
duct cell adenocarcinoma
duct cell carcinoma
duct dilator
duct ectasia
duct exploration
duct fistula
duct injury
duct lumen
duct of Cuvier
duct of epididymis
duct of Luschka
duct of Santorini
duct of Wirsung
duct stone
duct tumor
duct wall
ductal adenoma
ductal calculus
ductal cancer
ductal cannulation
ductal carcinoma
ductal carcinoma in situ
ductal cyst
ductal dilatation
ductal dilation
ductal ectasia
ductal hyperplasia
ductal obstruction
ductal sinus
ductal stricture
ductal system perforation
ductal-dependent lesion
ductal-dependent pulmonary circulation
ductile
ductile failure
ductile material
ductility

ductions and versions
ductless glands
DuctOcclud coil
ductogram
ductography
   pancreaticobiliary
     ductography
   peroral retrograde
     pancreaticobiliary
     ductography
duct-to-duct anastomosis
duct-to-mucosa anastomosis
ductus arteriosus
ductus choledochus
ductus clamp
ductus cochlearis
ductus deferens
ductus endolymphaticus
ductus lacrimalis
ductus perilymphatici
ductus perilymphaticus
ductus reuniens
ductus semicircularis
ductus semicircularis anterior
ductus semicircularis lateralis
ductus semicircularis posterior
ductus semicircularis superior
ductus spreader
ductus utriculosaccularis
Duddell membrane
Dudley hook
Dudley operation
Dudley rectal hook
Dudley rectal tenaculum hook
Dudley tenaculum
Dudley tenaculum hook
Dudley-Smith rectal speculum
Dudley-Smith speculum
Duecollement hemicolectomy
Duecollement maneuver
Duehr-Allen eye implant
Duet coronary stent
Duet glucose control monitor
Duett vascular sealing device
Duette basket
Duette catheter
Duette double lumen ERCP
   instrument
Duette probe
Duff debridement needle
Duffield cardiovascular scissors
Duffield scissors

Dufourmental flap
Dufourmental technique
Duggan rongeur
Duguid curved forceps
Duhamel colon operation
Duhamel operation
Duhamel procedure
Duhamel pull-through
   procedure of colon
Duehrssen incision
Duehrssen operation
Duehrssen tampon
Duehrssen vaginofixation
Dujovny microsuction
   dissection set
Duke bleeding time
Duke cannula
Duke pistol-grip cane
Duke pouch cutaneous urinary
   diversion
Duke trocar
Duke tube
Duke-Elder lamp
Duke-Elder operation
Duke-Elder ultraviolet light
Dukes carcinoma (A, B, C, or D)
Dukes classification of
   carcinoma
Dukes procedure
Dulaney antral cannula
Dulaney intraocular implant
   lens
Dulaney LASIK marker
Dulaney lens
Dulcolax bowel prep
dull aching pain
dull curettage
dull retractor
dull rotation forceps
dull to percussion abdomen
dulled sense of pain
dullness to percussion
dull-pointed forceps
dull-pronged retractor
Dulox sutures
Dumas pessary
Dumbach mini mesh
Dumbach regular mesh
Dumbach titanium mesh
dumbbell incision
dumbbell needle
dummy seeds

dummy sources in cesium
   implant
Dumon bronchoscope
Dumon laser bronchoscope
Dumon silicone stent
Dumon tracheobronchial stent
Dumon-Gilliard prosthesis
   introducer
Dumon-Gilliard prosthesis
   pushing tube
Dumon-Harrell bronchoscope
Dumon-Harrell tracheal tube
Dumont angular scissors
Dumont dissecting forceps
Dumont forceps
Dumont jeweler's forceps
Dumont retractor
Dumont scissors
Dumont Swiss dissecting
   forceps
Dumont thoracic scissors
Dumont tweezers
Dumontpallier pessary
dumping of barium meal
dumping stomach
dumping syndrome
dumpling aspect orange skin
   phenomenon
Duncan curet
Duncan dural film
Duncan endometrial biopsy
   curet
Duncan endometrial curet
Duncan fold
Duncan loop
Duncan position
Duncan shoulder brace
Duncan-Lovell modification
Dundas-Grant tube
Dunhill forceps
Dunhill hemostat
Dunlop elbow traction
Dunlop sleeve
Dunlop stripper
Dunlop thrombus stripper
Dunlop traction
Dunlop tractor
Dunn biopsy
Dunn decompressor
Dunn depressor
Dunn fracture device
Dunn operation

Dunn technique
Dunn tongue depressor
Dunn-Brittain foot arthrodesis
Dunn-Brittain foot stabilization
   technique
Dunn-Brittain operation
Dunn-Brittain triple arthrodesis
Dunn-Dautrey condylar head
   elevator
Dunn-Hess femoral component
Dunn-Hess osteotomy
Dunning curet
Dunning elevator
Dunning periosteal elevator
Dunnington operation
duobiotic
Duocondylar knee prosthesis
duo-decapolar catheter
duodenal adenocarcinoma
duodenal adenoma
duodenal artery
duodenal atresia
duodenal bulb
duodenal bulb deformity
duodenal clamp
duodenal compression
duodenal constriction
duodenal content examination
duodenal deformity
duodenal duplication
duodenal erosion
duodenal fistula
duodenal fluid collection
duodenal fold
duodenal foreign body
duodenal fossa
duodenal gland
duodenal hematoma
duodenal hernia
duodenal ileus
duodenal impression
duodenal loop
duodenal lumen
duodenal metastasis
duodenal mucosa
duodenal obstruction
duodenal opening
duodenal perforation
duodenal pin
duodenal polyp
duodenal recess
duodenal retractor

duodenal spasm
duodenal stasis
duodenal stump
duodenal stump leak
duodenal sweep
duodenal system perforation
duodenal tube
duodenal ulcer
duodenal ulceration
duodenal vein
duodenal villi
duodenal wall hamartoma
duodenal web
duodenectomy
duodenitis
duodenobiliary pressure
    gradient
duodenocaval fistula
duodenocholedochostomy
duodenocholedochotomy
duodenocolic
duodenocolic fistula
duodenocolic ligament
duodenocystostomy
duodenoduodenostomy
duodenoenterocutaneous
    fistula
duodenoenterostomy
duodenofiberscope
  Olympus
      duodenofiberscope
  Pentax FD-series
      duodenofiberscope
duodenogram
duodenography
duodenoileal bypass (DIB)
duodenoileostomy
duodenojejunal
duodenojejunal angle
duodenojejunal flexure
duodenojejunal fold
duodenojejunal fossa
duodenojejunal hernia
duodenojejunal junction
duodenojejunal obstruction
duodenojejunostomy
duodenolysis
duodenomesocolic fold
duodenopancreatectomy
duodenopyloric
duodenopyloric constriction
duodenorrhaphy

duodenoscope
  ACMI duodenoscope
  diagnostic duodenoscope
  Fujinon ED-series
      duodenoscope
  Fujinon FD-series
      duodenoscope
  GF-UM3 duodenoscope
  JF-200 duodenoscope
  JF-IT Olympus adult
      duodenoscope
  JF-IT20 duodenoscope
  JF-V10 duodenoscope
  large-channel therapeutic
      duodenoscope
  Olympus duodenoscope
  Olympus EW-series fiberoptic
      duodenoscope
  Olympus GIF-series
      duodenoscope
  Olympus JF-series video
      duodenoscope
  Olympus JF-V-series video
      duodenoscope
  Olympus JT-series video
      duodenoscope
  Olympus PJF-series pediatric
      duodenoscope
  Olympus video
      duodenoscope
  Pentax duodenoscope
  side-viewing duodenoscope
  standard duodenoscope
  therapeutic side-viewing
      duodenoscope
  video duodenoscope
duodenoscope cannula
duodenoscopy
duodenostomy
  Witzel duodenostomy
duodenotomy
duodenum
  C-loop of duodenum
  descending duodenum
  distal duodenum
  flexure of duodenum
  fold of duodenum
  inferior flexure of duodenum
  longitudinal fold of
      duodenum
  scarified duodenum
  superior flexure of duodenum

DuoDerm gel dressing
DuoDerm compression dressing
DuoDerm drain
DuoDerm dressing
DuoDerm hydrocolloid dressing
DuoDerm porous dressing
DuoDerm sustained
    compression bandage
Duo-Drive cortical bone screw
Duo-Drive cortical screw
Duo-Flow catheter
Duo-Klex artificial kidney
DuoLock curved tail closure
Duolock hip prosthesis
Duoloupe lens loupe
Duo-Patella knee prosthesis
Duo-Sonic stethoscope
Duostat rotating hemostatic
    valve
Duotrak blade
Duplay bursitis
Duplay hook
Duplay hypospadias repair
Duplay I technique
Duplay II technique
Duplay nasal speculum
Duplay operation
Duplay tenaculum
Duplay tenaculum forceps
Duplay tube
Duplay uterine tenaculum
Duplay uterine tenaculum
    forceps
Duplay-Lynch nasal speculum
Duplay-Lynch speculum
duplex placenta
duplex scanner
duplex scanning
duplex ultrasound
duplex-guided compression
duplication
    alimentary tract duplication
    central duplication
    complete duplication
    congenital duplication
    congenital hand duplication
    congenital thumb duplication
    cranial duplication
    duodenal duplication
    esophageal duplication
    fetal duplication
    gallbladder duplication

duplication (*continued*)
    gastric duplication
    incomplete duplication
    limb duplication
    Marks-Bayne technique for
        thumb duplication
    partial duplication
    preaxial thumb duplication
        (types I-IV)
    renal duplication
    symmetric thumb duplication
    thumb duplication
    trunk duplication
    tubular colonic duplication
    ureteral duplication
    Wassel thumb duplication
duplication anomaly
duplication cyst
duplication of organ
Duplicone silicone dental
    impression material
DuPont Cronex x-ray film
DuPont distal humeral plate
DuPont scanner
Dupuis cannula
Dupuy aeroplane splint
Dupuy any-angle splint
Dupuy cannulated reamer
Dupuy coaptation splint
Dupuy interference screw
Dupuy pituitary rongeur
Dupuy rainbow fracture frame
Dupuy rolled Colles splint
Dupuy-Dutemps blepharoplasty
Dupuy-Dutemps dacryostomy
Dupuy-Dutemps needle
Dupuy-Dutemps operation
DuPuy-Pott splint
Dupuytren amputation
Dupuytren contracture
Dupuytren enterotome
Dupuytren fascia
Dupuytren fracture
Dupuytren hydrocele
Dupuytren knife
Dupuytren operation
Dupuytren sign
Dupuytren splint
Dupuytren suture technique
Dupuytren sutures
Dupuytren tourniquet
Dupuytren's disease

Dupuy-Weiss needle
Dupuy-Weiss tonsillar needle
dura mater
Durabase soft rebase acrylic
durable medical equipment
DuraCast plaster bandage
Duracep biopsy forceps
Duracon knee implant
Duracon prosthesis
Durafill dental restorative
    material
Durafilm
Duraflow heart valve
Duragel lens
DuraGen absorbable dural graft
    matrix
DuraGen graft
DuraGen neurosurgical device
DuraGlide stone balloon
    catheter
DuraGlide stone removal
    balloon catheter
Dura-Guard patch
Durahesive skin barrier
Durahesive Wafer pouch
Dura-II concealable penile
    implant
Dura-II positionable penile
    prosthesis
Dura-Kold reusable compression
    ice wrap
dural arteriovenous fistula
dural arteriovenous
    malformation
dural cavernous sinus fistula
dural confluence of sinuses
dural covering
dural defect
dural ectasia
dural elevator
dural film sheeting
dural forceps
dural grafting
dural hook
dural hook knife
dural implant
dural incision
dural knife
dural needle
dural patch reconstruction
dural plate
dural protector

dural protector drill guide
dural repair
dural retractor
dural sac
dural scissors
dural separator
dural shunt syndrome
dural sinus
dural suction retractor
dural tenting suture
dural venous sinus injury
Duralay acrylic
Duraleve custom molded foot
    orthotic
Dura-Liner acrylic
DuraLite handle
DuraLite tube
Durallium implant
Duraloc acetabular cup
Duramer polyethylene
    component
Duran annuloplasty ring
Duran approach
Dura-Neb portable nebulizer
    pump
Duranest anesthetic agent
Duran-Houser wire splint
Durapatite bone replacement
    material
Durapatite graft
Durapatite implant
DuraPhase inflatable penile
    prosthesis
DuraPhase semirigid penile
    prosthesis
duraplasty
Durapore hypoallergenic tape
DuraPrep
Durapulse pacemaker
Durascope endoscope
Dur-A-Sil ear impression material
Durasoft 2 contact lens
Durasoft lens
Durasoft soft-compression
    reusable ice or heat wrap
Dura-Soft toric lens
Dura-Stick adhesive electrode
Durasul hip prosthesis
Durasul knee prosthesis
Dura-T contact lens
Dura-T lens
Duratec nursing home bed

Durathane cardiac device
Duray-Read chisel
Duray-Read gouge
Duray-Read osteotome
Duray-Ward osteotome
Duray-Wood chisel
Duerck node
Duredge knife
Duredge-Paufique knife
Durelon dental cement
Duret hemorrhage
Duret lesion
Durham flatfoot operation
Durham needle
Durham operation
Durham plasty for flatfoot
Durham tracheostomy tube
Durham tracheotomy trocar
Durham trocar
Durham tube
Durham-Caldwell operation
Durkan CTS gauge
Durman operation
Durnin angled director
Duromedics bileaflet mitral
    valve
Duromedics valve prosthesis
Duros leuprolide implant
Durotip scissors
durotomy
Duroziez sign
Durr nonpenetrating
    keratoplasty
Durr operation
Durrani dorsal vein complex
    ligation needle
Duryea retractor
dusky stoma
Dutch pessary
Dutcher body
Duthie reamer
duToit procedure
duToit rotator cuff procedure
duToit shoulder staple
duToit staple
duToit stapler
duToit-Roux arthroplasty
duToit-Roux capsulorrhaphy
duToit-Roux shoulder procedure
duToit-Roux staple
    capsulorrhaphy
Duval bag

Duval dermatome
Duval disposable dermatome
Duval forceps
Duval intestinal forceps
Duval irrigating syringe
Duval lung clamp
Duval lung forceps
Duval lung tissue forceps
Duval lung-grasping forceps
DuVal pancreatic drainage
DuVal pancreaticojejunostomy
Duval procedure
Duval Vital intestinal forceps
Duval-Allis forceps
Duval-Collin intestinal forceps
Duval-Coryllos rib shears
Duval-Crile forceps
Duval-Crile intestinal forceps
Duval-Crile lung forceps
Duval-Crile lung-grasping
    forceps
Duval-Crile tissue forceps
DuVal-Puestow
    pancreaticojejunostomy
Duval-Simon portable
    dermatome
Duval Vital intestinal forceps
Duvergier-Velter operation
Duvergier sutures
Duverney fissure
Duverney fracture
Duverney fracture of ilium
Duverney gland
Duverney plantar condylectomy
DuVries approach
DuVries condylectomy
DuVries deltoid ligament
    reconstruction technique
DuVries hammertoe repair
DuVries incision
DuVries lateral ankle
    reconstruction
DuVries needle
DuVries osteotomy
DuVries procedure
DuVries-Mann modified
    bunionectomy
Duyzings clasp
DVI pacemaker
DVI Simpson AtheroCath
DVI Simpson AtheroCath
    catheter

DVIU (direct vision internal
   urethrotomy)
DVT (deep vein thrombosis)
Dwar-Barrington resection
Dworacek-Farrior canal chisel
DWS (dorsal wrist syndrome)
Dwyer cable
Dwyer cancellous screw
Dwyer clawfoot operation
Dwyer clubfoot procedure
Dwyer collar
Dwyer device
Dwyer gouge
Dwyer incision
Dwyer instrument
Dwyer instrumentation and
   fusion
Dwyer operation for talipes
   equinovarus
Dwyer osteotomy
Dwyer procedure
Dwyer rod
Dwyer scoliosis procedure
Dwyer screw
Dwyer spinal mechanical stapler
Dwyer spinal screw
Dwyer staple
Dwyer-Hall plate
DXA densitometer
Dyban technique
Dycen pad
Dyck-Lambert classification
Dyclone anesthetic agent
dyclonine hydrochloride
   anesthetic agent
Dycor prosthetic foot
dye
   Ammon blue dye
   Berwick dye
   Cardio-Green dye
   carmine dye
   Congo red dye
   Evans blue dye
   excretion of dye
   flashlamp pulsed dye (FLPD)
     laser
   fluorescein dye
   indigo carmine dye
   injection of dye
   methylene blue dye
   prompt excretion of dye
   radiopaque dye

dye (*continued*)
   rapid emptying of dye
   residual dye
   Retrografin dye
dye allergy
dye dilution technique
dye injection
dye laser
dye sham intrarenal lesion
dye worker's carcinoma
dye yellow laser
Dymer excimer delivery probe
DynaBite biopsy forceps
Dynacor ear syringe
Dynacor enema cleansing kit
Dynacor Foley catheter
Dynacor leg bag
Dynacor suction catheter
Dynacor ulcer syringe
Dynacor vaginal irrigator set
Dynacor vaginal speculum
DynaDisc exercise equipment
Dynafabric material
Dynafill graft biomedium
   mineralized bone matrix
DynaFlex compression dressing
DynaFlex dressing
DynaFlex elastic bandage
DynaFlex Layer One padding
DynaFlex Layer Three bandage
DynaFlex Layer Two bandage
DynaFlex penile implant
DynaFlex penile prosthesis
Dyna-Flex wrap
DynaGraft granula
Dynagrip blade handle
Dynagrip handle
DynaGuard APM alternating
   pressure mattress
DynaHeat hot pack
DynaLator ultrasound unit
DynaLeap balloon material
Dynalink biliary self-expanding
   stent
Dynalyzer equipment
dynamic anchorage
dynamic aorta
dynamic axial fixator
dynamic bed
dynamic block
dynamic bolus tracking
   technique

dynamic bridging plate
dynamic cardiomyoplasty
dynamic compression
dynamic compression plate (DCP)
dynamic compression plate instrumentation
dynamic compression plate fixation
dynamic computed tomography
dynamic condylar screw (DCS)
dynamic condylar screw fixation
Dynamic cooling device
dynamic cystourethroscopy
Dynamic digit extensor tube
Dynamic elbow orthosis
dynamic facial skin lines
dynamic fluorescence video endoscopy
dynamic graciloplasty
dynamic hip screw
dynamic ileus
dynamic image
dynamic instability of wrist
Dynamic knee orthosis
dynamic line
dynamic lumbar stabilization
Dynamic Mesh craniomaxillofacial pre-angled connecting bar
Dynamic orthotic cranioplasty device
dynamic penile prosthesis
dynamic relation
dynamic repair
dynamic splint
dynamic splinting
Dynamic transverse traction device
dynamic urethral graciloplasty
dynamic wrinkle
Dynamic wrist orthosis
Dynamic Y stent
dynamization
dynamometer
    back, leg, and chest dynamometer
    Baseline dynamometer
    bicycle dynamometer
    Biodex isokinetic dynamometer
    bulb dynamometer

dynamometer (*continued*)
    Collins dynamometer
    computerized isokinetic dynamometer
    Cybex II isokinetic dynamometer
    electromechanical dynamometer
    hand dynamometer
    handheld dynamometer
    Harpenden handgrip dynamometer
    hydraulic hand dynamometer
    Isobex dynamometer
    Jamar dynamometer
    Jamar hydraulic hand dynamometer
    Lido Multi Joint II isokinetic dynamometer
    Micro FET isometric force dynamometer
    orthopedic dynamometer
    Padgett hydraulic hand dynamometer
    Preston dynamometer
    Smedley dynamometer
    Spark handheld dynamometer
    squeeze dynamometer
dynamoscope
dynamoscopy
DynaPak electrode kit
Dynaplex knee
DynaPulse 5000A ambulatory blood pressure monitor
Dynasplint knee extension unit
DynaSurg electric handpiece
Dynatrak handpiece
Dynatron 150 ultrasound
Dynatron 50, 125, 525 electrotherapy
Dynatron Mini 2000 electrotherapy
Dynatron TX 900 electrotherapy
Dynatronics Model 1620 laser
DynaWell medical compression device
DynaWraps wrap
Dynoptor ophthalmodynamometer
DyoBrite illuminator
DyoCam 550 arthroscopic video camera

DyoCam arthroscopic video camera
Dyonics arthroplasty bur
Dyonics arthroscope
Dyonics arthroscopic blade
Dyonics arthroscopic instrument
Dyonics basket forceps
Dyonics bur
Dyonics chondrotome
Dyonics cutter
Dyonics disposable arthroscope blade
Dyonics full-radius resector
Dyonics meniscal cutter
Dyonics meniscal trimmer
Dyonics meniscotome
Dyonics microsurgical instrument
Dyonics motorized meniscal shaver
Dyonics needle
Dyonics needle scope arthroscope
Dyonics rod lens arthroscope
Dyonics rod lens laparoscope
Dyonics shaver
Dyonics suction punch
Dyonics syringe injector
DyoPneumatic insufflator
DyoVac suction punch
dysarthric lesion
dysarthrosis
dyscephaly
dyschondroplasia
dyschromia (*pl.* dyschromias)
dysconjugate gaze (*also* disconjugate)
dyscrasic fracture
dysfunction
   bone marrow dysfunction
   chronic obstructive pulmonary dysfunction
   craniomandibular dysfunction (CMD)
   dental dysfunction
   ejaculatory dysfunction
   end organ dysfunction
   endothelial cell dysfunction
   erectile dysfunction
   esophageal body motor dysfunction

dysfunction (*continued*)
   extensor mechanism dysfunction
   facial neuromuscular dysfunction
   hepatic dysfunction
   hepatocellular synthetic dysfunction
   hypertonic uterine dysfunction
   late graft dysfunction
   minimal brain dysfunction (MBD)
   multiorgan system dysfunction
   multiple organ dysfunction (MOD)
   nasolacrimal dysfunction
   neurological dysfunction
   neuromotor dysfunction
   obstructive pulmonary dysfunction
   organ dysfunction
   organic dysfunction
   pancreatitis dysfunction
   pelvic floor dysfunction
   placental dysfunction
   postanesthetic central nervous system dysfunction
   postgastrectomy dysfunction
   postoperative renal dysfunction
   proximal myofascial dysfunction
   pulmonary dysfunction
   renal dysfunction
   sphincter of Oddi dysfunction
   superoxide-mediated endothelial cell dysfunction
   temporomandibular dysfunction (TMD)
   temporomandibular joint dysfunction (TMD, TMJ)
   vestibular dysfunction
   vocal dysfunction
dysfunctional
dysfunctional nasal valve
dysfunctional uterine bleeding
dysgenesis
   gonadal dysgenesis
   mixed gonadal dysgenesis
   pure gonadal dysgenesis

dysgnathic anomaly
dyskeratoma
dyskeratosis
  benign dyskeratosis
  benign intraepithelial
    dyskeratosis
  intraepithelial dyskeratosis
  malignant dyskeratosis
dyskeratosis congenita
dyskeratotic leukoplakia
dyskinesia
  biliary dyskinesia
dyskinetic and dystonic
  reactions
dyskinetic labor
dyskinetic reaction
dysmenorrhea
dysmenorrheal membrane
dysmorphic cranium
dysmorphism
  craniofacial dysmorphism
  facial dysmorphism
dysmorphology
  facial dysmorphology
  orbital dysmorphology
dysmotility
  esophageal dysmotility
dysmyogenic blepharoptosis
dysostosis
  acrofacial dysostosis
  cleidocranial dysostosis
  craniofacial dysostosis
  faciomandibular dysostosis
  mandibulofacial dysostosis
  maxillonasal dysostosis
  Nager acrofacial dysostosis
  orodigitofacial dysostosis
  otomandibular dysostosis
dysostosis multiplex
dysphagia
  benign dysphagia
  contractile ring dysphagia
  neurogenic dysphagia
  postoperative dysphagia
  postvagotomy dysphagia
  recurrent dysphagia
dysphagia lusoria
dysphasia
dysplasia
  anteroposterior dysplasia
  anteroposterior facial
    dysplasia

dysplasia (*continued*)
  asphyxiating thoracic
    dysplasia
  brachycephalofrontonasal
    dysplasia
  bronchopulmonary dysplasia
    (BPD)
  cervical dysplasia
  chondroectodermal dysplasia
  cleidocranial dysplasia
  condylar dysplasia
  congenital ectodermal
    dysplasia
  cortical dysplasia
  craniodiaphyseal dysplasia
  craniofacial dysplasia
  dentoalveolar dysplasia
  dentofacial dysplasia
  dentolabial dysplasia
  ectodermal dysplasia
  epiphyseal dysplasia
  epithelial dysplasia
  familial fibrous dysplasia
  familial white folded dysplasia
  fibromuscular dysplasia
  fibro-osseous dysplasia
  fibrous dysplasia
  florid osseous dysplasia
  focal cortical dysplasia
  focal osseous dysplasia
  frontonasal dysplasia
  hereditary bone dysplasia
  high-grade dysplasia
  hip dysplasia
  Holt-Oram atriodigital dysplasia
  internasal dysplasia
  low-grade dysplasia
  maxillomandibular dysplasia
  Mondini dysplasia
  monostotic fibrous dysplasia
  nasal dysplasia
  nasomaxillary dysplasia
  oculoauriculovertebral
    dysplasia
  oculodento-osseous dysplasia
  osseous dysplasia
  Robinow mesomelic dysplasia
  sphenoid dysplasia
  vertical dysplasia
  Wolfe breast dysplasia
  Wolfe classification of breast
    dysplasia

dysplasia dislocationdysplasia-
    associated lesion
dysplastic type
dysplastic valve
dyspneic
dysraphic malformation
dysrhythmia
dysrhythmic activity
dyssynchrony
dyssynergia
dyssynergic bladder
dystocia
    cervical dystocia
    placental dystocia
dystonia
dystonic movement
dystonic reactions
dystopia
    globe dystopia
    ocular dystopia
dystopic calcification
dystrophia
dystrophic calcification
dystrophic mineralization
dystrophic myotonia
dystrophic variant

Dystrophile exercise unit
dystrophy
    Dejerine-Landouzy
        dystrophy
    Duchenne-Landouzy
        dystrophy
    endothelial dystrophy
    limb-girdle dystrophy
    mucopolysaccharide keratin
        dystrophy
    muscular dystrophy
dysuria
debridement
    accurate debridement
    autolytic debridement
    burn debridement
    cavity debridement
    diagnostic arthroscopy and
        debridement
    enzymatic debridement
    epithelial debridement
    exploration and debridement
    serial debridement
    single-stage debridement
    wide debridement
    wound debridement

E

8-ball hemorrhage
8-ball hyphema
8-channel cross-sectional anal
    sphincter probe
8-hole miniplate
8-lumen catheter
8-lumen esophageal manometry
    catheter
8-lumen manometry catheter
8th cranial nerve
    (vesticulocochlear)
11th cranial nerve (accessory)
11th rib flank incision
11th rib transperitoneal incision
E
  fragment E
  immunoglobulin E (IgE)
E point
E wildcat orthodontic wire
E&J restrictor
E. Benson Hood Laboratories
    esophageal tube
E. Benson Hood Laboratories
    salivary bypass tube
E.CAM photon emission camera
E-2 foot prosthesis
EAB (elective abortion)
EAC (external auditory canal)
EAC catheter
Eagle arthroscope
Eagle spirometer
Eagle straight-ahead arthroscope
Eagle styloid process syndrome
Eagle syndrome
Eagle-Barrett syndrome
EaglePlug tapered-shaft
    punctum plug
Eagleton operation
EagleVision Freeman punctum
    plug
Eakin cohesive seal dressing
Eames technique
EAP (endoscopic access port)

ear anesthesia
ear applicator
ear basin
ear bistoury
ear block
ear bone
ear bougie
ear bowl
ear canal
ear cannula
ear cartilage
ear cartilage inflammation
ear cavity
ear clip
ear cup
ear curet
ear cut snare wire
ear dissector
ear elevator
ear forceps
ear forceps with suction
ear furuncle knife
ear instrument
ear instrument rack
ear knife
ear knife handle
ear lobule
ear loop
ear loupe
ear magnet
ear marker
ear mobilizer
ear operating instrument
ear oximeter
ear oximetry
ear pinna
ear pinna prosthesis
ear piston prosthesis
ear polyp forceps
ear polyp snare
ear probe
ear punch
ear punch forceps

ear rasp
ear reconstruction
ear replantation
ear rongeur
ear scissors
ear setback
ear shape
ear snare
ear snare wire
ear snare wire carrier
ear speculum
ear speculum holder
ear spoon
ear spoon and hook
ear suction adapter
ear suction tube
ear surgery
ear surgery Beaver blade
ear surgery blade
ear syringe
ear-dressing forceps
eardrum
eardrum elevator
ear-grasping forceps
Earle clamp
Earle hemorrhoidal clamp
Earle probe
Earle rectal probe
earlobe
    cleft earlobe
    deformity of earlobe
    incomplete cleft of earlobe
    ptotic earlobe
    resplitting of the earlobe
earlobe adipose tissue
earlobe composite graft
earlobe crease
earlobe keloid
earmold
    nonoccluding earmold
    open earmold
    perimeter earmold
    shell earmold
    skeleton earmold
    standard earmold
    vented earmold
ears, nose, and throat (ENT)
Easebak lumbar support cushion
Easi-Breathe inhaler
easily reducible hernia
EAST (Emory angioplasty vs.
    surgery trial)

East-Grinstead needle
East-Grinstead scissors
Eastman clamp
Eastman cystic duct forceps
Eastman dental cement
Eastman forceps
Eastman intestinal clamp
Eastman Kodak scanner
Eastman retractor
Eastman suction tube
Eastman tube
Eastman vaginal retractor
Easton cock-up splint
East-West retractor
East-West soft tissue retractor
Eastwood technique
Easy Access foot splint
Easy catheter
Easy Lok ankle brace
Easy Rider microcatheter
Easy Rider neurovascular
    catheter
Easy Up cushion
EasyChair massage chair
Easy-On elbow brace
easy-out retractor
EasyTrak coronary venous lead
Eatol plate arthroplasty
Eaton agent
Eaton closed reduction
Eaton implant arthroplasty
Eaton nasal speculum
Eaton prosthesis
Eaton speculum
Eaton trapezium finger joint
    replacement prosthesis
Eaton upper limb prosthesis
Eaton volar plate arthroplasty
Eaton-Littler ligament
    reconstruction
Eaton-Littler technique
Eaton-Malerich fracture-
    dislocation operation
Eaton-Malerich fracture-
    dislocation technique
Eaton-Malerich reduction
eave flap
Ebbehoj procedure
Eber forceps
Eber holder
Eber needle holder
Eber needle-holder forceps

Eberbusch ptosis correction
    procedure
Eberle contracture release
    technique
Eberle release
EBI bone stimulator
EBI external fixator
EBI SPF-2 implantable bone
    stimulator
EBI unit
EBL (endoscopic band ligation)
EBL (estimated blood loss)
Ebner gland
Ebner line
ebonation
Ebstein angle
Ebstein anomaly
Ebstein cardiac anomaly
Ebstein malformation
eburnated bone
eburnation
eburnized bone end
Eby band driver
E-C junction
EC-5000 excimer laser
E-CABG (endarterectomy and
    coronary artery bypass graft)
ECA-PCA bypass surgery
E-cath catheter
ECC (endocervical curettings)
ECCE (extracapsular cataract
    extraction)
Eccentric Y adjustable finger
    retractor
eccentric amputation
eccentric atrophy
eccentric drill guide
eccentric dynamic compression
    plate
eccentric fixation
eccentric hypertrophy
eccentric implantation
eccentric interocclusal record
Eccentric Isotac tibial guide
eccentric jaw position
eccentric jaw relation
Eccentric locked rib shears
eccentric maxillomandibular
    record
eccentric monocuspid tilting-
    disk prosthetic valve
eccentric occlusion

Eccentric syringe
Eccentric Y retractor
ecchondrotome
ecchymosis (*pl.* ecchymoses)
ecchymotic area
ecchymotic discoloration
ecchymotic rash
Eccocee ultrasound
eccrine acrospiroma
eccrine carcinoma
eccrine duct
eccrine gland
eccrine hidradenitis
eccrine spiradenoma
eccrine sweat glands
ECG (electrocardiogram)
ECG signal-averaging technique
ECG triggering unit
ECG-synchronized digital
    subtraction angiogram
echelon sutures
echinococcal cyst disease
echinococcal liver abscess
echinococcal liver cyst
echinococcosis
echinococcotomy
Echinococcus
echinococcus cyst
echinococcus liver cyst
Echlin bone rongeur
Echlin duckbill rongeur
Echlin laminectomy rongeur
Echlin rongeur forceps
Echlin-Luer rongeur
echo catheter
echo Doppler
echo formation
echo imaging
echo intensity
echo pattern
echo rephasing
echo reverberation
echo scan
echo scanner
echo score
echo texture
echo time
echo transponder electrode
    catheter
echo zone
echocardiogram
echocardiograph

echocardiographic assessment
echocardiographic probe
echocardiographic study
echocardiography
   2-dimensional
     echocardiography
   A-mode echocardiography
   Biosound Surgiscan
     echocardiography
   color-flow Doppler
     echocardiography
   contrast echocardiography
   cross-sectional
     echocardiography
   Doppler echocardiography
   sector scan echocardiography
   Siemens Sonoline SL-2
     echocardiography
   transesophageal
     echocardiography
   Ultramark 9 echocardiography
Echo-Coat ultrasound biopsy
   needle
echocolonoscope
   CF-UM3 echocolonoscope
   Olympus CF-UM3 flexible
     echocolonoscope
echo-dense valve
echoduodenoscope
   Olympus XJF-UM20
     echoduodenoscope
echoencephalogram
echoencephalography
echoendoscope
   GF-UM30P linear-oriented
     radial scanning
     echoendoscope
   linear-type echoendoscope
   mechanical
     longitudinal/sector
     scanning echoendoscope
   oblique-viewing
     echoendoscope
   Olympus echoendoscope
   Pentax linear scanning
     echoendoscope
   radial sector scanning
     echoendoscope
EchoEye ultrasound
echo-free space
echogenic area
echogenic liver

echogenic liver metastasis
echogenic mass
echogenic needle
echogenic pattern
echogenic sludge
echogenicity
echographic layer
echo-guided ultrasound
echolalia
   delayed echolalia
   immediate echolalia
   mitigated echolalia
Echols retractor
EchoMark angiographic catheter
EchoMark catheter
EchoMark salpingography
   catheter
echoplanar imaging
echoplanar magnetic resonance
   imaging
echo-poor areas of environment
echoscanner
EchoSeed brachytherapy
   seed/implant
Echosight Jansen-Anderson
   intrauterine catheter set
Echosight Patton coaxial
   catheter set
echo-signal shape
echo-spared area
Echotip Baker amniocentesis set
Echotip Dominion needle set
Echotip Kato-Asch needle set
ECI automatic reprocessor
ECIC bypass (extracranial-
   intracranial bypass)
Eck fistula
Eck fistula in reverse
Eckardt Heme-Stopper
   instrument
Eckardt temporary
   keratoprosthesis
Ecker fissure
Ecker-Kazanjian forceps
Ecker-Lotke-Glazer patellar
   tendon repair
Ecker-Lotke-Glazer tendon
   reconstruction technique
Ecker-Roopenian chisel
Eckert-Davis classification
Eckhoff forceps
Eckhout gastroplasty

Eckhout vertical gastroplasty
eclampsia
eclamptic toxemia
Eclipse Gel ankle brace
Eclipse holmium laser
Eclipse TENS unit
Eclipse TMR laser
ECMO (extracorporeal
    membrane oxygenation)
ECMO pump
EcoCheck oxygen monitor
Econo 90 traction unit
Econo-Float Water flotation
    mattress
Econolith device
Economo disease
economy line instrument
E-cotton bandage
ECRB (extensor carpi radialis
    brevis)
ECRL (extensor carpi radialis
    longus)
ECRL tendon
ECT (emission computerized
    tomography)
ECT (European compression
    technique)
ECT internal fracture fixation
ECT internal fracture fixation
    and bone screw
ECT pacemaker
ectasia (*also* ectasis)
    alveolar ectasia
    aortoannular ectasia
    artery ectasia
    corneal ectasia
    coronary artery ectasia
    distal ectasia
    duct ectasia
    ductal ectasia
    dural ectasia
    hypostatic ectasia
    iris ectasia
    mammary duct ectasia
    papillary ectasia
    scleral ectasia
    senile ectasia
    skyrocket capillary ectasia
    tubular ectasia
    vascular ectasia
ectasia of abdominal aorta
ectasia of aorta

ectasia of cornea
ectasia of sclera
ectasia of thoracic aorta
ectatic aneurysm
ectatic aortic valve
ectatic bronchus
ectatic carotid artery
ectatic dilation
ectatic emphysema
ectatic vascular lesion
ectatic vertebral artery
ectatic vessel
ectethmoid bones
ectocanthus
ectocolostomy
Ectocor pacemaker
ectocranial
ectocuneiform bone
ectocyst
ectoderm
ectodermal
ectodermal dysplasia
ectodermal tumor
ectopia
    bladder ectopia
    cerebellar ectopia
    crossed renal ectopia
    gallbladder ectopia
    macular ectopia
    renal ectopia
    testicular ectopia
    ureteral ectopia
ectopia lentis
ectopia of lens
ectopia vesicae
ectopic
ectopic ACTH syndrome
ectopic activity
ectopic antihelical folding
    deformity
ectopic anus
ectopic atrial pacemaker
ectopic atrial tachycardia
ectopic beat
ectopic bladder
ectopic bone
ectopic craniopharyngioma
ectopic cutaneous
    schistosomiasis
ectopic endometrial tissue
ectopic eruption
ectopic eyelash

ectopic focus
ectopic gastric mucosa
ectopic hyperparathyroidism
ectopic impulse
ectopic kidney
ectopic ossification
ectopic pacemaker
ectopic pancreas
ectopic parathormone
    production
ectopic parathyroid adenoma
ectopic pregnancy
ectopic rhythm
ectopic sebaceous gland
ectopic spleen
ectopic testis
ectopic tissue
ectopic ureter
ectopic ureterocele
ectopic varix
ectopy
ECTRA carpal tunnel instrument
ectropion of eyelid
ectropion repair
ectropion senilis
ECU (extensor carpi ulnaris)
ECU tendon
ECU tenodesis
eczematoid seborrhea
eczematous lesion
eczematous patch
EDAP lithotriptor
EDB (extensor digitorum brevis)
EDC (expected date of
    confinement)
EDCS pain management device
Eddey parotid retractor
Edebohls clamp
Edebohls incision
Edebohls kidney clamp
Edebohls operation
Edebohls position
Edelmann-Galton whistle
Edelstein scissors
edema
    angioneurotic edema
    antral edema
    Berlin edema
    brain edema
    brawny edema
    bullous edema
    bullous-like edema

edema (*continued*)
  butterfly pattern of perihilar
    edema
  cerebral edema
  constrictive edema
  corneal edema
  endothelial cell edema
  facial edema
  focal edema
  ileocecal edema
  inflammatory edema
  Iwanoff retinal edema
  labial edema
  laryngeal edema
  lower extremity edema
  lymphatic edema
  massive pulmonary
    hemorrhagic edema
  nephrotic edema
  neurogenic pulmonary edema
    (NPE)
  nonpitting edema
  palatal edema
  pedal edema
  penoscrotal edema
  pericholecystic edema
  periorbital edema
  peripapillary retinal edema
  peripheral extremity edema
  pitting edema
  postlaser edema
  prehepatic edema
  pretibial edema
  pulmonary edema
  purulent edema
  Reinke edema
  retropharyngeal edema
  stasis edema
  subglottic edema
  transient edema
  visceral edema
  Yangtze edema
edema glottidis
edematous
edematous change
Eden technique
Eden-Hybbinette arthroplasty
Eden-Hybbinette operation for
    shoulder dislocation
Eden-Hybbinette procedure
Eden-Hybbinette shoulder
    arthroplasty

Eden-Lange procedure
Eden-Lawson hysterectomy
Eden-Lawson operation
edentulous space
Eder cord blood collection
    device
Eder esophagoscope
Eder forceps
Eder gastroscope
Eder insufflator
Eder laparoscope
Eder photostrobe unit
Eder sigmoidoscope
Eder tongs
Eder-Chamberlin gastroscope
Eder-Cohn endoscope
Eder-Hufford esophagoscope
Eder-Hufford gastroscope
Eder-Palmer gastroscope
Eder-Palmer semiflexible
    fiberoptic endoscope
Eder-Puestow dilation
Eder-Puestow dilator
Eder-Puestow esophageal dilator
Eder-Puestow guidewire
Eder-Puestow wire
EDF cast
edge
    anastomotic edge
    cartilage edge
    chondral edge
    cut edge
    cutting edge
    feathered edge
    gaping wound edges
    incisal edge
    inferior edge
    inverted edge
    labioincisal edge (LIE)
    lateral edge
    ligament reflecting edge
    ligament shelving edge
    linguoincisal edge (LIE)
    liver edge
    ossified edge
    parallel to wound edges
    phonating edge
    Poupart ligament shelving
        edge
    raised edge
    reapproximate skin edges
    rounded edge

edge (*continued*)
    shearing edge
    shelving edge
    smooth liver edge
    spectral edge
    superior edge
    sutured parallel with wound
        edges
    thin edge
    wound edge
Edge blade
Edge coated blade
Edge coated needle electrode
Edge dilatation catheter
edge effect
Edge III hydrogel contact lens
Edge knee brace
edge scalloping deformity
edge strength
edge trimmed
edge undermined
EdgeAhead crescent knife
EdgeAhead phaco slit knife
edge-to-edge occlusion
edge-to-edge suture technique
edge-to-edge sutures
Edinburgh brain retractor
Edinburgh retractor
Edinburgh sutures
Edison fluoroscope
EDL (extensor digitorum
    longus)
Edlan vestibulotomy
Edlan-Mejchar operation
Edlich gastric lavage tube
Edlich lavage tube
Edlich tube lavage
EDM infusion catheter
Edmark mitral valve
Edmondson grading system for
    hepatocellular carcinoma
Edmondson-Steiner classification
Edna towel clamp
Edna towel forceps
EDQ (extensor digiti quinti)
edrophonium chloride
    anesthetic agent
Edslab applicator
Edslab catheter
Edslab cholangiography catheter
Edslab jaw spring clip
Edslab pressure gauge

EDTA Vacutainer tube
Edwards catheter
Edwards clamp
Edwards clip
Edwards diagnostic catheter
Edwards D-L modular fixator
Edwards double Softjaw clamp
Edwards graft
Edwards handleless clamp
Edwards heart valve
Edwards hook
Edwards implant
Edwards instrumentation
Edwards modular system sacral
     fixation device
Edwards parallel-jaw spring clip
Edwards patch
Edwards Prima Plus valve
Edwards procedure
Edwards prosthesis
Edwards raspatory
Edwards rectal hook
Edwards sacral screw
Edwards seamless heart valve
Edwards seamless prosthesis
Edwards septectomy
Edwards single Softjaw clamp
Edwards spring clamp
Edwards Teflon intracardiac
     prosthesis
Edwards Universal rod
Edwards Ventrac pulse generator
Edwards woven Teflon aortic
     bifurcation graft
Edwards-Barbaro T-shaped
     syringoperitoneal shunt
Edwards-Carpentier aortic valve
Edwards-Duromedics bileaflet
     heart valve
Edwards-Duromedics prosthetic
     valve
Edwards-Duromedics valve
Edwards-Levine hook
Edwards-Levine rod
Edwards-Levine sleeve
Edwards-Tapp arterial graft
Edwards-Verner raspatory
EEA (end-to-end anastomosis)
EEA Auto Suture
EEA Auto-Suture stapler
EEA circular stapler
EEA disposable loading unit

EEA stapler
EEA stapling device
EEG (electroencephalogram)
EEG activity
EEG and PSG instrumentation
EEG channel
EEG feedback
EEG record
EEG recording
EEG tracing
EEG wave
eel cobra tip
eel wire
EENT (eyes, ears, nose, and
     throat)
EF (ejection fraction)
EF slope
effaced cervix
effacement
effacement and dilatation
effacement of calyx
effacement of cervix
effacement of mucosa
effect parameter
effective
effective masking
effective setting expansion
effectiveness
effector operation
Effenberger contractor
Effenberger retractor
efferent artery
efferent duct
efferent glomerular arteriole
efferent limb
efferent loop
efferent nerve
efferent neuron
efferent vessel
effervescent
Effler double-ended dissector
Effler hiatal hernia repair
Effler operation
Effler tack
Effler-Groves cardiovascular
     forceps
Effler-Groves dissector
Effler-Groves forceps
Effler-Groves hook
Effler-Groves mode of Allison
     procedure
Effler-Groves operation

effleurage of uterus
effluent
effluent gas
effluxed clear urine
effused fluid
effusion
   cardiac effusion
   joint effusion
   loculated effusion
   loculated pleural effusion
   middle ear effusion (MEE)
   mucopurulent hemorrhagic
     effusion
   pericardial effusion
   pleural effusion
   suprapatellar effusion
effusion of joint
Efica CC dynamic air therapy
   unit
EFM (electronic fetal
   monitoring)
Efron jackknife classification
Eftekhar broken femoral stem
   technique
Efteklar clamp
Efteklar technique
Efteklar-Charnley hip prosthesis
E-G alloy
Egawa classification
EGD (esophagogastroduoden-
   oscopy)
Egemen keyhole suction-control
   device
EGF (epidermal growth factor)
egg membrane
eggcrate foam
eggcrate mattress
eggcrate positioner
eggcrate protector
Egger line
Eggers bone plate
Eggers contact splint
Eggers operation
Eggers plate
Eggers screw
Eggers splint
Eggers tendon transfer
eggshell aorta
eggshell calcification
eggshell nail
Eglis gland
Egnell breast pump

Egnell uterine aspirator
Egnell vacuum extractor
egress cannula
egress needle
EHL (extensor hallucis longus)
Ehmke ear prosthesis
Ehmke platinum Teflon implant
Ehmke platinum Teflon
   prosthesis
Ehrenritter ganglion
Ehrhardt forceps
Ehrhardt lid forceps
Ehrlich catheter
Ehrlich inner body
Ehrlich-Türck line
EHT electrode
     (electrohydrothermoelect-
     rode)
Eichelter-Schenk vena cava
    catheter
Eichen irrigating cannula
Eicher chisel
Eicher femoral prosthetic head
Eicher hip prosthesis
Eicher prosthesis
Eicher rasp
Eicher raspatory
Eicher tri-fin chisel
EIC-negative breast tumor
EID (emergency infusion
    device)
EID percutaneous central
    venous large-bore catheter
Eidemiller tunneler
EIE 150F operating microscope
EIE MiniEndo piezoelectric
    ultrasonic unit
Eifrig intraocular implant lens
Eifrig lens
Eigon CardioLoop recorder
Eigon disk
Eiken-Kizai hemodialysis blood
    tubing set
eikonometer
Eindhoven magnet
Einhorn chemotherapy regimen
Einhorn dilator
Einhorn esophageal dilator
Einhorn string test
Einhorn tube
Einthoven triangle
EIP (extensor indicis proprius)

EIP tendon
epiretinal delamination diamond knife
Eiselberg uterine scissors
Eiselberg-Mathieu needle holder
Eiselberg ligature scissors
Eisenberger technique
Eisenhammer speculum
Eisenmenger complex
Eisenstein clamp
Eisenstein forceps
Eisenstein hysterectomy forceps
Eissner prostatic cooler
Eitner operation
EJ bone marrow biopsy needle
ejaculation center
ejaculation disorder
ejaculatory duct
ejaculatory dysfunction
ejection click
ejection fraction (EF)
ejection murmur
ejection phase
ejection phase index
ejection rate
ejection shell image
ejection time
ejection-fraction image
Ejrup maneuver
EK-19 pad
Ekehorn operation
EKG (electrocardiogram)
EKG calipers
EKG monitor strip
EKG silence
Eklund technique
El Gamal cardiac device
El Gamal coronary bypass catheter
El Gamal guiding catheter
EL2-LS2 flexible video laparoscope
Ela Chorus DDD pacemaker
Ela pacemaker
Ela ventricular pacing lead
ELAFF (extended lateral arm free flap)
El-Ahwany humeral supracondylar fracture classification
Elan drill
Elan electrosurgical unit

Elan-E power drill
Elastafit tubing kit
Elastalloy esophageal endoprosthesis
Elastalloy esophageal stent
Elastalloy Ultraflex Strecker nitinol stent
ElastaTrac home lumbar traction unit
Elasta-Wrap elastic gauze
elastic adhesive bandage
elastic band
elastic band fixation
elastic band ligation
elastic bandage
elastic barrier
elastic bougie
elastic compression
elastic compression stockings
elastic deformation
elastic fibers
elastic foam bandage
elastic foam pressure dressing
elastic gauze
elastic hose
elastic impression material
elastic ligature
elastic line
elastic membrane
elastic modulus
elastic O ring
elastic orthosis
elastic plastic splint
elastic pulse
elastic recoil
elastic rubber band
elastic skin lines
elastic stable intramedullary nail
elastic sutures
elastic tissue
elastic traction
elastic-fiber fragmentation
elastic-hinge knee brace
elasticity of skin
elasticized compressive face garment
Elasticon bandage
elastic-thread ligature
Elastikon bandage
Elastikon dressing
Elastikon elastic tape
Elastikon elastic tape dressing

Elastikon wristlet dressing
Elasto dressing
Elast-O-Chain separator
ElastoGel cushions/pressure pads
ElastoGel hot/cold wrap
ElastoGel hydrogel dressing
ElastoGel hydrogel wound
    dressing
ElastoGel shoulder therapy wrap
Elasto-Link joint wrap
elastomer
   American Heyer-Schulte
     elastomer
   conventional silicone
     elastomer
   polyolefin elastomer
   silicone elastomer
elastomer shell
elastomeric impression material
elastomeric pump
Elastomull bandage
Elastomull dressing
Elastomull elastic gauze bandage
Elastoplast bandage
Elastoplast dressing
Elastoplast eye occlusor
Elastoplast pressure dressing
Elastopore dressing
Elastorc catheter guidewire
elastotic tissue
Elastylon glove
elbow
   baseball elbow
   Bateman denervation of knee
     or elbow
   boxer's elbow
   Boyd posterior bone block
     elbow
   capped elbow
   Coonrad total elbow
   Ewald total elbow
   Little Leaguer's elbow
   London total elbow
   Mazas hinge elbow
   McKee hinge elbow
   Morrey total elbow
   nursemaid's elbow
   Osborne lesion of elbow
   Pheasant elbow
   tennis elbow
   thrower's elbow
   Volz total elbow

elbow arthroplasty
elbow disarticulation
elbow dislocation
elbow extension splint
elbow flexion contracture
elbow flexion splint
elbow fracture
elbow hinge
elbow jerk
elbow joint
elbow magnet
elbow prosthesis
elbow reflex
elbow sleeve
elbow structure
elbowed bougie
elbowed catheter
Elbowlift suspension pad
elbow-wrist-hand orthosis
   (EWHO)
Elder classification of malignant
   melanoma
Eldridge-Green color vision light
Eldridge-Green lamp
Elecath catheter
Elecath circulatory support
   device
Elecath ECMO cannula
Elecath electrophysiologic
   stimulation catheter
Elecath pacemaker
Elecath thermodilution catheter
elective abortion (EAB)
elective aneurysmectomy
elective correction
elective cosmetic surgery (ECS)
elective dilatational
   tracheostomy
elective hernia repair
elective herniorrhaphy
elective laparotomy
elective lymph node dissection
   (ELND)
elective lymphadenectomy
elective neck dissection (END)
elective neck irradiation
elective repair
elective sigmoid resection
elective surgery
elective surgical procedure
elective therapy
electively fibrillated

electric activity
electric anesthesia
electric aspirator
electric aversion therapy
electric bed
electric bur
electric burn
electric calipers
electric capacity
electric cardiac pacemaker
electric cardioversion
electric casting machine
electric cautery
electric charge
electric coagulation
electric current
electric cutter
electric defibrillation
electric dermatome
electric differential therapy
electric drill
electric evacuator
electric field
electric generator
electric hair clippers
electric head lamp
electric impedance
electric implant
electric induction
electric irritability
electric knife
electric laryngofissure saw
electric meatotome
electric nerve stimulation
electric nerve stimulator
electric potential
electric probe
electric retinoscope
electric saw
electric shock
electric stimulation
electric stimulus
electric surgical clippers
electric syringe
electric therapy
electric tissue morcellator
electric trephine
electric, electrical
electrical activation abnormality
electrical artificial larynx
electrical brain stimulator
electrical burn

electrical catheter ablation
electrical heart position
electrical implant
electrical resistance detector
electrical sector scanner
electrical stimulation therapy
electrically driven bur
electricator coagulator
electricator electrosurgical unit
electricity-induced anesthesia
electroacoustic location
electroacupuncture device
Electro-Acuscope stimulator
electroanalgesia
electroanesthesia
Electro-Blend epilator
electrocardiogram (ECG, EKG)
electrocardiograph
electrocardiographic leads
electrocardiographic monitor
electrocardiographic
    transtelephonic monitor
electrocardiography
electrocardioscanner
electrocardioscope
electrocauterization
electrocauterize
electrocautery
    AmpErase electrocautery
    Aspen electrocautery
    bipolar electrocautery
    bleeding controlled with
        electrocautery
    Bovie electrocautery
    Bugbee electrocautery
    cystoscopic electrocautery
    Endo Clip monopolar
        electrocautery
    Fine micropoint
        electrocautery
    Geiger electrocautery
    Hildreth electrocautery
    hook electrocautery
    low-current electrocautery
    Malis electrocautery
    Mentor Wet-Field
        electrocautery
    Mira electrocautery
    monopolar electrocautery
    Mueller electrocautery
    multipolar electrocautery
    needlepoint electrocautery

electrocautery (*continued*)
  Neomed electrocautery
  ophthalmic electrocautery
  Op-Temp disposable
    electrocautery
  Parker-Heath electrocautery
  Prince electrocautery
  Rommel electrocautery
  Rommel-Hildreth
    electrocautery
  Schanz electrocautery
  Scheie electrocautery
  Todd electrocautery
  Valleylab electrocautery
  von Graefe electrocautery
  Wadsworth-Todd
    electrocautery
  wet-field electrocautery
  Ziegler electrocautery
electrocautery cautery
electrocautery knife
electrocautery pattern
electrocautery resection
electrocautery snaring
electrocautery unit
electrochemical detector
electrocholecystectomy
electrocholecystocausis
electrocoagulated bleeders
electrocoagulating biopsy forceps
electrocoagulation
  bipolar electrocoagulation
  direct current
    electrocoagulation
  endoscopic
    electrocoagulation
  monopolar electrocoagulation
  multipolar electrocoagulation
  pinpoint electrocoagulation
  snare electrocoagulation
  transendoscopic
    electrocoagulation
electrocoagulation diathermy
electrocoagulation necrosis
electrocoagulator
  Magielski electrocoagulator
electrocochleogram
electrocochleography
electroconductive cream
electroconization
electroconization of cervix
electroconvulsive therapy

electrocorticogram study
electrocorticography
electrocystoscope
electrode balloon
electrode catheter
electrode catheter ablation
electrode cream
electrode fixation
electrode gel
electrode glove
electrode impedance
electrode introducer
electrode migration
electrode pad
electrode placement
electrode potential
electrode response time
electrode sock
electrodermal response
electrodermatome
  Brown electrodermatome
  Padgett-Hood
    electrodermatome
electrodermatome sterile blade
Electrodes ball
Electrodes loop
Electrodes needle
Electrodes scalpel
electrodesiccate
electrodesiccated bleeding point
electrodesiccation
electrodesiccation and curettage
electrode-skin interface
electro-detachable balloon
electro-detachable platinum coil
electrodiagnostic testing
electrodialyzer
electrodiaphake
  LaCarrere electrodiaphake
electrodiaphane
electrodiaphanoscope
electrodiaphanoscopy
electrodispersive skin patch
Electrodyne cardiac monitor
Electrodyne defibrillator
Electrodyne pacemaker
electrodynogram
electroejaculation
  rectal probe
    electroejaculation
electroejaculator
  G&S electroejaculator

electroencephalic response
electroencephalogram (EEG)
electroencephalographic
electroencephalography
  biofeedback
    electroencephalograph
  BMSI 5000
    electroencephalograph
  cortical
    electroencephalogram
  Galileo evoked potential
    electroencephalograph
  Grass electroencephalograph
  intracerebral
    electroencephalogram
  isoelectric
    electroencephalogram
  Mingograf
    electroencephalograph
electroenterostomy
electroexcision
electrofulguration
electrofulguration hemostasis
electrogalvanic stimulation
electrogastroenterostomy
electrogastrogram
electrogastrography
electrogoniometer
electrogram
  Furman type II electrogram
  His bundle electrogram
electrohemostasis
electrohemostasis catheter
electrohydraulic
    cystolitholapaxy
electrohydraulic fragmentation
electrohydraulic lithotripsy (EHL)
electrohydraulic lithotripsy
    probe
electrohydraulic lithotriptor
electrohydraulic lithotriptor
    probe
electrohydraulic shock wave
    lithotripsy (ESWL)
electrohydraulic shock waves
electrohydrothermoelectrode
    (EH electrode)
electrokeratotomy
electrokymogram
electrokymography
Electro-Link joint wrap
ElectroLink TENS electrode

electrolithotripsy
electrolithotrity
electrolysis
electrolyte
electrolyte abnormality
electromagnet
  Hirschberg electromagnet
electromagnetic
electromagnetic flow meter
electromagnetic flow probe
electromagnetic flow transducer
electromagnetic flowmeter
electromagnetic focusing field
    probe
electromagnetic lithotriptor
electromagnetic radiation
    exposure
electromallet
electromechanical artificial
    heart
electromechanical dynamometer
electromechanical impactor
electromechanical morcellator
Electro-Mesh electrode
Electro-Mesh sleeve
electromicrokeratome
electromotive force
electromucotome
  Castroviejo electromucotome
  Steinhauser electromucotome
  Steinhauser-Castroviejo
    electromucotome
electromuscular sensibility
electromyogram
electromyogram (EMG)
electromyograph
electromyography
  conventional concentric
    electromyography
  laryngeal electromyography
electron beam
electron beam CT scanner
electron beam therapy
electron capture detector
electron gun
electron linear accelerator
electron microscope
electron microscopy
electron multiplier tube
electron probe x-ray
    microanalyzer
electron volt

electronarcosis agent
electroneurolysis
electroneuronography (ENOG)
electronic artificial larynx
electronic calipers
electronic component
electronic diaphragm pacing
electronic endoscope
electronic fetal monitoring
(EFM)
electronic flash generator
electronic goniometer
electronic infusion device
electronic knife
electronic larynx
electronic mass
electronic microanalyzer
electronic muscle stimulator
electronic nerve stimulator
electronic neurostimulation
electronic
ophthalmodynamometer
electronic pacemaker
electronic stethoscope
electronic stimulation
electronic stimulation of bone
growth
electronic stimulator
electronic summation device
electronic thermometer
electronic tonographer
electronic tonometer
electronic ureteral stimulator
electronically provoked
response
electronystagmograph (ENG)
electronystagmography
electro-oculogram (EOG)
electroparacentesis
electrophoresis
Agarose gel electrophoresis
gel electrophoresis
electrophoretic
electrophysiologic mapping
electrophysiologic monitoring
electrophysiologic study
electrophysiologic testing
electrophysiology
patch clamp
electrophysiology
electroresection
electroretinogram (ERG)

electroretinograph
electroretinography
electroscission
electroscope
Bruening electroscope
Haslinger electroscope
Electroscope disposable scissors
Electroscope scissors
electrosection
electroshield
Electroshield cyclindrical
conductive shield
Electroshield reusable sheath
electroshock
electrospinal orthosis (ESO)
electrostatic
electrostatic generator
electrostatic unit
electrostimulated graciloplasty
electrostimulation
Electrosurgery
bipolar electrosurgery
Electrosurgery forceps
Electrosurgery snare
electrosurgical biopsy forceps
electrosurgical cauterization
electrosurgical cord
electrosurgical current intensity
electrosurgical curved scissors
electrosurgical cutting knife
electrosurgical desiccation
electrosurgical dispersive pad
electrosurgical dissection
electrosurgical equipment
electrosurgical filter
electrosurgical fulguration
electrosurgical generator
electrosurgical knife
electrosurgical monopolar
spatula probe
electrosurgical needle
electrosurgical pencil
electrosurgical resectoscope tip
electrosurgical scaling
electrosurgical scalpel
electrosurgical snare
electrosurgical snare
polypectomy
electrosurgical spatula
electrosurgical unit (ESU)
electrotherapeutic sleep therapy
electrotherapy

electrotherm
electrotome
   infant electrotome
   McCarthy electrotome
   McCarthy miniature
     electrotome
   miniature electrotome
   Nesbit electrotome
   punctate electrotome
   Stern-McCarthy electrotome
electrotomy
electrotorque motor
electrourethrotome
Elekta stereotactic head frame
Elektrotom BiCut II coagulator
Elema pacemaker
Elema-Schonander pacemaker
Elema-Siemens AB pressure
   transducer
elementary fracture
elementary lesion
elephant cuff
elephant-ear clavicle splint
elephantiasis operation
elevated diaphragm
elevated hemodiaphragm
elevated lesion
elevated position
elevated pressure
elevated rim acetabular liner
elevated scapula
Elevath pacemaker
elevating forceps
elevating lens
elevation
   blanched cutaneous elevation
   chin elevation
   congenital scapular elevation
   diaphragmatic elevation
   disk elevation
   FAME midface elevation
   flap elevation
   heel elevation
   leg elevation
   medial elevation
   mucoperichondrial elevation
   periosteal elevation
   philtral column elevation
   scapular elevation
   sinus elevation
   ST segment elevation
   subgaleal elevation

elevation (*continued*)
   suborbital mimetic muscle
     elevation (SOMME)
   subperiosteal elevation
   transblepharoplasty
     subperiosteal midface
     elevation
   unilateral diaphragmatic
     elevation
elevation angle
elevation of diaphragm
elevation of extremity
elevation of skull fracture
elevation paresis
elevator (*see also* periosteal
   elevator)
   Abbott elevator
   Abbott table elevator
   Abraham elevator
   Adson elevator
   Adson periosteal elevator
   Adson-Love periosteal
     elevator
   Alexander elevator
   Alexander-Farabeuf elevator
   Allerdyce elevator
   Allis periosteal elevator
   amalgam plugger elevator
   Amerson bone elevator
   Anderson elevator
   angled elevator
   angular elevator
   Anthony elevator
   Antole-Condale elevator
   Apexo elevator
   Arenberg dural palpator
     elevator
   Artmann elevator
   Ashley cleft palate elevator
   Ashley elevator
   Aufranc periosteal elevator
   Aufricht elevator
   Aufricht nasal elevator
   Austin duckbill elevator
   Austin elevator
   Austin footplate elevator
   Austin right-angle elevator
   Bailey rib elevator
   ball-end elevator
   Ballenger elevator
   Ballenger septal elevator
   Ballenger-Hajek elevator

elevator (*continued*)
    Baron elevator
    Baron palate elevator
    Barsky elevator
    Batson-Carmody elevator
    beat-up periosteal elevator
    Behrend periosteal elevator
    Bellucci elevator
    Bennell elevator
    Bennett bone elevator
    Bennett elevator
    Berens lid elevator
    Berry-Lambert elevator
    Bethune elevator
    Bethune periosteal elevator
    Blair cleft palate elevator
    Blair elevator
    blunt elevator
    blunt periosteal elevator
    Boies nasal elevator
    Boies nasal fracture elevator
    Boies plastic surgery elevator
    bone elevator
    Bowen periosteal elevator
    Boyle uterine elevator
    brain elevator
    Bristow elevator
    Bristow periosteal elevator
    Bristow zygomatic elevator
    Brophy elevator
    Brophy periosteal elevator
    Brophy tooth elevator
    Brown bone elevator
    Brown elevator
    Brown tooth elevator
    Buck periosteal elevator
    Cameron elevator
    Cameron periosteal elevator
    Cameron-Haight elevator
    Cameron-Haight periosteal
        elevator
    Campbell elevator
    Campbell periosteal elevator
    Cannon-Rochester elevator
    Cannon-Rochester lamina
        elevator
    Carmody-Batson elevator
    Carroll elevator
    Carroll periosteal elevator
    Carroll-Legg periosteal
        elevator
    Carter elevator

elevator (*continued*)
    Carter eye elevator
    Carter submucous elevator
    caudal elevator
    Chandler bone elevator
    Chandler elevator
    Cheyne periosteal elevator
    chisel elevator
    Cinelli elevator
    Cinelli periosteal elevator
    cleft palate elevator
    Clevedent crossbar elevator
    Clevedent-Miller elevator
    clinic exolever elevator
    Cloward elevator
    Cloward osteophyte elevator
    Cloward periosteal elevator
    Cobb elevator
    Cobb periosteal elevator
    Cobb spinal elevator
    Cohen elevator
    Cohen periosteal elevator
    combined wire guide bone
        elevator
    Converse alar elevator
    Converse periosteal elevator
    Converse-MacKenty elevator
    Converse-MacKenty periosteal
        elevator
    Cooper elevator
    Cooper spinal fusion elevator
    Cordes-New elevator
    Cordes-New laryngeal punch
        elevator
    Coryllos periosteal elevator
    Coryllos-Doyen periosteal
        elevator
    costal elevator
    costal periosteal elevator
    Cottle alar elevator
    Cottle elevator
    Cottle graduated elevator
    Cottle nasal elevator
    Cottle periosteal elevator
    Cottle septal elevator
    Cottle septum elevator
    Cottle skin elevator
    Cottle-MacKenty elevator
    Cottle-MacKenty septal
        elevator
    Coupland elevator
    Cramer cleft palate elevator

elevator (*continued*)
  Crane elevator
  Crawford dural elevator
  Crego elevator
  Crego periosteal elevator
  Cronin cleft palate elevator
  Cronin palate elevator
  crossbar elevator
  Cryer dental elevator
  Cryer elevator
  Cryer root elevator
  curved periosteal elevator
  Cushing elevator
  Cushing little joker elevator
  Cushing periosteal elevator
  Cushing pituitary elevator
  Cushing staphylorrhaphy
    elevator
  Cushing-Hopkins periosteal
    elevator
  Darrach elevator
  Davidson periosteal elevator
  Davidson-Mathieu elevator
  Davidson-Mathieu-Alexander
    elevator
  Davidson-Mathieu-Alexander
    periosteal elevator
  Davidson-Sauerbruch elevator
  Davidson-Sauerbruch-Doyen
    elevator
  Davidson-Sauerbruch-Doyen
    periosteal elevator
  Davis periosteal elevator
  Dawson-Yuhl periosteal
    elevator
  Dawson-Yuhl-Key elevator
  Dean periosteal elevator
  DeJager elevator
  dental elevator
  Derlacki duckbill elevator
  Derlacki elevator
  dermal elevator
  D'Errico nerve elevator
  D'Errico periosteal elevator
  Desmarres elevator
  Desmarres lid elevator
  Dewar elevator
  Dingman elevator
  Dingman periosteal elevator
  Dingman zygoma elevator
  double club elevator
  double elevator

elevator (*continued*)
  double-ended elevator
  double-ended periosteal
    elevator
  Doyen costal elevator
  Doyen elevator
  Doyen periosteal elevator
  Doyen rib elevator
  drum elevator
  drumhead elevator
  duckbill elevator
  Dunn-Dautrey condylar head
    elevator
  Dunning elevator
  Dunning periosteal elevator
  dural elevator
  ear elevator
  eardrum elevator
  Ellik elevator
  endaural elevator
  Endotrac elevator
  ESI lighted suction elevator
  ethmoidal elevator
  Farabeuf elevator
  Farabeuf periosteal elevator
  Farrior-Shambaugh elevator
  Farris elevator
  Fay suction elevator
  Federspiel periosteal elevator
  fenestration elevator
  Ferris Smith elevator
  Fibre-Lite septal elevator
  file elevator
  Fiske periosteal elevator
  flap elevator
  Fomon elevator
  Fomon nostril elevator
  Fomon periosteal elevator
  footplate elevator
  fracture reducing elevator
  Frazier dural elevator
  Frazier elevator
  Frazier suction elevator
  Freer double elevator
  Freer double-ended elevator
  Freer double-ended septum
    elevator
  Freer elevator
  Freer nasoseptal elevator
  Freer periosteal elevator
  Freer septal elevator
  Freer single-ended elevator

elevator (*continued*)

Friedman elevator
Friedrich rib elevator
Gam-Mer periosteal elevator
Gill cleft palate elevator
Gillies elevator
Gillies zygoma elevator
Gillies zygomatic elevator
Gimmick elevator
Goldman elevator
Goldman septal elevator
Goodwillie periosteal elevator
Gorney septal suction
  elevator
Graham elevator
Graham scalene elevator
Guilford-Wright drum elevator
Guilford-Wright duckbill
  elevator
Haberman suction elevator
Haight periosteal elevator
Hajek elevator
Hajek-Ballenger elevator
Hajek-Ballenger septal
  elevator
Halle elevator
Halle nasal elevator
Halle septal elevator
Hamrick elevator
Hamrick suction elevator
hand surgery elevator
Hargis periosteal elevator
Harper periosteal elevator
Harrington spinal elevator
Hatt golf-stick elevator
hawk's beak elevator
Hayden elevator
Hayden palate elevator
Hayes phalangeal elevator
heavy elevator
Hedblom costal elevator
Hedblom elevator
Henahan elevator
Henner elevator
Henner endaural elevator
Herczel elevator
Herczel periosteal elevator
Herczel raspatory elevator
Herczel rib elevator
Hibbs chisel elevator
Hibbs costal elevator
Hibbs elevator

elevator (*continued*)

Hibbs periosteal elevator
Hibbs spinal fusion chisel
  elevator
hockey-stick elevator
Hoen elevator
Hoen periosteal elevator
Holly elevator
Hopkins elevator
Hopkins-Cushing periosteal
  elevator
Horsley elevator
Hough elevator
Hough hoe elevator
Hough spatula elevator
House drum elevator
House ear elevator
House elevator
House endaural elevator
House flap elevator
House Gimmick drum
  elevator
House Gimmick stapes
  elevator
House stapes elevator
House Teflon-coated elevator
Howorth elevator
Hudson double-ended
  elevator
Hudson elevator
Hu-Friedy elevator
Hulka-Kenwick uterine
  elevator
Hurd elevator
Hurd septal elevator
Hurd tonsil elevator
inclined-plane elevator
Iowa periosteal elevator
Iowa University elevator
Iowa University periosteal
  elevator
Jackson elevator
Jackson perichondrial
  elevator
Jacobson counter-pressure
  elevator
Jacobson elevator
Jannetta angular elevator
Jannetta duckbill elevator
Jannetta elevator
Jarit periosteal elevator
joker elevator

elevator (*continued*)

Jordan canal elevator
Jordan elevator
Jordan-Rosen elevator
Joseph elevator
Joseph nasal elevator
Joseph periosteal elevator
Joseph periosteotome
  elevator
Joseph-Killian elevator
Joseph-Killian septal elevator
J-periosteal elevator
Kahre-Williger periosteal
  elevator
Kartusch stimulus dissection
  elevator
Kennerdell-Maroon duckbill
  elevator
Key periosteal elevator
Killian double-ended elevator
Killian elevator
Killian septal elevator
Kilner elevator
Kinsella elevator
Kinsella periosteal elevator
Kirmisson elevator
Kirmisson periosteal elevator
Kleesattel elevator
Kleinert-Kutz elevator
Kocher elevator
Kocher periosteal elevator
Koenig elevator
Kos elevator
Krego elevator
Ladd elevator
Lambotte elevator
lamina elevator
Lamont elevator
Lane elevator
Lane periosteal elevator
Lange bone elevator
Langenbeck elevator
Langenbeck periosteal
  elevator
Lee-Cohen elevator
Lee-Cohen septal elevator
Lemmon sternal elevator
lemon squeezer obstetrical
  elevator
Lempert elevator
Lempert heavy elevator
Lempert narrow elevator

elevator (*continued*)

Lempert periosteal elevator
Lewin elevator
Lewis periosteal elevator
lid elevator
Lindholm-Stille elevator
lip elevator
Logan elevator
Logan periosteal elevator
long periosteal elevator
Louisville elevator
Love-Adson elevator
Love-Adson periosteal
  elevator
Lowis periosteal elevator
L-shaped elevator
lumbosacral fusion elevator
Luongo elevator
Luongo septal elevator
MacDonald periosteal elevator
MacKenty elevator
MacKenty periosteal elevator
MacKenty septal elevator
MacKenty-Converse periosteal
  elevator
Magielski elevator
malar elevator
Malis elevator
Matson elevator
Matson periosteal elevator
Matson rib elevator
Matson-Alexander elevator
Matson-Alexander rib elevator
McCabe elevator
McCollough elevator
McGee canal elevator
McGlamry elevator
McIndoe elevator
Mead periosteal elevator
Melt elevator
MGH elevator
MGH periosteal elevator
middle ear elevator
Miller dental elevator
Miller-Apexo elevator
Molt elevator
Molt periosteal elevator
Monks malar elevator
Moore bone elevator
Moore elevator
Moorehead elevator
mucoperiosteal elevator

elevator (*continued*)
- mucosa elevator
- Murphy-Lane bone elevator
- narrow elevator
- nasal elevator
- Netterville double-ended elevator
- Neurological Institute elevator
- Neurological Institute periosteal elevator
- neurosurgical elevator
- Norcross periosteal elevator
- Nordent oral surgery elevator
- Norrbacka bone elevator
- nostril elevator
- Obwegeser periosteal elevator
- Ohl periosteal elevator
- Oldberg elevator
- orthopedic elevator
- OSI extremity elevator
- osteophyte elevator
- Overholt double-ended elevator
- Overholt elevator
- Overholt periosteal elevator
- Pace periosteal elevator
- palate elevator
- palatorrhaphy elevator
- Paparella duckbill elevator
- Paparella elevator
- Paparella otologic surgery elevator
- Penfield elevator
- Pennington elevator
- Pennington septal elevator
- Pennington septum elevator
- perichondrial elevator
- periosteal elevator
- periosteum elevator
- Perkins elevator
- Phemister elevator
- Phemister raspatory elevator
- Pierce double-ended elevator
- Pierce elevator
- Pischel elevator
- pituitary elevator
- plastic surgery elevator
- Polcyn elevator
- Pollock sweetheart periosteal elevator
- Pollock zygoma elevator
- Pollock-Dingman elevator

elevator (*continued*)
- Poppen elevator
- Poppen periosteal elevator
- Potts dental elevator
- Potts elevator
- Presbyterian Hospital elevator
- Presbyterian Hospital staphylorrhaphy elevator
- pressure elevator
- Pritchard elevator
- Proctor elevator
- Proctor mucosal elevator
- Quervain elevator
- Ralks elevator
- Ramirez periosteal elevator
- Raney periosteal elevator
- Ray-Parsons-Sunday elevator
- Ray-Parsons-Sunday staphylorrhaphy elevator
- Read periosteal elevator
- Rhoton elevator
- rib elevator
- Richards-Cobb spinal elevator
- Richardson periosteal elevator
- right-angle elevator
- Rissler periosteal elevator
- Roberts-Gill periosteal elevator
- Rochester elevator
- Rochester laminar elevator
- Rochester spinal elevator
- Roger septal elevator
- Rolyan arm elevator
- root elevator
- Rosen angular elevator
- Rosen elevator
- round-tipped periosteal elevator
- Rowe bone elevator
- Rowe elevator
- Rubin-Lewis periosteal elevator
- Rudderman Frelevator fragment elevator
- Sabbatsberg septum elevator
- Sachs elevator
- Sauerbruch rib elevator
- Sauerbruch-Frey rib elevator
- Sayre double-end periosteal elevator
- Sayre double-ended elevator
- Sayre elevator

elevator (*continued*)
  Sayre periosteal elevator
  scalene elevator
  Scheer elevator
  Scheer knife elevator
  Schuknecht elevator
  Scott-McCracken elevator
  Scott-McCracken periosteal
    elevator
  screw elevator
  Sebileau elevator
  Sebileau periosteal elevator
  Sedillot elevator
  Sedillot periosteal elevator
  Seldin elevator
  septal elevator
  Sewall elevator
  Sewall ethmoidal elevator
  Sewall mucoperiosteal
    elevator
  Shambaugh elevator
  Shambaugh endaural elevator
  Shambaugh narrow elevator
  Shambaugh-Derlacki duckbill
    elevator
  Shambaugh-Derlacki elevator
  Shambaugh-Derlacki endaural
    elevator
  sharp elevator
  Shea elevator
  Silverstein dural elevator
  Sisson fracture-reducing
    elevator
  skin elevator
  skull elevator
  Slocum elevator
  SMIC periosteal elevator
  Smith-Petersen elevator
  soft tissue elevator
  Sokolec elevator
  Somers uterine elevator
  Soonawalla uterine elevator
  spinal elevator
  spinal fusion elevator
  spiral elevator
  Spurling periosteal elevator
  stapes elevator
  staphylorrhaphy elevator
  Steele periosteal elevator
  Stevens elevator
  Stille periosteal elevator
  Stille-Langenbeck elevator

elevator (*continued*)
  Stolte-Stille elevator
  Story orbital elevator
  straight elevator
  straight inclined plane elevator
  straight periosteal elevator
  stripper and elevator
  submucous elevator
  suction elevator
  Sumner elevator
  Sunday elevator
  Sunday staphylorrhaphy
    elevator
  Suraci zygoma hook elevator
  Swanson elevator
  Tabb ear elevator
  Tabb elevator
  Takahashi elevator
  Tarlov nerve elevator
  T-bar elevator
  Tenzel double-end periosteal
    elevator
  Tenzel elevator
  Tenzel periosteal elevator
  Tessier disimpaction elevator
  Tessier elevator
  T-handle elevator
  Tobolsky elevator
  tonsillar elevator
  tooth elevator
  Traquair periosteal elevator
  Tronzo elevator
  Turner cord elevator
  Turner elevator
  Turner periosteal elevator
  Urquhart periosteal elevator
  uterine elevator
  Veau elevator
  von Langenbeck periosteal
    elevator
  Wadia elevator
  Walker elevator
  Walker submucous elevator
  Ward elevator
  Ward periosteal elevator
  Warwick James elevator
  Watson-Jones elevator
  wedge elevator
  West blunt elevator
  Willauer-Gibbon periosteal
    elevator
  Williger elevator

elevator (*continued*)
Winter elevator
Woodson dental periosteal
elevator
Woodson elevator
Wright-Guilford drum elevator
Wurzelheber dental elevator
Yankauer periosteal elevator
zygoma elevator
elevator and dissector
elevator and raspatory
elevator and stripper
elevator disease
elevator extraction
elevator-curet
elevator-dissector
elevator-feeler
elevator-raspatory
elevator-stripper
elevatus deformity
elfin facies
Elgiloy clip
Elgiloy clip material
Elgiloy frame
Elgiloy frame of prosthetic valve
Elgiloy lead-tip pacemaker
Elgiloy metal alloy
Elgiloy pacemaker
Elgiloy-Heifitz aneurysm clip
Elgin table
Elias lid retractor
Eliasoph lid retractor
elimination disorder
elimination procedure
Eliminator ArthroWand
Eliminator biliary stent
Eliminator dilatation balloon
Eliminator nasal biliary catheter
set
Eliminator pancreatic stent
Eliminator PET biliary balloon
dilator
Eliminator stone extraction
basket
Elite dual-chamber rate-
responsive pacemaker
Elite Farley retractor
Elite guide catheter
Elite knee brace
Ellenbogen criteria for ideal
eyebrow position and
contour

Ellik bladder evacuator
Ellik elevator
Ellik evacuator
Ellik kidney stone basket
Ellik loop stone dislodger
Ellik meatotome
Ellik resectoscope
Ellik sound
Ellik stone basket
ellik'd (slang for removal of
bladder chips for Ellik
evacuator)
Ellik-Shaw obturator
Ellingson intraocular implant
lens
Ellingson lens
Elliot corneal trephine
Elliot eye trephine
Elliot femoral condyle blade plate
Elliot femoral condyle holder
Elliot femoral condyle plate
Elliot flap
Elliot gallbladder forceps
Elliot hemostatic forceps
Elliot knee plate
Elliot obstetrical forceps
Elliot operation
Elliot plate
Elliot position
Elliot treatment
Elliot trephination
Elliot trephine
Elliot trephine handle
Elliott blade plate
Elliott gallbladder forceps
Elliott hemostatic forceps
Elliott obstetrical forceps
ellipse
ellipsoid joint
ellipsoid of spleen
ellipsoidal articulation
ellipsoidal joint
elliptic, elliptical
elliptical amputation
elliptical anastomosis
elliptical biopsy
elliptical excision
elliptical excision technique
elliptical flap
elliptical incision
elliptical sagittal incision
elliptical scaphoid fossa

elliptical transverse skin paddle
elliptical uterine incision
Ellis buttress plate
Ellis classification
Ellis eye needle holder
Ellis foreign body needle
Ellis foreign body spud
Ellis foreign body spud needle
    probe
Ellis foreign body spud probe
Ellis holder
Ellis needle holder
Ellis operation
Ellis plate
Ellis probe
Ellis sign
Ellis skin traction technique
Ellis spud
Ellis technique
Ellis Vital needle holder
Ellis-Jones operation
Ellis-Jones peroneal tendon
    procedure
Ellis-Jones peroneal tendon
    technique
Ellison fixation staple
Ellison glenoid rim punch
Ellison knee procedure
Ellison lateral knee
    reconstruction
Ellison procedure
Ellison technique
Ellis-van Creveld syndrome
Ellman Surgitron electrosurgical
    unit
Ellsner gastroscope
Elmar artificial kidney
Elmed digital bipolar coagulator
Elmed Bi-Pol cutter
Elmed coagulation
Elmed diagnostic laparoscope
Elmed hysteroscope
Elmed operating laparoscope
Elmed peristaltic irrigation
    pump
Elmore tissue morcellator
Elmslie ankle reconstruction
Elmslie ligament repair
Elmslie modification of ankle
    reconstruction
Elmslie procedure
Elmslie-Cholmeley operation

Elmslie-Trillat patellar procedure
Elmslie-Trillat patellar tendon
    transplant
Elmslie-Trillat technique
El-Naggar-Nashold right-angled
    nucleus caudalis DREZ
    electrode
ELND (elective lymph node
    dissection)
Eloesser flap
Eloesser operation
elongated aorta
elongated gland
elongated S-incision
elongated uvula
elongation
elongation and torsion
elongation of thoracic aorta
ELP broach
ELP femoral prosthesis
ELP stem for hip arthroplasty
Elsahy technique
Elsberg brain-exploring cannula
Elsberg cannula
Elsberg incision
Elsberg ventricular cannula
Elschnig blepharorrhaphy
Elschnig bodies
Elschnig canthorrhaphy
Elschnig capsular forceps
Elschnig cataract knife
Elschnig central iridectomy
Elschnig corneal knife
Elschnig cyclodialysis forceps
Elschnig cyclodialysis spatula
Elschnig extrusion needle
Elschnig eye spoon
Elschnig fixation forceps
Elschnig forceps
Elschnig iridectomy
Elschnig keratoplasty
Elschnig knife
Elschnig lens scoop
Elschnig lens spoon
Elschnig lid retractor
Elschnig needle holder
Elschnig operation
Elschnig pearl
Elschnig pterygium knife
Elschnig refractor
Elschnig retractor
Elschnig scoop

Elschnig secondary membrane forceps
Elschnig spatula
Elschnig spoon
Elschnig tissue-grasping forceps
Elschnig trephine
Elschnig-O'Brien fixation forceps
Elschnig-O'Brien forceps
Elschnig-O'Brien tissue-grasping forceps
Elschnig-O'Connor fixation forceps
Elschnig-O'Connor forceps
Elschnig-Weber loupe
Elscint dual-detector cardiac camera
Elscint ESI-3000 ultrasound
Elscint Excel 905 scanner
Elscint MR scanner
Elscint Planar device
Elscint Twin CT scanner
Elta derma sterile impregnated hydrogel gauze pad
Elta Dermal hydrogel dressing
eluting stent
elution
Ely operation
Elysee Lasercare
EMA (epithelial membrane antigen)
E-Mac laryngoscope blade
EMB (endomyocardial biopsy)
Embarc bone repair material
embarrassed respiration
embedded tissue
embole
embolectomy
    arterial embolectomy
    balloon embolectomy
    catheter embolectomy
    direct embolectomy
    endarterectomy and embolectomy
    femoral embolectomy
    Fogarty arterial embolectomy
    pulmonary embolectomy
    Trendelenburg pulmonary embolectomy
embolectomy catheter
embolectomy curet
emboli (*sing.* embolus)
embolia

embolic aneurysm
embolic gangrene
embolic occlusion
embolic pneumonia
embolic shower
embolic thrombosis
embolism
    air embolism
    amniotic fluid embolism
    atheroma embolism
    bone marrow embolism
    capillary embolism
    catheter embolism
    cerebral air embolism
    cerebral embolism
    coronary embolism
    fat embolism
    gas embolism
    marrow embolism
    miliary embolism
    pantaloon embolism
    paradoxical embolism
    pulmonary embolism
    saddle embolism
    transfusion-related air embolism
    tumor embolism
    venous air embolism (VAE)
    venous embolism
embolization
    angiographic embolization
    arterial embolization
    cyanoacrylate embolization
    fat embolization
    hepatic artery embolization (HAE)
    pulmonary embolization
    renal arterial embolization
    selective arterial embolization
    Silastic bead embolization
    subselective embolization
    superselective microcoil embolization
    transhepatic embolization
    venous embolization
embolization coil
embolization treatment
embolized atheroma
embolomycotic aneurysm
embolus (*pl.* emboli)
    air embolus
    fat embolus

embolus (*continued*)
foam embolus
obturating embolus
polyurethane foam embolus
pulmonary embolus
riding embolus
straddling embolus
Embol-X arterial cannula
Embosphere microsphere
embrace reflex
embrasure
buccal embrasure
gingival embrasure
incisal embrasure
interdental embrasure
labial embrasure
lingual embrasure
occlusal embrasure
embrasure clasp
embrasure hook
embrasure space
embryo biopsy
embryo encapsulation
embryo reduction
embryoma
Embryon GIFT transfer catheter
Embryon GIFT transfer catheter set
Embryon HSG catheter
embryonal carcinoma
embryonal cell carcinoma
embryonal cyst
embryonal tumor
embryonic fixation syndrome
embryonic neural tube
embryonic sac
embryotomy
embryotomy knife
Emcee lens
EMED scanner
emedullate
emergency airway management
emergency appendectomy
emergency colonoscopy
emergency department thoracotomy (EDT)
emergency free flap
emergency indication
emergency infusion device (EID)
emergency laparotomy
emergency medicine

emergency operation
emergency oxygen mask assembly
emergency procedure
emergency room
emergency room thoracotomy
emergency surgery
emergency tracheal intubation
emergency tracheostomy
emergency tracheostomy set
emergency ventilation
emergency ventilation bronchoscope
emergent appendectomy
emergent herniorrhaphy
emergent intubation
emergent operation
emergent surgery
Emerson bronchoscope
Emerson cuirass respirator
Emerson postoperative ventilator
Emerson pump
Emerson respirator
Emerson restrictor
Emerson stripper
Emerson suction
Emerson suction tube
Emerson vein stripper
Emerson-Birtheez abdominal decompressor
Emerson-Segal Medimizer demand nebulizer
emery disk
Emery lens
Emesay suture button
Emesco 9NS handpiece
Emesco handpiece
emesis
emesis basin
emesis pan
emetic
EMG (electromyogram)
EMG (electromyograph)
EMG electrode
EMG stimulator
EMHI galvanic electrode stimulator
EMI CT scanner
EMI scan
EMI scanner
EMI unit

Emiks heart valve
eminectomy
eminence
  arcuata eminence
  articular eminence
  canine eminence
  collateral eminence
  cruciate eminence
  cruciform eminence
  deltoid eminence
  frontal eminence
  genital eminence
  hyperthenar eminence
  hypobranchial eminence
  hypopharyngeal eminence
  hypophysial eminence
  hypothenar eminence
  ileocecal eminence
  iliopectineal eminence
  iliopubic eminence
  intercondylar eminence
  intertubercular eminence
  malar eminence
  medial eminence
  nasal eminence
  orbital eminence
  parietal eminence
  pyramidal eminence
  retromylohyoid eminence
  temporomandibular joint
    articular eminence
  thenar eminence
  thyroid eminence
  triangular eminence
  zygomatic eminence
eminence of face
eminentia arcuata
eminentia triangularis
eminoplasty
Emir razor
Emir razor blade
emissary sphenoidal foramen
emissary vein
emission computerized
    tomography (ECT)
emission line
emission spectrometric detector
Emko foam
EMLA (eutectic mixture of local
    anesthetics)
EMLA anesthetic
Emmet forceps

Emmet hemostatic bag
Emmet needle
Emmet obstetrical forceps
Emmet obstetrical retractor
Emmet operation
Emmet ovarian trocar
Emmet probe
Emmet retractor
Emmet scissors
Emmet suture technique
Emmet sutures
Emmet tenaculum
Emmet tenaculum hook
Emmet trocar
Emmet uterine probe
Emmet uterine scissors
Emmet uterine tenaculum
Emmet uterine tenaculum hook
Emmet-Gellhorn pessary
Emmet-Murphy needle
emmetropia
Emmet-Studdiford
    perineorrhaphy
Emmett cervical tenaculum
Emory angioplasty vs. surgery
    trial (EAST)
Emory endoplastic
    electrosurgical dissector
Emory EndoPlastic retractor
Empac-Cavitron I&A unit
emphysematous
emphysematous gangrene
Empire needle
emplastrum
emprosthotonos position
empty can test
empty delta sign
empty movement
empty sella
empty sella syndrome
emptying time
empyema
  encapsulated empyema
  loculated empyema
  mastoid empyema
  putrid empyema
  thoracic empyema
empyema trocar
empyema tube
empyematic scoliosis
EMS 2000 neuromuscular
    stimulator

emulgent vein
emulsification
   fat emulsification
EMV grading of Glasgow coma
   scale
en bloc dissection
en bloc distal pancreatectomy
en bloc excision
en bloc lymphadenopathy
en bloc removal
en bloc resection
en bloc vulvectomy
en bloc, no touch technique
en chemise catheter
en coin fracture
en coup de sabre
en cuirasse
en face irradiation field
en face position
en face visualization
en masse
en rave fracture
enamel excrescence
enamel fracture
enamel knot
enamel margin
enamel matrix
enamel maturation
enamel membrane
enamel rod
enamel rod sheath
enarthrodial joint
encapsulated brain abscess
encapsulated breast implant
encapsulated empyema
encapsulated pleural fluid
encapsulated tumor
encapsulation
   embryo encapsulation
   peritoneal encapsulation
   tumor encapsulation
Encapsulon epidural catheter
Encapsulon sheath introducer
Encapsulon TFX-Medical
   bacterial filter
Encapsulon vessel dilator
encased heart
encased in plaster
encased screw
encatarrhaphy
encephalic angioma
encephalic region

encephaloarteriogram
encephalocele
encephalocentesis
encephalogram
encephalography
encephaloid gastric carcinoma
encephalomalacia
encephalomyelitis
encephalomyelopathy
encephalon
encephalopathies
encephalopathy
   clinical encephalopathy
   degenerative encephalopathy
   hepatic encephalopathy
   ischemic encephalopathy
   portal-systemic
      encephalopathy (PSE)
   portosystemic
      encephalopathy
   refractory encephalopathy
   subcortical encephalopathy
   traumatic progressive
      encephalopathy
encephalopuncture
encephalorrhagia
encephaloscope
encephaloscopy
encephalotrigeminal
   angiomatosis
encircling band
encircling clip
encircling cryoablation
encircling endocardial
   ventriculotomy
encircling explant
encircling operation for scleral
   buckle
encircling procedure for retinal
   detachment
encircling silicone tube
encircling tape ligature
encircling tube
Enclose anastomotic assist
   device
Encor lead
Encor pacemaker
Encore ceramic hip and knee
   joint replacement systems
Encore microptic powder-free
   latex surgical glove
encountered

encroach
encroachment
encrustation
encrusted pyelitis
encrusted tongue
encysted calculus
encysted hernia
encysted hydrocele
encysted intraabdominal
    collection
encysted pleurisy
END (elective neck dissection)
end artery
end colostomy
end exhalation
end expiration
end expiratory
end ileostomy
end inspiration
end organ dysfunction
end point
end stoma
end tube
endaortitis
endarterectomized
endarterectomy
    abdominal aortic
        endarterectomy
    aortoiliac endarterectomy
    aortoiliofemoral
        endarterectomy
    blunt eversion carotid
        endarterectomy
    carotid bifurcation
        endarterectomy
    carotid endarterectomy (CEA)
    carotid eversion
        endarterectomy
    carotid subclavian
        endarterectomy
    conventional endarterectomy
    coronary artery
        endarterectomy
    coronary endarterectomy
    distal endarterectomy
    eversion carotid
        endarterectomy
    eversion endarterectomy
    femoral endarterectomy
    gas endarterectomy
    iliac endarterectomy
    innominate endarterectomy

endarterectomy (*continued*)
    laser endarterectomy
    LeVeen endarterectomy
    manual core endarterectomy
    open endarterectomy
    profunda endarterectomy
    subclavian endarterectomy
    surgical endarterectomy
endarterectomy and coronary
        artery bypass graft (ECABG)
endarterectomy and
        embolectomy
endarterectomy dissector
endarterectomy loop
endarterectomy scissors
endarterectomy spatula
endarterectomy stripper
endarteritis
endaural approach
endaural curet
endaural elevator
endaural incision
endaural mastoid incision
endaural nystagmus
endaural retractor
endaural rongeur
endaural speculum
endaural surgery chisel
end-biting blunt-nosed rongeur
end-biting forceps
end-biting rongeur
end-cutting fissure bur
end-cutting reamer
end-diastolic murmur
end-diastolic pressure
end-diastolic volume
Endeavor nondetachable
        silicone balloon catheter
endemic Burkitt lymphoma
endemic goiter
end-end stapler
Ender femoral fracture
        technique
Ender fixation
Ender intramedullary nail
Ender nail
Ender nailing
Ender pin
Ender rod
endermic injection
Endermologie noninvasive body
        contouring device

end-fire transrectal probe
end-hits
end-hole balloon-tipped catheter
end-hole catheter
end-hole fluid-filled catheter
end-hole French catheter
end-hole pigtail catheter
end-hole ureteral catheter
Endius approach
Endius spinal camera
Endius spinal endoscope
end-loop colostomy
end-loop ileocolostomy
end-loop ileostomy
end-loop stoma
Endo Babcock grasper
Endo Babcock stapler
Endo Babcock surgical grasping
    device
Endo button
Endo Clip applier
Endo Clip ML/Surgiport System
    pack
Endo Clip monopolar
    electrocautery
Endo Dissect dissector
Endo GIA stapler
Endo GIA surgical clip
Endo Grasp device
Endo Hernia stapler
Endo hinged knee prosthesis
Endo Knot suture
Endo Multi-Mode stimulator
Endo rotating knee joint
    prosthesis
Endo Shears
Endo sled prosthesis
Endo Stitch suturing device
Endo Tip Storz trocar
Endo zoom lens camera
endoabdominal fascia
Endo-AID suction irrigation
endoalveolar crest
endoanal anastomosis
endoanal coil
endoanal ultrasound
endoaneurysmorrhaphy
endoaortic clamp
Endo-Assist blade
Endo-Assist cutting dissector
Endo-Assist disposable needle
    holder

Endo-Assist endoscopic forceps
Endo-Assist endoscopic knot
    pusher
Endo-Assist endoscopic ligature
    carrier
Endo-Assist endoscopic needle
    holder
Endo-Assist retractable blade
Endo-Assist retractable scalpel
Endo-Assist sponge aspirator
Endo-Avitene collagen
    hemostatic material
Endo-Avitene microfibrillar
    collagen hemostat
Endobag specimen bag
Endo-Bender bending device
endobiliary stent
endobrachial double-lumen tube
endobronchial anesthesia
endobronchial cancer
endobronchial fistula
endobronchial intubation
endobronchial intubation
    anesthetic technique
endobronchial tree
endobronchial tube
Endocam digital camera
Endocam endoscope
endocamera
    Olympus endocamera
    Polaroid instant endocamera
    Storz endocamera
endocapsular artificial lens
    intraocular lens
endocapsular balloon
endocardial balloon lead
endocardial bipolar pacemaker
endocardial cardiac lead
endocardial cushion defect
endocardial murmur
endocardial pacemaker
endocardial pressure
endocardial resection
endocardial sclerosis
endocardial screw
endocardial tumor
endocardial wire
endocardial-to-epicardial
    resection
endocardium
Endocare Horizon prostatic stent
Endocare nitinol stent

EndoCatch specimen retrieval instrument
EndoCath II device
endocavitary bladder diverticulectomy
endocavitary pelvic lymphadenectomy (ECPL)
endocavitary probe
endocavitary radiation therapy
Endocavity probe
Endocell endometrial cell collector
endocervical aspirator
endocervical biopsy
endocervical biopsy curet
endocervical biopsy punch
endocervical canal
endocervical culture
endocervical curet
endocervical curettage
endocervical curettings (ECC)
endocervical glands
endocervical lesion
endocervical mucosa
endocervical os
endocervical polyp
endocervical polypectomy
endocervical probe
endocervical smear
endocervix
endocholedochal
endochondral bone
endochondral bone deposit
endochondroma
Endoclose suture carrier
endocoagulator
EndoCoil biliary stent
EndoCoil esophageal stent
EndoCPB catheter
endocrine disorder
endocrine fracture
endocrine glands
endocrine imaging
endocrine neoplasia
endocrine surgery
Endocut cautery device
endodermal cyst
endodermal sinus
Endodissect reticulating dissecting instrument
endodontia
endodontic broach

endodontic bur
endodontic cavity
endodontic curet
endodontic endosseous implant
endodontic endosteal implant
endodontic file
endodontic irrigation
endodontic pin
endodontic plugger
endodontic reamer
endodontic technique
endodontitis
EndoDynamics suction polyp trap
endoesophageal MRI coil
endoesophageal prosthesis
endoesophageal stent
endoesophageal tube
EndoFix absorbable interference screw
Endoflex endoscopic retractor
Endoflex endoscopy instrument
Endo-Flo irrigator
endofluoroscopic technique
endoforehead
EndoForehead cannula
endoforehead lift
endoforehead-endomidface lift
endoforehead-periorbital-cheek lift
endoforeheadplasty
endogenous anastomosis
endogenous aneurysm
endogenous AV fistula
endogenous disease
Endo-GIA suture stapler
EndoGrasp device
Endo-Gripper endodontic handpiece
EndoHernia stapler
endoherniorrhaphy
endoilluminator
endolacrimal procedure
endolaryngeal brachytherapy mold
endolaryngeal lesion
Endo-Lase CO_2 laser
endolaser
endolaser probe
EndoLift device
EndoLive 3-D stereo video endoscope

Endoloop chromic ligature
   suture instrument
Endoloop sutures
EndoLumina bougie
endoluminal excision
endoluminal repair
endoluminal stent
endoluminal therapy
endolymphatic cavity
endolymphatic duct
endolymphatic fluid
endolymphatic sac
endolymphatic sac
   decompression
endolymphatic sac enlargement
   instrument
endolymphatic shunt tube
endolymphatic shunt tube
   introducer
endolymphatic space
endolymphatic subarachnoid
   shunt
endolymphatic tube
endomagnifier
EndoMate Grab Bag specimen
   retrieval bag
EndoMax advanced laparoscopic
   instrument
EndoMax endoscope
EndoMax endoscopic
   instrumentation
endometrectomy
endometrial ablation
endometrial ablator
endometrial adenocarcinoma
endometrial aspirator
endometrial biopsy
endometrial biopsy curet
endometrial cancer
endometrial cannula
endometrial carcinoma
endometrial cavity
endometrial chemical shift
   imaging
endometrial curet
endometrial forceps
endometrial glands
endometrial hyperplasia
endometrial implant
endometrial lesion
endometrial polyp
endometrial polyp forceps

endometrial resection
endometrial tissue
endometriosis
endometriotic implant
endometritis
endometrium
endomidface
endomidface lift
endomolare
endomyocardial
endomyocardial biopsy (EMB)
endomyocardial disease
endomyocardial fibrosis
endomysium
end-on mattress sutures
endonasal approach
endonasal
   dacryocystorhinostomy
endonasal disorder
endonasal fenestration
endonasal incision
endonasal rhinoplasty
endonerve stripper
endoneurolysis
endo-osseous dental implant
endo-osseous implant
Endopatch disposable surgical
   trocar
Endopath disposable surgical
   trocar
Endopath endoscopic linear
   cutter
Endopath hernia stapler
Endopath endoscopic
   articulating stapler
Endopath endoscopic stapler
Endopath endoscopic
   articulating linear cutter
Endopath endoscopic linear
   cutter
Endopearl bioabsorbable device
endoplasmic reticulum
endoplastic amputation
EndoPlastic retractor
Endo-Pool suction cannula
Endopore implant
Endopouch Pro specimen-
   retrieval bag
Endo-Probe endorectal probe
endoprosthesis
   acetabular endoprosthesis
   Atkinson endoprosthesis

endoprosthesis (*continued*)
  Austin Moore curved
    endoprosthesis
  Austin Moore straight-stem
    endoprosthesis
  Averett total hip
    endoprosthesis
  Bateman UPF II bipolar
    endoprosthesis
  Bi-Centric endoprosthesis
  biliary endoprosthesis
  Bio-Moore endoprosthesis
  Cathcart endoprosthesis
  Celestin endoprosthesis
  Centrax bipolar
    endoprosthesis
  crutched stick-type
    polyurethane
    endoprosthesis
  cuffed esophageal
    endoprosthesis
  double-lumen endoprosthesis
  double-pigtail endoprosthesis
  DoubleStent biliary
    endoprosthesis
  Elastalloy esophageal
    endoprosthesis
  expandable biliary
    endoprosthesis
  expandable metal mesh
    endoprosthesis
  femoral endoprosthesis
  IntraStent DoubleStent biliary
    endoprosthesis
  IntraStent DoubleStrut biliary
    endoprosthesis
  large-bore bile duct
    endoprosthesis
  Leinbach head and neck
    endoprosthesis
  Matchett-Brown hip
    endoprosthesis
  Medoc-Celestin
    endoprosthesis
  metatarsophalangeal
    endoprosthesis
  nonporous-coated
    endoprosthesis
  pancreatic endoprosthesis
  Passager endoprosthesis
  pigtail endoprosthesis
  plastic endoprosthesis

endoprosthesis (*continued*)
  Procter-Livingston
    endoprosthesis
  Ring-Derlan TM biliary
    endoprosthesis
  Schneider Wallstent biliary
    endoprosthesis
  self-expanding metallic
    endoprosthesis
  self-expandable stainless steel
    braided endoprosthesis
  self-expanding Wallstent
    endoprosthesis
  smooth endoprosthesis
  Thompson endoprosthesis
  tibial endoprosthesis
  Titan endoprosthesis
  transpapillary endoscopic
    endoprosthesis
  tumor-replacement
    endoprosthesis
  Unitrax modular
    endoprosthesis
  VIABIL biliary endoprosthesis
  Wallgraft endoprosthesis
  Wallstent biliary
    endoprosthesis
  Wilson-Cook endoprosthesis
endoprosthetic arthroplasty
endoprosthetic femoral head
    replacement
endoprosthetic flange
endopyelotomy
endorectal coil
endorectal coil magnetic
    resonance imaging
endorectal flap
endorectal ileal pull-through
    operation
endorectal ileoanal pull-through
    procedure
endorectal ileoanal pull-through
    technique
endorectal pull-through
    procedure
endorectal surface-coil MR
    imaging
endorectal ultrasound (ERU)
endorectal-pelvis phased-array
    coil
EndoRetract retractor
end-organ damage

Endosac seamless specimen
collection pouch
Endosac specimen bag
Endosample endometrial
sampling device
endoscope
AccuSharp endoscope
ACMI endoscope
Agee endoscope
AO indirect ophthalmoscope
Baggish hysteroscope
battery-powered endoscope
Benjamin pediatric
laryngoscope
cap-fitted endoscope
Cho 2-portal Dyonics
endoscope
Cho Dyonics two-portal
endoscope
Cilco ophthalmic endoscope
Circon-ACMI endoscope
Digiscope
disk endoscope
Dohlman endoscope
double-channel endoscope
Durascope endoscope
Eder-Cohn endoscope
Eder-Palmer semiflexible
fiberoptic endoscope
electronic endoscope
Endius spinal endoscope
Endocam endoscope
EndoLive 3-D stereo video
endoscope
EndoMax endoscope
end-viewing endoscope
ETB endoscope
EUM-series endoscope
EVIS EXERA endoscope
EVIS Q series endoscope
falloposcope
FG-series 2-channel endoscope
fiberoptic endoscope
Flexiblade laryngoscope
flexible endoscope
flexible fallopian tube
endoscope
Foroblique endoscope
forward-viewing endoscope
French-McCarthy endoscope
Fujinon endoscope
Futura resectoscope sheath

endoscope (*continued*)
Gaab endoscope
Gautier ureteroscope
GIF-HM endoscope
GIF-N-series fiberoptic
pediatric endoscope
GIF-XP endoscope
GIF-XQ endoscope
Hamou endoscope
Haslinger endoscope
Hopkins rod endoscope
InjecTx cystoscope
Jarit Rotator endoscope
JFB III endoscope
J-shaped endoscope
Kantor-Berci video
laryngoscope
Karl Storz Calcutript
endoscope
Karl Storz flexible endoscope
Kelly endoscope
Killian-Lynch laryngoscope
Kuda endoscope
large-channel endoscope
Lewy suspension laryngoscope
Lindholm operating
laryngoscope
Lowsley-Peterson endoscope
lung imaging fluorescence
endoscope
Machida flexible endoscope
magnetic resonance
endoscope
McCarthy endoscope
Messerklinger endoscope
MicroLap endoscope
MiniSite laparoscope
Morganstern continuous-flow
operating cystoscope
mother-baby endoscope
mother-daughter endoscope
Navigator flexible endoscope
near-infrared electronic
endoscope
Needlescoper endoscope
nonrigid endoscope
oblique-viewing endoscope
Olympus endoscope
Ono loupe for endoscope
ophthalmic endoscope
Ossoff-Karlen laryngoscope
Padgett endoscope

endoscope (*continued*)
   pediatric endoscope
   Pentax digital endoscope
   Pentax ultrasound endoscope
   Pentax video endoscope
   Pentax EndoNet digital
     endoscope
   Pentax flexible endoscope
   Pentax side-viewing
     endoscope
   percutaneous endoscope
   Pixie minilaparoscope
   rigid endoscope
   rigid intranasal endoscope
   ROAM right-angled
     endoscope
   Rockey endoscope
   Satellite ear endoscope
   semiflexible endoscope
   semirigid endoscope
   Sensatec endoscope
   side-viewing endoscope
   Simpson endoscope
   Sine-U-View nasal endoscope
   Sonde enteroscope
   Storz Sine-U-View endoscope
   stylet-scope endoscope
   Surgenomic endoscope
   TJF endoscope
   Toshiba video endoscope
   transpapillary endoscope
   TroCam endoscope
   UGI endoscope
   variable stiffness endoscope
   velolaryngeal endoscope
   video endoscope
   VideoHydro laparoscope
   Visicath endoscope
   Weerda endoscope
   Welch Allyn video endoscope
   Wolf endoscope
   Zeiss Endolive endoscope
endoscope impaction
endoscope-assisted
endoscope-assisted rectus
    abdominis muscle flap
    harvest
endoscope-assisted technique
endoscopic
   subperiosteal minimally
    invasive laser endoscopic
    (SMILE) face-lift

endoscopic abdominoplasty
   (muscle plication)
endoscopic access port (EAP)
endoscopic ampullary stenting
endoscopic anterior cruciate
   ligament reconstruction
endoscopic aspiration
   lumpectomy
endoscopic assisted facial
   implant insertion
endoscopic Babcock grasper
endoscopic band ligation (EBL)
endoscopic band ligator
endoscopic BICAP probe
endoscopic biliary
   decompression
endoscopic biliary drainage
endoscopic biliary stent
   placement
endoscopic biopsy
endoscopic biopsy forceps
endoscopic biopsy site
endoscopic bladder litholapaxy
endoscopic bladder neck
   suspension
endoscopic breast augmentation
endoscopic brow lift
endoscopic brow lift with
    simultaneous carbon
    dioxide laser resurfacing
endoscopic brush cytology
endoscopic cardiac surgery
endoscopic carpal tunnel
   decompression
endoscopic carpal tunnel
   release (ECTR)
endoscopic cholangiogram
endoscopic
   cholangiopancreatography
endoscopic color Doppler
endoscopic color Doppler
   ultrasonography
endoscopic connecting cord
endoscopic control
endoscopic craniectomy
endoscopic cystenterostomy
endoscopic cystoduodenostomy
endoscopic cystogastrostomy
endoscopic
   dacryocystorhinostomy
endoscopic decompression
endoscopic devolvulization

endoscopic dilation
endoscopic dissection
endoscopic dissector
endoscopic Doppler
    ultrasonography
endoscopic electrocoagulation
endoscopic electrode handle
endoscopic electrohydraulic
    lithotripsy
endoscopic electrosurgical
    cord
endoscopic esophagectomy
endoscopic esophagogastric
    variceal ligation
endoscopic ethmoidectomy
endoscopic examination
endoscopic extirpation
    cicatricial obliteration
endoscopic extraction
endoscopic extraction
    pancreatic duct stone
endoscopic face-lift
endoscopic finding
endoscopic fine-needle
    aspiration cytology
endoscopic fine-needle
    puncture
endoscopic fistulotomy
endoscopic flowprobe
endoscopic forceps
endoscopic forehead lift
endoscopic forehead-brow
    rhytidoplasty
endoscopic frontal craniotomy
endoscopic fulguration
endoscopic fundoplication
endoscopic gastrostomy
endoscopic grasping forceps
endoscopic guidance
endoscopic harvest
endoscopic healing
endoscopic heat probe
Endoscopic hemoclip device
endoscopic hemostasis
endoscopic hemostatic therapy
endoscopic image
endoscopic incision
endoscopic India ink injection
endoscopic injection
    sclerotherapy (EIS)
endoscopic injection therapy
endoscopic instrumentation

endoscopic intranasal frontal
    sinusotomy
endoscopic irrigator
endoscopic jejunostomy
endoscopic laser cautery
endoscopic laser therapy
endoscopic light source
endoscopic linear cutter
endoscopic magnet
endoscopic management
endoscopic manipulation
endoscopic mastopexy
endoscopic medial
    maxillectomy
endoscopic microwave
    coagulation
endoscopic mitral valve repair
endoscopic mucosal ablation
endoscopic mucosal procedure
endoscopic mucosal resection
    (EMR)
endoscopic mucosal technique
endoscopic muscle plication
endoscopic nasobiliary catheter
    drainage
endoscopic optical urethrotomy
endoscopic orbital
    decompression
endoscopic pancreatic drainage
endoscopic pancreatic duct
    sphincterotomy
endoscopic pancreatic stenting
endoscopic pancreatic therapy
endoscopic papillary balloon
    dilation
endoscopic papillotomy
endoscopic papillotomy and
    stenting
endoscopic parathyroidectomy
endoscopic photodynamic
    therapy
endoscopic photography
endoscopic plantar fasciotomy
endoscopic polypectomy
endoscopic procedure
endoscopic pulsed dye laser
    lithotripsy
endoscopic quadrature
    radiofrequency coil
endoscopic reflectance
endoscopic reflectance
    spectrophotometry

endoscopic removal
endoscopic retroflexion
endoscopic retrograde balloon
    dilatation
endoscopic retrograde biliary
    stenting
endoscopic retrograde
    cannulation
endoscopic retrograde
    cholangiogram (ERC)
endoscopic retrograde
    cholangiography
endoscopic retrograde
    cholangiopancreatogram
    (ERCP)
endoscopic retrograde
    cholangiopancreatography
    (ERCP)
endoscopic retrograde
    cholangiopancreatography
    catheter
endoscopic retrograde
    cholecystoendoprosthesis
endoscopic retrograde
    sclerotherapy
endoscopic retrograde
    sphincterotomy (ERS)
endoscopic route
endoscopic scissors
endoscopic sessile polypectomy
endoscopic sewing machine
endoscopic sigmoidopexy
endoscopic sinus surgery
endoscopic small bowel biopsy
endoscopic snare
endoscopic snare resection
endoscopic
    sphenoethmoidectomy
    with septoplasty
endoscopic sphenoidal biopsy
endoscopic sphincterectomy
endoscopic spinal fusion
endoscopic stent exchange
endoscopic sterilizing case
endoscopic stone disintegration
endoscopic stricturotomy
endoscopic strip craniectomy
endoscopic study
endoscopic subperiosteal
    forehead and midface lift
endoscopic subperiosteal
    forehead lift

endoscopic subperiosteal
    midface lift
endoscopic surgery
endoscopic suture-cutting
    forceps
endoscopic technique
endoscopic technology
endoscopic telescope
endoscopic threaded imaging
    port
endoscopic transaxillary breast
    augmentation (ETBA)
endoscopic transaxillary
    submuscular augmentation
    mammaplasty
endoscopic transesophageal
    fine-needle aspiration
endoscopic transpapillary
    cannulation
endoscopic transpapillary cyst
    drainage
endoscopic treatment
endoscopic trolley
endoscopic tube
endoscopic ultrasonographic
    imaging
endoscopic ultrasonography
endoscopic ultrasonography-
    guided cytology
endoscopic ultrasound
    evaluation
endoscopic variceal ligation
    (EVL)
endoscopic variceal
    sclerotherapy (EVS)
endoscopic video image
endoscopic video-assisted
    surgery
endoscopic visualization
endoscopic washing pipe
endoscopic-controlled
    lithotripsy
endoscopically assisted
    abdominoplasty
endoscopically assisted brow
    lift
endoscopically assisted harvest
endoscopically deliverable
    tissue-transfixing device
endoscopically harvested tissue
endoscopically performed
    longitudinal incision

endoscopic-assisted
    microsurgical technique
endoscopic-assisted technique
endoscopist
endoscopy
    advanced therapeutic
        endoscopy
    American Society for
        Gastrointestinal endoscopy
        (ASGE)
    anal endoscopy
    biliary endoscopy
    colorectal cancer endoscopy
    computerized electronic
        endoscopy
    dynamic fluorescence video
        endoscopy
    fiberoptic intraosseous
        endoscopy
    flexible fiberoptic endoscopy
    fluorescein endoscopy
    fluorescent electronic
        endoscopy
    gastrointestinal endoscopy
    high-altitude endoscopy
    high-magnification endoscopy
    intestinal endoscopy
    intragastric provocation under
        endoscopy
    intralacrimal endoscopy
    intraoperative biliary
        endoscopy
    intraventricular endoscopy
    laser-assisted spinal
        endoscopy
    lumbar epidural endoscopy
    lung-imaging fluorescent
        endoscopy
    nasal endoscopy
    outpatient endoscopy
    pancreatic endoscopy
    pancreaticobiliary endoscopy
    pediatric endoscopy
    percutaneous endoscopy
    peripartum endoscopy
    peroral endoscopy
    postsurgical endoscopy
    primary diagnostic endoscopy
    Savary gastrointestinal
        endoscopy
    sinus endoscopy
    small intestinal endoscopy

endoscopy (*continued*)
    surveillance endoscopy
    therapeutic endoscopy
    therapeutic upper endoscopy
    transcolonic endoscopy
    transesophageal endoscopy
    transnasal endoscopy
    transoral endoscopy
    UGI endoscopy
    ultra-high-magnification
        endoscopy
    upper alimentary endoscopy
    upper gastrointestinal
        endoscopy
    upper intestinal endoscopy
    video endoscopy
endoscopy browpexy
endoscopy complication
endoscopy procedure
EndoShears
EndoShield mask and goggles
endoskeletal prosthesis
endoskeleton
Endo-Sock bag
Endosoft reinforced cuffed tube
EndoSonics balloon dilatation
    catheter
endosonography instrument
endosonography-guided
    drainage
EndoSound endoscopic
    ultrasound
EndoSound endoscopic
    ultrasound catheter
EndoSound ultrasound probe
endospeculum
endospeculum forceps
endosseous blade implant
endosseous hydroxyapatite (HA)
    implant
endosseous implant
endosseous implant needle
    mandrel
endosseous vent implant
EndoStasis probe
Endostat calibration pod insert
Endostat disposable sterile fiber
Endostat fiber stripper
Endostat II bipolar/monopolar
    electrosurgical generator
endosteal implant
endosteal implant anchor

endosteum
EndoStitch laparoscopic
    suturing device
Endo-Suction sinus microstat set
Endotak C lead catheter
Endotak C transvenous lead
Endotak C tripolar pacing/
    sensing/defibrillation lead
Endotak Catheter lead catheter
Endotak defibrillator
Endotak DSP lead
Endotak Endurance EZ lead
Endotak Endurance Rx lead
Endotak Reliance defibrillator
    lead
Endotec spreader
Endotek machine
Endotek OM-3 Urodata monitor
Endotek UDS-1000 monitor
Endotek urodynamic monitor
endotemporal
endotemporal lift
endotemporal-endomidface lift
endothelial barrier
endothelial cancer
endothelial cell
endothelial cell basement
    membrane
endothelial cell dysfunction
endothelial cell edema
endothelial damage
endothelial denudation
endothelial dystrophy
endothelial injury
endothelial lining
endothelial lysis
endothelial relaxing factor
endothelial sarcoma
endothelial specular microscope
endothelial tissue
endothelialization
endothelialization of vascular
    graft
endotheliochorial placenta
endothelioma
endothelium
    continuous endothelium
    fenestrated endothelium
    vascular endothelium
Endo-therapy disposable biopsy
    forceps
endotherm knife

endothermy
endothoracic fascia
endothyropexy
EndoTip imaging port
endotoxic exposure
endotoxic shock
Endotrac cannula
Endotrac elevator
Endotrac obturator
Endotrac probe
Endotrac rasp
Endotrac retractor
endotracheal anesthesia
endotracheal cardiac output
    monitor
endotracheal catheter
endotracheal catheter forceps
endotracheal curet
endotracheal general anesthesia
endotracheal induction
endotracheal insufflation
endotracheal insufflation
    anesthesia
endotracheal intubation
endotracheal stripper
endotracheal suctioning
endotracheal tube
endotracheal tube brush
endotracheal tube cuff
endotracheal tube forceps
endotracheal tube placement
endotracheal tumor
endotriptor stone-crushing
    basket
Endotrol endotracheal tube
Endotrol tracheal tube
Endotron-Lipectron ultrasonic
    scalpel
Endo-Tube nasal jejunal feeding
    tube
endourologic treatment
endourological cold-knife
    incision
endourological therapy
endovaginal coil
endovaginal imaging
endovaginal transducer
endovascular aneurysm
endovascular approach
endovascular balloon occlusion
endovascular cardiopulmonary
    bypass

endovascular coagulation
endovascular coil
endovascular graft insertion
endovascular intervention
endovascular management
endovascular repair
endovascular stent
endovascular stent graft
endovascular stenting technique
endovascular surgery
endovascular therapy
endovasculitis
end-over-end running sutures
EndoVideo-Five endoscopic
    camera
EndoView camera
EndoWrist instrument
EndoZime sponge
endplate
    motor endplate
    vertebral endplate
endplate of vertebrae
end-sigmoid colostomy
end-stage disease
end-stage failure
end-stage fibro-fatty residuum
end-stage intestinal failure
end-stage
    lymphangiomyomatosis
end-stage renal disease (ESRD)
end-systolic murmur
end-systolic pressure
end-systolic volume
end-to-back bowel anastomosis
end-to-end anastomosis (EEA)
end-to-end enterostomy
end-to-end esophagogastrostomy
end-to-end
    esophagojejunostomy
end-to-end ileo-anal anastomosis
    without mucosal resection
end-to-end ileocolostomy
end-to-end intussuscepted
    pancreaticojejunostomy
end-to-end invaginating
end-to-end inverting
    pancreaticojejunostomy
end-to-end jejunoileal bypass
end-to-end microvascular
    anastomosis
end-to-end occlusion
end-to-end reconstruction

end-to-end reconstruction
    procedure
end-to-end reconstruction
    technique
end-to-end splenoadrenal
    anastomosis
end-to-end tendon repair
end-to-end venous anastomosis
end-to-side anastomosis
end-to-side arteriotomy
end-to-side
    choledochojejunostomy
end-to-side colostomy
end-to-side esophagogastrostomy
end-to-side
    esophagojejunostomy
end-to-side ileotransverse
    colostomy
end-to-side jejunoileal bypass
end-to-side nerve coaptation
end-to-side portacaval shunt
end-to-side reimplantation
end-to-side repair
end-to-side splenorenal shunt
end-to-side vasoepididymostomy
    technique
end-to-side vein bypass
Endur bonding material
Endura dilatation catheter
Endura dressing forceps
Endurance bone cement
EnduraSplint splint
Enduron acetabular liner
end-viewing endoscope
end-viewing gastroscope
end-weave anastomosis
Enertrax pacemaker
Enforcer SDS coronary stent
ENG (electronystagmograph)
Engel saw
Engel-Lysholm maneuver
Engelmann disease
Engelmann disk
Engelmann splint
Engelmann thigh splint
Engel-May nail
Engen palmar finger orthosis
Engen palmar wrist splint
Engh minimally invasive surgical
    instruments
Engh porous metal hip
    prosthesis

engine H-file
engine reamer
Engle plaster saw
Englehardt femoral prosthesis
Englert forceps
English anvil nail nipper
English brace
English cane
English clamp
English forceps
English hospital reflex percussor
English lock
English MacIntosh fiberoptic
    laryngoscope blade
English position
English rhinoplasty
English tissue forceps
English-McNab shoulder
    prosthesis
English-pattern tissue forceps
Engman disease
eng-organ failure
engorged collateral venous
    channels
engorged vasculature
engorgement
    vascular engorgement
    venous engorgement
    venule engorgement
engraftment
Engstrom multigas monitor
Engstrom respirator
EnGuard PFX lead electrode
enhanced external
    counterpulsation unit
enhanced scan
Enhanced Torque guiding
    catheter
enhancement gun
enhancement surgery
enhancer cushion
enhancing brain lesion
enhancing lesion
Enker brain retractor
Enker self-retaining brain
    retractor
enlarged adenoids
enlarged incision
enlarged mass
enlarged organ
enlarged parathyroid gland
enlarged uterus

enlargement of organ
enlarging bur
Enna classification
Enneking classification
Enneking rod
Enneking staging
Ennis forceps
ENOG (electroneuronography)
ensheathing callus
ensheathing trocar
ENSI syringe
ensiform appendix
ensiform cartilage
ensiform process
EnSite cardiac catheter
ENT (ear, nose, and threat)
ENT bite block
ENT chair
ENT electrode
ENT procedure instrument set
ENT speculum
ENT treatment unit
ENT wire crimper
Entact dilation and occlusion
    catheter
entangling technique
Entegra prosthesis
EnteraFlo enteral feeding pump
EnteraFlo enteral feeding tube
enteral feeding
enterectasis
enterectomy
enteric anastomosis
enteric cyst
enteric fistula
enteric intussusception
enteric isolation
enteric precautions
enteritis
Entero Vu contrast medium
enteroanastomosis
enterobiliary operation
enterocele
enterocele sac
enterocelectomy
enterocentesis
enterocholecystostomy
enterocholecystotomy
enterocleisis
enteroclysis
enteroclysis tube
enterocolectomy

enterocolic fistula
enterocolitis
enterocolostomy
enterocutaneous
enterocutaneous fistula
enterocystocele
enterocystoplasty
   Camey enterocystoplasty
   clam enterocystoplasty
   seromuscular
     enterocystoplasty
   sigmoid enterocystoplasty
enteroenteral fistula
enteroenteric fistula
enteroenterostomy
   Parker-Kerr end-to-end
     enteroenterostomy
   Parker-Kerr
     enteroenterostomy
   two-layer enteroenterostomy
enteroepiplocele
enterogastric reflex
enterogenital fistula
enterogenous
enterogenous cyst
enterohepatic circulation
enterohepatopexy
enteroinsular atresia
enterolith
enterolithiasis
enterolithotomy
enterolysis
enterolysis tube
enteromerocele
enteromesenteric
enteromesenteric occlusion
enteropancreatostomy
enteropathy
enteroperitoneal abscess
enteropexy
enteroplasty
enteroptosis
enteroptychia
enteroptychy
enterorrhaphy
   circular enterorrhaphy
enteroscope
   dedicated push enteroscope
   Goldberg MPC operative
     enteroscope
   Olympus enteroscope
   SIF10 Olympus enteroscope

enteroscope (*continued*)
   Sonde enteroscope
   video push enteroscope
enteroscopy
   intraoperative enteroscopy
   push enteroscopy
   push-type enteroscopy
   Roux-en-Y limb enteroscopy
   small bowel enteroscopy
   transgastrostomic
     enteroscopy
   video small-bowel
     enteroscopy
enterostomal therapy
enterostomy
   Bishop-Coop enterostomy
   double enterostomy
   end-to-end enterostomy
   gun-barrel enterostomy
   percutaneous enterostomy
   Witzel enterostomy
enterostomy clamp
enterotome
   Abraham enterotome
   Dupuytren enterotome
   laryngeal enterotome
   Lukens enterotome
enterotomy
   antimesenteric enterotomy
   inadvertent enterotomy
   longitudinal enterotomy
   Lukens enterotomy
   occult enterotomy
   small bowel enterotomy
enterotomy incision
enterotomy scissors
enterourethral fistula
enterovaginal fistula
enterovesical fistula
Enterra pacemaker
Enterra therapy
enthesis
enthetic
Entity pacemaker
entocuneiform bone
entomophthoramycosis
entoptic pulse
Entract stent
Entract stone retriever
entrapment
   catheter entrapment
   lateral canal entrapment

entrapment (*continued*)
  nerve entrapment
  peroneal nerve entrapment
  popliteal entrapment
  suprascapular nerve
    entrapment
  sural nerve entrapment
entrapment sack introducer
entrapment syndrome
entrapped gland
EnTre guidewire
Entrease variable depth punch
Entree disposable CO_2
  insufflation needle
Entree II cannula
Entree II trocar
Entree Plus cannula
Entree Plus trocar
Entrex small-joint arthroscopy
  instrument set
EntriFlex small-bowel feeding
  tube
EntriStar feeding tube
EntriStar percutaneous
  endoscopic gastrostomy
  (PEG) tube
entropion
  cicatricial entropion
  congenital entropion
  involuntary entropion
  Poulard entropion
entropion clamp
entropion forceps
entropion operation
entropion repair
entry point
entry zone lesion
enucleated
enucleation
  eye enucleation
  Foix enucleation
  leiomyoma enucleation
  surgical enucleation
enucleation compressor
enucleation neurotome
enucleation of cyst
enucleation of eye
enucleation of eyeball
enucleation procedure
enucleation scissors
enucleation scoop
enucleation snare

enucleation spoon
enucleation technique
enucleation wire snare
enucleator
  Banner snare enucleator
  Botvin-Bradford enucleator
  Botvin-Bradford eye
    enucleator
  Bradford snare enucleator
  Carpenter enucleator
  Castroviejo snare enucleator
  Foster snare enucleator
  Hardy bayonet enucleator
  Hardy enucleator
  Hardy microsurgical
    enucleator
  Marino rotatable
    transsphenoidal enucleator
  Meding tonsil enucleator
  prostatic enucleator
  Rhoton enucleator
  rotatable transsphenoidal
    enucleator
  snare enucleator
  tonsillar enucleator
  transsphenoidal enucleator
  Van Osdel tonsillar enucleator
  Young prostatic enucleator
enuresis
enuretic
envelope flap
envelope of discrepancy
envelope of tissue
Enviclusive semi-occlusive
  adhesive film dressing
Envinet gauze dressing
environment modification
environmental contamination
environmental decontamination
Envisan dextranomer pad
Envision endocavity probe
Envy catheter
enzymatic debridement
enzymatic decortication
enzymatic degradation
enzyme induction
EOC goniometer
EOG (electro-oculogram)
EOM (extraocular motion)
EOM (extraocular movement)
EOM (extraocular muscles)
epactal bones

epactal cartilages
epallobiosis
eparterial bronchus
epaulet flap
epaulet shoulder pad
EPB (extensor pollicis brevis)
ependyma
ependymoma
epi (slang for epinephrine)
EPI Sport epicondylitis clasp
epiaortic imaging technique
epiblepharon
epibulbar carcinoma
epic laser
epic microscope
epicanthal correction
epicanthal fold
epicanthal repair
epicanthic fold
epicanthoplasty
epicardial coronary artery
epicardial defibrillator patch
epicardial Doppler flow sector
    transducer
epicardial Doppler flow
    transducer
epicardial electrode
epicardial implantation of
    pacemaker electrode
epicardial lead
epicardial monitoring
epicardial pacemaker
epicardial pacing wire
epicardial retractor
epicardial sock electrode
epicardial space
epicardial surface
epicardiectomy
epicardiolysis
epicardium
Epicel skin graft material
epicerebral space
Epicon mesh
epicondylar avulsion fracture
epicondyle
    lateral epicondyle
    medial epicondyle
epicranial aponeurosis
epicranius muscle
epicritic sensorium
EPICS Profile flow cytometer
epicutaneous reaction

epicystotomy
EPID (electronic portal imaging
    device)
Epi-Derm silicone gel sheeting
epidermal actinic damage
epidermal atrophy
epidermal cancer
epidermal cyst
epidermal growth factor (EGF)
epidermal growth factor
    receptor
epidermal inclusion cyst
epidermal necrosis
epidermal nevus
epidermal ridges
epidermal sliding
epidermal testing
epidermatoplasty
epidermic graft
epidermidis
    stratum basale epidermidis
    stratum corneum epidermidis
    stratum germinativum
        epidermidis
    stratum granulosum
        epidermidis
    stratum lucidum epidermidis
    stratum spinosum epidermidis
epidermis
    hyperkeratotic epidermis
    hyperplastic epidermis
    thermally-altered epidermis
epidermization
epidermodysplasia
    verruciformis
epidermoid
epidermoid cancer
epidermoid carcinoma
epidermoid carcinoma in situ
epidermoid cyst
epidermoid resection
epidermoid tumor
epidermolysis
epidermolysis bullosa
epidermolysis bullosa
    dystrophica
epidermolysis bullosa simplex
epidermolysis simplex
epidermolytic hyperkeratosis
epidermolytic vesicant
epididymal sperm aspiration
epididymectomy

epididymidis
   globus major epididymidis
   globus minor epididymidis
epididymis (*pl.* epididymides)
   appendix of epididymis
   duct of epididymis
   lobule of epididymis
epididymis lesion
epididymodeferentectomy
epididymogram
epididymography
epididymoplasty
epididymorrhaphy
epididymotomy
epididymovasostomy
epidural abscess
epidural abscess evacuation
epidural administration
epidural anesthesia (EA)
epidural anesthetic
epidural block
epidural blockade
epidural blood patch
epidural blood patch anesthetic
   technique
epidural cavity
epidural electrode
epidural extramedullary lesion
epidural hematoma
epidural hemorrhage
epidural metastasis
epidural neural blockade
epidural opioid infusion
epidural peg electrode
epidural space
epidural steroid injection
epidural tumor evacuation
epidurally
epidurolysis
epiesophageal cancer
EpiE-Z Pen epinephrine injector
EpiE-Z Pen injection
epifascial injection
epifascicular epineurotomy
EpiFilm graft
EpiFilm otologic lamina dressing
EpiFlex heel and elbow protector
Epigard dressing
epigastric angle
epigastric artery
epigastric discomfort
epigastric flap

epigastric fold
epigastric fossa
epigastric hernia
epigastric herniorrhaphy
epigastric incision
epigastric inferior vein
epigastric pain
epigastric puncture
epigastric reflex
epigastric region
epigastric tenderness
epigastric vein
epigastrium
epigastrocele
epigastrorrhaphy
epiglottectomy
epiglottic cartilage
epiglottic hematoma
epiglottic reconstruction
epiglottidectomy
epiglottidis
epiglottis
epiglottis retractor
epiglottitis
epihyal bone
epikeratophakia
epikeratophakic keratoplasty
epilating forceps
epilation electrode
epilation forceps
epilation needle
epilator
   Electro-Blend epilator
   Epilot high-frequency needle-
     type epilator
   high-frequency tweezer-type
     epilator
   Removatron epilator
   Super Epitron high-frequency
     epilator
   Thermaderm epilator
   Trichodemolus epilator
epilepsy implant
epilepsy surgery
Epilock dressing
Epi-lock polyurethane foam
   wound dressing
Epilot high-frequency needle-
   type epilator
epimeric muscle
epimicroscope
epimyoepithelial island

epimyoepithelium
epinephrine
epineural repair
epineural suture technique
epineurial repair
epineurolysis
epineurotomy
  anterior epineurotomy
  epifascicular epineurotomy
  interfascicular epineurotomy
  local epineurotomy
epipapillary membrane
epipharynx
epiphenomena of dissection
epiphora
epiphrenic diverticulum
epiphyseal arrest
epiphyseal dysplasia
epiphyseal fracture
epiphyseal line
epiphyseal osteochondroma
epiphyseal plate
epiphyseal stapling
epiphyseal-diaphyseal fusion
epiphyses
epiphysial bar resection
epiphysial closure
epiphysial growth plate fracture
epiphysial plate injury
epiphysial slip fracture
epiphysial tibial fracture
epiphysiodesis
epiphysiolysis
epiphysis (*pl.* epiphyses)
  avulsion of epiphysis
  capital epiphysis
  femoral epiphysis
  Leadbetter epiphysis
  slipped capital femoral
    epiphysis
  slipped epiphysis
  slipping epiphysis
  stippled epiphysis
epiphysitis
epiplocele
epiploectomy
epiploenterocele
epiploic appendages
epiploic foramen
epiploic foramen of Winslow
epiploitis
epiplomerocele

epiplomphalocele
epiploon
epiplopexy
epiploplasty
epiplorrhaphy
epiplosarcomphalocele
epiploscheocele
epipteric bone
epiretinal membrane
episcleral artery
episcleral bleeder
episcleral circulation
episcleral explant
episcleral forceps
episcleral ganglion
episcleral lamina
episcleral space
episcleral tissue
episcleral vascular dilation
episcleral vein
Episeal wound dressing
episioperineoplasty
episioperineorrhaphy
episioplasty
episioproctotomy
episiorrhaphy
episiotomy
  Matsner episiotomy
  median episiotomy
  mediolateral episiotomy
  midline episiotomy
  ruptured episiotomy
episiotomy repair
episiotomy scar
episiotomy scissors
episodic pain
episodic paroxysmal hemicrania
  (EPH)
epispadias
epispadias-exstrophy complex
episquamous cells
EpiStar diode laser
Epistar subtraction angiogram
epistasis
Epistat double balloon
epistatic
epistaxis
epistaxis balloon
Epi-Stay device
epistropheus
epithelia (*pl.* of epithelium)
epithelial adaptation

epithelial attachment
epithelial atypia
epithelial barrier
epithelial basement membrane
epithelial breakdown
epithelial cancer
epithelial carcinoma
epithelial cast
epithelial cells
epithelial cicatrization
epithelial cuff
epithelial cyst
epithelial debridement
epithelial dysplasia
epithelial granuloma
epithelial inlay
epithelial inlay operation
epithelial invagination
epithelial lining
epithelial marker
epithelial membrane antigen
  (EMA)
epithelial migration
epithelial neoplasm
epithelial onlay operation
epithelial outlay operation
epithelial pearl
epithelial peg
epithelial proliferation
epithelial rest
epithelial rete peg
epithelial ridge
epithelial sarcoma (ES)
epithelial seam
epithelial sheath
epithelial sloughing
epithelial strand
epithelial tissue
epithelial turn-in flap
epithelialization
epithelialization technique
epithelialize
epithelial-myoepithelial (EME)
epithelial-myoepithelial carcinoma
epithelioid cell
epithelioid hemangioma
epithelioid sarcoma
epithelioid-cell sialadenitis
epithelioma
    basal cell epithelioma (BCE)
    Borst-Jadassohn type
      intraepidermal epithelioma

epithelioma (*continued*)
  Brooke epithelioma
  cystic adenoid epithelioma
  Ferguson-Smith epithelioma
  superficial basal cell
      epithelioma
  suprarenal epithelioma
epithelioma of Malherbe
epithelium (*pl.* epithelia)
  attachment epithelium
  autologous-cultured
      epithelium (ACE)
  Barrett epithelium
  buccal epithelium
  cornified epithelium
  crevicular epithelium
  cuboidal epithelium
  desquamating epithelium
  esophageal epithelium
  follicular epithelium
  hornified epithelium
  junctional epithelium
  keratinized epithelium
  noncornified epithelium
  nonhornified epithelium
  nonkeratinized epithelium
  parakeratinized epithelium
  pocket epithelium
  squamous epithelium
  stratified squamous
      epithelium
  sulcal epithelium
  sulcular epithelium
  urethral epithelium
  vestibular epithelium
epithelium-derived relaxation
    factor (EpDRF)
epithelization (variant of
    epithelialization)
epithesis
Epitome scalpel
EpiTouch laser
Epitrain active elbow support
Epitrain elastic elbow support
Epitrain elbow splint
Epitrain-N elbow support
epitrochlea
epitrochleoanconeus muscle
epituberculous infiltration
epitympanic recess
epitympanum
epivaginal connective tissue

epizootic abortion
EPL (extensor pollicis longus)
EPL (extracorporeal
    piezoelectric lithotriptor)
EPL tendon
Epley maneuver
E-point septal separation (EPSS)
eponychial fold
eponychium
Epoxy Die material
Epoxylite CBA dental resin
    cement
Eppendorf angiocatheter
Eppendorf cervical biopsy
    forceps
Eppendorf needle electrode
Eppendorf tube
Eppendorfer angiocatheter
Eppendorfer biopsy punch
Eppendorfer biopsy punch
    forceps
Eppendorfer cardiac catheter
Eppendorfer catheter
Eppendorfer cervical biopsy
    forceps
Eppendorfer punch
Eppendorfer uterine biopsy
    forceps
Epping epoxy
Eppright osteotomy
epsilon tip
epsilon wave
EPSS (E-point septal separation)
Epstein anomaly
Epstein blade
Epstein bone rasp
Epstein collar stud acrylic
    implant
Epstein collar stud acrylic lens
Epstein curet
Epstein down-biting curet
Epstein hammer
Epstein hemilaminectomy blade
Epstein hip dislocation
    classification
Epstein intraocular lens
Epstein lens implant
Epstein needle
Epstein nephrosis
Epstein neurological hammer
Epstein osteotome
Epstein posterior chamber lens

Epstein rasp
Epstein spinal fusion curet
Epstein-Copeland lens
Epstein-Thomas classification
ePTFE (expanded
    polytetrafluoroethylene)
    implant
ePTFE augmentation membrane
ePTFE graft prosthesis
ePTFE membrane
ePTFE vascular sutures (expanded
    polytetrafluoroethylene
    vascular sutures)
ePTFE ventricular shunt
    catheter
epulis-like lesion
epulosis
epulotic
epX suspension sleeve
equal and active bilaterally
equal and brisk reflexes
equal and symmetrical
    extremities
equal bilaterally
equal pulses bilaterally
equal reflexes bilaterally
equal sagittal flap
equalization
equator of eye
equatorial plane
Equen magnet
Equen stomach magnet
Equen-Neuffer knife
Equen-Neuffer laryngeal knife
equilateral hemianopia
equilibrating
equilibrating operation
equilibration
equilibratory ataxia
equilibratory coordination
equilibrium radionuclide
    angiogram
Equilizer short leg walking cast
equinocavovarus
equinocavus
equinovalgus
equinovalgus deformity
equinovarus
    Barr-Record operation for
        talipes equinovarus
    Bost operation for talipes
        equinovarus

equinovarus (*continued*)
 Dwyer operation for talipes
  equinovarus
 Heyman operation for talipes
  equinovarus
 Ingram operation for talipes
  equinovarus
 Lambrinudi operation for
  talipes equinovarus
 McCauley operation for
  talipes equinovarus
 Phelps operation for talipes
  equinovarus
 talipes equinovarus
 Turco operation for talipes
  equinovarus
 Verner operation for talipes
  equinovarus
 Zylik operation for talipes
  equinovarus
equinus
 forefoot equinus
 gastrocnemius equinus
 metatarsus equinus
 pes equinus
 talipes equinus
equinus deformity
equinus position
equipotential electrode
equipotential line
Equisetene sutures
equivalence point
equivalent fraction
equivalent retracting plane
equivocal diagnosis
equivocal response
equivocal symptom
Er:YAG laser
ERA resectoscope sheath
eradication
eradication therapy
eraser cautery
eraser-tip cautery
erasing of joint
erasing of vein
Erb point
Erb sign
Erbakan inferior fornix
  operation
Erbakan operation
Erb-Duchenne palsy
ERBE cryoprobe

Erben reflex
Erbotom F2 electrocoagulation
  unit
ERC (endoscopic retrograde
  cholangiogram)
ERCP (endoscopic retrograde
  cholangiopancreatography)
ERCP balloon extractor
ERCP cannula
ERCP cannulation
ERCP catheter
ERCP conventional prosthesis
ERCP dilator
ERCP equipment
ERCP guidewire
ERCP manometry
ERCP nasobiliary drain
ERCP sphincterotome
ERCPeel Away catheter
ERCP-guided biopsy
ERCP-induced splenic rupture
ErCr:YAG laser
Erdheim-Chester disease
ErecAid system for impotence
ErecAid vacuum erection device
erect position
erect spine
Erectek external erection device
erectile corpora
erectile dysfunction
erectile elements of the penis
erectile tissue
erection
 flexible erection
 intraoperative penile erection
 penile erection
 pharmacologically induced
  erection
 reflex erection
 reflexogenic erection
erector muscle
erector spinae retractor
erector-spinal reflex
ERG (electroretinogram)
ERG-Jet disposable contact
  lens
Ergo bipolar forceps
Ergo Cush back support
Ergo microaspirator
Ergo style flexion table
Ergoflex Premiere back support
ErgoForm contoured cold pack

Ergos O$_2$ pacemaker
Erhardt clamp
Erhardt ear speculum
Erhardt eyelid forceps
Erhardt forceps
Erhardt lid clamp
Erhardt lid forceps
Erhardt speculum
Eric Lloyd extractor
Eric Lloyd introducer
Erich alar cartilage relocation
Erich arch bar
Erich arch bar application and
    intermaxillary fixation
Erich arch malleable bar
Erich biopsy forceps
Erich dental arch bar
Erich facial fracture appliance
Erich facial fracture frame
Erich forceps
Erich laryngeal biopsy forceps
Erich maxillary splint
Erich nasal splint
Erich operation
Erich splint
Erich swivel
Erichsen ligature
Erich-Winter arch bar
Eri-Flo dialyzer
Eriksson brachial block
    technique
Eriksson cruciate reconstruction
Eriksson guide
Eriksson knee procedure
Eriksson knee prosthesis
Eriksson ligament technique
Eriksson muscle biopsy cannula
Eriksson-Paparella holder
erisiphake (see erysiphake)
Erlangen endoscopic
    sphincterotome
Erlangen magnetic colostomy
    device
Erlangen papillotome
Erlenmeyer flask deformity
Ermold needle holder
Ernest-McDonald soft
    intraocular lens
Ernst applicator
Ernst radium application
Ernst radium applicator
Ernst radium capsule

Ernst radium tandem
eroded incus
Erosa amnioscope
Erosa disposable hypodermic
    needle
Erosa-Spec vaginal speculum
E-rosette cell marker
E-rosette receptor
E-rosetting
erosion
    bony erosion
    cervical erosion
    corneal erosion
    crater-shaped erosion
    Dieulafoy erosion
    duodenal erosion
    gastric antral erosion
    gastric erosion
    implant erosion
    linear erosion
    notch-shaped erosion
    salt and pepper duodenal
        erosion
    saucer-shaped erosion
    superficial erosion
    V-shaped erosion
erosion desquamation
erosion of cervix
erosive anastomosis
erosive inflammation
erratic heart rhythm
ERS (endoscopic retrograde
    sphincterotomy)
ERU (endorectal ultrasound)
erupted incisor
erupted teeth
eruption cyst
Erx Avulsed Tooth kit
erysiphake
    Barraquer erysiphake
    Bell erysiphake
    Castroviejo erysiphake
    corneal erysiphake
    Dastoor erysiphake
    Dimitry erysiphake
    Dimitry-Bell erysiphake
    Dimitry-Thomas erysiphake
    Draeger high-vacuum
        erysiphake
    Esposito erysiphake
    Falcao erysiphake
    Flayol-Grant erysiphake

erysiphake (*continued*)
  Floyd-Grant erysiphake
  Harken erysiphake
  Harrington erysiphake
  Johnson erysiphake
  Johnson-Bell erysiphake
  Kara erysiphake
  L'Esperance erysiphake
  Maumenee erysiphake
  Maumenee-Park erysiphake
  New York erysiphake
  nucleus erysiphake
  Nugent erysiphake
  Nugent-Green-Dimitry
    erysiphake
  oval cup erysiphake
  Post-Harrington erysiphake
  right-angled erysiphake
  Sakler erysiphake
  Searcy erysiphake
  Searcy oval cup erysiphake
  Simcoe nucleus erysiphake
  Storz-Bell erysiphake
  Viers erysiphake
  Welsh erysiphake
  Welsh rubber bulb erysiphake
  Welsh Silastic erysiphake
erysiphake technique
erythematosa
  acne erythematosa
erythematous change
erythroderma
erythrodermatous lesion
Erythroflex catheter
Erythroflex hydromer-coated
  central venous catheter
erythroplakic lesion
ES (endoscopic sphincterotomy)
ES (epithelial sarcoma)
ESA acromioplasty electrode
ESA hook electrode
ESA Jet Stream ball electrode
ESA meniscectomy electrode
ESA Smillie electrode
escape beats
escape interval
escape of air
escape of gastroduodenal
  contents
escape pacemaker
escape rhythm
escaped ventricular contraction

Escapini cataract operation
Escapini operation
eschar
escharectomy
escharotomy
Eschenbach low vision
  rehabilitation guide
Eschenbach Optik lens
Eschmann endotracheal tube
  introducer
Escort defibrillator/pacer
  monitor
Escort balloon stone extractor
E-series bipolar forceps
E-series scissors
ESI bile block
ESI bite block
ESI laryngoscope
ESI lighted suction elevator
ESI mammaplasty retractor
ESI sigmoidoscope
ESKA Jonas Silicon-Silver
  semirigid penile prosthesis
ESKA-Buess esophageal tube
ESKA-Jonas silicone-silver penile
  prosthesis
Esmarch bandage
Esmarch bandage scissors
Esmarch operation
Esmarch plaster knife
Esmarch plaster scissors
Esmarch plaster shears
Esmarch probe
Esmarch roll dressing
Esmarch scissors
Esmarch shears
Esmarch tin bullet probe
Esmarch tourniquet
Esmarch tube
ESO (electrospinal orthosis)
esodic nerve
EsophaCoil biliary stent
EsophaCoil prosthesis
EsophaCoil self-expanding
  esophageal stent
esophageal ring
esophageal abscess
esophageal achalasia
esophageal adenocarcinoma
esophageal airway
esophageal anastomosis
esophageal A-ring

esophageal artery
esophageal atresia
esophageal balloon
esophageal balloon catheter
esophageal balloon dilator
esophageal band ligation
esophageal banding technique
esophageal biopsy
esophageal body motor
    dysfunction
esophageal bougie
esophageal bougienage
esophageal branch
esophageal B-ring
esophageal cancer
esophageal candidiasis
esophageal carcinoma
esophageal cardiogram
esophageal colic
esophageal compression
esophageal conductor
esophageal constriction
esophageal contractile ring
esophageal contraction ring
esophageal detection device
esophageal dilatation
esophageal dilation
esophageal dilation treatment
esophageal dilator
esophageal disorder
esophageal dissection
esophageal diverticulectomy
esophageal diverticulum
esophageal duplication
esophageal dysmotility
esophageal ectopic sebaceous
    gland
esophageal effect
esophageal epithelium
esophageal fistula
esophageal fistula closure
esophageal forceps
esophageal foreign body
esophageal fungal infection
esophageal glands
esophageal groove
esophageal hemangioma
esophageal hernia
esophageal hiatus
esophageal impression
esophageal infection
esophageal inflammation

esophageal inlet
esophageal introitus
esophageal intubation
esophageal lesion
esophageal Lewy body
esophageal lumen
esophageal manometry
esophageal manometry catheter
esophageal mass
esophageal measurement
esophageal mercury-filled
    bougie
esophageal mobilization
esophageal motility
esophageal motility disorder
esophageal mucosa
esophageal mucosal ring
esophageal muscular ring
esophageal myotomy
esophageal obstruction
esophageal obturator airway
esophageal perforation
esophageal perfusion catheter
esophageal peristaltic pressure
esophageal pill electrode
esophageal plexus
esophageal prosthesis
esophageal prosthetic
    placement
esophageal remnant
esophageal repair
esophageal resection
esophageal retractor
esophageal rupture
esophageal scissors
esophageal shears
esophageal shortening
esophageal shunt
esophageal sling procedure
esophageal sound
esophageal spasm
esophageal speculum
esophageal sphincter
esophageal sphincter pressure
esophageal sphincter
    relaxation
esophageal stenosis
esophageal stent
esophageal stethoscope
esophageal Strecker stent
esophageal stricture
esophageal tamponade

esophageal tear
esophageal temperature probe
esophageal transection
esophageal tube
esophageal tumor
esophageal ulcer
esophageal ulceration
esophageal variceal bleed
esophageal variceal bleeding
esophageal variceal
   sclerotherapy
esophageal varix (*pl.* varices)
esophageal vein
esophageal web
esophageal Z-Stent stent
esophageal-jejunal anastomosis
esophagectomy
  distal esophagectomy
  endoscopic esophagectomy
  Ivor Lewis esophagectomy
  Ivor Lewis 2-stage subtotal
   esophagectomy
  laparoscopic transhiatal
   esophagectomy
  laparoscopic-assisted
   esophagectomy
  Lewis-Tanner esophagectomy
  mediastinoscopy-assisted
   transhiatal esophagectomy
  minimally invasive
   esophagectomy
  near-total esophagectomy
  open esophagectomy
  subtotal esophagectomy
  thoracoabdominal
   esophagectomy
  thoracoscopic-assisted
   esophagectomy
  Torek esophagectomy
  total endoscopic
   esophagectomy
  total laparoscopic
   esophagectomy
  total thoracic esophagectomy
  transhiatal esophagectomy
   (THE)
  transsternal radical
   esophagectomy
  transthoracic esophagectomy
esophagectomy with
  thoracotomy
esophagobronchial fistula

esophagocardiomyotomy
esophagocolic anastomosis
esophagocologastrostomy
esophagocoloplasty
esophagocolostomy
esophagocutaneous fistula
esophagoduodenostomy
esophagoenterostomy
esophagoesophagostomy
esophagofiberscope
esophagofundopexy
esophagogastrectomy
  Ivor Lewis
   esophagogastrectomy
  thoracoabdominal
   esophagogastrectomy
esophagogastric
esophagogastric anastomosis
esophagogastric cancer
esophagogastric flap valve
esophagogastric fundoplasty
esophagogastric intubation
esophagogastric junction
esophagogastric mucosal
  junction
esophagogastric resection
esophagogastric tamponade
esophagogastric variceal
  bleeding
esophagogastric varix
esophagogastroanastomosis
esophagogastroduodenoscopy
  (EGD)
esophagogastrojejunostomy
esophagogastromyotomy
esophagogastropexy
esophagogastroplasty
esophagogastroscopy
  Abbott esophagogastroscopy
  intrathoracic
   esophagogastroscopy
  Johnson esophagogastroscopy
  Thal esophagogastroscopy
  Woodward
   esophagogastroscopy
esophagogastrostomy
  Abbott esophagogastrostomy
  cervical esophagogastrostomy
  Clagett Barrett
   esophagogastrostomy
  end-to-end
   esophagogastrostomy

esophagogastrostomy
  (*continued*)
  end-to-side
    esophagogastrostomy
  intrathoracic
    esophagogastrostomy
  Johnson esophagogastrostomy
  Thal esophagogastrostomy
  thoracic esophagogastrostomy
  Woodward
    esophagogastrostomy
esophagogram
  barium esophagogram
  water-soluble contrast
    esophagogram
esophagography
esophagoileostomy
esophagojejunal anastomosis
esophagojejunogastrostomosis
esophagojejunogastrostomy
esophagojejunoplasty
esophagojejunostomy
  end-to-end
    esophagojejunostomy
  end-to-side
    esophagojejunostomy
  loop esophagojejunostomy
  mechanical
    esophagojejunostomy
  mediastinal
    esophagojejunostomy
  Roux-en-Y
    esophagojejunostomy
  staples esophagojejunostomy
  transhiatal
    esophagojejunostomy
esophagolaryngectomy
esophagomediastinal fistula
esophagomyotomy
  circumferential
    esophagomyotomy
  Heller esophagomyotomy
  laparoscopic
    esophagomyotomy
  modified Heller
    esophagomyotomy
  open esophagomyotomy
  thoracic short
    esophagomyotomy
  thoracoscopic
    esophagomyotomy
esophagonasogastric tube

esophagopharynx
esophagoplasty
  balloon esophagoplasty
  behind-sternum column
    esophagoplasty
  Belsey esophagoplasty
  cervical esophagoplasty
  colic patch esophagoplasty
  colonic esophagoplasty
  gastric patch esophagoplasty
  gastric tube esophagoplasty
  Grondahl esophagoplasty
  Grondahl-Finney
    esophagoplasty
  intrathoracic esophagoplasty
  laparoscopic esophagoplasty
  one-stage posterior
    mediastinal esophagoplasty
  patch esophagoplasty
  pectoralis myocutaneous
    esophagoplasty
  pediatric esophagoplasty
  reverse gastric tube
    esophagoplasty
  single-step esophagoplasty
  subtotal esophagoplasty
  transmediastinal posterior
    esophagoplasty
esophagoplication
esophagoprobe
esophagoproximal gastrectomy
esophagopulmonary fistula
esophagorespiratory fistula
esophago-Roux-en-Y-jejunostomy
esophagorrhaphy
esophagosalivary reflex
esophagosalivary symptom
esophagoscope
  ACMI esophagoscope
  ACMI fiberoptic
    esophagoscope
  ballooning esophagoscope
  Blom-Singer esophagoscope
  Boros esophagoscope
  Broyles esophagoscope
  Bruening esophagoscope
  Chevalier Jackson
    esophagoscope
  child esophagoscope
  Denck esophagoscope
  Dohlman esophagoscope
  Eder esophagoscope

esophagoscope (*continued*)
Eder-Hufford esophagoscope
Eutaw-Hoffman esophagoscope
fiberoptic esophagoscope
folding esophagoscope
Foregger rigid esophagoscope
Foroblique esophagoscope
Foroblique fiberoptic esophagoscope
full-lumen esophagoscope
Haslinger esophagoscope
Holinger child esophagoscope
Holinger esophagoscope
Holinger infant esophagoscope
Hufford esophagoscope
infant esophagoscope
Jackson esophagoscope
Jackson full-lumen esophagoscope
Jackson standard full-lumen esophagoscope
Jasbee esophagoscope
Jesberg esophagoscope
Jesberg oval esophagoscope
Jesberg upper esophagoscope
J-scope esophagoscope
Kalk esophagoscope
Lell esophagoscope
LoPresti fiberoptic esophagoscope
Moersch esophagoscope
Mosher esophagoscope
Moure esophagoscope
Olympus esophagoscope
operating esophagoscope
optical esophagoscope
oval esophagoscope
oval-open esophagoscope
pediatric esophagoscope
Roberts esophagoscope
Roberts folding esophagoscope
Roberts oval esophagoscope
Roberts-Jesberg esophagoscope
Sam Roberts esophagoscope
Schindler esophagoscope
Schindler optical esophagoscope

esophagoscope (*continued*)
standard full-lumen esophagoscope
Storz esophagoscope
Storz operating esophagoscope
Storz optical esophagoscope
Storz pediatric esophagoscope
Tesberg esophagoscope
Tucker esophagoscope
Universal esophagoscope
upper esophagoscope
Yankauer esophagoscope
esophagoscopic cannula
esophagoscopic catheter
esophagoscopic forceps
esophagoscopic tube
esophagoscopy
fiberoptic esophagoscopy
video esophagoscopy
esophagospasm
esophagospasm dilator
esophagostoma
esophagostomy
cervical esophagostomy
palliative esophagostomy
esophagotome
esophagotomy
esophagotracheal fistula
esophagram
esophagus
abdominal esophagus
adenocarcinoma in Barrett esophagus
anastomosis of esophagus
aperistaltic esophagus
Barrett esophagus
bird's beak distal esophagus
brusque dilatation of esophagus
cardiac glands of esophagus
cervical esophagus
columnar-lined esophagus
corkscrew esophagus
dilatation of esophagus
distal esophagus
nutcracker esophagus
parrot-beak shape of distal esophagus
rosary-bead esophagus
stump of esophagus

esophagus (*continued*)
  thoracic esophagus
  Torek resection of thoracic
    esophagus
  tortuous esophagus
  upper esophagus
esotropia
ESP (extended supraplatysmal
    plane)
ESP dissection
ESP face-lift technique
ESP radiation reduction
    examination glove
Espocan combined
    spinal/epidural needle
Esposito erysiphake
essential telangiectasia
Esser eyelid operation
Esser graft
Esser implant
Esser inlay graft
Esser inlay operation
Esser operation
Esser prosthesis
Esser skin graft
Essex-Lopresti axial fixation
    technique
Essex-Lopresti calcaneal fracture
    classification
Essex-Lopresti calcaneal fracture
    technique
Essex-Lopresti classification
Essex-Lopresti fracture
Essex-Lopresti fracture reduction
Essex-Lopresti joint depression
    fracture
Essex-Lopresti maneuver
Essex-Lopresti open reduction
Essex-Lopresti reduction
    technique
Essig arch bar
Essig wire acrylic splint
Essig wiring
Essrig dissecting scissors
Essrig forceps
Essrig scissors
Essrig tissue forceps
Estecar prosthesis
Estes operation
Estes procedure
esthesiometer
esthetic appearance

esthetic breast reconstruction
esthetic CO_2 laser
esthetic dentistry
esthetic dentulous
esthetic denture
esthetic restoration
esthetic rhinoplasty
esthetic septorhinoplasty
esthetic surgery
esthetic Taylor mandibular angle
    implant
Estilux dental restorative
    material
estimated blood loss (EBL)
Estlander cheiloplasty
Estlander flap
Estlander flap cheiloplasty
Estlander operation
Estlander-Abbe flap
Estridge ventricular needle
Estring estradiol vaginal ring
Estring silicone vaginal ring
estrogen assay
estrogen receptor localization
estrogen-assisted colposcopy
estrogenic dependent
estrophy epispadias complex
ESWL (extracorporeal shock
    wave lithotripsy)
ESWT (extracorporeal shock
    wave therapy)
ET tube
ETB endoscope
Etch-Master instrument marker
Etch-Master kit
Ethalloy TruTaper cardiovascular
    needle
Ethalloy TruTaper needle
ethanol ablation
ethanol injection
ethanol injection therapy
ethanol-treated freeze-dried
    bone tissue
ether
ether anesthesia
ether anesthetic agent
ether bed
ether guard
Etheron augmentation
    mammography
Ethibond polybutilate-coated
    polyester sutures

Ethibond polyester sutures
Ethibond sutures
Ethicon needle
Ethicon clip
Ethicon disposable cannula
Ethicon disposable trocar
Ethicon endoscopic linear cutter
Ethicon endosurgery circular
    stapler
Ethicon mesh
Ethicon micropoint suture
Ethicon paste
Ethicon paste prosthesis
Ethicon Sabreloc sutures
Ethicon SAS (synthetic
    absorbable sutures)
Ethicon silk suture
Ethicon slip
Ethicon ST-4 straight taper-point
    needle
Ethicon staple
Ethicon sutures
Ethicon TG Plus needle
Ethicon TGW needle
Ethicon-Atraloc sutures
Ethiflex retention sutures
Ethiflex sutures
Ethiguard needle
Ethilon nylon sutures
Ethilon sutures
Ethi-pack sutures
Ethitek's automated protection
    manometer
ethmoid air cell
ethmoid angle
ethmoid antrum
ethmoid bone
ethmoid bulla
ethmoid canal
ethmoid cell
ethmoid cornu
ethmoid exenteration
ethmoid fistula
ethmoid plate
ethmoid punch forceps
ethmoid registration point
ethmoid sinus carcinoma
ethmoidal air cell
ethmoidal artery
ethmoidal bone
ethmoidal bulla
ethmoidal cells

ethmoidal chisel
ethmoidal crest
ethmoidal curet
ethmoidal elevator
ethmoidal exenteration forceps
ethmoidal fissure
ethmoidal foramen
ethmoidal forceps
ethmoidal fossa
ethmoidal groove
ethmoidal infundibulum
ethmoidal labyrinth
ethmoidal lamina cribrosa
ethmoidal mucosa
ethmoidal nerve
ethmoidal notch
ethmoidal ostium
ethmoidal periostitis
ethmoidal prechamber
ethmoidal process
ethmoidal punch
ethmoidal sinus
ethmoidal sinusitis
ethmoidal spine of Macalister
ethmoidal sulcus of Gegenbaur
ethmoidal sulcus of nasal bone
ethmoidal veins
ethmoidal-lacrimal fistula
ethmoid-Blakesley forceps
ethmoid-cutting forceps
ethmoidectomy
    anterior ethmoidectomy
    endoscopic ethmoidectomy
    external ethmoidectomy
    internal ethmoidectomy
    intranasal ethmoidectomy
    partial ethmoidectomy
    Riedel frontal ethmoidectomy
    total ethmoidectomy
    transantral ethmoidectomy
ethmoidolacrimal suture
ethmoidomaxillary
ethmoidomaxillary plate
ethmoidomaxillary suture
ethmoidotomy
ethocaine anesthetic agent
Ethox bite block
Ethox lavage tube
Ethox rectal tube
Ethox Surgi-Press pressure
    infuser
Ethrane anesthetic agent

Ethridge forceps
Ethridge hysterectomy forceps
Ethrone graft
Ethrone implant
Ethrone prosthesis
ethyl chloride anesthetic agent
ethyl cyanoacrylate glue
ethyl ether anesthetic agent
ethyl methacrylate
ethyl oxide anesthetic agent
ethyl vinyl ether anesthetic agent
ethylene anesthetic agent
ethylene oxide
ethylene oxide dressing
etidocaine hydrochloride
    anesthetic agent
etiological conclusion
etiology
E-to-A adapter
ETR (endoscopic carpal tunnel
    release)
E-type dental implant
EUA (examination under
    anesthesia)
EUB-405 ultrasound scanner
Eucerin soap
Euchidia technique
Eucotone monitor
EUE tonsillar snare
eugenic sterilization
eugnathic anomaly
EUM-series endoscope
eunuchism
eunuchoid gigantism
euplastic
Eureka collimator
Euro Precision Technology
    submicron lathe machine
Euro-Collins multiorgan
    perfusion kit
Euro-Med aspiration needle
Eurotech table
EUS-guided fine-needle
    aspiration
eustachian applicator
eustachian attachment
eustachian bougie
eustachian bur
eustachian canal
eustachian cartilage
eustachian catheter
eustachian muscle

eustachian probe
eustachian sound
eustachian tonsil
eustachian tube
eustachian valve
Eutaw-Hoffman esophagoscope
eutectic mixture of local
    anesthetics (EMLA)
euthyroid
Evac device
evacuating clot
evacuation
    CT-guided stereotactic
      evacuation
    digital rectal evacuation
    dilatation and evacuation
      (D&E)
    dilation and evacuation (D&E)
    epidural abscess evacuation
    epidural tumor evacuation
    fimbrial evacuation
    fluid evacuation
    hematobilia evacuation
    hematoma evacuation
    laser smoke evacuation
    rectal evacuation
    stool evacuation
    transsphenoidal evacuation
    uterine evacuation
evacuation disorder
evacuation of barium
evacuation of blood clots
evacuation of bowel
evacuation of clots
evacuation of subdural
    hematoma
evacuation procedure
evacuation proctography
evacuation score
evacuator
    Bard evacuator
    Bigelow evacuator
    bladder evacuator
    clot evacuator
    Creevy bladder evacuator
    Creevy evacuator
    Crigler evacuator
    Dentsply MVS evacuator
    electric evacuator
    Ellik bladder evacuator
    Ellik evacuator
    Ewald evacuator

evacuator (*continued*)
 high-volume evacuator
 Hutch evacuator
 ice clot evacuator
 Iglesias evacuator
 Kennedy-Cornwell bladder
  evacuator
 Laparofan smoke evacuator
 Laufe portable uterine
  evacuator
 Lavacuator gastric evacuator
 Lempert evacuator
 McCarthy bladder evacuator
 McCarthy evacuator
 McKenna evacuator
 oval-window piston evacuator
 Plume-Away evacuator
 Sklar evacuator
 smoke evacuator
 SmokEvac smoke evacuator
 Snyder Hemovac evacuator
 Storz bladder evacuator
 Storz evacuator
 Storz-Ellik evacuator
 suction evacuator
 Surgilase evacuator
 Thompson evacuator
 Timberlake evacuator
 Toomey bladder evacuator
 Toomey evacuator
 Urovac bladder evacuator
 uterine evacuator
evacuator tubing
evagination
Eva-Hewes reconstruction
evaluation
 acute physiologic assessment
  and chronic health
  evaluation
 acute physiology and chronic
  health evaluation (APACHE)
 angiodynagraphic evaluation
 angiographic evaluation
 anthropometric evaluation
 audiological evaluation
 baseline capacity evaluation
 clinical evaluation
 colonoscopic evaluation
 computerized muscle-joint
  evaluation
 cosmetic evaluation
 Cybex evaluation

evaluation (*continued*)
 cytologic evaluation
 diagnostic imaging evaluation
 Doppler pulse evaluation
 Dubowitz evaluation
 endoscopic ultrasound
  evaluation
 follow-up evaluation
 functional capacity evaluation
 genitourinary evaluation
 Glogau system of skin
  evaluation
 Harris hip evaluation
 hormonal evaluation
 infertility evaluation
 Iowa hip evaluation
 job capacity evaluation
 laparoscopic evaluation
 Larson hip evaluation
 mammographic evaluation
 manometric evaluation
 medical care evaluation
 mental status evaluation
 metabolic evaluation
 musculoskeletal evaluation
 neurodiagnostic evaluation
 neurologic evaluation
 neuroradiologic evaluation
 noninvasive evaluation
 pedicle evaluation
 physical capacity evaluation
 postoperative follow-up
  evaluation
 preoperative evaluation
 preoperative staging
  evaluation
 presurgical medical evaluation
 pretransplant evaluation
 pretreatment evaluation
 proctosigmoidoscopic
  evaluation
 radiographic evaluation
 radiologic evaluation
 roentgenographic evaluation
 serial radiographic evaluation
 sexual evaluation
 Smith physical capacities
  evaluation
 static evaluation
 status evaluation
 stent evaluation
 urological evaluation

evaluation (*continued*)
  uterine evaluation
  videoscopic evaluation
  videourodynamic evaluation
  visual function evaluation
  wake-up evaluation
  Wright-Giemsa evaluation
evaluation protocol
evaluative staging
evanescent
Evans ankle ligament repair
Evans ankle reconstruction
    technique
Evans articulator
Evans blue dye
Evans foot procedure
Evans forceps
Evans fusion
Evans intertrochanteric fracture
    classification
Evans operation
Evans procedure
Evans reconstruction
Evans staging of neuroblastoma
Evans Vital tissue forceps
Evans-Steptoe procedure
Evans-vital tissue forceps
Evazote cushioning material
Evazote foam
Eve-Neivert tonsillar wire
event
  acute cardiac event
  adverse event
  anatomic event
  cardiac event
  catastrophic event
  cerebral event
  cerebrovascular event
  fatal cardiac event
  intra-anesthetic event
  neuroelectric event
  precipitating noxious event
  soft event
  thromboembolic event
eventration
  diaphragmatic eventration
eventration disease
Everard Williams procedure
Everclear laryngeal mirror
Everday self-adhering urinary
    external catheter
Everest alloy

Everett eustachian catheter
Everett fallopian cannula
Everett fallopian catheter
Everett forceps
Everett-TeLinde operation
Evergreen Lasertek coagulator
Evergreen Lasertek laser
Evermed catheter
Eversbusch operation
Eversbusch ptosis operation
Evershears bipolar curved
    scissors
Evershears bipolar laparoscopic
    forceps
Evershears bipolar laparoscopic
    scissors
Evershears bipolar curved scissors
Evershears surgical instrument
    device
eversion carotid endarterectomy
eversion endarterectomy
eversion of organ
eversion operation
eversion orchiopexy
eversion osteotomy
eversion position
eversion stress test
eversion tape strapping
eversion technique
eversion-external rotation
    deformity
everted lid
everted nipple
everter (*see also* lid everter)
  Benke everter
  Berens everter
  Berens lid everter
  Berke double-end lid everter
  Keizer everter
  lid everter
  Luther-Peter lid everter
  Pess lid everter
  Schachne-Desmarres lid
    everter
  Siniscal-Smith lid everter
  Strubel lid everter
  Vail lid everter
  Walker lid everter
everter, evertor
everting interrupted suture
    technique
everting interrupted sutures

everting mattress sutures
everting sutures
Evert-O-Cath drug delivery
   catheter
Eves snare
Eves tonsillar knife
Eves tonsillar snare
Eves-Neivert tonsillar snare
Evipal anesthetic agent
EVIS endoscope
EVIS colonoscope
evisceration
   abdominal evisceration
   Burch evisceration
   drain site evisceration
   Ruedemann eye evisceration
   total abdominal evisceration
   upper abdominal evisceration
evisceration knife
evisceration of eyeball
evisceration of orbital contents
evisceration operation
evisceration spoon
evisceroneurotomy
EVL (endoscopic variceal
   ligation)
evoked action potential
evoked response
Evolution hip prosthesis
Evolution implant removal kit
Evolution XP scanner
EVS (endoscopic variceal
   sclerotherapy)
evulsion
Ewald capitellocondylar total
   elbow arthroplasty
Ewald elbow arthroplasty
Ewald elbow prosthesis
Ewald evacuator
Ewald forceps
Ewald gastroscope
Ewald lavage
Ewald prosthesis
Ewald stomach tube
Ewald tissue forceps
Ewald total elbow replacement
Ewald tube
Ewald-Hensler arthroscopic
   punch
Ewald-Hudson brain forceps
Ewald-Hudson clamp
Ewald-Hudson dressing forceps

Ewald-Hudson tissue forceps
Ewald-Walker kinematic knee
   arthroplasty
Ewald-Walker knee implant
Ewing capsular forceps
Ewing eye implant
Ewing forceps
Ewing lid clamp
Ewing operation
Ewing sarcoma
Ewing tumor
ex situ bench surgery
ex situ hepatectomy
ex situ in vivo procedure
ex situ-in situ hepatectomy
ex situ-in situ liver resection
ex situ-in situ technique
ex vacuo dilatation
ex vivo cannulation
ex vivo fertilization
ex vivo gene therapy
ex vivo perfusion
ex vivo technique
exacerbation of pain
exacerbation of symptoms
exact nature unknown
exam under anesthesia
examination
   abdominal examination
   anoscopic examination
   arthroscopic examination
   Ballard examination
   barium examination
   bench examination
   bile fluid examination
   bimanual examination
   bimanual pelvic examination
   bone marrow examination
   cardiac Doppler examination
   cardiac examination
   chest examination
   cineradiographic examination
   clinical examination
   colonoscopic examination
   colposcopic examination
   comparative radiographic
     examination
   contrast examination
   cystoscopic examination
   cytologic examination
   cytology examination
   dark-field examination

examination (*continued*)
  Denver Articulation Screening
    Examination (DASE)
  diascopic examination
  digital examination
  digital rectal examination
  Doppler flow probe
    examination
  double-contrast barium
    enema examination
  Dubowitz examination
  duodenal content
    examination
  endoscopic examination
  eye examination
  fiberoptic examination
  flashlight examination
  follow-up examination
  full-body cutaneous
    examination
  full-spine radiographic
    examination
  funduscopic examination
  gastric residue examination
  gray scale examination
  gross examination
  gynecological examination
  hand-held Doppler flow
    probe examination
  histologic examination
  histopathologic examination
  history and physical
    examination
  immunofluorescent
    examination
  laminogram examination
  laparoscopic examination
  limited examination
  LUS examination
  mediastinoscopic examination
  mental status examination
  motor examination
  neonate examination
  neurologic examination
  neurological examination
  neurological nerve
    conduction velocity
    examination
  neuro-ophthalmologic
    examination
  neurophysiologic examination
  neurotologic examination

examination (*continued*)
  newborn examination
  ophthalmic examination
  ophthalmoscopic examination
  oral peripheral examination
  otoscopic examination
  palpatory examination
  parasternal examination
  pathologic examination
  pathologic tissue examination
  pathology examination
  pelvic examination
  pericardial fluid examination
  peritoneal fluid examination
  peritoneoscopy examination
  photofluorographic
    examination
  physical examination
  planographic examination
  pleural fluid examination
  postmortem examination
  prior to examination
  proctoscopic examination
  proctosigmoidoscopic
    examination
  radial wrist examination
  radiologic examination
  radiological examination
  rectal examination
  rectovaginal examination
  reflex examination
  retinal examination
  self-breast examination
  sensory examination
  serial examinations
  serologic examination
  sideline examination
  slit-lamp examination
  small bowel followthrough
    examination
  soft x-ray examination
  speculum examination
  sterile examination
  sterile vaginal examination
  suboptimal examination
  supraclavicular examination
  suprasternal examination
  synovial fluid examination
  systemic examination
  tangent screen examination
  thermographic examination
  tomographic examination

examination (*continued*)
  transvaginal ultrasonographic
    examination
  ultrasound examination
  urethroscopic examination
  vaginal examination
  vaginorectal examination
  Wood light examination
examination insert tube
examination retractor
examination under anesthesia
    (EUA)
examine cholangiography
    catheter
examining arthroscope
examining gastroscope
examining hook
examining hysteroscope
examining lamp
examining light
examining stool
examining telescope
exarticulation
Excaliber handpiece
Excalibur introducer
excavated gastric carcinoma
excavated lesion
excavated tumor
excavating bur
excavation
  atrophic excavation
  glaucomatous excavation
  physiologic excavation
  pulpal excavations
  retinal excavation
  vesicouterine excavation
excavation of tumor
excavator
  Austin excavator
  Clev-Dent excavator
  dental excavator
  Farrior excavator
  Farrior oval-window
    excavator
  Farrior oval-window piston
    gauge excavator
  fenestration excavator
  Henry Schein excavator
  Hough excavator
  Hough oval-window
    excavator
  Hough whirlybird excavator

excavator (*continued*)
  Hough-Saunders excavator
  House excavator
  House-Hough excavator
  Lempert excavator
  Merlis obstetrical excavator
  middle ear excavator
  Nordent excavator
  oval-window excavator
  Paparella-Hough excavator
  PD excavator
  Schuknecht excavator
  Schuknecht whirlybird
    excavator
  sinus tympani excavator
  stapes excavator
  whirlybird excavator
  whirlybird stapes excavator
excavator hoe
Excel disposable biopsy forceps
Excel electric hospital bed
Excel Plus electrode
eXcel-DR needle
Excell polishing point
Exceltech imaging
excementosis (*pl.*
    excementoses)
  extension excementosis
  intraepithelial excementosis
  pronglike excementosis
  ultraterminal excementosis
excess overhang
excessive bleeding
excessive callus formation
excessive fluid retention
excessive lip support
excessive nasality
excessive overbite
excessive spacing
excessive supraorbital bossing
    (fullness)
exchange
  air exchange
  air-fluid exchange
  blood-gas exchange
  body-fluid exchange
  catheter exchange
  cation exchange
  chemical exchange
  endoscopic stent exchange
  fetal-maternal exchange
  fluid-gas exchange

exchange (*continued*)
  gas exchange
  gas-fluid exchange
  lens exchange
  multiple insert gas exchange
  plasma exchange
  pulmonary-gas exchange
  respiratory exchange
  saline implant exchange
  wire-guided balloon-assisted
    endoscopic biliary stent
    exchange
exchange diffusion
exchange guidewire
exchange technique
exchange transfusion
exchanger
  countercurrent heat
    exchanger
  heat and moisture exchanger
  heat/moisture exchanger
  HumidFilter heat and
    moisture exchanger
  hygroscopic heat and
    moisture exchanger
  moisture exchanger
  Portex ThermoVent heat and
    moisture exchanger
Excilon drain sponge
Excilon dressing sponge
Excilon IV sponge
ExciMed excimer laser
excimer
excimer cool laser
excimer gas laser
excimer laser
excimer laser coronary
  angioplasty
excimer laser photorefractive
  keratectomy
excimer ultraviolet laser
excised adenoids
excision
  abdominoperineal excision
  alar rim excision
  alar wedge excision
  anal fissure excision
  anoscopy with excision
  anterior port scalp excision
  Arlt pterygium excision
  Arlt-Jaesche excision
  Bartlett nail-fold excision

excision (*continued*)
  Bent shoulder excision
  Billroth tongue excision
  bone cyst excision
  Bose nail-fold excision
  cervical disk excision
  chalazion excision
  circumferential mesorectal
    excision
  clavicle excision
  cloverleaf excision
  cold snare excision
  complete circumferential
    mesorectal excision
  complete excision
  complete mesh excision
  Curtin plantar fibromatosis
    excision
  Dahlman diverticulum excision
  Das Gupta scapular excision
  direct crease excision
  direct supraciliary excision
  disk excision
  distal clavicular excision
  dorsal excision
  double V-Y plasty with paired
    inverted Burow triangle
    excisions
  elliptical excision
  en bloc excision
  endoluminal excision
  extended mesorectal excision
  extratemporal excision
  Feldman excision
  Ferciot excision
  Ferciot-Thomson excision
  flared-W excision
  Flatt excision
  funicular excision
  fusiform excision
  Gaillard-Thomas excision
  Gillespie wrist excision
  goiter excision
  hemivertebral excision
  hemorrhoid laser excision
  incomplete excision
  interdental excision
  intralesional excision
  inverted-T skin excision
  laser excision
  laser hemorrhoid excision
  local excision

excision (*continued*)
  L-shaped skin excision
  lunate excision
  marginal excision
  mass excision
  maxillary excision
  McKeever-Buck fragment
    excision
  mediastinal tumor excision
  meniscal excision
  mesorectal excision
  microlumbar disk excision
  modified fishtail excision
  Mohs excision
  M-plasty excision
  mucosal excision
  multiple surgical excisions
  neuroma excision
  operative excision
  osteocartilaginous excision
  partial excision
  partial mesh excision
  pentagonal block excision
  radical compartmental
    excision
  radical excision
  rectal excision
  regional excision
  retro-orbicularis ocular fat pad
    excision
  retropulsed bone excision
  ruptured disk excision
  sentinel node excision
  serial scar excisions
  shave excision
  sheet mesh excision
  simple excision
  St. Mark excision
  Stewart distal clavicular
    excision
  subperichondrial excision
  subtotal excision
  superficial excision
  surgical excision
  tangential excision
  Terwilliger excision
  Thompson excision
  through-and-through
    buttonhole fashion excision
  thymus gland excision
  total mesorectal excision
    (TME)

excision (*continued*)
  transanal excision
  ulnar head excision
  U-shaped skin excision
  vertical skin excision
  V-shaped skin excision
  wedge excision
  Weir excision
  wide excision
  wide local excision
  Wies entropion excision
  William microlumbar disk
    excision
  wound excision
  wrist excision
excision and biopsy
excision and cautery
excision and fulguration
excision and wedge biopsy
excision arthroplasty
excision biopsy
excision of cyst
excision of duct
excision of fissure
excision of joint
excision of lesion
excision of organ
excision of sinus
excision of tissue
excision of tumor
excisional arthrodesis
excisional biopsy
excisional biopsy procedure
excisional biopsy site
excisional biopsy technique
excisional cardiac surgery
excisional conization
excisional removal
excisional scar
excisional thoracoscopy
excision-curettage technique
excited skin syndrome
exclusion
  antral exclusion
  Devine antral exclusion
  hepatic vascular exclusion
    (HVE)
  intermittent vascular
    exclusion
  partial hepatic vascular
    exclusion (PHVE)
  subtotal gastric exclusion

exclusion (*continued*)
  total vascular exclusion
  vascular exclusion
  ventricular exclusion
exclusion bypass
exclusion clamp
excochleation
excoriated
excoriation
excrement
excrescence
  bony excrescence
  cauliflower excrescence
  enamel excrescence
  fluffy excrescences
  fungating excrescence
  fungous excrescence
  Lambl excrescence
  wart-like excrescence
excretion and secretion
excretion cystogram
excretion cystography
excretion of dye
excretion of protein
excretion pyelogram
excretion pyelography
excretion rate
excretion urogram
excretion urography
excretory cystogram
excretory duct
excretory function
excretory pyelogram
excretory urethrogram
excretory urogram
excretory urography
excruciating pain
excursion
  costal excursion
  diaphragmatic excursions
  dome excursion
  expansion and excursion
  eyelid excursion
  insertional excursion
  lateral excursion
  left lateral excursion
  protrusive excursion
  range of excursion
  respiratory excursion
  retrusive excursion
  right lateral excursion
  tendon excursion

exdwelling ureteral occlusion
  balloon catheter
exenterated orbit
exenteration
  anterior pelvic exenteration
  Brunschwig total pelvic
    exenteration
  ethmoid exenteration
  Iliff exenteration
  orbital exenteration
  organ exenteration
  pelvic exenteration
  pelvic organ exenteration
  petrous pyramid exenteration
  posterior exenteration
  posterior pelvic exenteration
  subtotal orbital exenteration
  supralevator pelvic
    exenteration
  total pelvic exenteration
exenteration forceps
exenteration of eye
exenteration of orbital contents
exenteration of pelvic organs
exenteration of sinus
exenteration spoon
exenterative
Exerball kit
exercise band
exercise imaging
exercise treadmill
exercise-associated acute renal
  failure
exeresis
exertional anterior
  compartment syndrome
exertional deep posterior
  compartment syndrome
Exeter bone lavage
Exeter intramedullary bone plug
Exeter ophthalmoscope
Ex-Fi-Re external fixation device
exfoliated
exfoliation syndrome
exfoliative
exfoliator
exit access
exit block
exit block murmur
eXit disposable puncture
  closure device
exit point

exit pupil
exit site
exit site infection
exit wound
Exmoor plastics aural grommet
Exner plexus
Exner rib shears
exocardial murmur
exoccipital bone
exocoelomic cavity
exocoelomic membrane
exocentric construction
exocervix
exocrine gland
exodontia
exogenous aneurysm
exogenous anticoagulant
    coagulation
exogenous disease
exogenous fibrin clot
exogenous reconstruction
exolever forceps
Exo-Overhead traction unit
exophthalmic goiter
exophthalmometer
    Hertel exophthalmometer
    Krahn exophthalmometer
    Luedde exophthalmometer
    Marco prism
        exophthalmometer
    Naugle orbitometer
        exophthalmometer
exophthalmometry
exophthalmos
exophytic adenocarcinoma
exophytic carcinoma
exophytic joint disease
exophytic lesion
exophytic mass
exoskeleton
Exo-Static cervical collar
Exo-Static overhead tractor
exostectomy
exostosectomy
exostosis (*pl.* exostoses)
    cartilaginous exostosis
    dental exostosis
    ivory exostosis
    metatarsal cuneiform
        exostosis
    osteocartilaginous exostosis
    osteochondral exostosis

exostosis (*continued*)
    subungual exostosis
    turret exostosis
exostosis bursata
exostosis cartilaginea
exostosis formation
exotropia
expandable access catheter
expandable biliary
    endoprosthesis
expandable blade
expandable breast implant
expandable cervical dilator
expandable esophageal stent
expandable intrahepatic
    portacaval shunt stent
expandable metal mesh
    endoprosthesis
expandable metallic stent
expandable olive
expandable prosthesis
Expandacell sponge
expanded free scalp flap
expanded lung
expanded
    polytetrafluoroethylene
    (ePTFE) implant
expanded
    polytetrafluoroethylene
    (EPTFE) sutures
expanded
    polytetrafluoroethylene
    vascular graft
expanded 2-flap method for
    microtia reconstruction
expander
    AccuSpan tissue expander
    Becker tissue expander
    BioDimensional tissue
        expander
    Biospan anatomical tissue
        expander
    Biospan breast tissue
        expander
    blood expander
    Cox-Uphoff International
        tissue expander (CUI tissue
        expander)
    Cox-Uphoff skin expander
    CUI tissue expander (Cox-
        Uphoff International tissue
        expander)

expander (*continued*)
  Dermamesh graft expander
  field expander
  Graether pupil expander
  Hespan plasma volume
    expander
  hetastarch plasma expander
  Hextend plasma volume
    expander
  Heyer-Schulte subcutaneous
    tissue expander
  Heyer-Schulte tissue expander
  Integra tissue expander
  McGhan Magna-Site tissue
    expander
  McGhan tissue expander
  Mentor Spectrum contour
    expander
  Mentor tissue expander
  Meshgraft skin expander
  plasma expander
  plasma volume expander
  PMT AccuSpan tissue
    expander
  PMT tissue expander
  Porex tissue expander
  Radovan subcutaneous tissue
    expander
  rectal expander
  Ruiz-Cohen round expander
  saline-filled expander
  self-inflating tissue expander
  Silastic HP tissue expander
  slow palatal expander
  soft tissue expander
  subcutaneous tissue expander
  subperiosteal tissue expander
    (STE)
  surgical skin graft expander
  Surgitek expander
  Surgitek T-Span tissue
    expander
  tissue expander
  T-Span tissue expander
  Versafil tissue expander
Expander mammary implant
expander pocket
expanding hematoma
expanding reamer
expanding retroperitoneal
  hematoma
Expand-O-Graft cutter

Expand-O-Graft disposable cutter
expansible infrastructure
  endosteal implant
expansible osseous neoplasm
expansile abdominal mass
expansile dilator
expansile forceps
expansile knife
expansile pulsation
expansile unilocular well-
  demarcated bone lesion
expansile valvulotome
expansion
  balloon expansion
  clonal expansion
  controlled expansion
  delayed expansion
  dental arch expansion
  dorsal expansion
  effective setting expansion
  field expansion
  hygroscopic expansion
  infarct expansion
  intraoperative skin expansion
  intravascular volume
    expansion
  investment expansion
  lateral extensor expansion
  linear thermal expansion
  maxillary expansion
  mercuroscopic expansion
  mesangial matrix expansion
  monoclonal expansion
  palatal expansion
  perceptual expansion
  plasma volume expansion
  rapid maxillary expansion
  repeated tissue expansion
  scalp expansion
  scalp tissue expansion
  secondary expansion
  serial expansion
  setting expansion
  skin expansion
  slow maxillary expansion
  stent expansion
  surgical-assisted rapid palatal
    expansion (SARPE)
  thermal coefficient expansion
  tissue expansion
  volume expansion
  wax expansion

expansion and activator therapy
expansion and excursion
expansion of chest
expansion of lung
expansion of arch
expansion plate appliance
expansion screw
expansive laminaplasty
expected date of confinement
  (EDC)
expelled afterbirth
expelled fetus
expelled flatus
expelled placenta
Expert bone densitometer
expiration and inspiration
expiration-inspiration ratio
expiratory curve
expiratory flow
expiratory flow rate
expiratory pressure
expiratory rhonchi
expiratory sounds
expiratory valve
expiratory wheezes
expired air collection
expirograph
  Godart expirograph
explant
  encircling explant
  episcleral explant
  Molteno episcleral explant
  posterior explant
  segmental explant
  sponge explant
explantation
  mammary prosthesis
    explantation
exploding head syndrome
Explora uterine curet
exploration
  abdominal exploration
  arthrotomy with exploration
  bilateral neck exploration
  bile duct exploration
  bronchotomy with
    exploration
  common bile duct
    exploration
  common duct exploration
  complete surgical exploration
  contralateral groin exploration

exploration (*continued*)
  duct exploration
  formal surgical exploration
  groin exploration
  intra-abdominal exploration
  laparoscopic common bile
    duct exploration
  laparoscopic transcystic
    common bile duct
    exploration (LTCBDE)
  laparoscopic transcystic duct
    exploration
  laparoscopically guided
    transcystic exploration
  Lynch frontal sinus
    exploration
  neck exploration
  open common bile duct
    exploration
  petrous pyramid air cell
    exploration
  remedial inguinal exploration
  routine bilateral neck
    exploration
  routine unilateral exploration
  sclerotomy with exploration
  standard neck exploration
  surgical exploration
  unilateral neck exploration
exploration and repair
exploratory biopsy
exploratory bougie
exploratory celiotomy
exploratory drive
exploratory incision
exploratory laparotomy
exploratory meatoantrotomy
exploratory operation
exploratory pneumonotomy
exploratory procedure
exploratory puncture
exploratory stroke
exploratory suction tip
exploratory surgery
exploratory thoracotomy
exploratory trephine
explorer
  disk explorer
  Hoen explorer
exploring cannula
exploring electrode
exploring needle

explosion fracture
explosion injury
explosive decompression
Expo eye dressing
Explorer pre-curved diagnostic
    EP catheter
expose retractor
exposed bone
exposed capsule
exposed organ
exposed tissue
exposing peritoneum
exposure
exposure keratitis
exposure keratopathy
exposure meter
Express balloon
express lens
Express OTW balloon catheter
Express PTCA catheter
Express stent
expressed skull fracture
expressor (*see also* lens
    expressor)
  Arroyo expressor
  Arruga eye expressor
  Arruga lens expressor
  Bagley-Wilmer lens expressor
  Berens lens expressor
  follicle lid expressor
  Fyodorov lens expressor
  Goldmann expressor
  Heath follicle expressor
  Heath lid expressor
  Hess tonsil expressor
  Heyner expressor
  hook expressor
  Hosford meibomian gland
      expressor
  intracapsular lens expressor
  iris expressor
  Kirby hook expressor
  Kirby intracapsular lens
      expressor
  Kirby lens expressor
  lens expressor
  lid expressor
  McDonald expressor
  Medallion lens expressor
  meibomian gland expressor
  nucleus expressor
  Osher nucleus stab expressor

expressor (*continued*)
  ring lens expressor
  Rizzuti eye expressor
  Rizzuti iris expressor
  Rizzuti lens expressor
  Smith lens expressor
  Smith lid expressor
  Stahl nucleus expressor
  tonsillar expressor
  Verhoeff lens expressor
  Wilmer-Bagley iris expressor
  Wilmer-Bagley lens expressor
expressor hook
expressor lens
expressor loop
expulsion
expulsion contraction
expulsion stent
expulsive hemorrhage
expulsive pain
exquisite pain
exquisite tenderness
exquisitely tender abdomen
EXS femoropopliteal bypass
    graft
EXS vascular graft
exsanguinate
exsanguinating hemorrhage
exsanguination
exsanguination tourniquet
    control
exsanguination transfusion
exsanguinotransfusion
exsect
exsection
exsector
exstrophy closure
exstrophy epispadias complex
exstrophy of bladder
exstrophy reconstruction
extended anatomical chin
extended anatomical high-
    profile malar implant
extended clasp
extended criteria donor (ECD)
extended end-to-end
    anastomosis
extended field irradiation therapy
extended frontal approach
extended iliofemoral approach
extended lateral arm free flap
    (ELAFF)

extended lateral arm free flap
  for head/neck
  reconstruction
extended left hepatectomy
extended left subcostal incision
extended liposuction
extended mandatory minute
  ventilation (EMMV)
extended mesh technique
extended mesorectal excision
extended multiplanar
  multivector face-lift
extended open-tip rhinoplasty
extended pelvic
  lymphadenectomy
extended position
extended posterior
  rhytidectomy
extended radical mastectomy
extended resection
extended right hemicolectomy
extended right hepatectomy
extended Ross procedure
extended round needle
extended sector ultrasonic probe
extended shoulder flap
extended subfrontal approach
extended sub-SMAS face-lift
extended supraplatysmal plane
  (ESP)
extended supraplatysmal plane
  (ESP) face-lift technique
Extended Wear self-adhering
  urinary external catheter
Extended Wear self-adhering
  urinary external catheter
  starter kit
extended-incision technique
extender
  autograft extender
  Kalish Duredge wire extender
  Küntscher nail extender
  Mentor penile prosthesis with
    rear-tip extender
  rear-tip extender
  Rousek extender
  Superstabilizer cemented
    stem extender
  Superstabilizer press-fit stem
    extender
  Sven Johansson extender
  Taq extender

Extendex tubing
Extend-It finger splint
extensibility
extensile approach
extension
  4th-blade extension
  angle of greatest extension
    (AGE)
  atlantooccipital extension
  attached gingiva extension
  Balfour 4th-blade extension
  Bardenheuer extension
  bifurcated drain extension
  Buck extension
  caliceal extension
  Centurion needleless catheter
    extensions
  clot extension
  Codivilla extension
  compression extension
  cranial extension
  deep brain extension
  distractive extension
  DOC guidewire extension
  extranodal extension
  extranodal tumor extension
  extrapancreatic extension
  extrascleral extension
  femoral-trunk extension
  finger-like extension
  flexion and extension
  flexion, abduction, external
    rotation, extension (fabere)
  footboard extension
  forced extension
  forceful extension
  full extension
  glottic extension
  greatest angle of extension
  groove extension
  head extension
  hip extension
  Hudson cerebellar extension
  infarct extension
  internal rotation in extension
  intrasellar extension
  Jackson-Pratt bifurcated drain
    extension
  knee extension
  lateral extension
  Linx guidewire extension
  LOC guidewire extension

extension (*continued*)
  local tumor extension
  lumbar extension
  nail extension
  needle extension
  NexGen offset stem extension
  Orascoptic loupe extension
  orbital extension
  paraplegia in extension
  resisted radial wrist extension
  ridge extension
  scalp extension
  Steinmann extension
  subependymal extension
  syringe extension
  thrombus extension
  tonsillar syringe extension
  wrist extension
extension base
extension bone clamp
extension bow
extension bridge
extension clamp
extension deformity
extension excementosis
extension fiber
extension for prevention
extension form
extension injury
extension instability
extension malposition
extension osteotomy
extension restriction
extension splint
extension teardrop fracture
extension traction
extension tractor
extension tube
extension tubing with
  connector
extension-type cervical spine
  injury
extensive debridement
extensive lymph node dissection
extensive posterior
  decompression
extensive resection
extensive-stage disease
extensor aponeurosis
extensor brevis flap
extensor carpi radialis brevis
  muscle (ECRB)

extensor carpi radialis longus
  (ECRL) muscle
extensor carpi radialis longus
  (ECRL) tendon
extensor carpi radialis longus
  flap
extensor carpi ulnaris (ECU)
  muscle
extensor carpi ulnaris (ECU)
  tendon
extensor digiti minimi muscle
extensor digiti minimi tendon
extensor digitorum brevis (EDB)
extensor digitorum communis
  tendon
extensor digitorum longus flap
extensor digitorum longus
  muscle
extensor digitorum muscle
extensor hallucis longus muscle
extensor indicis muscle
extensor indicis proprius (EIP)
  tendon
extensor mechanism dysfunction
extensor muscle
extensor pollicis brevis muscle
  (EPB)
extensor pollicis longus (EPL)
  muscle
extensor pollicis longus (EPL)
  tendon
extensor retinaculum
extensor retinaculum of ankle
extensor retinaculum of wrist
extensor tendon
extensor tendon injury
extensor tendon reconstruction
extensor tendon repair
extensor tenosynovectomy
extensor thrust reflex
extensor wad of three
exterior pelvic device
exteriorization colostomy
exteriorization of rectum
exteriorization of the umbilicus
exteriorize
exteriorized uterine repair
externa
  auris externa
  basis carinii externa
  benign necrotizing otitis
    externa (BNOE)

externa (*continued*)
  facies externa
  lamina externa
  malignant necrotizing otitis
    externa (MNOE)
  otitis externa
external acoustic foramen
external acoustic meatus
external anal sphincter muscle
external angle
external aperture of canaliculus
  of cochlea
external artery of nose
external asynchronous
  pacemaker
external auditory canal (EAC)
external auditory larynx
external axis of eye
external beam irradiation
external beam radiation therapy
external bevel incision
external bile drainage
external bile tract drainage
external biliary drainage
external biliary fistula
external biliary lavage
external bleeding
external branch of the superior
  laryngeal (EBSL) nerve
external calcaneoastragaloid
  ligament
external canal
external canthotomy
external canthus
external capsule
external cardiac massage
external carotid artery
external carotid nerve
external carotid vein
external chest compression
external clot
external collimator
external compression
external counterpressure device
external cruciate ligament
external demand pacemaker
external ear
external ear canal
external elastic lamina
external electrode
external ethmoidectomy
external fetal monitoring

external fixator
external frontal crest
external frontal sinusotomy
external functional
  neuromuscular stimulator
external geniculate body
external genitalia
external genitalia reconstruction
external genu of facial nerve
external hemipelvectomy
external hemorrhage
external hemorrhoid
external hemorrhoidectomy
external hernia
external iliac artery
external iliac lymph node
external iliac vein
external iliac vessel
external inflatable compressor
external inguinal ring
external intercostal muscles
external jugular vein
external landmark
external lateral ligament
external levator resection for
  ptosis
external levator resection to
  repair blepharoptosis
external ligament
external ligament of malleus
external ligament of mandibular
  articulation
external ligament of
  temporomandibular
  articulation
external ligament of
  temporomandibular joint
external mammary artery
external mammary vein
external mastoid process
external maxillary artery
external meatus
external mental crest
external monitor
external musculature
external nasal nerve
external nasal nerve block
external nasal splint
external nasal veins
external nose
external oblique aponeurosis
external oblique fascia

external oblique line
external oblique muscle
external oblique reflex
external oblique ridge
external obturator muscle
external occipital crest
external occipital protuberance
external orbital fracture
external orifice
external orthosis
external orthovoltage irradiation
external os
external osteotomy
external pacemaker
external palatine vein
external pancreatic fistula
external paralateronasal skin
    incision
external perineal fascia
external pharyngotomy
    approach
external photography
external pillar
external pin fixation
external pneumatic calf
    compression
external popliteal nerve
external proctotomy
external prosthesis
external pterygoid muscle
external pterygoid nerve
external pterygoid vein
external pudendal artery
external pudendal vein
external pudic vessel
external radial vein
external radiation therapy
external rectal sphincter
external rectus muscle
external rectus sheath
external ring
external rotation
external rotator
external salivary gland
external secretion
external semilunar cartilage
external shock wave lithotripsy
external sinusotomy
external skin tag
external spermatic artery
external spermatic fascia
external spermatic nerve

external sphenoid sinusotomy
external sphincter
external spinal fixation
external spinal skeletal fixator
external splint
external stripper
external table
external tachyarrhythmia control
external traction
external transthoracic
    pacemaker
external ureteral catheter
external urethral orifice
external urethral sphincter
external urethrotomy
external vacuum therapy
external vascular compression
    device
external vein stripper
external ventricular drainage
external version
external x-ray therapy
external-alignment compression
    jig
external-internal pacemaker
externalize
externally controlled pacemaker
externally releasable knot
externally rotated
externally supported Dacron
    graft
externofrontal retractor
extirpation
    Amreich vaginal extirpation
    dental pulp extirpation
    nodal extirpation
    pulp extirpation
    Rubbrecht extirpation
    sac extirpation
    surgical extirpation
extirpation of ganglion
extirpative defect
Extra Sport coronary guidewire
Extra View balloon
extra-abdominal anastomosis
extra-abdominal disease
extra-abdominal infective
    complication
extra-abdominal injury
extra-abdominal operation
extra-abdominal position
extra-alveolar crown

extra-anatomic bypass
extra-anatomic bypass
    procedure
extra-anatomic bypass technique
extra-anatomical renal
    revascularization technique
extra-arachnoid injection
extra-articular arthrodesis
extra-articular augmentation
extra-articular causes of wrist
    pain
extra-articular fracture
extra-articular graft
extra-articular hip fusion
extra-articular pain syndrome
extra-articular procedure
extra-articular reconstruction
extra-articular resection
extra-articular subtalar fusion
extra-articular subtalar joint
extra-articular technique
extra-axial brain tumor
extra-axial fluid collection
extra-axial injury
extrabursal approach
extracanthic diameter
extracapillary crescent formation
extracapsular
extracapsular ankylosis
extracapsular cataract extraction
    (ECCE)
extracapsular disease
extracapsular dissection
extracapsular extraction
extracapsular extraction of
    cataract
extracapsular eye forceps
extracapsular forceps
extracapsular fracture
extracapsular lens extraction
extracapsular metastasis
extracardiac graft
extracardiac right-to-left shunt
extracardiac shunt
extracellular matrix (ECM)
extracellular space
extracerebral factors
extracerebral fluid collection
extrachromic sutures
extraconal fat
extraconal fat compartment
extracoronal attachment

extracoronal retainer
extracorporeal anastomosis
extracorporeal bypass
extracorporeal circulation
extracorporeal CO_2 removal
    (ECOR)
extracorporeal exchange
    hypothermia
extracorporeal heart
extracorporeal irradiation
extracorporeal jamming knot
extracorporeal liver assist device
    (ELAD)
extracorporeal liver perfusion
extracorporeal membrane
    oxygenation (ECMO)
extracorporeal membrane
    oxygenator (ECMO)
extracorporeal perfusion
extracorporeal piezoelectric
    lithotriptor (EPL)
extracorporeal piezoelectric
    shock wave lithotripsy
extracorporeal procedure
extracorporeal pump
extracorporeal pump
    oxygenator
extracorporeal repair
extracorporeal shock wave
    lithotripsy (ESWL)
extracorporeal shock wave
    lithotriptor
extracorporeal surgery
extracorporeal technique
extracorporeal venous bypass
extracostal bundle
extracostal muscle
extracranial carotid artery
    disease
extracranial carotid circulation
extracranial carotid occlusive
    disease
extracranial mass lesion
extracranial meningioma
extracranial occlusive vascular
    disease
extracranial-intracranial bypass
    (ECIC bypass)
extracting forceps
extraction
    allograft extraction
    Arroyo cataract extraction

extraction (*continued*)
Arruga cataract extraction
bag extraction
Baker pyridine extraction
breech extraction
Burhenne biliary duct stone
 extraction
calculus extraction
cataract extraction
Chandler-Verhoeff lens
 extraction
comedo extraction
countercurrent extraction
cryocataract extraction
cryogenic cataract extraction
Daviel cataract extraction
dental extraction
elevator extraction
endoscopic extraction
extracapsular cataract
 extraction (ECCE)
extracapsular extraction
extracapsular lens extraction
1st-pass extraction
forceps extraction
foreign body extraction
harpoon extraction
intracapsular cataract
 extraction (ICCE)
intracapsular lens extraction
intraocular cataract extraction
Kirby cataract extraction
lactate extraction
laparoscopic stone
 extraction
lens extraction
liquid extraction
magnetic extraction
Malstrom extraction
manual extraction
Marshall-Taylor vacuum
 extraction
McIntyre intracapsular lens
 extraction
menstrual extraction
micro liquid extraction
partial breech extraction
podalic extraction
progressive extraction
rubber-band extraction
serial extraction
Smith cataract extraction

extraction (*continued*)
solid phase extraction
solvent extraction
spontaneous breech
 extraction
stone extraction
subtotal cataract extraction
suction extraction
systemic oxygen extraction
tooth extraction
total breech extraction
total cataract extraction
tumbling-technique cataract
 extraction
vacuum extraction
Vantos vacuum extraction
extraction atherectomy device
extraction balloon
extraction balloon technique
extraction bile duct stone
extraction flap
extraction forceps
extraction generator
extraction hook
extraction incision
extraction of calculus
extraction of cataract
extraction of kidney stone
extraction of lens
extraction of teeth
extraction of tooth
extraction of ureteral stone
extraction pancreatic stone
extraction pliers
extraction site
extraction space
extraction test
extractor (*see also*
 cryoextractor)
Amico extractor
Andrews comedo extractor
Applied Biosystems 340A
 nucleic acid extractor
Austin Moore extractor
ball extractor
Bellows cryoextractor
 extractor
Bilos pin extractor
Bird vacuum extractor
broach extractor
buccal fat extractor
cataract extractor

extractor (*continued*)
  cataract rotoextractor
    extractor
  Cherry extractor
  Cherry screw extractor
  Cilco extractor
  cloverleaf pin extractor
  comedo extractor
  cortex extractor
  Councill stone extractor
  Councill ureteral stone
    extractor
  deluxe FIN extractor
  DePuy extractor
  Dolan extractor
  driver-bender extractor
  Egnell vacuum extractor
  ERCP balloon extractor
  Eric Lloyd extractor
  Escort balloon stone
    extractor
  femoral head extractor
  femoral trial extractor
  fetal head extractor
  fetal vacuum extractor
  food extractor
  Gills-Welsh cortex extractor
  Glassman stone extractor
  Grieshaber extractor
  Hallach comedo extractor
  Hansen-Street driver-extractor
  hatchet extractor
  head extractor
  hoe extractor
  hooked extractor
  Intraflex intramedullary pin
    extractor
  Jarit comedo extractor
  Jewett bone extractor
  Kalish Duredge wire extractor
  Kelman extractor
  Ken driver-extractor
  Küntscher extractor
  Kobayashi vacuum extractor
  Krwawicz cataract extractor
  Lempert extractor
  Lewicky cortex extractor
  Lloyd nail extractor
  Look cortex extractor
  Luxator extractor
  magnetic extractor
  Malström vacuum extractor

extractor (*continued*)
  Mark II femoral component
    extractor
  Mark II tibial component
    extractor
  Massie extractor
  McDermott extractor
  McLaughlin extractor
  McNutt extractor
  McReynolds driver-extractor
  McReynolds extractor
  Mignon cataract extractor
  Mityvac extractor
  Moore extractor
  Moore hooked extractor
  Moore nail extractor
  Moore prosthesis extractor
  Moore-Blount extractor
  M-type extractor
  Murless fetal head extractor
  Murless head extractor
  Murless vector head extractor
  Rush extractor
  Rush pin driver-bender
    extractor
  Rush pin lead-filled head
    mallet with extractor
  Rutner stone extractor
  Saalfeld comedo extractor
  Schamberg comedo extractor
  Schamberg extractor
  Schneider extractor
  Schneider driver-extractor
  Schneider nail extractor
  Silastic cup extractor
  Silc extractor
  Simcoe cortex extractor
  Smirmaul nucleus extractor
  Smith-Petersen extractor
  Smith-Petersen nail extractor
  Soehendra stent extractor
  Southwick screw extractor
  stem extractor
  stone extractor
  Take-Out extractor
  T-C ring-handle pin and wire
    extractor
  Tender Touch extractor
  Thompson root extractor
  Torpin vectis extractor
  Trizol RNA extractor
  Troutman cataract extractor

extractor (*continued*)
  Unna comedo extractor
  Unna extractor
  ureteral stone extractor
  Vantos vacuum extractor
  Visitec cortex extractor
  Walton comedo extractor
  Walton extractor
  Welsh cortex extractor
  Wilson-Cook 8-wire basket
    stone extractor
  Zimmer extractor
  Zimmer driver-extractor
extractor hook
extractor injector
extractor nail drill
Extractor 3-lumen retrieval
  balloon catheter
Extractor triple-lumen retrieval
  balloon
extractor/injector cannula
extracutaneous vas fixation clamp
extradural abscess
extradural anesthesia
extradural anesthetic technique
extradural block
extradural compression
extradural cord compression
extradural defect
extradural exposure
extradural granulation
extradural hematoma
extradural hemorrhage
extradural metastatic disease
extradural space
extraesophageal reflux
extrafascial apicolysis
extrafascial hysterectomy
Extrafil breast implant
extrafollicular
extrahepatic abdominal
  carcinoma
extrahepatic bile duct
extrahepatic bile duct
  obstruction
extrahepatic biliary atresia
extrahepatic biliary cystic dilation
extrahepatic biliary obstruction
extrahepatic control
extrahepatic dissection
extrahepatic lesion
extrahepatic metastasis

extrahepatic nodal disease
extrahepatic obstruction
extrahepatic portal vein
  obstruction (HPO)
extrahepatic shunt
extrahepatic venous obstruction
extraintestinal complication
extralaryngeal approach
extralaryngeal muscle
extralaryngeal skeleton
extraluminal hemorrhage
extraluminal stripper
extralymphatic metastasis
extramammary disease
extramammary Paget disease
extramedullary alignment arch
extramedullary alignment guide
extramedullary involvement
extramedullary tibial alignment jig
extramucosal stitch
extramucosal tunnels
extramural lesion
extramural upper airway
  obstruction
extraneous electrode potential
extraneous movement
extranodal disease
extranodal extension
extranodal malignant lymphoma
extranodal non-Hodgkin
  lymphoma
extranodal tumor extension
extraoctave fracture
extraocular motion (EOM)
extraocular movement (EOM)
extraocular muscle involvement
extraocular muscles (EOM)
extraocular tension
extraoral appliance
extraoral approach
extraoral bone-anchored implant
extraoral defect
extraoral fracture appliance
extraoral incision
extraoral open reduction of
  mandible
extraoral sigmoid notch
  retractor
extraorbital disease
extraosseous
extraosseous chondrosarcoma
extrapancreatic extension

extrapelvic disease
extraperiosteal plombage
extraperiosteal pneumonolysis
extraperitoneal laparoscopic
    bladder neck suspension
extraperitoneal approach
extraperitoneal carbon dioxide
    insufflation
extraperitoneal cesarean section
extraperitoneal CO_2 insufflation
extraperitoneal endoscopic
    hernia repair
extraperitoneal endoscopic pelvic
    lymph node dissection
extraperitoneal fat
extraperitoneal laparoscopic
    herniorrhaphy
extraperitoneal space
extraperitoneal tissue
extrapetrosal drainage
extrapharyngeal approach
extrapharyngeal exposure
extrapleural anastomosis
extrapleural apicolysis
extrapleural fascia
extrapleural pneumonolysis
extrapleural pneumothorax
extrapleural resection of rib
extrapleural space
extrapolar region
extrapyramidal disease
extrapyramidal signs
extrapyramidal syndrome
extrasaccular hernia
ExtraSafe butterfly infusion needle
ExtraSafe catheter
ExtraSafe phlebotomy device
ExtraSafe syringe
extrascleral extension
extraskeletal chondroma
extraskeletal chondrosarcoma
extrasphincteric anal fistula
extra-stiff Amplatz wire
extra-stiff guidewire
extrastimulus technique
extra-support guidewire
extratemporal excision
extratesticular lesion
extrathoracic carotid subclavian
    bypass graft
extrathoracic metastasis
extrathoracic position

extrathoracic spread of cancer
extrathyroid invasion
extrauterine pelvic mass
extrauterine pregnancy
extravasated contract medium
extravasation
    fluid extravasation
    vascular extravasation
extravasation extremity
extravasation extrusion
extravasation feces
extravasation gas
extravasation injury
extravasation irrigation solution
extravasation of blood
extravasation of contrast medium
extravasation of urine
extravasation phenomenon
extravascular granulomatous
    features
extravascular space
extravelar muscle bundle
extraventricular drain
extravesical anastomosis
extravesical Lich approach
extravesical ureteral
    reimplantation technique
Extreme laser catheter
extreme lateral transcondylar
    approach
extreme Trendelenburg position
extremity abnormality
extremity amputation
extremity injury
extremity lesion
extremity malformation
extremity mobilization technique
extremity perfusion
extremity pump
extremity strength
ExtreSafe butterfly
ExtreSafe catheter
ExtreSafe lancet
ExtreSafe needle
ExtreSafe syringe
extrinsic allergic alveolitis
extrinsic bladder compression
extrinsic colon deformity
extrinsic compression
extrinsic defect
extrinsic denervation
extrinsic entrapment test

extrinsic environmental staining
extrinsic esophageal impression
extrinsic lesion
extrinsic mass
extrinsic mechanism
extrinsic muscle
extrinsic muscle of tongue
extrinsic muscle strength
extrinsic muscles of larynx
extrinsic nerve
extrinsic obstruction
extrinsic pathway
extrinsic pressure
extrinsic semiconductor
extrinsic sphincter
extruded disk
extruded disk fragment
extrusion
  bone graft extrusion
  centripetal extrusion
  disk extrusion
  extravasation extrusion
  implant extrusion
  oocyte extrusion
  placental extrusion
  sealer extrusion
  tube extrusion
  wire extrusion
extrusion balloon catheter
extrusion needle
extubation anesthetic technique
exuberant cicatrization
exuberant granulation
exudate
  acute inflammatory exudate
  circinate exudate
  conjunctival exudate
  cotton-wool exudate
  fatty exudate
  fibrinous exudate
  fluffy cotton-wool exudate
  foaming exudate
  gingival exudate
  hard exudate
  inflammatory exudate
  mucopurulent exudate
  pharyngeal exudate
  purulent exudate
  retinal exudate
  sanguineous exudate
  serous exudate
  soft exudate

exudate (*continued*)
  suppurative exudate
  tonsillar exudate
  waxy exudate
exudate disposal bag
exudation
  fibrinous exudation
  gingival exudation
  proteinaceous aqueous
    exudation
  purulent exudation
exudative ascites
exudative calcifying fasciitis
exudative granulomatous
    inflammation
exudative papulosquamous
    disease
exudative retinal detachment
exudative tonsillitis
ExuDerm hydrocolloid dressing
ExuDry absorptive dressing
exumbilication
eye
  appendages of the eye
  artificial eye
  asymmetric folds of eyes
  bagginess of eyes
  bony orbit of eye
  chamber of eye
  conformer for eye
  convergence of eyes
  cotton-ball hemorrhage of eye
  deorsumduction of eye
  dextroduction of eye
  enucleation of eye
  equator of eye
  exenteration of eye
  external axis of eye
  forced duction of eye
  globe of eye
  humor of eye
  lateral angle of eye
  levoduction of eye
  medial angle of eye
  patch eye
  raccoon eyes
  reform eye
  refraction of eye
  rudimentary eye
  schematic eye
  Snellen reform eye
  sphincter of eye

eye (*continued*)
  squinting eye
  vertical axis of eye
eye and ear cannula
eye aperture
eye bandage
eye blade
eye bottle rack
eye bubble
eye calipers
eye cautery
eye conformer
eye curet
eye cystitome
eye diathermy electrode
eye disease
eye displacement
eye drape
eye dressing
eye drill in arthrotomy
eye drops
eye enucleation
eye enucleation snare
eye evisceration spoon
eye examination
eye fixation forceps
eye fixation hook
eye forceps
eye heating pad
eye hook
eye implant (*see* implant)
eye implant conformer
eye infection
eye irrigator
eye knife
eye knife blade
eye knife box
eye knife guard
eye knife plastic box
eye lesion
eye loupe
eye magnet
eye motion
eye movement
eye movement artifact
eye muscle surgery
eye needle
eye needle holder
eye needle holder forceps
eye occluder
eye pad
eye pad dressing

eye patch
eye point
eye probe
eye protector
eye response
eye retractor
eye scissors
eye shield (*see* shield)
eye speculum
eye sphere implant
eye sphere introducer
eye spherical implant
eye spoon
eye spud
eye stitch scissors
eye surgery blade
eye suture forceps
eye suture scissors
eye sutures
eye tumor localization
eyeball
  avulsion of eyeball
  Bonnet enucleation of eyeball
  Critchett excision of anterior
    eyeball
  dimpling of eyeball
  enucleation of eyeball
  evisceration of eyeball
  shortening of eyeball
eyeball compression reflex
eyeball movement
eyeball under tension
eyebrow fixation
eyebrow height
eyebrow laceration
eyebrow lift
eyebrow ptosis
eyebrowpexy
eye-closure reflex
Eyecor camera
eyed needle
eyed obturator
eyed probe
eyed suture needle
eye-dressing forceps
eye-ear plane
EyeFix speculum
eye-fixation forceps
eyeglasses
eye-irrigating tip
eyelash loss
eyelash reflex

eyeless atraumatic suture needle
eyeless needle
eyeless suture needle
eyelet clasp
eyelet lag screw
eyelid
  Argyll Robertson strap
    operation for ectropion of
    eyelid
  crepitation in the lower
    eyelids
  ectropion of eyelid
  free margin of eyelid
  gray line of upper eyelid
  inelastic lower eyelid
  lateral commissure of eyelids
  lower eyelid
  medial commissure of eyelids
  upper eyelid
eyelid crease suture
eyelid excursion
eyelid forceps
eyelid fusion
eyelid invagination
eyelid laxity
eyelid margin
eyelid operation
eyelid ptosis
eyelid reconstruction
eyelid redundancy
eyelid resection
eyelid retractor
eyelid speculum
eyelid sphincter
eyelid sulcus placement
eyelid surgery
eyelid swelling
eyelid tightening
eyelid closure reflex
eyelidplasty
  double eyelidplasty
  double-fold line in double
    eyelidplasty
eyeline tattoo
Eye-Pak drape

eyepiece
  comparison eyepiece
  compensating eyepiece
  demonstration eyepiece
  huygenian eyepiece
  microscope eyepiece
  negative eyepiece
  positive eyepiece
  Ramsden eyepiece
  Storz eyepiece
  wide-field eyepiece
  Zeiss eyepiece
  Zeiss microscope eyepiece
eyepiece attachment
eyes, ears, nose, and throat
    (EENT)
eye width apart
Eyler elbow procedure
Eyler flexorplasty
Eyler operation
Eyler procedure
E-Z arm abduction orthosis
E-Z Cath catheter
E-Z Clean cautery tip
E-Z Clean laparoscopic
    electrode
E-Z Flap cranial flap fixation
E-Z Flex jaw exercising device
E-Z guide
EZ hand pump
E-Z hold catheter tube holder
E-Z Ject injector
E-Z syringe
EZ-Derm dressing
EZ-Derm porcine biosynthetic
    wound dressing
EZ-Derm temporary skin
    substitute
Ezeform splint
EZ-EM Cut biopsy needle
EZ-ON surgical bra
EZ-Trac orthopaedic suspension
    device
EZvue violet haptic 1-piece lens
Ezy Wrap shoulder immobilizer

1st cranial nerve
4-,6-,10-shooter Saeed multi-
band ligator
49er knee brace
4-A Magovern heart valve
4-A Magovern prosthesis
4-A Magovern valve prosthesis
4-in-1 cutting block
4M 30-degree arthroscope
4-prong rake retractor
4-strap
4 by 4 (4×4s)
4-bar linkage prosthetic knee
mechanism
4-bar polycentric knee
prosthesis
4-beam laser Doppler probe
4-bone SLAC (scapholunate
advanced collapse) wrist
reconstruction
4-bone SLAC wrist
reconstruction
4-chamber view of heart
4-corner midcarpal fusion
4-degrees-of freedom
manipulator
4-eye catheter
4-flanged nails
4-flap cleft palate repair
4-flap palatoplasty
4-flap procedure
4-flap Webster-Bernard
technique
4-flap Z-plasty
4-footed lens
4-gland hyperplasia
4-head camera
4-hole anteromedial Alta straight
plate
4-hole side plate
4-incision procedure
4-layer bandage
4-legged cage heart valve

4-loop iris clip implant
4-loop iris fixated implant
4-lumen polyvinyl manometric
catheter
4-lumen tube
4-mirror goniolens lens
4-part fracture
4-piece intraocular lens
4-place laminectomy
4-point biopsy
4-point cervical brace
4-point fixation
4-point fixation intraocular
lens
4-point gait
4-point spreader bag
4-port diamond placement
4-port procedure
4-port technique
4-portal technique
4-poster cervical brace
4-poster frame
4-prong finger speculum
4-prong finger splint
4-prong retractor
4-pronged liposuction cannula
4-pronged polyp grasper
4-quadrant biopsy
4-quadrant cervical punch biopsy
4-quadrant hemorrhoidectomy
4-sided cutting needle
4-tailed bandage
4-tailed dressing
4-tap screw
4th blade extension
4th branch anomaly
4th carpometacarpal joint
fracture
4th cranial nerve
4th parallel pelvic plane
4th ventricle
4th-degree radiation injury
4-vessel angiogram

4-vessel arteriogram
4-view chest-ray
4-wing catheter
4-wing drain
4-wing Malecot drain
4-wing Malecot retention
   catheter
5
  cranial nerve 5 (trigeminal)
  Medipain 5
5/500
  Alor 5/500
5000
  Abiomed BVAD 5000
    (biventricular assist device)
510-nm pigmented lesion dye
   laser
511-keV collimator
55 stapler
59
  Paloma Q-YAG 59
5C-T image
5-French angiographic catheter
5-French stiff catheter
5-prong rake blade
5th cranial nerve
5th intercostal space
5th metatarsal bone fracture
four by fours (4× 4s)
5-flap V-Y advancement
5-incision procedure
5-in-one repair
5-one knee ligament repair
5-one reconstruction
5-pin staple
5-port fan placement
5-prong rake blade retractor
FL Fischer bayonet scissors
FL Fischer microsurgical
   neurectomy bayonet
   scissors
F&R (force and rhythm)
FR Thompson hip prosthesis
FR Thompson rasp
Förster (see Foerster)
Foerster enucleation snare
Foerster iris forceps
F2 focal point
FA technique
FAB staging of carcinoma
   (French, American, British
   staging)

Fabco gauze bandage
Fabco gauze dressing
Fabco wrap
fabella (pl. fabellae)
fabellofibular ligament
fabere (flexion, abduction,
   external rotation, extension)
fabere abduction test
fabere extension text
fabere external rotation test
fabere fixation test
fabere sign
fabere-Patrick test
Fabian screw
fabricated implant
Fabry coagulator
Fabry disease
facelift
facelifting
face line
face mask
face presentation
face rest
face shield
face-bow
  adjustable axis face-bow
  Asher high-pull face-bow
face-bow record
face-down position
Face-It protective shield
face-lift (see facelift)
  composite facelift
  deep-plane facelift
  endoscopic facelift
  extended multiplanar
    multivector facelift
  extended sub-SMAS facelift
  FAME facelift
  open facelift
  SASMAS facelift
  secondary skin-only facelift
  sloughed facelift
  subcutaneous temporofacial
    facelift
  subcutaneous
    temporomandibular facelift
  subperiosteal facelift
  subperiosteal minimally
    invasive facelift
  subplatysmal facelift
  vertical facelift
  weekend facelift

facelift flap marker
facelift hematoma
facelift operation
facelift retractor
facelift retractor
facelift scissors
facelift technique
face-neck rejuvenation
    procedure
face-out, whole-body
    plethysmograph
face-shield headband
facet
    articular facet
    calcaneal facet
    clavicular facet
    corneal facet
    costal facet
    fibular facet
    inferior costal facet
    joint facet
    jump facet
    odd facet
    superior articular facet
    superior costal facet
    transverse costal facet
facet anomaly
facet cartilage
facet dislocation
facet eroder
facet excision technique
facet fracture stabilization
    wiring
facet fusion
facet joint injection
facet joint preparation
facet joints
facet of cornea
facet of the soft triangle
facet plane
facet rasp
facet raspatory
facet rhizotomy
facet subluxation
facet subluxation stabilization
    wiring
facet tropism
facetectomy
    O'Donoghue facetectomy
    partial facetectomy
faceted (*also* facetted)
faceted gallstone

faceted stone
face-to-pubes position
facial abrasions
facial aging
facial alloplastic implant
facial analysis
facial angle
facial animation
facial artery
facial artery musculomucosal
    (FAMM) flap
facial artery musculomucosal
    flap reconstruction
facial asymmetry
facial axis
facial bones
facial canal
facial causalgia
facial cleft
facial clefting
facial compression finger
    closure
facial compression skull cap
    closure
facial contour deformity
facial contouring
facial danger zones
facial deformity
Facial Disability Index (FDI)
facial disharmony
facial dysmorphism
facial dysmorphology
facial edema
facial erythema
facial esthetics
facial excursion measurement
facial expression
facial fascial layer
facial fracture
facial fracture appliance
facial fracture appliance dental
    arch bar
facial hamartoma
facial harmony
facial height
facial hemangioma
facial hemiatrophy
facial hemiatrophy of Romberg
facial hemihypertrophy
facial hemiplegia
Facial Impairment Scales for
    clefts

facial implant
facial inclination
facial landmark
facial lipodystrophy
facial mimetic muscle
facial mimetic musculature
facial mimic
facial moulage
facial muscle
facial nerve (cranial nerve 7)
facial nerve branches
facial nerve crossover
facial nerve decompression
facial nerve dissection
facial nerve dissector
facial nerve knife
facial nerve latency
facial nerve misdirection
facial nerve monitor
facial nerve palsy
facial nerve paralysis
facial nerve preservation
facial nerve rerouting
facial nerve resection
facial nerve root
facial nerve sacrifice
facial nerve sign
facial nerve stimulator
facial nerve weakness
facial nerve-preserving
    parotidectomy
facial neuralgia
facial neuromuscular
    dysfunction
facial node
facial palsy
facial paralysis
facial paralysis reconstruction
    with free muscle transfer
facial paralysis reconstruction
    with gracilis free muscle
    transfer
facial paralysis reconstruction
    with pectoralis minor
    muscle transfer
facial paralysis reconstruction
    with rectus abdominis
    muscle transfer
facial plane
facial plane angle
facial plastic surgery scissors
facial plastics garment

facial profile
facial prosthesis
facial prosthetic
facial reanimation
facial recess
facial reconstruction
facial regions
facial rejuvenation
facial restructuring
facial retaining ligaments
facial root
facial skin graft
facial sling
facial spasm
facial subcutaneous lift
facial support
facial surface of maxilla
facial symmetry
facial triangle
facial turnover flap
facial vein
facial weakness
facies
    adenoid facies
    Andy Gump facies
    cherubic facies
    elfin facies
    hound-dog facies
    Hutchinson facies
    leonine facies
    masklike facies
    moon-shaped facies
    myasthenic facies
    myopathic facies
    Potter facies
facies anterior corporis maxillae
facies anterior palpebrarum
facies anterior partis petrosae
facies antonina
facies articularis arytenoidea
    cricoideae
facies articularis cartilaginis
    arytenoideae
facies articularis ossis temporalis
facies articularis thyroidea
    cricoideae
facies bovina
facies contactus dentis
facies cranii
facies distalis dentis
facies externa
facies externa ossis frontalis

facies externa ossis parietalis
facies facialis dentis
facies inferior linguae
facies inferior partis petrosae
facies infratemporalis maxillae
facies interna
facies interna ossis frontalis
facies interna ossis parietalis
facies labialis
facies lateralis ossis zygomatici
facies lingualis dentis
facies maxillaris alae majoris
facies maxillaris ossis palatini
facies medialis cartilaginis
   arytenoideae
facies mesialis dentis
facies nasalis maxillae
facies nasalis ossis palatini
facies occlusalis dentis
facies orbitalis
facies orbitalis alae majoris
facies palatina
facies posterior cartilaginis
   arytenoideae
facies posterior palpebrarum
facies posterior partis petrosae
facies scaphoidea
facies temporalis
facies vestibularis dentis
facile reflex
facilitated angioplasty
facilitation
facilitative
faciobrachial hemiplegia
faciocervical
faciocraniosynostosis
faciolingual
faciolingual hemiplegia
faciomandibular dysostosis
facioplasty
facioplegia
facioscapulohumeral
facioscapulohumeral artery
faciostenosis
faciotelencephalic malformation
Facit uterine polyp forceps
FACScan flow cytometer
FACT (focused appendix
   computed tomography)
FACT catheter
FACT coronary balloon
   angioplasty catheter

FACT-HN (functional assessment
   of cancer therapy, head and
   neck)
factor
   angiogenesis factor
   antinuclear factor (ANF)
   autologous growth factor
      (AGF)
   basic fibroblastic growth
      factor (bFGF)
   blood coagulation factor
   Boltzmann factor
   chemotactic factor
   clotting factor
   coagulation factor
   colony-stimulating factor
      (CSF)
   contributing factor
   endothelial relaxing factor
   epidermal growth factor
      (EGF)
   epithelium-derived relaxation
      factor (EpDRF)
   extracerebral factors
   fibroblast growth factor (FGF)
   filling factor
   genetic factor
   granulocyte colony-
      stimulating factor (G-CSF)
   growth hormone-releasing
      factor (GHRF)
   hereditary factors
   inflammatory transcription
      factor
   inhibiting factor
   insulin-like growth factor
   intensification factor
   intrinsic factor
   macrophage-activating factor
      (MAF)
   macrophage-inhibiting factor
      (MIF)
   melanocyte-stimulating
      hormone-inhibiting factor
   migration-inhibiting factor
      (MIF)
   mitogenic factor (MF)
   nerve factor
   nerve growth factor (NGF)
   neurogenic factor
   osteoclast-activating factor
   platelet factor

factor (*continued*)
  platelet tissue factor
  platelet-activating factor (PAF)
  platelet-aggregating factor
    (PAF)
  platelet-derived growth factor
    (PDGF)
  prognostic factors
  recombinant human insulin-
    like growth factor (rhIGF)
  rheumatoid factor (RF)
  squamous cell carcinoma-
    inhibitory factor (SCCIF)
  sun protection factor (SPF)
  thyrotoxic complement-
    fixation factor
  transforming growth factor
    (TGF)
  tumor angiogenic factor
    (TAF)
  tumor lysis factor
  tumor necrosis factor
  vascular endothelial growth
    factor (VEGF)
factor replacement therapy
factor V Leiden mutation
Faden operation
Faden procedure
Faden retropexy
Faden strabismus operation
Faden sutures
Fader Tip ureteral stent
fadir (flexion, abduction,
  internal rotation) sign
Fager pituitary dissector
Fahey approach
Fahey hip pin
Fahey operation
Fahey pin
Fahey technique
Fahey-Compere pin
Fahey-O'Brien procedure
Fahey-O'Brien technique
Fahrenheit scale
failed anesthesia
failed back surgery syndrome
failed forceps delivery
failed intubation
failed nipple valve
failed procedure
failed surgery
fail-safe device

failure
  acute renal failure (ARF)
  acute respiratory failure
  anastomotic failure
  bone marrow failure
  brittle failure
  bypass failure
  cardiac failure (CF)
  cardiorespiratory failure
  chronic intestinal failure
  chronic renal failure (CRF)
  cocaine-induced respiratory
    failure
  congenital failure
  congestive cardiac failure
  congestive failure
  congestive heart failure (CHF)
  differentiation failure
  dilator placement failure
  ductile failure
  end-stage failure
  end-stage intestinal failure
  end-organ failure
  exercise-associated acute
    renal failure
  flap failure
  fold-flaw failure
  fulminant hepatic failure (FHF)
  functional intestinal failure
  graft failure
  Harrington rod
    instrumentation failure
  heart failure
  hepatic failure
  hepatorenal failure
  implant failure
  implantation failure
  instrumentation failure
  intestinal failure
  intubation failure
  irradiation failure
  kidney failure
  late graft failure
  late wound failure
  liver failure
  microcirculatory failure
  mixed failure
  multiorgan failure (MOF)
  multiorgan system failure
  multiple organ failure (MOF)
  multisystem organ failure
    (MSOF)

failure (*continued*)
  organ failure
  pacemaker failure
  postburn bone marrow failure
  postoperative hepatic failure
  postoperative liver failure
  posttraumatic renal failure
  pouch failure
  progressive failure
  progressive liver failure
  progressive respiratory failure
  pump failure
  renal failure
  respiratory failure
  sclerotherapy failure
  surgeon-dependent technique
    failure
  surgical failure
  suture failure
  technical failure
  ventricular failure
  ventricular heart failure
  wound failure
failure analysis (FA)
failure to awaken
failure to thrive
faint diastolic murmur
faint opacification
Fairbanks operation
Fairbanks technique
Fairbanks-Sever procedure
Fairbanks-Sever shoulder
  procedure
Fairdale orthodontic appliance
Fairline instruments
fait accompli
Fajersztajn sign
Falcao dissector
Falcao erysiphake
Falcao fixation forceps
Falcao suction dissection
Falcao suction dissector
falces (*sing.* falx)
falcial
falciform
falciform cartilage
falciform crest
falciform fold of fascia lata
falciform hymen
falciform ligament
falciform lobule
falciform margin

falciform process
falciform retinal fold
falcine region
Falcon coronary catheter
Falcon filter
Falcon lens
Falcon plastic flask
Falcon single-operator exchange
    balloon catheter
Falconer lobectomy
Falconer maneuver
Falconer rongeur
Falk appendectomy spoon
Falk clamp
Falk forceps
Falk lion-jaw forceps
Falk needle
Falk operation
Falk retractor
Falk spoon
Falk vaginal cuff
Falk vaginal cuff clamp
Falk vaginal retractor
Falk vesicovaginal fistula
    technique
Falk-Shukuris operation
falling palate
fallopian aqueduct
fallopian artery
fallopian canal
fallopian cannula
fallopian catheter
fallopian hiatus
fallopian neuritis
fallopian pregnancy
fallopian tube carcinoma
fallopian tube forceps
fallopian tube metastasis
fallopian tube repair prosthesis
fallopian tubes
falloposcope
falloposcopy
Fallot pentalogy
Fallot tetralogy
Fallot trilogy
Falope ring
Falope tubal sterilization ring
Falope-ring applicator
Falope-ring dilator
Falope-ring dual-incision
    instruments
Falope-ring guide kit

Falope-ring mini-laparotomy
   instruments
Falope-ring single-incision
   instruments
Falope-ring tubal occlusion
   band
Falope-ring tubal sterilization
false aneurysm
false ankylosis
false blepharoptosis
false bruit
false channel formation
false colonic obstruction
false cord carcinoma
false cords
false cyst
false diverticulum
false Dupuytren contracture
false ganglion
false hermaphroditism
false joint
false knot
false labor
false ligament
false membrane
false pregnancy
false ribs
false stricture
false sutures
false teeth
false vocal cord
false-negative
false-negative cholangiogram
false-positive
Falta triad
falx (*pl.* falces)
   aponeurotic falx
   inguinal falx
   ligamentous falx
falx cerebelli
falx cerebri
falx inguinalis
falx ligamentosa
falx of maxillary antrum
FAME facelift
FAME midface elevation
FAME midface lift
familial adenomatous polyposis
   (FAP)
familial aortic ectasia syndrome
familial atypical mole and
   melanoma (FAM-M)

familial atypical multiple mole
   melanoma syndrome
   (FAMMM)
familial breast cancer
familial cardiac myxoma
   syndrome
familial cholestasis syndrome
familial chondrodystrophy
familial colon cancer (FCC)
familial consequence
familial cutaneomucosal VM
familial defect
familial disease
familial disorder
familial dysautonomia
familial exudative
   vitreoretinopathy
familial fibrous dysplasia
familial hemiplegic migraine
familial HPT
familial hypocalciuric
   hypercalcemia
familial indication
familial multigland disease
familial neurilemmatosis
familial osteochondrodystrophy
familial paroxysmal
   rhabdomyolysis
familial polyposis syndrome
familial predisposition
familial tendency
familial white folded dysplasia
FAMM (facial artery
   musculomucosal)
FAMM flap
FAMMM (familial atypical mole
   and melanoma)
FAM-M syndrome
fan elevator retractor
fan flap
fan liver retractor
FANA (fluorescent antinuclear
   antibody test)
fan-beam collimator
fanning of toes
fanning-out technique
fan-shaped flap
Fansler anoscope
Fansler proctoscope
Fansler rectal speculum
Fansler speculum
Fansler-Frykman operation

Fansler-Ives anoscope
Fanta cataract operation
Fanta eye speculum
Fanta operation
Fanta speculum
fantascope
far field
far lateral inferior suboccipital
    approach
far point
far sight
far sutures
Farabeuf amputation
Farabeuf bone clamp
Farabeuf bone rasp
Farabeuf bone-holding forceps
Farabeuf double-ended retractor
Farabeuf elevator
Farabeuf forceps
Farabeuf operation
Farabeuf periosteal elevator
Farabeuf rasp
Farabeuf raspatory
Farabeuf retractor
Farabeuf saw
Farabeuf-Collin raspatory
Farabeuf-Lambotte bone-holding
    clamp
Farabeuf-Lambotte bone-holding
    forceps
Farabeuf-Lambotte clamp
Farabeuf-Lambotte forceps
Farabeur-Lambotte raspatory
Faraci punch
Faraci-Skillern punch
Faraci-Skillern sphenoid punch
Faraday law of induction
Faraday shield
Faraday shielded resonator
faradic current
faradic electrostimulation
faradic stimulation
Farah cystoscopic needle
far-and-near suture technique
far-and-near sutures
Farill operation
Farkas urethral speculum
Farley Elite spinal retractor
Farlow decompressor
Farlow snare
Farlow tongue depressor
Farlow tonsil snare

Farlow tonsillar snare
Farlow-Boettcher snare
Farlow-Boettcher tonsil snare
Farmer hallux valgus operation
Farmer operation
Farmer technique
farmer's skin
Farmingdale retractor
far-near sutures
Farnham forceps
Farnham nasal-cutting forceps
Faro coolbeam lamp
Farr retractor
Farr self-retaining retractor
Farr spring retractor
Farr wire retractor
Farre line
Farre tubercles
Farre white line
Farrell applicator
Farrell nasal applicator
Farrier flap exposure
    instruments
Farrier-Joseph nasal saw
Farrington forceps
Farrington nasal polyp forceps
Farrington septal forceps
Farrington septum forceps
Farrior angulated curet
Farrior anterior footplate pick
Farrior applicator
Farrior blunt palpator
Farrior bur
Farrior chuck handle
Farrior ear curet
Farrior ear speculum
Farrior excavator
Farrior flap exposure
    instruments
Farrior footplate pick
Farrior forceps
Farrior graft augmentation
Farrior knife
Farrior mushroom raspatory
Farrior otoplasty knife
Farrior oval ear speculum
Farrior oval speculum
Farrior oval-window excavator
Farrior oval-window pick
Farrior oval-window piston
    gauge excavator
Farrior posterior footplate pick

Farrior raspatory
Farrior septal cartilage stripper knife
Farrior sickle knife
Farrior speculum
Farrior suction applicator
Farrior triangular knife
Farrior wire crimper
Farrior wire-crimping forceps
Farrior-Derlacki chisel
Farrior-Dworacek canal chisel
Farrior-Joseph bayonet saw
Farrior-Joseph nasal saw
Farrior-McHugh ear knife
Farrior-McHugh knife
Farrior-Shambaugh elevator
Farris elevator
Farris tissue forceps
Fary anterior chamber maintainer
Fasanella cannula
Fasanella double-ended iris retractor
Fasanella iris retractor
Fasanella lacrimal cannula
Fasanella operation
Fasanella retractor
Fasanella-Servat blepharoptosis operation
Fasanella-Servat operation
Fasanella-Servat operation for lid ptosis
Fasanella-Servat ptosis correction procedure
Fasano test during rhizotomy
fascia (*pl.* fasciae)
  Adams excision of palmar fascia
  alar fascia
  angular tract of cervical fascia
  antebrachial fascia
  anterior rectus fascia
  aponeurotic fascia
  aryepiglottic fascia
  axillary fascia
  brachial fascia
  buccinator fascia
  buccopharyngeal fascia
  Buck fascia
  Camper fascia
  capsulopalpebral fascia
  cervical fascia

fascia (*continued*)
  circumflex iliac superficial fascia
  clavipectoral fascia
  Cloquet fascia
  Colles fascia
  coracocostal fascia
  cremaster fascia
  cremasteric fascia
  cribriform fascia
  crural fascia
  dartos fascia
  deep cervical fascia
  deep fascia
  deep perineal fascia
  deep temporal fascia (DTF)
  deltoid fascia
  Denonvilliers fascia
  dentate fascia
  dermis fascia
  diseased fascia
  dorsal aponeurotic fascia
  dorsal fascia
  dorsal interosseous fascia
  dorsal thoracic fascia
  Dupuytren fascia
  endoabdominal fascia
  endothoracic fascia
  external oblique fascia
  external perineal fascia
  external spermatic fascia
  extrapleural fascia
  fusion fascia
  Gerota fascia
  gluteal fascia
  graft of fascia
  hypothenar fascia
  inferior fascia
  infundibuliform fascia
  innominate fascia
  intermediate fascia
  internal abdominal fascia
  internal oblique fascia
  internal spermatic fascia
  interposing fascia
  investing fascia
  lacrimal fascia
  lateral oblique fascia
  lumbodorsal fascia
  masseteric fascia
  mastoid fascia
  orbital fasciae

fascia (*continued*)
  obturator fascia
  palmar fascia
  palpebral fascia
  paraspinous fascia
  parotid fascia
  pectineal fascia
  pectoral fascia
  perineal fascia
  perinephric fascia
  perirenal fascia
  perivesical fascia
  pharyngeal fascia
  pharyngobasilar fascia
  plantar fascia
  preparotid fascia
  prepubic fascia
  presacral fascia
  pretracheal fascia
  pubocervical fascia
  pubovesicocervical fascia
  rectovaginal fascia
  rectovesical fascia
  rectus fascia
  release of plantar fascia
  renal fascia
  Scarpa fascia
  Sibson fascia
  SMAS fascia
  spermatic fascia
  sternocleidomastoid fascia
  subcutaneous fascia
  subgaleal fascia
  subserous fascia
  subvesical fascia
  superficial abdominal fascia
  superficial facial fascia
  superficial fascia
  superficial perineal fascia
  superficial temporal fascia
  suprasternal fascia
  temporal fascia
  temporalis fascia
  temporalis superficialis fascia
  temporoparietal fascia
  Tenon fascia
  thenar fascia
  thoracic fascia
  thoracolumbar fascia
  thyrolaryngeal fascia
  transversalis fascia
  transverse fascia

fascia (*continued*)
  underlying fascia
  vesical fascia
  vesicovaginal fascia
  visceral fascia
  volar interosseous fascia
  Waldeyer fascia
fascia bulbi
fascia flap
fascia graft
fascia lata
fascia lata femoris
fascia lata graft
fascia lata heart valve
fascia lata implant
fascia lata prosthesis
fascia lata sling operation
fascia lata strip
fascia lata stripper
fascia needle
fascia of abdomen
fascia of Camper
fascia of Gallaudet
fascia stripper
fascia transversalis
fasciae (*sing.* fascia)
fascia-fat composite graft
fascial anchoring
fascial anchoring technique
fascial arthroplasty
fascial cleft
fascial closure
fascial colliculus
fascial cutter
fascial defect
fascial flap
fascial graft
fascial grafting
fascial hernia
fascial layer
fascial needle
fascial perforator
fascial planes
fascial plication
fascial press
fascial sarcoma
fascial sheath
fascial sling
fascial sling approach
fascial sling for facial paralysis
fascial sling procedure
fascial snare

fascial space
fascial stranding
fascial suspension
fascial-fatty layer
Fascian
fasciaplasty
fascia-splitting incision
fasciatome
 Lane fasciatome
 Luck fasciatome
 Masson fasciatome
 Moseley fasciatome
fascicle
 alveolar nerve fascicle
 muscle fascicle
 nerve fascicle
fascicular
fascicular graft
fascicular heart block
fascicular repair
fasciculated bladder
fasciculation
fasciculation potential
fasciculi (*sing.* fasciculus)
fasciculoventricular bypass
 tract
fasciculoventricular connection
fasciculus (*pl.* fasciculi)
 anterior cerebrospinal
  fasciculus
 cerebrospinal fasciculus
 medial longitudinal fasciculus
fasciculus aberrans of Monakow
fasciculus cuneatus
fasciculus gracilis
fasciculus lenticularis
fasciculus of Gowers
fasciculus of Rolando
fasciectomy
 limited fasciectomy
 Skoog fasciectomy
 Skoog incision in palmar
  fasciectomy
fasciitis
 exudative calcifying fasciitis
 infiltrative fasciitis
 necrotizing fasciitis (NF)
 nodular fasciitis
 palmar fasciitis
 plantar fasciitis
 proliferative fasciitis
 pseudosarcomatous fasciitis

fasciocutaneous
fasciocutaneous flap
fasciocutaneous free flap
fasciocutaneous island flap
fasciocutaneous perforator
fasciocutaneous vessel
fasciodesis
fasciogram
fascio-osteocutaneous flap
fascioplasty
fasciorrhaphy
fascioscapulohumeral
fasciotome
 Luck fasciotome
fasciotomy
 decompression fasciotomy
 double-incision fasciotomy
 endoscopic plantar
  fasciotomy
 Fronet fasciotomy
 multiple fasciotomies
 Nirschl fasciotomy
 percutaneous plantar
  fasciotomy
 plantar fasciotomy
 prophylactic fasciotomy
 Rorabeck fasciotomy
 single-incision fasciotomy
 Skoog fasciotomy
 Souttar iliac crest fasciotomy
 subcutaneous fasciotomy
 Yount fasciotomy
fasciovascular pedicle
fashion
 bread-loaf fashion
 Brooke fashion
 cork fashion
 crisscross fashion
 crossed sword fashion
 draped in a routine fashion
 Gillies fashion
 interrupted fashion
 inverted-T fashion
 isolated fashion
 performed in routine
  fashion
 Poppen fashion
 Pulvertaft fashion
 retrograde fashion
 simple interrupted fashion
 tumbling fashion
Fasplint splint

FAST balloon catheter (flow-assisted, short-term balloon catheter)
FAST balloon flotation catheter
fast neutron radiation therapy
FAST right heart cardiovascular catheter
fast twitch muscle
fast-absorbing catgut
FASTak suture anchor
fast-breeder reactor
Fastcure denture repair material
fastener
    ball fastener
    Brown-Mueller T-bar fastener
    Cath-Strip catheter fastener
    Intrafix tibial fastener
    NG strip nasal tube fastener
    Percu-Stay catheter fastener
    ROC XS suture fastener
    SmartPins fastener
    UC strip catheter tubing fastener
Fast-Fit vascular stocking
fast-flow arterial malformations
FastIn threaded anchor
Fastlok implantable staple
FastOut device
Fast-Pass endocardial lead
Fast-Pass lead pacemaker
Fast-Patch disposable defibrillation/electrocardiographic electrode
fast-pathway radiofrequency ablation
FasTrac guidewire
FasTrac hydrophilic-coated guidewire
FasTrac introducer
FasTracker infusion catheter
Fastrak scanner
Fastrak traction material
Fastrak traction strip dressing
fast-setting acrylic
fastSTART EMS neuromuscular stimulator
fastSTART HVPC pulsed stimulator
fast-track cardiac anesthesia
fast-twitch fatigable skeletal muscle
fast-twitch fibers

fat
    abdominal fat
    atrophy of fat
    bathtub deformity of facial fat
    body fat
    brown fat
    buccal fat
    central fat
    cervicofacial fat
    chyle fat
    descent of the cheek fat
    extraconal fat
    extraperitoneal fat
    fractionate and redistribute facial fat
    harvested fat
    Hoffa fat
    intraconal fat
    jowl fat
    laminar fat
    liquefaction of fat
    macroinjection of autologous fat
    masked fat
    mulberry fat
    orbital fat
    parapharyngeal fat
    pararenal fat
    perinephric fat
    periorbital fat
    perirenal fat
    Pitanguy fat
    preaponeurotic fat
    preperitoneal fat
    preplatysmal fat
    properitoneal fat
    protruding fat
    retro-orbicularis ocular fat (ROOF)
    stored fat
    subcutaneous fat
    subcuticular fat
    subepicardial fat
    suborbicularis oculi fat (SOOF)
    subplatysmal fat
    superficial fat
    white fat
FAT (function, appearance, time)
fat atrophy
fat augmentation
fat body of cheek

fat body of orbit
fat cell
fat cell graft
fat cell space
fat deposits
fat depot
fat embolism
fat embolization
fat embolus
fat emulsification
fat flap
fat fracture
fat graft
fat hernia
fat herniation
fat hypertrophy
fat injection
fat line
fat marrow
fat necrosis
fat pad
fat pad retractor
fat plane
fat towels
fat transplant
fatal cardiac event
fatal complications
fatal heart attack
fatal seizure
fatality rate
fat-density line
fatigability
fatigue fracture
fat-injection needles
Fat-O-Meter skinfold calipers
fat-pad retractor
fat-pad sign
fat-suppressed body coil
fat-suppression technique
fat-to-fat healing
FatTrack skinfold calipers
fatty ascites
fatty atrophy
fatty ball of Bichat
fatty capsule of kidney
fatty cardiopathy
fatty degeneration
fatty deposits
fatty exudate
fatty hernia
fatty humor
fatty hypertrophy

fatty infiltration
fatty liver
fatty marrow
fatty material
fatty tissue
fatty tumor
fauces
    anterior pillar of fauces
    pillar of fauces
faucet aspirator
Faucher stomach tube
faucial and lingual tonsillectomy
faucial arch
faucial area
faucial catheter
faucial cavity
faucial eustachian catheter
faucial paralysis
faucial reflex
faucial tonsil
faucial tonsillectomy
Fauer peritoneal clamp
Faught sphygmomanometer
Faulkner antral chisel
Faulkner antral curet
Faulkner antrum chisel
Faulkner antrum curet
Faulkner antrum gouge
Faulkner chisel
Faulkner curet
Faulkner double-end ring curet
Faulkner ethmoid curet
Faulkner ethmoidal curet
Faulkner folder
Faulkner nasal curet
Faulkner trocar
Faulkner trocar chisel
Faulkner-Browne chisel
faulty contact point
faulty eccentric occlusion
faulty valve action
faun tail nevus
Faure forceps
Faure peritoneal forceps
Faure uterine biopsy forceps
Fauvel forceps
Fauvel laryngeal forceps
Favaloro atrial retractor
Favaloro coronary scissors
Favaloro ligature carrier
Favaloro proximal anastomosis
    clamp

Favaloro retractor
Favaloro saphenous vein bypass
    graft
Favaloro scissors
Favaloro self-retaining sternal
    retractor
Favaloro sternal retractor
Favaloro tunneler
Favaloro-Morse rib spreader
Favaloro-Morse sternal spreader
Favaloro-Semb ligature carrier
Favorite clamp
Favre-Racouchot cyst
Fay suction elevator
Fay suction tube
Fazio-Montgomery cannula
Fazio-Montgomery tube
FB (fingerbreadths)
FB (foreign body)
FCR (flexor carpi radialis)
FCU (flexor carpi ulnaris)
FDB (flexor digitorum brevis)
FDDB (freeze-dried
    demineralized bone)
FDFG (free derma-fat graft)
FDI (Facial Disability Index)
FDL (flexor digitorum longus)
FDM (flexor digiti minimi)
FDP (flexor digitorum
    profundus)
FDP muscle
FDP tendon
FDQ (flexor digiti quinti)
FDS (flexor digitorum sublimis)
FDS (flexor digitorum
    superficialis)
FDS (flexor digitorum
    superficialis)
FDS muscle
FDS tendon
Feaster Dualens intraocular lens
Feaster dual-placement
    intraocular lens
Feaster hydrodissecting cannula
Feaster lens hook
Feaster lens manipulator
Feaster radial keratotomy knife
Feather carbon breakable blade
feather clamp
feather extended malar implant
feather knife
feather scalpel

feather the peel
feather the transition
feathered edge
feathered-edged proximal
    finishing line
feather-edged proximal finishing
    line
feathering technique
FeatherTouch automated rasp
FeatherTouch CO_2 laser
FeatherTouch SilkLaser
feature
    coarse facial features
    extravascular granulomatous
        features
    morphologic feature
    nondistinctive features
febrile convulsion
febrile reaction
febrile state
fecal abscess
fecal containment device (FCD)
fecal contents
fecal diversion
fecal diversion colostomy
fecal excretion
fecal fistula
fecal impaction
fecal incontinence
fecal marker
fecal material
fecal obstruction
fecal reservoir
fecal residue
fecalith
    appendiceal fecalith
fecalith obstruction
fecal-oral route
feces
    extravasation feces
    impacted feces
    incontinent of feces
    inspissated feces
    scybalous feces
feces and gas
Fechner intraocular implant
    lens
Fechner lens
Fechtner conjunctiva forceps
Fechtner intraocular lens
Fechtner ring forceps
fecopurulent

Federation of Gynecology and
    Obstetrics classification
Federici sign
Federov eye implant
Federov implant
Federov lens implant
Federov operation
Federov splenectomy
Federov type I lens implant
Federov type II lens implant
Federspiel cheek retractor
Federspiel needle
Federspiel periosteal elevator
Federspiel scissors
feeble pulse
feeder
    Brecht feeder
    Haberman feeder
    offset suspension feeder
    Rancho Los Amigos feeder
    suspension feeder
    Tumble Forms feeder
feeder-frond technique
feeding
    drip-tube feeding
    early enteral feeding
    enteral feeding
    forcible feeding
    GastroPort enteral feeding
    gastrostomy feeding
    gavage feeding
    hyperalimentation feeding
    intravenous feeding
    IV feeding
    jejunostomy elemental diet
        feeding
    jejunostomy tube feeding
    nasal feeding
    oral feeding
    postoperative regimen for oral
        early feeding (PROEF)
    tube feeding
feeding complication
feeding gastrostomy
feeding gastrostomy tube
feeding tube
feeding vessels
Fegerstra wire
Fehland clamp
Fehland intestinal clamp
Fehland intestinal forceps
Fehland right-angled colon clamp

Fehling TOP ejector punch
Feilchenfeld forceps
Feilchenfeld splinter forceps
Fein antral trocar
Fein antrum trocar
Fein cannula
Fein needle
Fein trocar
Feiss line
Feist-Mankin position
Feldbausch dilator
Feldman bur
Feldman excision
Feldman lid retractor
Feldman lip retractor
Feldman radial keratotomy
    marker
Feldman retractor
Feldstein blepharoplasty clip
Feleky instrument
Felig insulin pump
Fell sucker tip
felon
Felson silhouette sign
felt dressing
felt pads
felt patch
felt pledget
Felt shears
felt strip
felt-collar splint
felt-foam padding
felt-gauze pad
FelxiSeal fecal collector
female catheter
female catheter-dilator
female cystoscope
female hypospadias
female pseudohermaphroditism
female reproductive organs
female sound
female urethral syndrome
female urethroscope
female urinary pouch
fem-fem bypass (femoral-femoral
    bypass)
Fem-Flex II femoral cannula
feminization syndrome
feminizing genitoplasty
femoral 3-in-1 technique
femoral aligner
femoral AP-sizing guide

femoral arch
femoral arteriogram
femoral arteriography
femoral arteriotomy
femoral artery
femoral artery aneurysm
femoral artery approach
femoral artery cannula
femoral artery decannulation
femoral artery sheath
femoral artery-saphenous bulb
femoral bone
femoral broach
femoral bypass
femoral canal
femoral canal restrictor
femoral cerebral catheter
femoral circulation
femoral clamp
femoral component
femoral component pusher
femoral condyle
femoral condyle plate
femoral cortex
femoral cortical ring allograft
femoral crossover bypass
femoral cutaneous nerve
femoral diaphyseal fracture
femoral dislocation
femoral displacement
femoral distractor
femoral embolectomy
femoral endarterectomy
femoral endoprosthesis
femoral epiphysis
femoral fossa
femoral fracture
femoral graft
femoral guide pin
femoral guiding catheter
femoral head
femoral head driver
femoral head extractor
femoral head line
femoral head prosthesis
femoral head reamer
femoral head saw
femoral hemodialysis catheter
femoral hernia
femoral hernia repair
femoral herniorrhaphy
femoral impactor

femoral intermedullary guide
femoral intermuscular septum
femoral intertrochanteric
    fracture
femoral introducer sheath
femoral length
femoral ligament
femoral muscle
femoral neck
femoral neck fracture
femoral neck fracture reduction
femoral neck reamer
femoral neck retractor
femoral nerve
femoral nerve block
femoral nerve traction test
femoral nodes
femoral notch guide
femoral perfusion cannula
femoral plate
femoral plug
femoral prosthesis
femoral prosthesis fixation
femoral prosthetic broach
femoral prosthetic head
femoral prosthetic pusher
femoral pulse
femoral pusher
femoral rasp
femoral reflex
femoral resection
femoral resector
femoral septum
femoral shaft
femoral shaft fracture
femoral shaft rasp
femoral shaft reamer
femoral sheath
femoral shortening osteotomy
femoral sizer
femoral splint
femoral supracondylar fracture
femoral tensor
femoral torque
femoral trial extractor
femoral trials
femoral triangle
femoral vein
femoral vein cannulation
femoral vein decannulation
femoral vein-femoral artery
    bypass

femoral-femoral bypass (fem-fem bypass)
femoral-inguinal herniorrhaphy
femoral-peroneal in situ vein bypass graft
femoral-popliteal artery bypass
femoral-popliteal bypass (fem-pop bypass)
femoral-popliteal bypass graft (FPB graft)
femoral-popliteal occlusive disease
femoral-tibial bypass (fem-tib bypass)
femoral-tibial-peroneal bypass
femoral-trunk extension
femoroaxillary bypass
femorocele
femorodistal bypass
femorodistal reconstructive surgery
femorodistal vein graft
femorofemoral bypass
femorofemoral crossover bypass
femorofemoral crossover prosthesis
femoroiliac
femoroischial transplantation
femoropopliteal bypass
femoropopliteal bypass graft
femoropopliteal saphenous vein bypass
femoropopliteal vein
femorotibial bypass
FemoStop femoral artery compression arch
FemoStop femoral artery compression device
FemoStop inflatable pneumatic compression device
fem-pop bypass (femoral-popliteal bypass)
FemSoft urethral insert
fem-tib bypass (femoral-tibial bypass)
femtoliter (fL, fl)
femtomole
femur
  head of femur
  intercondylar notch of femur
  neck of femur

femur (*continued*)
  Osgood supracondylar osteotomy of femur
  round ligament of femur
  Schneider intramedullary fixation of femur
  shaft of femur
  shepherd's crook deformity of proximal femur
  Steide fracture of femur
  White procedure to shorten femur
  Zickel nailing of femur
fence
  Kirklin fence
  ligamentous facial fence
fence splint
fender fracture
fenestra (*pl.* fenestrae)
fenestra bone graft
fenestra choledocha
fenestra cochleae
fenestra implant
fenestra ovalis
fenestra prosthesis
fenestra rotunda
fenestra vestibuli
fenestrae (*sing.* fenestra)
fenestrated aneurysm clip
fenestrated blade forceps
fenestrated catheter
fenestrated compress
fenestrated compression plate
fenestrated cup biopsy forceps
fenestrated Drake clip
fenestrated drape
fenestrated ellipsoid spiked open span biopsy forceps
fenestrated endothelium
fenestrated Fontan operation
fenestrated forceps
fenestrated hymen
fenestrated lens scoop
fenestrated membrane
fenestrated septum
fenestrated sheath
fenestrated sheet
fenestrated spiked open span jumbo biopsy forceps
fenestrated sterile drape
fenestrated sterile field barrier
fenestrated tracheostomy tube

fenestrated tube
fenestrated valve
fenestrating
fenestration
    alveolar plate fenestration
    aortopulmonary fenestration
    apical fenestration
    atrophic fenestration
    baffle fenestration
    catheter-directed fenestration
    cusp fenestration
    cyst fenestration
    dental fenestration
    endonasal fenestration
    intercellular fenestration
    labyrinthine fenestration
    laparoscopic fenestration
    Lempert fenestration
    tracheal fenestration
fenestration bur
fenestration cavity
fenestration curet
fenestration elevator
fenestration excavator
fenestration hook
fenestration instruments
fenestration of semicircular canal
fenestration operation
fenestration procedure
fenestration saw
fenestrator
    Rosen fenestrator
fenestrometer
    Paparella fenestrometer
Fenger forceps
Fenger gall duct probe
Fenger gallbladder probe
Fenger gallstone probe
Fenger spiral gallstone probe
fentanyl anesthesia
fentanyl citrate
Fenton bolt
Fenton bulldog vulsellum
Fenton dilator
Fenton nail
Fenton operation
Fenton tibial bolt
Fenton uterine dilator
Fenwal hemapheresis pump
Fenzel hook
FEP-ringed Gore-Tex vascular
    graft

Ferciot excision
Ferciot splint
Ferciot technique
Ferciot wire guide
Ferciot-Thomson excision
Feree-Rand perimeter
Fergi needle
Fergus operation
Fergus percutaneous introducer
    kit
Ferguson abdominal scissors
Ferguson angiotribe
Ferguson angiotribe forceps
Ferguson basket
Ferguson bone clamp
Ferguson bone curet
Ferguson bone holder
Ferguson bone-holding forceps
Ferguson brain suction tube
Ferguson curet
Ferguson esophageal probe
Ferguson forceps
Ferguson gallstone scoop
Ferguson hemorrhoidectomy
Ferguson implant
Ferguson inguinal herniorrhaphy
Ferguson mouth gag
Ferguson needle
Ferguson probang
Ferguson probe
Ferguson retractor
Ferguson round-body needle
Ferguson scissors
Ferguson scoop
Ferguson stone basket
Ferguson suction
Ferguson suture needle
Ferguson technique
Ferguson tenaculum
Ferguson-Ackland mouth gag
Ferguson-Brophy mouth gag
Ferguson-Coley operation
Ferguson-Frazier suction tube
Ferguson-Gwathmey mouth gag
Ferguson-Metzenbaum scissors
Ferguson-Moon rectal retractor
Ferguson-Moon retractor
Ferguson-Smith epithelioma
Ferguson-Smith
    keratoacanthoma
Ferguson-Thompson-King
    osteotomy

Fergusson bone knife
Fergusson excision of maxilla
Fergusson incision
Fergusson knife
Fergusson operation
Fergusson speculum
Fergusson tubular vaginal
    speculum
Fericot tip-toe splint
Ferkel technique
Ferkel torticollis technique
fermentation tube
Fermit-N occlusal hole blockage
    material
fern test
Fernandez extensile anterior
    approach
Fernandez osteotomy
ferning technique
Fernstroem bladder retractor
Fernstroem-Stille retractor
Ferran awl
Ferrein canal
Ferrein foramen
Ferrein ligament
Ferrier gingival clamp
Ferrier coupler
Ferrier separator
Ferris biliary duct dilator
Ferris colporrhaphy forceps
Ferris common duct scoop
Ferris dilator
Ferris disposable bone marrow
    aspiration needle
Ferris filiform dilator
Ferris forceps
Ferris polyostomy wound
    dressing
Ferris Robb tonsillar knife
Ferris scoop
Ferris Smith bone-biting forceps
Ferris Smith cup rongeur
    forceps
Ferris Smith disk rongeur
Ferris Smith elevator
Ferris Smith forceps
Ferris Smith fragment forceps
Ferris Smith intervertebral disk
    rongeur
Ferris Smith knife
Ferris Smith needle holder
Ferris Smith operation

Ferris Smith orbital retractor
Ferris Smith pituitary rongeur
Ferris Smith punch
Ferris Smith retractor
Ferris Smith rongeur
Ferris Smith rongeur forceps
Ferris Smith tissue forceps
Ferris Smith-Gruenwald punch
Ferris Smith-Gruenwald rongeur
Ferris Smith-Gruenwald
    sphenoid punch
Ferris Smith-Halle bur
Ferris Smith-Halle sinus bur
Ferris Smith-Kerrison disk
    rongeur
Ferris Smith-Kerrison forceps
Ferris Smith-Kerrison
    laminectomy rongeur
Ferris Smith-Kerrison
    neurosurgical rongeur
Ferris Smith-Kerrison punch
Ferris Smith-Kerrison rongeur
Ferris Smith-Kerrison rongeur
    forceps
Ferris Smith-Lyman
    periosteotome
Ferris Smith-Sewall orbital
    retractor
Ferris Smith-Sewall refractor
Ferris Smith-Sewall retractor
Ferris Smith-Spurling disk
    rongeur
Ferris Smith-Spurling
    intervertebral disk forceps
Ferris Smith-Spurling rongeur
Ferris Smith-Takahashi forceps
Ferris Smith-Takahashi rongeur
Ferris tissue forceps
Ferris-Robb knife
Ferris-Robb tonsil knife
Ferrolite crown remover
ferromagnetic intracerebral
    aneurysm clip
ferromagnetic monitoring
    device
ferromagnetic silicone
ferromagnetic tamponade
ferrule
ferrule clamp
Ferry line
Ferszt dissecting hook
Ferszt ligature passer

fertilization
   ex vivo fertilization
   in vitro fertilization
   in vivo fertilization
fertilization age
fester
festooning
FET (finger extension test)
fetal abnormality
fetal age
fetal alcohol syndrome
fetal aspiration syndrome
fetal basiotripsy
fetal blood-sampling instrument
fetal bone fracture
fetal cardiac activity
fetal cardiac anomaly
fetal chest anomaly
fetal circulation
fetal cleidotomy
fetal cord
fetal cord clamp
fetal cranial diameter
fetal cranioclasis
fetal craniotomy
fetal cystic adenomatoid
   malformation
fetal death
fetal decelerations
fetal distress
Fetal Dopplex monitor
fetal drug therapy
fetal duplication
fetal face syndrome
fetal gastrointestinal anomaly
fetal giantism
fetal growth parameters
fetal growth retardation
fetal head
fetal head constraint
fetal head extractor
fetal head position
fetal heart
fetal heart rate monitor
fetal heart sounds (FHS)
fetal heart tones (FHT)
fetal hemorrhage
fetal hydantoin syndrome
fetal hydrops
fetal incontinence collector
fetal intracranial anatomy
fetal ischiopubiotomy

fetal lie
fetal liver biopsy
fetal liver transplantation
fetal lung maturity
fetal macrosomia
fetal malrotation
fetal membranes
fetal monitor
fetal movement
fetal pelvic disproportion
fetal placenta
fetal pole
fetal position
fetal reduction
fetal respiration
fetal rhythm
fetal scalp electrode
fetal skin biopsy
fetal small parts
fetal somatic activity
fetal stethoscope
fetal substantia nigra implants
fetal surgery
fetal thymus transplantation
fetal tissue
fetal tissue transplant
fetal vacuum extractor
fetal valproate syndrome
fetal vascular anomaly
fetal viability
fetal wastage
Fetalert fetal heart rate monitor
fetalis
   chondrodystrophia fetalis
   chondromalacia fetalis
   hydrops fetalis
fetalization
fetal-maternal exchange
fetal-maternal hemorrhage
FetalPulse Plus monitor
Fetasonde fetal monitor
Feth-R-Kath epidural catheter
fetogram
fetography
fetomaternal hemorrhage
fetopelvic disproportion
fetoplacental circulation
fetoscope
   Perell fetoscope
   Pinard fetoscope
fetoscopy
Fett carpal prosthesis

fetus
- expelled fetus
- full-term fetus
- harlequin fetus
- intrauterine fetus
- macerated fetus
- malformed fetus
- mummified fetus
- paper-doll fetus
- papyraceous fetus
- sireniform fetus

fetus expulsion
Feuerstein drainage tube
Feuerstein ear tube
Feuerstein myringotomy drain tube
Feuerstein split ventilation tube
FG diamond bur
FGF (fibroblast growth factor)
FG-series 2-channel endoscope
FGSM (Facial Grading System voluntary movement)
FHB (flexor hallucis brevis)
FHS (fetal heart sounds)
FHT (fetal heart tones)
FIA (fluorescent immunoassay)
fiber
- afferent fibers
- afferent nerve fiber
- alveolar crest fibers
- alveolar fibers
- anterior external arcuate fibers
- argyrophilic collagen fiber
- Bernheimer fibers
- braided polyester fiber
- Bruecke fibers
- bundle fiber
- CR Bard Urolase fiber
- carbon fiber
- circular fibers
- coated carbon fiber
- collagen fibers
- collagenous fibers
- deep transverse fibers
- dentinogenic fiber
- dentogingival fiber
- dentoperiosteal fiber
- elastic fibers
- Endostat disposable sterile fiber
- extension fiber

fiber (*continued*)
- fast-twitch fibers
- FiberLase flexible fiber
- Gerdy fibers
- Gratiolet radiating fibers
- Herxheimer fibers
- intermediate fiber
- interradicular fiber
- intrafusal fibers
- James fibers
- laser fiber
- Laserscope disposable Endostat fiber
- lattice fiber
- medullated nerve fiber
- Micro Link endoscope fiber
- micro-thin plastic fiber
- mooring fibers
- motor fibers
- Mueller fibers
- muscle fiber
- myelinated nerve fibers
- myelinated sensory nerve fiber
- myocardial fibers
- nerve cell fibers
- nerve fibers
- nonmedullated nerve fiber
- oblique fiber
- orbiculociliary fiber
- osteocollagenous fibers
- osteogenetic fibers
- Prolase fiber
- Prussak fibers
- Purkinje fibers
- Remak fibers
- reticular collagen fibers
- Ritter fibers
- Rosenthal fibers
- Sappey fibers
- Sharpey fibers
- Sharpy fibers
- skeletal muscle fibers
- slow-twitch fibers
- superficial transverse fibers
- sympathetic nerve fibers
- transverse fibers
- UltraLine Nd:YAG laser fiber
- unmyelinated nerve fibers
- Urolase Nd:YAG laser fiber
- Versatome laser fiber
- white fibers

fiber (*continued*)
  whorled collagen fibers
  yellow fibers
  zonular fibers
  zonule fibers
fiber bundle
fiber cell
fiber cleaver
fiber of Remak
fiber optic laryngoscopy
fiber tip modification
fibercolonoscope
fiberduodenoscope
  Machida fiberduodenoscope
    (FDS)
fiberendoscope
fibergastroscope
fiberglass bandage
fiberglass casting tape
fiberglass graft
fiberglass sleeve trocar
fiberglass staff
fiberhead hammer
fiber-illuminated
FiberLase flexible fiber
FiberLase laser
FiberLaser flexible beam
    delivery system for CO_2
    surgical lasers
Fiberlite microscope
fibermallet
fiberoptic anoscope
fiberoptic arthroscope
fiberoptic bronchoscope
fiberoptic bronchoscopy (FOB)
fiberoptic bronchoscopy
    anesthetic technique
fiberoptic bundle
fiberoptic cable
fiberoptic cable adapter
fiberoptic choledochoscope
fiberoptic cold light source
fiberoptic culdoscope
fiberoptic cystoscope
fiberoptic endoscope
fiberoptic endoscopy anesthetic
    technique
fiberoptic esophagoscope
fiberoptic esophagoscopy
fiberoptic examination
fiberoptic gastroscope
fiberoptic headlight

fiberoptic hysteroscope
fiberoptic injection
    sclerotherapy
fiberoptic instrument
fiberoptic intraosseous
    endoscopy
fiberoptic intubation
    procedure
fiberoptic laryngoscope
fiberoptic lens
fiberoptic light
fiberoptic light bundle
fiberoptic light cable
fiberoptic light carrier
fiberoptic light cord
fiberoptic light pipe
fiberoptic light projector
fiberoptic light source
fiberoptic lighted mirror
fiberoptic lighted suction tube
fiberoptic Lite-Piper cable
fiberoptic loupe
fiberoptic microscope
fiberoptic otoscope
fiberoptic oximeter catheter
fiberoptic panendoscope
fiberoptic panendoscopy
fiberoptic PCO_2 sensor
fiberoptic photographic sheath
fiberoptic pick
fiberoptic pressure catheter
fiberoptic probe
fiberoptic proctosigmoidoscope
fiberoptic retractor
fiberoptic right-angle telescope
fiberoptic sheath
fiberoptic sigmoidoscope
fiberoptic sigmoidoscopy
fiberoptic slide laryngoscope
fiberoptic smoke evacuating
    retractors
fiberoptic suction tube
fiberoptic surgical field
    illuminator
fiberoptic telescope
fiberoptic tracheal intubation
    anesthetic technique
fiberoptic tube
fiberoptic vaginal speculum
fiberoptic video glasses
fiberoptic videoendoscope
fiberoptics

fiberscope
  gastroduodenal fiberscope
  Hirschowitz fiberscope
  Hirschowitz gastroduodenal
    fiberscope
  nasopharyngeal fiberscope
  Olympus fiberscope
  Pentax fiberscope
  side-viewing fiberscope
  superfine fiberscope
fiberscopic transduodenal duct
    injection
fiber-splitting incision
FiberWire suture
Fibra Sonics phaco aspirator
Fibracol collagen alginate
    wound dressing
Fibracol collagen-alginate
    dressing
Fibrel collagen
Fibrel gelatin matrix implant
Fibre-Lite septal elevator
fibril
  anchoring fibril
  argyrophilic fibril
  collagen fibrils
  interodontoblastic collagen
    fibril
fibrillar mass of Flemming
fibrillar twitching
fibrillary contractions
fibrillary glia
fibrillary tremor
fibrillary waves
fibrillating action potentials
fibrillating waves
fibrillation
  atrial fibrillation
  auricular fibrillation
  cardiac fibrillation
  chronic atrial fibrillation
  continuous atrial fibrillation
  idiopathic ventricular
    fibrillation
  lone atrial fibrillation
  paroxysmal atrial fibrillation
    (PAF)
  synchronized fibrillation
  ventricular fibrillation (V-fib)
  ventricular
    tachycardia/ventricular
    fibrillation

fibrillation potential
fibrillation rhythm
fibrillation threshold
fibrillator subclavian-subclavian
    bypass
fibrillatory tremors
fibrils
fibrin bodies
fibrin calculus
fibrin deposit
fibrin film
fibrin film stent
fibrin foam
fibrin gel
fibrin glue
fibrin glue adhesive
fibrin glue polymer
fibrin matrix gel
fibrin peel
fibrin plug
fibrin sealant
fibrin sponge
Fibrindex test
fibrinogen
fibrinogenesis
fibrinoid necrosis
fibrinoid necrotizing
    inflammation
fibrinolysin coagulation
fibrinolytic hemorrhage
fibrinopurulent
fibrinopurulent inflammation
fibrinous adhesion
fibrinous bronchitis
fibrinous exudate
fibrinous exudation
fibrinous inflammation
fibrinous material
fibrinous pericarditis
fibrinous tissue
fibroadenoma
  intracanalicular fibroadenoma
  pericanalicular fibroadenoma
fibroadenomatous hyperplasia of
    prostate
fibroadenosis
fibroadipose tissue
fibroblast
  scar fibroblast
  wound fibroblast
fibroblast growth factor (FGF)
fibroblastic reaction

fibroblastic sarcoma
fibroblastic tissue
fibroblastoma
  perineural fibroblastoma
fibrocalcareous disease
fibrocalcareous scarring
fibrocalcific lesion
fibrocartilage
  circumferential fibrocartilage
  internal fibrocartilage
  interventricular fibrocartilage
  semilunar fibrocartilage
  white fibrocartilage
fibrocartilaginous
fibrocartilaginous disk
fibrocartilaginous joint
fibrocartilaginous material
fibrocaseous inflammation
fibrochondroma
fibrocystic breast disorder
fibrocystic change
fibrocystic complex
fibrocystic condition
fibrocystic disease
fibrocystic disorder
fibrocystic nodules
fibroelastic covering
fibroelastic membrane
fibroelastosis
fibroepithelial papilloma
fibroepithelial polyp
fibroepithelial polypoid
  anorectal lesion
fibroepithelioma
  premalignant fibroepithelioma
fibroepithelioma basal cell
  carcinoma
fibrofascial compartment
  syndrome
fibrofatty subcutaneous tissue
fibrofatty tissue
fibrofatty tumor
fibrofolliculoma
fibrogenic sarcoma
fibroglandular tissue
fibrogranuloma
fibrohistiocytic lesion
fibrohyaline nodule
fibrohyaline tissue
fibroid
  intramural fibroid
  pedunculated fibroid

fibroid (*continued*)
  prolapsed fibroid
  serosal fibroids
  uterine fibroid
fibroid adenoma
fibroid cataract
fibroid heart
fibroid hook
fibroid induration
fibroid inflammation
fibroid of uterus
fibroid tumor of uterus
fibroid uterus
fibroidectomy
  uterine fibroidectomy
fibrokeratoma
fibrolipoma
fibrolipomatous tissue
fibroma (*pl.* fibromas, fibromata)
  ameloblastic fibroma
  aponeurotic fibroma
  cementifying fibroma
  central fibroma
  central ossifying fibroma
  cystic fibroma
  desmoplastic fibroma
  giant cell fibroma
  intracanalicular fibroma
  juvenile ossifying fibroma
  malignant fibroma
  nasopharyngeal fibroma
  ossifying fibroma
  osteogenic fibroma
  periosteal fibroma
  peripheral ossifying fibroma
  senile fibroma
  telangiectatic fibroma
  traumatic fibroma
  uterine fibroma
fibroma cavernosum
fibroma cutis
fibroma molle
fibroma of nerve
fibroma pendulum
fibroma sarcomatosum
fibroma xanthoma
fibromatosis
  aggressive infantile
    fibromatosis
  central fibromatosis
  congenital fibromatosis
  digital fibromatosis

fibromatosis (*continued*)
   idiopathic fibromatosis
   palmar fibromatosis
fibromatosis gingivae
fibromectomy
fibrometer
fibromuscular dysplasia
fibromuscular hyperplasia
fibromuscular junction
fibromuscular stoma
fibromuscular walls
fibromusculoelastic lesion
fibromyalgia trigger point
fibromyelinic plaques
fibromyoma (*pl.* fibromyomas,
   fibromyomata)
fibromyomata uteri
fibromyomectomy
fibromyotomy
fibromyxomatous
fibromyxomatous connective
   tissue
fibromyxomatous lesion
fibromyxosarcoma
fibronectin
fibro-osseous
fibro-osseous ankylosis
fibro-osseous dysplasia
fibro-osseous flexor tendon
   canal
fibro-osseous lesion
fibro-osseous process
fibro-osseous tunnel
fibro-ossification
fibro-osteogenic myxoma
fibro-osteoma
fibropapilloma
fibroplasia
fibroplastic endocarditis
fibroproliferative membrane
fibrosarcoma
   ameloblastic fibrosarcoma
   fibrosarcoma infantile
      fibrosarcoma
   infantile fibrosarcoma
   odontogenic fibrosarcoma
fibrose
fibrosed hematoma
fibrosing myopathy
fibrosis
   endomyocardial fibrosis
   interstitial fibrosis

fibrosis (*continued*)
   myocardial fibrosis
   nodular subepidermal fibrosis
   pleural fibrosis
   pulmonary fibrosis
   replacement fibrosis
   subepidermal nodular fibrosis
   submucous fibrosis
fibrositis
fibrotic changes
fibrotic infiltration
fibrotic markings
fibrotic mitral valve
fibrotic scarring
fibrotic strands
fibrous adhesion
fibrous anal tags
fibrous ankylosis
fibrous appendix hepatis
fibrous band
fibrous bone lesion
fibrous capsular contracture
fibrous capsule
fibrous connective tissue
fibrous covering
fibrous dysplasia
fibrous dysplasia of jaws
fibrous goiter
fibrous hyperplasia
fibrous joint
fibrous loose body
fibrous membrane
fibrous nodule
fibrous nonunion
fibrous obliteration
fibrous organ
fibrous polly beak
fibrous polypoid lesion
fibrous process
fibrous renal capsule
fibrous repair
fibrous sac
fibrous sheath
fibrous thyroiditis
fibrous tissue
fibrous union
fibrous xanthoma
fibrovascular aponeurosis
fibrovascular hypertrophy
fibrovascular ingrowth
fibrovascular polyp
fibrovascular stroma

fibroxanthoma
fibula
   diastasis fibula
   distal fibula
   shaft of fibula
fibula donor site
fibula flap
fibula free flap
fibula osteoseptocutaneous
   flap
fibular artery
fibular bone
fibular collateral ankle sprain
fibular collateral ligament
fibular facet
fibular flap
fibular fracture
fibular head
fibular muscle
fibular neck
fibular nerve
fibular notch
fibular onlay strut graft
fibular osteocutaneous flap
fibular osteocutaneous free flap
fibular shaft
fibular strut graft
fibular tunnel syndrome
fibular veins
fibulocalcaneal
fibulotalar joint
Ficat procedure
Ficat staging for avascular
   necrosis (I-IV)
Fichman suture-cutting forceps
Fick halo
Fick measurement of cardiac
   output
Fick operation
Fick perforation of footplate
Fick position
Fick technique
Ficoll-Hypaque technique
fiddler neck
fiddle-string adhesions
FIDUS probe
field
   Barrier fenestrated sterile field
   bloodless field
   clear lung fields
   confrontation fields
   confrontation of visual fields

field (*continued*)
   contaminated field
   direct field
   draped operative field
   draped out of the field
   draping of field
   dry field
   electric field
   en face irradiation field
   far field
   Forel field
   Graefe electric field
   high-power field
   irradiation field
   isolated field
   lateral field
   lower margin of field
   lung fields
   magnetic field
   mantle field
   margin of field
   midlung field
   narrow field
   operative field
   parallel opposing tangential
     fields
   per high power field
   peripheral fields
   pulmonary fields
   quadrant field
   sterile field
   subdiaphragmatic fields
   surgical field
   tangential field
   temporal field
   upper mantle field
   wide field
Field blade
field block
field block anesthesia
field emission tube
field expander
field expansion
field gradient
field lock
field of dissection
field of vision (FOV)
field size
Field suction dissector
Field tourniquet
field-echo image
field-echo imaging

Fielding classification
Fielding femoral fracture
    classification
Fielding membrane
Fielding modification of Gallie
    technique
Fielding-Magliato
    subtrochanteric fracture
    classification
Field-Lee biopsy needle
field-of-view camera
fighter fracture
FIGO (International Federation
    of Gynecology and
    Obstetrics)
figure-8 cast
figure-8 dressing
figure-8 stitch
figure-4 position
figure-4 test
figure-of-8 bandage
figure-of-8 brace
figure-of-8 dressing
figure-of-8 suture technique
figure-of-8 sutures
fil D'Arion silicone tube
fil d'Arion tube
filament
    beaded filaments
    Charcot-Bottcher filament
    cytokeratin filament
    desmin filament
    neural filament
    Semmes-Weinstein pressure
        aesthesiometer filament
    vimentin filament
filament sutures
filament transformer
filamentary keratome
filamented form
filamentous adhesion
filamentous appendage
filamentous component
filamentous form
Filatov flap
Filatov keratoplasty
Filatov operation
Filatov spot
Filatov-Gillies flap
Filatov-Gillies tubed pedicle
Filatov-Marzinkowsky
    operation file

file
    Aagesen file
    bone file
    Charnley trochanter file
    endodontic file
    end-Z file
    Filatov-Marzinkowsky
        operation file
    Flexicut file
    Flex-R-File file
    Hedstrom file
    K root canal file
    Kerr K-Flex file
    K-Flexofile file
    Kleinert-Kutz bone file
    Lightspeed file
    master apical file (MAF)
    Miller bone file
    Mity Gates Glidden file
    Mity Hedstroem file
    Mity Turbo File
    nickel-titanium file
    Nordent bone file
    orthopedic bone file
    ProFile file
    pulp canal file
    Putti bone file
    root canal file
    S root canal file
    Schwed Flexicut file
    scrub file
    SMIC bone file
    SMIC periodontal file
    SureFlex nickel-titanium file
    surgical file
    taper hand file
file elevator
filet (see fillet)
filiform
    dog-legged filiforms
    LeFort filiform
    Rusch filiform
    stone dislodger filiform
    urethral filiforms
filiform bougie
filiform bougie probe
filiform catheter
filiform dressing
filiform follower (F&F)
filiform guide
filiform implantation
filiform Jackson bougie

filiform papillae
filiform pulse
filiform steel needle
filiform stone dislodger
filiform wart
filiforms and followers (F&F)
filiform-tipped catheter
filing first technique
filipuncture
fill breast implant
Fillauer bar
Fillauer dorsiflexion assist ankle
    joint
Fillauer ankle joint orthotic
Fillauer night splint
Fillauer ankle joint
Fillauer prosthesis liner
Fillauer Scottish Rite orthosis kit
Fillauer silicone suspension liner
Fillauer splint
filler
    Bio-Oss maxillofacial bone
        filler
    BonePlast bone void filler
    bovine-derived bone filler
    cellular wrinkle filler
    Cortoss bone filler
    CosmoPlast human collagen
        dermal filler
    Cutinova cavity wound filler
    omental filler
    OsteoSet bone filler
    paste filler
    ProOsteon implant 500
        coralline hydroxyapatite
        bone void filler
filler graft
fillet
fillet flap
fillet flap procedure
fillet local flap graft
fillet of foot free flap
filleted graft
filleting
Fillette joint
Fill-Hess Fragmatome
filling
    amalgam filling
    complete filling
    fragmentary filling
    rapid filling
    reflux filling

filling (*continued*)
    retrograde filling
    root-canal filling
    silicate filling
filling defect
filling factor
filling material
filling of bladder
filling of pulp canal
filling of right atrium
film alternator
film changer
film dosimetry
film oxygenator
film packs
film wound dressing
filmy adhesions
filmy tongue
filopodium (*pl.* filopodia)
filopressure
Filshie clip
Filshie clip minilaparotomy
        applicator
Filshie female sterilization clip
filter maintainer
filter mold
filter needle
filter paper
filter placement
Filter Security closed mini-
        pouch
filtered dual-sump drain
filtered mediastinal sump drain
filtered-back projection
filtering cicatrix
filtering operation
filtering procedure
filtration
    glomerular filtration
    rate of fluid filtration
filtration angle
filtration rate
filtration surgery
filtration-slit membrane
Filtryzer dialyzer
Filtzer corkscrew
Filtzer interbody rasp
fimbria (*pl.* fimbriae)
    ovarian fimbria
    uterine tube fimbria
fimbria ovarica
fimbrial evacuation

fimbrial repair kit
fimbriated end
fimbriated fold
fimbriated oviduct
fimbriectomy
  Kroener fimbriectomy
  Uchida fimbriectomy
fimbrioplasty
  Bruhat laser fimbrioplasty
fin
  catheter fin
  convertible fin
  convertible telescope and fin
  double-catheterizing fin
  prosthesis fin
final closure
final cone position
final consonant position
final diagnosis
final impression
final pathological diagnosis
final stage of labor
final-cut acetabular reamer
finder
  Carabelli lumen finder
  Damian lumen finder
  Dasco Pro angle finder
  full-view lumen finder
  gravity-driven angle finder
  hamate finder
  Hedwig lumen finder
  IMP femur finder
  lumen finder
  Moore direction finder
  pedicle finder
  Tucker vertebrated lumen
    finder
finding
  auscultatory findings
  compatible findings
  concurrent findings
  consistent findings
  copper-beaten finding
  cystoscopic findings
  diagnostic finding
  endoscopic finding
  focal finding
  incidental finding
  intraoperative ultrasound
    finding
  negative findings
  operative findings

finding (*continued*)
  paucity of findings
  pertinent findings
  positive finding
  positive x-ray finding
  variable findings
  x-ray findings
Findley folding pessary
fine arterial forceps
fine artery forceps
fine cautery
fine chromic sutures
fine crepitant rales
Fine crescent fixation ring
fine curet
fine dissecting forceps
Fine folding block
fine forceps
fine intestinal needle
fine line
Fine magnetic implant
fine manipulation
Fine micropoint cautery
Fine micropoint electrocautery
fine moist rales
fine motor
fine needle
fine olive bur
fine plain catgut
fine rales
Fine scissors
fine silk sutures
fine sutures
Fine suture-tying forceps
fine tissue forceps
fine tremor
fine-angled curet
fine-bore catheter
Fine-Castroviejo suturing
    forceps
fine-cup forceps
fine-dissecting forceps
fine-dissecting scissors
Fine-Gill corneal knife
fine-line tissue marker
fine-mesh dressing
fine-mesh gauze
fine-needle aspiration (FNA)
fine-needle aspiration biopsy
    (FNAB)
fine-needle aspiration cytology
    (FNAC)

fine-needle biopsy
fine-needle electrode
fine-needle percutaneous
 cholangiogram
fine-needle transhepatic
 cholangiogram
fine-pointed hemostat
Finesse cardiac device
Finesse guiding catheter
Finesse large-lumen guiding
 catheter
fine-stitch scissors
fine-suture scissors
Fine-Thornton scleral fixation
 ring
fine-tipped mosquito hemostat
fine-tipped up-and-down-angled
 bipolar forceps
fine-tissue forceps
fine-tooth clamp
fine-tooth forceps
fine-toothed clamp
fine-toothed forceps
fine-wire electrode
fine-wire speculum
finger
  articulations of fingers
  automatic finger
  avulsion of finger
  baseball finger
  bolster finger
  Brodie finger
  clawing of ring and little
   fingers
  clubbed finger
  clubbing of fingers
  denuded finger
  drop finger
  drumstick finger
  giant finger
  hammer finger
  hippocratic fingers
  index finger
  insane finger
  little finger
  lock finger
  long finger
  Lumbrical Plus finger
  lyre-shaped finger
  Madonna fingers
  mallet finger
  mechanical finger

finger (*continued*)
  middle finger
  palpating finger
  radial artery of index finger
  release of trigger finger
  ring finger
  rotational deformity of finger
  sausage finger
  snapping finger
  spade fingers
  spider finger
  spring finger
  stuck finger
  subcutaneous venous arch at
   root of fingers
  thumb finger
  trigger finger
  volar regions of fingers
  waxy finger
  web of fingers
  webbed fingers
  Zancolli capsulorrhaphy of
   fingers
finger agnosia
finger circumference gauge
finger contracture
finger cot
finger cuff
finger deformity
finger dilation
finger dissection
finger drop
finger extension clockspring
 splint
finger extension test (FET)
finger flap
finger flexion glove
finger flexion reflex
finger flexion splint
finger fracture dissection
finger fracture technique
finger gauze
finger goniometer
finger hook
finger jerk
finger joint arthroplasty
finger joint implant
finger loop
finger motion
finger plate
finger prick test
finger prosthesis

finger pulp
finger pursuit drift
finger rake retractor
finger reconstruction
finger replantation
finger retractor
finger ring cutter
finger ring saw
finger separator
finger splint
finger tamponade
finger vision
fingerbreadth (*pl.*
    fingerbreadths) (FB)
finger-cot dressing
finger-cot pack
finger-cot splint
finger-fillet flap
Finger Hugger splint
finger-like extension
finger-like villi
fingernail drill
fingerprint line
FingerPrint oximeter
finger-thumb reflex
fingertip
    Kleinert fingertip
    Kutler fingertip
    reimplantation of fingertip
    tingling of fingertips
fingertip amputation
fingertip dissection
fingertip fracture
fingertip injury
fingertip lesion
finger-to-nose
fingertrap suspension
fingertrap suture
finish bur
finish line
finishing ball reamer
finishing bur
finishing cup reamer
finishing knife
Fink biprong marker
Fink cataract aspirator
Fink cataract operation
Fink chalazion curet
Fink cul-de-sac cannula
Fink cul-de-sac irrigator
Fink curet
Fink fixation forceps

Fink forceps
Fink hook
Fink irrigator
Fink lacrimal retractor
Fink laryngoscope
Fink muscle hook
Fink muscle marker
Fink oblique muscle hook
Fink operation
Fink refractor
Fink retractor
Fink tendon tucker
Fink tendon-tucker forceps
Fink tucker
Fink valve
Finkelstein maneuver
Finkelstein sign for synovitis
Fink-Jameson forceps
Fink-Jameson oblique muscle
    forceps
Fink-Rowland keratome
Fink-Scobie hook
Fink-Weinstein 2-way syringe
Finn chamber
Finn chamber patch test device
Finn hinged knee replacement
Finn knee revision prosthesis
finned pacemaker lead
finned-stem punch
Finney gastroduodenostomy
Finney gastroenterostomy
Finney mask
Finney operation
Finney penile implant
Finney penile prosthesis
Finney prosthesis
Finney pyloroplasty
Finney-flexirod penile prosthesis
Finnoff laryngoscope
Finnoff transilluminator
Finochietto arterial clamp
Finochietto artery clamp
Finochietto bronchial clamp
Finochietto clamp
Finochietto clamp carrier
Finochietto forceps
Finochietto hand retractor
Finochietto infant rib contractor
Finochietto infant rib retractor
Finochietto laminectomy
    retractor
Finochietto lobectomy forceps

Finochietto needle
Finochietto needle holder
Finochietto operation
Finochietto retractor
Finochietto rib retractor
Finochietto rib spreader
Finochietto scissors
Finochietto spreader
Finochietto stirrup
Finochietto thoracic forceps
Finochietto thoracic scissors
Finochietto Vital needle holder
Finochietto-Billroth I
    gastrectomy
Finochietto-Billroth I
    gastrectomy technique
Finochietto-Bunnell test
Finochietto-Burford rib
    contractor
Finochietto-Burford rib spreader
Finochietto-Geissendorfer rib
    retractor
Finochietto-Stille rib spreader
Finsen carbon arc light
Finsen lamp
Finsen retractor
Finsen tracheal hook
Finsen wound hook
Finsen-Reya light
Finsterer myringotomy split
    tube
Finsterer operation
Finsterer suction tube
Finsterer sutures
Finsterer-Hofmeister operation
Finzi-Harmer operation
Firbracol collagen-alginate
    dressing
Fried-Hendel procedure
Firland nebulizer
Firlene eye magnet
firm cell mass
Firm D-Ring wrist support
firm lesion
firm tissue
firm uterus
FirmFlex custom orthosis
first arch syndrome
first branchial cleft sinus
first carpometacarpal joint
    fracture
first cone position

first dorsal metatarsal artery
first impression
first intention wound closure
first parallel pelvic plane
first ray surgery
First Response manual
    resuscitator
first rib resection via
    subclavicular approach
    technique
first rib shears
first stage of labor
first trimester of pregnancy
first web flap
first web space
FirstChoice pouch closed pouch
FirstChoice pouch post-
    operative drainable pouch
FirstChoice pouch urostomy
    pouch
first-degree burn (1st-degree
    burn)
first-degree hemorrhoid
first-degree radiation injury
first-degree sprain
first-grade fusion
first-line screening technique
first-pass extraction
first-pass nuclide rest and
    exercise angiogram
first-pass radionuclide
    angiogram
first-pass scintigraphy
first-pass technique
FirstSave automated external
    defibrillator
first-stage draining of liver
    abscess
first-stage procedure
first-stage repair
FirstStep mattress
FirstStep tibial osteotomy
    instruments
first-toe Jones repair
Firtel broach
Fisch bone drill irrigator
Fisch cutting bur
Fisch drill
Fisch dural hook
Fisch dural retractor
Fisch microcrurotomy scissors
Fischer arthrodesis

Fischer aspirative lipoplasty
Fischer curet technique
Fischer nasal rasp
Fischer needle
Fischer pneumothoracic needle
Fischer shunt
Fischer sign
Fischer syringe
Fischer tendon stripper
Fischer-Leibinger bur hole-
    mounted fixation device
Fischl dissecting forceps
Fischl forceps
Fischl skin hook
Fischmann angiotribe forceps
Fischmann urethroplasty
Fish antral probe
Fish cuneiform osteotomy
    technique
Fish forceps
Fish grasping forceps
Fish infusion cannula
Fish inlet
Fish nasal forceps
Fish nasal-dressing forceps
Fish sinus probe
Fisher Accumet pH meter
Fisher advancement flap
Fisher advancement forceps
Fisher bed
Fisher brace
Fisher cannula
Fisher capsular forceps
Fisher double-ended retractor
Fisher exact test
Fisher eye needle
Fisher fenestrated lid retractor
Fisher forceps
Fisher guide
Fisher half pin
Fisher iris forceps
Fisher knife
Fisher lid retractor
Fisher microcapillary tube
    reader
Fisher needle
Fisher operation
Fisher quartz cold generator
Fisher rasp
Fisher retractor
Fisher spoon
Fisher spud

Fisher technique
Fisher tonsil dissector
Fisher tonsil knife
Fisher tonsil retractor
Fisher tonsillar knife
Fisher tonsillar retractor
Fisher ventricular cannula
Fisher-Arlt forceps
Fisher-Arlt iris forceps
fisherman's knot
fisherman's pliers
Fisher-Nugent retractor
Fisher-Paykel resuscitator
Fisher-Smith spatula
fish-flesh consistency
Fishgold line
fishhook lead
fishhook needle
fish-mouth amputation
fish-mouth anastomosis
fish-mouth cervix
fish-mouth fracture
fish-mouth incision
fish-mouth mitral stenosis
fish-mouth suture
fishnet pattern
fish-scale gallbladder
fishtail chisel
fishtail deformity
fishtail raspatory
fishtail spatula
fishtail spatula raspatory
Fisk tractor
Fiskars scissors
Fiske periosteal elevator
Fisons indirect binocular
    ophthalmoscope
Fisons nebulizer
fissura (*pl.* fissurae)
fissura antitragohelicina
fissural cyst
fissure
    abdominal fissure
    anal fissure
    anterior median fissure
    antitragohelicine fissure
    auricular fissure
    azygos fissure
    calcarine fissure
    caudal transverse fissure
    cerebral fissure
    corneal fissure

fissure (*continued*)
dentate fissure
dorsal fissure
Duverney fissure
Ecker fissure
ethmoidal fissure
excision of fissure
fracture of superior orbital
  fissure
glaserian fissure
Henle fissures
horizontal fissure
inferior accessory fissure
inferior fissure
inferior orbital fissure
infraorbital fissure
interlobar fissure
interpalpebral fissure
intrahemispheric fissure
lateral cerebral fissure
linguogingival fissure
longitudinal cerebral fissure
major fissure
mandibular fissure
maxillary fissure
medial canthal fissure
median fissure
minor fissure
oblique fissure
oral fissure
orbital fissure
palatine bone fissure
palpebral fissure
Pansch fissure
parieto-occipital fissure
petro-occipital fissure
petrosquamous fissure
petrotympanic fissure
pharyngomaxillary fissure
portal fissure
posterior median fissure
pterygoid fissure
pterygomaxillary fissure
pterygopalatine fissure
rectal fissure
right sagittal fissure
Rolando fissure
sagittal fissure
Santorini fissure
Schwalbe fissure
sphenoidal fissure
sphenomaxillary fissure

fissure (*continued*)
sphenopalatine fissure
sphenopetrosal fissure
squamotympanic fissure
sternal fissure
superior orbital fissure
superior temporal fissure
sylvian fissure
tympanomastoid fissure
tympanosquamous fissure
umbilical fissure
vestibular fissure
zygomatic fissure
zygomaticosphenoid fissure
fissure bur
fissure cavity
fissure forceps
fissure fracture
fissure in ano
fissurectomy
fissured
fissured fracture
fissured tongue
fissuring
fist percussion
fistula (*pl.* fistulas, fistulae)
abdominal fistula
abdominal wall fistula
alveolar fistula
amphibolic fistula
anal fistula
anastomotic fistula
anorectal fistula
antecubital arteriovenous
  fistula
antroaural fistula
aortocaval fistula
aortoduodenal fistula
aortoenteric fistula
aortoesophageal fistula
aortogastric fistula
aortograft duodenal fistula
aortosigmoid fistula
arterial-arterial fistula
arterial-enteric fistula
arterial-portal fistula
arterioportal fistula
arterioportobiliary fistula
arteriosinusoidal penile fistula
arteriovenous fistula (AVF)
arteriovenous Gore-Tex fistula
  (AV Gore-Tex fistula)

fistula (*continued*)
- arteriovenous subclavian fistula
- aural fistula
- autocaval fistula
- AV fistula (arteriovenous fistula)
- AV Gore-Tex fistula (arteriovenous Gore-Tex fistula)
- benign duodenocolic fistula
- biliary fistula
- biliary-bronchial fistula
- biliary-cutaneous fistula
- biliary-duodenal fistula
- biliary-enteric fistula
- biliocystic fistula
- bilioenteric fistula
- biliopleural fistula
- bladder fistula
- blind fistula
- Blom-Singer tracheoesophageal fistula
- bowl fistula
- BP fistula
- brachioaxillary bridge graft fistula
- brachiosubclavian bridge graft fistula
- branchial fistula
- Brescia fistula
- Brescia-Cimino AV fistula
- Brescio-Cimino arteriovenous fistula
- bronchobiliary fistula
- bronchocutaneous fistula
- bronchoesophageal fistula
- bronchopleural fistula
- bronchopleurocutaneous fistula (BPCF)
- bronchopulmonary fistula
- calyceal fistula
- cameral fistula
- carotid-cavernous sinus fistula (CCSF)
- carotid-dural fistula
- cavernous sinus fistula
- cerebrospinal fluid fistula
- cervical fistula
- cervicovaginal fistula
- chole fistula
- cholecystenteric fistula

fistula (*continued*)
- cholecystocholedochal fistula
- cholecystocolic fistula
- cholecystocolonic fistula
- cholecystoduodenal fistula
- cholecystoduodenocolic fistula
- cholecystogastric fistula
- cholecystointestinal fistula
- choledochal-colonic fistula
- choledochocolonic fistula
- choledochoduodenal fistula
- choledochoenteric fistula
- chyle fistula
- Cimino arteriovenous fistula
- Cimino AV fistula
- Cimino fistula
- Cimino-Brescia arteriovenous fistula
- closure of fistula
- coccygeal fistula
- colobronchial fistula
- colocutaneous fistula
- cologastrocutaneous fistula
- coloileal fistula
- colonic fistula
- colorectal fistula
- colovaginal fistula
- colovesical fistula
- communicating fistula
- complete fistula
- complex anorectal fistula
- congenital pulmonary arteriovenous fistula
- congenital urethroperineal fistula
- controlled fistula
- corneal fistula
- coronary artery fistula (CAF)
- coronary artery-right ventricular fistula
- coronary fistula
- craniosinus fistula
- cutaneobiliary fistula
- cystogastric fistula
- dental fistula
- dialysis fistula
- dorsal enteric fistula
- duct fistula
- duodenal fistula
- duodenocaval fistula
- duodenocolic fistula

fistula (*continued*)

duodenoenterocutaneous fistula
dural arteriovenous fistula
dural cavernous sinus fistula
Eck fistula
endobronchial fistula
endogenous AV fistula
enteric fistula
enterocolic fistula
enterocutaneous fistula
enteroenteral fistula
enteroenteric fistula
enterogenital fistula
enterourethral fistula
enterovaginal fistula
enterovesical fistula
esophageal fistula
esophagobronchial fistula
esophagocutaneous fistula
esophagomediastinal fistula
esophagopulmonary fistula
esophagorespiratory fistula
esophagotracheal fistula
ethmoid fistula
ethmoidal-lacrimal fistula
external biliary fistula
external pancreatic fistula
extrasphincteric anal fistula
fecal fistula
forearm graft arteriovenous fistula
formation of fistula
gastric fistula
gastrocolic fistula
gastrocutaneous fistula
gastroduodenal fistula
gastroenteric fistula
gastrointestinal fistula
gastrointestinal-cutaneous fistula
gastrojejunocolic fistula
gastropleural fistula
genitourinary fistula
gingival fistula
Gore-Tex AV fistula
graft-enteric fistula
Gross tracheoesophageal fistula
hepatic artery-portal vein fistula
hepatic fistula

fistula (*continued*)

hepatopleural fistula
hepatoportal biliary fistula
high-flow arteriovenous fistula
horseshoe fistula
H-type tracheoesophageal fistula
iatrogenic arteriovenous fistula
ileocutaneous fistula
ileoduodenal fistula
ileosigmoid fistula
ileovesical fistula
incomplete fistula
inflammatory fistula
internal fistula
internal lacrimal fistula
intersphincteric anal fistula
intestinal fistula
intracranial arteriovenous fistula
intrahepatic arterial-portal fistula
intrahepatic AV fistula
intrahepatic spontaneous arterioportal fistula
intralabyrinthine fistula
intraocular fistula
jejunocolic fistula
labyrinthine fistula
lacrimal fistula
lacteal fistula
Latzko repair of vesicovaginal fistula
lymphatic fistula
mammary fistula
Mann-Bollman fistula
mesenteric arteriovenous fistula
mesenteric fistula
metroperitoneal fistula
mucous fistula
occluded fistula
open fistula
oral fistula
orbital fistula
oroantral fistula
orocutaneous fistula
orofacial fistula
oronasal fistula
palatal fistula

fistula (*continued*)
palatoalveolar fistula
pancreatic cutaneous fistula
pancreaticopleural fistula
pararectal fistula
parietal fistula
perianal fistula
perilymph fistula
perilymphatic fistula (PLF)
perineal urinary fistula
perineovaginal fistula
pharyngeal fistula
pharyngocutaneous fistula
pilonidal fistula
pleurobiliary fistula
pleuroesophageal fistula
postbiopsy renal AV fistula
postoperative pleurobiliary
    fistula
postradiation fistula
posttraumatic pancreatic-
    cutaneous fistula
preauricular fistula
primary arteriovenous fistula
pseudocystobiliary fistula
pulmonary arteriovenous
    fistula (PAF)
radiculomedullary fistula
rectal fistula
rectocutaneous fistula
rectolabial fistula
rectourethral fistula
rectourinary fistula
rectovaginal fistula
rectovesical fistula
rectovestibular fistula
rectovulvar fistula
renal fistula
renogastric fistula
respiratory-esophageal fistula
retroperitoneal fistula
reverse Eck fistula
salivary fistula
scleral fistula
sigmoid cutaneous fistula
sigmoidocutaneous fistula
sigmoidovesical fistula
solitary pulmonary
    arteriovenous fistula
spermatic fistula
spinal dural arteriovenous
    fistula

fistula (*continued*)
splanchnic AV fistula
splenic AV fistula
splenobronchial fistula
stercoral fistula
subclavian arteriovenous
    fistula
submental fistula
suprasphincteric fistula
sylvian fistula
synovial fistula
systemic arteriovenous fistula
TE fistula (tracheoesophageal
    fistula)
thigh graft arteriovenous
    fistula
Thiry fistula
Thiry-Vella fistula
thoracic duct fistula
thromboembolic fistula
thyroglossal fistula
tracheal fistula
tracheobiliary fistula
tracheobronchoesophageal
    fistula
tracheocutaneous fistula
tracheoesophageal fistula
transsphincteric anal fistula
traumatic fistula
ulcerogenic fistula
umbilical fistula
urachal fistula
ureteral fistula
ureterocolic fistula
ureterocutaneous fistula
ureteroduodenal fistula
ureteroperitoneal fistula
ureterouterine fistula
ureterovaginal fistula
urethrocavernous fistula
urethrocutaneous fistula
urethroperineal fistula
urethrorectal fistula
urethrovaginal fistula
urinary fistula
urinary-umbilical fistula
urinary-vaginal fistula
urogenital fistula
uteroperitoneal fistula
uterorectal fistula
uterovaginal fistula
vaginal fistula

fistula (*continued*)
  vaginocutaneous fistula
  vaginoperineal fistula
  vasocutaneous fistula
  Vella fistula
  venobiliary fistula
  vesical fistula
  vesicoabdominal fistula
  vesicoacetabular fistula
  vesicocervical fistula
  vesicocolic fistula
  vesicocutaneous fistula
  vesicoenteric fistula
  vesicointestinal fistula
  vesico-ovarian fistula
  vesicoperineal fistula
  vesicorectal fistula
  vesicosalpingovaginal fistula
  vesicoureteral fistula
  vesicouterine fistula
  vesicovaginal fistula
  vesicovaginorectal fistula
  vitelline fistula
  vulvorectal fistula
fistula auris congenita
fistula bimucosa
fistula funnel
fistula form
fistula hook
fistula in ano
fistula needle
fistula probe
fistula scissors
fistula takedown
fistula test
fistular closure
fistular formation
fistular hook
fistular knife
fistular needle
fistular probe
fistulation
  artificial fistulation
  postalveolar cleft palate
    fistulation (CPF)
  spreading fistulation
fistulatome
fistulectomy
fistulization
fistulizing surgery
fistuloenterostomy
fistulogram

fistulography
fistulotome
fistulotome knife
fistulotomy
  anal fistulotomy
  choledochoduodenal
    fistulotomy
  diathermic fistulotomy
  endoscopic fistulotomy
  laying-open fistulotomy
  Parks fistulotomy
  Parks method of anal
    fistulotomy
  Parks staged fistulotomy
fistulous tract
Fitch obturator
Fit-Lastic therapy band
fitness for general anesthesia
fitting
  immediate postsurgical fitting
    (IPSF)
Fitzgerald aortic aneurysm
    clamp
Fitzgerald aortic aneurysm
    forceps
Fitzgerald forceps
Fitzpatrick classification of sun-
    reactive skin types (types I-
    IV)
Fitzpatrick I and II patients
Fitzpatrick suction tube
Fitzpatrick sun-reactive skin
    type
Fitzwater forceps
Fitzwater ligature carrier
Fitzwater peanut sponge-holding
    forceps
Fixateur Interne rod
Fixateur Interne screw
fixation
  4-point fixation
  adjunctive screw fixation
  angled blade plate fixation
  anomalous fixation
  anterior internal fixation
  anterior metallic fixation
  anterior plate fixation
  anterior screw fixation
  anterior spinal fixation
  AO external fixation
  AO rigid fixation
  AO spinal internal fixation

fixation (*continued*)
APR cement fixation
arch bar fixation
Association for the Study of Internal Fixation (ASIF) plate
atlantoaxial rotatory fixation
autotrophic fixation
axial fixation
axis fixation
bar bolt fixation
Barr open reduction and internal fixation
Barr tibial fracture fixation
bicortical screw fixation
bifocal fixation
bifoveal fixation
binocular fixation
biodegradable plate fixation
biologic fixation
biphase external pin fixation
biphase pin fixation
blade plate fixation
bolt fixation
bone-ingrowth fixation
bridge plate fixation
brow fixation
capsular fixation
carbon dioxide fixation
catheter fixation
central fixation
cerclage wire fixation
cervical spine internal fixation
cervical spine screw-plate fixation
chest wall fixation
circumalveolar fixation
circumferential wire-loop fixation
circummandibular fixation
circumzygomatic fixation
closed reduction and internal fixation
closed reduction and percutaneous fixation (CRPF)
cloverleaf condylar-plate fixation
Cole tendon fixation
complement fixation
composite wiring fixation

fixation (*continued*)
compression plate fixation
condylar process fracture axial anchor screw fixation
condylar screw fixation
coracoclavicular screw fixation
coracoclavicular suture fixation
Cotrel-Dubousset fixation
Cotrel-Dubousset spinal rod fixation
cranial flap fixation
craniofacial fixation
cricoarytenoid fixation
crossed fixation
crossed K-wire fixation
Denham external fixation
Denham skeletal fixation
dens anterior screw fixation
Deverle fixation
Dimon-Hughston fracture fixation
dorsal plate and lag screw fixation
dorsal wire-loop fixation
dynamic compression-plate fixation
dynamic condylar-screw fixation
eccentric fixation
ECT internal fracture fixation
elastic band fixation
electrode fixation
Erich arch bar application and intermaxillary fixation
external pin fixation
external spinal fixation
eyebrow fixation
E-Z Flap cranial flap fixation
femoral prosthesis fixation
formalin fixation
fracture fixation
Galveston pelvic fixation
Gilmer intermaxillary fixation
Gouffon pin fixation
graft fixation
greenstick fixation
Guyton-Noyes fixation
Hackethal intramedullary bouquet fixation
half-pin fixation

fixation (*continued*)
  heart valve fixation
  hip fixation
  hook fixation
  hook-plate fixation
  iliac fixation
  Ilizarov external fixation
  Ilizarov internal fixation
  ingrowth fixation
  interference fit fixation
  interfragmentary wiring
    fixation
  intermaxillary fixation (IMF)
  internal fixation
  internal spinal fixation
  interosseous wire fixation
  interosseous wiring fixation
  intestinal fixation
  intramaxillary fixation
  intramedullary device fixation
  intramedullary fixation
  intramedullary rod fixation
  intramural fixation
  intraosseous fixation
  Kavanaugh-Brower-Mann
    fixation
  Kempf internal screw fixation
  key-free compression hip
    screw fixation
  Kirschner pin fixation
  Kirschner wire fixation
  Kronner external fixation
  Kronner skeletal fixation
  Kyle internal fixation
  LactoSorb resorbable
    craniomaxillofacial fixation
  lag screw fixation
  Lane plate for long-bone
    fixation
  line of fixation
  loop fixation
  lumbar pedicle fixation
  lumbar spine segmental
    fixation
  lumbar spine transpedicular
    fixation
  Luque loop fixation
  Luque rod fixation
  Luque-Galveston fixation
  Magerl posterior cervical
    screw fixation
  mandibular fixation

fixation (*continued*)
  mandibulomaxillary fixation
  Matta-Saucedo fixation
  maxillomandibular fixation
    (MMF)
  McIndoe and Reese alar
    cartilage suture fixation
  McKeever medullary clavicle
    fixation
  medial malleolus fixation
  medullary fixation
  medullary nail fixation
  metallic rod fixation
  microplate fixation
  microwave fixation
  miniplate fixation
  Modulock posterior spinal
    fixation
  monocular fixation
  multiple-point sacral fixation
  muscle fixation
  nail-plate fixation
  nasomandibular fixation
  near fixation
  neutralization plate fixation
  Nichols sacrospinous fixation
  nonresorbable fixation
  Obwegeser-Dalpont internal
    screw fixation
  occipitocervical fixation
  odontoid fracture internal
    fixation
  odontoid screw fixation
  open reduction and fixation
  open reduction and internal
    fixation (ORIF)
  open reduction with internal
    fixation (ORIF)
  OrthoFrame external fixation
  OrthoSorb pin fixation
  osseous fixation
  otosclerotic fixation
  parametrial fixation
  pedicle screw-rod fixation
  pedicular fixation
  pelvic fixation
  percutaneous fixation
  phalangeal fracture fixation
  Phemister acromioclavicular
    pin fixation
  pin-and-plaster fixation
  plate and screw fixation

fixation (*continued*)
plate fixation
plate-screw fixation
porous ingrowth fixation
posterior cervical fixation
posterior screw fixation
posterior segmental fixation
prophylactic skeletal fixation
prosthesis fixation
provisional fixation
pubic fixation
reduction and internal
    fixation
resorbable fixation
resorbable rigid fixation
restorative fixation
ReUnite hand fixation
ReUnite fixation
rigid fixation
rigid internal fixation (RIF)
rigid lag screw fixation
rigid plate fixation
rod fixation
rod sleeve fixation
Roger-Anderson pin fixation
role fixation
sacral pedicle screw fixation
sacral spine fixation
sacroiliac extension fixation
sacroiliac flexion fixation
sacrospinous ligament vaginal
    fixation
sacrum fusion screw fixation
Schneider fixation
scoliotic curve fixation
screw fixation
screw-and-plate fixation
screw-and-wire fixation
Searcy fixation
secondary fixation
segmental fixation
Seidel intramedullary fixation
semirigid fixation
skeletal fixation
skeletal pin fixation
SOF'WIRE spinal fixation
Spiessel internal screw
    fixation
spinal fixation
split fixation
spring fixation
standard formalin fixation

fixation (*continued*)
staple fixation
static fixation
Steinhauser internal screw
    fixation
Steinmann pin fixation
strut plate fixation
sublaminar fixation
sulcus fixation
surgical fixation
suture fixation
tantalum fixation
tantalum wire fixation
tension band fixation
tension-free scalp fixation
thin-wire Ilizarov fixation
titanium rigid fixation
transarticular wire fixation
transcalvarial suture fixation
transcapitellar wire fixation
transiliac rod fixation
transpedicular screw-rod
    fixation
transpedicular segmental
    fixation
transverse fixation
TSRH rod fixation
tunnel and sling fixation
Turvy internal screw fixation
visual fixation
wire fixation
wire loop fixation
Wolvek sternal approximation
    fixation
Zenker fixation
Zickel nail fixation
fixation anchor
fixation anomaly
fixation bandage
fixation base
fixation binocular forceps
fixation button
fixation delay
fixation device
fixation forceps
fixation graft
fixation hook
fixation in vivo
fixation jig
fixation object
fixation pick
fixation pin

fixation point
fixation reflex
fixation ring
fixation rod
fixation screw
fixation suture technique
fixation sutures
fixation target
fixation technique
fixation test
fixation twist hook
fixation with osteogenesis
fixation/anchor forceps
fixative solution
fixator
   Ace Unifix fixator
   Ace-Fischer external fixator
   Ace-Fischer fixator
   Agee Digit Widget mini-
      external fixator
   articulated external fixator
   Bay external fixator
   biplanar fixator
   Calandruccio external fixator
   circular external fixator
   Clyburn Colles fixator
   Clyburn Colles fracture fixator
   Clyburn dynamic Colles fixator
   DeBastiani external fixator
   dynamic axial fixator
   EBI external fixator
   Edwards D-L modular fixator
   external fixator
   external spinal skeletal fixator
   Herbert screw fixator
   Hex-Fix monolateral external
      fixator
   hinged articulated fixator
   Hoffmann external fixator
   Hoffmann Vital external
      fixator
   HTO fixator
   Ilizarov circulator external
      fixator
   Ilizarov external ring fixator
   Ilizarov fixator
   Ilizarov hybrid fixator
   Kessler external fixator
   Kronner external fixator
   mini-Hoffmann external
      fixator
   mini-Orthofix fixator

fixator (*continued*)
   Monofixateur external fixator
   Olerud internal fixator
   Orthofix monolateral femoral
      external fixator
   Oxford fixator
   Rennig dynamic wrist fixator
   Rezinian spinal fixator
   Roger Anderson external
      fixator
   spanning external fixator
   Stableloc Colles fracture
      external fixator
   Stuhler-Heise fixator
   Synthes external fixator
   Thomas fixator
   Vermont spinal fixator
   Wagner external fixator
fixator muscle of base of stapes
fixator muscles
fixed appliance
fixed arch bar
fixed bearing knee implant
fixed bridge
fixed cervical dilator
fixed deformity
fixed dressing
fixed expansion prosthesis
fixed femoral head prosthesis
fixed forceps
fixed maintainer space
fixed malleus
fixed mandibular implant (FMI)
fixed perfusion defect
fixed point
fixed ring retractor
fixed spasm
fixed support
fixed-angle AO bladeplate
fixed-dose patient-controlled
      analgesia (FDPCA)
fixed-offset guide
fixed-rate asynchronous atrial
      pacemaker
fixed-rate asynchronous
      ventricular pacemaker
fixed-rate pacemaker
fixed-wire balloon
fixing screw
fixing time
fixture
   implant fixture

FL pheresis (filtration
    leukapheresis)
fL, fl (femtoliter)
FL4 guide
flabby abdomen
flaccid dysarthria
flaccid skin
flaccidity
Flack node
flag flap
Flagg laryngoscope
Flagg stainless steel
    laryngoscope blade
flail chest
flail extremity
flail joint
flail mitral valve
flair
FLAIR image
Flajani operation
flame bur
flame hemorrhage
flame ionization detector
flame photometric detector
flame-shaped hemorrhage
flame-tip bur
flamingo antrostomy forceps
Flamm technique
flammable anesthetic
Flanagan gouge
Flanagan spinal fusion gouge
Flanagan-Burem graft
flange
    adhesive flange
    Callahan flange
    Coloplast flange
    ConQuest female continence
        system pressure pad with
        preattached flange
    ConQuest male continence
        system condom catheter
        with preattached flange
    dental flange
    endoprosthetic flange
    hip flange
    labial flange
    lingual flange
    mandibular lingual flange
    Scuderi-Callahan flange
    Syed template flange
flange of Syed template
flanged Teflon tube

flank approach
flank area
flank bone
flank dissection
flank gunshot wound
flank incision
flank incisional hernia
flank mass
flank pain
flank position
flank stripe
flank tenderness
flank wound
flankplasty
flank-strip sign on supine
    abdominal film
Flannery ear speculum
Flannery speculum
flap
    2nd toe wraparound flap
    3-paddle tensor fascia lata free
        flap
    3-square flap
    mutton chop flap
    turnover flap
    Abbe flap
    Abbe-Estlander flap
    Abbe lip flap
    Abbe-Estlander flap
    abdominal axial subcutaneous
        flap
    abdominal axial subcutaneous
        pedicle flap
    abdominal fasciocutaneous
        flap
    abdominal wall flap
    abdominothoracic flap
    abductor hallucis flap
    access flap
    adenoadipose flap
    adipofascial axial pattern
        cross-finger flap
    adipofascial flap
    adipofascial sural flap
    adipofascial turnover flap
    adipogenic growth factor-
        treated flaps
    advancement flap
    advancement of rectal flap
    allogenically vascularized
        prefabricated flap
    anconeus muscle flap

flap (*continued*)
  angiosomal flap
  Anita-Busch
    chondrocutaneous flap
  antegrade island flap
  anterior chest wall flap
  anterior helical rim free flap
  anterior skin flap
  anterolateral thigh flap
  anterolateral thigh free flap
  aponeurotic flap
  apron flap
  arc of rotation of
    fasciocutaneous flap
  Argamaso-Lewis composite
    flap
  arm flap
  arterial flap
  arterialized flap
  artery island flap
  Atasoy palmar flap
  Atasoy triangular
    advancement flap
  Atasoy volar V-Y flap
  Atasoy-Kleinert flap
  Atasoy-Kleinert volar V-Y
    advancement flap
  auricular rim-based reverse-
    flow-type of flap
  autologous tissue flaps
  axial advancement flap
  axial dorsal flap
  axial flag flap
  axial flap
  axial frontonasal flap
  axial pattern scalp flap
  axial pattern vascularized skin
    flap
  axial temporoparietal facial
    flap
  axial-based flap
  axillary flap
  Bakamjian flap
  Bakamjian pedicle flap
  Bakamjian tubed flap
  Banner flap
  base of flap
  Becker flap
  bell flap
  Berlin tulip flap
  Bernard flap
  biceps brachii flap

flap (*continued*)
  bicoronal scalp flap
  bilateral inferior epigastric
    artery flap (BIEF)
  bilateral pectoralis major
    muscle flap
  bilateral rotational flap
  bilateral V-Y Kutler flap
  bilobed fasciocutaneous flap
  bilobed flap
  bilobed skin flap
  bilobed transposition flap
  bipedicle delay flap
  bipedicle digital visor flap
  bipedicle dorsal flap
  bipedicle flap
  bipedicle mucoperiosteal flap
  bipedicle TRAM flap
  bipedicled delay flap
  bipedicled flap
  bladder flap
  Blaskovics flap
  Boari bladder flap
  Boari flap
  Boari-Kuss flap
  Boari-Ockerblad flap
  bone flap
  boomerang-shaped rectus
    abdominis
    musculocutaneous free flap
  brachioradialis flap
  bridge flap
  bridge pedicle flap
  broad-based type B Cormack-
    Lamberty pedicled
    fasciocutaneous flap
  buccal envelope flap
  buccal mucosal flap
  buccal musculomucosal flap
  buccinator myomucosal flap
  bulbocavernosus fat flap
  Bunnell bipedicle digital visor
    flap
  Bunnell bipedicle flap
  Bunnell flap
  buried de-epithelialized local
    flap
  buried dermal flap
  buried flap
  Burow flap
  bursal flap
  butterfly flap

flap (*continued*)

Byers flap
calvarium flap
candidiasis in facelift skin flap
canthomeatal flap
cartilage flap
caterpillar flap
cellulocutaneous flap
cervical flap
cervical humeral flap
cervical rotational flap
cervical tube flap
cervical visor flap
cervicofacial flap
Charretera flap
cheek advancement flap
cheek flap
cheek mucous-muscle flap
cheek rotation flap
cheek-lip flap
chest flap
Chinese flap
chondrocutaneous flap
circular flap
circular subcutaneous island
    flap
circumflex scapular flap
cleft margin flap
cocked-half flap
columellar flap
composite chondrocutaneous
    flap
composite flap
composite
    osteomyocutaneous
    preformed flap
compound flap
compound skin flap
conchal flap
conical flap
conjunctival flap
conjunctivo-Tenon flap
converging triangular flap
Converse flap
Converse scalping flap
Cormack-Lamberty
    fasciocutaneous flaps
    (types A-C)
corneal flap
coronoid flap
coverage flap
Crane flap

flap (*continued*)

craniotomy flap
Cronin-Matthews eave flap
cross flap
cross-arm flap
cross-finger flap
cross-leg flap
cross-leg skin flap
cross-lid flap
cross-lip flap
cross-lip pedicle flap
C-shaped scalp flap
cutaneoperiosteal flap
cutaneous flap
cutaneous forearm flap
Cutler flap
Cutler-Beard bridge flap
Cutler-Beard flap
Dandy myocutaneous scalp
    flap
Dardour flap
Dardour lateral flap
dartos fasciocutaneous flap
dartos musculocutaneous flap
decorticated flap
deep circumflex iliac artery-
    iliac crest flap
de-epithelialized local flap
de-epithelialized rectus
    abdominis muscle flap
de-epithelialized
    revascularized lateral
    intercostal flap
deflected skin flap
delay of flap
delayed flap
delayed skin flap
delayed transfer flap
deltoid flap
deltopectoral flap
deltoscapular flap
denuded and buried skin
    submental flap
dermal fat free flap
dermal fat pedicle flap
dermal pyramidal flap
dermoadipose flap
dermofat flap
developed flap
digastric muscle flap
digital flap
direct flap

flap (*continued*)

- direct transfer flap
- distal flap
- distal pedicle flap
- distal-based flap
- distal-based island flap
- distally based fasciocutaneous flap (DBFF)
- distant flap
- distant skin flap
- dorsal cross-finger flap
- dorsal flap
- dorsal pedicle TRAM flap
- dorsal rotation flap
- dorsal thoracic fascia free flap
- dorsal transposition flap
- dorsalis pedis flap
- double cross-lip flap
- double pedicle flap
- double pendulum flap
- double skin paddle fibular flap
- double V-Y flap
- double-ended flap
- double-paddle flap
- double-paddle island flap
- double-pedicle skin flap
- double-pedicle transverse rectus abdominis musculocutaneous flap
- Dufourmental flap
- eave flap
- Elliot flap
- elliptical flap
- Eloesser flap
- emergency free flap
- endorectal flap
- envelope flap
- epaulet flap
- epigastric flap
- epithelial turn-in flap
- equal sagittal flap
- Estlander flap
- Estlander-Abbe flap
- expanded free scalp flap
- extended lateral arm free flap (ELAFF)
- extended shoulder flap
- extensor brevis flap
- extensor carpi radialis longus flap
- extensor digitorum longus flap

flap (*continued*)

- extraction flap
- facial artery musculomucosal flap (FAMM flap)
- facial turnover flap
- FAMM flap (facial artery musculomucosal flap)
- fan flap
- fan-shaped flap
- fascia flap
- fascia lata flap
- fascial flap
- fasciocutaneous flap
- fasciocutaneous free flap
- fasciocutaneous island flap
- fascio-osteocutaneous flap
- fat flap
- fibula flap
- fibula free flap
- fibular osteoseptocutaneous flap
- fibular flap
- fibular osteocutaneous flap
- fibular osteocutaneous free flap
- Filatov flap
- Filatov-Gillies flap
- fillet flap
- fillet of foot free flap
- finger flap
- finger-fillet flap
- first web flap
- Fisher advancement flap
- flag flap
- flat flap
- fleur-de-lis flap
- fleur-de-lis forehead flap
- flexor carpi ulnaris flap
- foot fillet flap
- fascia lata flap
- foot 1st-web flap
- foramen ovale flap
- forearm flap
- forehead flap
- foreskin flap
- forked flap
- fornix-based conjunctival flap
- fornix-based flap
- free anterolateral thigh flap
- free arterialized venous forearm flap
- free bone flap

flap (*continued*)
  free composite flap
  free cutaneous lateral arm
    flap
  free expanded flap
  free facial flap
  free fasciocutaneous flap
  free fibular harvest flap
  free flap
  free forearm flap
  free groin flap
  free iliac bone crest flap
  free latissimus dorsi flap
  free microsurgical flap
  free microvascular flap
  free posterior interosseous
    flap
  free radial forearm flap
  free sensate flap
  free sequential flap
  free skin flap
  free temporal fascial flap
  free temporal flap
  free temporoparietal fascial
    flap
  free toe-to-finger hemipulp
    flap
  free toe-to-fingertip
    neurovascular flap
  free TRAM flap
  free transverse rectus
    abdominis
    musculocutaneous flap
  free vascularized flap
  French flap
  French sliding flap
  Fricke flap
  frontal bone flap
  frontogaleal flap
  full-thickness flap
  full-thickness periodontal flap
  fusiform flap
  fusiform island flap
  galea frontalis flap
  galea occipital flap
  galea periosteal flap
  galeal flap
  gastrocnemius flap
  gastrocnemius sliding flap
  gate flap
  gauntlet flap
  geometric nasal flap

flap (*continued*)
  Gilbert scapular flap
  Gillies fan flap
  Gillies flap
  Gillies up-and-down flap
  gingival flap
  glabellar bilobed flap
  glabellar rotation flap
  gluteal flap
  gluteal thigh flap
  gluteus maximus flap
  gluteus maximus
    musculocutaneous flap
  gluteus maximus
    myocutaneous flap
  gracilis flap
  gracilis muscle flap
  gracilis musculocutaneous
    flap
  great toe wraparound flap
  groin flap
  Gunderson conjunctival flap
  Gunter Von Noorden flap
  hand flap
  hemipulp flap
  hemitongue flap
  hinged corneal flap
  hinged flap
  horizontal bipedicle dermal
    flap
  horizontal flap
  horseshoe flap
  horseshoe-shaped flap
  horseshoe-shaped skin flap
  House sliding advancement
    flap
  Hueston spiral flap
  Hughes flap
  Hughes tarsoconjunctival flap
  HUMI cervical forceps skate
    flap
  hypogastric flap
  ideal flap
  iliac crest free flap
  iliac crest free osseous flap
  iliac crest osseous flap
  iliac crest osteocutaneous flap
  iliac crest osteomuscular flap
  iliac osteocutaneous flap
  iliac osteocutaneous free flap
  iliofemoral pedicle flap
  immediate flap

flap (*continued*)

immediate transfer flap
Imre sliding flap
inchworm flap
Indian flap
Indian forehead flap
Indian rotation flap
inferior flap
inferior gluteal flap
innervated free flap
innervated platysma flap
insensate flap
instep island flap
intercostal flap
interdigitated muscle flap
interdigitating skin flap
interdigitating triangular skin flap
interdigitating zigzag skin flap
internal oblique osteomuscular flap
interpolated flap
interpolation flap
intimal flap
intraoral flap
inverted horseshoe flap
inverted skin flap
I-shaped scalp flap
island fasciocutaneous flap
island flap
island leg flap
island pedicle flaps
island pedicle scalp flap
island skin flap
Italian distant flap
Italian flap
jejunal free flap
jejunum free flap
jump flap
jump skin flap
jumping man flap
Juri flap
Juri skin flap
Kapetansky flap
Karapandzic flap
Karydakis flap
Kazanjian flap
Kazanjian midline forehead flap
kite flap
Koerner flap
Kutler digital flap

flap (*continued*)

Kutler double lateral advancement flap
Kutler lateral V-Y advancement flap
Kutler V-Y flaps
Langenbeck flap
Langenbeck pedicle mucoperiosteal flap
laparoscopically harvested flap
lateral arm flap
lateral cartilage flap
lateral cutaneous thigh flap
lateral distally based fasciocutaneous flap
lateral intercostal flap
lateral supramalleolar flap
lateral thigh flap
lateral thigh free flap
lateral transverse thigh flap (LTTF)
lateral trapezius flap
lateral upper arm flap
latissimus dorsi flap
latissimus dorsi island flap
latissimus dorsi muscle flap
latissimus dorsi musculocutaneous flap
latissimus dorsi myocutaneous flap (LDMCF)
latissimus dorsi scapular bone flap
latissimus fasciocutaneous turnover flap
latissimus muscle flap
latissimus-scapular muscle flap
latissimus-serratus muscle flap
leg flap
Leibinger E-Z flap
LeMesurier rectangular flap
lifeboat flap
limbal-based flap
Limberg flap
Limberg local transposition flap
Limberg-type cutaneous flap
lined flap
lingual flap
lingual mucoperiosteal flap
lingual tongue flap

flap (*continued*)

Linton flap
lip flap
lip switch flap
lip-lip flap
Littler flap
Littler neurovascular island
    flap
liver flap
local flap
local muscle flap
local rotation flap
local skin flap
localized advancement flap
long rectangular flap
lower trapezius flap
lumbar periosteal turnover
    flap
lumbosacral back flap
lumbrical muscle flap
MacFee neck flap
Malaga flap
Maltese cross-patterned flap
maple leaf flap
marsupial flap
marsupial skin flap
masseter muscle flap
mastectomy skin flap
Mathieu island onlay flap
McCraw gracilis
    myocutaneous flap
McFarlane skin flap
McGregor forehead flap
medial cutaneous thigh flap
medial distally based
    fasciocutaneous flap
medial flap
medial forearm flap
medial plantar sensory flap
medial upper arm flap
median forehead flap
melolabial flap
mental V-Y island
    advancement island flap
mesiolabial bilobed
    transposition flap
microsurgical free flap
microvascular free flap
microvascular free posterior
    interosseous flap
midface avulsion flap
midline forehead flap

flap (*continued*)

Millard flap
Millard forehead flap
Millard island flap
Millard retroauricular and
    medial chondrocutaneous
    flap
Moberg advancement flap
Moberg volar advancement
    flap
modified dorsalis pedis
    myofascial flap
modified Singapore flap
monitor muscle flap
Monks-Esser flap
Monks-Esser island flap
Morrison neurovascular free
    flap
Morrison toe flap
moustache-like flap
mucochondrocutaneous flap
mucoperichondrial flap
mucoperiosteal flap
mucoperiosteal periodontal
    flap
mucoperiosteal sliding flap
mucosal periodontal flap
mucosal prelaminated flap
multistaged carrier flap
Munro Kerr bladder flap
muscle flap
muscle-periosteal flap
musculocutaneous flap
musculocutaneous free flap
musculofascial flap
musculotendinous flap
Mustarde lateral cheek
    rotation flap
Mustarde rotation-
    advancement flap
Mustarde rotational cheek
    flap
mutton chop flap
myocutaneous flap
myodermal flap
myofascial flap
myomucosal flap
Nahai tensor fascia lata flap
Nahai-Mathes fasciocutaneous
    flap (types A-C)
Nahigian butterfly flap
nape of neck flap

flap (*continued*)
 nasolabial flap
 nasolabial rotation flap
 Nassif parascapular flap
 Nataf lateral flap
 neck flap
 necrotic flap
 neurocutaneous flap
 neurocutaneous island flap
 neurosensorial free medial
    plantar flap
 neurosensory flap
 neurosensory island flap
 neurovascular free flap
 neurovascular island flap
 neurovascular island pedicle
    flap
 nutrient flap
 oblique flap
 Ochsenbein-Luebke flap
 Ockerblad-Boari flap
 omental flap
 omental transposition flap
 omocervical flap
 onlay island flap
 open flap
 opening flap
 Oriental V-Y flap
 Orticochea flap
 osseous flap
 osteocutaneous fillet flap
 osteocutaneous flap
 osteocutaneous scapular flap
 osteomusculocutaneous flap
 osteomyocutaneous flap
 osteoperiosteal flap
 osteoplastic bone flap
 osteoplastic flap
 over-and-out cheek flap
 palatal flap
 palatal island flap
 palatal mucoperiosteal flap
 palmar advancement flap
 palmar cross-finger flap
 palmar flap
 palmaris longus composite
    flap
 parasitic flap
 parabiotic flap
 paraextrophy skin flap
 paramedian forehead flap
 parascapular flap

flap (*continued*)
 parieto-occipital flap
 parrot beak flap
 partial-thickness flap
 pectoralis major flap
 pectoralis major
    myocutaneous flap
 pectoralis minor flap
 pectoralis myocutaneous flap
 pectoralis myofascial flap
 pedicle flap
 pedicle groin flap
 pedicle mucoperiosteal flap
 pedicled galeal frontalis flap
 pedicled latissimus flap
 pedicled mucosa flap
 pedicled myocutaneous flap
 pedicled pericranial flap
 pedicled tibial bone flap
 peg flap
 penile flap
 penile island flap
 perforator-based flap
 pericardial flap
 perichondrial flap
 pericoronal flap
 pericranial temporalis flap
 perineal artery axial flap
 perineal flap
 periodontal flap
 periosteal flap
 permanent pedicle flap
 peroneal island flap
 peroneus brevis flap
 peroneus longus flap
 pharyngeal flap
 platysma flap
 platysma myocutaneous flap
 Ponten fasciocutaneous flap
 postangioplasty intimal flap
 posterior auricular flap
 posterior flap
 posterior skin flap
 posterolateral flap
 pulp flap
 quadrapod flap
 quadrilobed flap
 racket-shaped flap
 radial forearm flap
 radial forearm osteocutaneous
    flap
 radial-based flap

flap (*continued*)

raised skin flap
RAM flap (rectus abdominis myocutaneous flap)
random cutaneous flap
random fasciocutaneous flap
random flap
random pattern flap
random temporoparietal fascial flap
random-pattern, palmar-based flap
rectangular flap
rectus abdominis flap
rectus abdominis free flap (RAFF)
rectus abdominis muscle flap
rectus abdominis myocutaneous flap (RAM)
rectus femoris fasciocutaneous flap
rectus femoris flap
rectus femoris musculocutaneous flap
rectus turnover flap
reflected skin flap
regional flap
remote pedicle flap
retinal flap
retroauricular free flap
retrograde perfused fasciocutaneous flap
retrograde-flow flap
reversal pedicle flap
reverse crossfinger flap
reverse digital artery flap
reverse digital artery island flap
reverse dorsal digital island flap
reverse flow island flap
reverse forearm island flap
reverse Karapandzic flap
reverse medial arm flap
reverse muscle flap
reversed digital artery flap
reversed dorsal digital flap
reversed extensor digitorum muscle island flap
reversed fasciosubcutaneous flap
reversed pedicle flap

flap (*continued*)

reverse-type mastoid fasciocutaneous flap
revolving-door island flap
rhomboid flap
rhomboid transposition flap
rope flap
rotation advancement flap
rotation flap
rotation of flap
rotation skin flap
rotation-advancement flap
rotational flap
rotator flap
Rubens breast flap
sandwich epicranial flap
sandwich flap
saphenous flap
sartorius flap
scalp sickle flap
scalping flap
scapula free flap
scapular flap
scapular island flap
scapular osteocutaneous flap
Scardino flap
Scarpa adipofascial flap
Schrudde rotational flap
scleral flap
scored alar mucocartilaginous flap
segmented flap
semilunar flap
sensate cutaneous flap
sensate flap
sensate medial plantar free flap
septal intranasal lining flap
sequential free flaps
serratus anterior flap
serratus anterior muscle flap
Sewell-Boyden flap
shaped glandular flap
shaped random pattern flap
short rectangular flap
shoulder flap
shutter flap
sickle flap
simple periodontal flap
simultaneous free flaps
single pedicle TRAM flap
single pedicle flap

flap (*continued*)

skate flap
skew flap
skin flap
sliding flap
SMAS-platysma flap
soft-tissue flap
soleus flap
spiral flap
split-thickness flap
split-thickness periodontal flap
steeple flap
Steichen neurovascular free
    flap
Stein-Abbe lip flap
Stein-Kazanjian flap
Stein-Kazanjian lower lip flap
Stenstrom foot flap
sternocleidomastoid flap
sternocleidomastoid
    musculocutaneous flap
sternocleidomastoid
    myocutaneous flap
subcapsular flap
subcutaneous flap
subcutaneous laterodigital
    reverse flap
subcutaneous pedicled flap
subcutaneous turnover flap
subgaleal flap
submental artery flap
submental island flap
submentonian dermo-fatty
    flap
subscapular flap
subscapular system free flap
superficial brachial flap
superior flap
superior gluteal flap
superiorly based Dardour
    lateral flap
superiorly based Nataf lateral
    flap
supramalleolar flap
supraorbital pericranial flap
supraperiosteal flap
sural artery flap
surgical flap
switch flap
synovial flap
Tagliacozzi flap
tailoring of flap

flap (*continued*)

tarsoconjunctival flap
temporal fascial flap
temporal island pedicle scalp
    flap
temporal muscle and fascia
    flap
temporalis fascia flap
temporalis flap
temporalis muscle flap
temporoparietal fascial flap
    (TPFF)
temporoparieto-occipital flap
temporoparieto-occipital
    rotation flap
tensor fascia femoris flap
tensor fascia lata muscle flap
Tenzel rotational cheek flap
Tenzel semicircular flap
Tham flap
thenar flap
thigh flap
Thom flap
thoracoacromial flap
thoracodorsal fascia flap
thoracoepigastric flap
toe fillet flap
toe pulp neurosensory flap
toe-to-thumb flap
tongue flap
TRAM flap
transposition flap
transverse abdominal island
    flap
transverse myocutaneous flap
transverse rectus abdominis
    muscle flap
trapezius flap
trapezius muscle
    myocutaneous flap
triangular advancement flap
triangular island flap
triceps flap
Truc flap
tube flap
tubed groin flap
tubed pedicle flap
tubed pedicle delayed groin
    flap
tubularized cecal flap
tumble flap
tumbler flap

flap (*continued*)
   tumbler skin flap
   tummy tuck flap
   tunnel flap
   turned-down tendon flap
   turnover flap
   turnover skin flap
   tympanomeatal flap
   tympanotomy flap
   unipedicled flap
   unpedicled flap
   unrepositioned flap
   up-and-down flap
   upper trapezius flap
   Urbaniak neurovascular free
      flap
   Urbaniak scapular flap
   U-shaped interdigitated
      muscle flap
   U-shaped scalp flap
   V flap
   Van Lint conjunctival flap
   Van Lint flap
   Vasconez tensor fasciae latae
      flap
   vascularity flap
   vascularized calvarial flap
   vascularized free flap
   vascularized island bone flap
   vascularized tibial bone flap
   vastus lateralis flap
   venous flap
   ventrum penis flap
   vermilion Abbe flap
   vertical bipedicle flap
   vertical flap
   visor flap
   volar flap
   volar tissue flap
   vomer flap
   von Brun flap
   von Langenbeck bipedicle
      mucoperiosteal flap
   von Langenbeck flap
   von Langenbeck palatal flap
   von Langenbeck pedicle flap
   Von Noorden flap
   V-Y advancement flap
   V-Y flap
   V-Y island flap
   V-Y Kutler flap
   V-Y mucosal flap

flap (*continued*)
   V-Y transposition flap
   waltzed flap
   waltzed skin flap
   Warren flap
   Washio skin flap
   web space flap
   Webster flap
   Weir pattern skin flap
   Widman flap
   winged V double flap
   Wookey flap
   Wookey neck flap
   wraparound flap
   wraparound neurovascular
      free flap
   Y flap
   Yotsuyanagi retroauricular
      chondrocutaneous flap
   Zimany bilobed flap
   Zimany flap
   Zitelli bilobed nasal flap
   Zovickian flap
flap advancement procedure
flap amputation
flap cannula
flap congestion
flap demarcator
flap dissector cannula
flap elevation
flap elevator
flap failure
flap graft
flap grafting
flap knife
flap knife dissector
flap maceration
flap meniscal tear
flap necrosis
flap of conjunctiva
flap of periosteum
flap operation
flap operation cataract
flap otoplasty
flap physiology
flap rotation
flap scissors
flap technique
flap tip
flap tracheostomy
flap valve after hiatal hernia
   repair

flap viability
flapless amputation
FlapMaker disposable
    microkeratome
flapping of conjunctiva
flapping sound
flapping tremor
flapping tremor sign
flapping valve syndrome
flap-type laceration
flap-valve mechanism
flared ABS tip
flared patch mes
flared spinal rod
flared W excision
flaring
    alar flaring
    labial flaring
    nasal flaring
    overzealous flaring
    reverse flaring
flaring apex
flaring of nostrils
flaring tool
flash burn
flash generator
flash ophthalmia
flash pan
flash stimulation
flash tube
flashlamp laser
flashlamp-pumped pulsed dye
    laser (FPPDL) 510 nm
flashlamp-pumped pulsed dye
    laser (FPPDL) 585 nm
flashlight examination
FlashPoint optical localizer
flask
    Dewar flask
    Falcon plastic flask
    tissue culture flask
    trap flask
flask closure
flask-shaped heart
flat abdomen
flat back curet
flat back deformity
flat bottom reservoir
flat brain spatula support
flat chest
flat condyloma
flat curve

flat depressed lesion
flat drill
flat electrocardiogram
flat elevated lesion
flat encephalogram
flat eye bandage
flat eye spud
flat feet
flat flap
flat hand
flat lip
flat pelvis
flat plate
flat plate of abdomen
flat spatula
flat spatula electrode
flat spatula needle
flat sutures
flat tenotomy hook
flat wart
flat wire coil stent
flat zonule separator
flat bladed nasal speculum
flat blade-tipped catheter
flat bottomed Kerrison rongeur
Flateau oval punch
flat-end cutter
flat-face appearance
flat-panel megavoltage imager
Flatt classification
Flatt driver
Flatt excision
Flatt finger prosthesis
Flatt implant
Flatt prosthesis
Flatt technique
Flatt thumb prosthesis
flattened
flattened duodenal fold
flattened irrigating cannula
flattened nose
flattening
    curvilinear flattening
flattening filter
flattening of T-wave
flat-tip electrode
flatulent
flatus
    expelled flatus
    passage of flatus
flatus tube insertion
flat-wire eye electrode

flava
  macula flava
flaval ligament
flavectomy
flaw
  perioral flaw
Flaxedil suture
Flaxedil sutures
Flayol-Grant erysiphake
fleck of barium
Fleck preparation
Fleet bowel prep
Fleet enema
fleeting chest pain
Fleischmann bursa
Fleischmann hygroma
Fleischner line
Fleisher corneal ring
Fleisher ring
Fleishner lines
Fleming conization instrument
Fleming conization of cervix
Fleming operation
Flemming
  fibrillar mass of Flemming
Flents breast comfort pack
flesh trabeculae of heart
Fletcher afterloading colpostat
Fletcher afterloading tandem
Fletcher AL tandem (afterloading
  tandem)
Fletcher dressing forceps
Fletcher forceps
Fletcher knife
Fletcher loading applicator
Fletcher sponge forceps
Fletcher tandem
Fletcher tonsil knife
Fletcher tonsillar knife
Fletcher-Delclos dome cylinder
Fletcher-Pierce cannula
Fletcher-Suit afterloading
  applicator
Fletcher-Suit afterloading
  tandem
Fletcher-Suit application
Fletcher-Suit applicator
Fletcher-Suit polyp forceps
Fletcher-Suit-Delclos colpostat
Fletcher-Van Doren forceps
Fletcher-Van Doren sponge-
  holding forceps

Fletcher-Van Doren uterine
  forceps
Fletcher-Van Doren uterine
  polyp forceps
Fletcher-Van Doren uterine
  polyp sponge-holding
  forceps
Fletching femoral hernia implant
  material
Fleurant bladder trocar
fleur-de-lis abdominoplasty
fleur-de-lis breast reconstruction
  pattern
fleur-de-lis flap
fleur-de-lis forehead flap
fleur-de-lis shape
fleur-de-lis-shaped skin paddle
Flex Foam brace
Flex Foam orthosis
Flex guidewire
Flex stent
flex-tip guidewire
Flex-Aid knuckle dressing
Flex-Cath double-lumen intra-
  aortic balloon catheter
Flexcon lens
FlexDerm wound dressing
flexed incision
flexed position
Flexfilm wound dressing
FlexFinder guidewire
Flex-Foot prosthesis
Flexguard tip catheter
Flexguide intubation
Flexguide intubation guide
Flexiblade laryngoscope
flexible angioscope
flexible aortic clamp
flexible arm microretractor
flexible aspiration needle
flexible bandage
flexible biopsy instrument
flexible biopsy needle
flexible blade osteotome
flexible bronchoscopic biopsy
  instrument
flexible cardiac valve
flexible catheter
flexible delivery device
flexible dental suction
flexible digital implant
flexible Dualens implant

flexible endoscope
flexible endoscopic surgery
flexible endosonography probe
flexible erection
flexible esophageal conductor
flexible fallopian tube endoscope
flexible fiberoptic
flexible fiberoptic
    bronchoscope
flexible fiberoptic endoscopy
flexible fiberoptic laryngoscopy
flexible fiberoptic
    sigmoidoscopy
flexible fluoropolymer contact
    lens
flexible foreign body forceps
flexible forward-viewing
    panendoscope
flexible fulgurating electrode
flexible gastroscope
flexible guidewire
flexible hinge suspension
flexible injection needle
flexible intramedullary nail
flexible laminar bone strip
flexible laparoscopic
    instruments
flexible laparoscopy
flexible metal catheter
flexible nasopharyngoscope
flexible neck rake retractor
flexible Olympus device
flexible optical biopsy forceps
flexible penile prosthesis
flexible pes planus
flexible probe
flexible pump
flexible radiothermal electrode
flexible reamer
flexible retractor
flexible retractor pressure clamp
flexible retractor sliding clamp
flexible rod penile implant
flexible round silicone rod
flexible rubber endoscopic tube
flexible rubber tube
flexible shaft retractor
flexible sigmoidoscope
flexible socket
flexible sound
flexible, steerable
    nasolaryngopharyngoscope

flexible steerable wire
flexible suction tube
flexible surface coil
flexible surface coil-type
    resonator
flexible tourniquet
flexible translimbal iris retractor
flexible tubing
flexible vascular clamp
flexible video laparoscope
flexible wire electrode
flexible-J guidewire
flexible-loop anterior chamber
    intraocular lens
flexible-loop posterior chamber
    intraocular lens
flexible-tip Bentsen guidewire
flexible-wire bundle reamer
Flexicair eclipse low-air-loss
    therapy unit
Flexicair II low-air-loss therapy
    unit bed
Flexicair low-air-loss bed
Flexicair MC3 low-air-loss
    therapy unit bed
Flexi-Cath double-lumen intra-
    aortic balloon catheter
Flexicath silicone subclavian
    cannula
Flexicon elastic gauze
Flexicon gauze bandage
Flexicon material
Flexicut file
Flexi-Flate inflatable penile
    prosthesis
Flexi-Flate penile implant
Flexiflo enteral feeding tube
Flexiflo enteral pump
Flexiflo feeding pump
Flexiflo Inverta-PEG gastrostomy
    kit
Flexiflo tube
Flexiflo Lap G laparoscopic
    gastrostomy kit
Flexiflo Lap J laparoscopic
    jejunostomy kit
Flexiflo over-the-guidewire
    gastrostomy kit
Flexiflo Sacks-Vine tube
Flexiflo Stomate low-profile
    gastrostomy tube
Flexiflo suction feeding tube

Flexiflo tap-fill enteral tube
Flexiflo Taptainer tube
Flexiflo tungsten-weighted
    feeding tube
Flexiflo Versa-PEG tube
FlexiGel gel sheet dressing
Flexigrid dressing
Flexilite conforming elastic
    bandage
Flexilite gauze bandage
Flexima biliary stent
Flexinet dressing
flexion
    angle of greatest flexion
        (AGF)
    forced flexion
    forceful flexion
    forward flexion
    full flexion
    gentle active flexion
    greatest angle of flexion
    neck flexion
    palmar flexion
    passive flexion
    plantar flexion
    wrist flexion
flexion, abduction, external
    rotation, extension (fabere)
flexion, abduction, internal
    rotation (fadir)
flexion and extension
flexion compression spine
    injury stabilization
flexion contracture
flexion crease
flexion deformity
flexion glove
flexion position
flexion reflex
flexion skin lines
flexion teardrop fracture
flexion-extension axis
flexion-extension injury
flexion-extension maneuver
flexion-extension plane
flexion-extension projection
flexion-extension reflex
flexion internal rotational
    deformity
Flexi-rod penile prosthesis
Flexi-rod semirigid penile
    prosthesis

Flexiscope arthroscope
Flexisplint
Flexisplint flexed-arm board
FlexiSport orthotic
Flexistone impression material
Flexitip catheter
Flexitone sutures
Flexi-Trak skin anchoring device
Flexi-Ty vessel band
Flexlase laser
Flexlens lens
FlexLite hinged knee support
Flexner-Worst iris claw lens
Flex-O-Jet aspirator
Flexon steel sutures
Flexon sutures
flexor canal
flexor carpi radialis, musculus
    (FCR)
flexor carpi radialis tendon
flexor carpi ulnaris flap
flexor carpi ulnaris muscle
flexor carpi ulnaris tendon
flexor carpi ulnaris, musculus
    (FCU)
flexor digiti minimi, musculus
    (FDM)
flexor digiti quinti, musculus
    (FDQ)
flexor digitorum brevis muscle
flexor digitorum brevis,
    musculus (FDB)
flexor digitorum longus muscle
flexor digitorum longus,
    musculus (FDL)
flexor digitorum profundus
    (FDP) muscle
flexor digitorum profundus
    (FDP) tendon
flexor digitorum profundus,
    musculus (FDP)
flexor digitorum sublimis,
    musculus (FDS)
flexor digitorum superficialis
    (FDS) muscle
flexor digitorum superficialis
    (FDS) tendon
flexor digitorum superficialis,
    musculus (FDS)
flexor hallucis brevis, musculus
    (FHB)
flexor hallucis longus muscle

flexor hallucis longus, musculus (FHL)
flexor hinge hand splint brace
flexor muscle
flexor origin
flexor origin syndrome
flexor pollicis brevis, musculus (FPB)
flexor pollicis longus (FPL) muscle
flexor pollicis longus (FPL) tendon
flexor pollicis longus abductorplasty
flexor pollicis longus, musculus (FPL)
flexor pollicis longus substitution maneuver
flexor retinaculum
flexor sheath
flexor tendon
flexor tendon adhesion
flexor tendon anastomosis
flexor tendon grafting
flexor tendon laceration
flexor tendon repair
flexor tendon rupture
flexor tendon sheath
flexor tenosynovitis
flexor tone
flexor wad of five
flexor zone
Flexoreamer
flexorplasty
    Bunnell modification of Steindler flexorplasty
    Eyler flexorplasty
    Steindler flexorplasty
FlexPosure endoscopic retractor
Flex-R-File file
Flex-Rite lumbar support
Flexseat cushion
Flexsteel retractor
Flexsteel ribbon retractor
FlexStent stent
FlexStrand cable
FlexTip intervertebral rongeur
flexure
    basicranial flexure
    caudal flexure
    cephalic flexure
    cervical flexure

flexure (*continued*)
    colic flexure
    dorsal flexure
    duodenojejunal flexure
    hepatic flexure
    iliac flexure
    left colonic flexure
    lumbar flexure
    mesencephalic flexure
    nuchal flexure
    pontine flexure
    right colonic flexure
    sacral flexure
    sigmoid flexure
    splenic flexure
flexure line
flexure of colon
flexure of duodenum
flexure of rectum
flexure skin lines
Flexxicon Blue catheter
Flexxicon Blue dialysis catheter
Flexxicon catheter
Flexxicon internal jugular catheter
Flexzan dressing
Flexzan Extra dressing
Flexzan foam wound dressing
Flexzan topical wound dressing
flicker-fusion frequency technique
flickering blockade
Flick-Gould technique
Flieringa fixation ring
Flieringa scleral ring
Flieringa-Kayser fixation ring
Flieringa-LeGrand fixation ring
Flint glass speculum
flip angle
flip-flap procedure
flip-flap technique
Flip-Flop pillow
FLOAM ankle stirrup brace
floating cartilage
floating catheter
floating disk heart valve
floating distal phalanx
floating forehead operation
floating gallbladder
floating gallstone
floating kidney
floating knee

floating lead
floating patella
floating premaxilla
floating ribs
floating spleen
floating table
floating thumb
floating umbilicus procedure
Flocare 500 feeding pump
floccular fossa
flocculonodular arteriovenous
    malformation
flocculonodular lobe
Flo-Fit cushion
Flo-Gard pump
FloMap guidewire
floor cells
floor fracture
floor of mouth (FOM)
floor of orbit
floor of orifice
floor-of-mouth closure
floor-of-mouth lesion
floor-standing surgical light
floppy disk
floppy guidewire
floppy mitral valve
floppy Nissen fundoplication
    procedure
floppy tip guidewire
floppy valve syndrome
floppy-tipped guide
floppy-tipped guidewire
floppy-type of Nissen
    fundoplication
Florentine iris
Florester vascular occluder
Flo-Rester device
Flo-Restors backbleeding control
    device
florid cutaneous papillomatosis
florid duct lesion
florid hyperplasia
florid osseous dysplasia
Florida back brace
Florida cervical brace
Florida contraflexion brace
Florida extension brace
Florida hyperextension brace
Florida post-fusion brace
Florida pouch
Florida spinal brace

Florida urinary pouch
floridic pain
floriform cataract
FloSeal matrix hemostatic
    sealant
Flo-Stat fluid monitor
flotation catheter
flotation gel pad
flotation rate
Flo-Tech prosthetic socket
Flo-Thru intraluminal shunt
Flo-Thru shunt
flow
    antegrade blood flow
    antegrade flow
    cerebral blood flow
    coronary blood flow
    diversion of blood flow
    Doppler color flow
    expiratory flow
    forced expiratory flow
    forearm flow
    free flow
    hepatic blood flow
    inadequate blood flow
    inspiratory flow
    laminar air flow
    laminar flow
    mucociliary flow
    operative mortality flow
    peak expiratory flow
    pulmonary flow
    rate of cerebral blood flow
        (rCBF)
    regional cerebral blood flow
    retrograde flow
    return flow
    reverse flow
    systemic blood flow
    vaginal flow
    venous flow
flow capacity
flow cytometer
flow detection technique
flow direction
flow interruption technique
flow mapping technique
flow of blood
flow of urinary stream
flow probe
flow rate
flow regulated suction tube

Flow Rider flow-directed
catheter
Flow Rider neurovascular
catheter
flow tract
flow volume
flow-assisted short-term balloon
catheter
flow-cytometry analysis
flow-directed balloon-tipped
catheter
flow-directed catheter
Flower bone
Flowers mandibular glove
Flowers mandibular Groove
implant
Flowers mandibular implants
FlowGel barrier material
FlowGun suction/irrigation
FloWire Doppler catheter
FloWire Doppler guidewire
flowmeter
   access peak flowmeter
   Astham Check peak
      flowmeter
   clinical electromagnetic
      flowmeter
   Dantec rotating disk
      flowmeter
   Dienco flowmeter
   Doppler flowmeter
   Doppler ultrasonic flowmeter
   Doppler ultrasound
      flowmeter
   electromagnetic flowmeter
   Gould electromagnetic
      flowmeter
   Heidelberg retinal flowmeter
   infrared laser-Doppler
      flowmeter
   laser Doppler flowmeter
   Life-Tech flowmeter
   mini-Wright peak flowmeter
   Narcomatic flowmeter
   Parks bidirectional Doppler
      flowmeter
   Personal Best peak flowmeter
   Pocketpeak peak flowmeter
   PreVent Pneumotach
      flowmeter
   pulsed Doppler ultrasonic
      flowmeter

flowmeter (*continued*)
   Statham flowmeter
   transit-time flowmeter
   Transonic flowmeter
   Wright peak flowmeter
flowmetry
   fluorescein flowmetry
   laser Doppler flowmetry
flow-on gradient-echo image
flow-oximetry catheter
flowprobe
flow-regulator clamp
Flowtron DVT compression
   device
Flowtron DVT prophylactic
   deep venous thrombosis
   unit
Flowtron DVT pump
Flowtron thigh-high device
FlowWire Doppler guidewire
Floxite mirror light
floxuridine in hepatic metastasis
Floyd loop cannula
Floyd needle
Floyd pneumothorax needle
Floyd-Barraquer speculum
Floyd-Barraquer wire speculum
Floyd-Grant erysiphake
fluctuant abscess
fluctuate
fluctuating
fluctuation
fluff
   Kerlix fluff
   sterile fluffs
   vitreous fluff
fluff dressing
fluffed gauze
fluffed gauze dressing
fluffs
fluffy compression dressing
fluffy cotton-wool exudate
fluffy excrescences
fluffy periostitis
fluffy-cuffed tube
Fluftex gauze rolls and sponge
Fluhrer bullet probe
Fluhrer rectal probe
fluid
   ascitic fluid
   bile-stained fluid
   bile-tinged fluid

fluid (*continued*)
  bloody peritoneal fluid
  body fluid
  bronchoalveolar lavage fluid
    (BALF)
  cerebrospinal fluid (CSF)
  chylous fluid
  cloudy fluid
  Dakin fluid
  Dialyflex dialysis fluid
  dialysis fluid
  diluting fluid
  disinfecting fluid
  effused fluid
  encapsulated pleural fluid
  endolymphatic fluid
  force fluids
  foul-smelling amniotic fluid
  free fluid
  halo test for cerebrospinal
    fluid (CSF) leak
  halo test for cerebrospinal
    fluid (CSF) rhinorrhea
  hydrocele fluid
  hyperalimentation fluid
  interarterial fluid
  intercellular fluid
  intestinal fluid
  intracellular fluid
  intravascular fluid
  intravenous fluid
  irrigation fluid
  joint fluid
  leakage of fluid
  loculated fluid
  lymphatic fluid
  meconium fluid
  meconium-stained amniotic
    fluid
  meniscal fluid
  milky fluid
  motor oil peritoneal fluid
  mucous fluid
  pericardial fluid
  perilymph fluid
  peritoneal fluid
  piggyback IV fluid
  pleural fluid
  prune-juice peritoneal fluid
  push fluids
  reaccumulation of fluid
  sanguineous fluid

fluid (*continued*)
  Schaudinn fluid
  seminal fluid
  serosanguineous fluid
  serous fluid
  spinal fluid
  sterile fluid
  straw-colored fluid
  subdural fluid
  subretinal fluid
  synovial fluid
  tapping of chest for fluid
  temporomandibular joint
    synovial fluid
  tissue fluid
  transcellular fluid
  transudation of fluid
  turbid fluid
  turbid milky fluid
  turbid peritoneal fluid
  ventricular fluid
  vitreous fluid
  Waldeyer fluid
fluid aspiration
fluid collection
fluid control trauma pad
fluid drainage
fluid evacuation
fluid extravasation
fluid formation
fluid intake
fluid loading anesthetic
    technique
fluid output
fluid pressure
fluid replacement
fluid reservoir
fluid retention
fluid volume
fluid wave
Fluid-Air Plus bed
fluid-filled balloon-tipped flow-
    directed catheter
fluid-filled catheter
fluid-filled pressure monitoring
    guidewire
fluid-filled sac
fluid-gas exchange
fluorescein angiogram
fluorescein angiography
fluorescein angioscopy
fluorescein dye

fluorescein endoscopy
fluorescein flowmetry
fluorescein fundus angioscopy
fluorescein instillation test
fluorescein string test
fluorescein strip
fluorescein uptake
fluorescence detector
fluorescence excitation filter
fluorescence fibergastroscope
fluorescence-guided smart laser
fluorescence microscope
fluorescence microscopy
fluorescent
fluorescent antibody
fluorescent antibody staining
    technique (FAST)
fluorescent antinuclear antibody
    test (FANA)
fluorescent electronic
    endoscopy
fluorescent imaging
fluorescent immunoassay (FIA)
fluorescent microscope
fluorescent optode technology
fluorescent probe
fluorescent ray
fluorescent scan
Fluorescite syringe
Fluoro Tip ERCP cannula
fluorography
fluorometer
    CytoFluor II fluorometer
    scanning fluorometer
fluorometric technique
Fluoropassiv thin-wall carotid
    patch graft
fluorophotometer
    Fluorotron Master
        fluorophotometer
    slit-lamp fluorophotometer
FluoroPlus angiogram
FluoroPlus Roadmapper digital
    fluoroscopy
fluoroptic thermometry probe
FluoroScan C-arm fluoroscope
FluoroScan C-arm fluoroscopy
fluoroscope
    C-arm fluoroscope
    Edison fluoroscope
    FluoroScan C-arm fluoroscope
    Xi-scan fluoroscope

fluoroscopic control
fluoroscopic foreign body
    forceps
fluoroscopic guidance
fluoroscopic imaging chair
fluoroscopic insertion
fluoroscopic monitor
fluoroscopic placement
fluoroscopic pushing technique
fluoroscopic study
fluoroscopic visualization
fluoroscopy
    2-plane fluoroscopy
    biplanar fluoroscopy
    biplane fluoroscopy
    cardiac fluoroscopy
    C-arm fluoroscopy
    FluoroPlus Roadmapper
        digital fluoroscopy
    FluoroScan C-arm fluoroscopy
    lateral fluoroscopy
    portable C-arm image
        intensifier fluoroscopy
    rapid scan fluoroscopy
    video fluoroscopy
fluoroscopy beam
fluoroscopy-guided balloon
    dilator
Fluorotome double-lumen
    sphincterotome
Fluorotron Master
    fluorophotometer
Fluosol artificial blood
Fluotec vaporizer
Fluothane anesthetic agent
flush aortogram
flush chamber
flush heparin lock
flush out kidneys
flush tube
flush with saline
flush with skin stoma
flush-and-bathe technique
flushing device
flushing of artery
flushing reservoir
flushing technique
flushing valve
flute cannula
flute needle
fluted finishing bur
fluted J-Vac drain

fluted reamer
fluted Sampson nail
fluted stem punch
fluted titanium nail
flute-ended right-angle drain
flutter
    alar flutter
    atrial flutter
    ventricular flutter
Flutter therapeutic device
Fluvog aspirator
Fluvog irrigator
flux
fluximetry
flying-T pelvic area
Flynn femoral neck fracture
    reduction
Flynn lens loop
Flynn scleral depressor
Flynn technique
Flynn-Richards-Saltzman
    technique
Flynt aortography needle
Flynt needle
FMA (Frankfort mandibular
    angle)
FMI (fixed mandibular implant)
FMIA (Frankfort mandibular
    incisor angle)
FN (facial nerve)
FNA (fine-needle aspiration)
FNA biopsy
FNA-21 syringe
FNAB (fine-needle aspiration
    biopsy)
FNAC (fine-needle aspiration
    cytology)
foam
    CarraSmart foam
    CIDA foam
    DermaMend foam
    eggcrate foam
    Emko foam
    Evazote foam
    fibrin foam
    hi-density foam
    Neoplush foam
    nonadherent foam
    open-celled foam
    Pedilen polyurethane foam
    polyethylene foam
    polystyrene foam

foam (*continued*)
    polyvinyl alcohol foam
    prosthetic foam
    PV foam
    Reston foam
    Reston polyurethane foam
    Temper foam
    tube foam
foam collar
foam cube
foam cube mattress
foam embolus
foam ring
foam rubber
foam rubber dressing
foam rubber graft
foam rubber stent
foam rubber vaginal stent
foam tape
foam tubing
foam wedge wheelchair
    cushion
foam wound dressing
foaming exudate
Foamtrac traction bandage
FOB (fiberoptic bronchoscopy)
Fobi pouch
focal abnormality
focal accumulation
focal and lateralizing neurologic
    signs
focal area of hemorrhage
focal atrophy
focal bleeding point
focal colonic mucosal ulcer
focal cortical dysplasia
focal defect
focal dermal hypoplasia
focal disease
focal edema
focal epithelial hyperplasia
focal fatty infiltration
focal finding
focal granulomatous
    inflammation
focal hemorrhage
focal image point
focal infarction
focal inflammation
focal keratosis
focal lesion
focal motor sign

focal nodular hyperplasia (FNH)
focal osseous dysplasia
focal parenchymal brain lesion
focal plane
focal point
focal splenic lesion
focal tenderness
focal tumor
focalizing signs
FocalSeal-R neurosurgical stent
foci (*sing.* focus)
foci of infection
focus (*pl.* foci)
   calcified focus
   ectopic focus
   Ghon focus
   hemorrhage focus
   metastatic focus
   midtemporal focus
   mirror focus
   spike focus
focus of atelectasis
focus of infection
Focus -PV balloon catheter
focused beam
focused grid
focused radiation therapy
focused, segmented ultrasound
   machine
Focustent coronary stent
Foerger airway
Foerster (*also* Förster)
Foerster abdominal retractor
Foerster abdominal ring
   retractor
Foerster capsulotomy knife
Foerster enucleation snare
Foerster eye forceps
Foerster forceps
Foerster gallbladder forceps
Foerster iris forceps
Foerster operation
Foerster photometer
Foerster snare
Foerster sponge forceps
Foerster sponge-holding
   forceps
Foerster surgical support
   brassiere
Foerster tissue forceps
Foerster uterine forceps
Foerster uveitis

Foerster-Ballenger forceps
Foerster-Bauer sponge-holding
   forceps
Foerster-Fuchs black spot
Foerster-Mueller forceps
Foerster-Penfield operation
Foerster-Van Doren sponge-
   holding forceps
fog reduction/elimination device
Fogarty adherent clot catheter
Fogarty anterior irrigation
   catheter
Fogarty arterial embolectomy
Fogarty arterial embolectomy
   catheter
Fogarty balloon
Fogarty balloon biliary catheter
Fogarty balloon catheter
Fogarty biliary balloon probe
Fogarty biliary probe
Fogarty bulldog clamp-applying
   forceps
Fogarty calibrator
Fogarty catheter
Fogarty clamp
Fogarty dilation catheter
Fogarty embolus catheter
Fogarty forceps
Fogarty gallstone catheter
Fogarty graft thrombectomy
   catheter
Fogarty Hydragrip clamp
Fogarty insert
Fogarty irrigation catheter
Fogarty occlusion catheter
Fogarty probe
Fogarty Thru-Lumen catheter
Fogarty vascular clamp
Fogarty venous irrigation
   catheter
Fogarty venous thrombectomy
   catheter
Fogarty-Chin catheter
Fogarty-Chin clamp
Fogarty-Chin extrusion balloon
   catheter
Fogarty-Chin peripheral
   dilatation catheter
Fogarty-Hydragrip insert
Fogarty-Softjaw insert
foil carrier
foil sheet

Foille dressing
Foimson biceps tendon repair
Foix enucleation
Folatex catheter
fold
  adipose fold
  AE fold (aryepiglottic fold)
  alar folds
  amniotic fold
  anterior axillary fold
  anterior mallear fold
  antihelical fold
  aryepiglottic fold (AE fold)
  axillary fold
  Bartlett nail fold
  breast folds
  bulboventricular fold
  caval fold
  cecal fold
  cholecystoduodenocolic
    fold
  ciliary folds
  circular fold
  circulator fold
  coarse folds
  conjunctival fold
  costocolic fold
  cuticular fold
  Dennie infraorbital fold
  Dennie-Morgan infraorbital
    folds
  Douglas fold
  Duncan fold
  duodenal fold
  duodenojejunal fold
  duodenomesocolic fold
  epicanthal fold
  epicanthic fold
  epigastric fold
  eponychial fold
  falciform retinal fold
  fimbriated fold
  flattened duodenal fold
  gastric folds
  gastric rugal fold
  gastropancreatic fold
  genital fold
  glossoepiglottic fold
  glossopalatine fold
  gluteal fold
  Guerin fold
  Hasner fold

fold (*continued*)
  haustral fold
  Heister fold
  helical fold
  hepatopancreatic fold
  horizontal folds
  Houston fold
  ileocecal fold
  ileocolic fold
  incudal fold
  inferior duodenal fold
  inferior rectal fold
  inferior transverse rectal
    fold
  inframammary fold
  infrapatellar synovial fold
  infraumbilical fold
  inguinal aponeurotic fold
  intercartilaginous fold
  interossicular fold
  interureteric fold
  iridial folds
  Kerckring folds
  Kohlrausch folds
  labial fold
  labiomental fold
  labioscrotal fold
  lacrimal fold
  laryngeal fold
  lateral glossoepiglottic fold
  lateral mallear fold
  lateral nail fold
  lateral nasal fold
  lateral umbilical folds
  longitudinal fold
  malar fold
  mallear fold
  malleolar folds
  mammary fold
  medial incudal fold
  medial umbilical fold
  median glossoepiglottic fold
  median thyrohyoid fold
  median umbilical fold
  medullary fold
  mesolateral fold
  mesonephric fold
  mesouterine fold
  middle umbilical fold
  Morgan fold
  mucobuccal fold
  mucolabial fold

fold (*continued*)
- mucosal folds
- mucosobuccal fold
- nail fold
- nasojugal fold
- nasolabial fold (NLF)
- neural fold
- Nelaton fold
- obturatoria stapedis fold
- opercular fold
- palatine folds
- palatoglossal fold
- palatopharyngeal fold
- palmate folds
- palpebral fold
- palpebronasal fold
- pancreaticogastric folds
- paraduodenal fold
- parietocolic fold
- parietoperitoneal fold
- Passavant fold
- patellar fold
- patellar synovial fold
- pharyngoepiglottic fold
- pleuroperitoneal fold
- presplenic fold
- pretarsal fold
- pterygomandibular fold
- Rathke folds
- rectal fold
- rectouterine fold
- rectovaginal fold
- rectovesical fold
- retinal fold
- retrotarsal fold
- right umbilical fold
- Rindfleisch folds
- roof of the nail fold
- rugal folds
- sacrogenital fold
- sacrouterine fold
- sacrovaginal fold
- sacrovesical fold
- salpingopalatine fold
- salpingopharyngeal fold
- Schultze fold
- semilunar conjunctival fold
- semilunar fold
- sentinel fold
- serosal fold
- sigmoid folds
- soft fold

fold (*continued*)
- soft tissue pinch-thickness at the inframammary fold (STPTIMF)
- spiral fold
- stapedial fold
- sublingual fold
- superior duodenal fold
- superior rectal fold
- synovial fold
- tail fold
- tarsal fold
- thickened folds
- thyrohyoid fold
- tonsillar fold
- transverse palatine folds
- transverse rectal folds
- transverse vesical fold
- Treves fold
- triangular fold
- umbilical fold
- urachal fold
- ureteric fold
- urogenital fold
- uterosacral fold
- uterovesical fold
- vaginal folds
- vascular fold
- Vater fold
- ventricular fold
- Veraguth fold
- vestibular fold
- villous fold
- vocal fold
- white dural fold

fold forceps
fold line
fold of colon
fold of cystic duct
fold of duodenum
fold of ear
fold of large intestine
fold of laryngeal nerve
fold of peritoneum
fold of rectum
fold of skin
fold of stomach
fold of tympanic membrane
fold of uterine tube
fold pattern
foldable intraocular lens
folded aluminum ear splint

folder
    Faulkner folder
    intraocular lens folder
fold-flaw failure
folding blade
folding emergency ventilation
    bronchoscope
folding esophagoscope
folding forceps
folding laryngoscope
folding lens
fold-over finger splint
Foley 3-way catheter
Foley acorn-bulb catheter
Foley bag
Foley balloon
Foley balloon catheter
Foley catheter
Foley cone-tip catheter
Foley forceps
Foley hemostatic bag
Foley operation
Foley plate
Foley pyeloplasty
Foley straight drain
Foley ureteropelvioplasty
Foley vas isolation forceps
Foley Y-plasty
Foley Y-type
    ureteropelvioplasty
Foley Y-V pyeloplasty
Foley-Alcock bag
Foley-Alcock bag catheter
Foley-Alcock catheter
Foley-Alcock hemostatic bag
Foley-Temp
foliate papillae
folium
    lingual folium
folium (pl. folia)
Folius muscle
follicle
    graafian follicle
    hair follicle
    Lieberkuhn follicles
    lingual follicle
    lingual lymph follicle
    lymphatic follicle
    Naboth follicles
    nabothian follicle
    ovarian follicle
follicle electrode

follicle expressor
follicle lid expressor
follicle stimulating hormone
    (FSH)
follicular abscess
follicular adenoma
follicular carcinoma
follicular cyst
follicular epithelium
follicular form
follicular hematoma
follicular inflammation
follicular infundibular cyst
follicular isthmus cyst
follicular keratosis
follicular lesion
follicular lymphoma
follicular membranes
follicular odontogenic cyst
follicular thyroid carcinoma
follicular ulcer
follicularis
    alopecia follicularis
    hydrosalpinx follicularis
    hyperkeratosis follicularis
    keratosis follicularis
folliculi (sing. folliculus)
    hydrops folliculi
    theca folliculi
folliculi lymphatici aggregati
folliculi lymphatici aggregati
    appendicis vermiformis
folliculi lymphatici gastrici
folliculi lymphatici lienales
folliculi lymphatici recti
folliculi lymphatici solitarii
    intestini crassi
folliculi lymphatici solitarii
    intestini tenuis
folliculitis
folliculitis cheloidalis
folliculitis decalvans
folliculitis nares perforans
folliculus (pl. folliculi)
Follmann balanitis
follow through (verb; see also
    follow-through)
follow up (verb; see also
    followup)
follower
    filiform follower
    filiforms and followers (F&F)

follower (*continued*)
  LeFort follower
  Rusch follower
follow-through (noun, adj; *see also* followthrough)
  peroral pneumocolon double-contrast followthrough
  small-bowel followthrough
followup
  postoperative followup
  postsurgical followup
followup (adj, noun; *see also* follow up)
followup care
followup evaluation
followup examination
followup procedure
followup studies
Foltz catheter
Foltz CSF-flushing reservoir
Foltz flushing reservoir
Foltz needle
Foltz reservoir
Foltz shunt
Foltz to-and-fro flusher
Foltz valve
Foltz-Overton cardiac catheter
Foltz-Overton shunt
FOM (floor of mouth)
Fome-Cuf endotracheal tube
Fome-Cuf laser kit
Fome-Cuf pediatric tracheostomy tube
Fomon angular scissors
Fomon chisel
Fomon chisel guard
Fomon dorsal scissors
Fomon double-edged knife
Fomon elevator
Fomon facelift scissors
Fomon graft augmentation
Fomon hook retractor
Fomon knife
Fomon lower lateral scissors
Fomon nasal chisel
Fomon nasal hook
Fomon nasal rasp
Fomon nasal retractor
Fomon nostril elevator
Fomon nostril retractor
Fomon operation
Fomon osteotome

Fomon periosteal elevator
Fomon periosteotome
Fomon rasp
Fomon raspatory
Fomon retractor
Fomon saberback scissors
Fomon scissors
Fomon upper lateral scissors
Fomon Vital dorsal scissors
Fonar Quad MRI scanner
Fonar Stand-Up MRI scanner
Fones technique
Fontan atriopulmonary anastomosis
Fontan fenestration closure
Fontan modification of Norwood procedure
Fontan operation
Fontan repair
Fontan tricuspid atresia
Fontana space
Fontan-Baudet procedure
fontanel (*variant of* fontanelle)
fontanelle
  anterior fontanelle
  anterolateral fontanelle
  bregmatic fontanelle
  Casser fontanelle
  casserian fontanelle
  cranial fontanelles
  frontal fontanelle
  Gerdy fontanelle
  mastoid fontanelle
  posterior occipital fontanelle
  posterolateral fontanelle
  posterotemporal fontanelle
  quadrangular fontanelle
  sagittal fontanelle
  sphenoidal fontanelle
  triangular fontanelle
fontanelle (*also* fontanel)
fontanelle flat
fontanelle open
Fontan-Kreutzer procedure
Fontan-Kreutzer repair
food bolus obstruction
food extractor
foot
  arcuate artery of foot
  articulations of foot
  Beachcomber prosthetic foot
  Bock foot

foot (*continued*)
  Charcot foot
  Cirrus composite prosthetic foot
  cleft foot
  ComfortWalk2 prosthetic foot
  common digital vein of foot
  diabetic foot
  dorsal artery of foot
  dorsal venous arch of foot
  drop foot
  Dycor prosthetic foot
  Foot-up ankle-foot orthosis for drop foot
  intercapitular vein of foot
  ischemic foot
  Kingsley Steplite foot
  lobster-claw foot
  Madura foot
  march foot
  Mendel dorsal reflex of foot
  Morand foot
  Morton foot
  multiaxis foot
  neuropathic foot
  perforating arteries of foot
  perforating ulcer of foot
  plantar aspect of foot
  rocker-bottom foot
  SACH foot
  sag foot
  single-axis Syme Dycor foot
  sole of foot
  spatula foot
  Sure-Flex prosthetic foot
  Syme amputation of foot
  Syme Dycor prosthetic foot
  tabetic foot
  taut foot
  trash foot
  trench foot
  Trowbridge TerraRound foot
  Vari-Flex prosthetic foot
foot bones
foot cradle
foot deformity
foot drape
foot drop night splint
foot fillet flap
foot first-web flap
foot holder
Foot Hugger foot support

Foot Levelers custom orthotic
Foot Levelers orthosis
foot magnet
foot model
foot orthotic device
foot pillow
foot pods of alar cartilage
foot rest
foot stabilizer
foot volumeter
Foot Waffle positioner
Foot Waffle prosthetic
foot yaws
foot-ankle brace
football knee
footboard extension
footdrop
footdrop brace
footling breech
footling breech presentation
footling delivery
footling presentation
footpiece
footplate
  Fick perforation of footplate
  Leyla footplate
  stapes footplate
footplate auger
footplate chisel
footplate elevator
footplate fragments
footplate hook
footplate pick
Foot-up ankle-foot orthosis for drop foot
forage core biopsy
forage procedure
foramen (*pl.* foramina)
  alveolar foramina
  anastomotic foramen
  anterior condyloid foramina
  anterior condyloid foramen
  anterior ethmoidal foramen
  anterior palatine foramen
  aortic foramen
  axillary foramen
  blind foramen
  Bochadalek foramen
  Botallo foramen
  Bozzi foramen
  caroticoclinoid foramen
  carotid foramen

foramen (*continued*)
  cecal foramen
  conjugate foramen
  cribroethmoid foramen
  emissary sphenoidal foramen
  epiploic foramen
  ethmoidal foramen
  external acoustic foramen
  Ferrein foramen
  frontal foramen
  Galen foramen
  great foramen
  greater palatine foramen
  greater sciatic foramen
  Huschke foramen
  Hyrtl foramen
  incisive foramen
  inferior dental foramen
  inferior orbital foramen
  infraorbital foramen
  infrapiriform foramen
  internal auditory foramen
  internal neurocranial foramen
  interventricular foramen
  intervertebral foramen
  jugular foramen
  lacerated foramen
  lateral foramen
  lesser palatine foramina
  lesser palatine foramen
  lesser sciatic foramen
  lingual foramen
  Luschka and Magendie
    foramen
  Luschka foramen
  Magendie foramen
  magnum foramen
  malar foramen
  mandibular foramen
  mastoid foramen
  maxillary foramen
  medial foramen
  meibomian foramen
  mental foramen
  mobile wad compartment of
    foramen
  Monro foramen
  Morgagni foramen
  multiple foramina
  nasal foramen
  nasopalatine foramen
  neural foramen

foramen (*continued*)
  nutrient foramen
  obturator foramen
  occipital foramen
  oculomotor foramen
  olfactory foramen
  optic foramen
  pacchionian foramen
  palatine foramen
  papillary foramen
  parietal foramen
  petrosal foramen
  pleuroperitoneal foramen
  posterior condyloid foramen
  posterior ethmoidal foramen
  postglenoid foramen
  rivinian foramen
  round foramen
  sacral foramen
  Scarpa foramen
  Schwalbe foramen
  sciatic foramen
  secundum foramen
  Soemmering foramen
  solitary foramen
  sphenoid emissary foramen
  sphenopalatine foramen
  sphenotic foramen
  Stensen foramen
  stylomastoid foramen
  superior maxillary foramen
  supraorbital foramen
  suprapiriform foramen
  teardrop foramen
  thyroid foramen
  transverse foramen
  venous foramen
  vertebral foramen
  vertebroarterial foramen
  Vesalius foramen
  Winslow foramen
  zygomatic foramen
  zygomaticofacial foramen
  zygomatico-orbital foramen
  zygomaticotemporal foramen
foramen apicis dentis
foramen cecum ossis frontalis
foramen compression test
foramen lacerum
foramen magnum
foramen magnum line
foramen mandibulae

foramen of Arnold
foramen of Bochdalek
foramen of Bochdalek hernia
foramen of Fallopio
foramen of Luschka
foramen of Monro
foramen of Morgagni
foramen of sclera
foramen of Winslow
foramen ovale
foramen ovale basis cranii
foramen ovale flap
foramen ovale ossis sphenoidalis
foramen rotundum
foramen sphenopalatinum
foramen spinosum
foramen stylomastoideum
foramen transversarium
foramen venae cavae
foramen-plugging forceps
foramina (*sing.* foramen; *see*
    foramen)
foramina for olfactory nerves
foramina nervosa
foramina of Scarpa
foraminal approach
foraminal hernia
foraminal herniation
foraminal punch
foraminotomy
Forane anesthetic agent
Forane general anesthetic
Forbes amputation
Forbes esophageal speculum
Forbes graft technique
Forbes modification of
    Phemister graft technique
Forbes procedure for tibial
    fracture nonunion
Forbes speculum
Forbes uterine-dressing forceps
force and rhythm (F&R)
Force balloon
Force balloon dilatation catheter
force fluids
force fulcrum retractor
Force FX generator
force line
force transducer
force-couple splint reduction
forced beat
forced displacement transducer

forced duction
forced duction of eye
forced duction test
forced exhalation
forced expiration
forced expiratory flow
forced expiratory spirogram
forced expiratory time
forced expiratory volume
forced extension
forced flexion
forced mandatory intermittent
    ventilation
forced movement
forced respiration
forced ventilation
forced-air active cooling device
forced-eye closure
forceful extension
forceful flexion
forceps (*see also* vulsellum)
    2-stream irrigating forceps
    2-toothed forceps
    3-armed basket forceps
    3-pronged forceps
    3-pronged grasping forceps
    Abbott-Mayfield forceps
    Abernaz strut forceps
    abscess forceps
    Absolok forceps
    ACMI forceps
    ACMI Martin endoscopic
      forceps
    ACMI Martin endoscopy
      forceps
    Acufex curved basket forceps
    Acufex rotary basket forceps
    Acufex straight basket forceps
    Acufex straight forceps
    AcuTouch tissue forceps
    Adair breast tenaculum
      forceps
    Adair tenaculum forceps
    Adair tissue forceps
    Adair tissue-holding forceps
    Adair uterine forceps
    Adair uterine tenaculum
      forceps
    Adair-Allis tissue forceps
    adenoid forceps
    Adler bone forceps
    Adler punch forceps

forceps (*continued*)

    Adler-Kreutz forceps
    adnexal forceps
    Adson arterial forceps
    Adson artery forceps
    Adson bayonet dressing forceps
    Adson bipolar forceps
    Adson brain forceps
    Adson clip-applying forceps
    Adson clip-introducing forceps
    Adson cranial rongeur forceps
    Adson dressing forceps
    Adson hemostatic forceps
    Adson hypophyseal forceps
    Adson microbipolar forceps
    Adson microdressing forceps
    Adson microtissue forceps
    Adson monopolar forceps
    Adson rongeur forceps
    Adson scalp clip-applying forceps
    Adson thumb forceps
    Adson tissue forceps
    Adson tooth forceps
    Adson Vital tissue forceps
    Adson-Biemer forceps
    Adson-Brown forceps
    Adson-Brown tissue forceps
    Adson-Callison tissue forceps
    Adson-Mixter neurosurgical forceps
    Adson Vital tissue forceps
    advancement forceps
    Aesculap forceps
    Akins valve re-do forceps
    Alabama University utility forceps
    Alderkreutz tissue forceps
    Alexander dressing forceps
    Alexander-Farabeuf forceps
    Allen intestinal forceps
    Allen uterine forceps
    Allen-Barkan forceps
    Allen-Braley forceps
    alligator crimper forceps
    alligator cup forceps
    alligator ear forceps
    alligator grasping forceps
    alligator nasal forceps
    alligator-type grasping forceps

forceps (*continued*)

    Allis delicate tissue forceps
    Allis intestinal forceps
    Allis Micro-Line pediatric forceps
    Allis thoracic forceps
    Allis tissue forceps
    Allis tissue-holding forceps
    Allis-Abramson breast biopsy forceps
    Allis-Adair intestinal forceps
    Allis-Adair tissue forceps
    Allis-Coakley tonsil forceps
    Allis-Coakley tonsillar forceps
    Allis-Coakley tonsil-seizing forceps
    Allis-Duval forceps
    Allis-Ochsner tissue forceps
    Allis-Ochsner tonsil forceps
    Allis-Ochsner tonsillar forceps
    Allison forceps
    Allis-Willauer tissue forceps
    Almeida forceps
    Alvis fixation forceps
    Ambrose eye forceps
    Ambrose suture forceps
    Amdur lid forceps
    Amenabar capsule forceps
    American Catheter Corp. biopsy forceps
    AMO phacoemulsification lens-folder forceps
    anastomosis forceps
    Andrews tonsil forceps
    Andrews tonsillar forceps
    Andrews tonsil-seizing forceps
    Andrews-Hartmann forceps
    aneurysm forceps
    Angell-James hypophysectomy forceps
    Angell-James punch forceps
    angiotribe forceps
    angled capsular forceps
    angled stone forceps
    angular forceps
    angulated forceps
    Anis capsulotomy forceps
    Anis corneal forceps
    Anis corneoscleral forceps
    Anis intraocular lens forceps
    Anis microsurgical tying forceps

forceps (*continued*)

Anis straight corneal forceps
Anis tying forceps
anterior capsule forceps
anterior forceps
anterior segment forceps
Anthony-Fisher forceps
antral forceps
aorta aneurysm forceps
aorta forceps
aortic aneurysm forceps
aortic forceps
aortic occlusion forceps
Apfelbaum bipolar forceps
Apple Medical bipolar forceps
application of obstetric
   forceps
applicator forceps
approximation forceps
Archer splinter forceps
Arrow articulation paper
   forceps
Arrowsmith fixation forceps
Arrowsmith-Clerf pin-closing
   forceps
Arroyo forceps
Arruga capsule forceps
Arruga curved capsular
   forceps
Arruga tip forceps
Arruga-Gill forceps
Arruga-McCool capsular
   forceps
Arruga-McCool capsule forceps
arterial forceps
artery forceps
Arthro Force basket cutting
   forceps
Arthur splinter forceps
articulating paper forceps
Asch nasal-straightening
   forceps
Asch septal forceps
Asch septal-straightening
   forceps
Asch septum-straightening
   forceps
Ash dental forceps
Ash septum-straightening
   forceps
Ashby fluoroscopic foreign
   body forceps

forceps (*continued*)

ASSI bipolar coagulating
   forceps
Athens forceps
Atra-grip forceps
atraumatic forceps
atraumatic tissue forceps
atraumatic visceral forceps
aural forceps
auricular appendage forceps
Austin forceps
Auto Suture forceps
Autraugrip tissue forceps
Auvard-Zweifel forceps
axis-traction forceps
Ayers chalazion forceps
Azar forceps
Azar intraocular forceps
Azar lens forceps
Azar tying forceps
Azar utility forceps
Babcock intestinal forceps
Babcock lung-grasping
   forceps
Babcock thoracic tissue
   forceps
Babcock thoracic tissue-
   holding forceps
Babcock tissue forceps
Babcock Vital intestinal
   forceps
Babcock Vital tissue forceps
Babcock-Beasley forceps
Babcock Vital atraumatic
   forceps
Babcock Vital intestinal
   forceps
Babcock Vital tissue forceps
baby Adson forceps
baby Allis forceps
baby Crile forceps
baby dressing forceps
baby hemostatic forceps
baby intestinal tissue forceps
baby Lane bone-holding
   forceps
baby Mikulicz forceps
baby Mixter forceps
baby mosquito forceps
baby Overholt forceps
baby tissue forceps
backbiting forceps

forceps (*continued*)
Backhaus towel forceps
Backhaus-Roeder forceps
Bacon cranial forceps
Bacon cranial rongeur forceps
Bacon rongeur forceps
Baer bone-cutting forceps
Bahnson-Brown tissue forceps
Bailey aortic valve-cutting
    forceps
Bailey chalazion forceps
Bailey-Williamson forceps
Bailey-Williamson obstetrical
    forceps
Bainbridge hemostatic forceps
Bainbridge intestinal forceps
Bainbridge resection forceps
Bainbridge thyroid forceps
Baird chalazion forceps
Baker tissue forceps
Ball forceps
Ballantine hysterectomy
    forceps
Ballantine-Peterson
    hysterectomy forceps
Ballen-Alexander forceps
Ballenger hysterectomy
    forceps
Ballenger sponge forceps
Ballenger sponge-holding
    forceps
Ballenger tonsil forceps
Ballenger tonsillar forceps
Ballenger tonsil-seizing
    forceps
Ballenger-Foerster forceps
Bane rongeur forceps
Bangerter muscle forceps
Banner forceps
Bansal LASIK forceps
Bard forceps
Bardeleben bone-holding
    forceps
Bard-Parker transfer forceps
Barkan iris forceps
Barlow forceps
Barnes-Crile hemostatic
    forceps
Barnes-Hill forceps
Barnes-Simpson obstetrical
    forceps
Baron forceps

forceps (*continued*)
Barracuda flexible cystoscopic
    hot biopsy forceps
Barraquer cilia forceps
Barraquer ciliary forceps
Barraquer conjunctiva
    forceps
Barraquer corneal forceps
Barraquer fixation forceps
Barraquer hemostatic
    mosquito forceps
Barraquer mosquito forceps
Barraquer suture forceps
Barraquer-Katzin forceps
Barraquer-Troutman corneal
    forceps
Barraquer-Troutman forceps
Barraquer-von Mandach
    capsule forceps
Barraquer-von Mandach clot
    forceps
Barraya tissue forceps
Barrett intestinal forceps
Barrett lens forceps
Barrett placenta forceps
Barrett tenaculum forceps
Barrett uterine tenaculum
    forceps
Barrett-Allen placenta
forceps
Barrett-Allen uterine forceps
Barrett-Allen uterine-elevating
    forceps
Barrett-Murphy intestinal
    forceps
Barrie-Jones angled crocodile
    forceps
Barron alligator forceps
Barsky forceps
Barton obstetrical forceps
basket forceps
basket-cutting forceps
basket-punch forceps
basket-type crushing forceps
Bauer dissecting forceps
Bauer sponge forceps
Baumberger forceps
Baumgartner forceps
Baum-Hecht tarsorrhaphy
    forceps
Bausch articulation paper
    forceps

forceps (*continued*)

bayonet bipolar electrosurgical forceps
bayonet bipolar forceps
bayonet molar forceps
bayonet monopolar forceps
bayonet root tip forceps
bayonet-type forceps
BB shot forceps
Bead ethmoid forceps
beaked cowhorn forceps
bean forceps
Beardsley forceps
bearing-seating forceps
Beasley-Babcock tissue forceps
Beaupre cilia forceps
Beaupre epilation forceps
Bechert lens-holding forceps
Bechert-McPherson tying forceps
Beck forceps
Beebe hemostatic forceps
Beebe wire-cutting forceps
Beer cilia forceps
Beer ciliary forceps
Behen ear forceps
Behrend cystic duct forceps
Bellucci ear forceps
Benaron scalp-rotating forceps
Bengolea artery forceps
Bennett cilia forceps
Bennett epilation forceps
Berens capsule forceps
Berens corneal transplant forceps
Berens muscle forceps
Berens muscle recession forceps
Berens ptosis forceps
Berens recession forceps
Berens suture forceps
Berens suturing forceps
Berger biopsy forceps
Bergeron pillar forceps
Bergh cilia forceps
Bergman-Forster sponge forceps
Bergman tissue forceps
Berke cilia forceps
Berke ptosis forceps
Berkeley Bioengineering ptosis forceps

forceps (*continued*)

Berkeley forceps
Bernard uterine forceps
Berne nasal forceps
Bernhard towel forceps
Berry uterine-elevating forceps
Best common duct stone forceps
Best gallstone forceps
Bettman-Noyes fixation forceps
Bevan gallbladder forceps
Bevan hemostatic forceps
Beyer rongeur forceps
B-H forceps
BiCoag bipolar laparoscopic forceps
Bierer ovum forceps
Bigelow forceps
Bill traction handle forceps
Billroth tumor forceps
Billroth uterine tumor forceps
Binkhorst lens forceps
binocular fixation forceps
biopsy forceps
biopsy punch forceps
biopsy specimen forceps
bipolar bayonet forceps
bipolar coagulating forceps
bipolar coagulation forceps
bipolar coagulation-suction forceps
bipolar coaptation forceps
bipolar cutting forceps
bipolar electrocautery forceps
bipolar eye forceps
bipolar forceps
bipolar irrigating forceps
bipolar laparoscopic forceps
bipolar long-shaft forceps
bipolar suction forceps
bipolar transsphenoidal forceps
Bircher-Ganske meniscal cartilage forceps
Bireks dissecting forceps
Birkett hemostatic forceps
Birks Mark II Colibri forceps
Birks Mark II grooved forceps
Birks Mark II microneedle-holder forceps

forceps (*continued*)
  Birks Mark II needle-holder
    forceps
  Birks Mark II straight forceps
  Birks Mark II suture-tying
    forceps
  Birks Mark II toothed forceps
  Birtcher endoscopic forceps
  Bishop tissue forceps
  Bishop-Harman dressing
    forceps
  Bishop-Harman foreign body
    forceps
  Bishop-Harman iris forceps
  Bishop-Harman tissue forceps
  bite biopsy forceps
  Bi-tec forceps
  biting forceps
  Björk diathermy forceps
  Björk-Stille diathermy forceps
  bladder forceps
  bladder specimen forceps
  Blade-Wilde ear forceps
  Blake dressing forceps
  Blake ear forceps
  Blake embolus forceps
  Blake gallstone forceps
  Blakesley ethmoid forceps
  Blakesley forceps
  Blakesley septal bone forceps
  Blakesley septal compression
    forceps
  Blakesley septal forceps
  Blakesley-Weil upturned
    ethmoid forceps
  Blakesley-Wilde ear forceps
  Blakesley-Wilde ethmoid
    forceps
  Blakesley-Wilde nasal forceps
  Blalock forceps
  Blalock-Kleinert forceps
  Blanchard hemorrhoid
    forceps
  Blanchard hemorrhoidal
    forceps
  Bland cervical traction
    forceps
  Bland vulsellum forceps
  Blaydes angled lens forceps
  Blaydes corneal forceps
  Blaydes lens-holding forceps
  blepharochalasis forceps

forceps (*continued*)
  Block-Potts intestinal forceps
  Blohmka tonsil forceps
  Blohmka tonsillar forceps
  Bloodwell tissue forceps
  Bloodwell vascular forceps
  Bloodwell vascular tissue
    forceps
  Bloodwell-Brown forceps
  Bloomberg lens forceps
  Blum forceps
  Blumenthal uterine dressing
    forceps
  blunt forceps
  Boer craniotomy forceps
  Boerma obstetrical forceps
  Boettcher arterial forceps
  Boettcher artery forceps
  Boettcher pulmonary artery
    forceps
  Boettcher tonsil artery
    forceps
  Boettcher tonsillar artery
    forceps
  Boettcher-Schnidt forceps
  Boies cutting forceps
  Bolton forceps
  Bonaccolto capsule fragment
    forceps
  Bonaccolto cup jaws forceps
  Bonaccolto fragment forceps
  Bonaccolto jeweler's forceps
  Bonaccolto jeweler's-type
    forceps
  Bonaccolto magnet tip
    forceps
  Bonaccolto utility forceps
  Bonaccolto utility pickup
    forceps
  Bond placenta forceps
  bone forceps
  bone punch forceps
  bone-biting forceps
  bone-cutting double-action
    forceps
  bone-cutting forceps
  bone-holding forceps
  bone-reduction forceps
  bone-splitting forceps
  Bonn European suturing
    forceps
  Bonn iris forceps

forceps (*continued*)
    Bonn peripheral iridectomy
        forceps
    Bonn suturing forceps
    Bonney tissue forceps
    Bores corneal fixation forceps
    Bores U-shaped forceps
    Boruchoff forceps
    Boston Lying-In cervical
        forceps
    Boston Lying-In cervical-
        grasping forceps
    Botvin iris forceps
    Botvin vulsellum forceps
    Bouchayer grasping forceps
    Bovie coagulating forceps
    Bovino scleral-spreading
        forceps
    bowel forceps
    Bowen suction loose body
        forceps
    box-joint forceps
    Boys-Allis tissue forceps
    Boys-Allis tissue-holding
        forceps
    Bozeman dressing forceps
    Bozeman LR dressing forceps
    Bozeman LR packing forceps
    Bozeman LR uterine-dressing
        forceps
    Bozeman uterine forceps
    Bozeman uterine-dressing
        forceps
    Bozeman uterine-packing
        forceps
    Bozeman-Douglas dressing
        forceps
    Bozeman-Douglas uterine-
        dressing forceps
    B-P transfer forceps
    Braasch bladder specimen
        forceps
    Bracken fixation forceps
    Bracken forceps
    Bracken iris forceps
    Bracken scleral fixation
        forceps
    Bracken tissue-grasping
        forceps
    Bracken-Forkas corneal
        forceps
    Bradford thyroid forceps

forceps (*continued*)
    Bradford thyroid traction
        vulsellum forceps
    brain clip forceps
    brain dressing forceps
    brain forceps
    brain spatula forceps
    brain tissue forceps
    brain tumor forceps
    Braithwaite forceps
    Brand passing forceps
    Brand shunt-introducing
        forceps
    Brand tendon forceps
    Brand tendon-holding forceps
    Brand tendon-passing
        forceps
    Brand tendon-tunneling
        forceps
    Braun uterine tenaculum
        forceps
    breast tenaculum forceps
    Brenner forceps
    Bridge deep-surgery forceps
    Bridge hemostatic forceps
    Bridge intestinal forceps
    Brigham 1×2 teeth forceps
    Brigham brain tumor forceps
    Brigham dressing forceps
    Brigham thumb tissue forceps
    broad-blade forceps
    Brock biopsy forceps
    bronchial biopsy forceps
    bronchial forceps
    bronchial-grasping forceps
    bronchoscopic biopsy forceps
    bronchoscopic forceps
    bronchoscopic rotation
        forceps
    bronchus forceps
    bronchus-grasping forceps
    Bronson-Magnion forceps
    Brophy dressing forceps
    Brophy tissue forceps
    Brown side-grasping forceps
    Brown thoracic forceps
    Brown tissue forceps
    Brown-Adson side-grasping
        forceps
    Brown-Adson tissue forceps
    Brown-Bahnson bayonet
        forceps

forceps (*continued*)
Brown-Buerger forceps
Brown-Cushing forceps
Brown-Swan forceps
Broyles optical forceps
Bruening cutting-tip forceps
Bruening ethmoid
exenteration forceps
Bruening nasal-cutting septal
forceps
Bruening nasal-cutting septum
forceps
Bruening septal forceps
Bruening septum forceps
Bruening-Citelli forceps
Brunner intestinal forceps
Brunner sigmoid anastomosis
forceps
Brunner tissue forceps
Brunschwig arterial forceps
Brunschwig artery forceps
Brunschwig viscera forceps
Brunschwig visceral forceps
Bryant nasal forceps
Buck foreign body forceps
Buerger-McCarthy bladder
forceps
Buerger-McCarthy forceps
Buie biopsy forceps
Buie rectal forceps
Buie specimen forceps
bulldog clamp-applier forceps
bulldog clamp-applying
forceps
bulldog forceps
bullet forceps
Bumpus specimen forceps
Bunim urethral forceps
Bunker forceps
Bunker modification of
Jackson laryngeal forceps
Buratto flap forceps
Buratto LASIK forceps
Buratto ophthalmic forceps
Burch biopsy forceps
Burford coarctation forceps
Burnham biopsy forceps
Burns bone forceps
Butler bayonet forceps
Bycep biopsy forceps
CL Jackson head-holding
forceps

forceps (*continued*)
CL Jackson pin-bending
costophrenic forceps
CL Jackson head-holding
forceps
CL Jackson pin-bending
costophrenic forceps
Cairns dissection forceps
Cairns hemostatic forceps
Cairns-Dandy hemostasis
forceps
Calibri forceps
Callahan fixation forceps
Callahan scleral fixation
forceps
Callison-Adson tissue forceps
Cameron-Miller type
monopolar forceps
Campbell ligature-carrier
forceps
Campbell ureteral catheter
forceps
Campbell ureteral forceps
Campbell urethral catheter
forceps
Cane bone-holding forceps
cannulated bronchoscopic
forceps
cannulated forceps
capsular forceps
capsule forceps
capsule fragment forceps
capsule-grasping forceps
capsulorhexis forceps (*also*
capsulorrhexis)
capsulotomy forceps
caput forceps
Carb-Bite tissue forceps
carbide-jaw forceps
Cardio-Grip iliac forceps
Cardio-Grip tissue forceps
cardiovascular forceps
cardiovascular tissue forceps
Cardona corneal prosthesis
forceps
Cardona threading lens
forceps
Carlens forceps
Carmalt artery forceps
Carmalt hemostatic forceps
Carmalt hysterectomy forceps
Carmalt splinter forceps

forceps (*continued*)

Carmalt thoracic forceps
Carmody forceps
Carmody thumb tissue forceps
Carmody tissue forceps
Carmody-Brophy forceps
carotid artery forceps
Carrel hemostatic forceps
Carrel mosquito forceps
Carroll bone-holding forceps
Carroll dressing forceps
Carroll tendon-passing forceps
Carroll tendon-pulling forceps
Carroll tissue forceps
Carroll-Adson dural forceps
Carroll-Adson forceps
cartilage forceps
cartilage-holding forceps
Cartman lens insertion forceps
caruncle forceps
Caspar alligator forceps
Cassidy-Brophy dressing forceps
Castaneda suture tag forceps
Castaneda vascular forceps
Castaneda-Mixter forceps
Castroviejo capsular forceps
Castroviejo capsule forceps
Castroviejo clip-applying forceps
Castroviejo cornea-holding forceps
Castroviejo corneoscleral forceps
Castroviejo corneoscleral suture forceps
Castroviejo cross-action capsular forceps
Castroviejo eye suture forceps
Castroviejo fixation forceps
Castroviejo lid forceps
Castroviejo scleral fold forceps
Castroviejo suture forceps
Castroviejo suturing forceps
Castroviejo transplant forceps
Castroviejo transplant-grafting forceps
Castroviejo tying forceps

forceps (*continued*)

Castroviejo wide-grip handle forceps
Castroviejo-Arruga capsule forceps
Castroviejo-Arruga forceps
Castroviejo-Colibri corneal forceps
Castroviejo-Furniss cornea-holding forceps
Castroviejo-Simpson forceps
Catalano capsular forceps
Catalano corneoscleral forceps
Catalano tying forceps
catheter forceps
catheter-introducing forceps
Cavanaugh-Wells tonsil forceps
center-action forceps
cephalic blade forceps
cervical biopsy forceps
cervical biopsy punch forceps
cervical forceps
cervical grasping forceps
cervical hemostatic forceps
cervical punch forceps
cervical traction forceps
cervix forceps
cervix-holding forceps
cesarean forceps
chalazion forceps
Chamberlen obstetrical forceps
Championniere forceps
Chandler iris forceps
Chandler spinal-perforating forceps
Chang bone-cutting forceps
Chaput tissue forceps
Charnley suture forceps
Charnley wire-holding forceps
Charnley-Riches arterial forceps
Cheatle sterilizer forceps
Cheatle sterilizing forceps
Cheron uterine dressing forceps
Cherry forceps
Cherry-Adson forceps
Cherry-Kerrison rongeur forceps

forceps (*continued*)

Chester sponge forceps
Chevalier Jackson
   bronchoesophagoscopy
   forceps
Chevalier Jackson forceps
chicken-bill rongeur forceps
Child clip-applying forceps
Child intestinal forceps
Child-Phillips forceps
Children's Hospital dressing
   forceps
Children's Hospital intestinal
   forceps
Childs-Phillips forceps
Chimani pharyngeal forceps
Choyce intraocular lens
   forceps
Choyce lens forceps
Choyce lens-inserting forceps
Christopher-Stille forceps
Chubb tonsil forceps
Chubb tonsillar forceps
Cicherelli rongeur forceps
Cilco lens forceps
cilia forceps
cilia suture forceps
Circon Tripolar forceps
circular cup bronchoscopic
   biopsy forceps
Citelli punch forceps
Citelli-Bruening ear forceps
Civiale forceps
clamp forceps
clamp-carrier forceps
Clark capsule fragment
   forceps
Clark ligator scissor forceps
Clark-Guyton forceps
Clark-Verhoeff capsule
   forceps
claw forceps
Clayman corneal forceps
Clayman lens forceps
Clayman lens-holding forceps
Clayman lens-inserting
   forceps
Clayman suturing forceps
Clayman-Kelman intraocular
   lens forceps
Clayman-McPherson tying
   forceps

forceps (*continued*)

cleft palate forceps
Clemetson uterine forceps
Clerf forceps
Clevedent forceps
Cleveland bone-cutting
   forceps
clip forceps
clip-applying aneurysm
   forceps
clip-applying forceps
clip-bending forceps
clip-cutting forceps
clip-introducing forceps
clip-removing forceps
closed iris forceps
closer forceps
closing forceps
clot forceps
coagulating forceps
coagulating-suction forceps
coagulation forceps
Coakley tonsillar forceps
Coakley-Allis tonsillar forceps
coaptation bipolar forceps
coarctation forceps
coated biopsy forceps
Cobaugh eye forceps
Codman fallopian tube forceps
Codman ovary forceps
Cohen corneal forceps
Cohen nasal-dressing forceps
cold biopsy forceps
cold cup biopsy forceps
cold cup forceps
Coleman-Taylor IOL forceps
Colibri corneal forceps
Colibri corneal utility forceps
Colibri eye forceps
Colibri-Pierse forceps
Colibri-Storz corneal forceps
College forceps
Coller arterial forceps
Coller artery forceps
Coller hemostatic forceps
Colley tissue forceps
Colley traction forceps
Collier hemostatic forceps
Collier-Crile hemostatic
   forceps
Collier-DeBakey hemostatic
   forceps

forceps (*continued*)
Collin dressing forceps
Collin intestinal forceps
Collin lung-grasping forceps
Collin mucous forceps
Collin ovarian forceps
Collin tissue forceps
Collin tongue forceps
Collin tongue-seizing forceps
Collin uterine-elevating
forceps
Collin-Duval intestinal forceps
Collin-Duval-Crile intestinal
forceps
Collin-Pozzi uterine forceps
Collis microutility forceps
Collis-Maumenee corneal
forceps
Coloviras-Rumel thoracic
forceps
Colver tonsil forceps
Colver tonsillar pillar-grasping
forceps
Colver tonsil-seizing forceps
Colver-Coakley tonsil
forceps
Colver-Coakley tonsillar
forceps
common duct stone forceps
common duct-holding forceps
common McPherson forceps
compression forceps
Cone wire-twisting forceps
conjunctival fixation forceps
conjunctival forceps
connector forceps
contact compressive forceps
continuous clip forceps
Cook flexible biopsy forceps
Cooley anastomosis forceps
Cooley aortic forceps
Cooley arterial occlusion
forceps
Cooley auricular appendage
forceps
Cooley cardiovascular forceps
Cooley coarctation forceps
Cooley CSR forceps
Cooley curved forceps
Cooley double-angled jaw
forceps
Cooley graft forceps

forceps (*continued*)
Cooley iliac forceps
Cooley multipurpose forceps
Cooley neonatal vascular
forceps
Cooley patent ductus forceps
Cooley pediatric aortic
forceps
Cooley peripheral vascular
forceps
Cooley tangential pediatric
forceps
Cooley tissue forceps
Cooley vascular forceps
Cooley vascular tissue forceps
Cooley-Baumgarten aortic
forceps
Cooley-Derra anastomosis
forceps
Cope lung forceps
Coppridge grasping forceps
Coppridge urethral forceps
Corbett bone-cutting forceps
Cordes esophagoscopy
forceps
Cordes-New forceps
Cordes-New laryngeal punch
forceps
Corey ovum forceps
Corey placental forceps
Corgill-Hartmann forceps
cornea-holding forceps
corneal fixation forceps
corneal forceps
corneal prosthesis forceps
corneal splinter forceps
corneal transplant forceps
corneal utility forceps
corneal-suturing forceps
cornea-suturing forceps
corneoscleral forceps
corneoscleral suturing forceps
Cornet forceps
coronary artery forceps
Corson myoma forceps
Corwin tonsillar forceps
Corwin tonsillar hemostatic
forceps
Cottle biting forceps
Cottle insertion forceps
Cottle lower lateral forceps
Cottle tissue forceps

forceps (*continued*)
  Cottle-Arruga cartilage
    forceps
  Cottle-Jansen rongeur forceps
  Cottle-Kazanjian bone-cutting
    forceps
  Cottle-Kazanjian nasal forceps
  Cottle-Kazanjian nasal-cutting
    forceps
  Cottle-Walsham septum
    straightening forceps
  Cottle-Walsham septum-
    straightening forceps
  cowhorn tooth-extracting
    forceps
  Cozean angled lens forceps
  Cozean bipolar forceps
  Cozean implantation forceps
  Cozean-McPherson angled
    lens forceps
  Cozean-McPherson tying
    forceps
  Crafoord arterial forceps
  Crafoord bronchial forceps
  Crafoord coarctation forceps
  Crafoord pulmonary forceps
  Crafoord-Sellors hemostatic
    forceps
  Craig nasal-cutting forceps
  Craig septal forceps
  Craig septum bone-cutting
    forceps
  Craig septum-cutting forceps
  Craig tonsil-seizing forceps
  cranial forceps
  cranial rongeur forceps
  cranium clip-applying forceps
  Crawford fascial forceps
  Crawford-Knighton forceps
  Creevy biopsy forceps
  Crenshaw caruncle forceps
  Crile arterial forceps
  Crile gall duct forceps
  Crile hemostatic forceps
  Crile Micro-Line artery
    forceps
  Crile-Barnes hemostatic
    forceps
  Crile-Duval lung-grasping
    forceps
  Crile-Rankin forceps
  crimper closer forceps

forceps (*continued*)
  crimper forceps
  crimping forceps
  Crockard ligament grasping
    forceps
  Crockard odontoid peg-
    grasping forceps
  crocodile biopsy forceps
  crocodile forceps
  cross-action capsular forceps
  cross-action forceps
  Crossen puncturing
    tenaculum forceps
  crural nipper forceps
  Cryer Universal forceps
  CSF shunt connector forceps
  CSF shunt-introducing forceps
  Cukier nasal forceps
  Cullen obstetrical forceps
  Culler eye forceps
  Culler fixation forceps
  Cullom septal forceps
  cup biopsy forceps
  cup forceps
  cup-biting forceps
  cupped forceps
  cup-shaped curet forceps
  cup-shaped ear forceps
  cup-shaped forceps
  cup-shaped inner ear forceps
  cup-shaped middle ear
    forceps
  curet forceps
  Curtis tissue forceps
  curved dissecting forceps
  curved forceps
  curved iris forceps
  curved knot-tying forceps
  curved Maryland forceps
  curved microbipolar forceps
  curved micromonopolar
    forceps
  curved tying forceps
  curved-tip jeweler's bipolar
    forceps
  Cushing bayonet forceps
  Cushing bipolar forceps
  Cushing bipolar neurosurgical
    forceps
  Cushing brain forceps
  Cushing cranial rongeur
    forceps

forceps (*continued*)
    Cushing decompression
        forceps
    Cushing dressing forceps
    Cushing monopolar forceps
    Cushing thumb forceps
    Cushing tissue forceps
    Cushing Vital tissue forceps
    Cushing-Brown tissue forceps
    Cushing-Gutsch dressing
        forceps
    Cushing-Gutsch tissue
        forceps
    Cushing-Taylor carbide-jaw
        forceps
    Cutler forceps
    cutting forceps
    cylindrical-object forceps
    cystic duct forceps
    cystoscopic forceps
    Czerny tenaculum forceps
    Dahlgren skull-cutting forceps
    Dahlgren-Hudson cranial
        forceps
    Daicoff needle-pulling forceps
    Daicoff vascular forceps
    Dale femoral-popliteal
        anastomosis forceps
    Dallas lens-inserting forceps
    D'Allesandro serial suture-
        holding forceps
    Dan chalazion forceps
    Danberg forceps
    Danberg iris forceps
    Dandy arterial forceps
    Dandy hemostatic forceps
    Dandy scalp forceps
    Dandy scalp hemostatic
        forceps
    Dandy-Kolodny hemostatic
        forceps
    Dan-Gradle ciliary forceps
    Dartigues kidney-elevating
        forceps
    Dartigues uterine-elevating
        forceps
    Davidson pulmonary vessel
        forceps
    Davis bayonet forceps
    Davis capsular forceps
    Davis coagulating forceps
    Davis diathermy forceps

forceps (*continued*)
    Davis monopolar bayonet
        forceps
    Davis sterilizing forceps
    Davis thoracic tissue forceps
    Davol rongeur forceps
    Dawson-Yuhl rongeur forceps
    Dawson-Yuhl-Kerrison
        rongeur forceps
    Dawson-Yuhl-Leksell rongeur
        forceps
    De Alvarez forceps
    De Juan forceps
    Dean tonsillar forceps
    Dean tonsillar hemostatic
        forceps
    Dean-Shallcross tonsil-seizing
        forceps
    DeBakey aortic forceps
    DeBakey arterial forceps
    DeBakey Autraugrip forceps
    DeBakey dissecting forceps
    DeBakey tangential occlusion
        forceps
    DeBakey thoracic forceps
    DeBakey tissue forceps
    DeBakey vascular forceps
    DeBakey vascular tissue
        forceps
    DeBakey-Bahnson forceps
    DeBakey-Bainbridge vascular
        forceps
    DeBakey-Beck multipurpose
        forceps
    DeBakey-Colovira-Rumel
        thoracic forceps
    DeBakey-Coloviras-Rumel
        thoracic forceps
    DeBakey-Cooley anastomosis
        forceps
    DeBakey-Cooley
        cardiovascular forceps
    DeBakey-Derra anastomosis
        forceps
    DeBakey-Diethrich coronary
        artery forceps
    DeBakey-Diethrich vascular
        forceps
    DeBakey-Kelly hemostatic
        forceps
    DeBakey-Liddicoat vascular
        forceps

forceps (*continued*)
  DeBakey-Mixter thoracic
    forceps
  DeBakey-Pean cardiovascular
    forceps
  DeBakey-Rankin hemostatic
    forceps
  DeBakey-Reynolds
    anastomosis forceps
  DeBakey-Rumel thoracic
    forceps
  DeBakey-Semb forceps
  Decker microsurgical forceps
  Deddish-Potts intestinal
    forceps
  deep-surgery forceps
  deep-vessel forceps
  Defourmental rongeur forceps
  DeLee cervical forceps
  DeLee cervix-holding forceps
  DeLee dressing forceps
  DeLee obstetrical forceps
  DeLee ovum forceps
  DeLee shuttle forceps
  DeLee spoon tissue forceps
  DeLee uterine forceps
  DeLee uterine packing
    forceps
  DeLee uterine-packing
    forceps
  DeLee-Simpson forceps
  delicate thumb-dressing
    forceps
  Delrin locking-handle forceps
  Demarest septal forceps
  DeMartel appendix forceps
  DeMartel scalp flap forceps
  DeMartel scalp forceps
  DeMartel-Wolfson closing
    forceps
  DeMartel-Wolfson intestinal-
    holding forceps
  Demel wire-tightening forceps
  Demel wire-twisting forceps
  Dench ear forceps
  Denis Browne tonsillar
    forceps
  Dennen forceps
  Dennis forceps
  Dennis intestinal forceps
  dental dressing forceps
  dental forceps

forceps (*continued*)
  depilatory dermal forceps
  Derf forceps
  DermaCare electrosurgical
    forceps
  Derra cardiovascular forceps
  Derra urethral forceps
  Derra-Cooley forceps
  D'Errico bayonet pituitary
    forceps
  D'Errico dressing forceps
  D'Errico hypophyseal forceps
  D'Errico tissue forceps
  Desjardins gallstone forceps
  Desjardins kidney pedicle
    forceps
  Desmarres chalazion forceps
  Desmarres lid forceps
  DeTakats-McKenzie brain clip-
    applying forceps
  DeTakats-McKenzie clip-
    applying forceps
  DeVilbiss cranial forceps
  DeVilbiss rongeur forceps
  DeWecker forceps
  DeWeese axis traction forceps
  DeWeese axis traction
    obstetrical forceps
  Dewey obstetrical forceps
  Diaflex grasping forceps
  diathermic forceps
  diathermy forceps
  Dieffenbach forceps
  diener forceps
  Dieter malleus forceps
  Diethrich right-angled
    hemostatic forceps
  dilating forceps
  Dingman bone-holding
    forceps
  disimpaction forceps
  disk forceps
  diskectomy forceps
  disposable forceps
  dissecting forceps
  dissection forceps
  divergent outlet forceps
  Dixon flamingo forceps
  Dixon-Lovelace hemostatic
    forceps
  Dixon-Thorpe vitreous foreign
    body forceps

forceps (*continued*)
Docktor tissue forceps
Dodick lens-holding forceps
Dodick Nucleus Cracker
forceps
Dodrill forceps
dolphin dissecting forceps
dolphin grasping forceps
dolphin-billed grasping
forceps
dolphin-type atraumatic
forceps
Donberg iris forceps
donor button forceps
Dorsey bayonet forceps
double-action bone-cutting
forceps
double-action hump forceps
double-action rongeur forceps
double-articulated
bronchoscopic forceps
double-concave forceps
double-concave rat-tooth
forceps
double-cupped forceps
double-ended needle forceps
double-ended suture forceps
double-ended tissue forceps
double-fixation forceps
double-pronged forceps
double-spoon biopsy forceps
double-spoon forceps
Douglas cilia forceps
Douglas ciliary forceps
Douglas eye forceps
Doyen gallbladder forceps
Doyen intestinal forceps
Doyen towel forceps
Doyen uterine forceps
Doyen vulsellum forceps
Draeger forceps
dressing forceps
Drews cilia forceps
Drews ciliary forceps
Drews intraocular forceps
Drews intraocular lens
forceps
Drews-Sato tying forceps
Dreyfus prosthesis forceps
drill guide forceps
duckbill forceps
Duguid curved forceps

forceps (*continued*)
dull rotation forceps
dull-pointed forceps
Dumont dissecting forceps
Dumont jeweler's forceps
Dumont Swiss dissecting
forceps
Dunhill forceps
Duplay tenaculum forceps
Duplay uterine tenaculum
forceps
Duracep biopsy forceps
dural forceps
Duval intestinal forceps
Duval lung forceps
Duval lung tissue forceps
Duval lung-grasping forceps
Duval-Allis forceps
Duval-Collin intestinal forceps
Duval-Crile intestinal forceps
Duval-Crile lung forceps
Duval-Crile lung-grasping
forceps
Duval-Crile tissue forceps
Duval Vital intestinal forceps
DynaBite biopsy forceps
Dyonics basket forceps
ear forceps
ear polyp forceps
ear punch forceps
ear-dressing forceps
ear-grasping forceps
Eastman cystic duct forceps
Eber needle-holder forceps
Echlin rongeur forceps
Ecker-Kazanjian forceps
Eckhoff forceps
Eder forceps
Edna towel forceps
Effler-Groves cardiovascular
forceps
Ehrhardt lid forceps
Eisenstein hysterectomy
forceps
electrocoagulating biopsy
forceps
electrosurgery forceps
electrosurgical biopsy forceps
elevating forceps
Elliot gallbladder forceps
Elliot hemostatic forceps
Elliot obstetrical forceps

forceps (*continued*)
Elliott gallbladder forceps
Elliott hemostatic forceps
Elliott obstetrical forceps
Elschnig capsular forceps
Elschnig cyclodialysis forceps
Elschnig fixation forceps
Elschnig secondary
  membrane forceps
Elschnig tissue-grasping
  forceps
Elschnig-O'Brien fixation
  forceps
Elschnig-O'Brien tissue-
  grasping forceps
Elschnig-O'Connor fixation
  forceps
Elschnig-O'Connor forceps
Emmet obstetrical forceps
end-biting forceps
Endo-Assist endoscopic
  forceps
endometrial forceps
endometrial polyp forceps
endoscopic biopsy forceps
endoscopic forceps
endoscopic grasping forceps
endoscopic suture-cutting
  forceps
endospeculum forceps
Endo-therapy disposable
  biopsy forceps
endotracheal catheter forceps
endotracheal tube forceps
Endura dressing forceps
Englert forceps
English tissue forceps
English-pattern tissue forceps
Ennis forceps
entropion forceps
epilating forceps
epilation forceps
episcleral forceps
Eppendorfer biopsy punch
  forceps
Eppendorfer cervical biopsy
  forceps
Eppendorfer uterine biopsy
  forceps
Ergo bipolar forceps
Erhardt eyelid forceps
Erhardt lid forceps

forceps (*continued*)
Erich biopsy forceps
Erich laryngeal biopsy
  forceps
Ernest-McDonald soft
  intraocular lens-folding
  forceps
Ernest-McDonald soft IOL
  folding forceps
E-series bipolar forceps
esophageal forceps
esophagoscopic forceps
Essrig tissue forceps
ethmoid punch forceps
ethmoidal exenteration
  forceps
ethmoidal forceps
ethmoid-cutting forceps
Ethridge hysterectomy
  forceps
Evans Vital tissue forceps
Everett forceps
Evershears bipolar
  laparoscopic forceps
Ewald tissue forceps
Ewald-Hudson brain forceps
Ewald-Hudson dressing
  forceps
Ewald-Hudson tissue forceps
Ewing capsule forceps
Excel disposable biopsy
  forceps
exenteration forceps
exolever forceps
expansile forceps
extracapsular eye forceps
extracapsular forceps
extracting forceps
extraction forceps
eye fixation forceps
eye forceps
eye needle holder forceps
eye suture forceps
eye-dressing forceps
eye-fixation forceps
eyelid forceps
Foerster iris forceps
Facit uterine polyp forceps
Falcao fixation forceps
Falk lion-jaw forceps
fallopian tube forceps
Farabeuf bone-holding forceps

forceps (*continued*)
  Farabeuf-Lambotte bone-holding forceps
  Farnham nasal-cutting forceps
  Farrington nasal polyp forceps
  Farrington septal forceps
  Farrington septum forceps
  Farrior wire-crimping forceps
  Farris tissue forceps
  Faure peritoneal forceps
  Faure uterine biopsy forceps
  Fauvel laryngeal forceps
  Fechtner conjunctiva forceps
  Fechtner ring forceps
  Fehland intestinal forceps
  Feilchenfeld splinter forceps
  fenestrated blade forceps
  fenestrated cup biopsy forceps
  fenestrated ellipsoid spiked open span biopsy forceps
  fenestrated forceps
  fenestrated spiked open span jumbo biopsy forceps
  Fenger forceps
  Ferguson angiotribe forceps
  Ferguson bone-holding forceps
  Ferris colporrhaphy forceps
  Ferris Smith bone-biting forceps
  Ferris Smith cup rongeur forceps
  Ferris Smith fragment forceps
  Ferris Smith rongeur forceps
  Ferris Smith tissue forceps
  Ferris Smith-Kerrison rongeur forceps
  Ferris Smith-Spurling intervertebral disk forceps
  Ferris Smith-Takahashi forceps
  Ferris tissue forceps
  Fichman suture-cutting forceps
  fine arterial forceps
  fine artery forceps
  fine dissecting forceps
  fine forceps
  Fine suture-tying forceps
  fine tissue forceps
  Fine-Castroviejo suturing forceps

forceps (*continued*)
  fine-cup forceps
  fine-dissecting forceps
  fine-tipped up-and-down-angled bipolar forceps
  fine-tissue forceps
  fine-tooth forceps
  fine-toothed forceps
  Fink fixation forceps
  Fink tendon-tucker forceps
  Fink-Jameson oblique muscle forceps
  Finochietto lobectomy forceps
  Finochietto thoracic forceps
  Fischl dissecting forceps
  Fischmann angiotribe forceps
  Fish grasping forceps
  Fish nasal forceps
  Fish nasal-dressing forceps
  Fisher advancement forceps
  Fisher capsular forceps
  Fisher iris forceps
  Fisher-Arlt forceps
  Fisher-Arlt iris forceps
  fissure forceps
  Fitzgerald aortic aneurysm forceps
  Fitzwater peanut sponge-holding forceps
  fixation binocular forceps
  fixation forceps
  fixation-anchor forceps
  fixed forceps
  flamingo antrostomy forceps
  Fletcher dressing forceps
  Fletcher sponge forceps
  Fletcher-Suit polyp forceps
  Fletcher-Van Doren sponge-holding forceps
  Fletcher-Van Doren uterine forceps
  Fletcher-Van Doren uterine polyp forceps
  Fletcher-Van Doren uterine polyp sponge-holding forceps
  flexible foreign body forceps
  flexible optical biopsy forceps
  fluoroscopic foreign body forceps
  Foerster eye forceps

forceps (*continued*)

Foerster gallbladder forceps
Foerster iris forceps
Foerster sponge forceps
Foerster sponge-holding
    forceps
Foerster tissue forceps
Foerster uterine forceps
Foerster-Ballenger forceps
Foerster-Bauer sponge-holding
    forceps
Foerster-Mueller forceps
Foerster-Van Doren sponge-
    holding forceps
Fogarty bulldog clamp-
    applying forceps
fold forceps
folding forceps
Foley vas isolation forceps
foramen-plugging forceps
Forbes uterine-dressing
    forceps
foreign body cystoscopy
    forceps
foreign body eye forceps
foreign body forceps
foreign body-retrieving
    forceps
Foerster iris forceps
forward-grasping forceps
Foss cardiovascular forceps
Foss clamp forceps
Foss intestinal clamp forceps
Foster-Ballenger forceps
Fox bipolar electrocautery
    forceps
Fox bipolar forceps
Fox cartilage forceps
Fox tissue forceps
Fraenkel cutting-tip forceps
Fraenkel double-articulated-tip
    forceps
fragment forceps
Francis chalazion forceps
Francis spud chalazion
    forceps
Francis-Gray forceps
Frangenheim biopsy punch
    forceps
Frangenheim hook forceps
Frangenheim hook-punch
    forceps

forceps (*continued*)

Fraenkel cutting-tip forceps
Fraenkel esophagoscopy
    forceps
Fraenkel laryngeal forceps
Fraenkel tampon forceps
Frankfeldt grasping forceps
Fraser forceps
Freer septal forceps
Freer-Gruenwald forceps
Freer-Gruenwald punch
    forceps
French-pattern forceps
Fricke arterial forceps
Friedman rongeur forceps
Fry nasal forceps
Fraenkel cutting-tip forceps
Fraenkel esophagoscopy
    forceps
Fraenkel laryngeal forceps
Fraenkel tampon forceps
Fuchs capsular forceps
Fuchs capsule forceps
Fuchs capsulotomy forceps
Fuchs extracapsular forceps
Fuchs iris forceps
Fujinon biopsy forceps
Fulpit tissue forceps
Furniss cornea-holding
    forceps
Furniss intestinal forceps
Furniss polyp forceps
Furniss-Castroviejo forceps
Furniss-Clute forceps
Furniss-Rizzuti forceps
Gabriel Tucker forceps
Gafco-Halsted forceps
galea forceps
gall duct forceps
gallbladder forceps
gallstone forceps
Gambale-Merrill bone-cutting
    forceps
Gam-Mer bone-cutting forceps
Gardner bone forceps
Gardner hysterectomy forceps
Garland hysterectomy forceps
Garrigue uterine-dressing
    forceps
Garrison forceps
Gaskin fragment forceps
gastrointestinal forceps

forceps (*continued*)

Gaure peritoneal forceps
Gauss hemostatic forceps
Gavin-Miller colon forceps
Gavin-Miller intestinal forceps
Gavin-Miller tissue forceps
Gaylor uterine biopsy forceps
Gaylor uterine specimen forceps
Geissendorfer uterine forceps
Gelfilm forceps
Gelfoam pressure forceps
Gellhorn uterine biopsy forceps
Gelpi hysterectomy forceps
Gelpi-Lowrie hysterectomy forceps
Gemini gall duct forceps
Gemini hemostatic forceps
Gemini Mixter forceps
Gemini thoracic forceps
general tissue forceps
general wire forceps
Gerald bayonet microbipolar neurosurgical forceps
Gerald bipolar forceps
Gerald brain forceps
Gerald dressing forceps
Gerald monopolar forceps
Gerald straight microbipolar neurosurgical forceps
Gerald tissue forceps
Gerbode cardiovascular tissue forceps
GI forceps
GIA forceps
Gifford fixation forceps
Gifford iris forceps
Gilbert cystic duct forceps
Gildenberg biopsy forceps
Gill curved iris forceps
Gill incision-spreading forceps
Gill iris forceps
Gill-Arruga capsular forceps
Gill-Chandler iris forceps
Gillespie obstetrical forceps
Gill-Fuchs capsular forceps
Gill-Hess iris forceps
Gillies dissecting forceps
Gillies tissue forceps
Gillquist-Oretorp-Stille forceps
Gill-Safar forceps

forceps (*continued*)

Gill-Welsh capsular forceps
Ginsberg tissue forceps
giraffe biopsy forceps
Girard corneoscleral forceps
Glassman noncrushing pickup forceps
Glassman pickup forceps
Glassman-Allis common duct-holding forceps
Glassman-Allis intestinal forceps
Glassman-Allis miniature intestinal forceps
Glassman-Allis noncrushing common duct forceps
Glassman-Allis noncrushing intestinal forceps
Glassman-Allis noncrushing tissue-holding forceps
Glassman-Babcock forceps
Glenn diverticular forceps
Glenn diverticulum forceps
Glenner hysterectomy forceps
Glenner vaginal hysterectomy forceps
glenoid-reaming forceps
globular object forceps
Glover anastomosis forceps
Glover coarctation forceps
Glover curved forceps
Glover infundibular rongeur forceps
Glover patent ductus forceps
Glover rongeur forceps
Glover spoon-shaped forceps
goiter forceps
goiter vulsellum forceps
goiter-seizing forceps
Gold deep-surgery forceps
Gold hemostatic forceps
Goldman-Kazanjian nasal forceps
Goldmann capsulorrhexis forceps
Gomco forceps
Good obstetrical forceps
Goodhill tonsillar forceps
Goodhill tonsillar hemostatic forceps
Goodyear-Gruenwald forceps
Gordon bead forceps

forceps (*continued*)

Gordon cilia forceps
Gordon ciliary forceps
Gordon uterine forceps
Gordon uterine vulsellum forceps
Gordon vulsellum forceps
Grabow forceps
Gradle cilia forceps
Gradle ciliary forceps
Graefe curved iris forceps
Graefe dressing forceps
Graefe eye-fixation forceps
Graefe fixation forceps
Graefe iris forceps
Graefe nonmagnetic fixation forceps
Graefe straight iris forceps
Graefe tissue forceps
Graefe tissue-grasping forceps
Grafco-Halsted forceps
grasping and cutting forceps
grasping biopsy forceps
grasping forceps
grasping tripod forceps
Gray arterial forceps
Gray cystic duct forceps
Grayson forceps
Grayton forceps
Grazer blepharoplasty forceps
Green capsular forceps
Green chalazion forceps
Green fixation forceps
Green suction tube forceps
Green tissue-grasping forceps
Green-Armytage forceps
Green-Armytage hemostatic forceps
Greene tube-holding forceps
Greenwood bipolar coagulation-suction forceps
Gregory forceps
Greven alligator forceps
Grey Turner forceps
Grieshaber diamond-coated forceps
Grieshaber internal limiting membrane forceps
Grieshaber iris forceps
Grieshaber manipulator forceps
Griffiths-Brown forceps

forceps (*continued*)

grooved tying forceps
Gross dressing forceps
Gross hyoid-cutting forceps
Gross sponge forceps
Grotting forceps
Gruenwald bayonet-dressing forceps
Gruenwald dissecting forceps
Gruenwald dressing forceps
Gruenwald Durogrip forceps
Gruenwald ear forceps
Gruenwald nasal forceps
Gruenwald nasal-cutting forceps
Gruenwald nasal-dressing forceps
Gruenwald tissue forceps
Gruenwald-Bryant forceps
Gruenwald-Bryant nasal forceps
Gruenwald-Bryant nasal-cutting forceps
Gruenwald-Jansen forceps
Gruenwald-Love neurosurgical forceps
Gruppe wire prosthesis-crimping forceps
Gruppe wire-crimping forceps
Guggenheim adenoid forceps
Guggenheim adenoidal forceps
guide forceps
Guilford-Wright forceps
guillotome forceps
Guist fixation forceps
Gunderson bone forceps
Gunderson muscle forceps
Gunderson muscle recession forceps
Gunderson recession forceps
Gunnar-Hey roller forceps
Guppe forceps
Gusberg uterine forceps
Gutgemann auricular appendage forceps
Gutglass cervix hemostatic forceps
Gutglass hemostatic cervical forceps
Gutierrez-Najar grasping forceps

forceps (*continued*)
 Guyton suturing forceps
 Guyton-Clark capsule
  fragment forceps
 Guyton-Clark fragment
  forceps
 Guyton-Noyes fixation forceps
 Haberer gastrointestinal
  forceps
 Haberer intestinal forceps
 Haberer-Gili forceps
 Hagenbarth clip-applying
  forceps
 Haig Ferguson obstetrical
  forceps
 Haig obstetrical forceps
 Haig-Ferguson obstetrical
  forceps
 Hajek antral punch forceps
 Hajek sphenoid punch
  forceps
 Hajek-Koffler bone punch
  forceps
 Hajek-Koffler punch forceps
 Hajek-Koffler sphenoidal
  forceps
 Hajek-Koffler sphenoidal
  punch forceps
 Hakler forceps
 Halberg contact lens forceps
 Hale obstetrical forceps
 Halifax placement forceps
 Hallberg forceps
 hallux forceps
 Halsey mosquito forceps
 Halsted arterial forceps
 Halsted curved mosquito
  forceps
 Halsted hemostatic forceps
 Halsted hemostatic mosquito
  forceps
 Halsted Micro-Line arterial
  forceps
 Halsted Micro-Line artery
  forceps
 Halsted mosquito forceps
 Halsted-Swanson tendon-
  passing forceps
 Hamby clip-applying forceps
 Hamilton deep-surgery
  forceps
 hammer forceps

forceps (*continued*)
 Hank-Dennen obstetrical
  forceps
 Hannahan forceps
 Hardy bayonet dressing
  forceps
 Hardy bayonet neurosurgical
  bipolar forceps
 Hardy microbipolar forceps
 Hardy microsurgical bayonet
  bipolar forceps
 harelip forceps
 Harken cardiovascular forceps
 Harken-Cooley forceps
 Harman fixation forceps
 Harms corneal forceps
 Harms microtying forceps
 Harms suture-tying forceps
 Harms tying forceps
 Harms utility forceps
 Harms vessel forceps
 Harms-Tubingen tying forceps
 Harrington clamp forceps
 Harrington lung-grasping
  forceps
 Harrington thoracic forceps
 Harrington vulsellum forceps
 Harrington-Mayo forceps
 Harrington-Mayo tissue
  forceps
 Harrington-Mixter clamp
  forceps
 Harrington-Mixter forceps
 Harrington-Mixter thoracic
  forceps
 Harris suture-carrying forceps
 Harrison bone-holding
  forceps
 Hartmann alligator forceps
 Hartmann ear forceps
 Hartmann ear polyp forceps
 Hartmann ear-dressing
  forceps
 Hartmann hemostatic forceps
 Hartmann hemostatic
  mosquito forceps
 Hartmann mosquito forceps
 Hartmann mosquito
  hemostatic forceps
 Hartmann nasal polyp forceps
 Hartmann nasal-cutting
  forceps

forceps (*continued*)
Hartmann nasal-dressing
 forceps
Hartmann tonsillar punch
 forceps
Hartmann uterine biopsy
 forceps
Hartmann-Citelli alligator
 forceps
Hartmann-Citelli ear punch
 forceps
Hartmann-Corgill ear forceps
Hartmann-Gruenwald forceps
Hartmann-Gruenwald nasal-
 cutting forceps
Hartmann-Herzfeld ear
 forceps
Hartmann-Noyes nasal-
 dressing forceps
Hartmann-Proctor ear forceps
Hartmann-Weingärtner ear
 forceps
Hartmann-Wullstein ear
 forceps
Haslinger tip forceps
Hasner lid forceps
Hasson bullet-tip forceps
Hasson grasping forceps
Hasson needle-nose forceps
Hasson ring forceps
Hasson spike-tooth forceps
Haugh ear forceps
Hawkins cervical biopsy
 forceps
Hawks-Dennen obstetrical
 forceps
Hayes anterior resection
 forceps
Hayes Martin forceps
Hayes-Olivecrona forceps
Hayton-Williams forceps
Healy gastrointestinal forceps
Healy intestinal forceps
Healy suture-removing
 forceps
Healy uterine biopsy forceps
Heaney hysterectomy forceps
Heaney tissue forceps
Heaney-Ballantine
 hysterectomy forceps
Heaney-Kantor hysterectomy
 forceps

forceps (*continued*)
Heaney-Rezek hysterectomy
 forceps
Heaney-Simon hysterectomy
 forceps
Heaney-Stumf forceps
Heath chalazion forceps
Heath clip-removing forceps
Heath nasal forceps
Hecht fascia lata forceps
Heermann alligator ear
 forceps
Heermann alligator forceps
Heermann ear forceps
Hegenbarth clip forceps
Hegenbarth clip-applying
 forceps
Hegenbarth clip-removing
 forceps
Hegenbarth-Michel clip-
 applying forceps
Heidelberg fixation forceps
Heifitz cup serrated ring
 forceps
Heiming kidney stone forceps
Heiss arterial forceps
Heiss hemostatic forceps
Heiss vulsellum forceps
Heller biopsy forceps
Hemoclip-applying forceps
hemorrhoid forceps
hemorrhoidal forceps
hemostasis clip-applying
 forceps
hemostasis forceps
hemostatic cervical forceps
hemostatic cervix forceps
hemostatic clip-applying
 forceps
hemostatic forceps
hemostatic neurosurgical
 forceps
hemostatic tissue forceps
hemostatic tonsillar forceps
hemostatic tracheal forceps
Hendren cardiovascular
 forceps
Hendren pediatric forceps
Henke punch forceps
Henrotin uterine vulsellum
 forceps
Henrotin vulsellum forceps

forceps (*continued*)

Henry cilia forceps
Herff membrane-puncturing forceps
Herget biopsy forceps
Hermann bone-holding forceps
Herrick kidney forceps
Hersh LASIK retreatment forceps
Hertel kidney stone forceps
Hertel rigid dilator stone forceps
Hertel rigid kidney stone forceps
Hertel stone forceps
Herz meniscal tendon forceps
Herzfeld ear forceps
Hess capsule forceps
Hess capsule iris forceps
Hess iris forceps
Hess-Barraquer forceps
Hess-Barraquer iris forceps
Hessburg lens-inserting forceps
Hess-Gill eye forceps
Hess-Gill iris forceps
Hess-Horwitz iris forceps
Hevesy polyp forceps
Heyman nasal forceps
Heyman nasal-cutting forceps
Heyman-Knight nasal dressing forceps
Heyner forceps
Heywood-Smith dressing forceps
Heywood-Smith gallbladder forceps
Heywood-Smith sponge-holding forceps
Hibbs biting forceps
Hibbs bone-cutting forceps
Hibbs bone-holding forceps
high forceps
Hildebrandt uterine hemostatic forceps
Hildyard nasal forceps
Himalaya dressing forceps
Hinderer cartilage forceps
Hinderer cartilage-holding forceps

forceps (*continued*)

Hirsch hypophysis punch forceps
Hirschman hemorrhoidal forceps
Hirschman jeweler's forceps
Hirschman lens forceps
Hirst obstetrical forceps
Hirst placental forceps
Hirst-Emmet obstetrical forceps
Hirst-Emmet placental forceps
Hodge obstetrical forceps
Hoen alligator forceps
Hoen bayonet forceps
Hoen dressing forceps
Hoen grasping forceps
Hoen hemostatic forceps
Hoen scalp forceps
Hoen tissue forceps
Hoffmann ear forceps
Hoffmann ear punch forceps
Hoffmann-Pollock forceps
holding forceps
Holinger specimen forceps
hollow-object forceps
Holmes fixation forceps
Holth punch forceps
Holzbach hysterectomy forceps
hook basket forceps
hook forceps
Hopkins aortic forceps
Horsley bone-cutting forceps
Horsley-Stille bone-cutting forceps
Horsley-Stille rib shears forceps
Hosemann choledochus forceps
Hosford-Hicks forceps
Hosford-Hicks transfer forceps
Hoskins beaked Colibri forceps
Hoskins fine straight forceps
Hoskins fixation forceps
Hoskins microstraight forceps
Hoskins miniaturized micro straight forceps
Hoskins straight microiris forceps
Hoskins suture forceps

forceps (*continued*)
   Hoskins-Dallas intraocular
      lens-inserting forceps
   Hoskins-Luntz forceps
   Hoskins-Skeleton fine forceps
   Hoskins-Skeleton grooved
      broad-tipped forceps
   host tissue forceps
   hot biopsy forceps
   hot flexible forceps
   hot Sampler disposable hot
      biopsy forceps
   Hough alligator forceps
   House alligator crimper
      forceps
   House alligator forceps
   House alligator grasping
      forceps
   House alligator strut forceps
   House crimper forceps
   House cup forceps
   House ear forceps
   House Gelfoam pressure
      forceps
   House grasping forceps
   House miniature forceps
   House oval-cup forceps
   House pressure forceps
   House strut forceps
   House-Dieter eye forceps
   Housepian clip-applying
      forceps
   House-Wullstein cup ear
      forceps
   House-Wullstein cup forceps
   House-Wullstein ear forceps
   House-Wullstein forceps
   House-Wullstein oval cup
      forceps
   Howard closing forceps
   Howard tonsil forceps
   Howard tonsillar forceps
   Howard tonsil-ligating forceps
   Howmedica Microfixation
      System forceps
   Hoxworth forceps
   Hoyt deep-surgery forceps
   Hoyt hemostatic forceps
   Hoytenberger tissue forceps
   Hubbard corneoscleral
      forceps
   Huber forceps handle

forceps (*continued*)
   Hudson brain forceps
   Hudson cranial forceps
   Hudson cranial rongeur
      forceps
   Hudson dressing forceps
   Hudson rongeur forceps
   Hudson tissue forceps
   Hudson tissue-dressing
      forceps
   Hufnagel mitral valve forceps
   Hufnagel mitral valve-holding
      forceps
   Hulka clip forceps
   Hulka tenaculum forceps
   Hulka-Kenwick forceps
   Hulka-Kenwick uterine-
      elevating forceps
   Hulka-Kenwick uterine-
      manipulating forceps
   hump forceps
   Hunt angled serrated ring
      forceps
   Hunt angled-tip forceps
   Hunt bipolar forceps
   Hunt chalazion forceps
   Hunt grasping forceps
   Hunt tumor forceps
   Hunt vessel forceps
   Hunter splinter forceps
   Hunt-Yasargil pituitary forceps
   Hurd bone forceps
   Hurd bone-cutting forceps
   Hurd septal bone-cutting
      forceps
   Hurd septal forceps
   Hurd septum-cutting forceps
   Hurdner tissue forceps
   Hurteau forceps
   Hyde corneal forceps
   Hyde double-curved corneal
      forceps
   hyoid-cutting forceps
   hypogastric artery forceps
   hypophyseal forceps
   hypophysectomy forceps
   hysterectomy forceps
   Ilg capsular forceps
   Ilg curved micro tying forceps
   Ilg curved microtying forceps
   Ilg insertion forceps
   iliac forceps

forceps (*continued*)
Iliff blepharochalasis forceps
IM Jaws alligator forceps
Imperatori laryngeal forceps
implant forceps
implantation forceps
Inamura small incision capsulorrhexis forceps
infant biopsy forceps
infundibular forceps
infundibular rongeur forceps
Ingraham-Fowler clip-applying forceps
inlet forceps
insertion forceps
instrument-grasping forceps
instrument-handling forceps
insulated bayonet forceps
insulated forceps
insulated monopolar forceps
insulated tissue forceps
intervertebral disk forceps
intervertebral disk rongeur forceps
intestinal anastomosis forceps
intestinal closing forceps
intestinal forceps
intestinal holding forceps
intestinal tissue forceps
intestinal tissue-holding forceps
intracapsular lens forceps
intraocular forceps
intraocular irrigating forceps
intraocular lens forceps
intrathoracic forceps
introducing forceps
Iowa membrane forceps
Iowa membrane-puncturing forceps
Iowa State fixation forceps
Iowa State forceps
Iowa-Mengert membrane forceps
iris bipolar forceps
iris forceps
iris tissue forceps
Iselin forceps
isolation forceps
I-tech intraocular foreign body forceps
I-tech splinter forceps

forceps (*continued*)
I-tech tying forceps
IV disk forceps (intravertebral disk forceps)
Jackson alligator forceps
Jackson alligator grasping forceps
Jackson approximation forceps
Jackson biopsy forceps
Jackson broad staple forceps
Jackson button forceps
Jackson conventional foreign body forceps
Jackson cross-action forceps
Jackson cylindrical object forceps
Jackson cylindrical-object forceps
Jackson double-concave rat-tooth forceps
Jackson double-prong forceps
Jackson down-jaw forceps
Jackson dressing forceps
Jackson dull rotation forceps
Jackson dull pointed forceps
Jackson endoscopic forceps
Jackson fenestrated peanut-grasping forceps
Jackson flexible upper lobe bronchus forceps
Jackson forward-grasping forceps
Jackson globular object forceps
Jackson head-holding forceps
Jackson hemostatic forceps
Jackson hollow-object forceps
Jackson infant biopsy forceps
Jackson infant forceps
Jackson laryngeal applicator forceps
Jackson laryngeal basket forceps
Jackson laryngeal forceps
Jackson laryngeal punch forceps
Jackson laryngeal ring-rotation forceps
Jackson laryngeal rotation forceps
Jackson laryngeal-dressing forceps

forceps (*continued*)
Jackson laryngeal-grasping
    forceps
Jackson laryngofissure forceps
Jackson papilloma forceps
Jackson pin-bending
    costophrenic forceps
Jackson punch forceps
Jackson ring-jaw globular
    object forceps
Jackson ring-jaw forceps
Jackson ring-rotation forceps
Jackson rotation forceps
Jackson sharp-pointed
    rotation forceps
Jackson side-curved forceps
Jackson sister-hook forceps
Jackson tendon-seizing forceps
Jackson tracheal forceps
Jackson tracheal hemostatic
    forceps
Jackson triangular-punch
    forceps
Jacob capsule fragment
    forceps
Jacob uterine vulsellum
    forceps
Jacob vulsellum forceps
Jacobs biopsy forceps
Jacobs capsular fragment
    forceps
Jacobs vulsellum forceps
Jacobson bipolar forceps
Jacobson dressing forceps
Jacobson forceps
Jacobson hemostatic forceps
Jacobson microdressing
    forceps
Jacobson mosquito forceps
Jaffe capsulorrhexis forceps
Jaffe suturing forceps
Jager meniscal forceps
Jako laryngeal forceps
Jako microlaryngeal cup
    forceps
Jako microlaryngeal grasping
    forceps
James wound-approximation
    forceps
Jameson muscle forceps
Jameson muscle recession
    forceps

forceps (*continued*)
Jameson recession forceps
Jameson strabismus forceps
Jameson tracheal muscle
    forceps
Jameson tracheal muscle
    recession forceps
Jannetta alligator grasping
    forceps
Jannetta bayonet forceps
Jannetta microbayonet
    forceps
Jansen bayonet dressing
    forceps
Jansen bayonet ear forceps
Jansen bayonet forceps
Jansen bayonet nasal forceps
Jansen dissecting forceps
Jansen dressing forceps
Jansen ear forceps
Jansen monopolar forceps
Jansen nasal-dressing forceps
Jansen thumb forceps
Jansen-Gruenwald forceps
Jansen-Middleton nasal-cutting
    forceps
Jansen-Middleton punch
    forceps
Jansen-Middleton septal
    forceps
Jansen-Middleton septotomy
    forceps
Jansen-Middleton septum-
    cutting forceps
Jansen-Mueller forceps
Jansen-Struyken septal forceps
Jarcho tenaculum forceps
Jarcho uterine tenaculum
    forceps
Jarell forceps
Jarit brain forceps
Jarit microsuture tying forceps
Jarit mosquito forceps
Jarit sterilizer forceps
Jarit tendon-pulling forceps
Jarit tube-occluding forceps
Jarit wire-pulling forceps
Jarit-Allis tissue forceps
Jarit-Crafoord forceps
Jarit-Dandy forceps
Jarit-Liston bone-cutting
    forceps

forceps (*continued*)

Jarvis hemorrhoid forceps
Javerts placental forceps
Javerts polyp forceps
Jayles forceps
Jensen intraocular lens
  forceps
Jensen lens forceps
Jensen lens-inserting forceps
Jerald forceps
Jervey capsular fragment
  forceps
Jervey iris forceps
Jesberg grasping forceps
jeweler's bipolar forceps
jeweler's pickup forceps
John Hopkins gall duct
  forceps
John Hopkins hemostatic
  forceps
John Hopkins serrefine
  forceps
John Weiss forceps
Johns Hopkins gall duct
  forceps
Johns Hopkins gallbladder
  forceps
Johns Hopkins hemostatic
  forceps
Johns Hopkins occluding
  forceps
Johns Hopkins serrefine
  forceps
Johnson brain tumor forceps
Johnson ptosis forceps
Johnson thoracic forceps
Jones hemostatic forceps
Jones IMA forceps
Jones towel forceps
Joplin bone-holding forceps
Jordan strut forceps
Judd strabismus forceps
Judd suture forceps
Judd-Allis intestinal forceps
Judd-Allis tissue forceps
Judd-DeMartel gallbladder
  forceps
Juers crimper forceps
Juers lingual forceps
Juers-Lempert rongeur
  forceps
jugum forceps

forceps (*continued*)

Julian splenorenal forceps
Julian thoracic artery forceps
Julian thoracic forceps
Julian thoracic hemostatic
  forceps
Julian-Damian thoracic
  forceps
jumbo biopsy forceps
jumbo forceps
Jurasz laryngeal forceps
K/S-Allis forceps
Kadesky forceps
Kahler biopsy forceps
Kahler bronchial biopsy
  forceps
Kahler bronchial forceps
Kahler bronchoscopic forceps
Kahler bronchus-grasping
  forceps
Kahler laryngeal biopsy
  forceps
Kahler laryngeal forceps
Kahler polyp forceps
Kahn tenaculum forceps
Kalman occluding forceps
Kalman tube-occluding
  forceps
Kalt capsular forceps
Kalt capsule forceps
Kansas University corneal
  forceps
Kantor forceps
Kantrowitz dressing forceps
Kantrowitz thoracic forceps
Kantrowitz tissue forceps
Kapp applying forceps
Kapp-Beck forceps
Karl Storz forceps
Karp aortic punch forceps
Katena forceps
Katzin-Barraquer Colibri
  forceps
Katzin-Barraquer corneal
  forceps
Kaufman ENT forceps
Kaufman insulated forceps
Kazanjian bone-cutting
  forceps
Kazanjian cutting forceps
Kazanjian nasal forceps
Kazanjian nasal hump forceps

forceps (*continued*)

Kazanjian nasal hump-cutting forceps
Kazanjian nasal-cutting forceps
Kazanjian-Cottle forceps
Keeler extended round tip forceps
Keeler intraocular foreign body grasping forceps
Keen Edge disposable biopsy forceps
Kelly artery forceps
Kelly dressing forceps
Kelly hemostatic forceps
Kelly ovum forceps
Kelly placenta forceps
Kelly polypus forceps
Kelly tissue forceps
Kelly urethral forceps
Kelly-Gray uterine forceps
Kelly-Murphy hemostatic forceps
Kelly-Murphy hemostatic uterine vulsellum forceps
Kelly-Rankin forceps
Kelman implantation forceps
Kelman intraocular forceps
Kelman irrigator forceps
Kelman-McPherson corneal forceps
Kelman-McPherson microtying forceps
Kelman-McPherson suture forceps
Kelman-McPherson tissue forceps
Kelman-McPherson tying forceps
Kennedy uterine vulsellum forceps
Kennedy vulsellum forceps
Kennerdell bayonet forceps
Kent forceps
keratotomy forceps
Kern bone-holding forceps
Kern-Lane bone-holding forceps
Kerrison forceps
Kershner one-step micro capsulorrhexis forceps
Kevorkian uterine biopsy forceps

forceps (*continued*)

Kevorkian-Younge biopsy forceps
Kevorkian-Younge cervical biopsy forceps
Kevorkian-Younge uterine biopsy forceps
Khodadad microclip forceps
kidney pedicle forceps
kidney stone forceps
kidney-elevating forceps
Kielland obstetrical forceps
Kielland-Luikart obstetrical forceps
Killian septal compression forceps
Killian septal forceps
Killian-Jameson forceps
King tissue forceps
King wound forceps
King-Prince muscle forceps
King-Prince recession forceps
Kingsley grasping forceps
Kirby capsular forceps
Kirby corneoscleral forceps
Kirby eye tissue forceps
Kirby fixation forceps
Kirby intracapsular lens forceps
Kirby iris forceps
Kirby lens forceps
Kirby tissue forceps
Kirby-Arthus fixation forceps
Kirby-Bracken iris forceps
Kirkpatrick tonsil forceps
Kirschner-Ullrich forceps
Kirwan bipolar electrosurgical forceps
Kirwan coaptation ophthalmic bipolar forceps
Kirwan iris curved ophthalmic bipolar forceps
Kirwan iris straight ophthalmic bipolar forceps
Kirwan jeweler's curved ophthalmic bipolar forceps
Kirwan jeweler's insulated straight ophthalmic bipolar forceps
Kirwan-Adson ophthalmic bipolar forceps

forceps (*continued*)

Kirwan-Nadler-style
  coaptation ophthalmic
  bipolar forceps
Kirwan-Tenzel ophthalmic
  bipolar forceps
Kitner goiter forceps
Kitner thyroid-packing
  forceps
Kjelland obstetrical forceps
Kjelland-Barton forceps
Kjelland-Luikart obstetrical
  forceps
KleenSpec forceps
Kleinert-Kutz bone-cutting
  forceps
Kleinert-Kutz rongeur forceps
Kleinert-Kutz tendon forceps
Kleinert-Kutz tendon retriever
  forceps
Kleinert-Kutz tendon-passing
  forceps
Kleinert-Kutz tendon-
  retrieving forceps
Kleppinger bipolar forceps
KLI bipolar forceps
KLI monopolar forceps
Knapp trachoma forceps
Knapp-Luer trachoma forceps
Knight nasal forceps
Knight nasal septum-cutting
  forceps
Knight nasal-cutting forceps
Knight polyp forceps
Knight septal forceps
Knight septum-cutting
  forceps
Knight turbinate forceps
Knighton-Crawford forceps
Knight-Sluder nasal forceps
Knolle lens implantation
  forceps
Knolle-Shepard lens forceps
Knolle-Volker lens-holding
  forceps
knot-holding forceps
knotting forceps
Kustner uterine tenaculum
  forceps
Koby cataract forceps
Kocher arterial forceps
Kocher artery forceps

forceps (*continued*)

Kocher hemostatic forceps
Kocher intestinal forceps
Kocher kidney-elevating
  forceps
Kocher Micro-Line intestinal
  forceps
Kocher-Ochsner hemostatic
  forceps
Koeberle forceps
Koenig vascular forceps
Koerte gallstone forceps
Koffler septal forceps
Koffler septum bone forceps
Koffler septum forceps
Koffler-Lillie septal forceps
Koffler-Lillie septum forceps
Kogan endospeculum forceps
Kolb bronchial forceps
Kolb bronchus forceps
Kolodny forceps
Korte gallstone forceps
Kos crimper forceps
Kraff intraocular utility
  forceps
Kraff lens-inserting forceps
Kraff suturing forceps
Kraff tying forceps
Kraff-Osher lens forceps
Kraff-Utrata capsulorrhexis
  forceps
Kraff-Utrata intraocular utility
  forceps
Kraff-Utrata tear capsulotomy
  forceps
Kramer forceps
Kratz lens-inserting forceps
Krause biopsy forceps
Krause esophagoscopy
  forceps
Krause punch forceps
Krause Universal forceps
Kremer fixation forceps
Kremer two-point fixation
  forceps
Kronfeld micropin forceps
Kronfeld suture forceps
Kronfeld suturing forceps
Kroenlein hemostatic forceps
Krukenberg pigment spindle
  forceps
Kuhne coverglass forceps

forceps (*continued*)
Kuhnt capsule forceps
Kuhnt fixation forceps
Kulvin-Kalt forceps
Kulvin-Kalt iris forceps
Kurze microbiopsy forceps
Kurze micrograsping forceps
Kurze pickup forceps
Küstner uterine tenaculum forceps
Kwapis interdental forceps
Loew-Beer forceps
Loewenberg forceps
Laborde forceps
Lahey arterial forceps
Lahey dissecting forceps
Lahey gall duct forceps
Lahey goiter vulsellum forceps
Lahey goiter-seizing forceps
Lahey hemostatic forceps
Lahey lock arterial forceps
Lahey thoracic forceps
Lahey thyroid tenaculum forceps
Lahey thyroid tissue traction forceps
Lahey thyroid traction forceps
Lahey thyroid traction vulsellum forceps
Lahey-Babcock forceps
Lahey-Pean forceps
Lahey-Sweet dissecting forceps
Lajeune hemostatic forceps
Lalonde delicate hook forceps
Lalonde extra fine skin hook forceps
LaLonde skin hook forceps
Lambert chalazion forceps
Lambert-Kay anastomosis forceps
Lambotte bone-holding forceps
Lambotte fibular forceps
Lancaster-O'Connor forceps
lancet-shaped biopsy forceps
Landers vitrectomy lens forceps
Landolt spreading forceps
Landon forceps
Lane bone-holding forceps

forceps (*continued*)
Lane gastrointestinal forceps
Lane intestinal forceps
Lane screw-holding forceps
Lane tissue forceps
Lang iris forceps
Lange approximation forceps
Langenbeck bone-holding forceps
laparoscopic forceps
Laplace forceps
large-angled forceps
LaRoe undermining forceps
Larsen tendon forceps
Larsen tendon-holding forceps
laryngeal applicator forceps
laryngeal basket forceps
laryngeal biopsy forceps
laryngeal bronchial grasping forceps
laryngeal curet forceps
laryngeal forceps
laryngeal grasping forceps
laryngeal punch forceps
laryngeal rotation forceps
laryngeal sponging forceps
laryngofissure forceps
laser microlaryngeal cup forceps
laser microlaryngeal grasping forceps
laser ovary forceps
Lauer forceps
Laufe divergent outlet forceps
Laufe obstetrical forceps
Laufe uterine polyp forceps
Laufe-Barton obstetrical forceps
Laufe-Barton-Kjelland obstetrical forceps
Laufe-Barton-Kjelland-Piper obstetrical forceps
Laufe-Piper obstetrical forceps
Laufe-Piper uterine polyp forceps
Laufman forceps
Laurer forceps
Laval advancement forceps
Lawrence deep forceps
Lawrence hemostatic forceps
Lawton forceps

forceps (*continued*)

Lawton-Schubert biopsy forceps
Lawton-Wittner cervical biopsy forceps
Lazar microsuction forceps
Leader vas isolation forceps
Leahey chalazion forceps
Leahey marginal chalazion forceps
Leahey suture forceps
Leasure nasal forceps
Leaver sclerotomy forceps
Lebsche forceps
Ledhey forceps
Lee delicate hemostatic forceps
Lees arterial forceps
Lees nontraumatic forceps
Lefferts bone-cutting forceps
Leibinger plate-holding forceps
Leigh capsule forceps
Lejeune thoracic forceps
Leksell rongeur forceps
Leland-Jones forceps
Lemmon-Russian forceps
Lemoine forceps
Lempert rongeur forceps
lens forceps
lens implant forceps
lens implantation forceps
lens loop forceps
lens-threading forceps
Leo Schwartz sponge-holding forceps
Leonard deep forceps
Leriche hemostatic forceps
Leriche tissue forceps
LeRoy clip-applying forceps
LeRoy scalp clip-applying forceps
Lester fixation forceps
Lester muscle forceps
Levenson tissue forceps
Levora fixation forceps
Levret forceps
Lewin bone-holding forceps
Lewin spinal-perforating forceps
Lewis septal forceps

forceps (*continued*)

Lewis tonsillar hemostatic forceps
Lewis ureteral stone isolation forceps
Lewkowitz lithotomy forceps
Lewkowitz ovum forceps
Lewkowitz placental forceps
Lexer tissue forceps
Leyro-Diaz thoracic forceps
lid forceps
Lieberman suturing forceps
Lieberman tying forceps
Lieberman-Pollock double corneal forceps
Lieb-Guerry forceps
ligamenta flava forceps
ligament-grasping forceps
ligamentum flavum forceps
ligamentum-grasping forceps
ligature forceps
ligature-carrying aneurysm forceps
ligature-carrying forceps
Lillehei valve forceps
Lillehei valve-grasping forceps
Lillie intestinal forceps
Lillie tissue-holding forceps
Lillie-Killian septal bone forceps
Lillie-Killian septal forceps
Lindsay-Rea forceps
Lindstrom lens-insertion forceps
lingual forceps
Linnartz forceps
Linn-Graefe iris forceps
lion forceps
lion-jaw bone-holding forceps
lion-jaw forceps
Lister conjunctival forceps
Liston bone-cutting forceps
Liston-Key bone-cutting forceps
Liston-Key-Horsley forceps
Liston-Littauer bone-cutting forceps
Liston-Stille bone-cutting forceps
lithotomy forceps
Litt forceps
Littauer bone-cutting forceps

forceps (*continued*)

Littauer cilia forceps
Littauer ear polyp forceps
Littauer ear-dressing forceps
Littauer nasal-dressing forceps
Littauer-Liston bone-cutting forceps
Littauer-West cutting forceps
Littlewood tissue forceps
Livernois lens-holding forceps
Livernois pickup and folding forceps
Livingston forceps
Llobera fixation forceps
Llorente dissecting forceps
Lloyd-Davies occlusion forceps
lobectomy forceps
lobe-grasping forceps
lobe-holding forceps
Lobell splinter forceps
Lobenstein-Tarnier forceps
lobster bone-reduction forceps
Lockwood intestinal forceps
Lockwood tissue forceps
Lockwood-Allis intestinal forceps
Lockwood-Allis tissue forceps
Loew-Beer forceps
Loewenberg forceps
Lombard-Beyer rongeur forceps
London tissue forceps
Long hysterectomy forceps
Long Island College Hospital placenta forceps
long tissue forceps
long-jaw basket forceps
loop-type snare forceps
loop-type stone-crushing forceps
loose body forceps
loose body suction forceps
Lordan chalazion forceps
Lore subglottic forceps
Lore suction tip-holding forceps
Lore suction tube-holding forceps
Lothrop ligature forceps
Love-Gruenwald alligator forceps

forceps (*continued*)

Love-Gruenwald pituitary forceps
Love-Kerrison rongeur forceps
Lovelace bladder forceps
Lovelace gallbladder traction forceps
Lovelace hemostatic forceps
Lovelace lung-grasping forceps
Lovelace thyroid traction vulsellum forceps
Lovelace tissue forceps
Lovelace traction lung forceps
Lovelace traction tissue forceps
low forceps
low outlet forceps
lower anterior forceps
lower forceps
lower lateral forceps
Lowis intervertebral disk forceps
Lowis IV disk rongeur forceps
Lowman bone-holding forceps
Lowsley grasping forceps
Lowsley prostatic forceps
Lowsley prostatic lobe-holding forceps
Lowsley-Luc forceps
Luc ethmoid forceps
Luc nasal-cutting forceps
Luc septum forceps
Luc septum-cutting forceps
Lucae bayonet dressing forceps
Lucae bayonet ear forceps
Lucae bayonet tissue forceps
Lucae dissecting forceps
Lucae dressing forceps
Lucae ear forceps
Luer curet forceps
Luer hemorrhoidal forceps
Luer rongeur forceps
Luer-Whiting rongeur forceps
Luhr plate-holding forceps
Luikart obstetrical forceps
Luikart-Bill forceps
Luikart-Kjelland obstetrical forceps

forceps (*continued*)

Luikart-McLane obstetrical forceps
Luikart-Simpson obstetrical forceps
lung forceps
lung tissue forceps
lung-grasping forceps
Lutz septal forceps
Lutz septal ridge forceps
Lutz septal ridge-cutting forceps
Lynch cup-shaped curette forceps
Lynch laryngeal forceps
Lyon forceps
MacCarty forceps
MacGregor conjunctival forceps
Machemer diamond-dust-coated foreign body forceps
Machemer diamond-dusted forceps
MacKenty tissue forceps
McQuigg-Mixter forceps
Madden forceps
Madden-Potts intestinal forceps
Madden-Potts tissue forceps
Magielski coagulating forceps
Magielski tonsil forceps
Magielski tonsil-seizing forceps
Magielski-Heermann strut forceps
Magill catheter forceps
Magill catheter-introducing forceps
Magill endotracheal forceps
Maier dressing forceps
Maier polyp forceps
Maier sponge forceps
Maier uterine forceps
Maier uterine-dressing forceps
Mailler colon forceps
Mailler cut-off forceps
Mailler intestinal forceps
Mailler rectal forceps
Maingot hysterectomy forceps
Malis angled bayonet forceps
Malis angled-up bipolar forceps

forceps (*continued*)

Malis bipolar coagulation forceps
Malis bipolar cutting forceps
Malis bipolar irrigating forceps
Malis cup forceps
Malis jeweler bipolar forceps
Malis titanium microsurgical forceps
Malis-Jensen bipolar forceps
Malis-Jensen microbipolar forceps
malleus forceps
mammary-coronary tissue forceps
Manche LASIK forceps
mandibular forceps
Manhattan Eye & Ear suturing forceps
Mann forceps
Manning forceps
Mansfield forceps
Mantis retrograde forceps
March-Barton forceps
Marcuse forceps
marginal chalazion forceps
Market forceps
Markwalder rib forceps
Marshik tonsillar forceps
Marshik tonsil-seizing forceps
Martin bipolar coagulation forceps
Martin cartilage forceps
Martin meniscal forceps
Martin nasopharyngeal biopsy forceps
Martin nasopharyngeal forceps
Martin thumb forceps
Martin tissue forceps
Martin uterine tenaculum forceps
Maryan biopsy punch forceps
Masket forceps
Masterson hysterectomy forceps
Mastin goiter forceps
Mastin muscle forceps
mastoid rongeur forceps
Mathieu forceps
Mathieu foreign body forceps

forceps (*continued*)

Mathieu tongue forceps
Mathieu tongue-seizing forceps
Mathieu urethral forceps
matte black forceps
Maumenee capsule forceps
Maumenee corneal forceps
Maumenee cross-action capsule forceps
Maumenee straight-action capsule forceps
Maumenee Suregrip forceps
Maumenee tissue forceps
Maumenee-Colibri corneal forceps
Max Fine tying forceps
Max forceps
maxillary disimpaction forceps
maxillary forceps
maxillary fracture forceps
Maxum Carr-Locke angled forceps
Maxum reusable endoscopic forceps
Mayer forceps
Mayfield aneurysm forceps
Mayfield applying forceps
Mayo bone-cutting forceps
Mayo kidney pedicle forceps
Mayo tissue forceps
Mayo ureter isolation forceps
Mayo-Blake gallstone forceps
Mayo-Harrington forceps
Mayo-Ochsner forceps
Mayo-Pean forceps
Mayo-Robson gastrointestinal forceps
Mayo-Robson intestinal forceps
Mayo-Russian gastrointestinal forceps
Mazzariello-Caprini stone forceps
Mazzocco flexible lens forceps
McCain TMJ forceps
McCarthy visual hemostatic forceps
McCarthy-Alcock hemostatic forceps

forceps (*continued*)

McClintock placenta forceps
McClintock uterine forceps
McCollough strabismus forceps
McCollough suturing forceps
McCollough tying forceps
McCoy septal forceps
McCoy septum-cutting forceps
McCullough strabismus forceps
McCullough suture forceps
McCullough suture-tying forceps
McCullough suturing forceps
McCullough utility forceps
McDonald lens-folding forceps
McGannon lens forceps
McGee wire-closure forceps
McGee wire-crimping forceps
McGee-Paparella wire-crimping forceps
McGee-Priest wire forceps
McGee-Priest wire-closure forceps
McGee-Priest wire-crimping forceps
McGee-Priest-Paparella closure forceps
McGill forceps
McGivney hemorrhoidal forceps
McGravey tissue forceps
McGregor conjunctival forceps
McGuire marginal chalazion forceps
McHenry tonsillar artery forceps
McHenry tonsillar forceps
McIndoe bone-cutting forceps
McIndoe dissecting forceps
McIndoe dressing forceps
McIndoe rongeur forceps
McIntosh suture-holding forceps
McKay ear forceps
McKenzie brain clip-applying forceps
McKenzie clip-applying forceps

forceps (*continued*)

McKenzie grasping forceps
McKernan forceps
McKernan-Adson forceps
McKernan-Potts forceps
McLane obstetrical forceps
McLane pile forceps
McLane-Luikart obstetrical
  forceps
McLane-Tucker obstetrical
  forceps
McLane-Tucker-Kjelland
  forceps
McLane-Tucker-Luikart forceps
McLean capsule forceps
McLean muscle-recession
  forceps
McLean ophthalmological
  forceps
McLearie bone forceps
McNealey-Glassman-Babcock
  forceps
McNealey-Glassman-Babcock
  viscera-holding forceps
McNealey-Glassman-Babcock
  visceral forceps
McNealey-Glassman-Mixter
  ligature-carrying aneurysm
  forceps
McPherson angled forceps
McPherson bent forceps
McPherson corneal forceps
McPherson irrigating forceps
McPherson lens forceps
McPherson microbipolar
  forceps
McPherson microcorneal
  forceps
McPherson microiris forceps
McPherson microsuture
  forceps
McPherson straight bipolar
  forceps
McPherson suture-tying
  forceps
McPherson suturing forceps
McPherson tying forceps
McPherson tying iris forceps
McPherson-Castroviejo
  forceps
McPherson-Pierse
  microcorneal forceps

forceps (*continued*)

McPherson-Pierse
  microsuturing forceps
McQueen vitreous forceps
McQuigg forceps
McQuigg-Mixter bronchial
  forceps
McWhorter tonsillar forceps
Meacham-Scoville forceps
Mead forceps
meat forceps
meat-grasping forceps
mechanical finger forceps
mechanical forceps
Medicon wire-twister forceps
Medicon-Jackson rectal
  forceps
Medicon-Packer mosquito
  forceps
medium forceps
Meeker deep-surgery forceps
Meeker gallbladder forceps
Meeker hemostatic forceps
Meeker intestinal forceps
meibomian expressor forceps
meibomian forceps
Meltzer adenoid punch
  forceps
membrane forceps
membrane-puncturing forceps
Mendel ligature forceps
Mendez multi-purpose LASIK
  forceps
Mengert membrane-
  puncturing forceps
meniscal basket forceps
Mentor-Maumenee Suregrip
  forceps
Merlin stone forceps
Merriam forceps
Merz hysterectomy forceps
Metico forceps
Metzel-Wittmoser forceps
Metzenbaum tonsillar forceps
Metzenbaum-Tydings forceps
MGH uterine vulsellum
  forceps
MGH vulsellum forceps
Michel clip-applying forceps
Michel clip-removing forceps
Michel tissue forceps
Michigan intestinal forceps

forceps (*continued*)
    Michigan University intestinal
        forceps
    Micrins forceps
    micro-Allis forceps
    microarterial forceps
    microbayonet forceps
    microbiopsy forceps
    microbipolar forceps
    MicroBite forceps
    microbronchoscopic grasping
        forceps
    microbronchoscopic tissue
        forceps
    microclamp forceps
    microclip forceps
    micro-Colibri forceps
    microcorneal forceps
    microcup pituitary forceps
    microdissecting forceps
    microdressing forceps
    microextractor forceps
    micro-Halsted arterial forceps
    micro-jeweler's monopolar
        forceps
    microlaryngeal grasping
        forceps
    Micro-Line artery forceps
    microneedle holder forceps
    microneurosurgery forceps
    Micro-One dissecting forceps
    micropin forceps
    Microsnap hemostatic forceps
    microsurgery biopsy forceps
    microsurgical grasping
        forceps
    microsurgical tying forceps
    microsuture forceps
    microsuture-tying forceps
    Microtek cupped forceps
    microtip bipolar forceps
    microtip bipolar jeweler's
        forceps
    microtissue forceps
    Micro-Two forceps
    microtying eye forceps
    microtying forceps
    microutility forceps
    microvascular clamp-applying
        forceps
    microvascular forceps
    microvascular tying forceps

forceps (*continued*)
    Microvasive disposable
        alligator-shaped forceps
    Microvasive radial jaw biopsy
        forceps
    midcavity forceps
    middle ear forceps
    middle ear strut forceps
    Mighty Bite Zimmon lateral
        biopsy cup forceps
    Mikulicz peritoneal forceps
    Mikulicz tonsillar forceps
    Miles punch biopsy forceps
    Milex forceps
    Miller articulating forceps
    Miller bayonet forceps
    Miller rectal forceps
    Millin capsule forceps
    Millin capsule-grasping
        forceps
    Millin ligature-guiding forceps
    Millin lobe-grasping forceps
    Millin prostatectomy forceps
    Millin T-shaped angled forceps
    Millin T-shaped forceps
    Mill-Rose biopsy forceps
    Mill-Rose RiteBite biopsy
        forceps
    Mill-Rose Surebrite biopsy
        forceps
    Mills tissue forceps
    miniature forceps
    miniature intestinal forceps
    mini-micro forceps
    Mitchell-Diamond biopsy
        forceps
    mitral forceps
    mitral valve-holding forceps
    Mixter arterial forceps
    Mixter baby hemostatic
        forceps
    Mixter full-curve forceps
    Mixter gall duct forceps
    Mixter gallbladder forceps
    Mixter gallstone forceps
    Mixter mosquito forceps
    Mixter pediatric hemostatic
        forceps
    Mixter thoracic forceps
    Mixter-McQuigg forceps
    Mixter-O'Shaughnessy
        dissecting forceps

forceps (*continued*)
Mixter-O'Shaughnessy hemostatic forceps
Mixter-O'Shaughnessy ligature forceps
Mixter-O'Shaughnessy dissecting and ligature forceps
Mixter-Paul arterial forceps
Mixter-Paul hemostatic forceps
Moberg forceps
Moberg-Stille forceps
modified Younge forceps
Moehle corneal forceps
Moersch bronchoscopic forceps
Moersch bronchoscopic specimen forceps
Molt pedicle forceps
Monod punch forceps
monopolar coagulating forceps
monopolar forceps
monopolar insulated forceps
monopolar tissue forceps
Montenovesi cranial forceps
Montenovesi cranial rongeur forceps
Moody fixation forceps
Moolgaoker forceps
Moore lens-inserting forceps
Morgenstein blunt forceps
Moritz-Schmidt laryngeal forceps
Morris forceps
Morson forceps
Mosher ethmoid punch forceps
mosquito forceps
mosquito hemostatic forceps
Mount intervertebral disk forceps
Mount intervertebral disk rongeur forceps
Mount-Mayfield aneurysm forceps
Mount-Mayfield forceps
Mount-Olivecrona forceps
mouse-tooth forceps
Moynihan gall duct forceps
Moynihan intestinal forceps

forceps (*continued*)
Moynihan kidney pedicle forceps
Moynihan towel forceps
Moynihan-Navratil forceps
MPC coagulation forceps
Muck tonsillar forceps
mucous forceps
mucus forceps
Mueller forceps
Mueller-Markham patent ductus forceps
Muir hemorrhoidal forceps
Muldoon meibomian forceps
Multibite multiple sample biopsy forceps
multipurpose forceps
multitoothed cartilage forceps
Mundie placenta forceps
Murless head extractor forceps
Murphy tonsillar forceps
Murphy-Pean hemostatic forceps
Murray forceps
muscle forceps
Museholdt nasal-dressing forceps
Museux tenaculum forceps
Museux uterine forceps
Museux uterine vulsellum forceps
Museux vulsellum forceps
Museux-Collins uterine vulsellum forceps
Musial tissue forceps
Mustarde forceps
Myerson bronchial forceps
Myerson laryngeal forceps
Myerson miniature laryngeal biopsy forceps
Myles hemorrhoidal forceps
Myles nasal forceps
Myles nasal-cutting forceps
Nadler bipolar coaptation forceps
Naegele obstetrical forceps
nail-cutting forceps
nail-extracting forceps
nail-pulling forceps
Nakao Ejector biopsy forceps
nasal alligator forceps

forceps (*continued*)
    nasal bone forceps
    nasal cartilage-holding forceps
    nasal cutting forceps
    nasal forceps
    nasal hump forceps
    nasal hump-cutting forceps
    nasal insertion forceps
    nasal lower lateral forceps
    nasal needle holder forceps
    nasal polyp forceps
    nasal polypus forceps
    nasal septal forceps
    nasal-cutting forceps
    nasal-dressing forceps
    nasal-grasping forceps
    nasal-packing forceps
    nasopharyngeal biopsy
        forceps
    Natvig wire-twister forceps
    needle forceps
    needle-holder forceps
    Negus tonsillar forceps
    Negus-Green forceps
    Nelson lung forceps
    Nelson lung-dissecting
        forceps
    Nelson tissue forceps
    Nelson-Martin forceps
    neonatal vascular forceps
    nephrolithotomy forceps
    Neubauer foreign body
        forceps
    Neubauer vitreous
        microextractor forceps
    Neubuser tube-seizing forceps
    neurosurgical dressing
        forceps
    neurosurgical forceps
    neurosurgical ligature forceps
    neurosurgical suction forceps
    neurosurgical tissue forceps
    neurovascular forceps
    Neuwirth-Palmer forceps
    Neville-Barnes forceps
    Nevins dressing forceps
    Nevins tissue forceps
    Nevyas lens forceps
    New biopsy forceps
    New Orleans Eye & Ear
        Hospital fixation forceps
    New Orleans forceps

forceps (*continued*)
    New tissue forceps
    New York Eye and Ear fixation
        forceps
    New York Eye and Ear
        Hospital fixation forceps
    Newman tenaculum forceps
    Newman uterine tenaculum
        forceps
    Nicola forceps
    Niedner dissecting forceps
    NIH mitral valve forceps
    NIH mitral valve-grasping
        forceps
    Niro bone-cutting forceps
    Niro wire-twisting forceps
    Nisbet eye forceps
    Nisbet fixation forceps
    Nissen cystic forceps
    Nissen gall duct forceps
    Noble iris forceps
    noncrushing common duct
        forceps
    noncrushing forceps
    noncrushing intestinal forceps
    noncrushing pickup forceps
    noncrushing tissue-holding
        forceps
    nonfenestrated forceps
    nonmagnetic dressing forceps
    nonmagnetic forceps
    nonmagnetic tissue forceps
    nonperforating towel forceps
    nonslipping forceps
    nontoothed forceps
    nontraumatizing forceps
    nontraumatizing viscera
        forceps
    nontraumatizing visceral
        forceps
    Nordan tying forceps
    Nordan-Colibri forceps
    Norris sponge forceps
    Norwood forceps
    Noto dressing forceps
    Noto ovum forceps
    Noto polypus forceps
    Noto sponge forceps
    Noto sponge-holding forceps
    Novak fixation forceps
    Noyes ear forceps
    Noyes nasal forceps

forceps (*continued*)

Noyes nasal-dressing forceps
Nugent fixation forceps
Nugent rectus forceps
Nugent superior rectus
    forceps
Nugent utility forceps
Nugowski forceps
Nussbaum intestinal forceps
Nyhus-Potts intestinal forceps
Nystroem tumor forceps
Oberhill obstetrical forceps
O'Brien fixation forceps
O'Brien tissue forceps
O'Brien-Elschnig forceps
obstetrical forceps
occluding forceps
occlusion forceps
Ochsner artery forceps
Ochsner cartilage forceps
Ochsner forceps
Ochsner hemostatic forceps
Ochsner tissue forceps
Ochsner-Dixon arterial
    forceps
Ockerblad forceps
O'Connor biopsy forceps
O'Connor eye forceps
O'Connor grasping forceps
O'Connor iris forceps
O'Connor lid forceps
O'Connor sponge forceps
O'Connor-Elschnig fixation
    forceps
O'Dell spicule forceps
odontoid peg-grasping forceps
O'Gawa suture forceps
O'Gawa suture-fixation
    forceps
O'Gawa tying forceps
O'Gawa-Castroviejo forceps
O'Gawa-Castroviejo tying
    forceps
Ogura cartilage forceps
Ogura tissue forceps
O'Hanlon forceps
O'Hara forceps
Oldberg intervertebral disk
    forceps
Oldberg pituitary rongeur
    forceps
Olivecrona aneurysm forceps

forceps (*continued*)

Olivecrona clip-applying and
    removing forceps
Olivecrona clip-applying
    forceps
Olivecrona rongeur forceps
Olivecrona-Toennis clip-
    applying forceps
Olsen bayonet monopolar
    forceps
Olympus alligator-jaw
    endoscopic forceps
Olympus basket-type
    endoscopic forceps
Olympus biopsy forceps
Olympus endoscopic biopsy
    forceps
Olympus Endo-Therapy
    disposable biopsy forceps
Olympus FB-series biopsy
    forceps
Olympus FG-series forceps
Olympus FS-K-series
    endoscopic suture-cutting
    forceps
Olympus FS-series endoscopic
    suture-cutting forceps
Olympus grasping rat-tooth
    forceps
Olympus hot biopsy forceps
Olympus magnetic extractor
    forceps
Olympus minisnare forceps
Olympus pelican-type
    endoscopic forceps
Olympus rat-tooth endoscopic
    forceps
Olympus reusable oval cup
    forceps
Olympus rubber-tip
    endoscopic forceps
Olympus shark-tooth
    endoscopic forceps
Olympus tripod-type
    endoscopic forceps
Olympus W-shaped
    endoscopic forceps
Ombredanne forceps
optical biopsy forceps
oral forceps
oral rongeur forceps
Orr forceps

forceps (*continued*)

Orr gall duct forceps
orthopedic forceps
O'Shaughnessy arterial forceps
Osher bipolar coaptation
  forceps
Osher capsular forceps
Osher conjunctival forceps
Osher foreign body forceps
Osher haptic forceps
Osher superior rectus forceps
ossicle-holding forceps
Ossoff-Karlan laser forceps
Ostrom antrum punch-tip
  forceps
Ostrom punch forceps
otologic cup forceps
Otto tissue forceps
Oughterson forceps
outlet forceps
oval cup forceps
ovary forceps
Overholt clip-applying forceps
Overholt dissecting forceps
Overholt thoracic forceps
Overholt-Geissendoerfer
  arterial forceps
Overholt-Geissendoerfer
  dissecting forceps
Overholt-Mixter dissecting
  forceps
Overstreet endometrial polyp
  forceps
Overstreet polyp forceps
ovum forceps
Pace-Potts forceps
Packer mosquito forceps
packing forceps
Page tonsillar forceps
Palmer biopsy drill forceps
Palmer biopsy forceps
Palmer cutting forceps
Palmer grasping forceps
Palmer ovarian biopsy forceps
Palmer-Drapier forceps
Pang biopsy forceps
Pang nasopharyngeal forceps
Panje-Shagets
  tracheoesophageal fistula
  forceps
papilloma forceps
parametrium forceps

forceps (*continued*)

Park lens implantation forceps
Parker fixation forceps
Parker-Kerr forceps
partial-occlusion forceps
Passarelli 1-pass
  capsulorrhexis forceps
passing forceps
patent ductus forceps
Paterson brain clip forceps
Paterson laryngeal forceps
Paton anterior chamber lens
  implant forceps
Paton capsular forceps
Paton corneal forceps
Paton corneal transplant
  forceps
Paton extra-delicate forceps
Paton suturing forceps
Paton tying forceps
Paton stitch removing forceps
Patterson bronchoscopic
  forceps
Patterson specimen forceps
Paufique suture forceps
Paulson infertility microtissue
  forceps
Paulson infertility microtying
  forceps
Pauwels fracture forceps
Pavlo-Colibri corneal forceps
Payman intraocular forceps
Payne-Ochsner arterial
  forceps
Payne-Pean arterial forceps
Payne-Rankin arterial forceps
Payne-Rankin forceps
Payr forceps
Payr pylorus forceps
Pean arterial forceps
Pean hemostatic forceps
Pean hysterectomy forceps
Pean intestinal forceps
Pean sponge forceps
peanut forceps
peanut sponge-holding
  forceps
peanut-fenestrated forceps
peanut-grasping forceps
peapod bead-type forceps
peapod intervertebral disk
  forceps

forceps (*continued*)
pediatric forceps
pedicle forceps
Peet mosquito forceps
Peet splinter forceps
pelican biopsy forceps
Pelkmann foreign body
    forceps
Pelkmann gallstone forceps
Pelkmann sponge forceps
Pelkmann uterine forceps
Pelkmann uterine-dressing
    forceps
pelvic reduction forceps
pelvic tissue forceps
Pemberton forceps
Penfield suture forceps
Penfield watchmaker suture
    forceps
Penn-Anderson scleral fixation
    forceps
Pennington hemorrhoidal
    forceps
Pennington hemostatic
    forceps
Pennington tissue forceps
Pennington tissue-grasping
    forceps
Percy intestinal forceps
Percy tissue forceps
Percy-Wolfson gallbladder
    forceps
Perdue tonsillar hemostat
    forceps
Perez-Castro forceps
perforating forceps
peripheral blood vessel
    forceps
peripheral iridectomy forceps
peripheral vascular forceps
peritoneal forceps
Perman cartilage forceps
Perone LASIK flap forceps
Perritt fixation forceps
Perritt lens forceps
Perry forceps
Peters tissue forceps
Peyman intraocular forceps
Peyman vitreous-grasping
    forceps
Peyman-Green vitreous
    forceps

forceps (*continued*)
Pfau polyp forceps
Pfister-Schwartz basket
    forceps
phalangeal forceps
Phaneuf arterial forceps
Phaneuf artery forceps
Phaneuf hysterectomy forceps
Phaneuf peritoneal forceps
Phaneuf uterine artery
    forceps
Phaneuf vaginal forceps
Phillips fixation forceps
Phillips swan neck forceps
phimosis forceps
Phipps forceps
phrenicectomy forceps
physician's pickup forceps
physician's splinter forceps
pickup forceps
pickup noncrushing forceps
Pierse Colibri forceps
Pierse corneal Colibri-type
    forceps
Pierse corneal forceps
Pierse fixation forceps
Pierse tip forceps
Pierse-Colibri corneal utility
    forceps
Pierse-Hoskins forceps
Pigott forceps
Pike jawed forceps
pile forceps
pillar forceps
pillar-grasping forceps
Pilling forceps
Pilling-Liston bone utility
    forceps
pin-bending forceps
pinch forceps
pin-seating forceps
Piper obstetrical forceps
Piranha uteroscopic biopsy
    forceps
Pischel micropin forceps
Pistofidis cervical biopsy
    forceps
Pitanguy forceps
Pitha foreign body forceps
Pitha urethral forceps
pituitary forceps
pituitary rongeur forceps

forceps (*continued*)
placement forceps
placenta forceps
placenta previa forceps
placental forceps
plain forceps
plain thumb forceps
plain tissue forceps
plastic forceps
plate-holding forceps
platform forceps
pleurectomy forceps
Pley capsule forceps
Pley extracapsular forceps
Pley forceps
Plondke uterine forceps
Plondke uterine-elevating
    forceps
point forceps
Polaris reusable forceps
Polk placental forceps
Polk sponge forceps
Pollock double corneal
    forceps
polyp forceps
polypus forceps
Poppen intervertebral disk
    forceps
Porter duodenal forceps
Post forceps
posterior forceps
postnasal sponge forceps
Potter sponge forceps
Potter tonsillar forceps
Potts bronchial forceps
Potts bulldog forceps
Potts coarctation forceps
Potts fixation forceps
Potts intestinal forceps
Potts patent ductus forceps
Potts thumb forceps
Potts-Nevins dressing forceps
Potts-Smith bipolar forceps
Potts-Smith dressing forceps
Potts-Smith monopolar forceps
Potts-Smith tissue forceps
Poutasse renal artery forceps
Pozzi tenaculum forceps
Pratt hemostatic forceps
Pratt tissue forceps
Pratt T-shaped hemostatic
    forceps

forceps (*continued*)
Pratt vulsellum forceps
Pratt-Smith hemostatic
    forceps
Pratt-Smith tissue-grasping
    forceps
Precisor Direct Bite biopsy
    forceps
Prentiss forceps
prepuce forceps
Presbyterian Hospital forceps
pressure forceps
Preston ligamentum flavum
    forceps
Price-Thomas bronchial
    forceps
Primbs suturing forceps
Prince advancement forceps
Prince muscle forceps
Prince trachoma forceps
proctological biopsy forceps
proctological forceps
proctological grasping forceps
proctological polyp forceps
Proctor phrenectomy forceps
Proctor phrenicectomy
    forceps
prostatectomy forceps
prostatic forceps
prostatic lobe forceps
prostatic lobe-holding forceps
Proud adenoidectomy forceps
Providence Hospital arterial
    forceps
Providence Hospital artery
    forceps
Providence Hospital classic
    forceps
Providence Hospital
    hemostatic forceps
ptosis forceps
pulmonary artery forceps
pulmonary vessel forceps
punch forceps
Puntenney tying forceps
Puntowicz arterial forceps
pupil spreader/retractor
    forceps
Pean arterial forceps
Pean GI forceps
Pean hemostatic forceps
Pean hysterectomy forceps

forceps (*continued*)

Pean intestinal forceps
Pean sponge forceps
QSA dressing forceps
quadripolar cutting forceps
Quervain cranial forceps
Quervain cranial rongeur forceps
Quevedo conjunctival forceps
Quevedo fixation forceps
Quevedo suturing forceps
Quinones uterine-grasping forceps
Quinones-Neubauer uterine-grasping forceps
Quire finger forceps
Quire foreign body forceps
Quire mechanical finger forceps
Raaf forceps
Raaf-Oldberg intervertebral disk forceps
Radial Jaw biopsy forceps
Radial Jaw bladder biopsy forceps
Radial Jaw hot biopsy forceps
Radial Jaw single-use biopsy forceps
Raimondi scalp hemostatic forceps
Ralks ear forceps
Ralks splinter forceps
Ralks wire-cutting forceps
Rampley sponge forceps
Rand forceps
Randall kidney stone forceps
Randall stone forceps
Raney clip forceps
Raney rongeur forceps
Raney scalp clip-applying forceps
Raney straight coagulating forceps
Rankin arterial forceps
Rankin hemostatic forceps
Rankin-Crile hemostatic forceps
Rankin-Kelly hemostatic forceps
Rankow forceps
Rapp forceps

forceps (*continued*)

Rappazzo intraocular foreign body forceps
Ratliff-Blake gallstone forceps
Ratliff-Mayo gallstone forceps
rat-tooth forceps
Ray kidney stone forceps
reach-and-pin forceps
Read forceps
recession forceps
rectal biopsy forceps
rectal forceps
Reese advancement forceps
Reese muscle forceps
Reich-Nechtow hypogastric artery forceps
Reich-Nechtow hysterectomy forceps
Reill forceps
Reiner-Knight ethmoid-cutting forceps
Reinhoff arterial forceps
Reisinger lens-extracting forceps
renal artery forceps
Resano sigmoid forceps
resection intestinal forceps
retrieval forceps
Reul coronary forceps
reverse-action hypophysectomy forceps
Rezek forceps
Rhein capsulorrhexis cystitome forceps
Rhein fine foldable lens-insertion forceps
Rhoton bipolar forceps
Rhoton cup forceps
Rhoton dural forceps
Rhoton grasping forceps
Rhoton microcup forceps
Rhoton microdissecting forceps
Rhoton microtying forceps
Rhoton microvascular forceps
Rhoton ring tumor forceps
Rhoton tissue forceps
Rhoton transsphenoidal bipolar forceps
Rhoton tying forceps
Rhoton-Adson dressing forceps

forceps (*continued*)

Rhoton-Adson tissue forceps
Rhoton-Cushing tissue forceps
Rhoton-Tew bipolar forceps
rib rongeur forceps
Riba-Valeira forceps
Rica clip-applying forceps
Rica hemostatic forceps
Rica-Adson forceps
Rich forceps
Richards tonsil-grasping forceps
Richards tonsillar forceps
Richards tonsil-seizing forceps
Richards-Andrews forceps
Riches artery forceps
Riches diathermy forceps
Richmond forceps
Richter suture clip-removing forceps
Richter-Heath clip-removing forceps
ridge forceps
Ridley forceps
Rienhoff arterial forceps
right-angle forceps
rigid biopsy forceps
rigid kidney stone forceps
ring forceps
ringed formed forceps
Ringenberg stapedectomy forceps
ring-rotation forceps
ring-tip forceps
Ripstein arterial forceps
Ripstein tissue forceps
Ritch-Krupin-Denver eye valve insertion forceps
RiteBite biopsy forceps
Ritter forceps
Rizzuti double-prong forceps
Rizzuti fixation forceps
Rizzuti scleral forceps
Rizzuti superior rectus forceps
Rizzuti-Furness cornea-holding forceps
Rizzuti-Verhoeff forceps
Robb tonsillar forceps
Robb tonsillar sponge forceps
Roberts arterial forceps
Roberts bronchial forceps

forceps (*continued*)

Roberts hemostatic forceps
Robertson tonsillar forceps
Robertson tonsil-seizing forceps
Roberts-Singley dressing forceps
Roberts-Singley thumb forceps
Robson intestinal forceps
Rochester gallstone forceps
Rochester oral tissue forceps
Rochester Russian tissue forceps
Rochester tissue forceps
Rochester-Carmalt hemostatic forceps
Rochester-Carmalt hysterectomy forceps
Rochester-Davis forceps
Rochester-Ewald tissue forceps
Rochester-Harrington forceps
Rochester-Mixter artery forceps
Rochester-Mixter gall duct forceps
Rochester-Mueller forceps
Rochester-Ochsner hemostat forceps
Rochester-Pean hysterectomy forceps
Rochester-Pean hysterectomy forceps
Rochester-Rankin arterial forceps
Rochester-Rankin hemostatic forceps
Rochester-Russian forceps
Rockey forceps
Roeder towel forceps
Roeltsch forceps
Roger vascular-toothed hysterectomy forceps
Rogge sterilizing forceps
Rolf jeweler's forceps
Rolf utility forceps
roller forceps
ronguer forceps (*see also* rongeur)
Ronis cutting forceps
Rose disimpaction forceps

forceps (*continued*)
  rotating forceps
  rotation forceps
  Roubaix forceps
  round punch forceps
  round-handled forceps
  Rovenstine catheter-
    introducing forceps
  Rowe bone-drilling forceps
  Rowe disimpaction forceps
  Rowe glenoid-reaming forceps
  Rowe maxillary forceps
  Rowe modified-Harrison
    forceps
  Rowe-Harrison bone-holding
    forceps
  Rowe-Killey forceps
  Rowland double-action
    forceps
  Rowland double-action hump
    forceps
  Rowland hump forceps
  Rowland nasal hump forceps
  Royce forceps
  rubber-dam clamp forceps
  rubber-shod forceps
  Rubin-Wright forceps
  Rudd Clinic hemorrhoidal
    forceps
  Ruel forceps
  Rugby deep-surgery forceps
  Rugelski arterial forceps
  Rumel dissecting forceps
  Rumel lobectomy forceps
  Rumel rubber forceps
  Rumel thoracic forceps
  Rumel thoracic-dissecting
    forceps
  Ruskin bone-cutting forceps
  Ruskin bone-splitting forceps
  Ruskin rongeur forceps
  Ruskin-Liston bone-cutting
    forceps
  Ruskin-Rowland bone-cutting
    forceps
  Russ tumor forceps
  Russ vascular forceps
  Russell hysterectomy forceps
  Russell David forceps
  Russian Pean forceps
  Russian thumb forceps
  Russian tissue forceps

forceps (*continued*)
  Rycroft tying forceps
  S&T LaLonde hook forceps
  Sachs tissue forceps
  Saenger ovum forceps
  Saenger placental forceps
  Sajou laryngeal forceps
  Sam Roberts bronchial biopsy
    forceps
  Samuels hemoclip-applying
    forceps
  Sanders vasectomy forceps
  Sanders-Castroviejo suturing
    forceps
  Sandt suture forceps
  Sandt utility forceps
  Santy dissecting forceps
  Santy ring-end forceps
  Saqalain dressing forceps
  Sarot artery forceps
  Sarot intrathoracic forceps
  Sarot pleurectomy forceps
  Satellight needle holder
    forceps
  Satinsky forceps
  Satterlee advancement
    forceps
  Satterlee muscle forceps
  Sauer outer ring forceps
  Sauer suture forceps
  Sauer suturing forceps
  Sauerbruch pickup forceps
  Sauerbruch rib forceps
  Sawtell arterial forceps
  Sawtell gallbladder forceps
  Sawtell hemostatic forceps
  Sawtell tonsillar forceps
  Sawtell-Davis tonsillar
    hemostat forceps
  scalp clip forceps
  scalp clip-applying forceps
  scalp forceps
  Scanlan laparoscopic forceps
  Scanzoni forceps
  Schaaf foreign body forceps
  Schaedel towel forceps
  Schaefer fixation forceps
  Schanzioni craniotomy
    forceps
  Scharff bipolar forceps
  Schatz utility forceps
  Scheer crimper forceps

forceps (*continued*)

Scheie-Graefe fixation forceps
Scheinmann esophagoscopy forceps
Scheinmann laryngeal forceps
Schepens forceps
Schick forceps
Schindler peritoneal forceps
Schlesinger cervical punch forceps
Schlesinger intervertebral disk forceps
Schlesinger meniscus-grasping forceps
Schlesinger rongeur forceps
Schnidt gall duct forceps
Schnidt thoracic forceps
Schnidt tonsillar forceps
Schnidt tonsillar hemostatic forceps
Schnidt-Rumpler forceps
Schoenberg intestinal forceps
Schoenberg uterine forceps
Schoenberg uterine-elevating forceps
Scholten endomyocardial biopsy forceps
Schroeder tissue forceps
Schroeder uterine tenaculum forceps
Schroeder uterine vulsellum forceps
Schroeder vulsellum forceps
Schroeder-Braun uterine forceps
Schroeder-Braun uterine tenaculum forceps
Schroeder-Van Doren tenaculum forceps
Schubert cervical biopsy forceps
Schubert uterine biopsy forceps
Schubert uterine biopsy punch forceps
Schubert uterine tenaculum forceps
Schumacher biopsy forceps
Schutz forceps
Schwartz clip-applying forceps
Schwartz multipurpose forceps

forceps (*continued*)

Schwartz obstetrical forceps
Schwartz temporary clamp-applying forceps
Schweigger capsular forceps
Schweigger capsule forceps
Schweigger extracapsular forceps
Schweizer cervix-holding forceps
Schweizer uterine forceps
scissors forceps
scleral twist-grip forceps
sclerectomy punch forceps
Scobee-Allis forceps
Scott lens-insertion forceps
Scoville brain forceps
Scoville brain spatula forceps
Scoville clip-applying forceps
Scoville-Greenwood bayonet neurosurgical bipolar forceps
Scoville-Greenwood forceps
Scoville-Hurteau forceps
screw-holding forceps
Scudder intestinal forceps
Scuderi bipolar coagulating forceps
Searcy capsular forceps
Searcy capsule forceps
Segond hysterectomy forceps
Segond tumor forceps
Segond-Landau hysterectomy forceps
Seiffert esophagoscopy forceps
Seiffert laryngeal forceps
Seitzinger tripolar cutting forceps
seizing forceps
Seletz foramen-plugging forceps
self-opening forceps
self-retaining bone forceps
Selman nonslip tissue forceps
Selman peripheral blood vessel forceps
Selman tissue forceps
Selman vessel forceps
Selverstone embolus forceps
Selverstone intervertebral disk forceps

forceps (*continued*)

Selverstone rongeur forceps
Semb bone forceps
Semb bone-cutting forceps
Semb bone-holding forceps
Semb dissecting forceps
Semb ligature forceps
Semb ligature-carrying
    forceps
Semb rib forceps
Semb rongeur forceps
Semb-Ghazi dissecting forceps
Semken bipolar forceps
Semken dressing forceps
Semken infant forceps
Semken microbipolar
    neurosurgical forceps
Semken thumb forceps
Semken tissue forceps
Semken-Taylor forceps
Semmes dural forceps
Senn forceps
Senning cardiovascular forceps
Senturia forceps
septal bone forceps
septal compression forceps
septal forceps
septal ridge forceps
septum-cutting forceps
septum-straightening forceps
sequestrum forceps
serrated conjunctival forceps
serrated forceps
serrefine forceps
Sewall brain clip-applying
    forceps
Seyfert forceps
Shaaf eye forceps
Shaaf foreign body forceps
Shallcross cystic duct forceps
Shallcross gallbladder forceps
Shallcross hemostatic forceps
Shallcross nasal forceps
Shallcross nasal-packing
    forceps
Shallcross-Dean gall duct
    forceps
Shapshay-Healy laryngeal
    alligator forceps
Shark forceps
Shark disposable biopsy
    forceps

forceps (*continued*)

shark-tooth forceps
sharp-pointed forceps
Shearer chicken-bill forceps
sheathed flexible gastric
    forceps
sheathed flexible gastroscopic
    forceps
Sheehy ossicle-holding
    forceps
Sheets lens forceps
Sheets-McPherson angled
    forceps
Sheets-McPherson tying
    forceps
Sheinmann laryngeal forceps
Shepard bipolar forceps
Shepard curved intraocular
    lens forceps
Shepard intraocular lens
    forceps
Shepard intraocular lens-
    inserting forceps
Shepard lens forceps
Shepard tying forceps
Shepard-Reinstein intraocular
    lens forceps
Shields forceps
Shoemaker intraocular lens
    forceps
short-tooth forceps
Shuppe biting forceps
Shuster suture forceps
Shuster tonsillar forceps
Shutt Aggressor forceps
Shutt alligator forceps
Shutt basket forceps
Shutt B-scoop forceps
Shutt grasping forceps
Shutt Mantis retrograde
    forceps
Shutt Mini-Aggressor forceps
Shutt retrograde forceps
Shutt shovel-nosed forceps
Shutt suction forceps
shuttle forceps
side-biting Stammberger
    punch forceps
side-curved forceps
side-cutting basket forceps
side-grasping forceps
side-lip forceps

forceps (*continued*)
Siegler biopsy forceps
sigmoidoscope biopsy forceps
Silcock dissection forceps
silicone rod and sleeve forceps
silicone sponge forceps
Silver endaural forceps
Simcoe implantation forceps
Simcoe lens-inserting forceps
Simcoe nucleus forceps
Simcoe posterior chamber forceps
Simcoe superior rectus forceps
Simons stone-removing forceps
Simpson obstetrical forceps
Simpson-Braun obstetrical forceps
Simpson-Luikart forceps
Simpson-Luikart obstetrical forceps
Sims-Maier sponge and dressing forceps
single-tooth forceps
Singley intestinal forceps
Singley intestinal tissue forceps
Singley tissue forceps
Singley-Tuttle dressingforceps
Singley-Tuttle intestinal forceps
Singley-Tuttle tissue forceps
Sinskey intraocular lens forceps
Sinskey microtying forceps
Sinskey-McPherson forceps
Sinskey-Wilson forceps
Sinskey-Wilson foreign body forceps
sinus biopsy forceps
Sisson forceps
sister-hook forceps
Skeleton fine forceps
Skene tenaculum forceps
Skene uterine forceps
Skene vulsellum forceps
Skillern phimosis forceps
Skillman arterial forceps
Skillman hemostatic forceps
Skillman mosquito forceps

forceps (*continued*)
Skillman prepuce forceps
skin forceps
sleeve-spreading dilating forceps
sleeve-spreading forceps
sliding capsular forceps
sliding capsule forceps
Sluder-Ballenger tonsillar punch forceps
small bone-cutting forceps
small cup biopsy forceps
Smart chalazion forceps
Smart nonslipping chalazion forceps
Smellie obstetrical forceps
Smith & Nephew Richards bipolar forceps
Smith grasping forceps
Smith lion-jaw forceps
Smith obstetrical forceps
Smith-Leiske cross-action intraocular lens forceps
Smith-Petersen forceps
Smithwick clip-applying forceps
Smithwick-Hartmann forceps
smooth dressing forceps
smooth tissue forceps
smooth-tipped jeweler's forceps
smooth-tooth forceps
Snellen entropion forceps
Snowden-Pencer forceps
Snyder corneal spring forceps
Snyder deep-surgery forceps
Somers uterine forceps
Somers uterine-elevating forceps
Songer tonsillar forceps
Soonawalla vasectomy forceps
Sopher ovum forceps
Sourdille forceps
Spaleck forceps
Sparta micro iris forceps
Sparta micro-iris forceps
spatula forceps
specimen forceps
speculum forceps
Spence rongeur forceps
Spence-Adson clip-introducing forceps

forceps (*continued*)

Spencer biopsy forceps
Spencer chalazion forceps
Spencer plication forceps
Spencer rongeur forceps
Spencer-Wells arterial forceps
Spencer-Wells chalazion forceps
Spencer-Wells hemostatic forceps
Spero meibomian expressor forceps
Spero meibomian forceps
Spetzler forceps
sphenoidal punch forceps
spicule forceps
spinal perforating forceps
spinal rongeur forceps
spinal-perforating forceps
spiral forceps
splaytooth forceps
splinter forceps
splitting forceps
sponge forceps
sponge-and-dressing forceps
sponge-holding forceps
sponging forceps
spoon forceps
spoon-shaped forceps
spreading forceps
spring-handled forceps
Spurling intervertebral disk forceps
Spurling IV disk forceps
Spurling rongeur forceps
Spurling tissue forceps
Spurling-Kerrison forceps
Spurling-Kerrison rongeur forceps
square specimen forceps
squeeze-handle forceps
SSW forceps
ST Lalonde hook forceps
St. Clair forceps
St. Clair-Thompson abscess forceps
St. Clair-Thompson adenoidal forceps
St. Clair-Thompson peritonsillar abscess forceps
St. Martin eye forceps

forceps (*continued*)

St. Martin suturing forceps
St. Vincent tube-clamping forceps
St. Vincent tube-occluding forceps
Stamm bone-cutting forceps
Stammberger side-biting punch forceps
standard arterial forceps
standard artery forceps
stapedectomy forceps
stapes forceps
staple forceps
Stark vulsellum forceps
Starr fixation forceps
Staude tenaculum forceps
Staude uterine tenaculum forceps
Staude-Jackson tenaculum forceps
Staude-Moore uterine tenaculum forceps
Stavis fixation forceps
Steinmann intestinal forceps
Steinmann intestinal grasping forceps
Steinmann tendon forceps
Stephens soft IOL-inserting forceps
sterilizer forceps
sterilizing forceps
sternal punch forceps
Stern-Castroviejo locking forceps
Stern-Castroviejo suturing forceps
Stevens fixation forceps
Stevens iris forceps
Stevenson alligator forceps
Stevenson cupped-jaw forceps
Stevenson grasping forceps
Stevenson microsurgical forceps
Stieglitz splinter forceps
Stille gallstone forceps
Stille kidney forceps
Stille rongeur forceps
Stille tissue forceps
Stille-Adson forceps
Stille-Babcock forceps
Stille-Barraya intestinal forceps

forceps (*continued*)

Stille-Barraya intestinal-
grasping forceps
Stille-Barraya vascular forceps
Stille-Björk forceps
Stille-Crafoord forceps
Stille-Crile forceps
Stille-Halsted forceps
Stille-Horsley bone-cutting
forceps
Stille-Horsley rib forceps
Stille-Liston bone forceps
Stille-Liston bone-cutting
forceps
Stille-Liston rib-cutting
forceps
Stille-Luer rongeur forceps
Stille-Russian forceps
Stille-Waugh forceps
Stiwer biopsy forceps
Stiwer bone-holding forceps
Stiwer dressing forceps
Stiwer sponge forceps
Stiwer tissue forceps
Stolte capsulorrhexis forceps
Stone clamp-applying forceps
Stone intestinal forceps
Stone tissue forceps
stone-crushing forceps
stone-extraction forceps
stone-grasping forceps
Stoneman forceps
Storey gall duct forceps
Storey thoracic forceps
Storey-Hillar dissecting
forceps
Storz biopsy forceps
Storz bronchoscopic forceps
Storz capsular forceps
Storz ciliary forceps
Storz corneal forceps
Storz curved forceps
Storz cystoscopic forceps
Storz esophagoscopic forceps
Storz grasping biopsy forceps
Storz kidney stone forceps
Storz plate-holding forceps
Storz miniature forceps
Storz nasopharyngeal biopsy
forceps
Storz optical biopsy forceps
Storz sinus biopsy forceps

forceps (*continued*)

Storz stone-crushing forceps
Storz stone-extraction forceps
Storz-Bonn suturing forceps
Storz-Ultrata forceps
strabismus forceps
straight coagulating forceps
straight forceps
straight knot-tying forceps
straight line bayonet forceps
straight Maryland forceps
straight microbipolar forceps
straight micromonopolar
forceps
straight single tenaculum
forceps
straight tying forceps
straight-end cup forceps
straight-tip bipolar forceps
straight-tip jeweler's bipolar
forceps
Strassburger tissue forceps
Strassmann uterine forceps
Strassmann uterine-elevating
forceps
Stratte forceps
Strelinger catheter-
introducing forceps
Stringer catheter-introducing
forceps
Stringer newborn throat
forceps
Strow corneal forceps
Struempel ear alligator
forceps
Struempel ear punch forceps
Struempel-Voss ethmoidal
forceps
Struempel-Voss nasal forceps
Strully dressing forceps
Strully tissue forceps
strut forceps
Struyken ear forceps
Struyken nasal forceps
Struyken nasal-cutting forceps
Struyken turbinate forceps
Styles forceps
subglottic forceps
suction forceps
Suker iris forceps
superior rectus forceps
SureBite biopsy forceps

forceps (*continued*)

Sutherland vitreous forceps
Sutherland-Grieshaber forceps
suture and tying forceps
suture clip forceps
suture forceps
suture tag forceps
suture-carrying forceps
suture-holding forceps
suture-pulling forceps
suture-tying forceps
suture-tying platform forceps
suturing forceps
Swan-Brown arterial forceps
Sweet clip-applying forceps
Sweet dissecting forceps
Sweet ligature forceps
synovium biopsy forceps
Szuler vascular forceps
Szultz corneal forceps
tack-and-pin forceps
Takahashi cutting forceps
Takahashi ethmoid forceps
Takahashi ethmoidal forceps
Takahashi iris retractor
    forceps
Takahashi nasal forceps
Takahashi neurological
    forceps
Takahashi neurosurgical
    forceps
Take-apart forceps
tampon forceps
Tamsco forceps
tangential forceps
taper-jaw forceps
Tarnier axis-traction forceps
Tarnier obstetrical forceps
Taylor dissecting forceps
Taylor tissue forceps
Taylor-Cushing dressing
    forceps
Teale tenaculum forceps
Teale uterine forceps
Teale uterine vulsellum
    forceps
Teale vulsellum forceps
Tekno forceps
tenaculum forceps
tenaculum-reducing forceps
tendon forceps
tendon-holding forceps

forceps (*continued*)

tendon-passing forceps
tendon-pulling forceps
tendon-retrieving forceps
tendon-seizing forceps
tendon-tunneling forceps
Tennant intraocular lens
    forceps
Tennant lens forceps
Tennant titanium suturing
    forceps
Tennant tying forceps
Tennant-Colibri corneal
    forceps
Tennant-Maumenee forceps
Tennant-Troutman superior
    rectus forceps
Tenzel bipolar forceps
Terson capsule forceps
Terson extracapsular forceps
Tessier disimpaction device
    forceps
Thackray dental forceps
Therma Jaw hot urologic
    forceps
Theurig sterilizer forceps
Thomas Allis tissue forceps
Thomas fixation forceps
Thomas shot compression
    forceps
Thomas uterine tissue-
    grasping forceps
Thompson hip prosthesis
    forceps
Thoms tissue forceps
Thoms tissue-grasping forceps
Thoms-Allis intestinal forceps
Thoms-Allis tissue forceps
Thoms-Gaylor biopsy forceps
Thoms-Gaylor uterine forceps
thoracic artery forceps
thoracic forceps
thoracic hemostatic forceps
thoracic tissue forceps
Thorek gallbladder forceps
Thorek-Mixter gall duct
    forceps
Thorek-Mixter gallbladder
    forceps
Thornton episcleral forceps
Thornton fixation forceps
Thornton intraocular forceps

forceps (*continued*)

Thorpe conjunctival forceps
Thorpe corneal forceps
Thorpe corneoscleral forceps
Thorpe fixation forceps
Thorpe foreign body forceps
Thorpe-Castroviejo corneal
    forceps
Thorpe-Castroviejo fixation
    forceps
Thorpe-Castroviejo vitreous
    foreign body forceps
Thrasher intraocular forceps
Thrasher lens implant forceps
throat forceps
thumb forceps
thumb tissue forceps
thumb-dressing forceps
Thurston-Holland fragment
    forceps
thyroid forceps
thyroid traction forceps
Tickner tissue forceps
Tiemann bullet forceps
Tiger Shark forceps
Tilley dressing forceps
Tilley-Henckel forceps
Tischler cervical biopsy
    forceps
Tischler cervical biopsy
    punch forceps
Tischler cervical forceps
Tischler-Morgan uterine
    biopsy forceps
tissue dressing forceps
tissue forceps
tissue-grasping forceps
tissue-holding forceps
tissue-spreading forceps
titanium microsurgical bipolar
    forceps
Tivnen tonsillar forceps
Tivnen tonsil-seizing forceps
Tobey ear forceps
Tobold laryngeal forceps
Tobold-Fauvel forceps
Tobold-Fauvel grasping
    forceps
Toennis tumor-grasping
    forceps
Toennis-Adson forceps
Tomac forceps

forceps (*continued*)

tongue forceps
tongue-seizing forceps
tonsil forceps
tonsil-holding forceps
tonsillar abscess forceps
tonsillar artery forceps
tonsillar forceps
tonsillar hemostatic forceps
tonsillar needle holder
    forceps
tonsillar pillar grasping
    forceps
tonsillar punch forceps
tonsil-ligating forceps
tonsil-seizing forceps
tonsil-suturing forceps
Tooke corneal forceps
Toomey forceps
toothed forceps
toothed thumb forceps
toothed tissue forceps
tooth-extracting forceps
toothless forceps
Torchia capsular forceps
Torchia lens implantation
    forceps
Torchia microbipolar forceps
Torchia tissue forceps
Torchia tying forceps
Torchia-Colibri forceps
Torres cross-action forceps
torsion forceps
towel clip forceps
towel forceps
Tower muscle forceps
Townley tissue forceps
tracheal forceps
tracheal hemostatic forceps
trachoma forceps
traction forceps
transfer forceps
transplant-grafting forceps
transsphenoidal bipolar
    forceps
transsphenoidal forceps
traumatic grasping forceps
triangular punch forceps
tripod grasping forceps
Troeltsch dressing forceps
Troeltsch ear forceps
Trotter forceps

forceps (*continued*)

Trousseau dilating forceps
Troutman corneal forceps
Troutman microsurgery forceps
Troutman rectal forceps
Troutman superior rectus forceps
Troutman tying forceps
Troutman-Barraquer-Colibri forceps
Troutman-Barraquer corneal fixation forceps
Troutman-Barraquer corneal forceps
Troutman-Barraquer iris forceps
Troutman-Llobera fixation forceps
Troutman-Llobera Flieringa forceps
Troutman-Llobera-Flieringa forceps
Truline forceps
Trush grasping forceps
Trylon hemostatic forceps
T-shaped forceps
tube-occluding forceps
tubing clamp forceps
tubing forceps
tubing introducer forceps
Tubinger gallstone forceps
tubular forceps
Tucker bead forceps
Tucker hallux forceps
Tucker reach-and-pin forceps
Tucker staple forceps
Tucker tack and pin forceps
Tucker-McLane axis-traction forceps
Tucker-McLane obstetrical forceps
Tucker-McLane-Luikart forceps
Tudor-Edwards bone-cutting forceps
Tuffier arterial forceps
tumor forceps
tumor-grasping forceps
turbinate forceps
Turnbull adhesion forceps
Turner-Babcock tissue forceps

forceps (*continued*)

Turner-Warwick stone forceps
Turner-Warwick-Adson forceps
Turrell biopsy forceps
Turrell rectal biopsy forceps
Turrell specimen forceps
Turrell-Wittner rectal biopsy forceps
Turrell-Wittner rectal forceps
Tuttle dressing forceps
Tuttle obstetrical forceps
Tuttle thoracic forceps
Tuttle thumb forceps
Tuttle tissue forceps
Tuttle-Singley thoracic forceps
Twisk forceps
Tydings tonsil forceps
Tydings-Lakeside tonsillar forceps
Tydings-Lakeside tonsil-seizing forceps
tying forceps
tympanoplasty forceps
Tyrrell foreign body forceps
Ullrich bone-holding forceps
Ullrich dressing forceps
Ullrich-Aesculap forceps
Ullrich-St. Gallen forceps
Ultrata capsulorrhexis forceps
unipolar hand-switching needle-point electrocautery forceps
Universal forceps
University forceps
University of Kansas corneal forceps
University of Michigan Mixter thoracic forceps
upbiting biopsy forceps
upbiting cup forceps
up-cupped forceps
upcurved basket forceps
upper universal forceps
Uppsala gall duct forceps
upturned forceps
upward bent forceps
Urbantschitsch nasal forceps
ureteral catheter forceps
ureteral isolation forceps
ureteral stone forceps
urethral forceps

forceps (*continued*)

U-shaped forceps
uterine artery forceps
uterine biopsy forceps
uterine biopsy punch forceps
uterine forceps
uterine manipulating forceps
uterine polyp forceps
uterine specimen forceps
uterine tenaculum forceps
uterine vulsellum forceps
uterine-dressing forceps
uterine-elevating forceps
uterine-grasping forceps
uterine-holding forceps
uterine-manipulating forceps
uterine-packing forceps
utility forceps
Utrata capsulorrhexis forceps
V. Mueller biopsy forceps
V. Mueller bone-cutting
    forceps
V. Mueller laser Backhaus
    towel forceps
V. Mueller laser Crile micro-
    arterial forceps
V. Mueller laser micro-Allis
    forceps
V. Mueller laser Rhoton
    microtying forceps
V. Mueller laser Singley tissue
    forceps
V. Mueller nonperforating
    towel forceps
V. Mueller tying forceps
V. Mueller-Vital laser Babcock
    forceps
V. Mueller-Vital laser Potts-
    Smith forceps
vaginal hysterectomy forceps
Valin forceps
van Buren bone-holding
    forceps
van Buren forceps
van Buren sequestrum forceps
Van Doren uterine biopsy
    punch forceps
Van Doren uterine forceps
Van Mandach capsule
    fragment and clot forceps
Van Ruben forceps
Van Struyken nasal forceps

forceps (*continued*)

Vander Pool sterilizer forceps
Vanderbilt arterial forceps
Vanderbilt deep-vessel forceps
Vanderbilt forceps
Vanderbilt University
    hemostatic forceps
Vanderbilt University vessel
    forceps
Vannas fixation forceps
Vantage tube-occluding
    forceps
Vantec grasping forceps
Varco gallbladder forceps
Varco thoracic forceps
vas isolation forceps
vascular forceps
vascular tissue forceps
vasectomy forceps
Vaughn sterilizer forceps
vectis cesarean forceps
vectis cesarean section
    forceps
vectis forceps
vena cava forceps
vena caval forceps
Verbrugge bone-holding
    forceps
Verhoeff capsule forceps
Verhoeff cataract forceps
vertical forceps
vessel clip-applying forceps
vessel forceps
vessel pediatric forceps
vessel peripheral forceps
Vick-Blanchard forceps
Vick-Blanchard hemorrhoidal
    forceps
Vickerall round ringed forceps
Vickers ring-tip forceps
Victor-Bonney forceps
Vigger-5 eye forceps
Virtus splinter forceps
viscera-holding forceps
visceral forceps
vise forceps
visual hemostatic forceps
Vital general tissue forceps
Vital intestinal forceps
Vital lung-grasping forceps
Vital needle-holder forceps
Vital tissue forceps

forceps (*continued*)
 Vital-Adson tissue forceps
 Vital-Babcock tissue forceps
 Vital-Cushing tissue forceps
 Vital-Duval intestinal forceps
 Vital-Evans pelvic tissue
   forceps
 Vital-Potts-Smith forceps
 Vital-Wangensteen tissue
   forceps
 vitreous-grasping forceps
 Vogler hysterectomy forceps
 Vogt toothed capsular forceps
 vomer forceps
 vomer septal forceps
 von Graefe fixation forceps
 von Graefe iris forceps
 von Graefe tissue forceps
 Von Mandach capsule
   fragment forceps
 Von Mandach clot forceps
 von Petz forceps
 Voris-Oldberg intervertebral
   disk forceps
 Voris-Oldberg IV disk rongeur
   forceps
 Vorse tube-occluding forceps
 Vorse-Webster forceps
 VPI-Ambrose resectoscope
   forceps
 vulsella forceps
 vulsellum forceps
 Wachtenfeldt clip-applying
   forceps
 Wachtenfeldt clip-removing
   forceps
 Wadsworth lid forceps
 Wainstock eye suturing
   forceps
 Waldeau fixation forceps
 Waldenstrom laryngeal
   forceps
 Waldeyer forceps
 Walker forceps
 Wallace cesarean forceps
 Walsh tissue forceps
 Walsham nasal forceps
 Walsham septal forceps
 Walsham septum-
   straightening forceps
 Walter splinter forceps
 Walther tissue forceps

forceps (*continued*)
 Walton meniscal forceps
 Walton-Allis tissue forceps
 Walton-Liston forceps
 Walton-Schubert uterine
   biopsy forceps
 Walzl hysterectomy forceps
 Wangensteen intestinal
   forceps
 Wangensteen tissue forceps
 Warthen forceps
 watchmaker forceps
 Watson duckbill forceps
 Watson tonsil-seizing forceps
 Watson-Williams ethmoid-
   biting forceps
 Watson-Williams nasal forceps
 Watson-Williams polyp
   forceps
 Watzke forceps
 Waugh dissection forceps
 Waugh dressing forceps
 Waugh tissue forceps
 Waugh-Brophy forceps
 wave-tooth forceps
 Weaver chalazion forceps
 Weck hysterectomy forceps
 Weck rectal biopsy forceps
 Weck towel forceps
 Weck uterine biopsy forceps
 Weck-Harms forceps
 Weeks eye forceps
 Weiger-Zollner forceps
 Weil ear forceps
 Weil ethmoidal forceps
 Weil-Blakesley ethmoidal
   forceps
 Weiner uterine biopsy forceps
 Weingartner ear forceps
 Weisenbach forceps
 Weisman uterine tenaculum
   forceps
 Weiss forceps
 Welch Allyn anal biopsy
   forceps
 Weller cartilage forceps
 Weller meniscal forceps
 Wells forceps
 Welsh ophthalmological
   forceps
 Welsh pupil spreader-retractor
   forceps

forceps (*continued*)

Welsh pupil-spreader forceps
Wertheim hysterectomy forceps
Wertheim uterine forceps
Wertheim vaginal forceps
Wertheim-Cullen compression forceps
Wertheim-Cullen hysterectomy forceps
Wertheim-Cullen kidney pedicle forceps
Wertheim-Cullen pedicle forceps
Wertheim-Navratil forceps
West nasal-dressing forceps
Westermark uterine dressing forceps
Westermark-Stille forceps
Westmacott dressing forceps
Westphal gall duct forceps
Westphal hemostatic forceps
Wheeler plaque forceps
Wheeler vessel forceps
White tonsil forceps
White tonsil hemostat forceps
White tonsillar forceps
White tonsil-seizing forceps
White-Lillie tonsil forceps
White-Oslay prostatic forceps
White-Oslay prostatic lobe-holding forceps
White-Smith forceps
Whitney superior rectus forceps
Wickman uterine forceps
Wiener hysterectomy forceps
Wies chalazion forceps
Wiet otologic cup forceps
Wikstroem artery forceps
Wilde ear forceps
Wilde ethmoidal exenteration forceps
Wilde ethmoidal forceps
Wilde intervertebral disk forceps
Wilde laminectomy forceps
Wilde nasal-cutting forceps
Wilde nasal-dressing forceps
Wilde septal forceps
Wilde-Blakesley ethmoidal forceps

forceps (*continued*)

Wilder dilating forceps
Wilde-Troeltsch forceps
Wilkerson intraocular lens-insertion forceps
Willauer intrathoracic forceps
Willauer-Allis thoracic forceps
Willauer-Allis thoracic tissue forceps
Willauer-Allis tissue forceps
Willett placenta previa forceps
Willett placental forceps
Willett scalp flap forceps
Williams diskectomy forceps
Williams gastrointestinal forceps
Williams intestinal forceps
Williams splinter forceps
Williams tissue forceps
Williams uterine forceps
Williams vessel-holding forceps
Williamsburg forceps
Wills Hospital ophthalmic forceps
Wills Hospital ophthalmology forceps
Wills Hospital utliity forceps
Wills utility forceps
Wilmer iris forceps
Wilson vitreous foreign body forceps
Wilson-Cook biopsy forceps
Wilson-Cook bronchoscope biopsy forceps
Wilson-Cook colonoscope biopsy forceps
Wilson-Cook gastroscope biopsy forceps
Wilson-Cook grasping forceps
Wilson-Cook hot biopsy forceps
Wilson-Cook retrieval forceps
Wilson-Cook tripod retrieval forceps
Winter ovum forceps
Winter placental forceps
Winter-Nassauer placental forceps
wire prosthesis-crimping forceps

forceps (*continued*)

wire-closure forceps
wire-crimper forceps
wire-crimping forceps
wire-pulling forceps
wire-twisting forceps
Wittner uterine biopsy
    forceps
Wolf biopsy forceps
Wolf biting basket forceps
Wolf cataract delivery
    forceps
Wolf curved basket forceps
Wolf eye forceps
Wolfe uterine cuff forceps
Wolfson forceps
Woodward hemostatic
    forceps
Woodward thoracic artery
    forceps
Woodward thoracic
    hemostatic forceps
Woodward-Potts intestinal
    forceps
Worth advancement forceps
Worth muscle forceps
Worth strabismus forceps
wound forceps
wound-clip forceps
Wright-Rubin forceps
Wrigley forceps
W-shape forceps
Wullstein ear forceps
Wullstein tympanoplasty
    forceps
Wullstein-House cup-shaped
    forceps
Wullstein-Paparella forceps
Wylie tenaculum forceps
Wylie uterine forceps
Wylie uterine tenaculum
    forceps
X-long cement forceps
Yankauer ethmoid forceps
Yankauer ethmoid-cutting
    forceps
Yankauer-Little tube forceps
Yasargil angled forceps
Yasargil applying forceps
Yasargil artery forceps
Yasargil bipolar forceps
Yasargil clip-applying forceps

forceps (*continued*)

Yasargil flat serrated ring
    forceps
Yasargil microvessel clip-
    applying forceps
Yasargil neurosurgical bipolar
    forceps
Yasargil straight forceps
Yeoman rectal biopsy forceps
Yeoman uterine biopsy
    forceps
Yeoman uterine forceps
Yeoman-Wittner rectal biopsy
    forceps
Yeoman-Wittner rectal forceps
Young intestinal forceps
Young lobe forceps
Young prostatectomy forceps
Young prostatic forceps
Young tongue forceps
Young tongue-seizing forceps
Younge uterine biopsy
    forceps
Younge uterine forceps
Younge-Kevorkian forceps
Z-clamp hysterectomy forceps
Zenker dissecting and ligature
    forceps
Zenker forceps
Zeppelin obstetrical forceps
Ziegler cilia forceps
Ziegler ciliary forceps
Zimmer-Hoen forceps
Zimmer-Schlesinger forceps
Zollinger multipurpose tissue
Zollinger multipurpose tissue
    forceps
Zweifel angiotribe forceps
forceps delivery
forceps extraction
forceps guard
forceps handle
forceps jar
forceps maneuver
forceps operation
forceps point
forceps removal
forceps tip
forcible feeding
forcipressure
Ford clamp
Ford Hospital ventricular cannula

Ford stethoscope
Ford triangulation technique
Ford-Deaver retractor
Fordyce disease
Fordyce granules
Fordyce spots
fore-and-aft splint
fore-and-aft suture technique
forearm aluminum shelf crutch
forearm amputation
forearm and metacarpal splint
forearm flap
forearm flow
forearm fracture
forearm graft arteriovenous
    fistula
forearm splint
forearm tourniquet
forebrain bundle
Forect I, II lesion
Foredom-Oster vibrator
forefoot amputation
forefoot arthroplasty
forefoot equinus
forefoot valgus
forefoot varus
Foregger bronchoscope
Foregger laryngoscope
Foregger rigid esophagoscope
Foregger tube
Foregger-Racine adapter
foregut malformation
forehead animation
forehead asymmetry
forehead convexity
forehead elevation and fixation
    with percutaneous
    microscrews
forehead flap
forehead lift
forehead lifting
forehead positioner
forehead prominence
forehead reconstruction
forehead rhytids
forehead wrinkling
forehead-brow complex
forehead-nose position
forehead-plasty
foreign body (FB)
foreign body aspiration
foreign body bur

foreign body contamination
foreign body curet
foreign body cystoscopy forceps
foreign body extraction
foreign body eye forceps
foreign body eye spud
foreign body forceps
foreign body giant cell
foreign body granuloma
foreign body impaction
foreign body in organ
foreign body locator
foreign body loop
foreign body magnet
foreign body needle
foreign body obstruction
foreign body passed
foreign body probe
foreign body reaction
foreign body removal
foreign body removed
foreign body remover
foreign body retained
foreign body rhinitis
foreign body screw
foreign body seen on x-ray
foreign body spud
foreign body trauma
foreign body-retrieving forceps
foreign substance
Forel commissure
Forel decussation
Forel field
Forel space
forequadrant incision
forequarter amputation
ForeRunner coronary sinus
    guiding catheter
Forerunner defibrillator
foreskin flap
Forest-Hastings technique
Forestier disease
fork
    3-prong fork
    aluminum alloy fork
    Bezold-Edelman tuning fork
    broadbill hemostat with push
        fork
    crus guide fork
    double-pronged fork
    Gardiner-Brown neurological
        tuning fork

fork (*continued*)

Gardiner-Brown tuning fork
Hardy 3-prong fork
Hardy implant fork
Hartmann tuning fork
implant fork
Jannetta double-pronged fork
Jarit tuning fork
knife and fork
Leasure tuning fork
magnesium tuning forks
McCabe crus guide fork
neurological tuning fork
Okonek-Yasargil tumor fork
Penn tuning fork
Ralks tuning fork
Rhoton 3-prong fork
Rica tuning fork
Riverbank Laboratories tuning
   fork
Rydel-Seiffert tuning fork
SMIC tuning fork
Sugita fork
tuning fork
fork hammer
forked flap
forked tongue
forked T-tube
forked uvula
Forker retractor
forklike stump
form

Amoena breast form
arch form
breast-mound form
cystic form
Discrene breast form
Dow Corning external breast
   form
extension form
filamented form
filamentous form
fistula form
follicular form
hematoma form
mastopexy form
Nearly Me breast form
nonfilamented form
occlusal form
retention form
Roth arch form
segmented forms

form (*continued*)

Spenco external breast form
spherical-shaped form
stab form
Trulife silicone breast form
Vestibulator positioning
   tumble forms
Yours Truly asymmetrical
   external breast form
Formad kidney
formal hemipelvectomy
formal hepatic resection
formal laparotomy
formal protocol
formal surgical exploration
formaldehyde catgut sutures
formalin fixation
formalin-fixed speculum
formation

abscess formation
adhesion formation
anastomotic stricture
   formation
anterior synechia formation
antiantibody formation
aspergilloma formation
balloon cell formation
bas-fond formation
blood vessel formation
bone formation
branching tubule formation
bubble formation
bunion formation
callous formation
callus formation
cancellous formation
cataract formation
chiasma formation
cloacal formation
clot formation
coagulum formation
colloid formation
colony formation
concept formation
crater formation
cutaneous capillary
   formation
cyclops formation
dentinoid formation
echo formation
excessive callus formation
exostosis formation

formation (*continued*)
- extracapillary crescent formation
- false channel formation
- fistular formation
- fluid formation
- gallstone formation
- gender identity formation
- germinal center formation
- Gothic arch formation
- hemostatic plug formation
- heterotopic bone formation
- identity formation
- ileostomy formation
- image formation
- impulse formation
- inflammatory pseudotumor formation
- intramembranous formation
- keloid formation
- kerion formation
- ketone body formation
- knot formation
- lappet formation
- localized plaque formation
- mesencephalic reticular formation
- micelle formation
- midbrain reticular formation
- neocartilage formation
- neointima formation
- new bone formation
- osteophyte formation
- pannus formation
- paramedian pontine reticular formation
- periosteal new bone formation
- pontine paramedian reticular formation
- posterior synechia formation
- procallus formation
- pseudoaneurysm formation
- pseudocyst formation
- pseudojoint formation
- pseudopod formation
- reaction formation
- reticular formation
- root formation
- rouleaux formation
- sac formation
- scar formation

formation (*continued*)
- sequestrum formation
- seroma formation
- somite formation
- sparsity of bone formation
- spikelike formation
- spore formation
- spur formation
- star formation
- stone granuloma formation
- stricture formation
- struvite crystal formation
- symptom formation
- synechia formation
- thrombus formation
- trellis formation
- twin formation
- valve formation
- web formation

formation of fistula
Formatray mandibular splint
formed nonirrigating cystotome
Formex barium catheter
FormFlex lens
FormFlex lens loop
forming wires
formocresol pulpotomy
forniceal invasion
fornix (*pl.* fornices)
- body of fornix
- cerebral fornix
- commissure of fornix
- conjunctival fornix
- crus of fornix
- lateral fornix
- pillar of fornix
- superior fornix
- vaginal fornix

fornix approach
fornix cerebri
fornix conjunctivae
fornix longus of Forel
fornix of superior conjunctiva
fornix pharyngis
fornix sacci lacrimalis
fornix-based conjunctival flap
fornix-based flap
Foroblique bronchoscope
Foroblique bronchoscopic telescope
Foroblique cystoscope
Foroblique cystourethroscope

Foroblique endoscope
Foroblique esophagoscope
Foroblique fiberoptic
     esophagoscope
Foroblique lens
Foroblique panendoscope
Foroblique resectoscope
Foroblique telescope
Forrester brace
Forrester cervical collar brace
Forrester clamp
Forrester collar
Forrester head halter
Forrester head splint
Forrester splint
Forrester-Brown head halter
Forschheimer spots
Forster (see Foerster)
Förster (see Foerster)
Fort bougie
Fort urethral bougie
FortaDerm dressing
FortaGen mesh
Forte instrument
Fortin finger test
Fortuna syringe
forward bending
forward displacement
forward flexion
forward mandibular distraction
forward masking
forward movement
forward subluxation
forward triangle technique
forward-bending maneuver
forward-cutting knife
forward-grasping forceps
forwarding probe
forward-viewing endoscope
forward-viewing scope
Fosler splint
Fosnaugh nail biopsy
Foss anterior resection clamp
Foss bifid gallbladder retractor
Foss bifid retractor
Foss biliary retractor
Foss cardiovascular clamp
Foss cardiovascular forceps
Foss clamp
Foss clamp forceps
Foss forceps
Foss gallbladder retractor

Foss intestinal clamp
Foss intestinal clamp forceps
Foss retractor
fossa (pl. fossae)
   amygdaloid fossa
   antecubital fossa
   anterior cranial fossa
   articular surface of
        mandibular fossa
   axillary fossa
   Bichat fossa
   Biesiadecki fossa
   Broesike fossa
   canine fossa
   central fossa
   cerebral fossa
   Claudius fossa
   conchal fossa
   condylar fossa
   condyloid fossa
   coronoid fossa
   cranial fossa
   crural fossa
   Cruveilhier fossa
   cubital fossa
   digastric fossa
   distal fossa
   distal triangular fossa (DTF)
   duodenal fossa
   duodenojejunal fossa
   elliptical scaphoid fossa
   epigastric fossa
   ethmoidal fossa
   femoral fossa
   floccular fossa
   fusiform fossa
   gallbladder fossa
   Gerdy hyoid fossa
   glenoid fossa
   greater supraclavicular fossa
   Gruber-Landzert fossa
   Hartmann fossa
   hepatic fossa
   hyaloid fossa
   hypophyseal fossa
   iliac fossa
   iliacosubfascial fossa
   iliopectineal fossa
   incisive fossa
   inferior duodenal fossa
   infraclavicular fossa
   infraduodenal fossa

fossa (*continued*)
  infraspinous fossa
  infratemporal fossa
  inguinal fossa
  innominate fossa
  intercondylar fossa
  intercondyloid fossa
  interpeduncular fossa
  intrabulbar fossa
  ischioanal fossa
  ischiorectal fossa
  Jobert de Lamballe fossa
  Jonnesco fossa
  jugular fossa
  juxta-auricular fossa
  lacrimal fossa
  lacrimal sac fossa
  Landzert fossa
  lateral bulbar fossa
  lateral inguinal fossa
  lesser supraclavicular fossa
  lingual fossa (LF)
  Malgaigne fossa
  mandibular fossa
  mastoid fossa
  maxillary fossa
  medial inguinal fossa
  Merkel fossa
  mesentericoparietal fossa
  mesiolingual fossa (MLF)
  middle cranial fossa
  middle fossa
  Mohrenheim fossa
  Morgagni fossa
  mylohyoid fossa
  nasal fossa
  navicular fossa
  obturator fossa
  Ogura fossa
  olecranon fossa
  omoclavicular fossa
  oral fossa
  ovarian fossa
  paraduodenal fossa
  parajejunal fossa
  pararectal fossa
  paravesical fossa
  pelvic fossa
  petrosal fossa
  piriform fossa
  pituitary fossa
  popliteal fossa

fossa (*continued*)
  posterior cranial fossa
  posterior fossa
  preauricular fossa
  prostatic fossa
  pterygoid fossa
  pterygomaxillary fossa
  pterygopalatine fossa
  radial fossa
  radius fossa
  renal fossa
  retroduodenal fossa
  retromandibular fossa
  retromolar fossa
  rhomboid fossa
  Rosenmueller fossa
  saccular fossa
  scaphoid fossa
  sigmoid fossa
  sphenomaxillary fossa
  splenic fossa
  subarcuate fossa
  subcecal fossa
  subinguinal fossa
  sublingual fossa
  submandibular fossa
  submaxillary fossa
  subpyramidal fossa
  subscapular fossa
  subsigmoid fossa
  superior duodenal fossa
  supraclavicular fossa
  supramastoid fossa
  supraspinatus fossa
  supraspinous fossa
  suprasternal fossa
  supratonsillar fossa
  supravesical fossa
  sylvian fossa
  temporal fossa
  temporal-pterygomaxillary
    fossa
  temporomandibular joint
    fossa
  tibiofemoral fossa
  tonsillar fossa
  Treitz fossa
  triangular fossa
  trochlear fossa
  umbilical fossa
  urachal fossa
  Velpeau fossa

fossa (*continued*)
  vermian fossa
  Waldeyer fossa
  zygomatic fossa
fossa curet
fossa navicularis auriculae
fossa of anthelix
fossa of lacrimal gland
fossa of lacrimal sac
fossa of Rosenmueller
fossa triangularis auriculae
fossula (*pl.* fossulae)
Foster bed
Foster defibrillator
Foster fracture frame
Foster frame
Foster needle holder
Foster scissors
Foster snare
Foster snare enucleator
Foster sutures
Foster turning frame
Foster-Ballenger forceps
Foster-Ballenger nasal speculum
Foster-Ballenger speculum
Foster-Gillies needle holder
Fothergill operation
Fothergill stitch
Fothergill sutures
Fothergill-Donald operation
Fothergill-Hunter operation
Fothergill-Shaw operation
Fotofil dental restorative
  material
Fotona Novalis ER:YAG laser
Fotona Novalis R ruby laser
Foucher epiphysial injury
  classification
Fould entropion operation
Fould operation
Fouli tourniquet
foul-smelling amniotic fluid
fountain decussation
fountain decussation of Meynert
Fountain design prosthesis
Fountain infusion catheter
fountain syringe
fourchette
Fourier transform
Fourier-acquired steady-state
  technique (FAST)
Fournier disease

Fournier gangrene
Fournier teeth
Fournier test
Fournier tip
FOV (field of vision)
fovea (*pl.* foveae)
  pterygoid fovea
  sublingual fovea
  submandibular fovea
  superior fovea
fovea ethmoidalis
fovea nuchae
fovea of condyloid process
foveal ligament
foveal vision
foveated chest
foveolar gastric mucosa
foveolar reflex
Foville tract
Fowler angular incision
Fowler double-end curet
Fowler dressing
Fowler incision
Fowler maneuver
Fowler operation
Fowler position
Fowler procedure for
  boutonnière deformity
Fowler self-retaining retractor
Fowler sound
Fowler technique
Fowler thoracoplasty
Fowler urethral sound
Fowler-Murphy treatment
Fowler-Philip approach
Fowler-Philip incision
Fowler-Stephens maneuver
Fowler-Stephens orchiopexy
Fowler-Stephens procedure
Fowler-Weir incision
Fowler-Zollner knife
Fowles dislocation technique
Fowles open reduction
Fowles technique
Fox aluminum eye shield
Fox balloon
Fox bipolar electrocautery
  forceps
Fox bipolar forceps
Fox blepharoplasty
Fox cartilage forceps
Fox clavicle splint

Fox clavicular splint
Fox conformer
Fox curet
Fox dermal curet
Fox entropion operation
Fox eye conformer
Fox eye implant
Fox eye shield
Fox eye speculum
Fox eyelid implant
Fox graft
Fox hydrostatic irrigator
Fox I&A unit
Fox implant
Fox internal fixation device
Fox irrigator
Fox operation
Fox postnasal balloon
Fox prosthesis
Fox scissors
Fox speculum
Fox sphere implant
Fox spherical eye implant
Fox splint
Fox tissue forceps
Fox wrench
Fox-Blazina knee procedure
Fox-Blazina prosthesis
FPB (femoral-popliteal bypass)
FPB (flexor pollicis brevis)
FPL (flexor pollicis longus)
FPL muscle
FPL tendon
fps (frames per second)
Frackelton fascial needle
Frackelton needle
Frackelton wire threader
fraction fever
fractional anesthesia
fractional area change (FAC)
fractional biopsy
fractional culture
fractional curettage
fractional D&C (fractional
    dilatation and curettage)
fractional dilation and
    curettage
fractional epidural anesthesia
fractional spinal anesthesia
fractional sterilization
fractionate and redistribute
    facial fat

fractionated external beam
    irradiation
fractionated high-dose rate
fractionated radiation therapy
fractionated radiotherapy
fractionation
  dose fractionation
fractionation rate
fractionation with
    chemotherapy
fractionation without
    chemotherapy
Fractomed splint
Fractura Flex bandage
Fractura Flex cast
Fractura Flex elastic bandage
fracture
  2-part fracture
  3-part fracture
  4-part fracture
  4th carpometacarpal joint
    fracture
  5th metatarsal bone fracture
  abduction-external rotation
    fracture
  acetabular rim fracture
  acute fracture
  agenetic fracture
  alveolar process fracture
  alveolar socket wall fracture
  anatomic fracture
  Anderson-Hutchins unstable
    tibial shaft fracture
  angulation fracture
  angulated fracture
  ankle mortise fracture
  anterior column fracture
  anterior cranial fossa
    fracture
  anterior fracture
  anterolateral compression
    fracture
  apex fracture
  apophyseal fracture
  apophysial fracture
  arch fracture
  articular fracture
  articular mass separation
    fracture
  articular pillar fracture
  Atkin epiphysial fracture
  atlantal fracture

fracture (*continued*)

atlas-axis combination fracture
atrophic fracture
aviator's fracture
avulsion chip fracture
avulsion fracture
axial loading fracture
axis fracture
axis-atlas fracture
backfire fracture
banana fracture
Bankart fracture
Barton fracture
Barton-Smith fracture
basal neck fracture
basal skull fracture
baseball finger fracture
basicervical fracture
basilar femoral neck fracture
basilar fracture
basilar skull fracture
beak fracture
bedroom fracture
bending fracture
Bennell fracture
Bennett comminuted fracture
Bennett fracture
bent fracture
bicondylar T-shaped fracture
bicondylar Y-shaped fracture
bicycle spoke fracture
bilateral condylar fracture
bimalleolar ankle fracture
bimalleolar fracture
birth fracture
blow-in fracture
blow-out fracture
boot-top fracture
Bosworth fracture
both-bone fracture
both-column fracture
bowing fracture
bowing of fracture
boxer's fracture
bronchial fracture
bucket-handle fracture
buckle fracture
bumper fracture
bumper-fender fracture
bunk-bed fracture

fracture (*continued*)

Burkhalter-Reyes method of phalangeal fracture
burst fracture
bursting fracture
butterfly fracture
buttonhole fracture
calcaneal avulsion fracture
calcaneal displaced fracture
capillary fracture
capitate fracture
capitellar fracture
carpal bone stress fracture
carpal fracture
carpometacarpal joint fracture
cartwheel fracture
cementum fracture
central fracture
cephalomedullary nail fracture
cerebral palsy pathological fracture
cervical spine fracture
cervicotrochanteric displaced fracture
Chance fracture
Chance lumbar spine fracture
Chance vertebral fracture
Chaput fracture
chauffeur's fracture
Chiene test for femoral neck fracture
chip fracture
chiropractic treatment of fracture
chisel fracture
chondral fracture
Chopart fracture
circumferential fracture
clavicular birth fracture
clay-shoveler's fracture
cleavage fracture
closed diaphyseal fracture
closed fracture
closed reduction of fracture
closed skull fracture
closed-break fracture
coccyx fracture
Colles fracture
combined flexion-distraction injury and burst fracture

fracture (*continued*)

combined radial-ulnar-humeral fracture
comminuted fracture
comminuted intraarticular fracture
comminuted orbital fracture
comminuted skull fracture
complete fracture
complex fracture
complex simple fracture
complicated fracture
composite fracture
compound comminuted fracture
compound fracture
compound skull fracture
compressed fracture
compression fracture
condylar femoral fracture
condylar fracture
condylar process fracture
congenital fracture
contrecoup fracture
coracoid fracture
corner fracture
coronal split fracture
coronoid process fracture
cortical fracture
Cotton ankle fracture
Cotton fracture
cough fracture
crack fracture
cranial fracture
craniofacial disjunction fracture
crown fracture
crown-root fracture
crush fracture
crushed eggshell fracture
crushing fracture
Danis-Weber fracture
dashboard fracture
de Quervain fracture
debridement of compound skull fracture
deferred fracture
Delbet splint for heel fracture
dens fracture
dentate fracture
dentoalveolar fracture
depressed fracture

fracture (*continued*)

depressed skull fracture
depression fracture
derby hat fracture
Desault fracture
Descot fracture
diacondylar fracture
diametric pelvic fracture
diaphysial fracture
diastatic fracture
diastatic skull fracture
dicondylar fracture
die punch fracture
direct fracture
dishpan fracture
dislocation fracture
displaced fracture
displaced malar fracture
displaced zygomatic fracture
displacement of fracture
distal femoral epiphysial fracture
distal humeral fracture
distal radial fracture
distraction of fracture
dog-leg fracture
dome fracture
donor radius fracture
double fracture
Dupuytren fracture
Duverney fracture
dyscrasic fracture
elbow fracture
elementary fracture
elevation of skull fracture
en coin fracture
en rave fracture
enamel fracture
endocrine fracture
epicondylar avulsion fracture
epiphyseal fracture
epiphysial growth plate fracture
epiphysial slip fracture
epiphysial tibial fracture
Essex-Lopresti fracture
Essex-Lopresti joint depression fracture
explosion fracture
expressed skull fracture
extension teardrop fracture
external orbital fracture

fracture (*continued*)

extra-articular fracture
extracapsular fracture
extraoctave fracture
facial fracture
fat fracture
fatigue fracture
femoral diaphyseal fracture
femoral fracture
femoral intertrochanteric
    fracture
femoral neck fracture
femoral shaft fracture
femoral supracondylar
    fracture
fender fracture
fetal bone fracture
fibular fracture
fighter fracture
finger fracture
fingertip fracture
first carpometacarpal joint
    fracture
fishmouth fracture
fissure fracture
fissured fracture
flexion teardrop fracture
floor fracture
forearm fracture
frontal sinus fracture
fronto-orbitonasoethmoidal
    fracture
Frykman classification of
    hand fractures
Frykman fracture
Gaenslen fracture
Galeazzi fracture
gamekeeper's thumb fracture
Garden femoral neck
    fracture
glabellar fracture
glenoid rim fracture
Gosselin fracture
greater trochanteric femoral
    fracture
greater tuberosity fracture
greenstick fracture
greenstick LeFort fracture
grenade-thrower fracture
growing fracture
Guerin fracture
Guggenheim fracture

fracture (*continued*)

gunshot fracture
Gustilo scoring for open
    fractures (types II, IIIA, IIIB,
    IIIC)
Gustilo-Anderson open
    clavicular fracture
gutter fracture
Hahn-Steinthal fracture
hairline fracture
hamate tail fracture
hangman's fracture
Hawkins fracture
hay baler's fracture
head-splitting humeral
    fracture
healed fracture
healing fracture
healing of fracture
hemicondylar fracture
hemi-LeFort fracture (I, II,
    etc.)
Henderson fracture
Hermodsson fracture
hickory-stick fracture
high-energy fracture
Hill-Sachs fracture
hip fracture
hockey-stick fracture
Hoffa fracture
Hohl fracture
Holstein-Lewis fracture
hoop stress fracture
horizontal fracture
horizontal maxillary fracture
horizontal oblique fracture
humeral fracture
humeral head-splitting
    fracture
humeral physeal fracture
humeral shaft fracture
humeral supracondylar
    fracture
Hutchinson fracture
hyoid bone fracture
iatrogenic fracture
ice skater fracture
ileofemoral wing fracture
impacted fracture
implant fracture
impression fracture
impure blow-out fracture

fracture (*continued*)
    incomplete compound
        fracture
    incomplete fracture
    indirect fracture
    inflammatory fracture
    infraction fracture
    infraorbital fracture
    insufficiency fracture
    intercondylar femoral fracture
    intercondylar fracture
    intercondylar humeral
        fracture
    intercondylar tibial fracture
    internal fixation of fracture
    interperiosteal fracture
    intertrochanteric femoral
        fracture
    intertrochanteric 4-part
        fracture
    intertrochanteric fracture
    intra-articular fracture
    intra-articular proximal tibial
        fracture
    intracapsular fracture
    intraoperative fracture
    intraorbital fracture
    intraperiosteal fracture
    intraperitoneal fracture
    intrauterine fracture
    inverted-Y fracture
    ipsilateral acetabular fracture
    ipsilateral femoral neck
        fracture
    ipsilateral femoral shaft
        fracture
    ipsilateral pelvic fracture
    ipsilateral tibial fracture
    irreducible fracture
    jaw fracture
    Jefferson fracture
    joint depression fracture
    Jones fracture
    juxtacortical fracture
    Key-Conwell classification of
        pelvic fracture
    knee fracture
    Knight and North
        classification of malar
        fractures (groups I-VI)
    Kocher fracture
    Kocher-Lorenz fracture

fracture (*continued*)
    laminar fracture
    lap seatbelt fracture
    laryngeal cartilage fracture
    lateral condylar humeral
        fracture
    lateral mass fracture
    Laugier fracture
    lead-pipe fracture
    LeFort classification of
        maxillary fractures (I, II, III)
    LeFort fibular fracture
    LeFort mandibular fracture
    LeFort-Wagstaffe fracture
    lesser trochanter fracture
    leverage fracture
    line of fracture
    linear fracture
    linear skull fracture
    Lisfranc foot fracture
    Lisfranc fracture
    long bone fracture
    longitudinal fracture
    loose fracture
    lorry-driver fracture
    low lumbar spine fracture
    low-energy fracture
    lower frontal bone fracture
    lower-extremity fracture
    lumbar spine burst fracture
    lumbosacral junction fracture
    lunate fracture
    Maisonneuve fibular fracture
    Maisonneuve fracture
    major fracture
    malar complex fracture
    malar fracture
    Malgaigne fracture
    Malgaigne pelvic fracture
    malleolar fracture
    mallet fracture
    malunion of fracture
    malunited calcaneus fracture
    malunited forearm fracture
    malunited fracture
    malunited radial fracture
    mandibular body fracture
    mandibular condyle fracture
    mandibular ramus fracture
    mandibular symphysis
        fracture
    manipulation of fracture

fracture (*continued*)

manual reduction of fracture
march fracture
marginal fracture
marginal ridge fracture
Martin screw for hip fracture
maternal fracture
maxillary fracture
maxillofacial fracture
medial orbital wall fracture
mesiodistal fracture
metacarpal fracture
metacarpal head fracture
metacarpal neck fracture
metacarpal shaft fracture
metaphysial tibial fracture
metatarsal fracture
midface fracture
midfacial fracture
midfoot fracture
midshaft fracture
milkman fracture
minimally displaced fracture
missed fracture
Moberg-Gedda fracture
molar tooth fracture
monomalleolar ankle fracture
Monteggia forearm fracture
Monteggia fracture
Montercaux ankle fracture
Montercaux fracture
Moore fracture
Mouchet fracture
multangular ridge fracture
multilevel fracture
multiple fractures
multiray fracture
nasal fracture
nasal-septal fracture
nasoethmoidal fracture
nasoethmoidal-orbital fracture
nasomaxillary fracture
naso-orbital fracture
navicular fracture
naviculocapitate fracture
neck fracture
Neer classification of shoulder
    fractures
neoplastic fracture
neurogenic fracture
neuropathic fracture
nightstick fracture

fracture (*continued*)

nonarticular distal radial
    fracture
noncomminuted fracture
noncontiguous fracture
nondisplaced crack fracture
nondisplaced fracture
nonphyseal fracture
nonrotational burst fracture
nonunion fracture
nonunion of fracture
nonunited fracture
nutcracker fracture
oblique fracture
obturator avulsion fracture
occipital condyle fracture
occipital fracture
occult fracture
occult scaphoid fracture
odontoid condyle fracture
odontoid fracture
odontoid neck fracture
Ogden classification of
    fractures
old fracture
olecranon fracture
one-part fracture
open fracture
open reduction of fracture
open skull fracture
open-book fracture
orbital blow-in fracture
orbital blow-out fracture
orbital floor fracture
orbital fracture
orbital rim fracture
orbital roof fracture
orbital wall fracture
osteochondral slice fracture
osteoporotic compression
    fracture
osteoporotic fracture
outlet strut fracture
pacemaker lead fracture
Pais fracture
palatal alveolar fracture
palate fracture
pancraniomaxillofacial
    fracture
panfacial fracture
parasymphyseal fracture
paratrooper fracture

fracture (*continued*)
parry fracture
partial union of fracture
patellar sleeve fracture
Patey fracture
pathologic compression
    fracture
pathologic fracture
pathologic fracture pedicle
    fracture
Pauwels fracture
pelvic avulsion fracture
pelvic fracture
pelvic ring fractures
pelvic straddle fracture
penetrating fracture
penetration fracture
PER fracture (pronation,
    external rotation fracture)
perforating fracture
periarticular fracture
perilunate fracture
periprosthetic fracture
peritrochanteric fracture
pertrochanteric fracture
petrous pyramid fracture
phalangeal diaphysial fracture
phalangeal fracture
physeal fracture
Piedmont fracture
pillion fracture
pillow fracture
pilon ankle fracture
pilon fracture
ping-pong fracture
Pipkin fracture
pisiform fracture
plafond fracture
plaque fracture
plastic bowing fracture
plateau fracture
Poland classification of
    fractures
pond fracture
porcelain fracture
Posada fracture
posterior arch fracture
posterior bow femoral
    fracture
posterior column fracture
posterior element fracture
posterior fracture

fracture (*continued*)
posterior ring fracture
posterior wall fracture
postirradiation fracture
postoperative fracture
Pott ankle fracture
Pott fracture
pressure fracture
profundus artery fracture
pronation, external rotation
    fracture (PER fracture)
pronation-abduction fracture
pronation-eversion fracture
proper alignment and
    apposition of fracture
prosthetic fracture
proximal femoral fracture
proximal humeral fracture
proximal tibial metaphysial
    fracture
pure blow-out fracture
pylon fracture
pyramidal fracture
Quervain fracture
radial head fracture
radial neck fracture
radial styloid fracture
realigned fracture
reduced fracture
reduction of fracture
refracture following fracture
resecting fracture
reverse Barton fracture
reverse Bennett fracture
reverse Colles fracture
reverse Monteggia fracture
reverse Bennett fracture
Richards external fixation
    device for fractures
ring fracture
ring-disrupting fracture
Riseborough-Radin
    classification of humeral
    fractures
Rolando fracture
roof fracture
root fracture
rotation fracture
rotational burst fracture
sacral fracture
sacroiliac fracture
sacrum fracture

fracture (*continued*)

sagittal slice fracture
Salter fracture (I-VI)
Salter-Harris fracture (I-IV)
Sarmiento osteotomy for
    intertrochanteric fracture
scaphoid fracture
Schatzker fracture
scotty-dog fracture
seatbelt fracture
secondary fracture
Secund fracture
segmental fracture
segmented fracture
Segond fracture
Seinsheimer classification of
    subtrochanteric fractures
sentinel spinous process
    fracture
septal fracture
SER fracture (supination,
    external rotation fracture)
SER-IV fracture
SEX fracture (supination,
    external rotation fracture)
shaft fracture
shear fracture
Shepherd fracture
short oblique fracture
shoveler's fracture
sideswipe elbow fracture
sideswipe fracture
silver-fork fracture
simple comminuted fracture
simple fracture
simple skull fracture
single fracture
skier fracture
Skillern fracture
skull fracture
sleeve fracture
slice fracture
slot fracture
Smith fracture
sourcil fracture
spinal compression fracture
spinal fracture
spine fracture
spinous process fracture
spiral fracture
spiral oblique fracture
splintered fracture

fracture (*continued*)

split fracture
split-heel fracture
splitting fracture
spontaneous fracture
sprain fracture
sprinter's fracture
stable burst fracture
stable fracture
stairstep fracture
stellate fracture
stellate skull fracture
step-off fracture
Stieda fracture
straddle fracture
strain fracture
stress fracture
strut fracture
subcapital fracture
subcutaneous fracture
subperiosteal fracture
subtrochanteric femoral
    fracture
subtrochanteric fracture
supination, external rotation
    fracture (SER fracture, SEX
    fracture)
supination-adduction fracture
supination-eversion fracture
supination-external rotation
    fracture
supracondylar fracture
supracondylar humeral
    fracture
supracondylar Y-shaped
    fracture
supraorbital fracture
surgical neck fracture
symphyseal fracture
T fracture
talar avulsion fracture
talar neck fracture
talar osteochondral fracture
tarsal bone fracture
T-condylar fracture
teacup fracture
teardrop fracture
telescoping septal fracture
temporal bone fracture
tension fracture
terminal tuft fracture
testis fracture

fracture (*continued*)

thoracic spine fracture
thoracolumbar burst fracture
thoracolumbar spine fracture
through-and-through fracture
thrower fracture
thumb fracture
tibial bending fracture
tibial condyle fracture
tibial diaphysial fracture
tibial fracture
tibial open fracture
tibial plafond fracture
tibial plateau fracture
tibial shaft fracture
tibial triplane fracture
tibial tuberosity fracture
Tile-Pennal classification of
  pelvic ring fractures
Tillaux-Chaput fracture
Tillaux-Kleiger fracture
toddler fracture
tongue fracture
tonus fracture
tooth fracture
torsion fracture
torsional fracture
torus fracture
trabecular bone fracture
tracheal fracture
traction fracture
trampoline fracture
transcapitate fracture
transcervical femoral
  fracture
transcervical fracture
transchondral fracture
transcondylar fracture
transepiphyseal fracture
transhamate fracture
transiliac fracture
translational fracture
transsacral fracture
transscaphoid dislocation
  fracture
transscaphoid fracture
transtriquetral fracture
transverse comminuted
  fracture
transverse facial fracture
transverse fracture
transverse maxillary fracture

fracture (*continued*)

transversely oriented endplate
  compression fracture
trapezial fracture
trapezium fracture
transverse process fracture
traumatic fracture
Trillaux fracture
trimalar fracture
trimalleolar ankle fracture
trimalleolar fracture
triplane fracture
triplane tibial fracture
tripod fracture
triquetral fracture
Tronzo classification of
  trochanteric fractures
trophic fracture
T-shaped fracture
tuft fracture
type C pelvic ring fracture
type I, II, III, IIIA, IIIB, IIIC
  open fracture
ulnar fracture
uncinate process fracture
undisplaced fracture
unicondylar fracture
unilateral condylar fracture
unilateral fracture
unimalleolar fracture
unstable fracture
unstable zygomatic complex
  fracture
ununited fracture
vertebra plana fracture
vertebral body fracture
vertebral stable burst fracture
vertebral wedge compression
  fracture
vertical fracture
vertical oblique pattern
  fracture
vertical shear fracture
vertical tooth fracture
Volkmann fracture
wagon wheel fracture
Wagstaffe fracture
Walther fracture
Watson-Jones repair of ankle
  fracture
Weber classification of
  fractures

fracture (*continued*)
    wedge compression fracture
    wedge fracture
    wedge-shaped uncomminuted
        tibial plateau fracture
    western boot in open fracture
    Wilkin classification of radial
        neck fractures
    willow fracture
    Wilson fracture
    Winquist-Hansen classification
        of femoral fractures
    Y-shaped fracture
    Y-T fracture
    zygoma fracture
    zygomatic arch fracture
    zygomatic body fracture
    zygomatic complex fracture
    zygomatic maxillary complex
        fracture
    zygomaticomaxillary fracture
    zygomatico-orbital fracture
fracture alignment
fracture appliance (*see*
    appliance)
fracture at the rhinion
fracture band
fracture bar
fracture bed
fracture blister
fracture bowing
fracture bracing
fracture by contrecoup
fracture callus
fracture chip
fracture chisel
fracture classification
fracture disease
fracture dislocation
fracture en coin
fracture en rave
fracture fixation
fracture fixation device
fracture fragment
fracture fragments
fracture frame
fracture frame (*see* frame)
fracture fusion
fracture gap
fracture healing
fracture line
fracture medialization

fracture nail
fracture of bone
fracture of cartilage
fracture of hook of the hamate
fracture of superior orbital
    fissure
fracture position
fracture reduced
fracture reducing elevator
fracture reduction
fracture repair
fracture site
fracture splint
fracture stabilization
fracture table
fracture union
fracture with cross union
fracture with delayed union
fracture with malunion
fracture with nonunion
fractured bone
fracture-dislocation (*see also*
    fracture; dislocation)
    atlantoaxial fracture-
        dislocation
    Bennett fracture-dislocation
    carpometacarpal fracture-
        dislocation
    closed reduction of fracture-
        dislocation
    Galeazzi fracture-dislocation
    Lisfranc fracture-dislocation
    Monteggia fracture-dislocation
    open reduction of fracture-
        dislocation
    pedicolaminar fracture-
        dislocation
    perilunate fracture-dislocation
    posterior fracture-dislocation
    tarsometatarsal fracture-
        dislocation
    thoracolumbar spine fracture-
        dislocation
    tibial plateau fracture-
        dislocation
    transcapitate fracture-
        dislocation
    transhamate fracture-
        dislocation
    transtriquetral fracture-
        dislocation
    unstable fracture-dislocation

fracture-dislocation (*continued*)
  volar plate arthroplasty
    technique fracture-
    dislocation
fracture-dislocation reduction
fracturing the stricture
Fraenkel (*also* Fränkel)
Fraenkel appliance
Fraenkel cutting-tip forceps
Fraenkel double-articulated-tip
  forceps
Fraenkel esophagoscopy forceps
Fraenkel exercises
Fraenkel forceps
Fraenkel headband
Fraenkel laryngeal forceps
Fraenkel line
Fraenkel neurologic deficit
  classification
Fraenkel sign
Fraenkel sinus probe
Fraenkel speculum
Fraenkel tampon forceps
Fraenkel white line
Fragen anterior commissure
  microlaryngoscope
Fragen carrier
Fragen laryngoscope
Fragen laryngoscope fiberoptic
  light
Fragen scope
fragility
fragmatic buttress
fragmatome
  CooperVision fragmatome
  Fill-Hess fragmatome
  Girard fragmatome
fragmatome flute syringe
fragmatome tip
fragmatome tip with ultrasound
  spatula
fragment
  articular fragment
  avascular fragment
  avulsed fragment
  bone fragment
  bony fragment
  butterfly fracture fragment
  butterfly fragment
  capital fragment
  catheter fragment
  caudal fragment

fragment (*continued*)
  cephalad fragment
  chondral fragment
  clavicular fracture fragment
  condylar fragment
  cortical fragment
  decidual fragment
  disk fragment
  distal fragment
  extruded disk fragment
  footplate fragments
  fracture fragment
  free disk fragment
  free-floating cartilaginous
    fragment
  glistening fragments
  hinged fragment
  Hoskins razor blade fragment
  hypervascular fragment
  loose fragment
  lower fragment
  metallic fragment
  osteochondral fragment
  placental fragment
  realignment of fracture
    fragments
  removal of placental
    fragments
  residual fragment
  retained placental fragment
  shell fragment
  shrapnel fragment
  sternal fragment
  trapdoor fragment
  tuberosity fragment
  wedge-shaped uncomminuted
    fragment
fragment forceps
fragment of bone
fragment of placenta
fragment pared with motor saw
fragment splintered to pieces
fragment wound
fragmentary filling
fragmentation
  elastic-fiber fragmentation
  electrohydraulic fragmentation
  graft fragmentation
  laser-induced fragmentation
  multiple fragmentations
  stone fragmentation
  ultrasonic fragmentation

fragmentation probe
fragmentation process
fragmentation/aspiration
    handpiece
Frahur cartilage clamp
Frahur clamp
Frahur scissors
Fraley syndrome
frameless stereotactic guidance
Framer finger extension bow
Framer splint
Framer tendon passer
Framer tendon-passing needle
frames per second (fps)
framework
    implant framework
    neural crest mesenchymal
        connective tissue
        framework
    osteocartilaginous framework
Francer porcelain powder
Franceschetti coreoplasty
    operation
Franceschetti corepraxy
    operation
Franceschetti corneal trephine
Franceschetti deviation
    operation
Franceschetti keratoplasty
Franceschetti pupil deviation
    operation
Franceschetti syndrome
Franceschetti trephine
Franceschetti-Jadassohn
    syndrome
Franceschetti-type freeblade
Francis chalazion forceps
Francis forceps
Francis knife spud
Francis spud
Francis spud chalazion forceps
Francis-Gray forceps
Francis-Gray wire crimper
Francke needle
Franco operation
Franco triflange ventilation
    tube
Frangenheim biopsy punch
    forceps
Frangenheim forceps
Frangenheim hook forceps
Frangenheim hook punch

Frangenheim hook-punch
    forceps
Frangenheim laparoscope
Frangenheim-Goebell-Stoeckel
    fascia lata suspension
frank breech
frank breech presentation
frank dislocation
frank fronds
Frank gastrostomy
frank hemorrhage
Frank intrabiliary rupture
Frank operation
frank perforation
Frank permanent gastrotomy
    technique
Frank procedure
frank prolapse
Frank sign
Frank technique of dilation
Frank XYZ orthogonal lead
Franke syndrome
Franke tabes operation
Franke technique
Franke triad
Fränkel (see Fraenkel)
Fraenkel (also Fränkel)
Fraenkel appliance
Fraenkel cutting-tip forceps
Fraenkel esophagoscopy forceps
Fraenkel laryngeal forceps
Fraenkel neurologic deficit
    classification
Fraenkel speculum
Fraenkel tampon forceps
Fraenkel white line
Frankenhauser ganglion
Frankfeldt diathermy snare
Frankfeldt grasping forceps
Frankfeldt hemorrhoidal needle
Frankfeldt needle
Frankfeldt rectal snare
Frankfeldt sigmoidoscope
Frankfeldt snare
Frankfort horizontal light line
Frankfort horizontal line
Frankfort horizontal plane
Frankfort mandibular angle
    (FMA)
Frankfort mandibular incision
    angle (FMIA)
Frankfort mandibular plane

Franklin liver puncture needle
Franklin malleable retractor
Franklin rectractor
Franklin-Silverman biopsy
  cannula
Franklin-Silverman biopsy
  needle
Franklin-Silverman cannula
Franklin-Silverman curet
Franklin-Silverman prostatic
  biopsy needle
Frank-Starling curve
Franseen liver biopsy needle
Franseen rectal curet
Franz abdominal retractor
Franz monophasic action
  potential catheter
Franzen needle guide
Franz-O'Rahilly classification
frappage therapy
Fraser decompressor
Fraser depressor
Fraser forceps
Fraser Harlake respirometer
Fraser syndrome
Frater intracardiac retractor
Frater retractor
Frater sutures
Fraunfelder no-touch technique
Fraunhofer lines
Frazier aspirating tube
Frazier brain suction tube
Frazier brain-exploring cannula
Frazier brain-exploring trocar
Frazier Britetrac nasal suction
  tube
Frazier cannula
Frazier cerebral retractor
Frazier cordotomy hook
Frazier cordotomy knife
Frazier dural elevator
Frazier dural guide
Frazier dural hook
Frazier dural scissors
Frazier dural separator
Frazier elevator
Frazier fiberoptic suction tube
Frazier hook
Frazier incision
Frazier insulated suction tube
Frazier knife
Frazier laminectomy retractor

Frazier lighted retractor
Frazier modified suction tube
Frazier nasal suction tip
Frazier nasal suction tube
Frazier needle
Frazier nerve hook
Frazier operation
Frazier osteotome
Frazier pituitary capsulectomy
  knife
Frazier retractor
Frazier scissors
Frazier separator
Frazier skin hook
Frazier straight suction tube
Frazier stylet
Frazier suction
Frazier suction elevator
Frazier suction tip
Frazier suction tip aspirator
Frazier suction tube
Frazier suction tube obturator
Frazier trocar
Frazier tube
Frazier ventricular cannula
Frazier ventricular needle
Frazier-Adson clamp
Frazier-Adson osteoplastic clamp
Frazier-Adson osteoplastic flap
  clamp
Frazier-Fay retractor
Frazier-Ferguson aspirating tube
Frazier-Ferguson ear suction
  tube
Frazier-Paparella mastoid suction
  tube
Frazier-Paparella mastoid tube
Frazier-Paparella suction tube
Frazier-Paparella tube
Frazier-Sachs clamp
Frazier-Spiller operation
Frechet extended scalp
  reduction
Freckner operation
Fred Thompson broach
Frederick needle
Frederick pneumothoracic
  needle
Frederick pneumothorax needle
Frederick-Miller tube
Fredet-Ramstedt operation
Fredet-Ramstedt pyloromyotomy

Fredricks mammary prosthesis
Fredricks mammary support
Fredrickson
    hyperlipoproteinemia
    classification
Fredrickson-Levy-Lees
    classification
free abdominal air
free air
free anterolateral thigh flap
free arterialized venous forearm
    flap
free autogenous
    corticocancellous iliac bone
    graft
free autogenous pearl fat graft
free band of colon
free body
free bone flap
free bone graft
free bone reconstruction
free composite flap
free composite graft
free cutaneous lateral arm flap
free cutaneous nerve graft
free dermal fat graft (FDFG)
free disk fragment
free expanded flap
free facial flap
free fasciocutaneous flap
free fat graft
free fibular harvest flap
free fillet extremity flap for
    reconstruction
free flap
free flap for burn scar revision
free flap procedure
free flap reconstruction
free flap vaginoplasty
free flow
free fluid
free forearm flap
free fragment disk
free fragment herniation
free gastric margin
free gingival margin
free gracilis muscle harvest
free gracilis muscle
    reconstruction
free graft
free groin flap
free groin transplant

free gum margin
free iliac bone crest flap
free implant
free induction decay
free induction signal
free jejunal graft
free latissimus dorsi flap
free ligature
free ligature sutures
free ligature suture technique
free mandibular movement
free margin of eyelid
free microsurgical flap
free microvascular flap
free muscle graft
free muscle transfer
free non-vascularized composite
    nail graft
free of disease
free of obstruction
free omental flap transfer
free peritoneal air
free posterior interosseous flap
free prosthesis
free radial forearm flap
free sensate flap
free sequential flap
free skin flap
free skin graft
free sponge
free temporal fascial flap
free temporal flap
free temporoparietal fascial flap
free tenotomy
free tie
free tissue transfer (FTT)
free tissue transfer
    reconstruction
free toe-to-finger hemipulp flap
free toe-to-fingertip
    neurovascular flap
free TRAM flap
free transplantation of nipple
free transverse rectus abdominis
    musculocutaneous flap
free vascularized flap
free-beam coagulation
free-body analysis
free-body spinal fusion
Freebody-Bendall-Taylor fusion
    technique
freed by blunt dissection

freed by sharp dissection
freed up
Freedom arthritis support
Freedom dental unit
Freedom external catheter
Freedom knife
Freedom stimulator
Freedom splint
Freedom catheter
Freedom palm guard
Freedom stent
Freedom thumb spica cast
Freedom T-tap leg bag kit
FreeDop portable Doppler unit
free-floating cartilaginous fragment
Free-Flow system prosthesis
Freegenol cement
free-hand allograft valve
free-hand knife
free-hand suturing technique
freeing of adhesions
freeing up of adhesions
freely mobile
freely movable
Freeman cannula
Freeman calcaneal fracture classification
Freeman capsular polisher
Freeman clamp
Freeman cookie-cutter areolar marker
Freeman facelift retractor
Freeman femoral component
Freeman leukotome
Freeman modular total hip prosthesis
Freeman operation
Freeman polisher
Freeman positioning cannula
Freeman punctum plug
Freeman resurfacing technique
Freeman retractor
Freeman rhytidectomy scissors
Freeman scissors
Freeman total hip replacement
Freeman transorbital leukotome
Freeman-Samuelson knee prosthesis
Freeman-Schepens scissors
Freeman-Sheldon syndrome

Freeman-Swanson knee prosthesis
Freemont spinal sphygmomanometer
Freenseen liver biopsy needle
Freenseen rectal curet
Freer bone chisel
Freer chisel
Freer dissection
Freer dissector
Freer double elevator
Freer double-end elevator
Freer double-ended elevator
Freer double-ended septum elevator
Freer double-pronged hook
Freer dural dissector
Freer dural retractor
Freer elevator
Freer elevator-dissector
Freer gouge
Freer hook
Freer knife
Freer lacrimal chisel
Freer mucosa knife
Freer nasal chisel
Freer nasal gouge
Freer nasal knife
Freer nasal spatula
Freer nasal submucous knife
Freer nasoseptal elevator
Freer periosteal elevator
Freer periosteotome
Freer retractor
Freer septal elevator
Freer septal forceps
Freer septal knife
Freer single-ended elevator
Freer skin hook
Freer skin retractor
Freer spatula
Freer submucous chisel
Freer submucous instrument
Freer submucous retractor
free-revascularized autograft
Freer-Gruenwald forceps
Freer-Gruenwald punch forceps
Freer-Ingal nasal knife
Freer-Ingal nasal submucous knife
Freer-Ingal septal knife
Freer-Ingal submucous knife

free-root insertion technique
Freer-Sachs dissector
free-skin patch graft
free-spinning probe
free-standing implant
free-standing single crown
free-standing stent
Freestyle aortic root
    bioprosthesis
Freestyle CAPD catheter adapter
Freestyle valve
free-tie sutures
free-toe transfer
Freeway catheter
Freeway speculum
Freeway-Graves speculum
freeze-dried allograft
freeze-dried bone allograft
freeze-dried bone graft
freeze-dried demineralized bone
    (FDDB)
freeze-dried graft
freeze drying
freezing point osmometer
Freezor cryocatheter
Freiberg cartilage knife
Freiberg disease
Freiberg hip retractor
Freiberg knife
Freiberg meniscectomy knife
Freiberg nerve root retractor
Freiberg retractor
Freiberg traction
Freiberg tractor
Freiburg biopsy set
Freiburg Injecttimer
Freiburg mediastinoscope
Freidenwald-Guyton sling
Freidenwald-Guyton snare
Freidrich-Ferguson retractor
Freimuth curet
Freimuth ear curet
Freitag stent
Frejka cast
Frejka hip pillow
Frejka jacket
Frejka orthosis
Frejka pillow
Frejka pillow splint
Frejka splint
Frejka traction
Frekatheter vena cava catheter

Frelex lens
fremitus
    friction fremitus
    pectoral fremitus
    pleural fremitus
    tactile fremitus
frena (*sing.* frenum)
French angiographic catheter
French bougie
French brain retractor
French Brown-Buerger cystoscope
French catheter
French catheter gauge
French catheter scale
French chest tube
French chisel
French Cope loop nephrostomy
    catheter
French curve out-of-plane
    catheter
French cystoscope
French dilator
French double-lumen catheter
French elbow osteotomy
French flap
French Foley catheter
French fracture technique
French Gesco catheter
French hook spatula
French in-plane guiding catheter
French Schneider catheter
French lacrimal dilator
French lacrimal probe
French lacrimal spatula
French lock
French MBIH catheter
French mushroom-tipped catheter
French needle
French needle holder
French operation
French pigtail nephrostomy
    catheter
French plane
French position
French red-rubber Robinson
    catheter
French retractor
French Robinson catheter
French rod bender
French SAL catheter
French scale for sizing tubular
    instruments

French shaft catheter
French sheath
French Silastic Foley catheter
French sizing of catheter
French skin flap operation
French sliding flap
French sound
French spring-eye needle
French S-shaped brain retractor
French S-shaped retractor
French steel sound
French stent
French supracondylar fracture
    operation
French sutures
French Swan-Ganz balloon
French Teflon pyeloureteral
    catheter
French tripolar His catheter
French, American, British
    staging of carcinoma (FAB)
French-Daid introducer
French-eye needle
French-eye needle holder
French-eye Vital needle holder
French-following metal sound
French-Hanks uterine dilator
French-Iglesias resectoscope
French-line abdominoplasty
French-McCarthy endoscope
French-McCarthy panendoscope
French-McRea dilator
French-pattern eye spatula
French-pattern forceps
French-pattern lacrimal probe
French-pattern osteotome
French-pattern raspatory
French-pattern spatula
French-Stern-McCarthy
    retractor
French-Wappler cystoscope
Frenckner curet
Frenckner-Stille curet
Frenckner-Stille punch
frenectomy
frenoplasty
frenotomy
Frenta enteral feeding bag
frenula (*sing.* frenulum)
frenuloplasty
frenulum (*pl.* frenula)
    lingual frenulum

frenulum epiglottidis
frenulum labii inferioris
frenulum labii superioris
frenulum linguae
frenulum of clitoris
frenulum of inferior lip
frenulum of lower lip
frenulum of penis
frenulum of superior lip
frenulum of tongue
frenulum of upper lip
frenum (*pl.* frena)
    labial frenum
    lingual frenum
frenum of tongue
Frenzel ear operating head
Frenzel lenses
Frenzel maneuver
frequency
    angular frequency
    defined frequency
    high frequency
    infrasonic frequency
    input frequency
    low frequency
    supersonic frequency
frequency doubled
        neodymium:yttrium-
        aluminum-garnet laser
frequency-difference
        interferential current
        therapy
Fresenius dialysis machine
Fresenius Euro-Collins kit
Fresenius filter
Fresgen frontal sinus probe
fresh autologous de-
        epithelialized dermis
fresh bleeding
fresh blood clot
fresh extrapelvic ovarian
        transplantation
fresh frozen allograft
fresh frozen plasma
Fresnel goggles
Fresnel lens
Fresnel lens pusher
Fresnel manipulating hook
Fresnel membrane
Fresnel prism
Fresnel zone plate
Freund anomaly

Freund hysterectomy
Freund operation
Frey eye implant
Frey syndrome
Frey tunneled eye implant
Freyer drain
Freyer operation
Freyer suprapubic drain
Frey-Freer bur
Frey-Sauerbruch rib shears
friability
friable cervix
friable clot
friable mucosa
friable tissue
friable vessel
Friatec implant
Friatec manual arthroscopy
    instrument
fricative sounds
Fricke arterial forceps
Fricke bandage
Fricke dressing
Fricke eyelid operation
Fricke flap
Fricke operation
Fricke scrotal dressing
Frickman I operation
Frickman II operation
friction burn
friction fremitus
friction knot
friction lock pin
friction rub
friction sound
friction trauma-associated
    leukoplakia
friction-fit adapter
friction-reduced segmented
    table
Friede operation
Friedenwald funduscope
Friedenwald operation
Friedenwald ophthalmoscope
Friedenwald ptosis operation
Friedenwald-Guyton operation
Friedewald approximation
Friedlander incision marker
Friedman bone rongeur
Friedman clip
Friedman elevator
Friedman hand-held Hruby lens

Friedman knife guide
Friedman olive-tip vein
    stripper
Friedman perineal retractor
Friedman manipulator
Friedman rasp
Friedman retractor
Friedman rongeur forceps
Friedman splint brace
Friedman sutures
Friedman tantalum clip
Friedman vaginal retractor
Friedman vein stripper
Friedman-Otis bougie
Friedman-Otis bougie à boule
Friedreich ataxia
Friedreich foot operation
Friedreich sign
Friedreich tabes
Friedrich clamp
Friedrich operation
Friedrich raspatory
Friedrich rib elevator
Friedrich-Ferguson retractor
Friedrich-Petz clamp
Friedrich-Petz machine resector
Friend aspirating tube
Friend catheter
Friend-Hebert catheter
Friesner ear knife
Friesner ear perforator
Friesner knife
Frigitronics colposcope
Frigitronics cryoextractor
Frigitronics cryophake
Frigitronics cryoprobe
Frigitronics cryostylet
Frigitronics cryosurgical unit
Frigitronics disposable
    cryosurgical stylet
Frigitronics freeze-thaw
    cryopexy probe
Frigitronics cryoextractor
Frigitronics probe
Frigitronics retinal probe unit
Frigitronics vitrector
Frimberger-Karpiel 12 o'clock
    papillotome
Frimberger-Karpiel 12 o'clock
    sphincterotome
fringe joint
Fritsch abdominal retractor

Fritsch catheter
Fritsch operation
Fritsch retractor
Fritsch uterine douche
Fritz aspirator
Fritz automatic drainage
    treatment unit
Fritz vitreous transplant needle
frog cortex remover
frog splint
frogleg position
frog-leg projection
frog-leg splint
frog-leg view
frog-legged position
froglike position
Froehlich syndrome
Frohm mouth gag
Frohse arcade
Froimson biceps procedure
Froimson procedure
Froimson splint
Froimson technique
Froimson-Oh repair
Frolova primary palatoplasty
Froment sign
Fromm triangle orthopaedic
    device
Frommel operation
Frommer dilator
frondlike filling defect
Fronet fasciotomy
front build-up eye implant
front wall needle
frontal abscess
frontal angle of parietal bone
frontal antrotomy
frontal antrum
frontal arteriovenous
    malformation
frontal artery
frontal belly of the
    occipitofrontal muscle
frontal bone advancement
frontal bone advancement with
    strip craniectomy
frontal bone flap
frontal bone resorption
frontal bone squama
frontal border
frontal bossing
frontal brachycephaly

frontal branch
frontal cephalocele
frontal cortical approach
frontal craniotomy
frontal crest
frontal diploic vein
frontal eminence
frontal fontanelle
frontal foramen
frontal furrow
frontal gyrectomy
frontal gyrus
frontal hamulus
frontal irrigation
frontal leads
frontal lift
frontal lisp
frontal lobe
frontal lobotomy
frontal margin
frontal mirror
frontal nerve
frontal notch
frontal ostium
frontal paranasal sinus
frontal plagiocephaly
frontal plane correction
frontal process of maxilla
frontal projection
frontal recess
frontal region
frontal release sign
frontal resorption
frontal segment
frontal sinus aperture
frontal sinus bougie
frontal sinus cannula
frontal sinus cavity
frontal sinus chisel
frontal sinus curet
frontal sinus dilator
frontal sinus fracture
frontal sinus growth
frontal sinus mucocele
frontal sinus operation
frontal sinus probe
frontal sinus rasp
frontal sinus septoplasty
frontal sinus wash tube
frontal sinusitis
frontal sinusotomy
frontal suture

frontal vein
frontal view
frontal zygomatic suture line
frontalis
    alopecia liminaris frontalis
    apertura sinus frontalis
    crista frontalis
    facies externa ossis frontalis
    facies interna ossis frontalis
    foramen cecum ossis frontalis
    galea frontalis
    gyrus frontalis
    hamulus frontalis
    spina frontalis
    spina nasalis ossis frontalis
    torus frontalis
frontalis hyperactivity
frontalis muscle
frontalis muscle paralysis
frontalis nerve
frontalis sling
frontalis sling procedure
frontalis sling technique
frontalis snare
frontalis suspension
front-entry guide
frontoanterior position
frontocaudal
frontocentral region
frontocranial
frontocranial remodeling
frontodextra posterior
frontodextra transversa
frontoethmoidal cephalocele
frontoethmoidal
        meningoencephalocele
frontoethmoidal
        sphenoidectomy
frontoethmoidal suture
frontogaleal flap
frontoglabellar wrinkle
frontolacrimal suture
frontolateral laryngectomy
frontomalar suture
frontomaxillary suture
frontomental diameter
frontonasal duct
frontonasal dysplasia
frontonasal process
frontonasal suture
fronto-occipital diameter
fronto-orbital advancement

fronto-orbital remodeling
fronto-orbital rim
fronto-orbitonasoethmoidal
        fracture
frontoparietal area
frontoparietal arteriovenous
        malformation
frontoparietal region
frontoparietal suture
frontoposterior position
frontosphenoid suture
frontotemporal approach
frontotemporal craniotomy
frontotemporal craniotomy
        incision
frontotransverse position
frontozygomatic suture
frontozygomatic suture line
front-tap reflex
front-viewing scope
Frosh procedure for ingrown
        nail
frost anesthesia
Frost operation
Frost procedure
Frost scissors
Frost stitch
Frost sutures
Frosted Flex earmold material
Frost-Lang operation
frown incision
frown line
frozen hand
frozen knee joint
frozen section
frozen section diagnosis
frozen shoulder
frozen tissue
Fruehevald splint
Frumin valve
Fry nasal forceps
Frydman catheter
Frye aspirator
Frye portable aspirator
Frykholm bone rongeur
Frykholm goniometer
Frykholm rongeur
Frykman classification of hand
        fractures
Frykman distal radius fracture
        classification
Frykman fracture

Frykman radial fracture
    classification
FSD colpostat
F-series dialyzer
FSH (follicle stimulating
    hormone)
FTO eye patch
FTSG (full-thickness skin
    graft)
FTT (free tissue transfer)
Fuchs canthorrhaphy operation
Fuchs capsule forceps
Fuchs capsulotomy forceps
Fuchs crypt
Fuchs extracapsular forceps
Fuchs forceps
Fuchs iris bombe transfixion
    operation
Fuchs iris forceps
Fuchs keratome
Fuchs lancet-type keratome
Fuchs operation
Fuchs position
Fuchs retinal detachment
    syringe
Fuchs 2-way eye syringe
fugitive swelling
Fugo blade
Fugo plasma knife
Fuji dental cement
Fujica camera
Fujica gastrocamera
Fujinon gastroscope
Fujinon biopsy forceps
Fujinon colonoscope
Fujinon diagnostic laparoscope
Fujinon disposable injector
Fujinon bronchoscope
Fujinon video colonoscope
Fujinon duodenoscope
Fujinon endoscope
Fujinon flexible bronchoscope
Fujinon flexible
    choledochoscope
Fujinon flexible endoscope
Fujinon flexible ENT scope
Fujinon flexible fiberoptic
    laparoscope
Fujinon flexible hysteroscope
Fujinon flexible lower GI
    endoscope
Fujinon flexible sigmoidoscope

Fujinon flexible upper GI
    endoscope
Fujinon forceps
Fujinon variceal injector
Fujita snake retractor
Fujita suction cannula
Fukala operation
Fukasaku pupil snapper hook
Fukuda humeral head retractor
Fukusaku spatula
Fukushima C-clamp
Fukushima dissector
Fukushima malleable brain
    spatula
Fukushima monopolar malleable
    coagulator
Fukushima retractor
Fukushima rongeur
Fukushima-Giannotta curet
Fukushima-Giannotta dissector
Fukushima-Giannotta needle
    holder
Fukushima-Giannotta scissors
fulcrum line
Fulford procedure
fulgurating electrode
fulgurating unit
fulguration
    cystoscopic fulguration
    destruction of lesion by
        fulguration
    electrosurgical fulguration
    endoscopic fulguration
    excision and fulguration
    indirect fulguration
    Keating-Hart fulguration
fulguration electrode
fulguration of bleeding points
Fulkerson osteotomy
full axillary dissection
full breech presentation
full diagnostic laparoscopy
full extension
full flexion
full function
full occlusal splint
full pack
full range of motion
full weightbearing (FWB)
full-blown infection
full-body cutaneous examination
full-circle goniometer

full-column barium enema
full-curve sound
full-curved clamp
Fuller bivalve trach tube
Fuller operation
Fuller perianal shield
Fuller rectal dressing
Fuller shield
Fuller shield dressing
Fuller shield rectal dressing
Fuller silicone sponge
Fuller tube
Fullerview flexible iris retractor
full-face peel
FullFlow catheter
FullFlow perfusion dilation
    catheter
full-hand splint
full-intensity needle
full-jacketed bullet wound
full-leg circumferential
    lipoplasty
full-lumen esophagoscope
full-radius resector
full-radius synovial resector
full-spectrum breast
    augmentation
full-spine radiographic
    examination
full-term delivery
full-term fetus
full-term infant
full-thickness burn
full-thickness defect
full-thickness flap
full-thickness flap loss
full-thickness graft
full-thickness implant
full-thickness periodontal flap
full-thickness prosthesis
full-thickness rectal aspiration
full-thickness skin graft (FTSG)
full-thickness skin rhytidectomy
full-time occlusion eye patch
full-view lumen finder
full-wave rectifier
full weightbearing exercises
fully aroused
fully automatic, atrioventricular
    universal dual-channel
    pacemaker
fully automatic pacemaker

fully constrained
    tricompartmental knee
    prosthesis
fulminant hepatic failure (FHF)
fulminant invasive infection
fulminant mediastinitis
fulminating appendicitis
fulminating disease
fulmination
Fulpit forceps
Fulpit tissue forceps
Fulton deep-surgery scissors
Fulton laminectomy rongeur
Fulton mouth gag
Fulton pediatric scissors
Fulton retractor
Fulton rongeur
Fulton scissors
Ful-Vue ophthalmoscope
Ful-Vue spot retinoscope
Ful-Vue streak retinoscope
function
  barrier function
  cardiac function
  cardiovascular function
  cerebral function
  circulatory system function
  cortical function
  detrusor function
  diminished function
  excretory function
  full function
  gallbladder function
  graft function
  hemispheric functions
  House-Brackmann
    classification for facial
    nerve function
  impaired function
  kidney function
  labyrinthine function
  liver function
  motor and sensory function
  motor function
  muscle function
  neurological function
  occlusal function
  organically impaired brain
    function
  profundus function
  pulmonary function
  pyramidal function

function (*continued*)
  renal function
  respiratory function
  sensory functions
  shunt function
  speech-motor function
  unimpaired function
  velopharyngeal function
  vestibular function
function of joint
function study
functional activity
functional assessment of cancer
    therapy-head and neck
    (FACT-HN)
functional blepharoplasty
functional blindness
functional capacity classification
functional capacity evaluation
functional cardiac murmur
functional change
functional condition
functional congestion
functional cystic duct
    obstruction
functional death
functional disorder
functional electronic peroneal
    brace
functional endoscopic sinus
    surgery (FESS)
functional fracture brace
functional illness
functional intestinal failure
functional jaw orthopedics
functional lift
functional lymph node
    dissection
functional magnetic resonance
    imaging (fMRI)
functional malposition
functional mandibular
    movement
functional neck dissection
functional neurosurgery
functional occlusal harmony
functional occlusal registration
functional orthodontic therapy
functional orthotic
functional palatorrhaphy
functional pinch
functional position

functional prepubertal
    castration syndrome
functional range of motion
functional reconstruction
functional repair
functional resting position splint
functional rhinoplasty
functional sphincter
functional splint
functional stricture
functional technique
functional veloplasty
functioning allograft
fundal angioscopy
fundal camera
fundal coating lens
fundal glands
fundal height
fundal laser lens
fundal placenta
fundal plication
fundal portion of uterus
fundal to cervical end
fundal varices
fundal-focalizing lens
fundamental cause
fundectomy
fundi (*sing.* fundus)
fundi intact
fundic gland
fundic mucosa
fundic-antral junction
fundoplasty
  270-degree laparoscopic
    posterior fundoplasty
  anterior fundoplasty
  Belsey IV fundoplasty
  esophagogastric fundoplasty
  Gomez fundoplasty
  Hill fundoplasty
  laparoscopic esophagogastric
    fundoplasty
  Nissen fundoplasty
  posterior fundoplasty
  Thal fundoplasty
  Thal-Nissen fundoplasty
  Toupet fundoplasty
fundoplication
  Belsey Mark II fundoplication
  Belsey Mark IV 240-degree
    fundoplication
  Belsey partial fundoplication

fundoplication (*continued*)
 Belsey two-thirds wrap
   fundoplication
 Collis-Nissen fundoplication
 Dor anterior fundoplication
 endoscopic fundoplication
 floppy-type of Nissen
   fundoplication
 Guarner wrap fundoplication
 Heller myotomy with Dor
   fundoplication
 herniated fundoplication
 high-resistance fundoplication
 Hill gastropexy
   fundoplication
 Hunter technique for Toupet
   fundoplication
 intrathoracic Nissen
   fundoplication
 laparoscopic anterior partial
   fundoplication
 laparoscopic
   esophagogastroplasty
   with Nissen fundoplication
 laparoscopic Nissen and
   Toupet fundoplication
 laparoscopic Nissen
   fundoplication (LNF)
 low-resistance fundoplication
 microlaparoscopic Nissen
   fundoplication
 modified Belsey
   fundoplication
 Nissen 360-degree
   transabdominal
   fundoplication
 Nissen 360-degree wrap
   fundoplication
 Nissen fundoplication
 Nissen-Rossetti fundoplication
 open fundoplication
 open Nissen fundoplication
   (ONF)
 redo fundoplication
 Rossetti modification of
   Nissen fundoplication
 slipped Nissen fundoplication
 Thal fundoplication
 total fundoplication
 Toupet fundoplication
 Toupet hemifundoplication
   fundoplication

fundoplication (*continued*)
 transthoracic Nissen
   fundoplication
 twisted fundoplication
 uncut Collis-Nissen
   fundoplication
 videoscopic fundoplication
fundus (*pl.* fundi)
 bald gastric fundus
 gallbladder fundus
 gastric fundus
 tessellated fundus
 uterine fundus
fundus camera
fundus contact lens
fundus focalizing lens
fundus gland
fundus photography
fundus rotation gastroplasty
funduscope
 Friedenwald funduscope
funduscopic examination
funduscopy
fundusectomy
fundus-retinal camera
fungal infection
fungating excrescence
fungating lesion
fungating mass
fungating sore
fungating tumor
fungating wound
fungiform papillae
fungoid
fungus excrescence
fungus ball
funic reduction
funicular artery
funicular excision
funicular graft
funicular hernia
funicular hydrocele
funicular inguinal hernia
funicular repair
funicular sutures
funiculopexy
funiculus (*pl.* funiculi)
funiculus spermaticus
funnel chest
funnel chest deformity
funnel deformity
funnel stitch

funnel-shaped pelvis
Funsten supination splint
Furacin dressing
Furacin gauze
Furacin gauze dressing
Furacin gauze holder
furcate placenta
Furlong tendon stripper
Furlow closure
Furlow cylinder inserter
Furlow cylinder passer
Furlow double Z-plasty
Furlow double-opposing Z-plasty
Furlow double-opposing Z-plasty palatoplasty
Furlow double-reversing Z-plasty
Furlow inserter
Furlow introducer
Furlow needle holder
Furlow procedure
Furlow-Fisher modification of Virag 1 operation
Furman type II electrogram
Furniss anastomosis clamp
Furniss cornea-holding forceps
Furniss polyp forceps
Furniss-Clute anastomosis clamp
Furniss-Clute duodenal clamp
Furniss-Clute pin
Furniss-McClure-Hinton clamp
Furniss anastomosis
Furniss anastomotic clamp
Furniss catheter
Furniss clamp
Furniss cornea-holding forceps
Furniss female catheter
Furniss forceps
Furniss incision
Furniss otoplasty
Furniss polyp forceps
Furniss sutures
Furniss ureterointestinal anastomosis
Furniss-Castroviejo forceps
Furniss-Clute anastomosis clamp
Furniss-Clute clamp
Furniss-Clute duodenal clamp
Furniss-Clute forceps
Furniss-Clute pin
Furniss-McClure-Hinton clamp
Furniss-Rizzuti forceps

furrier's sutures
furrow
    corneal marginal furrow
    digital furrow
    frontal furrow
    gluteal furrow
    mentolabial furrow
    nasal-labial furrow
    orbital-palpebral furrow
    palpebral furrow
    sagittal furrow
    Schmorl furrow
    shoulder of furrow
    transverse furrow
furrowed tongue
furuncle
furuncular otitis
furunculosis
fused bifocal lens
fused commissures
fused hips
fused kidney
fused teeth
fused vertebrae
fused vulva
fused-tip catheter
fuser pump
fusiform aneurysm
fusiform bougie
fusiform cataract
fusiform deformity
fusiform dilatation
fusiform excision
fusiform flap
fusiform fossa
fusiform gyrus
fusiform island flap
fusiform lobule
fusiform muscle
fusiform plication
fusiform scar
fusiform skin revision
fusiform swelling
fusiform widening of abdominal aorta
fusiform widening of duct
fusion
    1st-grade fusion
    2nd-grade fusion
    2-stage hip fusion
    3rd-grade fusion
    4-corner midcarpal fusion

fusion (*continued*)
 Abbott-Fisher-Lucas hip fusion
 Adams-Horwitz ankle fusion
 Adkins spinal fusion
 Albee fusion
 Albee spinal fusion
 amplitude of fusion
 Anderson ankle fusion
 ankle fusion
 anterior cervical diskectomy
  and fusion
 anterior cervical fusion (ACF)
 anterior lumbar vertebral
  interbody fusion
 anterior spinal fusion
 atlantoaxial fusion
 atlantoccipital fusion
 autograft fusion
 Bailey-Badgley cervical spine
  fusion
 binaural fusion
 binocular fusion
 Blair fusion
 Bosworth fusion
 Bosworth spinal fusion
 Bradford fusion
 Brittain fusion
 Brooks-Jenkins fusion
 Brooks-type fusion
 calcaneotibial fusion
 central fusion
 centric fusion
 cervical fusion
 cervical interbody fusion
 cervical spine posterior fusion
 Chandler hip fusion
 Charnley compression fusion
 Charnley compression-type
  knee fusion
 Chuinard-Peterson ankle
  fusion
 clothespin H spinal fusion
 Cloward anterior spinal fusion
 Cloward back fusion
 Coltart calcaneotibial fusion
 commissural fusion
 convex fusion
 Copeland-Howard
  scapulothoracic fusion
 Davis fusion
 Dewar posterior cervical
  fusion

fusion (*continued*)
 diaphyseal-epiphyseal fusion
 DIP fusion
 diskectomy with Cloward
  fusion
 distal interphalangeal fusion
 distal tibiofibular fusion
 dowel spinal fusion
 Dwyer instrumentation and
  fusion
 endoscopic spinal fusion
 epiphyseal-diaphyseal fusion
 Evans fusion
 extra-articular hip fusion
 extra-articular subtalar fusion
 eyelid fusion
 facet fusion
 flicker fusion
 fracture fusion
 free-body spinal fusion
 Gallie spinal fusion
 Gallie subtalar ankle fusion
 Gill-Manning-White fusion
 Glissane ankle fusion
 Goldner anterior fusion
 Goldstein spine fusion
 Hall facet fusion
 hammer toe correction with
  interphalangeal fusion
 Harrington spinal fusion
 Harris-Smith cervical fusion
 Henry-Geist spinal fusion
 H-graft fusion
 Hibbs spinal fusion
 Hibbs-Jones spinal fusion
 hip fusion
 Hodgson spine fusion
 Horwitz-Adams ankle fusion
 in situ spinal fusion
 interbody fusion
 interbody spinal fusion
 interfacet wiring and fusion
 intertransverse fusion
 intra-articular knee fusion
 joint fusion
 Kellogg-Speed lumbar spinal
  fusion
 Kellogg-Speed spinal fusion
 King intraarticular hip fusion
 knee fusion
 labial fusion
 lateral fusion

fusion (*continued*)
 long segment spinal fusion
 low cervical spine fusion
 lumbar spinal fusion
 lumbar vertebral interbody
  fusion
 lumbosacral fusion
 lunotriquetral fusion
 MacNab-Dall spinal fusion
 mitral valve fusion
 müllerian duct fusion
 Moe spinal fusion
 motor fusion
 multilevel spinal fusion
 naviculocuneiform fusion
 occipitocervical fusion
 Overton spinal fusion
 pantalar fusion
 pericardial fusion
 peripheral fusion
 posterior cervical fusion
 posterior lumbar interbody
  fusion (PLIF)
 posterior spinal fusion
 posterior-interbody lumbar
  spinal fusion
 posterior-lateral lumbar spinal
  fusion
 posterolateral interbody
  fusion
 posterolateral lumbosacral
  fusion
 radiocarpal fusion
 radiolunate fusion
 radioscaphoid fusion
 robertsonian fusion
 Robinson cervical spine
  fusion
 Robinson-Southwick spinal
  fusion
 Roger cervical spine fusion
 Roger spinal fusion
 root fusion
 sacral spine fusion
 scaphocapitate fusion
 scaphoid-capitate fusion
 scapulothoracic fusion
 Schneider hip fusion
 selective thoracic spine fusion
 sensory fusion
 short segment spinal fusion
 Simmons cervical spine fusion

fusion (*continued*)
 single-level spinal fusion
 small joint fusion
 Smith-Peterson sacroiliac joint
  fusion
 Smith-Robinson anterior
  fusion
 Smith-Robinson cervical
  fusion
 Smith-Robinson interbody
  fusion
 Soren ankle fusion
 spinal fusion
 splenogonadal fusion
 Stamm hip fusion
 Stamm procedure for intra-
  articular hip fusion
 symmetric vertebral fusion
 talocalcaneal fusion
 talonavicular fusion
 thoracic facet fusion
 thoracic spinal fusion
 thumb fusion
 tibiofibular fusion
 tibiotalar fusion
 tibiotalocalcaneal fusion
 tissue fusion
 trapeziometacarpal fusion
 triscaphe fusion
 upper cervical spine fusion
 urethrohymenal fusion
 vertebral fusion
 Watkins spinal fusion
 Watson
  scaphotrapeziotrapezoidal
  fusion
 White posterior ankle fusion
 whole-arm fusion
 Wilson ankle fusion
 Wiltberger fusion
 Wiltse bilateral lateral fusion
 Winter convex fusion
 wrist fusion
 Zielke instrument for scoliosis
  spinal fusion
fusion area
fusion cage
fusion complex
fusion defect
fusion faculty
fusion fascia
fusion frame

fusion grade
fusion implantation
fusion in situ
fusion instruments
fusion nonunion rate
fusion of bone
fusion of joint
fusion operation
fusion peptide
fusion plate
fusion procedure
fusion reflex
fusion stiffness
fusion technique
fusion tube
fusion welding
fusion-free position
fusospirochetal stomatitis
Futch cannula
Futcher line

Futura resectoscope sheath
Futura splint
Futuro splint
Futuro wrist brace
Futuro wrist support
FWB (full weightbearing)
FyBron alginate dressing
FyBron calcium alginate
    dressing
Fyodorov dipstick
Fyodorov eye implant
Fyodorov 4-loop iris clip
    intraocular lens
Fyodorov lens expressor
Fyodorov type I, II intraocular
    lens
Fyodorov type I, II lens implant
Fyodorov-Sputnik contact
    intraocular lens
FZ (frontozygomatic)

G
...

Gaab endoscope
Gabarro graft
Gabarro operation
Gabarro retractor
Gabbay-Frater suture guide
Gabor probe
Gabriel proctoscope
Gabriel syringe
Gabriel Tucker bougie
Gabriel Tucker forceps
Gabriel Tucker tube
Gaenslen fracture
Gaenslen incision
Gaenslen procedure
Gaenslen sign
Gaenslen split-heel incision
Gafco-Halsted forceps
Gaffee speculum
Gaffney ankle prosthesis
Gaffney joint
gag reflex
Gage sign
Gaillard operation
Gaillard-Arlt sutures
Gaillard-Thomas excision
gait
    4-point gait
    antalgic gait
    ataxic gait
    calcaneal gait
    cerebellar gait
    lurching gait
    spastic gait
gait lock splint
gait lock splint brace (GLS)
gait plate
gaiter brace
galactocele
galactophorous canals
galactophorous duct
galactoplania
galactorrhea
galactostasis

Galand disk lens
Galand in-the-bag lens
Galand-Knolle modified J-loop
    intraocular lens
Galant abdominal reflex
Galant abdominal response
Galante hip guide
Galante hip prosthesis
Galaxy pacemaker
Galbiati bilateral fetal
    ischiopubiotomy
galea
    aponeurotic galea
    aponeurotica galea
    tendinous galea
galea aponeurosis plication
galea aponeurotica
galea forceps
galea frontalis advancement
galea frontalis flap
galea occipital flap
galea periosteal flap
galea-frontalis-occipitalis release
galeal flap
galeal forceps
galeal scoring technique
galeaplasty
Galeati gland
Galeazzi fracture of radius
Galeazzi fracture-dislocation
Galeazzi patellar operation
Galeazzi sign
Galen anastomosis
Galen bandage
Galen dressing
Galen foramen
Galen vein
Galen ventricle
galenic venous malformation
galeoperiosteum
Galetti articulator
Galezowski dilator
Galezowski lacrimal dilator

Galilean loupe
Galilean microscope
Galileo evoked potential
    electroencephalograph
Galileo rigid hysteroscope
Galin intraocular lens implant
Galin lens spatula
Galin silicone bleb cup
gall duct dilator
gall duct forceps
gall duct obstruction
gall duct probe
gall duct scoop
gall duct spoon
Gall-Addison uterine
    manipulator
Gallagher antral frontal
    raspatory
Gallagher antral rasp
Gallagher bipolar mapping probe
Gallagher rasp
Gallagher trocar
gallamine anesthetic agent
Gallannaugh bone plate
gallbladder (GB)
    bifurcation of gallbladder
    bilobed gallbladder
    body of gallbladder
    calcified gallbladder
    calculous gallbladder
    Courvoisier gallbladder
    dilated gallbladder
    distended gallbladder
    fish-scale gallbladder
    floating gallbladder
    hourglass gallbladder
    hydrops of gallbladder
    inflamed gallbladder
    mobile gallbladder
    multiseptate gallbladder
    perforated gallbladder
    phrygian cap of gallbladder
    porcelain gallbladder
    stasis gallbladder
    strawberry gallbladder
    thick-walled gallbladder
    wandering gallbladder
gallbladder aspirator
gallbladder bed
gallbladder calculus
gallbladder cancer
gallbladder cannula

gallbladder carcinoma
gallbladder colic
gallbladder contraction
gallbladder distention
gallbladder duplication
gallbladder ectopia
gallbladder ejection rate
gallbladder films
gallbladder forceps
gallbladder fossa
gallbladder function
gallbladder fundus
gallbladder ileus
gallbladder inflammation
gallbladder neck
gallbladder operation
gallbladder perforation
gallbladder plate
gallbladder retractor
gallbladder ring clamp
gallbladder scan
gallbladder scissors
gallbladder scoop
gallbladder series
gallbladder shadow
gallbladder spoon
gallbladder stone
gallbladder trocar
gallbladder tube
gallbladder wall
gallbladder wall abscess
gallbladder-vena cava line
Gallie atlantoaxial fusion
    technique
Gallie cryoenucleator
Gallie fascia needle
Gallie fusion-using cable
Gallie herniorrhaphy
Gallie needle
Gallie operation
Gallie procedure
Gallie spinal fusion
Gallie subtalar ankle fusion
Gallie technique
Gallie tendon passer
Gallie transplant
Gallie wiring technique
Gallie-LeMesurier operation
Gallini bone marrow aspiration
    needle
gallium-aluminum-arsenide laser
gallop rhythm

Galloway electrode
Gallows splint
gallows-type retractor
gallstone
    asymptomatic gallstone
    bilirubin pigment gallstone
    black pigment gallstone
    brown pigment gallstone
    cholesterol gallstone
    dissolving gallstone
    faceted gallstone
    floating gallstone
    innocent gallstone
    mixed-cholesterol gallstone
    mulberry gallstone
    pigmented gallstone
    radiolucent gallstone
    retained gallstone
    silent gallstone
    symptomatic gallstone
gallstone basket
gallstone colic
gallstone dilator
gallstone disease
gallstone forceps
gallstone formation
gallstone ileus
gallstone migration
gallstone obstruction
gallstone probe
gallstone scoop
GALT (gut-associated lymphoid
    tissue)
Galt aspirating cannula
Galt drill
Galt saw
Galt skull trephine
Galt trephine
Galton ear whistle
Galton whistle
galvanic cautery
galvanic current
galvanic electrode stimulator
galvanic eye current controller
galvanic probe
galvanic response
galvanic skin response
galvanic stimulation
galvanocaustic amputation
galvanocaustic snare
galvanocautery
galvanoionization

galvanometer
galvanosurgery
galvanotonic contractions
Galveston metacarpal brace
Galveston pelvic fixation
Galveston plate
Galveston splint
Galveston technique
Gambale-Merrill bone-cutting
    forceps
Gambee anastomosis
Gambee stitch
Gambee suture technique
Gambee sutures
Gambro catheter
Gambro dialyzer
Gambro filter
Gambro freezing bag
Gambro Lundia plate
Gambro Lundia Minor
    hemodialyzer
Gambro oxygenator
Gambro-Lundia coil dialyzer
gamekeeper's thumb dislocation
gamekeeper's thumb fracture
gamete intrafallopian transfer
    (GIFT)
gamete manipulation
Gamgee dressing
Gamgee tissue
gamma camera
gamma globulin
gamma irradiation
gamma knife
gamma locking nail for hip
gamma loop disorder
gamma probe
gamma probe localization
gamma ray
gamma scintillation camera
gamma transverse colon loop
gamma trochanteric locking nail
gamma well counter
gamma-detecting probe
gamma-ray counter
Gamna nodules
Gamna-Gandy nodule
Gamophen sutures
Gandy-Gamna nodule
gangliated nerve
gangliectomy
gangliolysis

ganglion (*pl.* ganglia, ganglions)
  aberrant ganglion
  acousticofacial ganglion
  Acrel ganglion
  Andersch ganglion
  aorticorenal ganglion
  Arnold ganglion
  Auerbach ganglion
  auricular ganglion
  basal ganglia
  Bezold ganglion
  Blandin ganglion
  Bochdalek ganglion
  Bock ganglion
  cardiac ganglion
  carotid ganglion
  celiac ganglion
  cephalic ganglion
  cervical ganglion
  cervicothoracic ganglion
  cervicouterine ganglion
  ciliary ganglion
  Cloquet ganglion
  coccygeal ganglion
  cochlear ganglion
  compound ganglion
  Corti ganglion
  diffuse ganglion
  dorsal root ganglion
  Ehrenritter ganglion
  episcleral ganglion
  extirpation of ganglion
  false ganglion
  Frankenhauser ganglion
  Ganser ganglion
  Gasser ganglion
  gasserian ganglion
  geniculate ganglion
  glossopharyngeal ganglion
  hypogastric ganglion
  hypoglossal ganglion
  inferior cervical ganglion
  inferior ganglion
  inferior mesenteric ganglion
  intercarotid ganglion
  intermediate ganglion
  interpeduncular ganglion
  interventricular ganglion
  intervertebral ganglion
  intracranial ganglion
  jugular ganglion
  Kuttner ganglion

ganglion (*continued*)
  lacrimal ganglion
  Langley ganglion
  Laumonier ganglion
  Lee ganglion
  lingual ganglion
  Lobstein ganglion
  Loetwig ganglion
  Ludwig ganglion
  lumbar ganglion
  Luschka ganglion
  Meckel ganglion
  Meissner ganglion
  mesenteric ganglion
  middle cervical ganglion
  motor roots of submandibular
    ganglion
  Mueller ganglion
  nasociliary ganglion
  nephrolumbar ganglion
  nodose ganglion
  oculomotor ganglion
  olfactory ganglion
  optic ganglion
  otic ganglion
  parasympathetic ganglion
  paravertebral ganglion
  pelvic ganglion
  periosteal ganglion
  petrosal ganglion
  pharyngeal branch of
    pterygopalatine ganglion
  phrenic ganglion
  prevertebral ganglia
  prevertebral ganglion
  primary ganglion
  prostatic ganglion
  pterygopalatine ganglion
  recurrent ganglion
  renal ganglia
  Remak ganglion
  renal ganglion
  Ribes ganglion
  sacral ganglion
  sacral ganglia
  Scarpa ganglion
  Schacher ganglion
  Schmiedel ganglion
  semilunar ganglion
  simple ganglion
  solar ganglion
  sphenomaxillary ganglion

ganglion (*continued*)
  sphenopalatine ganglion
  spinal ganglion
  spiral ganglion
  splanchnic ganglion
  stellate ganglion
  sublingual ganglion
  submandibular ganglion
  submaxillary ganglion
  superior carotid ganglion
  superior cervical ganglion
  superior ganglion
  superior mesenteric ganglion
  superior vagal ganglion
  suprarenal ganglion
  sympathetic ganglia
  synovial ganglion
  terminal ganglion
  thoracic ganglia
  thyroid ganglion
  trigeminal ganglion
  Troisier ganglion
  tympanic ganglion
  upper ganglion
  vagal ganglion
  Valentin ganglion
  vallecula for petrosal ganglion
  ventricular ganglion
  vertebral ganglion
  vestibular ganglion
  Vieussens ganglion
  Walther ganglion
  Wrisberg ganglion
  wrist ganglion
ganglion block
ganglion blockage
ganglion blocker
ganglion cyst
ganglion hook
ganglion impar block
ganglion injection needle
ganglion knife
ganglion of Mueller
ganglion of nerve
ganglion of vagus
ganglion scissors
ganglionated chain
ganglionectomy
ganglioneurofibroma
ganglioneuroma
ganglionic blockade
ganglionic blocking agent

ganglionic branches
ganglionic center
ganglionic glioma
ganglionic saliva
ganglionostomy
ganglioside
gangliosympathectomy
gangrene
  appendiceal gangrene
  arteriosclerotic gangrene
  circumscribed gangrene
  cold gangrene
  cutaneous gangrene
  decubital gangrene
  diabetic gangrene
  disseminated gangrene
  dry gangrene
  embolic gangrene
  emphysematous gangrene
  Fournier gangrene
  gas gangrene
  hemorrhagic gangrene
  hospital gangrene
  hot gangrene
  humid gangrene
  incipient gangrene
  inflammatory gangrene
  mammary gangrene
  Meleney synergistic gangrene
  mephitic gangrene
  moist gangrene
  nosocomial gangrene
  oral gangrene
  Pott gangrene
  pressure gangrene
  primary gangrene
  progressive bacterial
     synergistic gangrene
  progressive gangrene
  secondary gangrene
  senile gangrene
  static gangrene
  symmetric gangrene
  thrombotic gangrene
  traumatic gangrene
  venous gangrene
  wet gangrene
  white gangrene
gangrenous granulomatous
   inflammation
gangrenous hernia
gangrenous organ

gangrenous rhinitis
gangrenous stomatitis
Ganley splint
Ganley technique
Gannetta dissector
Gans cyclodialysis
Gans cyclodialysis cannula
Gans eye cannula
Ganser diverticulum
Ganser ganglion
Gant arthrodesis
Gant clamp
Gant gallbladder retractor
Gant hemostat
Gant hip osteotomy
Gant line
Gant operation
Gant osteotomy
Gant probe
Gant rectal probe
gantry
gantry angle
gantry stretcher
Gantzer muscle
granulosity
Ganz-Edwards coronary infusion
    catheter
Ganzfeld electroretinograph
Ganzfeld stimulator
gap arthroplasty
gap bleed
gap depth
gap junction
gap migration
gaping wound
gaping wound edges
Garceau approach
Garceau bougie
Garceau catheter
Garceau cheilectomy
Garceau cheilotomy
Garceau clubfoot procedure
Garceau tendon technique
Garceau ureteral catheter
Garceau-Brahms clubfoot
    procedure
Garcia aorta clamp
Garcia endometrial biopsy
    set
Garcia-Novito eye implant
Garcia-Rock endometrial biopsy
    curet

Garcia-Rock endometrial suction
    curet
Garcin syndrome
Garden procedure
garden spade deformity
Gardiner-Brown neurological
    tuning fork
Gardiner-Brown tuning fork
Gardlok neurosurgical sponge
Gardner bone chisel
Gardner bone forceps
Gardner chair
Gardner chisel
Gardner head holder
Gardner headrest
Gardner hysterectomy forceps
Gardner meningocele repair
Gardner needle
Gardner needle holder
Gardner operation
Gardner shoulder approach
Gardner skull clamp
Gardner suture needle
Gardner tongs
Gardner-Wells fixation frame
Gardner-Wells headrest
Gardner-Wells skull tongs
Gardner-Wells tongs
Gardner-Wells traction tongs
Garfield-Holinger laryngoscope
gargle
    rectal gargle
gargoylism
Gariel pessary
Gariot articulator
Garland clamp
Garland forceps
Garland hysterectomy clamp
Garland hysterectomy forceps
Garlock spur crusher
Garner balloon shunt
Garney rubber band applicator
Garren gastric bubble
Garren-Edwards balloon
Garren-Edwards gastric balloon
Garren-Edwards gastric bubble
Garretson bandage
Garretson dressing
Garrett dilator
Garrett orientation line
Garrett peripheral vascular
    retractor

Garrett vascular dilator
Garrett vein passer
Garrigue forceps
Garrigue speculum
Garrigue uterine-dressing forceps
Garrigue vaginal retractor
Garrigue vaginal speculum
Garrigue weighted vaginal
    speculum
Garrison forceps
Garrison knife
Garrison rongeur
Garron spatula
garrote tourniquet
Gartland humeral supracondylar
    fracture classification
Gartland Universal radial
    fracture classification
Gartner cyst
Gartner duct
Gartner tonometer
gartnerian cyst
gas abscess
gas analyzer
gas anesthetic
gas cautery
gas chromatography
gas collection
gas cylinder
gas density line
gas discharge lamp
gas embolism
gas endarterectomy
gas exchange
gas gangrene
gas gangrene antitoxin
gas insufflation
gas insufflator
gas laser
Gas-Lyte aspirator
gas machine
gas pack
gas pattern
gas sterilization
gas tube
gas volume
gaseous agent
gaseous cholecystitis
gaseous decompression
gaseous dilatation
gaseous distention
gaseous injection

gaseous laparoscopy
gas-fluid exchange
gas-forming liver abscess
Gaskell clamp
Gaskin fragment forceps
gasless endoscopic
    thyroidectomy
gasless laparoscopic
    hysterectomy
gasless laparoscopy
gas-liquid chromatography
Gasparotti bevel tip
Gass cataract-aspirating cannula
Gass cervical punch
Gass corneoscleral punch
Gass dye applicator
Gass endarterectomy spatula
Gass hook
Gass I&A unit
Gass muscle hook
Gass neurosurgical light
Gass punch
Gass retinal detachment cannula
Gass retinal detachment hook
Gass scleral marker
Gass scleral punch
Gass sclerotomy punch
Gass vitreous-aspirating cannula
Gasser ganglion
gasserectomy
gasserian ganglion block
gasserian ganglion blockade
gasserian ganglion hook
gasserian ganglionectomy
gas-solid chromatography
gastralgia
gastrectomy
    antecolic gastrectomy
    anterior gastrectomy
    Aquirre gastrectomy
    Balfour gastrectomy
    Bancroft-Plenk gastrectomy
    Billroth gastrectomy
    Billroth I partial gastrectomy
    Billroth II gastrectomy
    Braun-Jaboulay gastrectomy
    Connell gastrectomy
    curative radical total
      gastrectomy
    distal gastrectomy
    distal with excision of ulcer
      gastrectomy

gastrectomy (*continued*)
  esophagoproximal
    gastrectomy
  Finochietto-Billroth I
    gastrectomy
  hand-assisted laparoscopic
    gastrectomy
  high subtotal gastrectomy
  Hofmeister gastrectomy
  Hofmeister-Billroth II
    gastrectomy
  Horsley gastrectomy
  Japanese-style gastrectomy
  limited gastrectomy
  Maki pylorus-preserving
    gastrectomy
  Mikulicz gastrectomy
  near-total gastrectomy
  Nissen gastrectomy
  palliative total gastrectomy
  pancreatic-preserving total
    gastrectomy
  partial gastrectomy (PG)
  Pauchet gastrectomy
  Payr gastrectomy
  Polya gastrectomy
  proximal gastrectomy
  pylorus-preserving
    gastrectomy (PPG)
  Pean-Billroth I gastrectomy
  radical gastrectomy
  radical total gastrectomy
  reverse gastrectomy
  Roux-en-Y gastrectomy
  Schoemaker gastrectomy
  Schoemaker-Billroth II
    gastrectomy
  segmental gastrectomy
  standardized curative radical
    total gastrectomy
  subtotal gastrectomy
  total gastrectomy
  video-assisted gastrectomy
  von Haberer gastrectomy
  von Haberer-Aquirre
    gastrectomy
  von Haberer-Finney
    gastrectomy
gastrectomy specimen
gastric acidity
gastric adenocarcinoma
gastric air bubble

gastric analysis
gastric antral erosion
gastric arteries
gastric arteriovenous
  malformation
gastric aspiration tube
gastric atony
gastric atrophy
gastric balloon
gastric balloon implantation
gastric bed metastasis
gastric bubble
gastric bypass (GBP)
gastric bypass operation
gastric bypass procedure (GBP)
gastric calculus
gastric cancer
gastric carcinoma
gastric cardia
gastric clamp
gastric coin removal
gastric compression
gastric contents
gastric cytology
gastric decompression
gastric dilatation
gastric dilation
gastric distention
gastric duplication
gastric duplication cyst
gastric emptying
gastric emptying procedure
  (GEP)
gastric emptying scan
gastric epithelial cell infiltration
gastric erosion
gastric fistula
gastric fluid aspiration
gastric folds
gastric foreign body
gastric freezing
gastric fundal wrap
gastric fundus
gastric gavage
gastric glands
gastric hemorrhage
gastric hernia
gastric hypersecretion
gastric impression
gastric insufflation
gastric lavage
gastric lavage tube

gastric leiomyoma resection
gastric loop bypass
gastric MALT lymphoma
gastric margin
gastric motility disorder
gastric mucosa
gastric mucosal barrier
gastric mucosal pattern
    classification
gastric neurectomy
gastric non-Hodgkin
    lymphoma
gastric notch
gastric omentum
gastric outlet
gastric outlet obstruction
gastric partitioning
gastric patch esophagoplasty
gastric perforation
gastric pit
gastric plexus
gastric pouch
gastric pressure
gastric procedure
gastric pull-through procedure
gastric pull-up procedure
gastric pylorus
gastric reduction surgery
gastric resection
gastric resection retractor
gastric residue examination
gastric rugae
gastric rugal fold
gastric rupture
gastric sclerosis
gastric secretion
gastric shield
gastric sling muscle
gastric stapling procedure
gastric stoma
gastric stump
gastric stump carcinoma
gastric suction
gastric surface of spleen
gastric tear
gastric tube
gastric tube esophagoplasty
gastric tumor
gastric ulcer
gastric ulceration
gastric valve tightening
    procedure

gastric valve tightening
    technique
gastric variceal bleeding
gastric varices
gastric veins
gastric vena caval shunt
gastric volvulus
gastric washings
gastrinoma
gastrin-secreting non-beta islet
    cell tumor
gastrocamera
gastrocardiac syndrome
Gastroccult
gastrocele
gastrocnemius equinus
gastrocnemius flap
gastrocnemius muscle
gastrocnemius reflex
gastrocnemius sliding flap
gastrocolic fistula
gastrocolic ligament
gastrocolic omentum
gastrocolic reflex
gastrocolitis
gastrocolostomy
gastrocolotomy
gastrocolpotomy
gastrocs (*slang for*
    gastrocnemius muscles)
gastrocutaneous fistula
gastrodiaphanoscopy
gastrodiaphany
gastroduodenal anastomosis
gastroduodenal artery
gastroduodenal complication
gastroduodenal contents
gastroduodenal fiberscope
gastroduodenal fistula
gastroduodenal lumen
gastroduodenal mucosa
gastroduodenal tube
gastroduodenal ulcer
gastroduodenectomy
gastroduodenitis
gastroduodenopancreatectomy
gastroduodenoscopy
    Billroth gastroduodenoscopy
gastroduodenostomy
    Billroth I gastroduodenostomy
    Finney gastroduodenostomy
    Jaboulay gastroduodenostomy

gastroduodenostomy (*continued*)
  vagotomy and antrectomy
    with gastroduodenostomy
gastroendoscopy
gastroenteric
gastroenteric fistula
gastroenteroanastomosis
gastroenterocolostomy
gastroenterogenous cyst
gastroenterologist
gastroenteropancreatic (GEP)
gastroenteroplasty
gastroenteroptosis
gastroenterostomy
  Balfour gastroenterostomy
  Billroth gastroenterostomy
  Billroth I gastroenterostomy
  Billroth II gastroenterostomy
  Braun-Jaboulay
    gastroenterostomy
  Courvoisier
    gastroenterostomy
  Finney gastroenterostomy
  Heineke-Mikulicz
    gastroenterostomy
  Hofmeister
    gastroenterostomy
  laparoscopic
    gastroenterostomy
  percutaneous
    gastroenterostomy
  Polya gastroenterostomy
  prophylactic
    gastroenterostomy
  Roux gastroenterostomy
  Roux-en-Y gastroenterostomy
  Schoemaker
    gastroenterostomy
  short-limb Roux-en-Y
    gastroenterostomy
  side-to-side gastroenterostomy
  transomental posterior
    gastroenterostomy
  truncal vagotomy and
    gastroenterostomy
  von Haberer
    gastroenterostomy
  von Haberer-Finney
    gastroenterostomy
  Wölfler gastroenterostomy
gastroenterostomy catheter
gastroenterostomy clamp

gastroenterostomy
  intussusception
gastroenterostomy stoma
gastroenterostomy tube
gastroenterotomy
gastroepiploic arcade
gastroepiploic artery
gastroepiploic branch
gastroepiploic lymph node
gastroepiploic vein
gastroepiploic vessels
gastroesophageal hernia
gastroesophageal incompetence
gastroesophageal junction
gastroesophageal reflux
gastroesophageal reflux disease
  (GERD)
gastroesophageal sphincter
gastroesophageal variceal plexus
gastroesophagostomy
gastrofiberscope
gastrogalvanization
gastrogastrostomy
gastrogavage
gastrogram
gastrography
gastrohepatic
gastrohepatic ligament
gastrohepatic omentum
gastroileac augmentation
gastroileal anastomosis
gastroileal reflex
gastroileitis
gastroileostomy
gastrointestinal (GI)
gastrointestinal anastomosis
  (GIA)
gastrointestinal biopsy
gastrointestinal bleed
gastrointestinal bleeding
gastrointestinal carcinoma
gastrointestinal clamp
gastrointestinal complication
gastrointestinal condition
gastrointestinal continuity
gastrointestinal disease
gastrointestinal endoscopy
gastrointestinal fistula
gastrointestinal forceps
gastrointestinal instrument
gastrointestinal intubation
gastrointestinal lesion

gastrointestinal malignancy
gastrointestinal metastasis
gastrointestinal mucosa
gastrointestinal needle
gastrointestinal perforation
gastrointestinal resection
gastrointestinal series
gastrointestinal spasm
gastrointestinal stoma
gastrointestinal surgery
gastrointestinal surgical gut
    sutures
gastrointestinal surgical linen
    sutures
gastrointestinal surgical silk
    sutures
gastrointestinal
    symptomatology
gastrointestinal tract
gastrointestinal tube
gastrointestinal ulcer
gastrointestinal-cutaneous fistula
gastrojejunal anastomosis
gastrojejunal loop obstruction
    syndrome
gastrojejunal ulcer
gastrojejunocolic
gastrojejunocolic fistula
gastrojejunostomy
    antecolic gastrojejunostomy
    antecolic long-loop
        isoperistaltic
        gastrojejunostomy
    anterior gastrojejunostomy
    antiperistaltic
        gastrojejunostomy
    Billroth gastrojejunostomy
    Billroth II gastrojejunostomy
    compression button
        gastrojejunostomy
    Dragstedt vagotomy and
        gastrojejunostomy
    Hofmeister antecolic
        gastrojejunostomy
    isoperistaltic
        gastrojejunostomy
    loop gastrojejunostomy
    Mayo gastrojejunostomy
    Moynihan gastrojejunostomy
    no-loop gastrojejunostomy
    partial inferior retrocolic end-
        to-side gastrojejunostomy

gastrojejunostomy (*continued*)
    partial superior retrocolic
        end-to-side
        gastrojejunostomy
    percutaneous endoscopic
        gastrojejunostomy
    Polya gastrojejunostomy
    prophylactic
        gastrojejunostomy
    retrocolic end-to-side
        gastrojejunostomy
    Roscoe-Graham anterior
        gastrojejunostomy
    Roux-en-Y
        gastrojejunostomy
    total retrocolic end-to-side
        gastrojejunostomy
gastrojejunostomy tube
gastrolienal ligament
gastrolysis
gastromegaly
gastromotor insufficiency
gastromyotomy
gastronesteostomy
gastropancreatic fold
gastropancreatic ligament
gastropancreatic reflex
gastropancreatic vagovagal
    reflex
gastroparesis
    postvagotomy gastroparesis
gastropathy
    indomethacin-induced
        gastropathy
gastropexy
    anterior gastropexy
    Belsey Mark IV gastropexy
    belt loop gastropexy
    Boerema anterior gastropexy
    circumcostal gastropexy
    Hill posterior gastropexy
    incisional gastropexy
    laparoscopic-assisted
        gastropexy
    percutaneous anterior
        gastropexy
    posterior diaphragmatic
        gastropexy
    T-fastener gastropexy
    T-tack gastropexy
gastrophotography
gastrophrenic ligament

gastroplasty
  adjustable ring gastroplasty
  Albert-Lembert gastroplasty
  banded gastroplasty
  Collis gastroplasty
  Collis-Nissen gastroplasty
  Eckhout gastroplasty
  Eckhout vertical gastroplasty
  fundus rotation gastroplasty
  Gomez gastroplasty
  Gomez horizontal gastroplasty
  greater curvature banded
    gastroplasty
  hand-assisted laparoscopic
    vertical-banded gastroplasty
  horizontal gastroplasty
  Kuzmak gastroplasty
  laparoscopic gastroplasty
  Laws gastroplasty
  layer-to-layer gastroplasty
  Mason gastroplasty
  Mason vertical-banded
    gastroplasty
  O'Leary gastroplasty
  O'Leary lesser curvature
    gastroplasty
  open vertical banded
    gastroplasty
  silicone elastomer ring
    vertical gastroplasty
  Stamm gastroplasty
  tubular vertical gastroplasty
  unbanded gastroplasty
  V-banded gastroplasty
  vertical ring gastroplasty
    (VRG)
  vertical Silastic ring
    gastroplasty
  vertical-banded gastroplasty
    (VBG)
  V-Y gastroplasty
gastroplasty stapler
gastropleural fistula
gastroplication
Gastro-Port feeding tube
gastroptosis
gastropylorectomy
gastropyloric
gastrorrhaphy
gastrorrhea
gastrorrhexis
gastroschisis

gastroscope
  ACMI examining gastroscope
  ACMI fiberoptic gastroscope
  ACMI gastroscope
  Benedict gastroscope
  Benedict operating
    gastroscope
  Bernstein gastroscope
  Bernstein modification
    gastroscope
  Cameron gastroscope
  Cameron omni-angle
    gastroscope
  Chevalier Jackson gastroscope
  disposable-sheath flexible
    gastroscope
  Eder gastroscope
  Eder-Chamberlin gastroscope
  Eder-Hufford gastroscope
  Eder-Palmer gastroscope
  Ellsner gastroscope
  end-viewing gastroscope
  Ewald gastroscope
  examining gastroscope
  fiberoptic gastroscope
  flexible gastroscope
  Fujinon gastroscope
  GFC gastroscope
  GTF-A gastroscope
  Herman-Taylor gastroscope
  Hirschowitz fiberscope
    gastroscope
  Housset-Debray gastroscope
  Janeway gastroscope
  Jenning-Streifeneder
    gastroscope
  Kelling gastroscope
  Mancke flex-rigid
    gastroscope
  Olympus gastroscope
  operating gastroscope
  pediatric gastroscope
  Pentax gastroscope
  peroral gastroscope
  Schindler gastroscope
  Sielaff gastroscope
  Taylor gastroscope
  Tomenius gastroscope
  Universal gastroscope
  Wolf-Henning gastroscope
  Wolf-Knittlingen gastroscope
  Wolf-Schindler gastroscope

gastroscopy
  drainage gastroscopy
  high-magnification
    gastroscopy
  infrared transillumination
    gastroscopy
  Stamm-Senn gastroscopy
  Stamm-Seu gastroscopy
gastrosoleus muscle
gastrosphincteric pressure
    gradient
gastrosplenic ligament
gastrosplenic omentum
gastrostogavage
gastrostolavage
gastrostoma
gastrostomy
  AEI button for replacement
    gastrostomy
  Bates gastrostomy
  Beck gastrostomy
  Beck-Jianu gastrostomy
  Billroth gastrostomy
  Billroth I gastrostomy
  Billroth II gastrostomy
  button one-step gastrostomy
  Depage-Janeway gastrostomy
  Dragstedt feeding
    gastrostomy
  drainage gastrostomy
  dual percutaneous
    endoscopic gastrostomy
  endoscopic gastrostomy
  feeding gastrostomy
  Frank gastrostomy
  Gauderer-Ponsky-Izant PEG
    gastrostomy
  Glassman gastrostomy
  Janeway gastrostomy
  Kader gastrostomy
  laparoscopic gastrostomy
  Marwedel gastrostomy
  Microvasive one step button
    gastrostomy
  palliative gastrostomy
  Partipilo gastrostomy
  percutaneous endoscopic
    gastrostomy (PEG)
  percutaneous gastrostomy
  Russell gastrostomy
  Russell percutaneous
    endoscopic gastrostomy

gastrostomy (*continued*)
  Sachs-Vine feeding
    gastrostomy
  Spivack gastrostomy
  Ssabanejew-Frank gastrostomy
  Stamm gastrostomy
  Surgitek one-step
    percutaneous endoscopic
    gastrostomy
  tube gastrostomy
  ultrasound-assisted
    percutaneous endoscopic
    gastrostomy
  venting percutaneous
    gastrostomy
  Witzel gastrostomy
gastrostomy button
gastrostomy feeding
gastrostomy feeding tube
gastrostomy plug
gastrostomy pump
gastrostomy scarring
gastrostomy scoop
gastrostomy tube
gastrosuccorrhea
gastrotome
gastrotomy
  anterior gastrotomy
  Depage Janeway gastrotomy
  Hahn gastrotomy
  Mikulicz gastrotomy
Gatch bed
gate clamp
gate clip
gate control
gate flap
gated blood pool angiogram
gated blood pool scan
gated nuclear angiogram
gated pool scan
gated pool test
gated radionuclide angiogram
gated technique
gated test
Gatellier incision
Gatellier operation
Gatellier-Chastang ankle
    approach
Gatellier-Chastang incision
Gatellier-Chastang posterolateral
    approach
Gates-Glidden bur

Gates-Glidden drill
Gatlin gun drill guide
Gator drape
Gator meniscal cutter
Gator resector
Gatron nerve stimulator
Gau gastric balloon
Gaubatz rib retractor
Gaucher splenomegaly
Gauder Silicon PEG catheter
Gauderer-Ponsky catheter
Gauderer-Ponsky PEG operation
Gauderer-Ponsky-Izant PEG
    gastrostomy
gauge
Gauge curved chisel
Gaulian knife guide
Gault cochleopalpebral reflex
gauntlet anesthesia
gauntlet bandage
gauntlet flap procedure
gauntlet graft
gauntlet splint
Gaur balloon distention
    technique
Gaure peritoneal forceps
Gauss hemostatic forceps
Gauss sign
gaussian line
Gauthier retractor
Gautier ureteroscope
Gauvain brace
gauze (*see also* bandage)
    absorbable gauze
    absorbent gauze
    Adaptic gauze
    adhesive gauze
    Aquaphor gauze
    Aureomycin gauze
    Avant Gauze nonwoven gauze
    Bettman gauze
    BIPP ribbon gauze
    cellulose gauze
    collodion gauze
    cotton gauze
    Cover-Roll adhesive gauze
    Curafil hydrogel impregnated
        gauze
    dry sterile gauze
    dry textile gauze
    Elasta-Wrap elastic gauze
    elastic gauze

gauze (*continued*)
    fine-mesh gauze
    finger gauze
    Flexicon elastic gauze
    fluffed gauze
    Furacin gauze
    Gelfoam gauze
    GraftCyte gauze
    impregnated gauze
    Intersorb fine mesh gauze
    Intersorb absorbent roll
        stretch gauze
    Intersorb wide mesh gauze
    iodoform gauze
    KBM absorbent gauze
    Kerlix gauze
    Kling elastic gauze
    Kling gauze
    KomForm coated gauze
    Mersilene gauze
    nonstick gauze
    Nuform gauze
    Owen rayon gauze
    Oxycel gauze
    packed with gauze
    PanoGauze hydrogel-
        impregnated gauze
    paraffin-impregnated gauze
    petrolatum-impregnated
        gauze
    plain gauze
    rayon gauze
    Ray-Tec gauze
    Safe-Wrap gauze
    sodium chloride-impregnated
        gauze
    Sof-Form conforming gauze
    Sta-tite elastic roll gauze
    sterile absorbent gauze
    surgical gauze
    surgical steel gauze
    Surgicel gauze
    Surgitube tubular gauze
    tantalum gauze
    Teletrast gauze
    Telfa gauze
    Topper nonadherent gauze
    trailer gauze
    TransiGel hydrogel-
        impregnated gauze
    tube gauze
    uterus packed with gauze

gauze (*continued*)
  Vaseline-coated gauze
  White Plume absorbent gauze
  woven cotton gauze
  Xeroform gauze
  zinc gelatin impregnated gauze
  gauze bandage (*see also*
    gauze, gauze dressing)
gauze dissection
gauze dissector sponge
gauze dressing (*see also*
  bandage, gauze)
gauze neck tie
gauze pack
gauze packer
gauze packing
gauze pad
gauze pad carrier
gauze rosebud sponge
gauze scissors
gauze sponge
gauze stent
gauze stent dressing
gauze strip
gauze tissue bag
gauze wick
Gauztape bandage
Gauztex bandage
Gauztex dressing
gavage
  gastric gavage
  nasal gavage
gavage feeding
gavage tube
Gavard muscle
Gavello operation
Gavin-Miller clamp
Gavin-Miller colon forceps
Gavin-Miller intestinal forceps
Gavin-Miller tissue forceps
gavinofixation
Gavriliu gastric tube
Gay glands
Gayet operation
Gaylor forceps
Gaylor punch
Gaylor tenaculum
Gaylor uterine biopsy forceps
Gaylor uterine specimen forceps
Gaylor-Alexander punch
Gaylord pneumatic tourniquet
Gaynor-Hart position

Gaza operation
Gazayerli endoscopic retractor
Gazayerli knot pusher
Gazayerli-Mediflex retractor
gaze
  conjugate gaze
  disconjugate gaze
Gazelle balloon dilatation
  catheter
GB (gallbladder)
G-banding technique
G-bevel cannula
GBP (gastric bypass)
GC (general closure)
GC filling instrument
GC needle
GC syringe
G-CSF (granulocyte colony-
  stimulating factor)
GE 9800 high-resolution CT
  scanner
GE Advance PET scanner
GE CT Advantage scanner
GE CT Max scanner
GE CT Pace scanner
GE Genesis CT scanner
GE GN 500-MHz scanner
GE HiSpeed Advantage helical
  CT scanner
GE MR Max scanner
GE MR Signa scanner
GE MR Vectra scanner
GE Omega 500-MHz scanner
GE pacemaker
GE single-axis SR-230
  echoplanar scanner
GE Spiral CT scanner
GEA graft
gear shift pedicle probe
Geckeler screw
GEE oculoplethysmography
Geenan cytology brush
Geenan Endotorque guide
Geenan Endotorque guidewire
Geenan Endotorque wire
Geenan graduated dilation
  catheter
Geenan pancreatic stent
Gee-OPG
  (oculoplethysmography)
Gehrung pessary
Geibel blade plate

Geiger cautery
Geiger counter
Geiger electrocautery
Geiger-Downes cautery
Geiger-Mueller counter
Geiger-Mueller detector
Geiger-Mueller tube
Geissendorfer forceps
Geissendorfer rib retractor
Geissendorfer uterine forceps
Geissler tube
Geissler-Pluecker tube
gel barrier
gel bleeds
gel cast
Gel Clean
gel cushion
gel electrophoresis
gel pack
gel pad
gel suspension sleeve
gel wound dressing
Gelastic bed
gelatin compression body
gelatin compression boot
gelatin sponge
gelatin sponge pad
gelatin-covered mesh stent
gelatiniform carcinoma
gelatinous acute inflammation
gelatinous capsule
gelatinous carcinoma
gelatinous compression boot
gelatinous disk
gelatinous film
gelatinous infiltration
gelatinous marrow
gelatinous material
gelatinous sponge
gelatinous tissue
gelatin-resorcin-formalin tissue
    glue
GelBand arm band
Gelcast
Geldmacher tendon-passing
    probe
gel-filled implant
gel-filled prosthesis
Gelfilm cap
Gelfilm dressing
Gelfilm forceps
Gelfilm plate

Gelfilm retinal implant
Gelfilm retinal orbital implant
GelFlex wrist support
Gelfoam cookie
Gelfoam cube
Gelfoam dressing
Gelfoam forceps
Gelfoam gauze
Gelfoam pack
Gelfoam packing
Gelfoam pad
Gelfoam pledget
Gelfoam powder
Gelfoam pressure forceps
Gelfoam punch
Gelfoam sponge
Gelfoam strip
Gelfoam torpedo
Gel-Foam Ultra-Wedge cushion
Gelfoam-soaked pledget
Gell and Coombs classification
Gellhorn forceps
Gellhorn pessary
Gellhorn punch
Gellhorn uterine biopsy forceps
Gellhorn uterine biopsy punch
Gellman instrumentation
Gellquist scissors
GellyComb bed
Gelman procedure
Gelocast cast material
Gelocast dressing
Gelocast Unna boot
gelotripsy
Gelpi abdominal retractor
Gelpi forceps
Gelpi hysterectomy forceps
Gelpi perineal retractor
Gelpi retractor
Gelpi self-retaining retractor
Gelpi vaginal retractor
Gelpi-Lowrie forceps
Gelpi-Lowrie hysterectomy
Gelpi-Lowrie hysterectomy
    forceps
Gelpi-Lowrie retractor
gel-saline mammary implant
gel-saline Surgitek prosthesis
Gelseal vascular patch
Gelsoft vascular graft
Gel-Sole shoe insert
Gel-Syte wound dressing

gel-treated scars
Gelweave vascular graft
Gely sutures
Gem defibrillator
Gem DR implantable
    defibrillator
Gembase dental cement
Gemcem dental cement
Gemcore dental cement
gemellary pregnancy
gemellus muscle
geminate teeth
Gemini clamp
Gemini cup
Gemini DDD pacemaker
Gemini forceps
Gemini gall duct forceps
Gemini hemostatic forceps
Gemini hip system prosthesis
Gemini Mixter forceps
Gemini pacemaker
Gemini paired helical wire
    basket
Gemini syringe
Gemini thoracic forceps
genal glands
Gendelach sphenoid punch
gender identity formation
gender reassignment
gene induction
gene mapping
gene replacement therapy
Genell biopsy curet
GeneraBloc bite block
general anatomy
general anesthesia (GA)
general anesthetic technique
general cataract
general closure (GC)
general closure needle
general closure sutures
general endotracheal anesthesia
    (GET)
general eye surgery sutures
general inhalation anesthesia
general insufflation anesthesia
general laparoscopic surgical
    procedure
general operating scissors
general probe
general retractor
general surgery

general thoracic surgery
general thrust manipulation
general tissue forceps
general utility scissors
general wire forceps
generalized atrophic benign
    epidermolysis bullosa
    (GABEB)
generalized chondromalacia
generalized cortical hyperostosis
generalized fatigue
generalized maculopapular rash
generalized malignancy
generalized metastasis
generalized osteoarthritis (GOA)
generalized pain
generalized scleroderma
generalized tenderness
generalized weakness
generalized xanthelasma
Generation II knee brace
Genesis 2000 carbon dioxide
    laser
Genesis arthroplasty hardware
Genesis diamond blade
Genesis knee prosthesis
Genesis lens
Genesis unicompartmental knee
Genestone 190 lithotripter
genetic abnormality
genetic amniocentesis
genetic anomaly
genetic approach
genetic condition
genetic defect
genetic diagnosis
genetic disease
genetic factor
genetic lesion
genetic markers
genetic pattern
genetic risk
genetic structures
genetic therapy
genetically at risk
gene-transfer therapy
genial advancement plate
genial apophysis
genial hypertrophy
genial tubercle
genicular anastomosis
genicular artery

genicular branch
genicular veins
geniculate
geniculate bodies
geniculate body
geniculate ganglion
geniculocalcarine tract
geniculum of facial canal
geniculum of facial nerve
geniocheiloplasty
genioglossus muscle
geniohyoglossus muscle
geniohyoid muscle
geniohyoid space
genioplasty
    advancement genioplasty
    alloplastic augmentation
        genioplasty
    augmentation genioplasty
    centering genioplasty
    jumping genioplasty
    lengthening genioplasty
    osseous genioplasty
    reduction genioplasty
    reduction-advancement
        genioplasty
    sliding genioplasty
    staged genioplasty
genioplasty procedure
Genisis dual-chamber
    pacemaker
Genisis pacemaker
genital area
genital carcinoma
genital duct
genital eminence
genital fold
genital gland
genital neoplasia
genital papulosquamous lesion
genital reconstruction
genital swelling
genitalia
genitofemoral nerve
genitoplasty
    feminizing genitoplasty
    masculinizing genitoplasty
Genitor mini-intrauterine
    insemination cannula
genitospinal center
genitourinary anomaly
genitourinary cancer

genitourinary evaluation
genitourinary fistula
genitourinary region
genitourinary tract
genodermatology
genodermatosis
Genotropin pen
Gensini angiocatheter
Gensini cardiac device
Gensini catheter
Gensini coronary arteriography
    catheter
Gensini Teflon catheter
gentamicin implant
Gentell alginate wound dressing
Gentell foam wound dressing
Gentell hydrogel dressing
Gentell isotonic saline wet
    dressing
gentian violet marking pen
gentle active flexion
gentle compression
gentle exercise
gentle rocking motion
Gentle Threads interference
    screws
Gentle Threads resorbable
    interference screws
Gentle Touch colostomy
    appliance
gentle traction
Gentle-Flo suction catheter
GentleLASE laser
GentleLASE Plus laser
GentleYAG laser
genu (pl. genua)
genu corporis callosi
genu impressum
genu nervi facialis
genu of facial canal
genu recurvatum
genu valgum
genu valgum deformity
genu valgus
genu varum
genu varum deformity
genucubital position
genufacial position
Genupak tampon
genupectoral position
Genutrain knee brace
Genutrain knee support

geographic landmarks
geographic tongue
Geomedic arthroplasty
Geomedic femoral condyle prosthesis
Geomedic femoral pusher
Geomedic jig
Geomedic knee prosthesis
Geomedic prosthesis
Geomedic total knee prosthesis
geometric broken line closure (GBLC)
Geometric knee prosthesis
geometric nasal flap
geopatellar-type knee replacement
Georgariou operation
George Washington strut
George Winter elevator torque technique
Georgia valve
Georgiade breast prosthesis
Georgiade fixation device
Georgiade intraoral traction
Georgiade rasp
Georgiade visor
Georgiade visor cervical traction
Gerald bayonet microbipolar neurosurgical forceps
Gerald bipolar forceps
Gerald brain forceps
Gerald clamp
Gerald dressing forceps
Gerald monopolar forceps
Gerald straight microbipolar neurosurgical forceps
Gerald tissue forceps
Gerber space maintainer
Gerber test
Gerbode annuloplasty
Gerbode cardiovascular tissue forceps
Gerbode dilator
Gerbode forceps
Gerbode mitral dilator
Gerbode mitral valvulotome
Gerbode mitral valvulotomy dilator
Gerbode modified Burford rib spreader
Gerbode patent ductus clamp
Gerbode rib spreader

Gerbode sternal retractor
Gerbode valve dilator
GERD (gastroesophageal reflux disease)
Gerdy fibers
Gerdy fontanelle
Gerdy hyoid fossa
Gerdy interauricular loop
Gerdy knee tubercle
Gerdy tubercle
Gerhardt sign
Gerhardt table
Gerhardt triangle
geriatric anesthesia
Geristore dental implant
Geristore repair material
Gerlach tonsil
germ line
Germafect
Germain needle holder
German A-O hip compression screw
germ-free environment
germinal center formation
germinal infection
germinal layer
germinal matrix
germinal matrix hemorrhage
germinal membrane
germinal rod
germ-laden air
geroderma
geromorphism
Gerota capsule
Gerota fascia
Gerow Small-Carrion penile implant
Gerow-Harrington heart-shaped distal end retractor
Gerster bone clamp
Gerster fracture appliance
Gerster traction bar
Gerster traction device
Gersuny operation
Gerzog bone hammer
Gerzog bone mallet
Gerzog ear knife
Gerzog hammer
Gerzog knife
Gerzog mallet
Gerzog mastoid mallet
Gerzog nasal speculum

Gerzog speculum
Gerzog-Ralks ear knife
Gerzog-Ralks knife
Gesco aspirator
Gesco cannula
Gesco catheter
Gess cannula tip
gestant anomaly
gestation
gestational age
gestational diabetes
gestational period
gestational sac
gestational size
gestational weeks
gesticulatory tic
GET anesthesia (general
    endotracheal anesthesia)
Getty decompression technique
Getty technique for spinal
    stenosis
Getz crown
Getz root canal pin
Geuder corneal needle
Geuder implanter
Geuder keratoplasty needle
GFC gastroscope
GFH alloy
GFS Mark II inflatable penile
    prosthesis
GFX coronary stent
Ghajar guide
Ghazi rib retractor
Gherini-Kauffman endo-
    otoprobe
Gherini-Kauffman endo-
    otoprobe laser
Ghon complex
Ghon focus
Ghon lesion
Ghon primary lesion
Ghon tubercle
Ghormley double cannula
Ghormley operation
ghost ophthalmoscope
ghost pain
ghost vessels
ghoul hand
GHRF (growth hormone-
    releasing factor)
GI (gastrointestinal)
GI bleed

GI clamp
GI forceps
GI pop-off silk sutures
GI silk sutures
GIA (gastrointestinal
    anastomosis)
GIA circular stapler
GIA forceps
GIA II loading unit
GIA instrument
GIA staple
GIA stapler
GIA stapling device
Giampapa sutures
Giampapa suturing technique
Giannestras metatarsal
    procedure
Giannestras modification of
    Lapidus technique
Giannestras procedure
Giannestras step-down
    procedure
Giannestras turnbuckle
Giannini needle holder
Gianotti-Crosti syndrome
giant cell adenocarcinoma
giant cell arteritis
giant cell carcinoma
giant cell fibroma
giant cell granuloma
giant cell hyaline angiopathy
giant cell lesion
giant cell tumor
giant condyloma acuminatum
giant congenital nevus
giant fibroadenoma of the breast
giant finger
giant follicle lymphoma
giant pigmented nevus
giant swelling
giantism
Gianturco coil
Gianturco expandable metallic
    biliary stent
Gianturco expanding metallic
    stent
Gianturco metal urethral stent
Gianturco occlusion coil
Gianturco prosthesis
Gianturco steel coil
Gianturco stent
Gianturco sutures

Gianturco wool-tufted wire coil
Gianturco zigzag stent
Gianturco Z-stent
Gianturco-Roehm bird's nest vena caval filter
Gianturco-Roehm vena cava filter
Gianturco-Rosch self-expandable biliary Z stent
Gianturco-Rosch Z-stent
Gianturco-Roubin flexible coil stent
Gianturco-Roubin FlexStent coronary stent
Gianturco-Roubin stent
Gianturco-Wallace-Anderson coil
Giardet corneal transplant scissors
Gibbon catheter
Gibbon hernia
Gibbon hydrocele
Gibbon indwelling ureteral stent
Gibbon stent
Gibbon ureteral stent
Gibbon urethral catheter
Gibbs eye punch
gibbus deformity
Gibney bandage
Gibney boot
Gibney dressing
Gibney fixation bandage
Gibney perispondylitis
Gibney strapping
Gibralter headrest
Gibson anterior chamber irrigator
Gibson approach
Gibson bandage
Gibson dressing
Gibson eye irrigator
Gibson I&A unit
Gibson incision
Gibson inner ear shunt
Gibson irrigator
Gibson long vertical relaxing incision
Gibson murmur
Gibson operation
Gibson principle
Gibson splint
Gibson stone dislodger
Gibson sutures

Gibson vestibule
Gibson-Balfour abdominal retractor
Gibson-Balfour retractor
Gibson-Foley incision
Gibson-Gibson posterior muscle-cutting incision
Gibson-type incision
Giebel blade plate
Giedion syndrome
Gierke respiratory bundle
Giertz rib guillotine
Giertz rib shears
Giertz rongeur
Giertz-Shoemaker rib shears
Giertz-Shoemaker shears
Giertz-Stille rib shears
Giertz-Stille scissors
Giesy ureteral dilatation balloon
Gifford applicator
Gifford corneal applicator
Gifford corneal curet
Gifford curet
Gifford delimiting keratotomy operation
Gifford fixation forceps
Gifford forceps
Gifford holder
Gifford iris forceps
Gifford keratotomy
Gifford maneuver
Gifford mastoid retractor
Gifford needle holder
Gifford operation
Gifford reflex
Gifford retractor
Gifford scalp retractor
Gifford sign
Gifford-Galassie reflex
Gifford-Jansen mastoid retractor
GIF-HM endoscope
GIF-N-series fiberoptic pediatric endoscope
GIFT (gamete intrafallopian transfer)
gift wrap suture technique
GIF-XP-series endoscope
GIF-XQ endoscope
GIF-XQ fiberoptic instrument
GIF-XQ-series endoscope
gigahertz
gigantism

gigantomastia
gigantosoma
Gigli operation
Gigli pubiotomy
Gigli saw
Gigli solid-handle saw
Gigli spiral saw wire
Gigli wire saw
Gigli-saw blade
Gigli-saw conductor
Gigli-saw guide
Gigli-saw handle
Gigli-saw wire
Gigli-Strully saw
Gilbert balloon catheter
Gilbert catheter
Gilbert cystic duct forceps
Gilbert forceps
Gilbert pediatric balloon
    catheter
Gilbert pediatric catheter
Gilbert plug-sealing catheter
Gilbert prosthesis
Gilbert scapular flap
Gilbert sign
Gilbert stage shoulder
    abduction
Gilbert-Graves speculum
Gilbert-Tamai-Weiland technique
Gilbert-type Bardex Foley
    catheter
Gilchrist disease
Gilchrist procedure
Gildenberg biopsy forceps
Gilfillan humeral prosthesis
Giliberty acetabular prosthesis
Giliberty cup hip prosthesis
Giliberty device
Giliberty prosthesis
Giliberty total hip prosthesis
Gill biopsy brush
Gill blade
Gill cleft palate elevator
Gill corneal knife
Gill counterpressor
Gill curved iris forceps
Gill double I&A cannula
Gill double Luer-Lok cannula
Gill dropfoot procedure
Gill forceps
Gill I respirator
Gill incision spreader

Gill incision-spreading forceps
Gill intraocular implant lens
Gill iris forceps
Gill iris knife
Gill knife
Gill laminectomy
Gill lesion
Gill massive sliding graft
Gill needle
Gill needle holder
Gill operation
Gill pop-up arcuate diamond knife
Gill pressor counter
Gill procedure
Gill renal tourniquet
Gill respirator
Gill scissors
Gill shoulder arthrodesis
Gill sinus cannula
Gill sliding graft technique
Gill-Arruga capsular forceps
Gill-Chandler iris forceps
Gilles operation
Gillespie obstetrical forceps
Gillespie operation
Gillespie wrist excision
Gillette brace
Gillette joint orthosis
Gillette joint prosthesis
Gillette modification of ankle-
    foot orthosis
Gill-Fine corneal knife
Gill-Fuchs capsular forceps
Gill-Fuchs forceps
Gill-Hess blade
Gill-Hess forceps
Gill-Hess iris forceps
Gill-Hess knife
Gill-Hess mules
Gill-Hess scissors
Gilliam operation
Gilliam suspension of uterus
Gilliam uterine suspension
Gilliam-Doleris operation
Gilliam-Doleris uterine
    suspension
Gillies approach
Gillies bone graft
Gillies bone hook
Gillies cocked hat procedure
Gillies construction of
    replacement thumb

Gillies dissecting forceps
Gillies dural hook
Gillies ectropion graft
Gillies elevation procedure
Gillies elevator
Gillies fan flap
Gillies fashion
Gillies flap
Gillies forceps
Gillies graft
Gillies hook
Gillies horizontal dermal suture
Gillies implant
Gillies incision
Gillies nasal hook
Gillies needle holder
Gillies operation
Gillies prosthesis
Gillies scar correction operation
Gillies scissors
Gillies single-hook skin retractor
Gillies skin hook
Gillies suture scissors
Gillies tissue forceps
Gillies up-and-down flap
Gillies zygoma elevator
Gillies zygoma hook
Gillies zygomatic elevator
Gillies zygomatic hook
Gillies-Converse skin hook
Gillies-Dingman hook
Gillies-Dingman tenaculum hook
Gillies-Fry operation
Gillies-Kilner operation
Gillies-Millard cocked-hat
  technique
Gillies-Millard technique
Gillies-Sheehan needle holder
Gill-Jonas modification of
  Norwood procedure
Gill-Jonas procedure
Gill-Manning decompression
  laminectomy
Gill-Manning-White fusion
Gill-Manning-White
  spondylolisthesis technique
Gillmore needle
Gillquist approach
Gillquist suction curet
Gillquist suction tube
Gillquist-Oretorp-Stille dilator
Gillquist-Oretorp-Stille forceps

Gillquist-Oretorp-Stille knife
Gillquist-Oretorp-Stille needle
  holder
Gillquist-Oretorp-Stille probe
Gillquist-Stille arthroplasty
  suction tube
Gills intraocular implant lens
Gills lens
Gills technique
Gill-Safar forceps
Gill-Stein arthrodesis of wrist
Gill-Stein operation
Gill-Stein radiocarpal arthrodesis
Gills-Welsh cortex extractor
Gills-Welsh irrigating cannula
Gill-Thomas locator
Gill-Welsh aspirating cannula
Gill-Welsh capsular forceps
Gill-Welsh capsular polisher
Gill-Welsh curet
Gill-Welsh double cannula
Gill-Welsh guillotine port
Gill-Welsh knife
Gill-Welsh lens loop
Gill-Welsh olive-tip cannula
Gill-Welsh scissors
Gill-Welsh spatula
Gill-Welsh-Morrison lens loop
Gill-Welsh-Vannas angled
  microscissors
Gill-Welsh-Vannas capsulotomy
  scissors
Gilman-Abrams gastric tube
Gilman-Abrams tube
Gilmer dental splint
Gilmer intermaxillary fixation
Gilmer splint
Gilmer tooth splint
Gilmer wire
Gilmer wiring
Gilmore intraocular implant lens
Gilmore lens
Gilmore probe
Gillquist arthroscopy
Gillquist incision
Gillquist procedure
Gil-Vernet dissection
Gil-Vernet ileocecal cystoplasty
Gil-Vernet ileocecal cystoplasty
  urinary diversion
Gil-Vernet lumbotomy retractor
Gil-Vernet operation

Gil-Vernet procedure
Gil-Vernet pyelolithotomy
Gil-Vernet renal sinus retractor
Gil-Vernet retractor
Gil-Vernet technique
Gimbel fountain cannula
Gimbel glove
Gimbel stabilizing ring
Gimbernat ligament
Gimmick elevator
gingiva (*pl.* gingivae)
gingival anatomy
gingival augmentation
gingival cartilage
gingival cavity
gingival clamp
gingival crevice
gingival deformity
gingival embrasure
gingival esthetics
gingival exudate
gingival exudation
gingival finishing line
gingival fistula
gingival flap
gingival hemorrhage
gingival incision
gingival inflammation
gingival lancet
gingival ligament
gingival line
gingival margin
gingival massage
gingival mucosa
gingival point
gingival position
gingival space
gingival sulcus
gingival trough
gingivectomy
    chemosurgical gingivectomy
    Ochsenbein gingivectomy
gingivectomy knife
gingivitis
    cotton-roll gingivitis
    desquamative gingivitis
    leukemic hyperplastic
        gingivitis
    marginal gingivitis
    menstruation gingivitis
gingivobuccal groove
gingivobuccal sulcus

gingivodental ligament
gingivoglossitis
gingivolabial groove
gingivolabial incision
gingivolabial sulcus
gingivolingual groove
gingivolingual sulcus
gingivo-osseous
gingivoperiosteoplasty
gingivoplasty
gingivostomatitis
ginglymoid joint
Gingrass-Messer pin
Ginsberg forceps
Ginsberg tissue forceps
Gio-occlusive dressing
Giordano operation
Giordano sphincter
GIP/Medi-Globe needle
giraffe biopsy forceps
Girard anterior chamber needle
Girard cataract-aspirating needle
Girard corneoscleral forceps
Girard corneoscleral scissors
Girard forceps
Girard Fragmatome probe
Girard irrigating cannula
Girard irrigating tip
Girard keratoprosthesis
Girard keratoprosthesis
        operation
Girard needle
Girard phacofragmatome
Girard phacofragmatome needle
Girard probe
Girard procedure
Girard scleral ring
Girard synechia spatula
Girard ultrasonic unit
Girard-Swan knife
Girard-Swan knife-needle
Girard-Swan needle
girdle
    Ace halo pelvic girdle
    compression girdle
    limb girdle
    Lipo-Medi girdle
    male compression girdle
    pectoral girdle
    pelvic girdle
    shoulder girdle
girdle anesthesia

Girdlestone excision of femoral
   head and neck
Girdlestone hip resection
Girdlestone joint resection
Girdlestone laminectomy
Girdlestone resection
Girdlestone resection arthroplasty
Girdlestone-Taylor operation for
   claw toes
Girdlestone-Taylor procedure
Girdner probe
Gironcoli hernia
Gish micro YAG laser
Gissane angle
Gissane spike
Gissane spike nail
GIST (gastrointestinal stromal
   tumor)
Gittes operation
Gittes procedure
Gittes technique
Gittes-Loughlin bladder neck
   suspension
Gittes-Loughlin procedure
Giuffrida-Ruggieri stigma
Givner eye retractor
Givner lid retractor
Gizmo catheter
glabella
glabellar bilobed flap
glabellar cease
glabellar crease
glabellar fracture
glabellar frown line
glabellar laxity
glabellar line
glabellar rasp
glabellar region
glabellar rhytids
glabellar rotation flap
glabellar wrinkle
glabelloalveolar line
glabrous skin
Glacier ceramic 4-in-1 knee
   cutting guide
GLAD (glenolabral articular
   disruption of shoulder)
gladiolus bone
Gladstone-Putterman
   transmarginal rotation
   entropion clamp
glairy mucus

gland
abnormally hyperplastic gland
accessory adrenal gland
accessory gland
accessory parotid gland
accessory suprarenal gland
accessory thyroid gland
achroacytosis of lacrimal
   gland
acid gland
acinar gland
acinous gland
admaxillary gland
adrenal glands
aggregate gland
agminate gland
albarran gland
alveolar gland
anal gland
anterior lingual gland
apical gland
apocrine gland
apocrine sweat glands
areola of mammary gland
areolar gland
arteriococcygeal gland
arytenoid glands
axillary gland
axillary sweat gland
Bartholin glands
Bartholin, Skene, and urethral
   glands (BSU glands)
Bauhin glands
Baumgarten gland
Blandin and Nuhn glands
Blandin glands
Boerhaave gland
Bowman glands
brachial gland
bronchial glands
Bruch gland
Brunner glands
buccal glands
bulbocavernous glands
bulbourethral glands
cardiac glands
carotid gland
celiac glands
ceruminous gland
cervical glands
cheek glands
Ciaccio glands

gland (*continued*)
- ciliary glands
- circumanal glands
- Cobelli glands
- coccygeal glands
- coil gland
- compound gland
- conglobate gland
- contralateral parathyroid gland
- Cowper glands
- cutaneous gland
- dominant gland
- drainage of gland
- ductless glands
- duodenal gland
- Duverney gland
- Ebner gland
- eccrine gland
- eccrine sweat glands
- ectopic sebaceous gland
- Eglis gland
- elongated gland
- endocervical glands
- endocrine glands
- endometrial glands
- enlarged parathyroid gland
- entrapped gland
- esophageal ectopic sebaceous gland
- esophageal glands
- exocrine gland
- external genitalia, Bartholin, urethral, and Skene glands
- external salivary gland
- fossa of lacrimal gland
- fundal glands
- fundic gland
- fundus gland
- Galeati gland
- gastric glands
- Gay glands
- genal glands
- genital gland
- Gley glands
- glossopalatine gland
- greater vestibular gland
- gustatory glands
- Guerin gland
- Harder glands
- harderian glands
- Haver glands

gland (*continued*)
- Havers gland
- haversian gland
- hematopoietic gland
- hemolymph glands
- Henle glands
- hibernating gland
- holocrine gland
- hypercellular gland
- hyperplastic gland
- incision and drainage of gland
- inferior gland
- inferior parathyroid gland
- inferior thyroid gland
- inguinal gland
- internal salivary gland
- interstitial gland
- intestinal glands
- intraepithelial glands
- ipsilateral gland
- jugular gland
- Knoll glands
- Krause gland
- labial glands
- labial minor salivary gland
- lacrimal gland
- lactiferous gland
- laryngeal glands
- lesser vestibular gland
- Lieberkuhn gland
- lingual gland
- Littre glands
- lobe of pituitary gland
- lobe of thyroid gland
- Luschka gland
- lymph gland
- major salivary glands
- malar glands
- mammary glands
- mandibular gland
- Manz gland
- marrow-lymph gland
- master gland
- maxillary gland
- Meibom gland
- meibomian glands
- merocrine gland
- mesenteric gland
- milk gland
- minor salivary glands
- mixed glands
- mixed tumor of salivary gland

gland (*continued*)
  molar glands
  Moll glands
  Montgomery glands
  mucilaginous gland
  muciparous gland
  mucoparous gland
  mucous glands
  mucus-secreting gland
  Mery gland
  Naboth glands
  nabothian gland
  nasal glands
  nondominant gland
  Nuhn glands
  odoriferous gland
  oil glands
  olfactory glands
  pacchionian glands
  palatal gland
  palatine glands
  palpebral glands
  parathyroid gland
  paraurethral glands
  parotid gland
  pectoral glands
  peptic gland
  perspiratory gland
  Peyer glands
  pharyngeal glands
  pileous gland
  pineal gland
  pituitary gland
  Poirier glands
  prehyoid gland
  preputial gland
  prostate gland
  pyloric gland
  racemose gland
  remnant gland
  retrosternal gland
  Rivinus gland
  Rosenmueller gland
  salivary gland
  sebaceous glands
  seminal gland
  sentinel gland
  seromucous glands
  serous glands
  Serres glands
  sexual gland
  Skene glands

gland (*continued*)
  solitary gland
  splenolymph glands
  Stahr gland
  sublingual glands
  sublingual salivary gland
  submandibular gland
  submandibular salivary gland
  submaxillary gland
  submaxillary salivary gland
  submental glands
  substernal gland
  sudoriferous glands
  sudoriparous glands
  superior lacrimal gland
  superior parathyroid gland
  superior thyroid gland
  supernumerary gland
  suprahyoid gland
  suprarenal glands
  Suzanne gland
  sweat glands
  swollen glands
  synovial gland
  target gland
  tarsal gland
  tarsoconjunctival glands
  Theile glands
  thymus gland
  thyroid gland
  tortuosity of glands
  tracheal gland
  trachoma gland
  trigeminal gland
  tubular gland
  Tyson glands
  urethral gland
  uterine gland
  vaginal gland
  vesical gland
  vestibular gland
  von Ebner glands
  vulvovaginal glands
  Woelfer gland
  Waldeyer glands
  Wasmann gland
  Weber gland
  Wepfer gland
  Wolfring glands
  Zeiss glands
gland appearance
gland removal

gland size
gland volume
glandilemma
glands of mouth
glandular abscess
glandular atrophy
glandular cancer
glandular carcinoma
glandular foramen of tongue
glandular fossa of frontal bone
glandular hypertrophy
glandular hypospadias
glandular massage
glandular neoplasm
glandular odontogenic cyst
glandular tissue
glanduloplasty (*variant of*
    glanuloplasty)
glans clitoridis
glans of penis
glans penis
glanuloplasty
Glaser laminectomy retractor
Glaser retractor
glaserian fissure
Glasgold Wafer chin implant
Glasgow coma scale
Glasgow sign
Glass abdominal retractor
glass hand
glass hand operation
glass ionomer cement
glass ionomer restorative material
glassblower's cataract
Glasscock dressing
Glasscock ear dressing
Glasscock scissors
Glasscock-House knife
Glasser fixation screw
Glasser gastrostomy tube
Glassman anterior resection
    clamp
Glassman basket
Glassman bowel atraumatic
    clamp
Glassman brush
Glassman clamp
Glassman forceps
Glassman gastroenterostomy
    clamp
Glassman gastrointestinal clamp
Glassman gastrostomy

Glassman grasper
Glassman intestinal clamp
Glassman liver-holding clamp
Glassman noncrushing
    gastroenterostomy clamp
Glassman noncrushing
    gastrointestinal clamp
Glassman noncrushing
    instruments
Glassman noncrushing pickup
    forceps
Glassman pickup forceps
Glassman scissors
Glassman stone extractor
Glassman-Allis clamp
Glassman-Allis common duct-
    holding forceps
Glassman-Allis forceps
Glassman-Allis intestinal forceps
Glassman-Allis miniature
    intestinal forceps
Glassman-Allis noncrushing
    common duct forceps
Glassman-Allis noncrushing
    intestinal forceps
Glassman-Allis noncrushing
    tissue-holding forceps
Glassman-Babcock forceps
glassy cell carcinoma
glassy membrane
glassy swelling
Glat hand drill
Glattelast elastic knee support
glaucoma
    absolute glaucoma
    angle-closure glaucoma
    closed-angle glaucoma
    congestive glaucoma
    narrow-angle glaucoma
    neovascular glaucoma
    open-angle glaucoma
    wide-angle glaucoma
glaucoma drainage device
glaucoma knife
glaucoma pencil
glaucoma surgery
glaucomatous cataract
glaucomatous excavation
glaucomatous halo
Gleason headband
Gleason prostatic carcinoma
    score

Gleason rasp
Gleason raspatory
Gleason score of prostatic
  carcinoma
Gleason speculum
Gleason staging of prostate
  cancer
Gledhill technique
Glegg nasal polyp snare
Glen Anderson technique
Glen Anderson
  ureteroneocystostomy
Glenn anastomosis
Glenn diverticular forceps
Glenn diverticulum forceps
Glenn operation
Glenn procedure
Glenn shunt
Glenner forceps
Glenner hysterectomy forceps
Glenner retractor
Glenner vaginal hysterectomy
  forceps
Glenner vaginal retractor
glenohumeral articulation
glenohumeral dislocation repair
glenohumeral joint
glenohumeral joint dislocation
glenohumeral ligaments
glenoid cavity
glenoid drill
glenoid drill guide
glenoid fin broach
glenoid fixation screw
glenoid fossa
glenoid fossa of temporal bone
glenoid labrum
glenoid ligaments
glenoid point
glenoid process
glenoid punch
glenoid rim fracture
glenoid-reaming forceps
glenoplasty
Gley glands
glial membrane
glial sheath
Glick instrument
glide
  acentric glide
  Hessburg intraocular lens
    glide

glide (*continued*)
  intraocular lens glide
  mandibular glide
  mushroom walker glide
  Pearce intraocular glide
  Sheets intraocular glide
  Sheets lens glide
Glidecath hydrophilic coated
  catheter
Glidewire catheter
Glidewire Gold surgical
  guidewire
Glidewire Gold surgical
  guidewire
Glidex coated Percuflex
  catheter
gliding hinge joint
gliding joint
gliding motion
gliding movement
gliding prosthesis
gliding-hole-first technique
glioma
  ganglionic glioma
  infiltrating glioma
  nasal glioma
  peripheral glioma
  telangiectatic glioma
glioma sarcomatosum
glioneuroma
gliosarcoma
gliotic membrane
glissade
  hernia en glissade
Glissane ankle fusion
glissement
  hernia par glissement
Glisson capsule
Glisson sling
Glisson sling splint
Glisson snare
glistening fragments
glistening transparent meninges
global force applicator
global hypoperfusion
Global stent Freedom stent
Global stent V-Flex stent
Global total shoulder implant
globe dystopia
globe of eye
globe prolapsus pessary
globe retropulsion

globular abdomen
globular collection
globular object forceps
globulin
  antihemophilic globulin (AHG)
  antithymocyte globulin (ATG)
  gamma globulin
  immune globulin
  intramuscular immune
    globulin
  intravenous immune globulin
globulomaxillary cyst
globus abdominalis
globus hystericus
globus major epididymidis
globus minor epididymidis
globus of heel
globus pallidus
Glolite infrared light
glomangioma
glomangiomatous osseous
    malformation syndrome
glomangiosis
Glomark fluorescent skin marker
glomectomy
glomerular arteriole
glomerular basement membrane
glomerular capsule
glomerular extracellular matrix
glomerular filtration rate (GFR)
glomerular hyperfiltration
glomerular infiltration
glomerular macrophage
    infiltration
glomerular nephritis
glomerular neutrophil
    infiltration
glomerular tip lesion
glomerulocapsular nephritis
glomerulonephritis
glomerulus (pl. glomeruli)
glomus arteriovenous
    malformation
glomus body
glomus jugulare tumor
glomus tumor
Glori post-keloid surgery
    pressure earrings
glossectomy
  Commando glossectomy
  Commando radical
    glossectomy

glossectomy (continued)
  partial glossectomy
  subtotal glossectomy
  total glossectomy
glossitis
  atrophic glossitis
  benign migratory glossitis
  Clarke-Fournier glossitis
  Hunter glossitis
  idiopathic glossitis
  median rhomboid glossitis
  Moeller glossitis
  rhomboid glossitis
glossitis areata exfoliativa
glossitis desiccans
glossitis migrans
glossocele
glossodynia
glossodynia exfoliativa
glossoepiglottic
glossoepiglottic fold
glossohyal
glossoncus
glossopalatine ankylosis
glossopalatine arch
glossopalatine fold
glossopalatine gland
glossopalatine muscle
glossopexy
glossopharyngeal breathing
glossopharyngeal ganglion
glossopharyngeal muscle
glossopharyngeal nerve (cranial
    nerve 9)
glossopharyngeal nerve block
glossopharyngeal nerve sign
glossopharyngeal neurotomy
glossoplasty
glossorrhaphy
glossosteresis
glossotomy
  labiomandibular glossotomy
  median labiomandibular
    glossotomy
  midline sagittal glossotomy
Glo-Tip ERCP catheter
glottal area
glottal chink
glottic carcinoma
glottic chink
glottic closure
glottic extension

glottic larynx
glottic prosthesis
glottic spasm
glottic squamous cell carcinoma
glottic stenosis
glottidis
   edema glottidis
   rima glottidis
   spasmus glottidis
   vestibulum glottidis
glottis (*pl.* glottides)
glottitis
glove
glove anesthesia
Glove drain
gloved-fist technique
Glove-n-Gel amniotome
Glove-n-Gel amniotomy kit
Glover anastomosis forceps
Glover auricular clamp
Glover auricular-appendage
   clamp
Glover bulldog clamp
Glover coarctation clamp
Glover coarctation forceps
Glover curved clamp
Glover curved forceps
Glover dilator
Glover forceps
Glover infundibular rongeur
   forceps
Glover modification of Brock
   aortic dilator
Glover patent ductus clamp
Glover patent ductus forceps
Glover rongeur
Glover rongeur forceps
Glover spoon anastomosis clamp
Glover spoon-shaped
   anastomosis clamp
Glover spoon-shaped forceps
Glover suction tube
Glover suture technique
Glover vascular clamp
Glover-DeBakey clamp
glover's sutures
Glover-Stille clamp
gloving
   double gloving
gloving technique
GLR (gravity lumbar reduction)
glucagonoma syndrome

Gluck incision
Gluck rib shears
Gluck shears
Glucolet lancet device
GlucoScan monitor
glucose 6-phosphate
   dehydrogenase
glue
   Aron Alpha glue
   BioGlue glue
   Biolex wound glue
   butyl cyanoacrylate glue
   CoSeal fibrin glue
   CoStasis fibrin glue
   cyanoacrylate glue
   ethyl cyanoacrylate glue
   fibrin glue
   gelatin-resorcin-formalin tissue
    glue
   Histoacryl glue
   hydroxyapatite fibrin glue
   K-Simplex glue
   methyl cyanoacrylate glue
   methyl methacrylate glue
   Tisseel fibrin glue
   Tisseel surgical glue
   tissue glue
glue patch
glue patch leak
glued-on hard contact lens
glue-in sutures
glueophytes (*slang*)
glutaraldehyde-tanned bovine
   carotid artery graft
glutaraldehyde-tanned bovine
   heart valve
glutaraldehyde-tanned porcine
   heart valve
gluteal artery
gluteal banana roll
gluteal bonnet
gluteal cleft
gluteal fascia
gluteal flap
gluteal fold
gluteal furrow
gluteal hernia
gluteal line
gluteal muscle
gluteal nerve
gluteal reflex
gluteal thigh flap

gluteal veins
gluteal vessels
gluteofemoral
gluteus maximus
gluteus maximus flap
gluteus maximus
    musculocutaneous flap
gluteus maximus myocutaneous
    flap
gluteus minimus
glycerin syringe
glycerin-preserved graft
glyceryl guaiacolate
glyceryl methacrylate
glyceryl trinitrate
glycine
glycocalyx-enclosed biofilm
glycogen infiltration
glycolic acid
glycolic acid peeling
glycolic skin peel
glycosialorrhea
glycosuria
Glynn-Neibauer technique
GM (gingival margin)
GM alloy
gnarled enamel
gnathalgia
gnathic index
gnathion
gnathitis
gnathodynamometer
gnathodynia
gnathography
gnathologic instrument
gnathologic orthopedics
gnathological splint
gnathoplasty
gnathoschisis
gnathostatic cast
gnathostomatics
gnawing pain
gnawing sensation
GOA (generalized osteoarthritis)
Gobble Plus removal instrument
Gobin-Weiss loop
goblet incision
Goddio disposable cannula
Godelo dilator
Godina vessel-fixation
    instrument
Godwin tumor

Goebel procedure
Goebel-Frangenheim-Stoeckel
    operation
Goebel-Stoeckel operation
Goebel-Stoeckel sling
Goebel-Stoeckel snare
Goebel-Stoeckel-Frangenheim
    procedure
Goeckerman light therapy
Goelet double-ended retractor
Goelet retractor
Goethe sutures
Goetz bipolar electrode
Goetz cardiac device
Goffe colporrhaphy
Goffe operation
Goffman blue eye garter shield
Goffman occluder
Gohrbrand cardiac dilator
Gohrbrand dilator
Gohrbrand valvulotome
Goidnich bone plate
goiter
    aberrant goiter
    adenomatous goiter
    colloid goiter
    congenital goiter
    cystic goiter
    diffuse colloid goiter
    diffuse multimodular goiter
    diffuse toxic non-nodular
        goiter
    endemic goiter
    exophthalmic goiter
    fibrous goiter
    multinodular goiter
    nodular goiter
    nontoxic goiter
    papillomatous goiter
    parenchymatous goiter
    substernal goiter
    suffocative goiter
    thyrotoxic goiter
    toxic goiter
goiter clamp
goiter dissector
goiter excision
goiter forceps
goiter hook
goiter ligature carrier
goiter recurrence
goiter retractor

goiter scissors
goiter tenaculum
goiter vulsellum forceps
goiter-seizing forceps
Golaski graft
Golaski-UMI vascular prosthesis
gold bur
gold crown
Gold deep-surgery forceps
gold ear marker
gold eye implant
gold eyelid implant
Gold forceps
Gold hemostatic forceps
gold knife
gold needle
gold pessary
gold plate technique
Gold portable CO_2 laser
Gold Probe bipolar hemostasis
    catheter
Gold Probe electrohemostasis
    catheter
gold ring
gold saw
gold seed implantation
    technique
gold sphere eye implant
gold strip
gold weight and wire spring
    implant material
Goldbacher anoscope
Goldbacher anoscope speculum
Goldbacher needle
Goldbacher proctoscope
Goldbacher rectal needle
Goldbacher speculum
Goldberg MPC mediastinoscope
Goldberg MPC operative
    enteroscope
Goldberg technique
Goldblatt clamp
Goldblatt hypertension
Goldblatt kidney
Golden sign
Goldenberg Snarecoil bone
    marrow biopsy needle
gold-handled chuck
Goldman bar
Goldman cartilage punch
Goldman chisel
Goldman classification

Goldman curet
Goldman elevator
Goldman guarded chisel
Goldman guillotine nerve knife
Goldman hook
Goldman knife
Goldman knife guide
Goldman nasal tip
    reconstruction
Goldman nerve
Goldman punch
Goldman saw
Goldman scissors
Goldman score of cardiovascular
    risk
Goldman septal elevator
Goldman septal scissors
Goldman serrated knife
Goldman Universal nerve hook
Goldman-Fox gum scissors
Goldman-Fox knife
Goldman-Fox probe
Goldman-Fox wound
    debridement scissors
Goldman-Kazanjian forceps
Goldman-Kazanjian nasal
    forceps
Goldman-Kazanjian rongeur
Goldman-McNeill blepharostat
Goldmann applanation
    tonometer
Goldmann capsulorrhexis
    forceps
Goldmann expressor
Goldmann goniolens
Goldmann kinetic technique
Goldmann knife needle
Goldmann macular contact lens
Goldmann multimirror lens
Goldmann multimirrored lens
    implant
Goldmann perimeter
Goldmann perimetry
Goldmann static technique
Goldmann 3-mirror gonioscopy
    lens
Goldmann tonometer
Goldmann-Favre syndrome
Goldmann-Larson foreign body
Gold Mules eye implant
Goldner anterior fusion
Goldner modification

Goldner reconstruction
Goldner-Clippinger technique
Goldner-Hayes procedure
gold-paneled chisel
gold-plated bandage scissors
Goldscheider disease
Goldsmith operation
Goldstein anterior chamber
cannula
Goldstein anterior chamber
irrigator
Goldstein anterior chamber
syringe
Goldstein anterior chamber-
irrigating cannula
Goldstein curet
Goldstein eye syringe
Goldstein irrigating cannula
Goldstein irrigator
Goldstein lacrimal cannula
Goldstein lacrimal sac retractor
Goldstein lacrimal syringe
Goldstein approximator clamp
Goldstein mucosa speculum
Goldstein retractor
Goldstein septal speculum
Goldstein speculum
Goldstein spinal fusion
technique
Goldstein spine fusion
Goldstein syringe
Goldthwait bar
Goldthwait brace
Goldthwait fracture appliance
Goldthwait fracture frame
Goldthwait operation
Goldthwait procedure
Goldthwait sign
Goldthwait-Hauser procedure
Goldwasser suture carrier
golf tee hollow titanium cannula
golf tee UAL cannula
golf tee-shaped polyvinyl
prosthesis
golf-club eye spud
golfer's skin
Golgi cells
Golgi complex
Golgi corpuscles
Golgi device
Golgi membranes
Golgi-Mazzoni corpuscles

Goligher extraperitoneal
ileostomy
Goligher ileostomy
Goligher modification of the
Berkeley-Bonney retractor
Goligher retractor
Goligher retractor frame
Goligher speculum
Goligher sternal-lifting retractor
Goll tract
Goltz syndrome
Golub EKG lead
GoLytely bowel prep
gomangioma of ear
Gomco aspirator
Gomco bell
Gomco bell clamp
Gomco bloodless circumcision
clamp
Gomco circumcision clamp
Gomco drain
Gomco ENT treatment unit
Gomco forceps
Gomco hemostat
Gomco portable suction
aspirator
Gomco suction
Gomco suction aspirator
Gomco suction tube
Gomco technique
Gomco thermotic pump
Gomco thoracic drainage pump
Gomco umbilical cord clamp
Gomco uterine aspirator
Gomco-Bell clamp
Gomez fundoplasty
Gomez gastric retractor
Gomez gastroplasty
Gomez horizontal gastroplasty
Gomez retractor
Gomez-Marquez lacrimal
operation
gomphosis
gonad shield
gonadal agenesis
gonadal aplasia
gonadal complication
gonadal dysgenesis
gonadal endocrine disorder
gonadal veins
gonadectomy
gonadotropin

gonads
gonarthrotomy
Gonda reflex
gonial angle
Gonin cautery
Gonin marker
Gonin operation
Gonin-Amsler scleral marker
Gonin-Amsler scleral marker
  scissors
goniocraniometry
goniofocalizing lens
goniogram
  Becker goniogram
goniolaser
  Thorpe four-mirror goniolaser
goniolens
  4-mirror goniolens
  Allen-Thorpe goniolens
  Barkan goniolens
  Cardona focalizing goniolens
  Goldmann goniolens
  Koeppe goniolens
  PF Lee pediatric goniolens
  single-mirror goniolens
  Thorpe 4-mirror goniolens
  Thorpe-Castroviejo goniolens
  Zeiss goniolens
goniometer
  Bailliart goniometer
  Carroll finger goniometer
  Conzett goniometer
  digital goniometer
  electronic goniometer
  EOC goniometer
  finger goniometer
  Frykholm goniometer
  full-circle goniometer
  Grafco goniometer
  international standard
    goniometer
  Jarit finger goniometer
  Mottgen goniometer
  orthopedic goniometer
  Osborne goniometer
  Polk finger goniometer
  Polk goniometer
  Sammons biplane goniometer
  Sceratti goniometer
  Sedan goniometer
  Thole goniometer
  Tomac goniometer

goniometer (*continued*)
  two-arm goniometer
  Universal goniometer
  Zimmer goniometer
gonion
  soft tissue gonion
goniophotography
gonioprism
  Jacob-Swan gonioprism
  Posner diagnostic gonioprism
  Posner gonioprism
  Posner surgical gonioprism
goniopuncture
goniopuncture knife
gonioscope
  Allen-Thorpe gonioscope
  Barkan gonioscope
  Heine gonioscope
  Jacob-Swan gonioscope
  Koeppe gonioscope
  Maine gonioscope
  Nevada gonioscope
  Richards-Schaefer gonioscope
  Sussman 4-mirror gonioscope
  Thorpe surgical gonioscope
  Troncoso gonioscope
  Zeiss Formair gonioscope
gonioscopic implant
gonioscopic lens
gonioscopic prism
gonioscopy
gonioscopy lens
goniotomy
  Barkan goniotomy
goniotomy knife
goniotomy knife cannula
goniotomy needle holder
gonococcal flexor tenosynovitis
Gonzalez specialized dissecting
    cannula
Gooch mastoid retractor
Gooch retractor
Gooch splint
Good antral rasp
Good forceps
Good frontal raspatory
Good obstetrical forceps
Good rasp
Good retractor
Good scissors
Good speculum
Good tonsillar scissors

Goodale-Lubin cardiac catheter
Goodale-Lubin catheter
Goodall-Power operation
Goode knife
Goode Magne-Splint magnetic
    nasal splint
Goode nasal splint
Goode tube
Goode T-tube
Goode T-tube ventilating tube
Goode tube
Goodell dilator
Goodell sign
Goodell uterine dilator
Goodell-Power operation
Goode-Magne nasal airway splint
Goodfellow cannula
Goodfellow frontal sinus cannula
Goodhill cautery
Goodhill double-end curet
Goodhill forceps
Goodhill hook
Goodhill knife
Goodhill prosthesis
Goodhill retractor
Goodhill strut introducer
Goodhill tonsillar forceps
Goodhill tonsillar hemostatic
    clamp
Goodhill tonsillar hemostatic
    forceps
Goodhill-Down knife
Goodhill-Pynchon tonsillar
    suction tube
Goodhill-Pynchon tube
Goodley cervical traction
Good-Reiner tonsil scissors
Goodwillie periosteal elevator
Goodwin bone clamp
Goodwin clamp
Goodwin technique
Goodwin-Hohenfellner
    technique
Goodwin-Scott technique
Goodyear retractor
Goodyear tonsillar knife
Goodyear tonsillar retractor
Goodyear uvula retractor
Goodyear-Gruenwald forceps
Goosen vascular punch
gooseneck chisel
gooseneck deformity

gooseneck light
gooseneck rongeur
gooseneck sign
gooseneck snare
Gordon approach
Gordon arm splint
Gordon bead forceps
Gordon cilia forceps
Gordon elementary body
Gordon joint injection
    technique
Gordon reflex
Gordon splint
Gordon stethoscope
Gordon syndrome
Gordon technique
Gordon uterine forceps
Gordon uterine vulsellum
    forceps
Gordon vulsellum forceps
Gordon-Bronstrom technique
Gordon-Taylor hindquarter
    amputation
Gordon-Taylor technique
Gore cast liner
Gore Resolut regenerative tissue
    membrane
Gore SAM patch material
Gore subcutaneous
    augmentation material
    (SAM)
Gore suture passer
Gore thyroplasty device
Gore-Tex alloplastic material
Gore-Tex aortofemoral (AF)
    fistula
Gore-Tex artificial knee
    ligament
Gore-Tex augmentation material
    (GTAM)
Gore-Tex augmentation
    membrane (GTAM)
Gore-Tex AV fistula
Gore-Tex baffle
Gore-Tex bifurcated vascular
    graft
Gore-Tex cardiovascular patch
Gore-Tex catheter
Gore-Tex closure
Gore-Tex cushion
Gore-Tex DualMesh
Gore-Tex DualMesh Plus

Gore-Tex FEP-Ringed vascular graft
Gore-Tex jump graft
Gore-Tex knee prosthesis
Gore-Tex ligament
Gore-Tex limb
Gore-Tex lip augmentation
Gore-Tex membrane
Gore-Tex mesh
Gore-Tex MycroMesh
Gore-Tex MycroMesh Plus
Gore-Tex nasal implant
Gore-Tex patch
Gore-Tex periodontal material
Gore-Tex peritoneal catheter
Gore-Tex prosthesis
Gore-Tex regenerative material
Gore-Tex SAM facial implant
Gore-Tex shunt
Gore-Tex soft-tissue patch
Gore-Tex stretch vascular graft
Gore-Tex strips
Gore-Tex surgical membrane
Gore-Tex sutures
Gore-Tex tapered vascular graft
Gore-Tex tube
Gore-Tex vascular graft
Gore-Tex vascular implant
Gore-Tex vascular prosthesis
Gore-Tex waterproof cast liner
gorget
   Anthony gorget
   grooved gorget
   Teale gorget
Gorlin catheter
Gorlin cyst
Gorlin pacing catheter
Gorlin syndrome
Gorlin-Chaudhry-Moss syndrome
Gorney dissector
Gorney face-lift scissors
Gorney rhytidectomy scissors
Gorney septal scissors
Gorney septal suction elevator
Gorney turbinate scissors
Gorsch needle
Gorsch sigmoidoscope
Goshgarian transpalatal bar
gossamer silk sutures
Gosselin fracture
Gosset abdominal retractor
Gosset appendectomy retractor

Gosset self-retaining retractor
gossypiboma
Gothic arch formation
gothic palate
Gott butterfly heart valve
Gott cannula
Gott implant
Gott low-profile prosthesis
Gott malleable retractor
Gott mitral valve prosthesis
Gott shunt
Gott tube
Gott valve
Gott-Balfour blade
Gott-Daggett heart valve prosthesis
Gott-Daggett shunt
Gottesman splash shield
Gott-Harrington blade
Gottlieb epithelial attachment
Gottschalk middle ear aspirator
Gottschalk nasostat
Gottschalk operation
Gottschalk saw
Gottschalk transverse saw
Gouffon hip pin
Gouffon pin fixation
gouge
   Abbott gouge
   Alexander bone gouge
   Alexander mastoid gouge
   Andrews mastoid gouge
   annulus gouge
   antral gouge
   AO gouge
   Army bone gouge
   Army pattern bone gouge
   arthroplasty gouge
   Aufranc arthroplasty gouge
   Ballenger gouge
   Bishop mastoid gouge
   Boley dental gouge
   bone gouge
   Bowen gouge
   Buck-Gramco gouge
   Campbell arthroplasty gouge
   Campbell gouge
   Capner gouge
   Cave scaphoid gouge
   Charnley gouge
   Cobb spinal gouge
   Codman bone gouge

gouge (*continued*)

Compere gouge
concave gouge
Cooper spinal fusion gouge
Crane gouge
curved gouge
Derlacki gouge
Dix gouge
Dontrix gouge
Duray-Read gouge
Dwyer gouge
Faulkner antrum gouge
Flanagan spinal fusion gouge
Freer nasal gouge
Gam-Mer gouge
grooved eye gouge
Guy model nasal gouge
Heermann gouge
Hibbs bone gouge
Hibbs spinal fusion gouge
hip arthroplasty gouge
hip gouge
Hoen lamina gouge
Holmes cartilage gouge
Hough gouge
hump gouge
Jewett gouge
Kelley gouge
Kezerian gouge
Killian gouge
Kuhnt gouge
lacrimal sac gouge
Lahey Clinic spinal fusion gouge
Lahey gouge
lamina gouge
Lexer gouge
Lillie gouge
long-handle offset gouge
Lucas gouge
Mannerfelt gouge
Martin hip gouge
mastoid gouge
Metzenbaum gouge
Meyerding curved gouge
Meyerding gouge
Moe gouge
Moore gouge
Moore spinal fusion gouge
Morgenstein gouge
Murphy bone gouge
nasal hump gouge

gouge (*continued*)

Neivert rocking gouge
Newport cartilage gouge
Nicola gouge
orthopedic gouge
Parkes hump gouge
Partsch bone gouge
Pilling gouge
Pitanguay-McIndoe gouge
Putti arthroplasty gouge
Read gouge
Rica mastoid gouge
Richards-Cobb spinal gouge
Richards-Hibbs gouge
Rowen spinal fusion gouge
Rubin gouge
scaphoid gouge
Schuknecht gouge
semicircular gouge
septal gouge
Sheehan gouge
SMIC mastoid gouge
Smith-Petersen arthroplasty gouge
Smith-Peterson bone gouge
Smith-Peterson curved gouge
spinal fusion gouge
spinal gouge
spud gouge
Stacke gouge
Stagnara gouge
Stille bone gouge
Stille-pattern bone gouge
surgical gouge
swan gouge
swan-neck gouge
tendon gouge
tissue gouge
Todd foreign body gouge
trough gouge
Troutman gouge
Troutman mastoid gouge
tubular gouge
Turner spinal gouge
U Xacto gouge
US Army gouge
Ultra-Cut Cobb spinal gouge
Ultra-Cut Hibbs gouge
vomerine gouge
Walton foreign body gouge
Watson-Jones bone gouge
West bone gouge

gouge (*continued*)
  West nasal gouge
  Xacto gouge
  Zielke scoliosis gouge
  Zimmer gouge
gouge spud
Gougerot-Sjogren syndrome
Gould electromagnetic
    flowmeter
Gould intraocular implant lens
Gould PentaCath thermodilution
    catheter
Gould gastric motility measuring
    device
Gould pressure monitor
Gould procedure
Gould Statham pressure
Gould Statham pressure
    transducer
Gould sutures
Gould-Brush 8-channel recorder
Goulet retractor
Gouley catheter
Gouley dilator
Gouley guide
Gouley tunneled urethral sound
Gouley urethral sound
Gouley whalebone filiform
    catheter
Goulian blade
Goulian dermatome
Goulian knife
Goulian mammaplasty
Goulian mastopexy
Goulian procedure to harvest
    skin graft
Goulter device
goundou facial deformity
gout
gouty arthritis
gouty tophus
Geotz catheter
Govons pituitary curet
Gowen decompression tube
Gowers maneuver
Gowers sign
Gowers tract
gowning technique
Goyrand hernia
GPRVS (giant prosthetic
    reinforcement of the
    visceral sac)

GPRVS hernioplasty
GPX rotary instrument
graafian cyst
graafian follicle
graafian ovules
graafian vesicle
grab bar
grabbing technique
Graber appliance
Graber-Duvernay hip
    procedure
Grabow forceps
Grace plate 4-hold adapter
Gracey curet
gracilis flap
gracilis free muscle transfer
gracilis muscle
gracilis muscle flap
gracilis muscle transposition
gracilis musculocutaneous flap
gracilis myocutaneous vaginal
    reconstruction
graciloplasty
  double dynamic graciloplasty
  double-wrap graciloplasty
  dynamic graciloplasty
  dynamic urethral graciloplasty
  electrostimulated
      graciloplasty
  single dynamic graciloplasty
  stimulated graciloplasty
  unstimulated graciloplasty
grade IV Baker scale contracture
graded exposure
graded spinal anesthesia
gradient
  A-a gradient (alveolar-arterial
      gradient)
  alveolar-arterial oxygen
      gradient
  alveolocapillary partial
      pressure gradient
  aortic pressure gradient
  aortic valve gradient
  biliary-duodenal pressure
      gradient
  Doppler pressure gradient
  duodenobiliary pressure
      gradient
  field gradient
  gastrosphincteric pressure
      gradient

gradient (*continued*)
  hepatic venous pressure gradient
  intracavitary pressure gradient
  mitral valve gradient
  peak systolic gradient
  peak transaortic valve gradient
  peak-to-peak systolic gradient
  pressure gradient
  pullback pressure gradient
  pulmonary valve gradient
  temperature gradient
  transaortic valve gradient
  transcapillary hydrostatic pressure gradient
  transmural hydrostatic pressure gradient
gradient coil
gradient index lens
gradient-echo MR imaging
gradient-recalled echo image
gradiometer
Gradle cilia forceps
Gradle corneal trephine
Gradle electrode
Gradle eyelid retractor
Gradle forceps
Gradle keratoplasty
Gradle needle electrode
Gradle operation
Gradle refractor
Gradle retractor
Gradle scissors
Gradle stitch scissors
Gradle tonometer
Gradle trephine
gradual weightbearing
gradual withdrawal
graduated catheter
graduated compress
graduated pitcher
graduated sound
graduated tenotomy
graduated-sized catheter
gradient-echo MR image
Gradwohl sternal bone marrow aspirator
Graefe (*also* von Graefe)
Graefe cataract knife
Graefe cautery
Graefe curved iris forceps
Graefe cystitome

Graefe cystoscope
Graefe cystotome
Graefe disease
Graefe dressing forceps
Graefe electric field
Graefe eye speculum
Graefe eye-fixation forceps
Graefe fixation forceps
Graefe flexible cystotome
Graefe hook
Graefe incision
Graefe instrument
Graefe iris forceps
Graefe iris hook
Graefe iris knife
Graefe iris needle
Graefe knife
Graefe knife-needle
Graefe mules
Graefe muscle hook
Graefe needle
Graefe nonmagnetic fixation forceps
Graefe operation
Graefe scarifier
Graefe scissors
Graefe sickle knife
Graefe sign
Graefe speculum
Graefe spot
Graefe strabismus hook
Graefe straight iris forceps
Graefe test
Graefe tissue forceps
Graefe tissue-grasping forceps
Graefenberg ring (*also* Gräfenberg)
Graether buttonhook
Graether collar button
Graether mushroom hook
Graether pupil expander
Graether refractor
Graether retractor
Graf cervical cordotomy knife
Grafco breast pump
Grafco cannula
Grafco colostomy bag
Grafco cotton tip applicator
Grafco eye shield
Grafco goniometer
Grafco head mirror
Grafco ileostomy bag

Grafco incontinence clamp
Grafco laryngeal mirror
Grafco magnet
Grafco Martin laryngectomy
   tube
Grafco ophthalmoscope
Grafco otoscope
Grafco percussion hammer
Grafco perineal lamp
Grafco pinwheel
Grafco tourniquet
Grafco umbilical cord clamp
Grafco-Halsted forceps
Gräfenberg ring (*also*
   Graefenberg)
graft (*see also* implant, patch,
   prosthesis, valve)
  3-vein graft
  accordion graft
  acellular muscle graft
  acetabular augmentation graft
  acrylic graft
  activated graft
  add-on graft
  adipodermal graft
  adipose graft
  adrenal medulla graft
  advancement flap graft
  Advanta graft
  alar batten graft
  Albee bone graft
  albumin-coated vascular graft
  albuminized woven Dacron
   tube graft
  aldehyde-tanned bovine
   carotid artery graft
  AlloDerm acellular dermal
   graft
  AlloDerm cellular dermal graft
  AlloDerm dermal graft
  AlloDerm onlay graft
  AlloDerm processed tissue
   graft
  AlloDerm spacer graft
  AlloDerm universal dermal
   tissue graft
  allogeneic graft
  allogenic graft
  allogenous graft
  AlloMatrix injectable putty
   bone graft substitute
  alveolar bone graft

graft (*continued*)
  alveolar cleft graft
  amnion graft
  anastomosed graft
  animal graft
  aortic aneurysm graft
  aortic tube graft
  aortocoronary bypass graft
  aortocoronary snake graft
  aortofemoral bypass graft
   (AFBG)
  aortohepatic arterial graft
  aortovein bypass graft
  Apligraf
  araldehyde-tanned bovine
   carotid artery graft
  Aria graft
  arterial graft
  arteriovenous Gore-Tex graft
   (AV Gore-Tex graft)
  Atrium Advanta graft
  Atrium hemodialysis graft
  augmentation graft
  auricular cartilage graft
  auricular composite graft
  autochthonous graft
  autodermic graft
  autoepidermic graft
  autogenetic graft
  autogenous bone graft
  autogenous cartilage graft
  autogenous corticocancellous
   graft
  autogenous fat graft
  autogenous nerve graft
  autogenous vein graft
  autologous fat graft
  autologous iliac crest bone graft
  autologous rib bone graft
  autologous vein graft
  autoplastic graft
  AV Gore-Tex graft
   (arteriovenous Gore-Tex
   graft)
  avascular graft
  axillobifemoral bypass graft
  Baker composite graft
  Banks bone graft
  Bard Composix mesh graft
  Bard PTFE graft
  Bard Sperma Tex preshaped
   mesh graft

graft (*continued*)

Bard Visilex mesh graft
batten graft
B-B graft
Berens graft
bifurcated vascular graft
bifurcation graft
bilateral myocutaneous graft
Biobrane glove graft
Biobrane substitute skin graft
Biocoral graft
Biograft bovine heterograft
BioGran resorbable synthetic
  bone graft
BioGran synthetic graft
Bionit vascular graft
Bio-Oss bone filler graft
BioPolyMeric femoropopliteal
  bypass graft
BioPolyMeric vascular graft
Björk-Shiley graft
Blair-Brown skin graft
bolus ties over graft
bone autogenous graft
bone chip graft
bone graft
bone marrow graft
bone peg graft
BonePlast graft
bone-retinaculum-bone
  autograft graft
bone-tendon-bone graft
bone-to-bone graft
Bonfiglio bone graft
Boplant graft
bovine graft
bovine pericardium dural
  graft
Boyd bone graft
brachiosubclavian bridge graft
branched vascular graft
Braun skin graft
Braun-Wangensteen graft
brephoplastic graft
Brescia-Cimino graft
Brett bone graft
bridge graft
buccal mucosa graft
buttress grafts
B-W graft
bypass graft
bypass vein graft

graft (*continued*)

cable graft
cadaveric graft
Calcitite bone graft
calvarial bone graft
calvarial free bone graft
Campbell graft
cancellous and cortical bone
  graft
cancellous cellular bone graft
cancellous chip bone graft
cancellous insert graft
cantilever graft
cantilevered bone graft
cap graft
Carbo-Seal cardiovascular
  composite graft
Cardiopass graft
cardiovascular patch graft
carotid-vertebral vein bypass
  graft
cartilage graft
cartilaginous autologous thin
  septal graft
cartilaginous graft
carved cartilage graft
cavum conchal cartilage graft
cephalic trim cap graft
cephalic vein graft
chessboard skin graft
chip graft
chondromucosal graft
Clancy patellar tendon graft
clip graft
clothespin graft
cobra-hood technique for
  transecting graft
Codivilla bone graft
collagen graft
collagen-impregnated knitted
  Dacron velour graft
Collagraft bone graft matrix
combined penetrating and
  lamellar corneal graft
compilation autogenous vein
  graft
composite auricular graft
composite biodegradable skin
  graft
composite inlay antral and
  nasal bone graft
composite rib graft

graft (*continued*)

- composite skin graft
- composite valve graft
- compound graft
- compressed Ivalon patch graft
- concealer graft
- conchal cartilage graft
- conchal cartilage-ethmoid bone graft
- conchal tip graft
- conjunctival patch graft
- connective tissue graft
- convex cartilage graft
- Cooley woven Dacron graft
- coralline PBHA bone graft
- coralline porous block hydroxyapatite bone graft
- corneal graft
- coronary artery bypass graft (CABG)
- cortical bone graft
- cortical strut graft
- corticocancellous block graft
- corticocancellous bone graft
- Corvita endoluminal graft
- Corvita endovascular graft
- costal cartilage graft
- costochondral graft (CCG)
- Cotton cartilage graft
- Cragg endoluminal graft
- cranial bone graft
- Creech aorto-iliac graft
- crescent corneal graft
- cross-facial nerve graft
- cross-leg bypass graft
- crossover graft
- crushed cartilage graft
- Cryolife valvular graft
- cultured epithelial autograft
- cultured mucosal graft
- cutis graft
- cymba conchal cartilage graft
- Cymetra tissue replacement graft
- Dacron knitted graft
- Dacron onlay patch graft
- Dacron patch graft
- Dacron preclotted graft
- Dacron Sauvage graft
- Dacron tightly woven graft
- Dacron tube graft
- Dacron tubular graft

graft (*continued*)

- Dacron velour graft
- Dacron weave-knit graft
- Dacron-covered stent graft
- Daniel iliac bone graft
- Dardik Biograft vein graft
- Dardik human graft
- Dardik umbilical graft
- Davis muscle-pedicle graft
- de-aired graft
- DeBakey graft
- defatted skin graft
- delayed graft
- Dembone graft
- demineralized bone graft
- Dermagraft graft
- dermal fat graft
- dermal graft
- dermic graft
- dermis patch graft
- dermis-fat graft
- dermofat graft
- devitalized bone graft
- diamond inlay bone graft
- Diastat vascular access graft
- diced cartilage graft
- Distaflo bypass graft
- distal femoropopliteal bypass graft
- distal nerve graft
- Doherty graft
- donor iliac Y graft
- dorsal onlay graft
- dorsal vein patch graft
- double graft
- double papilla graft
- double papilla pedicle graft
- double-barreled fibular bone graft
- double-end graft
- double-ended graft
- double-thickness Sheen graft
- double velour knitted graft
- Douglas mesh skin graft
- Douglas skin graft
- dowel bone graft
- Dragstedt skin graft
- drums of skin graft
- dual onlay cortical bone graft
- dual inlay bone graft
- DualMesh biomaterial graft
- dual-onlay bone graft

graft (*continued*)
  dual-onlay graft
  DuraGen graft
  Durapatite graft
  earlobe composite graft
  Edwards Teflon intracardiac
    patch graft
  Edwards woven Teflon aortic
    bifurcation graft
  Edwards-Tapp arterial graft
  endarterectomy and coronary
    artery bypass graft (E-CABG)
  endothelialization of vascular
    graft
  endovascular stent graft
  epidermic graft
  EpiFilm graft
  Esser inlay graft
  Esser skin graft
  Ethrone graft
  expanded
    polytetrafluoroethylene
    vascular graft
  EXS femoropopliteal bypass
    graft
  EXS vascular graft
  externally supported Dacron
    graft
  extra-articular graft
  extracardiac graft
  extrathoracic carotid
    subclavian bypass graft
  facial skin graft
  fascia graft
  fascia lata graft
  fascia-fat composite graft
  fascial graft
  fascicular graft
  fat cell graft
  fat graft
  Favaloro saphenous vein
    bypass graft
  femoral graft
  femoral-peroneal in situ vein
    bypass graft
  femoral-popliteal bypass graft
    (FPB graft)
  femorodistal vein graft
  femoropopliteal bypass graft
  fenestra bone graft
  FEP-ringed Gore-Tex vascular
    graft

graft (*continued*)
  fiberglass graft
  fibular onlay strut graft
  fibular strut graft
  filler graft
  fillet local flap graft
  filleted graft
  fixation graft
  Flanagan-Buren graft
  flap graft
  Fluoropassiv thin-wall carotid
    patch graft
  foam rubber graft
  Fox graft
  free autogenous
    corticocancellous iliac bone
    graft
  free autogenous graft
  free autogenous pearl fat graft
  free bone graft
  free composite graft
  free cutaneous graft
  free cutaneous nerve graft
  free dermal-fat graft (FDFG)
  free fat graft
  free graft
  free jejunal graft
  free muscle graft
  free non-vascularized
    composite nail graft
  free skin graft
  free skin patch graft
  freeze-dried bone graft
  freeze-dried graft
  full-thickness skin graft (FTSG)
  funicular graft
  Gabarro graft
  gauntlet graft
  GEA graft
  Gelsoft vascular graft
  Gelweave vascular graft
  Gill massive sliding graft
  Gillies bone graft
  Gillies ectropion graft
  glutaraldehyde-tanned bovine
    graft
  glycerin-preserved graft
  Golaski graft
  Gore-Tex bifurcated vascular
    graft
  Gore-Tex FEP-Ringed vascular
    graft

graft (*continued*)

Gore-Tex jump graft
Gore-Tex stretch vascular graft
Gore-Tex tapered vascular graft
Gore-Tex vascular graft
Goulian procedure to harvest
  skin graft
graft preparation graft
Grafton bone graft
Grafton DMB bone graft
gull-wing concha composite
  graft
H.Vantage graft
hair replacement graft
hair-bearing graft
Haldeman bone graft
Hancock pericardial valve
  graft
Hancock vascular graft
Hapset hydroxyapatite bone
  graft plaster
hard palate mucosa graft
Harman bone graft
Harris superior acetabular
  graft
Harrison interlocked mesh
  graft
Haven skin graft
Healos bone graft substitute
  material
Hedrocel bone substitute graft
Hemashield collagen-
  enhanced graft
Hemashield vascular graft
hemicylindrical bone graft
hemicylindrical graft
Henderson onlay bone graft
Henry bone graft
heterodermic graft
heterogenous graft
heterologous graft
heteroplastic graft
heterospecific graft
heterotrophic graft
Hey-Groves-Kirk bone graft
H-graft bone graft
Hibbs graft
Hoaglund bone graft
homogeneous graft
homogenous bone graft
homogenous graft
homograft graft

graft (*continued*)

homologous graft
homoplastic graft
Horton-Devine dermal graft
HTO Wedge tissue allograft
human umbilical vein bypass
  graft (HUV bypass graft)
Huntington bone graft
HUV bypass graft (human
  umbilical vein bypass graft)
Hybrid graft
hydroxyapatite block graft
hyperplastic graft
IEA graft
iliac crest bone graft
iliac graft
IMA graft
implantation graft
Impra bypass graft
Impra Flex vascular graft
Impra microporous PTFE
  vascular graft
Impra vascular graft
Impra vein graft
in situ tricortical iliac crest
  block bone graft
Inclan graft
infusion graft
inlay bone graft
insert graft
interbody bone graft
intercalary bone graft
Intercede graft
InterGard heparin vascular
  graft
internal mammary artery graft
internal mammary graft
internal thoracic artery graft
  (ITA graft)
InterPore graft
interposition Dacron graft
interposition graft
interposition of graft
interposition saphenous vein
  graft
interspecific graft
intracranial-extracranial nerve
  graft
intracranial-intratemporal
  nerve graft
intramedullary-spongiosa graft
intramedullary bone graft

graft (*continued*)
Ionescu-Shiley pericardial
  valve graft
Ionescu-Shiley pericardial
  xenograft
Ionescu-Shiley vascular graft
island graft
isogeneic graft
isogenic graft
isologous graft
isoplastic graft
ITA graft (internal thoracic
  artery graft)
Ivalon compressed patch graft
Ivalon sponge graft
Jeb graft
Judet graft
jump graft
Kebab graft
Keystone graft
Kiel graft
Kimura cartilage graft
kinking of graft
knitted Dacron arterial graft
knitted graft
knitted Teflon graft
Koenig graft
Krause graft
Krause-Wolfe graft
Kutler V-Y flap graft
lamellar corneal graft
lamellar graft
Langenskiöld bone graft
lateral pedicle graft
latex sponge graft
lay-on graft
Lee anterosuperior iliac sine
  graft
Lee bone graft
left internal mammary artery
  graft (LIMA graft)
LifeCell AlloDerm acellular
  dermal graft
ligament graft
LIMA graft (left internal
  mammary artery graft)
linear graft
load-bearing graft
loop forearm graft
Lo-Por vascular graft
lyophilized bone graft
lyophilized dura graft

graft (*continued*)
lyophilized graft
mandrel graft
mandril graft
Mangoldt epithelial graft
Marlex mesh graft
Marquez-Gomez conjunctival
  graft
marsupial graft
Massie sliding graft
massive sliding graft
matchstick graft
Matti-Russe bone graft
mattressed onlay graft
McFarland bone graft
McFarland tibia graft
McIndoe inlay graft
McIndoe skin graft
McMaster bone graft
Meadox bifurcated graft
Meadox Microvel arterial graft
Meadox Microvel double-
  velour Dacron graft
Meadox Microvel double-
  velour knitted Dacron
  arterial graft
Meadox Microvel graft
Meddox vascular graft
Mediform dural graft
Medtronic AneuRx stent graft
medullary bone graft
Meek island sandwich graft
Mersilene graft
mesenteric bypass graft
mesh skin graft
meshed graft
meshed split-thickness skin
  graft
metatarsal free vascularized
  graft
methyl methacrylate graft
Meyerding bone graft
Meyers quadratus muscle-
  pedicle bone graft
Microknit patch graft
Microknit vascular graft
microvascular graft
Microvel double velour graft
Microvel graft
Millesi interfascicular grafts
Millesi nerve graft
Milliknit graft

graft (*continued*)

mitral valve homograft graft
modified graft
modified Peck onlay graft
morcellized bone graft
mucoperiosteal periodontal graft
mucosal graft
mucosal periodontal graft
mucous membrane graft
Mueller patellar tendon graft
Mules graft
multi-layered graft
multivisceral graft
murine graft
muscle graft
muscular graft
mushroom corneal graft
Mustarde graft
MycroMesh biomaterial
myocutaneous graft
nerve cable graft
nerve graft
neuromuscular pedicle graft
neurovascular island graft
Nicoll bone graft
Nicoll cancellous bone graft
Nicoll cancellous insert graft
nonisometric graft
nonpenetrating corneal graft
nonvalved graft
nonvascularized bone graft (NVBG)
nonvascularized fibular strut graft
Ollier thick split free graft
Ollier-Thiersch graft
omental graft
omental skin graft
onlay bone graft
onlay cortical graft
onlay graft
onlay tip graft
oral mucosa graft
organ graft
orthotopic bone graft
orthotropic bone graft
osseous graft
osteoarticular graft
osteocartilaginous graft
osteochondral graft
OsteoGen bone graft

graft (*continued*)

osteoperiosteal bone graft
Ostrup vascularized rib graft
outer table graft
overlay cantilever bone graft
Overton dowel graft
Padgett mesh skin graft
Paladon graft
papilla graft
papillary pedicle graft
Papineau bone graft
Papineau cancellous graft
paraffin graft
Paritene mesh graft
partial-thickness graft
particulate cancellous bone graft
patch graft
patent graft
pattern-cut corneal graft
pedicle fat graft
pedicle graft
pedicled cartilage graft
pedicled skin graft
peg bone graft
peg graft
pelvic peritoneal graft
penetrating corneal graft
penetrating graft
pentagon lobule graft
perichondrial graft
perichondrocutaneous graft
Peri-guard vascular graft
PerioGlas synthetic bone graft
periosteal graft
Perma-Flow coronary bypass graft
PermaMesh graft
PermaSeal dialysis access graft
Phemister onlay bone graft
pie-crusting skin graft
pigskin graft
pinch skin graft
plasma TFE graft
plasma TFE vascular graft
Plexiglas graft
plumping graft
Plystan graft
polyethylene graft
Poly-Plus Dacron vascular graft
polytetrafluoroethylene graft (PTFE graft)

graft (*continued*)

polytetrafluoroethylene
membrane graft
polyurethane graft
polyvinyl graft
porcine graft
porcine xenograft
portacaval H graft
postage-stamp skin graft
postauricular graft
powdered bone graft
preclotted graft
preputial island graft
primary bone graft
primary contraction of skin
graft
primary skin graft
ProOsteon 500 bone implant
graft
prop graft
prophylactic bone graft
Proplast graft
prosthetic arterial graft
prosthetic patch graft
portacaval H graft
proud graft
PTFE endovascular graft
PTFE Gore-Tex graft
punch graft
Rapidgraft arterial vessel
substitute
Rastelli graft
rectangular cartilage graft
reduced-size graft
rejected graft
rejection of graft
reoperative coronary artery
bypass graft (rCABG)
replacement graft
Repliform graft
revascularized bone graft
Reverdin epidermal free graft
Reverdin skin graft
reversed left saphenous vein
bypass graft
reverse-flow vascularized
bone graft
revision of graft
rib costochondral dorsal onlay
graft
rib graft
rigid graft

graft (*continued*)

ring graft
Robinson vein graft
rolled graft
roof-patch graft
rope graft
rotational flap graft
Russe bone graft
Russe inlay bone graft
Ryerson bone graft
sagittal cartilage graft
sandwiched iliac bone graft
saphenous graft
saphenous vein bypass graft
(SVBG)
saphenous vein interposition
graft
saphenous vein patch graft
Sauvage arterial graft
Sauvage Dacron graft
Sauvage filamentous velour
graft
Sauvage vein graft
Sauvage-Bionit graft
scapula crest pedicled bone
graft
scotty-dog graft
seamless arterial graft
seamless graft
secondary contraction of skin
graft
Seddon nerve graft
seed graft
segmental graft
segmental tendon graft
sentinel skin paddle graft
septal cartilage graft
septal chondromucosal graft
sequential graft
Sheen tip graft
sheet graft
shell graft
shield-type graft
Shiley Tetraflex vascular graft
sieve graft
Silastic graft
Silovi saphenous vein bypass
graft
Silovi saphenous vein graft
Siloxane graft
single onlay cortical bone
graft

graft (*continued*)
- skate graft
- skin graft
- skip graft
- sleeve graft
- slice graft
- sliding inlay bone graft
- sliver bone graft
- snake graft
- Solvang graft
- Soto-Hall bone graft
- Sparks mandrel graft
- Speed osteotomy and bone graft
- Speed osteotomy graft
- Sperma-Tex preshaped mesh
- split calvarial graft
- split skin graft
- split-thickness graft
- split-thickness skin graft
- sponge graft
- spongiosa bone graft
- spreader graft
- St. Jude composite valve graft
- stainless steel graft
- Stark graft
- stent graft
- step graft
- straight graft
- straight tubular graft
- strut graft
- subdermal graft
- subepithelial connective tissue graft
- Supramid graft
- sural nerve cable graft
- Surgipro Prolene mesh
- SurgiSis mesh graft
- swaging graft
- syngeneic graft
- synthetic bone graft
- synthetic graft
- Tait graft
- take of the graft
- Talent stent graft
- Tanner-Vandeput graft
- tantalum mesh graft
- tarsoconjunctival composite graft
- Taylor-Townsend-Corlett iliac crest bone graft
- Teflon graft

graft (*continued*)
- temporalis fascia graft
- temporofacial graft
- tendon graft
- Tevdek graft
- thick-split graft
- Thiersch medium-split free graft
- Thiersch skin graft
- Thiersch thin-split free graft
- Thiersch-Duplay tube graft
- thin-split graft
- Thomas extrapolated bar graft
- Thoralon biomaterial
- thrombosed graft
- tip graft
- tissue graft
- toboggan-shaped septal cartilage columella-tip graft
- Transcyte skin substitute graft
- transplanted stamp graft
- transposition of graft
- Trelex mesh graft
- T-shaped graft
- tube flap graft
- tube graft
- tube pedicle graft
- tubed free skin graft
- tubular graft
- Tudor-Thomas graft
- tumbler graft
- tunnel graft
- twin-barreled fibular graft
- umbilical graft
- umbilical vein graft
- umbrella graft
- underlay fascial graft
- underlayer cantilever bone graft
- undermineralized bone graft
- Unigraft bone graft material
- Unilab Surgibone
- unilateral aortofemoral graft
- unmeshed split-thickness skin graft
- USCI Sauvage graft
- Usher Marlex mesh graft
- vaginal graft
- valise handle graft
- valved graft
- Van Millingen graft
- Varivas loop graft

graft (*continued*)
Varivas R vein graft
Vascu-Guard bovine
    pericardial surgical patch
vascular graft
vascularized bone graft
    (VBG)
vascularized metaphyseal
    bone graft
vascularized scapular bone
    graft
vascularized tendon graft
Vasculour II DeBakey graft
Vascutek gelseal vascular graft
Vascutek knitted vascular
    graft
Vascutek woven vascular graft
Vectra vascular access
vein graft
vein patch graft
Velex woven Dacron vascular
    graft
velour collar graft
velour graft
VenaFlow vascular graft
venous graft
venous interposition graft
ventriculoarterial graft
Verdan graft
Veri-Soft graft
Vitagraft vascular graft
Vitallium graft
Vivosil graft
Weary patch graft
Weaveknit vascular graft
Weavenit patch graft
Weck-cel graft
wedge graft
Weiland iliac crest bone graft
Wesolowski bypass graft
Wesolowski Teflon graft
Wesolowski vascular graft
Wheeler graft
white graft
Whitecloud-LaRocca fibular
    strut graft
whole bone transplant graft
whole lobar graft
Wilson bone graft
Wilson-Jacobs patellar graft
Windson-Insall-Vince bone graft
wire mesh graft

graft (*continued*)
Wolf full-thickness free graft
Wolfe graft
Wolfe-Kawamoto bone graft
Wolfe-Kawamoto iliac graft
Wolfe-Krause graft
woven Dacron graft
XenoDerm graft
xenogeneic graft
Xenotech graft
Y-shaped graft
Zenith AAA endovascular graft
Zenotech graft
zooplastic graft
Z-plasty local flap graft
Graft ACE fixed-wire balloon
    catheter
graft anastomosis
graft atrophy
graft bed
graft blade plate
graft board
graft carrier spoon
graft clamp
graft clotting
graft contamination
graft cup
graft donor site
graft driver
graft expulsion
graft failure
graft fixation
graft fragmentation
graft function
graft harvest
graft harvesting
graft impingement
graft implantation
graft infection
graft interstice
graft measuring instrument
graft occlusion
graft of fascia
graft of nerve
graft of organ
graft of tendon
graft patency
graft placement
graft preparation graft
graft rejection
graft resorption
graft sensation

graft site
graft spatulation
graft strength
graft structure
graft suction tube
graft surveillance
graft survival
graft tamp
graft thrombectomy
graft thrombosis
graft treatment
graft vasculopathy
graft versus host
graft weight
Graftac absorbable skin tack
Graftac skin stapler
GraftAssist vein and graft holder
GraftAssist vein graft holder
GraftCyte dressing
GraftCyte gauze
GraftCyte gauze wound dressing
GraftCyte hydrating mist
GraftCyte moist dressing
GraftCyte moist wound dressing
GraftCyte post-surgical shampoo
grafted kidney rejection
grafted skin
graft-enteric fistula
graft-host interface
grafting
   2-step grafting
   alveolar grafting
   areolar grafting
   autogenous bone grafting
   autogenous grafting
   bone grafting
   cartilage grafting
   cranial bone grafting
   dermal grafting
   dermis-fat grafting
   dural grafting
   fascial grafting
   flap grafting
   flexor tendon grafting
   hair grafting
   Mangoldt epithelial grafting
   mucosal grafting
   nipple grafting
   one-stage grafting
   onlay bone grafting
   onlay grafting
   osseous grafting

grafting (*continued*)
   simultaneous grafting
   skin grafting
GraftJacket tendon repair
GraftJacket tissue matrix
GraftJacket ulcer repair matrix
Graftmaster device
Grafton bone graft
Grafton bone grafting material
Grafton DMB bone graft
Graftpatch
graft-seeker catheter
graft-seeking catheter
Graftskin
graft-versus-host disease (GVHD)
   (grades 1-4)
graft-versus-host reaction
Graham blunt hook
Graham cardiovascular scissors
Graham catheter
Graham Clark silicone sponge
Graham closure of ulcer
Graham dural hook
Graham elevator
Graham muscle hook
Graham nerve hook
Graham omental patch
Graham operation
Graham patch
Graham pediatric scissors
Graham plication
Graham rib contractor
Graham scalene elevator
Graham scissors
Graham Steell murmur
Graham-Kerrison punch
Graham-Roscie operation
Gram-Mer bipolar coagulator
gram-negative bacteremia
gram-negative microorganism
gram-positive bacteremia
gram-positive microorganism
Grams nylon nonabsorbable
   sutures
Grams polypropylene
   nonabsorbable sutures
Grams silk nonabsorbable sutures
Granberry decompressor
Granberry hyperextension
   fracture frame
Granberry splint
Granberry tongue depressor

Grancher triad
grand mal
grand multiparity
granddaughter cyst
Grandon cannula
Grandon cortex extractor
Grandon radial marker
Grandon T-incision marker
GraNee needle
Granger articulator
Granger line
Granger sign
Granger x-ray view
granny knot sutures
Grant abdominal aortic
    aneurysmal clamp
Grant aneurysmal clamp
Grant aortic aneurysm clamp
Grant dural separator
Grant gallbladder retractor
Grant holder
Grant needle holder
Grant operation
Grant retractor
Grant separator
Grantham electrode
Grantham femur fracture
    classification
Grantham lobotomy electrode
Grantham lobotomy needle
Grant-Ward operation
GranuFoam
granular bed
granular cell layer
granular cell myeloblastoma
granular cell myoblastoma
granular cell schwannoma
granular cell tumor
granular degeneration
granular kidney
granular layer
granular reticulum
granulating wound
granulation
    arachnoid granulations
    extradural granulation
    exuberant granulation
    healing by granulation
    pacchionian granulation
    red granulation
    Reilly granulations
    toxic granulation

granulation phase
granulation stenosis
granulation tissue
granulation tube
granule
    Birbeck granule
    Fordyce granules
    Interpore granule
    juxtaglomerular granules
    lamellar granule
    Langerhans cell granule
    Langley granules
    membrane-coating granule
    mucigen granule
    ProOsteon Implant 500
        granule
granulocyte colony-stimulating
        factor (G-CSF)
granuloma
    actinic granuloma
    apical granuloma
    caseating granuloma
    central giant cell granuloma
    eosinophilic granuloma
    epithelial granuloma
    foreign body granuloma
    giant cell granuloma
    histiocytic granuloma
    inflammatory granuloma
    Langerhans cell eosinophilic
        granuloma
    laryngeal granuloma
    lethal midline granuloma
    lipoid granuloma
    lipophagic granuloma
    lymphomatoid granuloma
    malignant granuloma
    midline lethal granuloma
    midline malignant reticulosis
        granuloma
    necrotizing granuloma
    noncaseating granuloma
    pyogenic granuloma
    reticulohistiocytic granuloma
    sarcoidal granuloma
    silica granuloma
    silicone granuloma
    swimming pool granuloma
    ulcerated granuloma
    ulcerating granuloma
granuloma annulare
granuloma faciale

granuloma gangrenescens
granuloma gluteale infantum
granuloma pyogenicum
granuloma telangiectaticum
granulomatosa
  cheilitis granulomatosa
  Miescher cheilitis
    granulomatosa
granulomatosa cheilitis
granulomatosis
  bronchocentric
    granulomatosis
  Langerhans cell
    granulomatosis
  Wegener granulomatosis
granulomatous angiitis
granulomatous cheilitis
granulomatous dermal infiltrate
granulomatous disease
granulomatous inflammation
granulomatous inflammatory
  reaction
granulomatous lesion
granulomatous lining
granulomatous mastitis
granulomatous reaction
granulomatous rosacea
granulomatous sialadenitis
granulomatous slack skin
granulomatous tenosynovitis
granulomatous tissue
granulomatous vasculitis
granulosa
  appendicitis granulosa
granulosa cell carcinoma
granulosa-theca cell tumor
granulosity
Grapper instrument
Graseby anesthesia pump
Graser diverticulum
grasp reflex
grasp response
grasp strength
grasper
  3-pronged grasper
  4-pronged polyp grasper
  Acufex linear grasper
  atraumatic curved grasper
  Blakesley grasper
  bowel grasper
  Endo Babcock grasper
  endoscopic Babcock grasper

grasper (*continued*)
  Glassman grasper
  Hansen grasper
  Hasson grasper
  laparoscopic grasper
  Lion's Claw grasper
  Lion's Paw grasper
  loose body grasper
  MetraGrasp ligament grasper
  Polaris reusable grasper
  polyp grasper
  Shutt grasper
  Storz cholangiograsper
  tripod grasper
  Wickham-Miller triradiate
    optical kidney stone grasper
grasper-cutter
  Questus Leading Edge
    arthroscopic grasper-cutter
grasping and cutting forceps
grasping biopsy forceps
grasping clamp
grasping forceps
grasping forceps tip
grasping punch
grasping reflex
grasping technique
grasping tripod forceps
Grass electroencephalograph
Grass Model S9 stimulator
Grass pressure recording device
Grass muscle stimulator
Grass visual pattern generator
Grass-Cranley phleborheogram
Grasshopper positioner
grass-line ligature
grating in joint
grating pain
grating sensation
grating sound
Gratiolet radiating fibers
Gratloch wire bender
grattage
grattage of conjunctiva
Graves bivalve speculum
Graves Britetrac vaginal
  speculum
Graves Coldlite speculum
Graves open-side vaginal
  speculum
Graves scapula
Graves technique

Graves vaginal speculum
gravid uterus
gravida (1, 2, 3, etc.)
gravidarum
   chloasma gravidarum
   hyperemesis gravidarum
   striae gravidarum
gravimetric technique
gravitating hemorrhage
gravitation abscess
gravitational line
gravitational particle collection
gravitational shock
gravitational skin lines
gravitational ulcer
gravity cystography
gravity displacement sterilizer
gravity drainage
gravity infusion cannula
gravity line
gravity lumbar reduction (GLR)
gravity-free position
Gravlee umbilical gun
Gravlee washings
Gravlee-Jetz washer
Grawitz tumor
Gray arterial forceps
Gray bone drill
Gray clamp
Gray cystic duct forceps
Gray drill
Gray flexible intramedullary
   reamer
Gray forceps
gray induration
gray infiltration
gray line of upper eyelid
gray matter
gray patch
Gray resectoscope
gray scale examination
Gray surgical retractor
grayish tissue
grayline incision
gray-scale imaging
gray-scale ultrasonography
gray-scale ultrasound
Grayson corneal forceps
Grayson ligament
Grayton corneal forceps
Grazer abdominoplasty
Grazer blepharoplasty forceps

graduated Garrett dilator
grease gun injury
great adductor muscle
great anterior radicular artery
great auricular nerve
great cardiac vein
great cerebral vein
great cistern
great foramen
Great Ormand Street
   tracheostomy
Great Ormond Street pediatric
   tracheostomy tube
great saphenous vein
great toe implant
great toe sign
great toe transplant
great toe wraparound flap
great transverse commissure
great vessels
great wing of sphenoid bone
greater alar cartilage
greater arc injury of the carpus
greater arterial circle of iris
greater circle of iris
greater circulation
greater curvature
greater curvature banded
   gastroplasty
greater curvature of stomach
greater curvature ulcer
greater curve position
greater horn of hyoid bone
greater ischiatic notch
greater multangular bone
greater occipital nerve block
greater omentum
greater palatine artery
greater palatine canal
greater palatine foramen
greater palatine groove
greater palatine nerve
greater palatine sulcus of maxilla
greater palatine sulcus of
   palatine bone
greater pectoral muscle
greater pelvis
greater peritoneal cavity
greater peritoneal sac
greater petrosal nerve
greater petrosal nerve hiatus
greater psoas muscle

greater rhomboid muscle
greater sacrosciatic notch
greater saphenous vein
greater saphenous vein ligation
    and stripping
greater sciatic foramen
greater sciatic notch
greater splanchnic nerve
greater superficial nerve
greater superficial petrosal
    nerve
greater supraclavicular fossa
greater trochanter
greater trochanter muscle
greater trochanteric femoral
    fracture
greater tubercle
greater tuberosity fracture
greater tympanic spine
greater vestibular gland
greater wing of sphenoid
greater zygomatic muscle
greatest angle of extension
greatest angle of flexion
greatest gluteal muscle
Greck ileostomy bag
Greco cutting block
Greeley technique for
    gynecomastia reduction
Green automatic corneal
    trephine
green Bovie
green braided sutures
Green bulldog clamp
Green calipers
Green capsular forceps
Green cataract knife
Green chalazion forceps
Green clamp
Green corneal curet
Green corneal dissector
Green corneal knife
Green corneal marker
Green curet
Green dissector
Green double spatula
Green eye calipers
Green eye dissector
Green eye needle holder
Green eye shield
Green eye spatula
Green eye speculum

Green fixation forceps
Green goiter retractor
Green holder
Green hook
Green knife
green laser
Green lens scoop
Green lens spatula
Green lid clamp
green Mersilene sutures
green monofilament
    polyglyconate sutures
Green mouth gag
Green muscle hook
Green needle holder
Green operation
Green optical crater marker
Green pendulum scalpel
Green procedure
Green refractor
Green replacer spatula
Green resectoscope
Green retractor
Green scapular procedure
Green scleral resection knife
Green scoop
Green shield
Green Sleeve compression
    device
Green spatula
Green strabismus hook
Green suction tube forceps
Green suction tube-holding
    clamp
Green thyroid retractor
Green tissue-grasping forceps
Green trephine
Green tube-holding forceps
Green tucker
Green-Armytage cesarean
    section hemostat
Green-Armytage hemostatic
    forceps
Green-Armytage operation
Green-Armytage polythene rod
Green-Armytage reamer
Green-Armytage syringe
Green-Banks procedure
Greenberg bar
Greenberg clamp
Greenberg instrument holder
Greenberg Maxi-Vise adapter

Greenberg retractor frame
Greenberg retractor set
Greenberg Universal retractor
Greenberg-Sugita retractor
Greene endocervical curet
Greene endocervical uterine
  curet
Greene intraocular implant lens
Greene lens
Greene needle
Greene placental curet
Greene retractor
Greene sign
Greene tube-holding forceps
Greene uterine curet
Greenfield caval catheter
Greenfield filter
Greenfield inferior vena caval
  filter
Greenfield needle
Greenfield spinocerebellar
  ataxia classification
Greenfield titanium inferior
  vena cava (IVC) filter
Greenfield vena caval filter
Green-Gould needle
Green-Grice transfer
Greenhow incision
Greenhow-Rodman incision
Green-Kenyon corneal marker
Greenough microscope
Green-Sewall mouth gag
greenstick fixation
greenstick fracture
greenstick fracture splint
greenstick LeFort fracture
greenstick medialization
Greenville gastric bypass
Greenwald Control Tip
  cystoscopic electrode
Greenwald cutting loop
Greenwald flexible endoscopic
  electrode
Greenwald needle
Greenwald retractor
Greenwald Roth Grip-Tip suture
  guide
Greenwald sound
Greenwood bipolar coagulation-
  suction forceps
Greenwood spinal trephine
Greenwood trephine

Greer EZ Access drainage
Gregg cannula
Gregoir-Lich procedure
Gregory baby profunda clamp
Gregory bulldog clamp
Gregory carotid bulldog clamp
Gregory external clamp
Gregory forceps
Gregory instruments for in situ
  saphenous vein bypass
Gregory Pell sectioning
  technique
Gregory stay suture clamp
Gregory stay sutures
Gregory vascular miniature
  clamp
Greidman splint
Greig cephalopolysyndactyly
  syndrome
Greiling gastroduodenal tube
Greissinger foot prosthesis
Greissinger Multi-Axis joint
  implant
grenade-thrower fracture
grenz ray
grenz ray therapy
grenz zone
Greulich-Pyle atlas
Greulich-Pyle bone age
Greulich-Pyle technique
Greven alligator forceps
Grey Turner forceps
Grey Turner sign
Grice incision
Grice lift
Grice procedure for talipes valgus
Grice retractor
Grice suture needle
Grice-Green arthrodesis of
  subtalar joint
Grice-Green procedure for
  talipes valgus
grid
  Amsler grid
  Bernell grid
  Bucky grid
  focused grid
  Hirji-Callandar grid
  oscillating grid
  radiographic grid
  Shar-Tek foot positioning grid
  Wetzel grid

gridiron incision
Gridley intraocular lens
Grierson tendon stripper
Grieshaber air pump
Grieshaber Balfour retractor
Grieshaber blade
Grieshaber calibrated corneal
  trephine
Grieshaber corneal needle
Grieshaber corneal trephine
Grieshaber diamond-coated
  forceps
Grieshaber extractor
Grieshaber eye knife
Grieshaber eye needle
Grieshaber eye needle holder
Grieshaber flexible iris retractor
Grieshaber holder
Grieshaber internal limiting
  membrane forceps
Grieshaber iris forceps
Grieshaber iris needle
Grieshaber keratome
Grieshaber knife
Grieshaber manipulator
Grieshaber manipulator forceps
Grieshaber microbipolar
  coagulator
Grieshaber needle holder
Grieshaber ophthalmic needle
Grieshaber ruby knife
Grieshaber self-retaining retractor
Grieshaber spring wire retractor
Grieshaber 3-function
  manipulator
Grieshaber trephine
Grieshaber 2-function
  manipulator
Grieshaber ultrasharp knife
Grieshaber vertical cutting
  scissors
Grieshaber vitrectomy tip
Grieshaber vitreous scissors
Grieshaber wire retractor
Grieshaber-Balfour retractor
Griesinger sign
Griesinger symptom
Griesinger syndrome
Griffen Roux-en-Y bypass
Griffin dressing
Griffiths incision
Griffith-Brown forceps

Grigor fiberoptic guiding catheter
Grillo patch
grimace test for knee pain
Grimelius technique
Grimsdale operation
GRIN lens
grind test
grinding movement
grinding test of Apley
Grinfeld cannula
grip strength
Gripper acetabular cup prosthesis
Gripper needle
Grip-Tip suture guide
griseotomy
  circular griseotomy
Gristina-Webb total shoulder
  arthroplasty
Gritti amputation
grittiness
Gritti-Stokes amputation
Gritti-Stokes knee amputation
gritty tumor
Grizzard subretinal cannula
Gruentzig balloon dilation
Gruentzig technique
Gruning eye magnet (see
  Gruening)
Gruntzig (see Gruentzig)
Groenholm lid retractor
Groenholm refractor
Groenholm retractor
Groff electrosurgical knife
groin dissection
groin exploration
groin flap
groin hernia
groin incision
groin puncture
Grollman catheter
Grollman pigtail catheter
Grollman pulmonary artery-
  seeking catheter
Gromley-Russell cannula
grommet
  Exmoor plastics aural
    grommet
  Shah grommet
  Shepard grommet
  Silastic grommet
  Szulc grommet
  Twardon grommet

grommet bone liner
grommet drain tube
grommet myringotomy tube
grommet tube
grommet ventilating tube
Grondahl esophagoplasty
Grondahl-Finney
    esophagogastroplasty
Grondahl-Finney esophagoplasty
Groningen button
Groningen voice prosthesis
groove
    alar facial groove
    alar groove
    alveolabial groove
    alveolingual groove
    alveolobuccal groove
    anterior auricular groove
    anterior interventricular
      groove
    anterior palatine groove
    arterial groove
    atrioventricular groove
    auriculoventricular groove
    bicipital groove
    Blessig groove
    carotid groove
    cavernous groove
    chiasmatic groove
    corneal lamellar groove
    costal groove
    deltopectoral groove
    digastric groove
    distal oblique groove (DOG)
    esophageal groove
    ethmoidal groove
    gingivobuccal groove
    gingivolabial groove
    gingivolingual groove
    greater palatine groove
    hamular groove
    Harrison groove
    inferior petrosal groove
    infragluteal groove
    inframalar groove
    infraorbital groove
    interatrial groove
    intercondylar groove
    intercostal groove
    intermandibular groove
    intermuscular groove
    interosseous groove

groove (*continued*)
    intertubercular groove
    interventricular groove
    intraorbital groove
    labial groove
    labiomental groove
    lacrimal groove
    laryngotracheal groove
    lateral bicipital groove
    Liebermeister groove
    limbal groove
    linear groove
    lingual development groove
      (LDG)
    lingual groove (LG)
    linguogingival groove
    Lucas groove
    marionette groove
    mastoid groove
    median groove
    meningeal groove
    mesiobuccal developmental
      groove (MBDG)
    mesiolingual developmental
      groove (MLDG)
    mesiolingual groove (MLG)
    musculospiral groove
    mylohyoid groove
    nail groove
    nasofacial groove
    nasolabial groove
    nasolacrimal groove
    nasomaxillary groove
    nasopalatine groove
    nasopharyngeal groove
    obturator groove
    occipital groove
    olfactory groove
    oval-form colonic groove
    palatine groove
    palatomaxillary groove
    palatovaginal groove
    paraglenoid groove
    pectoral groove
    peroneal groove
    pharyngeal grooves
    pharyngotympanic groove
    popliteal groove
    posterior auricular groove
    preauricular groove
    pterygopalatine groove
    radial groove

groove (*continued*)
- Schmorl groove
- Sibson groove
- sinus groove
- skin grooves
- Sondergaard groove
- spindle colonic groove
- spiral groove
- subclavian groove
- subcostal groove
- supra-acetabular groove
- transverse anthelicine groove
- transverse nasal groove
- ulnar groove
- uncinate groove
- urethral groove
- venous groove
- Verga lacrimal groove
- vertebral groove
- vertical groove
- vomeral groove
- vomerine groove
- vomerovaginal groove
- Waterston groove

groove extension
groove for nasal nerve
groove for radial nerve
groove of crus of the helix
groove of lacrimal bone
groove of nail matrix
groove sutures
grooved director
grooved director dilator
grooved eye gouge
grooved gorget
grooved incision
grooved piece
grooved silicone implant
grooved silicone sponge
grooved tying forceps
grooving reamer
Groshong catheter
Groshong double-lumen
    catheter
Groshong shunt
gross adenopathy
gross appearance
Gross brain spatula
Gross coarctation clamp
Gross coarctation occlusion
    clamp
Gross curet

gross cystic disease
gross deformity
gross description
Gross dressing forceps
Gross ductus spreader
Gross ear curet
Gross ear hook
Gross ear spoon
Gross ear spud
gross examination
Gross forceps
Gross hook
Gross hyoid-cutting forceps
Gross iris retractor
gross lesion
gross manipulation
gross motor
Gross operation
Gross patent ductus retractor
Gross probe
Gross retractor
Gross spatula
Gross sponge forceps
Gross spoon
Gross spreader
Gross spud
Gross spur crusher
Gross tracheoesophageal fistula
gross tumor
Grossan nasal irrigator tip
Grosse-Kempf bone drill
Grosse-Kempf femoral nail
Grosse-Kempf interlocking nail
Grosse-Kempf nail
Grosse-Kempf tibial nail
Grosse-Kempf tibial technique
grossly
Gross-Pomoranz-Walkins retractor
Grotena abdominal support
Grotting forceps
ground plate
ground-glass appearance
ground-glass lesion
ground-glass pattern
grounding pad
group fascicular repair
Grover Atra-grip clamp
Grover auricular appendage
    clamp
Grover meniscotome
Grover meniscus knife
Groves-Goldner technique

growing fracture
growing point
growing tumor
growth
  asymmetric
    maxillomandibular growth
  axonal growth
  basicranial sagittal growth
  cancerous growth
  cartilaginous growth
  catch-up growth
  chondromatous growth
  condylar growth
  crack growth
  cranial growth
  electronic stimulation of bone
    growth
  facial growth
  frontal sinus growth
  hamartomatous growth
  intrauterine growth
  malignant growth
  neoplastic growth
  new growth
  osteocartilaginous growth
  pedunculated growth
  vegetation growth
growth arrest
growth arrest line
growth hormone-releasing
    factor (GHRF)
growth plate abscess
growth plate complex
growth retardation
Gruber bougie
Gruber ear speculum
Gruber hernia
Gruber medicated bougie
Gruber sutures
Gruber-Landzert fossa
Gruca hip reamer
Gruca stabilization
Gruening eye magnet
Gruentzig arterial balloon
    catheter
Gruentzig balloon angiography
    catheter
Gruentzig balloon catheter
    angioplasty
Gruentzig balloon dilation
Gruentzig balloon dilator
Gruentzig Dilaca catheter

Gruentzig dilating catheter
Gruentzig dilatation of renal
    arteries
Gruentzig femoral stiffening
    cannula
Gruentzig PTCA technique
Gruentzig steerable catheter
Gruentzig technique
Gruenwald bayonet-dressing
    forceps
Gruenwald dissecting forceps
Gruenwald dressing forceps
Gruenwald Durogrip forceps
Gruenwald ear forceps
Gruenwald nasal forceps
Gruenwald nasal punch
Gruenwald nasal-cutting forceps
Gruenwald nasal-dressing
    forceps
Gruenwald neurosurgical
    rongeur
Gruenwald pituitary rongeur
Gruenwald punch
Gruenwald retractor
Gruenwald rongeur
Gruenwald tissue forceps
Gruenwald-Bryant nasal forceps
Gruenwald-Bryant nasal-cutting
    forceps
Gruenwald-Jansen forceps
Gruenwald-Love intervertebral
    disk rongeur
Gruenwald-Love neurosurgical
    forceps
grumose
grumose material
Gruning (see Gruening)
grunting maneuver
grunting respirations
Gruppe forceps
Gruppe wire crimper
Gruppe wire prosthesis
Gruppe wire prosthesis-
    crimping forceps
Gruppe wire-crimping forceps
Grynfelt hernia
Grynfelt triangle
gryphosis
gryposis
Gräfenberg ring (see
    Graefenberg)
GS-9 blade

GS-9 needle
GSA-9 blade
GSB elbow prosthesis
GSB knee prosthesis
GTAM (Gore-Tex augmentation material)
GTAM (Gore-Tex augmentation membrane)
GTF-A gastroscope
GU irrigant dressing
guaiac test
Guangzhou prosthetic valve
guard
    Action Eyes and Albany eye guards
    Albany eye guard
    BandageGuard half-leg guard
    cannula guard
    cataract knife guard
    cervical drill guard
    chisel guard
    Cloward cervical drill guard
    Codman skull perforator guard
    drill guard
    ether guard
    eye knife guard
    Fomon chisel guard
    forceps guard
    Freedom Palm guard
    Heansen keratome guard
    Horsley guard
    intracardiac sucker guard
    Joseph guard
    keratome guard
    Kneed-It knee guard
    laser-assisted intrastromal keratomileusis cannula eye guard
    LASIK eye guard
    McDavid ankle guard
    McDavid hinged knee guard
    Midax Rex bur guard
    mouth guard
    Omed vented instrument guard
    palm guard
    Peri-Guard vascular graft guard
    pin guard
    plastic mouth guard
    Progressive palm guard

guard (continued)
    scalpel guard
    Somatics mouth guard
    Stacke chisel guard
    Storz Teflon forceps guard
    tip guard
    tooth guard
    Twist-Lock drill guard
    Ullrich drill guard
    UltraPower bur guard
    Wright-Rubin forceps guard
guarded chisel
guarded irrigating cystotome
guarded osteotome
guarded postoperative period
guarded prognosis
Guardian catheter
Guardian pacemaker
guarding
    abdominal guarding
    involuntary guarding
    muscle guarding
    voluntary guarding
guarding of muscle
guarding sign
Guardsman femoral interference screw
Guarner wrap fundoplication
gubernaculum
    chorda gubernaculum
    Hunter gubernaculum
gubernaculum dentis
Gubler line
Gudden commissure
Gudden tract
Gudebrod sutures
Guedel airway
Guedel laryngoscope
Guedel laryngoscope blade
Guedel rubber airway
Guedel-Negus laryngoscope
Guell laser-assisted intrastromal keratomileusis (LASIK) cannula
Guéneau de Mussy point
Guepar (Group for Utilization and Study of Articular Prostheses)
Guepar hinge-knee prosthesis
Guepar II hinged knee prosthesis
Guepar knee prosthesis

Guepar prosthesis
Guepar total knee prosthesis
Guerin fold
Guerin fracture
Guerin gland
Guerin lock
Guerrant-Cochran splint
Guest needle
Guggenheim adenoid forceps
Guggenheim fracture
Guggenheim scissors
Guggenheim-Schuknecht
     scissors
Guglielmi detachable coil
Guhl classification
Guhl technique
Guibor canalicular tube
Guibor canaliculus intubation
     set
Guibor Expo eye bubble
Guibor Expo flat eye bandage
Guibor eye tube
Guibor lacrimal drain
Guibor shield
Guibor Silastic intubation set
Guibor Silastic tube
guidance
     endoscopic guidance
     fluoroscopic guidance
     frameless stereotactic
          guidance
     laparoscopic guidance
     magnetic imaging guidance
     stereotactic guidance
     ultrasound guidance
     video-laparoscopic guidance
guidance image
Guidant balloon
Guidant CRM pacemaker
Guidant defibrillator
Guidant guidewire
Guidant coronary stent
Guidant pacemaker
Guidant stent
Guidant CPI device
guide (see also needle guide,
     saw guide)
     Accu-Line chamfer resection
          guide
     acetabular angle guide
     acetabular guide
     acetabular shell guide

guide (continued)
     ACL drill guide
     ACL guide
     ACS LIMA guide
     Acufex alignment guide
     Acufex drill guide
     Adapteur multifunctional drill
          guide
     adjustable anterior guide
     Adson drill guide
     Adson Gigli-saw guide
     Adson saw guide
     Adson-Shaefer dural guide
     AFB needle guide
          (aortofemoral bypass
          needle guide)
     AGC dual-pivot resection
          guide
     Alvarado orthopedic guide
     Amplatz tube guide
     anterior cruciate ligament
          drill guide
     anterior femoral resection
          guide
     antirotation guide
     AO stopped-drill guide
     AOR guide
     Arani guide
     Arrow true torque wire guide
     Arthrex drill guide
     Arthrex tibial tunnel guide
     Asta-Cath female catheter
          guide
     Bailey Gigli-saw guide
     Barraquer wire guide
     barrel guide
     basal ganglia guide
     Blair Gigli-saw guide
     Blair saw guide
     bone guide
     Borchard bone wire guide
     Borchard Gigli-saw guide
     bougie guide
     Bow & Arrow cannulated drill
          guide
     bronchoscopic guide
     bronchoscopic instrument
          guide
     Brown-Roberts-Wells CT
          stereotaxic guide
     BRW CT stereotaxic guide
     Bullseye femoral guide

guide (*continued*)
- Benique catheter guide
- Caldwell guide
- cartilage guide
- catheter guide
- CCK femoral stem provisional guide
- chamfer guide
- Clayman intraocular guide
- Cloward drill guide
- Cloward guide
- Codman guide
- Concept tibial guide
- condylar guide
- Cone guide
- contoured anterior spinal plate drill guide
- Cook stereotaxic guide
- Cooper basal ganglia guide
- Cooper guide
- Cooper nasal ganglia guide
- core wire guide
- Cor-Flex guide
- Cor-Flex wire guide
- Cosman-Nashold spinal stereotaxic guide
- Cottle bone guide
- Cottle cartilage guide
- Cottle knife guide
- Crockard sublaminar wire guide
- cruciate ligament guide
- Cushing Gigli-saw guide
- Cushing saw guide
- custom drill guide
- Dap II biopsy needle guide
- Davis saw guide
- disposable measuring guide
- distal femoral cutting guide
- drill guide
- dural protector drill guide
- eccentric drill guide
- Eriksson guide
- extramedullary alignment guide
- E-Z guide
- femoral AP-sizing guide
- femoral intermedullary guide
- femoral notch guide
- Ferciot wire guide
- filiform guide
- Fisher guide

guide (*continued*)
- fixed-offset guide
- FL4 guide
- Flexguide intubation guide
- floppy-tipped guide
- Franzen needle guide
- Frazier dural guide
- Friedman knife guide
- front-entry guide
- Gabbay-Frater suture guide
- Galante hip guide
- Gatlin gun drill guide
- Gaulian knife guide
- Geenan Endotorque guide
- Ghajar guide
- Gigli-saw guide
- glenoid drill guide
- Goldman knife guide
- Gouley guide
- Greenwald Grip-Tip suture guide
- Greenwald Roth Grip-Tip suture guide
- Grip-Tip suture guide
- guidepin guide
- gutter guide
- Guyon catheter guide
- Guyon curved catheter guide
- hand-held drill guide
- Harris hip guide
- Harris precoat neck osteotomy guide
- Harris-Galante hip guide
- Harrison forked-type strut guide
- Harrison guide
- Hewson ligament drill guide
- Hewson ligament guide
- hip alignment guide
- hollow needle guide
- House strut guide
- House wire guide
- Howell tibial guide
- humeral cutting guide
- IM/EM tibial resection guide
- image guide
- instrument guide
- Interson biopsy needle guide
- intramedullary guide
- Iowa pudendal needle guide
- Iowa trumpet forceps guide
- Iowa trumpet needle guide

guide (*continued*)

Jonesco bone wire guide
Joseph saw guide
Kazanjian guide
Kendrick Gigli-saw guide
Kleegman needle guide
Lebsche saw guide
Lebsche wire saw guide
LeFort filiform guide
Levin drill guide
ligature guide
Lipscomb-Anderson drill guide
long nail-mounted drill guide
L-resection guide
Lunderquist guide
Lunderquist-Ring torque guide
Maggi disposable biopsy
    needle guide
mandrin guide
measuring guide
microdrilling guide
MOD femoral drill guide
Modny guide
mold guide
Morrissey Gigli-saw guide
Mueller catheter guide
Mumford Gigli-saw guide
nasal cartilage guide
needle guide
Neivert knife guide
occlusal guide
Oshukova collapsible bougie
    guide
Palmer cruciate ligament
    guide
patellar drill guide
patellar reamer guide
patellar resection guide
Pilot suturing guide
Pilotip catheter guide
pin guide
Poppen Gigli-saw guide
protector guide
ProTrac ACL tibial guide
Puddu drill guide
pudendal needle guide
punch guide
Rand-Wells
    pallidothalamectomy guide
Raney Gigli-saw guide
rear-entry ACL drill guide
Reece osteotomy guide

guide (*continued*)

Rhinelander guide
Richards adjustable-angle
    guide
Richards barrel guide
Richards calibrated-tip
    threaded guide
Richards drill guide
Richards stationary-angle guide
Rosenburg drill guide
Roth Grip-Tip suture guide
Roth urethral suture guide
Savary-Gilliard wire guide
saw guide
Scanlan ligature guide
scaphoid screw guide
Schlesinger Gigli-saw guide
Sheets lens guide
Slick stylette endotracheal
    tube guide
Slidewire extension guide
Staden pin guide
stapes wire guide
stationary angle guide
Stewart cruciate ligament
    guide
Stewart ligament guide
Stille Gigli-saw guide
stoma-centering guide
straight catheter guide
strut guide
surgical instrument guide
suture guide
targeting drill guide
Teale lithotomy gorget guide
telescopic view guide
telescoping guide
TFE-coated wire guide
tibial cutter guide
tibial resection guide
tissue anchor guide (TAG)
Todd stereotaxic guide
Todd-Heyer cannula guide
Todd-Wells stereotaxic guide
torque guide
Tracer hybrid wire guide
true torque wire guide
trumpet needle guide
Tucker vertebrated guide
tunnel drill guide
Unis Universal guide
Urbanski strut guide

guide (*continued*)
  Uslenghi drill guide
  Van Buren catheter guide
  Wilson-Cook standard wire
    guide
  wire guide
guide catheter
guide forceps
guide pin (*see* pin)
guide plane
guide sutures
guidewire (*see* wire)
guided bone regeneration
guided fine-needle aspiration
guided tissue regeneration
guided transcutaneous biopsy
guided-needle aspiration
  cytology
Guidefather catheter
guidepin guide
guidewire
  ACS HI-Torque Balance
    Middleweight guidewire
  Athlete coronary guidewire
  Bard Commander PTCA
    guidewire
  Bentson guidewire
  cannula with pre-loaded
    guidewire
  catheter guidewire
  Conceptus Robust guidewire
  Cross-it guidewire
  Doppler guidewire
  Extra Sport coronary
    guidewire
  FasTrac guidewire
  FlexFinder guidewire
  floppy guidewire
  FloWire Doppler guidewire
  Geenan Endotorque
    guidewire
  Glidewire Gold surgical
    guidewire
  HyTek guidewire
  Intercept-Vascular guidewire
  Lumina guidewire
  Lunderquist guidewire
  Magnum guidewire
  Mailman coronary guidewire
  Microvasive Glidewire
    guidewire
  Mirage guidewire

guidewire (*continued*)
  Mustang steerable guidewire
  Phantom cardiac guidewire
  Prima laser guidewire
  QuickSilver hydrophilic-
    coated guidewire
  Radiofocus Glidewire
    guidewire
  RotaWire guidewire
  silk guidewire
  SilverSpeed hydrophilic
    guidewire
  Sniper Elite hydrophilic
    guidewire
  steerable guidewire
  Storq guidewire
  Suretac guidewire
  Terumo guidewire
  TherOx infusion guidewire
  TomCat PTCA guidewire
  Ultra-Select guidewire
  VascuLink vascular access
    guidewire
  VertiGraft textured allograft
    bone guidewire
  WaveWire guidewire
  Whisper guidewire
  Zebra exchange guidewire
guidewire and mini-snare
  technique
guidewire exchange technique
guidewire manipulation
guidewire perforation
Guidi canal
guiding cannula
guiding catheter
guiding plane
guiding sheath
Guild-Pratt rectal speculum
Guild-Pratt speculum
Guilford brace
Guilford ear scissors
Guilford scissors
Guilford sickle knife
Guilford stapedectomy
Guilford-Schuknecht scissors
Guilford-Schuknecht wire-
    cutting scissors
Guilford-Wright bivalve
  speculum
Guilford-Wright bur
Guilford-Wright bur saw

Guilford-Wright clip
Guilford-Wright crurotomy knife
Guilford-Wright curet
Guilford-Wright cutting block
Guilford-Wright double-edged knife
Guilford-Wright drum elevator
Guilford-Wright duckbill elevator
Guilford-Wright elevator knife
Guilford-Wright flap knife
Guilford-Wright footplate pick
Guilford-Wright forceps
Guilford-Wright incudostapedial knife
Guilford-Wright meatal retractor
Guilford-Wright middle ear instrument
Guilford-Wright prosthesis
Guilford-Wright roller knife
Guilford-Wright scissors
Guilford-Wright stapes pick
Guilford-Wright suction tube
Guilford-Wright Teflon wire piston
Guilford-Wright wire cutter
Guilford-Wullstein bur saw
Guilland sign
Guillian knife
guillotine
    Ballenger-Sluder guillotine
    Charnley femoral inlay guillotine
    Derra guillotine
    Giertz rib guillotine
    hemostatic tonsillar guillotine
    Lilienthal rib guillotine
    lingual guillotine
    Molt guillotine
    Molt-Storz guillotine
    Myles guillotine
    Poppers tonsillar guillotine
    rib guillotine
    Sauer guillotine
    Sauerbruch rib guillotine
    Sluder tonsillar guillotine
    Sluder-Sauer tonsil guillotine
    SMIC tonsillar guillotine
    Storz guillotine
    tonsil guillotine
    tonsillar guillotine
    Van Osdel guillotine

guillotine adenotome
guillotine amputation
guillotine amputation of appendix
guillotine amputation of cervix
guillotine cutting tip
guillotine incision
guillotine needle biopsy
guillotine scissors
guillotine technique
guillotine vitrectomy instrument
guillotine-type cutter
guillotome forceps
Guimaraes implantable contact lens manipulator
Guimaraes ophthalmic flap spatula
Guist enucleation hemostat
Guist enucleation scissors
Guist eye implant
Guist eye speculum
Guist fixation forceps
Guist forceps
Guist scissors
Guist speculum
Guist sphere eye implant
Guist sphere implant
Guist-Black eye speculum
Guiteras irrigation
Guiteras nozzle irrigator
Guiteras urethroscope
Gulani triple function LASIK cannula
Guleke bone rongeur
Guleke-Stookey operation
Gull renal epistaxis
Gullstrand lens
Gullstrand lens loupe
Gullstrand ophthalmoscope
Gullstrand slit lamp
Gullstrand-Zeiss lens loupe
gull-wing concha composite graft
gull-wing incision
gull-wing pattern
gum elastic bougie introducer
gum lancet
gum line
Gum Machine oral irrigator
gum massage
gum resection
gum scissors

Gumby technique for thumb
   casting
gummatous necrosis
gummy smile
gums
gun
   Arthrex meniscal dart gun
   Auto-Suture TA-50 staple gun
   Bard bioptic gun
   Bard Biopty gun
   BD gun
   Biofix arrow gun
   biopsy gun
   Biopty gun
   Bone Injection gun
   caulking gun
   cement gun
   Cobe staple gun
   Cook biopsy gun
   coring biopsy gun
   electron gun
   EnhanCement gun
   Gravlee umbilical gun
   Harris cement gun
   Heaf gun
   heat gun
   introducer gun
   Lidge cement gun
   Mentor injector gun
   Messing root canal gun
   modified caulking gun
   Moss T-anchor needle
     introducer gun
   Promag biopsy gun
   Reflex gun
   seam-sealer gun
   Shunn gun
   skin gun
   spring-loaded biopsy gun
   staple gun
   surgical stapling biopsy gun
gun-barrel enterostomy
Gunderson bone forceps
Gunderson conjunctival flap
Gunderson muscle forceps
Gunderson muscle recession
   forceps
Gunderson recession forceps
Gunderson-Sosin classification
Gunderson-Sosin modification
Gundry cannula
Gunn closing sign

Gunnar-Hey roller forceps
Gunning jaw splint
gunpowder lesion
gunshot fracture
gunshot wound
GunSlinger shoulder orthosis
Gunston arthroplasty
Gunston knee prosthesis
Gunston polycentric knee
   prosthesis
Gunston-Hult knee prosthesis
Gunter Von Noorden flap
Gunter Von Noorden incision
Gunther Tulip vena cava MRI
   filter
Gurd procedure
Gurd resection
gurgling bowel sounds
gurgling rales
gurney
Gusberg cervical biopsy curet
Gusberg cervical cone curet
Gusberg endocervical biopsy
   curet
Gusberg endocervical biopsy
   punch
Gusberg endocervical curet
Gusberg hysterectomy clamp
Gusberg punch
Gusberg uterine forceps
Gussenbauer clamp
Gussenbauer operation
Gussenbauer suture technique
Gussenbauer sutures
gusset-type patch
gustatory anesthesia
gustatory glands
gustatory lacrimation
gustatory rhinorrhea
Gustilo fracture score
Gustilo knee prosthesis
Gustilo puncture wound
   classification
Gustilo scoring for open
   fractures (types II, IIIA, IIIB,
   IIIC)
Gustilo-Anderson classification
Gustilo-Anderson open
   clavicular fracture
Gustilo-Anderson open fracture
   classification
Gustilo-Kyle total hip

Gustilo-Kyle total knee
gut
  artificial gut
  blind gut
  lumen of gut
  postanal gut
  preoral gut
  primitive gut
  ribbon gut
  silkworm gut
gut and colon clamp
gut chromic sutures
gut clamp
gut plain sutures
gut sutures
gut wool
gut-associated lymphoid tissue
  (GALT)
Gutgeman auricular appendage
  clamp
Gutgemann auricular appendage
  clamp
Gutgemann auricular appendage
  forceps
Gutglass cervix hemostat
Gutglass cervix hemostatic
  forceps
Gutglass hemostat
Gutglass hemostatic cervical
  forceps
Guthrie eye-fixation hook
Guthrie fixation hook
Guthrie iris hook
Guthrie muscle
Guthrie retractor
Guthrie skin hook
Guthrie-Smith bed
Gutierrez-Najar grasping forceps
Guttaform dental impression
  material
gutta-percha
gutta-percha point
gutter
  abdominal gutter
  lateral gutter
  left gutter
  paracolic gutter
  pelvic gutter
  right gutter
gutter finger splint
gutter fracture
gutter guide

gutter speculum
gutter splint
guttering of bone
Guttmann arthrodesis
Guttmann obstetrical retractor
Guttmann retractor
Guttmann subtalar arthrodesis
Guttmann technique
Guttmann vaginal retractor
Guttmann vaginal speculum
guttural duct
guttural pulse
guttural rales
guttural sound
Gutzeit dacryostomy operation
Guy gouge
Guy knife
Guy nasal gouge
guy steadying sutures
guy sutures
Guy tenotomy knife
Guyon amputation
Guyon ankle amputation
  technique
Guyon bougie
Guyon canal
Guyon canal release
Guyon canal syndrome
Guyon catheter guide
Guyon clamp
Guyon curettage
Guyon curved catheter guide
Guyon dilating bougie
Guyon dilating sound
Guyon dilator
Guyon exploratory bougie
Guyon kidney clamp
Guyon operation
Guyon sound
Guyon ureteral catheter
Guyon urethral sound
Guyon vessel clamp
Guyon-Benique sound
Guyon-Benique urethral sound
Guyon-Benique sound
Guyon-Pean clamp
Guyon-Pean vessel clamp
guy-steading sutures
Guyton corneal transplant
  trephine
Guyton electrode
Guyton forceps

Guyton operation
Guyton ptosis operation
Guyton scissors
Guyton sutures
Guyton suturing forceps
Guyton trephine
Guyton-Clark capsule fragment
    forceps
Guyton-Clark forceps
Guyton-Clark fragment forceps
Guyton-Friedenwald sutures
Guyton-Lundsgaard cataract
    knife
Guyton-Lundsgaard keratome
Guyton-Lundsgaard scalpel
Guyton-Lundsgaard sclerotome
Guyton-Maumenee speculum
Guyton-Noyes fixation
Guyton-Noyes fixation forceps
Guyton-Park eye speculum
Guyton-Park lid speculum
Guyton-Park speculum
Guyuron procedure
Guzman-Blanco epiglottic
    retractor
Guzman-Blanco epiglottis
    retractor
Gueneau de Mussy point
Guerin fold
Guerin fracture
Guerin gland
Guerin lock
GVHD (graft-versus-host disease)
Gwathmey ether hook
Gwathmey oil-ether anesthesia
Gwathmey suction tube
Gwathmey-Yankauer ether inhaler
Gyn-A-Lite speculum illuminator
Gyn-A-Lite vaginal speculum
Gynaspir vacuum curettage
gynecoid pelvis
gynecologic anesthesia
gynecologic disorder
gynecologic laparoscopy
gynecologic, gynecological
gynecological carcinoma
gynecological cryosurgery
gynecological examination
gynecological malignancy
gynecological procedure
gynecological surgery
gynecology instrument set

gynecomastia
    surgical classification of
        gynecomastia
        (grades 1, 2A, 2B, 3)
Gynefold pessary
Gynefold prolapse pessary
Gynefold retrodisplacement
    pessary
GyneLase diode laser
GyneSys diagnostic catheter
Gynex angle hook
Gynex Emmett tenaculum
Gynex endospeculum
Gynex extended-reach needle
Gynex iris hook
Gyno Sampler endometrial
    sampling device
gynoplastics
gynoplasty
Gynos perineometer
GynoSampler endometrial
    aspirator
Gypsona cast
Gypsona plaster dressing
Gypsona rapid-setting cast
    material
gyrectomy
gyri (*sing.* gyrus)
    preinsular gyri
    transverse temporal gyri
gyri breves insulae
gyri cerebri
gyri insulae
gyri of cerebrum
gyri orbitales
gyri profundi cerebri
gyri temporales transversi
gyri transitivi cerebri
gyriform carcinoma
gyrose area
gyrous area
gyrus (*sing.* gyri)
    angular gyrus
    anterior central gyrus
    cingulate gyrus
    dentate gyrus
    frontal gyrus
    fusiform gyrus
    Heschl gyrus
    inferior frontal gyrus
    infracalcarine gyrus
    lingual gyrus

gyrus (*continued*)
  middle frontal gyrus
  parahippocampal gyrus
  postcentral gyrus
  precentral gyrus
  quadrate gyrus
  subcallosal gyrus
  subcollateral gyrus
  superior frontal gyrus
  superior occipital gyrus
  superior temporal gyrus
  supracallosal gyrus
  supramarginal gyrus
  temporal gyrus
  uncinate gyrus
gyrus dentatus
gyrus fasciolaris
gyrus fornicatus
gyrus frontalis
gyrus fusiformis
gyrus geniculi
gyrus hippocampi
gyrus limbicus

gyrus lingualis
gyrus longus insulae
gyrus marginalis
gyrus of Broca
gyrus of insula
gyrus olfactorius lateralis of
    Retzius
gyrus olfactorius medialis of
    Retzius
gyrus paracentralis
gyrus parahippocampalis
gyrus paraterminalis
gyrus postcentralis
gyrus precentralis
gyrus rectus
gyrus subcallosus
gyrus supracallosus
gyrus supramarginalis
gyrus temporalis inferior
gyrus temporalis medius
gyrus temporalis superior
gyrus uncinatus
Gysi articulator

H1 catheter
Haab after-cataract knife
Haab eye knife
Haab eye magnet
Haab knife needle
Haab needle
Haab reflex
Haab scleral resection knife
Haab-Grieshaber knife
Haag slit lamp
Haagensen staging of breast cancer (A, B, etc.)
Haagensen test
Haagensen triple biopsy of breast
Haag-Streit keratometer
Haag-Streit light
Haag-Streit ophthalmometer
Haag-Streit slit lamp
Haas dislocation operation
Haas operation
habenula
habenular commissure
Haber syndrome
Haberer abdominal spatula
Haberer gastrointestinal forceps
Haberer intestinal clamp
Haberer spatula
Haberman feeder
Haberman suction elevator
habitual abortion
habitual dislocation
habitual occlusion
habitual temporomandibular joint luxation
habituation
habitus
  body habitus
Hachinski ischemic scale
Hacker hypospadias
Hackethal intramedullary bouquet fixation
Hackethal stacked nailing technique

HA-coated hip implant
HA-coated Micro-Vent implant
HA-coated root-form dental implant
Haddad-Riordan wrist arthrodesis
Hadeco ES100VX mini Doppler
Hadeco Minidop Doppler
Hader bar clip
Hader dental attachment
Hader implant bar
Hadju-Cheney syndrome
Hadju-Cheney acro-osteolysis syndrome
Hadlock table
Hadow balloon
Haefliger cleaver
Haeggstrom antral trocar
Haelan tape
Haemogram blood loss monitor
Haemolite
  Cell Saver Haemolite
Haemonetics cell saver
Haemonetics Cell Saver 5
Haemoson ultrasound Doppler
Haenig irrigating scissors
Haering esophageal prosthesis
Haering tube
Haftelast self-adhering bandage
Hagan surface suction tube
Hagar probe
Hagedorn cheiloplasty
Hagedorn needle
Hagedorn operation
Hagedorn operation suture needle
Hagedorn-Le Mesurier method of cleft lip repair
Hagenbarth clip-applying forceps
Hagerty operation
Haggitt classification
Hagie hemostat
Hagie hip pin
Hagie pin
Hagie pin nail

Hagie T-stack
Haglund deformity
Haglund plaster scissors
Haglund scissors
Haglund speculum
Haglund spreader
Haglund vaginal speculum
Haglund-Stille plaster spreader
Haglund-Stille vaginal speculum
Hagner bag
Hagner bag catheter
Hagner catheter
Hagner hemostatic bag
Hagner operation
Hagner urethral bag
Hague cataract lamp
Hague lamp
Hahn bone nail
Hahn cannula
Hahn cleft
Hahn gastrotomy
Hahn operation
Hahn screw
Hahnenkratt dental clasp
Hahnenkratt aspirator
Hahnenkratt lingual bar
Hahnenkratt orthodontic wire
Hahnenkratt retainer
Hahnenkratt root canal pin
Hahnenkratt temporary crown
Hahn-Steinthal fracture
Haid cervical plate
Haid Universal bone plate
Haidinger brush
Haig Ferguson obstetrical
    forceps
Haig obstetrical forceps
Haight anastomosis
Haight baby retractor
Haight operation
Haight pediatric rib spreader
Haight periosteal elevator
Haight pulmonary retractor
Haight-Finochietto rib retractor
Haight-Finochietto rib spreader
Haik eye implant
Haimovici arteriotomy scissors
Haines arachnoid dissector
Haines-Zancolli test
hair ball
hair bulb
hair collar sign

hair follicle
hair grafting
hair papilla
hair replacement graft
hair shaft
hair transplant punch
hair-bearing area
hair-bearing graft
hair-bearing reconstruction
hairline fracture
hairline incision
hairline of brow
hair-matrix carcinoma
hairpin loop
hairy hamartoma
hairy leukoplakia (HL)
hairy mole
hairy nevus
hairy cell leukemia
Hajek antral punch forceps
Hajek cannula
Hajek chisel
Hajek downbiting rongeur
Hajek elevator
Hajek forceps
Hajek hammer
Hajek incision
Hajek mallet
Hajek operation
Hajek punch
Hajek retractor
Hajek rongeur
Hajek septal chisel
Hajek sphenoid punch forceps
Hajek upbiting rongeur
Hajek-Ballenger dissector
Hajek-Ballenger elevator
Hajek-Ballenger septal dissector
Hajek-Ballenger septal elevator
Hajek-Claus punch
Hajek-Claus rongeur
Hajek-Koffler bone punch
Hajek-Koffler bone punch
    forceps
Hajek-Koffler forceps
Hajek-Koffler laminectomy
    rongeur
Hajek-Koffler punch forceps
Hajek-Koffler sphenoidal
    rongeur
Hajek-Skillern punch
Hajek-Skillern sphenoidal punch

Hajek-Tieck nasal speculum
Hakanson technique
Håkansson bone rongeur
Håkansson-Olivecrona rongeur
Hakim catheter
Hakim reservoir
Hakim shunt
Hakim tube
Hakim valve
Hakim-Cordis pump
Hakko catheter
Hakme technique
Halban culdoplasty
Halberg clip
Halberg contact lens forceps
Halberg indirect ophthalmoscope
Halberg trial clip occluder
Haldane tube
Haldane-Priestly tube
Haldeman bone graft
Hale obstetrical forceps
Hales piesimeter
half-and-half nail
half-axial projection
half-body irradiation
half-circle plate
half-curved clamp
half-hitch knot
half-hitch sutures
half-intensity needle
half-moon retractor
half-mouth technique
half-pin fixation
half-ring leg splint
half-ring Thomas splint
half-shell cast
half-thickness
half-value
Halifax fine adjustment
     instrument
Halifax interlaminar clamp
Halifax placement forceps
Hall arthrotome
Hall band intrauterine device
Hall bur
Hall craniotome
Hall dermatome
Hall double-hole spinal stapler
Hall drill
Hall driver
Hall facet fusion
Hall in-and-out craniotome

Hall intrauterine device
Hall large bone instrument
Hall mastoid bur
Hall Micro-Aire drill
Hall Neurairtome drill
Hall neurosurgical craniotome
Hall neurotome
Hall Orthairtome drill
Hall Osteon drill
Hall Osteon drill system kit
Hall Osteon irrigation kit
Hall prosthetic heart valve
Hall sacral anchor
Hall sagittal saw
Hall self-holding introducer
Hall large bone instrument
Hall sign
Hall spinal screw
Hall step-down drill
Hall sternal saw
Hall Surgairtome drill
Hall Surgairtome II drill
Hall valve
Hall valvulotome
Hall Versipower drill
Hall Versipower oscillating saw
Hall Versipower reamer
Hall Versipower reciprocating saw
Hallberg biliointestinal bypass
Hallberg forceps
Hall-Chevalier stripper
Halle bone curet
Halle chisel
Halle curet
Halle dura knife
Halle elevator
Halle ethmoidal curet
Halle infant nasal speculum
Halle knife
Halle needle
Halle point
Halle speculum
Halle trigeminus knife
Halle vascular spatula
Haller ansa
Haller circle
Haller layer of choroid
Haller membrane
Haller plexus
Hallermann-Streiff syndrome
Hallermann-Streiff-François
     syndrome

Halle-Tieck nasal speculum
Hallin carotid endarterectomy
    shunt
Hall-Kaster disk prosthetic valve
Hall-Kaster heart valve
Hall-Kaster mitral valve
    prosthesis
Hall-Kaster tilting disk valve
    prosthesis
Hall-Morris biphase screw
Hallpike maneuver
Hallpike-Blackmore ear
    microscope
Hallpike-Dix maneuver
Hall-Relton frame
Hall-Serge aerotome
hallucis longus laceration
hallux abductus
hallux dolorosa
hallux extensus
hallux forceps
hallux malleus
hallux rigidus
hallux valgus
hallux varus
Hall-Zimmer saw
halo
    Ace low-profile MR halo
    Ace Mark III halo
    Bremer halo
    Brown-Roberts-Wells head
        ring halo
    cranial halo
    Fick halo
    glaucomatous halo
    Houston halo
    Lerman non-invasive halo
    Mark III halo
halo blue nevus
halo body cast
halo brace
halo cast
Halo catheter
halo cervical orthosis
halo deformity
halo femoral traction device
halo fracture frame
halo gravity traction device
halo head frame
halo hoop device
halo melanoma
halo nevus

halo retractor
halo ring
halo test for cerebrospinal fluid
    (CSF) rhinorrhea
halo traction
halo traction device
halo tractor
halo vest
halo vision
Halo XP catheter
halo-femoral traction
halogen coaxial
    ophthalmoscope
halogen exam light
halogen ophthalmoscope
halogen otoscope
halogenated agent
halogenated volatile anesthetic
halo-Ilizarov distraction
    instrumentation
halo-pelvic traction
halo-ring adapter
halothane anesthetic agent
halo-to-bale traction
halo-vest orthosis
Halpin operation
Halsey eye needle holder
Halsey forceps
Halsey mosquito forceps
Halsey nail scissors
Halsey needle
Halsey Vital needle holder
Halsey-Webster needle holder
Halsted arterial forceps
Halsted clamp
Halsted curved mosquito forceps
Halsted forceps
Halsted hemostat
Halsted incision
Halsted inguinal herniorrhaphy
Halsted law
Halsted ligament
Halsted maneuver
Halsted mastectomy
Halsted Micro-Line artery forceps
Halsted mosquito hemostat
Halsted mules
Halsted operation
Halsted radical mastectomy
Halsted strabismus scissors
Halsted straight mosquito clamp
Halsted sutures

Halsted-Bassini hernia repair
Halsted-Ferguson operation
Halsted-Meyer incision
Halsted-Swanson tendon-passing
    forceps
Halsted-Willy Meyer incision
halter (*see also* head halter)
    Cerva Crane halter
    deluxe head halter
    DePuy head halter
    Diskard head halter
    disposable head halter
    Forrester head halter
    Forrester-Brown head halter
    head halter
    neck-wrap halter
    Repro head halter
    standard head halter
    TMJ halter
    Zimfoam head halter
    Zimmer head halter
    Zyler head halter
halter traction
Halverson classification
Halverson-McVay hernia
    classification
hamartoma
    angiomatous lymphoid
        hamartoma
    Becker hair hamartoma
    duodenal wall hamartoma
    facial hamartoma
    hairy hamartoma
    intrapulmonary hamartoma
    neuromuscular hamartoma
    pancreatic hamartoma
hamartomatous gastric polyp
hamartomatous growth
Hamas technique
Hamas total wrist
Hamas upper limb prosthesis
hamate
    body of the hamate
    hook of the hamate
    pole of the hamate
hamate bone
hamate finder
hamate tail fracture
Hamazaki-Wesenberg body
Hamby brain retractor
Hamby clip-applying forceps
Hamby forceps

Hamby retractor
Hamby right-angle clip applier
Hamby rod
Hamby twist drill
Hamby-Hibbs retractor
Hamer scalpel
Hamilton bandage
Hamilton decompressor
Hamilton deep-surgery forceps
Hamilton pelvic traction screw
    tractor
Hamilton tongue depressor
Hamilton ventilator
Hamilton-Forewater amniotomy
    hook
Hamilton-Steward catheter
Hamis sutures
Hamm fulgurating electrode
Hamm resectoscope electrode
Hamman click
Hamman crunch
Hamman sign
hammer
    Babinski percussion hammer
    Bakelite hammer
    Baylor hammer
    Berliner neurosurgical hammer
    Berliner percussion hammer
    Boxwood hammer
    Buck neurological hammer
    Buck percussion hammer
    Carroll aluminum hammer
    cervical/lumbar hammer
    Chandler hammer
    Cloward hammer
    Crane hammer
    Dejerine percussion hammer
    Dejerine-Davis percussion
        hammer
    Epstein neurological hammer
    fiberhead hammer
    fork hammer
    Gerzog bone hammer
    Grafco percussion hammer
    Hajek hammer
    Hibbs hammer
    House tapping hammer
    intranasal hammer
    Kirk orthopedic hammer
    Küntscher hammer
    Lucae bone hammer
    MacAusland bone hammer

hammer (*continued*)
    Meyerding aluminum hammer
    Millet test hammer
    Neef hammer
    neurological percussion
        hammer
    nylon head hammer
    orthopedic hammer
    percussion hammer
    Quisling intranasal hammer
    Rabiner neurological hammer
    Ralks hammer
    rawhide bone hammer
    reflex hammer
    Rica bone hammer
    rotatory hammer
    Rush hammer
    shatter hammer
    slide hammer
    sliding hammer
    SMIC bone hammer
    Smith-Petersen hammer
    standard-pattern hammer
    stapes tapping hammer
    surgical hammer
    tack hammer
    tapping hammer
    Taylor percussion hammer
    Taylor reflex hammer
    Traube neurological hammer
    Tromner percussion hammer
    vibratory hammer
    Wagner hammer
    Wartenberg neurological
        hammer
    White hammer
    Williger hammer
hammer finger
hammer forceps
hammer nose
hammertoe correction
hammertoe correction with
    interphalangeal fusion
hammertoe repair
Hammersmith heart valve
Hammersmith mitral prosthesis
Hammersmith mitral valve
    prosthesis
Hammersmith prosthesis
hammertoe deformity
hammer-type acupuncture
    needle

hammock bandage
hammock dressing
hammock ligament
hammock nephropexy
hammock pupil
hammocking of valve
hammock-method nephropexy
Hammond alloy
Hammond blade
Hammond bunionectomy
Hammond operation
Hammond orthodontic splint
Hammond winged retractor blade
Hamou colpomicrohysteroscope
Hamou contact
    microhysteroscope
Hamou endoscope
Hamou hysteroscope
Hampton electrosurgical unit
Hampton hump
Hampton line
Hampton maneuver
Hampton needle holder
Hampton operation
Hampton small bowel operation
Hamrick elevator
Hamrick suction dissector
Hamrick suction elevator
hamstring ligament
    augmentation
hamstring muscle
hamstring tendon
hamstrung knee
hamular groove
hamular notch
hamular procedure
hamular process
hamulus
    frontal hamulus
    lacrimal hamulus
    pterygoid hamulus
    sulcus of pterygoid hamulus
hamulus of ethmoid bone
hamulus of hamate bone
hamulus ossis hamati
hamulus pterygoideus
Hanafee catheter
Hanafee catheter tip
Hanastome microkeratome
Hanau articulator
Hancke-Vilman biopsy handle
    instrument

Hancock amputation
Hancock aortic prosthetic valve
Hancock aortic punch
Hancock bioprosthetic heart
    valve
Hancock coronary perfusion
Hancock embolectomy catheter
Hancock fiberoptic catheter
Hancock heterograft heart valve
Hancock hydrogen detection
    catheter
Hancock luminal
    electrophysiologic
    recording catheter
Hancock operation
Hancock porcine xenograft
Hancock temporary cardiac
    pacing wire
Hancock thermodilution
    catheter
Hancock valve
Hancock vascular graft
Hancock wedge-pressure
    catheter
hand and arm scrub
hand block
hand brace
hand brush dispenser
hand cautery
hand chuck
hand cock-up sling
hand cock-up snare
hand cock-up splint
hand dynamometer
hand ear perforator
hand exercise ball
hand flap
hand helper device
hand perforator
hand replantation
hand retractor
hand saw
hand scrub
hand signal
hand steadiness
hand strength test
hand surgery elevator
hand surgery osteotome
hand surgery rasp
hand table
hand trephine
hand tubing roller

hand ventilation
Handages
Hand-Aid arterial wrist support
Hand-Aid strapping material
hand-assisted laparoscopic
    colectomy
hand-assisted laparoscopic
    gastric bypass
hand-assisted laparoscopic live-
    donor nephrectomy
hand-assisted laparoscopic
    surgery (HALS)
hand-assisted laparoscopic
    vertical-banded gastroplasty
hand-assisted laparoscopy
hand-control cautery
hand-crimped stent
handcutting instrument
Handeze fingerless glove
hand-held Doppler flow probe
    examination
handheld drill guide
handheld dynamometer
handheld exploring electrode
    probe
handheld eye magnet
handheld fundus camera
handheld Hruby lens
handheld mapping probe
handheld nebulizer
handheld retractor
handheld rotary prism
handheld trephine
Handi-Hook
Handisol phototherapy device
handle (*see also* traction handle)
    Acufex handle
    autopsy blade handle
    autopsy handle
    Bard-Parker handle
    Bard-Parker knife handle
    Barton traction handle
    bayonet handle
    Beaver blade chuck handle
    Beaver blade handle
    Beaver chuck handle
    Beaver handle
    Beaver knife handle
    Beaver surgical blade handle
    Bill axis traction handle
    blade handle
    Bovie chuck-type handle

handle
    BP surgical handle
    bronchoscopic forceps handle
    Bruening esophagoscopy
        forceps handle
    Castroviejo-Kalt traction handle
    cautery handle
    Charnley brace handle
    chuck handle
    Cloward cross-bar handle
    Cloward double-hinge
        cervical retractor handle
    Cloward dowel handle
    cord handle
    Corwin knife handle
    Cottle knife handle
    Cottle modified knife handle
    Cottle protected knife handle
    DuraLite handle
    Dynagrip blade handle
    Dynagrip handle
    ear knife handle
    Elliot trephine handle
    endoscopic electrode handle
    Farrior chuck handle
    forceps handle
    Gigli-saw handle
    Hardy lateral knife handle
    hexagonal handle
    hook-on battery handle
    hook-on laryngoscope handle
    House knife handle
    House myringotomy knife
        handle
    Huber forceps handle
    insulated knife handle
    interchangeable punch handle
    Jackson bronchoscopic
        forceps handle
    Jackson forceps handle
    Jackson Universal handle
    Klein Delrin Luer-Lok handle
    knife handle
    knurled handle
    laryngeal knife handle
    laryngeal mirror handle
    laryngoscope battery handle
    Luikart-Bill traction handle
    Lynch laryngeal knife handle
    malleus handle
    Marino rotatable
        transsphenoidal knife handle

handle (*continued*)
    Marlow Primus handle
    measurement control handle
    Morse instrument handle
    myringotomy knife handle
    obstetrical traction handle
    Ortho-Grip silicone rubber
        handle
    Parker-Bard handle
    protected knife handle
    rotary scissors with cigar
        handle
    rotary scissors with loop
        handle
    rotatable transsphenoidal
        knife handle
    Rusch laryngoscope handle
    safety handle
    saw handle
    scalpel handle
    scaphoid spoon handle
    slotted handle
    Sluder Universal handle
    Stiwer scalpel handle
    stone basket screw-mounted
        handle
    Storz ear knife handle
    Strully Gigli-saw handle
    surgical handle
    surgical knife handle
    Thera-Band handle
    Tip-Trol handle
    T-pin handle
    traction handle
    tympanum perforator handle
    Universal chuck handle
    Universal handle
    Universal mirror handle
    Universal nasal instrument
        handle
    V. Mueller Tip-Trol handle
    V. Mueller Universal handle
    Welch Allyn battery handle
    Welch Allyn cord handle
handle of malleus
handle traction
handleless clamp
Handley incision
Handley lymphangioplasty
Handley operation
handmade anastomosis
hand-mounted stent

hand-sewn anastomosis
hand-sutured closure
hand-sutured ileoanal
  anastomosis
hand-switching electrocautery
  pencil
HandTact instrument set
Handtrol electrosurgical pencil
handwasher machine
Handy II articulator
Handy non-mydriatic video
  fundus camera
Handy-Buck extension tractor
Handy-Buck traction
Hanely-McDermitt pelvimeter
Haney clamp
Haney needle driver
Hanger prosthesis
hanging arm cast
hanging cast
hanging columella
hanging drop
hanging heart
hanging hip operation
hanging panniculus
hanging skin
hanging toe operation
hanging-drop technique
hanging-weight method for
  reducing dislocated shoulder
hangman's fracture
hangnail
Hanhart syndrome
Hank uterine dilator
Hank-Bradley uterine dilator
Hank-Dennen obstetrical
  forceps
Hankin reduction
Hanks uterine dilator
Hanks-Bradley uterine dilator
Hanley rectal bladder procedure
Hann filter
Hanna classification of head and
  neck defects (classes A, B, C)
Hanna splint
Hanna trephine
Hannahan bur
Hannahan forceps
Hannon endometrial curet
Hannover canal
Hannover classification
Hannover needle holder

Hans Rudolph 3-way valve
Hansatome microkeratome
Hansen fracture classification
Hansen grasper
Hansen keratome
Hansen-Street anchor plate
Hansen-Street driver-extractor
Hansen-Street intramedullary nail
Hansen-Street intramedullary rod
Hansen-Street pin
Hansen-Street plate
Hansen-Street self-broaching nail
Hanslik patellar prosthesis
Hapex bioactive material
haploscope
Hapsburg jaw
Hapsburg lip
Hapset bone graft plaster
  material
Hapset hydroxyapatite bone
  graft plaster
haptens
haptic area implant
haptic area lens
haptic loupe
haptic plate lens
haptic-fixated intraocular lens
haptics
haptocholangiostomy
Hara gallbladder inflammation
  classification
Hara infiltration block
Harada-Ito procedure
hard adhesions
hard calculus
hard cancer
hard cataract
hard cleft palate
hard contact lens
hard exudate
hard indurated colon mass
hard lens
hard mallet
hard metal disease
hard pad disease
hard palate cancer
hard palate dissection
hard palate mucosa graft
hard palate retractor
hard socket
hard sore
hard subcutaneous node

hard tissue replacement (HTR)
hard tissue replacement-
    malleable facial implant
hard ulcer
Hardcastle tarsometatarsal joint
    injury classification
hardening of artery walls
Harder glands
harderian glands
Hardesty tendon hook
Hardesty tenotomy hook
Hardinge lateral approach
Hardinge technique
hard-soft palate junction
Hardt osteotome
Hardy 3-prong fork
Hardy bayonet curet
Hardy bayonet dressing forceps
Hardy bayonet enucleator
Hardy bayonet modification of
    Bronson-Ray
Hardy bivalve speculum
Hardy dissector
Hardy enucleator
Hardy hypophysial curet
Hardy implant fork
Hardy lateral knife handle
Hardy lensometer
Hardy microbipolar forceps
Hardy microcuret
Hardy microdissector
Hardy microsurgical bayonet
    bipolar forceps
Hardy microsurgical enucleator
Hardy modification of Bronson-
    Ray curet
Hardy pituitary dissector
Hardy pituitary spoon
Hardy retractor
Hardy rongeur
Hardy sellar punch
Hardy speculum
Hardy suction tube
Hardy transsphenoidal mirror
Hardy-Cushing speculum
Hardy-Duddy speculum
Hardy-Duddy vaginal retractor
Hardy-Duddy weighted vaginal
    speculum
Hardy-Rand-Rittler plate
Hardy-Sella pump
Hare compact traction splint

Hare splint device
Hare traction device
Hare traction splint
harelip forceps
harelip needle
harelip operation
harelip suture technique
harelip sutures
Harewood suspension
    procedure
Hargin antral trocar
Hargin antrum trocar
Hargin trocar
Hargis periosteal elevator
Hark operation for talipes valgus
Harken auricular clamp
Harken ball heart valve
Harken cardiovascular forceps
Harken clamp
Harken erysiphake
Harken forceps
Harken heart needle
Harken prosthetic valve
Harken retractor
Harken spreader
Harken valve
Harken valvulotome
Harken-Cooley forceps
Harken-Starr valve
harlequin deformity
harlequin fetus
harlequin orbit
Harm posterior cervical plate
Harman approach
Harman bone graft
Harman deltoid procedure
Harman eye dressing
Harman fixation forceps
Harman incision
Harman cataract operation
Harman-Fahey technique
Harmon cervical approach
Harmon chisel
Harmon hip reconstruction
Harmon incision
Harmon modified posterolateral
    approach
Harmon operation
Harmon shoulder approach
Harmon transfer technique
Harmonic hemorrhoidectomy
Harmonic scalpel

Harmonic scissors
Harmonic sutures
harmonious retinal
  correspondence
Harms cage
Harms corneal forceps
Harms microtying forceps
Harms probe
Harms suture-tying forceps
Harms trabeculotomy probe
Harms utility forceps
Harms vessel forceps
Harms-Dannheim trabeculotomy
  operation
Harms-Moss anterior thoracic
  instrumentation
Harms-Tubingen tying forceps
Harold Crowe drill nail
Harold Hayes eustachian bougie
Harpenden handgrip
  dynamometer
Harpenden skinfold calipers
Harper cervical laminectomy
  punch
Harper periosteal elevator
Harper rongeur
Harper-Warren incision
harpoon suture anchor
Harrah lung clamp
Harrell Y stent
Harriluque sublaminar wiring
  modification
Harriluque technique
Harrington bladder retractor
Harrington Britetrac retractor
Harrington clamp forceps
Harrington deep surgical scissors
Harrington distraction
  instrumentation
Harrington dual square-ended
  rod
Harrington erysiphake
Harrington esophageal
  diverticulectomy
Harrington flat wrench
Harrington hernia repair
Harrington hook clamp
Harrington hook driver
Harrington lung-grasping
  forceps
Harrington operation
Harrington overlapping closure

Harrington pedicle hook
Harrington retractor
Harrington rod
Harrington rod instrumentation
  distraction outrigger device
Harrington rod instrumentation
  failure
Harrington scissors
Harrington spinal elevator
Harrington spinal fusion
Harrington splanchnic retractor
Harrington spreader
Harrington strut
Harrington sutures
Harrington sympathectomy
  retractor
Harrington thoracic forceps
Harrington tonometer
Harrington total hip arthroplasty
Harrington vulsellum forceps
Harrington-Allison repair
Harrington-Carmalt clamp
Harrington-Deaver retractor
Harrington-Kostuik distraction
  device
Harrington-Kostuik
  instrumentation
Harrington-Mayo forceps
Harrington-Mayo rib shears
Harrington-Mayo scissors
Harrington-Mayo tissue forceps
Harrington-Mixter clamp
  forceps
Harrington-Mixter thoracic
  clamp
Harrington-Mixter thoracic
  forceps
Harrington-Pemberton retractor
Harrington-Pemberton
  sympathectomy retractor
Harris anterolateral approach
Harris band
Harris brace-type reamer
Harris broach
Harris catheter
Harris cemented hip prosthesis
Harris center-cutting acetabular
  reamer
Harris condylocephalic rod
Harris dissector
Harris drip
Harris femoral head gauge

Harris forceps
Harris growth arrest line
Harris hip guide
Harris hip nail
Harris hip prosthesis
Harris hip screw
Harris incision
Harris intramedullary nail
Harris lateral approach
Harris line
Harris prosthesis
Harris modified J-loupe
    intraocular lens
Harris nail
Harris operation
Harris plate
Harris precoat prosthesis
Harris punch
Harris reamer
Harris rigid intraocular lens
Harris segregator
Harris separator
Harris sling
Harris snare
Harris superior acetabular graft
Harris suture-carrying forceps
Harris sutures
Harris tonsillar knife
Harris total hip prosthesis
Harris trephine
Harris tube
Harris uterine injector (HUI)
Harris uterine injector catheter
Harris-Beath flatfoot procedure
Harris-Beath operation for
    talipes valgus
Harris-Beath technique
Harris-Beath x-ray view
Harris-Galante cup
Harris-Galante porous metal hip
    prosthesis
Harris-Galante porous-coated
    femoral component
Harris-Kronner uterine
    manipulator/injector
    (HUMI)
Harris-Mueller procedure
Harris-Norton hip reamer
Harrison bone-holding forceps
Harrison capsular knife
Harrison chalazion retractor
Harrison curet

Harrison fetal bladder stent
Harrison forked-type strut guide
Harrison groove
Harrison guide
Harrison implant
Harrison interlocked mesh
    dressing
Harrison interlocked mesh graft
Harrison interlocking mesh
    prosthesis
Harrison knife
Harrison myringoplasty knife
Harrison prosthesis
Harrison retractor
Harrison scarifying curet
Harrison scissors
Harrison speculum
Harrison sulcus
Harrison suture-removing
    scissors
Harrison tucker
Harrison-Nicolle polypropylene
    pegs
Harrison-Shea curet
Harrison-Shea knife
Harris-Sinskey microlens hook
Harris-Smith anterior interbody
    drill
Harris-Smith cervical fusion
harsh murmur
harsh respiration
Harstein iris cryoretractor
Hart extension finger splint
Hart pediatric 3-mirror lens
Hart splint
Hartel guideline
Hartel technique
Harting body
Hartinger Coincidence
    refractometer
Hartley implant
Hartley mammary prosthesis
Hartley-Krause operation
Hartmann adenoidal curet
Hartmann catheter
Hartmann clamp
Hartmann closure
Hartmann colostomy
Hartmann curet
Hartmann ear speculum
Hartmann fossa
Hartmann hemostat

Hartmann hemostatic mosquito
forceps
Hartmann knife
Hartmann mastoid rongeur
Hartmann mosquito forceps
Hartmann nasal conchotome
Hartmann operation
Hartmann point
Hartmann pouch
Hartmann procedure
Hartmann punch
Hartmann reconstruction
technique
Hartmann resection
Hartmann rongeur
Hartmann solution
Hartmann speculum
Hartmann tonsillar dissector
Hartmann tonsillar punch
Hartmann tonsillar punch
forceps
Hartmann tuning fork
Hartmann uterine biopsy
forceps
Hartmann-Citelli alligator
forceps
Hartmann-Citelli ear punch
Hartmann-Citelli ear punch
forceps
Hartmann-Citelli punch
Hartmann-Corgill ear forceps
Hartmann-Gruenwald forceps
Hartmann-Gruenwald nasal-
cutting forceps
Hartmann-Herzfeld ear forceps
Hartmann-Herzfeld ear rongeur
Hartmann-Herzfeld rongeur
Hartmann-Noyes nasal-dressing
forceps
Hartmann-Proctor ear forceps
Hartmann-Weingartner ear
forceps
Hartmann-Wullstein ear forceps
Hartstein iris cryoretractor
Hartstein irrigating iris retractor
Hartstein irrigator
Hartstein retractor
Hartzler coronary dilation
catheter
Hartzler angioplasty balloon
Hartzler balloon catheter
Hartzler dilatation catheter

Hartzler Micro catheter
Hartzler Micro angioplasty
balloon
Hartzler Micro balloon for
coronary angioplasty
Hartzler rib retractor
Hartzler ultra low-profile
catheter
Harvard manometer
Harvard dual-syringe pump
Harvard cannula
Harvard manometer
Harvard microbore intravenous
extension set
Harvard needle
Harvard PCA pump
harvest
bone harvest
double rectus harvest
endoscope-assisted rectus
abdominis muscle flap
harvest
endoscopic harvest
endoscopically assisted
harvest
free gracilis muscle harvest
graft harvest
in situ graft harvest
open method harvest
tissue harvest
harvest organ
harvest tissue
harvested fat
harvester
QuickDraw bone harvester
Harvester bipolar scissors
harvesting
autograft harvesting
donor island harvesting
graft harvesting
in situ graft harvesting
stem-cell marrow harvesting
harvesting an organ
harvesting skin
Harvey Stone clamp
Harvey Stone hemostat
Harvey wire-cutting scissors
Hashimoto struma
Hashmat shunt
Hashmat-Waterhouse shunt
Haslinger bronchoscope
Haslinger electroscope

Haslinger endoscope
Haslinger esophagoscope
Haslinger head holder
Haslinger headrest
Haslinger laryngoscope
Haslinger palate retractor
Haslinger retractor
Haslinger tip forceps
Haslinger tonsil hemostat
Haslinger tracheobronchoesophago-
    scope
Haslinger tracheoscope
Haslinger uvula retractor
Hasner fold
Hasner lid
Hasner lid forceps
Hasner operation
Hasner valve
Hass hip osteotomy
Hass procedure
Hass technique
Hassab operation
Hassall body
Hassall-Henle wart
Hassan catheter
Hassan-type port
Hassmann-Brunn-Neer elbow
    technique
Hasson balloon uterine elevator
    cannula
Hasson blunt port
Hasson blunt-end cannula
Hasson bullet-tip forceps
Hasson cannula
Hasson grasper
Hasson grasping forceps
Hasson laparoscope
Hasson laparoscopic trocar
Hasson needle-nose forceps
Hasson open laparoscopy
    cannula
Hasson retractor
Hasson ring forceps
Hasson spike-tooth forceps
Hasson stable access cannula
Hasson technique
Hasson trocar
Hasson uterine manipulator
Hasson-Eder laparoscope cannula
Hasson-Eder laparoscopy
    cannula

Hastings bipolar
    hemiarthroplasty
Hastings frame
Hastings open reduction
Hastings procedure
Hasund appliance
Hatafuku fundus onlay patch
    esophageal repair
Hatch catheter
Hatch chisel
Hatch clamp
Hatcher operation
Hatcher pin
hatchet extractor
hatchet head deformity
Hatfield bone curet
HA-threaded hexlock implant
Hatt golf-stick elevator
Hatt spoon
Haultain operation
haunch bone
Hauser bunionectomy
Hauser heel cord procedure
Hauser knee procedure
Hauser operation
Hauser patellar realignment
    technique
Hauser patellar tendon
    procedure
Hauser transplant
Hausmann vascular clamp
haustra (*sing.* haustrum)
haustra coli
haustral fold
haustral markings
haustral pattern
haustral segmentation
haustration
haustrum (*plur.* haustra)
Haven hook
Haven skin graft
Haven skin graft hook
Haver glands
Haverfield brain cannula
Haverfield hemilaminectomy
    retractor
Haverfield retractor
Haverfield-Scoville
    hemilaminectomy retractor
Haverfield-Scoville retractor
Haverhill clamp
Haverhill dermal abrader

Haverhill ear operation
Haverhill needle
Haverhill-Mack clamp
Havers gland
haversian bone
haversian canal
haversian gland
haversian lamella
haversian space
Havlicek spiral cannula
Havlicek trocar
Hawkeye suture needle
Hawkins breast localization
    needle
Hawkins cervical biopsy forceps
Hawkins cervix conization
    cautery
Hawkins forceps
Hawkins fracture
Hawkins inside-out
    nephrostomy technique
Hawkins line
Hawkins needle
Hawkins procedure
Hawkins sign
Hawkins single-stick technique
Hawkins talar fracture
    classification
Hawkins-Akins needle
hawk's beak elevator
Hawks-Dennen obstetrical
    forceps
Hawley appliance
Hawley bite plate
Hawley retainer
Hawley table
Haws-type brachydactyly
Hawthorne effect
hay baler's fracture
Hay lateral approach
Hayden curet
Hayden elevator
Hayden footplate pick
Hayden palate elevator
Hayden probe
Hayden tonsil curet
Hayden tonsillar curet
Hayek oscillator
Hayem icterus
Hayes anterior resection clamp
Hayes anterior resection forceps
Hayes colon clamp

Hayes intestinal clamp
Hayes Martin forceps
Hayes Martin incision
Hayes phalangeal elevator
Hayes retractor
Hayes vaginal speculum
Hayes-Olivecrona forceps
Hayman dilator
Haynes brain cannula
Haynes cannula
Haynes operation
Haynes pin
Haynes retractor
Haynes scissors
Haynes-Griffin mandible splint
Haynes-Griffin mandibular splint
Haynes Stellite implant metal
    prosthesis
Hays finger retractor
Hays hand retractor
Hayton-Williams forceps
Hayton-Williams mouth gag
HBIG (hepatitis B
    immunoglobulin)
HBO (hyperbaric oxygen)
HBO-induced angiogenesis
HD Secura dialyzer
HD2 prosthesis
HD2 total hip prosthesis
HDI ultrasound
HDR intracavitary radiation
    therapy
HEA (hemorrhages, exudates,
    and aneurysms)
head
    Austin Moore head
    Biolox ball head
    Biolox ceramic femoral head
    Bruening-Storz diagnostic
        head
    Bruening-Work diagnostic head
    bulldog head
    cobalt-chromium head
    condylar head
    condyle head
    contra-angle head
    coupling head
    crowning of infant's head
    DePuy hip prosthesis with
        Scuderi head
    Eicher femoral prosthetic
        head

head (*continued*)
femoral head
femoral prosthetic head
fetal head
fibular head
Frenzel ear operating head
hourglass head
humeral head
Judet femoral prosthetic head
Lexan head
malleus head
mandibular head
Matroc femoral head
metacarpal head
metatarsal head
molding of head
Morse head
MRI probe head
Naden-Rieth femoral
    prosthetic head
oblique head
Omniflex head
Oxinium femoral head
pointed head
radial head
Rhoton-Merz rotatable
    coupling head
rotatable coupling head
saddle head
Series-II humeral head
steeple head
Storz-Bruening diagnostic
    head
subluxed radial head
talus head
Thompson femoral head
tower head
transverse head
Vitox femoral head
Work-Bruening diagnostic
    head
Ziramic femoral head
Zirconia orthopedic
    prosthetic head
Zyranox femoral head
head and neck in extended
    position
head and neck reconstruction
head brace
head circumference
head coil
head compression

head dependent position
head-down presentation
head drape
head extended
head extension
head extractor
head fixation device
head fracture frame
head halter (*see* halter)
head halter cervical traction
head halter traction
head harness
head holder (*see* holder)
head lamp
head of condyloid process of
    mandible
head of femur
head of humerus
head of malleus
head of pancreas
head of radius
head of talus
Head paradoxical reflex
head ring
head sling
head spoon separator
head tilt
head trauma
head-turn technique
head, eyes, ears, nose, and throat
    (HEENT)
head-at-risk signs
headband-and-mirror set
head-bobbing doll syndrome
head holder (*see also* holder)
    3-point head holder
    AMSCO head holder
    Bayless neurosurgical head
        holder
    CBI stereotactic head holder
    crown-of thorns head holder
    Derlacki-Juers head holder
    Gardner head holder
    Haslinger head holder
    integrated head holder
    Juers-Derlacki Universal head
        holder
    Malcolm-Rand carbon-
        composite head holder
    Mayfield head holder
    Mayfield radiolucent head
        holder

head holder (*continued*)
 Mayfield skull-pin head holder
 Mayfield tic head holder
 Mayfield-Kees head holder
 Methodist Hospital head holder
 neurosurgical head holder
 Paparella monkey-head holder
 Parkinson head holder
 pin head holder
 pinion head holder
 radiolucent cranial pin head
  holder
 Storz head holder
 Sugita head holder
 Universal head holder
 VBH head holder
 Veley head holder
 Vogel-Bale-Hohner head holder
headhunter catheter
headhunter visceral angiography
  catheter
headlight
 coaxial headlight
 direct-focus headlight
 fiberoptic headlight
 high beam fiberoptic
  headlight
 Storz headlight
 surgeon's headlight
 Welch Allyn headlight
headlight (*see* light)
head-low incision
headrest
 adjustable headrest
 Adson headrest
 Brown-Roberts-Wells headrest
 Craig headrest
 doughnut headrest
 Gardner headrest
 Gardner-Wells headrest
 Gibralter headrest
 Haslinger headrest
 horseshoe headrest
 Lempert rongeur headrest
 Light headrest
 Light-Veley headrest
 Mayfield pediatric horseshoe
  headrest
 Mayfield radiolucent headrest
 Mayfield swivel horseshoe
  headrest
 Mayfield-Kees headrest

headrest (*continued*)
 McConnell orthopedic
  headrest
 Multipoise headrest
 neurosurgical headrest
 pin headrest
 pinion headrest
 Richards headrest
 Roberts headrest
 Sam Roberts headrest
 Shea headrest
 Storz adjustable headrest
 Veley headrest
head-splitting humeral fracture
head-turning reflex
head-up tilt position
healed by first intention
healed by second intention
healed fracture
healed scar
Healey revision acetabular
  component
healing
 delayed healing
 delayed wound healing
 endoscopic healing
 fat-to-fat healing
 fracture healing
 per primam healing
 per secundam healing
 proliferative phase of wound
  healing
 remodeling phase of wound
  healing
 scarless fetal wound healing
 substrate phase of wound
  healing
 wound healing
healing biopsy incision
healing by first intention
healing by granulation
healing by second intention
healing by third intention
healing fracture
healing incision site
healing of fracture
healing per primam intentionem
healing per secundam intentionem
healing ridge
healing screw
healing wound
Healon injection cannula

Healon irrigant

Healos bone graft substitute material

Healos synthetic bone grafting material

Healthdyne apnea monitor

Healthdyne pulse oximeter

Healthdyne ventilator

Healthflex orthotic

HealthShield antimicrobial mediastinal wound drainage catheter

HealthShield catheter

HealWell Cub plantar fasciitis night splint

Healy gastrointestinal forceps

Healy intestinal forceps

Healy suture-removing forceps

Healy uterine biopsy forceps

Heaney bulldog-jaw needle holder

Heaney clamp

Heaney curet

Heaney endometrial biopsy curet

Heaney hysterectomy forceps

Heaney hysterectomy retractor

Heaney needle holder

Heaney operation

Heaney retractor

Heaney sutures

Heaney technique

Heaney tissue forceps

Heaney uterine curet

Heaney vaginal hysterectomy

Heaney vaginal retractor

Heaney Vital needle holder

Heaney-Ballantine hysterectomy forceps

Heaney-Kantor hysterectomy forceps

Heaney-Rezek hysterectomy forceps

Heaney-Simon hysterectomy forceps

Heaney-Simon hysterectomy retractor

Heaney-Simon vaginal retractor

Heaney-Stumf forceps

Hearn needle

heart

    4-chamber view of heart

    3-chambered heart

    abdominal heart

heart (*continued*)

    air-driven artificial heart

    Akutsu artificial heart

    ALVAD artificial heart

    apex of heart

    armored heart

    artificial heart

    athlete's heart

    Baylor total artificial heart

    beer heart

    boat-shaped heart

    bony heart

    boot-shaped heart

    catheterization of heart

    cervical heart

    clockwise rotation of heart

    conduction system of heart

    contour of heart

    contracted heart

    crisscross heart

    crux of heart

    decompression of heart

    decortication of heart

    defibrillated heart

    denervated heart

    diaphragmatic surface of heart

    digitalization of heart

    electromechanical artificial heart

    encased heart

    extracorporeal heart

    fetal heart

    fibroid heart

    flask-shaped heart

    flesh trabeculae of heart

    hanging heart

    Hershey total artificial heart

    hypoplastic heart

    icing heart

    implantable artificial heart

    infundibulum of heart

    interventricular sulcus of heart

    intracorporeal heart

    irritable heart

    Jarvik

    Jarvik artificial heart

    Liotta total artificial heart

    Mahaim bundle in heart

    mechanical heart

    mush heart

heart (*continued*)
Norwood operation for hypoplastic left-sided heart
open heart
orthotopic biventricular artificial heart
orthotopic univentricular artificial heart
paracorporeal heart
parchment heart
pear-shaped heart
Penn State artificial heart
Phoenix total artificial heart
project sites of heart
prosthetic heart
pumping heart
RTV total artificial heart
smoker's heart
soldier's heart
sternocostal surface of heart
sulcus of heart
Symbion artificial heart
Symbion Jarvik artificial heart
Symbion total artificial heart
Symbion/CardioWest total artificial heart
total artificial heart
transverse sulcus of heart
triatrial heart
trilocular heart
University of Akron artificial heart
Utah total artificial heart
wandering heart
heart and hand syndrome
heart anomaly
heart attack
heart block
heart border
heart bypass
heart catheterization
heart chamber
heart clot
heart defect
heart disease
heart donor
heart failure
Heart Laser
heart massage
heart monitor
heart murmur
heart muscle

heart needle
heart orifices
heart pacemaker
heart pacemaker leads
heart position
heart prosthesis
heart pump
heart rate
heart rhythm
heart shock
heart silhouette
heart size
heart sounds
heart surgery
heart synchronized ventilation
heart tissue
heart tones
heart transplant
heart transplantation
heart valve (*see* graft, implant, prosthesis, valve)
heart valve fixation
heart valve prosthesis
heart valve replacement
heartbeat
multifocal heartbeats
heart-lung bypass
heart-lung machine
heart-lung resuscitator
heart-lung transplant
heart-lung transplantation
HeartMate implantable ventricular assist device
HeartMate portable pump
Heartport endoaortic clamp
heat cautery
heat exposure
heat gun
heat pad
heat radiation
heat sensation
heat therapy
heat-moister exchanger
heated tracheostomy collar
heater probe unit (HPU)
heater-probe coagulation
heat-expandable stent
Heath anterior chamber syringe
Heath chalazion curet
Heath chalazion forceps
Heath chalazion knife
Heath clip

Heath clip-removing forceps
Heath clip-removing scissors
Heath curet
Heath dilator
Heath dissector
Heath expressor
Heath follicle expressor
Heath lid expressor
Heath mallet
Heath mules
Heath nasal forceps
Heath operation
Heath punctum dilator
Heath suture scissors
Heath suture-cutting scissors
Heath trephine flap dissector
Heath wire cutter
Heath wire-cutting scissors
Heaton inguinal herniorrhaphy
Heaton operation
HeatProbe device
heat-vulcanized silicone
    elastomer implants
heavy body impression material
heavy cross-slot screwdriver
heavy elevator
heavy gauge sutures
heavy metal injection
heavy monofilament sutures
heavy retention sutures
heavy septal scissors
heavy silk retention suture
heavy silk retention sutures
heavy silk sutures
heavy skin
heavy twill belt
heavy weighted speculum
heavy wire sutures
heavy-angled scissors
heavy-bodies material
heavy-duty pliers with side-cutter
heavy-gauge sutures
heavy-ion irradiation
heavy-ion mammography
Heberden anomaly
Heberden disease
Heberden nodes
Heberden rheumatism
hebosteotomy
hebotomy
Hebra blade
Hebra chalazion curet

Hebra corneal curet
Hebra fixation hook
Hebra hook
Hecht fascia lata forceps
Heck disease
Hedblom costal elevator
Hedblom elevator
Hedblom raspatory
Hedblom retractor
Hedblom rib retractor
hedger's cataract
Hedley procedure
Hedrocel bone substitute
    material
Hedrocel bone substitute
    material graft
Hedstrom file
Hedwig introducer
Hedwig lumen finder
heel
    anterior heel
    basketball heels
    black-dot heel
    cracked heel
    globus of heel
    policeman's heel
    rubber walking heel
    SACH heel
    solid ankle cushioned heel
      (SACH)
    Telson hinged walking heel
    Thomas heel
    torque heel
    walking heel
    wedge adjustable cushioned
      heel (WACH)
    wedge heel
heel and toe of anastomosis
heel bone
heel cord lengthening
heel cup
heel cushion
heel elevation
Heel Free splint
Heel Hugger therapeutic heel
    stabilizer
heel lift
heel pad
heel pillow
heel sleeve
heel spur
heel tap test

heel tendon
Heelbo decubitus elbow protector
Heelbo decubitus heel protector
Heelbo decubitus protector
Heelbo protector
Heeler inflatable heel protector
heel-in-armpit method to reduce
    dislocated shoulder
heel-to-crown
heel-toe anastomosis
heel-to-ear maneuver
HEENT (head, eyes, ears, nose,
    and throat)
Heermann alligator ear forceps
Heermann alligator forceps
Heermann chisel
Heermann ear forceps
Heermann gouge
Heermann incision
Heffernan nasal speculum
Heffernan speculum
Heffington lumbar seat
Hefke-Turner sign
Hegar bougie
Hegar dilator
Hegar needle
Hegar needle holder
Hegar operation
Hegar rectal dilator
Hegar sign
Hegar uterine dilator
Hegar-Baumgartner needle
Hegar-Baumgartner needle holder
Hegar-Goodell dilator
Hegar-Mayo-Seeley needle holder
Hegar-Olsen needle holder
Hegemann scissors
Hegenbarth clip
Hegenbarth clip forceps
Hegenbarth clip-applying forceps
Hegenbarth clip-removing forceps
Hegenbarth-Adams clip
Hegenbarth-Michel clip-applying
    forceps
Hahnenkratt matrix band
Heiberg-Esmarch maneuver
Heidbrink expiratory spill valve
Heidelberg fixation forceps
Heidelberg laser tomographic
    scanner
Heidelberg retinal flowmeter
Heidenhain crescents

Heidenhain law
Heidenhain rods
Heifitz aneurysm clip
Heifitz carotid occluder
Heifitz cerebral aneurysm clamp
Heifitz clamp
Heifitz clip
Heifitz clip applier
Heifitz cup serrated ring forceps
Heifitz ingrown nail procedure
Heifitz microclip
Heifitz operation
Heifitz retractor
Heifitz skull perforator
Heifitz spatula
Heifitz technique
Heifitz tongs
Heifitz traction tongs
Heifitz-Weck clip
height of mandibular ramus
height of palate
Heiming kidney stone forceps
Heimlich chest drainage valve
Heimlich heart valve
Heimlich maneuver
Heimlich operation
Heimlich tube
Heimlich valve
Heimlich Vygon pneumothorax
    valve
Heimlich-Gavriliu gastric tube
Heine rongeur
Heine cyclodialysis
Heine gonioscope
Heine operation
Heine penlight
Heineke colon resection
Heineke operation
Heineke-Mikulicz
    gastroenterostomy
Heineke-Mikulicz herniorrhaphy
Heineke-Mikulicz hypospadias
    operation
Heineke-Mikulicz incision
Heineke-Mikulicz operation
Heineke-Mikulicz pyloroplasty
Heinig procedure
Heinkel sigmoidoscope
Heinkel-Semm dilator instrument
Heinkel-Semm laparoscopy
    instruments
Heinz body

Heinz-Ehrlich body
Hieshima balloon occluder
Heisrath operation
Heiss arterial forceps
Heiss hemostatic forceps
Heiss mastoid retractor
Heiss soft tissue retractor
Heiss vulsellum forceps
Heister diverticulum
Heister fold
Heister mallet
Heister mouth gag
Heister valve
Heitz-Boyer clamp
Heitz-Boyer operation
Helal flap arthroplasty
Helanca prosthesis
Helanca seamless tube prosthesis
Held bundle
Held decussation
Helfrick anal retractor
Helfrick anal ring retractor
Helfrick retractor
helical axis of motion
helical catheter
helical coil
helical coil stent
helical computed tomographic
    angiogram
helical crease
helical crus
helical CT scanner
helical fold
helical PTCA dilatation catheter
helical rim
helical surgery
helical suture technique
helical sutures
helical tube saw
helical-ridged ureteral stent
helical-tip halo catheter
helicine arteries of penis
helicine artery
helicoid endosseous implant
helicoid endosteal implant
Heliodorus bandage
heliotrope eruption
Helistat absorbable collagen
    sponge
helium anesthetic agent
helium insufflation
helium-cadmium diagnostic laser

helium-filled balloon catheter
helium-neon aiming laser
helium-neon laser (He-Ne laser)
helix (pl. helices)
    auricular helix
    caudal helix
    crus of helix
    groove of crus of the helix
    segmental loss of helix
    spine of helix
    tail of helix
helix balloon
helix endocervical curet
helix knot pusher
helix of ear
Helix PTCA dilatation catheter
helix uterine biopsy curet
Heller biopsy forceps
Heller cardiomyotomy
Heller esophagomyotomy
Heller myotomy
Heller myotomy with Dor
    fundoplication
Heller operation
Heller probe
Heller-Belsey operation
Heller-Dor operation
Heller-Nissen operation
Hellstrom pyeloplasty
Helmholtz coil
Helmholtz double-surface coil
Helmholtz keratometer
Helmholtz line
Helmholtz ophthalmoscope
Helmholtz speculum
Helmont speculum
Helmstein balloon
heloma
Helsper laryngectomy button
Helsper tracheostoma vent
Helsper tracheostomy vent tube
Helveston Big Barbie retractor
Helveston Great Big Barbie
    retractor
Helveston scleral marking ruler
Helveston hook
Helweg bundle
Helweg tract
Hemaduct wound drain
Hemaflex PTCA sheath with
    obturator
Hemaflex pure collagen hemostat

Hemaflex sheath
Hemagard collection tube
hemagglutination
hemal arch
hemal node
hemangiectasia
hemangiectasis
hemangiectatic hypertrophy
hemangioendothelioma
  kaposiform
    hemangioendothelioma
  malignant
    hemangioendothelioma
  spindle cell
    hemangioendothelioma
hemangioendothelioma
  tuberosum multiplex
hemangiofibroma
hemangioma (*pl.* hemangiomas,
  hemangiomata)
  adnexal hemangioma
  ameloblastic hemangioma
  arteriovenous hemangioma
  capillary hemangioma
  cavernous hemangioma
  central hemangioma
  cervicofacial hemangioma
  cherry hemangioma
  choroidal hemangioma
  circumscribed choroidal
    hemangioma (CCH)
  congenital hemangioma
  congenital subglottic
    hemangioma
  craniofacial hemangioma
  deep hemangioma
  epithelioid hemangioma
  esophageal hemangioma
  facial hemangioma
  hypertrophic hemangioma
  intramuscular hemangioma
  involuting flat hemangioma
  laryngeal hemangioma
  lumbar hemangioma
  mixed hemangioma
  port-wine hemangioma
  sclerosing hemangioma
  scrotal hemangioma
  senile hemangioma
  spider hemangioma
  strawberry hemangioma
  subcutaneous hemangioma

hemangioma (*continued*)
  subglottic hemangioma
  superficial hemangioma
  synovial hemangioma
  verrucous hemangioma
hemangioma birthmark
hemangioma planum extensum
hemangioma simplex
hemangioma-thrombocytopenia
  syndrome
hemangiomatosis
  Osler hemangiomatosis
  Parkes-Weber
    hemangiomatosis
  thrombocytopenic
    hemangiomatosis
hemangiomatous tissue
hemangiopericytoma
  benign hemangiopericytoma
  borderline malignant
    hemangiopericytoma
  congenital
    hemangiopericytoma
  malignant
    hemangiopericytoma
hemangiosarcoma
hemapheresis
Hemaquet catheter introducer
Hemaquet introducer
Hemaquet PTCA sheath with
  obturator
Hemaquet sheath
Hemaquet sheath introducer
Hemarrest patch
hemarthrosis
Hemashield collagen-enhanced
  graft
Hemashield vascular graft
hematapostema
hematobilia evacuation
hematocele
  parametric hematocele
  retrouterine hematocele
hematocephalus
hematogenic metastasis
hematogenic shock
hematogenous contamination
hematogenous metastasis
hematogenous spread of cancer
hematoid carcinoma
hematologic complication
hematologic disorder

hematoma
  acute subdural hematoma
  aneurysmal hematoma
  aortic intramural hematoma
  axillary hematoma
  basal ganglia hematoma
  bladder flap hematoma
  bowel wall hematoma
  cerebellar hematoma
  chronic subdural hematoma
  communicating hematoma
  corpus luteum hematoma
  dissecting intramural hematoma
  duodenal hematoma
  epidural hematoma
  epiglottic hematoma
  evacuation of subdural
    hematoma
  expanding hematoma
  expanding retroperitoneal
    hematoma
  extradural hematoma
  face-lift hematoma
  fibrosed hematoma
  follicular hematoma
  interhemispheric subdural
    hematoma
  interstitial loculated hematoma
  intracerebral hematoma
  intracranial hematoma
  intrahepatic hematoma
  intramural hematoma
  intraparenchymal hematoma
  isodense subdural hematoma
  mesenteric hematoma
  nasopharyngeal hematoma
  orbital hematoma
  organized hematoma
  para-aortic hematoma
  parenchymal hematoma
  perianal hematoma
  periaortic mediastinal
    hematoma
  pericardial hematoma
  peridiaphragmatic hematoma
  perigraft hematoma
  perinephric hematoma
  periorbital hematoma
  perirenal hematoma
  postoperative hematoma
  puerperal hematoma
  pulsatile hematoma

hematoma (*continued*)
  rectal sheath hematoma
  rectus sheath hematoma
  renal hematoma
  retrobulbar hematoma
  retroperitoneal hematoma
  retropharyngeal hematoma
  retroplacental hematoma
  retrouterine hematoma
  sciatic nerve palsy hematoma
  septal hematoma
  solid visceral hematoma
  spectacle hematoma
  spinal hematoma
  subcapsular renal hematoma
  subchorionic hematoma
  subcutaneous hematoma
  subdural hematoma
  subfascial hematoma
  subgaleal hematoma
  subgluteal hematoma
  sublingual hematoma
  submembranous placental
    hematoma
  submental hematoma
  subperiosteal hematoma
  subungual hematoma
  sylvian hematoma
  traumatic intracranial
    hematoma
  umbilical cord hematoma
  wound hematoma
  wrap hematoma
hematoma aspiration
hematoma auris
hematoma drainage
hematoma evacuation
hematoma form
hematopoiesis
hematopoietic gland
hematopoietic metastasis
hematopoietic tissue
hematorrhea
Hemex prosthetic valve
hemiacidrin irrigation
hemiacrosomia
hemiageusia
hemianesthesia
hemiarthroplasty
  Bateman hemiarthroplasty
  DePuy Porocoat
    hemiarthroplasty

hemiarthroplasty (*continued*)
  Hastings bipolar
    hemiarthroplasty
  I-beam hip hemiarthroplasty
  large humeral head
    hemiarthroplasty
  McKeever-MacIntosh
    hemiarthroplasty
  Neer hemiarthroplasty
  prosthetic hemiarthroplasty
  Smith-Petersen
    hemiarthroplasty
hemiatrophy
hemiazygos vein
hemiblock
hemibody irradiation
hemibody radiation therapy
hemic calculus
hemic murmur
hemic systole
hemicircular incision
hemiclavicular line
hemicolectomy
  Decollement hemicolectomy
  extended right
    hemicolectomy
  hand-assisted laparoscopic
    hemicolectomy
  laparoscopic left
    hemicolectomy
  laparoscopic-assisted
    hemicolectomy
  left hemicolectomy
  right hemicolectomy
  standard right hemicolectomy
hemicondylar fracture
hemicorporectomy
hemicorticectomy
hemicrania
hemicraniectomy
hemicraniosis
hemicraniotomy
hemicylindrical bone graft
hemicylindrical graft
hemicystectomy
hemidecortication
hemidiaphragm
hemidiaphragm rupture
hemidystrophy
hemiectromelia
hemielliptica
hemifacial atrophy

hemifacial hypertrophy
hemifacial microsomia (HFM, HM)
hemifacial microsomia anomaly
hemifacial spasm
hemi-Fontan operation
hemi-Fontan procedure
hemifundoplication
  laparoscopic posterior
    hemifundoplication
hemigastrectomy
hemigigantism
hemiglossal
hemiglossectomy
hemignathia
hemihepatectomy
hemihepatic vascular occlusion
hemihydranencephaly
hemihyperplasia
hemihypertrophy
hemihypoplasia
hemi-implant
  Swanson hemi-implant
hemi-interpositional implant
hemi-Koch procedure
hemilaminectomy
  complete lateral
    hemilaminectomy
  lumbar hemilaminectomy
  partial hemilaminectomy
  Scoville hemilaminectomy
  unilateral hemilaminectomy
hemilaminectomy blade
hemilaminectomy prong
hemilaminectomy retractor
hemilaryngectomy
hemi-LeFort fracture (I, II, etc.)
hemilingual atrophy
hemiliver
hemimacroglossia
hemimandible reconstruction
hemimandibular hyperplasia
hemimandibulectomy
hemimastectomy
hemimaxillectomy
hemimelia
hemimyelocele
hemimyelomeningocele
heminasal defect
heminephrectomy
heminephroureterectomy
hemiorchiectomy
hemipagus

hemipancreatectomy
hemipancreaticosplenectomy
hemiparalysis
hemiparesis
hemipelvectomy
  complete internal
    hemipelvectomy
  external hemipelvectomy
  formal hemipelvectomy
  internal hemipelvectomy
  partial internal hemipelvectomy
hemipelvis
hemiphalangectomy
hemiplegia
hemiplegic rigidity
hemipulp flap
hemipylorectomy
hemiresection interposition
  arthroplasty
hemiscrotectomy
hemisect
hemisection
hemiseptum of interalveolar
  bone
hemisphere
  cerebellar hemisphere
  cerebral hemisphere
  dominant hemisphere
  lateral hemispheres
hemisphere eye implant
hemisphere of brain
hemispherectomy
hemispheric disconnection
  syndrome
hemispheric functions
hemispherical pusher
hemisphincter
hemistrumectomy
hemithoracic duct
hemithoracicus
hemithorax
hemithyroidectomy
hemitongue flap
hemitransfixion incision
hemivertebra
hemivertebral excision
hemivulvectomy
hemi-Koch procedure
Hemmer connection sleeve
Hemmer connector flusher
Hemobahn endovascular
  prosthesis

Hemo-Cath catheter
Hemoccult negative
Hemoccult positive
Hemoclear dialyzer
hemoclip (*see also* clip)
  Samuels-Weck Hemoclip
  Weck Hemoclip
hemoclip applier
hemoclip cartridge base
hemoclip clamp
hemoclip-applying forceps
hemoculture negative
hemodialysis
hemodialysis catheter
hemodialysis treatment
hemodialysis tube
hemodialyzer
  coil hemodialyzer
  Dow hollow-fiber hemodialyzer
  Gambro hemodialyzer
  hollow-fiber hemodialyzer
  parallel plate hemodialyzer
  Redy hemodialyzer
hemodiaphragm
hemodynamic collapse
hemodynamic instability
hemodynamic maneuver
hemodynamic monitoring
hemodynamic support
hemodynamics
hemoendothelial placenta
hemofiltration
  continuous arteriovenous
    hemofiltration (CAVH)
  continuous venovenous
    hemofiltration
hemofiltration therapy
Hemoject injection catheter
Hemoject needle
hemologic parameters
Hem-o-lok clip
Hem-o-lok polymer ligating clip
hemolymph glands
hemolysis
hemolytic disease
hemolytic splenomegaly
hemolytic uremic syndrome
hemolyzed serum
Hemopad
hemoperfusion
Hemophan membrane
hemophilic arthropathy

hemopneumothorax
hemoptysis
Hemopump
hemorrhage
  8-ball hemorrhage
  abdominal hemorrhage
  accidental hemorrhage
  active hemorrhage
  adrenal hemorrhage
  alveolar hemorrhage
  aneurysmal hemorrhage
  antepartum hemorrhage
  arachnoid hemorrhage
  arterial hemorrhage
  bilateral adrenal hemorrhage
  bladder hemorrhage
  blot hemorrhage
  blot-and-dot hemorrhage
  brainstem hemorrhage
  brisk hemorrhage
  capillary hemorrhage
  capsuloganglionic
    hemorrhage
  catheter-induced pulmonary
    artery hemorrhage
  cerebellar hemorrhage
  cerebral hemorrhage
  choroidal hemorrhage
  colonic diverticular
    hemorrhage
  colorectal hemorrhage
  concealed hemorrhage
  conjunctival hemorrhage
  diffuse pulmonary alveolar
    hemorrhage
  disk drusen hemorrhage
  diverticular hemorrhage
  dot hemorrhage
  dot-and-blot hemorrhage
  Duret hemorrhages
  epidural hemorrhage
  expulsive hemorrhage
  exsanguinating hemorrhage
  external hemorrhage
  extradural hemorrhage
  extraluminal hemorrhage
  fetal hemorrhage
  fetal-maternal hemorrhage
  fetomaternal hemorrhage
  fibrinolytic hemorrhage
  flame hemorrhage
  flame-shaped hemorrhage

hemorrhage (*continued*)
  focal hemorrhage
  frank hemorrhage
  gastric hemorrhage
  germinal matrix hemorrhage
  gingival hemorrhage
  gravitating hemorrhage
  hepatic hemorrhage
  Icelandic form of intracranial
    hemorrhage
  intermediate hemorrhage
  internal hemorrhage
  intestinal hemorrhage
  intra-abdominal arterial
    hemorrhage
  intra-abdominal hemorrhage
  intra-alveolar hemorrhage
  intracapsular hemorrhage
  intracerebral hemorrhage
  intracranial hemorrhage
  intraluminal hemorrhage
  intramedullary hemorrhage
  intramural intestinal
    hemorrhage
  intraocular hemorrhage
  intraoperative hemorrhage
  intraparenchymal hemorrhage
  intrapartum hemorrhage
  intraperitoneal hemorrhage
  intraplaque hemorrhage
  intraventricular hemorrhage
  laryngeal hemorrhage
  lobar hemorrhage
  lower gastrointestinal
    hemorrhage
  massive hemorrhage
  mediastinal hemorrhage
  meningeal hemorrhage
  mesencephalic hemorrhage
  nasal hemorrhage
  nasopharyngeal hemorrhage
  neonatal intracranial
    hemorrhage
  neonatal intraventricular
    hemorrhage
  nonaneurysmal
    perimesencephalic
    subarachnoid hemorrhage
  ochre hemorrhage
  oropharyngeal hemorrhage
  pancreatitis-related
    hemorrhage

hemorrhage (*continued*)

parenchymatous intracerebral hemorrhage
perianeurysmal hemorrhage
perinephric space hemorrhage
periventricular-intraventricular hemorrhage
petechial hemorrhage
placental hemorrhage
pontine hemorrhage
postextraction hemorrhage
postgastrectomy hemorrhage
postoperative hemorrhage
postpartum hemorrhage
postpolypectomy hemorrhage
posttraumatic hemorrhage
posttreatment hemorrhage
preplacental hemorrhage
preretinal hemorrhage
primary hemorrhage
profuse hemorrhage
pulmonary hemorrhage
punctate hemorrhage
recurrent hemorrhage
recurring hemorrhage
refractory variceal hemorrhage
renal cyst hemorrhage
reperfusion-induced hemorrhage
retinal hemorrhage
retinopathy hemorrhage
retrobulbar hemorrhage
retroperitoneal hemorrhage
retropharyngeal hemorrhage
round hemorrhage
salmon-patch hemorrhage
scleral hemorrhage
secondary hemorrhage
signal hemorrhage
slit hemorrhage
splinter hemorrhage
spontaneous renal hemorrhage
sternocleidomastoid hemorrhage
stigmata of recent hemorrhage (SRH)
stress ulcer hemorrhage
subarachnoid hemorrhage
subcapsular hemorrhage

hemorrhage (*continued*)

subchorial hemorrhage
subchorionic hemorrhage
subconjunctival hemorrhage
subcortical hemorrhage
subdural hemorrhage
subependymal hemorrhage
subepithelial hemorrhage
subgaleal hemorrhage
subhyaloid hemorrhage
subintimal hemorrhage
submucosal gastric hemorrhage
submucosal hemorrhage
subperiosteal hemorrhage
subretinal hemorrhage
suprachoroidal hemorrhage
syringomyelic hemorrhage
thalamic-subthalamic hemorrhage
torrential hemorrhage
transplacental hemorrhage
traumatic hemorrhage
unavoidable hemorrhage
upper GI hemorrhage
uterine hemorrhage
variceal hemorrhage
venous hemorrhage
vitreal hemorrhage
vitreous breakthrough hemorrhage
vitreous hemorrhage
white-centered hemorrhage
yellow-ochre hemorrhage
hemorrhage control
hemorrhage focus
hemorrhage per rhexis
hemorrhagic
hemorrhagic angiomyolipoma
hemorrhagic ascites
hemorrhagic bulla
hemorrhagic complication
hemorrhagic condition
hemorrhagic cyst
hemorrhagic endovasculitis
hemorrhagic familial angiomatosis
hemorrhagic gangrene
hemorrhagic infarction
hemorrhagic inflammation
hemorrhagic laryngitis
hemorrhagic lesion

hemorrhagic metastasis
hemorrhagic pyoderma
  gangrenosum
hemorrhagic radiation injury
hemorrhagic rash
hemorrhagic shock
hemorrhagic stroke
hemorrhagic telangiectasia
hemorrhagic transformation
hemorrhea
hemorrhoid
  1st-degree hemorrhoid
  2nd-degree hemorrhoid
  3rd-degree hemorrhoid
  combined hemorrhoids
  cutaneous hemorrhoid
  external hemorrhoid
  injection of hemorrhoid
  internal hemorrhoid
  ligation of hemorrhoid
  lingual hemorrhoid
  Lord dilation of hemorrhoid
  mixed hemorrhoids
  mucocutaneous hemorrhoid
  necrotic hemorrhoid
  prolapsed hemorrhoid
  prolapsing internal hemorrhoid
  rectal hemorrhoid
  strangulated hemorrhoid
  thrombosed hemorrhoid
  thrombosed internal and
    external hemorrhoid
hemorrhoid cryotherapy
hemorrhoid forceps
hemorrhoid infrared
  photocoagulation
hemorrhoid laser excision
hemorrhoid sclerotherapy
hemorrhoid vaporization
hemorrhoidal arteries
hemorrhoidal banding
hemorrhoidal clamp
hemorrhoidal forceps
hemorrhoidal ligator
hemorrhoidal needle
hemorrhoidal nerves
hemorrhoidal plexus
hemorrhoidal prolapse
hemorrhoidal skin tags
hemorrhoidal tags
hemorrhoidal veins
hemorrhoidal vessels

hemorrhoidectomy
  2-quadrant
    hemorrhoidectomy
  3-quadrant
    hemorrhoidectomy
  4-quadrant
    hemorrhoidectomy
  ambulatory
    hemorrhoidectomy
  anoderm-preserving
    hemorrhoidectomy
  Buie hemorrhoidectomy
  closed hemorrhoidectomy
  diathermy hemorrhoidectomy
  Doppler-guided artery ligation
    hemorrhoidectomy
  external hemorrhoidectomy
  Ferguson hemorrhoidectomy
  Harmonic hemorrhoidectomy
  internal hemorrhoidectomy
  laser hemorrhoidectomy
  ligation hemorrhoidectomy
  limited hemorrhoidectomy
  Longo hemorrhoidectomy
  Lord hemorrhoidectomy
  Milligan-Morgan
    hemorrhoidectomy
  modified Whitehead
    hemorrhoidectomy
  Morinaga hemorrhoidectomy
  nonmucosal
    hemorrhoidectomy
  open hemorrhoidectomy
  Parks hemorrhoidectomy
  radical hemorrhoidectomy
  rubber band hemorrhoidectomy
  scissors-excision
    hemorrhoidectomy
  semiopen hemorrhoidectomy
  St. Mark hemorrhoidectomy
  stapled hemorrhoidectomy
hemorrhoidolysis
hemosialemesis
hemosiderin
hemospermia
hemostasis
  chemical hemostasis
  complete hemostasis
  electrofulguration hemostasis
  endoscopic hemostasis
  immaculate hemostasis
  meticulous hemostasis

hemostasis (*continued*)
    proactive hemostasis
    secured hemostasis
hemostasis accomplished
hemostasis attained
hemostasis clip
hemostasis clip-applying forceps
hemostasis forceps
hemostasis scalp clip
hemostasis secured
hemostasis silver clip
hemostat
    Actifoam active hemostat
    Actifoam hemostat
    Adair hemostat
    Adson hemostat
    Allis hemostat
    angulated-vein hemostat
    Avitene Ultrafoam collagen
        hemostat
    Avtifoam active hemostat
    Bardex hemostat
    Berne hemostat
    blackened hemostat
    Block gastric hemostat
    Blohmka tonsil hemostat
    Blohmka tonsillar hemostat
    Blotts hemostat
    blunt-nose hemostat
    Boettcher hemostat
    Bolder hemostat
    Bovie coagulating-current
        hemostat
    Bovie cutting-current
        hemostat
    broadbill hemostat
    Brown-Buerger hemostat
    bulldog hemostat
    Carmalt hemostat
    Charnley-Barnes hemostat
    Coakley tonsil hemostat
    Collastat microfibrillar
        collagen hemostat
    Collier-DeBakey hemostat
    Colver tonsil hemostat
    Corwin tonsillar hemostat
    Crafoord hemostat
    Crile gall duct hemostat
    curved hemostat
    curved Kelly hemostat
    curved mosquito hemostat
    Dandy scalp hemostat

hemostat (*continued*)
    Davis tonsillar hemostat
    Dean tonsil hemostat
    Deaver hemostat
    Dunhill hemostat
    Endo-Avitene microfibrillar
        collagen hemostat
    fine-pointed hemostat
    fine-tipped mosquito
        hemostat
    Gant hemostat
    Gomco hemostat
    Green-Armytage cesarean
        section hemostat
    Guist enucleation hemostat
    Gutglass cervix hemostat
    Hagie hemostat
    Halsted hemostat
    Halsted mosquito hemostat
    Hartmann hemostat
    Harvey Stone hemostat
    Haslinger tonsil hemostat
    Hemaflex pure collagen
        hemostat
    Hemopad sterile absorbably
        collagen hemostat
    hemostatic eraser
    Hemotene absorbable
        collagen hemostat
    Hopkins hemostat
    Hugh Young hemostat
    Instat collagen absorbable
        hemostat
    Instat microfibrillar collagen
        hemostat
    Jackson tracheal hemostat
    Judson-Bruce hemostat
    Kelly hemostat
    Kocher hemostat
    Kolodny scalp hemostat
    Lahey hemostat
    Lewin tonsil hemostat
    Lewis hemostat
    Lothrop hemostat
    Lowsley hemostat
    Maier hemostat
    Maingot hemostat
    Massachusetts hemostat
    Mathrop hemostat
    Mayfield aneurysm hemostat
    Mayo hemostat
    Mayo-Ochsner hemostat

hemostat (*continued*)
Mayo-Pean hemostat
McWhorter hemostat
McWhorter tonsillar hemostat
Meigs hemostat
Michel clip hemostat
microfibrillar collagen
   hemostat
Mixter hemostat
mosquito hemostat
Nu-Knit absorbable hemostat
Ochsner hemostat
Ormco orthodontic hemostat
orthopedic hemostat
Oxycel hemostat
Peat hemostat
Percy hemostat
Perdue tonsillar hemostat
Providence Hospital hemostat
Raimondi hemostat
Rankin hemostat
Rankin-Crile hemostat
Rankin-Kelly hemostat
Richardson hemostat
Rochester-Carmalt hemostat
Rochester-Ochsner hemostat
Rochester-Pean hemostat
Rumel bronchial hemostat
Sawtell hemostat
Sawtell-Davis hemostat
scalp hemostat
Schnidt tonsillar hemostat
Shallcross tonsillar hemostat
Smedberg hemostat
Snyder hemostat
Spongostan hemostat
straight hemostat
straight mosquito hemostat
Surgicel fibrillator absorbable
   hemostat
Surgicel Nu-Knit absorbable
   hemostat
Thrombogen absorbable
   hemostat
tonsillar hemostat
tracheal hemostat
Weitlaner hemostat
Westphal hemostat
Woodward hemostat
hemostat technique
hemostatic agent
hemostatic bag

hemostatic catheter
hemostatic cervical forceps
hemostatic cervix forceps
hemostatic clamp
hemostatic clip
hemostatic clip applier
hemostatic clip-applying forceps
hemostatic collodion
hemostatic eraser
hemostatic forceps
hemostatic ligatures
hemostatic material
hemostatic neurosurgical
   forceps
hemostatic occlusive leverage
   device
hemostatic plug formation
hemostatic puncture closure
   device
hemostatic sponge
hemostatic staple line
hemostatic suture technique
hemostatic sutures
hemostatic thoracic clamp
hemostatic tissue forceps
hemostatic tonometer
hemostatic tonsillar forceps
hemostatic tonsillar guillotine
hemostatic tonsillectome
hemostatic tracheal forceps
Hemostatix scalpel
Hemostatix scalpel blade
Hemotene absorbable collagen
   hemostat
hemothorax
Hemovac drain
Hemovac suction
Hemovac suction device
Hemovac suction tube
Hemovac treatment unit
Hemovac tube
Hemovac unit
Henahan elevator
Henschke colpostat
hen-cluck stertor
Hendel guided osteotome
Henderson approach
Henderson approximator
Henderson arthrodesis
Henderson chisel
Henderson clamp approximator
Henderson classification

Henderson fracture
Henderson graft
Henderson hip arthrodesis
Henderson lag screw
Henderson onlay bone graft
Henderson operation
Henderson posterolateral
    approach
Henderson posteromedial
    approach
Henderson reamer
Henderson retractor
Henderson self-retaining
    retractor
Henderson skin incision
Henderson technique
Henderson-Haggard inhaler
Hendler unitunnel technique
Hendon venoclysis cannula
Hendren blade
Hendren cardiovascular clamp
Hendren cardiovascular forceps
Hendren ductus clamp
Hendren megaureter clamp
Hendren pediatric forceps
Hendren pediatric retractor blade
Hendren retractor blade
Hendren ureteral clamp
Hendrickson drain
Hendrickson hemostatic bag
Hendrickson lithotrite
Hendrickson stone crusher
Hendrickson suprapubic drain
He-Ne laser (helium-neon laser)
Henke forceps tip
Henke punch forceps
Henke punch forceps tip
Henke space
Henke tonsillar dissector
Henke triangle
Henke-Stille conchotome
Henle ampulla
Henle body
Henle elastic membrane
Henle fenestrated membrane
Henle fiber layer
Henle fissures
Henle glands
Henle ligament
Henle loop
Henle membrane
Henle sphincter

Henle spine
Henley carotid retractor
Henley dilator
Henley retractor blade
Henley subclavian artery clamp
Henley vascular clamp
Hennebert reflex
Henner endaural elevator
Henner endaural retractor
Henning cardiac dilator
Henning cast spreader
Henning dilator
Henning inside-to-outside
    technique
Henning instrument set
Henning mallet
Henning meniscal retractor
Henning plaster spreader
Henning sign
Henny laminectomy rongeur
Henny rongeur
Henrotin retractor
Henrotin speculum
Henrotin uterine vulsellum
    forceps
Henrotin vaginal speculum
Henrotin vulsellum forceps
Henrotin weighted vaginal
    speculum
Henry acromioclavicular
    technique
Henry anterior strap approach
Henry anterolateral approach
Henry approach
Henry bone graft
Henry cilia forceps
Henry extensile approach
Henry femoral herniorrhaphy
Henry hernia
Henry incision
Henry instrument tray
Henry master knot
Henry operation
Henry posterior interosseous
    nerve approach
Henry posterior interosseous
    nerve exposure
Henry radial approach
Henry repair of femoral hernia
Henry resection
Henry Schein excavator
Henry Schein filling instrument

Henry splenectomy
Henry technique
Henry-Geist operation
Henry-Geist spinal fusion
Henschke ovoid
Henschke seed applicator
Henschke-Mauch knee
Henschke-Mauch lower limb
 prosthesis
Hensen body
Hensen duct
Hensen plane
Hensen duct
Henton needle
Henton suture hook
Henton suture needle
Henton tonsillar hook
Henton tonsillar needle
Henton tonsillar suture hook
Henton tonsillar suture needle
HEPA filter
Hepacon cannula
Hepacon catheter
Hepacon shunt
Hepamed-coated Wiktor stent
heparin arterial filter
heparin irrigation
heparin lock
heparin lock introducer
heparin needle
heparin sodium
heparin well
heparinase
heparin-bonded Bott-type tube
heparin-bonded tube
heparin-coated catheter
heparin-coated Palmaz-Schatz
 stent
heparin-coating guidewire
heparin-flushing needle
heparinization procedure
heparinized saline
heparinized solution infusion
HepatAssist bioartificial liver
hepatectomize
hepatectomy
  cadaveric donor hepatectomy
  central hepatectomy
  concomitant hepatectomy
  Dono hepatectomy
  donor hepatectomy
  ex situ hepatectomy

hepatectomy (*continued*)
  ex situ-in situ hepatectomy
  extended left hepatectomy
  extended right hepatectomy
  laparoscopic hepatectomy
  laparoscopic-assisted
   hepatectomy (LAH)
  LCVP-aided hepatectomy
  LCVP-assisted hepatectomy
  left hepatectomy
  limited hepatectomy
  living donor partial
   hepatectomy
  local hepatectomy
  partial hepatectomy
  recipient hepatectomy
  regional hepatectomy
  right lobe hepatectomy
  segmental hepatectomy
  simultaneous segmental
   hepatectomy
  standardized hepatectomy
  subsegmental hepatectomy
  subtotal hepatectomy
  total left hepatectomy
  triple lobe hepatectomy
  wedge hepatectomy
hepatic abscess
hepatic adenoma
hepatic allograft
hepatic architecture
hepatic arterial infusion (HAI)
hepatic arterial therapy
hepatic artery
hepatic artery embolization (HAE)
hepatic artery infusion pump
hepatic artery ligation
hepatic artery-portal vein fistula
hepatic bed
hepatic blood flow
hepatic calculus
hepatic cecum
hepatic cell carcinoma
hepatic circulation
hepatic colorectal metastasis
hepatic complication
hepatic decompensation
hepatic distention
hepatic diverticulum
hepatic duct
hepatic duct calculus
hepatic dullness

hepatic dysfunction
hepatic encephalopathy
hepatic failure
hepatic fistula
hepatic flexure
hepatic fossa
hepatic hemorrhage
hepatic hilum
hepatic injury
hepatic ligament
hepatic lobe
hepatic lobectomy
hepatic lobule
hepatic margin
hepatic mass lesion
hepatic necrosis
hepatic obstruction
hepatic outflow block
hepatic outflow tract
hepatic parasitic cyst
hepatic perfusion
hepatic plexus
hepatic radicles
hepatic resection
hepatic resectional surgery
hepatic rupture
hepatic segments
hepatic transplant
hepatic transplantation
hepatic triad
hepatic trinity
hepatic tumor
hepatic vascular exclusion (HVE)
hepatic vascular isolation
    technique
hepatic vein catheterization
hepatic veins
hepatic venous outflow
    obstruction
hepatic venous pressure gradient
hepatic venous web disease
hepatic web
hepatic web dilation
hepaticocholangiocholecysto-
    enterostomy
hepaticocholangiogastrostomy
hepaticocholangiojejunostomy
hepaticocholedochostomy
hepaticocutaneous jejunostomy
hepaticocystoduodenostomy
hepaticocystojejunostomy
hepaticodochotomy

hepaticoduodenostomy
hepaticoenterostomy
hepaticogastrostomy
hepaticojejunostomy
    Hepp-Couinaud
        hepaticojejunostomy
    mucosa-to-mucosa Roux-en-Y
        hepaticojejunostomy
    Roux-en-Y
        hepaticojejunostomy
    wide mucosa-to-mucosa Roux-
        en-Y hepaticojejunostomy
hepaticolenticular degeneration
hepaticolithectomy
hepaticolithotomy
hepaticolithotripsy
hepaticoportoenterostomy
hepaticopulmonary
hepaticostomy
hepaticotomy
hepatic-renal angle
hepatitis B immunoglobulin
    (HBIG)
hepatitis virus
hepatization
hepatobiliary imaging
hepatobiliary scan
hepatobiliary scintigraphy
hepatobiliary surgery
hepatocele
hepatocellular adenoma
hepatocellular cancer
hepatocellular carcinoma (HCC)
hepatocellular synthetic
    dysfunction
hepatocholangiocystoduodenos-
    tomy
hepatocholangioduodenostomy
hepatocholangioenterostomy
hepatocholangiogastrostomy
hepatocholangiostomy
hepatocholedochostomy
hepatocirrhosis
hepatocolic ligament
hepatocystic duct
hepatocystocolic ligament
hepatocyte transplantation
hepatodiaphragmatic adhesions
hepatoduodenal ligament
hepatoduodenal reflection
hepatoduodenostomy
hepatoenterostomy

hepatofugal porto-systemic
venous shunt
hepatogastric ligament
hepatogastroduodenal ligament
hepatogastrostomy
hepatogenic
hepatojejunal anastomosis
hepatojejunostomy
complex hepatojejunostomy
high hepatojejunostomy
hilar hepatojejunostomy
intracystic hepatojejunostomy
laparoscopic
hepatojejunostomy
palliative hepatojejunostomy
pediatric hepatojejunostomy
peripheral hepatojejunostomy
Roux-en-Y hepatojejunostomy
side-to-side hepatojejunostomy
simple hepatojejunostomy
hepatojugular reflux
hepatolenticular disease
hepatolithectomy
hepatolithotomy
hepatoma
hepatomegalia
hepatomegaly
hepatopancreatic ampulla
hepatopancreatic fold
hepatopexy
hepatophrenic ligament
hepatopleural fistula
hepatoportal biliary fistula
hepatoportoenterostomy
hepatoptosis
hepatorenal angle
hepatorenal bypass
hepatorenal disease
hepatorenal failure
hepatorenal ligament
hepatorenal pouch
hepatorenal syndrome
hepatorrhaphy
hepatosplenomegaly
hepatostomy
hepatotomy
hepatotoxicity
hepatoumbilical ligament
Hepp-Couinaud biliary tract
procedure
Hepp-Couinaud
hepaticojejunostomy

heptadactyly
herald patch
Herbert Adams coarctation
clamp
Herbert alphanumeric
classification system for
scaphoid fractures (types
A1, A2, B1-4, C, D1, D2)
Herbert bone screw
Herbert knee prosthesis
Herbert knife
Herbert operation
Herbert prosthesis
Herbert scaphoid bone screw
Herbert scaphoid screw
Herbert sclerotomy knife
Herbert screw
Herbert screw fixator
Herbert-Whipple bone screw
Herbert-Whipple screw
Hercules plaster shears
Hercules power injector
Hercules scissors
Herculon sutures
Herczel dissector
Herczel periosteal elevator
Herczel raspatory
Herczel raspatory elevator
Herczel rib elevator
Herczel rib raspatory
hereditary ataxia
hereditary bone dysplasia
hereditary breast cancer
hereditary cancer syndrome
hereditary deforming
chondrodysplasia
hereditary disease
hereditary disorder
hereditary factors
hereditary flat adenoma
syndrome
hereditary hemorrhagic
angioma
hereditary hemorrhagic
telangiectasia
hereditary neuropathic
amyloidosis
hereditary nonpolyposis colon
cancer (HNPCC)
hereditary nonpolyposis colon
carcinoma (HNPCC)
hereditary predisposition

hereditary tendency
Herff clamp
Herff clip
Herff membrane-puncturing
   forceps
Herget biopsy forceps
Hering canal
Hering duct
Hering-Breuer reflex
heritable connective tissue
   disease
herloon hernia balloon trocar
Hermann bone-holding forceps
Herman-Taylor gastroscope
hermaphrodite
hermaphroditism
   bilateral hermaphroditism
   false hermaphroditism
   spurious hermaphroditism
   synchronous
      hermaphroditism
   transverse hermaphroditism
   unilateral hermaphroditism
hermetically sealed pacemaker
Hermodsson fracture
Hermodsson internal rotation
   technique
Hernandez-Ros bone staple
Herndon procedure
Herndon-Heyman operation for
   talipes valgus
Herndon-Heyman procedure
hernia (*pl.* hernias, herniae)
   abdominal hernia
   abdominal incisional hernia
   abdominal wall hernia
   acquired hernia
   adiposa hernia
   amniotic hernia
   anterior iliac obturator hernia
   antevesical hernia
   aperture of inguinal hernia
   axial hiatal hernia
   Barth hernia
   Beclard hernia
   Bergmann hernia
   bilateral inguinal hernia (BIH)
   bilocular femoral hernia
   Birkett hernia
   bladder hernia
   Bochdalek hernia
   broad ligament hernia

hernia (*continued*)
   cecal hernia
   cerebral hernia
   Cheatle-Henry hernia
   Cloquet hernia
   combined hiatal hernia
   complete hernia
   concealed hernia
   concentric hernia
   congenital diaphragmatic
      hernia (CDH)
   congenital hernia
   Cooper hernia
   crural hernia
   cystic hernia
   diaphragmatic hernia
   direct hernia
   direct inguinal hernia
   diverticular hernia
   double-loop hernia
   dry hernia
   duodenal hernia
   duodenojejunal hernia
   easily reducible hernia
   encysted hernia
   epigastric hernia
   esophageal hernia
   external hernia
   extrasaccular hernia
   fascial hernia
   fat hernia
   fatty hernia
   femoral hernia
   flank incisional hernia
   foraminal hernia
   funicular hernia
   funicular inguinal hernia
   gangrenous hernia
   gastric hernia
   gastroesophageal hernia
   Gibbon hernia
   Gironcoli hernia
   gluteal hernia
   Goyrand hernia
   groin hernia
   Gruber hernia
   Grynfelt hernia
   Henry hernia
   Henry repair of femoral
      hernia
   Hesselbach hernia
   Hey hernia

hernia (*continued*)
 hiatal hernia
 hiatus hernia
 high operation for femoral hernia
 Hill repair of hiatal hernia
 Holthouse hernia
 iliacosubfascial hernia
 in recto hernia
 incarcerated hernia
 incisional hernia
 incomplete hernia
 indirect hernia
 indirect inguinal hernia
 infantile hernia
 inguinal hernia
 inguinocrural hernia
 inguinofemoral hernia
 inguinolabial hernia
 inguinoproperitoneal hernia
 inguinoscrotal hernia
 inguinosuperficial hernia
 interior mesogastric hernia
 intermuscular hernia
 internal hernia
 interparietal hernia
 intersigmoid hernia
 interstitial hernia
 intestinal hernia
 intraepiploic hernia
 intrailiac hernia
 intrapelvic hernia
 iris hernia
 irreducible hernia
 ischiatic hernia
 ischiorectal hernia
 Jodd repair of postoperative ventral hernia
 Kunster hernia
 Kronlein hernia
 labial hernia
 Larrey hernia
 Laugier hernia
 left inguinal hernia (LIH)
 Lesgaft hernia
 lesser sac hernia
 levator hernia
 Littre hernia
 Littre-Richter hernia
 lower operation for femoral hernia

hernia (*continued*)
 lower quadrant abdominal incisional hernia
 lumbar hernia
 Madden repair of incisional hernia
 Malgaigne hernia
 Maydl hernia
 meningeal hernia
 mesenteric hernia
 mesocolic hernia
 midline incisional hernia
 Morgagni hernia
 Morgagni-Larrey type hernia
 mucosal hernia
 multiorgan hernia
 muscle hernia
 nontraumatic hernia
 oblique hernia
 oblique inguinal hernia
 obturator hernia
 omental hernia
 orbital hernia
 ovarian hernia
 pannicular hernia
 pantaloon hernia
 pantaloon inguinal hernia
 par glissement hernia
 paraduodenal hernia
 paraesophageal diaphragmatic hernia
 paraesophageal hernia
 paraesophageal hiatal hernia
 parahiatal hernia
 paraileostomal hernia
 paraperitoneal hernia
 parapubic hernia
 parasaccular hernia
 parastomal hernia
 paraumbilical hernia
 parietal hernia
 parumbilical hernia
 pectineal crural hernia
 pectineal hernia
 pediatric hernia
 pericolostomy hernia
 perineal hernia
 peritoneal hernia
 peritoneopericardial diaphragmatic hernia
 peritoneopericardial hernia
 perivesical hernia

hernia (*continued*)
Petit hernia
pleuroperitoneal hernia
port site hernia
posterior labial hernia
posterior vaginal hernia
primary indirect inguinal
    hernia
properitoneal hernia
properitoneal inguinal hernia
pudendal hernia
pulsion hernia
radical operation for hernia
rectal hernia
recurrent hernia
recurrent incisional hernia
reducible hernia
reduction of hernia
retrocecal hernia
retrocolic hernia
retrograde hernia
retroperitoneal hernia
retropubic hernia
retrosternal hernia
retrovaginal hernia
Richter hernia
Rieux hernia
right inguinal hernia (RIH)
Rokitansky hernia
rolling hernia
rolling hiatal hernia
saddlebag hernia
sciatic hernia
scrotal hernia
secondary hernia
Serafini hernia
short esophagus type hiatal
    hernia
sliding abdominal hernia
sliding esophageal hiatal hernia
sliding hernia
sliding hiatal hernia
sliding inguinal hernia
sliding-type hiatal hernia
slip hernia
slipped hernia
spigelian hernia
Spigelius hernia
spontaneous lateral ventricle
    hernia
spontaneous ventrolateral
    hernia

hernia (*continued*)
stoma hernia
strangulated hernia
strangulated incisional hernia
strangulated inguinal hernia
strangulated paraesophageal
    hernia
subdiaphragmatic hernia
subpubic hernia
superior lumbar hernia
suprapubic hernia
supravesical hernia
synovial hernia
thyroidal hernia
tonsillar hernia
TRAM flap hernia
transient hiatal hernia
transmesenteric hernia
traumatic diaphragmatic hernia
Treitz hernia
trocar site hernia
true hernia
tunicary hernia
umbilical hernia
unilateral hernia
urinary bladder hernia
uterine hernia
vaginal hernia
vaginolabial hernia
Velpeau hernia
ventral hernia
ventrolateral hernia
vesicle hernia
vitreous hernia
voluminous hernia
von Bergmann hernia
wound hernia
Wutzer hernia
hernia adiposa
hernia defect
hernia en bissac
hernia en glissade
hernia foraminis ovalis
hernia in recto
hernia incarceration
hernia incision
hernia metastasis
hernia par glissement
hernia paralysis
hernia pouch
hernia repair
hernia retractor

hernia rupture
hernia sac
hernia stapler
hernial aneurysm
hernial canal
hernial protrusion
hernial sac
Herniamesh surgical mesh
Herniamesh surgical plug
herniated disk
herniated fat pad
herniated fundoplication
herniated nucleus pulposus
herniation
  brain herniation
  cardiac herniation
  caudal transtentorial
    herniation
  central herniation
  cerebral herniation
  cervical midline disk
    herniation
  cingulate herniation
  cisternal herniation
  diaphragmatic herniation
  disk herniation
  fat herniation
  foraminal herniation
  free fragment herniation
  intercervical disk herniation
  intervertebral disk herniation
  intestinal herniation
  lumbar disk herniation
  midline disk herniation
  nucleus pulposus herniation
  posterolateral herniation
  rostral transtentorial
    herniation
  sphenoidal herniation
  subfalcial herniation
  synovial herniation
  tentorial herniation
  thoracic disk herniation
  tonsillar herniation
  transtentorial herniation
  traumatic cervical disk
    herniation
  uncal herniation
  ureteroneocystostomy
    herniation
  visceral herniation
  vitreous herniation

herniation of brain
herniation of disk
herniation of muscle
herniation of nucleus pulposus
herniation pit
hernioappendectomy
hernioenterotomy
hernioid
herniolaparotomy
herniology
hernioplasty
  abdominal midline incisional
    hernioplasty
  classical Judd-Mayo overlap
    midline incisional
    hernioplasty
  GPRVS hernioplasty
  incisional hernioplasty
  ischiatic hernioplasty
  Judd-Mayo overlap midline
    incisional hernioplasty
  laparoscopic hernioplasty
  Lictenstein tension-free
    hernioplasty
  massive incisional hernioplasty
  McVay hernioplasty
  mesh plug hernioplasty
  midline incisional hernioplasty
  modified Shouldice
    hernioplasty
  modified TAPP hernioplasty
  overlap midline incisional
    hernioplasty
  prosthetic incisional
    hernioplasty
  Shouldice hernioplasty
  tension-free hernioplasty
  transabdominal preperitoneal
    hernioplasty
herniopuncture
herniorrhaphy
  Adden herniorrhaphy
  Allison herniorrhaphy
  Andrews inguinal
    herniorrhaphy
  Anson-McVay femoral
    herniorrhaphy
  Anson-McVay herniorrhaphy
  Anson-McVay inguinal
    herniorrhaphy
  anterior inguinal
    herniorrhaphy

herniorrhaphy (*continued*)
  Babcock inguinal
    herniorrhaphy
  Banks-Michel herniorrhaphy
  Bassini herniorrhaphy
  Bassini inguinal
    herniorrhaphy
  Belsey herniorrhaphy
  Berkowitz-Bellis
    herniorrhaphy
  Bloodgood inguinal
    herniorrhaphy
  Brenner inguinal
    herniorrhaphy
  Cattell herniorrhaphy
  Czerny herniorrhaphy
  diaphragmatic herniorrhaphy
  elective herniorrhaphy
  emergent herniorrhaphy
  epigastric herniorrhaphy
  extraperitoneal laparoscopic
    herniorrhaphy
  femoral herniorrhaphy
  femoral-inguinal
    herniorrhaphy
  Ferguson inguinal
    herniorrhaphy
  Gallie herniorrhaphy
  Halsted inguinal
    herniorrhaphy
  Halsted-Bassini herniorrhaphy
  Heaton inguinal
    herniorrhaphy
  Heineke-Mikulicz
    herniorrhaphy
  Henry femoral herniorrhaphy
  Hill hiatus herniorrhaphy
  Hill-type hiatus herniorrhaphy
  imbrication herniorrhaphy
  inguinal herniorrhaphy
  inlay inguinal herniorrhaphy
  laparoscopic total
    extraperitoneal
    herniorrhaphy
  LaRoque herniorrhaphy
  Lichtenstein herniorrhaphy
  Lotheissen herniorrhaphy
  Macewen herniorrhaphy
  Madden herniorrhaphy
  Madden incisional
    herniorrhaphy
  Mayo herniorrhaphy

herniorrhaphy (*continued*)
  McVay herniorrhaphy
  mesh herniorrhaphy
  modified Bassini
    herniorrhaphy
  modified McVay
    herniorrhaphy
  Ogilvie femoral
    herniorrhaphy
  Ogilvie herniorrhaphy
  open herniorrhaphy
  pants-over-vest herniorrhaphy
  Ponka herniorrhaphy
  primary inguinal
    herniorrhaphy
  Shouldice inguinal
    herniorrhaphy
  sutureless laparoscopic
    extraperitoneal inguinal
    herniorrhaphy
  Tanner herniorrhaphy
  totally extraperitoneal
    inguinal herniorrhaphy
  transabdominal laparoscopic
    herniorrhaphy
  umbilical herniorrhaphy
  ventral herniorrhaphy
  vest-over-pants herniorrhaphy
  vest-over-pants inguinal
    herniorrhaphy
  Wangensteen herniorrhaphy
herniorrhaphy incision
herniotome
  Cooper herniotome
herniotome knife
herniotomy
  Petit herniotomy
herpes desquamans
herpes digitalis
herpes facialis
herpes genitalis
herpes labialis
herpes mentalis
herpes simplex virus
herpes virus
herpes zoster virus
herpesvirus
herpetic paronychia
herpetic ulcer
herpetic whitlow
herpetiform
herpetoid lesion

Herrick kidney clamp
Herrick kidney forceps
Herrick kidney pedicle clamp
Herrick lacrimal plug
Herrick pedicle clamp
Herrick silicone lacrimal implant
Herring lateral pillar
Herring tube
Hersbury anterior chamber
    intraocular lens
Hersh LASIK retreatment forceps
Hersh LASIK retreatment spatula
Hershey left ventricular assist
    device
Hershey total artificial heart
Hertel bougie
Hertel bougie-urethrotome
Hertel exophthalmometer
Hertel kidney stone forceps
Hertel nephrostomy speculum
Hertel rigid dilator stone forceps
Hertel rigid kidney stone forceps
Hertel speculum
Hertel stone forceps
Hertel urethrotome
hertz units (Hz)
Hertzler baby retractor
Hertzler baby rib retractor
Hertzler baby rib spreader
Hertzler rib retractor
Hertzler rib spreader
Hertzog intraocular lens
Hertzog lens spatula
Hertzog pliable probe
Herxheimer fibers
Herz meniscal tendon forceps
Herzfeld ear forceps
Herzmark fracture frame
Herzmark hyperextension frame
Hespan plasma volume
    expander
Hess capsule forceps
Hess capsule iris forceps
Hess expressor
Hess eyelid operation
Hess iris forceps
Hess lens scoop
Hess lens spoon
Hess nerve root retractor
Hess ptosis operation
Hess scoop
Hess spoon

Hess tonsil expressor
Hess-Barraquer iris forceps
Hessburg corneal shield
Hessburg eye shield
Hessburg intraocular lens
Hessburg intraocular lens glide
Hessburg lacrimal needle
Hessburg lens-inserting forceps
Hessburg needle
Hessburg vacuum trephine
Hessburg-Barron vacuum
    trephine
Hesselbach hernia
Hesselbach ligament
Hesselbach triangle
Hesseltine clamp
Hesseltine umbilical cord clamp
Hesseltine umbiliclip
Hess-Gill eye forceps
Hess-Gill iris forceps
Hess-Horwitz iris forceps
hetastarch plasma expander
heteroautoplasty
heterochromic cataract
heterocladic anastomosis
heterodermic graft
heterogeneous attenuation
heterogeneous keratoplasty
heterogenetic antigen
heterogenic
heterogenote
heterogenous graft
heterograft
    autogenous fascial heterograft
    bovine heterograft
    porcine heterograft
heterograft implant
heterograft prosthesis
heterograft valve
heterologous graft
heterologous insemination
heterologous material
heterologous tissue
hetero-osteoplasty
heterophoric position
heteroplasia
heteroplastic graft
heteroplasty
heterospecific graft
heterotopic bone formation
heterotopic graft
heterotopic ossification

heterotopic pancreas
heterotopic pregnancy
heterotopic replantation
heterotopic tissue
heterotopic transplant
heterotopic transplantation
heterotransplant
heterotransplantation
heterotrophic bone graft
Hetzel-Dent grading scale
Heubner artery
Heuser membrane
Hevesy polyp forceps
Hewlett-Packard ultrasound
Hewlett-Packard biplane probe
Hewlett-Packard color flow
    imager
Hewlett-Packard defibrillator
Hewlett-Packard ear oximeter
Hewlett-Packard earlobe
    oximeter
Hewlett-Packard Echo-Doppler
    machine
Hewlett-Packard omniplane probe
Hewlett-Packard scanner
Hewlett-Packard transducer
Hewlett-Packard ultrasound
Hewson breakaway pin
Hewson drill
Hewson ligament drill guide
Hewson ligament guide
Hewson ligature passer
Hewson passer
Hewson suture passer
Hewson-Richards reamer
hex bar
hex implant
hex procedure
hex screw (hexagon)
hexagon screw
hexagon snare
hexagonal handle
hexagonal handle osteotome
hexagonal wrench
hexapolar catheter
Hexascan computerized
    dermatology handpiece
Hexascan mode
Hexcel cast
Hexcel cast dressing
Hexcel total condylar knee
    system prosthesis

Hexcel total condylar prosthesis
Hexcelite cast
Hexcelite intermediate phase
    casting
Hexcelite long-arm cast
Hexcelite mesh
Hexcelite sheet splint
Hexcelite thermoplastic cast
Hex-Fix monolateral external
    fixator
Hex-Fix Universal swivel clamp
hexhead bolt
hexhead nail
hexhead pin
hexhead screw
hexhead screwdriver
hexlock implant
hexobarbital anesthetic agent
Hextend plasma volume
    expander
hexylcaine hydrochloride
    anesthetic agent
Hey amputation
Hey hernia
Hey internal derangement
Hey ligament
Hey operation
Hey skull saw
Heyer valve
Heyer-Pudenz valve
Heyer-Robertson suprapubic
    drain
Heyer-Schulte antisiphon device
Heyer-Schulte biopsy clamp
Heyer-Schulte brain retractor
Heyer-Schulte breast implant
Heyer-Schulte breast prosthesis
Heyer-Schulte catheter
Heyer-Schulte chin prosthesis
Heyer-Schulte clamp
Heyer-Schulte disposal bag
Heyer-Schulte dural film
    sheeting
Heyer-Schulte hydrocephalus
    shunt
Heyer-Schulte implant
Heyer-Schulte Jackson Pratt
    wound-drainage reservoir
Heyer-Schulte lens implant
Heyer-Schulte malar prosthesis
Heyer-Schulte mammary
    prosthesis

Heyer-Schulte microscope
Heyer-Schulte muscle biopsy clamp
Heyer-Schulte exudate bag
Heyer-Schulte prosthesis
Heyer-Schulte PVC kit
Heyer-Schulte Rayport muscle biopsy clamp
Heyer-Schulte retractor
Heyer-Schulte rhinoplasty implant
Heyer-Schulte shunt
Heyer-Schulte silicone kit
Heyer-Schulte silicone sphere
Heyer-Schulte Small-Carrion sizing set
Heyer-Schulte subcutaneous tissue expander
Heyer-Schulte testicular prosthesis
Heyer-Schulte tissue expander
Heyer-Schulte valve
Heyer-Schulte wedge-suction reservoir
Heyer-Schulte wound drain
Heyer-Schulte-Fischer ventricular cannula
Heyer-Schulte-Ommaya CSF reservoir
Heyer-Schulte-Pudenz cardiac catheter
Heyer-Schulte-Spetzler lumbar peritoneal shunt
Hey-Groves fascia lata technique
Hey-Groves ligament reconstruction technique
Hey-Groves needle
Hey-Groves operation
Hey-Groves-Kirk bone graft
Hey-Groves-Kirk technique
Heyman capsule
Heyman clubfoot procedure
Heyman forceps
Heyman nasal forceps
Heyman nasal scissors
Heyman nasal-cutting forceps
Heyman operation
Heyman operation for talipes equinovarus
Heyman procedure for genu recurvatum
Heyman septum-cutting rongeur

Heyman-Herndon clubfoot procedure
Heyman-Herndon operation
Heyman-Herndon release
Heyman-Herndon tarsometatarsal release for clubfoot
Heyman-Herndon-Strong technique
Heyman-Knight nasal dressing forceps
Heyman-Paparella angular scissors
Heyman-Paparella scissors
Heyner curet
Heyner dilator
Heyner double cannula
Heyner expressor
Heyner forceps
Heyner double needle
Heywood-Smith dressing forceps
Heywood-Smith gallbladder forceps
Heywood-Smith sponge-holding forceps
HF dialyzer
HF infrared laser
H-file
H-flap incision
HG Multilock hip prosthesis
HGM argon green laser
HGM intravitreal laser
HGM ophthalmic laser
HGM krypton yellow and green laser
HGP II acetabular component
HGP II acetabular cup
H-graft bone graft
H-graft fusion
HGSIL (high-grade squamous intraepithelial lesion)
HH shunt for neonatal hydrocephalus
HH open-ended alimentation catheter
HH Rickham cerebrospinal fluid reservoir
HH shunt introducer
Hi Speed pulse lavage
hiatal hernia
hiatal insufficiency

hiatopexy
hiatoplasty
hiatus
  accessory maxillary hiatus
  adductor hiatus
  aortic hiatus
  basilic hiatus
  Breschet hiatus
  diaphragmatic hiatus
  esophageal hiatus
  fallopian hiatus
  greater petrosal nerve hiatus
  lesser petrosal nerve hiatus
  maxillary hiatus
  saphenous hiatus
  semilunar hiatus
hiatus ethmoidalis
hiatus hernia
hiatus of canal for greater
    petrosal nerve
hiatus of canal for lesser
    petrosal nerve
hiatus of facial canal
hiatus of fallopian canal
Hibbs approach
Hibbs arthrodesis
Hibbs biting forceps
Hibbs blade
Hibbs bone chisel
Hibbs bone curet
Hibbs bone gouge
Hibbs bone-cutting forceps
Hibbs bone-holding forceps
Hibbs chisel elevator
Hibbs clamp
Hibbs costal elevator
Hibbs foot procedure
Hibbs fracture appliance
Hibbs fracture frame
Hibbs gag
Hibbs graft
Hibbs hammer
Hibbs hip arthrodesis
Hibbs laminectomy retractor
Hibbs mallet
Hibbs mouth gag
Hibbs onlay graft fusion of
    lumbar spine
Hibbs operation
Hibbs osteotome
Hibbs periosteal elevator
Hibbs procedure

Hibbs retractor blade
Hibbs self-retaining laminectomy
    retractor
Hibbs self-retaining retractor
Hibbs spinal curet
Hibbs spinal fusion
Hibbs spinal fusion chisel
    elevator
Hibbs spinal fusion gouge
Hibbs spinal retractor blade
Hibbs sponge
Hibbs technique
Hibbs-Jones spinal fusion
Hibbs-Spratt spinal fusion curet
hibernating gland
hibernating myocardium
Hibiclens cleansers
Hibiclens scrub
Hibiclens skin cleanser
Hibistat cleansers
Hibistat scrub
Hibitane cleansers
Hibitane tincture
Hickman indwelling catheter
Hickman indwelling right atrial
    catheter
Hickman line
Hickman percutaneous
    introducer
Hickman Silastic semipermanent
    central line
Hickman tunneled catheter
Hickman-Broviac catheter
hickory-stick fracture
Hicks contraction
Hicks lugged plate
Hicks sign
Hicks version
HIDA scan of gallbladder and
    liver
Hidalgo catheter
hidradenitis axillaris of Verneuil
hidradenitis suppurativa
hidradenoma
  clear cell hidradenoma
  cystic hidradenoma
  nodular hidradenoma
  papillary hidradenoma
  solid hidradenoma
hidrocystoma
Hiebert esophageal suture spoon
Hiebert vascular dilator

Hieshima coaxial catheter
Higbee speculum
Higbee vaginal speculum
Higgenson syringe
Higgins bag
Higgins catheter
Higgins hemostatic bag
Higgins incision
Higgins operation
Higgins technique
Higgins ureterointestinal
    anastomosis
Higginson irrigation syringe
Higgs spike operation for
    hammertoe correction
high attenuation
high beam fiberoptic headlight
high cellularity
high endothelial venule
High Flex bubble oxygenator
high flux dialyzer
high forceps
high frenum attachment
high frequency
high frequency oscillatory
    ventilator
high hepatojejunostomy
high incision
high intraluminal pressure
high intrauterine insemination
high lateral tension
    abdominoplasty
high ligation
high lip line
high lithotomy
high median nerve palsy
high neurological lesion
high occlusion
high operation for femoral hernia
high output ileostomy
high point of cupid's bow
high pressure zone (HPZ)
high saphenous vein ligation
high small-bowel obstruction
high smile line
high spinal anesthesia
high stirrups position
high subtotal gastrectomy
high threshold receptor
high tibial osteotomy
high ulnar nerve palsy
high-altitude endoscopy

high-amplitude shock wave
high-amplitude sucking technique
high-capacity drain
high-capacity silicone drain
high-compliance latex balloon
high-diameter dilator
high-dose chemotherapy
high-dose radioiodine therapy
high-dose therapy
high-energy fracture
high-energy laser
higher than heart, legs elevated
highest concha
highest intercostal artery
highest intercostal vein
Highet-Sander modified criteria
    of MacKinnon and Dellon
    for sensory recovery
    following nerve repair
Highet-Sander modified criteria
    of Zachary and Holmes for
    sensory recovery following
    nerve repair
high-fidelity catheter
high-fidelity micromanometric
    catheter
high-field open MRI scanner
high-flow arterial malformation
high-flow arterial stenosis
high-flow arteriovenous fistula
high-flow arteriovenous
    malformation
high-flow cannula
high-flow catheter
high-flow coaxial cannula
high-flow regulator
high-flux dialysis membrane
high forceps delivery
high forceps operation
high-frequency cord
high-frequency focused transducer
high-frequency jet ventilation
    (HFJV)
high-frequency jet ventilator
high-frequency miniature probe
high-frequency miniprobe
high-frequency oscillation
    ventilator
high-frequency oscillatory
    ventilation (HFOV)
high-frequency percussive
    ventilation

high-frequency positive-pressure
   ventilation (HFPPV)
high-frequency tweezer-type
   epilator
high-frequency ventilation (HFV)
high-grade dysplasia
high-grade MALT lymphoma
high-grade obstruction
high-grade squamous
   intraepithelial lesion
high-humidity tracheostomy
   collar
high-humidity tracheostomy
   mask
high-humidity tracheostomy
   shield
high-impedance, low-threshold
   lead
high-intensity lesion
high-intensity light bundle
high-kV technique
Highlight spectral indirect
   ophthalmoscope
highly selective vagolysis
highly selective vagotomy
high-magnification colonoscopy
high-magnification endoscopy
high-magnification gastroscopy
high-mandibular plane-angle
   skeletal structure
Highmore abscess
Highmore antrum
Highmore body
high-pitched bowel sounds
high-power field
high-pressure anesthesia
high-pressure chamber
high-resistance fundoplication
high-resolution conventional
   static scanner
high-resolution image
high-resolution linear array
   transducer
high-resolution multileaf
   collimator
high-resolution probe
high-resolution real-time scanner
high-riding patella
high-risk angioplasty
high-risk needle (HR needle)
high-risk papillary cancer
high-sensitivity collimator

high-speed bur
high-speed dermabrader
high-speed diamond 3-tiered
   depth cutting bur
high-speed diamond wheel bur
high-speed drill
high-speed electrical tissue
   morcellator
high-speed microdrill
high-speed rotation dynamic
   angioplasty catheter
high-speed rotational
   atherectomy
high-speed steel bur
high-speed tungsten carbide bur
high-speed 2-grit bur
high-speed wrist slip joint
high-tension sutures technique
   to suture
high-torque bur
high-torque guidewire
high-torque wire
high-voltage electron
   microscope
high-voltage therapy
high-volume evacuator
Hilton sutureless infusion
   cannula
hila (sing. hilum)
Hilal coil
Hilal microcoil
Hilal modified headhunter
   catheter
hilar adenopathy
hilar biopsy
hilar carcinoma
hilar clamp
hilar dance
hilar fullness
hilar hepatojejunostomy
hilar lymph nodes
hilar mass
hilar node
hilar plate
hilar prominence
hilar region
hilar shadow
hilar structure
Hildebrandt uterine hemostatic
   forceps
Hildreth cautery
Hildreth coagulator

Hildreth electrocautery
Hildreth electrode
Hildreth ocular cautery
Hildreth tip
Hildyard nasal forceps
Hiles intraocular lens
Hiles lens
Hi-level bandage scissors
Hilgenreiner angle
Hilgenreiner brace
Hilgenreiner horizontal Y line
Hilgenreiner line
Hilgenreiner splint
Hilgenreiner-Perkins line
Hilger facial nerve stimulator
Hilger nerve stimulator
Hilger tracheal tube
Hilger tube
hili (*sing.* hilus)
Hill antireflux operation
Hill cluster harvest technique
Hill fundoplasty
Hill gastropexy fundoplication
Hill hiatal herniorrhaphy
Hill hiatus hernia operation
Hill hiatus hernia repair
Hill hiatus herniorrhaphy
Hill median arcuate repair
Hill nasal raspatory
Hill operation
Hill posterior gastropexy
Hill procedure
Hill raspatory
Hill rectal retractor
Hill repair of hiatal hernia
Hill retractor
Hill sign
Hill stitch scissors
Hill sutures
Hill-Allison operation
Hill-Bosworth saw
Hill-Ferguson rectal retractor
Hill-Ferguson retractor
Hillis eyelid retractor
Hillis lid retractor
Hillis perforator
Hillis refractor
Hillis retractor
Hillis-Mueller maneuver
Hill-Nahai-Vasconez-Mathes
    technique
Hill-Sachs deformity

Hill-Sachs fracture
Hill-Sachs lesion
Hill-Sachs shoulder dislocation
Hill-Sachs shoulder lesion
Hill-type hiatus herniorrhaphy
Hi-Lo tracheal tube
Hilsinger tonsillar knife
Hilton laryngeal saccule
Hilton muscle
Hilton sac
Hilton self-retaining infusion
    cannula
Hilton white line
hilum (*pl.* hila)
    hepatic hilum
    left hilum
    right hilum
    splenic hilum
hilus (*pl.* hili)
    kidney hilus
    lung hilus
    pulmonary hilus
hilus of ovary
Himalaya dressing forceps
Himmelstein pulmonary
    valvulotome
Himmelstein sternal retractor
Himmelstein valvulotome
Hinchey diverticulitis grade
    classification
H-incision
hind kidney
hindbrain deformity
Hinderer cartilage forceps
Hinderer cartilage-holding forceps
Hinderer lower nasal base
    implant
Hinderer malar prosthesis
Hinderer prosthesis
hindfoot amputation
hindfoot deformity
hindfoot orthosis
hindfoot ulcer
hindquarter amputation
Hines-Anderson
    pyeloureteroplasty
hinge
    Camber axis hinge
    Compass hinge
    Dee elbow hinge
    elbow hinge
    implant hinge

hinge (*continued*)
  Ishizuki hinge
  Kinematic rotating hinge
  Kudo hinge
  Lacey rotating hinge
  London elbow hinge
  offset hinge
  Pritchard-Walker elbow hinge
  Rancho swivel hinge
  rotating hinge
  Scheier hinge
  Silastic HP Swanson flexible
    toe hinge
  Souter hinge
  TM5 hinge
  triaxial hinge
  Volz elbow hinge
  Wadsworth hinge
  Weser dental hinge
hinge articulator
hinge axis
hinge joint
hinge movement
hinge osteotomy
hinge position
hinge-axis movement
hinge-axis point
hinged articulated fixator
hinged articulation
hinged articulator
hinged cast
hinged constrained knee
    prosthesis
hinged corneal flap
hinged flap
hinged fragment
hinged great toe replacement
    prosthesis
hinged implant
hinged implant prosthesis
hinged skin hook
hinged Thomas splint
hinged total knee prosthesis
hinged-leaflet aortic valve
hinged-leaflet vascular
    prosthesis
hinged-loop snare wire
hinge-knee prosthesis
hingeless heart valve prosthesis
Hingson-Edwards needle
Hingson-Ferguson needle
Hinkle-James rectal speculum

Hinman procedure
Hinman syndrome
Hinsberg operation
hip
  3-dimensional interlocking
    hip (TDI hip)
  Abbott arthrodesis of hip
  abduction contraction of hip
  adduction contracture of hip
  adductor tenotomy with total
    hip
  Amstutz total hip
  anthropometric total hip
  Autophor total hip
  Batchelor osteotomy of hip
  Bio-Groove hip
  Biomet hip
  bipolar total hip
  Brunswick total hip
  ceramic total hip
  CFS total hip (contoured
    femoral stem total hip)
  Christiansen total hip
  CLS total hip
  congenital dislocated hip
    (CDH)
  congenital dysplasia of hip
    (CDH)
  contracture of hip
  Corin total hip
  DuaLock total hip
  fused hips
  Gamma locking nail for hip
  Gemini hip
  Gustilo-Kyle total hip
  Harris total hip
  Howmedica PCA textured hip
  Indiana conservative hip
  internal rotation contracture
    of hip
  Johnson-Iowa total hip
  Leinbach head and neck total
    hip
  Link anatomical hip
  Link total hip
  McCarroll osteotomy hip
  McCutchen hip
  Mittlemeir ceramic total hip
  Mueller total hip
  nailing of hip
  PCA hip
  PCA total hip

hip (*continued*)
Precision Osteolock total hip
Precoat Plus total hip
Protasul prosthetic hip
Ring-Moore total hip
Sarmiento osteotomy of hip
snapping hip
Spectron total hip
Stanmore total hip
Sugioki osteotomy of hip
TDI hip (3-dimensional interlocking hip)
Techmedica total hip
transient osteoporosis of hip
Tronzo approach to hip
Tronzo lateral approach to hip
Tronzo total hip
Urist-Matchett-Brown total hip
HIP (homograft incus prosthesis)
hip abduction
hip adduction
hip alignment guide
hip arthrodesis
hip arthroplasty
hip arthroplasty gouge
hip bone
hip cup prosthesis
hip deformity
hip disarticulation
hip disarticulation prosthesis
hip dislocation
hip dysplasia
hip extension
hip fixation
hip flange
hip flexion contracture
hip fracture
hip fusion
hip gouge
hip guidance orthosis
hip joint
hip musculature
hip nail
hip nailing
hip pin
hip pinning
hip pointer
hip prosthesis
hip reduction
hip replacement
hip retractor
hip rotation

hip rotationplasty
hip ruler
hip screw
hip skid
hip spica cast
hip spica dressing
Hi-Per cardiac device
Hi-Per Flex exchange guidewire
Hi-Per Flex exchange wire
hip-knee orthosis
hip-knee-ankle orthosis
hip-knee-ankle-foot orthosis (HKAFO)
Hippel (*see also* von Hippel)
Hippel keratoplasty
Hippel operation
Hippel trephine
hippocampus
Hippocrates bandage
Hippocrates manipulation
hippocratic fingers
Hippocratic maneuver
hippocratic splash
hippocratic succussion
hippocratic wreath
Hiram Kite 3-part cast for clubfoot
Hirano bodies in hippocampus
Hirano polypectomy
Hircoe denture base material
Hirsch hypophysial punch
Hirsch hypophysis punch forceps
Hirsch mucosal clamp
Hirschberg electromagnet
Hirschberg magnet
Hirschberg reflex
Hirschberg sign for pyramidal tract disease
Hirschfield eye light
Hirschman anoscope
Hirschman anoscope rectal speculum
Hirschman anoscope with obturator
Hirschman clamp
Hirschman forceps
Hirschman hemorrhoidal forceps
Hirschman hook
Hirschman hooked cannula
Hirschman intraocular implant lens

Hirschman iris hook
Hirschman iris spatula
Hirschman jeweler's forceps
Hirschman lens
Hirschman lens forceps
Hirschman lens manipulator
Hirschman lens spatula
Hirschman nasoendoscope
Hirschman pile clamp
Hirschman proctoscope
Hirschman proctoscope with
    obturator
Hirschman retractor
Hirschman spatula
Hirschman speculum
Hirschman-Martin proctoscope
Hirschowitz fiberscope
Hirschowitz fiberscope
    gastroscope
Hirschowitz gastroduodenal
    fiberscope
Hirschowitz gastroduodenal
    scope
Hirschowitz gastroscope
Hirschsprung disease
Hirschtick utility shoulder splint
Hirst obstetrical forceps
Hirst operation
Hirst placental forceps
Hirst-Emmet obstetrical forceps
Hirst-Emmet placental forceps
His band
His bundle ablation
His bundle catheter
His bundle electrogram
His bundle heart block
His bundle recording
His canal
His catheter
His line
His perivascular space
His plane
His potential
His spindle
His-Haas operation
His-Haas procedure for long
    thoracic nerve palsy
HiSpeed CT scanner
His-Purkinje conduction
Hiss bunionectomy
His-Tawara bundle
His-Tawara node

histiocytic cytophagic
    panniculitis
histiocytic granuloma
histiocytic response
histiocytoma
    angiomatoid fibrous
        histiocytoma (AFH)
    benign fibrous histiocytoma
    cutaneous fibrous
        histiocytoma
    lipoid histiocytoma
    malignant fibrous histiocytoma
histiocytomatosis
histiocytosis
    benign cephalic histiocytosis
    juvenile xanthogranuloma
        histiocytosis
    Langerhans cell histiocytosis
    nodular histiocytosis
    skin-limited histiocytosis
Histoacryl glue adhesive
histochromatosis
histocompatibility
histocompatible
histogram mode
histoincompatibility
histologic assessment
histologic diagnosis
histologic examination
histologic lesion
histologic tooth repair
histological assessment
histological diagnosis
histologically benign
histologically malignant
histologically normal
histology
histopathologic diagnosis
histopathologic examination
histophysiology
historrhexis
Hitachi convex ultrasound probe
Hitachi convex-convex biplane
    probe
Hitachi CT Scanner
Hitachi MRI scanner
Hitachi fingertip ultrasound
    probe
Hitachi linear ultrasound probe
Hitachi Open MRI System scanner
Hitachi transrectal ultrasound
    probe

Hitachi transvaginal ultrasound
    probe
Hitachi ultrasound
Hitchcock biceps procedure
Hitchcock stereotactic
    immobilization frame
Hitchcock tendon technique
hitchhiker's thumb
HiTec insufflator
Hi-Top foot/ankle brace
Hi-Torque Flex-T guidewire
Hi-Torque Floppy exchange
    guidewire
Hi-Torque Floppy guide catheter
Hi-Torque floppy guidewire
Hi-Torque Floppy intermediate
    guidewire
Hi-Torque intermediate
    guidewire
Hi-Torque screw
Hi-Torque standard guidewire
Hitselberger sign
Hitselberger-McElveen neural
    dissector
Hittenberger prosthesis
HIV classification
HIZ (high intensity zone)
    lesion
HKAFO (hip-knee-ankle-foot
    orthosis)
HKAFO prosthesis
HLA complex
HMTV (human mammary tumor
    virus)
HNPCC syndrome
Huerthle adenoma
Huerthle cell tumor
Ho:YAG (holmium:yttrium-
    aluminum-garnet) laser
Ho:YAG laser angioplasty
Hoaglund bone graft
Hoaglund sign
Hobbs dilatation balloon
    catheter
Hobbs needle
Hobbs polypectomy snare
Hobbs stent set
Hobbs stone basket
hobnail liver
Hochenegg operation
hockey-stick catheter
hockey-stick deformity

hockey-stick elevator
hockey-stick fracture
hockey-stick incision
hockey-stick tricuspid valve
Hodge intestinal decompression
    tube
Hodge maneuver
Hodge obstetrical forceps
Hodge pessary
Hodge plane
Hodgen hip splint
Hodgen leg splint
Hodgen splint
Hodgkin disease
Hodgkin lymphoma
Hodgson approach
Hodgson hypospadias repair
Hodgson spine fusion
Hodgson technique
Hodgson-Tuksu tumble flap
    hypospadias repair
Hodor-Dobbs procedure
hoe
    excavator hoe
    Hough excavator hoe
    Hough hoe
    Hough-Saunders stapes hoe
    Joe's hoe
    middle ear hoe
    monangle hoe
    Nordent hoe
    stapes hoe
hoe extractor
Hoefer laser densitometer
Hoefflin suture passer
Hoen alligator forceps
Hoen bayonet forceps
Hoen cannula
Hoen dressing forceps
Hoen dural separator
Hoen elevator
Hoen explorer
Hoen gouge
Hoen grabber
Hoen grasping forceps
Hoen hemilaminectomy
    retractor
Hoen hemostatic forceps
Hoen hook
Hoen intervertebral disk
    rongeur
Hoen lamina gouge

Hoen laminectomy rongeur
Hoen laminectomy scissors
Hoen needle
Hoen nerve hook
Hoen periosteal elevator
Hoen periosteal raspatory
Hoen pituitary rongeur
Hoen plate
Hoen raspatory
Hoen retractor
Hoen rongeur
Hoen scalp forceps
Hoen scalp retractor
Hoen scissors
Hoen separator
Hoen skull plate
Hoen tissue forceps
Hoen ventricular cannula
Hoen ventricular needle
Hoesel needle holder
Hoff towel clamp
Hoffa fat
Hoffa fracture
Hoffa operation
Hoffa tendon shortening
Hoffa-Lorenz operation
Hoffa fat pad
Hoffer corneal marker
Hoffer forward-cutting knife
    cannula
Hoffer intraocular implant lens
Hoffer knife
Hoffer lens
Hoffer procedure
Hoffer ridge of lens implant
Hoffer ridged intraocular lens
Hoffer ridged lens implant
Hoffman-Mohr procedure
Hoffman jejunoplasty
Hoffman transfixion pin
Hoffmann apex fixation pin
Hoffmann approach
Hoffmann biopsy punch
Hoffmann clamp
Hoffmann claw toe
Hoffmann duct
Hoffmann ear forceps
Hoffmann ear punch
Hoffmann ear punch forceps
Hoffmann ear rongeur
Hoffmann external fixation
    device

Hoffmann external fixator
Hoffmann eye implant
Hoffmann compact external
    fixation component
Hoffmann ligament clamp
Hoffmann mini-lengthening
    fixation device
Hoffmann panmetatarsal head
    resection
Hoffmann pin
Hoffmann punch
Hoffmann reconstruction of
    forefoot
Hoffmann scleral fixation pick
Hoffmann screw
Hoffmann sign
Hoffmann traction device
Hoffmann transfixion pin
Hoffmann-Clayton procedure
Hoffmann-Keller-Lapidus
    procedure
Hoffmann-Osher-Hopkins plaster
    knife
Hoffmann-Pollock forceps
Hoffmann-Vidal external fixation
    device
Hoffrel transesophageal probe
Hofmeister anastomosis
Hofmeister antecolic
    gastrojejunostomy
Hofmeister drainage bag
Hofmeister endometrial biopsy
    curet
Hofmeister gastrectomy
Hofmeister gastroenterostomy
Hofmeister operation
Hofmeister procedure
Hofmeister technique
Hofmeister-Billroth II
    gastrectomy
Hofmeister-Finsterer operation
Hofmeister-Polya anastomosis
Hofmeister-Polya operation
Hogan-Converse graft
    augmentation
Hogan dacryocystostomy
Hogan keratoplasty
Hogan operation
Hogan test
Hoguet hernia repair
Hoguet maneuver
Hoguet operation

Hoguet pantaloon hernia repair
Hohl classification
Hohl fracture
Hohl tibial condylar fracture
   classification
Hohl-Luck tibial plateau fracture
   classification
Hohl-Moore classification
Hohl-Moore technique
Hohmann bone lever
Hohmann bunionectomy
Hohmann clamp
Hohmann operation
Hohmann osteotome
Hohmann procedure
Hohmann retractor
Hohmann tennis elbow
   procedure
Hohmann-Aldinger bone lever
Hohn catheter
Hohn central venous catheter
Hohn vessel dilator
Hoke arthrodesis of foot and
   ankle
Hoke flatfoot procedure
Hoke incision
Hoke operation
Hoke operation for talipes
   valgus
Hoke osteotome
Hoke procedure
Hoke spoon
Hoke technique
Hoke 3-level incision
Hoke triple talus arthrodesis
Hoke-Kite technique
Hoke-Martin traction
Hoke-Martin tractor
Hoke-Miller procedure
Hoke-Roberts spoon
hoku point
Holcomb gastric tourniquet
Hold-and-Hold immobilizer
Hold-and-Hold positioner
Holdaway line
Holdaway ratio
Holden line
Holden uterine curet
holder (*see also* head holder,
   needle holder)
   Alabama-Green needle eye
     holder

holder (*continued*)
   Allen well leg holder
   Alvarado surgical knee holder
   Andrews rigid chest support
     holder
   Anspach leg holder
   Arruga eye holder
   arthroscopic ankle holder
   arthroscopic leg holder
   Bard leg bag holder
   Barraquer curved holder
   Baumgartner holder
   Baumgartner dental holder
   Bethea sheet holder
   Birks Mark II micro cross-
     action holder
   Björk-Shiley heart valve
     holder
   blade holder
   bladebreaker holder
   Bodkin thread holder
   bone graft holder
   Bookler swivel-ball
     laparoscopic instrument
     holder
   Bovie holder
   Boyce holder
   Bunt forceps holder
   Bunt instrument holder
   Castroviejo blade holder
   Castroviejo razor blade holder
   Castroviejo razor holder
   catheter guide holder
   catheter leg tube holder
   catheter waist tube holder
   Cath-Secure catheter holder
   Chaffin-Pratt percolator
     hanger holder
   Charnley trochanter holder
   Circon leg holder
   clamp holder
   Collins leg holder
   Comfit endotracheal tube
     holder
   Cottle instrument tray and
     spring holder
   Craig headrest holder
   Crockard suction tube holder
   Dale Foley catheter holder
   Dale Foley catheter legband
     holder
   Dale gastrostomy tube holder

holder (*continued*)

Dale nasal dressing holder
Dale secondary wound dressing and holder
Dale tapeless wound dressing holder
Dale tracheostomy tube holder
Dean knife holder
Dees holder
DeMartel-Wolfson clamp holder
Derf holder
Derlacki ossicle holder
DeRoyal catheter tube holder
Drummond hook holder
ear speculum holder
Eber holder
Elliot femoral condyle holder
Ellis holder
Eriksson-Paparella holder
Ferguson bone holder
foot holder
Furacin gauze holder
Gambro dialyzer holder
Gifford holder
GraftAssist vein and graft holder
Grant holder
Green holder
Greenberg instrument holder
Grieshaber holder
hook holder
House-Urban bone holder
House-Urban holder
House-Urban temporal bone holder
Huang vein holder
instrument holder
I-tech cannula holder
Jacobson holder
Jarcho tenaculum holder
Jarit forceps holder
Jarit wire holder
Jordan-Caparosa holder
Juers-Derlacki holder
Lapides holder
laryngoscope chest support holder
laryngoscope holder
leg holder
Lenny Johnson surgical-assist knee holder

holder (*continued*)

Leonard Arms instrument holder
Lewy chest holder
Lewy laryngoscope holder
limb holder
lion-jaw bone holder
Lundia dialyzer holder
Margraf beam aligning film holder
Marquette 3-channel laser holder
Mason leg holder
mat holder
Mathieu holder
Mayo holder
microstaple holder
mirror holder
Murray holder
Neo-Fit neonatal endotracheal tube holder
nerve holder
Neumann razor blade fragment holder
OSI arthroscopic well-leg leg holder
pin holder
Portmann speculum holder
Posilok instrument holder
prosthetic valve holder
Quinn holder
razor blade holder
Reverdin holder
Rica forceps holder
Rinn XCP film holder
rod holder
Schaefer sponge holder
Schlein shoulder holder
Schmidt rod holder
Shea speculum holder
sheet holder
Sims sponge holder
speculum holder
spring holder
Steinmann holder
Stenstrom nerve holder
sterile forceps holder
Surcan knee holder
Surcan leg holder
SurgAssist surgical leg holder
surgical-assist leg holder
suture holder

holder (*continued*)
  Swiss blade holder
  swivel joint suture holder
  Taylor catheter holder
  temporal bone holder
  tenaculum holder
  Texas Scottish Rite Hospital
    hook holder
  The tracheostomy tube holder
  Thomas long-term
    endotracheal tube holder
  Tomac vest-style holder
  Trake-Fit tracheal tube holder
  trochanter holder
  Universal speculum holder
  Vacutainer holder
  valve holder
  Vital Cooley general tissue
    holder
  Watanabe pin holder
  Watson heart valve holder
  Weck instrument holder
  Wehbe arm holder
  Weisenbach sterile forceps
    holder
  well-leg holder
  Wister forceps holder
  Worcester instrument holder
  Young rubber dam holder
  Young-Millin holder
  Zollinger leg holder
holding clip
holding forceps
hold-relax technique
Holdsworth spinal fracture
    classification
hole
  acetabular seating hole
  bur hole
  drill hole
  drilled bur hole
  Hough hole
  tibial peg holes
  transosseous holes
hole punch set
hole-in-one technique
Holinger anterior commissure
    laryngoscope
Holinger applicator
Holinger aspirating tube
Holinger bougie
Holinger bronchoscope

Holinger bronchoscopic magnet
Holinger bronchoscopic
    telescope
Holinger cannula
Holinger child esophagoscope
Holinger curved scissors
Holinger dissector
Holinger endarterectomy
    dissector
Holinger endoscopic magnet
Holinger esophagoscope
Holinger forceps
Holinger hook-on folding
    laryngoscope
Holinger hourglass anterior
    commissure laryngoscope
Holinger hourglass laryngoscope
Holinger infant bougie
Holinger infant bronchoscope
Holinger infant esophageal
    speculum
Holinger infant esophagoscope
Holinger infant laryngoscope
Holinger laryngeal dissector
Holinger laryngoscope
Holinger magnet
Holinger modified Jackson
    laryngoscope
Holinger needle
Holinger open-end aspirating
    tube
Holinger scissors
Holinger slotted laryngoscope
Holinger specimen forceps
Holinger speculum
Holinger telescope
Holinger tube
Holinger ventilating fiberoptic
    bronchoscope
Holinger-Garfield laryngoscope
Holinger-Hurst bougie
Holinger-Jackson bronchoscope
Holladay posterior capsular
    polisher
Holladay-Binkhorst equation
Hollande solution
Hollenhorst plaque
Holley vascular stripper
HolliGard seal closed stoma
    pouch
Hollister bag
Hollister belt

Hollister bridge suture bolster
Hollister catheter
Hollister circumcision device
Hollister clamp
Hollister collecting device
Hollister colostomy bag
Hollister colostomy irrigator
Hollister disposable Convex
    insert
Hollister drainage bag
Hollister external catheter
Hollister First Choice pouch
Hollister Holligard pouch
Hollister irrigator drain
Hollister Karaya ostomy pouch
Hollister Karaya seal pouch
Hollister laryngoscope
Hollister loop colostomy set
Hollister medial adhesive
    bandage
Hollister ostomy pouch
Hollister self-adhesive catheter
Hollister tube
Hollister urostomy bag
Hollister wound exudate absorber
hollow cannula
hollow chisel
hollow cutter
hollow fiber capillary dialyzer
hollow filter dialyzer
hollow Lucite pessary
hollow needle
hollow needle guide
hollow organ
hollow Silastic disk heart valve
hollow sphere eye implant
hollow sphere implant
hollow sphere orbital implant
hollow sphere prosthesis
hollow sunken orbit
hollow visceral injury
hollow visceral tonometer
hollow viscus
hollow viscus injury
hollow-fiber dialyzer
hollow-fiber hemodialyzer
hollow-object forceps
Holman lung retractor
Holman retractor
Holman-Mathieu cannula
Holman-Mathieu salpingography
    cannula

Holmes cartilage gouge
Holmes chair
Holmes chisel
Holmes fixation forceps
Holmes gouge
Holmes nasopharyngoscope
Holmes operation
Holmes scissors
holmium laser
holmium laser lithotriptor
holmium:YAG laser
holmium:yttrium-argon-garnet
    laser
Holocaine anesthetic agent
holocrine gland
Holofx Oxford retroillumination
    cataract camera
Hologic densitometer
Hologic scanner
Hologic dual-energy x-ray
    absorptiometry scanner
holography
holoprosencephalic
    malformation
holoprosencephaly
holosystolic murmur
Holscher nerve retractor
Holscher nerve root retractor
Holscher root retractor
Holstein-Lewis fracture
holster
Holt nail
Holt nail plate
Holt self-retaining catheter
Holter connector
Holter distal atrial catheter
Holter distal catheter passer
Holter distal peritoneal catheter
Holter elliptical valve
Holter high-pressure valve
Holter in-line shunt filter
Holter introducer
Holter lumboperitoneal catheter
Holter medium-pressure valve
Holter mini-elliptical valve
Holter monitor
Holter pump
Holter pump clamp
Holter shunt
Holter straight valve
Holter traction
Holter tube

Holter tubing
Holter valve
Holter ventricular catheter
Holter ventriculostomy reservoir
Holter-Hausner catheter
Holter-Hausner valve
Holter-Rickham ventriculostomy
reservoir
Holter-Salmon-Rickham
ventriculostomy reservoir
Holter-Selker ventriculostomy
reservoir
Holth corneoscleral punch
Holth cystoscope
Holth cystotome
Holth iridencleisis
Holth operation
Holth punch
Holth punch forceps
Holth punch sclerectomy
Holth scleral punch
Holth sclerectomy
Holth sclerectomy punch
Holthouse hernia
Holth-Rubin punch
Holt-Oram atriodigital dysplasia
Holt-Oram syndrome
Holtz corneoscleral punch
Holtz ear curet
Holtz endometrial curet
Holzer stain
Holz procedure
Holzbach abdominal retractor
Holzbach hysterectomy forceps
Holzheimer mastoid retractor
Holzheimer skin retractor
Holzknecht space
Holzknecht stomach
Homan retractor
Homans sign
homatropine dilatation
home uterine activity monitor
homeograft
homeo-osteoplasty
homeostasis
homeotransplant
Homer localization needle
Homerlok needle
Homestretch lumbar traction
Homiak radium colpostat
Homochron monitor
homocladic anastomosis

homogeneity
homogeneous ablation
homogeneous component
homogeneous graft
homogenizer
homogenous bone graft
homogenous graft
homogenous keratoplasty
homogenous tooth
transplantation
homogenous transplant
homograft
cadaveric homograft
Cryolife homograft
cryopreserved aortic
homograft
denatured homograft
homovital homograft
living homograft
pulmonary homograft
homograft aortic valve
replacement
homograft cadaver
homograft graft
homograft implant
homograft implant material
homograft prosthesis
homograft reaction
homograft rejection
homograft valve
homokeratoplasty
homologous anaphylaxis
homologous artificial
insemination
homologous graft
homoplastic
homoplastic graft
homoplasty
homotopic transplantation
homotransplant
homotransplantation
homovital homograft
Honan balloon
Honan cuff
Honan eye-pressure reducer
Honan manometer
Honan pressure reducer
honeycomb appearance
honeycomb cystitis
honeycomb lesion
honeycomb lung
honeycomb pattern

Honeywell recorder
Honore-Smathers tube
Hood-Kirklin incision
Hood dermatome
Hood dissector
Hood headlight
Hood Laboratories Eccovision
  acoustic rhinometer
Hood manual dermatome
Hood operation
Hood procedure
Hood stoma stent
Hood technique
hooded transilluminator
Hood-Graves speculum
Hood-Graves vaginal speculum
hooding of the upper lid skin
Hood-Kirkland incision
Hood-Westaby T-Y stent
hook (*see also* buttonhook)
  2-prong dural hook
  2-pronged dural hook
  Abramson hook
  Adson angular hook
  Adson blunt dissecting hook
  Adson blunt hook
  Adson brain hook
  Adson dissecting hook
  Adson dissector hook
  Adson dural hook
  Adson knot tier hook
  Adson sharp hook
  Allport incus hook
  Amenabar discission hook
  anchor hook
  Anderson suture pusher and
    double hook
  Angle vessel hook
  angled discission hook
  APRL hooks (Army Prosthetics
    Research Laboratory hooks)
  Army Prosthetics Research
    Laboratory hooks (APRL
    hooks)
  Arruga extraction hook
  Ashbell hook
  attic hook
  Aufranc hook
  Azar lens hook
  ball nerve hook
  ball-end hook
  ball-tip nerve hook

hook (*continued*)
  Bane hook
  Barr crypt hook
  Barr fistula hook
  Barr hook
  Barr rectal fistular hook
  Barsky hook
  Barton double hook
  Barton hook
  Bellucci hook
  bent hook
  Berens hook
  Berens scleral hook
  Bethune hook
  Bethune nerve hook
  biangled hook
  bifid hook
  Billeau ear hook
  Birks Mark II hook
  Blair hook
  Blair palate hook
  blunt dissecting hook
  blunt hook
  blunt iris hook
  blunt nerve hook
  boat hook
  Bobechko sliding barrel hook
  Boettcher hook
  Boettcher tonsil hook
  Boettcher tonsillar hook
  bone hook
  Bonn hook
  Bonn iris hook
  Bonn microiris hook
  Bose hook
  Bose tracheal hook
  Bose tracheostomy hook
  Boyes-Goodfellow hook
  Bozeman hook
  brain hook
  Braun decapitation hook
  Braun hook
  Braun obstetrical hook
  Braun-Jardine-DeLee hook
  Brown hook
  Brown suture hook
  Brown tissue hook
  Bryant mitral hook
  Buck hook
  Burch hook
  buttonhook
  buttressed hook

hook (*continued*)
calvarial hook
canted finger hook
Carroll bone hook
Carroll skin hook
Caspar hook
caudal hook
cautery hook
Chavasse squint hook
Chavasse strabismus hook
Chernov hook
Chernov tracheostomy hook
Clayman iris hook
cleft palate sharp hook
closed Cotrel-Dubousset hook
Cloward cautery hook
Cloward dural hook
Cloward hook
coarctation hook
cold knife hook
Collier-Martin hook
Colver examining hook
Colver examining retractor
hook
Colver hook
Colver retractor hook
compression hook
Converse hinged skin hook
Converse hook
Converse skin hook
cordotomy hook
corkscrew dural hook
corneal hook
Cotrel-Dubousset closed
hook
Cottle double hook
Cottle nasal hook
Cottle skin hook
Cottle tenaculum hook
Cottle-Joseph hook
cranial Jacobs hook
Crawford canaliculus hook
Crawford hook
Crile nerve hook
Crile single hook
crochet hook
crura hook
crypt hook
Culler rectus muscle hook
curved hook
curved nerve hook
Cushing dural hook

hook (*continued*)
Cushing gasserian ganglion
hook
Cushing hook
Cushing nerve hook
cystic hook
Daily fixation hook
Dandy hook
Dandy nerve hook
Davis hook
Day hook
DeBakey valve hook
decapitation hook
delicate skin hook
DePuy nerve hook
destructive obstetrical hook
Dingman zygoma hook
Dingman zygomatic hook
discission hook
dissecting hook
dissection hook
dissector hook
distraction hook
Dohlman hook
Dohlman incus hook
double hook
double-fixation hook
double-pronged Cottle hook
double-pronged Fomon hook
double-pronged hook
double-tenaculum hook
down-angle hook
downsized circular laminar
hook
Doyen rib hook
Drews hook
Drews-Sato suture-pickup
hook
Drummond hook
Dudley hook
Dudley rectal hook
Dudley rectal tenaculum hook
Dudley tenaculum hook
Duplay hook
dural hook
ear hook
ear spoon and hook
Edwards hook
Edwards rectal hook
Edwards-Levine hook
Effler-Groves hook
embrasure hook

hook (*continued*)

Emmet tenaculum hook
Emmet uterine tenaculum hook
examining hook
expressor hook
extraction hook
extractor hook
eye fixation hook
eye hook
Feaster lens hook
fenestration hook
Fenzel hook
Ferszt dissecting hook
fibroid hook
finger hook
Fink hook
Fink muscle hook
Fink oblique muscle hook
Fink-Scobie hook
Finsen tracheal hook
Finsen wound hook
Fisch dural hook
fistula hook
fistular hook
fixation hook
fixation twist hook
flat tenotomy hook
Fomon nasal hook
footplate hook
Frazier cordotomy hook
Frazier dural hook
Frazier nerve hook
Frazier skin hook
Freer double-pronged hook
Freer hook
Freer skin hook
Fresnel manipulating hook
Fukasaku pupil snapper hook
ganglion hook
Gass muscle hook
Gass retinal detachment hook
gasserian ganglion hook
Gillies bone hook
Gillies dural hook
Gillies nasal hook
Gillies skin hook
Gillies zygoma hook
Gillies zygomatic hook
Gillies-Converse skin hook
Gillies-Dingman tenaculum hook

hook (*continued*)

goiter hook
Goldman Universal nerve hook
Goodhill hook
Graefe iris hook
Graefe muscle hook
Graefe strabismus hook
Graether mushroom hook
Graham blunt hook
Graham dural hook
Graham muscle hook
Graham nerve hook
Green muscle hook
Green strabismus hook
Gross ear hook
Guthrie eye-fixation hook
Guthrie fixation hook
Guthrie iris hook
Guthrie skin hook
Gwathmey ether hook
Gynex angle hook
Gynex iris hook
Hall modified Moe hook
Hamilton-Forewater amniotomy hook
Hardesty tendon hook
Hardesty tenotomy hook
Harrington pedicle hook
Harris-Sinskey microlens hook
Haven skin graft hook
Hebra fixation hook
Helveston hook
Henton suture hook
Henton tonsillar hook
Henton tonsillar suture hook
hinged skin hook
Hirschman iris hook
Hoen nerve hook
Hosmer Dorrance hook
Hough hook
House 90-degree hook
House crural hook
House footplate hook
House incus hook
House oval-window hook
House plate hook
House strut hook
House tragus hook
Humby hook
Hunkeler ball-point hook
incus hook

hook (*continued*)
- instant skin hook
- intermediate CD hook
- intracapsular lens expressor hook
- intraocular hook
- iris hook
- irrigating iris hook
- Isola spinal implant system hook
- IUD removal hook
- Jackson tracheal hook
- Jacobson blunt hook
- Jacobs cranial hook
- Jaeger strabismus hook
- Jaffe iris hook
- Jaffe lens-manipulating hook
- Jaffe microlens hook
- Jaffe-Maltzman hook
- Jako fine ball-tip hook
- Jako-Kleinsasser ball-tip hook
- Jameson muscle hook
- Jameson strabismus hook
- Jannetta hook
- Jardine hook
- Jarit bone hook
- Jarit palate hook
- jaw hook
- Johnson skin hook
- Jordan hook
- Joseph nasal hook
- Joseph sharp skin hook
- Joseph single-prong hook
- Joseph skin hook
- Joseph tenaculum hook
- Juers hook
- Katena boat hook
- Keene compression hook
- Kelly tenaculum hook
- Kelly uterine tenaculum hook
- Kelman irrigation hook
- Kelman manipulator hook
- Kennerdell muscle hook
- Kennerdell nerve hook
- Kennerdell-Maroon hook
- Kennerdell-Maroon-Jameson hook
- Kilner goiter hook
- Kilner sharp hook
- Kilner skin hook
- Kimball nephrostomy hook
- Kincaid right-angle hook

hook (*continued*)
- Kirby double-fixation muscle hook
- Kirby intracapsular lens expressor hook
- Kirby lens expressor hook
- Kirby muscle hook
- Klapp tendon hook
- Kleinert-Kutz hook
- Kleinert-Kutz skin hook
- Kleinsasser hook
- Klemme dura hook
- Klintskog amniotomy hook
- Knapp iris hook
- Knodt hook
- Kobayashi hook
- Kratz iris push-pull hook
- Krayenbuehl dural hook
- Krayenbuehl nerve hook
- Krayenbuehl vessel hook
- Kuglen hook
- Kuglen iris hook
- Kuglen manipulating iris hook
- Küntscher nail-extracting hook
- Lahey Clinic dura hook
- Lahey hook
- Lambotte bone hook
- laminar CD hook
- Lange fistula hook
- Lange plastic surgery hook
- Laqua black line retinal hook
- large ball nerve hook
- Leader iris hook
- Leader vas hook
- Leatherman alar hook
- Leatherman child spinal hooks
- Leatherman compression hook
- Leinbach olecranon hook
- lens expressor hook
- lens hook
- Levy-Kuglen iris hook
- Lewicky microlens hook
- lid hook
- lid-retracting hook
- ligature hook
- Lillie attic hook
- Lillie ear hook
- Linton vein hook
- long blunt nerve hook
- long palate hook

hook (*continued*)
Lordan muscle-splitting hook
Loughnane prostatic hook
Lucae hook
lyre-shaped finger hook
Madden sympathectomy hook
Magielski hook
Maidera-Stern suture hook
Malgaigne patellar hook
Malis nerve hook
Manson double-ended
    strabismus hook
Marino rotatable
    transsphenoidal right-angle
    hook
Marlen airing hook
Martin rectal hook
Maumenee iris hook
Mayo fibroid hook
McIntyre irrigating iris hook
McMahon nephrostomy hook
McReynolds hook
Meyerding double-ended
    retractor with skin hook
Meyerding skin hook
microball hook
microiris hook
microlens hook
micronerve hook
microscopic hook
microsurgical ear hook
microvessel hook
middle ear hook
Millard double hook
Millard thimble hook
Miltex tenaculum hook
mitral hook
Miya hook
Moe alar hook
Moe-style spinal hook
Morrison skin hook
Moss hook
multispan fracture hook
Murphy ball-end hook
muscle hook
nasal hook
nasal polyp hook
Neivert nasal polyp hook
Neivert polyp hook
nephrostomy hook
nerve hook
nerve pull hook

hook (*continued*)
neutral hook
New tracheal hook
New tracheostomy hook
New tracheotomy hook
Newell nucleus hook
Newhart incus hook
Newman hook
Nova hook
Nugent iris hook
oblique muscle hook
O'Brien rib hook
obstetrical decapitating hook
obstetrical hook
Ochsner hook
O'Connor flat tenotomy hook
O'Connor muscle hook
O'Connor tenotomy hook
Oesch hook
open CD hook
ophthalmic hook
Osher irrigating implant hook
Osher-Fenzel hook
oval-window hook
Pajot decapitating hook
palate hook
palate pusher hook
patellar hook
Paul tendon hook
PCL-oriented placement
    marking hook
Peacock rhizotomy hook
pear-shaped nerve hook
pediatric CD hook
pediatric TSRH hook
pedicle CD hook
pedicle hook
Penn swivel hook
Pickrell hook
plain ear hook
posterior palate hook
Praeger iris hook
Pratt crypt hook
Pratt cystic hook
Pratt rectal hook
prostatic hook
Rainin iris hook
Rainin lens hook
Ramsbotham decapitating
    hook
Rappazzo iris hook
rectal crypt hook

hook (*continued*)

rectal hook
rectus muscle hook
retinal detachment hook
retractor hook
Rhoton nerve hook
ribbed hook
Rica cerumen hook
Richards bone hook
right-angle hook
Rizzuti lens hook
Robinson hook
Rolf muscle hook
Rosser crypt hook
rotatable transsphenoidal
    right-angle hook
rubber-shod hook
Russian fixation hook
Russian 4-pronged fixation
    hook
Sachs dural hook
Sadler bone hook
Saunders-Paparella stapes
    hook
Scanlan micronerve hook
Scanlan microvessel hook
Scheer hook
Schnitman skin hook
Schuknecht footplate hook
Schuknecht stapes hook
Schwartz cervical tenaculum
    hook
Schwartz expression hook
scleral hook
scleral twist fixation hook
Scobee muscle hook
Scobee oblique muscle hook
Scoville blunt hook
Scoville curved hook
Scoville curved nerve hook
Scoville dural hook
Scoville nerve hook
Scoville retractor hook
Searcy fixation hook
Selby hook
Selverstone cordotomy hook
Shambaugh endaural hook
Shambaugh fistula hook
Shambaugh microscopic hook
sharp hook
Sharpley hook
Shea fenestration hook

hook (*continued*)

Shea fistular hook
Shea footplate hook
Shea oblique hook
Shea stapes hook
Sheets iris hook
Shepard reversed iris hook
Shutt hook
side-opening laminar hook
Simon fistula hook
single hook
Sinskey iris hook
Sinskey lens-manipulating
    hook
Sinskey microlens hook
Sisson spring hook
skin graft hook
skin hook
Skin-Cottle hook
sliding barrel hook
Sluder sphenoidal hook
Smellie crochet hook
Smellie obstetrical hook
SMIC cerumen hook
Smith expressor hook
Smith lid hook
Smith lid-retracting hook
Smithwick blunt nerve hook
Smithwick dissector hook
Smithwick ganglion hook
Smithwick nerve hook
Smithwick sympathectomy
    hook
spatula hook
Speer suture hook
split-finger hook
spring hook
square-ended hook
squint hook
St. Martin-Franceschetti
    secondary cataract hook
Stallard scleral hook
stapes hook
Stevens muscle hook
Stevens tenotomy hook
Stevens traction hook
Stewart crypt hook
Stewart rectal hook
Stille coarctation hook
Storz iris hook
Storz twist hook
strabismus hook

hook (*continued*)

  straight dural hook
  straight nerve hook
  Strandell-Stille tendon hook
  Strully dural twist hook
  strut bar hook
  strut hook
  Suraci elevator hook
  suture hook
  suture pickup hook
  swivel hook
  sympathectomy hook
  Tauber ligature hook
  tenaculum hook
  tendon hook
  Tennant anchor lens-insertion hook
  Tennant iris hook
  tenotomy hook
  Texas Scottish Rite Hospital trial hook
  Toennis dural hook
  Tomas iris hook
  Tomas suture hook
  tonsillar hook
  tonsillar suture hook
  Torchia lens hook
  Torchia-Kuglen hook
  Torrence steel hook
  tracheal hook
  tracheostomy hook
  tracheotomy hook
  tragus House hook
  Trautman hook
  triple hook
  TSRH buttressed laminar hook
  TSRH circular laminar hook
  TSRH pedicle hook
  tubal hook
  twist fixation hook
  Tyrrell iris hook
  Tyrrell skin hook
  Tyrrell tympanic membrane hook
  UCLA hook
  Universal nerve hook
  University of Kansas hook
  up-angle hook
  Updegraff hook
  uterine tenaculum hook
  V. Mueller blunt hook
  valve hook

hook (*continued*)

  vas hook
  Visitec angled lens hook
  Visitec corneal suture manipulating hook
  Visitec double iris hook
  Visitec straight lens hook
  Volkmann bone hook
  Volkmann vas hook
  von Graefe muscle hook
  von Graefe strabismus hook
  von Szulec hook
  Wagener ear hook
  Walsh hook
  Weary nerve hook
  Weiss hook
  Welch Allyn hook
  Wiener corneal hook
  Wiener scleral hook
  Wiener suture hook
  Wilder foreign body hook
  Wilder lens hook
  Yankauer hook
  Yasargil spring hook
  Zaufel-Jansen ear hook
  Zielke bifid hook
  Zoellner stapes hook
  zygoma hook
  Zylik-Joseph hook
hook approximator
hook basket forceps
hook blocker
hook cautery
hook distractor
hook electrocautery
hook expressor
hook fixation
hook forceps
Hook hemi-harness shoulder immobilizer
hook holder
hook impactor
hook knife
hook manipulator
hook of the hamate
hook pusher
hook retractor
hook rotary scissors
hook scissors
hook spatula
hook with spatula
hooked catheter

hooked extractor
hooked intramedullary nails
hooked knife
hooked medullary nail
hooked nail
hooked needle
hooked wire localization
hook-end intramedullary pin
hook-lying position
hook-nail deformity
hook-on battery handle
hook-on bronchoscope
hook-on folding laryngoscope
hook-on laryngoscope handle
hook-plate fixation
hook-type dermal curet
hook-type eye implant
hookwire needle
hoop stress fracture
Hooper deep surgery scissors
Hooper pediatric scissors
Hoopes corneal marker
Hope murmur
Hope processor
Hope resuscitation bag
Hope resuscitator
Hope sign
Hopener clamp
Hopf disease
Hopf keratosis
Hopkins aortic clamp
Hopkins aortic forceps
Hopkins aortic occlusion clamp
Hopkins arthroscope
Hopkins clamp
Hopkins dilator
Hopkins direct-vision telescope
Hopkins elevator
Hopkins endoscopy telescope
Hopkins forceps
Hopkins forward-oblique
    telescope
Hopkins hemostat
Hopkins Hospital periosteal
    raspatory
Hopkins hysterectomy clamp
Hopkins rod lens
Hopkins lateral telescope
Hopkins lens
Hopkins nasal endoscopy
    telescope
Hopkins operation

Hopkins pediatric telescope
Hopkins drainage catheter
Hopkins periosteal raspatory
Hopkins plaster knife
Hopkins raspatory
Hopkins retrospective telescope
Hopkins rigid telescope
Hopkins rod
Hopkins rod endoscope
Hopkins rod lens telescope
Hopkins sigmoidoscope
Hopkins telescope
Hopkins-Cushing periosteal
    elevator
Hopmann polyp
Hopp anterior commissure
    laryngoscope blade
Hopp laryngoscope
Hopp laryngoscope blade
Hoppenfeld-Deboer approach
Hoppenfeld-Deboer technique
Hopp-Morrison laryngoscope
hordeolum eye implant
Horgan center blade
Horgan operation
Horgan retractor
Horgan-Coryllos-Moure rib
    shears
Horgan-Wells rib shears
Hori technique
Horico diamond instrument
Horico disk
Horizon stent
Horizon surgical ligating and
    marking clip
horizontal atrophy
horizontal bipedicle dermal flap
horizontal canal
horizontal drain attachment
    device
horizontal fissure
horizontal flap
horizontal flexible bar retractor
horizontal folds
horizontal fracture
horizontal gastroplasty
horizontal growth phase
horizontal incision
horizontal lid laxity
horizontal limb
horizontal mattress suture
    technique

horizontal mattress sutures
horizontal maxillary
  advancement
horizontal maxillary fracture
horizontal oblique fracture
horizontal osteotomy
horizontal overlap
horizontal plane
horizontal plate of palatine bone
horizontal position
horizontal projection
horizontal resorption
horizontal retractor
horizontal rhytids
horizontal ring curet
horizontal sternotomy
horizontal sutures
horizontal tract
horizontal tube
horizontal tube attachment device
horizontal-shaped skin paddle
horizontovertical laryngectomy
hormonal evaluation
hormone
  adrenocorticotropic hormone
    (ACTH)
  follicle stimulating hormone
    (FSH)
  melanocyte-stimulating
    hormone
  pituitary growth hormone
  placental growth hormone
  recombinant human growth
    hormone (rhGH)
  synthetic human growth
    hormone
horn
  Ammon horn
  cicatricial horn
  cutaneous horn
  lateral ventricle horn
  lesser horn
  mucosal horn
  posterior horn
  sebaceous horn
  warty horn
horn cells
Horn endo-otoprobe laser
horn of clitoris
horn of lateral ventricle
horn of spinal cord
horn of uterus

Horner muscle
Horner operation
Horner ptosis
Horner pupil
Horner syndrome
Horner-Trantas spots
hornified epithelium
hornpipe position
horny spine
horopter
  Vieth-Mueller horopter
horsehair sutures
horseshoe abscess
horseshoe fistula
horseshoe flap
horseshoe headrest
horseshoe heel pad
horseshoe incision
horseshoe kidney
horseshoe Le Fort I osteotomy
horseshoe magnet
horseshoe placenta
horseshoe pregnancy
horseshoe sutures
horseshoe tear
horseshoe tourniquet
horseshoe-shaped flap
horseshoe-shaped incision
horseshoe-shaped pad
horseshoe-shaped skin flap
Horsley anastomosis
Horsley bone cutter
Horsley bone knife
Horsley bone rongeur
Horsley bone wax
Horsley bone-cutting forceps
Horsley cranial bone rongeur
Horsley cranial rongeur
Horsley dural knife
Horsley dural separator
Horsley elevator
Horsley gastrectomy
Horsley guard
Horsley operation
Horsley pyloroplasty
Horsley rongeur
Horsley separator
Horsley spine cutter
Horsley sutures
Horsley trephine
Horsley wax
Horsley-Clarke stereotactic frame

Horsley-Stille bone-cutting
　　forceps
Horsley-Stille rib shears
Horsley-Stille rib shears forceps
Horton-Devine dermal graft
Horton-Devine operation
Horvath operation
Horwitz-Adams ankle
　　arthrodesis
Horwitz-Adams ankle fusion
Horwitz-Adams operation
hose
　　antiembolic hose
　　delivery hose
　　elastic hose
　　Juzo hose
　　Linton elastic hose
　　TED hose
　　thromboembolic disease hose
Hosel needle holder
Hosel retractor
Hosemann choledochus forceps
Hosemann choledochus knife
hose-pipe appearance of
　　terminal ileum
Hosford double-ended lacrimal
　　dilator
Hosford eye dilator
Hosford foreign body spud
Hosford lacrimal dilator
Hosford meibomian gland
　　expressor
Hosford spud
Hosford-Hicks forceps
Hosford-Hicks needle
Hosford-Hicks transfer forceps
Hoskins beaked Colibri forceps
Hoskins fine straight forceps
Hoskins fixation forceps
Hoskins microstraight forceps
Hoskins miniaturized micro-
　　straight forceps
Hoskins nylon suture laser lens
Hoskins razor blade fragment
Hoskins razor fragment blade
Hoskins straight microiris
　　forceps
Hoskins suture forceps
Hoskins-Barkan goniotomy
　　infant lens
Hoskins-Castroviejo corneal
　　scissors

Hoskins-Dallas intraocular
　　lens-inserting forceps
Hoskins-Drake implant
Hoskins-Luntz forceps
Hoskins-Skeleton fine forceps
Hoskins-Skeleton grooved broad-
　　tipped forceps
Hoskins-Westcott tenotomy
　　scissors
Hosmer above-knee rotator
Hosmer Dorrance fracture
　　bracing
Hosmer Dorrance hook
Hosmer elbow prosthesis
Hosmer single-axis locking knee
Hosmer voluntary control 4-bar
　　knee orthosis
Hosmer Walk prosthesis
Hosmer weight-activated
　　locking knee prosthesis
Hosmer-Dorrance voluntary
　　control 4-bar knee
　　mechanism
hospital bed
hospital bucket
hospital course
hospital gangrene
hospital monitoring
hospitalization
Hossli suction tube
host tissue forceps
hostile abdomen
hot abscess
hot biopsy forceps
hot biopsy technique
hot compress
hot cone
hot conization
hot defect
hot flexible forceps
hot gangrene
hot heel sign
hot infusion
hot knife
hot lesion
hot line
hot moist compresses
hot moist pack
hot nodule
hot pack
hot pad
hot patella sign

Hot Sampler disposable hot
  biopsy forceps
hot snare
hot spot
hot wet pack
Hotchkiss ear suction tube
Hotchkiss operation
Hotchkiss-McManus PAS
  technique
hot-cold lysis
hot cross bun skull
hot-knife conization
Hotsy cautery
Hotsy Totsy cautery
hot-tip laser
hot-tipped catheter
hot-wire pneumotachometer
hot-wire respirometer
Hotz ear applicator
Hotz ear curet
Hotz ear probe
Hotz entropion operation
Hotz procedure
Hotz-Anagnostakis operation
Hotz-type alveolar molding plate
Hough alligator forceps
Hough anterior crurotomy nipper
Hough auger
Hough bed
Hough chisel
Hough crurotomy nipper
Hough crurotomy saw
Hough curet
Hough drape
Hough drum scraper
Hough ear forceps
Hough elevator
Hough excavator
Hough excavator hoe
Hough fascial knife
Hough footplate auger
Hough footplate pick
Hough gouge
Hough hoe
Hough hoe elevator
Hough hook
Hough incision knife
Hough middle ear instrument
Hough operation
Hough osteotome
Hough oval-window excavator
Hough pick

Hough scissors
Hough spatula
Hough spatula elevator
Hough stapedectomy
Hough stapedectomy footplate
  pick
Hough stapedial footplate auger
Hough Teflon cutter
Hough tendon knife
Hough tympanoplasty knife
Hough whirlybird excavator
Hough whirlybird knife
Hough-Boucheron ear speculum
Hough-Cadogan suction tube
Hough-Derlacki mobilizer
Hough-Powell digitizer
Hough-Rosen knife
Hough-Saunders excavator
Hough-Saunders stapes hoe
Houghton rongeur
Houghton-Akroyd fracture
  technique
Houghton-Akroyd open
  reduction
Hough-Wullstein bur saw
Hough-Wullstein crurotomy saw
  bur
Hough-Wullstein saw
Hounsfield unit
hourglass anterior commissure
  laryngoscope
hourglass bladder
hourglass chest
hourglass deformity
hourglass dressing
hourglass gallbladder
hourglass head
hourglass membrane
hourglass murmur
hourglass nasal deformity
hourglass stomach
Hourin tonsil needle
House 90-degree hook
House adapter
House advancement anoplasty
House alligator crimper forceps
House alligator forceps
House alligator grasping forceps
House alligator scissors
House alligator strut forceps
House-Pulec otic-periotic shunt
House angular knife

House blade
House block
House bur
House calipers
House calipers strut
House chisel
House crimper forceps
House crural hook
House cup forceps
House curet
House cutting block
House detachable blade
House dissecting scissors
House dissector
House drum elevator
House ear curet
House ear elevator
House ear forceps
House ear knife
House ear separator
House endaural elevator
House endolymphatic shunt
House endolymphatic shunt
    tube
House endolymphatic shunt
    tube introducer
House excavator
House flap anoplasty
House flap elevator
House footplate chisel
House footplate hook
House Gelfoam pressure forceps
House Gimmick drum elevator
House Gimmick stapes elevator
House grade facial palsy
House grasping forceps
House guide
House hammer
House hand-held double-end
    retractor
House hand-held retractor
House hook
House implant
House incudostapedial joint
    knife
House incus hook
House incus replacement
    prosthesis
House irrigator
House knife blade
House knife handle
House lacrimal dilator

House lancet
House lancet knife
House malleus nipper
House measuring rod
House middle ear instrument
House middle ear mirror
House miniature forceps
House myringoplasty knife
House myringotomy knife
House myringotomy knife
    handle
House needle
House neurovascular clip
House obtuse pick
House oiler tip
House ophthalmic blade
House oval-cup forceps
House oval-window hook
House oval-window pick
House pick
House piston
House piston prosthesis
House piston wire
House plate hook
House pressure forceps
House prosthesis
House reconstruction
House retractor
House rod
House round knife
House scissors
House separator
House shunt
House shunt tube
House sickle knife
House sliding advancement flap
House speculum
House stainless steel mesh
    prosthesis
House stapedectomy
House stapes curet
House stapes elevator
House stapes needle
House stapes piston
House stapes speculum
House stapes wire prosthesis
House sterilizing box
House strut calipers
House strut forceps
House strut guide
House strut hook
House strut pick

House sucker irrigator
House suction adapter
House suction irrigator
House suction tube
House suction tube adapter
House suction-irrigator tube
House tantalum prosthesis
House tapping hammer
House technique
House Teflon cutting block
House Teflon-coated elevator
House tragus hook
House T-tube irrigator
House tube
House tympanoplasty curet
House tympanoplasty knife
House wire
House wire guide
House wire loop
House wire stapes prosthesis
House wire-fat prosthesis
House-Barbara needle
House-Barbara pick
House-Barbara shattering needle
House-Baron suction tube
House-Bellucci alligator scissors
House-Bellucci-Shambaugh
    alligator scissors
House-Bellucci-Shambaugh
    scissors
House-Billeau ear loop
House-Brackmann classification
    for facial nerve function
House-Brackmann facial
    weakness scale
House-Brackmann grade (I-V)
House-Brackmann scoring
House-Buck curet
House-Crabtree dissector
House-Crabtree dissector pick
House-Delrin cutting block
House-Derlacki chisel
House-Dieter eye forceps
House-Dieter malleus nipper
House-Dieter nipper
House-Hough excavator
House-Paparella stapes curet
Housepian aneurysm clip
Housepian clip-applying forceps
Housepian sellar punch
House-Radpour suction tube
House-Radpour suction-irrigator

House-Rosen needle
House-Rosen utility knife
House-Saunders middle ear
    curet
House-Sheehy knife curet
House-Stevenson suction tube
House-Stevenson suction-
    irrigator
House-Urban bone holder
House-Urban dissector
House-Urban ear marker
House-Urban gold ear marker
House-Urban holder
House-Urban marker
House-Urban middle fossa
    retractor
House-Urban oiler tip
House-Urban retractor
House-Urban rotary dissector
House-Urban temporal bone
    holder
House-Urban tip
House-Urban tube
House-Urban vacuum rotary
    dissector
House-Urban-Pentax camera
House-Urban-Stille camera
House-Wullstein cup ear forceps
House-Wullstein cup forceps
House-Wullstein ear forceps
House-Wullstein forceps
House-Wullstein oval cup
    forceps
House-Wullstein perforating bur
Housset-Debray gastroscope
Houston fold
Houston halo
Houston halo cervical support
Houston halo cervical traction
Houston halo traction
Houston halo traction collar
Houston muscle
Houston nasal osteotome
Houston operation
Houston osteotomy
Houston shoulder arthrodesis
Houston valve
Houtz endometrial curet
Hovanian procedure
Hovanian transfer technique
Hovius canal
Hovius circle

Hovius membrane
Hovius plexus
Howard abrader
Howard basket
Howard closing forceps
Howard corneal abrader
Howard Jones needle
Howard spinal curet
Howard spinal stone dislodger
Howard spiral dislodger
Howard stone basket
Howard stone dislodger
Howard technique
Howard tonsil forceps
Howard tonsillar forceps
Howard tonsil-ligating forceps
Howard-DeBakey aortic
    aneurysm clamp
Howard-Flaherty spiral dislodger
Howard-Flaherty spiral stone
    dislodger
Howard-Schatz laser
Howard-Schatz laser technique
Howarth nasal raspatory
Howell tibial guide
Howell biliary aspiration needle
Howell biopsy aspiration needle
Howell coronary scissors
Howell rotatable papillotome
Howell rotatable
    sphincterotome
Howell tunable diaphragm
    stethoscope
Howell-Jolly bodies
Howland lock
Howmedica Centrax head
    replacement
Howmedica cerclage
Howmedica Duracon implant
Howmedica instruments
Howmedica Kinematic II knee
    prosthesis
Howmedica lag screw
Howmedica Luer screw
Howmedica microfixation forceps
Howmedica microfixation plate
    cutter
Howmedica monotube
Howmedica monotube external
    rotator
Howmedica orthopedic
    prosthesis

Howmedica PCA textured hip
Howmedica plate
Howmedica prosthesis
Howmedica screw
Howmedica Simplex P cement
Howmedica surgical
    instruments
Howmedica total condylar knee
    replacement
Howmedica Universal
    compression screw
Howmedica Universal total knee
    prosthesis
Howorth approach
Howorth elevator
Howorth operation
Howorth osteotome
Howorth procedure
Howorth prosthesis
Howorth retractor
Howorth toothed retractor
Howse-Coventry hip prosthesis
Howse-Coventry prosthesis
Howse-Coventry screw
Howship-Romberg sign
Howtek scanner
Hoxworth clip
Hoxworth forceps
Hoya objective refractometer
Hoyer anastomosis
Hoyer lift
Hoyer lift sling
Hoyer snare
Hoyt deep-surgery forceps
Hoyt hemostatic forceps
Hoytenberger tissue forceps
HPC guidewire
HPU (heater probe unit)
HR needle (high-risk needle)
Hruby contact implant
Hruby contact lens
Hruby laser
Hryntschak catheter
H-shaped anal anastomosis
H-shaped capsular incision
H-shaped ileal pouch
H-shaped ileal pouch-anal
    anastomosis
H-shaped plate
HSS knee prosthesis
HSS total condylar knee
    prosthesis

HTO fixator
HTO wedge tissue allograft
HTR (hard tissue replacement)
HTR-MFI chin implant
HTR-MFI curved implant
HTR-MFI implant
HTR-MFI malar implant
HTR-MFI onlay facial
    augmentation implant
HTR-MFI paranasal implant
HTR-MFI premaxillary implant
HTR-MFI ramus implant
HTR-MFI straight implant
H-type tracheoesophageal fistula
Huang Universal arm retractor
Huang vein holder
hub saw
Hubbard airplane vent tube
Hubbard bolt
Hubbard corneoscleral forceps
Hubbard electrode
Hubbard plate
Hubbard retractor
Hubbard tank
Hubbard tub
Hubbard-Nylok bolt
Hubbell intraocular implant lens
Huber forceps handle
Huber needle
Huber needle for translumbar
    aortogram
Huber point needle
Huber probe
Huber procedure
Huber technique
Huchard sign
Huckstep intramedullary
    compression nail
Huco diamond knife
Hudgins salpingography cannula
Hudson adapter
Hudson all-clear nasal cannula
Hudson bone retractor
Hudson brace bur
Hudson brace with bur
Hudson brain forceps
Hudson cerebellar attachment
Hudson cerebellar attachment drill
Hudson cerebellar extension
Hudson clamp
Hudson conical bur
Hudson cranial bur

Hudson cranial drill
Hudson cranial forceps
Hudson cranial rongeur
Hudson cranial rongeur forceps
Hudson double-ended elevator
Hudson dressing forceps
Hudson drill
Hudson Lifesaver resuscitator
Hudson line
Hudson retractor
Hudson rongeur
Hudson rongeur forceps
Hudson tissue forceps
Hudson tissue-dressing forceps
Hudson TLSO brace
Hudson-type oxygen mask
Hudson-Jones knee cage brace
Hudson-Stahli line
Hueck ligament
Hueston finger amputation
Hueston flap procedure
Hueston spiral flap
Hueter bandage
Hueter incision
Hueter line
Hueter maneuver
Hueter perineal dressing
Hueter sign
Hueter-Mayo operation
Huey scissors
Huey suture scissors
Huffman infant vaginal
    speculum
Huffman infant vaginoscope
Huffman speculum
Huffman vaginoscope
Huffman-Graves adolescent
    vaginal speculum
Huffman-Graves speculum
Huffman-Graves vaginal
    speculum
Huffman-Huber infant
    urethrotome
Huffman-Huber infant
    vaginoscope
Huffman-Huber vaginoscope
Hufford esophagoscope
Hufnagel aortic clamp
Hufnagel ascending aortic clamp
Hufnagel caged-ball heart valve
Hufnagel clamp
Hufnagel commissurotomy knife

Hufnagel disk heart valve
Hufnagel disk heart valve
    prosthesis
Hufnagel forceps
Hufnagel implant
Hufnagel knife
Hufnagel low-profile heart
    prosthesis
Hufnagel mitral valve forceps
Hufnagel mitral valve-holding
    forceps
Hufnagel needle holder
Hufnagel operation
Hufnagel prosthesis
Hufnagel prosthetic valve
Hufnagel valve
Hufnagel valve prosthesis
Hufnagel valve-holding clamp
Hufnagel-Kay heart valve
Hufnagel-Ryder needle holder
Hu-Friedy dental bur
Hu-Friedy elevator
Hu-Friedy PermaSharp sutures
Hu-Friedy suction tip aspirator
Huger diamond-back nasal
    scissors
Huggins operation
Hugh Young adrenalectomy
Hugh Young hemostat
Hugh Young incision
Hugh Young pedicle clamp
Hughes eye implant
Hughes eye reconstruction
Hughes eyelid operation
Hughes flap
Hughes fulguration electrode
Hughes implant
Hughes modification of Burch
    technique
Hughes operation
Hughes tarsoconjunctival flap
Hughston button for meniscal
    repair
Hughston classification
Hughston knee jerk test
Hughston knee view on x-ray
Hughston patellar procedure
Hughston patellar transplant
Hughston procedure
Hughston quadriceps
    reconstruction
Hughston technique

Hughston test
Hughston view
Hughston-Degenhardt
    reconstruction
Hughston-Hauser procedure
Hughston-Jacobson lateral
    compartment
    reconstruction
Hughston-Jacobson technique
Huguier sinus
HUI (Harris uterine injection)
HUI catheter
HUI device for tubal lavage
HUI uterine injector
Huibregtse biliary stent
Huibregtse-Katon ERCP catheter
Huibregtse-Katon needle knife
Huibregtse-Katon papillotome
Huibregtse-Katon
    sphincterotome
Hui-Linscheid procedure
Hulbert electrosurgical knife
Hulbert endo-electrode set
Hulka cannula
Hulka clip
Hulka clip applier
Hulka clip forceps
Hulka tenaculum
Hulka tenaculum forceps
Hulka uterine cannula
Hulka uterine manipulator
Hulka uterine tenaculum
Hulka-Clemens clip
Hulka-Kenwick uterine elevator
Hulka-Kenwick uterine-elevating
    forceps
Hulka-Kenwick uterine-
    manipulating forceps
Hulten-Stille cannula
human immunodeficiency virus
human lymphocyte antigens
human lyophilized dura
    cystoplasty
human mammary tumor virus
    (HMTV)
human papilloma virus
human tissue collagen matrix
human tissue polymer
human umbilical vein bypass
    graft (HUV bypass graft)
Humby alar cartilage relocation
Humby hook

Humby knife
Humby operation
Hume aortic clamp
humeral approach
humeral articulation
humeral bone
humeral cutting guide
humeral fracture
humeral head
humeral head-splitting fracture
humeral impactor
humeral line
humeral physeal fracture
humeral reamer
humeral retractor
humeral saw
humeral shaft
humeral shaft fracture
humeral supracondylar fracture
humeroperoneal neuromuscular
    disease
humeroradial articulation
humeroulnar articulation
humeroulnar joint
humerus
    amputation through surgical
        neck of humerus
    capitulum of humerus
    head of humerus
    nutrient arteries of humerus
    shaft of humerus
    surgical neck of humerus
humerus splint
HUMI cannula
HUMI catheter
HUMI cervical forceps
HUMI device for tubal lavage
HUMI injector
HUMI uterine manipulator
Hummelsheim operation
Hummelsheim procedure
Hummer microdebrider
humor
    aqueous humor
    fatty humor
    vitreous humor
humor of eye
humoral immunity
hump
    biparietal hump
    bone hump
    buffalo hump

hump (*continued*)
    dorsal hump
    dowager hump
    dromedary hump
    Hampton hump
    nasal hump
hump forceps
hump gouge
hump removal
humpback deformity
humpback deformity of
    scaphoid
Humphrey automatic
    keratometer
Humphrey automatic refractor
Humphrey coronary sinus-
    sucker suction tube
Humphrey coronary sinus
    suction
Humphrey coronary sinus
    suction tube
Humphrey coronary sinus-
    sucker suction tube
Humphrey eye instruments
Humphrey lens analyzer
Humphrey perimeter
Humphrey retinal imager
Humphrey vision analyzer
Humphries aortic aneurysm
    clamp
Humphries aortic clamp
Humphries reverse-curve aortic
    clamp
Humphry ligament
Hungerford technique
Hunkeler ball-point hook
Hunkeler frown incision marker
Hunkeler intraocular lens
Hunkeler lightweight intraocular
    lens implant
Hunner ulcer
Hunsaker jet ventilation tube
Hunstad infusion needle
Hunstad system for tumescent
    anesthesia
Hunt angiographic trocar
Hunt angled serrated ring
    forceps
Hunt angled-tip forceps
Hunt arachnoid dissector
Hunt atrophy
Hunt bipolar forceps

Hunt bladder retractor
Hunt chalazion forceps
Hunt chalazion scissors
Hunt colostomy clamp
Hunt dissector
Hunt grasping forceps
Hunt metal sound
Hunt needle
Hunt neuralgia
Hunt operation
Hunt reaction
Hunt retractor
Hunt sound
Hunt syndrome
Hunt test
Hunt trocar
Hunt tumor forceps
Hunt vessel forceps
Hunter balloon
Hunter canal
Hunter curet
Hunter dural separator
Hunter glossitis
Hunter gubernaculum
Hunter large uterine curet
Hunter ligament
Hunter line
Hunter 1-piece all-PMMA
    intraocular lens
Hunter open cord tendon
    implant
Hunter operation
Hunter rod
Hunter separator
Hunter Silastic rod
Hunter splinter forceps
Hunter syndrome
Hunter technique for Toupet
    fundoplication
Hunter tendon prosthesis
Hunter tendon rod
Hunter uterine curet
hunterian ligation
hunterian perforator
Hunter-Satinsky clamp
Hunter-Schreger line
Hunter-Sessions balloon
Hunter-Sessions vena cava-
    occluding balloon catheter
Hunt-Hess neurological
    classification
Huntington bone graft

Huntington chorea
Huntington disease
Huntington operation
Huntington technique
Huntington tibial technique
Hunt-Lawrence pouch
Hunt-Reich secondary cannula
Hunt-Yasargil pituitary forceps
Hupp retractor
Hupp tracheal retractor
Hurd bipolar diathermy
    electrode
Hurd bone forceps
Hurd bone-cutting forceps
Hurd dissector
Hurd electrode
Hurd elevator
Hurd pillar retractor
Hurd retractor
Hurd septal bone-cutting
    forceps
Hurd septal elevator
Hurd septal forceps
Hurd septum-cutting forceps
Hurd suture needle
Hurd tonsil dissector
Hurd tonsil elevator
Hurd tonsil knife
Hurd tonsillar dissector
Hurd tonsillar pillar retractor
Hurd turbinate electrode
Hurd-Morrison dissector
Hurdner tissue forceps
Hurd-Weder tonsil dissector
Hurler syndrome
Hurler-Scheie syndrome
Hurricaine local anesthetic
Hurson flexible pressure clamp
Hurson flexible retractor
Hurson flexible sliding clamp
Hurst bougie
Hurst bullet-tip dilator
Hurst bullet-tip esophageal
    dilator
Hurst esophageal bougie
Hurst esophageal dilator
Hurst mercury bougie
Hurst mercury dilator
Hurst mercury-filled bougie
Hurst mercury-filled dilator
Hurst mercury-filled esophageal
    bougie

Hurst-Maloney dilator
Hurst-Tucker pneumatic dilator
Hurteau forceps
Hurthle adenoma
Hurthle cell tumor
Hurtig dilator
Hurwitt catheter
Hurwitz catheter
Hurwitz clamp
Hurwitz dialysis catheter
Hurwitz esophageal clamp
Hurwitz gastrostomy tube
Hurwitz intestinal clamp
Hurwitz thoracic trocar
Hurwitz trocar
Huschke auditory teeth
Huschke canal
Huschke cartilage
Huschke foramen
Huschke ligament
Huschke valve
Huse cannula
Husen button for meniscal repair
Husk mastoid rongeur
Husk bone rongeur
Hustead epidural needle
Hutch bladder diverticulum
Hutch evacuator
Hutch operation
Hutch ureteral reflux operation
Hutchins biopsy needle
Hutchinson crescentic notch
Hutchinson facies
Hutchinson fracture
Hutchinson freckle
Hutchinson iris retractor
Hutchinson patch
Hutchinson sign
Hutchinson-Gilford disease
Hutchinson-Gilford progeria
Hutchinson-Gilford syndrome
Hutchison syndrome
HUV bypass graft (human
    umbilical vein bypass graft)
Huxley layer
Huxley membrane
Huxley respirator
Huxley sheath
Huygens eyepiece
huygenian eyepiece
Huzly applicator
Huzly aspirator

Huzly irrigator
Huzly tampon applicator
HV splint
HVF ventilator
hyaline articular cartilage
hyaline basement membrane
hyaline body
hyaline cartilage
hyaline degeneration
hyaline membrane disease
hyaline membrane syndrome
hyalinization
hyaloid artery
hyaloid body
hyaloid canal
hyaloid fossa
hyaloid membrane
hyaloid posterior membrane
hyaloid vessel
Hyams catheter
Hyams conization
Hyams conization technique
Hyams meatus clamp
Hyams operation
Hyams scleral knife
Hybbinette-Eden operation
hybrid fixation of hip
    replacement component
hybrid prosthesis
hybridization-subtraction
    technique
hybridoma technique
hybrid-type implant
hyCURE collagen hemostatic
    wound dressing
hyCURE hydrolyzed protein
    powder and exudate
    absorber
hyCURE wound care powder
hydatid cyst
hydatid cyst intrahepatic rupture
hydatid liver cyst
hydatid disease
hydatid of Morgagni
hydatid pregnancy
hydatidiform mole
hydatidostomy
Hyde frog irrigating cannula
Hyde astigmatism ruler
Hyde corneal forceps
Hyde double-curved corneal
    forceps

Hyde irrigator and aspirator unit
Hyde needle holder
Hyde shunt
hydraclip
hydraclip clamp
Hydracon contact lens
HydraGran absorption dressing
Hydragrip clamp
Hydragrip clamp insert
Hydrajaw insert
hydrarthrosis
hydrasoft contact lens
Hydrasorb foam wound dressing
hydrated pyelogram
hydration and turgor
hydration therapy
hydraulic dissection
hydraulic hand dynamometer
hydraulic incontinent prosthesis
hydraulic knee
hydraulic knee unit prosthesis
hydraulic vein stripper
Hydro Plus coated guidewire
hydroactive dressing
HydroBlade keratome
HydroBrush keratome
Hydrocal cast material
Hydro-Cast dental mold
HydroCath central venous
    catheter
hydrocele
    cervical hydrocele
    Dupuytren hydrocele
    encysted hydrocele
    funicular hydrocele
    Gibbon hydrocele
    Maunoir hydrocele
    noncommunicating
        hydrocele
    Nuck hydrocele
    scrotal hydrocele
    Volkmann operation for
        hydrocele
hydrocele colli
hydrocele feminae
hydrocele fluid
hydrocele of Nuck
hydrocele repair
hydrocele trocar
hydrocelectomy
    Andrews hydrocelectomy
    Lord hydrocelectomy

hydrocephalus
    H-H neonatal shunt for
        hydrocephalus
hydrocephalus shunt
hydrocephalus shunt
    instruments
Hydrocol dressing
Hydrocol sacral wound dressing
Hydrocollator gel pack
Hydrocollator heating unit
Hydrocollator pad
Hydrocollator steam packs
hydrocolloid dressing
hydrocolloid impression
    material
hydrocolloid occlusive dressing
hydrocurve contact lens
hydrocurve intraocular lens
    implant
HydroDerm transparent dressing
hydrodissection tip
hydrofiber dressing
Hydroflex inflatable penile
    prosthesis
Hydroflex penile implant
Hydroflex penile implant rod
Hydroflex penile prosthesis
Hydroflex penile semirigid
    implant
Hydrofloss electronic oral
    irrigator
HydroFlow technique
Hydrogel dressing
Hydrogel expansile intraocular
    lens
Hydrogel wound dressing
Hydrogel-coated PTCA balloon
    catheter
Hydrogel alginate
Hydrojet aspirator
HydroKeratome
Hydrolyser microcatheter
hydrolysis
    ATP hydrolysis
    intragastric hydrolysis
    urea hydrolysis
hydrolysis of solution
hydrolysis of surfactant
Hydromer coated polyurethane
    stent
Hydromer grafted catheter
Hydron burn bandage

Hydron lens
hydronephrosis
hydroperitoneum
hydropertubation
hydrophilic contact lens
hydrophilic dilator
hydrophilic filter media
hydrophilic gel
hydrophilic polymer dressing
hydrophilic polymer-coated
    steerable guidewire
hydrophilic polyurethane foam
    dressing
hydrophilic semipermeable
    absorbent polyurethane
    foam dressing
hydrophilic-coated guidewire
hydropic nephrosis
hydropigenous nephritis
HydroPlus stent
hydropolymer dressing
hydrops abdominis
hydrops fetalis
hydrops folliculi
hydrops of gallbladder
hydrops of pleura
hydrops spurius
hydrosalpinx follicularis
hydrosalpinx simplex
hydrostatic bag
hydrostatic balloon
hydrostatic balloon catheter
hydrostatic balloon dilation
hydrostatic decompression
hydrostatic dilator
hydrostatic dissector
hydrostatic irrigator
hydrostatic pressure
hydrothorax
hydrotubation
hydroureter
hydroureteral nephrosis
Hydroview intraocular lens
hydroxyapatite (HA)
    Calcitite hydroxyapatite
    nonresorbable
        hydroxyapatite
    porous hydroxyapatite
hydroxyapatite adhesive
hydroxyapatite arthropathy
hydroxyapatite block graft
hydroxyapatite ceramic material

hydroxyapatite
    chondrocalcinosis
hydroxyapatite coated implant
hydroxyapatite fibrin glue
hydroxyapatite implant material
hydroxyapatite ocular implant
hydroxyapatite orbital implant
hydroxyapatite ossicular
    prosthesis
hydroxyapatite-coated implant
hydroxyethyl methacrylate
hydroxyproline
hydroxypropyl methylcellulose
HyFil hydrogel dressing
Hyflex X-File instrument
hyfrecation
hyfrecator
    Birtcher hyfrecator
hyfrecator-coagulator
Hyginet elastic dressing retainer
Hyginet outer expandable
    netting
hygroma
    cervical hygroma
    cystic hygroma
    Fleischmann hygroma
    subdural hygroma
hygroma colli cysticum
hygromatous
hygroscopic expansion
hygroscopic heat and moisture
    exchanger
hygroscopic technique
Hylaform viscoelastic gel
Hylamer acetabular line
hymen
    cribriform hymen
    denticular hymen
    falciform hymen
    fenestrated hymen
    imperforate hymen
    intact hymen
    lunar hymen
    rigid hymen
    septate hymen
hymenal band
hymenal cyst
hymenal membrane
hymenal orifice
hymenal ring
hymenal syndrome
hymenectomy

hymenoplasty
hymenorrhaphy
hymenotomy
Hynes pharyngoplasty
Hynes-Anderson dismembered
    pyeloplasty
hyoepiglottic ligament
hyoglossal membrane
hyoglossal muscle
hyoglossus muscle
hyoid advancement
hyoid arch
hyoid bone
hyoid bone fracture
hyoid bone resection
hyoid branchial arch
hyoid bursa
hyoid cartilage
hyoid myotomy
hyoid region
hyoid syndrome
hyoid-cutting forceps
hyomandibular cleft
hyothyroid ligament
hyothyroid membrane
Hypafix retention tape
Hypafix tape
hyparterial bronchus
hypaxial muscle
hyperabduction maneuver
hyperactive bowel sounds
hyperactive carotid sinus reflex
hyperactive glabellar muscle
hyperactive muscle
hyperactive reflex
hyperacute graft-versus-host
    disease
hyperacute phase
hyperaerated chest
hyperalimentation
    parenteral hyperalimentation
hyperalimentation catheter
hyperalimentation feeding
hyperalimentation fluid
hyperalimentation solution
hyperalimentation therapy
hyperalimentation tubing
hyperbaric anesthesia
hyperbaric chamber
hyperbaric local anesthetic
hyperbaric oxygen (HBO)
hyperbaric oxygen therapy

hyperbaric oxygen-induced
    angiogenesis
hyperbaric spinal anesthesia
hypercellular gland
hypercholesterolemic
    splenomegaly
Hyperclens soap
HyperControl elbow brace
hyperdactyly
hyperdense brain lesion
hyperdistended abdomen
hyperdivergent facial pattern
hyperdivergent patient
hyperdivergent skeletal pattern
hyperdynamic circulation
hyperechoic
hyperemesis gravidarum
hyperemia
hyperemic membranes
hyperesthesia
    cervical hyperesthesia
    laryngeal hyperesthesia
    sensory hyperesthesia
hypereuryopia
Hyperex thoracic orthosis
hyperextension
    cruciform anterior spinal
        hyperextension (CASH)
hyperextension brace
hyperextension deformity
hyperextension fracture frame
hyperextension-hyperflexion
    injury
hyperfiltration
    capillary hyperfiltration
    glomerular hyperfiltration
    renal hyperfiltration
hyperfiltration injury
Hyperflex flexible guidewire
Hyperflex tracheostomy tube
hyperfractionated total body
    irradiation
hyperfunctional facial lines
hyperfunctional facial rhytids of
    the forehead
hyperfunctional glabellar line
Hypergel dressing
Hypergel hydrogel wound
    dressing
Hypergel wound dressing
hyperintense brain lesion
hyperintense mass

Hyperion LTK laser
hyperirritability
hyperkeratosis
  epidermolytic hyperkeratosis
  subungual hyperkeratosis
hyperkeratosis congenita
hyperkeratosis figurata
  centrifuga atrophica
hyperkeratosis follicularis
hyperkeratosis penetrans
hyperkeratotic epidermis
hyperkeratotic lesion
hyperkinetic facial lines
hyperlucent lung
hypermastia
hypermature cataract
hypermelanosis
  linear and whorled nevoid
    hypermelanosis
  nevoid hypermelanosis
hypermobile mucosa
hypermobility
  temporomandibular joint
    hypermobility
hypernephroid carcinoma
hypernephroma
hyperopia
hyperopic
hyperosmolar coma
hyperostosis
  ankylosing hyperostosis
  diffuse idiopathic sclerosing
    hyperostosis (DISH)
  diffuse idiopathic skeletal
    hyperostosis
  generalized cortical
    hyperostosis
  infantile cortical hyperostosis
  reactive hyperostosis
  subpontic hyperostosis
hyperostosis corticalis
  deformans
hyperostosis corticalis
  generalisata
hyperostosis cranii
hyperparathyroidism
  ectopic hyperparathyroidism
  primary hyperparathyroidism
hyperparotidism
hyperpathia
hyperperfusion injury
hyperphalangism

hyperphoria
hyperpigmentation
  centrofacial
    hyperpigmentation
  cutaneous hyperpigmentation
  postpeel hyperpigmentation
  postsclerotherapy
    hyperpigmentation
hyperpigmented lesion
hyperpituitarism
hyperpituitary gigantism
hyperplasia
  4-gland hyperplasia
  adenomatous hyperplasia
  asymmetric hyperplasia
  atypical hyperplasia (AH)
  atypical melanocytic
    hyperplasia
  basal cell hyperplasia
  benign hyperplasia
  benign prostatic hyperplasia
    (BPH)
  cementum hyperplasia
  condylar hyperplasia
  congenital adrenal hyperplasia
  congenital sebaceous
    hyperplasia
  coronoid hyperplasia
  cystic hyperplasia
  ductal hyperplasia
  endometrial hyperplasia
  fibromuscular hyperplasia
  fibrous hyperplasia
  florid hyperplasia
  focal epithelial hyperplasia
  focal nodular hyperplasia
    (FNH)
  hemimandibular hyperplasia
  idiopathic gingival
    hyperplasia
  inferior pole hyperplasia
  inflammatory fibrous
    hyperplasia
  inflammatory papillary
    hyperplasia
  intimal hyperplasia
  intraductal hyperplasia
  juxtaglomerular cell
    hyperplasia
  lipoid hyperplasia
  lobar hyperplasia
  lobular hyperplasia

hyperplasia (*continued*)
  lymphoid hyperplasia
  medication-induced
    hyperplasia
  moderate hyperplasia
  multigland hyperplasia
  multiglandular parathyroid
    hyperplasia
  multiple gland hyperplasia
  neoplastic hyperplasia
  papillary hyperplasia
  parathyroid hyperplasia
  parotid lymph node
    hyperplasia
  polyclonal hyperplasia
  pseudocarcinomatous
    hyperplasia
  pseudoepitheliomatous
    hyperplasia
  sebaceous hyperplasia
  senile sebaceous hyperplasia
  solid hyperplasia
  sporadic multigland
    hyperplasia
  sporadic multiple gland
    parathyroid hyperplasia
  squamous hyperplasia
  stent-induced intimal
    hyperplasia
  stromal hyperplasia
  Swiss-cheese hyperplasia
  thyroid hyperplasia
  tissue hyperplasia
  trilobar hyperplasia
  verrucous hyperplasia
hyperplastic chondrodystrophy
hyperplastic cyst
hyperplastic cystadenoma
hyperplastic epidermis
hyperplastic epithelial lesion
hyperplastic gastric polyp
hyperplastic gland
hyperplastic graft
hyperplastic inflammation
hyperplastic laryngitis
hyperplastic lesion
hyperplastic membrane
hyperplastic mucosa
hyperplastic polyp
hyperplastic rhinosinusitis
hyperplastic tissue
hyperplastic tumor

hyperreflexia
hyperreflexic bladder
hyperresonance to percussion
hyperresonant abdomen
hypersecretion
hypersensitive xiphoid
  syndrome
hypersensitivity
hypersensitivity skin testing
hypersplenia
hypersplenism
hypertelorism
  canthal hypertelorism
  Munro classification of orbital
    hypertelorism (types A-D)
  orbital hypertelorism
  pseudo-orbital hypertelorism
hypertension
  ambulatory venous
    hypertension
  Goldblatt hypertension
  intracranial hypertension
  lithotripsy-induced
    hypertension
  portal hypertension
  postoperative hypertension
  postural hypertension
  pulmonary hypertension
  renovascular hypertension
  venous hypertension
hypertension and impotency
hypertensive arteriopathy
hypertensive arteriosclerosis
hypertensive heart disease
hypertensive lower esophageal
  sphincter
hypertensive pulmonary
  vascular disease
hypertensive therapy
hypertensive vascular disease
hyperthenar eminence
hyperthermia of anesthesia
hyperthermia therapy
hyperthermic isolated limb
  perfusion (HILP)
hyperthyroid
hyperthyroidism
hypertonia
  lip hypertonia
hypertonic bladder
hypertonic muscle
hypertonic solution

hypertonic sphincter
hypertonic uterine dysfunction
hypertrophic angioma
hypertrophic burn scar
hypertrophic cardiomyopathy
(HCM)
hypertrophic catarrh
hypertrophic cicatrix
hypertrophic gastritis
hypertrophic granulation tissue
hypertrophic hemangioma
hypertrophic laryngitis
hypertrophic osteoarthropathy
hypertrophic port-wine stain
hypertrophic pyloric stenosis
hypertrophic rosacea
hypertrophic scar
hypertrophic scarring
hypertrophic spur
hypertrophica
  acne hypertrophica
  tenosynovitis hypertrophica
hypertrophied papilla
hypertrophy
  asymmetric septal
    hypertrophy (ASH)
  benign prostatic hypertrophy
  biatrial hypertrophy
  bilateral masseteric
    hypertrophy
  Billroth hypertrophy
  breast hypertrophy
  cardiac hypertrophy
  compensatory hypertrophy
  complementary hypertrophy
  concentric hypertrophy
  eccentric hypertrophy
  fat hypertrophy
  fatty hypertrophy
  fibrovascular hypertrophy
  genital hypertrophy
  glandular hypertrophy
  hemangiectatic hypertrophy
  hemifacial hypertrophy
  labial hypertrophy
  limb hypertrophy
  masseter muscle hypertrophy
  masseteric hypertrophy
  mixed hypertrophy
  myocardial hypertrophy
  prostatic hypertrophy
  skeletal hypertrophy

hypertrophy (*continued*)
  submucosal gland
    hypertrophy
  unilateral facial hypertrophy
  unilateral hypertrophy
  ventricular hypertrophy
  virginal hypertrophy
hypertropia
hypervascular fragment
hyperventilation maneuver
hyperventilation procedure
hyperventilation syndrome
hypesthesia
  bilateral hypesthesia
  pinwheel hypesthesia
  stocking-and-glove-type
    hypesthesia
hypesthesia and paralysis
hyphema
  8-ball hyphema
  anterior chamber hyphema
hypnosis anesthesia
hypnotic agents
hypnotic effect
hypoactive bowel sounds
hypoactive bowel tones
hypoactive deep tendon reflexes
hypoactive movements
hypoactive reflex
hypobaric anesthesia
hypobaric spinal anesthesia
hypobranchial eminence
hypocalcification
hypochondriac region
hypochondriac region of
    abdomen
hypochondrium
    (*pl.* hypochondria)
hypocondylar
hypocontractile
hypocystomy
hypocystotomy
hypodactyly
hypodense brain lesion
hypodermatoclysis
hypodermatomy
hypodermic implantation
hypodermic injection
hypodermic microscope
hypodermic needle
hypodermic syringe
hypodermic tablet

hypodermoclysis
hypoechoic lesion
hypoesthesia
hypofunction
hypogastric arteries
hypogastric artery forceps
hypogastric artery ligation
hypogastric branch of
    iliohypogastric nerve
hypogastric flap
hypogastric ganglion
hypogastric nerve
hypogastric plexus
hypogastric plexus block
    anesthesia technique
hypogastric pressure
hypogastric region
hypogastric vein
hypogastric vessel
hypogenesis
hypoglossal canal
hypoglossal facial nerve
    anastomosis
hypoglossal facial transfer
    procedure
hypoglossal ganglion
hypoglossal nerve
    (cranial nerve 12)
hypoglossal nerve sign
hypoglossal paralysis
hypoglossal plexus
hypoglossal-facial
    neuroanastomosis
hypoglossal-to-facial nerve transfer
hypoglossia
hypoglossia-hypodactylia
    syndrome
hypoglossia-hypodactyly syndrome
hypoglottis
hypognathous
hypokalemia
hypokinesia
hypokinesis
hypolipoproteinemia
hypomastia with ptosis
hypomelanosis
    congenital circumscribed
        hypomelanosis
    idiopathic guttate
        hypomelanosis
hypomeric muscle
hyponychia

hyponychium
hyponychon
hypoparathyroidism
hypoperfusion
    global hypoperfusion
    regional hypoperfusion
    splanchnic hypoperfusion
    spreading hypoperfusion
    systemic hypoperfusion
hypophalangism
hypopharyngeal carcinoma
hypopharyngeal diverticulum
hypopharyngeal eminence
hypopharyngeal lipoma
hypopharyngeal squamous cell
    carcinoma
hypopharyngeal stenosis
hypopharyngoscope
hypopharynx
hypophysial duct
hypophysial forceps
hypophysial fossa
hypophysial portal circulation
hypophysection
hypophysectomy
    partial central
        hypophysectomy
    stereotaxic
        hypophysectomy
    total hypophysectomy
    transethmoidal
        hypophysectomy
    transsphenoidal
        hypophysectomy
    unilateral hypophysectomy
hypophysectomy forceps
hypophysectomy instruments
hypophysial curet
hypophysial eminence
hypophysis
    infundibulum of hypophysis
    pharyngeal hypophysis
    tentorium of hypophysis
hypopigmentation
    cutaneous
        hypopigmentation
    postinflammatory
        hypopigmentation
    postpeel hypopigmentation
hypopigmented macular
    eruption
hypopituitarism

hypoplasia
  aortic hypoplasia
  breast hypoplasia
  cartilage-hair hypoplasia
  condylar hypoplasia
  focal dermal hypoplasia
  lingual hypoplasia
  malar hypoplasia
  mandibular condylar
    hypoplasia
  mandibular hypoplasia
  maxillary hypoplasia
  maxillary-zygomatic
    hypoplasia
  midface hypoplasia
  midfacial hypoplasia
  soft tissue hypoplasia
  thenar muscle hypoplasia
  thumb hypoplasia
  zygomaticomaxillary
    hypoplasia
hypoplastic chondrodystrophy
hypoplastic heart
hypoplastic kidney
hypoplastic left heart repair
hypoplastic left heart syndrome
hypoplastic mandible
hypoplastic mandibular body
hypoplastic thumb
hypoplastic tuberous breast
hypoplastic urethra
hypoplastic valve
hypopyon operation
hyporeflexic bladder
hyposomia
hypospadias
  balanic hypospadias
  distal hypospadias
  female hypospadias
  glandular hypospadias
  Hacker hypospadias
  midpenile hypospadias
  penile hypospadias
  penoscrotal hypospadias
  perineal hypospadias
  pseudovaginal hypospadias
hypospadias operation
hypospadias repair
hypospray jet injection needle
hypostasis
hypostatic abscess
hypostatic ectasia

hypostatic splenization
hypotelorism
  ocular hypotelorism
  orbital hypotelorism
hypotension
  induced hypotension
  orthostatic hypotension
  postural hypotension
  vascular hypotension
hypotensive agents
hypotensive anesthesia
hypotensive surgery
hypothalamic area
hypothalamic-hypophysial portal
    circulation
hypothalamic-hypophysial-
    ovarian-endometrial axis
hypothalamic-pituitary-adrenal
    axis
hypothalamic-pituitary-ovarian
    axis
hypothalamic-pituitary-testicular
    axis
hypothalamotomy
hypothalamus
hypothenar eminence
hypothenar fascia
hypothenar hammer syndrome
hypothenar muscles
hypothenar septum
hypothenar space
hypothermal
hypothermia
  drug-induced hypothermia
  extracorporeal exchange
    hypothermia
  intraoperative core
    hypothermia
  surface cooling hypothermia
hypothermia anesthetic
    technique
hypothermia blanket
hypothermia cap
hypothermia mattress
hypothermic anesthesia
hypothermic effect
hypothermic hepatic
    perfusion
hypothermic mattress
hypothermic procedure
hypothermic surgery
hypothermic technique

hypothermy
hypothyroid ligament
hypothyroidism
hypotonic bladder
hypotonic colon
hypotonic duodenography
hypotonic muscle
hypotonicity
hypotony
hypotympanotomy
hypotympanum
hypovolemic shock
hypoxemia
hypoxia and anoxia
hypsibrachycephalic
hypsicephalic
hypsicephaly
hypsiconchous
hypsiloid angle
hypsiloid cartilage
hypsistaphylia
hypsistenocephalic
hypocephalus
hyrax appliance
Hyrtl anastomosis
Hyrtl foramen
Hyrtl loop
Hyrtl nerve
Hyrtl sphincter
Hyskon distending medium
Hyskon irrigation solution
hysterectomy
  abdominal hysterectomy
  abdominovaginal
   hysterectomy
  Bonney abdominal
   hysterectomy
  Bonney hysterectomy
  cesarean hysterectomy
  chemical hysterectomy
  classic abdominal Semm
   hysterectomy
  Delaplane hysterectomy
  Doyen hysterectomy
  Doyen vaginal hysterectomy
  Eden-Lawson hysterectomy
  extrafascial hysterectomy
  Freund hysterectomy
  gasless laparoscopic
   hysterectomy
  Gelpi-Lowry hysterectomy
  Heaney vaginal hysterectomy

hysterectomy (*continued*)
  laparoscopic Doderlein
   hysterectomy
  laparoscopic radical
   hysterectomy
  laparoscopically assisted
   vaginal hysterectomy (LAVH)
  laparoscopic-assisted vaginal
   hysterectomy
  Lash hysterectomy
  Latzko radical abdominal
   hysterectomy
  Latzko radical hysterectomy
  Mayo hysterectomy
  Mayo-Ward hysterectomy
  Meigs radical hysterectomy
  Meigs-Wertheim hysterectomy
  modified radical hysterectomy
  Mueller vaginal hysterectomy
  obstetrical hysterectomy
  paravaginal hysterectomy
  pelviscopic intrafascial
   hysterectomy
  Porro cesarean hysterectomy
  Porro hysterectomy
  Pean hysterectomy
  radical abdominal
   hysterectomy
  radical vaginal hysterectomy
  Ries-Wertheim hysterectomy
  Schauta radical vaginal
   hysterectomy
  Spalding-Richardson
   hysterectomy
  Spaulding-Richardson
   hysterectomy
  subtotal hysterectomy
  supracervical hysterectomy
  supravaginal hysterectomy
  TeLinde hysterectomy
  total abdominal hysterectomy
   (TAH)
  total hysterectomy
  vaginal hysterectomy
  Ward-Mayo vaginal
   hysterectomy
  Wertheim hysterectomy
hysterectomy clamp
hysterectomy forceps
hysterectomy kit
hysterectomy knife
hysterectomy retractor

hysterectomy scissors
hysteresis of pacemaker
hysteresis rate of pacemaker
hysterical anesthesia
hysterocolpectomy
hysterocolposcope
hysterofiberscope
    Olympus flexible
        hysterofiberscope
hysteroflator
    Lindeman hysteroflator
hysterogram
hysterography
hysterolysis
hysteromyomectomy
hysteromyotomy
hystero-oophorectomy
hysteropexy
    abdominal hysteropexy
    Abell hysteropexy
    Alexander-Adams
        hysteropexy
    Baldy-Webster hysteropexy
    Davis hysteropexy
    Simpson hysteropexy
    subperitoneal Baldy-Webster
        hysteropexy
hysteroplasty
hysterorrhaphy
hysterosalpingectomy
    laparoscopic
        hysterosalpingectomy
hysterosalpingogram (HSG)
hysterosalpingography
hysterosalpingography
    catheter
hysterosalpingo-oophorectomy
hysterosalpingorrhaphy
hysterosalpingostomy

hysteroscope
    ACMI hysteroscope
    ACMI Micro-H hysteroscope
    AMSCO hysteroscope
    Baggish hysteroscope
    Circon ACMI hysteroscope
    contact hysteroscope
    diagnostic hysteroscope
    Elmed hysteroscope
    examining hysteroscope
    fiberoptic hysteroscope
    Fujinon flexible
        hysteroscope
    Galileo rigid hysteroscope
    Hamou hysteroscope
    Karl Storz 15 French flexible
        hysteroscope
    MicroSpan hysteroscope
    Olympus hysteroscope
    OPERA Star hysteroscope
    Scopemaster contact
        hysteroscope
    Storz hysteroscope
    Valle hysteroscope
    Van der Pas hysteroscope
hysteroscope sheath
hysteroscopic insufflator
hysteroscopic surgery
hysteroscopy
hysterotomy
hysterotrachelectomy
hysterotracheloplasty
hysterotrachelorrhaphy
hysterotrachelotomy
Hy-Tape adhesive
Hy-Tape latex-free surgical tape
Hy-Tape surgical tape
HyTek guidewire
Hz (hertz units)

I bolt
I marker
I&A (irrigation and aspiration)
I&A coaxial cannula
I&A instrument
I&A kit
I&A machine
I&D (incision and drainage)
I&O (in and out; intake and output)
I/E ratio (inspiratory/expiratory ratio)
I-131 (radioactive iodine)
I-131 uptake
I-A unit (irrigate-aspirate unit)
IAB catheter (intra-aortic balloon catheter)
IABP (intra-aortic balloon pump)
Iamin Gel wound dressing
Iamin hydrating gel wound dressing
IAN (inferior alveolar nerve)
iatrogenic arteriovenous fistula
iatrogenic bowel injury
iatrogenic cholesteatoma
iatrogenic deformity
iatrogenic disease
iatrogenic fracture
iatrogenic hernia defect
iatrogenic hypothyroidism
iatrogenic immunosuppression
iatrogenic infection
iatrogenic nasal stenosis
iatrogenic perforation
iatrogenic tension pneumothorax
iatrogenic transmission
iatrogenic trauma
iatrogenic ureteral injury
iatrotechnique
IBD (inflammatory bowel disease)
I-beam
   Jergesen I-beam
I-beam cement punch

I-beam hemiarthroplasty hip prosthesis
I-beam hip hemiarthroplasty
I-beam hip operation
I-beam nail
I-beam press-fit punch
IBF knee instrument
IBF total knee instrumentation
IBM blood cell processor
IBS (inflammatory bowel syndrome) nerve
IBSL (internal branch of superior laryngeal) nerve
ICA (internal carotid artery)
ICAO (internal carotid artery occlusion)
Icarex mirror reflex lens camera
ICCE (intracapsular cataract extraction)
ICD (intercanthal distance)
ice clot evacuator
ice skater fracture
Ice Wedge hot/cold therapy wrap
iced cystogram
iced saline
iced saline lavage
iced saline solution
Icelandic form of intracranial hemorrhage
icepick-type scar
ice-tong calipers
icing heart
ICLH (Imperial College, London Hospital)
ICLH arthroplasty
ICLH double-cup arthroplasty
ICP (intracranial pressure)
ICP Camino bolt
ICP catheter
ICP monitor
ICP-T fiberoptic ICP monitoring catheter
ICR (intracavitary radium)

ICS plate
ICSI (intracytoplasmic sperm
    injection)
ICSI IVF (intracytoplasmic
    sperm injection for in vitro
    fertilization)
ictal abnormality
ICV reservoir
IDC (interdigitating dendritic
    cell)
IDD (intraluminal duodenal
    diverticulum)
Ideal arch wire
Ideal automatic tourniquet
Ideal cardiac device
ideal occlusion
Ideal tourniquet
Ideberg glenoid fracture
    classification
identical pattern
identical plane dose
identical point
identifiable electrical activity
identified and ligated
Identifit hip prosthesis
Identity pacemaker
identity formation
IDET procedure
idioglossia
idioglottic
idiographic approach
idiomuscular contractility
idiomuscular contraction
idionodal rhythm
idiopathic
idiopathic adult intussusception
idiopathic bone cavity
idiopathic brown induration
idiopathic dilation
idiopathic eczematous disease
idiopathic enlargement
idiopathic facial paralysis
idiopathic fibromatosis
idiopathic gingival hyperplasia
idiopathic glossitis
idiopathic guttate
    hypomelanosis
idiopathic hypertrophic
    subaortic stenosis (IHSS)
idiopathic ileocecal
    intussusception
idiopathic megacolon

idiopathic multiple hemorrhagic
    sarcoma
idiopathic multiple pigmented
    hemorrhagic sarcoma
idiopathic obstruction
idiopathic peptic ulcer disease
idiopathic preretinal membrane
idiopathic ventricular fibrillation
idiopathic/tobacco-associated
    leukoplakia
idiosyncratic allergic reaction
idioventricular rhythm
IDIS angiography (intraoperative
    digital subtraction
    angiography)
IEA graft
IFC pheresis (intermittent-flow
    centrifugation pheresis)
I-Flow nerve block infusion kit
IgA (immunoglobulin A)
IgE (immunoglobulin E)
Iglesias continuous-flow
    resectoscope
Iglesias dilator
Iglesias electrode
Iglesias evacuator
Iglesias fiberoptic resectoscope
Iglesias microlens resectoscope
ignipuncture
IHSS (idiopathic hypertrophic
    subaortic stenosis)
IKI catgut sutures
Ikuta clamp approximator
Ikuta fixation device
ILA stapler
ILA stapling device
ILA surgical stapler
ILAC target
ILA-series stapling device
ileal arteries
ileal biopsy
ileal bladder
ileal colostomy
ileal conduit
ileal conduit urinary diversion
ileal inflammation
ileal inflow tract
ileal J-pouch
ileal loop
ileal loop stoma
ileal perforation
ileal pouch surgery

ileal pouch-anal anastomosis (IPAA)
ileal pouch-distal rectal
    anastomosis
ileal pull-through operation
ileal pull-through procedure
ileal resection
ileal reservoir
ileal reservoir construction
ileal S-pouch
ileal stasis
ileal transverse colostomy
ileal varices
ileal veins
ileal W-pouch
ileal-sigmoid anastomosis
ileectomy
ileitis
    abdominal ileitis
    distal ileitis
    regional ileitis
ileoanal anastomosis
ileoanal endorectal pull-through
    operation
ileoanal pouch
ileoanal pouch procedure
ileoanal pull-through procedure
ileoanal reservoir
ileoascending colostomy
ileobladder cystoscopy
ileobladderoscopy
ileocecal bladder
ileocecal bladder construction
ileocecal cystoplasty
ileocecal edema
ileocecal eminence
ileocecal fold
ileocecal junction
ileocecal pouch
ileocecal valve
ileocecocystoplasty bladder
    augmentation
ileocecostomy
ileocecum
ileocolectomy
ileocolic artery
ileocolic fold
ileocolic intussusception
ileocolic lymph nodes
ileocolic plexus
ileocolic resection
ileocolic vein
ileocolitis ulcerosa chronica

ileocolonic pouch urinary
    diversion
ileocolonic resection
ileocolostomy
    end-loop ileocolostomy
    end-to-end ileocolostomy
    LeDuc-Camey ileocolostomy
ileocolotomy
ileocutaneous fistula
ileocystoplasty
    Camey ileocystoplasty
    clam ileocystoplasty
    LeDuc-Camey ileocystoplasty
    T-type ileocystoplasty
ileocystostomy
    cutaneous ileocystostomy
ileoduodenal fistula
ileoduodenotomy
ileoentectropy
ileoesophagostomy
ileofemoral deep vein thrombosis
ileofemoral wing fracture
ileogastric reflex
ileoileal anastomosis
ileoileal intussusception
ileoileostomy
ileojejunal bypass
ileojejunitis
ileoloopogram
ileoneocystostomy
ileopancreatostomy
ileopexy
ileoproctostomy
ileorectal anastomosis (IRA)
ileorectostomy
ileorrhaphy
ileoscopy
ileosigmoid anastomosis
ileosigmoid colostomy
ileosigmoid fistula
ileosigmoid knot
ileosigmoidostomy
ileostogram
ileostomy
    Bishop-Koop ileostomy
    blow-hole ileostomy
    Brooke ileostomy
    continent ileostomy
    cutaneous ileostomy
    defunctioning loop ileostomy
    Dennis-Brooke ileostomy
    diversionary ileostomy

ileostomy (*continued*)
  diverting loop ileostomy
  double-barreled ileostomy
  end ileostomy
  end-loop ileostomy
  Goligher extraperitoneal
    ileostomy
  high output ileostomy
  incontinent ileostomy
  J-loop ileostomy
  Koch continent ileostomy
  Koch reservoir ileostomy
  loop ileostomy
  loop-end ileostomy
  permanent ileostomy
  permanent loop ileostomy
  pouched ileostomy
  split ileostomy
  temporary loop ileostomy
  terminal ileostomy
  Turnbull end-loop ileostomy
ileostomy appliance
ileostomy bag
ileostomy closure
ileostomy construction
ileostomy effluent
ileostomy formation
ileostomy pouch
ileostomy reversal
ileostomy sac
ileostomy spout
ileostomy stenosis
ileostomy stoma
ileostomy without colectomy
ileotomy
ileotransverse colon
    anastomosis
ileotransverse colostomy
ileotransverse colotomy
ileotransversotomy
ileoureterostomy
  Bricker ileoureterostomy
ileovesical anastomosis
ileovesical fistula
ileovesicostomy
  incontinent ileovesicostomy
ileum
  distal ileum
  hose-pipe appearance of
    terminal ileum
  jejunalization of the ileum
  terminal ileum

ileus
  adhesive ileus
  adynamic ileus
  duodenal ileus
  dynamic ileus
  gallbladder ileus
  gallstone ileus
  mechanical ileus
  meconium ileus
  occlusive ileus
  paralytic ileus
  postoperative ileus
  reflex ileus
  reflexive ileus
  reflex-type ileus
ileus following abdominal
    surgery
Ilfeld brace
Ilfeld splint
Ilfeld-Gustafson splint
Ilg capsular forceps
Ilg curved microtying forceps
Ilg insertion forceps
Ilg lens loupe
Ilg microneedle holder
Ilg needle
Ilg needle holder
Ilg probe
iliac artery
iliac artery aneurysm
iliac artery angioplasty
iliac artery stent
iliac autograft
iliac bifurcation
iliac bone
iliac buttressing procedure
iliac chain
iliac clamp
iliac colon
iliac crest
iliac crest biopsy
iliac crest bone aspiration
iliac crest bone graft
iliac crest bone graft
    stabilization
iliac crest free flap
iliac crest free osseous flap
iliac crest osseous flap
iliac crest osteocutaneous flap
iliac crest osteomuscular flap
iliac crest resection
iliac endarterectomy

iliac fixation
iliac flexure of colon
iliac forceps
iliac fossa
iliac graft
iliac graft separator
iliac lymph nodes
iliac muscle
iliac osteocutaneous flap
iliac osteocutaneous free flap
iliac region
iliac screw
iliac spine
iliac vein
iliac vessels
iliac wing resection
iliac-femoral cannula
iliacosubfascial fossa
iliacosubfascial hernia
Iliff approach
Iliff blepharochalasis forceps
Iliff clamp
Iliff dacryoattachment for
  Stryker saw
Iliff exenteration
Iliff eyelid repair
Iliff lacrimal probe
Iliff lacrimal trephine
Iliff procedure to correct ptosis
Iliff ptosis operation
Iliff trephine
Iliff-Haus operation
Iliff-Park speculum
Iliff-Wright fascia needle
ilioabdominal
iliococcygeal muscle
iliocolotomy
iliocostal muscle
iliocostal space
iliocostalis dorsi muscle
iliocostalis lumborum muscle
iliofemoral approach
iliofemoral ligament
iliofemoral pedicle flap
iliofemoral triangle
iliohypogastric nerve
iliohypogastric nerve block
iliohypogastric neuralgia
ilioinguinal acetabular approach
ilioinguinal artery
ilioinguinal incision
ilioinguinal nerve

ilioinguinal nerve block
ilioinguinal neuralgia
ilioinguinal vein
ilioinguinal-iliohypogastric nerve
  block (INB)
iliolumbar artery
iliolumbar vein
iliolumbocostoabdominal
iliopectinate line
iliopectineal arch
iliopectineal bursa
iliopectineal eminence
iliopectineal fossa
iliopectineal line
iliopopliteal bypass
iliopsoas bursa
iliopsoas muscle
iliopsoas sign
iliopubic eminence
iliosacral articulation
iliosacral screw
iliotibial band (ITB)
iliotibial band graft
  augmentation
iliotibial tract
iliotrochanteric ligament
ilium
  ala of ilium
  Duverney fracture of ilium
ilium bone
ilium crest
ilium microvascular transfer
Ilizarov bone-lengthening
  technique
Ilizarov bone-straightening
  technique
Ilizarov circular external
  fixator
Ilizarov circulator external
  fixator
Ilizarov device
Ilizarov distractor
Ilizarov external fixation
Ilizarov external ring fixator
Ilizarov frame
Ilizarov hybrid fixator
Ilizarov internal fixation
Ilizarov leg-lengthening
  procedure
Ilizarov limb-lengthening
  technique
Ilizarov procedure

Ilizarov ring
Ilizarov screw
Ilizarov technique
Illi intracranial fixation device
Illinois needle
Illouz aspirative lipoplasty
Illouz liposuction technique
Illouz modified tip
Illouz original liposuction
   technique
Illouz procedure
Illouz standard tip
Illouz suction cannula
Illumen-8 guiding catheter
Illumen-9 guiding catheter
Illumina Pro series laparoscopic
   laser
illuminated nasal speculum
illuminated probe
illuminated speculum
illuminated suction needle
illuminated ureter probe
illuminating stylet
illumination probe
illuminator (*see also*
   transilluminator)
  Barkan illuminator
  Britetrac illuminator
  Bush ureteral illuminator
  Cogent XL illuminator
  DyoBrite illuminator
  fiberoptic surgical field
     illuminator
  Gyn-A-Lite speculum
     illuminator
  intramedullary illuminator
  Light Commander xenon
     illuminator
  Luxo surgical illuminator
  Mammo Mask illuminator
  Novar oral illuminator
  Pelosi illuminator
  Pilling fiberoptic illuminator
  slit illuminator
  speculum illuminator
  suspended operating
     illuminator
  ureteral illuminator
  XL illuminator
illuminator ear unit
illuminator head unit
Ilopan disposable syringe

ILP (intralesional laser
   photocoagulation)
ILS (intraluminal stapler)
ILUS catheter
ILVEN (inflammatory linear
   verrucous epidermal nevus)
IM Jaws alligator forceps
IM nail
IM tendon stripper
IM/EM tibial resection guide
IMA (internal mammary artery,
   inferior mesenteric artery)
IMA graft
IMA retractor
IMA scissors
IMAB (internal mammary artery
   bypass)
image
  2nd-echo image
  2C-L image
  3-dimensional image
  4C-T image
  5C-T image
  A-mode image
  AP-T image
  axial spin-echo image
  B-mode image
  body image
  cross-sectional image
  DG-L image
  DG-T image
  dynamic image
  ejection shell image
  ejection-fraction image
  endoscopic image
  endoscopic video image
  field-echo image
  flow-on gradient-echo image
  fluid-attenuated inversion
     recovery image
  gradient-recalled echo image
  gradient-echo MR image
  guidance image
  hard-copy image
  high-resolution image
  intermediate-weighted MR
     images
  mirror image
  MP-L image
  MP-T image
  multiplanar image
  MV-T image

image (*continued*)
  planar image
  point-counting image
  pulsed Doppler images
  Purkinje images
  radiographic image
  readable image
  real-time echo-planar image
  real-time multiplanar image
  sagittal spin-echo image
  short-pulse repetition
    time/echo time image
  single-slice gradient-echo image
  spin-echo image
  static image
  surface-projection rendering
    image
  T1-weighted spin-echo image
  T2-weighted spin-echo image
  thin-section axial image
  tomographic images
  transmission image
  ultrasound image
  video image
  x-ray image
image acquisition
image analysis
image compression
image converter
Image custom external breast
  prosthesis
image formation
image guide bundle
image intensification
image intensifier
image interpretation
image Orthicon tube
image point
image registration
image subtraction
Imagecath rapid exchange
  angioscope
image-guided breast biopsy
  (GBB)
image-guided fine-needle
  aspiration biopsy
image-guided pancreatic core
  aspiration
image-guided stereotactic brain
  biopsy
image-guided surgery (IGS)
image-processing unit

ImagerTorque selective catheter
image-related screening
  technique
imaginary line
imaging densitometer
imaging modality
imaging procedure
imaging staging
imaging strategy
imaging study
imaging technique
imaging-angioplasty balloon
  catheter
Imagyn microlaparoscope
Imagyn surgical stapler
Imatron C-100 system for heart
  studies
Imatron C-100 system for high-
  resolution body imaging
Imatron C-100 Ultrafast CT
  scanner
Imatron Fastrac C-100 cine x-ray
  CT scanner
imbalance
  occlusal imbalance
  orofacial muscle imbalance
imbedded microtransducer
imbricated sutures
imbricating layer
imbricating stitch
imbricating sutures
imbrication
  capsular imbrication
  MacNab line for facet
    imbrication
  medial capsular imbrication
  medialis obliquus imbrication
  platysmal imbrication
  retinal imbrication
imbrication face-lift
imbrication herniorrhaphy
imbrication lines of von Ebner
IMC (internal mammary chain)
IMCOR implant
IMED Gemini volumetric
  controller
IMED Gemini volumetric pump
IMED infusion device
IMED infusion pump
Imex antepartum monitor
Imex OB Doppler
Imex scleral implant

IMF (inframammary fold, intermaxillary fixation)
immaculate hemostasis
immature bone
immature cataract
immature dentinoma
immature labor
immature ovarian teratoma
immature scar
immeasurable fluid loss
ImmEdge Pen
immediate amputation
immediate breast reconstruction
immediate echolalia
immediate extension technique
immediate fit prosthesis
immediate flap
immediate hypersensitivity
immediate impression implant
Immediate Load implant
immediate postoperative prosthesis (IPOP)
immediate postsurgical fitting (IPSF)
immediate transfer flap
immediate transfusion
immediately (stat)
Immergut suction tube
Immergut suction-coagulation tube
immersible video camera
immersion technique
imminent abortion
imminent death
Immix bioabsorbable implant
immobile
immobility
immobilization
    cast immobilization
    cervical immobilization
    postoperative immobilization
    rigid cervical immobilization
    shoulder immobilization
    sling immobilization
    spica cast immobilization
    sternal-occipital-mandibular immobilization
    tooth immobilization
    Treponema pallidum immobilization
    Webril immobilization

immobilization jacket
immobilization of joint
immobilized extremity
immobilized in cast
immobilized in plaster cast
immobilized joint
immobilized knee
immobilizer
    arm and shoulder immobilizer
    Comfort wrist immobilizer
    C-splint immobilizer
    Ezy Wrap shoulder immobilizer
    Hold-and-Hold immobilizer
    Hook hemi-harness shoulder immobilizer
    Kapp surgical knee immobilizer
    knee immobilizer
    long leg immobilizer
    Neutral WEDGE immobilizer
    OEC knee immobilizer
    Olympic immobilizer
    QuickCast wrist immobilizer
    shoulder abduction immobilizer
    sternal-occipital-mandibular immobilizer (SOMI)
    sterno-occipitomanubrial immobilizer
    Trimline knee immobilizer
    Velpeau shoulder immobilizer
    Watco knee immobilizer
    Westfield-style acromioclavicular immobilizer
    Zinco Gunslinger shoulder immobilizer
immobilizing bandage
immobilizing dressing
immotile cilia syndrome
immovable bandage
immovable joint
immune adherence
immune complex
immune deficiency
immune globulin
immune modulation
immune response
immune system anatomy
immune-mediated coagulation disorder

immunity
  active immunity
  adaptive immunity
  cell-mediated immunity
  humoral immunity
  innate immunity
  passive immunity
  tumor-specific transplantation
    immunity (TSTI)
immunity reaction
immunization
immuno-inflammation
immunoassay
  fluorescent immunoassay (FIA)
immunobiology
immunocompetent cell
immunocompetent site
immunocompetent squamous
    cell cancer model
immunocompetent tissue therapy
immunocompromised patient
immunocytochemical approach
immunodeficiency
immunodepressed patient
immunoelectro-osmophoresis
immunoelectrophoresis
immunofiltration
immunofluorescence
immunofluorescent examination
immunofluorescent microscopy
immunofluorescent stain
immunogenicity
immunoglobulin
  hepatitis B immunoglobulin
    (HBIG)
  salivary immunoglobulin
  secretory immunoglobulin
immunoglobulin A (IgA)
immunoglobulin E (IgE)
immunoglobulin G (IgG)
immunohistochemical study
immunohistochemical technique
immunologic classification
immunologic complication
immunologic memory
immunologic suppression
immunologic workup
immunological competence
immunomodulating effect
immunomodulation
immunoperoxidase stain
immunoproliferative lesion

immunoprophylaxis
immunoradiometric analysis
    (IRMA)
immunoreactive
immunoreactivity
immunostainer
immunosuppressant
immunosuppressed patient
immunosuppression
  drug-induced
    immunosuppression
  iatrogenic
    immunosuppression
immunosuppressive agent
immunosuppressive therapy
immunosurveillance
immunotherapy
Imount instruments
IMP Femur Finder
IMP Universal lateral positioner
IMPA (incisal mandibular plane
    angle)
impact glove
impact injury
Impact modular porous
    prosthesis
impacted calculus
impacted cerumen
impacted fecal material
impacted feces
impacted foreign body
impacted fracture
impacted molar
impacted stone
impacted stool
impacted teeth
impaction
  basket impaction
  bony impaction
  ceruminal impaction
  dental impaction
  endoscope impaction
  fecal impaction
  foreign body impaction
  LeFort I impaction
  mesioangular impaction
  mucoid impaction
  posterior impaction
  stone impaction
  stool impaction
impaction lesion
impaction point

impactor
  Austin Moore impactor
  Biomet impactor
  Bio-Moore stem impactor
  bone impactor
  Cloward bone graft impactor
  Cloward dowel impactor
  Cohort spinal impactor
  cup impactor
  electromechanical impactor
  femoral impactor
  hook impactor
  humeral impactor
  Kuenstcher impactor
  lateral gutter impactor
  Moe impactor
  mushroom impactor
  orthopedic impactor
  Raylor bone impactor
  rotating air impactor
  rotating arm impactor
  shell impactor
  Smith-Petersen impactor
  spinal impactor
  spondylophyte impactor
  tibial impactor
  vertebral body impactor
impactor plate
impactor rod
impactor-extractor
impaired ability
impaired function
impaired regeneration syndrome
impaired sensation
impaired vision
impairment
  cardiac impairment
  kidney impairment
  motor impairment
  neurological impairment
  partial impairment
  sensory impairment
impalement injury
impassable obstruction
impassable scar tissue
impassable stricture
impedance
  acoustic impedance
  electric impedance
  electrode impedance
  input impedance
impedance electrode

impedance matching
impedance plethysmography
  (IPG)
impediment
impending infarction
impending stroke
Imperatori antral wash bottle
Imperatori laryngeal forceps
Imperatori laryngeal speculum
imperceptible pulse
imperfect closure
imperforate anus
imperforate hymen
impermeable dressing
impermeable junction
impermeable stricture
Impersol catheter
Impex aspiration and injection
  needle
Impex diamond radial
  keratotomy knife
Impex/Lerner foldable lens
  removing set
impingement
  graft impingement
  nerve impingement
impingement rod
impingement sign
impingement syndrome
ImplaMed gold screw
implant (*see also* implant, graft,
  lens patch, prosthesis, valve)
  2-piece implant
  3D Accuscan facial implant
  3i implant
  3M implant
  3M mammary implant
  4-loop iris clip implant
  4-loop iris fixated implant
  accessory eye implant
  accordion implant
  acorn-shaped eye implant
  acorn-shaped implant
  acrylic ball eye implant
  acrylic conformer eye implant
  acrylic eye implant
  Acticon neosphincter implant
  Acuflex intraocular lens
    implant
  adhesive silicone implant
  adjustable breast implant
  adjustable saline breast implant

implant (*continued*)
  adrenal medullary implants
  Advent implant
  Aequalis humeral head
    implant
  afterloading implant
  AGC knee implant
  alar-columella implant
  Allen eye implant
  Allen orbital implant
  Allen Supramid implant
  Allen-Brailey intraocular lens
    implant
  Allen-Braley lens implant
  alloplastic facial implant
  alloplastic implants
  Alpar implant
  Alpar intraocular lens implant
  Alpha 1 penile implant
  amelogen dental implant
  AMO intraocular lens implant
  AMO scleral implant
  anatomical Tobin malar
    prosthetic implant
  anchor endosteal implant
  anterior chamber acrylic
    implant
  anterior subperiosteal implant
  AO/ASIF orthopedic implant
  Appolionio eye lens implant
  Arenberg-Denver inner-ear
    valve implant
  Arion implant
  Arnett LeFort implant
  Arroyo implant
  Arruga eye implant
  Arruga movable eye implant
  Arruga-Moura-Brazil orbital
    implant
  arthroplastic implant
  articulated chin implant
  artificial joint implant
  Ascension implant
  Ashworth-Blatt implant
  Aspheric lens implant
  A-type dental implant
  augmentation with implant
  autologous implant
  Avanta soft skeletal implant
  Azar eye implant
  Baerveldt glaucoma implant
  Baerveldt seton implant

implant (*continued*)
  bag-gel implant
  BAK/C cervical interbody
    fusion implant
  Balnetar implant
  Bannon-Klein implant
  Bard implant
  Barkan infant lens implant
  Barraquer implant
  Bechert intraocular lens
    implant
  Bechtol implant
  Becker implant
  Beekhuis-Supramid
    mentoplasty augmentation
    implant
  Berens conical eye implant
  Berens orbital implant
  Berens pyramidal eye
    implant
  Berens sphere eye implant
  Berens-Rosa eye implant
  Berens-Rosa scleral implant
  Bicon dental implant
  Bicoral implant
  Bietti eye implant
  bifocal eye implant
  bilumen implant
  bilumen mammary implant
  Binder submalar implant
  Binkhorst collar stud lens
    implant
  Binkhorst eye implant
  Binkhorst 4-loop iris-fixated
    implant
  Binkhorst intraocular lens
    implant
  Binkhorst lens implant
  Binkhorst 2-loop intraocular
    lens implant
  BioCare implant
  Biocell anatomical
    reconstructive mammary
    implant
  Biocell RTV breast implant
  Biocell RTV saline-filled breast
    implant
  Biocell smooth surface
    implant
  Biocell textured implant
  Biocell textured shell surface
    implant

implant (*continued*)

Biocell textured surface implant
Bioceram 2-stage series endosteal dental implant
Biocoral implant
BioCurve saline-filled breast implant
Biodel implant
biodimensional saline-filled implant
Bio-eye hydroxyapatite ocular implant
Biofix biodegradable implant
Bio-Gide dental implant
BioHorizon implant
Biomatrix ocular implant
Biomet custom implant
Bionix SmartNail bioresorbable implant
bioresorbable implant
Bio-Vent implant
Biovert ceramic implant
bivalve nasal splint implant
blade endosteal implant
blade-form implant
Blair-Brown implant
Boberg-Ans lens implant
Bonaccolto eye implant
Bonaccolto orbital implant
bone implant
BoneSource implant
Bosker transmandibular implant
bovine collagen implant
bovine implant
Boyd orbital implant
Branemark endosteal implant
Branemark osseointegration implant
Braun implant
breast implant
Brink peripyriform implant
Brown-Dohlman corneal implant
Brown-Dohlman eye implant
Brown-Dohlman Silastic corneal implant
buildup eye implant
Bunker implant
calcification of breast implant
Calcitek implant

implant (*continued*)

calcium phosphate ceramic implant
candle vaginal cesium implant
carbon implant
cardiovascular implant
Cardona focalizing fundus lens implant
Cardona goniofocalizing implant
carpal lunate implant
Carrion-Small penile implant
cartilage implant
Cartwright implant
Castroviejo acrylic eye implant
Celestin implant
celluloid implant
ceramic endosteal implant
CeraOne abutment implant
Charnley implant
Chatzidakis implant
cheek implant
chessboard implant
chin implant
Choyce eye implant
Choyce Mark eye implant
chromium-cobalt alloy implant
Clarion multi-strategy cochlear implant
Clayman lens implant
cobalt-chromium implant
cobalt-chromium-molybdenum alloy metal implant
cobalt-chromium-tungsten-nickel alloy metal implant
Coburn anterior chamber intraocular lens implant
Coburn Mark eye implant
cochlear implant
Codere orbital floor implant
cohesive anatomic silicone gel breast implants
collagen implant
collagen meniscus implant
columella implant
Combi-40 cochlear implant
Complete implant
complete subperiosteal implant
complete-arch blade endosteal implant

implant (*continued*)
  Compliant pre-stress bone
    implant
  condylar implant
  conical eye implant
  contact shell implant
  Contigen Bard cochlear
    implant
  Contigen Bard collagen implant
  Continuum knee system
    implant
  Contour Profile saline breast
    implant
  Contour Profile silicone
    breast implant
  conventional reform eye
    implant
  conventional shell-type eye
    implant
  Cooper implant
  Copeland intraocular lens
    implant
  Corail HA-coated stem hip
    implant
  Core-Vent implant
  corneal eye implant
  Corning implant
  corrected cosmetic contact
    shell eye implant
  cosmetic contact shell implant
  Cox-Uphoff implant
  Crete-Manche implant
  Cronin mammary implant
  CUI columellar implant
  CUI dorsal implant
  CUI malar implant
  CUI rhinoplasty implant
  curl-back shell eye implant
  curvilinear chin implant
  Custodis implant
  custom-contoured implant
  Cutler eye implant
  cylinder-type implant
  Dacron implant
  Dacron-backed implant
  Dannheim eye implant
  Davis implant
  DCS implant (dorsal column
    stimulator/stimulation
    implant)
  DeBakey implant
  defibrillator implant

implant (*continued*)
  Deflux system implant
  dental implant
  DePuy orthopedic implant
  Dermostat orbital implant
  DeWecker eye implant
  Doherty eye implant
  Doherty sphere eye implant
  Doherty spherical eye implant
  Donnheim implant
  dorsal columella implant
  dorsal column stimulator
    implant (DCS implant)
  double-lumen breast implant
  double-plate Molteno implant
  double-stem implant
  Dow Corning implant
  Dragstedt implant
  D-shaped implant
  dual-chambered implant
  dual-compartment gel-
    inflatable mammary
    implant
  dummy sources in cesium
    implant
  Duracon knee implant
  Dura-II concealable penile
    implant
  dural implant
  Durapatite implant
  Duros leuprolide implant
  DynaFlex penile implant
  Edwards implant
  Edwards Teflon intracardiac
    implant
  Ehmke platinum Teflon
    implant
  electric implant
  encapsulated breast implant
  endodontic endosseous
    implant
  endodontic endosteal implant
  endometrial implant
  endometriotic implant
  endo-osseous dental implant
  Endopore implant
  endosseous blade implant
  endosseous vent implant
  endosteal implant
  epilepsy implant
  Epstein collar stud acrylic
    implant

implant (*continued*)

Epstein lens implant
Esser implant
esthetic Taylor mandibular angle implant
Ethrone implant
E-type dental implant
Ewald-Walker knee implant
Ewing eye implant
expandable breast implant
expansible infrastructure endosteal implant
extended anatomical high-profile malar implant
Extrafil breast implant
extraoral bone-anchored implant
eye implant
eye sphere implant
eye spherical implant
fabricated implant
facial alloplastic implant
facial implant
fascia lata implant
feather extended malar implant
Federov eye implant
Federov lens implant
Federov type I lens implant
Federov type II lens implant
fenestra implant
Ferguson implant
fetal substantia nigra implants
Fibrel gelatin matrix implant
fill breast implant
Fine magnetic implant
finger joint implant
Finney penile implant
fixed bearing knee implant
fixed mandibular implant (FMI)
Flatt implant
flexible digital implant
flexible Dualens implant
flexible rod penile implant
Flexi-Flate penile implant
Flexi-rod II penile implant
Flowers mandibular groove implant
Flowers mandibular implants
Flowers tear trough implant
Fox eye implant
Fox eyelid implant
Fox sphere implant

implant (*continued*)

Fox spherical eye implant
free implant
free-standing implant
Frey eye implant
Frey tunneled eye implant
Friatec implant
front build-up eye implant
full-thickness implant
Fyodorov eye implant
Galin intraocular lens implant
Garcia-Novito eye implant
gel-filled implant
Gelfilm retinal implant
Gelfilm retinal orbital implant
gel-saline mammary implant
gentamicin implant
Geristore dental implant
Gerow penile implant
Gillies implant
Glasgold Wafer chin implant
glass sphere eye implant
Global total shoulder implant
gold eye implant
gold eyelid implant
gold eyelid load implant
gold implant
gold sphere eye implant
Goldmann multi-mirrored lens implant
gonioscopic implant
Gore-Tex nasal implant
Gore-Tex (SAM) facial implant
Gore-Tex vascular implant
Gott implant
great toe implant
Greissinger multi-axis joint implant
grooved silicone implant
Guist sphere eye implant
Guist sphere implant
HA-coated hip implant
HA-coated Micro-Vent implant
HA-coated root-form dental implant
Haik eye implant
Haik implant
haptic area implant
hard tissue replacement-malleable facial implant
Harris implant
Harrison implant

implant (*continued*)
Hartley implant
HA-threaded hexlock implant
heat-vulcanized silicone
  elastomer implants
helicoid endosseous implant
helicoid endosteal implant
hemi-interpositional implant
hemisphere eye implant
Herrick silicone lacrimal
  implant
heterograft implant
hex implant
hexlock implant
Heyer-Schulte breast implant
Heyer-Schulte lens implant
Heyer-Schulte rhinoplasty
  implant
HIHA tendon implant
Hinderer lower nasal base
  implant
hinged implant
histoclasia implant
Hoffer ridged lens implant
Hoffmann eye implant
hollow sphere eye implant
hollow sphere implant
hollow sphere orbital implant
homograft implant
hook-type eye implant
hordeolum eye implant
Hoskins-Drake implant
House implant
Howmedica Duracon implant
Hruby contact implant
Hufnagel implant
Hughes eye implant
Hunkeler lightweight
  intraocular lens implant
Hunter open cord tendon
  implant
hybrid-type implant
Hydrocurve intraocular lens
  implant
Hydroflex penile implant
Hydroflex penile semirigid
  implant
hydroxyapatite ocular implant
hydroxyapatite orbital implant
hydroxyapatite-coated implant
Imcor implant
Imex scleral implant

implant (*continued*)
immediate impression implant
Immediate Load implant
Implantech Binder implant
Implantech facial implant
Implantech Flowers implant
Implantech Mittelman implant
Implantech Terino implant
Imtec premounted threaded
  implant
IMZ endosteal implant
inflatable implant
inflatable penile implant
inflated implant
inlay implant
Insall-Burstein intracondylar
  total knee implant
Intacs corneal ring implant
integral implant
Integral Omniloc implant
Intermedics intraocular lens
  implant
Interpore implant
Interpore osteointegrated
  implant
interstitial implant
intracochlear implant
intramuscular gluteal implant
intraocular lens implant
intraorbital implant
intraosseous implant
intraperiosteal implant
IOptex laser intraocular lens
  implant
Iovision implant
Iowa orbital implant
iridium implant
iridium wire implant
ITI dental implant
ITI type-F endosseous implant
ITI Bonefit endosseous
  implant
Ivalon eye implant
Ivalon Lucite orbital eye
  implant
Ivalon sponge eye implant
Ivalon sponge implant
Jardon-Straith chin implant
Jardon-Straith nasal implant
joint implant
Jonas implant
Jordan eye implant

implant (*continued*)
K implant
Keragen implant
Kerato-Gel implant
Kerato-Lens implant
Kinetik great toe implant
King orbital implant
Klockner implant
Koenig total great toe implant
Koeppe gonioscopic lens implant
Koeppe intraocular lens implant
Kratz implant
Kratz-Sinskey intraocular lens implant
Krause-Wolfe implant
Kryptok bifocal lens implant
Lacey total knee implant
LaminOss implant
Landegger orbital implant
LaPorte great toe implant
LaPorte total toe implant
large-pore polyethylene implant
Lash-Loeffler implant
Lawrence 1st metatarsophalangeal joint implant
Lemoine eye implant
Lemoine orbital implant
lens implant
Levitt eye implant
Lifecath peritoneal implant
Lifecore Restore wide diameter implant
Lincoff eye implant
Lincoff scleral sponge implant
Linkow blade implant
liposuction fat fillant implant
Little intraocular lens implant
Liverpool elbow implant
loptex laser intraocular lens implant
Lovac fundus contact lens implant
Lovac 6-mirror gonioscopic lens implant
low bleed implants
low-profile breast implant
Lucite eye implant
Lucite sphere implant

implant (*continued*)
Luhr implant
lumbar anterior root stimulator implant
lunate implant
lymphoma implant
MacIntosh implant
Maestro implant
magnetic eye implant
magnetic implant
malar implant
malleable facial implant
mammary implant
Marlex mesh implant
McCannel implant
McCutchen hip implant
McGhan breast implant
McGhan Biocell anatomical breast implant
McGhan eye implant
McGhan facial implant
Medallion intraocular lens implant
MedDev gold eyelid implant
Medical Optics eye implant
Medical Optics intraocular lens implant
Medpor biomaterial implant
Medpor facial implant
Medpor malar implant
Medpor reconstructive implant
Medpor surgical implant
Melauskas acrylic orbital implant
Meme mammary implant
Meniscus Arrow implant
Mentor breast implant
Mentor malleable semirigid penile implant
Mentor Siltex implant
meridional implant
Mersilene implant
meshed ball implant
mesostructure implant
metacarpophalangeal implant
metal hemi-toe implant
metal orthopedic implant
metal-backed acetabular component hip implant
metallic implant
metastatic implant

implant (*continued*)
  methyl methacrylate beads
    implant
  methyl methacrylate eye
    implant
  Micro-Lok implant
  Microvel implant
  Micro-Vent implant
  middle ear implant
  Miller-Galante total knee
    implant
  Mini-Matic implant
  Miragel implant
  Mittelman implant
  Mittelman prejowl-chin
    implants
  mobile bearing knee implant
  modular implant
  Molteno double-plate implant
  Molteno drainage eye implant
  monostructure implant
  motility eye implant
  mucosal implant
  Mueller shield eye implant
  Muhlberger orbital implant
  Mules eye implant
  Mules sphere eye implant
  multichannel cochlear implant
  nasal dorsal implant
  needle endosseous implant
  needle endosteal implant
  Neer II total shoulder system
    implant
  neoplastic port site implant
  NeuFlex metacarpophalangeal
    joint implant
  NeuroControl Freehand
    implant
  NexGen knee implant
  Nexus implant
  Niebauer implant
  Niebauer-Cutter implant
  Nobel Biocare implant
  Nobelpharma implant
  Nocito eye implant
  nonautologous implant
  NovaGold breast implant
  Nucleus cochlear implant
  Nucleus multichannel
    cochlear implant
  Octa-Hex implant
  Oculo-Plastik ocular implant

implant (*continued*)
  Ollier-Thiersch implant
  O'Malley self-adhering lens
    implant
  Omniloc dental implant
  onlay implant
  OP-1 implant (osteogenic
    protein 1)
  Ophtec occlusion implant
  optic implant
  oral implant
  orbital floor implant
  orbital implant
  ORC posterior chamber
    intraocular lens implant
  Organon percutaneous implant
  orthotic attachment implant
  Osseodent dental implant
  osseointegrated cylinder
    implant
  osseointegrated oral implant
  Osseotite dental implant
  Osseotite 2-stage procedure
    implant
  osseous implant
  Osteo implant
  OsteoGen HA dental implant
  Osteogen resorbable
    osteogenic bone-filling
    implant
  osteointegrated dental implant
  Osteoplate implant
  Padgett implant
  Panje implant
  paraffin implant
  Paragon implant
  Partnership implant
  Pasqualini implant
  patch implant
  patella-resurfacing implant
  patient-matched implant
  peanut eye implant
  Pearce posterior chamber
    intraocular lens implant
  Pearce vaulted-Y lens implant
  pectoralis muscle implant
  pedicle implant
  penile implant
  percutaneous dorsal column
    stimulator implant
  perigingival implant
  Periotest implant

implant (*continued*)

permanent implant
permucosal endosteal implant
PhacoFlex foldable intraocular
    lens implant
piggyback implant
pin endosseous implant
pin implant
PIP Hydrogel breast implants
Pisces implant
planar mesh implant
planoconvex eye implant
plastic ball eye implant
plastic implant
plastic sphere eye implant
plastic sphere implant
Platina intraocular lens implant
platinum eyelid implant
Plexiglas eye implant
Plexiglas implant
Plystan implant
PMI implant
Polaris adjustable spinal cage
    implant
polyethylene eye implant
polyethylene sphere implant
polyglycolide implant
polylactide implant
polymer tooth replica implant
polymethyl methacrylate
    implant
Polystan implant
polytetrafluoroethylene
    implant
polyurethane implant
polyurethane-coated silicone
    breast implant
polyvinyl implant
polyvinyl sponge implant
Porex implant
Porex Medpor implant
Porex PHA implant
porous polyethylene implant
post implant
posterior chamber lens
    implant
Precision eye implant
Precision Cosmet intraocular
    lens implant
premandible implant
press-fit implant
processed carbon implant

implant (*continued*)

ProOsteon synthetic bone
    implant
Proplast facial implant
Proplast nasal implant
Proplast preformed facial
    implant
Proplast preformed implant
Proplast-Teflon disk implant
prosthetic implant
Protek joint implant
PTFE-containing implant
pyramidal eye implant
Radin-Rosenthal implant
radiocarpal implant
radium implant
Radovan breast implant
ramus blade implant
ramus endosteal implant
Rastelli implant
Rayner-Choyce eye implant
RBM implant
reduced-height implants
reform eye implant
reform implant
removable implant
Replace system tapered implant
Restore bone implant
Restore dental implant
Restore orthobiologic soft-
    tissue implant
Restore RBM implant
Restore threaded implant
retinal Gelfilm implant
Reuter bobbin implant
Reverdin implant
reverse-shape eye implant
reverse-shape implant
rhinoplasty implant
Ridley anterior chamber
    implant
Ridley anterior chamber lens
    implant
Ridley Mark II lens implant
Rizzo dorsal implant
Roberts dental implant
Rodin implant
Rodin orbital implant
root-form dental implant
Rosa-Berens orbital implant
Ruedemann eye implant
Ruiz plano fundus lens implant

implant (*continued*)
  SAM facial implant
  SACH implant
  saline breast implant
  saline-filled anatomical breast
    implant
  saline-filled round breast
    implant
  Sargon implant
  Sauerbruch implant
  Schepens hollow hemisphere
    implant
  Schocket tube implant
  scleral buckle eye implant
  scleral buckler implant
  scleral eye implant
  screw-type implant
  Screw-Vent implant
  Seeburger implant
  seed implant
  self-tapping screw-type
    implant
  semishell eye implant
  Septopal implant
  serrefine implant
  Severin implant
  Sgarlato hammertoe implant
  Shearing posterior chamber
    intraocular lens implant
  shelf-type implant
  shell eye implant
  shell-type eye implant
  Shepard intraocular lens
    implant
  SHIP hammertoe implant
  SHIP-Shaw rod hammertoe
    implant
  Sichel movable implant
  Sichel movable orbital
    implant
  Sichel orbital implant
  Silastic chin implant
  Silastic corneal eye implant
  Silastic Cronin implant
  Silastic eye implant
  Silastic finger implant
  Silastic midfacial malar
    implant
  Silastic penile implant
  Silastic rhinoplasty implant
  Silastic scleral buckler eye
    implant

implant (*continued*)
  Silastic scleral buckler implant
  Silastic silicone rubber
    implant
  Silastic subdermal implant
  Silastic testicular implant
  Silastic toe implant
  silicone buckling implant
  silicone button eye implant
  silicone elastomer rubber ball
    implant
  silicone eye implant
  silicone gel breast implant
  silicone gel implant
  silicone gel-filled breast
    implant (SGBI)
  silicone gel-filled mammary
    implant (SGMI)
  silicone meshed motility
    implant
  silicone nasal strut implant
  silicone pad eye implant
  silicone rod implant
  silicone sleeve eye implant
  silicone sponge implant
  silicone strip eye implant
  silicone textured mammary
    implant
  silicone tire eye implant
  silicone-filled anatomical
    breast implant
  silicone-filled breast implant
  silicone-filled mammary
    implant
  silicone-filled round breast
    implant
  siloxane implant
  Siltex mammary implant
  Simaplast implants
  Simcoe eye implant
  Simcoe intraocular lens
    implant
  single-chambered saline
    implant
  single-channel cochlear
    implant
  single-stage screw implant
  single-tooth subperiosteal
    implant
  Sinskey lens implant
  Sinterlock implant
  sizing implants

implant (*continued*)
 sleeve implant
 sling-like taping around the implant
 Small-Carrion Silastic rod for penile implant
 SmartScrew bioabsorbable implant
 Smith orbital floor implant
 smooth staple implant
 Snellen conventional reform eye implant
 Snellen eye implant
 soft silicone sphere implant
 SoftForm facial implant
 SoftForm implant
 solid silicone buttock implant
 solid silicone with Supramid mesh implant
 Spectra-System implant
 Spectrum Designs facial implant
 spermatocele implant
 sphere eye implant
 spherical eye implant
 Sphero Flex implant
 spiral endosseous implant
 spiral endosteal implant
 Spline Twist microtextured titanium implant
 split-thickness implant
 sponge implant
 stainless steel implant
 STA-peg implant
 Star/Vent 1-stage dental screw implant
 Startanius blade implant
 Steri-Oss endosteal dental implant
 stock implant
 Stone eye implant
 Straith chin implant
 Straith nasal implant
 Strampelli implant
 S-type dental implant
 subdermal implant
 submucosal implant
 submuscular implant
 subpectoral implant
 subperiosteal implant
 SuperCat self-tapping implant
 superficial implant

implant (*continued*)
 Supramid mesh implant
 Supramid-Allen implant
 supraperiosteal implant
 surface eye implant
 surface implant
 surgibone implant
 Surgicel implant
 Surgitek Flexi-Flate penile implant
 Surgitek mammary implant
 Sustain HA-coated screw implant
 Sustain hydroxyapatite biointegrated dental implant
 Swanson carpal lunate implant
 Swanson carpal scaphoid implant
 Swanson finger joint implant
 Swanson great toe implant
 Swanson implant
 Swanson metacarpophalangeal implant
 Swanson radial head implant
 Swanson radiocarpal implant
 Swanson Silastic implant
 Swanson small joint implant
 Swanson trapezium implant
 Swanson ulnar head implant
 Swanson wrist joint implant
 Swede-Vent self-tapping external hex implant
 Swiss MP joint implants
 Syed template implant
 Syed-Neblett implant
 synthetic implant
 tantalum eye implant
 tantalum mesh eye implant
 tantalum mesh implant
 tapered Micro-Vent implant
 Taper-Lock external hex implant
 tear trough style implant
 teardrop-shaped breast implant
 Techmedica implant
 Teflon mesh implant
 Teflon orbital floor implant
 tendon implant
 Tennant Anchorflex lens implant

implant (*continued*)
    Tensilon implant
    Terino anatomical chin implant
    testicular implant
    Tevdek implant
    textured saline breast implant
    TG Osseotite implant
    TheraSeed implant
    thick-walled Dacron-backed implant
    Thiersch implant
    ThreadLoc implant
    TiMesh patient-configured titanium craniomaxillofacial implant
    TiO-Blast dental implant
    tire eye implant
    titanium alloy implant
    titanium plasma sprayed dental implant
    titanium-sprayed IMZ implant
    TMI implant
    Tobin anatomical malar prosthetic implant
    tobramycin-impregnated PMMA implant
    total top implant
    Townley implant
    transmandibular implant (TMI)
    transosseous implant
    transosteal implant
    trapezium implant
    trial implant
    Trilucent breast implant
    triplant implant
    triple lumen implant
    Troncoso gonioscopic lens implant
    Troncoso implant
    Troutman eye implant
    Troutman implant
    Troutman magnetic implant
    tunneled eye implant
    tunneled implant
    Twist implant
    Twist Ti implant
    Ultex lens implant
    unicompartmental knee implant
    Unilab Surgibone implant
    Universal wrist implant

implant (*continued*)
    universal subperiosteal implant
    ureteral implant
    Uribe orbital implant
    Usher Marlex mesh implant
    U-type dental implant
    VA magnetic implant
    VA magnetic orbital implant
    Varigray lens implant
    Varilux lens implant
    vascular bundle implant
    vent implant
    vent-plate implant
    Vitallium eye implant
    Vitek interpositional implant
    Vitrasert intraocular implant
    Vivosil implant
    VoCoM thyroplasty implant
    Volk conoid implant
    Walter Reed implant
    WasherLoc implant
    Weavenit implant
    Weber hip implant
    Weck-cel implant
    Weil implant
    Weil-modified Swanson implant
    Wheeler eye implant
    Wheeler sphere eye implant
    Wheeler spherical eye implant
    wire mesh eye implant
    wire mesh implant
    Wolfe implant
    Wolfe-Krause implant
    Zang metatarsal cap implant
    Zeichner implant
    Zest subperiosteal implant
    Zoladex implant
    Zyderm collagen implant
    Zyplast implant
implant abutment
implant alloy aluminum
implant anchor
implant arthroplasty
implant biocompatibility
implant biodegradation
implant blank
implant button
implant cataract lens
implant cervix
implant collar

implant conformer
implant contouring
implant deflation
implant elastomer shell
implant entry
implant erosion
implant extrusion
implant failure
implant fatigue
implant fixture
implant forceps
implant fork
implant fracture
implant frame
implant framework
implant gingival sulcus
implant hinge
implant infrastructure
Implant Innovations titanium
    screw
implant lens
implant magnet
implant malposition
implant material
implant mesostructure
implant metal
implant migration
implant model
implant neck
implant placement
implant post
implant reaction
implant removal
implant restoration
implant rippling
implant screw
implant shelf
implant site dilator
implant sleeve
implant sponge
implant stage
implant structure
implant substructure interspace
implant substructure strut
implant superstructure attachment
implant superstructure connector
implant superstructure frame
implant superstructure neck
implant surgery
implant surgical splint
implant surgical splint
    superstructure

implant survival rate
implant template
implant tire
implant/flap reconstruction
implantable artificial heart
implantable atrial defibrillator
implantable bone growth
    stimulator
implantable cardiac pulse
    generator
implantable cardioverter/
    defibrillator catheter
implantable cardioverter-
    defibrillator/atrial
    tachycardia pacing
implantable defibrillator
implantable drug infusion
    pump
implantable infusion port
implantable loop recorder
implantable neural stimulator
implantable osmotic pump
implantable pacemaker
implantable pain modality
implantable silicone
    microballoon
implantable vascular access
    device (IVAD)
implantation
    circumferential implantation
    cornual implantation
    cortical implantation
    displacement implantation
    eccentric implantation
    filiform implantation
    fusion implantation
    gastric balloon implantation
    graft implantation
    hypodermic implantation
    interstitial implantation
    intraocular lens implantation
    intrusive implantation
    mesh implantation
    metastatic implantation
    muscle implantation
    needle tract implantation
    nerve implantation
    parenchymatous implantation
    periosteal implantation
    placental implantation
    radioactive seed implantation
    radon seed implantation

implantation (*continued*)
  real-time 3-D biplanar
    transperineal prostate
    implantation
  screw implantation
  Sewell internal mammary
    implantation
  silk implantation
  stent implantation
  subcutaneous implantation
  subdural grid implantation
  submuscular implantation
  subpectoral implantation
  subpectoral-subserratus
    muscle implantation
  superficial implantation
  surgical implantation
  Surgicel implantation
  tension-free mesh
    implantation
  teratic implantation
  tubouterine implantation
  ureter implantation
  ureterovesical implantation
implantation bleeding
implantation cyst
implantation failure
implantation forceps
implantation graft
implantation metastasis
implantation of pacemaker
implantation of radioactive
  isotopes
implantation of radium
implantation of ureter into
  rectum
implantation phase
implantation response
implantation site
implantation technique
implantation test
implant-bearing surface
implant-bone interface
implant-cement interface
Implantech facial implant
Implantech Flowers implant
Implantech Mittelman implant
Implantech SE-100 smoke
  aspiration tip
Implantech Terino implant
implanted electrode
implanted infusion pump

implanted pacemaker
implanted pump
implanted suture technique
implanted sutures
implanted tube
implanter
  Geuder implanter
  Wallner interstitial prostate
    implanter
implanting radioactive sources
implant-layering process
implantodontics
implantodontist
implantodontology
implantologist
implantology
implant-related complications
  (IRC)
implant-supported fixed
  prosthesis
Implast adhesive
Implast bone cement adhesive
Implens intraocular implant lens
Implens intraocular lens
impotence
impotency
Impra bypass graft
Impra vascular graft
Impra collagen-impregnated
  Dacron prosthesis
Impra Flex vascular graft
Impra graft
Impra microporous PTFE
  vascular graft
Impra peritoneal catheter
Impra vascular graft
Impra vein graft
impregnated dressing
impregnated electrode
impregnated gauze
Impregum impression material
impression
  cardiac impression
  cleft palate impression
  dental impression
  denture impression
  digitate impression
  duodenal impression
  esophageal impression
  extrinsic esophageal
    impression
  final impression

impression (*continued*)
first impression
gastric impression
mandibular impression
maxillary impression
modeling plastic impression
preliminary impression
prepared cavity impression
renal impression
suprarenal impression
surgical bone impression
trigeminal impression
impression fracture
impression material syringe
impression preparation
impression technique
impression tonometer
improved condition
improved Webb stripper
improvement
impulse
apical impulse
cardiac impulse
ectopic impulse
irresistible impulse
nerve impulse
neural impulse
pacing impulse
point of maximal impulse
(PMI)
impulse formation
Imre canthoplasty
Imre flap operation
Imre lateral canthoplasty
Imre lid operation
Imre sliding flap
Imre treatment
Imtec BioBarrier membrane
Imtec premounted threaded
implant
IMV (intermittent mandatory
ventilation)
IMZ endosteal implant
IMZ-type restoration
in
in ano
in extremis
in recto hernia
in situ bypass
in situ dissection
in situ graft harvest
in situ hypothermic perfusion

in situ procedure
in situ reconstruction
in situ spinal fusion
in situ squamous cell carcinoma
in situ tricortical iliac crest
block bone graft
in situ uterine repair
in situ valve scissors
in situ valve-cutter kit
in toto
in utero exposure
in utero murine craniofacial
surgery
in utero repair
in vitro fertilization
in vitro fertilization
micropipette
in vitro-growth palatal mucosa
sheet
in vivo fertilization
inactivating agent
inactive condition
inactive electrode
inadequacy
inadequate blood flow
inadequate bowel prep
inadequate cardiac output
inadequate dilation
inadequate pelvis
inadequate surgery
inadvertent enterotomy
inadvertent laceration
inadvertent venous injury
Inahara shunt
Inahara-Pruitt vascular shunt
Inamura small incision
capsulorrhexis forceps
in-and-out catheterization
inborn error of metabolism
incandescent endoscope lamp
incandescent sheath
incarcerated
incarcerated hernia
incarcerated omentum
incarcerated placenta
InCare brace
incarnative
Incavo wire passer
incentive spirometry
Incert bioabsorbable
implantable sponge
Incert sponge

incessant movements
inchworm flap
incident exposure
incident point
incidental appendectomy
incidental finding
incidental murmur
incidental rupture
incipient cataract
incipient gangrene
incisal angle
incisal cavity
incisal edge
incisal embrasure
incisal guidance angle
incisal mandibular plane angle
   (IMPA)
incisal margin
incisal point
incisal quadrant view
incisal surface of tooth
incise and drain
incise drape
incised
   central sutures incised
incised pretarsal dermis
incised wound
incisiolabial
incisiolingual
incision
   3-armed stellate incision
   11th rib flank incision
   11th rib transperitoneal incision
   ab externo incision
   ab interno incision
   abdominal incision
   abdominal wall incision
   abdominoinguinal incision
   abdominothoracic incision
   access incision
   Agnew-Verhoeff incision
   alar incision
   Alexander incision
   Amussat incision
   angular incision
   anterior hairline incision
   anterior incision
   anterior pillar incision
   anterolateral thoracotomy
      incision
   anteromedial incision
   aortotomy incision

incision (*continued*)
   appendectomy incision
   apron skin incision
   apron U-shaped incision
   arcuate incision
   areolar incision
   arteriotomy incision
   Auvray incision
   axillary incision
   backcut incision
   Banks-Laufman incision
   Bar incision
   Bardenheuer incision
   Battle incision
   battledore incision
   Battle-Jalaguier-Kammerer
      incision
   bayonet incision
   bayonet-type incision
   belt-approach incision
   Bergmann incision
   Bergmann-Israel incision
   Bevan abdominal incision
   bicoronal incision
   bifrontal incision
   bikini skin incision
   bilateral subcostal incision
   bilateral transabdominal
      incision
   bisubcostal incision
   bivalved elliptical incision
   Blair incision
   blepharoplasty incision
   Bosworth-Shawler incision
   boutonniere incision
   bowling-pin incision
   Boyd incision
   Boyd posterior incision
   Brackin incision
   breast incision
   Brock incision
   Brockman incision
   Brunner modified incision
   Brunner palmar incision
   Bruser lateral incision
   Bruser skin incision
   bucket-handle incision
   Buck-Gramcko incision
   bur-hole incision
   Burns-Haney incision
   Burwell-Scott modification of
      Watson-Jones incision

incision (*continued*)

buttonhole incision
buttonhole skin incision
Caldwell-Luc incision
capsular incision
cautery incision
Cave incision
celiotomy incision
cervical incision
cesarean section incision
Chamberlain incision
Chang-Miltner incision
Charnley incision
Cheatle-Henry incision
Cherney abdominal incision
Cherney lower transverse
   abdominal incision
Chernez incision
chevron-shaped incision
Chiene incision
choledochotomy incision
chord incision
Cincinnati incision
circular guillotine incision
circular incision
circumareolar incision
circumcisional incision
circumcorneal incision
circumferential incision
circumferentiating skin
   incision
circumlimbal incision
circumlimbar incision
circumlinear incision
circumoral incision
circumscribing incision
circum-umbilical incision
clamshell incision
classical incision
classical transverse incision
clavicular incision
clean and dry incision
clitoral incision
Clute incision
Codman incision
Coffey incision
Cohen uterine incision
collar incision
Colonna-Ralston incision
colpotomy incision
confirmatory incision
conjunctival incision

incision (*continued*)

Conley neck incision
Conley radical neck incision
Connell incision
contoured pretragal incision
corneal incision
corneoscleral incision
corollary incision
coronal incision
corridor incision
cortical incision
Cottle incision
Courvoisier incision
Couvelaire incision
Crawford incision
crease incision
crescent incision
crescentic-shaped incision
crevicular incision
Crile incision
crisscrossing abdominal wall
   incisions
crosshatch incision
cross-shaped incision
cross-tunneling incision
crow's foot incision
crucial incision
cruciate incision
Cubbins incision
culdotomy incision
Curtin incision
curved incision
curved longitudinal incision
curved periscapular incision
curved-downward incision
curvilinear incision
curvilinear skin incision
curving incision
cutdown incision
Czerny incision
darting incision
Davis-Geck incision
Davis-Rockey incision
de Quervain incision
Deaver skin incision
decompression incision
deepened incision
deltoid-splitting incision
deltopectoral incision
Depage incision
diamond-shaped incision
Dührssen incision

incision (*continued*)
    donor incision
    dorsal linear incision
    dorsal longitudinal incision
    dorsal lumbotomy incision
    dorsal supine incision
    dorsal transverse incision
    dorsolateral incision
    dorsomedial incision
    double incision
    double-Y incision
    dry incision
    dumbbell incision
    dural incision
    DuVries incision
    Dwyer incision
    Edebohls incision
    elliptical incision
    elliptical sagittal incision
    elliptical uterine incision
    Elsberg incision
    endaural incision
    endaural mastoid incision
    endonasal incision
    endoscopic incision
    endoscopically performed
       longitudinal incision
    endotragal incision
    endourological cold-knife
       incision
    enlarged incision
    enterotomy incision
    epigastric incision
    exploratory incision
    extended left subcostal
       incision
    external bevel incision
    external paralateronasal skin
       incision
    extraction incision
    extraoral incision
    fascia-splitting incision
    Fergusson incision
    fiber-splitting incision
    fishmouth incision
    flank incision
    flexed incision
    forequadrant incision
    Fowler angular incision
    Fowler-Philip incision
    Fowler-Weir incision
    Frazier incision

incision (*continued*)
    frontotemporal craniotomy
       incision
    frown incision
    Furniss incision
    Gaenslen split-heel incision
    Gatellier incision
    Gatellier-Chastang incision
    Gibson long vertical relaxing
       incision
    Gibson-Foley incision
    Gibson-Gibson posterior
       muscle-cutting incision
    Gibson-type incision
    Gillies incision
    Gilquist incision
    gingival incision
    gingivolabial incision
    Gluck incision
    goblet incision
    Graefe incision
    grayline incision
    Greenhow incision
    Greenhow-Rodman incision
    Grice incision
    gridiron incision
    Griffith incision
    groin incision
    grooved incision
    guillotine incision
    gull-wing incision
    Gunter Von Noorden incision
    hairline incision
    Hajek incision
    Halsted incision
    Halsted-Meyer incision
    Halsted-Willy Meyer incision
    Handley incision
    Harman incision
    Harmon incision
    Harper-Warren incision
    Harris incision
    Hayes Martin incision
    head-low incision
    healing biopsy incision
    Heermann incision
    Heineke-Mikulicz incision
    hemicircular incision
    hemitransfixion incision
    Henderson skin incision
    Henry incision
    hernia incision

incision (*continued*)

herniorrhaphy incision
H-flap incision
Higgins incision
high incision
hockey-stick incision
Hoke incision
Hoke 3-level incision
Hood-Kirkland incision
horizontal incision
horseshoe incision
horseshoe-shaped incision
H-shaped capsular incision
Hueter incision
Hugh Young incision
ilioinguinal incision
inferior conjunctival fornix
   incision
infraclavicular incision
inframammary incision
infraorbital incision
infraumbilical incision
inguinal incision
initial incision
inner bevel incision
intercartilaginous incision
internal bevel incision
intestinal incision
intra-areolar incision
intracapsular incision
intranasal intercartilaginous
   incision
intraoral incision
intraperitoneal incision
inverse bevel incision
inverted bevel incision
inverted-T incision
inverted-U abdominal incision
inverted-U incision
inverted-Y incision
Jackson incision
Jalaguier incision
Jergesen incision
Joel-Cohen abdominal incision
J-shaped incision
J-shaped skin incision
Kammerer incision
Kammerer-Battle incision
Kehr incision
keratome incision
Kerr incision
keyhole incision

incision (*continued*)

Killian incision
Kuenster incision
Kocher biliary tract incision
Kocher collar incision
Kocher collar thyroidectomy
   incision
Kocher incision
Koenig-Schaefer incision
Lahey incision
lamellar incision
Lamm incision
Langenbeck incision
Lanz incision
laparotomy incision
LaRoque herniorrhaphy
   incision
lateral flank incision
lateral incision
lateral rectus incision
lateral to the incision
lateral utility incision
lazy M incision
lazy C incision
lazy H incision
lazy S incision
lazy Z incision
L-curved incision
Lempert incision
Leslie incision
Lilienthal incision
limbal incision
line incision
linear incision
linear skin incision
linear transverse incision
Linton incision
lip-splitting incision
Loeffler-Ballard incision
long oblique incision
longhorn-shaped incision
longitudinal incision
longitudinal midline incision
Longuet incision
low incision
low midline incision
low transverse incision
low-collar incision
lower lip-splitting incision
lower midline incision
lower uterine segment incision
low-flying bird incision

incision (*continued*)
  low-segment transverse
    incision
  L-shaped capsular incision
  Ludloff incision
  lumboiliac incision
  Lyman incision
  Lynch incision
  MacFee incision
  Mackenrodt incision
  malar incision
  Mallard incision
  Manske-McCarroll-Swanson
    incision
  marginal incision
  Martin incision
  Mason incision
  mastectomy incision
  mastoid incision
  Mayfield incision
  Maylard incision
  Mayo-Robson incision
  McArthur incision
  McBurney appendectomy
    incision
  McIndoe incision
  McKissock incision
  McLaughlin incision
  McLaughlin-Ryder incision
  McMahon-Laird incision
  McVay incision
  meatal incision
  medial incision
  medial parapatellar incision
  median appendectomy incision
  median incision
  median parapatellar incision
  median sternotomy incision
  Meisterschnitt incision
  Mercedes incision
  Meyer hockey-stick incision
  Meyer-Halsted incision
  midabdominal transverse
    incision
  midaxillary line incision
  midline abdominal incision
  midline incision
  midline lower abdominal
    incision
  midline oblique incision
  midline sternum-splitting
    incision

incision (*continued*)
  midline upper abdominal
    incision
  midsternum-splitting incision
  Mikulicz incision
  minilaparotomy incision
  modified Gibson incision
  modified Weber-Fergusson
    incision
  Morison incision
  Morris incision
  Moynihan incision
  multiple-port incision
  Munro Kerr incision
  muscle-splitting incision
  myringotomy incision
  Nagamatsu incision
  nasal incision
  near-edge of incision
  Nicola incision
  non-rib-spreading
    thoracotomy incision
  Ober incision
  oblique incision
  oblique inguinal incision
  oblique relaxing incision
  Obwegeser incision
  Ollier incision
  omega-shaped incision
  operative incision
  orbicular incision
  original incision
  Orr incision
  oval incision
  ovarian incision
  overlapping incision
  palmar incision
  paracostal incision
  parainguinal incision
  parallel incision
  parallel-transverse incision
  paramedian appendectomy
    incision
  paramedian incision
  paramuscular incision
  parapatellar incision
  pararectus incision
  parasagittal incision
  parascapular incision
  paraumbilical incision
  paravaginal incision
  Parker incision

incision (*continued*)
  parumbilical incision
  Penduloff incision
  penile-scrotal incision
  penoscrotal incision
  perianal incision
  periareolar incision
  perilimbal incision
  perineal incision
  peripatellar incision
  perirectal incision
  periscapular incision
  peritoneal incision
  periumbilical incision
  Perthes incision
  Pfannenstiel incision
  Phemister incision
  Picot incision
  planar incision
  plantar longitudinal incision
  plaque incision
  pleuropericardial incision
  popliteal incision
  port incision
  postauricular incision
  posterior hemicircular
    incision
  posterior incision
  posterior stab incision
  posterior transthoracic
    incision
  posterolateral
    costotransversectomy
    incision
  posterolateral incision
  preauricular incision
  precut incision
  Pridie incision
  primary access incisions
  Pringle incision
  proximal incision
  puboxyphoid incision
  Pulvertaft fishmouth incision
  puncture incision
  pyelotomy incision
  Pean incision
  Quervain incision
  racquet incision
  racquet-shaped incision
  radial incision
  radial skin incision
  Ragnault incision

incision (*continued*)
  Rambo endaural incision
  recently healed surgical
    incision
  rectus incision
  rectus muscle-splitting incision
  rectus sheath incision
  recumbent incision
  relaxing incision
  releasing incision
  relief incision
  relieving incision
  Rethi incision
  retroauricular incision
  retrotragal incision
  reverse bevel incision
  reverse Y incision
  right rectus incision
  right upper paramedian
    incision
  right-sided submandibular
    transverse incision
  rim incision
  Risdon extraoral incision
  Risdon pretragal incision
  Robertson incision
  Rockey-Davis appendectomy
    incision
  Rodman mastectomy incision
  Rollet incision
  Rosen incision
  Roux-en-Y incision
  Roux-en-Y jejunal loop incision
  Ruddy incision
  Rush incision
  Russe incision
  S incision
  saber incision
  saber-cut incision
  saber-slash incision
  salmon backcut incision
  Salus incision
  Sanders incision
  Sanger incision
  saw incision
  scalp incision
  Schobinger incision
  Schuchardt relaxing incision
  scoring incision
  scratch incision
  scratch-type incision
  scrotal incision

incision (*continued*)

Sellheim incision
semicircular incision
semiflexed incision
semilunar incision
semishelving incision
serpentine incision
S-flap incision
Shambaugh endaural incision
sharp incision
Shea incision
Shea-Hough incision
shelving incision
shield incision
Shoepinger incision
shoulder-strap incision
Silvio incision
Simon incision
single midline extraperitoneal
  incision
Singleton incision
sinuous incision
skin incision
skin-crease incision
skinfold incision
skin-knife incision
skinline incision
skived incision
Sloan abdominal incision
slot incision
slot-type rim incision
smile incision
smiling incision
Smith-Petersen incision
Souttar craniotomy incision
Souttar skin incision
spindle-shaped incision
spiral incision
split incision
split-heel incision
S-shaped incision
St. Mark incision
stab incision
stab-wound incision
stairstep transcolumellar
  incision
standard clavicular incision
standard Kocher incision
standard retroperitoneal flank
  incision
stellate incision
stepladder incision

incision (*continued*)

steri-stripped incision
sternal-splitting incision
sternotomy incision
Stewart incision
stocking-seam incision
Strombeck mammaplasty
  incision
straight incision
subciliary incision
subcostal flank incision
subcostal incision
subcostal transperitoneal
  incision
subinguinal incision
sublabial incision
submammary incision
submental incision
suboccipital incision
subtrochanteric incision
subumbilical incision
supracervical incision
supraciliary incision
suprapubic appendectomy
  incision
suprapubic incision
suprapubic Pfannenstiel
  incision
supraumbilical incision
surgical incision
Sutherland-Rowe incision
Swan incision
tangential incision
temporal incision
tennis-racket incision
tepee incision
Thomas-Warren incision
thoracicoabdominal incision
thoracoabdominal incision
thoracotomy incision
tracheal incision
transacromial incision
transaxillary incision
transection incision
transfixation incision
transmeatal incision
transmeatal tympanoplasty
  incision
transpubic incision
transrectus incision
transurethral laser incision
transverse abdominal incision

incision (*continued*)

transverse appendectomy
   incision
transverse incision
transverse mastectomy incision
transverse skin incision
trap incision
trapdoor incision
trapezoidal incision
trifurcate incision
T-shaped incision
T-tube incision
Turner-Warwick incision
Uchida incision
umbilical skin-knife incision
unilateral subcostal incision
upper abdominal midline
   incision
upper midline incision
upright Y incision
upward-gaze incision
U-shaped incision
uterine incision
utility-type incision
vermis incision
vertical bur-hole incision
vertical elliptical incision
vertical incision
vertical lateral parapatellar
   incision
vertical midline incision
vertical uterine incision
Vischer lumboiliac incision
volar midline oblique incision
volar transverse incision
volar zig-zag finger incision
von Langenbeck incision
Von Noorden incision
V-shaped incision
Wagner skin incision
Ward-Hendrick incision
Warren incision
Watson-Jones incision
web space incision
Weber-Fergusson incision
Weber-Fergusson-Longmire
   incision
wedge incision
Weir incision
Westin-Hall incision
Wheeler incision
Whipple incision

incision (*continued*)

wide skin incision
Wies entropion incision
Wilde incision
Willy Meyer incision
Willy Meyer mastectomy
   incision
Wise breast incision
W-shaped incision
xiphoid-to-os pubis incision
xiphoid-to umbilicus incision
xiphoid-to-pubis midline
   abdominal incision
xiphoid-to-umbilicus incision
Y incision
Y-double incision
York-Mason incision
Y-shaped incision
Y-type incision
Y-V-plasty incision
Z-flap incision
zigzag finger incision
zigzag incision
Z-plasty incision
Z-shaped incision
incision and drainage (I&D)
incision and drainage of abscess
incision and drainage of bursa
incision and drainage of gland
incision and packing
incision and packing of wound
incision and removal of calculus
incision and resuture of wound
incision carried down
incision clean and dry
incision closed anatomically
incision closed in layers
incision closed musculofascially
incision closure
incision curved downward
incision curved periscapularly
incision dilator
incision extended bilaterally
incision healed per primam
   intentionem
incision healed per secundam
   intentionem
incision into organ or tissue
incision knife
incision line
incision of organ or tissue
incision retractor

incision scissors
incision site
incision spreader
incision widened
incisional biopsy
incisional corporoplasty
incisional gastropexy
incisional hernia
incisional hernioplasty
incisional infiltration
incisional joint
incisional metastasis
incisional pain
incisional scar
incisional site draining
incision-halving technique
incisionless otoplasty
incisioproximal
incisive canal
incisive duct
incisive foramen
incisive fossa of mandible
incisive fossa of maxilla
incisive muscle of lower lip
incisive muscle of upper lip
incisive papilla
incisive sutures
incisor
    erupted incisor
    mandibular incisor
    maxillary incisor
    shovel-shaped incisor
Incisor arthroscopic blade
incisor point
incisura (pl. incisurae)
incisura angularis ventriculi
incisura cardiaca ventriculi
incisura Santorini
incisural dissection
incisural space
incisural ulcer
incisure
    sagittal incisure
Inclan graft
Inclan-Ober procedure
Inclan-Ober scapula procedure
inclination
    condylar guide inclination
    facial inclination
    lateral condylar inclination
    lingual inclination
inclination angle

inclination guidewire
inclined-plane elevator
inclusion body disease
inclusion cyst
inclusion disease
incompatibility
incompatible blood transfusion
incompatible bone marrow
incompetence
    aortic incompetence
    cervical incompetence
    gastroesophageal
        incompetence
    lip incompetence
    palatal incompetence
    urethral incompetence
    valvular incompetence
    velopharyngeal incompetence
        (VPI)
incompetency
incompetent aortic valve
incompetent atrioventricular valve
incompetent cervix
incompetent esophageal
        sphincter
incompetent foramen ovale
incompetent ileocecal valve
incompetent mitral valve
incompetent perforator
incompetent pulmonic valve
incompetent sphincter
incompetent tricuspid valve
incompetent upper lip
incompetent valve
incompetent vein
incomplete abortion
incomplete amputation
incomplete atrioventricular
        dissociation
incomplete A-V dissociation
incomplete breech position
incomplete cleft of earlobe
incomplete cleft palate
incomplete colonoscopy
incomplete compound fracture
incomplete dislocation
incomplete duplication
incomplete excision
incomplete facial paralysis
incomplete fistula
incomplete fracture
incomplete hernia

induced sleep
induced tension pneumothorax
induction
  anesthetic induction
  complementary induction
  dorsal induction
  electric induction
  endotracheal induction
  enzyme induction
  Faraday law of induction
  gene induction
  labor augmentation induction
  lysogenic induction
  magnetic induction
  menstrual cycle induction
  negative control enzyme
    induction
  neuromuscular system
    electric induction
  ovulation induction
  pain induction
  positive control enzyme
    induction
  rapid-sequence induction (RSI)
  remission induction
  Spemann induction
  sputum induction
  superovulation induction
induction anesthetic technique
induction chemotherapy
induction of anesthesia
induction of labor
inductive resistance
InDura catheter
InDura pump
indurated border
indurated mass
indurated papule
induration
  brawny induration
  cyanotic induration
  fibroid induration
  Froriep induration
  gray induration
  idiopathic brown induration
  laminate induration
  parchment induration
  penile induration
  phlebitic induration
  plastic induration
  red induration
induration and swelling

industrial exposure
indwelling catheter
indwelling catheter program
  (ICP)
indwelling Foley catheter
indwelling nonvascular shunt
indwelling stent
indwelling subclavian catheter
indwelling transcutaneous
  vascular access device
indwelling ureteral stent
indwelling venous catheter
inelastic compression garment
inelastic impression material
inelastic lower eyelid
Inerpan dressing
Inerpan flexible burn dressing
inevitable abortion
infant
  full-term infant
  liveborn infant
  stillborn infant
infant abdominal retractor
infant abduction splint
infant Ambu resuscitator
infant biopsy forceps
infant bougie
infant bronchoscope
infant catheter
infant cystoscope
infant dilator
infant electrotome
infant esophagoscope
infant eye speculum
infant eyelid retractor
infant feeding tube
infant female catheter
infant Karickhoff laser lens
infant male catheter
infant nasal cannula assembly
infant rib retractor
infant rib shears
infant rib spreader
infant sound
infant telescope
infant 3-mirror laser lens
infant urethral sound
infant urethrotome
infant urethrotome blade
infant vaginal speculum
infant vaginoscope
infant vascular clamp

infant ventilation monitor
infantile apertognathia
infantile aphasia
infantile articulation
infantile cataract
infantile choriocarcinoma
   syndrome
infantile condition
infantile cortical hyperostosis
infantile embryonal carcinoma
infantile fibrosarcoma
infantile hernia
infantile organ
infantile perseveration
infantile vascular tumor
infarct expansion
infarct extension
infarct-avid scintigraphy
infarctectomy
infarcted bowel
infarcted scar
infarcted transverse colon
infarction
   acute myocardial infarction
     (AMI)
   anterolateral infarction
   anteroseptal myocardial
     infarction (AMI)
   cardiac infarction
   cerebral infarction
   focal infarction
   hemorrhagic infarction
   impending infarction
   intestinal infarction
   lacunar infarction
   mesenteric infarction
   myocardial infarction (MI)
   posterior infarction
   posterolateral infarction
   postmyocardial infarction
   renal infarction
   rule out myocardial infarction
     (ROMI)
   subendocardial infarction
   subendocardial myocardial
     infarction (SEMI)
infarctive lesion
In-Fast cystourethropexy
infected case
infected collection
infected incisional site
infected organ

infected wound
infecting organism
infection calculus
infectious complication
infectious disease
infectious etiology
infectious hepatitis virus
infectious lymphadenopathy
infectious mononucleosis
infectious papilloma virus
infectious process
infective disorder
infective endocarditis
infective extra-abdominal
   complication
inferior accessory fissure
inferior arcuate bundle
inferior alveolar artery
inferior alveolar nerve (IAN)
inferior alveolar nerve block
inferior alveolar nerve fascicle
inferior alveolar neurovascular
   bundle
inferior alveolar vein
inferior angle of parietal bone
inferior artery
inferior border of mandible
inferior cantholysis
inferior cardiac cervical nerve
inferior carotid triangle
inferior cerebellar arteries
inferior cerebellar veins
inferior cerebral veins
inferior cervical ganglion
inferior clunial nerves
inferior colliculus
inferior complete closed
   dislocation
inferior complete compound
   dislocation
inferior concha
inferior conjunctival fornix
   incision
inferior constrictor pharyngeal
   muscle
inferior costal facet
inferior crus of greater alar
   cartilage of nose
inferior crus of lateral canthal
   tendon
inferior deep cervical node
inferior dental arch

inferior dental foramen
inferior dental thrombosis
inferior displacement
inferior duodenal fold
inferior duodenal fossa
inferior duodenal recess
inferior edge
inferior epigastric artery
inferior ethmoidal concha
inferior extensor retinaculum
inferior extradural approach
inferior fascia
inferior fissure
inferior flap
inferior flexure of duodenum
inferior frontal gyrus
inferior ganglion
inferior ganglion of
    glossopharyngeal nerve
inferior ganglion of vagus
inferior gemellus muscle
inferior gland
inferior gluteal artery
inferior gluteal flap
inferior gluteal nerve
inferior gluteal veins
inferior horn of thyroid cartilage
inferior labial artery
inferior labial veins
inferior lacrimal canaliculus
inferior lacrimal duct
inferior laryngeal artery
inferior laryngeal cavity
inferior laryngeal nerve
inferior laryngeal vein
inferior laryngotomy
inferior lateral cutaneous nerve
    of arm
inferior lip
inferior lip of pons
inferior longitudinal muscle of
    tongue
inferior longitudinal scar
inferior malposition
inferior marginotomy
inferior maxilla
inferior maxillary bone
inferior meatal antrostomy
inferior meatus
inferior mesenteric artery (IMA)
inferior mesenteric ganglion
inferior nasal concha

inferior nasal nerve
inferior nasal venule of retina
inferior nerve
inferior oblique (IO)
inferior oblique muscle
inferior omental recess
inferior ophthalmic vein
inferior orbital fissure
inferior orbital foramen
inferior palpebral arch
inferior palpebral vein
inferior pancreaticoduodenal
    arteries
inferior parathyroid gland
inferior parietal lobe
inferior pedicle
inferior pedicle inverted-T
    procedure
inferior pelvic aperture
inferior petrosal groove
inferior petrosal sinus
inferior pharyngeal constrictor
inferior phrenic arteries
inferior phrenic vein
inferior pole hyperplasia
inferior pole of thyroid
inferior pole peritonsillar abscess
inferior posterior serratus muscle
inferior rectal artery
inferior rectal fold
inferior rectal nerves
inferior rectal vein
inferior rectus (IR)
inferior rectus muscle
inferior retinacular lateral
    canthoplasty
inferior retrognathia
inferior root of ansa cervicalis
inferior sagittal sinus
inferior suprarenal artery
inferior surface
inferior surface of tongue
inferior tarsal muscle
inferior tarsus
inferior teeth
inferior temporal venule of retina
inferior thoracic aperture
inferior thyroid artery
inferior thyroid gland
inferior thyroid notch
inferior thyroid vein
inferior tracheotomy

inferior transvermian approach
inferior transverse ligament
inferior transverse rectal fold
inferior turbinal crest of maxilla
inferior turbinal crest of palatine bone
inferior turbinate bone
inferior turbinate concha
inferior tympanic artery
inferior ulnar artery
inferior vein
inferior vena cava
inferior vena cava catheter
inferior vena cava clip
inferior vena cava interruption
inferior vena cava ligation
inferior vena cava reconstruction
inferior vena cava umbrella filter
inferior venacavography
inferior vertebral notch
inferior vesical artery
inferior vessels
inferior vestibular nucleus
inferior wall
inferior-lateral endonasal transsphenoidal approach
inferior-superior zygomatic arch radiograph
inferoapical defect
inferolateral aspect
inferomedial aspect
inferomedian
inferonasally
inferoposterior
inferosuperior axial projection
inferosuperior projection
inferosuperior tangential projection
inferotemporal
infertility detection
infertility evaluation
infiltrate
  corneal infiltrate
  creeping infiltrates
  granulomatous dermal infiltrate
  lung infiltrate
  lymphomatous infiltrate
  multifocal lymphocytic infiltrate
  parenchymal infiltrate
  patchy infiltrate
  strandy infiltrate

infiltrated duct cell carcinoma
infiltrated with Xylocaine
infiltrating adenocarcinoma
infiltrating carcinoma
infiltrating duct adenocarcinoma
infiltrating ductal carcinoma
infiltrating ductal cell carcinoma
infiltrating glioma
infiltrating lobular carcinoma
infiltration
  adipose infiltration
  bacterial mucosal infiltration
  bone marrow infiltration
  brachial plexus infiltration
  calcareous infiltration
  cellular infiltration
  choroidal infiltration
  colonic infiltration
  diffuse fatty infiltration
  epituberculous infiltration
  fatty infiltration
  fibrotic infiltration
  focal fatty infiltration
  gastric epithelial cell infiltration
  gelatinous infiltration
  glomerular infiltration
  glomerular macrophage infiltration
  glomerular neutrophil infiltration
  glycogen infiltration
  gray infiltration
  incisional infiltration
  leukemic infiltration
  leukocyte infiltration
  leukocytic infiltration
  lipomatous infiltration
  local infiltration
  local tissue infiltration
  lymphocytic infiltration
  lymphoid infiltration
  massive malignant infiltration
  mononuclear cell infiltration
  neutrophilic infiltration
  panmucosal inflammatory cell infiltration
  paraneural infiltration
  parenchyma infiltration
  patchy infiltration
  peribronchiolar lymphocyte infiltration

infiltration (*continued*)
  pericapsular fat infiltration
  perineural infiltration
  plasma cell portal infiltration
  pulmonary infiltration
  root infiltration
  sanguineous infiltration
  stringy infiltration
  superwet preoperative
    subcutaneous infiltration
  tuberculous infiltration
  tumor infiltration
infiltration analgesia
infiltration anesthesia
infiltration anesthetic technique
infiltration block
infiltration cannula
infiltrative basal cell carcinoma
infiltrative carcinoma
infiltrative fasciitis
infiltrative local anesthesia
infiltrative process
infiltrator
  Klein infiltrator
Infiniti catheter
Infinity modular hip prosthesis
inflamed appendix
inflamed diverticulum
inflamed gallbladder
inflamed organ
inflamed ulcer
inflammation
  active chronic inflammation
  acute and chronic
    inflammation
  acute hemorrhagic
    inflammation
  acute inflammation
  adhesive inflammation
  allergic inflammation
  alterative inflammation
  atrophic inflammation
  bronchial inflammation
  bullous granulomatous
    inflammation
  caseous inflammation
  calcified granulomatous
    inflammation
  cardinal signs of inflammation
  cartilage inflammation
  caseating granulomatous
    inflammation

inflammation (*continued*)
  catarrhal inflammation
  cavitating inflammation
  central zone inflammation
  cervical inflammation
  chronic inflammation
  chronic jejunal inflammation
  circumscribed inflammation
  confluent inflammation
  croupous inflammation
  cystic acute inflammation
  cystic chronic inflammation
  cystic granulomatous
    inflammation
  degenerative inflammation
  diffuse acute inflammation
  diffuse chronic inflammation
  disseminated inflammation
  ear cartilage inflammation
  erosive inflammation
  esophageal inflammation
  exanthematous inflammation
  exudative granulomatous
    inflammation
  fibrinoid necrotizing
    inflammation
  fibrinopurulent inflammation
  fibrinous inflammation
  fibrocaseous inflammation
  fibroid inflammation
  focal granulomatous
    inflammation
  focal inflammation
  follicular inflammation
  gallbladder inflammation
  gangrenous granulomatous
    inflammation
  gelatinous acute
    inflammation
  gingival inflammation
  granulomatous inflammation
  hemorrhagic inflammation
  hyperplastic inflammation
  ileal inflammation
  immuno-inflammation
  interstitial inflammation
  intralobular inflammation
  ischemic ocular inflammation
  localized inflammation
  membranous acute
    inflammation
  microbiliary inflammation

inflammation (*continued*)
  miliary granulomatous
    inflammation
  mucosal inflammation
  multifocal inflammation
  myocardial inflammation
  necrotic inflammation
  necrotizing granulomatous
    inflammation
  neutrophilic inflammation
  nonlocalized inflammation
  nonnecrotizing
    granulomatous
    inflammation
  obliterative inflammation
  ocular inflammation
  organizing inflammation
  ossifying inflammation
  pelvic inflammation
  periodontal inflammation
  perirectal inflammation
  portal eosinophilic
    inflammation
  portal tract inflammation
  prepatellar bursa
    inflammation
  production inflammation
  proliferative inflammation
  pseudomembranous acute
    inflammation
  purulent inflammation
  pustular inflammation
  recurrent inflammation
  retrodiskal
    temporomandibular joint
    pad inflammation
  sanguineous inflammation
  sclerosing inflammation
  serofibrinous inflammation
  serous acute inflammation
  serous inflammation
  spinal inflammation
  subacute inflammation
  suppurative chronic
    inflammation
  suppurative acute
    inflammation
  suppurative granulomatous
    inflammation
  suppurative inflammation
  transmural inflammation
  transudative inflammation

inflammation (*continued*)
  traumatic inflammation
  ulcerative inflammation
  urate-associated inflammation
  uremic inflammation
  vaginal inflammation
  vesicular acute inflammation
  vesicular granulomatous
    inflammation
inflammation and swelling
inflammatory arteritis
inflammatory arthropathy
inflammatory atrophy
inflammatory bowel disease (IBD)
inflammatory bowel syndrome
  (IBS)
inflammatory breast carcinoma
inflammatory carcinoma
inflammatory cavity
inflammatory cell
inflammatory change
inflammatory condition
inflammatory cyst
inflammatory disease
inflammatory edema
inflammatory exudate
inflammatory fibroid polyp
inflammatory fibrous
  hyperplasia
inflammatory fistula
inflammatory fracture
inflammatory gangrene
inflammatory granuloma
inflammatory lesion
inflammatory linear verrucous
  epidermal nevus (ILVEN)
inflammatory mass
inflammatory membrane
inflammatory oncotaxis
inflammatory pain
inflammatory papillary
  hyperplasia
inflammatory papillomatosis
inflammatory pelvic disease (IPD)
inflammatory perforation
inflammatory problem
inflammatory process
inflammatory pseudotumor
  formation
inflammatory reaction
inflammatory response
inflammatory rupture

inflammatory sinus tract
inflammatory tissue
inflammatory transcription
    factor
inflammatory zone
inflatable catheter
inflatable cuff
inflatable elbow splint
inflatable Foley bag catheter
inflatable implant
inflatable mammary prosthesis
inflatable Mentor penile
    prosthesis
inflatable penile implant
inflatable penile prosthesis
inflatable penile prosthesis with
    reservoir
inflatable splint
inflatable thoracic lumbosacral
    orthosis
inflatable tourniquet cuff
inflatable tracheal tube cuff
inflatable urinary incontinence
    prosthesis
inflated balloon
inflated eardrum
inflated implant
inflated tourniquet
inflation of bulb
inflation of tourniquet
inflation reflex
inflator
    Bonney inflator
    Bonney retrograde inflator
    LeVeen inflator
    Ogden-Senturia eustachian
        inflator
    rapid cuff inflator
inflow cannula
inflow control
inflow occlusion
inflow of arterial blood
inflow tract
infra-areolar scar
infra-auricular mass
infra-axillary
infrabony pocket
infrabony pocket curettage
infrabrow scar
infrabulge clasp
infracalcarine gyrus
infracartilaginous

infraciliary line
infraclavicular fossa
infraclavicular incision
infraclavicular region
infraclavicular triangle
infraclinoid aneurysm
infracostal line
infracrestal pocket
infracted turbinate
infraction fracture
infraction of turbinate
infracubital bypass
infraduction
infraduodenal fossa
infraglenoid
infraglottic carcinoma
infraglottic cavity
infraglottic space
infraglottic squamous cell
    carcinoma
infragluteal groove
infraguide tip
infrahepatic arteriography
infrahepatic arteriography and
    infusion
infrahepatic caval anastomosis
infrahyoid artery
infrahyoid muscles
infrahyoid strap muscle
infrainguinal bypass
infralabyrinthine air cell
infralabyrinthine approach
inframalar groove
inframammary approach
inframammary crease
inframammary crease-to-nipple
    distance (IMC-N)
inframammary distance
inframammary fold (IMF)
inframammary incision
inframammary region
inframammary scar
inframandibular
inframaxillary
inframaxillism
inframesocolic space
infranodal extrasystole
infraoccipital nerve
infraocclusion
infraorbital anesthesia
infraorbital artery
infraorbital block

infraorbital branch of interior maxillary artery
infraorbital branch of maxillary nerve
infraorbital canal
infraorbital fissure
infraorbital foramen
infraorbital fracture
infraorbital groove
infraorbital groove of maxilla
infraorbital incision
infraorbital injection
infraorbital margin
infraorbital nerve
infraorbital nerve block
infraorbital plate
infraorbital region
infraorbital ridge of maxilla
infraorbital rim
infraorbital space
infraorbital space abscess
infraorbital sulcus
infraorbital sulcus of maxilla
infraorbital sutures
infraorbital tear trough
infraorbitomeatal line
infrapalpebral sulcus
infrapatellar fat body
infrapatellar fat pad
infrapatellar synovial fold
infrapatellar tendon rupture
infrapiriform foramen
infrapopliteal bypass
infrapopliteal transluminal angioplasty
infrared applicator
infrared coagulation
infrared coagulator
infrared laser-Doppler flowmeter
infrared light-emitting diode
infrared liver scanner
infrared microscope
infrared photocoagulation
infrared spectrophotometry
infrared therapy
infrared transillumination gastroscopy
infrared-beam diode laser
infrarenal aorta
infrarenal aortic reconstruction
infrarenal endograft placement

infrarenal node
infrarenal template procedure
infrascapular region
infrasonic frequency
Infrasonics ventilator
infraspinatus muscle
infraspinatus reflex
infraspinatus tendon
infraspinous fossa
infraspinous muscle
infrasternal angle
infrasternal angle of thorax
infratemporal crest
infratemporal fossa
infratemporal fossa approach
infratemporal region
infratemporal space
infratemporal surface of maxilla
infratemporal wall
infratentorial arteriovenous malformation
infratentorial supracerebellar approach
infratrochlear branch of ophthalmic nerve
infratrochlear nerve
infraumbilical fold
infraumbilical incision
infraumbilical position
infrazygomatic crest
infrequent menstruation
infrequent pulse
Infumed pump
infundibula (*sing.* infundibulum)
infundibula of kidney
infundibular cell
infundibular forceps
infundibular punch
infundibular resection
infundibular rongeur
infundibular rongeur forceps
infundibular ventricular septal defect
infundibular wedge resection
infundibulectomy
   Brock infundibulectomy
infundibulectomy rongeur
infundibuliform fascia
infundibuliform recess
infundibulopelvic ligament
infundibulum (*pl.* infundibula)
infundibulum of fallopian tube

infundibulum of heart
infundibulum of hypophysis
infundibulum of urinary bladder
infundibulum of uterine tube
Infusaid catheter
Infusaid chemotherapy pump
Infusaid hepatic pump
Infusaid infusion pump
Infusaid needle
Infusaid pump
Infusaid pump for drug infusion
infusate
Infuse-a-Port catheter
Infuse-a-Port port
Infuse-a-Port pump
infusible pressure infusion bag
infusing solutions
infusion
   analgesic infusion
   chronic subcutaneous infusion
   cold infusion
   colloid infusion
   computer-assisted controlled
     infusion (CACO)
   crystalloid infusion
   drip infusion
   drug infusion
   epidural opioid infusion
   heparinized solution infusion
   hepatic arterial infusion (HAI)
   hot infusion
   infrahepatic arteriography and
     infusion
   Infusaid pump for drug
     infusion
   intravariceal infusion
   intravenous infusion
   isolated infusion
   IV infusion
   lipid infusion
   mesenteric vasodilator infusion
   nerve block infusion
   saline infusion
   target-controlled infusion
     (TCO)
   triple-lumen infusion
   vasodilator infusion
infusion cannula
infusion catheter
infusion chemotherapy
infusion cholangiography
infusion device

infusion drip
infusion graft
infusion nephrotomography
infusion of antibiotics
infusion of chemotherapeutic
   agent
infusion port
infusion pump
infusion pyelogram
infusion pyelography
infusion rate
infusion site
infusion suction vitreous
   cutter
infusion technique
infusion tube
infusion/infiltration cannula
infusional chemotherapy
infusion-withdrawal pump
infusor (*see* infuser)
Ingals cannula
Ingals flexible silver cannula
Ingals nasal speculum
Ingals rectal injection cannula
Ingals speculum
Inge lamina spreader
Inge laminectomy retractor
Inge procedure
Inge retractor
Inge spreader
Ingelman-Sundberg gracilis
   muscle procedure
Ingersoll adenoid curet
Ingersoll tonsil needle
Ingersoll tonsillar needle
ingestion of barium
ingestion of drugs
Inglis reconstruction
Inglis triaxial total elbow
   arthroplasty
Inglis-Cooper technique
Inglis-Ranawat-Straub approach
Inglis-Ranawat-Straub technique
Ingraham infant skull punch
Ingraham-Fowler clip-applying
   forceps
Ingraham-Fowler cranium clip
Ingraham-Fowler tantalum clip
Ingram bony bridge resection
Ingram catheter
Ingram operation for talipes
   equinovarus

Ingram operation for talipes valgus
Ingram procedure
Ingram regimen
Ingram technique
Ingram trocar
ingress tube
ingress/egress cannula
ingrown hair
ingrown nail
ingrown toenail
ingrowth
   bone ingrowth
   bony ingrowth
   fibrovascular ingrowth
   porous ingrowth
   squamous epithelial ingrowth
   squamous ingrowth
ingrowth fixation
inguinal adenopathy
inguinal aponeurotic fold
inguinal approach
inguinal area
inguinal artery
inguinal canal
inguinal canal dissection
inguinal crest
inguinal falx
inguinal field block
inguinal fossa
inguinal gland
inguinal hernia
inguinal hernia repair
inguinal herniorrhaphy
inguinal incision
inguinal ligament
inguinal lymph node
inguinal lymph node metastasis
inguinal lymphadenectomy
inguinal nerve
inguinal node dissection
inguinal nodes
inguinal perivascular block
inguinal reflex
inguinal region
inguinal ring
inguinal sphincter
inguinal triangle
inguinal-femoral node dissection
inguinoabdominal
inguinocrural hernia
inguinodynia

inguinofemoral hernia
inguinolabial hernia
inguino
inguinoproperitoneal hernia
inguinoscrotal hernia
inguinosuperficial hernia
inhalant anesthesia
inhalation aerosol
inhalation agent
inhalation analgesia
inhalation anesthesia
inhalation anesthetic technique
inhalation breath unit
inhalation cannula
inhalation mask anesthesia
inhalation pneumonia
inhalation therapy
inhalation tuberculosis
inhalational anesthesia
inhalator
   OIC emergency oxygen inhalator
   Oxy-Quik Mark IV oxygen inhalator
inherent extensibility of skin
inherent filter
inherent risk
inherited abnormality
inherited cancer syndrome
inherited disorder
inherited genetic defect
inherited tendency
inhibit blood clots
inhibit labor
inhibiting factor
inhibition sign
inhibitor
   shoulder subluxation inhibitor (SSI) brace
inhibitory
in-hospital mortality rate
initial colostomy
initial consonant position
initial diagnosis
initial dose
initial incision
initial incision retractor
initial manifestation
initial masking
initial necrosectomy
initial occlusive contact
initial operation

initial preparation
initial primary pathogen
initial resection
initial screening procedure
initial syphilitic lesion
initial systemic chemotherapy
initial therapy
initial treatment
initial venous shunt
injectable collagen
Injectate probe
injecting contrast medium
injection
  air injection
  block injection
  blood patch injection
  bolus injection
  Brown-Sequard injection
  cervical nerve root injection
  ciliary injection
  circumcorneal injection
  collagen injection
  conjunctival injection
  continuous subcutaneous
    insulin injection
  contrast injection
  corticoid injection
  depot intramuscular injection
  dermal injection
  dermal route of injection
  double injection
  dye injection
  endermic injection
  endoscopic India ink
    injection
  epidural steroid injection
  EpiE-Z Pen injection
  epifascial injection
  ethanol injection
  extra-arachnoid injection
  facet joint injection
  fat injection
  fiberscopic transduodenal
    duct injection
  gaseous injection
  hand injection
  heavy metal injection
  hypodermic injection
  infraorbital injection
  intra-amniotic saline injection
  intra-arterial injection
  intra-articular injection

injection (*continued*)
  intracardiac injection
  intracavernosal injection
  intracavernous injection
  intracordal silicone injection
  intracutaneous injection
  intracytoplasmic sperm
    injection (ICSI)
  intradermal injection
  intralesional injection
  intralesional steroid injection
  intramuscular injection
  intraosseous injection
  intraperitoneal injection
  intrapulpal injection
  intratendinous injection
  intrathecal injection
  intratumoral injection
  intravariceal injection
  intravascular injection
  intravenous injection
  intraventricular injection
  intravitreal injection
  ipsilateral injection
  isotope injection
  local injection
  lumbar facet injection
  lumbar nerve root injection
  manual injection
  marrow injection
  mental block injection
  microdroplet liquid silicone
    injections
  Microfil injection
  nasopalatine injection
  nerve root injection
  nerve root sleeve injection
  paracervical injection
  paramagnetic contrast
    injection
  paravariceal injection
  parenchymal route of injection
  parenchymatous injection
  percutaneous ethanol injection
  peribulbar injection
  perinephric air injection
  periocular injection
  peroneal tendon sheath
    injection
  pituitrin uterine injection
  power injection
  retrobulbar injection

injection (*continued*)
  retrograde injection
  root injection
  route of injection
  saline injection
  sclerosing injection
  selective injection
  sensitizing injection
  serial injection
  serial scar injections
  sham injection
  Silastic injection
  silicone injection
  steroid injection
  straight AP pelvic injection
  subarachnoid injection
  subconjunctival injection
  subcutaneous injection
  tangential colonic submucosal
    injection
  tendon aspiration and injection
  test injection
  transduodenal fiberscopic
    duct injection
  trigger point injection
  ultrasonographically-guided
    injection
  Van Lint injection
  vocal cord injection
  Zyderm collagen injection
injection cannula
injection electrode catheter
injection gold probe
injection injury
injection mass
injection molding
injection needle
injection of air
injection of bursa
injection of contrast medium
injection of drug
injection of dye
injection of hemorrhoids
injection of local anesthetic
injection of radiopaque material
injection of varices
injection port
injection sclerotherapy
injection site
injection study
injection technique
injection therapy

injection volume
Injectoflex respirator jet
injector
  Amplatz injector
  auto injector
  automatic twin syringe
    injector
  Bioject jet injector
  Cordis injector
  Dermo-Jet high pressure
    injector
  Dyonics syringe injector
  extractor injector
  Fujinon disposable injector
  Fujinon variceal injector
  Harris uterine injector (HUI)
  Hercules power injector
  Medrad angiographic injector
  Medrad automated power
    injector
  Medrad contrast medium
    injector
  Medrad injector
  Medrad Mark IV angiographic
    injector
  Medrad power angiographic
    injector
  Miller ratchet injector
  Mill-Rose esophageal injector
  modified Mark IV R-wave-
    triggered power injector
  Olympus injector
  power injector
  pressure injector
  Rhino Rocket injector
  Rowden uterine manipulator
    injector (RUMI)
  Teflon injector
  Tubex injector
  uterine injector
  Viamonte-Hobbs dye injector
  Virag injector
injured axon
injured limb
injured organ
injured tissue
injury
  1st-degree radiation injury
  2nd-degree radiation injury
  3rd-degree radiation injury
  4th-degree radiation injury
  acceleration injury

injury (*continued*)

acceleration/deceleration injury
acute phase of burn injury
Ajmalin liver injury
anal sphincter injury
anterior abdominal injury
arterial injury
associated injury
avulsion flap injury
avulsion injury
axial compression injury
axillary vascular injury
axonal injury
axonometric injury
backstroke injury
basement membrane zone injury
bifurcation injury
bile duct injury
birth injury
blast injury
blunt carotid injury (BCI)
blunt injury
blunt liver injury
blunt torso injury
bowel injury
brachial plexus traction injury
brain injury
breaststroke injury
burn injury
calcaneal apophysis occult compression injury
Callahan extension of cervical injury
carotid injury
catastrophic brain injury
cerebral injury
cervical cord injury
closed brachial plexus injury
closed degloving injury
closed head injury (CHI)
closed injury
closed soft tissue injury
clotheslines injury
cold injury
cold intolerance after fingertip injury
complement-induced lung injury
compression injury
concomitant spinal cord injury

injury (*continued*)

contrecoup injury
cord injury
cotton roll injury
cribriform plate injury
crush injury
crushed chest injury
crushing injury
cutaneous burn injury
deceleration injury
decompensation injury
degloving injury
dentinoblastic injury
destructive injury
diaphragm injury
diaphragmatic injury
duct injury
dural venous sinus injury
endothelial injury
epiphysial plate injury
explosion injury
extension injury
extension-type cervical spine injury
extensor tendon injury
extra-abdominal injury
extra-axial injury
extravasation injury
extremity injury
fingertip injury
flexion-extension injury
geriatric injury
grease gun injury
head injury
hemorrhagic radiation injury
hepatic injury
hollow visceral injury
hollow viscus injury
hyperextension-hyperflexion injury
hyperfiltration injury
hyperperfusion injury
iatrogenic bowel injury
iatrogenic ureteral injury
impact injury
impalement injury
inadvertent venous injury
injection injury
innominate vascular injury
intestinal radiation injury
intimal injury
intra-abdominal injury

injury (*continued*)
  intracranial injury
  intraoperative inadvertent
    venous injury
  intrathoracic injury
  irradiation injury
  ischemia and reperfusion injury
  ischemia-reperfusion injury
  ischemic liver injury
  isolated arterial injury
  isolated liver injury
  isolated venous injury
  jamming injury
  joint injury
  kidney injury
  kneecapping injury
  lateral compression injury
  left-sided injury
  lethal injury
  levator injury
  liver injury
  major vascular injury
  maxillofacial injury
  medication-induced injury
  microwave radiation injury
  mild traumatic brain injury
    (mTBI)
  minor injury
  minor splenic injury
  missile injury
  multihit injury
  nail injury
  needlestick injury
  nerve crush injury
  nerve injury
  neurologic injury
  nonsevered injury
  obstetric brachial plexus
    injury
  obstetrical traction injury
  obturator nerve injury
  occult compression injury
  occult diaphragmatic injury
  open head injury
  organ-specific pattern of
    injury
  osteochondral injury
  paint-gun injury
  pediatric injury
  penetrating liver injury
  penetrating thoracoabdominal
    injury

injury (*continued*)
  penile injury
  percutaneous injury (PI)
  perigenicular vascular injury
  perinatal injury
  peripheral nerve injury
  peroneal injury
  pronation injury
  pronation-abduction injury
  pronation-eversion injury
  pronation-eversion external
    rotation injury
  proximal subclavian injury
  radial mutilation injury
  radiation injury
  recurrent nerve injury
  related injury
  renal injury
  reperfusion injury
  retroclavicular injury
  right-sided injury
  ring avulsion injury
  rotator cuff injury
  seat belt injury
  self-induced injury
  severe traumatic brain injury
  severity of injury
  snow-plow injury
  soft structure injury
  soft-tissue extremity injury
  sphincter injury
  spinal cord injury
  splenic injury
  steering-wheel injury
  stretch injury
  subclavian injury
  subendocardial injury
  subepicardial injury
  suction injury
  supination injury
  supination-eversion injury
  supination-external rotation
    injury
  supination-inversion rotation
    injury
  supination-plantar flexion
    injury
  swimming injury
  tampon injury
  tattoo injury
  tendon injury
  thermal injury

injury (*continued*)
  thoracic inlet vascular injury
  thoracoabdominal injury
  through-and-through avulsion
    injury
  torso injury
  transfusion-related acute lung
    injury (TRALD)
  transfusion-related lung injury
    (TRLI)
  translation injury
  traumatic brain injury (TBI)
  traumatic injury
  trifurcation injury
  trocar injury
  trocar-related injury
  twisting injury
  ureteral injury
  urinary tract injury
  valgus-external rotation injury
  vascular injury
  venous injury
  ventilator-induced lung injury
    (VILI)
  visceral injury
  viscus injury
  volar plate injury
  whiplash injury
  wringer injury
  zone of injury
injury prevention
Injury Severity Score (ISS)
injury site
ink
  Bonney blue ink
inlay
  composite inlay
  corneal inlay
  direct method for making
    inlays
  epithelial inlay
  porcelain inlay
inlay bone graft
inlay graft
inlay implant
inlay inguinal herniorrhaphy
inlay mold
inlay restoration
inlet
  anterior sagittal pelvic inlet
  Berry rotating inlet
  esophageal inlet

inlet (*continued*)
  Fish inlet
  pelvic inlet
  thoracic inlet
  transverse diameter of inlet
  transverse pelvic inlet
inlet allotransplantation
inlet cannula
inlet forceps
inlet views
in-line blood gas monitor
in-line perfusion
in-line venous pressure monitor
innate immunity
inner aspect
inner bevel incision
inner callus
inner canthus
inner core for outside housing
inner ear ablation
inner ear tack procedure
inner fibrous layer
inner hamstring
inner layer
inner limiting membrane
inner lip plate
inner pillar
inner quadrant
inner surface
inner table bones of skull
inner table of frontal bone
inner table of skull
inner thigh lift
inner thighplasty (string
    technique)
innermost intercostal muscles
innermost membrane of meninges
innervated free flap
innervated muscles
innervated platysma flap
innervation
  areas of innervation
  cutaneous innervation
  reciprocal innervation
  segmental innervation
  striated muscle innervation
innervation apraxia
innervation of head and neck
innervation problem
Innervision MR scanner
Innervision ventricular catheter
innocent gallstone

innocent murmur
innocuous lump
innocuous tumor
Innomed bone curet
innominate aneurysm
innominate artery compression
    syndrome
innominate artery reconstruction
innominate bone resection
innominate cartilage
innominate endarterectomy
innominate fascia
innominate fossa
innominate fossa of auricle
innominate line
innominate osteotomy
innominate vascular injury
innominate veins
Innova pelvic floor stimulator
Innovar anesthetic agent
innovative therapy
INO (internuclear
    ophthalmoplegia)
Inokuchi vascular stapler
inoperable cancer
inoperable carcinoma
inoperable condition
inoperable malignancy
inoperable patient
inoperable tumor
inorganic dental cement
inorganic murmur
Inoue balloon catheter
Inoue self-guiding balloon
input device
input frequency
input impedance
input layer
input shunt
input stage
input terminal
input voltage
Inrad fine-needle prostate
    aspiration kit
Inro surgical nail
Inronail fingernail prosthesis
Inronail toenail prosthesis
Insall anterior cruciate ligament
    reconstruction
Insall approach
Insall ligament reconstruction
    technique

Insall patellar injury classification
Insall procedure
Insall-Burstein arthroplasty
Insall-Burstein intracondylar
    knee implant
Insall-Burstein intracondylar
    total knee implant
Insall-Burstein knee prosthesis
Insall-Burstein prosthesis
Insall-Burstein total knee
    prosthesis
Insall-Burstein total knee
    replacement
Insall-Burstein-Freeman knee
    arthroplasty
Insall-Burstein-Freeman total knee
Insall-Burstein-Freeman total
    knee instrumentation
Insall-Hood posterior cruciate
    reconstruction
insemination
    artificial insemination
    artificial intravaginal
        insemination
    cervical insemination
    cup insemination
    direct intraperitoneal
        insemination
    heterologous insemination
    high intrauterine insemination
    homologous artificial
        insemination
    intrafollicular insemination
    intratubal insemination
    intrauterine insemination
    Makler insemination
    subzonal insemination
    therapeutic insemination
    washed intrauterine
        insemination
insemination swim-up technique
insensate flap
insensible fluid output
insert graft
insert mattress sutures
insert tube
inserted and positioned
inserter (also insertor)
    AMO-PhacoFlex lens and
        inserter
    Buck femoral cement
        restrictor inserter

inserter (*continued*)
  cement restrictor inserter
  cement spacer inserter
  Cody tack inserter
  DDT lock screw inserter
  deluxe FIN pin inserter
  diaphragm inserter
  Furlow cylinder inserter
  Kirschner wire inserter
  Lehner inserter
  Massie inserter
  Moon-Robinson prosthesis
    inserter
  Prodigy lens inserter
  Robinson-Moon prosthesis
    inserter
  Shaffner orthopedic inserter
  spacer inserter
  Storz inserter
  subperiosteal glass bead
    inserter
  tack inserter
  Texas Scottish Rite Hospital
    hook inserter
  twist-in drain tube inserter
  Tytan tube inserter
  ventilation inserter
inserter tack
insertion
  anatomic insertion
  anomalous insertion
  aponeurosis of insertion
  axillary insertion
  biliary endoprosthesis
    insertion
  bronchoscopy with insertion
  buttonhole puncture
    technique for hemodialysis
    needle insertion
  catheter insertion
  caval insertion
  cervical radium insertion
  cesium insertion
  cystoradium insertion
  depth of insertion (DOI)
  endoscopic assisted facial
    implant insertion
  endovascular graft insertion
  flatus tube insertion
  fluoroscopic insertion
  intracavitary radium insertion
  jejunal tube insertion

insertion (*continued*)
  J-tube insertion
  laminaria insertion
  marginal insertion
  myringotomy and grommet
    insertion
  path of insertion
  PEG insertion
  percutaneous catheter
    insertion
  percutaneous endoscopic
    gastrostomy insertion
  percutaneous pin insertion
  radium insertion
  reflected from insertion
  rerouting insertion
  retrograde catheter insertion
  route of insertion
  Rush rod insertion
  screw insertion
  subcilial blepharoplasty malar
    implant insertion
  subclavian central venous
    catheter insertion
  tandem insertion
  tendinous insertion
  tendon insertion
  tensor insertion
  tibial insertion
  transjugular insertion
  uterine radium insertion
  vaginal radium insertion
  velamentous insertion
  wire insertion
insertion forceps
insertion loss
insertion of cannula
insertion of catheter
insertion of fixation device
insertion of metal plate
insertion of nail
insertion of pacemaker
insertion of pack
insertion of pin
insertion of prosthesis
insertion of radioactive material
insertion of radium
insertion of screw
insertion of tampon
insertion of traction device
insertion of T-tube
insertion of tube

insertion of vaginal pack
insertion of vascular prosthesis
insertion of wire
insertion point
insertion tandem
insertion technique
insertional excursion
insertor (*see* inserter)
inside diameter
inside-out technique
inside-the-needle catheter
    (INC)
inside-the-needle infusion
    catheter
inside-to-outside technique
inspection, palpation,
    percussion, and
    auscultation (IPAA)
InspiraEase device
inspiratory dyspnea
inspiratory flow rate
inspiratory force
inspiratory murmur
inspiratory muscles
inspiratory pressure
inspiratory respiration
inspiratory rib cage depression
inspiratory sounds
inspiratory spasm
inspiratory stridor
inspiratory vapor concentration
inspiratory wheezing
inspiratory/expiratory ratio (I/E
    ratio)
inspired oxygen
inspired ventilation (VI)
Inspiron device
Inspiron small inspiratory
    training device
inspissated cerumen
inspissated feces
Innsbruck electrode
instability
    anterolateral rotatory
        instability (ALRI)
    anteromedial rotatory
        instability (AMRI)
    atlantoaxial instability
    cardiac instability
    carpal instability
    dorsal intercalated segmental
        instability (DISI)

instability (*continued*)
    dorsal intercalated segmental
        instability (DISI) deformity
    extension instability
    hemodynamic instability
    joint instability
    ligamentous instability
    lunotriquetral instability
    membrane instability
    neurological instability
    perilunar instability (PLI)
    progressive perilunar
        instability (stages I-IV)
    rotational instability
    rotatory instability
    scapholunate instability
    volar intercalated segmental
        instability (VISI)
instability of joint
installation procedure
Instand Response technology
    generator
instant cold pack
instant delivery
instant skin hook
instantaneous axis of rotation
instantaneous pressure
InstaScan scanner
Instat collagen absorbable
    hemostat
InStent balloon-expandable stent
instep island flap
instillation
    contrast material instillation
    intratracheal instillation
    intravesical instillation
    lavage instillation
    local instillation
instillation of anesthesia
instillation of anesthetic
instillation of contrast medium
instillation of diagnostic media
instillation therapy
instillator
instrument
    3M filling instrument
    A13 Sequel programmable
        behind-the-ear hearing
        instrument
    ablative instrument
    Abradabloc dermabrasion
        instrument

instrument (*continued*)
abrading instrument
accessory instrument
Accu-Line distal femoral
   resection instrument
Accu-Line patellar instrument
AccuSharp instrument
activating adjusting
   instrument (AAI)
Acufex arthroscopic
   instrument
Acufex microsurgical
   instrument
acupuncture instrument
adapted instrument
adenoid instrument
Alcon Surgical instrument
Alvarado Orthopedic
   Research instrument (AOR
   instrument)
American Hydron instrument
American Optical Company
   instrument
American V. Mueller urological
   instrument
Anis microsurgical eye
   instrument
anterior cervical disk
   interbody fusion instrument
antrum instrument
AO Reichert scientific
   instrument
AOR instrument
arterial oscillator
   endarterectomy instrument
arthroscopic instrument
Arthrotek Ellipticut hand
   instrument
Ascon instrument
ASSI dual-ended surgical
   instrument
ASSI nasal and sinus
   instrument
atrial instrument
attempted passage of
   instrument
Ausman microsurgery
   instrument
Austin middle ear instrument
Austin Moore bone-measuring
   instrument
Austin Moore instrument

instrument (*continued*)
Austin-Moore bone measuring
   instrument
Auto-Suture EEA instrument
Ayerst instrument
BabyBeat ultrasound
   instrument
BackBiter instrument
Backlund stereotactic
   instrument
back-stopped laser instrument
Bausch-Lomb instrument
Bechert microsurgery
   instrument
bibeveled cutting instrument
binocular instrument
Biomer microsuturing
   instrument
Biomet instrument
Biomet total knee instrument
biopsy instrument
Birtcher electrosurgical
   instrument
blackened laser instrument
Blackwood suture instrument
blood sampling instrument
bone abduction instrument
bone biopsy instrument
brain surgery instrument
C.W. Mayo instrument
Carl Zeiss instrument
cervical disk instrument
cervical range-of-motion
   instrument
Cheshire-Poole-Yankauer
   suction instrument
chiropractic adjusting
   instrument
Clarke stereotactic instrument
cleft palate instrument
Cloward laminectomy
   instrument
Cobb spinal instrument
Collis TDR instrument
conization instrument
contour-facilitating instrument
Cooley neonatal instrument
Corex instrument
cradling instrument
cranial operating instrument
cryosurgical instrument
CSF shunt instrument

instrument (*continued*)
  currycomb instrument
  Cushing brain instrument
  cutdown instrument
  Daisy I&A instrument
  Dawson-Yuhl spinal
    instrument
  Delcom filling instrument
  dermal instrument
  diamond instrument
  Diamond-Lite cardiovascular
    instrument
  Diamond-Lite titanium
    instrument
  Digitate microsurgical
    instrument
  digitized instrument
  dilation instrument
  direct laryngeal operating
    instrument
  disposable instrument
  Dix double-ended
    instrument
  Dolphin instrument
  Dualine digital hearing
    instrument
  Duette double lumen ERCP
    instrument
  Dwyer instrument
  Dyonics arthroscopic
    instrument
  Dyonics microsurgical
    instrument
  ear instrument
  ear operating instrument
  economy line instrument
  Endoflex endoscopy
    instrument
  Endoloop chromic ligature
    suture instrument
  endolymphatic sac
    enlargement instrument
  EndoMax advanced
    laparoscopic instrument
  endosonography instrument
  Fairline instrument
  falloposcope endoscopic
    instrument
  Falope-ring dual-incision
    instrument
  Falope-ring mini-laparotomy
    instrument

instrument (*continued*)
  Falope-ring single-incision
    instrument
  Farrier flap exposure
    instrument
  fenestration instrument
  fetal blood-sampling
    instrument
  fiberoptic instrument
  Fleming conization
    instrument
  flexible biopsy instrument
  flexible bronchoscopic biopsy
    instrument
  flexible laparoscopic
    instrument
  Freer submucous instrument
  French scale for sizing tubular
    instrument
  fusion instrument
  gastrointestinal instrument
  GIA instrument
  GIF-XQ fiberoptic instrument
  Glassman noncrushing
    instrument
  gnathologic instrument
  Graefe instrument
  graft measuring instrument
  Guilford-Wright instrument
  Guilford-Wright middle ear
    instrument
  Guilford-Wullstein instrument
  guillotine vitrectomy
    instrument
  Halifax fine adjustment
    instrument
  Hall large bone instrument
  Hall surgical instrument
  hand surgery instrument
  handcutting instrument
  Heinkel-Semm dilator
    instrument
  Heinkel-Semm laparoscopy
    instrument
  Henry Schein filling instrument
  Heyer-Schulte hydrocephalus
    shunt instrument
  Heyer-Schulte shunt
    instrument
  Horico diamond instrument
  Hough middle ear instrument
  House middle ear instrument

instrument (*continued*)
  Howmedica surgical
    instrument
  Humphrey eye instrument
  hydrocephalus shunt
    instrument
  hypophysectomy instrument
  I&A instrument
  Imount instrument
  inadequately sterilized
    instrument
  indirect contact with
    contaminated instrument
  interbody fusion instrument
  interchangeable ear
    instrument
  intracanal instrument
  intraocular instrument
  intraorbital tumor instrument
  IOLAB titanium instrument
  ionization instrument
  Iowa trumpet instrument
  Jackson bronchoscopic
    instrument
  Jackson laryngeal instrument
  Jacobson microsurgery
    instrument
  Jannetta microneurosurgery
    instrument
  Jewett nail instrument
  Johnson Endobag instrument
  Jordan middle ear instrument
  Jordan strut-measuring
    instrument
  JP instrument (Jackson-Pratt)
  K x-ray fluorescence
    instrument
  Kapp surgical instrument
  Keeler cryosurgical
    instrument
  Kellman instrument
  Kimberley diamond
    instrument
  Kirkland instrument
  Kirschner surgical instrument
  Kitner blunt dissecting
    instrument
  Kitner instrument
  Kleinsasser laryngeal
    microsurgery instrument
  Kuntschner nail instrument
  knot-tying instrument

instrument (*continued*)
  Krwawicz cataract
    cryosurgical instrument
  Kurze microneurosurgery
    instrument
  Ladmore plastic filling
    instrument
  Lahey Clinic instrument
  laminectomy instrument
  laparoscope instrument
  laparoscopy dilation
    instrument
  LapTie endoscopic knot-tying
    instrument
  LDS instrument
  Lempert instrument
  Lewicky instrument
  ligature-passing instrument
  Lorie tonsillar suture
    instrument
  Luikart Iconoclast blunt
    dissection instrument
  Luongo instrument
  Lusk instrument
  MacKinnon-Dellon
    Diskriminator instrument
  Malis bipolar instrument
  Marlow instrument
  Matsuda titanium surgical
    instrument
  McCabe measuring
    instrument
  McCall instrument
  McElroy instrument
  McGee middle ear instrument
  mechanical radial-scanning
    instrument
  Medicon instrument
  Micro-Aire instrument
  Micro-Aire pneumatic power
    instrument
  micro-Doppler instrument
  microlaryngeal instrument
  Micromedics surgical
    instrument
  Midas Rex pneumatic
    instrument
  Millet neurological test
    instrument
  mini-driver instrument
  Mitek SuperAnchor instrument
  Monarch bleaching instrument

instrument (*continued*)

Monogram total knee instrument
multipurpose instrument
myoma fixation instrument
Nakayama instrument
nasal instrument
nasal plastic instrument
National instrument
Neoknife electrosurgical instrument
Neuro-Trace instrument
Newport medical instrument
Nicolet Compass electromyography instrument
Nordent filling instrument
Nucleotome diskectomy instrument
Nucleotome Endoflex instrument
oblique forward-viewing instrument
obstetrical instrument
Obwegeser orthognathic surgery instrument
Olympus GIF-XQ fiberoptic instrument
Orthair bunionectomy instrument
Orthair orthopedic instrument
Ortho-Athrex instrument
orthopedic cutting instrument
OrthoVise orthopaedic instrument
Paparella middle ear instrument
passage of instrument
pencil-grip instrument
piercing instrument
pistol-grip instrument
Plastibell compression instrument
plugging instrument
point-search instrument
Polaris reusable laparoscopic instrument
polytome instrument
Precision tack instrument
pulsed-range gated Doppler instrument
Quinton suction biopsy instrument

instrument (*continued*)

Rancho external fixation instrument
reciprocal planing instrument
reduction instrument
Reichert refracting instrument
Retinomax refractometry instrument
Rizzuti-Bonaccolto instrument
Rizzuti-Fleischer instrument
Rizzuti-Kayser-Fleischer instrument
Rizzuti-Lowe instrument
Rizzuti-Maxwell instrument
Rizzuti-Soemmering instrument
Rosen middle ear instrument
Rosenberg gynecomastia dissection instrument
rotary cutting instrument
Ruggles surgical instrument
Rumex titanium instrument
Rusch nephrostomy instrument
Rush pin instrument
Rush rod instrument
Safco diamond instrument
Salinger reduction instrument
Sauer-Wiener intranasal instrument
Scheer middle ear instrument
Schlesinger instrument
Schneider PTCA instrument
Schuknecht middle ear instrument
ScoliTron instrument
screwdriver instrument
Semmes-Weinstein monofilament instrument
Sharpoint cutting instrument
Shea middle ear instrument
Shriners Hospital instrument
single-beveled cutting instrument
single-plane instrument
single-reference-point instrument
slotted instrument
small-diameter endosonographic instrument
Smith-Miller-Patch cryosurgical instrument

instrument (*continued*)

Snowden-Pencer laparoscopic cholecystectomy instrument
solid-state instrument
spark-gap instrument
spring-loaded biopsy instrument
stapling instrument
Stat aspirating instrument
Stat cutting instrument
Steele filling instrument
stereotaxic instrument
sterilized instrument
sternal instrument
Storz arthroscopy operating instrument
Storz flexible biopsy instrument
Storz gynecological instrument
Storz otolaryngological instrument
Storz proctoscopic instrument
Storz urological instrument
strut measuring instrument
strut measuring instrument
successful passage of instrument
suction biopsy instrument
Sutcliffe laser shield and retracting instrument
Sutherland rotatable microsurgery instrument
suturing instrument
tattooing instrument
tendon-tucking instrument
Tessier craniofacial instrument
test handle instrument
Thomas Kapsule instrument
Todd-Wells stereotaxic instrument
tonsil-suturing instrument
Townley anatomic instrument
trocar tunneling instrument
tunneling instrument
Ultra-Cut Cobb spinal instrument
Ultra-Cut surgical instrument
ultrasonic bone-cutting instrument

instrument (*continued*)

Unitech instrument
ureteral visualization instrument
Uroloop instrument
vertebral body biopsy instrument
Vickers microsurgical instrument
viewing instrument
Vilex plastic surgery instrument
Wallach minifreezer cryosurgical instrument
Welch Allyn instrument
Wiener-Sauer intranasal tear-sac operation instrument
Wiet graft-measuring instrument
Wigand endoscopic instrument
Wood-Doig vacuum biopsy instrument
Wright-Guilford middle ear instrument
Yankauer eustachian instrument
Yasargil neurological instrument
Yasargil-Aesculap instrument
Zeiss instrument
Zeiss ophthalmological instrument
instrument basket
instrument birth
instrument coding tape
instrument cradle
instrument guide
instrument holder
Instrument Makar biodegradable interference screw
instrument marker
instrument polish
instrument rack
instrument retrieval container
instrument roll
instrument set
instrument stabilizer pad
instrument stand
instrument sterilizer
instrument sterilizing case
instrument table

instrument, sponge, and needle count
instrumental compression
instrumental dilation
instrumental perforation
instrumentation
  Accolade surgical instrumentation
  Accu-Line knee instrumentation
  advanced breast biopsy instrumentation (ABBI)
  anterior distraction instrumentation
  AO interior fixation instrument
  AO notched instrumentation
  ArthoPlastics ankle instrumentation
  Baxter V. Mueller laparoscopic instrumentation
  biofeedback instrumentation
  Caspar anterior instrumentation
  compression U-rod instrumentation
  Cotrel-Dubousset instrumentation (CDI)
  Cotrel-Dubousset pedicle screw instrumentation
  Cotrel-Dubousset pedicular instrumentation
  Cotrel-Dubousset spinal instrumentation
  craniofacial instrumentation
  distraction instrumentation
  double Zielke instrumentation
  Dwyer instrumentation
  dynamic compression plate instrumentation
  Edwards instrumentation
  EEG and PSG instrumentation
  EndoMax endoscopic instrumentation
  endoscopic instrumentation
  Gellman instrumentation
  halo-Ilizarov distraction instrumentation
  Harms-Moss anterior thoracic instrumentation
  Harrington distraction instrumentation
  Harrington instrumentation

instrumentation (*continued*)
  Harrington rod instrumentation
  Harrington spinal instrumentation
  incremental instrumentation
  Insall-Burstein-Freeman total knee instrumentation
  insufficient instrumentation
  interspinous segmental spinal instrumentation
  Jacobs locking hook spinal rod instrumentation
  Karl Storz instrumentation
  Louis instrumentation
  L-rod instrumentation
  lumbosacral spine transpedicular instrumentation
  Luque segmental spinal instrumentation
  Luque semirigid segmental spinal instrumentation
  Microvasive instrumentation
  Midas Rex instrumentation
  minimal instrumentation
  modular instrumentation
  Moss instrumentation
  Moss-Miami spinal instrumentation
  Mueller laparoscopic instrumentation
  multiple hook assembly instrumentation
  Ortholoc IM instrumentation
  Passport instrumentation
  posterior distraction instrumentation
  posterior hook-rod spinal instrumentation
  Putti-Platt instrumentation
  Russell-Taylor interlocking nail instrumentation
  sacral spine modular instrumentation
  sacral spine Universal instrumentation
  segmental spinal instrumentation
  Smith-Richards instrumentation
  Stefee spinal instrumentation
  stereotactic instrumentation

instrumentation (*continued*)
  Stryker power instrumentation
  TAG instrumentation
  urethral instrumentation
  Zielke pedicular
    instrumentation
  Zimmer intramedullary knee
    instrumentation
instrumentation failure
instrument-grasping forceps
instrument-handling forceps
insufficiency
  abdominal wall insufficiency
  aortic insufficiency
  aortic valve insufficiency
  cerebrovascular insufficiency
  coronary insufficiency
  degenerative mitral valve
    insufficiency
  gastromotor insufficiency
  hiatal insufficiency
  mitral insufficiency
  myocardial insufficiency
  palatal insufficiency
  placental insufficiency
  pulmonic insufficiency
  superficial valvular
    insufficiency
  uteroplacental insufficiency
  valvular insufficiency
  velar insufficiency
  velopharyngeal insufficiency
    (VPI)
  venous insufficiency
insufficiency fracture
insufficient instrumentation
insufficient jaw grading
insufficient lip support
insufflated peritoneal cavity
insufflation
  air insufflation
  carbon dioxide insufflation
  constant flow insufflation
  cranial insufflation
  endotracheal insufflation
  extraperitoneal carbon
    dioxide insufflation
  extraperitoneal CO_2
    insufflation
  gas insufflation
  gastric insufflation
  helium insufflation

insufflation (*continued*)
  intraperitoneal carbon
    dioxide insufflation
  intraperitoneal CO_2
    insufflation
  methylene blue insufflation
  perirenal insufflation
  peritoneal insufflation
  presacral insufflation
  retroperitoneal gas
    insufflation
  Rubin tubal insufflation
  talc insufflation
  thoracoscopic talc insufflation
  tubal insufflation
insufflation anesthesia
insufflation anesthetic
  technique
insufflation device
insufflation of fallopian tubes
insufflation of lungs
insufflation of stomach
insufflation of uterus
insufflation pressure
insufflation test set
insufflator
  Bonney insufflator
  Buckstein colonic insufflator
  colonic insufflator
  Dench insufflator
  DyoPneumatic insufflator
  Eder insufflator
  gas insufflator
  HiTec insufflator
  hysteroscopic insufflator
  Kelly insufflator
  Kidde tubal insufflator
  laparoscopic insufflator
  laparoscopy insufflator
  Reuben insufflator
  Semm insufflator
  Sieger insufflator
  Snowden-Pencer insufflator
  Stille insufflator
  Storz Laparoflator insufflator
  tubal insufflator
  tube insufflator
  variable flow insufflator
  Venturi insufflator
  Weber colonic insufflator
  Weber insufflator
  Wisap insufflator

Insuflon catheter
Insuflon insulin delivery device
insular carcinoma
insular sclerosis
insular scotoma
insulated bayonet forceps
insulated cautery
insulated curved scissors
insulated electrode needle
insulated knife handle
insulated monopolar forceps
insulated straight scissors
insulated suction tube
insulated tissue forceps
insulin coma therapy
insulin pen pump
insulin shock therapy
insulin-induced lipohypertrophy
insulin-like growth factor
InSurg common bile duct (CBD)
    basket
InSurg laparoscopic
    instrumentation
InSurg laparoscopic stone basket
InSync cardiac stimulator
inSync miniform
Insyte AutoGuard catheter
In-Tac bone anchor
Intacs corneal ring implant
Intacs intrastromal corneal ring
intact anastomosis
intact bone structure
intact canal wall technique
intact catheter
intact hymen
intact membrane
intact motor tract
intact rib cage
intact skin sutures
intact tissues
intact tonsils
Intact xenograft prosthetic
    valve
intake and output (I&O)
Intec implantable defibrillator
Integra artificial skin
Integra catheter
Integra balloon
Integra tissue expander
integral asepsis
integral dose
integral fiberoptic sheath

integral implant
Integral Interlok femoral
    prosthesis
integral intraoral bilateral
    posterior mesostructure
Integral Omniloc implant
integral uniformity scintillation
    camera
integrated electromyogram
integrated head holder
integrating microscope
integrative mastoplasty
Integriderm mattress
Integris scanner
Integris cardiovascular imaging
Integris imager
Integrity acetabular cup
Integrity acetabular cup prosthesis
Integrity acetabular cup screw
Integrity pacemaker
Integrity neutral liner
InteguDerm dressing
integument
integumentary barrier
Intellicath pulmonary artery
    catheter
Intelligent dressing
Intelliject pump
intense concentration
intensification factor
intensified radiographic imaging
    system scanner
intensifier
intensifying screen
intensity
    echo intensity
    electrosurgical current
        intensity
    luminous intensity
    maximal intensity
intensive treatment
intent
intention
    healed by first intention
    healed by second intention
    healed by third intention
    healing by first intention
    healing by second intention
    healing by third intention
intention spasm
intentional marker
intentional replantation

intentionem
  healing per secundam
    intentionem
  incision healed per primam
    intentionem
  incision healed per secundam
    intentionem
  per primam intentionem
  per secundam intentionem
interalveolar bone crater
interalveolar distance
interalveolar septum
interalveolar space
interannular segment
interaortic balloon pump
interarch distance
interarterial fluid
interarticular cartilage
interarticular joint
interarytenoid muscle
interarytenoid notch
interarytenoid space
interatrial conduction delay
interatrial groove
interatrial septal defect
interatrial septum
interauditory canal tomogram
interaural attenuation
interauricular loop
interauricular septum
interbody bone graft
interbody circular rasp
interbody fusion
interbody fusion instruments
interbody fusion rasp
interbody graft tamp
interbody rasp
interbody spinal fusion
intercalary allograft
intercalary bone graft
intercalary graft
intercalary resection
intercalated defect
intercalated disk
intercalated duct
intercalated duct lumen
intercalated joint
intercalation
intercanthal distance (ICD)
intercanthic diameter
intercapillary nephrosclerosis
intercapital veins

intercapitular vein of foot
intercapitular vein of hand
intercarotid ganglion
intercarpal articulation
intercarpal joint synchondrosis
intercartilaginous fold
intercartilaginous incision
intercartilaginous rim
intercartilaginous rima
intercavernous sinus
Interceed absorbable adhesion
    barrier
Interceed adhesion barrier
Interceed barrier material
intercellular bridges
intercellular canaliculus
intercellular fenestration
intercellular fluid
intercellular layer
intercellular matrix process
intercellular space
intercellular substance
intercellular tissue space
Intercept vascular guidewire
interceptive occlusal contact
interceptive orthodontic
    manipulation
interceptive orthodontics
Intercept vascular guidewire
intercervical disk herniation
interchangeable ear
    instruments
interchangeable forceps tips
interchangeable laryngeal
    forceps tips
interchangeable punch handle
interchangeable vein stripper
interchondral articulation
interclavicular notch
intercondylar eminence
intercondylar femoral fracture
intercondylar fossa
intercondylar fracture
intercondylar groove
intercondylar humeral fracture
intercondylar line
intercondylar notch
intercondylar notch of femur
intercondylar process
intercondylar space
intercondylar tibial fracture
intercondyloid fossa

intercoronary anastomosis
intercostal anesthesia
intercostal artery
intercostal articulation
intercostal block
intercostal bundle
intercostal catheter
intercostal drain
intercostal flap
intercostal fossa block
intercostal groove
intercostal margin
intercostal membrane
intercostal muscle
intercostal nerve block
intercostal nerve block
   anesthetic technique
intercostal nerves
intercostal retraction
intercostal space
intercostal tenderness
intercostal trocar
intercostal tube
intercostal vein
intercostal vessels
intercostalis externus muscle
intercostalis internus muscle
intercostobrachial nerves
intercricothyroidotomy
intercricothyrotomy
intercristal space
intercuspal position
intercuspation
interdental denudation
interdental embrasure
interdental excision
interdental knife
interdental ligament
interdental ligation
interdental lisp
interdental resection
interdental space
interdental splint
interdental wire
interdermal buried sutures
interdigital ligament
interdigital spaces
interdigitated muscle flap
interdigitating coil stent
interdigitating dendritic cell
   (IDC)
interdigitating skin flap

interdigitating triangular skin
   flap
interdigitating zigzag skin flap
interdigitation
interdomal sutures
interelectrode distance
interendognathic sutures
interface
   acoustic interface
   bioacrylic interface
   bone-cement interface
   bone-implant interface
   cement interface
   cement-bone interface
   cup-cement interface
   electrode-skin interface
   graft-host interface
   implant-bone interface
   implant-cement interface
   long-term bone-
     instrumentation interface
   metal interface
   pin-bone interface
   prosthesis interface
   prosthesis-cement interface
   soft-tissue interface
   structural interface
Interface arterial blood filter
interfacet wiring and fusion
interfacial canals
interfacial surface tension
interfascial approach
interfascial space
interfascicular epineurotomy
interfemoral
interference barrier filter
interference fit fixation
interference microscope
interference modification
interference screw
interference screw technique
interferential stimulator
interferential therapy
interfering artifact
interforniceal approach
interfragmentary compression
interfragmentary lag screw
interfragmentary plate
interfragmentary wiring
interfragmentary wiring fixation
InterGard collagen graft
InterGard heparin vascular graft

InterGard knitted
intergluteal cleft
intergluteal sulcus
intergonial angle
interhemispheric approach
interhemispheric derivation
interhemispheric subdural
    hematoma
interilioabdominal amputation
interincisal angle
interincisal distance
interincisal opening
interinnominoabdominal
    amputation
interior chest wall
interior maxillary branch of
    external carotid artery
interior mesogastric hernia
interior of tumor excavated
interlacing blood vessels
interlacing ligatures
interlamellar space
interlaminar clamp
interlaminar procedure
interlesional therapy
Interlink threaded lock cannula
interlobar arteries of kidney
interlobar fissure
interlobar notch
interlobar veins of kidney
interlobular arteries of kidney
interlobular arteries of liver
interlobular bile
interlobular duct
interlobular veins of kidney
interlobular veins of liver
interlocked mesh prosthesis
interlocking detachable coil
interlocking ligatures
interlocking sound
interlocking suture technique
interlocking sutures
Interlok primary femoral
    component
interloop abscess
intermandibular groove
intermaxillary bone
intermaxillary fixation (IMF)
intermaxillary relation
intermaxillary sutures
intermaxillary traction
intermaxillary wire

intermediary amputation
intermediary movement
intermediate amputation
intermediate bundle
intermediate callus
intermediate carcinoma
intermediate hook
intermediate dorsal cutaneous
    nerve
intermediate fascia
intermediate fiber
intermediate ganglion
intermediate hemorrhage
intermediate junction
intermediate laryngeal cavity
intermediate layer
intermediate line
intermediate nerve
intermediate operation
intermediate plexus
intermediate restoration
intermediate restoration
    material (IRM)
intermediate sacral crest
intermediate splint
intermediate string
intermediate supraclavicular
    nerves
intermediate sutures
intermediate tendon of
    diaphragm
intermediate zone
intermediate-weighted MR images
Intermedics atrial
    antitachycardia pacemaker
Intermedics Cyberlith X
    multiprogrammable
    pacemaker
Intermedics intraocular lens
Intermedics intraocular lens
    implant
Intermedics intraocular radius
    gauge
Intermedics intraocular
    tonometer
Intermedics lithium-powered
    pacemaker
Intermedics Marathon dual-
    chamber rate-responsive
    pacemaker
Intermedics knee prosthesis
Intermedics pacemaker

Intermedics phaco and I-A kits
Intermedics phaco I&A unit
Intermedics pulse generator
Intermedics Quantum
   pacemaker
Intermedics Quantum
   programmable pulse
   generator
Intermedics Quantum unipolar
   pacemaker
Intermedics Stride pacemaker
Intermedics Thinlith II
   pacemaker
intermenstrual bleeding
intermenstrual pain
intermenstrual spotting
intermesenteric abscess
intermesenteric arterial
   anastomosis
intermetacarpal articulation
intermetatarsal articulation
intermetatarsal ligament
intermittent catheterization
intermittent claudication
intermittent demand ventilation
intermittent extremity pump
intermittent flow machine
intermittent inflow occlusion
intermittent mandatory
   ventilation (IMV)
intermittent mechanical
   ventilation
intermittent pain
intermittent pneumatic
   compresssion (IPC)
intermittent positive pressure
   breathing (IPPB)
intermittent positive pressure
   ventilation (IPPV)
intermittent subclavian vein
   obstruction
intermittent sutures
intermittent therapy
intermittent traction
intermittent vascular exclusion
intermuscular groove
intermuscular hernia
intermuscular membrane
intermuscular septum
internal abdominal fascia
internal abdominal ring
internal acoustic orifice

internal anal sphincter
internal anatomy
internal auditory artery
internal auditory canal
internal auditory foramen
internal auditory vein
internal bevel incision
internal branch
internal branch of the superior
   laryngeal (IBSL) nerve
internal calcaneoastragaloid
   ligament
internal callus
internal canthus
internal capsule
internal carotid artery
internal carotid nerve
internal carotid venous plexus
internal cerebral veins
internal cervical device
internal clot
internal crucial ligament
internal decompression
internal decompression trocar
internal defatting
internal derangement (ID)
internal drainage
internal ear prosthesis
internal elastic membrane
internal ethmoidectomy
internal female genital organ
internal fiberoptic cable
internal fibrocartilage
internal fistula
internal fixating device
internal fixation device
internal fixation of fracture
internal fixation, closed
   reduction
internal hemipelvectomy
internal hemorrhage
internal hemorrhoid
internal hemorrhoidal
   complex
internal hemorrhoidectomy
internal hernia
internal iliac artery
internal iliac vein
internal inguinal ring
internal intercostal muscles
internal intussusception
internal jugular vein

internal jugular vein cannulation anesthetic technique
internal jugular vein catheterization anesthetic technique
internal jugular vein puncture anesthetic technique
internal jugular vein puncture technique
internal juncture
internal lacrimal fistula
internal lateral ligament
internal male genital organ
internal mammary artery (IMA)
internal mammary artery bypass (IMAB)
internal mammary artery catheter
internal mammary artery graft
internal mammary artery pedicled fasciocutaneous island flap reconstruction of breast
internal mammary graft
internal mammary lymphoscintigraphy (IML)
internal mammary node biopsy
internal mammary plexus
internal mastopexy
internal maxillary artery
internal maxillary vein
internal monitor
internal neurocranial foramen
internal neurolysis
internal nucleus hydrodelineation needle
internal oblique aponeurosis
internal oblique fascia
internal oblique line
internal oblique muscle
internal oblique osteomuscular flap
internal obturator muscle
internal occipital crest
internal occipital ridge
internal os
internal pillars
internal plexus
internal proctotomy
internal pterygoid muscle
internal pudendal artery
internal pudendal vein
internal radiation therapy

internal rectal artery
internal rectal nerve
internal rectal sphincter
internal respiration
internal rotation
internal rotation contracture of hip
internal rotation deformity
internal rotation in extension
internal rotator
internal salivary gland
internal spermatic artery
internal spermatic fascia
internal spermatic vessels
internal sphincter
internal sphincterotomy
internal spinal fixation
internal spiral sulcus
internal surface
internal table
internal thoracic artery
internal thoracic artery graft (ITA graft)
internal thoracic lymphatic plexus
internal thoracic vein
internal thyroarytenoid muscle
internal tibial torsion (ITT)
internal tibial torsion brace
internal traction
internal urethral orifice
internal urethral sphincter
internal urethrotomy
internal vein stripper
internal vein stripping
internal version
internal zygomatic foramen of Meckel
internasal dysplasia
internasal suture
International cancer of cervix classification
International Federation of Gynecology and Obstetrics (FIGO)
International Federation of Gynecology and Obstetrics classification
international stage classification
international standard goniometer

internipple inframammary fold
   distance (IN-IMF distance)
internodal tract
internuclear ophthalmoplegia
   (INO)
interocclusal clearance
interocclusal record
interocclusal rest space
interodontoblastic collagen fibril
interorbital space
interosseous anterior nerve
interosseous artery
interosseous border
interosseous cartilage
interosseous crest
interosseous cruris nerve
interosseous dorsalis nerve
interosseous groove
interosseous knife
interosseous ligament
interosseous margin
interosseous membrane
interosseous muscle
interosseous nerve
interosseous posterior nerve
interosseous talocalcaneal
   ligament
interosseous veins
interosseous wire
interosseous wire fixation
interosseous wiring
interosseous wiring fixation
interossicular fold
interpalpebral fissure
interpalpebral suture
interpalpebral zone
interpapillary ridges
interparietal bone
interparietal hernia
interparietal sulcus
interparietal suture
interpedicular joint space
interpeduncular cistern
interpeduncular fossa
interpeduncular fossa lesion
interpeduncular ganglion
interpelviabdominal amputation
interperiosteal fracture
interphalangeal
   distal interphalangeal (IP)
   proximal interphalangeal (PIP)
interphalangeal amputation

interphalangeal articulation
interphalangeal joint (IPJ)
interphalangeal joint dislocation
interplate cranial sutures
interpleural analgesia
interpleural anesthesia
interpleural anesthetic
   technique
interpleural block
interpleural space
interpolated flap
interpolation flap
Interpore block
Interpore bone replacement
   material
Interpore ceramic material
Interpore graft
Interpore granule
Interpore implant
Interpore osteointegrated
   implant
Interpore porous hydroxyapatite
   block
Interpore preshaped wedge
interposing fascia
interposition
   colonic interposition
   incus interposition
   jejunal interposition
   soft-tissue interposition
   temperoparietal facial flap
      interposition
   tissue interposition
interposition arthroplasty
interposition Dacron graft
interposition graft
interposition membrane
interposition mesocaval shunt
interposition of colon
interposition of graft
interposition of uterus
interposition operation
interposition saphenous vein
   graft
interposition uterine suspension
interpositional arthroplasty
interpositional elbow
   arthroplasty
interpositional gap arthroplasty
interpositional shoulder
   arthroplasty
Interpret ultrasound catheter

interprismatic space
interproximal bone
interproximal reduction
interproximal space
interpubic disk
interpupillary distance (IPD)
interpupillary line
interradicular abscess
interradicular alveoloplasty
interradicular artery
interradicular fiber
interradicular lesion
interradicular osseous defect
interradicular septum
interradicular space
interrupted aortic arch
interrupted black silk sutures
interrupted chromic catgut
    sutures
interrupted chromic sutures
interrupted cotton sutures
interrupted far-near sutures
interrupted fashion
interrupted fine silk sutures
interrupted Lembert sutures
interrupted mattress sutures
interrupted near-far sutures
interrupted plain catgut sutures
interrupted pledgeted suture
interrupted respiration
interrupted silk sutures
interrupted suture technique
interrupted sutures
interrupted vertical mattress
    sutures
interscalene approach
interscalene block
interscalene block anesthetic
    technique
interscalene blockade
interscalene brachial plexus
    block
interscapular amputation
interscapular reflex
interscapular region
interscapulothoracic amputation
Interseal acetabular cup
intersection syndrome
intersegmental table
interseptal osteoclasia
intersheath space
intersigmoid hernia

intersigmoid recess
Intersorb absorptive burn pad
Intersorb fine mesh gauze
Intersorb 6-ply absorbent roll
    stretch gauze
Intersorb wide mesh gauze
interspace narrowing
interspace width marker
interspecific graft
intersphenoidal synchondrosis
intersphincteric abscess
intersphincteric anal fistula
intersphincteric anorectal space
interspinal line
interspinal muscles
interspinal muscles of thorax
interspinal plane
interspinous cable
interspinous pseudarthrosis
interspinous segmental spinal
    instrumentation
interspinous segmental spinal
    instrumentation technique
interstice
  graft interstice
interstitial atrophy
interstitial fibrosis
interstitial gland
interstitial hernia
interstitial implant
interstitial implantation
interstitial inflammation
interstitial irradiation
interstitial loculated hematoma
interstitial markings
interstitial photodynamic therapy
interstitial pneumonia
interstitial radiation
interstitial radiation therapy
interstitial spaces
interstitial therapy
interstitial tissues
intertarsal articulation
interthalamic commissure
interthoracoscapular amputation
intertragic notch
intertransverse fusion
intertransverse muscles
intertriginous area
intertrochanteric crest
intertrochanteric femoral
    fracture

intertrochanteric 4-part fracture
intertrochanteric fracture
intertrochanteric line
intertrochanteric plate
intertrochanteric ridge
intertuberal diameter
intertubercular eminence
intertubercular groove
intertubercular line
intertubercular plane
intertubular tissue
interureteric fold
interureteric ridge
interval appendectomy
interval improvement
interval operation
intervening tissues
intervention
   angiographic intervention
   cardiac intervention
   endovascular intervention
   medical intervention
   neurosurgical intervention
   operative intervention
   prophylactic angiographic
     intervention
   supportive intervention
   surgical intervention
   therapeutic intervention
interventional cardiac
   catheterization
interventional cardiologist
interventional catheter
interventional option
interventional procedure
interventional radiology
interventional technique
interventional therapy
interventricular artery
interventricular cartilage
interventricular conduction
   defect
interventricular disk
interventricular fibrocartilage
interventricular foramen
interventricular ganglion
interventricular groove
interventricular heart block
interventricular notch
interventricular septal defect
   (IVSD)
interventricular septal rupture

interventricular septum
interventricular space
interventricular sulcus of heart
interventricular vein
intervertebral body
intervertebral cartilage
intervertebral curet
intervertebral disk
intervertebral disk forceps
intervertebral disk herniation
intervertebral disk rongeur
intervertebral disk rongeur
   forceps
intervertebral foramen
intervertebral ganglion
intervertebral punch
intervertebral spreader
intervertebral vein
intervillous circulation
intervillous lacuna
interwoven bundle
intestinal adhesions
intestinal allograft
intestinal anastomosis
intestinal anastomosis clamp
intestinal anastomosis forceps
intestinal anastomotic leakage
intestinal arterial arcade
intestinal arteries
intestinal atony
intestinal atresia
intestinal bag
intestinal biopsy
intestinal bleeding
intestinal bypass procedure
intestinal calculus
intestinal clamp
intestinal closing forceps
intestinal contents
intestinal decompression
intestinal decompression trocar
intestinal diversion conduit
intestinal diverticulum
intestinal endoscopy
intestinal failure
intestinal fistula
intestinal fixation
intestinal flora
intestinal fluid
intestinal glands
intestinal hemorrhage
intestinal hernia

intestinal herniation
intestinal holding forceps
intestinal incision
intestinal infarction
intestinal intussusception
intestinal ischemic disorder
intestinal loop
intestinal lumen
intestinal motility disorder
intestinal mucosa
intestinal needle
intestinal obstruction
intestinal occlusion clamp
intestinal occlusion retractor
intestinal perforation
intestinal peritoneum
intestinal plication needle
intestinal polyp
intestinal prolapse
intestinal radiation injury
intestinal resection
intestinal resection clamp
intestinal ring clamp
intestinal scissors
intestinal secretions
intestinal stasis
intestinal surgery
intestinal sutures
intestinal tissue forceps
intestinal tissue-holding forceps
intestinal tract
intestinal transplantation
intestinal trocar
intestinal tube
intestinal vaginoplasty
intestinal villi
intestinal web
intestinointestinal reflex
in-the-bag lens
in-the-ear listening device
intima
    tunica intima
intimal arteriosclerosis
intimal dehiscence
intimal flap
intimal hyperplasia
intimal injury
intimal layer
intimal thickening
Intimax biliary catheter
Intimax cholangiography
    catheter

Intimax occlusion catheter
Intimax vascular catheter
intimectomy knife
intra-abdominal abscess
intra-abdominal adhesions
intra-abdominal arterial
    hemorrhage
intra-abdominal bleeding
intra-abdominal contents
intra-abdominal disease
intra-abdominal exploration
intra-abdominal hemorrhage
intra-abdominal ileal reservoir
intra-abdominal injury
intra-abdominal laser procedure
intra-abdominal lesion
intra-abdominal mass
intra-abdominal procedure
intra-abdominal surgery
intra-abdominal vasectomy
intra-abdominal viscera
intra-alveolar hemorrhage
intra-alveolar pocket
intra-alveolar root
intra-amniotic saline injection
intra-anal wart
intra-anesthetic event
intra-aortic balloon
intra-aortic balloon assist device
intra-aortic balloon catheter
intra-aortic balloon
    counterpulsation
intra-aortic balloon pump (IABP)
intra-aortic balloon pumping
    (IABP)
intra-aortic counterpulsation
    balloon
intra-areolar incision
intra-arterial cannula
intra-arterial chemotherapy
    (IAC)
intra-arterial chemotherapy
    catheter
intra-arterial digital subtraction
    angiography
intra-arterial injection
intra-arterial therapy
intra-articular anesthetic
    technique
intra-articular arthrodesis
intra-articular cartilage
intra-articular fracture

intra-articular injection
intra-articular knee fusion
intra-articular loose body
intra-articular procedure
intra-articular proximal tibial
    fracture
intra-articular reconstruction
intra-atrial baffle
intra-atrial conduction defect
intra-auricular muscle
intra-axial brain tumor
intrabony defect
intrabony lesion
intrabony pocket
intrabulbar fossa
intracameral
intracanal instrument
intracanalicular fibroadenoma
intracanalicular fibroma
intracanalicular irradiation
intracanalicular papilloma
intracapsular ankylosis
intracapsular cataract extraction
    (ICCE)
intracapsular dissection
intracapsular fracture
intracapsular hemorrhage
intracapsular incision
intracapsular lens
intracapsular lens expressor
intracapsular lens expressor
    hook
intracapsular lens extraction
intracapsular lens forceps
intracapsular lens loupe
intracapsular lens spoon
intracapsular metastasis
intracapsular rupture
intracapsular
    temporomandibular joint
    arthroplasty
intracapsular tumor removal
intracapsularly
intracardiac cannula
intracardiac catheter
intracardiac injection
intracardiac needle holder
intracardiac patch
intracardiac patch prosthesis
intracardiac phonocardiography
intracardiac pressure
intracardiac retractor

intracardiac shunt
intracardiac sucker guard
intracardiac suction tube
intracardiac sump tube
intracardiac vent
intracardial shunt
intracartilaginous
Intracath catheter
intracavernosal injection
intracavernous injection
intracavitary afterloading
    applicator
intracavitary anesthesia
intracavitary application
intracavitary cesium therapy
intracavitary gynecologic
    applicator
intracavitary pressure gradient
intracavitary radiation
intracavitary radiation boost
    therapy
intracavitary radium (ICR)
intracavitary radium insertion
intracavitary therapy
Intracell mechanical muscle
    device
Intracell myofascial trigger-point
    device
intracellular fluid
intracellular keratinization
intracerebral arteriovenous
    malformation
intracerebral bleed
intracerebral depth electrode
intracerebral electrode
intracerebral
    electroencephalogram
intracerebral hematoma
intracerebral hemorrhage
intracerebral inoculation
intracerebral vascular
    malformation
intracerebrovascular accident
intracervical bag
intracervical device (ICD)
intracervical pack
intrachondrial bone
intracisternal puncture
intracochlear implant
IntraCoil nitinol stent
intraconal fat
intraconal fat compartment

intraconal lesion
intracondylar
Intracone intramedullary reamer
intracordal silicone injection
intracordal Teflon injection set
intracorneal lens
intracoronal retainer
intracoronary Doppler flow
     wire
intracoronary guiding catheter
intracoronary perfusion catheter
intracoronary stent
intracoronary thrombolysis
intracorporeal anastomosis
intracorporeal heart
intracorporeal injection therapy
intracorporeal knot
intracorporeal knotting
     technique
intracorporeal laser lithotripsy
intracorporeal lithotripsy
intracorporeal shock wave
     lithotripsy
intracranial anatomy
intracranial aneurysm
intracranial arteriovenous fistula
intracranial arteriovenous
     malformation
intracranial bleeding
intracranial bruit
intracranial calcification
intracranial cavity
intracranial circulation
intracranial dural vascular
     anomaly
intracranial ganglion
intracranial hematoma
intracranial hemorrhage
intracranial hypertension
intracranial injury
intracranial lesion
intracranial mass lesion
intracranial metastasis
intracranial neoplasm
intracranial pressure (ICP)
intracranial pressure catheter
intracranial pressure catheter
     monitor
intracranial pressure monitor
     (ICP monitor)
intracranial pressure monitor
     screw

intracranial pressure monitoring
intracranial pressure monitoring
     device
intracranial tumor
intracranial vascular
     malformation
intracranial-extracranial nerve
     graft
intracranial-intratemporal nerve
     graft
intracristal space
intractable pain
intractable ulcer
intracutaneous injection
intracutaneous reaction
intracuticular
intracuticular nylon sutures
intracuticular running sutures
intracuticular stitch
intracuticular sutures
intracystic hepatojejunostomy
intracystic papilloma
intracytoplasmic sperm
     injection (ICSI)
intradermal anesthetic
intradermal injection
intradermal mattress suture
     technique
intradermal mattress sutures
intradermal nevus
intradermal polyglactic acid
     suture
intradermal reaction
intradermal sutures
intradermal tattooing technique
intradermic sutures
intradiscal electrothermal
     therapy (IDET)
IntraDop intraoperative Doppler
IntraDop probe
Intraducer peritoneal cannula
Intraducer peritoneal catheter
intraductal cancer
intraductal carcinoma
intraductal cholangioscopy
intraductal hyperplasia
intraductal imaging catheter
intraductal ultrasound
intraductal ultrasound probe
intradural abscess
intradural approach
intradural dissection

intradural extramedullary lesion
intradural retractor
intradural tumor surgery
intraepidermal bulla
intraepidermal carcinoma
intraepidermal vesiculation
intraepiploic hernia
intraepithelial carcinoma
intraepithelial dyskeratosis
intraepithelial glands
intraepithelial neoplasia
intraepithelial nonkeratizing
    carcinoma
intraepithelial vessels
intrafascial space
intrafascicular sutures
Intrafix tibial fastener
Intraflex intramedullary pin
Intraflex intramedullary pin
    extractor
Intraflex intramedullary pins
intrafollicular insemination
intrafusal fibers
intragastric anastomosis
intragastric balloon
intragastric bubble
intragastric cannula
intragastric continuous pH-meter
intragastric drip
intragastric hydrolysis
intragastric provocation under
    endoscopy
intraglandular fluid collection
intraglandular stone
intrahaustral contraction ring
intrahemispheric fissure
intrahepatic abscess
intrahepatic anatomy
intrahepatic arterial-portal fistula
intrahepatic atresia
intrahepatic AV fistula
intrahepatic bile duct
intrahepatic biliary cystic
    dilation
intrahepatic biliary duct
intrahepatic block
intrahepatic
    cholangiojejunostomy
intrahepatic control
intrahepatic ductal dilation
intrahepatic hematoma
intrahepatic lesion

intrahepatic metastasis
intrahepatic radicle
intrahepatic spontaneous
    arterioportal fistula
intrahepatic stone
intrailiac hernia
intrajugular process of temporal
    bone
intralabyrinthine fistula
intralacrimal endoscopy
intralacrimal surgery
intralesional corticosteroid
intralesional excision
intralesional injection
intralesional laser
    photocoagulation (ILP)
intralesional steroid injection
intralesional therapy
intraligamentary anesthesia
intraligamentary syringe
intraligamentous ectopic
    pregnancy
intraligamentous pregnancy
intralingual cyst of foregut
    origin
intralobular duct
intralobular inflammation
intralocular
intraluminal cyst
intraluminal duodenal
    diverticulum (IDD)
intraluminal filling defect
intraluminal foreign body
intraluminal gas
intraluminal hemorrhage
intraluminal intubation
intraluminal mass
intraluminal pressure
intraluminal probe
intraluminal radiation therapy
intraluminal reference electrode
intraluminal stapler
intraluminal stone
intraluminal stripper
intraluminal sutures
intraluminal tube
intraluminal tube prosthesis
intraluminal ultrasound
intramammary abscess
intramastoid abscess
intramaxillary fixation
intrameatal electrode

Intramed angioscopic valve
intramedullary (IM) nail
intramedullary and spongiosa graft
intramedullary anesthesia
intramedullary arteriovenous malformation
intramedullary alignment rod
intramedullary bar
intramedullary bone graft
intramedullary broach
intramedullary canal
intramedullary canal plug
intramedullary catheter
intramedullary demyelination
intramedullary device
intramedullary device fixation
intramedullary drill
intramedullary fixation
intramedullary fixation device
intramedullary graft
intramedullary guide
intramedullary hemorrhage
intramedullary illuminator
intramedullary Kuntscher nail
intramedullary lesion
intramedullary nail
intramedullary nailing
intramedullary pin
intramedullary reamer
intramedullary rod
intramedullary rod fixation
intramedullary Rush rod
intramedullary skeletal kinetic distractor nail (ISKD)
intramedullary supracondylar multihole nail
intramedullary tumor biopsy
intramedullary wire
intramembranous formation
intramembranous space
intramesenteric abscess
intramucosal insert
intramucosal metastasis
intramural abscess
intramural air dissection
intramural aneurysm
intramural artery
intramural blood perfusion
intramural colonic air
intramural diverticulum
intramural esophageal rupture

intramural extramucosal lesion
intramural fibroid
intramural fistulous tract
intramural fixation
intramural hematoma
intramural intestinal hemorrhage
intramural involvement
intramural leiomyomata
intramural pregnancy
intramuscular abscess
intramuscular administration
intramuscular anesthetic
intramuscular glands of tongue
intramuscular gluteal implant
intramuscular hemangioma
intramuscular immune globulin
intramuscular injection
intramuscular preanesthetic medication anesthetic technique
intramuscular venous malformation
Intran disposable intrauterine pressure measurement catheter
Intran intrauterine pressure measurement catheter
intranasal analgesic
intranasal anesthesia
intranasal antral speculum
intranasal application
intranasal approach
intranasal bivalve splint
intranasal block
intranasal bone lever
intranasal darts
intranasal ethmoidectomy
intranasal hammer
intranasal intercartilaginous incision
intranasal packing
intranasal punch
intranasal saw
intranasal sinus surgery
intranasal sinusotomy
intranasal splint
intranasal tube
in-transit disease
in-transit metastasis
intranuclear inclusion
intraocular administration
intraocular balloon

intraocular cannula
intraocular cataract extraction
intraocular contents
intraocular fistula
intraocular forceps
intraocular foreign biopsy
intraocular hemorrhage
intraocular hook
intraocular instruments
intraocular irrigating forceps
intraocular lens (IOL)
intraocular lens cannula
intraocular lens dislocation
intraocular lens folder
intraocular lens forceps
intraocular lens glide
intraocular lens implant
intraocular lens implantation
intraocular muscles
intraocular pressure (IOP)
intraocular scissors
intraocular tension
intraocular tension recorder
intraoperative assessment
intraoperative bile sample
intraoperative biliary endoscopy
intraoperative biopsy
intraoperative bleeding
intraoperative blood loss
intraoperative bowel lavage
intraoperative bowel
    preparation
intraoperative cavernous nerve
    stimulation
intraoperative cholangiogram
intraoperative colonic lavage
intraoperative complication
intraoperative computer-assisted
    spinal orientation technique
intraoperative confirmation
intraoperative contamination
intraoperative core body
    temperature
intraoperative core hypothermia
intraoperative death
intraoperative digital subtraction
    angiography
intraoperative dynamic
    cholangiography
intraoperative enteroscopy
intraoperative fluid management
intraoperative fracture

intraoperative frozen section
intraoperative hemorrhage
intraoperative imaging
intraoperative inadvertent
    venous injury
intraoperative interpretation
intraoperative lymphatic mapping
intraoperative monitor
intraoperative morbidity
intraoperative MRI
intraoperative neurophysiologic
    monitoring
intraoperative normothermia
intraoperative parathyroid
    hormone monitoring
intraoperative penile erection
intraoperative plateletpheresis
intraoperative procedure
intraoperative radiation
intraoperative rupture
intraoperative skin expansion
intraoperative spatial
    confirmation
intraoperative stress relaxation
intraoperative touch prep
    cytology
intraoperative transcranial
    Doppler monitoring
intraoperative tumor staging
intraoperative ultrasonic probe
intraoperative ultrasonography
    (IOUS)
intraoperative ultrasound (IOUS)
intraoperative urine output
intraoperative vascular accident
intraoperative verification
IntraOptics intraocular lens
IntraOptics lensometer
intraoral access
intraoral anesthesia
intraoral antrostomy
intraoral approach
intraoral cancer
intraoral cone
intraoral cone irradiation
intraoral cyst
intraoral flap
intraoral fracture appliance
intraoral incision
intraoral Kaposi sarcoma
intraoral lesion
intraoral lining deficiency

intraoral meloplasty
intraoral mucosal defect
intraoral projection
intraoral stent
intraoral titanium mandibular
    distraction device
intraoral wire
intraorbital anesthesia
intraorbital foreign body
intraorbital fracture
intraorbital groove
intraorbital implant
intraorbital surgery
intraorbital tumor instruments
intraosseous abscess
intraosseous ameloblastoma
intraosseous anesthesia
intraosseous bone lesion
intraosseous carcinoma
intraosseous cyst
intraosseous fixation
intraosseous ganglion cyst
intraosseous implant
intraosseous injection
intraosseous lesion
intraosseous needle
intraosseous therapy
intraosseous venography
intraparavariceal procedure
intraparenchymal digital
    dissection
intraparenchymal hematoma
intraparenchymal hemorrhage
intraparietal sulcus
intraparietal sulcus of Turner
intraparotid mesenchymal tumor
intraparotideal metastasis
intrapartum death
intrapartum hemorrhage
intrapartum monitor
intrapelvic hernia
intrapelvic kidney pelvis
intrapelvic protrusion
intrapericardial
    aorticopulmonary shunt
intraperiosteal fracture
intraperiosteal implant
intraperitoneal abscess
intraperitoneal adhesions
intraperitoneal air
intraperitoneal anesthesia
intraperitoneal anesthetic

intraperitoneal carbon dioxide
    insufflation
intraperitoneal cavity
intraperitoneal chemotherapy
intraperitoneal CO_2 insufflation
intraperitoneal drug
    administration
intraperitoneal endometrial
    metastatic disease
intraperitoneal fracture
intraperitoneal hemorrhage
intraperitoneal hyperthermic
    chemotherapy (IPHC)
intraperitoneal hyperthermic
    perfusion
intraperitoneal incision
intraperitoneal injection
intraperitoneal migration of
    pacemaker
intraperitoneal onlay mesh
intraperitoneal perforation
intraperitoneal position
intraperitoneal pregnancy
intraperitoneal procedure
intraperitoneal radiation therapy
intraperitoneal technique
intraperitoneal transfusion
intraperitoneal viscus
intraperitoneal viscus rupture
intrapharyngeal space
intraplaque hemorrhage
intrapleural block
intrapleural catheter
intrapleural catheter placement
intrapleural chemotherapy
intrapleural pneumonolysis
intrapleural rupture
intrapleural sealed drainage unit
intra-prostatic stent
intrapulmonary hamartoma
intrapulmonary metastasis (IPM)
intrapulmonary shunt
intrapulpal anesthesia
intrapulpal injection
intrapyretic amputation
intrarectal ultrasonography
intrarenal reflux
intrarenal vein
intraretinal microangiopathy
intraretinal microvascular
    abnormalities (IRMA)
Intrascan ultrasound

intrascrotal pain
intrasellar extension
intrasellar lesion
intraseptal alveoloplasty
IntraSite gel dressing
IntraSite gel wound dressing
intraspinal administration
intraspinal anesthesia
intraspinal block
intraspinal therapy
IntraStent biliary stent
intratendinous injection
intratentorial supracerebellar
    approach
intrathecal administration
intrathecal analgesic
intrathecal anesthesia
intrathecal anesthetic
intrathecal cannulation
    anesthetic technique
intrathecal contrast material
intrathecal injection
intrathecal morphine anesthetic
    technique
intrathecal opioid labor
    analgesia
intrathecal space
intrathecal therapy
intrathecally
intrathoracic anastomosis
intrathoracic bleeding
intrathoracic disease
intrathoracic
    esophagogastroscopy
intrathoracic
    esophagogastrostomy
intrathoracic esophagoplasty
intrathoracic forceps
intrathoracic gas volume
intrathoracic injury
intrathoracic Nissen
    fundoplication
intrathoracic position
intrathoracic pressure variations
intrathoracic stomach
intrathoracic thyroid
intrathyroid cartilage
intratip lobule
intratracheal anesthesia
intratracheal instillation
intratracheal intubation
intratracheal tube

intratreatment
intratrochlear nerve
intratubal insemination
intratumoral injection
intraurethral coil
intraurethral prostatic bridge
    catheter
intrauterine amputation
intrauterine balloon cannula
intrauterine balloon-type
    cannula
intrauterine cannula
intrauterine catheter
intrauterine clotting
intrauterine contraceptive
    device (IUCD)
intrauterine curettage
intrauterine device (IUD)
intrauterine fetus
intrauterine foreign body
intrauterine fracture
intrauterine gestation
intrauterine growth
intrauterine growth retardation
    (IUGR)
intrauterine insemination
intrauterine insemination
    cannula
intrauterine insemination
    catheter
intrauterine pack
intrauterine pessary
intrauterine pressure
intrauterine pressure catheter
intrauterine pressure monitor
intrauterine probe
intrauterine radium application
intrauterine transfusion
intravaginal ring
intravaginal space
intravaginal therapy
intravariceal infusion
intravariceal injection
intravasation
    venous intravasation
intravascular catheter electrode
intravascular coagulation
intravascular coagulopathy
intravascular Doppler-tipped
    guidewire
intravascular endothelial
    proliferative lesion

intravascular fluid
intravascular fluid therapy
intravascular foreign body
intravascular injection
intravascular mass
intravascular pressure
intravascular stent
intravascular ultrasound catheter
intravascular volume expansion
intravelar veloplasty
intravenous (IV)
intravenous accurate control
    device
intravenous administration
intravenous analgesic
intravenous anesthesia
intravenous anesthetic
intravenous angiocardiography
intravenous antibiotic therapy
intravenous block anesthesia
intravenous bolus
intravenous bolus injection of
    contrast medium
intravenous cannulation
intravenous cannulation
    anesthetic technique
intravenous catheter
intravenous cholangiogram
    (IVC)
intravenous cholangiography
    (IVC)
intravenous cholecystography
intravenous contrast material
intravenous digital subtraction
    imaging
intravenous dose
intravenous drip
intravenous feeding
intravenous fluid
intravenous hydration therapy
intravenous immune globulin
intravenous infusion
intravenous injection
intravenous intubation
intravenous lead
intravenous line
intravenous needle
intravenous ozone therapy
intravenous pacing catheter
intravenous Pitocin drip
intravenous pyelogram (IVP)
intravenous pyelography

intravenous regional anesthesia
    (IVRA)
intravenous sedation anesthesia
intravenous tension
intravenous therapy
intravenous transfusion
intravenous tubing roller
intravenous ultrasound catheter
intravenous urogram
intravenous urography
intraventricular aberration
intraventricular conduction
    delay (IVCD)
intraventricular endoscopy
intraventricular hemorrhage
intraventricular injection
intraventricular pressure
intraventricular pressure
    monitoring catheter
intraventricular therapy
intravesical alum irrigation
intravesical anastomosis
intravesical chemotherapy
intravesical instillation
intravesical prostatic tissue
intravesical space
intravitreal cryoprobe
intravitreal delivery
intravitreal injection
intravitreal laser
Intrepid balloon catheter
Intrepid percutaneous
    transluminal coronary
    angioplasty catheter
Intrepid PTCA catheter
intrinsic brainstem lesion
intrinsic compression
intrinsic defect
intrinsic factor
intrinsic fibroblastic activity
intrinsic mass
intrinsic minus deformity
intrinsic minus hand
intrinsic minus position
intrinsic muscle of tongue
intrinsic muscles of larynx
intrinsic plus deformity
intrinsic pressure
intrinsic transverse connector
intrinsicoid deflection
intrinsicplasty
    Zancolli lasso intrinsicplasty

Intro Deuce double-lumen
   introducer
introducer (*see also* sphere
   introducer)
ACS percutaneous introducer
Allen eye introducer
Allen sphere introducer
Allen spherical eye introducer
Angestat hemostasis
   introducer
Angetear tear-away introducer
Atkinson introducer
Avanti introducer
Balkin introducer
Cardak percutaneous catheter
   introducer
Carter sphere introducer
Carter spherical eye
   introducer
catheter introducer
Check-Flo introducer
Ciaglia percutaneous
   tracheostomy introducer
Cook introducer
Cook micropuncture
   introducer
Cook Peel-Away introducer
Cope-Saddekni introducer
Davol pacemaker introducer
Desilets introducer
Desilets-Hoffman catheter
   introducer
Desilets-Hoffman introducer
Desilets-Hoffman
   micropuncture introducer
Desilets-Hoffman pacemaker
   introducer
Dumon-Gilliard prosthesis
   introducer
electrode introducer
Encapsulon sheath introducer
endolymphatic shunt tube
   introducer
entrapment sack introducer
Eric Lloyd introducer
Eschmann endotracheal tube
   introducer
Excalibur introducer
eye sphere introducer
FasTrac introducer
French-Daid introducer
Furlow introducer

introducer (*continued*)
   Goodhill strut introducer
   gum elastic bougie introducer
   Hall self-holding introducer
   Hedwig introducer
   Hemaquet catheter introducer
   Hemaquet sheath introducer
   heparin lock introducer
   H-H shunt introducer
   Hickman percutaneous
      introducer
   Holter introducer
   House endolymphatic shunt
      tube introducer
   Implantaid cardiac lead
      introducer
   Input PS introducer
   Intro Deuce double-lumen
      introducer
   Littleford introducer
   Littleford-Spector introducer
   LPS Peel-Away introducer
   Maryfield introducer
   metallic sphere introducer
   Micropuncture Peel-Away
      introducer
   Morgan vent tube introducer
   Moss T-anchor needle
      introducer
   Mullins catheter introducer
   Mullins transseptal introducer
   Neuroguide peel-away
      catheter introducer
   Nottingham introducer
   peel-away introducer
   Pennine-O'Neil urinary
      catheter introducer
   percutaneous lead introducer
   permanent lead introducer
   pull-apart introducer
   Ramses diaphragm introducer
   Razi cannula introducer
   Richardson polyethylene tube
      introducer
   shunt-tube introducer
   silicone introducer
   Speck introducer
   sphere introducer
   split-sheath introducer
   stent introducer
   Storz vent tube introducer
   subclavian introducer

introducer (*continued*)
  SupraFoley suprapubic
    introducer
  Taut percutaneous introducer
  Touhy-Borst side-arm
    introducer
  tube introducer
  Tuohy-Bost introducer
  Tuohy-Bost micropuncture
    introducer
  UMI transseptal catheter
    introducer
  Uni-Shunt with reservoir
    introducer
  USCI introducer
  ventricular catheter
    introducer
  Weaver trocar introducer
  Wellwood-Ferguson
    introducer
introducer catheter
introducer for spheres
introducer gun
introducer sheath
introducing forceps
introduction of radiopaque
  substance
introduction of radium
introitus
  esophageal introitus
  neovaginal introitus
  nonmarital introitus
  nulliparous introitus
  parous introitus
  relaxed introitus
  virginal introitus
Introl bladder neck support
  prosthesis
intrusive implantation
intrusive surgery
intubation
  altercursive intubation
  aqueductal intubation
  blind nasotracheal intubation
  bronchoscope-guided
    intubation
  catheter-guided endoscopic
    intubation
  double-lumen intubation
  emergency tracheal
    intubation
  emergent intubation

intubation (*continued*)
  endobronchial intubation
  endotracheal intubation
  esophageal intubation
  esophagogastric intubation
  failed intubation
  Flexguide intubation
  gastrointestinal intubation
  intraluminal intubation
  intratracheal intubation
  intravenous intubation
  lighted stylet-guided oral
    intubation
  mainstem intubation
  nasal intubation
  nasoendotracheal intubation
  nasogastric intubation
  nasotracheal intubation
  O'Dwyer intubation
  oral endotracheal intubation
  oral intubation
  oral lighted-stylet intubation
  orotracheal intubation
  pyloric intubation
  rapid sequence induction
    intubation
  silicone intubation
  suction and intubation
  terminal ileum intubation
  total time to intubation (TTI)
  tracheal intubation
  translaryngeal tracheal
    intubation
  tube intubation
intubation and suction
intubation anesthesia
intubation anesthetic technique
intubation failure
intubation laryngoscope
intubation set
intubation tube
intubationist
intubator
intumescence
intumescent cataract
intussuscepted bowel
intussusception
  adult intussusception
  appendiceal intussusception
  bowel intussusception
  cecal intussusception
  cecocolic intussusception

intussusception (*continued*)
  colocolic intussusception
  colonic intussusception
  enteric intussusception
  gastroenterostomy
    intussusception
  idiopathic adult
    intussusception
  idiopathic ileocecal
    intussusception
  ileocolic intussusception
  ileoileal intussusception
  internal intussusception
  intestinal intussusception
  pediatric intussusception
  rectorectal intussusception
  reduction of intussusception
  retrograde intussusception
  sigmoid-rectal intussusception
  small bowel idiopathic
    intussusception
  stomal intussusception
intussusceptum
invaginated membrane
invaginated nipple
invaginated stump
invaginating
  end-to-end invaginating
invaginating anastomosis
invaginating suture technique
invagination
  basilar invagination
  epithelial invagination
  eyelid invagination
  Oehlers invagination
  skin envelope invagination
  stomal invagination
  stump invagination
invagination of umbilicus
invagination technique
invasion
  advanced local invasion
  blood vessel invasion (BVI)
  cancer invasion
  capsular invasion
  chest wall invasion
  extrathyroid invasion
  forniceal invasion
  laryngotracheal invasion
  local invasion
  lymph vessel invasion (LVI)
  lymphatic invasion

invasion (*continued*)
  lymphovascular invasion
  margin invasion
  microscopic invasion
  mucosal invasion
  perineural invasion
  serosal invasion
  submucosal invasion
  tumor invasion
  vascular invasion
  venous invasion
  wall invasion
invasion keratitis
invasive adenocarcinoma
invasive breast cancer
invasive breast carcinoma
invasive carcinoma
invasive ductal cancer
invasive ductal carcinoma
invasive fungal infection
invasive hemodynamic
    monitoring
invasive lesion
invasive lobular carcinoma
invasive localization
invasive pressure measurement
invasive procedure
invasive technique
invasive therapy
invasive tumor
inverse bevel incision
inverse symmetry
inverse-ratio ventilation
inversion
  nipple inversion
  penile skin inversion
inversion ankle stress x-ray
inversion appendectomy
inversion deformity
inversion operation
inversion position
inversion sprain
inversion time
inversion-ligation appendectomy
inverted bevel incision
inverted buttoned device
inverted cone bur
inverted ductal papilloma
inverted edge
inverted horseshoe flap
inverted jackknife position
inverted knot sutures

inverted schneiderian papilloma
inverted skin flap
inverted sutures
inverted teardrop areola
  deformity
inverted testis
inverted T-scar
inverted T-wave
inverted U-pouch ileal reservoir
inverted uterus
inverted V-sign
inverted-L osteotomy
inverted-T fashion
inverted-T incision
inverted-T scar
inverted-T skin excision
inverted-U abdominal incision
inverted-U incision
inverted-Y fracture
inverted-Y incision
inverter
  appendix inverter
  Barrett appendix inverter
  Mayo-Boldt appendix inverter
  Mayo-Kelly appendix inverter
  Wangensteen tissue inverter
inverting appendiceal stump
inverting knot technique
inverting papilloma
inverting sutures
invertor
Investa sutures
investing cartilage
investing fascia
investment expansion
involuntary contraction
involuntary entropion
involuntary guarding
involuntary movement
involuntary muscle
involuted phase
involuting flat hemangioma
involution cyst
involution of uterus
involutional blepharoptosis
involutional ovarian changes
involvement
  bifurcation involvement
  border involvement
  celiac nodal involvement
  diffuse breast involvement
  extramedullary involvement

involvement (*continued*)
  extraocular muscle
    involvement
  intramural involvement
  liver involvement
  local involvement
  lymph involvement
  lymph node involvement
  lymphatic involvement
  macroscopic involvement
  mammary involvement
  margin resection involvement
  massive involvement
  mesocolic involvement
  metastatic involvement
  nerve involvement
  nervous system involvement
  nodal involvement
  node involvement
  portal node involvement
  pulmonary involvement
  regional involvement
  regional node involvement
  retinal involvement
  rib involvement
  segmental involvement
  serosal involvement
  skin involvement
  subdiaphragmatic
    involvement
  trifurcation involvement
inward movement
inward rotation
INX stainless steel stent
Inyo nail
IO (inferior oblique)
Ioban antimicrobial incise drape
Ioban drape
Ioban Steri-Drape
Iocare titanium needle
iodine catgut sutures
iodine cup
iodized oil study
iodized surgical gut sutures
iodo prep
iodochromic catgut suture
Iodoflex absorptive dressing
Iodoflex solid gel pad
iodoform gauze packer
iodoform gauze packing
iodohippurate sodium I-131
  renogram

iodophor solution
iodophor Steri-Drape
iodophor-impregnated adhesive
 wrap
Iodosorb absorptive dressing
iodoventriculogram
iodoventriculography
Iogel intraocular lens
iohexol contrast medium
iohexol CT scan
IOL (intraocular lens)
IOLAB Azar intraocular lens
IOLAB intraocular lens
IOLAB irrigating needle
IOLAB lens
IOLAB Slimfit lens
IOLAB taper-cut needle
IOLAB taper-point needle
IOLAB titanium instrument
IOLAB titanium needle
ion laser
ion microscope
ion pump
ion therapy
Ionescu (*also* Jonnesco)
Ionescu fossa
Ionescu operation
Ionescu sympathectomy
Ionescu tri-leaflet valve
Ionescu tri-leaflet valve
 procedure
Ionescu valve
Ionescu-Shiley aortic valve
 prosthesis
Ionescu-Shiley artificial cardiac
 valve
Ionescu-Shiley bioprosthetic
 valve
Ionescu-Shiley bovine
 pericardial valve
Ionescu-Shiley heart valve
Ionescu-Shiley low-profile
 prosthetic valve
Ionescu-Shiley pericardial patch
Ionescu-Shiley pericardial valve
Ionescu-Shiley pericardial valve
 graft
Ionescu-Shiley pericardial
 xenograft
Ionescu-Shiley porcine
 heterograft heart valve
Ionescu-Shiley prosthesis

Ionescu-Shiley standard
 pericardial prosthetic valve
Ionescu-Shiley valve
Ionescu-Shiley vascular graft
Ionguard titanium modular head
 component
ionic surgery
ionization counter
ionization instrument
ionizing irradiation
ionizing radiation
ionotherapy
ion-selective electrode
ion-specific field effect
 transducer
iontophoresis electrode
iontophoretic applicator
IOP (intraocular pressure)
Ioptex intraocular lens
Ioptex laser intraocular lens
 implant
Ioptex TabOptic lens
Iotec trocar
Iovision implant
Iowa forceps
Iowa hip component
Iowa hip evaluation
Iowa implant
Iowa membrane forceps
Iowa membrane-puncturing
 forceps
Iowa needle guide
Iowa orbital implant
Iowa periosteal elevator
Iowa pudendal needle guide
Iowa State fixation forceps
Iowa State forceps
Iowa total hip prosthesis
Iowa trumpet forceps guide
Iowa trumpet instrument
Iowa trumpet needle guide
Iowa University elevator
Iowa University periosteal
 elevator
Iowa-Mengert membrane
 forceps
IP (interphalangeal)
IP joint
IPAS flexible cannula
IPAS syringe
IPAT (integrated parallel
 acquisition technique)

IPC (intermittent pneumatic compression)
IPD (inflammatory pelvic disease, interpupillary distance)
IPG (impedance plethysmography)
IPJ (interphalangeal joint)
IPOP cast dressing (immediate postoperative prosthesis cast dressing)
IPPA (inspection, palpation, percussion, and auscultation)
IPPB (intermittent positive pressure breathing)
IPSF (immediate postsurgical fitting)
ipsilateral acetabular fracture
ipsilateral adrenalectomy
ipsilateral aspect
ipsilateral common carotid artery
ipsilateral contraction
ipsilateral ear
ipsilateral femoral neck fracture
ipsilateral femoral shaft fracture
ipsilateral gland
ipsilateral hand deformity
ipsilateral injection
ipsilateral mentalis muscle
ipsilateral nerve root lesion
ipsilateral nonreversed greater saphenous vein bypass
ipsilateral pelvic fracture
ipsilateral portal vein obstruction
ipsilateral reflex
ipsilateral rhinorrhea
ipsilateral thyroid lobectomy
ipsilateral tibial fracture
ipsilateral total lobe and contralateral subtotal lobectomy
IR (inferior rectus)
Irby head frame
IRC (implant-related complications)
Irex Exemplar ultrasound
iridectomesodialysis
iridectomize

iridectomy
  antiglaucoma peripheral iridectomy
  argon laser iridectomy
  basal iridectomy
  Bethke iridectomy
  buttonhole iridectomy
  Castroviejo iridectomy
  central iridectomy
  Chandler iridectomy
  Cleasby iridectomy
  complete iridectomy
  Elschnig central iridectomy
  laser iridectomy
  optic iridectomy
  optical iridectomy
  patent iridectomy
  peripheral iridectomy
  preliminary iridectomy
  pupil-to-root iridectomy
  sector iridectomy
  simple iridectomy
  stenopeic iridectomy
  superior sector iridectomy
  surgical iridectomy
  therapeutic iridectomy
  Ziegler iridectomy
iridectomy operation
iridectomy scar
iridectomy scissors
iridencleisis
  Holth iridencleisis
iridesis
iridial folds
iridial tent
iridic muscles
iridium implant
iridium needle
iridium needle holder
iridium prosthesis
iridium wire implant
iridium-192 loaded stent
iridocapsular fixation lens
iridocapsular implant cataract lens
iridocapsular intraocular lens
iridocapsulectomy
iridocapsulotomy
  Berens iridocapsulotomy
iridocapsulotomy scissors
iridocorneal angle
iridocorneal endothelial syndrome

iridocorneal epithelial syndrome
iridocorneosclerectomy
iridocyclectomy
iridocystectomy
iridodesis
iridodialysis
   anterior iridodialysis
   Bonzel iridodialysis
   posterior iridodialysis
iridodialysis spatula
iridolenticular
iridomesodialysis
iridoplasty
iridosclerotomy
iridostasis
iridotomy
   Abraham iridotomy
   Castroviejo radial iridotomy
   laser iridotomy
   peripheral iridotomy
   radial iridotomy
   superior iridotomy
iridotomy scissors
iris
   cloudy iris
   dehiscence of iris
   Florentine iris
   greater arterial circle of iris
   greater circle of iris
   lesser arterial circle of iris
   lesser circle of iris
   reposited iris
   stretching of iris
iris atrophy
iris bipolar forceps
iris bombé
iris ciliary body
iris claw lens
iris contracture
iris coronary stent
iris crypt
iris dehiscence
iris dialysis
iris diastasis
iris disposable retractor
iris ectasia
iris expressor
iris fixation intraocular lens
iris fixation lens
iris forceps
iris hernia
iris hook

iris hook cannula
iris inclusion operation
iris knife
iris knife-needle
iris lens manipulator
iris microforceps
iris microscissors
iris miniature scissors
iris needle
Iris Oculight SLx MicroPulse
   laser
iris pillars
iris pillars were reposited
iris plane intraocular lens
iris prolapse
iris protrusion
iris replacer
iris reposited
iris repositor
iris retractor
IRIS scanner
iris scissors
iris scraped free
iris spatula
iris stretching
iris stretching operation
iris suture microforceps
iris tissue forceps
iris transfixation
iris-clip intraocular lens
iris-supported intraocular lens
iritis
iritomy
IRMA (immunoradiometric
   assay, intraretinal
   microvascular abnormality)
Iron Intern retractor
irradiated cells
irradiated surgical defects
irradiation
   abdominal irradiation
   abdominopelvic irradiation
   adjuvant irradiation
   betatron irradiation
   breast irradiation
   cardiac irradiation
   cataract irradiation
   cesium irradiation
   charged-particle irradiation
   childhood thyroid irradiation
   cobalt-60 irradiation
   convergent beam irradiation

irradiation (*continued*)
cranial irradiation
craniospinal irradiation
definitive irradiation
elective neck irradiation
external beam irradiation
external orthovoltage
    irradiation
extracorporeal irradiation
fractionated external beam
    irradiation
gamma irradiation
half-body irradiation
heavy-ion irradiation
hemibody irradiation
hyperfractionated total body
    irradiation
interstitial irradiation
intracanalicular irradiation
intraoral cone irradiation
ionizing irradiation
linearly polarized near-
    infrared irradiation
local irradiation
long-wave irradiation
low-dose irradiation
lymph node irradiation
lymphoid irradiation
mantle irradiation
mediastinal irradiation
nD:YAG laser irradiation
neuraxis irradiation
para-aortic node irradiation
partial-breast irradiation
pelvic irradiation
periaortic irradiation
postoperative irradiation
prophylactic irradiation
selective irradiation
single-fraction total body
    irradiation
surface irradiation
therapeutic irradiation
total axial node irradiation
total body irradiation
total lymphoid irradiation
total nodal irradiation
ultraviolet blood irradiation
UV irradiation
whole abdominopelvic
    irradiation
whole body irradiation

irradiation (*continued*)
whole brain irradiation
whole-abdomen irradiation
whole-pelvis irradiation
irradiation and chemotherapy
irradiation and surgery
irradiation cataract
irradiation cystitis
irradiation damage
irradiation effect
irradiation failure
irradiation field
irradiation injury
irradiation menses
irradiation process
irradiation pulse
irradiation rate
irradiation respirations
irradiation sterilization
irradiation therapy
irreducible fracture
irreducible hernia
irregular amputated mucosal
    pattern
irregular bleeding
irregular border
irregular calcification
irregular cervix
irregular contractions
irregular defects
irregular heart rhythm
irregular intervals
irregularity
    cardiac irregularity
    cyclic irregularity
    luminal irregularity
irregularly irregular rhythm
irregularly shaped body
irresectable disease
irreversible brain damage
irreversible coma
irreversible condition
irreversible disability
irreversible disorder
irreversible hydrocolloid
    impression material
irrigated bladder
irrigated with normal saline
    solution
irrigated with saline solution
irrigating bronchoscope
irrigating cannula

irrigating catheter
irrigating contact Goldmann
 lens
irrigating cord
irrigating curet
irrigating cystotome
irrigating Dilaprobe
irrigating eye spatula
irrigating iris hook
irrigating lens loop
irrigating lens manipulator
irrigating mushroom retractor
irrigating notched spatula
irrigating probe
irrigating sheath
irrigating solution
irrigating tip
irrigating tube
irrigating uterine curet
irrigating valve
irrigating vectis
irrigating vectis loop
irrigating-aspirating cannula
irrigating-aspirating tip
irrigating-positioning needle
irrigation
 acetohydroxamic acid
  irrigation
 antibiotic irrigation
 bacitracin irrigation
 bronchoscopy with irrigation
 caloric irrigation
 canal irrigation
 chamber irrigation
 closed irrigation
 continuous bladder irrigation
 continuous irrigation
 copious irrigation
 curettage and irrigation
 debridement and irrigation
 endodontic irrigation
 frontal irrigation
 Guiteras irrigation
 hemiacidrin irrigation
 heparin irrigation
 intravesical alum irrigation
 Meditron bipolar generator
  with irrigation
 on-table irrigation
 oral irrigation
 pulse lavage irrigation
 pulsed irrigation

irrigation (*continued*)
 rectal pulsed irrigation
 rectum irrigation
 saline irrigation
 sinus irrigation
 tendon sheath irrigation
 whole-gut irrigation
 wound irrigation
irrigation and aspiration (I&A)
irrigation and curettage
irrigation burn
irrigation catheter
irrigation fluid
irrigation of bladder
irrigation of nose
irrigation of sinuses
irrigation solution
irrigation syringe
irrigation techniques
irrigation-aspiration core
irrigator
 anterior chamber irrigator
 antral irrigator
 Barraquer irrigator
 Baumrucker clamp irrigator
 B-H anterior chamber irrigator
 Bishop-Harman anterior
  chamber irrigator
 Buie rectal irrigator
 Carabelli irrigator
 Creevy irrigator
 DeVilbiss eye irrigator
 Doss automatic percolator
  irrigator
 Dougherty eye irrigator
 Endo-Flo irrigator
 endoscopic irrigator
 eye irrigator
 Fink cul-de-sac irrigator
 Fisch bone drill irrigator
 Fox hydrostatic irrigator
 Gibson anterior chamber
  irrigator
 Gibson eye irrigator
 Goldstein anterior chamber
  irrigator
 Guiteras nozzle irrigator
 Hartstein irrigator
 Hollister colostomy irrigator
 House sucker irrigator
 House suction irrigator
 House T-tube irrigator

irrigator (*continued*)
Huzly irrigator
Hydrofloss electronic oral irrigator
hydrostatic irrigator
HydroSurg laparoscopic irrigator
Irrijet irrigator
Kelman irrigator
Kemp rectal irrigator
Lamb irrigator
laser-assisted intrastromal keratomileusis flap irrigator
LASIK flap irrigator
Lukens double-channel irrigator
McKenna irrigator
Moncrieff anterior chamber irrigator
nasal irrigator
Nezhat irrigator
olive-tipped irrigator
ophthalmic irrigator
Ortholav pulsed irrigator
percolator irrigator
Perry ostomy irrigator
Pro Pulse irrigator
Radpour irrigator
Radpour-House suction irrigator
Randolph irrigator
rectal irrigator
Rollet anterior chamber irrigator
Shambaugh irrigator
Shea irrigator
sinus irrigator
stainless irrigator
Stopko irrigator
Stryker suction irrigator
suction irrigator
Thornwald antral irrigator
Thornwald irrigator
Valentine irrigator
Vidaurri irrigator
Water Pik irrigator
Wells irrigator
Younge irrigator
Zerowet irrigator
Zimmer suction irrigator
irrigator-suction tube
Irrigo syringe
Irrijet DS wound irrigation device

Irrijet irrigator
irritable bladder
irritable bowel syndrome
irritable colon
irritable heart
irritable joint
irritable lesion
irritable stricture
irritant
irritative lesion
irritative reaction
Irrivac syringe
Irvine corneal scissors
Irvine I&A unit
Irvine operation
Irvine probe-point scissors
Irvine-Gass syndrome
Irving operation
Irving sterilization operation
Irving technique of tubal ligation
Irving tubal ligation
Irwin operation
Irwin pelvic osteotomy
Irwin technique
IS artificial cardiac valve
IS joint knife (incudostapedial joint knife)
Isaacs aspiration syringe
Isaacs-Ludwig arteriole
Isaacson classification (IC)
ischemia
    distal ischemia
    hand ischemia
    midgut ischemia
    myocardial ischemia
    subendocardial ischemia
    wound ischemia
ischemia and reperfusion injury
ischemia-guided medical therapy
ischemic aortic disease
ischemic bowel
ischemic compression
ischemic contracture
ischemic disease
ischemic encephalopathy
ischemic foot
ischemic heart disease
ischemic liver injury
ischemic necrosis
ischemic neuropathy

ischemic ocular inflammation
ischemic reflex
ischemic time
ischemic ulatrophy
ischemic-tourniquet technique
ischiadic nerve
ischial bone
ischial brace
ischial containment socket
ischial pressure sore
ischial ramus
ischial spines
ischial tuberosity
ischial weightbearing brace
ischial weightbearing leg brace
ischial weightbearing prosthesis
ischial-gluteal weightbearing
    socket
ischiatic hernia
ischiatic hernioplasty
ischiatic notch
ischiatic scoliosis
ischiectomy
ischioanal fossa
ischiocapsular ligament
ischiocavernous muscle
ischiococcygeal
ischiodymia
ischiofemoral arthrodesis
ischiogluteal
ischiohebotomy
ischiopubic ramus
ischiopubiotomy
    fetal ischiopubiotomy
    Galbiati bilateral fetal
        ischiopubiotomy
ischiorectal abscess
ischiorectal anorectal space
ischiorectal fossa
ischiorectal fossa plane
ischiorectal hernia
ischiosacral
ischiovertebral
ischium
iseiconic lens (*also* iseikonic
    lens)
iseikonic lens (*also* iseiconic
    lens)
Iselin forceps
I-shaped scalp flap
ishemic muscular atrophy
Ishihara color test

Ishihara cautery
Ishihara IV slit lamp
Ishihara plate
Ishihara pseudoisochromatic
    plate
Ishizuki hinge
ISI laparoscopic instruments
island
    attached island
    bone island
    bony island
    cartilage island
    epimyoepithelial island
    Langerhans island
    mucosal island
    myoepithelial cell island
    Reil island
    septocutaneous island
    septofasciocutaneous island
    skin island
    teres major skin island
island adipofascial flap in
        Achilles tendon resurfacing
island fasciocutaneous flap
island flap
island frontalis muscle transfer
island graft
island leg flap
island of Reil
island pedicle flaps
island pedicle scalp flap
island skin flap
island-flap procedure
islands of Langerhans
islet cell cancer
islet cell tumor
islet structures
islets of Langerhans
isoantibody
isobaric anesthesia
isobaric spinal anesthesia
isobaric transition
Isobex dynamometer
isocentric oblique
isocentric technique
isochromatic plate
Isocon camera
isodense subdural hematoma
isodense with surrounding
    tissues
isodiametric bipolar screw-in
    lead

isodose curve
isodose line
isodosimetry
isoechoic
isoeffect curve
isoelastic pelvic prosthesis
isoelastic rip clamp
isoelectric
    electroencephalogram
isoelectric line
isoelectric point
isoenzyme
IsoFlex pacing lead
Isoflow pump
isogeneic graft
isogenic graft
isognathus
isograft
isohydric cycle
isokinetic collection
Isola spinal implant system
    anchor
Isola spinal implant system
    component
Isola spinal implant system eye
    rod
Isola spinal implant system hook
Isola spinal implant system iliac
    screw
Isola vertebral screw
Isola wire
isolated and tagged
isolated annuloplasty
isolated arterial injury
isolated dislocation
isolated episode
isolated fashion
isolated field
isolated heat perfusion
isolated hepatic perfusion
isolated iliac artery aneurysm
isolated infusion
isolated limb perfusion (ILP)
isolated liver injury
isolated metastatic tumor
isolated naso-ocular cleft
isolated perfusion
isolated premature beats
isolated procedure
isolated sphenoid sinusitis
isolated unilateral cleft
    lip/alveolus (UCLA)

isolated venous injury
isolation and asepsis
isolation and identification
isolation bag
isolation face mask
isolation forceps
isolation perfusion therapy
isolation technique
isolator
    surgical isolator
    Vickers isolator
Isolator blood culture
Isolator lysis-centrifugation tube
isolette
isologous graft
Isomet saw
isometer
Isometer bone graft placement
    site detector
isometric point
isometric strain gauge
isometric technique
isometric transition
isoperistaltic anastomosis
isoperistaltic gastrojejunostomy
isoperistaltic jejunostomy
isoplastic graft
Isoprene plastic splint
isotonic machine
isotope bone scan
isotope calibrator
isotope injection
isotope localization
isotope scanning
isotope scanning studies
isotope studies
isotope therapy
isotopes
isotopic pulse generator
    pacemaker
isotransplantation
isotropic disk
isovolumic contractor
Israel blunt rake retractor
Israel camera
Israel decompressor
Israel depressor
Israel dissector
Israel nasal rasp
Israel operation
Israel rake retractor
Israel rasp

Israel raspatory
Israel retractor
Israel suction tube
Israel tongue depressor
Israel tonsillar dissector
Israel tube
Isse endo brow instrument
Istanbul flap for phallic
   reconstruction
I-Stat cautery
isthmectomy
   thyroid isthmectomy
isthmorrhaphy
isthmus
   aortic isthmus
   Kroenig isthmus
   thyroid isthmus
   velopharyngeal isthmus
isthmus of fallopian tube
isthmus of uterus
isthmus tubae uterinae
ITA graft (internal thoracic
   artery graft)
Italian distant flap
Italian flap
Italian operation
Italian rhinoplasty
Itard eustachian catheter
ITB (iliotibial band)
ITC radiopaque balloon catheter
I-tech cannula
I-tech cannula holder
I-tech cannula tray
I-tech intraocular foreign body
   forceps
I-tech needle holder
I-tech splinter forceps
I-tech tying forceps
I-tech Castroviejo bladebreaker
I-Temp cautery
iterative reconstruction
ITI dental implant
ITI endosseous implant
Ito needle
Ito nevus
Ito procedure
Itrel I unipolar pulse generator
Itrel II quadripolar pulse
   generator
ITT (internal tibial torsion)
IUCD (intrauterine
   contraceptive device)

IUD (see intrauterine device)
IUD bow
IUD coil
IUD dislodged
IUD removed hook
IUD spotting
IUD string
IUGR (intrauterine growth
   retardation)
IUI disposable cannula
IV (intravenous, intervertebral)
IV administration
IV administration of medication
IV anesthesia
IV angiocardiography
IV antibiotic
IV bolus injection of contrast
   material
IV catheter
IV cholangiography
IV cocktail
IV contrast medium
IV discontinued
IV disk (intravertebral disk)
IV disk forceps (intravertebral
   disk forceps)
IV disk rongeur (intravertebral
   disk rongeur)
IV drip
IV feeding
IV fluid therapy
IV hydration
IV infusion
IV line
IV needle
IV pyelogram
IV pyelography
IV stand
IV therapy
IV transfusion
IV urography
IVAC device
IVAC infusion pump
IVAC machine
IVAC pump
IVAC ventilator
IVAC volumetric infusion pump
Ivalon compressed patch graft
Ivalon dressing
Ivalon embolic sponge
Ivalon eye implant
Ivalon graft

Ivalon implant
Ivalon Lucite orbital eye
    implant
Ivalon material
Ivalon patch
Ivalon prosthesis
Ivalon rectopexy
Ivalon sponge
Ivalon sponge eye implant
Ivalon sponge graft
Ivalon sponge implant
Ivalon sponge rectopexy
Ivalon sponge wrap
Ivalon sponge-wrap operation
Ivalon sutures
Ivalon wire coil
Ivan laryngeal applicator
Ivan nasopharyngeal applicator
IVC (intravenous
    cholangiogram, intravenous
    cholangiography)
IVC ligation
IVC occlusion
IVC reconstruction
IVCD (intraventricular
    conduction delay)
Iverson dermabrader
Ives anoscope

Ives proctoscope
Ives rectal speculum
Ives speculum
Ives-Fansler anoscope
Ivor Lewis esophagectomy
Ivor Lewis esophagogastrectomy
Ivor Lewis 2-stage subtotal
    esophagectomy
Ivor-Lewis resection
ivory bones
ivory exostosis
ivory membrane
Ivory rubber dam clamp
IVP (intravenous pyelogram)
IVSD (interventricular septal
    defect)
IVT percutaneous catheter
    introducer sheath
IVUS catheter
Ivy bleeding time
Ivy loop
Ivy loop wiring
Ivy mastoid rongeur
Ivy needle holder
Ivy rongeur
Ivy wire
Ivy wire loops
Iwanoff retinal edema

J exchange guidewire
J loop technique
J needle
J orthogonal electrode
J pad
J Rosen guidewire
J&J Band-Aid sterile drape
J&J dressing
J/cm^2 (joules per square centimeter)
J-24 cervical orthosis
J-35 hyperextension orthosis
J-45 contraflexion orthosis
J-55 postfusion orthosis
Jabaley scissors
Jabaley Supercut scissors
Jabaley-Stille scissors
Jabaley-Stille Supercut scissors
Jaboulay amputation
Jaboulay button
Jaboulay gastroduodenostomy
Jaboulay operation
Jaboulay pyloroplasty
Jaboulay-Doyen-Winkleman operation
Jaboulay-Doyen-Winkleman technique
JACE hand continuous passive motion unit
JACE-STIM electrical stimulator
JACE-STIM electrotherapy unit
jacket
  body jacket
  Bonchek-Shiley cardiac jacket
  Boston soft body jacket
  Calot jacket
  cervicothoracic jacket
  cuirass jacket
  Daily cooling jacket
  Frejka jacket
  Immobilization jacket
  Kalot jacket
  Kydex body jacket

jacket (*continued*)
  Lexan jacket
  Low Profile plastic body jacket
  Medtronic cardiac cooling jacket
  Minerva back jacket
  Minerva plaster jacket
  Minerva plastic jacket
  Orthoplast jacket
  plaster-of-Paris jacket
  Raney jacket
  Risser wedging jacket
  Royalite body jacket
  Sayre jacket
  Willock respiratory jacket
  Wilmington plastic jacket
jacket-type chest dressing
jackknife position
Jackman coronary sinus electrode catheter
Jackson alligator forceps
Jackson alligator grasping forceps
Jackson-Parker classification of Hodgkin disease
Jackson anterior commissure laryngoscope
Jackson appliance
Jackson applicator
Jackson approximation forceps
Jackson aspirating tube
Jackson atomizer
Jackson battery cord
Jackson biopsy forceps
Jackson bistoury
Jackson bite block
Jackson bone clamp
Jackson bone-extension clamp
Jackson bone-holding clamp
Jackson bougie
Jackson broad staple forceps
Jackson bronchial dilator

Jackson bronchoscope
Jackson bronchoscopic forceps
  handle
Jackson bronchoscopic
  instrument
Jackson button forceps
Jackson cane-shaped tracheal
  tube
Jackson cane-shaped tube
Jackson clamp
Jackson cone-shaped tracheal
  tube
Jackson conventional foreign
  body forceps
Jackson costophrenic
  bronchoscope
Jackson crib
Jackson cross-action forceps
Jackson cylindrical object
  forceps
Jackson dilator
Jackson double-concave rat-
  tooth forceps
Jackson double-ended retractor
Jackson double-prong forceps
Jackson down-jaw forceps
Jackson dressing forceps
Jackson dull rotation forceps
Jackson dull-pointed forceps
Jackson elevator
Jackson endoscopic forceps
Jackson esophageal bougie
Jackson esophageal dilator
Jackson esophageal scissors
Jackson esophageal shears
Jackson esophagoscope
Jackson fenestrated peanut-
  grasping forceps
Jackson fiberoptic slide
  laryngoscope
Jackson flexible upper lobe
  bronchus forceps
Jackson forceps handle
Jackson forward-grasping
  forceps
Jackson full-lumen
  bronchoscope
Jackson full-lumen
  esophagoscope
Jackson full-lumen standard
  bronchoscope
Jackson globular object forceps

Jackson goiter retractor
Jackson head-holding forceps
Jackson hemostat
Jackson hemostatic forceps
Jackson hold-holding forceps
Jackson hollow-object forceps
Jackson hook
Jackson imaging table
Jackson incision
Jackson infant biopsy forceps
Jackson infant forceps
Jackson intervertebral disk
  rongeur
Jackson knife
Jackson lacrimal intubation set
Jackson laryngeal applicator
Jackson laryngeal applicator
  forceps
Jackson laryngeal atomizer
Jackson laryngeal basket forceps
Jackson laryngeal forceps
Jackson laryngeal instruments
Jackson laryngeal punch forceps
Jackson laryngeal ring-rotation
  forceps
Jackson laryngeal rotation
  forceps
Jackson laryngeal scissors
Jackson laryngeal-dressing
  forceps
Jackson laryngeal-grasping
  forceps
Jackson laryngectomy tube
Jackson laryngofissure forceps
Jackson laryngoscope
Jackson laryngostat
Jackson magnification ruler set
Jackson membrane
Jackson open-end aspirating
  tube
Jackson orthogonal catheter
Jackson papilloma forceps
Jackson perichondrial elevator
Jackson pin-bending
  costophrenic forceps
Jackson probe
Jackson punch
Jackson punch forceps
Jackson radiopaque bougie
Jackson retractor
Jackson ring jaw globular object
  forceps

Jackson ring-jaw forceps
Jackson ring-rotation forceps
Jackson rod
Jackson rotation forceps
Jackson scalpel
Jackson scissors
Jackson self-retaining goiter retractor
Jackson sharp-pointed rotation forceps
Jackson shears
Jackson side-curved forceps
Jackson silver tracheostomy tube
Jackson sister-hook forceps
Jackson sliding laryngoscope
Jackson speculum
Jackson spinal surgery table
Jackson sponge carrier
Jackson square punch tip
Jackson standard bronchoscope
Jackson standard full-lumen esophagoscope
Jackson standard laryngoscope
Jackson staple bronchoscope
Jackson steel-stem woven filiform bougie
Jackson syndrome
Jackson tenaculum
Jackson tendon-seizing forceps
Jackson tracheal bistoury knife
Jackson tracheal bougie
Jackson tracheal dilator
Jackson tracheal forceps
Jackson tracheal hemostat
Jackson tracheal hemostatic forceps
Jackson tracheal hook
Jackson tracheal knife
Jackson tracheal retractor
Jackson tracheal scalpel
Jackson tracheal tenaculum
Jackson tracheal tube
Jackson tracheoscope
Jackson tracheotomic bistoury
Jackson tracheotomy set
Jackson triangular brass dilator
Jackson triangular-punch forceps
Jackson tube
Jackson turbinate scissors
Jackson Universal handle

Jackson vaginal retractor
Jackson vaginal speculum
Jackson veil
Jackson velvet-eye aspirating tube
Jackson warning stop tube
Jackson-Babcock operation
Jackson-Moore shears
Jackson-Mosher cardiospasm dilator
Jackson-Mosher dilator
Jackson-Plummer dilator
Jackson-Pratt bifurcated drain extension
Jackson-Pratt catheter
Jackson-Pratt dissector
Jackson-Pratt drain
Jackson-Pratt wound drain
Jackson-Pratt large-volume suction reservoir
Jackson-Pratt reservoir
Jackson-Pratt round PVC drain
Jackson-Pratt silicone flat drain
Jackson-Pratt silicone round drain
Jackson-Pratt suction drain
Jackson-Pratt suction reservoir
Jackson-Pratt suction tube
Jackson-Pratt T-tube drain
Jackson-Rees endotracheal tube
Jackson-Trousseau dilator
Jacob capsule fragment forceps
Jacob clamp
Jacob key
Jacob membrane
Jacob tenaculum
Jacob ulcer
Jacob uterine tenaculum
Jacob uterine vulsellum forceps
Jacob vulsellum forceps
Jacobaeus operation
Jacobaeus procedure
Jacobaeus thoracoscope
Jacobs biopsy forceps
Jacobs capsular fragment forceps
Jacobs chuck
Jacobs chuck adapter
Jacobs chuck and key
Jacobs chuck drill
Jacobs clamp
Jacobs distraction rod

Jacobs locking hook spinal rod
Jacobs locking-hook spinal rod
  instrumentation
Jacobs locking-hook spinal rod
  technique
Jacobs snap-lock chuck
Jacobs T-handled chuck
Jacobs uterine tenaculum
Jacobs vulsellum forceps
Jacobson anastomosis
Jacobson bayonet-shaped
  scissors
Jacobson bipolar forceps
Jacobson bladder retractor
Jacobson blood vessel probe
Jacobson blunt hook
Jacobson bulldog clamp
Jacobson cartilage
Jacobson clamp
Jacobson counter-pressure
  elevator
Jacobson curet
Jacobson dressing forceps
Jacobson elevator
Jacobson endarterectomy spatula
Jacobson goiter retractor
Jacobson hemostatic forceps
Jacobson holder
Jacobson hook
Jacobson knife
Jacobson knot tier
Jacobson microbulldog clamp
Jacobson microdressing forceps
Jacobson microscissors
Jacobson microsurgery
  instrument
Jacobson modified vessel
  clamp
Jacobson mosquito forceps
Jacobson needle holder
Jacobson nerve
Jacobson organ
Jacobson plexus
Jacobson probe
Jacobson punch
Jacobson reflex
Jacobson retinitis
Jacobson retractor
Jacobson scissors
Jacobson spatula
Jacobson spring-handled needle
  holder

Jacobson spring-handled
  scissors
Jacobson suture pusher
Jacobson technique
Jacobson vas deferens probe
Jacobson vessel clamp
Jacobson vessel knife
Jacobson vessel punch
Jacobson Vital needle holder
Jacobson-Potts vessel clamp
Jacobs-Palmer laparoscope
Jacob-Swan gonioprism
Jacob-Swan gonioscope
Jacob-Swan gonioscopic prism
Jacob-Swan goniotomy pliers
Jacoby heel splint
Jacod syndrome
Jacobs cranial hook
Jacquart facial angle
Jacquemier sign
Jacques catheter
Jacques gastric tube
Jacques stomach tube
Jaeger bone plate
Jaeger hook
Jaeger keratome
Jaeger keratome knife
Jaeger knife
Jaeger lid plate
Jaeger lid plate retractor
Jaeger lid retractor
Jaeger metal lid plate
Jaeger reading chart
Jaeger retractor
Jaeger strabismus hook
Jaeger-Hamby procedure
Jaeger-Whiteley catheter
Jaesche operation
Jaesche-Arlt operation
Jaffe bone disease
Jaffe capsulorrhexis forceps
Jaffe Cilco lens
Jaffe disease
Jaffe eyelid speculum
Jaffe hook
Jaffe intraocular spatula
Jaffe iris hook
Jaffe laser blepharoplasty and
  facial resurfacing set
Jaffe lens
Jaffe lens spatula
Jaffe lens-manipulating hook

Jaffe lid retractor
Jaffe microlens hook
Jaffe needle holder
Jaffe ocular implant lens
Jaffe 1-piece intraocular lens
Jaffe procedure
Jaffe retractor
Jaffe scissors
Jaffe speculum
Jaffe suturing forceps
Jaffe wire lid retractor
Jaffe-Bechert nucleus rotator
Jaffe-Givner lid retractor
Jaffe-Maltzman hook
Jaffe-Maltzman lens manipulator
Jaeger meniscal forceps
Jahnke anastomosis clamp
Jahnke-Barron heart support net
Jahnke-Cook-Seeley clamp
Jahss maneuver
Jahss osteotomy
Jahss position
Jahss procedure
Jaime lacrimal operation
Jako biopsy
Jako clamp
Jako facial nerve monitor
Jako fine ball-tip hook
Jako knife
Jako knot pusher
Jako laryngeal forceps
Jako laryngeal knife
Jako laryngeal microforceps
Jako laryngeal microinstrument
Jako laryngeal microscissors
Jako laryngeal mirror
Jako laryngeal needle holder
Jako laryngeal probe
Jako laryngeal suction tube
Jako laryngoscope
Jako laser aspirating tube
Jako laser retractor
Jako laser trocar
Jako microlaryngeal cup forceps
Jako microlaryngeal grasping
    forceps
Jako microlaryngeal scissors
Jako microlaryngoscope
Jako monitor
Jako nerve monitor
Jako probe
Jako suction tube

Jako suspension otoscope
Jakob reverse pivot shift sign
Jakob technique
Jako-Cherry laryngoscope
Jako-Kleinsasser ball-tip hook
Jako-Kleinsasser knife
Jako-Kleinsasser microforceps
Jako-Kleinsasser microscissors
Jako-Pilling laryngoscope
Jalaguier cleft lip repair
Jalaguier incision
Jalaguier-Reverdin needle
Jamar dynamometer
Jamar hydraulic hand
    dynamometer
Jamar hydraulic pinch gauge
James accessory tract
James atrionodal bypass tract
James bundle
James fibers
James intranodal tract
James lumbar peritoneal
    catheter
James position
James wound-approximation
    forceps
Jameson calipers
Jameson dissecting scissors
Jameson eye calipers
Jameson facelift scissors
Jameson forceps
Jameson hook
Jameson muscle clamp
Jameson muscle forceps
Jameson muscle hook
Jameson muscle recession
    forceps
Jameson needle
Jameson needle holder
Jameson operation
Jameson recession forceps
Jameson strabismus forceps
Jameson strabismus hook
Jameson strabismus needle
Jameson tracheal muscle forceps
Jameson tracheal muscle
    recession forceps
Jameson-Werber scissors
Jameson-Metzenbaum scissors
jamming injury
jamming knot
Jamshidi adult needle

Jamshidi liver biopsy needle
Jamshidi muscle needle biopsy
Jamshidi-Kormed bone marrow biopsy needle
Janacek reimplantation set
Janecki-Nelson shoulder girdle resection
Janelli clip
Janes fracture appliance
Janes fracture frame
Janeway gastroscope
Janeway gastrostomy
Janeway lesion
Janeway sphygmomanometer
Janeway spots
Janko clamp
Jannetta alligator grasping forceps
Jannetta aneurysm neck dissector
Jannetta angular elevator
Jannetta angular knife
Jannetta bayonet forceps
Jannetta bayonet needle holder
Jannetta bayonet scissors
Jannetta bayonet-shaped needle holder
Jannetta bayonet-shaped scissors
Jannetta dissector
Jannetta double-pronged fork
Jannetta duckbill elevator
Jannetta elevator
Jannetta hook
Jannetta knife
Jannetta microbayonet forceps
Jannetta microneurosurgery instrument
Jannetta microvascular decompression procedure
Jannetta needle holder
Jannetta posterior fossa retractor
Jannetta probe
Jannetta sterilizing rack
Jannetta storage rack
Jannetta vascular decompression of 5th nerve
Jannetta-Kurze dissecting scissors
Jansen bayonet dressing forceps
Jansen bayonet ear forceps
Jansen bayonet forceps
Jansen bayonet nasal forceps

Jansen bayonet rongeur
Jansen bone curet
Jansen clamp
Jansen curet
Jansen disease
Jansen dissecting forceps
Jansen dressing forceps
Jansen ear forceps
Jansen ear rongeur
Jansen mastoid raspatory
Jansen mastoid retractor
Jansen mastoid rongeur
Jansen monopolar forceps
Jansen mouth gag
Jansen nasal-dressing forceps
Jansen operation
Jansen periosteotome
Jansen rongeur
Jansen scalp retractor
Jansen scissors
Jansen test
Jansen thumb forceps
Jansen-Cottle rongeur
Jansen-Gifford mastoid retractor
Jansen-Gruenwald forceps
Jansen-Middleton nasal-cutting forceps
Jansen-Middleton punch forceps
Jansen-Middleton rongeur
Jansen-Middleton scissors
Jansen-Middleton septal forceps
Jansen-Middleton septal punch
Jansen-Middleton septotomy forceps
Jansen-Middleton septum-cutting forceps
Jansen-Mueller forceps
Jansen-Newhart mastoid probe
Jansen-Sluder mouth gag
Jansen-Struyken septal forceps
Jansen-Wagner mastoid retractor
Jansen-Zaufel bone rongeur
Jansey procedure
Jansky classification
Jantene operation
Japanese approach
Japanese Bruening anastigmatic aural magnifier
Japanese cancer classification
Japanese classification for gastric carcinoma (JCGC)
Japanese standard operation

Japanese suction tip
Japanese-style gastrectomy
Japanese-style
    lymphadenectomy
Japanese-style operation
Japas foot procedure
Japas procedure
Jarabak archwire
Jarcho tenaculum
Jarcho tenaculum forceps
Jarcho tenaculum holder
Jarcho uterine tenaculum
Jarcho uterine tenaculum
    forceps
Jardine hook
Jardon eye shield
Jardon-Straith chin implant
Jardon-Straith nasal implant
Jari renal sinus retractor
Jarit air injection cannula
Jarit anterior resection clamp
Jarit bipolar coagulator
Jarit bladebreaker
Jarit bone hook
Jarit brain forceps
Jarit cartilage clamp
Jarit comedo extractor
Jarit cross-action retractor
Jarit disposable cannula
Jarit disposable trocar
Jarit dissecting scissors
Jarit endarterectomy scissors
Jarit finger goniometer
Jarit flat-top scissors
Jarit forceps holder
Jarit hand surgery osteotome
Jarit intestinal clamp
Jarit lacrimal cannula
Jarit lower lateral scissors
Jarit mallet
Jarit meniscal clamp
Jarit microstitch scissors
Jarit microsurgery scissors
Jarit microsurgical needle holder
Jarit microsuture tying forceps
Jarit mosquito forceps
Jarit PEER retractor
Jarit palate hook
Jarit periosteal elevator
Jarit peripheral vascular scissors
Jarit pin cutter
Jarit plaster knife

Jarit plaster shears
Jarit renal sinus retractor
Jarit reverse adenoid curet
Jarit rotator
Jarit rotator endoscope
Jarit spring-wire retractor
Jarit sterilizer forceps
Jarit sternal needle holder
Jarit stitch scissors
Jarit tendon-pulling forceps
Jarit 3-prong cast spreader
Jarit tube-occluding forceps
Jarit tuning fork
Jarit utility shears
Jarit wire holder
Jarit wire-pulling forceps
Jarit-Allis tissue forceps
Jarit-Crafoord forceps
Jarit-Dandy forceps
Jarit-Deaver retractor
Jarit-Graves vaginal speculum
Jarit-Kerrison laminectomy
    rongeur
Jarit-Liston bone-cutting forceps
Jarit-Mason cast breaker
Jarit-Pederson vaginal speculum
Jarit-Poole abdominal suction
    tube
Jarit-Ruskin bone rongeur
Jarit-Yankauer suction tube
Jarjavay muscle
Jarvik-7 mechanical pump
Jarvis clamp
Jarvis hemorrhoid forceps
Jarvis hemorrhoidal forceps
Jarvis operation
Jarvis pile clamp
Jarvis snare
Jatene arterial switch procedure
Jatene arterial switch valve
Jatene-Macchi prosthetic valve
Javal keratometer
Javal ophthalmometer
Javerts placental forceps
Javerts polyp forceps
Javid bypass clamp
Javid bypass shunt
Javid bypass tube
Javid carotid artery bypass
    clamp
Javid carotid artery clamp
Javid carotid clamp

Javid carotid shunt
Javid catheter
Javid clamp
Javid endarterectomy shunt
Javid internal carotid shunt
Javid shunt
Javid tube
jaw
   angle of jaw
   bird-beak jaw
   cleft jaw
   Cox regression analysis of
      partially edentulous jaw
   crackling jaw
   fibrous dysplasia of jaws
   Hapsburg jaw
   lower jaw
   lumpy jaw
   multiple exostoses of jaw
   parrot jaw
   progonoma of jaw
   ramus of jaw
   receding lower jaw
   upper jaw
   wired jaw
   wiring of jaw
jaw fracture
jaw grading
jaw hook
jaw jerk reflex
jaw joint
jaw movement
jaw protrusion
jaw radiograph
jaw reflex
jaw relation
jaw relation record
jaw repositioning
jaw rongeur
jaw separation
jaw splint
jaw spreader
jaw spring clip
jaw stabilization
jaw thrust maneuver
jawbone
jawline
jaw-neck resection
jaw-to-jaw position
jaw-winking phenomenon
Jayles forceps
Jazbi dissector

Jazbi nasal instrument set
Jazbi suction tonsillar dissector
Jazbi tonsil dissector
Jazbi tonsillar dissector
JB catheter
JB-1 catheter
Jefferson fracture
Jefferson retractor
Jefferson self-retaining retractor
Jeffrey introducer set
Jeffrey radial fracture
   classification
Jeffrey technique
Jehle coronary perfusion
   catheter
jejunal and ileal veins
jejunal arteries
jejunal biopsy
jejunal bypass
jejunal diverticulum
jejunal feeding tube
jejunal free flap
jejunal interposition
jejunal interposition of Henle
   loop
jejunal limb
jejunal loop
jejunal mucosa
jejunal pouch
jejunal Roux-en-Y loop
jejunal tube insertion
jejunal ulcer
jejunal veins
jejunal villi
jejunalization of the ileum
jejunectomy
jejunocecostomy
jejunocholecystostomy
jejunocolic fistula
jejunocolostomy
jejunoileal anastomosis
jejunoileal bypass (JIB)
jejunoileal bypass reversal
   procedure
jejunoileal bypass reversal
   technique
jejunoileal bypass surgery
jejunojejunal anastomosis
jejunojejunostomy
jejunopexy
jejunoplasty
jejunorrhaphy

jejunostomy
  afferent jejunostomy
  antecolic jejunostomy
  anterior jejunostomy
  antiperistaltic jejunostomy
  decompression jejunostomy
  endoscopic jejunostomy
  hepaticocutaneous
    jejunostomy
  isoperistaltic jejunostomy
  laparoscopic jejunostomy
  loop jejunostomy
  needle catheter jejunostomy
  posterior jejunostomy
  Roscoe-Graham jejunostomy
  Witzel jejunostomy
  Witzel tunnel for feeding
    jejunostomy
jejunostomy elemental diet
  feeding
jejunostomy tract
  choledochoscopy
jejunostomy tube
jejunostomy tube feeding
jejunotomy
jejunum free flap
jejunum loop
Jelco catheter
Jelco intravenous catheter
Jelco intravenous stylet
Jelco needle
Jelenko arch bar
Jelenko arch bar application
Jelenko bar
Jelenko facial fracture appliance
Jelenko pliers
Jelenko splint
Jelks operation
jelly dressing
jelly-like mass
Jelm catheter
Jelm 2-way catheter
Jelonet dressing
Jena colposcope
Jena-Schiotz tonometer
Jendrassik maneuver
Jenkins chisel
Jennings Loktite mouth gag
Jennings mouth gag
Jennings-Skillern mouth gag
Jenning-Streifeneder gastroscope
Jenny mammary prosthesis

Jensen capsular polisher
Jensen classification
Jensen diamond polisher
Jensen intraocular lens forceps
Jensen lens forceps
Jensen lens-inserting forceps
Jensen operation
Jensen polisher
Jensen procedure
Jensen scratcher
Jensen ties
Jensen transposition procedure
Jensen transposition surgery for
  lateral rectus paresis
Jensen-Thomas I&A cannula
Jerald forceps
Jergesen I-beam
Jergesen incision
Jergesen reamer
Jergesen tube
jerking eye movements
jerking musculature
jerky movements
Jerne technique
Jervey capsular fragment forceps
Jervey iris forceps
Jesberg aspirating tube
Jesberg bronchoscope
Jesberg clamp
Jesberg esophagoscope
Jesberg forceps
Jesberg grasping forceps
Jesberg infant bronchoscope
Jesberg laryngectomy clamp
Jesberg oval esophagoscope
Jesberg scope
Jesberg tube
Jesberg upper esophagoscope
Jesco scissors
Jesse-Stryker saw
jet douche
jet humidifier
jet lesion
jet nebulizer
jet pilot position
jet stylet
jet ventilation
jet ventilation anesthetic
  technique
Jetco spray cannula
Jeter lag screw
Jeter position screw

Jewel AF implantable
    defibrillator
Jewel atrial fibrillation dual
    chamber device
jeweler's bipolar forceps
jeweler's microforceps
jeweler's pickup forceps
Jewett and Whitmore
    classification
Jewett bar
Jewett bone chip packer
Jewett bone extractor
Jewett classification of bladder
    carcinoma
Jewett contraflexion orthosis
Jewett double-angle osteotomy
    plate
Jewett driver
Jewett electrode
Jewett fracture appliance
Jewett frame
Jewett gouge
Jewett hip nail
Jewett nail
Jewett nail overlay plate
Jewett nail plate
Jewett operation
Jewett orthosis
Jewett pickup screw
Jewett plate
Jewett postfusion orthosis
Jewett prosthesis
Jewett reamer
Jewett screw
Jewett slotted plate
Jewett socket reamer
Jewett sound
Jewett thoracolumbosacral
    orthosis
Jewett urethral sound
Jewett uterine dilator
Jewett uterine sound
Jewett-Benjamin cervical
    orthosis
J-guidewire
J-hook electrosurgical probe
Jianu-Beck operation
jib
JIB (jejunoileal bypass)
jig
    Ace-Hershey halo jig
    chamfer jig

jig (*continued*)
    Charnley tibial onlay jig
    cutting jig
    external-alignment
        compression jig
    extramedullary tibial
        alignment jig
    fixation jig
    Geomedic jig
    Osteonics jig
    Plexiglas jig
    precompression jig
    tibial resection jig
jigsaw blade
Jimmy dislodger
Jimmy dissector
Jinotti dual-purpose catheter
J-junction
JL catheter
JL-4 catheter (Judkins left, 4 cm)
JL-5 catheter (Judkins left, 5 cm)
J-loop electrode
J-loop ileostomy
J-loop posterior chamber
    intraocular lens
J-loop posterior chamber lens
J-loop technique
J-Maxx stent
JMS injection needle
Joal lens
Jobe sign
Jobe-Glousman capsular shift
    procedure
Jobe-Patt splint
Jobert de Lamballe fossa
Jobert de Lamballe operation
Jobert de Lamballe sutures
Jobert suture technique
Jobert sutures
Jobson-Horne cotton applicator
Jobson-Horne probe
Jobson-Pynchon decompressor
Jobson-Pynchon tongue
    depressor
Jobst air band
Jobst appliance
Jobst athrombotic pump
Jobst boot
Jobst bra
Jobst compression garment
Jobst compression unit
Jobst dressing

Jobst elastic stocking
Jobst extremity pump
Jobst glove
Jobst mammary support
    dressing
Jobst postoperative air-boot
Jobst pressure garment
Jobst prosthesis
Jobst sleeve
Jobst stockings
Jobst stocking prosthesis
Jobst dressing
Jobst-Stride support stockings
Jobst-Stridette support stockings
Jocath coronary balloon
    catheter
Jodd repair of postoperative
    ventral hernia
Joel scanning electron
    microscope
Joel-Baker anastomosis
Joel-Baker tube
Joel-Cohen abdominal incision
Joe's hoe
Joe's hoe retractor
Jography angiographic catheter
Joguide coronary guiding
    catheter
Johannson hip nail
Johannson lag screw
Johannson-Stille cystotomy
    trocar
Johannson-Stille lag screw
Johanson urethroplasty
John Green calipers
John Green pendulum scalpel
John Weiss forceps
John Wobig entropion repair
Johner-Wruhs tibial fracture
    classification
Johns Hopkins bulldog clamp
Johns Hopkins coarctation
    clamp
Johns Hopkins gall duct forceps
Johns Hopkins gallbladder
    forceps
Johns Hopkins gallbladder
    retractor
Johns Hopkins hemostatic
    forceps
Johns Hopkins modified Potts
    clamp

Johns Hopkins needle holder
Johns Hopkins occluding
    forceps
Johns Hopkins retractor
Johns Hopkins serrefine forceps
Johns Hopkins stone basket
Johns Hopkins tube
Johnson & Johnson Band-Aid
    sterile drape
Johnson & Johnson biliary stent
Johnson & Johnson coronary
    stent
Johnson & Johnson dressing
Johnson & Johnson gauze
    sponge
Johnson & Johnson non-stick
    pads
Johnson & Johnson PFC
    cruciate-substituting insert
Johnson & Johnson tourniquet
Johnson & Johnson waterproof
    tape
Johnson basket
Johnson brain tumor forceps
Johnson canaliculus wire
Johnson cervical thoracic
    orthosis
Johnson cheek retractor
Johnson coagulation suction
    tube
Johnson dental band
Johnson double cannula
Johnson Endobag instrument
Johnson erysiphake
Johnson esophagogastroscopy
Johnson esophagogastrostomy
Johnson evisceration knife
Johnson gauze sponge
Johnson hook
Johnson hook retractor
Johnson intestinal tube
Johnson knife
Johnson needle holder
Johnson operation
Johnson pelvic fracture
    technique
Johnson position
Johnson procedure
Johnson pronator advancement
Johnson prostatic needle holder
Johnson ptosis forceps
Johnson ptosis knife

Johnson ptotic knife
Johnson retractor
Johnson screwdriver
Johnson skin hook
Johnson spatula
Johnson splint
Johnson staple technique
Johnson stone basket
Johnson stone dislodger
Johnson technique
Johnson thoracic forceps
Johnson tonsillar punch
Johnson total hip stabilization
   orthosis
Johnson tube
Johnson twin-wire appliance
Johnson ureteral basket
Johnson ureteral stone basket
Johnson ventriculogram
   retractor
Johnson-Bell erysiphake
Johnson-Iowa total hip
Johnson-Kerrison punch
Johnson-Spiegel procedure
Johnson-Tooke corneal knife
Johnston buttonhole procedure
Johnston clamp
Johnston dilator
Johnston gastrostomy plug
Johnston infant dilator
Johnston LASIK flap applanator
Johnston plug
Johnston pursestring suture
   technique
joint
  AC joint
  Ackerman bar joint
  acromioclavicular joint
  Allman classification of AC
    joint
  amphiarthrodial joint
  amphidiarthrodial joint
  ankle joint
  anterior intraoccipital joint
  arthrodial joint
  artificial hip joint (AHJ)
  astragalonavicular joint
  atlantoaxial joint
  atlanto-occipital joint
  axial rotation joint
  ball-and-socket joint
  bar joint

joint (*continued*)
  biaxial joint
  bicondylar joint
  bilocular joint
  Brodie joint
  Budin joint
  butt joint
  Cam Lock knee joint
  capitolunate joint
  capitular joint
  capsular joint
  capsule of
    temporomandibular joint
  cartilaginous joint
  Charcot joint
  Chopart joint
  Clutton joint
  coccygeal joint
  cochlear joint
  composite joint
  compound joint
  condyloid joint
  costochondral joint
  costotransverse joint
  costovertebral joint
  cotyloid joint
  cranial suture joint
  cricoarytenoid joint
  cricothyroid joint
  Cruveilhier joint
  CUI joint
  cuneiform joint
  Delrin joint
  dentoalveolar joint
  derangement of joint
  diarthrodial joint
  DIP joint
  dislocated joint
  dislocation of joint
  distal interphalangeal joint
  double-action ankle joint
  effusion of joint
  elbow joint
  ellipsoidal joint
  enarthrodial joint
  erasing of joint
  excision of joint
  external ligament of
    temporomandibular joint
  extra-articular subtalar joint
  facet joints
  false joint

joint (*continued*)
  fibrocartilaginous joint
  fibrous joint
  fibulotalar joint
  Fillauer dorsiflexion assist
    ankle joint
  Fillauer PDC ankle joint
  Fillette joint
  flail joint
  fringe joint
  frozen knee joint
  function of joint
  fusion of joint
  Gaffney joint
  ginglymoid joint
  glenohumeral joint
  gliding hinge joint
  gliding joint
  grating in joint
  Greissinger joint
  Grice-Green arthrodesis of
    subtalar joint
  high-speed wrist slip joint
  hinge joint
  hip joint
  humeroulnar joint
  immobilization of joint
  immobilized joint
  immovable joint
  incisional joint
  incudomalleal joint
  incudomalleolar joint
  incudostapedial joint
  instability of joint
  Integrated Ankle orthotic
    ankle joint
  interarticular disk of
    temporomandibular joint
  interarticular joint
  intercalated joint
  intercarpal joint
  interphalangeal joint (IPJ)
  IP joint
  irritable joint
  jaw joint
  Klenzak double-channeled
    ankle joint
  Klenzak knee joint
  knee joint
  lateral atlantoaxial joint
  lavage of joint
  ligamentous joint

joint (*continued*)
  Lisfranc joint
  locked joint
  locking of joint
  loosening of prosthetic joint
  lumbosacral joint
  lunotriquetral joint
  Luschka joints
  malleo-incudal joint
  mandibular joint
  manipulation of joint
  manubriosternal joint
  MCP joint
  membrane of joint
  meniscus of acromioclavicular
    joint
  meniscus of
    temporomaxillary joint
  metacarpophalangeal joint
  Metasul joint
  metatarsal cuneiform joint
  metatarsal joint
  metatarsophalangeal joint
  midcarpal joint
  midcervical apophyseal joint
  mixed joint
  mortise of joint
  movable joint
  multiaxial joint
  natural joint
  neurocentral joint
  nonsynovial joint
  Oklahoma ankle joint
  Ottoback modular knee joint
  Ottoback children's hydraulic
    knee joint
  peg-and-socket joint
  Perstein joint
  petro-occipital joint
  PIP joint
  pisotriquetral joint
  pivot joint
  plane joint
  polyaxial joint
  posterior intraoccipital joint
  proximal interphalangeal joint
  radiocarpal joint
  radiohumeral joint
  radiolunate joint
  radioulnar joint
  replacement of joint
  rotary joint

joint (*continued*)

rotation joint
sacrococcygeal joint
sacroiliac joint
saddle joint
scaphotrapeziotrapezoid joint
    (STT joint)
scapuloclavicular joint
screw joint
septic joint
shoulder joint
SI joint
silicone rubber joint
simple joint
single sleeve bar joint
socket joint
spheroid joint
spiral joint
sprain of joint
stabilization of joint
Steiger joint
sternal joint
sternoclavicular joint
sternocostal joint
stiffening of joint
stiffness of joints
stifle joint
STT joint
    (scaphotrapeziotrapezoid
    joint)
subtalar joint
surgical immobilization of
    joint
suture joint
swollen and painful joints
swollen joints
synarthrodial joint
synchondrodial joint
syndesmodial joint
synovial joint
T rotating joint
talocrural joint
talonavicular joint
tarsal joint
Tamarack flexure joint
temporomandibular joint
temporomandibular joint
    (TMJ) syndrome
temporomaxillary joint
thigh joint
tibiofibular joint
tibiotalar joint

joint (*continued*)

transitional lumbosacral joint
transverse tarsal joint
triscaphe joint
trochoid joint
ulnocarpal joint
uncovertebral joint
uniaxial joint
unilocular joint
unstable joint
vector lunate joint
von Gies joint
wedge-and-groove joint
wrist joint
xanthoma of joint
xiphisternal joint
zygapophyseal joint
joint abnormality
joint ankylosis
joint arthrodesis
joint arthroplasty
joint aspiration
joint branch
joint capsule
joint cartilage
joint cavity
joint cinch
joint click
joint contracture
joint crepitus
joint deformity
joint depression fracture
joint disarticulation
joint disease
joint dislocation
joint distraction cuff
joint effusion
joint facet
joint fluid
joint fusion
joint implant
joint injury
joint instability
joint jack
joint knife
joint line
joint line pain
joint manipulation
joint mice
joint mobilization
joint motion
joint mouse

joint movement
joint oil
joint pain
joint position
joint position sense
joint protection training
joint reconstruction
joint repair
joint replacement
joint rheumatoid arthritis
joint sepsis
joint socket
joint space
joint space narrowing
joint spring splint
joint stiffening
joint surface
joint swelling
joint tenderness
joint toilet
joint trauma
jointed vein stripper
Joint-Jack finger splint
joints of Luschka
Jo-Kath catheter
joker (endarterectomy
    instrument)
joker dissector
joker elevator
Jolly dilator
Jolly prostatic scissors
Jolly test
Jolly uterine dilator
Jonas implant
Jonas modification of Norwood
    procedure
Jonas silicone-silver penile
    prosthesis
Jonas silver penile prosthesis
Jonas-Graves speculum
Jonas-Graves vaginal speculum
Jonell countertraction finger
    splint
Jonell countertraction
    metacarpal splint
Jonell finger splint
Jonell thumb splint
Jones abduction frame
Jones adenoid curet
Jones ankle procedure
Jones arm splint
Jones bunionectomy

Jones canaliculus dilator
Jones cervical knife
Jones clamp
Jones closure
Jones curet
Jones dilator
Jones dissecting scissors
Jones dressing
Jones 1st-toe repair
Jones forceps
Jones forearm splint
Jones fracture
Jones hammertoe operation
Jones hemostatic forceps
Jones IMA diamond knife
Jones IMA epicardial retractor
Jones IMA forceps
Jones IMA needle holder
Jones IMA scissors
Jones keratome
Jones knee procedure
Jones knife
Jones lacrimal canaliculus
    dilator
Jones metacarpal splint
Jones nasal splint
Jones operation
Jones pin
Jones position
Jones punctum dilator
Jones Pyrex tube
Jones repair of first toe
Jones resection arthroplasty
Jones retractor
Jones scissors
Jones splint
Jones suspension traction
Jones sutures
Jones tear duct tube
Jones technique
Jones tenodesis
Jones tenosuspension
Jones thoracic clamp
Jones toe procedure
Jones toe repair
Jones towel clamp
Jones towel forceps
Jones traction splint
Jones tube
Jones tube procedure
Jones-Barnes-Lloyd-Roberts
    classification

Jones-Barnett technique
Jones-Brackett approach
Jones-Brackett technique
Jonesco bone wire guide
Jonesco wire suture needle
Jones-Politano technique
Jonge position
Jonnesco (*see* Ionescu)
Jonnson maneuver
Joplin bone-holding forceps
Joplin bunionectomy
Joplin operation
Joplin stripper
Joplin technique
Joplin tendon passer
Joplin tendon stripper
Joplin toe prosthesis
Jordan bur
Jordan canal elevator
Jordan canal incision knife
Jordan capsule knife
Jordan dilator
Jordan elevator
Jordan eye implant
Jordan hook
Jordan implant
Jordan knife
Jordan middle ear instrument
Jordan needle
Jordan perforating bur
Jordan stapedectomy knife
Jordan strut forceps
Jordan strut-measuring
    instrument
Jordan wire loop dilator
Jordan-Caparosa holder
Jordan-Day cutting bur
Jordan-Day dermatome
Jordan-Day drill
Jordan-Day fenestration bur
Jordan-Day polishing bur
Jordan-Hermann chisel
Jordan-Rosen curet
Jordan-Rosen elevator
Jorgensen technique
Jorgenson dissecting scissors
Jorgenson gallbladder scissors
Jorgenson retractor
Jorgenson thoracic scissors
Joseph angular knife
Joseph antral perforator
Joseph bayonet saw

Joseph bistoury knife
Joseph button knife
Joseph button-end knife
Joseph cervical knife
Joseph chisel
Joseph clamp
Joseph double-edged knife
Joseph elevator
Joseph guard
Joseph hook
Joseph knife
Joseph measuring ruler
Joseph nasal elevator
Joseph nasal hook
Joseph nasal knife
Joseph nasal rasp
Joseph nasal raspatory
Joseph nasal saw
Joseph nasal scissors
Joseph nasal splint
Joseph operation
Joseph perforator
Joseph periosteal elevator
Joseph periosteal raspatory
Joseph periosteotome
Joseph periosteotome elevator
Joseph punch
Joseph rasp
Joseph raspatory
Joseph rhinoplasty
Joseph ruler
Joseph saw
Joseph saw guide
Joseph saw protector
Joseph septal bar
Joseph septal clamp
Joseph septal fracture appliance
Joseph septal frame
Joseph septal splint
Joseph serrated scissors
Joseph sharp skin hook
Joseph single-prong hook
Joseph skin hook
Joseph skin hook retractor
Joseph split
Joseph tenaculum
Joseph tenaculum hook
Joseph wound retractor
Josephberg probe
Joseph-Farrier saw
Joseph-Killian elevator
Joseph-Killian septal elevator

Joseph-Maltz angular nasal saw
Joseph-Maltz knife
Joseph-Maltz nasal saw
Joseph-Maltz scissors
Josephson catheter
Josephson quadpolar mapping
    electrode
Josephson quadripolar catheter
Joseph-Stille saw
Joseph-Verner raspatory
Joseph-Verner saw
Jostent coronary stent graft
Jostent stent
Jostra arterial blood filter
Jostra cardiotomy reservoir
Jostra catheter
joule counter
joule unit
jowl fat
jowl reduction lipectomy
joystick retractor
JP instruments (*see* Jackson-
    Pratt)
J-periosteal elevator
J-point
J-point treadmill test
J-pouch
JR catheter
JR-4 catheter (Judkins right, 4 cm)
JR-5 catheter (Judkins right, 5 cm)
J-scope esophagoscope
J-sella deformity
J-shaped anal anastomosis
J-shaped endoscope
J-shaped freer
J-shaped I&A cannula
J-shaped ileal pouch
J-shaped ileal pouch-anal
    anastomosis
J-shaped incision
J-shaped reservoir
J-shaped skin incision
J-shaped tube
J-stent
J-stripper
JT interval
J-tip guidewire
J-tip wire
J-tipped exchange guidewire
J-tipped guidewire
J-tipped wire
J-tube insertion

J-type maneuver
Judd cannula
Judd clamp
Judd cystoscope
Judd female urethrocystoscope
Judd forceps
Judd hernia repair
Judd operation
Judd pyloroplasty
Judd pyloroplasty technique
Judd strabismus forceps
Judd suture forceps
Judd trocar
Judd-Allis clamp
Judd-Allis forceps
Judd-Allis intestinal forceps
Judd-Allis intestinal retractor
Judd-Allis tissue forceps
Judd-DeMartel forceps
Judd-DeMartel gallbladder
    forceps
Judd-Mason bladder retractor
Judd-Mason prostatic retractor
Judd-Mason retractor
Judd-Mayo overlap midline
    incisional hernioplasty
Judet approach
Judet arthrogram
Judet arthroplasty
Judet dissector
Judet femoral prosthetic head
Judet graft
Judet hip
Judet hip prosthesis
Judet hip x-ray view
Judet impactor
Judet impactor for acetabular
    component
Judet impactor for acetabular
    cup
Judet operation
Judet press-fit hip prosthesis
Judet prosthesis
Judet strut
Judet x-ray view
Judkins cardiac catheterization
    technique
Judkins coronary catheter
    (left/right)
Judkins curved catheter
Judkins femoral catheterization
    technique

Judkins guiding catheter
Judkins left (JL) catheter
Judkins left 4 (JL4) catheter
Judkins left coronary catheter
Judkins right (JR) catheter
Judkins right coronary catheter
Judkins selective coronary
    arteriography
Judkins technique for coronary
    arteriogram
Judkins torque-control catheter
Judkins USCI catheter
Judkins-4 guiding catheter
Judkins-Sones technique of
    cardiac catheterization
Judson-Bruce hemostat
Judson-Smith manipulator
Juers crimper
Juers crimper forceps
Juers ear curet
Juers hook
Juers lingual forceps
Juers wire crimper
Juers-Derlacki holder
Juers-Derlacki Universal head
    holder
Juers-Lempert endaural
    rongeur
Juers-Lempert forceps
Juers-Lempert rongeur
Juers-Lempert rongeur forceps
Juevenelle clamp
jugal bone
jugal point
jugal sutures
jughandle roentgenogram
jughandle view
jugomasseteric mutilation
jugomaxillary point
jugular arch
jugular bulb anomaly
jugular bulb catheter placement
    assessment
jugular bulb decompression
jugular chain lymph node
jugular compression maneuver
jugular crest of great wing of
    sphenoid bone
jugular duct
jugular floor
jugular foramen
jugular fossa

jugular ganglion of
    glossopharyngeal nerve
jugular gland
jugular lymph nodes
jugular nerve
jugular notch of sternum
jugular pulse
jugular sign
jugular technique
jugular trunk
jugular vein dissection
jugular venography
jugular venous arch
jugular venous catheter
jugular wall
jugulodigastric nodes
jugulodigastric region
jugulo-omohyoid node
jugum (pl. juga)
jugum forceps
Juhn trap
Juhn tympanocentesis trap
Julian cystoresectoscope
Julian needle holder
Julian splenorenal forceps
Julian thoracic artery forceps
Julian thoracic forceps
Julian thoracic hemostatic
    forceps
Julian Vital needle holder
Julian-Damian clamp
Julian-Damian thoracic forceps
Julian-Fildes clamp
jumbo biopsy
jumbo biopsy forceps
jumbo forceps
jump facet
jump flap
jump graft
jump skin flap
jumper-knee position
jumper's knee
jumping genioplasty
jumping man flap
junction
    alar-facial junction
    anorectal junction
    aortic sinotubular junction
    atrioventricular junction
    atypical junction
    cardioesophageal junction
    cavohepatic junction

junction (*continued*)
  choledochoduodenal junction
  choledochopancreatic ductal
    junction
  chondroethmoidal junction
  corneoscleral junction
  cortical medullary junction
  costochondral junction
  cystic duct-infundibulum
    junction
  cystic-choledochal junction
  dentinocemental junction
  dentoepithelial junction
  dentogingival junction
  dermoepidermal junction
  duodenojejunal junction
  E-C junction
  esophagogastric junction
  esophagogastric mucosal
    junction
  fibromuscular junction
  fundic-antral junction
  gap junction
  gastroesophageal junction
  hard-soft palate junction
  ileocecal junction
  impermeable junction
  intermediate junction
  lid-cheek junctions
  manubriogladiolar junction
  manubriosternal junction
  mucocutaneous junction
  mucogingival junction
  myoneural junction
  nasolabial junction
  neuroeffector junction
  neuromuscular junction
  nexus-type junction
  osteochondral junction
  pancreaticobiliary ductal
    junction
  pontomedullary junction
  prostatovesicular junction
  pyloroduodenal junction
  rectosigmoid junction
  sacrococcygeal junction
  sclerocorneal junction
  sclerolimbal junction
  scotoma junction
  sinotubular junction
  squamocolumnar junction
  sternoclavicular junction

junction (*continued*)
  sternomanubrial junction
  tracheoesophageal junction
  ureteropelvic junction (UPJ)
  ureterovesical junction (UVJ)
  uterovesical junction (UVJ)
  vermilion-skin junction
  xiphomanubrial junction
junction obstruction
junctional arrhythmia
junctional cavity
junctional complex
junctional dilatation
junctional dilation
junctional epithelium
junctional nevus
junctional pacemaker
junctional rhythm
junctional tachycardia
junctional tissue
juncturae tendineae
juncture stricture
Jung microtome knife
Jung muscle
Jung-Schaffer lens
Junker inhaler
Junod boot
Junod procedure
Jurasz laryngeal forceps
Jurgan pin
Jurgan pin ball
Jurgan pin ball pin protector
Juri flap
Juri degree of male pattern
    baldness
Juri skin flap
Jurkat T-cell line
jutting mandible
Juvara procedure
juvenile angiofibroma
juvenile carcinoma
juvenile embryonal carcinoma
juvenile melanoma
juvenile nasopharyngeal
    angiofibroma
juvenile ossifying fibroma
juvenile polyps
juvenile reflex
juvenile xanthogranuloma
juvenile xanthogranuloma
    histiocytosis
juxta-anal colostomy

juxta-articular ankylosis
juxta-articular nodule
juxta-auricular fossa
juxtabrow skin
juxtacapillary receptor
juxtacortical chondroma
juxtacortical fracture
juxtacortical osteogenic
    sarcoma
juxtacubital reconstruction
juxtaglomerular body
juxtaglomerular cell hyperplasia
juxtaglomerular complex
juxtaglomerular granules
juxtapapillary diverticulum
juxtapose

juxtaposition
juxtapyloric ulcer
juxtaregional lymph node
juxtarestiform body
Juzo hose
Juzo shrinker
Juzo stocking for
    thrombophlebitis
Juzo stockings
J-Vac bulb suction reservoir
J-Vac catheter
J-Vac closed wound drain
J-Vac closed wound drainage
J-Vac drain
J-Vac suction reservoir
J-wire

K blade
K cell
K dissector sponge
K implant
K pack
K pad
K reamer
K root canal file
k space
K stylet
K wire
K wire driver
K wire (Kirschner wire)
K wire placement
K x-ray fluorescence instrument
Kader fishhook needle
Kader gastrostomy
Kader intestinal spatula
Kader needle
Kader operation
Kader-Senn gastrotomy
    technique
Kader-Senn operation
Kadesky forceps
Kadir Hi-Torque guidewire
Kaessmann nail
KAFO (knee-ankle-foot orthosis)
KAFO prosthesis
Kager fat pad
Kager triangle
Kahler biopsy forceps
Kahler bronchial biopsy forceps
Kahler bronchial forceps
Kahler bronchoscopic forceps
Kahler bronchus-grasping
    forceps
Kahler double-action tip
Kahler laryngeal biopsy forceps
Kahler laryngeal forceps
Kahler polyp forceps
Kahn cannula
Kahn dilator
Kahn dissecting scissors

Kahn tenaculum
Kahn tenaculum forceps
Kahn traction tenaculum
Kahn trigger cannula
Kahn trigger tenaculum
Kahn uterine cannula
Kahn uterine dilator
Kahn uterine trigger cannula
Kahn-Graves vaginal speculum
Kairos pacemaker
Kaiser speculum
Kajava classification of
    supernumerary nipples and
    breasts
Kalamarides dural retractor
Kalamchi classification
Kal-Dermic sutures
Kalginate alginate wound
    dressing
Kalginate calcium alginate
    wound dressing
Kalinowski ear speculum
Kalinowski perforator
Kalinowski rasp
Kalinowski-Verner ear speculum
Kalinowski-Verner rasp
Kalisinski ureteral procedure
Kalish Duredge wire cutter
Kalish Duredge wire extender
Kalish Duredge wire extractor
Kalk electrode
Kalk esophagoscope
Kalk palpitation probe
Kall modification of Silverman
    needle
Kallassy ankle support
Kallassy brace
Kallassy orthosis
Kallmann syndrome
Kalman filter
Kalman needle holder
Kalman occluding forceps
Kalman tube-occluding forceps

Kalos pacemaker
Kalt capsule forceps
Kalt corneal needle
Kalt eye needle
Kalt eye needle holder
Kalt eye spoon
Kalt needle
Kalt needle holder
Kalt needle holder clamp
Kalt spoon
Kalt suture technique
Kalt sutures
Kalt vein needle
Kalt Vital needle holder
Kalt-Arruga needle holder
Kaltostat Fortex dressing
Kaltostat hydrofiber wound
   packing
Kaltostat wound dressing
Kaltostat wound packing
Kaltostat wound packing dressing
Kaltostat wound packing
   material
Kambin instrumentation
Kambin-Gellman
   instrumentation
Kamdar microscissors
Kamerling lens
Kaminsky catheter
Kaminsky stent
Kammerer incision
Kammerer-Battle incision
Kanavel brain-exploring cannula
Kanavel cock-up splint
Kanavel conductor
Kanavel exploring cannula
Kanavel sign
Kanavel splint
Kanavel table
Kanavel-Senn retractor
Kane obstetrical clamp
Kane umbilical clamp
Kane umbilical cord clamp
Kaneda anterior spinal
   instrumentation
Kaneda anterior spine
   stabilizing device
Kaneda distraction device
Kaneda distractor
Kaneda rod
kangaroo feeding pump
kangaroo ligature

kangaroo silicone gastrostomy
   feeding tube
kangaroo tendon
kangaroo tendon sutures
Kangnian acupuncture needle
Kansas University corneal
   forceps
Kantor circumcision
Kantor circumcision clamp
Kantor forceps
Kantor sign
Kantor-Berci video laryngoscope
Kantrowitz clamp
Kantrowitz dressing forceps
Kantrowitz hemostatic clamp
Kantrowitz pacemaker
Kantrowitz thoracic clamp
Kantrowitz thoracic forceps
Kantrowitz tissue forceps
Kantrowitz vascular dissecting
   scissors
Kantrowitz vascular scissors
Kapandji laparoscopic
   technique
Kapel elbow dislocation
   technique
Kapel elbow procedure
Kapel technique
Kapetansky flap
Kaplan cardinal line
Kaplan cold-punch resectoscope
Kaplan needle
Kaplan oblique line
Kaplan open reduction
Kaplan PenduLaser laser
Kaplan PenduLaser surgical laser
Kaplan resectoscope
Kaplan technique
Kaplan tracheostomy needle
Kaplan-Feinstein comorbidity
   grade
Kaposi sarcoma of mastoid
Kaposi varicelliform eruption
kaposiform
   hemangioendothelioma
Kapp applying forceps
Kapp clamp
Kapp clip
Kapp microarterial clamp
Kapp microclamp
Kappa pacemaker
Kappa test

Kapp-Beck bronchial clamp
Kapp-Beck coarctation clamp
Kapp-Beck colon clamp
Kapp-Beck forceps
Kapp-Beck serration
Kapp-Beck-Thomson clamp
Kappeler maneuver
Kaps operating microscope
Kara cataract-aspirating cannula
Kara erysiphake
Kara needle
Karakousis-Vezeridis procedure
Karakousis-Vezeridis resection
Karamar-Mailatt tarsorrhaphy
    clamp
Karapandzic flap
Karapandzic technique
Karaya adhesive
Karaya adhesive appliance
Karaya adhesive ileostomy
    appliance
Karaya dressing
Karaya electrode
Karaya ring ileostomy appliance
Karaya seal ileostomy appliance
Karaya seal ileostomy stomal
    bag
Karaya seal pouch
Karaya self-adhesive conductive
    material
Karickhoff diagnostic lens
Karickhoff double cannula
Karickhoff keratoscope
Karickhoff laser lens
Karl Ilg instruments
Karl Storz 15 French flexible
    hysteroscope
Karl Storz Calcutript endoscope
Karl Storz coagulator
Karl Storz flexible endoscope
Karl Storz instrumentation
Karl Storz light source
    connector
Karl Storz lithotriptor
Karl Storz-Lutzeyer lithotriptor
Karlin instrument
Karlin microknife
Karlin spinal table
Karman cannula
Karmen catheter
Karmody vascular spring
    retractor

Karmody venous scissors
Karnofsky rating scale
    classification
Karnofsky tumor grading (1 to
    100)
Karp aortic punch
Karp aortic punch forceps
Karras angiography needle
Kartagener syndrome
Kartagener triad
Kartch pigtail probe
Kartchner carotid artery clamp
Kartusch stimulus dissection
    elevator
Kartush insulated retractor
Kartush tympanic membrane
    patcher
Karwetsky U-bow activator
Karydakis flap
Kasabach-Merritt phenomenon
Kasabach-Merritt syndrome
Kasai operation
Kasai peritoneal venous shunt
Kasai portoenterostomy
Kasai procedure
Kasai procedure for biliary
    atresia
Kasdan retractor
Kashiwagi calcaneal resection
Kaslow gastrointestinal tube
Kaslow intestinal tube
Kaslow irrigation tube
Kaslow stomach tube
Kaster mitral valve prosthesis
Katena boat hook
Katena cannula
Katena double-edged sapphire
    blade
Katena forceps
Katena iris spatula
Katena ring
Katena speculum
Katena trephine
Katena Vannas scissors
Katena-Barron trephine
Kates forefoot arthroplasty
Kates-Kessel-Kay technique
Kato thick smear technique
Katon catheter
Katsch chisel
Katz-Berci optical stylet
Katzeff cartilage scissors

Katzen infusion wire
Katzen long balloon dilatation
   catheter
Katzenstein rectal cannula
Katzin corneal transplant
   scissors
Katzin operation
Katzin transplant scissors
Katzin trephine
Katzin-Barraquer Colibri forceps
Katzin-Barraquer corneal
   forceps
Katzin-Long balloon
Katzin-Troutman scissors
Kaufer tendon technique
Kaufer type II retractor
Kauffman sign
Kauffman test
Kauffman-White classification
Kaufman adapter
Kaufman catheter
Kaufman clamp
Kaufman clip applier
Kaufman ENT forceps
Kaufman vitrector
Kaufman anti-incontinence
   prosthesis
Kaufman incontinence device
Kaufman incontinence
   procedure
Kaufman incontinence
   prosthesis
Kaufman insulated forceps
Kaufman kidney clamp
Kaufman male urinary
   incontinence prosthesis
Kaufman operation
Kaufman penile prosthesis
Kaufman prosthesis
Kaufman syringe
Kaufman retractor
Kaufman urinary incontinence
   prosthesis
Kaufman vitrector
Kaufman vitreophage
Kavanaugh-Brower-Mann
   fixation
Kawaii-Yamamoto procedure
Kawamoto technique
Kay aortic anastomosis clamp
Kay aortic clamp
Kay tricuspid valvuloplasty

Kay-Cross oxygenator
Kay-Cross suction tip suction
   tube
Kaye antihelix operation
Kaye blepharoplasty scissors
Kaye face-lift scissors
Kaye fine-dissecting scissors
Kaye minimal-incision anterior
   approach
Kaye tamponade balloon
Kay-Lambert clamp
Kayser-Fleischer ring
Kay-Shiley disk prosthetic valve
Kay-Shiley disk valve prosthesis
Kay-Shiley heart valve
Kay-Shiley mitral valve
Kay-Shiley valve prosthesis
Kay-Suzuki disk prosthesis
Kay-Suzuki disk valve prosthesis
Kay-Suzuki heart valve
Kay-Suzuki valve prosthesis
Kazangia-Converse facial
   fracture classification
Kazangia-Converse mandibular
   fracture classification
Kazanjian action-type osteotome
Kazanjian bar
Kazanjian bone-cutting forceps
Kazanjian button
Kazanjian cutting forceps
Kazanjian flap
Kazanjian guide
Kazanjian midline forehead flap
Kazanjian nasal cutting scissors
Kazanjian nasal forceps
Kazanjian nasal hump forceps
Kazanjian nasal hump-cutting
   forceps
Kazanjian nasal splint
Kazanjian nasal-cutting forceps
Kazanjian operation
Kazanjian osteotome
Kazanjian scissors
Kazanjian shears
Kazanjian splint
Kazanjian T-bar
Kazanjian tooth button
Kazanjian vestibuloplasty
Kazanjian vestibulotomy
Kazanjian wire
Kazanjian-Cottle forceps
Kazanjian-Goldman rongeur

K-Blade keratome
K-Blade microsurgical blade
K-Blade super-sharp blade
KBM absorbent gauze
KBM cotton ball
KCP phacoemulsifier
K-curet
KD chin prosthesis
KDF-2.3 intrauterine
   insemination cannula
Keane Mobility bed
Kearney side-notch intraocular
   lens
Kearns bag catheter
Kearns bladder dilator
Kearns dilator
Keates intraocular implant lens
Keating-Hart fulguration
Keating-Hart treatment
KED (Kendrick extrication
   device)
keel
  McNaught keel
  Montgomery laryngeal keel
keel operation
keel stent
keel tip
keeled chest
Keeler cryoextractor
Keeler cryophake
Keeler cryoprosthesis
Keeler cryosurgical instrument
Keeler cryosurgical unit
Keeler extended round-tip
   forceps
Keeler fiberoptic headlight
Keeler intraocular foreign body
   grasping forceps
Keeler intravitreal scissors
Keeler knife
Keeler lamp
Keeler lancet tip
Keeler loupe
Keeler micro spear tip
Keeler microscissors
Keeler ophthalmoscope
Keeler panoramic lens
Keeler panoramic loupe
Keeler panoramic surgical
   telescope
Keeler polarizing
   ophthalmoscope

Keeler prism
Keeler prosthesis
Keeler Pulsair noncontact
   tonometer
Keeler puncture tip
Keeler razor tip
Keeler retinoscope
Keeler retractable blade
Keeler round tip
Keeler ruby knife
Keeler spotlight lens loupe
Keeler triple-facet tip
Keeler ultrasonic cataract
   removal lancet
Keeler wide-angle lens loupe
Keeler-Amoils curved cataract
   probe
Keeler-Amoils glaucoma probe
Keeler-Amoils long-shank retinal
   probe
Keeler-Amoils microcurved
   cataract probe
Keeler-Amoils ophthalmic
   cryosystem
Keeler-Amoils ophthalmic long-
   shank probe
Keeler-Amoils ophthalmic
   Machemer retinal probe
Keeler-Amoils ophthalmic
   straight cataract probe
Keeler-Amoils ophthalmic
   vitreous probe
Keeler-Amoils-Machemer retinal
   probe
Keeler-Fison tissue retractor
Keeler Galilean surgical loupe
Keeler Konan Specular
   microscope
Keeler-Rodger iris retractor
Keeley vein stripper
keen edge disposable biopsy
   forceps
Keen operation
Keene compression hook
Keene obturator
Keene self-sealing sleeve and
   obturator
keeper tendon
Kees aneurysm set
Kees clip applier
Kegel exercises
Kegel perineometer

Kehr gallbladder tube
Kehr incision
Kehr operation
Kehr sign
Kehr technique
Kehr T-tube
Kehr tube
Keisler lacrimal cannula
Keith abdominal needle
Keith bundle
Keith drain
Keith node
Keith scissors
Keith-Flack node
Keith-Wagener hypertensive
    retinopathy classification (I-
    IV)
Keith-Wagener retinopathy
Keith-Wagener-Barker
    hypertensive classification
    (KWB classification)
Keitzer infant urethrotome
Keizer everter
Keizer eye retractor
Keizer lid retractor
Keizer-Lancaster eye speculum
Keizer-Lancaster lid retractor
Kel retractor
Kelami classification
Kelar microscope
kelectome
Kelikian foot dressing
Kelikian knee surgery
Kelikian tendon transfer
    procedure
Kelikian-Clayton-Loseff
    technique
Kelikian-McFarland procedure
Kelikian-Riashi-Gleason patellar
    tendon repair
Kelikian-Riashi-Gleason
    technique
Kellam-Waddel classification
Kellan hydrodissection cannula
Kellan sutureless incision blade
Keller arthroplasty
Keller bunion osteotomy
Keller bunionectomy
Keller cephalometric device
Keller hallux rigidus operation
Keller hallux valgus operation
Keller operation

Keller osteotomy
Keller procedure
Keller resection arthroplasty
Keller-Blake half-ring leg splint
Keller-Blake leg splint
Keller-Madlener operation
Kelley gouge
Kelling gastroscope
Kelling-Madlener procedure
Kellman cystotome
Kellman instrument
Kellman irrigation-aspiration
    core
Kellman-Elschnig cyclodialysis
    spatula
Kellogg tongue depressor
Kellogg-Speed fusion technique
Kellogg-Speed lumbar spinal
    fusion
Kellogg-Speed operation
Kellogg-Speed spinal fusion
Kelly abdominal retractor
Kelly adenotome
Kelly artery forceps
Kelly clamp
Kelly combined packer and
    tucker
Kelly curet
Kelly cystoscope
Kelly dilator
Kelly direct-vision adenotome
Kelly dressing forceps
Kelly endoscope
Kelly fistular scissors
Kelly hemostat
Kelly hemostatic forceps
Kelly hook
Kelly insufflator
Kelly intestinal needle
Kelly operation
Kelly orifice dilator
Kelly ovum forceps
Kelly panendoscope
Kelly placenta forceps
Kelly plication
Kelly plication suture
Kelly polypus forceps
Kelly proctoscope
Kelly punch
Kelly rectal speculum
Kelly retractor
Kelly scissors

Kelly sigmoidoscope
Kelly speculum
Kelly sphincter dilator
Kelly sphincteroscope
Kelly sutures
Kelly technique
Kelly tenaculum hook
Kelly tissue forceps
Kelly tube
Kelly tucker
Kelly urethral forceps
Kelly urinary incontinence
    operation
Kelly uterine dilator
Kelly uterine scissors
Kelly uterine tenaculum
Kelly uterine tenaculum hook
Kelly-Deming operation
Kelly-Descemet membrane
    punch
Kelly-Gray uterine curet
Kelly-Gray uterine forceps
Kelly-Kennedy modification
Kelly-Kennedy operation
Kelly-Kennedy sutures
Kelly-Kennedy vaginal plication
Kelly-Littauer stitch scissors
Kelly-Murphy hemostatic forceps
Kelly-Murphy hemostatic uterine
    vulsellum forceps
Kelly-Rankin forceps
Kelly-Sims vaginal retractor
Kelly-Stoeckel operation
Kelman anterior chamber
    intraocular lens
Kelman aspirator
Kelman cannula
Kelman cryoextractor
Kelman cryophake
Kelman cryostylet
Kelman cryosurgical unit
Kelman cyclodialysis
Kelman cyclodialysis cannula
Kelman cystitome knife
Kelman cystotome
Kelman dipstick
Kelman extractor
Kelman flexible tripod lens
Kelman forceps
Kelman I&A unit
Kelman II 3-point fixation rigid
    tripod intraocular lens

Kelman implantation forceps
Kelman intraocular forceps
Kelman intraocular implant
    lens
Kelman intraocular lens
Kelman iris retractor
Kelman irrigation hook
Kelman irrigation-aspiration tip
Kelman irrigator
Kelman irrigator forceps
Kelman keratome
Kelman lens
Kelman manipulator hook
Kelman Multiflex intraocular lens
Kelman needle
Kelman Omnifit intraocular lens
Kelman operation
Kelman lens
Kelman phacoemulsification
    (KPE)
Kelman phacoemulsifier
Kelman Quadraflex anterior
    chamber intraocular lens
Kelman Quadraflex intraocular
    lens
Kelman retractor
Kelman S-flex intraocular lens
Kelman speculum
Kelman tip
Kelman-Cavitron I&A unit
Kelman-McPherson corneal
    forceps
Kelman-McPherson microtying
    forceps
Kelman-McPherson suture
    forceps
Kelman-McPherson tissue
    forceps
Kelman-McPherson tying
    forceps
keloid formation
keloid of cornea
keloid scar
keloid tumor
keloidal blastomycosis
keloidal folliculitis
keloidal scarring
keloplasty
kelotomy
Kelsey pile clamp
Kelsey-Fry bone awl
Kelvin body

Kelvin pacemaker
Kelvin scale
Kemp rectal irrigator
Kemp trocar
Kempf internal screw fixation
Ken driver
Ken driver-extractor
Ken plate
Ken screwdriver
Ken sliding nail
Kendall endotracheal tube cuff
Kendall pump
Kendall sequential compression
 device
Kendrick extrication device
 (KED)
Kendrick Gigli-saw guide
Kendrick method below-knee
 amputation
Kendrick procedure
Kendrick technique
Kendrick-Sharma-Hassler-
 Herndon technique
Kennan cervical punch
Kennedy bar
Kennedy classification
Kennedy forceps
Kennedy ligament augmentation
 device (Kennedy LAD)
Kennedy ligament technique
Kennedy procedure
Kennedy sinus pack
Kennedy spillproof cup
Kennedy urinary incontinence
 operation
Kennedy uterine vulsellum
 forceps
Kennedy vulsellum forceps
Kennedy-Cornwell bladder
 evacuator
Kennedy-Losee modification
Kennedy-Pacey operation
Kennerdell bayonet forceps
Kennerdell medial orbital
 retractor
Kennerdell muscle hook
Kennerdell nerve hook
Kennerdell spatula
Kennerdell-Maroon dissector
Kennerdell-Maroon duckbill
 elevator
Kennerdell-Maroon hook

Kennerdell-Maroon orbital
 retractor
Kennerdell-Maroon orbital
 retractor set
Kennerdell-Maroon orbital
 tumor instruments
Kennerdell-Maroon probe
Kennerdell-Maroon-Jameson
 hook
Kenny-Howard splint
Kensey atherectomy catheter
Kent bundle
Kent bundle ablation
Kent forceps
Kent-His bundle
Kenwood laparotomy sponge
Keofeed feeding tube
Keolar implant material
Keracor laser
Keragen implant
keratectomy
 Castroviejo keratectomy
 excimer laser photorefractive
  keratectomy
 photorefractive keratectomy
  (PRK)
 phototherapeutic
  keratectomy
 superficial keratectomy
keratectomy operation
keratectomy scissors
keratin pearl
keratinization
keratinized cell
keratinized epithelium
keratinized tissue
keratinizing epithelial
 odontogenic cyst
keratinizing epithelial
 odontogenic tumor
keratinizing squamous cell
 carcinoma
keratinocyte
keratinous cyst
keratinous sheet
keratitis
 band keratitis
 deep keratitis
 exposure keratitis
 invasion keratitis
 ribbonlike keratitis
 xerotic keratitis

keratitis lesion
keratitis-deafness cornification
　　disorder
keratoacanthoma
　Ferguson-Smith
　　keratoacanthoma
　nodulo-vegetating
　　keratoacanthoma
　solitary keratoacanthoma
　subungual keratoacanthoma
　　(SUKA)
keratocentesis operation
keratocoagulation
keratoconjunctivitis
keratoconjunctivitis sicca
keratocyst
keratocyte
keratoderma blennorrhagica
keratoderma climactericum
Kerato-Gel implant
keratolens
Kerato-Lens implant
keratoleptynsis
keratolysis
keratolytic agent
keratoma
keratome
　Agnew keratome
　Atkinson keratome
　Bard-Parker keratome
　Beaver blade keratome
　Berens partial keratome
　Castro-Martinez keratome
　Castroviejo angled keratome
　Czermak keratome
　Daily keratome
　Draeger modified keratome
　filamentary keratome
　Fink-Rowland keratome
　Fuchs lancet-type keratome
　Grieshaber keratome
　Guyton-Lundsgaard keratome
　Hansen keratome
　HydroBlade keratome
　HydroBrush keratome
　Jaeger keratome
　Jones keratome
　Kelman keratome
　Kirby keratome
　Kirby-Duredge keratome
　Lancaster keratome
　Landolt keratome

keratome (*continued*)
　Lichtenberg keratome
　Martinez keratome
　Martinez-Castro keratome
　McCaslin wave-edge keratome
　McReynolds pterygium
　　keratome
　McReynolds-Castroviejo
　　keratome
　pterygium keratome
　Rowland keratome
　SatinSlit keratome
　Storz keratome
　Storz-Duredge keratome
　Thomas keratome
　UltraShaper keratome
　UniShaper single-use
　　keratome
　Wiener keratome
keratome blade
keratome guard
keratome incision
keratometer
　Autoref keratometer
　Bausch & Lomb manual
　　keratometer
　Canon auto refraction
　　keratometer
　Canon automatic keratometer
　Haag-Streit keratometer
　Helmholtz keratometer
　Humphrey automatic
　　keratometer
　Javal keratometer
　manual keratometer
　Marco manual keratometer
　Osher surgical keratometer
　Storz keratometer
　surgical keratometer
　Terry keratometer
　Topcon keratometer
keratometer lens
keratometry
keratomileusis
keratopachyderma
keratopathy
keratophakic keratoplasty
keratoplasty
　allopathic keratoplasty
　Arroyo keratoplasty
　Arruga keratoplasty
　autogenous keratoplasty

keratoplasty (*continued*)
Durr nonpenetrating
keratoplasty
epikeratophakic keratoplasty
Filatov keratoplasty
Franceschetti keratoplasty
Gradle keratoplasty
heterogeneous keratoplasty
Hippel keratoplasty
Hogan keratoplasty
homogenous keratoplasty
Imre keratoplasty
keratophakic keratoplasty
lamellar keratoplasty
lamellar refractive
keratoplasty
layered keratoplasty
Magitot keratoplasty
Morax keratoplasty
nonpenetrating keratoplasty
optic keratoplasty
optical keratoplasty
partial keratoplasty
Paufique keratoplasty
penetrating keratoplasty
perforating keratoplasty
photorefractive keratoplasty
punctate epithelial
keratoplasty
refractive keratoplasty
Sourdille keratoplasty
superficial lamellar
keratoplasty
tectonic keratoplasty
thermal keratoplasty
total keratoplasty
keratoplasty scissors
keratoprosthesis
Cardona keratoprosthesis
Choyce keratoprosthesis
Eckardt temporary
keratoprosthesis
Girard keratoprosthesis
Lander wide-field temporary
keratoprosthesis
PHEMA keratoprosthesis
keratoscope
Bright-Ring keratoscope
Karickhoff keratoscope
Klein self-luminous
keratoscope
Placido keratoscope

keratoscope (*continued*)
Polack keratoscope
van Loonen operating
keratoscope
wire-loop keratoscope
keratoscopy
keratosis (*pl.* keratoses)
actinic keratosis
focal keratosis
follicular keratosis
Hopf keratosis
papillary keratosis
seborrheic keratosis
senile keratosis
solar keratosis
keratosis blennorrhagica
keratosis climactericum
keratosis follicularis
keratosis labialis
keratosis obliterans
keratosis obturans
keratosis senilis
keratostomy
keratotic lesion
keratotic papilloma
keratotic papule
keratotomy
arcuate transverse keratotomy
astigmatic keratotomy
delimiting keratotomy
Gifford keratotomy
laser keratotomy
radial keratotomy (RK)
refractive keratotomy
Ruiz trapezoidal keratotomy
Terry keratotomy
trapezoidal keratotomy
keratotomy forceps
keratotomy knife
KeraVision Intacs intracorneal
ring
Kerckring folds
Kerckring nodule
Kerckring valve
kerion formation
Kerley A, B, C lines
Kerlix bandage
Kerlix cast pad
Kerlix conforming bandage
dressing
Kerlix fluff
Kerlix gauze

Kerlix laparotomy sponge
Kerlix packing sponge
Kerlix rolls
Kerlix super sponge
Kerlix wrap
Kern bag
Kern bone clamp
Kern bone-holding clamp
Kern bone-holding forceps
Kern miniforceps
Kern technique
Kernahan-Elsahy classification
    for cleft lip and palate
Kernan-Jackson coagulating
    bronchoscope
Kerner dental mirror
kernicterus
Kern-Lane bone-holding forceps
Kernohan grading of malignant
    astrocytoma of spinal cord
Kernohan notch
Kernohan system of glioma
    classification
Kerr abduction splint
Kerr cesarean section
Kerr clip
Kerr clip applier
Kerr electrotorque drill
Kerr hand drill
Kerr incision
Kerr K-Flex file
Kerr motor
Kerr Permplastic material
Kerr rongeur
Kerr sign
Kerr splint
Kerrison bone punch
Kerrison cervical rongeur
Kerrison forceps
Kerrison laminectomy punch
Kerrison laminectomy rongeur
Kerrison lumbar rongeur
Kerrison mastoid rongeur
Kerrison microrongeur
Kerrison punch
Kerrison retractor
Kerrison technique
Kerrison-Costen ear rongeur
Kerrison-Ferris Smith rongeur
Kerrison-Jacoby punch
Kerrison-Morgenstein rongeur
Kerrison-Rhoton sella punch

Kerrison-Schwartz rongeur
Kerrison-Spurling rongeur
Kershner
Kersting colostomy clamp
Kesling appliance
Kessel osteotomy plate
Kessel-Bonney extension
    osteotomy
Kessel-Bonney procedure
Kesselring aspirative lipoplasty
Kesselring curet technique
Kessler external fixator
Kessler metacarpal distractor
Kessler operation
Kessler podiatry rasp
Kessler prosthesis
Kessler repair
Kessler stitch
Kessler suture repair of tendon
Kessler sutures
Kessler traction frame
Kessler upper limb prosthesis
Kessler-Kleinert suture
Kestenbaum eye procedure
Kestler ambulatory head traction
Kestler ambulatory head tractor
Ketac cement
Ketac liner
ketoacidosis
ketone bodies
ketone body formation
ketoprofen analgesic therapy
Kety-Schmidt inert gas
    saturation technique
Keuch pupil dilator
Kevlar gloves
Kevlar material
Kevorkian biopsy punch
Kevorkian endocervical curet
Kevorkian endometrial curet
Kevorkian punch biopsy
Kevorkian uterine biopsy
    forceps
Kevorkian-Younge biopsy curet
Kevorkian-Younge biopsy
    forceps
Kevorkian-Younge cervical
    biopsy forceps
Kevorkian-Younge endocervical
    biopsy curet
Kevorkian-Younge uterine
    applicator

Kevorkian-Younge uterine
    biopsy forceps
Kevorkian-Younge uterine curet
key
    Allen-type hex key
    chuck key
    Jacob key
    Jacob chuck and key
    Universal hand drill with
        chuck key
key chuck
Key knee arthrodesis
Key operation
Key periosteal elevator
key pinch
key point
Key rasp
key ridge
key stitch
Key-Conwell pelvic fracture
    classification
keyed filling device
keyed supracondylar plate
Keyes bone-splitting chisel
Keyes cutaneous biopsy punch
Keyes cutaneous punch
Keyes cutaneous trephine
Keyes dermal punch
Keyes dermatologic punch
Keyes lithotrite
Keyes punch biopsy
Keyes skin punch
Keyes vulvar punch
Keyes-Ultzmann syringe tube
Keyes-Ultzmann-Luer cannula
key-free compression hip screw
    fixation
key-free compression screw
keyhole approach
keyhole coronary bypass
    procedure
keyhole deformity
keyhole incision
keyhole laminectomy
keyhole punch
keyhole pupil
keyhole shape
keyhole surgery
keyhole tenodesis technique
keyhole-shaped craniectomy
key-in-lock maneuver
key-in-lock rotation

KeyMed advanced esophageal
    dilator set
KeyMed dilator
KeyMed disposable variceal
    injection needle
KeyMed esophageal tube
KeyMed unit
key-slot patella tendon transfer
Keystone graft
keystone ligament
Keystone splint
Keystone technique
Keystone viewer
Kezerian chisel
Kezerian curet
Kezerian gouge
Kezerian osteotome
KF ring
K-Flexofile tip
K-Flexofile file
K-Gar umbilical clamp
Khafagy modified ileocecal
    cystoplasty urinary
    diversion
Khan-Jaeger clamp
Khodadad clamp
Khodadad clip
Khodadad microclamp
Khodadad microclip
Khodadad microclip forceps
Khodadoust line
Khouri hydrodissection cannula
kibisitome cystotome
Kibrick test for infertility
Kibrick-Isojima test for infertility
Kickaldy-Willis hip arthrodesis
Kicker Pavlik harness brace
Kidd cystoscope
Kidd trocar
Kidd tube
Kidde atomizer
Kidde cannula technique
Kidde Flex-i-Tip
Kidde insufflator
Kidde nebulizer
Kidde tourniquet
Kidde tourniquet cuff
Kidde tubal insufflator
Kidde uterine cannula
Kidde-Robbins tourniquet
Kidner foot procedure
Kidner lesion

Kidner operation
Kidner podiatric procedure
Kidner removal of accessory
    navicular bone
Kidner technique
kidney abscess
kidney adenocarcinoma
kidney adenoma
kidney anomaly
kidney biopsy
kidney carbuncle
kidney clamp
kidney colic
kidney failure
kidney function
kidney hilus
kidney impairment
kidney injury
kidney internal splint
kidney internal splint/stent
    (KISS)
kidney internal splint/stent
    catheter (KISS catheter)
kidney internal stent
kidney internal stent catheter
kidney pedicle clamp
kidney pedicle forceps
kidney pelvectomy
kidney pelvis
kidney perfused and cooled
kidney perfusion pump
kidney position
kidney punch
kidney recipient
kidney rest
kidney retractor
kidney scan
kidney shadow
kidney stone
kidney stone forceps
kidney suture needle
kidney suturing needle
kidney tissue
kidney transplant
kidney-elevating forceps
kidneys, ureters, bladder (KUB)
kidney-sparing operation
Kido suprapubic trocar
Kiel classification of non-
    Hodgkin lymphoma
Kiel graft
Kielland (see Kjelland)

Kienbock disease
Kienbock dislocation
Kienbock disease
Kienbock dislocation
Kiene bone tamp
Kiernan space
Kiesselbach area
Kiesselbach plexus
Kiesselbach triangle
Kifa catheter
Kifa clip
Kifia catheter
Kilfoyle humeral medial
    condylar fracture
    classification
Killey molar retractor
Killian antral cannula
Killian antrum cannula
Killian bronchoscope
Killian bundle
Killian chisel
Killian cutting forceps tip
Killian dehiscence
Killian dissector
Killian double-articulated
    forceps tip
Killian double-ended elevator
Killian forceps tip
Killian frontal sinus chisel
Killian frontal sinus operation
Killian frontoethmoidectomy
    procedure
Killian gouge
Killian incision
Killian knife
Killian laryngeal spatula
Killian nasal cannula
Killian nasal speculum
Killian operation
Killian probe
Killian rectal speculum
Killian rongeur
Killian septal compression
    forceps
Killian septal elevator
Killian septal forceps
Killian septal speculum
Killian suction tube
Killian tonsil knife
Killian washing tube
Killian-Claus chisel
Killian-Eicken cannula

Killian-Freer operation
Killian-Halle nasal speculum
Killian-Jameson forceps
Killian-King goiter retractor
Killian-Lynch laryngoscope
Killian-Lynch suspension
  laryngoscope
Killian-Reinhard chisel
Killip classification of heart
  disease (I, II, etc.)
Killip wire
Killip-Kimball heart failure
  classification
Kilner chisel
Kilner elevator
Kilner goiter hook
Kilner malar lever
Kilner mouth gag
Kilner nasal retractor
Kilner needle holder
Kilner operation
Kilner retractor
Kilner scissors
Kilner sharp hook
Kilner skin hook
Kilner skin hook retractor
Kilner suture carrier
Kilner-Dott mouth gag
Kilner-Doughty mouth gag
Kilner-Doughty plate
Kilp lens
Kilpatrick retractor
Kimball catheter
Kimball hook
Kimball nephrostomy hook
Kimmelstiel-Wilson lesion
Kimny catheter
Kimpton vein spreader
Kimpton-Brown tube
Kimray thermodilution
Kimray-Greenfield antiembolus
  filter
Kimray-Greenfield vena caval
  filter
Kimura cartilage graft
Kimura platinum spatula
KinAir bed
KinAir III, TC low-air-loss bed
KinAir IV mattress
Kinast indirect reduction
Kincaid right-angle hook
Kindt artery clamp

Kindt carotid artery clamp
Kindt carotid clamp
Kinematic rotating-hinge total
  knee prosthesis
Kinematic total knee prosthesis
Kinematic rotating hinge
Kinematic rotating-hinge knee
  prosthesis
Kinematic rotating-hinge total
  knee
Kinemax Plus knee prosthesis
kineplastic amputation
kineplasty
kinesthetic disorder
KineTec hip CPM machine
kinetic continuous passive
  motion device
kinetic CPM device
kinetic rehabilitation device
Kinetik great toe implant
kinetocardiogram
kinetocardiography
King adenoidal punch
King umbrella closure
King brace
King cardiac bioptome
King cardiac device
King catheter
King cervical brace
King clamp
King connector adapter
King corneal trephine
King fluff rolls and sponge
King goiter retractor
King goiter self-retaining
  retractor
King guiding catheter
King hip fusion procedure
King implant
King interlocking device
King intra-articular hip fusion
King multipurpose catheter
King multipurpose coronary
  graft catheter
King needle
King open reduction
King operation
King orbital implant
King punch
King retractor
King self-retaining goiter
  retractor

King suture needle
King technique
King tissue forceps
King traction
King trephine
King type IV curve posterior
correction
King vocal cord operation
King wound forceps
King-Armstrong unit
King-Hurd retractor
King-Hurd tonsil dissector
King-Prince knife
King-Prince muscle forceps
King-Prince recession forceps
King-Richards dislocation
technique
King-Richards operation
Kingsley grasping forceps
Kingsley orthodontic plate
Kingsley splint
King-Steelquist hindquarter
amputation
kinked aorta
kinking of duct
kinking of graft
kinking of ureter
kink-resistant catheter
kink-resistant peritoneal
catheter
Kinsella periosteal elevator
Kinsella-Buie lung clamp
Kinsey atherectomy
Kinsey atherectomy catheter
Kinsey rotation atherectomy
extrusion angioplasty
kiotome
kiotomy
Kirby angulated iris spatula
Kirby capsular forceps
Kirby cataract extraction
Kirby cataract knife
Kirby corneoscleral forceps
Kirby curved zonular separator
Kirby cylindrical zonular
separator
Kirby double-ball separator
Kirby double-fixation muscle
hook
Kirby expressor
Kirby eye tissue forceps
Kirby fixation forceps

Kirby flat zonule separator
Kirby hook
Kirby hook expressor
Kirby intracapsular expressor
with curved zonular
separator
Kirby intracapsular lens
expressor
Kirby intracapsular lens
expressor hook
Kirby intracapsular lens forceps
Kirby intracapsular lens loupe
Kirby intracapsular lens
separator
Kirby intracapsular lens spoon
Kirby intracapsular scoop
Kirby intraocular lens loupe
Kirby iris forceps
Kirby iris spatula
Kirby keratome
Kirby knife
Kirby lens dislocator
Kirby lens expressor
Kirby lens expressor hook
Kirby lens forceps
Kirby lens loupe
Kirby lens spoon
Kirby lid retractor
Kirby muscle hook
Kirby operation
Kirby retractor
Kirby scissors
Kirby separator
Kirby sliding technique
Kirby spatula
Kirby spoon
Kirby sutures
Kirby tissue forceps
Kirby-Arthus fixation forceps
Kirby-Bracken iris forceps
Kirby-Duredge keratome
Kirby-Duredge knife
Kirchner diverticulum
Kirchner retractor
Kirchner wire
Kirk amputation
Kirk bone hammer
Kirk mallet
Kirk orthopedic hammer
Kirk thigh amputation
technique
Kirkaldy-Willis hip arthrodesis

Kirkaldy-Willis operation
Kirkheim-Storz urethrotome
Kirkland cement
Kirkland cement dressing
Kirkland curet
Kirkland instrument
Kirkland knife
Kirkland periodontal pack
Kirklin atrial retractor
Kirklin fence
Kirklin sternal awl
Kirkpatrick tonsil forceps
Kirmisson operation
Kirmisson periosteal elevator
Kirmisson periosteal raspatory
Kirner deformity
Kirsch laser
Kirschenbaum foot positioner
Kirschenbaum retractor
Kirschner abdominal retractor
Kirschner abdominal self-
    retaining retractor
Kirschner bone drill
Kirschner boring wire
Kirschner bow
Kirschner device
Kirschner femoral canal plug
Kirschner guiding probe
Kirschner interlocking
    intramedullary nail
Kirschner hip replacement
Kirschner operation
Kirschner pin fixation
Kirschner skeletal traction
Kirschner surgical instrument
Kirschner sutures
Kirschner TOD plate
Kirschner total hip replacement
Kirschner total shoulder
    prosthesis
Kirschner traction
Kirschner traction bow nut
Kirschner self-centering captive-
    head bipolar component
Kirschner wire (K-wire)
Kirschner wire cutter
Kirschner wire drill
Kirschner wire fixation
Kirschner wire inserter
Kirschner wire pin
Kirschner wire placement
Kirschner wire splint

Kirschner wire spreader
Kirschner wire tightener
Kirschner wire traction
Kirschner wire traction bow
Kirschner wire tractor
Kirschner-Balfour abdominal
    retractor
Kirschner-Ullrich forceps
Kirwan bipolar coagulator
Kirwan bipolar electrosurgical
    forceps
Kirwan coaptation ophthalmic
    bipolar forceps
Kirwan cranioblade
Kirwan iris curved ophthalmic
    bipolar forceps
Kirwan iris straight ophthalmic
    bipolar forceps
Kirwan jeweler's curved
    ophthalmic bipolar forceps
Kirwan jeweler's insulated
    straight ophthalmic bipolar
    forceps
Kirwan-Adson ophthalmic
    bipolar forceps
Kirwan-Nadler coaptation
    ophthalmic bipolar forceps
Kirwan-Tenzel ophthalmic
    bipolar forceps
Kirwin cystoscope
Kisch reflex
Kish urethral catheter
Kish urethral illuminated
    catheter set
Kishi lens
KISS catheter (kidney internal
    splint/stent catheter)
kissing balloon angioplasty
kissing balloon technique
kissing spine syndrome
kissing stent
kissing ulcer
Kistner button
Kistner dissector
Kistner plastic tracheostomy
    tube
Kistner plastic tube
Kistner probe
Kistner tracheal button
Kistner tracheostomy tube
Kite corrective cast
kite flap

Kitner blunt dissecting
   instrument
Kitner blunt dissector
Kitner clamp
Kitner dissecting scissors
Kitner dissection
Kitner dissector
Kitner goiter forceps
Kitner instrument
Kitner retractor
Kitner sponge
Kitner thyroid-packing forceps
Kittner dissector
Kiwisch bandage
KJ (knee jerk)
Kjelland (*also* Kielland)
Kjelland blade
Kjelland obstetrical forceps
Kjelland operation
Kjelland-Barton forceps
Kjelland-Luikart obstetrical
   forceps
Kjelland rotation
Klaff septal speculum
Klapp tendon hook
Klatskin cholangiocarcinoma
Klatskin liver biopsy needle
Klatskin tumor
Klause antrum punch
Klause-Carmody antrum punch
Klebanoff common duct bougie
Klebanoff common duct sound
Klebanoff gallstone scoop
kleeblattschädel deformity
kleeblattschädel anomaly
kleeblattschädel
   craniosynostosis
kleeblattschädel syndrome
Kleegman cannula
Kleegman dilator
Kleegman needle guide
KleenSpec disposable anoscope
KleenSpec disposable
   laryngoscope
KleenSpec disposable
   sigmoidoscope
KleenSpec disposable speculum
KleenSpec disposable vaginal
   speculum
KleenSpec forceps
KleenSpec laryngoscope
KleenSpec otoscope adapter

KleenSpec otoscope tip
KleenSpec sigmoidoscope
KleenSpec speculum
KleenSpec vaginal speculum
Kleesattel elevator
Kleesattel raspatory
Kleiger closure
Klein 1-hole infiltrator tip
Klein cannula tip
Klein curved cannula
Klein Delrin Luer-Lok handle
Klein infiltration needle
Klein infiltrator
Klein multihole infiltrator tip
Klein pump
Klein punch
Klein self-luminous keratoscope
Klein technique
Klein transseptal introducer
   sheath
Klein ventilation tube
Kleinert dynamic traction splint
Kleinert fingertip
Kleinert modification
Kleinert operation
Kleinert repair
Kleinert rubber-band splint
Kleinert splint
Kleinert sutures
Kleinert technique
Kleinert tendon passer
Kleinert volar pedicle procedure
Kleinert volar pedicle splint
Kleinert volar V-Y plasty
Kleinert-Kutz bone cutter
Kleinert-Kutz bone file
Kleinert-Kutz bone rongeur
Kleinert-Kutz bone-cutting
   forceps
Kleinert-Kutz clamp
Kleinert-Kutz clamp
   approximator
Kleinert-Kutz dissector
Kleinert-Kutz elevator
Kleinert-Kutz hook
Kleinert-Kutz hook retractor
Kleinert-Kutz microclip
Kleinert-Kutz rasp
Kleinert-Kutz rongeur forceps
Kleinert-Kutz skin hook
Kleinert-Kutz synovectomy
   rongeur

Kleinert-Kutz tendon forceps
Kleinert-Kutz tendon retriever
Kleinert-Kutz tendon retriever
    forceps
Kleinert-Kutz tendon-passing
    forceps
Kleinert-Kutz tendon-retrieving
    forceps
Kleinert-Kutz tenotomy scissors
Kleinert-Ragnell retractor
Kleinsasser anterior commissure
    laryngoscope
Kleinsasser hook
Kleinsasser knife
Kleinsasser laryngeal
    microscissors
Kleinsasser laryngeal
    microsurgery instruments
Kleinsasser laryngoscope
Kleinsasser lens loop
Kleinsasser microlaryngeal
    scissors
Kleinsasser operating
    laryngoscope
Kleinsasser probe
Kleinsasser retractor
Kleinsasser-Riecker
    laryngoscope
Kleinschmidt appendectomy
    clamp
Kleinschmidt technique
Klein-Tolentino ring
Klemme appendectomy
    retractor
Klemme dura hook
Klemme gasserian ganglion
    retractor
Klemme laminectomy retractor
Klemme locked intramedullary
    nail
Klemme retractor
Klenzak brace
Klenzak double-channeled ankle
    joint
Klenzak double-upright splint
Klenzak knee joint
Klenzak orthosis
Klenzak splint
Kleppinger bipolar forceps
Klevas clamp
KLI bipolar forceps
KLI dual control assembly

KLI insufflator
KLI laparoscopy console
KLI laprocator laparoscope
KLI monopolar forceps
Klima-Rosegger sternal needle
Klima-Rosegger trocar
Klinefelter syndrome
Kliners alar retractor
Kling adhesive dressing
Kling bandage
Kling cervical brace
Kling conform dressing
Kling elastic
Kling elastic gauze
Kling gauze bandage
Kling gauze dressing
Kling sponge
Kling-Richards operation
Klinikum Berlin tubing clamp
Klinkenberg-Loth scissors
Klintmalm clamp
Klippel retractor set
Klippel-Feil anomaly
Klippel-Feil deformity
Klippel-Trenaunay syndrome
Klippel-Trenaunay-Weber
    syndrome
Klockner implant
Klondike bed
Kloti vitreous cutter
KLS Centre-Drive screw
KLS-Martin Centre-Drive screw
KLS-Martin modular neuro kit
KMC femoral stem prosthesis
KMP femoral stem prosthesis
K-nail
Knapp blade
Knapp cataract knife
Knapp cyclodialysis spatula
Knapp cystotome
Knapp eye speculum
Knapp flap operation
Knapp forceps
Knapp iris hook
Knapp iris knife
Knapp iris knife needle
Knapp iris probe
Knapp iris repositor
Knapp iris scissors
Knapp iris spatula
Knapp knife-needle
Knapp lacrimal sac retractor

Knapp lens loupe
Knapp lens scoop
Knapp lid operation
Knapp needle
Knapp operation
Knapp probe
Knapp procedure
Knapp pterygium operation
Knapp retractor
Knapp scoop
Knapp spatula
Knapp speculum
Knapp spoon
Knapp strabismus scissors
Knapp trachoma forceps
Knapp-Culler speculum
Knapp-Imre lid operation
Knapp-Luer trachoma forceps
Knapp-Wheeler-Reese operation
knee action
knee anatomy
knee arthroplasty
knee bend
knee bolster
knee bone
knee brace splint
knee cage brace
knee cap
knee dislocation
knee extension
knee extension orthosis
knee fracture
knee fusion
knee immobilized
knee immobilizer
knee immobilizer splint
knee jerk (KJ)
knee joint
knee ligament
knee brace
knee motion
knee orthosis
knee plate
knee positioner
knee prosthesis
knee replacement
knee replacement surgery
knee retractor
knee salvage
knee splint
knee stiffness
knee support

knee swelling
knee wedge
knee-ankle orthosis
knee-ankle-foot orthosis (KAFO)
knee-bearing prosthesis
knee-capping injury
knee-chest position
knee-elbow position
knee-foot-ankle orthosis
knee-jerk reflex
kneeling position
kneeling-squatting position
knife (*see also* knife-dissector,
    knife-needle, scalpel)
Abraham tonsil knife
abscess knife
acetabular knife
ACL graft knife
Adson blunt knife
Adson dural knife
Adson sharp knife
Agnew canaliculus knife
A-K diamond knife
Alcon A-OK crescent knife
Alcon A-OK
    phacoemulsification slit
    knife
Alcon A-OK ShortCut knife
Alcon surgical knife
Aleman meniscotomy knife
Alexander otoplasty knife
Allen-Barkan knife
Allen-Hanbury knife
Amenabar knife
amputating knife
amputation knife
Anderson double-end knife
angle knife
angular knife
antral knife
appendotome knife
arachnoid knife
Arbuckle antral knife
Arenberg endolymphatic sac
    knife
Armour dural knife
arthroscopy knife
Arthro-Lok knife
Asico multi-angled diamond
    knife
Atkins tonsil knife
Atkins tonsillar knife

knife (*continued*)

Atkinson eye knife
Austin dental knife
Austin dissection knife
Austin sickle knife
Ayerst knife
Ayre cone knife
Ayre-Scott cervical cone knife
Ayre-Scott knife
backcutting knife
backward-cutting knife
Bailey round knife
Bailey-Glover-O'Neill
  commissurotomy knife
Bailey-Morse mitral knife
Ballenger cartilage knife
Ballenger mucosa knife
Ballenger nasal knife
Ballenger nose knife
Ballenger septal knife
Ballenger swivel knife
banana knife
Banner enucleation knife
Bard-Parker surgical knife
Barkan goniotomy knife
Barker Vacu-tome suction
  knife
Barnhill adenoid knife
Baron ear knife
Barraquer corneal knife
Barraquer keratoplasty knife
Barrett uterine knife
Barth mastoid knife
bayonet knife
Beard cataract knife
Beard lid knife
Beaver blade cataract knife
Beaver blade discission knife
Beaver cataract knife
Beaver ear knife
Beaver goniotomy needle
  knife
Beaver tonsillar knife
Beaver Xstar knife
Beck tonsillar knife
Beck-Schenck tonsil knife
Beer canaliculus knife
Beer cataract knife
Bellucci lancet knife
Berens cataract knife
Berens corneal knife
Berens glaucoma knife

knife (*continued*)

Berens iris knife
Berens keratoplasty knife
Berens ptosis knife
Berens sclerotomy knife
Billeau ear knife
Bircher meniscus knife
Bishop-Harman knife
bistoury knife
blade knife
bladebreaker knife
Blair cleft palate knife
Blair-Brown knife
Blair-Brown skin graft knife
Blake gingivectomy knife
Blount knife
Bock knife
Bodenham-Blair skin graft
  knife
Bodenham-Humby skin graft
  knife
Bodian discission knife
Bonta mastectomy knife
Bosher commissurotomy knife
Bovie knife
Bowman eye knife
brain knife
Braithwaite skin graft knife
Brock commissurotomy knife
Brock mitral valve knife
Brock pulmonary valve knife
Brophy bistoury knife
Brophy cleft palate knife
Brown cleft palate knife
Brown-Blair skin graft knife
Brun bone knife
Buck dissecting knife
Buck ear knife
Buck myringotome knife
Buck myringotomy knife
Bucy cordotomy knife
Burford-Lebsche sternal knife
button knife
button-end knife
button-nosed knife
Caltagirone skin graft knife
canal knife
canaliculus knife
Canfield tonsil knife
Canfield tonsillar knife
capsular knife
Carpenter knife

knife (*continued*)
Carter septal knife
cartilage knife
cast knife
Castroviejo bladebreaker knife
Castroviejo discission knife
Castroviejo ophthalmic knife
Castroviejo twin knife
Castroviejo-Wheeler discission knife
cataract knife
catlin amputating knife
cautery knife
Cave cartilage knife
Celita Elite knife
Celita Sapphire knife
cervical cone knife
cervical cordotomy knife
cervical knife
chalazion knife
chisel knife
circle knife
cirsotome knife
clasp knife
cleft palate knife
coagulating knife
Cobbett skin graft knife
cold coning knife
cold knife
cold-cone knife
Collin amputating knife
Collin amputation knife
Collings electrosurgery knife
Colver tonsillar knife
commissurotomy knife
Concept arthroscopic knife
cone biopsy knife
conization knife
Converse nasal knife
cordotomy knife
corneal knife
cornea-splitting knife
Cornman dissecting knife
Cottle double-edged knife
Cottle double-edged nasal knife
Cottle nasal knife
Crescent plaster knife
Crile cleft palate knife
Crile gasserian ganglion knife
Cronin palate knife
Crosby knife

knife (*continued*)
crypt knife
Culbertson canal knife
Curdy sclerotome knife
Curran eye knife
curved knife
Cushing dural hook knife
Cushing dural knife
Cusick eye knife
Cusick goniotomy knife
cutting Bovie knife
Cyberknife
Czermak eye knife
Daily eye knife
Davidoff cordotomy knife
Daviel chalazion knife
Davis tonsillar knife
Day tonsillar knife
Dean capsulotomy knife
Dean curved eye knife
Dean iris knife
Dean needle knife
Dean tonsillar knife
deep knife
DeLee laparotrachelotomy knife
Dench ear knife
dental knife
DePalma knife
Derf ear knife
Derlacki capsular knife
Derlacki capsule knife
Dermot-Pierse ball-tipped knife
Derra commissurotomy knife
Derra guillotine knife
D'Errico laminar knife
Desmarres iris knife
Desmarres paracentesis knife
Deutschman cataract knife
Devonshire knife
Diamatrix trapezoidal diamond knife
diamond blade knife
diamond knife
diamond phaco knife
diamond-dusted knife
Diamontek knife
diathermia knife
diathermy knife
Dieffenbach knife
Dintenfass ear knife

knife (*continued*)
Dintenfass-Chapman ear knife
discission knife
dissection knife
dissector knife
double-edged knife
double-edged sickle knife
double-ended flap knife
Douglas tonsillar knife
Down epiphyseal knife
Downing cartilage knife
drum elevator knife
Dupuytren knife
dural hook knife
dural knife
Duredge knife
Duredge-Paufique knife
ear furuncle knife
ear knife
EdgeAhead crescent knife
EdgeAhead phaco slit knife
epiretinal delamination
    diamond knife
electric knife
electrocautery knife
electronic knife
electrosurgical cutting knife
electrosurgical knife
Elschnig cataract knife
Elschnig corneal knife
Elschnig pterygium knife
embryotomy knife
endotherm knife
Equen-Neuffer laryngeal
    knife
Esmarch plaster knife
Eves tonsillar knife
evisceration knife
expansile knife
eye knife
facial nerve knife
Farrior otoplasty knife
Farrior septal cartilage
    stripper knife
Farrior sickle knife
Farrior triangular knife
Farrior-McHugh ear knife
Farrior-McHugh knife
feather knife
Fergusson bone knife
Ferris Robb tonsillar knife
Ferris Smith knife

knife (*continued*)
Ferris-Robb tonsil knife
Fine-Gill corneal knife
finishing knife
Fisher tonsil knife
Fisher tonsillar knife
fistular knife
fistulotome knife
flap knife
Fletcher tonsil knife
Fletcher tonsillar knife
Foerster capsulotomy knife
Fomon double-edged knife
forward-cutting knife
Fowler-Zollner knife
Frazier cordotomy knife
Frazier pituitary capsulectomy
    knife
Freedom knife
free-hand knife
Freer mucosa knife
Freer nasal knife
Freer nasal submucous knife
Freer septal knife
Freer-Ingal nasal knife
Freer-Ingal nasal submucous
    knife
Freer-Ingal septal knife
Freer-Ingal submucous knife
Freiberg cartilage knife
Freiberg meniscectomy knife
Friesner ear knife
Fugo plasma knife
gamma knife
Gamon eye knife
Gandhi knife
ganglion knife
Garrison knife
Gerzog ear knife
Gerzog-Ralks ear knife
Gill corneal knife
Gill iris knife
Gill pop-up arcuate diamond
    knife
Gill-Fine corneal knife
Gill-Hess knife
Gill-Welsh knife
gingivectomy knife
Girard-Swan knife
Glasscock-House knife
glaucoma knife
gold knife

knife (*continued*)

Goldman guillotine nerve knife
Goldman serrated knife
Goldman-Fox knife
goniopuncture knife
goniotomy knife
Goodhill knife
Goodhill-Down knife
Goodyear tonsillar knife
Goulian knife
Graefe cataract knife
Graefe cystitome knife
Graefe iris knife
Graefe sickle knife
Graf cervical cordotomy knife
Green cataract knife
Green corneal knife
Green scleral resection knife
Grieshaber eye knife
Grieshaber ruby knife
Grieshaber ultrasharp knife
Groff electrosurgical knife
Grover meniscus knife
Guilford sickle knife
Guilford-Wright crurotomy knife
Guilford-Wright double-edged knife
Guilford-Wright elevator knife
Guilford-Wright flap knife
Guilford-Wright incudostapedial knife
Guilford-Wright roller knife
Guy tenotomy knife
Guyton-Lundsgaard cataract knife
Haab after-cataract knife
Haab eye knife
Haab scleral resection knife
Haab-Grieshaber knife
Halle dura knife
Halle trigeminus knife
Harmonic scalpel
Harris tonsillar knife
Harrison capsular knife
Harrison myringoplasty knife
Harrison-Shea knife
Hartmann knife
Heath chalazion knife
Herbert sclerotomy knife
herniotome knife

knife (*continued*)

Hilsinger tonsillar knife
Hoffer knife
Hoffmann-Osher-Hopkins plaster knife
hook knife
hooked knife
Hopkins plaster knife
Horsley bone knife
Horsley dural knife
Hosemann choledochus knife
hot knife
Hough fascial knife
Hough incision knife
Hough tendon knife
Hough tympanoplasty knife
Hough whirlybird knife
Hough-Rosen knife
House angular knife
House ear knife
House incudostapedial joint knife
House lancet knife
House myringoplasty knife
House myringotomy knife
House round knife
House sickle knife
House tympanoplasty knife
House-Rosen utility knife
Huco diamond knife
Hufnagel commissurotomy knife
Hulbert electrosurgical knife
Hundley knee knife
Hurd tonsil knife
Hyams scleral knife
hysterectomy knife
Impex diamond radial keratotomy knife
incision knife
incudostapedial joint knife
incudostapedial knife
interdental knife
interosseous knife
intimectomy knife
iris knife
IS joint knife (incudostapedial joint knife)
Jackson tracheal bistoury knife
Jackson tracheal knife
Jacobson vessel knife

knife (*continued*)

Jaeger keratome knife
Jako laryngeal knife
Jako-Kleinsasser knife
Jannetta angular knife
Jarit plaster knife
Johnson evisceration knife
Johnson ptosis knife
Johnson ptotic knife
Johnson-Tooke corneal knife
joint knife
Jones cervical knife
Jones IMA diamond knife
Jordan canal incision knife
Jordan capsule knife
Jordan stapedectomy knife
Joseph angular knife
Joseph bistoury knife
Joseph button knife
Joseph button-end knife
Joseph cervical knife
Joseph double-edged knife
Joseph nasal knife
Joseph-Maltz knife
Jung microtome knife
Katens-Ruby knife
Keeler ruby knife
Keeler-Meyer diamond knife
Kelman cystitome knife
keratotomy knife
Killian tonsil knife
Killian tonsillar knife
King-Prince knife
Kirby cataract knife
Kirby-Duredge knife
Kirkland knife
Kleinsasser knife
Knapp cataract knife
Knapp iris knife
Koos vessel knife
Korte plaster knife
Kratz-Ziegler knife
Krause ear knife
Kreissl meatotomy knife
Krull acetabular knife
Kyle crypt knife
Ladd knife
lamina knife
Lancaster eye knife
Lance knife
lancet knife
Landolt eye knife

knife (*continued*)

Lang eye knife
Lange blade knife
Lange cartilage knife
Langenbeck flap knife
Langenbeck resection knife
Lanigan cartilage knife
laparotrachelotomy knife
laryngeal knife
Laseredge microsurgical knife
Lebsche sternal knife
Lebsche thoracic knife
Lee cartilage knife
Lee-Cohen knife
Leksell gamma knife
Leland tonsillar knife
Leland-Jones tonsillar knife
Lempert paracentesis knife
lenticular knife
lid knife
Lieb-Guerry eye knife
ligamentum teres knife
ligature knife
Lillie tonsillar knife
Lindvall meniscectomy knife
Lindvall-Stille meniscal knife
Lipschiff knife
Lister knife
Liston amputating knife
Liston amputation knife
Liston phalangeal knife
Lorez ultra-sharp knife
Lothrop tonsillar knife
Lowe microtome knife
Lowe-Breck cartilage knife
Lowe-Breck meniscectomy
  knife
Lowell glaucoma knife
Lucae ear perforation knife
Lundsgaard knife
Lundsgaard-Burch knife
Lynch obtuse-angle laryngeal
  knife
Lynch right-angle knife
Lynch straight knife
Lynch tonsillar knife
MacCallum knife
Machemer scleral knife
Machemer sclerotomy knife
MacKenty cleft palate knife
Magielski bayonet canal knife
Magielski canal knife

knife (*continued*)
  Maltz angle knife
  Maltz button-end knife
  Maltz cartilage knife
  Mandelbaum ear knife
  Marcks knife
  margin-finishing knife
  Martinez corneal dissector
    knife
  mastectomy knife
  mastoid knife
  Maumenee eye knife
  Maumenee goniotomy knife
  Mayo knife
  McCabe canal knife
  McCabe dissector knife
  McCarthy diathermic knife
  McCaslin knife
  McGee tympanoplasty knife
  McHugh facial nerve knife
  McHugh flap knife
  McHugh-Farrior canal knife
  McKeever cartilage knife
  McMurray tenotomy knife
  McPherson-Wheeler eye knife
  McPherson-Ziegler iris knife
  McPherson-Ziegler microiris
    knife
  McReynolds pterygium knife
  McReynolds-Castroviejo
    pterygium knife
  Mead lancet knife
  meatotomy knife
  meniscal knife
  meniscectomy knife
  Mercer cartilage knife
  Merrifield knife
  Metzenbaum septum knife
  Metzger infant knife
  Meyer Swiss diamond lancet
    knife
  Meyer Swiss diamond wedge
    knife
  Meyhoeffer eye knife
  Micra knife
  microblade knife
  microiris knife
  micrometer knife
  microsurgical knife
  microvessel knife
  Midas Rex knife
  middle ear canal knife

knife (*continued*)
  middle ear capsule knife
  middle ear knife
  Miller tonsillar knife
  Millette tonsil knife
  Millette-Tydings knife
  Miltex ligature knife
  Mitchell cartilage knife
  mitral knife
  mitral stenosis knife
  Moebius cataract knife
  Monahan-Lewis knife
  Monocorps knife
  Monocorps milium knife
  Moorehead ear knife
  Morgenstein periosteal knife
  Mori knife
  Moritz-Schmidt knife
  mucosa knife
  mucus knife
  Murphy plaster knife
  myelotomy knife
  Myocure knife
  myringoplasty knife
  myringotome knife
  myringotomy knife
  nasal knife
  nasal swivel knife
  Neff meniscus knife
  Neivert tonsillar knife
  Nelson Rocker knife
  Neoflex bendable knife
  Neoflex electrocautery knife
  neurosurgical knife
  Newman uterine knife
  Niedner commissurotomy
    knife
  Nordent periodontic knife
  Nunez-Nunez mitral stenosis
    knife
  obtuse-angle knife
  O'Connor hex probe knife
  O'Connor left-curve knife
  O'Connor meniscotomy knife
  O'Connor probe knife
  O'Connor retrograde knife
  O'Connor right-curve knife
  O'Connor straight knife
  Oertli razor bladebreaker
    knife
  Olivecrona trigeminus knife
  Olk membrane peeler knife

knife (*continued*)

O'Malley knife
operating knife
ophthalmic knife
Optima diamond knife
Orandi knife
Orban knife
Oretorp meniscectomy knife
Oretorp retractable knife
orthopedic knife
Osher diamond knife
Osher micrometer cataract
  knife
oval knife
Pace hysterectomy knife
Page tonsillar knife
Paparella canal knife
Paparella incudostapedial
  joint knife
Paparella sickle knife
Paparella-House knife
paracentesis knife
Parasmillie knife
Parker serrated discission
  knife
Parker tenotomy knife
Paton corneal knife
Paufique corneal knife
Paufique graft knife
Paufique keratoplasty knife
Paufique lamellar knife
Paufique-Duredge knife
periodontal knife
Phaco-4 diamond step knife
phalangeal knife
Philadelphia tonsil knife
pick knife
pituitary capsulectomy knife
plaster cast knife
plaster knife
platelet-shaped knife
Politzer angular ear knife
Politzer ear knife
Politzer-Ralks knife
Pope rectal knife
Potter modified knife
Potter sickle knife
Potts expansile knife
Prince knife
pterygium knife
ptosis knife
pull knife

knife (*continued*)

pulmonary valve knife
Quantum enhancement knife
Questus Leading Edge
  sheathed arthroscopy knife
radial keratotomy knife
Ralks ear knife
Ramsbotham knife
Rayport dural knife
razor blade knife
Reese ptosis knife
Rehne skin graft knife
Reiner ear knife
Reiner plaster knife
retrograde knife
retrograde-cutting hook-
  shaped knife
reversible knife
Rhein diamond knife
Rhein clear corneal diamond
  knife
Rica trigeminal knife
Richardson right-angle ear
  knife
Ridlon plaster knife
right-angle knife
Rish cartilage knife
Rizzuti scleral knife
Rizzuti-Spizziri cannula knife
Robb tonsillar knife
Robertson tonsillar knife
Robinson flap knife
Rochester mitral stenosis
  knife
rocker knife
Roentgen knife
Roger septal knife
roller knife
Rosen cartilage knife
Rosen ear incision knife
Rosen incision knife
round ruby knife
Rowland eye knife
Royce bayonet ear knife
Royce ear knife
ruby diamond knife
ruby knife
Ryerson tenotome knife
Salenius meniscus knife
sapphire knife
Sarot knife
SatinCrescent implant knife

knife (*continued*)
SatinShortCut implant knife
SatinSlit implant knife
Sato corneal knife
Sato eye knife
scarifier knife
Schanz knife
Scheer elevator knife
Scheie goniopuncture knife
Scheie goniotomy knife
Scholl meniscus knife
Schuknecht roller knife
Schuknecht sickle knife
Schultze embryotomy knife
Schwartz cordotomy knife
scimitar-blade knife
scleral resection knife
sclerotomy knife
scalp knife
Seiler conization knife
Seiler tonsillar knife
Sellor mitral valve knife
semilunar cartilage knife
septal knife
serrated fine-cutting knife
serrated knife
Sexton bayonet ear knife
Sexton ear knife
Shaffer eye knife
Shaffer modification of Barkan knife
Shambaugh knife
Shambaugh-Derlacki knife
Shambaugh-Lempert knife
sharp knife
Sharpoint microsurgical knife
Sharpoint slit knife
Shaw knife
Shea incision knife
Sheehy canal knife
Sheehy myringotomy knife
Sheehy round knife
Sheehy-House knife
Sherman knife
ShortCut knife
Sichel iris knife
sickle knife
sickle middle-ear knife
sickle tonsillar knife
sickle-shaped House knife
sickle-shaped knife
Silver knife

knife (*continued*)
Silverstein round knife
Silverstein sickle knife
Simon fistula knife
Simons cleft palate knife
Sims knife
skin graft knife
skin knife
skiving knife
slit blade knife
Sluder tonsillar knife
SMIC sternal knife
Smillie cartilage knife
Smillie meniscal cartilage knife
Smillie meniscus knife
Smith cataract knife
Smith cordotomy knife
Smith-Fisher cataract knife
Smith-Green cataract knife
Somers tonsillar knife
Speed-Sprague knife
sphenoidal knife
Spizziri cannula knife
stapedectomy knife
stapedius tendon knife
DBO free-hand diamond knife
Stecher arachnoid knife
sternal knife
Stern-McCarthy knife
Stevens eye knife
Stevens tissue knife
Stewart cartilage knife
stiletto knife
Stilli knife
stitch-removing knife
Storz cataract knife
Storz folding-handle ear knife
Storz sheath-handle ear knife
Storz-Duredge cataract knife
Storz-Duredge steel cataract knife
straight cutting knife
straight tympanoplasty knife
Strayer meniscal knife
Stryker cartilage knife
Stryker-School meniscal knife
submucous knife
suction knife
Suker spatula knife
Swan discission knife
Swan spade-type needle knife

knife (*continued*)
  Swanson knife
  swift-cut phaco incision knife
  swivel knife
  sword knife
  Tabb double-ended flap knife
  Tabb ear knife
  Tabb myringoplasty knife
  Tabb pick knife
  Taylor knife
  tendon knife
  tenotomy knife
  teres knife
  testing drum knife
  thermal knife
  Thiersch skin graft knife
  Thomas knife
  Thornton T-incision diamond
    knife
  Thorpe foreign body knife
  Tiemann Meals tenolysis knife
  Tobold laryngeal knife
  Tonnis dura knife
  tonsillar knife
  Tooke angled corneal knife
  Tooke iris knife
  Tooke-Johnson corneal knife
  Torchia corneal knife
  tracheal bronchial knife
  tracheal knife
  trifacet knife
  trigeminal knife
  triple-edge diamond-blade
    knife
  Troutman corneal knife
  Troutman-Tooke corneal knife
  Tubby tenotomy knife
  turbinate knife
  Tweedy canaliculus knife
  twin knife
  Tydings tonsil knife
  tympanoplastic knife
  tympanoplasty knife
  U.S. Army-pattern knife
  Ullrich fistula knife
  Ullrich uterine knife
  UltraCision ultrasonic knife
  Unicat knife
  Unigraft knife
  Unitome knife
  upward-cutting triangular
    knife

knife (*continued*)
  uterine knife
  vacutome knife
  valvotomy knife
  Van Osdel tonsillar knife
  Vannas abscess knife
  Vaughan abscess knife
  vessel knife
  Vic hair transplant knife
  Vic Vallis running hair knife
  Victor blood lancet knife
  Virchow brain knife
  Virchow cartilage knife
  Virchow skin graft knife
  Visitec circular knife
  Visitec crescent knife
  Visitec phaco slit knife
  Visitec stiletto knife
  vitreous knife
  V-lance eye knife
  Wagner knife
  Walb knife
  Walker-Lee eye knife
  Wallace-Maloney knife
  Walton ear knife
  Watson skin grafting knife
  wave-edge knife
  Weber canaliculus knife
  Weber eye knife
  Weber iris knife
  Webster skin graft knife
  Weck knife
  Weck-blade knife
  Weiss eye knife
  Weiss-pattern knife
  Weitter plaster knife
  Wheeler discission knife
  Wheeler iris knife
  Wheeler malleable-shape knife
  whirlybird knife
  Wiener eye knife
  Wilder cystitome knife
  Wilder eye knife
  Williams cartilage knife
  Wolf chisel knife
  Wolf draw knife
  Wolf meniscal knife
  Woodruff spatula knife
  Wright-Guilford double-edged
    knife
  Wright-Guilford elevator knife
  Wright-Guilford flap knife

knife (*continued*)
  Wright-Guilford
    incudostapedial knife
  Wright-Guilford roller knife
  Wullstein double-edged knife
  Wullstein ear knife
  X-Acto utility knife
  X-knife
  Yamanda myelotomy knife
  Yankauer salpingeal knife
  Yasargil arachnoid knife
  Yund ligamentum teres knife
  Ziegler iris knife
knife and scissors dissection
knife blade
knife cannula cystotome
knife conization
knife cystitome
knife cystotome
knife dissector
knife electrode
knife handle
knife spud
knife-dissector
  Martinez knife-dissector
knife-edged finishing line
Knifelight surgical knife
Knifelight surgical light
knife-needle
  Girard-Swan knife-needle
  Graefe knife-needle
  iris knife-needle
  Knapp knife-needle
  McCaslin knife-needle
  Parker knife-needle
  Swan knife-needle
  Ziegler iris knife-needle
  Ziegler knife-needle
Knight-North classification of
    malar fractures (groups
    I-VI)
Knight brace
Knight nasal forceps
Knight nasal scissors
Knight nasal septum-cutting
    forceps
Knight nasal-cutting forceps
Knight needle
Knight polyp forceps
Knight septal forceps
Knight septum-cutting forceps
Knight turbinate forceps

Knighton hemilaminectomy self-
    retaining retractor
Knighton-Crawford forceps
Knighton-Kerrison punch
Knight-Sluder nasal forceps
Knight-Taylor-Williams spinal
    orthosis
Knight-Taylor brace
Knight-Taylor orthosis
Knight-Taylor
    thoracolumbosacral
    orthosis
knitted Dacron arterial graft
knitted graft
knitted prosthesis
knitted sewing ring
knitted Teflon graft
knitted Teflon prosthesis
knitted vascular prosthesis
knobby process
knocked-down shoulder
knock-knee deformity
Knodt distraction rod
Knodt hook
Knodt rod
Knodt rod fusion of spine
Knoll glands
Knoll refraction technique
Knolle anterior chamber
    irrigating cannula
Knolle cannula
Knolle capsular polisher
Knolle capsule polisher
Knolle cystitome
Knolle dipstick
Knolle intraocular lens
Knolle irrigating loop with I&A
    tip
Knolle lens
Knolle lens cortex spatula
Knolle lens gauge
Knolle lens implantation forceps
Knolle lens nucleus spatula
Knolle lens speculum
Knolle needle holder
Knolle polisher
Knolle posterior capsule
    polisher
Knolle-Kelman cannulated
    cystotome
Knolle-Kelman sharp cystotome
Knolle-Pearce cannula

Knolle-Pearce irrigating lens
   loop
Knolle-Pearce lens loop
Knolle-Shepard lens forceps
Knolle-Volker lens-holding
   forceps
knot
   Aberdeen knot
   Ahern knot
   bow-tie knot
   capstan knot
   clinch knot
   clove-hitch knot
   curved-needle surgeon knot
   double knot
   enamel knot
   externally releasable knot
   extracorporeal jamming knot
   false knot
   fisherman's knot
   friction knot
   granny knot
   half-hitch knot
   Henry master knot
   ileosigmoid knot
   intracorporeal knot
   jamming knot
   Kitano knot
   laparoscopic extracorporeal
      knot
   one-handed knot
   partial-throw surgeon knot
   primitive knot
   reef knot
   Roeder loop knot
   sailor's knot
   secure intracorporeal knot
   self-tightening slip knot
   square knot
   stay knot
   surgeon's knot
   surgical knot
   syncytial knots
   Tim knot
   Topel knot
   Tripier operation throw
      square knot
   true knot
   vital knot
   wire knot
knot formation
knot holding capacity (KHC)

knot of Henry
knot pusher
knot pusher-tier
knot tier
knot tying
knot-holding forceps
Knott technique
knotting forceps
knot-tying instrument
Knowles bandage scissors
Knowles hip pin
Knowles pin nail
Knowles scissors
knuckle of bowel
knuckle of choroid
knuckle of colon
knuckle of tube
knuckle pad
knuckle-binder splint
knurled CD rod (Cotrel-
   Dubousset rod)
knurled Cotrel-Dubousset rod
knurled handle
Knutsson penile clamp
Knutsson urethrography clamp
Knuttsen bending film
Koagamin dressing
Ko-Airan maneuver
Koala intrauterine pressure
   catheter
Koala vascular clamp
Kobak needle
Kobayashi hook
Kobayashi retractor
Kobayashi vacuum extractor
Kobelt tube
Koby cataract
Koby cataract forceps
Koch ileostomy
Koch node
Koch nucleus hydrolysis needle
Koch phaco manipulator
Koch phaco manipulator/
   splitter
Koch pouch cutaneous urinary
   diversion
Koch pouch modified
   procedure
Koch shoulder reduction
Koch technique
Kocher anastomosis
Kocher approach

Kocher arterial forceps
Kocher artery forceps
Kocher biliary tract incision
Kocher bladder retractor
Kocher bladder spatula
Kocher blade retractor
Kocher bone retractor
Kocher brain spoon
Kocher bronchocele sound
Kocher clamp
Kocher classification
Kocher collar incision
Kocher collar thyroidectomy
    incision
Kocher curved L approach
Kocher depressor
Kocher dilatation ulcer
Kocher dissector
Kocher elevator
Kocher forceps
Kocher fracture
Kocher fracture of capitellum
Kocher gallbladder retractor
Kocher goiter director
Kocher goiter dissector
Kocher goiter self-retaining
    retractor
Kocher grooved director
Kocher hemostat
Kocher hemostatic forceps
Kocher incision
Kocher intestinal clamp
Kocher intestinal forceps
Kocher kidney-elevating forceps
Kocher lateral J approach
Kocher maneuver
Kocher Micro-Line intestinal
    forceps
Kocher operation
Kocher periosteal dissector
Kocher periosteal elevator
Kocher point
Kocher probe
Kocher raspatory
Kocher reflex
Kocher retractor
Kocher scissors
Kocher self-retaining goiter
    retractor
Kocher shoulder reduction
Kocher sound
Kocher spoon

Kocher ulcer
Kocher ureterosigmoidostomy
    procedure
Kocher-Crotti goiter retractor
Kocher-Crotti self-retaining
    goiter retractor
Kocher-Gibson posterolateral
    approach
kocherization
Kocher-Langenbeck approach
Kocher-Langenbeck exposure
Kocher-Langenbeck retractor
Kocher-Lorenz fracture
Kocher-McFarland arthroplasty
    approach
Kocher-McFarland hip
    arthroplasty
Kocher-Ochsner hemostatic
    forceps
Kocher-Osborn hip arthroplasty
Kocher-Wagner retractor
Koch-Julian sphincterotome
Koch-Mason dressing
Kock continent ileostomy
Kock ileal reservoir
Kock nipple
Kock operation
Kock pouch
Kock pouch modified procedure
Kock reservoir
Kock reservoir ileostomy
Kocks operation for uterine
    prolapse
Koeberle forceps
Koeberle operation
Koenig (*also* König)
Koenig disease
Koenig elevator
Koenig graft
Koenig grooved director
Koenig metatarsal broach
Koenig MPJ prosthesis
Koenig nail-splitting scissors
Koenig operation
Koenig probe
Koenig raspatory
Koenig retractor
Koenig rod
Koenig technique
Koenig total great toe implant
Koenig vascular forceps
Koenig vein retractor

Koenig-Schaefer approach
Koenig-Schaefer incision
Koenig-Schaefer medial
    approach
Koenig-Stille scissors
Koenig-Wittek operation
Koeppe diagnostic lens
Koeppe goniolens
Koeppe gonioscope
Koeppe gonioscopic lens
Koeppe gonioscopic lens
    implant
Koeppe intraocular lens implant
Koeppe lamp
Koeppe nodule
Koerner flap
Koerte (*also* Körte)
Koerte abdominal spatula
Koerte gallstone forceps
Koerte plaster knife
Koerte retractor
Koerte-Ballance operation
Koerte-Wagner retractor
Koester nodule
Koffler operation
Koffler septal forceps
Koffler septum bone forceps
Koffler septum forceps
Koffler-Hajek laminectomy
    rongeur
Koffler-Hajek sphenoidal punch
Koffler-Lillie septal forceps
Koffler-Lillie septum forceps
Kogan endocervical speculum
Kogan endospeculum
Kogan endospeculum forceps
Kogan urethra speculum
Koh ultramicro instrument
Kohler disease
Kohler line
Kohlman urethral dilator
Kohlrausch folds
Kohlrausch veins
KOI diamond knife
koilocytotic
Koken nasal stent
Kokowicz raspatory
Kolb bronchus forceps
Kolb trocar
Kole procedure
Kollagen dressing
Koln clip

Kolodny clamp
Kolodny forceps
Kolodny scalp hemostat
Komai stereotactic head frame
Kommerell diverticulum
Konan SP8000 noncontact
    specular microscope
Kondoleon operation
Kondoleon-Sistrunk
    elephantiasis procedure
Konica scanner
Konig (*see* Koenig)
Konigsberg catheter
Konigsberg microtransducer
Konno operation
Konno procedure
Konno repair
Kono operation
Kono patch enlargement of
    ascending aorta
Konon aortic valve replacement
Kontron balloon
Kontron balloon catheter
Kontron electrode
Kontron intra-aortic balloon
Kontron intra-aortic balloon
    pump
Koontz hernia needle
Koos vessel knife
Kopan breast lesion localization
    needle
Kopetzy sinus bur
Koplik sign
Koplik spot
Koranyi auscultation
Koranyi percussion
Koranyi sign
Kormed disposable liver biopsy
    needle
Korn Cage knee
Korn Cage knee brace
Körner (*see* Korner)
Korner (*also* Körner)
Korotkoff sound
Korsakoff disease
Koranyi auscultation
Koranyi percussion
Koranyi sign
Körte (*see* Koerte)
Kos attic cannula
Kos chisel
Kos crimper forceps

Kos curet
Kos ear suction tube
Kos elevator
Kos middle ear instrument
Kos pick
Koslowski hip nail
Koslowski microforceps
Kostuik rod
Kostuik screw
Kostuik-Harrington device
Kostuik-Harrington spinal
    instrumentation
Koutsogiannis procedure
Kowa automatic fundus lens
Kowa FM-500 laser flare meter
Kowa hand-held slit lamp
Kowa Optimed slit lamp
Kowa slit lamp
Koylon foam rubber dressing
Koyter muscle
K-pad hot pack
KPE (Kelman
    phacoemulsification)
K-Pratt dilator
Kronig area
Kronig cesarean section
Kronig isthmus
Kronig percussion
Kronig technique
Kronlein hemostatic forceps
Kronlein hernia
Kronlein operation
Kronlein orbitotomy
Kronlein-Berke operation
Kronlein-Berke retractor
Krackow blade staple
Krackow maneuver
Krackow point
Krackow suture
Kraff capsular polisher
Kraff capsule polisher curet
Kraff cortex cannula
Kraff intraocular implant lens
Kraff intraocular utility forceps
Kraff lens-inserting forceps
Kraff nucleus lens loop
Kraff nucleus splitter
Kraff suturing forceps
Kraff tying forceps
Kraff-Osher lens forceps
Kraff-Utrata capsulorrhexis
    forceps

Kraff-Utrata intraocular utility
    forceps
Kraff-Utrata tear capsulotomy
    forceps
Krahn exophthalmometer
Krakau tonometer
Kramer bivalve ear speculum
Kramer direct-vision telescope
Kramer ear speculum
Kramer forceps
Kramer operating laryngoscope
Kramer speculum
Kramer syringe
Kramer telescope
Kramer-Craig-Noel osteotomy
Kramp scissors
Kraske operation
Kraske parasacral approach
Kraske position
Kraske procedure
Krasky retractor
Krasnov implant cataract lens
Kratz aspirating speculum
Kratz cystotome
Kratz diamond-dusted needle
Kratz elliptical-style lens
Kratz implant
Kratz intraocular implant lens
Kratz iris push-pull hook
Kratz lens-inserting forceps
Kratz modified J-loop intraocular
    lens
Kratz polisher
Kratz posterior chamber
    intraocular lens
Kratz scratcher
Kratz-Barraquer wire lid
    speculum
Kratz-Jensen polisher
Kratz-Jensen scratcher
Kratz-Johnson intraocular lens
Kratz-Johnson modified J-loop
    intraocular lens
Kratz-Sinskey intraocular lens
    implant
Kratz-Ziegler knife
Kraupa operation
Krause angular oval punch
Krause antral trocar
Krause arm rest
Krause biopsy forceps
Krause cannula

Krause corpuscle
Krause denervation
Krause ear knife
Krause ear polyp snare
Krause ear snare
Krause esophagoscopy forceps
Krause forceps tip
Krause gland
Krause graft
Krause laryngeal snare
Krause nasal polyp snare
Krause nasal snare
Krause nasal snare cannula
Krause operation
Krause oval punch tip
Krause punch
Krause punch forceps
Krause punch forceps tip
Krause respiratory bundle
Krause square-basket tip
Krause through-cutting forceps
    tip
Krause transverse suture
Krause trocar
Krause Universal forceps
Krause valve
Krause ventricle
Krause-Davis spatula
Krause-Wolfe graft
Krause-Wolfe implant
Krause-Wolfe operation
Krause-Wolfe prosthesis
Krawkow-Cohn technique
Krawkow-Thomas-Jones technique
Krayenbuehl dural hook
Krayenbuehl nerve hook
Krayenbuehl vessel hook
Krego elevator
Kreibig operation
Kreiker blepharochalasis
Kreiker operation
Kreischer bone chisel
Kreiselman incubator
Kreiselman packer
Kreiselman resuscitation unit
Kreiselman resuscitator
Kreiselman unit
Kreissl meatotomy knife
Kremer excimer laser
Kremer fixation forceps
Kremer triple-optical zone
    corneal marker

Kremer 2-point fixation forceps
Krempen-Craig-Sotelo tibial
    nonunion technique
Krempen-Silver-Sotelo nonunion
    operation
Kretschmer retractor
Kreuscher bunionectomy
Kreuscher operation
Kreuscher scissors
Kreuscher semilunar cartilage
    scissors
Kreutzmann cannula
Kreutzmann trocar
Krieberg operation
Krieger wide-field fundus lens
Krimer operation
Krinsky-Prince accommodation
    ruler
Kristellar vaginal retractor
Kristeller maneuver
Kristeller retractor
Kristeller speculum
Kristeller technique
Kristeller vaginal retractor
Kristeller vaginal speculum
Kristiansen eyelet lag screw
Kristiansen screw
Kroener fimbriectomy
Kroener operation
Krol esophageal dilator
Krol-Koski tracheal dilator
Kromayer lamp
Kromayer mercury vapor light
Kron bile duct dilator
Kron bile duct probe
Kron gall duct dilator
Kron gall duct probe
Kronecker aneurysm needle
Kronendonk pin
Kroner tubal ligation
Kronfeld electrode
Kronfeld eyelid retractor
Kronfeld micropin forceps
Kronfeld pin
Kronfeld retractor
Kronfeld surface electrode
Kronfeld suture forceps
Krönig area
Krönig cesarean section
Krönig isthmus
Krönig percussion
Krönig technique

Krönlein hemostatic forceps
Krönlein hernia
Krönlein operation
Krönlein orbitotomy
Krönlein procedure
Krönlein-Berke operation
Krönlein-Berke retractor
Kronner external fixation
Kronner external fixation device
Kronner external fixator
Kronner skeletal fixation
Kronner uterine
    manipulator/injector
Kropp cystourethroplasty
Kropp operation
Kropp procedure
Krosnick vesicourethral
    suspension clamp
Krukenberg amputation
Krukenberg arm
Krukenberg hand
Krukenberg hand
    reconstruction
Krukenberg operation
Krukenberg pigment spindle
    forceps
Krukenberg procedure
Krukenberg spindle
Krukenberg tumor
Krukenberg veins
Krull acetabular knife
Krumeich-Barraquer
    microkeratome
Krupin eye disk
Krupin glaucoma valve
Krupin valve with disk
Krupin-Denver eye valve
Krwawicz cataract cryosurgical
    instrument
Krwawicz cataract extractor
Krwawicz cataract lens
Krwawicz cryoextractor
Kry-Med 300 cryoprobe
Kry-Med cryopexy unit
Kryostik
Kryptok bifocal lens
Kryptok bifocal lens implant
krypton (red) laser
krypton laser
krypton laser with Hexascan
krypton red laser
krypton ventilation imaging

KSO brace
K-Sponge hydrocellulose sponge
K-Temp thermometer
K-Thermia blanket
K-Thermia equipment
K-Thermia OR cart
K-Thermia pad
KTP laser
KTP laser probe
KTP/532 laser
K-Tube
KUB (kidneys, ureters, bladder)
KUB x-ray
Kuda endoscope
Kuda laparoscope
Kuda retractor
Kudo elbow component
Kudo hinge
Kuettner technique
Kugel anastomosis
Kugel approach
Kugel artery
Kugel hernia patch
Kugel hernia repair
Kugel mesh
Kugel patch
Kugelberg reconstruction
Kugelberg-Welander disease
Kuglen angled lens manipulator
Kuglen hook
Kuglen iris hook
Kuglen irrigating lens
    manipulator
Kuglen lens manipulator
Kuglen lens retractor
Kuglen manipulating iris hook
Kuglen refractor
Kuglen retractor
Kuglen straight lens manipulator
Kuhlman brace
Kuhlman cast cutter
Kuhlman cervical brace
Kuhlman cervical traction
Kuhlman cervical traction device
Kuhlman Kast Kutter
Kuhlman traction
Kuhn endotracheal tube
Kuhn mask
Kuhn tube
Kuhn-Bolger angled curet
Kuhne coverglass forceps
Kuhnt capsule forceps

Kuhnt dacryostomy
Kuhnt eyelid operation
Kuhnt fixation forceps
Kuhnt forceps
Kuhnt gouge
Kuhnt intermediary tissue
Kuhnt operation
Kuhnt postcentral vein
Kuhnt tarsectomy
Kuhnt-Helmbold operation
Kuhnt-Junius repair
Kuhnt-Szymanowski ectropion
    repair procedure
Kuhnt-Szymanowski eyelid
    operation
Kuhnt-Szymanowski operation
Kuhnt-Szymanowski procedure
Kuhnt-Szymanowski technique
Kuhnt-Thorpe operation
Kulchitsky cell carcinoma
Kulenkampff anesthesia
Kulvin-Kalt iris forceps
Kulvin-Kalt mules
Kumar applicator
Kumar spica cast technique
Kumar-Cowell-Ramsey
    technique
Kumpe catheter
Kundin wound measurement
    gauge
Kuntscher cloverleaf nail
Kuntscher drill
Kuntscher driver
Kuntscher extractor
Kuntscher femur guide pin
Kuntscher hammer
Kuntscher impactor
Kuntscher intramedullary nail
Kuntscher nail
Kuntscher nail driver
Kuntscher nail extender
Kuntscher nail instrument
Kuntscher nail set
Kuntscher nail-extracting hook
Kuntscher pin
Kuntscher reamer
Kuntscher rod
Kuntscher shaft reamer
Kuntscher technique
Kuntscher traction device
Kuntscher-Hudson brace
Kurer anchor

Kurkenberg sponge
Kurlander orthopedic wrench
Kurosaka bone screw
Kurosaka cannulated screw
Kurosaka extremity screw
Kurosaka interference fixation
    screw
Kurosaka interference-fit screw
Kursteiner canals
Kurten vein stripper
Kurten wire brush
Kurzbauer position
Kurze dissecting scissors
Kurze dissector
Kurze forceps
Kurze microbiopsy forceps
Kurze microdissector
Kurze micrograsping forceps
Kurze microneurosurgery
    instruments
Kurze microscissors
Kurze pickup forceps
Kurze scissors
Kurze suction tube
Kurze suction-irrigator
Kurze suction-irrigator tube
Kurzweil reading machine
Kuschner-Tandatnick curet
Kuschner-Tandatnick
    endometrial biopsy
Kuschner-Tandatnick
    endometrial biopsy curet
Kushner-Tandatnick endometrial
    biopsy curet
Kussmaul breathing
Kussmaul pulse
Kussmaul respirations
Kussmaul sign
Kuster hernia
Küstner (*see* Kustner)
Kustner (*also* Küstner)
Kuster operation
Kustner incision
Kustner operation
Kustner sign
Kustner suture
Kustner tenaculum
Kustner uterine inversion
    correction
Kustner uterine tenaculum
    forceps
Kutler amputation

Kutler digital flap
Kutler double lateral advancement flap
Kutler finger amputation technique
Kutler fingertip
Kutler lateral V-Y advancement flap
Kutler V-Y flap graft
Kuttner blunt dissection
Kuttner dissector
Kuttner ganglion
Kuttner wound stretcher
Kutzmann clamp
Kuyper-Murphy sternal retractor
Kuzmak gastric banding
Kuzmak gastroplasty
Kwapis interdental forceps
Kwapis ligature carrier
Kwapis subcondylar retractor
KWB classification (Keith-Wagener-Barker hypertensive classification)
Kwitko conjunctival spreader
Kwitko intraocular implant lens
Kwitko lens spatula
Kwitko operation

K-Y pliers
Kydex body jacket
Kydex brace
Kyle applicator
Kyle crypt knife
Kyle ear applicator
Kyle internal fixation
Kyle nasal speculum
Kyle speculum
Kyle-Gustilo classification
Kyle-Gustilo-Premer classification
kymogram
kymography
Kyoto-Barrett-Boyes perfusion technique
kyphectomy
  Sharrard kyphectomy
Kypher sutures
kyphos resection
kyphoscoliosis
kyphosis brace
kyphosis correction
kyphosis creation
kyphotic angle
kyphotic deformity
kyphotic pelvis

L approach
l or L (liter)
L stylet
LA cervical orthosis
LT Jones tear duct tube
L/S ratio (lecithin/sphingomyelin ratio)
LA/Ao ratio (left atrial/aortic)
Laband syndrome
Labbe gastrotomy technique
Labbe operation
Labbe triangle
Labbe vein
Labbe gastrotomy technique
Labbe operation
Labbe triangle
Labbe vein
labia (*sing.* labium)
labia major
labia majora
labia minor
labia minora
labial and lingual arches
labial angle
labial arch
labial arteries
labial artery
labial assimilation
labial bar
labial branches
labial cavity
labial cleft
labial commissure
labial curve
labial edema
labial embrasure
labial filter
labial flange
labial flaring
labial fold
labial frenum
labial fusion
labial gingiva

labial glands
labial groove
labial hernia
labial hypertrophy
labial lamina
labial line
labial minor salivary gland
labial movement
labial nerves
labial notch
labial occlusion
labial pad
labial pit
labial region
labial splint
labial stent
labial sulcus
labial surface
labial swelling
labial teeth
labial torque
labial tubercle
labial veins
labial vestibule
labial wire
labial-buccal sulcus
labialism
labialization
labicolumellar crease incision
labiectomy
labioalveolar
labioaxiogingival
labiocervical
labiochorea
labioclination
labiocolumellar crease
labiodental area
labiodental sulcus
labiogeniomandibular mutilation
labiogingival (LAG)
labioglossolaryngeal paralysis
labioglossomandibular approach
labioglossopharyngeal nerve

labiograph
labioincisal edge (LIE)
labioincisal line angle
labiolingual plane
labiolingual splint
labiolingual technique
labiolingually
labiomandibular approach
labiomandibular glossotomy
labiomandibular ligament
labiomarginal sulcus
labiomental amputation
labiomental fold
labiomental groove
labionasal
labiopalatal amputation
labiopalatine
labioplacement
labioplasty
labioproximal
labioscrotal fold
labioscrotal swelling
labiotenaculum
labioversion
labium (*pl.* labia)
labium inferius oris
labium mandibulare
labium maxillare
labium oris
labium superior oris
labor
   arrest of labor
   atonic labor
   augmentation of labor
   complicated labor
   desultory labor
   dry labor
   dyskinetic labor
   false labor
   final stage of labor
   first stage of labor
   immature labor
   induced labor
   induction of labor
   inhibit labor
   obstructed labor
   Pitocin augmentation of labor
   postponed labor
   premature labor
   prodromal labor
   protracted labor
   spontaneous labor

labor (*continued*)
   stage of labor
   termination of labor
   threatened labor
   trial of labor
   true labor
labor augmentation
labor augmentation induction
labor pain
labor terminated
Laborde dilator
Laborde forceps
Laborde tracheal dilator
labored breathing
labored respiration
labrale inferius
labrale superioris
labrale superius
labrum (*pl.* labra)
labyrinth
   bony labyrinth
   ethmoidal labyrinth
   Ludwig labyrinth
   membranous labyrinth
   Minotaur labyrinth
   osseous labyrinth
   otic labyrinth
   renal labyrinth
   Santorini labyrinth
   vestibular labyrinth
labyrinth curet
labyrinth membrane
labyrinth of brain
labyrinthectomy
labyrinthine angiospasm
labyrinthine aplasia
labyrinthine arteries
labyrinthine cryptococcosis
labyrinthine fenestration
labyrinthine fistula
labyrinthine function
labyrinthine gusher
labyrinthine hydrops
labyrinthine membrane
labyrinthine nystagmus
labyrinthine ossification
labyrinthine righting reflex
labyrinthine segment
labyrinthine surgery
labyrinthine symptoms
labyrinthine torticollis
labyrinthine veins

labyrinthine vertigo
labyrinthitis
  circumscribed labyrinthitis
  congenital luetic labyrinthitis
  diffuse serous labyrinthitis
  diffuse suppurative
    labyrinthitis
  obliterative labyrinthitis
  suppurative labyrinthitis
  viral labyrinthitis
labyrinthotomy
  transmeatal labyrinthotomy
LAC (long-arm cast)
LaCarrere electrode
LaCarrere electrodiaphake
LaCarrere operation
lace sutures
lacerated foramen
lacerated perineum
lacerated tendon
lacerated wound
laceration
  aortic laceration
  avulsed laceration
  birth canal laceration
  bladder laceration
  brain laceration
  burst-type laceration
  canalicular laceration
  central stellate laceration
  cervical laceration
  chevron laceration
  concurrent hepatic laceration
  conjunctival laceration
  corneal laceration
  corneoscleral laceration
  diaphragm laceration
  diaphragmatic laceration
  eyebrow laceration
  flap-type laceration
  flexor tendon laceration
  hallucis longus laceration
  inadvertent laceration
  lid margin laceration
  liver laceration
  longitudinal laceration
  lower pole laceration
  minor laceration
  parenchymal laceration
  perineal laceration
  peripheral laceration
  rectal laceration

laceration (*continued*)
  scalp laceration
  splenic laceration
  stellate laceration
  superficial laceration
  tarsal laceration
  tendon laceration
  tentorial laceration
  through-and-through
    laceration
  traumatic lacerations
  vaginal laceration
  vascular laceration
  vermilion laceration
laceration of organ
Lacey prosthesis
Lacey rotating hinge
Lacey total knee implant
Lachman maneuver
Lachman tear
Lachman-MacIntosh test
lachrymal (*see* lacrimal)
lacidem sutures
lacinate ligament
laciniate ligament
Lack tongue retractor
Lacricath lacrimal duct catheter
lacrimal abscess
lacrimal angle duct anomaly
lacrimal artery
lacrimal awl
lacrimal balloon catheter
lacrimal bone
lacrimal calculus
lacrimal canal
lacrimal canaliculus
lacrimal canaliculus dilator
lacrimal cannula
lacrimal caruncle
lacrimal chisel
lacrimal crest
lacrimal dilator
lacrimal duct
lacrimal duct probe
lacrimal fascia
lacrimal fistula
lacrimal fold
lacrimal fossa
lacrimal ganglion
lacrimal gland repair
lacrimal groove of maxilla
lacrimal hamulus

lacrimal intubation probe
lacrimal irrigating cannula
lacrimal lake
lacrimal margin
lacrimal needle
lacrimal nerve
lacrimal osteotome
lacrimal papilla
lacrimal point
lacrimal probe
lacrimal process
lacrimal punctum
lacrimal retractor
lacrimal sac bur
lacrimal sac chisel
lacrimal sac fossa
lacrimal sac gouge
lacrimal sac retractor
lacrimal sac rongeur
lacrimal sound
lacrimal stent
lacrimal sulcus of lacrimal bone
lacrimal sulcus of maxilla
lacrimal surgery
lacrimal syringe
lacrimal trephine
lacrimal tube
lacrimal veins
lacrimation reflex
lacrimation test
lacrimoauriculodentodigital
    (LADD) syndrome
lacrimoconchal suture
lacrimoethmoidal suture
lacrimomaxillary suture
lacrimonasal duct
lacrimoturbinal suture
lactate extraction
lactate solution
lactated Ringer solution
lactating breast
lacteal cataract
lacteal fistula
lacteal sinus
lactic dehydrogenase
lactiferous duct
lactiferous gland
lactiferous sinus
Lactomer absorbable
    subcuticular skin staple
Lactomer copolymer absorbable
    stapler

Lactomer skin staple material
LactoScrew suture anchor
LactoSorb copolymer
LactoSorb resorbable
    craniomaxillofacial fixation
LactoSorb resorbable fixation
    device
lacuna (*pl.* lacunae)
lacuna magna
lacuna musculorum
lacuna skull
lacuna vasorum
lacunae of Morgagni
lacunar abscess
lacunar infarct
lacunar infarction
lacunar ligament
LAD (left anterior descending
    artery, ligament
    augmentation device)
LADAR (laser detection and
    ranging)
LADD
    (lacrimoauriculodentodigital)
Ladd band
Ladd calipers
Ladd clamp
Ladd elevator
Ladd intracranial pressor sensor
Ladd intracranial pressure
    monitor
Ladd intracranial pressure
    sensor
Ladd knife
Ladd lid clamp
Ladd operation
Ladd pressure monitor
Ladd procedure
Ladd procedure for malrotation
    of bowel
Ladd raspatory
LADD syndrome
Ladmore plastic filling
    instrument
Laennec cirrhosis
Laennec sign
Laerdal infant resuscitator
Lafayette skinfold calipers
LaForce adenotome
LaForce adenotome blade
LaForce hemostatic
    tonsillectome

LaForce knife spud
LaForce tonometer
LaForce tonsillectome
LaForce tonsillectomy
LaForce-Grieshaber adenotome
LaForce-Stevenson adenotome
LaForce-Storz adenotome
lag dilation
lag screw fixation
lag screw technique of
    interfragmentary
    compression
lag technique
lag time
Lagleyze eyelid operation
Lagleyze needle
Lagleyze-Trantas operation
lagophthalmos
Lagrange eye scissors
Lagrange humeral supracondylar
    fracture classification
Lagrange modification of Arruga
    operation
Lagrange modification of Berens
    operation
Lagrange operation
Lagrange sclerectomy
Lagrange sclerectomy scissors
Lagrange-Letoumel hip
    prosthesis
Lagrange-Letoumel hip socket
    prosthesis
Lahey (*see also* Lahey Clinic)
Lahey arterial forceps
Lahey bag
Lahey bronchial clamp
Lahey Carb-Edge scissors
Lahey carrier
Lahey catheter
Lahey clamp
Lahey Clinic (*see also* Lahey)
Lahey Clinic dura hook
Lahey Clinic instruments
Lahey Clinic nerve root retractor
Lahey Clinic osteotome
Lahey Clinic rectal scissors
Lahey Clinic retractor
Lahey Clinic skull trephine
Lahey Clinic spinal fusion gouge
Lahey Clinic thin osteotome
Lahey delicate scissors
Lahey dissecting forceps

Lahey dissecting scissors
Lahey drain
Lahey forceps
Lahey gall duct forceps
Lahey goiter retractor
Lahey goiter tenaculum
Lahey goiter vulsellum forceps
Lahey goiter-seizing forceps
Lahey gouge
Lahey hemostat
Lahey hemostatic forceps
Lahey hook
Lahey incision
Lahey ligature carrier
Lahey ligature passer
Lahey lock arterial forceps
Lahey needle
Lahey operating scissors
Lahey operation
Lahey osteotome
Lahey retractor
Lahey scissors
Lahey sutures
Lahey tenaculum
Lahey tenaculum forceps
Lahey thoracic clamp
Lahey thoracic forceps
Lahey thyroid clamp
Lahey thyroid retractor
Lahey thyroid scissors
Lahey thyroid tenaculum
Lahey thyroid tenaculum forceps
Lahey thyroid tissue traction
    forceps
Lahey thyroid traction forceps
Lahey thyroid traction vulsellum
    forceps
Lahey trephine
Lahey tube
Lahey Y-tube
Lahey-Babcock forceps
Lahey-Metzenbaum dissecting
    scissors
Lahey-Pean forceps
Lahey-Sweet dissecting forceps
LAI (labioincisal)
LAI knee prosthesis
LAID laser
Laidley cystoscope
Laidley double-catheterizing
    cystoscope
Laimer-Haeckerman area

Laing concentric hip cup
Laing osteotomy plate
Laird cyclodialysis spatula
Laird-McMahon anorectoplasty
laissez-faire lid operation
Lajeune hemostatic forceps
Lakeside nasal scissors
Lallemand body
Lallemand-Trousseau body
Lalonde bone clamp
Lalonde delicate hook forceps
Lalonde tendon approximator
Lam modification of Jones
    procedure
Lam operation
Lamaze childbirth technique
Lamaze method of childbirth
Lamaze technique
Lamb cannula
Lamb irrigator
Lamb transfer
Lambda Omni Stanicor
    pacemaker
Lambda pacemaker
lambda suture line
lambda wave
lambdoid margin
lambdoid suture line
lambdoid synostosis deformity
lambdoid synostotic
    plagiocephaly
lambdoidal suture
Lambert aortic clamp
Lambert chalazion forceps
Lambert forceps
Lambert-Eaton myasthenic
    syndrome
Lambert-Kay anastomosis
    forceps
Lambert-Kay aorta clamp
Lambert-Kay clamp
Lambert-Kay vascular clamp
Lambert-Lowman bone clamp
Lambert-Lowman chisel
Lambone demineralized laminar
    bone
Lambone freeze-dried bone
Lambotte bone hook
Lambotte bone-holding clamp
Lambotte bone-holding forceps
Lambotte chisel
Lambotte clamp

Lambotte elevator
Lambotte fibular forceps
Lambotte osteotome
Lambotte rasp
Lambotte raspatory
Lambotte rib raspatory
Lambotte splitting chisel
Lambotte-Henderson osteotome
Lambrinudi operation for talipes
    equinovarus
Lambrinudi splint
Lambrinudi technique
Lambrinudi triple arthrodesis
lamella (pl. lamellae)
lamellar blade
lamellar bone
lamellar cataract
lamellar corneal graft
lamellar corneal transplant
lamellar crystalline inclusions
lamellar exfoliation
lamellar graft
lamellar granule
lamellar incision
lamellar refractive keratoplasty
lamellated bone
lamina
    alar lamina
    basal lamina
    basilar lamina
    Bowman lamina
    cribrous lamina
    deep lamina
    dentogingival lamina
    episcleral lamina
    external elastic lamina
    fusca lamina
    labial lamina
    osseous spiral lamina
    palatine lamina
    parietal lamina
    posterior lamina
    proper lamina
    pterygoid lamina
    suprachoroid lamina
    thyroid lamina
    vestibular lamina
    visceral lamina
lamina (pl. laminae)
lamina affixa
lamina cribrosa
lamina dissector

lamina dura
lamina dura-like appearance
lamina elevator
lamina externa
lamina gouge
lamina interna
lamina knife
lamina medialis
lamina papyracea
lamina profunda
lamina propria
lamina spread
lamina spreader
lamina superficialis fasciae
    cervicalis
lamina-bud stage
laminagraph
laminagraphy
laminaplasty
    expansive laminaplasty
    Tsuji laminaplasty
laminar air flow
laminar air flow unit
laminar bone
laminar C-D hook
laminar cortex posterior aspect
laminar dissector
laminar fat
laminar flow
laminar fracture
laminaria cervical tent
laminaria insertion
laminaria seaweed obstetrical
    cervical dilator
laminaria seaweed obstetrical
    dilator
laminaria tent
laminate induration
laminated clot
laminectomy
    4-place laminectomy
    cervical spine laminectomy
    decompression laminectomy
    decompressive laminectomy
    Gill laminectomy
    Gill-Manning decompression
        laminectomy
    Girdlestone laminectomy
    keyhole laminectomy
    lumbar laminectomy
    multilevel laminectomy
    radial laminectomy

laminectomy (*continued*)
    subtotal laminectomy
    thoracic laminectomy
laminectomy blade
laminectomy chisel
laminectomy frame
laminectomy instrument
laminectomy punch
laminectomy raspatory
laminectomy retractor
laminectomy retractor blade
laminectomy rongeur
laminectomy scissors
laminectomy self-retaining
    retractor
laminectomy shears
laminectomy wedge sponge
Laminex needle
laminoforaminotomy
laminogram examination
laminograph
laminography
LaminOss implant
laminotomy
laminotomy and diskectomy
Lamis Autofuse infusion pump
Lamis patella clamp
Lamitrode lead
Lamm incision
Lamont elevator
Lamont nasal raspatory
Lancaster eye knife
Lancaster eye magnet
Lancaster eye speculum
Lancaster keratome
Lancaster knife
Lancaster lid speculum
Lancaster magnet
Lancaster operation
Lancaster sclerotome
Lancaster speculum
Lancaster transilluminator
Lancaster-O'Connor forceps
Lancaster-O'Connor speculum
lance (*see also* lancet)
Lance knife
Lancefield classification
Lanceford porous metal hip
    prosthesis
lanceolate deformity
lancet (*see also* lance, lancet
    knife)

lancet blade
lancet knife (*see also* lance, lancet)
lancet sutures
lancet-shaped biopsy forceps
lancet-shaped electrode
Lanchner operation
lancinating pain
Lancisi muscle
Lancisi nerve
Lancisi sign
Landau dilator
Landau pelvic access trocar
Landau speculum
Landau trocar
Landau vaginal retractor
Landegger orbital implant
Landers wide-field temporary keratoprosthesis
Landers biconcave lens
Landers contact lens
Landers irrigating vitrectomy ring
Landers vitrectomy lens forceps
Landers vitrectomy ring
Landers-Foulk lens
Landers-Foulks prosthesis
Landers-Foulks temporary keratoprosthesis lens
Landmark midline catheter
landmark preserved
Landolt bodies
Landolt C ring
Landolt cannula
Landolt enucleation scissors
Landolt eye knife
Landolt eyelid reconstruction
Landolt keratome
Landolt operation
Landolt pituitary speculum
Landolt ring
Landolt spreader
Landolt spreading forceps
Landon colpostat
Landon forceps
Landon narrow-bladed retractor
Landry vein light
Landry vein light venoscope
Landry-Guillain-Barre syndrome
Landsmeer ligaments
Landstrom arcuate incision marker

Landstrom astigmatic marker
Landstrom muscle
Landzert fossa
Lane band
Lane bone lever
Lane bone screw
Lane bone-holding clamp
Lane bone-holding forceps
Lane catheter
Lane cleft palate needle
Lane dissector
Lane elevator
Lane fasciatome
Lane fracture plate
Lane gastroenterostomy clamp
Lane gastrointestinal forceps
Lane intestinal clamp
Lane intestinal forceps
Lane mouth gag
Lane operation
Lane periosteal elevator
Lane periosteal raspatory
Lane plate for long-bone fixation
Lane procedure
Lane raspatory
Lane rectal catheter
Lane retractor
Lane rongeur
Lane screwdriver
Lane screw-holding forceps
Lane suture needle
Lane suturing needle
Lane tissue forceps
Lane towel clamp
Lane ureteral meatotomy electrode
Lane-Lannelongue operation
Lang dissector
Lang eye knife
Lang eye speculum
Lang iris forceps
Lang jet adjustor kit
Lang knife
Lang scoop
Lang speculum
Lang sutures
Lang-Jamar skinfold calipers
Lange antral punch
Lange antrum punch
Lange approximation forceps
Lange blade
Lange blade knife

Lange bone elevator
Lange bone retractor
Lange cartilage knife
Lange fistula hook
Lange metatarsus varus
    procedure
Lange mouth gag
Lange operation
Lange plastic surgery hook
Lange position
Lange punch
Lange retractor
Lange skin-fold calipers
Lange speculum
Lange tendon lengthening
Lange tendon lengthening and
    repair
Lange tendon repair
Lange-Converse nasal root
    rongeur
Lange-Converse rongeur
Lange-Hofmann bone lever
Lange-Hohmann bone retractor
Langenbeck amputation
Langenbeck bone-holding
    forceps
Langenbeck elevator
Langenbeck flap
Langenbeck flap knife
Langenbeck forceps
Langenbeck incision
Langenbeck knife
Langenbeck metacarpal
    amputation saw
Langenbeck metacarpal saw
Langenbeck needle holder
Langenbeck operation
Langenbeck palatorrhaphy
Langenbeck pedicle
    mucoperiosteal flap
Langenbeck periosteal elevator
Langenbeck periosteal raspatory
Langenbeck periosteal retractor
Langenbeck raspatory
Langenbeck repair
Langenbeck resection knife
Langenbeck retractor
Langenbeck saw
Langenbeck with pharyngeal
    flap palatorrhaphy
Langenbeck-Cushing vein
    retractor

Langenbeck-Green retractor
Langenbeck-Mannerfelt retractor
Langenbeck-O'Brien raspatory
Langenbeck-Ryder needle holder
Langendorff perfusion
Langenskiold bone graft
Langenskiold fusion
Langenskiold bone graft
Langenskiold fusion of growth
    plate
Langenskiold hip osteotomy
Langenskiold procedure
Langenskiold technique
Langer axillary arch
Langer cleavage line
Langer lines
Langer muscle
Langerhans cell eosinophilic
    granuloma
Langerhans cell granule
Langerhans cell granulomatosis
Langerhans cell histiocytosis
Langerhans cells
Langerhans island
Langerhans-type giant cells
Lange-Wilde snare
Langinate impression material
Langley ganglion
Langley granules
Langley nerves
Lanigan cartilage knife
Lannelongue operation
Lannu anterior chamber lens
Lanz incision
Lanz line
Lanz low-pressure cuff
    endotracheal tube
Lanz operation
Lanz point
Lanz pressure regulating valve
Lanz tracheostomy tube
lap count
lap pack
lap pad
lap seatbelt fracture
lap sheet
lap sponge
lap tapes
Lap Vacu-Irrigator
laparoscope
    wolf laparoscope
laparectomy

laparoaminoscopy
laparocele
laparocholecystotomy
laparocolectomy
laparocolostomy
laparocolotomy
laparocystectomy
laparocystidotomy
laparoenterostomy
laparoenterotomy
laparogastroscopy
laparogastrostomy
laparogastrotomy
laparohepatotomy
laparohysterectomy
laparohystero-oophorectomy
laparohysteropexy
laparohysterosalpingo-
    oophorectomy
laparohysterotomy
laparoileotomy
Laparomed cholangiogram device
Laparomed suture-applier device
laparomyomectomy
laparomyositis
laparonephrectomy
laparorrhaphy
LaparoSAC single-use cannula
LaparoSAC single-use obturator
LaparoSAC single-use obturator
    and cannula
LaparoSAC trocar
laparosalpingectomy
laparosalpingo-oophorectomy
laparosalpingotomy
laparoscope
    ACMI laparoscope
    American Medical source
        laparoscope
    AMS autoclavable laparoscope
    Cabot diagnostic laparoscope
    Cabot operating laparoscope
    Circon ACMI diagnostic
        laparoscope
    Daniel double-punch laser
        laparoscope
    Dyonics rod lens laparoscope
    Eder laparoscope
    Elmed diagnostic laparoscope
    Elmed operating laparoscope
    flexible video laparoscope
    Frangenheim laparoscope

laparoscope (*continued*)
    Fujinon diagnostic laparoscope
    Fujinon flexible fiberoptic
        laparoscope
    Fujinon operating
        laparoscope
    Hasson laparoscope
    Jacobs-Palmer laparoscope
    KLI laparoscope
    Kuda laparoscope
    Lent laparoscope
    Marlow diagnostic laparoscope
    Marlow operating laparoscope
    Menghini-Wildhirt
        laparoscope
    MiniSite laparoscope
    offset operating laparoscope
    Olympus diagnostic
        laparoscope
    Olympus operating
        laparoscope
    Polaris laparoscope
    Richard Wolf Medical
        Instruments diagnostic
        laparoscope
    Richard Wolf Medical
        Instruments operating
        laparoscope
    Ruddock laparoscope
    Sharplav laparoscope
    Solos endoscopy diagnostic
        laparoscope
    Stoltz laparoscope
    Storz operating laparoscope
    Surgiview multi-use
        disposable laparoscope
    Wildhirt laparoscope
    Wisap diagnostic laparoscope
    Wisap operating laparoscope
    Wolf insufflation laparoscope
    Ziskie operating laparoscope
laparoscope instrument
laparoscope lens warmer
laparoscopic adjustable silicone
    gastric banding
laparoscopic adrenalectomy
laparoscopic Allis clamp
laparoscopic anterior partial
    fundoplication
laparoscopic appendectomy (LA)
laparoscopic approach
laparoscopic artery ligation

laparoscopic assistance
laparoscopic autopsy
laparoscopic bariatric surgery
laparoscopic bilioenteric
    anastomosis
laparoscopic bladder neck
    suture suspension
    procedure
laparoscopic bowel resection
laparoscopic Burch procedure
laparoscopic bypass procedure
laparoscopic cannula
laparoscopic cardiomyotomy
laparoscopic celiac plexus pain
    block
laparoscopic cholecystectomy
    (LC)
laparoscopic cholecystotomy
laparoscopic clip application
laparoscopic colectomy
laparoscopic colorectal cancer
    surgery
laparoscopic colposuspension
    technique
laparoscopic common bile duct
    exploration
laparoscopic cyst decortication
laparoscopic Doderlein
    hysterectomy
laparoscopic dismembered
    pyeloplasty
laparoscopic dissection and
    manipulation
laparoscopic distal
    pancreatectomy
laparoscopic donor
    nephrectomy (LDN)
laparoscopic Doppler probe
laparoscopic Dorr anti-reflux
    surgery
laparoscopic esophageal
    myomectomy
laparoscopic esophagogastric
    fundoplasty
laparoscopic
    esophagogastroplasty with
    Nissen fundoplication
laparoscopic esophagomyotomy
laparoscopic esophagoplasty
laparoscopic evaluation
laparoscopic examination
laparoscopic extracorporeal knot

laparoscopic feeding tube
    replacement
laparoscopic fenestration
laparoscopic forceps
laparoscopic gallbladder removal
laparoscopic gas
laparoscopic gastric banding
laparoscopic gastric bypass
laparoscopic gastroenterostomy
laparoscopic gastroplasty
laparoscopic gastrostomy
laparoscopic grasper
laparoscopic guidance
laparoscopic Hassab operation
laparoscopic Heller myotomy
laparoscopic hepatectomy
laparoscopic hepatojejunostomy
laparoscopic hernioplasty
laparoscopic
    hysterosalpingectomy
laparoscopic insufflator
laparoscopic intracorporeal
    ultrasonography (LICU)
laparoscopic jejunostomy
laparoscopic laser
    cholecystectomy (LLC)
laparoscopic left hemicolectomy
laparoscopic liver biopsy
laparoscopic lymph node
    dissection procedure
laparoscopic lymph node
    dissection technique
laparoscopic lymphocelectomy
laparoscopic lysis of adhesion
laparoscopic management
laparoscopic needle
    colposuspension
laparoscopic needle driver
laparoscopic Nissen-Toupet
    fundoplication
laparoscopic Nissen
    fundoplication (LNF)
laparoscopic Nissen
    fundoplication with
    esophageal lengthening
laparoscopic orchiopexy
laparoscopic para-aortic lymph
    node sampling
laparoscopic para-aortic lymph
    node sampling procedure
laparoscopic para-aortic lymph
    node sampling technique

laparoscopic-assisted living
  donor nephrectomy
laparoscopic-assisted procedure
laparoscopic-assisted small
  bowel resection
laparoscopic-assisted vaginal
  hysterectomy
laparoscopic-assisted vaginal
  hysteroscopy (LAVH)
laparoscopy
  2nd-look laparoscopy
  ambulatory gynecologic
    laparoscopy
  bedside laparoscopy
  closed laparoscopy
  diagnostic laparoscopy
  double-puncture laparoscopy
  flexible laparoscopy
  full diagnostic laparoscopy
  gaseous laparoscopy
  gasless laparoscopy
  gynecologic laparoscopy
  hand-assisted laparoscopy
  laser laparoscopy
  mandatory laparoscopy
  needle laparoscopy
  open laparoscopy
  pelvic laparoscopy
  revision laparoscopy
  single-port laparoscopy
  single-puncture laparoscopy
  therapeutic laparoscopy
  Z-technique in laparoscopy
laparoscopy cannula
laparoscopy dilation instrument
laparoscopy insufflator
laparoscopy-assisted colectomy
laparoscopy-guided subhepatic
  cholecystostomy
LaparoSonic coagulating shears
laparosplenectomy
laparosplenotomy
Laparostat with fiber diversion
laparotome
laparotomy
  elective laparotomy
  emergency laparotomy
  exploratory laparotomy
  formal laparotomy
  negative laparotomy
  open laparotomy
  pelvic laparotomy

laparotomy (*continued*)
  routine laparotomy
  staging laparotomy
  standard midline laparotomy
laparotomy incision
laparotomy pack
laparotomy pad
laparotomy sponge
laparotomy sponge ring
laparotrachelotomy
laparotrachelotomy knife
laparotyphlotomy
laparouterotomy
Lapides catheter
Lapides collecting bag
Lapides elastic belt
Lapides holder
Lapides ileostomy bag
Lapides needle
Lapides needle holder
Lapides procedure
Lapides technique
Lapides tube
Lapides urological procedure
Lapidus alternating air-pressure
  mattress
Lapidus bed
Lapidus bunionectomy
Lapidus hammertoe technique
Lapidus technique
Laplace forceps
Laplace liver retractor
Laplace retractor
LaPorta great toe implant
LaPorte total toe implant
lappet formation
L-approach
Lapras catheter
Lapra-Ty sutures
Lapro-Clip ligating clip
Lapro-Loop device
LapTie endoscopic knot-tying
  instrument
Lapwall laparotomy sponge
Laqua black line retinal hook
lardaceous organ
lardaceous tissue
Lardennois button
Laredo-Bard needle
Lares dental handpiece
large antral cannula
large ball nerve hook

large bowel
large bowel curet
large cell carcinoma
Large clamp
large diameter handpiece
large for gestational age (LGA)
large intestine
large mask airway
large nail spicule bur
large physiological cup
large self-retaining retractor
large uterine curet
Large vena cava clamp (Alfred
    M. Large)
Large vena caval clamp
large vessel vasculitis
large-angled forceps
large-bore bile duct
    endoprosthesis
large-bore cannula
large-bore catheter
large-bore gastric lavage tube
large-bore heat probe
large-bore imaging system
    scanner
large-bore magnet
large-bore needle
large-bore slotted aspirating
    needle
large-bowel obstruction
large-caliber nonabsorbable
    suture
large-cell lymphoma
large-channel endoscope
large-channel therapeutic
    duodenoscope
large-core needle aspiration
    biopsy
large-core technique
large-diameter bougie
large-diameter optics intraocular
    lens
large-droplet fatty liver
large humeral head
    hemiarthroplasty
large-loop electrode
large-lumen catheter
large-particle biopsy
large-pore polyethylene implant
large-volume round silicone drain
large-volume suction reservoir
Larmon forefoot arthroplasty

Larmon forefoot procedure
LaRocca lacrimal tube
LaRocca nasolacrimal tube
LaRoe undermining forceps
LaRoque hernia repair
LaRoque herniorrhaphy
LaRoque herniorrhaphy incision
LaRoque sutures
LaRoque-Branson hernia repair
Laroyenne operation
Larrey amputation
Larrey bandage
Larrey dressing
Larrey hernia
Larrey operation
Larrey point
Larrey space
Larry director
Larry grooved director
Larry probe
Larry rectal director
Larry rectal probe
Larsen syndrome
Larsen tendon forceps
Larsen tendon-holding forceps
Larson anterior cruciate
    augmentation
Larson hip evaluation
Larson ligament reconstruction
Larson syndrome
Larson technique
Lortat-Jacob hepatic resection
laryngeal adhesion
laryngeal aditus
laryngeal anesthesia
laryngeal angioleiomyoma
laryngeal anomaly
laryngeal aperture
laryngeal applicator
laryngeal applicator forceps
laryngeal artery
laryngeal atomizer
laryngeal atresia
laryngeal basket forceps
laryngeal biopsy forceps
laryngeal blastomycosis
laryngeal block
laryngeal bronchial grasping
    forceps
laryngeal burn
laryngeal cancer
laryngeal cannula

laryngeal carcinoid
laryngeal carcinoma
laryngeal cartilage
laryngeal cartilage fracture
laryngeal cavity
laryngeal chondroma
laryngeal chondroradionecrosis
laryngeal chorea
laryngeal cleft
laryngeal commissure
laryngeal cramp
laryngeal crisis
laryngeal curet forceps
laryngeal cyst
laryngeal dilator
laryngeal dissector
laryngeal diversion
laryngeal drop operation
laryngeal edema
laryngeal electromyography
laryngeal enterotome
laryngeal epilepsy
laryngeal fold
laryngeal forceps tip
laryngeal framework surgery
laryngeal glands
laryngeal granuloma
laryngeal grasping forceps
laryngeal hemangioma
laryngeal hemorrhage
laryngeal hyperesthesia
laryngeal image biofeedback
laryngeal keel operation
laryngeal knife
laryngeal knife handle
laryngeal lancet
laryngeal lipoma
laryngeal mask
laryngeal mask airway (LMA)
laryngeal mask insertion
    anesthetic technique
laryngeal melanosis (LM)
laryngeal mirror
laryngeal mirror handle
laryngeal motor paralysis
laryngeal mucosa
laryngeal neoplasm
laryngeal nerve
laryngeal neuroendocrine
    carcinoma
laryngeal obstruction
laryngeal oscillation

laryngeal papillomatosis
laryngeal paraganglioma
laryngeal paresthesia
laryngeal perichondritis
laryngeal plexus
laryngeal polyp
laryngeal pouch
laryngeal probe
laryngeal prominence
laryngeal prosthesis
laryngeal punch
laryngeal punch forceps
laryngeal reconstruction
laryngeal reflex
laryngeal region
laryngeal release
laryngeal repair
laryngeal respiration
laryngeal retractor
laryngeal rotation forceps
laryngeal saccular cyst
laryngeal saccule of Hilton
laryngeal saw
laryngeal scissors
laryngeal sensory paralysis
laryngeal sinus
laryngeal snare
laryngeal spasm
laryngeal speculum
laryngeal sponge carrier
laryngeal sponging forceps
laryngeal stenosis
laryngeal stent
laryngeal stridor
laryngeal stuttering
laryngeal swab
laryngeal syncope
laryngeal syringe
laryngeal tension
laryngeal trocar
laryngeal tube
laryngeal tuberculosis
laryngeal vein
laryngeal ventricle
laryngeal vestibule
laryngeal web
laryngeal-bronchial telescope
laryngectomy
    American laryngectomy
    anterior partial laryngectomy
    Chevalier Jackson
        laryngectomy

laryngectomy (*continued*)
  frontolateral laryngectomy
  horizontovertical
    laryngectomy
  narrow-field laryngectomy
  near-total laryngectomy
  partial laryngectomy
  salvage laryngectomy
  subtotal laryngectomy
  subtotal supraglottic
    laryngectomy (SSL)
  supracricoid laryngectomy
  supracricoid partial
    laryngectomy
  supraglottic laryngectomy
  total laryngectomy
  vertical partial laryngectomy
  wide-field total laryngectomy
laryngectomy clamp
laryngectomy saw
laryngectomy tube
larynges (*pl.* of larynx)
laryngismus
laryngismus stridulus
laryngitic
laryngitis
  acute laryngitis
  acute supraglottic laryngitis
  chronic hyperplastic laryngitis
  chronic laryngitis
  chronic subglottic laryngitis
  croupous laryngitis
  hemorrhagic laryngitis
  hyperplastic laryngitis
  hypertrophic laryngitis
  membranous laryngitis
  spasmodic laryngitis
  traumatic laryngitis
laryngitis sicca
laryngitis stridulosa
laryngocele
  symptomatic laryngocele
  ventricular laryngocele
laryngocentesis
laryngoesophagectomy
laryngofissure with tracheotomy
laryngofissure forceps
laryngofissure profilometer
laryngofissure retractor
laryngofissure saw
laryngofissure scissors
laryngofissure shears

Laryngoflex reinforced
  endotracheal tube
laryngogram
laryngograph
laryngography
laryngology
laryngomalacia
laryngonasopharyngoscope
  Berci-Ward
    laryngonasopharyngoscope
laryngoparalysis
laryngopathy
laryngopharyngeal cavity
laryngopharyngeal recess
laryngopharyngeal reflex
laryngopharyngeal sensation
laryngopharyngectomy
  partial laryngopharyngectomy
    (PLP)
  total laryngopharyngectomy
    (TLP)
laryngopharyngitis
laryngopharyngoesophagectomy
laryngopharyngoscope
  Berci-Ward
    laryngopharyngoscope
  Proctor
    laryngopharyngoscope
  Storz laryngopharyngoscope
laryngopharynx
laryngophthisis
laryngoplasty
laryngoplegia
laryngoptosis
laryngopyocele
laryngorrhaphy
laryngoscope
  adult laryngoscope
  adult reverse-bevel
    laryngoscope
  Albert-Andrews laryngoscope
  Andrews infant laryngoscope
  anesthetist's folding
    laryngoscope
  anterior commissure
    laryngoscope
  Atkins-Tucker shadow-free
    laryngoscope
  baby Miller laryngoscope
  Belscope laryngoscope
  Benjamin binocular slimline
    laryngoscope

laryngoscope (*continued*)
  Benjamin pediatric operating
    laryngoscope
  Benjamin-Lindholm
    microsuspension
    laryngoscope
  Bizzarri-Guiffrida laryngoscope
  Briggs laryngoscope
  Broyles anterior commissure
    laryngoscope
  Broyles optical laryngoscope
  Broyles wasp-waist
    laryngoscope
  Bullard intubating
    laryngoscope
  Burton laryngoscope
  Chevalier Jackson
    laryngoscope
  Clerf laryngoscope
  commissure laryngoscope
  Dedo laryngoscope
  Dedo laser laryngoscope
  Dedo-Jako laryngoscope
  Dedo-Pilling laryngoscope
  direct laryngoscope
  disposable laryngoscope
  dual distal-lighted
    laryngoscope
  ESI laryngoscope
  fiberoptic laryngoscope
  fiberoptic slide laryngoscope
  Fink laryngoscope
  Finnoff laryngoscope
  Flagg laryngoscope
  Flexiblade laryngoscope
  folding laryngoscope
  Foregger laryngoscope
  Fragen laryngoscope
  Garfield-Holinger
    laryngoscope
  Guedel laryngoscope
  Guedel-Negus laryngoscope
  Haslinger laryngoscope
  Holinger anterior commissure
    laryngoscope
  Holinger hook-on folding
    laryngoscope
  Holinger hourglass anterior
    commissure laryngoscope
  Holinger hourglass
    laryngoscope
  Holinger infant laryngoscope

laryngoscope (*continued*)
  Holinger modified Jackson
    laryngoscope
  Holinger slotted laryngoscope
  Holinger-Garfield
    laryngoscope
  Hollister laryngoscope
  hook-on folding laryngoscope
  Hopp laryngoscope
  Hopp-Morrison laryngoscope
  hourglass anterior
    commissure laryngoscope
  intubation laryngoscope
  Jackson anterior commissure
    laryngoscope
  Jackson fiberoptic slide
    laryngoscope
  Jackson laryngoscope
  Jackson standard
    laryngoscope
  Jako laryngoscope
  Jako-Cherry laryngoscope
  Jako-Pilling laryngoscope
  Kantor-Berci video
    laryngoscope
  Killian-Lynch suspension
    laryngoscope
  KleenSpec disposable
    laryngoscope
  Kleinsasser anterior
    commissure laryngoscope
  Kleinsasser operating
    laryngoscope
  Kleinsasser-Riecker
    laryngoscope
  Kramer operating
    laryngoscope
  laser laryngoscope
  Lewy anterior commissure
    laryngoscope
  Lewy suspension
    laryngoscope
  Lindholm operating
    laryngoscope
  Lundy laryngoscope
  Lynch suspension
    laryngoscope
  Machida fiberoptic
    laryngoscope
  Machida laryngoscope
  Magill laryngoscope
  Mantel laryngoscope

laryngoscope (*continued*)
  Miller laryngoscope
  mirror laryngoscope
  multipurpose laryngoscope
  Negus laryngoscope
  optical laryngoscope
  Ossloff-Karlan laser
    laryngoscope
  Ossloff-Karlan-Dedo
    laryngoscope
  Ossloff-Karlan-Jako
    laryngoscope
  Ossloff-Karlan laser
    laryngoscope
  pencil-handled laryngoscope
  polio laryngoscope
  reverse-bevel laryngoscope
  Rica anesthetic laryngoscope
  Rica anterior commissure
    laryngoscope
  Rica infant laryngoscope
  Riecker-Kleinsasser
    laryngoscope
  Roberts self-retaining
    laryngoscope
  rotating laryngoscope
  Rusch laryngoscope
  Sam Roberts self-retaining
    laryngoscope
  Sanders intubation
    laryngoscope
  self-retaining laryngoscope
  shadow-free laryngoscope
  Shapshay-Healy operating
    laryngoscope
  Shapshay-Healy phonatory
    laryngoscope
  Siker mirror laryngoscope
  sliding laryngoscope
  slotted laryngoscope
  SMIC anterior commissure
    laryngoscope
  standard Jackson
    laryngoscope
  standard laryngoscope
  Stange laryngoscope
  Storz anterior commissure
    laryngoscope
  Storz infection ventilation
    laryngoscope
  Storz-Hopkins laryngoscope
  Storz-Riecker laryngoscope

laryngoscope (*continued*)
  straight-blade laryngoscope
  suspension laryngoscope
  Tucker anterior commissure
    laryngoscope
  Tucker mid-lighted optic slide
    laryngoscope
  Tucker slotted laryngoscope
  Tucker-Holinger laryngoscope
  Tucker-Jake laryngoscope
  wasp-waist laryngoscope
  Weerda distending operating
    laryngoscope
  Welch Allyn Kleenspec
    laryngoscope
  Welch Allyn laryngoscope
  Wisconsin laryngoscope
  Wis-Foregger laryngoscope
  Wis-Hipple laryngoscope
  Yankauer laryngoscope
laryngoscope battery handle
laryngoscope blade
laryngoscope chest support
    holder
laryngoscope folding blade
laryngoscope holder
laryngoscope profilometer
laryngoscopic view
laryngoscopic visualization
laryngoscopist
laryngoscopy
  Broyles laryngoscopy
  direct laryngoscopy
  fiberoptic laryngoscopy
  flexible fiberoptic
    laryngoscopy
  indirect laryngoscopy
  laser laryngoscopy
  microdirect laryngoscopy
  mirror-image laryngoscopy
  suspension laryngoscopy
laryngoscopy anesthetic
    technique
laryngospasm
laryngospastic reflex
laryngostat
  Jackson laryngostat
  Lewy laryngostat
  Priest wasp-waist laryngostat
  Proctor laryngostat
  Proctor-Hellens laryngostat
  Roman laryngostat

laryngostenosis
laryngostomy
laryngostroboscope
　Nagashima
　　laryngostroboscope
laryngotomy
　inferior laryngotomy
　median laryngotomy
　subhyoid laryngotomy
　superior laryngotomy
　thyrohyoid laryngotomy
　transepiglottic laryngotomy
laryngotracheal diversion
laryngotracheal groove
laryngotracheal invasion
laryngotracheal reconstruction
　(LTR)
laryngotracheal stenosis
laryngotracheal trauma
laryngotracheitis
laryngotracheobronchitis
laryngotracheobronchoscopy
laryngotracheoesophageal
　cleft
laryngotracheoplasty (LTP)
laryngotracheoscopy
laryngotracheostomy
laryngotracheotomy
larynx (*pl.* larynges)
　American artificial larynx
　arch of larynx
　artificial larynx
　chondromalacia of larynx
　Cooper-Rand intraoral
　　artificial larynx
　electrical artificial larynx
　electronic artificial larynx
　electronic larynx
　external auditory larynx
　extrinsic muscles of larynx
　glottic larynx
　intrinsic muscles of larynx
　neuroendocrine tumor of
　　larynx
　neurofibroma of larynx
　Nu-Vois artificial larynx
　pneumatic artificial larynx
　saccule of larynx
　sesamoid cartilage of larynx
　supraglottic larynx
　Vicq d'Azyr operation of
　　larynx

larynx (*continued*)
　web of larynx
　Xomed intraoral artificial
　　larynx
Lasag contact lens
Lasag laser
Laschal suture scissors
LaseAway laser
Lasegue maneuver
Lasegue sign
laser
　2-joule erbium laser
　AccuLase excimer laser
　AcuBlade robotic laser
　acupuncture laser
　Aesculap argon ophthalmic
　　laser
　Aesculap excimer laser
　Aesculap-Meditec excimer
　　laser
　Albarran laser
　alexandrite laser
　alexandrite long-pulsed laser
　AMO laser
　Arago argon laser
　argon blue laser
　argon green laser
　argon ion laser
　argon laser
　argon pump dye laser
　argon tunable dye laser
　argon-krypton laser
　argon-fluoride laser
　argon-krypton laser
　argon-pumped tunable dye
　　laser
　ArthroGuide carbon dioxide
　　laser
　ArthroProbe laser
　Articu-Lase laser
　atheroablation laser
　Athos laser
　Aura desktop laser
　Aurora diode laser
　balloon-centered argon laser
　Biophysic laser
　Britt argon laser
　Britt argon pulsed laser
　Britt krypton laser
　Britt pulsed argon laser
　Candela pulsed dye laser
　carbon dioxide laser

laser (*continued*)
Cardona laser
Carl Zeiss YAG laser
Cavitron laser
char-free carbon-dioxide laser
Chromaser dermatology laser
Chrys surgical CO_2 laser
Cilco argon laser
Cilco Frigitronics laser
Cilco Hoffer Laseridge laser
Cilco krypton laser
Cilco Lasertek argon laser
Cilco YAG laser
ClearView CO_2 laser
CO_2 Heart Laser 2 laser
CO_2 laser
CO_2 Sharplan laser
Coherent laser
Coherent argon laser
Coherent carbon dioxide laser
Coherent CO_2 surgical laser
Coherent EPIC laser
Coherent Medical YAG laser
Coherent Novus Omni
    multiwavelength laser
Coherent radiation argon laser
Coherent UltraPulse laser
Coherent Versapulse
cold beam laser
continuous wave CO_2 laser
continuous wave laser
continuous-wave argon laser
continuous-wave diode laser
Contour laser
CoolGlide laser
cool-tip laser
CoolTouch Nd:YAG laser
Cooper argon laser
Cooper LaserSonics laser
CooperVision argon laser
CooperVision YAG laser
copper bromide laser
copper vapor laser
copper vapor pulsed laser
coumarin pulsed dye laser
coumarin-flashlamp-pumped
    pulsed-dye laser
Crystalase alexandrite DP laser
Crystalase erbium 2 laser
Crystalase erbium laser
Culpolase laser
Cynosure laser

laser (*continued*)
Derma laser
Derma K combination laser
DermaLase laser
DioLite laser
Diomed surgical diode laser
Dornier endourology laser
Dynatronics laser
Eclipse holmium laser
Eclipse TMR laser
Endo-Lase CO_2 laser
Epic laser
EpiLaser hair removal laser
EpiStar diode laser
EpiTouch laser
Er:YAG laser
Erbium-YAG laser
ErCr:YAG laser
esthetic CO_2 laser
Evergreen Lasertek laser
ExciMed excimer laser
excimer cool laser
excimer gas laser
excimer laser
excimer ultraviolet laser
FeatherTouch CO_2 laser
FiberLase laser
flashlamp pulsed Nd:YAG
    laser
flashlamp pumped pulsed dye
    laser
flashlamp-excited long-pulse
    alexandrite laser
flashlamp-excited pulsed dye
    laser
flashlamp-pulsed Nd:YAG
    laser
flashlamp-pumped pulsed dye
    laser (FPPDL)
Flexlase 600 laser
fluorescence-guided smart
    laser
Fotona Novalis ER:YAG laser
Fotona Novalis R ruby laser
frequency doubled
    neodymium:yttrium-
    aluminum-garnet laser
gallium-aluminum-arsenide
    laser
gas laser
Genesis 2000 carbon dioxide
    laser

laser (*continued*)
  GentleLASE laser
  GentleLASE Plus laser
  GentleYAG laser
  Gherini-Kauffman endo-
    otoprobe laser
  Gish micro YAG laser
  Gold portable CO_2 laser
  green laser
  GyneLase diode laser
  Heart Laser
  helium-neon aiming laser
  He-Ne laser (helium-neon
    laser)
  Heraeus LaserSonics laser
  HF infrared laser
  HGM argon green laser
  HGM intravitreal laser
  HGM ophthalmic laser
  HGM krypton yellow and
    green laser
  high-energy laser
  holmium laser
  holmium:YAG laser
  holmium:yttrium-argon-garnet
    laser
  Horn endo-otoprobe laser
  Hoskins nylon suture laser
    laser
  hot-tip laser
  Howard-Schatz laser
  Hruby laser
  Hyperion LTK laser
  IL MED laser
  Illumina Pro series
    laparoscopic laser
  infrared-beam diode laser
  intravitreal laser
  ion laser
  Iris Oculight laser
  Kaplan PenduLaser laser
  Kaplan PenduLaser surgical
    laser
  Keracor laser
  KIP laser
  Kirsch laser
  Kremer excimer laser
  krypton red laser
  KTP laser
  Lambda dye laser
  Lasag laser
  LaseAway laser

laser (*continued*)
  LaseAway Smooth Touch laser
  Laser Lancet laser
  Laserex Era YAG laser
  LaserHarmonic laser
  LaserSonics laser
  Lasertek laser
  Lasertek YAG laser
  Lassag laser
  Lastec System angioplasty
    laser
  Lateralase laser
  lateral-firing laser
  Lightblade laser
  liquid organic dye laser
  low-energy laser
  Lumonics YAG laser
  Luxar NovaPulse CO_2 laser
  MC-700 multi-wavelength
    ophthalmic laser
  MCM smart Laser
  Medilas Nd:YAG surgical laser
  Meditec laser
  MedLite Q-Switched YAG laser
  MEL 60 scanning laser
  MEL 70 flying spot laser
  Microlase transpupillary diode
    laser
  MicroProbe ophthalmic laser
  microsecond pulsed
    flashlamp pumped dye
    laser
  mid-infrared pulsed laser
  Mira laser
  Mochida CO_2 Medi-Laser laser
  mode-locked laser
  Moeller laser
  Molectron laser
  MultiLase Nd:YAG surgical
    laser
  Myriadlase Side-Fire laser
  Nanolas Nd:YAG laser
  NaturaLase Er:YAG laser
  NaturaLase Erbium laser
  Nd:YAG laser
  Nd:YLF laser
  neodymium laser
  neodymium:yttrium-lithium-
    fluoride photodisruptive
    laser
  Neurolase microsurgical CO_2
    laser

laser (*continued*)

Nidek EC-5000 excimer laser
NovaLine excimer laser
NovaPulse CO_2 laser
Novascan scanning headpiece laser
Novatec LightBlade laser
Novulase 660 laser
OcuLight ophthalmic laser
oculocutaneous laser
OmniMed argon-fluoride excimer laser
OmniPulse holmium laser
OmniPulse-MAX holmium laser
Ophthalas argon/krypton laser
Ophthalas krypton laser
Opmilas surgical laser
Opmilas CO_2 laser
Opmilas CO_2 multipurpose laser
orange dye laser
orthogonal laser
OtoLam laser
Palomar laser
Paragon laser
PBI copper vapor laser
PC EDO ophthalmic office laser
Pegasus Nd:YAG surgical laser
photoDerm laser
photodisrupting laser
PhotoGenica laser
Photon laser
PhotoPoint laser
photovaporizing laser
Polaris Nd:YAG laser
Polytec ruby laser
potassium titanyl phosphate laser
Prima laser
Prolase lateral firing Nd:YAG laser
Prostalase laser
pulsed dye laser
pulsed metal vapor laser
pulsed tunable dye laser
pulsed yellow dye laser
PulseMaster laser
Pulsolith pulsed-dye laser
pumped dye laser

laser (*continued*)

Q-LAS YAG laser
QS alexandrite laser
QS Nd:YAG laser
QS ruby laser
QS ruby/YAG laser
Q-switched alexandrite laser
Q-switched Er:YAG laser
Q-switched Nd:YAG laser
Q-switched neodymium:YAG laser
Q-switched ruby laser
Q-switched ruby/YAG laser
red laser
red-beam laser
resurfacing laser
RevitaLase erbium cosmetic laser
rhodamine laser
rotational ablation laser
ruby laser
scanning excimer laser
ScleroLaser
Scleroplus dye laser
Sharplan argon laser
Sharplan CO_2 laser
Sharplan Nd:YAG surgical laser
Sharplan flashscan surgical laser
SharpLase Nd:YAG laser
SideFire laser
Silhouette endoscopic laser
SilkLaser aesthetic CO_2 laser
SilkTouch laser
SITE argon laser
Skinlight Er:YAG laser
Skinlight YAG laser
SLT laser
smart laser
Smoothbeam laser
SoftLight laser
Spectranetics laser
Spectra-Physics argon laser
Spectra-Physics microsurgical laser
spectroscopy-directed laser
Spectrum K1 laser
Spectrum ruby laser
SPTL vascular lesion laser
Star X carbon dioxide laser
stereotactic laser
stereotaxic laser

laser (*continued*)

Storz laser
Summit excimer laser
Summit Omnimed excimer laser
Summit SVS laser
Summit Excimed laser
Surgica laser
surgical laser
Surgicenter CO_2 laser
Surgilase high-powered CO_2 laser
Surgilase Nd:YAG laser
SurgiLight OptiVision YAG laser
Surgipulse CO_2 laser
Tactilaze angioplasty laser
Takata laser
TEC positioning laser
thulium-holmium:YAG laser
tissue welding by laser
TKS laser
Topaz CO_2 laser
tracker-assisted laser
transpupillary laser
Tru-Pulse CO_2 skin resurfacing laser
tunable dye laser
tunable flashlamp-excited pulsed dye laser
UltraFine erbium laser
UltraLine laser
UltraPulse CO_2 laser
UltraPulse surgical laser
ultrapulsed laser
Unilase CO_2 laser
UroGold laser
Urolase CO_2 laser
Urolase fiber laser
V-beam pulsed dye laser
V-beam vascular laser
veinLase captured-pulse laser
VersaLight laser
VersaPulse holmium laser
visual endoscopically controlled laser
Visulas argon C laser
Visulas Hd:YAG laser
Visulas Nd:YAG laser
Visulas YAG C laser
VISX excimer laser
Waterlase Millennium laser
Wild laser

laser (*continued*)

Xanar CO_2 laser
XeCl excimer laser
YAG laser
yttrium-aluminum-garnet laser (YAG laser)
Zeiss laser
Zeiss Visulas laser
Zyoptix laser
laser ablation
laser angioplasty
laser arthroscopy
laser balloon
laser beam
laser biliary lithotripsy
laser catheter
laser cavity
laser cervical conization
laser coagulation
laser coagulation vaporization procedure (LCVP)
laser conization
laser delivery catheter
laser diode
laser dissection technique
laser Doppler flowmetry
laser Doppler fluximetry
laser Doppler perfusion monitor
laser Doppler velocimeter
laser endarterectomy
laser endoforeheadplasty
laser excision
laser festoon reduction
laser fiber
laser flare meter
laser flow cytometer
laser fume absorber
laser hair removal
laser hair transplantation
laser Heaney needle holder
laser hemorrhoid excision
laser hemorrhoidectomy
laser holography
laser in situ keratomileusis (LASIK)
laser incisional blepharoplasty
laser intraocular lens
laser iridectomy
laser iridotomy
laser Julian needle holder
laser keratotomy
Laser Lancet laser

laser laparoscopic
  cholecystectomy (LLC)
laser laparoscopic vagotomy
laser laparoscopy
laser laryngoscope
laser laryngoscopy
laser lens
laser lithotriptor
laser lithotriptor basket
laser lower lid transconjunctival
  blepharoplasty
laser manipulation
laser meloplasty
laser microlaryngeal cup forceps
laser microlaryngeal grasping
  forceps
laser microprobe
laser microscope
laser microsurgery
laser mirror
laser optometer
laser ovary forceps
laser palatoplasty
laser partial nephrectomy
laser photoablation
laser photocoagulation
laser photovaporization
laser plume
laser probe
laser procedure
laser radiation
laser recanalization
laser resurfacing
laser rod
laser scalpel
laser shield
laser skin resurfacing
laser smoke evacuation
laser speckle
laser stapedectomy
laser stapedotomy
laser stereolithography process
laser surgery
laser taper
laser therapy
laser tip
laser tissue weld
laser tissue welding
laser trabeculoplasty
Laser Trach wrapped
  endotracheal tube
laser treatment

laser tubal scissors
laser tweezers
laser uterosacral nerve ablation
laser vaporization
laser welding
laser-adjustable lens
laser-assisted appendectomy
laser-assisted balloon angioplasty
laser-assisted in situ
  keratomileusis (LASIK)
laser-assisted intrastromal
  keratomileusis cannula
laser-assisted intrastromal
  keratomileusis cannula eye
  guard
laser-assisted intrastromal
  keratomileusis flap irrigator
laser-assisted microanastomosis
  (LAMA)
laser-assisted spinal endoscopy
laser-assisted uvulopalatoplasty
  (LAUP)
laser-balloon angioplasty
laser-balloon procedure
laserbrasion
Laserdish electrode
Laserdish pacing lead
laser-Doppler flowmetry probe
laser-Doppler Periflux probe
Laseredge microsurgical knife
laser-evoked potential
Laserex Era YAG laser
laser-filtering surgery
Laserflex intraocular lens
Laserflo laser Doppler monitor
Laserflow blood perfusion
  monitor
Laserflow BPM2 real time
  cerebral perfusion monitor
  monitor
Laserflow Doppler probe
LaserHarmonic laser
Laseridge Optics lens
laser-induced fragmentation
laser-induced intracorporeal
  shock wave lithotripsy
lasering
laseroscopy
Laserscope
Laserscope disposable Endostat
  fiber
LaserSonics laser

LaserSonics Nd:YAG LaserBlade
 scalpel
LaserSonics Paragon laser
LaserSonics SurgiBlade
Lasertek laser
Lasertek YAG laser
Laser-Trach endotracheal tube
lasertripsy
Lasertubus tracheal tube
Lasette laser finger perforator
LASH (left anterior superior
 hemiblock)
Lash hysterectomy
Lash operation
Lash procedure
lash reflex
Lash technique
Lash-Loeffler penile implant
 material
Lash-Loeffler penile prosthesis
Lash-Masler penile prosthesis
Lash-Moser prosthesis
LASIK (laser in situ
 keratomileusis) procedure
LASIK eye guard
LASIK flap irrigator
lasing medium
Lassag Micropter II laser
lasso snare
Lassus technique
LAST coronary bypass
 procedure
Lastac coronary angioplasty
Lastac system angioplasty laser
Latarjet nerve
Latarjet vein
latch key lid
late abortion
late-term abortion
late complication
late decelerations
late graft dysfunction
late graft failure
late infection rate
late phase reaction
late wound failure
latent cancer
latent carcinoma
latent pacemaker
latent period
latent reflex
lateral abdominal region

lateral aberrant thyroid
 carcinoma
lateral aberration
lateral abscess
lateral accessory ligament of
 Henle
lateral alveolar abscess
lateral ampullary nerve
lateral angle of eye
lateral antebrachial cutaneous
 nerve
lateral anterior position
lateral anterior x-ray position
lateral aperture
lateral approach
lateral arm flap
lateral aspect
lateral aspiration
lateral atlantoaxial joint
lateral band
lateral bicipital groove
lateral bulbar fossa
lateral canal entrapment
lateral canthal raphe
lateral cantholysis
lateral canthopexy
lateral canthoplasty
lateral canthotomy
lateral canthus
lateral capsule
lateral cartilage flap
lateral cartilage of nose
lateral cathotomy
lateral central palmar space
lateral cephalogram
lateral cerebral aperture
lateral cerebral fissure
lateral cerebral sulcus
lateral cervical node dissection
lateral circumflex artery of thigh
lateral circumflex femoral artery
lateral collateral ligaments
lateral column
lateral commissure of eyelids
lateral compartment
 reconstruction
lateral compression
lateral compression injury
lateral condylar humeral fracture
lateral condylar inclination
lateral condylar pole of the TMJ
lateral condyle

lateral constriction phenomenon
lateral conus
lateral cricoarytenoid muscle
lateral crural convexity (LAC)
lateral crural spanning suture
lateral crural steal (LCS)
lateral crus of greater alar
    cartilage
lateral curvature of spine
lateral cutaneous nerve
lateral cutaneous thigh flap
lateral cyst
lateral decubitus position
lateral deltoid splitting approach
lateral deviation on opening
lateral displacement
lateral distally based
    fasciocutaneous flap
lateral dorsal cutaneous nerve
lateral edge
lateral electrical spine
    stimulation (LESS)
lateral epicondyle
lateral excursion
lateral extension
lateral extensor expansion
lateral extracavitary approach
lateral facial cleft
lateral facial cleft deformity
lateral femoral cutaneous nerve
lateral field
lateral flank incision
lateral fluoroscopy
lateral foramen
lateral fornix
lateral fusion
lateral galea aponeurotica
lateral Gatellier-Chastung
    approach
lateral geniculate body
lateral glossoepiglottic fold
lateral ground bundle
lateral guide pin
lateral gutter
lateral gutter impactor
lateral head extraoral radiography
lateral hemifacial lesion
lateral hemispheres
lateral horn of hyoid bone
lateral incisal guide angle
lateral incision
lateral inferior genicular artery

lateral inguinal fossa
lateral intercostal flap
lateral internal pelvic reservoir
lateral J approach
lateral jaw projection
lateral joint line
lateral joint space
lateral Kocher approach
lateral lacunae of cranial dura
    mater
lateral ligament
lateral ligament of
    temporomandibular
    articulation
lateral lithotomy
lateral lobes of prostate
lateral mallear fold
lateral mallear ligament
lateral malleolus
lateral mamillary nucleus of Rose
lateral mandibulectomy
lateral mass fracture
lateral mastoid bone
lateral maxillary ligament
lateral meniscus
lateral microlens telescope
lateral movement
lateral nail fold
lateral nasal artery
lateral nasal fold
lateral neck crease
lateral nystagmus
lateral oblique fascia
lateral oblique jaw
    roentgenogram
lateral oblique projection of
    mandible
lateral oblique radiograph
lateral oblique transcranial view
lateral occlusion
lateral oral commissure
lateral orbitotomy
lateral osteotome
lateral osteotomy
lateral palpebral arteries
lateral palpebral commissure
lateral palpebral raphe
lateral pancreaticojejunostomy
lateral parotidectomy
lateral pedicle graft
lateral perforation
lateral pharyngeal space

lateral pharyngotomy
lateral pinch
lateral plantar artery
lateral plantar nerve
lateral position
lateral positioner
lateral posterior nasal arteries
lateral presentation
lateral process
lateral projection
lateral prone position
lateral pterygoid muscle
lateral pterygoid nerve
lateral pterygoid plate
lateral ramus roentgenogram
lateral rectus (LR)
lateral rectus capitis
lateral rectus incision
lateral rectus muscle
lateral rectus position
lateral rectus resection
lateral recumbent position
lateral region
lateral relation
lateral retractor
lateral sacral arteries
lateral sacral veins
lateral scar
lateral screw
lateral sinus
lateral sinus radiograph
lateral skull radiograph
lateral skull roentgenogram
lateral spinothalamic
lateral striate arteries
lateral sulcus
lateral superior genicular artery
lateral supraclavicular nerves
lateral supramalleolar flap
lateral surface of zygomatic bone
lateral tarsal arteries
lateral tarsal strip procedure
lateral thigh flap
lateral thigh free flap
lateral thoracic artery
lateral thoracic vein
lateral thorax
lateral thyrohyoid ligament
lateral TMJ ligament
lateral to the incision
lateral transverse thigh flap
    (LTTF)

lateral trap suture
lateral trapezius flap
lateral trim of the adenoid
lateral umbilical folds
lateral upper arm flap
lateral upper lip vermilion
    border
lateral utility incision
lateral vector lifts
lateral ventricle
lateral ventricle horn
lateral version of uterus
lateral views
lateral wall of sphenoid bone
lateral wall retractor
lateral window technique
lateral x-ray view
Lateralase laser
lateral-firing laser
laterality
lateralization
lateralizing
lateral-lateral pouch
laterally reflected
lateroaortic lymph node
    dissection
lateroaortic metastasis
laterocollateral ligament
laterofacial cleft
laterognathia
laterognathism
lateromedial oblique projection
lateropharyngeal space
laterotrusive movement
late-stage disease
latex bag
latex balloon
latex band
latex catheter
latex closure
latex drain
latex O band
latex prosthesis
latex sponge graft
latex tube
Latham appliance
Lathbury application
Lathbury cotton applicator
lathe-cut polymethyl
    methacrylate intraocular
    lens
lathing procedure

Latis catheter
latis dual-lumen graft-cleaning
    catheter
latissimus dorsi breast
    reconstruction
latissimus dorsi island flap
latissimus dorsi muscle flap
latissimus dorsi
    musculocutaneous flap
latissimus dorsi myocutaneous
    flap (LDMCF)
latissimus dorsi procedure
latissimus dorsi segmental
    musculovascular pedicle
latissimus dorsi/scapular bone
    flap
latissimus fasciocutaneous
    turnover flap
latissimus muscle flap
latissimus-scapular muscle flap
latissimus-serratus muscle flap
Latram mastectomy procedure
Latrobe soft palate retractor
lats (slang for latissimus)
Latson multipurpose catheter
lattice degeneration
lattice fiber
lattice retinal degeneration
lattice space
Lattimer Silastic testicular
    prosthesis
Latzko cesarean section
Latzko closure
Latzko colpocleisis
Latzko fistula repair
Latzko operation
Latzko partial colpocleisis
Latzko radical abdominal
    hysterectomy
Latzko radical hysterectomy
Latzko repair of vesicovaginal
    fistula
Latzko vesicovaginal fistula
    repair
Lauenstein procedure
Lauenstein wrist procedure
Lauenstein x-ray projection
Lauer forceps
Laufe aspirating curet
Laufe cervical dilator
Laufe divergent outlet forceps
Laufe obstetrical forceps

Laufe portable uterine evacuator
Laufe retractor
Laufe uterine polyp forceps
Laufe-Barton obstetrical forceps
Laufe-Barton-Kjelland obstetrical
    forceps
Laufe-Barton-Kjelland-Piper
    obstetrical forceps
Laufe-Novak diagnostic curet
Laufe-Novak gynecologic curet
Laufe-Piper obstetrical forceps
Laufe-Piper uterine polyp
    forceps
Laufe-Randall gynecologic curet
Laufman forceps
Lauge-Hansen ankle
    classification
Lauge-Hansen ankle fracture
    classification
Laugier fracture
Laugier hernia
Laumonier ganglion
Launois-Cléret deformity
LAUP (laser-assisted
    uvulopalatoplasty)
Laurell technique
Lauren gastric carcinoma
    classification
Laurens operation
Laurens-Alcatel nuclear powered
    pacemaker
Laurer forceps
Laurus needle driver
LAV (lymphadenopathy-
    associated virus)
Lavacuator gastric evacuator
lavage
    abdominal lavage
    bowel lavage
    bronchial lavage
    bronchoalveolar lavage (BAL)
    colonic lavage
    continuous pericardial lavage
    continuous postoperative
        closed lavage
    copious lavage
    copious peritoneal lavage
    diagnostic peritoneal lavage
        (DPL)
    Edlich tube lavage
    Ewald lavage
    Exeter bone lavage

lavage (*continued*)
   external biliary lavage
   gastric lavage
   Hi Speed pulse lavage
   HUMI device for tubal lavage
   iced saline lavage
   intraoperative bowel lavage
   intraoperative colonic lavage
   PEG lavage (polyethylene
     glycol lavage)
   peritoneal lavage
   pleural lavage
   polyethylene glycol lavage
   pulsatile pressure lavage
   saline lavage
   tracheal lavage
lavage and suction
lavage bowel preparation
lavage instillation
lavage of bronchi
lavage of joint
lavage of pleura
lavage of sinus
lavage of stomach
lavage solution
lavaged with sterile saline
lavaging catheter
Laval advancement forceps
LaVeen ascites shunt
LaVeen helical stripper
LaVeen inflation syringe
law of denervation
Lawford speculum
Lawrence Add-A-Cath
Lawrence deep forceps
Lawrence first
     metatarsophalangeal joint
     implant
Lawrence hemostatic forceps
Lawrence position
Lawrie modified circumflex
   scissors
Laws gastroplasty
Lawson operation
Lawson-Thornton plate
Lawton corneal scissors
Lawton forceps
Lawton microneedle holder
Lawton scissors
Lawton-Balfour self-retaining
   retractor
Lawton-Schubert biopsy forceps

Lawton-Wittner cervical biopsy
   forceps
laxity
   aponeurotic laxity
   eyelid laxity
   glabellar laxity
   horizontal lid laxity
   ligamentous laxity
   musculofascial laxity
   orbicularis laxity
   skin laxity
   submental laxity
laxity of cheeks
Layden infant lens
layer
   aponeurotic layer
   barrier layer
   basal layer
   Bergmann layer
   Bowman layer
   cambrium layer
   closed in anatomic layers
   closed in layers
   cornified layer
   cremasteric layer
   deep layer
   Dermanet wound contact
     layer
   echographic layer
   echo-poor layer
   facial fascial layer
   fascial layer
   fascial-fatty layer
   germinal layer
   granular cell layer
   granular layer
   Henle fiber layer
   hidden layer
   Huxley layer
   imbricating layer
   incision closed in layers
   individual layers
   inner fibrous layer
   inner layer
   input layer
   intercellular layer
   intermediate layer
   intimal layer
   meningeal layer
   mesothelial cell layer
   molecular external layer
   muscular layer

layer (continued)
   musculoaponeurotic layer
   musculofascial layers
   nerve fiber bundle layer
   neural retinal layer
   nuclear external layer
   Ollier layer
   orbital layer
   outer fibrous layer
   outer layer
   outermost layer
   papyraceous layer
   parakeratotic layer
   parietal layer
   plexiform external layer
   posterior layer
   pretracheal layer
   prevertebral layer
   Sattler layer
   seromuscular layer
   serosal layer
   serous layer
   silica-carbon layer
   skin layers
   SMAS layer
   subdermal layer
   submucous layer
   superficial layers
   suprachoroid layer
   surface cell layer
   visceral layer
   Weil basal layer
layer of tissue
layer technique
layered closure
layered keratoplasty
layer-to-layer gastroplasty
laying-open fistulotomy
Layman decompressor
Layman tongue depressor
Layman-Storz snare
lay-on graft
Lazar microsuction forceps
Lazaro da Silva technique
   colostomy
Lazarus-Nelson technique
lazy bowel
lazy-M incision
lazy-C incision
lazy-H incision
lazy-S incision
lazy-Z incision

L-buttress plate
LCA (left coronary artery)
L-Cath peripherally inserted
   neonatal catheter
LCC (lung compression clamp)
LCP disease (Legg-Calve-Perthes
   disease)
LCS (lateral crural steal)
L-curved incision
LCVP-aided hepatectomy
LCVP-aided hepatic resection
LCVP-aided technique
LCVP-assisted hepatectomy
LCVP-assisted major liver
   resection
LCX, LCx (left circumflex artery)
LDA stapler
LDF stapler
LDMCF (latissimus dorsi
   myocutaneous flap)
LDN technique
LDR intracavitary radiation
   therapy
LDS applier
LDS clip
LDS clip applier
LDS instrument
LDS stapler
LDU brace
Le Bag urinary pouch
Le Dran suture technique
LeFort classification
LeFort II osteotomy
LeFort suture technique
LeFort-Neugebauer operation
Leach technique
Leach-Igou osteotomy
Leach-Igou step-cut medial
   osteotomy
lead
lead apron
lead artifact
lead block
lead bra
lead eye shield
lead hand
lead line
lead pellet marker
lead placement
lead plate
lead shield
lead strip

lead sutures
Leadbetter cystourethroplasty
Leadbetter epiphysis
Leadbetter hip manipulation
Leadbetter maneuver
Leadbetter modification
    technique
Leadbetter operation
Leadbetter procedure
Leadbetter-Politano operation
Leadbetter-Politano procedure
Leadbetter-Politano ureteral
    implant prosthesis
Leadbetter-Politano ureteral
    reimplantation
Leadbetter-Politano
    ureteroneocystotomy
Leadbetter-Politano
    ureterovesical
    reimplantation
Leadbetter-Politano
    ureterovesicoplasty
Leader forceps
Leader hook
Leader iris hook
Leader vas hook
Leader vas isolation forceps
Leader-Kohlman dilator
lead-filled head mallet
lead-filled mallet
lead-pipe colon
lead-pipe fracture
lead-shot tie suture
leaf (pl. leaves)
leaf gauge
leaf splint
leaflet
    aortic valve leaflet
    cardiac valve leaflets
    doming of mitral valve leaflet
    hammocking of posterior
        mitral leaflet
    triangular resection of
        leaflet
leaflet prolapse
leaflet retractor
leaflet thickening
leaflet tip
leaflike villi
leaf-spring brace
Leahey chalazion forceps
Leahey clamp

Leahey marginal chalazion
    forceps
Leahey operation
Leahey suture forceps
leak
    anastomotic stump leak
    bile leak
    cerebrospinal fluid leak
    chylous leak
    cystic duct stump leak
    duodenal stump leak
    glue patch leak
    mask leak
    pancreatic stump leak
    periprosthetic leak
    postoperative anastomotic
        leak
    Roux limb stump leak
    Seidel test for aqueous fluid
        leak
    stump leak
    trocar gas leak
leak point pressure
leakage
    anastomotic leakage
    bile leakage
    biliary leakage
    cervical leakage
    chylous leakage
    corneal leakage
    intestinal anastomotic leakage
    local leakage
    silicone implant leakage
    silicone leakage
    tube leakage
leakage of fluid
leakage rate
Leake Dacron mandible
    prosthesis
leaking about shunt site
leaking aneurysm
leaky valve
LEAP (lower extremity
    amputation prevention)
    monofilament test
leapfrog position
least-wrinkled fill volume
Leasure aspirator
Leasure nasal forceps
Leasure round punch tip
Leasure tracheal retractor
Leasure tuning fork

Leather antegrade valve
leather bottle stomach
leather orthosis
leather restraint
Leather retrograde valve
Leather valve cutter
Leather venous valvulotome
Leather-Carmody scissors
Leather-Karmody in-site valve
   scissors
Leatherman alar hook
Leatherman child spinal hooks
Leatherman compression hook
Leatherman trochanteric
   retractor
Leaver sclerotomy forceps
leaves (*sing.* leaf)
leaves of broad ligament
leaves of dura
leaves of mesentery
LeBag ileocolic urinary reservoir
LeBerne treatment table
Leboyer delivery technique
Leboyer technique
Lebsche chisel
Lebsche forceps
Lebsche knife
Lebsche punch
Lebsche raspatory
Lebsche rongeur
Lebsche saw guide
Lebsche shears
Lebsche sternal chisel
Lebsche sternal knife
Lebsche sternal punch
Lebsche sternal shears
Lebsche thoracic knife
Lebsche wire saw
Lebsche wire saw guide
lecithin/sphingomyelin ratio
   (L/S ratio)
LeCocq brace
Lecompte maneuver
lecture-scope
LeDentu suture technique
LeDentu sutures
Ledhey forceps
Ledor pigtail catheter
LeDran sutures
LeDuc anastomosis
LeDuc technique
LeDuc-Camey ileocolostomy

LeDuc-Camey ileocystoplasty
Lee-Westcott needle
Lee anterosuperior iliac sine
   graft
Lee bone graft
Lee bronchus clamp
Lee cartilage knife
Lee cryoprobe
Lee delicate hemostatic forceps
Lee diamond bur
Lee double-ended retractor
Lee ganglion
Lee graft
Lee knife
Lee lingual button
Lee microvascular clamp
Lee needle
Lee procedure
Lee reconstruction
Lee technique
Lee-Cohen elevator
Lee-Cohen knife
Lee-Cohen septal elevator
Leeds-Keio ligament prosthesis
LEEP conization
Lees arterial forceps
Lees clamp
Lees nontraumatic forceps
Lees vascular clamp
Lees wedge resection clamp
Lefevre gastrectomy technique
Leff alloy
Leff stethoscope
Lefferst rib shears
Lefferts bone-cutting forceps
Lefferts rib spreader
LeFort amputation
LeFort bougie
LeFort catheter
LeFort classification of maxillary
   fractures (I, II, III)
LeFort colpocleisis
LeFort dilator
LeFort fibular fracture
LeFort filiform
LeFort filiform bougie
LeFort filiform guide
LeFort follower
LeFort fracture (I, II or III)
LeFort I apertognathia repair
LeFort I impaction
LeFort I maxillary reconstruction

LeFort III advancement osteotomy
LeFort III craniofacial disjunction
LeFort III facial advancement
LeFort II midface osteotomy
LeFort I osteotomy
LeFort male catheter
LeFort maxillary osteotomy
LeFort operation
LeFort osteotomy
LeFort osteotomy procedure
LeFort partial colpocleisis
LeFort procedure (I, II, III)
LeFort sound
LeFort speculum
LeFort sutures
LeFort urethral catheter
LeFort urethral sound
LeFort urethral speculum
LeFort urethral ultrasound
LeFort uterine prolapse repair
LeFort uterine sound
LeFort-Wagstaffe fracture
LeFort-Wehrbein-Duplay hypospadias repair
left anterior descending artery (LAD)
left anterior oblique position
left atrial isolation procedure
left atrium to distal arterial aortic bypass
left atrium to femoral artery circulatory bypass
left axis deviation
left bundle branch block
left cardiac catheterization
left colectomy
left colic artery
left colic vein
left colon
left colonic flexure
left coronary angiogram
left coronary artery
left coronary catheter
left coronary cinearteriogram
left decubitus position
left diaphragm
left dominant coronary circulation
left dorsoanterior
left dorsoposterior

left 5th intercostal space
left frontal craniotomy (LFC)
left gastric artery
left gastric vein
left gastroepiploic artery
left gastroepiploic vein
left gutter
left heart bypass
left heart catheter
left heart catheterization
left hemicolectomy
left hemodiaphragm
left hepatectomy
left hepatic duct
left hilum
left hypogastric nerve
left inferior pulmonary vein
left inguinal hernia (LIH)
left intercostal space
left internal mammary artery graft (LIMA graft)
left Judkins catheter
left lateral bending
left lateral decubitus position
left lateral excursion
left lateral position
left lateral projection
left lateral region
left lobe
left long leg brace
left lower lobe (LLL)
left lower quadrant (LLQ)
left main bronchus
left mentoanterior position (LMA position)
left mentoposterior position (LMP position)
left mentotransverse position (LMT position)
left occipitoanterior position (LOA position)
left occipitoposterior position (LOP position)
left occipitotransverse position (LOT position)
left posterior oblique
left pulmonary artery
left radical groin dissection
left rhomboid muscle
left rotation
left sacroanterior position (LSA position)

left sacroposterior position (LSP
    position)
left scapuloanterior position
    (LScA position)
left scapuloposterior position
    (LScP position)
left segmental colectomy
left superficial temporal artery
    to middle cerebral artery
    anastomosis
left superior pulmonary vein
left suprarenal vein
left testicular vein
left umbilical vein
left upper lobe (LUL)
left upper lobe bronchus
left upper quadrant (LUQ)
left venous angle
left ventricle
left ventricular
left ventricular assist device
    (LVAD)
left ventricular bypass pump
left ventricular cineangiogram
left ventricular clamp catheter
left ventricular end-diastolic
    pressure
left ventricular inflow tract
left ventricular outflow tract
left ventricular sump catheter
left ventricular transvenous lead
left-curved scissors
left-handed cornea scissors
left-sided colorectal obstruction
left-sided injury
left-side-down position
left-to-right shunt
left-to-right subtotal
    pancreatectomy
leg brace
leg cast
leg elevation
leg extension splint
leg flap
leg holder
leg motion
leg positioner
leg raising
leg rigidly extended
leg roll
leg splint
leg-block anesthesia

Legend pacemaker
Legg operation
Legg osteotome
Legg-Calve-Perthes disease (LCP
    disease)
Legg-Perthes disease
legholder
leg-holding device
leg-length discrepancy
leg-length measurement
Legueu bladder retractor
Legueu kidney retractor
Legueu spatula
Lehman aortographic catheter
Lehman cardiac device
Lehman catheter
Lehman pancreatic manometry
    catheter
Lehman syringe
Lehman technique
Lehman ventriculography
    catheter
Lehner II inserter
Lehner II loader
Leib-Guerry cataract implant
    lens
Leibinger 3-D bone plate
Leibinger E-Z flap
Leibinger Micro Dynamic mesh
Leibinger Micro Plus plate
Leibinger Micro Plus screw
Leibinger Micro System plate
    cutter
Leibinger Micro System plate-
    holding forceps
Leibinger plate
Leibinger plating
Leibinger Würzburg plate
Leibinger Würzburg screw
Leibolt technique
Leica microscope
Leica vibrating knife microtome
Leicaflex camera
Leiden mutation
Leigh capsule forceps
Leigh zonule lens stripper
Leighton needle
Leinbach device
Leinbach head and neck
    endoprosthesis
Leinbach head and neck total
    hip

Leinbach hip prosthesis
Leinbach olecranon hook
Leinbach olecranon screw
Leinbach osteotome
Leinbach prosthesis
Leinbach screw
leiomyoma (*pl.* leiomyomas,
   leiomyomata)
leiomyoma enucleation
leiomyomata uteri
leiomyosarcoma
Leios pacemaker
Leisegang colposcope
Leishman classification
Leiske intraocular lens
Leiske Optiflex lens
Leiske Physioflex intraocular lens
Leiter cystoscope
Leiter tube
Leitz microtome
Leitz microscope
Leivers blade
Leivers mouth gag
Lejeune applicator
Lejeune cotton applicator
Lejeune scissors
Lejeune thoracic forceps
Lejour breast reduction
Lejour mammaplasty
Lejour mastoplasty
Lejour technique
Lejour-type reduction
Leksell bone rongeur
Leksell cardiovascular rongeur
Leksell director
Leksell D-shaped stereotactic
   frame
Leksell forceps
Leksell frame
Leksell gamma knife
Leksell grooved director
Leksell laminectomy rongeur
Leksell punch
Leksell rongeur forceps
Leksell stereotactic device
Leksell stereotactic gamma unit
Leksell stereotaxic frame
Leksell sternal approximator
Leksell sternal spreader
Leksell technique
Leksell trephine
Leksell-Elekta stereotactic frame

Leksell-Stille thoracic rongeur
Leksell-Stille thoracic
   cardiovascular rongeur
Leland refractor
Leland tonsillar knife
Leland-Jones clamp
Leland-Jones forceps
Leland-Jones peripheral vascular
   clamp
Leland-Jones tonsillar knife
Leland-Jones vascular clamp
Lell bite block
Lell esophagoscope
Lell laryngofissure saw
Lell tracheal tube
LeMaitre biliary catheter
LeMaitre valvulotome
LeMaitre-Bookwalter dilator
Lem-Blay circumcision clamp
LeMesurier operation
LeMesurier rectangular flap
LeMesurier repair
Lemmon blade
Lemmon contractor
Lemmon intimal dissector
Lemmon needle holder
Lemmon rib approximator
Lemmon rib contractor
Lemmon rib spreader
Lemmon self-retaining sternal
   retractor
Lemmon sternal approximator
Lemmon sternal elevator
Lemmon sternal retractor
Lemmon sternal spreader
Lemmon-Russian forceps
Lemoine eye implant
Lemoine forceps
Lemoine orbital implant
Lemoine-Searcy anchor
Lemoine-Searcy fixation anchor
   loop
Lemole atrial valve self-retaining
   retractor
Lemole mitral valve retractor
lemon squeezer obstetrical
   elevator
Lempert bone curet
Lempert bone rongeur
Lempert bur
Lempert diamond-dust polishing
   bur

Lempert elevator
Lempert endaural curet
Lempert endaural rongeur
Lempert evacuator
Lempert excavator
Lempert extractor
Lempert fenestration
Lempert fenestration bur
Lempert fine curet
Lempert forceps
Lempert heavy elevator
Lempert incision for radical
    tympanoplasty
Lempert instrument
Lempert knife
Lempert malleus cutter
Lempert malleus nipper
Lempert malleus punch
Lempert narrow elevator
Lempert operation
Lempert paracentesis knife
Lempert perforator
Lempert periosteal elevator
Lempert procedure
Lempert punch
Lempert retractor
Lempert rongeur
Lempert rongeur forceps
Lempert rongeur headrest
Lempert sutures
Lempert-Beckman-Colver
    endaural speculum
Lempert-Colver endaural
    speculum
Lempert-Colver retractor
Lempert-Colver speculum
Lempert-Juers rongeur
Lempert-Storz lens
Lempert-Storz lens loupe
Lempert-Storz loupe
Lempka stripper
Lempka vein stripper
Lems lens
Lenard ray tube
Lenart-Kullman technique
length of mandible
length of palate
lengthening
    Allan bone lengthening
    Anderson tibial lengthening
    cord lengthening
    distraction lengthening

lengthening (*continued*)
    heel cord lengthening
    Lange tendon lengthening
    laparoscopic Nissen
        fundoplication with
        esophageal lengthening
    levator-Müeller complex
        lengthening
    palate lengthening
    penile lengthening
    step-cut lengthening
    tendon Achilles lengthening
        (TAL)
    tendon lengthening
    V-Y advancement for
        columellar lengthening
lengthening genioplasty
lengthening of bone
lengthening of tendon
Lennander operation
Lennarson suction tube
Lennert classification
Lennert lesion
Lennhoff sign
Lenox Hill knee brace
Lenox Hill knee orthosis
Lenox Hill Spectralite knee
    brace
lens (*pl.* lenses)
    1-plate haptic silicone
        intraocular lens
    2-Optifit toric lens
    3M intraocular lens
    3-footed lens intraocular
        lens
    3-mirror contact lens
    3-mirror intraocular lens
    3-piece acrylic intraocular lens
    3-piece modified J-loop
        intraocular lens
    3-piece silicone intraocular
        lens
    3-point fixation intraocular
        lens
    4-footed lens
    4-mirror goniolens lens
    4-piece intraocular lens
    4-point fixation intraocular
        lens
    Abraham contact lens
    Abraham iridectomy laser lens
    Abraham iridectomy lens

lens (*continued*)

Abraham peripheral button
  iridotomy lens
Abraham YAG laser lens
AC lens
AccuGel lens
achromatic lens
acrylic lens
AcrySof foldable intraocular
  lens
Acuvue bifocal lens
Acuvue disposable contact
  lens
Acuvue lens
Adaptar no-line contact lens
Adaptar contact lens
adherent lens
Advent Flurofocon contact lens
AIRLens contact lens
Albarran lens
Alcon intraocular lens
Alien WildEyes lens
Allen-Braley intraocular lens
all-PMMA 1-piece C-loop
  intraocular lens
Alpar lens
Amenabar lens
Amercal-Shepard intraocular
  lens
American intraocular lens
American Medical Optics
  intraocular lens
AMO Advent contact lens
AMO Array foldable
  intraocular lens
AMO intraocular lens
AMO Sensar intraocular lens
AMO Sensar posterior
  chamber intraocular lens
Amsoft lens
Anis posterior chamber
  capsule intraocular lens
Anis staple implant cataract
  lens
Anis staple lens
anterior chamber intraocular
  lens
Appolionio implant cataract
  lens
Aquasight lens
Arnott 1-piece all-PMMA
  intraocular lens

lens (*continued*)

Array foldable intraocular lens
Array multifocal intraocular
  lens
Arruga lens
Artisan phakic intraocular lens
aspheric cataract lens
aspheric viewing lens
aspherical ophthalmoscopic
  lens
auxiliary lens
Azar flexible-loop anterior
  chamber intraocular lens
Azar Mark II intraocular lens
Azar Tripod implant cataract
  lens
bag-fixated intraocular lens
Bagolini lens
Baikoff lens
bandage soft contact lens
Barkan gonioscopic lens
Barkan goniotomy lens
Barkan infant lens
Barkan operating lens
Barnes-Hind lens
Baron intraocular lens
Barraquer J-loop intraocular
  lens
Barrett hydrogel intraocular
  lens
Bausch & Lomb Optima lens
Bausch & Lomb lens
Beale intraocular implant lens
Bechert 1-piece all-PMMA
  intraocular lens
Beebe lens
biconcave contact lens
biconvex intraocular lens
bicylindrical lens
Bietti implant cataract lens
bifocal intracorneal lens
Binkhorst collar stud
  intraocular lens
Binkhorst mustache lens
  intraocular lens
Binkhorst modified J-loops
  intraocular lens
Binkhorst 2-loop lens
Binkhorst-Fyodorov lens
biomicroscopic indirect lens
Bi-Soft contact lens
bispherical lens

lens (*continued*)
  bitoric lens
  Bloodshot WildEyes lens
  Boberg lens
  Boberg-Ans intraocular lens
  Boston Envision lens
  Bowling lens
  Boyd intraocular implant lens
  Boys-Smith laser lens
  Brücke lens
  Bron implant cataract lens
  Bunker intraocular implant lens
  Burian-Allen contact lens
  Byrne expulsive hemorrhage
    lens
  Byron intraocular implant lens
  capsular-style lens
  Capsulform lens
  Cardona fiberoptic diagnostic
    lens
  Carl Zeiss lens
  cast-molded PMMA
    intraocular lens
  catadioptric lens
  cataract lens
  CeeOn heparinized
    intraocular lens
  Centra-Flex lens
  central retinal lens
  CGI-1 contact lens
  Charles contact lens
  Charles intraocular lens
  Charles irrigating lens
  Chiroflex lens
  Choyce anterior chamber lens
  Choyce implant cataract lens
  Choyce Mark intraocular lens
  Choyce-Tennant lens
  Choyce Mark VIII lens
  Ciba Soft lens
  Ciba Thin lens
  Cilco intraocular lens
  Cilco MonoFlex PMMA lens
  Cilco Optiflex intraocular lens
  Cilco posterior chamber
    intraocular lens
  Cilco Slant lens
  Cilco-Simcoe II lens
  Cilco-Sonometrics lens
  CIMA flex foldable silicone
    lens
  ClariFlex intraocular lens

lens (*continued*)
  Clayman intraocular implant
    lens
  Clayman intraocular lens
  Clayman-Kelman lens
  C-loop posterior chamber lens
  closed-loop intraocular lens
  Coburn equiconvex lens
  Coburn intraocular lens
  Coburn-Storz intraocular lens
  Cogan-Boberg-Ans lens
  Collamer intraocular lens
  Collamer 1-piece lens
  Comberg contact lens
  compressible acrylic
    intraocular lens
  compression-molded PMMA
    intraocular lens
  concave lens
  concavoconcave lens
  concavoconvex lens
  condensing lens
  conoid lens
  contact bandage lens
  contact lens
  contact low-vacuum lens
  converging lens
  convex lens
  convexity of lens
  convexoconcave lens
  Cooper lens
  CooperVision J-loop
    intraocular lens
  CooperVision PMMA-ACL Flex
    lens
  CooperVision-Cilco-Kelman
    multiflex all-PMMA
    intraocular lens
  CooperVision-Cilco-Novaflex
    anterior chamber
    intraocular lens
  Copeland anterior chamber
    intraocular lens
  Copeland radial loop
    intraocular lens
  Copeland radial panchamber
    intraocular lens
  Copeland radial panchamber
    UV lens
  coquille plano lens
  Cosmet lens
  Crookes lens

lens (*continued*)

crystalline lens
CSI lens
cylindrical lens
Danker-Wohlk contact lens
Darin intraocular implant lens
decentered lens
diagnostic fiberoptic lens
Dickerson intraocular implant lens
diopter lens
direct gonioscopic lens
discission of lens
disk lens intraocular lens
dispersing lens
Donnheim lens
Drews intraocular implant lens
Dubroff radial loop intraocular lens
Dulaney intraocular implant lens
Duragel lens
Durasoft contact lens
Durasoft toric lens
Dura-T contact lens
E-clips prescription computer lens
ectopia of lens
Edge III hydrogel contact lens
Eifrig intraocular implant lens
elevating lens
Ellingson intraocular implant lens
Emcee lens
Emery lens
endocapsular artificial lens intraocular lens
Epstein collar stud acrylic lens
Epstein intraocular lens
Epstein posterior chamber lens
Epstein-Copeland lens
ERG-Jet disposable contact lens
Ernest-McDonald soft intraocular lens
Eschenback Optik lens
etafilcon A disposable contact lens
European in-the-bag lens
express lens
expressor lens
extended-wear soft contact lens

lens (*continued*)

extraction of lens
EZ.1 multifocal contact lens
EZVue violet haptic intraocular lens
F/M base curve contact lens
Falcon lens
Feaster Dualens intraocular lens
Feaster dual-placement intraocular lens
Fechner intraocular implant lens
Fechner lens
Fechtner intraocular lens
fiberoptic lens
Flexcon lens
flexible fluoropolymer contact lens
flexible-loop anterior chamber intraocular lens
flexible-loop posterior chamber intraocular lens
Flexlens lens
Flexner-Worst iris claw lens
Focus Night & Day contact lens
foldable intraocular lens
folding lens
FormFlex formocresol lens
FormFlex intraocular lens
Foroblique lens
Frelex lens
Fresnel lens
Friedman hand-held Hruby lens
fundal coating lens
fundal laser lens
fundal focalizing lens
fundus contact lens
fundus focalizing lens
fused bifocal lens
Fyodorov 4-loop iris clip intraocular lens
Fyodorov type I, II intraocular lens
Fyodorov-Sputnik contact intraocular lens
Galand disk lens
Galand in-the-bag lens
Galand-Knolle modified J-loop intraocular lens

lens (*continued*)

Galin intraocular implant lens
Genesis lens
Gentex PDQ polycarbonate lens
Gill intraocular implant lens
Gills intraocular implant lens
Gilmore intraocular implant lens
glued-on hard contact lens
Goldmann macular contact lens
Goldmann multimirror lens
Goldmann 3-mirror gonioscopy lens
goniofocalizing lens
goniolens
goniolens lens
gonioscopic lens
gonioscopy lens
Gould intraocular implant lens
gradient index lens
Greene intraocular implant lens
Gridley intraocular lens
GRIN lens
Gullstrand lens
hand-held Hruby lens
haptic area lens
haptic plate lens
haptic-fixated intraocular lens
hard contact lens
hard lens
Harris modified J-loop intraocular lens
Harris rigid quadriped intraocular lens
Hart pediatric 3-mirror lens
Hersbury anterior chamber intraocular lens
Hertzog intraocular lens
Hessburg intraocular lens
Hiles intraocular lens
Hirschman intraocular implant lens
Hoffer intraocular implant lens
Hoffer ridged intraocular lens
Hopkins II rod lens
Hoskins nylon suture laser lens

lens (*continued*)

Hoskins-Barkan goniotomy infant lens
Hruby contact lens
Hubbell intraocular implant lens
Hunkeler intraocular lens
Hunter 1-piece all-PMMA intraocular lens
Hydracon contact lens
Hydrasoft contact lens
Hydrocurve contact lens
Hydrocurve lens
Hydrogel expansile intraocular lens
Hydron lens
hydrophilic contact lens
Hydrosight lens
Hydroview intraocular lens
IMMA lens
implant cataract lens
Implens intraocular implant lens
Implens intraocular lens
infant Karickhoff laser lens
infant 3-mirror laser lens
Interflux intraocular lens
Intermedics intraocular lens
Interspace YAG laser lens
in-the-bag lens
intracapsular lens
intracorneal lens
intraocular lens (IOL)
IntraOptics intraocular lens
Iogel intraocular lens
Iolab Azar intraocular lens
Iolab intraocular lens
Iolab lens
IOLAB Slimfit lens
Ioptex intraocular lens
Irene lens
iridocapsular fixation lens
iridocapsular implant cataract lens
iridocapsular intraocular lens
iris claw lens
iris fixation intraocular lens
iris fixation lens
iris plane intraocular lens
iris-clip intraocular lens
iris-supported intraocular lens

lens (*continued*)

irrigating contact Goldmann lens
iseiconic (*see* iseikonie)
iseiconic lens
Iwata-Ricky gonioscopic lens
Jaffe Cilco lens
Jaffe lens
Jaffe ocular implant lens
Jaffe 1-piece all-PMMA intraocular lens
J-Flex posterior chamber lens
J-loop posterior chamber intraocular lens
J-loop posterior chamber lens
Joal lens
Jung-Schaffer lens
Kamerling Capsular 90 lens
Kamerling 1-piece all-PMMA intraocular lens
Karickhoff diagnostic lens
Karickhoff laser lens
Kearney side-notch intraocular lens
Keates intraocular implant lens
Keeler panoramic lens
Kelman anterior chamber intraocular lens
Kelman flexible tripod lens
Kelman II 3-point fixation rigid tripod intraocular lens
Kelman intraocular implant lens
Kelman intraocular lens
Kelman Multiflex II intraocular lens
Kelman Omnifit II intraocular lens
Kelman Omnifit intraocular lens
Kelman CapSul lens
Kelman Quadraflex anterior chamber intraocular lens
Kelman Quadraflex intraocular lens
Kelman S-flex intraocular lens
keratometer lens
Kilp lens
Kishi lens
Knolle intraocular lens
Koeppe diagnostic lens
Koeppe gonioscopic lens

lens (*continued*)

Koteline bifocal lens
Kowa automatic fundus lens
Kraff intraocular implant lens
Krasnov implant cataract lens
Kratz elliptical-style lens
Kratz intraocular implant lens
Kratz modified J-loop intraocular lens
Kratz posterior chamber intraocular lens
Kratz-Johnson intraocular lens
Kratz-Johnson modified J-loop intraocular lens
Krieger wide-field fundus lens
Krwawicz cataract lens
Kryptok bifocal lens
Kwitko intraocular implant lens
Landers biconcave lens
Landers contact lens
Landers-Foulks temporary keratoprosthesis lens
Lannu anterior chamber lens
large-diameter optics intraocular lens
Lasag contact lens
laser lens
laser-adjustable lens
Laserflex intraocular lens
Laseridge Optics lens
lathe-cut polymethyl methacrylate intraocular lens
Layden infant lens
Leib-Guerry cataract implant lens
Leiske intraocular lens
Leiske Optiflex lens
Leiske Physioflex intraocular lens
Lempert-Storz lens
Lems lens
Lester notch intraocular lens
Levick 1-piece all-PMMA intraocular lens
Lewicky intraocular lens
Lieb-Guerry cataract implant lens
Lieb-Guerry cataract lens
ligament of lens
Lindstrom Centrex lens

lens (*continued*)
Lindstrom modified J-loop, 3-piece reverse PMMA optic intraocular lens
Liteflex intraocular lens
Little lens
Little-Arnott tripod intraocular lens
long-wearing contact lens
loop-fixated intraocular lens
Lovac fundal contact lens
Lovac gonioscopic lens
low-power optics for myopic correction lens
Lynell intraocular lens
Machemer flat lens
Machemer infusion contact lens
Machemer magnifying vitrectomy lens
macular contact lens
Mainster retina laser lens
Mainster Ultra Field PRP laser lens
Mainster wide-field lens
Mainster-HM retinal laser lens
Mainster-S retinal laser lens
Mainster-WF retinal laser lens
Maltese cross lens
Mandelkorn suture lysis lens
Manschot intraocular implant lens
March laser lens
Mark IX lens
McCannel intraocular implant lens
McGhan intraocular lens
McGhan-3M intraocular lens
McIntyre intraocular implant lens
McLean prism contact lens
McLean prismatic fundus laser lens
Medallion lens
Medicornea Kratz intraocular lens
Meditech bandage contact lens
Mehta intraocular lens
MemoryLens foldable intraocular lens
meniscal lens

lens (*continued*)
meniscal posterior concave intraocular lens
Mentor ORC MemoryLens lens
meter lens
Michelis intraocular implant lens
MiniQuad XL lens
modified C-loop intraocular lens
modified J-loop, posterior chamber intraocular lens
Momosi spider lens intraocular lens
Monoflex lens
Morgan therapeutic lens
Multi-Optics lens
multiple-piece intraocular lens
narrow lens
needling of lens
Neolens lens
New Orleans lens
NewVues lens
Nikon aspheric lens
Nikon SMZ 2T magnifying lens
Nivita lens
Nokrome bifocal lens
Nova Aid lens
Nova Curve lens
Nova Soft II lens
Novaflex intraocular lens
NuVue lens
objective lens
Oculaid lens
ocular Gamboscope lens
O'Malley-Pearce-Luma lens
Omnifit intraocular lens
omnifocal lens
open lens
open-loop intraocular lens
Ophtec lens
Optical Radiation intraocular lens
Optiflex intraocular lens
Optima contact lens
Opti-Vu lens
Opt-Visor lens
ORC anterior chamber intraocular lens
ORC posterior chamber intraocular lens

lens (*continued*)

orthoscopic lens
O'Shea lens
Osher pan-fundus lens
Osher surgical posterior pole lens
Osher-Fresnel intraocular lens
Packard intraocular lens
Palmer lens
Palmer-Buono contact lens
panchamber UV lens
Pannu II intraocular lens
Pannu intraocular lens
PanoView Optics lens
parfocal defraction lens
PC-IOL lens
Pearce posterior chamber intraocular lens
Pearce Tripod cataract lens
Pearce Tripod intraocular lens
Pearce Tripod lens
Pearce-Keates bifocal intraocular lens
pediatric Karickhoff laser lens
pediatric 3-mirror laser lens
periscopic lens
Permalens lens
Perspex CQ intraocular lens
Perspex CQ-Shearing-Simcoe-Sinskey lens
Peyman special optics for low vision lens
Peyman wide-field lens
Peyman-Green vitrectomy lens
Peyman-Tennant-Green lens
PhacoFlex II intraocular lens
Phakic 6 lens
Pharmacia Intermedics ophthalmic intraocular lens
Pharmacia intraocular lens
Pharmacia Visco J-loop lens
piggyback contact lens
plano lens
planoconcave lens
planoconvex nonridge lens
plastic lens
Platina clip implant cataract lens
Platina clip lens
plus power lens

lens (*continued*)

PMMA contact lens
PMMA hard contact lens
PMMA intraocular lens
Pointer 1-piece all-PMMA intraocular lens
polypropylene intraocular lens
Posner diagnostic lens
posterior chamber intraocular lens
posterior convex intraocular lens
Precision Cosmet lens
prismatic contact lens
prismatic gonioscopic lens
prismatic goniotomy lens
Prokop intraocular lens
prosthetic lens
punctal lens (*also* punktal)
punktal lens (*also* punctal)
QuadPediatric fundus lens
Rappazzo intraocular lens
Rayner lens
Rayner-Choyce intraocular lens
Red Reflex Lens Systems lens
refraction of lens
reserve intraocular lens
retroscopic lens
Revolution lens
Ridley implant cataract lens
right-angle lens
right-angled telescopic lens
rigid gas-permeable contact lens
rigid intraocular lens
Ritch contact lens
Ritch nylon suture laser lens
Ritch trabeculoplasty laser lens
Rodenstock panfundus lens
Roussel-Frankhauser contact lens
Ruiz fundal contact lens
Ruiz fundal laser lens
Ruiz plano fundal lens
Sableflex anterior chamber intraocular lens
sapphire lens
SaturEyes contact lens
Sauflon contact lens

lens (*continued*)

Sauflon PW hydrophilic contact lens
Schachar implant cataract lens
Scharf implant cataract lens
Scharff lens
sclerosed lens
SeeQuence disposable contact lens
SeeQuence disposable lens
self-stabilizing vitrectomy lens
Sensar foldable acrylic posterior chamber intraocular lens
semiflexible intraocular lens
semirigid intraocular lens
Severin intraocular lens
Severin multiple closed-loop intraocular lens
shagreen lesions of lens
Shah-Shah intraocular lens
Shearing intraocular implant lens
Shearing J-Loop intraocular lens
Shearing posterior chamber intraocular lens
Shearing S-style anterior chamber intraocular lens
Sheets closed-loop posterior chamber intraocular lens
Sheets intraocular lens
Shepard flexible anterior chamber intraocular lens
short C-loop intraocular lens
Siepser intraocular lens
Signet Optical lens
silica contact lens
silicone elastomer lens
Silsoft extended wear contact lens
silvered contact lens
Simcoe anterior chamber lens
Simcoe C-loop intraocular lens
Simcoe intraocular implant lens
Simcoe posterior chamber lens
SingleStitch PhacoFlex lens
Sinskey intraocular lens
Sinskey J-loop intraocular lens

lens (*continued*)

Sinskey posterior chamber intraocular lens
Sinskey posterior chamber lens
Slant haptic intraocular lens
Slimfit lens
Smith intraocular implant lens
Snellen soft contact lens
Soflens contact lens
SoFlex lens
soft contact lens
soft intraocular lens
soft lens
Softcon contact lens
SoftSITE multifocal contact lens
Sola Optical USA spectralite high-index lens
Sola VIP lens
Soper cone hard contact lens
Sovereign bifocal lens
Spectralite Transitions lens
spherocylindrical lens
Sputnik-Federov lens
Staar foldable intraocular lens
Staar implantable contact lens
Staar toric lens
Stableflex lens
Stankiewicz iris clip intraocular lens
Starr polyamide loop intraocular lens
Stein intraocular implant lens
Stokes lens
Storz capsular blue intraocular lens
Straatsma intraocular implant lens
Strampelli implant cataract lens
Super Field NC slit lamp lens
Supramid lens
Surefit anterior chamber intraocular lens
Surefit intraocular lens
Surevue contact lens
Surgidev intraocular lens
Surgidev Leiske anterior chamber intraocular lens
Sutherland lens
Tano double-mirror peripheral vitrectomy lens

lens (*continued*)

T-contact lens
Tennant Anchorflex anterior chamber intraocular lens
Tennant intraocular implant lens
Thorpe 4-mirror goniolaser lens
Thorpe gonioprism lens
Thorpe plastic lens
Tillyer bifocal lens
T-lens therapeutic contact lens
Tolentino prism lens
Tolentino vitrectomy lens
Topcon aspheric lens
toric intraocular lens
Touchlite zoom lens
tripod intraocular lens
Trokel lens
Trokel-Peyman laser lens
Troncoso tubular lens
Trupower aspherical lens
Truvision Omni lens
Ultex bifocal lens
Ultra mag lens
Ultra view SP slit lamp lens
UltraCon rigid gas permeable contact lens
ultraviolet-blocking intraocular lens
uniplanar intraocular lens
Univision low-vision microscopic lens
Urrets-Zavalia retinal surgical lens
uvea-fixated intraocular lens
uvea-supported intraocular lens
Uvex lens
UVR-absorbing intraocular lens
Varigray lens
Varilus Infinity lens
Varilus Plus lens
Vest lens
Viscolens lens
Vision Tech lens
Visitec Company lens
Volk conoid lens
Volk conoid ophthalmic lens
Volk high-resolution aspherical lens

lens (*continued*)

Volk Panretinal lens
Volk QuadrAspheric fundal lens
Volk Super Quad 160 pan retinal lens
Volk SuperField aspherical lens
Volk SuperPupil NC lens
Wang lens
Ward-Lempert lens
water fissures in lens
Weber-Elschnig lens
Wesley Jessen lens
Wild lens
Wise iridotomy laser lens
Wise sphincterotomy laser lens
Worst gonioprism contact lens
Worst intraocular lens
Worst lobster-claw lens
Worst Medallion lens
Yalon intraocular lens
Yannuzzi fundus laser lens
Youens lens
Zeiss aspheric lens
Zeiss-Gullstrand lens
Ziski iris clip intraocular lens
Zoeffle soft intraocular lens
lens aberration
lens cannula
lens capsule
lens clip
lens delivered by tumbling procedure
lens delivered intracapsularly
lens dislocation
lens elevated
lens enucleation scoop
lens exchange
lens expressor (*see* expressor)
lens expressor hook
lens extracted
lens extraction
lens forceps
lens glide cutter
lens hook
lens implant
lens implant forceps
lens implantation forceps
lens lane

lens lasso
lens loupe forceps
lens loupe (*see also* loop, loupe)
lens manipulator
lens mitral heart valve
lens opacification
lens opacity
lens prism
lens pusher
lens removal
lens scoop
lens spatula
lens spoon
lens suture technique
lensed fiber-tip laser delivery
    catheter
lenses (*see* lens)
   Aquaflex contact lenses
   decentration of lenses
   EZvue violet haptic one-piece
    lenses
   Frenzel lenses
   Sinskey blue loop intraocular
    lenses
Lens-Eze inserter
Lensmeter lensometer
lensometer
   Allergan-Humphrey
    lensometer
   AMO lensometer
   Carl Zeiss lensometer
   Coburn lensometer
   Hardy lensometer
   IntraOptics lensometer
   LensCheck Advanced Logic
    lensometer
   Lensmeter lensometer
   Marco lensometer
   Reichert lensometer
   Reichert-Lenschek advanced
    logic lensometer
   Topcon LM P5 digital
    lensometer
   Zeiss LA 110 projection
    lensometer
lens-threading forceps
Lent laparoscope
Lent photolaparoscope
Lente silver nitrate probe
lenticular bone
lenticular carcinoma
lenticular cataract

lenticular degeneration
lenticular knife
lenticular loop
lenticular process
lenticular process of incus
lentigo (*pl.* lentigines)
lentigo maligna melanoma
lentigo senilis
lentigo simplex
Lentulo spiral drill
Lentz tracheotomy tube
Leon cobra cannula
Leon cobra tip
Leonard catheter
Leonard deep forceps
Leonard tube
Leonard-George position
Leone expansion screw
Leone eye procedure
Leopold operation
Lepird procedure
L'Episcopo hip reconstruction
L'Episcopo operation
L'Episcopo-Zachary shoulder
    procedure
Lepley-Ernst tracheal tube
leptomeningeal anastomosis
leptomeningeal carcinoma
leptomeningeal metastasis
leptomeningeal space
leptomeninges
Leptos pacemaker
Lere bone mill
Leriche hemostatic forceps
Leriche operation
Leriche spatula
Leriche tissue forceps
Leri-Weill disease
Leri-Weill syndrome
Lerman hinge brace
Lerman non-invasive halo
Lermoyez nasal punch
LeRoy clip-applying forceps
LeRoy disposable scalp clip
LeRoy infant scalp clip
LeRoy scalp clip-applying
    forceps
LeRoy ventricular catheter
LeRoy-Raney scalp clip
LES (lower esophageal
    sphincter)
Leser-Trelat sign

Lesgaft hernia
Lesgaft space
Lesgaft triangle
lesion architecture
lesion arrangement
lesion consistency
lesion distribution
lesion evolution
lesion identification
lesion margination
lesion milked out
lesion morphology
lesion of organ
lesion of tissue
lesion resected
lesion size
Leslie incision
Leslie-Ryan anterior axillary
    approach
L'Esperance erysiphake
L'Esperance needle
Lespinasse sutures
LESS (lateral electrical spine
    stimulation)
lesser alar cartilage
lesser arc injury of the carpus
lesser arterial circle of iris
lesser circle of iris
lesser curvature of stomach
lesser curvature ulcer
lesser ganglion of Meckel
lesser horn of hyoid bone
lesser multangular bone
lesser occipital nerve
lesser omentum
lesser ovarian vein
lesser palantine arteries
lesser palatine artery
lesser palatine canal
lesser palatine foramen
lesser palatine foramina
lesser palatine nerves
lesser pancreas
lesser peritoneal cavity
lesser peritoneal sac
lesser petrosal nerve
lesser petrosal nerve hiatus
lesser resection
lesser sac approach
lesser sac hernia
lesser sac technique
lesser sciatic foramen

lesser sciatic notch
lesser superficial petrosal nerve
lesser supraclavicular fossa
lesser trochanter
lesser trochanter fracture
lesser tubercle
lesser vestibular gland
lesser wing of sphenoid
lesser zygomatic muscle
Lester fixation forceps
Lester Jones operation
Lester Jones tube
Lester lens manipulator
Lester Martin modification of
    Duhamel procedure
Lester muscle forceps
Lester notch intraocular lens
Lester-Burch eye speculum
Lester-Jones operation
lethal concentration
lethal damage
lethal injury
lethal midline granuloma
Letournel acetabular fracture
    bone plate
Letournel approach
Letournel fracture plate
Letournel guideline
Letournel-Judet acetabular
    fracture classification
Letournel-Judet approach
letterbox technique
leucotomy (see leukotomy)
leukemia
leukemic hyperplastic gingivitis
leukemic infiltration
leukocyte infiltration
leukocytic infiltration
leukodontia
leukoedema
Leukofix surgical tape
Leukoflex surgical tape
leukokeratosis
leukokeratosis nicotina palati
leukoma
LeukoNet filter
leukonychia
leukopenia
leukoplakia
leukoplakia buccalis
leukoplakia lingualis
Leukopor surgical tape

leukorrhea
Leukos pacemaker
Leukosilk surgical tape
leukotome
  Bailey leukotome
  Dorsey transorbital leukotome
  Freeman transorbital
    leukotome
  Lewis leukotome
  Love leukotome
  McKenzie leukotome
  Nosik transorbital leukotome
  Tworek transorbital
    leukotome
leukotomy
Leukotrap red cell collector
Leung endoscopic nasal biliary
    drainage set
Leung thumb loss classification
Leurs nasal rasp
Leusch atraumatic obturator
Levant stone dislodger
Levant stone dislodger basket
LeVasseur-Merrill retractor
levator anguli oris muscle
levator ani muscle
levator ani syndrome
levator aponeurosis repair
levator aponeurosis surgery
levator check ligament
levator complex
levator costae muscle
levator dehiscence
levator disinsertion
levator glandulae thyroidea
    muscle
levator hernia
levator injury
levator labii superioris alaeque
    nasi muscle
levator labii superioris muscle
levator muscle of angle of mouth
levator nerve
levator palatini muscle
levator resection
levator scapulae syndrome
levator sling
levator snare
levator span
levator veli palatini muscle
levator-Mueller complex
    lengthening

LeVeen catheter
LeVeen dialysis shunt
LeVeen endarterectomy
LeVeen inflator
LeVeen peritoneal shunt
LeVeen peritoneovenous shunt
LeVeen valve
level of anesthesia
level of awareness
level of consciousness
level of pain
Levenson tissue forceps
lever
  Alexander bone lever
  Austin Moore-Murphy bone
    lever
  Bennett bone lever
  bone lever
  Bristow lever
  Buck-Gramcko bone lever
  Charnley femoral lever
  Cottle bone lever
  Hohmann bone lever
  Hohmann-Aldinger bone lever
  intranasal bone lever
  Kilner malar lever
  Lane bone lever
  Lange-Hofmann bone lever
  Murphy bone lever
  Murphy-Lane lever
  Tager lever
  Torpin obstetrical lever
  Verbrugge-Mueller bone lever
  Wagner bone lever
  Watson-Jones bone lever
lever pessary
leverage fracture
lever-type screwdriver
Levick 1-piece all-PMMA
    intraocular lens
Levin drill guide
Levin duodenal tube
Levin electrode
Levin tube
Levin tube catheter
Levin-Davol tube
Levine dislocation operation
Levine foreign body spud
Levine gradation of cardiac
    murmurs (*grades 1-6*)
Levine hip dislocation operation
Levine shunt

Levine sign
Levine-Harvey classification
Levinthal surgery retractor
Levis arm splint
Levitt eye implant
levobupivacaine anesthetic
levocardia
levocardiogram
levoduction of eye
levogram
levophase of angiogram
Levora fixation forceps
levorotatory scoliosis
levotransposed position
levotransposition of great
    arteries (L-transposition of
    great arteries)
Levret forceps
Levret maneuver
Levy-Rappel foot orthosis
Levy articulating retractor
Levy mold orthotics
Levy perineal retractor
Levy-Kuglen iris hook
Levy-Kuglen lens manipulator
Levy-Okun stripper
Lewicky cortex extractor
Lewicky formed cystotome
Lewicky instrument
Lewicky intraocular lens
Lewicky IOL spatula
Lewicky microlens hook
Lewicky needle
Lewicky self-retaining chamber
    maintainer
Lewicky threaded infusion
    cannula
Lewin baseball finger splint
Lewin bone clamp
Lewin bone-holding clamp
Lewin bone-holding forceps
Lewin bunion dissector
Lewin sesamoidectomy
    dissector
Lewin spinal-perforating forceps
Lewin splint
Lewin tonsil hemostat
Lewin tonsil screw
Lewin-Stern finger splint
Lewin-Stern thumb splint
Lewis cystometer
Lewis decompressor

Lewis dental mirror
Lewis expandable adjustable
    prosthesis
Lewis forceps
Lewis hemostat
Lewis intercalary resection
Lewis intramedullary device
Lewis laryngectomy tube
Lewis lead on ECG
Lewis lens loupe
Lewis lens scoop
Lewis leukotome
Lewis loupe
Lewis mouth gag
Lewis nail
Lewis nasal raspatory
Lewis operation
Lewis Pair-Pak needle
Lewis periosteal elevator
Lewis periosteal raspatory
Lewis position
Lewis rasp
Lewis raspatory
Lewis recording cystometer
Lewis retractor
Lewis scoop
Lewis septal forceps
Lewis snare
Lewis suspension device
Lewis tongue depressor
Lewis tonsillar hemostatic
    forceps
Lewis tonsillar screw
Lewis tonsillar snare
Lewis tube
Lewis ureteral stone isolation
    forceps
Lewis uvula retractor
Lewis-Chekofsky femur
    resection
Lewis-Leigh positive-pressure
    nonrebreathing valve
Lewis-Resnik punch
Lewis-Tanner esophagectomy
Lewis-Tanner procedure
Lewis-Tanner subtotal
    esophagectomy and
    reconstruction
Lewit stretch technique
Lewkowitz lithotomy forceps
Lewkowitz ovum forceps
Lewkowitz placental forceps

Lewy anterior commissure
  laryngoscope
Lewy bodies
Lewy chest holder
Lewy laryngoscope
Lewy laryngoscope holder
Lewy laryngostat
Lewy suspension device
Lewy suspension laryngoscope
Lewy Teflon glycerin-mixture
  injection needle
Lewy Teflon glycerin-mixture
  syringe
Lewy-Holinger Teflon injection
  needle
Lewy-Rubin needle
Lewy-Rubin Teflon glycerin-
  mixture injection needle
Lexan head
Lexan jacket
Lexer chisel
Lexer dissecting scissors
Lexer gouge
Lexer operation
Lexer osteotome
Lexer scissors
Lexer tissue forceps
Lexer-Durotip dissecting scissors
Leycom volume conductance
  catheter
Leydig drain
Leyla footplate
Leyla self-retaining brain
  retractor
Leyla self-retaining tractor bar
Leyla-Yasargil self-retaining
  retractor
Leyro-Diaz thoracic forceps
Lezinski Flex-HA PORP ossicular
  chain prosthesis
Lezius suction tube
LF (lingual fossa)
LFA (low-friction arthroplasty)
L-form osteotomy
LG bundle
LGA (large for gestational age)
LGSIL (low-grade squamous
  intraepithelial lesion)
L-hook electrosurgical probe
Libbe lower bowel evacuation
  device
Liberty CMC thumb brace

Liberty One splint
Libman-Sacks lesion
Lich extravesical technique
Lich operation
Lich procedure
lichen planus verrucosus
lichenified lesions
lichenoid amyloidosis
lichenoid graft-versus-host disease
Lich-Gregoir anastomosis
Lich-Gregoir kidney transplant
  surgery
Lich-Gregoir repair
Lich-Gregoir technique
Lich-Gregoire repair in kidney
  transplant surgery
Lichtenberg carbide-jaw needle
  holder
Lichtenberg corneal trephine
Lichtenberg keratome
Lichtenberg needle holder
Lichtenberg trephine
Lichtenstein hernial repair
Lichtenstein herniorrhaphy
Lichtenstein inguinal hernia repair
Lichtenstein mesh repair
Lichtenstein operation
Lichtman classification of
  Kienböck disease (stages I,
  II, IIIA, IIIB, IV)
Lichtman technique
Lichtwicz abdominal trocar
Lichtwicz antral cannula
Lichtwicz antral needle
Lichtwicz antral trephine
Lichtwicz antral trocar
Lichtwicz-Bier antral needle
LICO disposable penlight
LICO Hertel exophthalmometer
Lictenstein tension-free
  hernioplasty
lid block anesthesia
lid clamp
lid dermabrader
lid elevator
lid everter (*see* everter)
lid expressor
lid forceps
lid hook
lid knife
lid lag
lid margin

lid margin laceration
lid operation
lid plasty
lid plate
lid ptosis
lid ptosis operation
lid reflex
lid retraction
lid retractor
lid scalpel
lid speculum
lid surgery
lid suture operation
lid-cheek junctions
Liddicoat aortic valve retractor
Liddle aorta clamp
Liddle aortic clamp
LidFix speculum
lid-fracturing blepharoplasty
Lidge cement gun
Lidge reducer sleeve
lid-loading technique
Lido lift
Lido Multi Joint II isokinetic
    dynamometer
lidocaine drip
lidocaine hydrochloride
    anesthetic agent
lidocaine jelly
lid-retracting hook
lid-sharing technique
LIE (labioincisal edge,
    linguoincisal edge)
Lieberkühn crypts
Lieberkühn follicles
Lieberkühn gland
Lieberman abrader
Lieberman aspirating speculum
Lieberman forceps
Lieberman K-wire speculum
Lieberman MicroFinger
    manipulator
Lieberman phaco crusher
Lieberman proctoscope
Lieberman sigmoidoscope
Lieberman sigmoidoscope with
    swinging window
Lieberman suturing forceps
Lieberman tying forceps
Lieberman wire aspirating
    speculum with V-shape
    blades

Lieberman-Pollock double
    corneal forceps
Liebermeister groove
Lieb-Guerry cataract implant
    lens
Lieb-Guerry cataract lens
Lieb-Guerry eye knife
Lieb-Guerry forceps
Liebolt arthrodesis
Liebolt operation
Liebolt radioulnar technique
Liebreich probe
lienal artery
lienal vein
lienculus
lienectomy
lienocolic
lienopancreatic
lienophrenic
lienorenal ligament
Lieppman cystitome
Lieppman microcystitome
Lieppman sharp cystitome
Lieppman spatula
Lierberman K-Wire speculum
Liesegang flexible hysteroscope
Lieutaud body
lifeboat flap
LifeCare PCA3 Infusion System
    (PCA3)
Lifecare ventilator
Lifecath catheter
Lifecath peritoneal implant
Lifecore Restore wide diameter
    implant
LifeJet high-flow chronic dialysis
    catheter
Lifeline electrode
Life-Lok clamp
Lifemask infant resuscitator
Lifemed cannula
Lifemed catheter
Lifemed heterologous heart
    valve
Lifepak cardiac monitor
Lifepak defibrillator
LifePort infusion set
Lifesaver disposable resuscitator
    bag
life-saving form of therapy
life-saving suction tube
Lifestream centrifugal pump

Lifestream coronary dilatation
  catheter
Lifestream coronary dilation
  catheter
life-support measure
life-sustaining measure
life-sustaining procedure
Life-Tech flowmeter
life-threatening cancer
life-threatening complication
life-threatening condition
lift
  arm lift
  bicoronal forehead lift
  biplanar forehead lift
  breast lift
  brow lift
  brow-forehead lift
  buttocks lift
  canthal lift
  cervicofacial face lift
  chair lift
  chin lift
  corner mouth lift
  coronal brow lift
  coronal lift
  deep plane face-lift
  deep-plane lift
  Easy Pivot patient lift
  endoforehead lift
  endoforehead-endomidface
    lift
  endoforehead-periorbital-
    cheek lift
  endomidface lift
  endoscopic brow lift
  endoscopic forehead lift
  endoscopic subperiosteal
    forehead and midface lift
  endoscopic subperiosteal
    forehead lift
  endoscopic subperiosteal
    midface lift
  endoscopically assisted brow
    lift
  endotemporal lift
  endotemporal-endomidface lift
  eyebrow lift
  face lift
  facial subcutaneous lift
  FAME midface lift
  forehead lift

lift (*continued*)
  frontal lift
  functional lift
  Grice lift
  heave and lift
  heel lift
  HI-LOW power lift
  Hoyer lift
  inner thigh lift
  lateral vector lifts
  Lido lift
  M/L lift
  mask lift
  midface lift
  mirror lift
  modified anterior hairline
    forehead lift
  MTE dynamic lift
  neck lift
  open coronal brow lift
  palatal lift
  platform lift
  pneumatic chair lift
  Sabina lift
  scalp lift
  shoe lift
  subperiosteal brow lift
  subperiosteal malar cheek lift
  subperiosteal mid-face lift
  temporomandibular
    endoscopic lift
  thigh lift
  transblepharoplasty forehead
    lift
  transcoronal eyebrow lift
lift sheet
lift vector
lift-and-cut biopsy
Liga surgical clip
Ligaclip
Ligaclip MCA multiple-clip applier
Ligaclip surgical clip
ligament
  accessory collateral ligament
  accessory ligament
  acromioclavicular ligament
  acromiocoracoid ligament
  Adams advancement of round
    ligaments
  adipose ligament
  advancement of round
    ligament

ligament (*continued*)
  alar ligament
  Alexander shortening of
    round ligaments
  annular ligament
  anterior annular ligament
  anterior cruciate ligament
    (ACL)
  anterior ligament
  anterior mallear ligament
  anterior suspensory ligament
  anterior talocalcaneal
    ligament
  anterior talofibular ligament
  anterolateral ligament
  apical dental ligament
  arcuate ligaments
  arcuate popliteal ligament
  arcuate pubic ligament
  Arnold ligament
  axis ligament
  Berry ligament
  Bertin ligament
  bifurcated ligament
  Bigelow ligament
  brachioradial ligament
  Brodie ligament
  Broyle ligament
  calcaneofibular ligament
  calcaneonavicular ligament
  Caldani ligament
  Campbell ligament
  capitolunate ligament
  capsular ligament
  cardinal ligaments
  carpometacarpal ligament
  caudal ligament
  check ligament
  cholecystoduodenal ligament
  ciliary ligament
  circular dental ligament
  Cleland cutaneous ligament
  Cleland ligament
  collateral ligaments
  Colles ligament
  conoid ligament
  contracture of ligament
  Cooper ligaments
  coracoacromial ligament
  coracoclavicular ligament
  coracohumeral ligament
  coronary ligaments

ligament (*continued*)
  costoclavicular ligament
  costotransverse ligament
  cotyloid ligament
  Cowper ligament
  cricoarytenoid ligament
  cricothyroarytenoid ligament
  cricothyroid ligament
  cricotracheal ligament
  cruciate ligaments
  crural ligament
  cuneiform ligament
  cuneonavicular ligament
  deep transverse ligament
  deltoid ligament
  dentate ligament
  denticulate ligament
  dentoalveolar ligament
  detachment of ligament
  dorsal calcaneocuboid
    ligament
  dorsal carpal ligament
  dorsal intercarpal ligament
  dorsal ligament
  dorsal radiocarpal ligament
  dorsal radioulnar ligament
  dorsal talonavicular ligament
  duodenocolic ligament
  external calcaneoastragaloid
    ligament
  external cruciate ligament
  external lateral ligament
  external ligament
  fabellofibular ligament
  facial retaining ligaments
  falciform ligament
  femoral ligament
  Ferrein ligament
  fibular collateral ligament
  flaval ligament
  foveal ligament
  gastrocolic ligament
  gastrohepatic ligament
  gastrolienal ligament
  gastropancreatic ligament
  gastrophrenic ligament
  gastrosplenic ligament
  Gimbernat ligament
  gingival ligament
  gingivodental ligament
  glenohumeral ligaments
  glenoid ligaments

ligament (*continued*)
  Gore-Tex artificial knee
    ligament
  Gore-Tex ligament
  Grayson ligament
  Halsted ligament
  hammock ligament
  Henle ligament
  hepatic ligament
  hepatocolic ligament
  hepatocystocolic ligament
  hepatoduodenal ligament
  hepatogastric ligament
  hepatogastroduodenal
    ligament
  hepatophrenic ligament
  hepatorenal ligament
  hepatoumbilical ligament
  Hesselbach ligament
  Hey ligament
  Hueck ligament
  Humphry ligament
  Hunter ligament
  Huschke ligament
  hyoepiglottic ligament
  hyothyroid ligament
  hypothyroid ligament
  iliofemoral ligament
  iliotrochanteric ligament
  incudal ligament
  inferior transverse ligament
  infundibulopelvic ligament
  inguinal ligament
  interdental ligament
  interdigital ligament
  intermetatarsal ligament
  internal calcaneoastragaloid
    ligament
  internal crucial ligament
  internal lateral ligament
  interosseous ligament
  interosseous talocalcaneal
    ligament
  ischiocapsular ligament
  keystone ligament
  knee ligament
  labiomandibular ligament
  lacinate ligament
  laciniate ligament
  lacunar ligament
  Landsmeer ligaments
  lateral collateral ligaments

ligament (*continued*)
  lateral ligament
  lateral mallear ligament
  lateral maxillary ligament
  lateral thyrohyoid ligament
  lateral TMJ ligament
  laterocollateral ligament
  leaves of broad ligament
  levator check ligament
  lienorenal ligament
  Lisfranc ligament
  Lockwood ligament
  long external lateral ligament
  long plantar ligament
  longitudinal ligament
  lunotriquetral interosseous
    ligament (LTIL)
  lunotriquetral ligament
  mallear ligament
  mammillo-accessory ligament
  maxillary ligament
  medial collateral ligament
    (MCL)
  medial ligament
  medial palpebral ligament
  medial puboprostatic
    ligaments
  medial talocalcaneal ligament
  median arcuate ligament
  median thyrohyoid ligament
  meniscofemoral ligament
  middle umbilical ligament
  mucosal suspensory ligament
  nasolabial ligament
  nasomandibular ligament
  natatory ligament
  nephrocolic ligament
  nuchal ligament
  oblique popliteal ligament
  oblique retinacular ligament
  olecranon ligament
  Osborne ligament
  ovarian ligament
  palmar beak ligament
  palmar ligaments
  palmar radioulnar ligament
  pancreaticosplenic ligament
  patellar ligament
  pectinate ligament
  pectineal ligament
  peridental ligament
  peri-implant ligament

ligament (*continued*)
   periodontal ligament (PDL)
   Petit ligament
   petroclinoid ligament
   phrenicocolic ligament
   phrenicoesophageal ligament
   phrenicolienal ligament
   phrenicosplenic ligament
   phrenoesophageal ligament
   pisohamate ligament
   pisometacarpal ligament
   plantar calcaneocuboid
      ligament
   plantar ligaments
   posterior annular ligament
   posterior cruciate ligament
   posterior false ligament
   posterior incudal ligament
   posterior leaf of broad
      ligament
   posterior ligament
   posterior suspensory ligament
   posterior talocalcaneal
      ligament
   Poupart inguinal ligament
   proper ligament
   pubocapsular ligament
   pubocervical ligament
   pubofemoral ligament
   puboprostatic ligament
   pubovesical ligament
   pulmonary ligament
   radial collateral ligament
   radiocarpal ligament
   radioscapholunate ligament
   rectouterine ligament
   reflex ligament
   rhomboid ligament
   Robert ligament
   round ligament
   ruptured ligament
   sacrogenital ligament
   sacrospinous ligament
   sacrotuberous ligament
   sacrouterine ligament
   Sappey ligament
   scapholunate interosseous
      ligament
   scapholunate ligament
   Scarpa ligament
   shelving edge of Poupart
      ligament

ligament (*continued*)
   shelving portion of ligament
   short calcaneocuboid
      ligament
   short plantar ligament
   shortening of round ligament
   shortening of sacrouterine
      ligament
   Soemmering ligament
   sphenomandibular ligament
   spiral ligament
   splenocolic ligament
   splenorenal ligament
   sprain of ligament
   spring ligament
   sternoclavicular ligament
   sternocostal ligament
   Struthers ligament
   Stryker Dacron prosthetic
      ligament
   stylohyoid ligament
   stylomandibular ligament
   superior astragalonavicular
      ligament
   superior incudal ligament
   superior mallear ligament
   suspensory ligament
   sutural ligament
   talocalcaneal ligament
   talocalcaneonavicular
      ligament
   talofibular ligament
   talonavicular ligament
   tarsometatarsal ligament
   tear of ligament
   temporomandibular ligament
   tendinotrochanteric ligament
   thyroepiglottic ligament
   thyrohyoid ligament
   tibial collateral ligament
   tibiocollateral ligament
   tibiofibular ligament
   Toldt ligament
   torn ligament
   transseptal ligament
   transverse acetabular ligament
   transverse carpal ligament
   transverse humeral ligament
   transverse ligament
   transverse metacarpal
      ligament
   transverse metatarsal ligament

ligament (*continued*)
  transverse scapular ligament
  trapezoid ligament
  Treitz ligament
  triangular ligament
  true collateral ligament
  ulnar collateral ligament
  ulnar ligament
  ulnocarpal ligament
  umbilical ligament
  uteropelvic ligaments
  uterosacral ligament
  vaginal ligaments
  Valsalva ligaments
  ventricular ligament
  vesicouterine ligament
  vestibular ligament
  vocal ligament
  volar beak ligament
  volar carpal ligament
  volar ligament
  volar radiocarpal ligament
  web ligament
  Weitbrecht ligament
  Whitnall ligament
  Wieger ligament
  Winslow ligament
  Wrisberg ligament
  yellow ligament
  Zenotech synthetic ligament
  Zinn ligament
  zygomatic ligament
  zygomatic osteocutaneous
    ligament
  zygomatic retaining ligament
ligament augmentation
ligament augmentation device
    (LAD)
ligament button
ligament clamp
ligament graft
ligament of Henry
ligament of incus
ligament of knee
ligament of lens
ligament of malleus
ligament of Struthers
ligament of Toldt
ligament of Treitz
ligament of Wrisburg
ligament reconstruction
ligament reflecting edge

ligament reinsertion
ligament shelving edge
ligamenta (*sing.* ligamentum)
ligamenta flava forceps
ligamental anesthesia
ligamental mucosa
ligament-grasping forceps
ligamentous ankylosis
ligamentous calcification
ligamentous facial fence
ligamentous falx
ligamentous instability
ligamentous joint
ligamentous laxity
ligamentous strain
ligamentous structure
ligamentum (*pl.* ligamenta)
ligamentum flavum forceps
ligamentum teres femoris
ligamentum teres knife
ligamentum venosum
ligamentum-grasping forceps
Ligamentus Ankle orthotic
Ligamentus Ankle orthosis
ligand adhesive
Ligapak sutures
Lig-A-Ring separator
ligated and amputated
ligated and retracted
ligated and sectioned
ligated and transected
ligated with silk
ligated with transfixion sutures
ligate-divide-staple technique
ligating and dividing stapler
ligation
  aneurysm clip ligation
  artery ligation
  auricular ligation
  band ligation
  Bardenheuer ligation
  Barron hemorrhoid ligation
  Barron ligation
  bidirectional ligation
  bile duct ligation
  Blalock-Taussig shunt ligation
  bleeding site ligation
  common bile duct ligation
  Desault ligation
  direct ligation
  distal ligation
  elastic band ligation

ligation (*continued*)
  endoscopic band ligation (EBL)
  endoscopic esophagogastric
    variceal ligation
  endoscopic variceal ligation
    (EVL)
  esophageal band ligation
  hepatic artery ligation
  high ligation
  high saphenous vein ligation
  hunterian ligation
  hypogastric artery ligation
  inferior vena cava ligation
  interdental ligation
  Irving tubal ligation
  IVC ligation
  Kroner tubal ligation
  laparoscopic artery ligation
  laparoscopic tubal ligation
  laparoscopic varix ligation
  Linton radical vein ligation
  Linton subfascial ligation
  low ligation
  modified Irving-type tubal
    ligation
  open retroperitoneal high
    ligation
  Parkland tubal ligation
  parotid duct ligation
  parotid ligation
  patent ductus arteriosus
    ligation
  pedicle ligation
  pole ligation
  Pomeroy tubal ligation
  postureteral ligation
  rubber-band hemorrhoid
    ligation
  rubber-band ligation
  sigmoid sinus ligation
  sling ligation
  spermatic vein ligation
  stripping and ligation
  stump ligation
  surgical ligation
  suture ligation
  teeth ligation
  tooth ligation
  tracheal ligation
  transesophageal varix ligation
  transgastric ligation
  Trendelenburg vein ligation

ligation (*continued*)
  tubal ligation
  Uchida tubal ligation
  variceal band ligation
  varicocele ligation
  varicose vein stripping and
    ligation
  varix ligation
  vessel ligation
ligation and stripping
ligation device
ligation hemorrhoidectomy
ligation of artery
ligation of bleeders
ligation of hemorrhoid
ligation of vas deferens
ligation of vein
ligation of vessels
ligation suture technique
ligation sutures
ligator
  Arrequi laparoscopic knot
    pusher ligator
  Barron hemorrhoidal ligator
  Centrix PDQ ligator
  Clarke-Reich ligator
  DDV ligator
  endoscopic band ligator
  Gigator hemorrhoidal ligator
  hemorrhoidal ligator
  Lurz-Goltner ligator
  McGivney hemorrhoidal
    ligator
  RapidFire multiple band
    ligator
  rubber band ligator
  Rudd Clinic hemorrhoidal
    ligator
  Saeed 6-Shooter multi-band
    ligator
  Saeed multi-band ligator
  Saeed variceal ligator
  Salvatore umbilical cord
    ligator
  Sanford ligator
  Scanlan ligator
  Speedband multiple band
    ligator
  Stiegmann-Goff Clearvue
    endoscopic ligator
  Tucker hemorrhoidal ligator
  Twist-Mate ligator

ligature (*see also* sutures)
  anchor with suture ligature
  catgut ligature
  chain ligature
  chromic ligature
  Desault ligature
  elastic ligature
  elastic-thread ligature
  encircling tape ligature
  Erichsen ligature
  free ligature
  grass-line ligature
  hemostatic ligature
  interlacing ligature
  interlocking ligature
  kangaroo ligature
  McGraw elastic ligature
  Mersilene tape ligature
  occluding ligature
  orthodontic ligature
  plastic ligature
  Potts ligature
  provisional ligature
  proximal ligature
  pursestring ligature
  soluble ligature
  Speedband ligature
  steel ligature
  suboccluding ligature
  Surgiwip suture ligature
  suture ligature
  Tahoe Surgical Instruments ligature
  tape ligature
  terminal ligature
  wire ligature
ligature cannula
ligature carrier (*see also* carrier, ligature passer)
  Braun ligature carrier
  Cardio-Grip ligature carrier
  Cave-Rowe ligature carrier
  Cooley ligature carrier
  DeBakey ligature carrier
  deep ligature carrier
  Deschamps ligature carrier
  Favaloro ligature carrier
  Favaloro-Semb ligature carrier
  Fitzwater ligature carrier
  Kwapis ligature carrier
  Lahey ligature carrier
  linear in-line ligature carrier

ligature carrier (*continued*)
  Madden ligature carrier
  Mayo goiter ligature carrier
  Miya hook ligature carrier
  Raz double-prong ligature carrier
  Tauber ligature carrier
  Wangensteen deep ligature carrier
  Wangensteen ligature carrier
  Yasargil ligature carrier
  Young ligature carrier
ligature cutter
ligature director
ligature forceps
ligature guide
ligature hook
ligature knife
ligature needle
ligature passer (*see also* passer, ligature carrier)
ligature scissors
ligature set
ligature sutures
ligature tie wire
ligature tucker
ligature wire
ligature-carrying aneurysm forceps
ligature-carrying forceps
ligatureless bracket
ligature-locking pliers
ligature-passing instrument
ligature-tying pliers
light amplification
light and accommodation
light body impression material
light carrier
light coagulation
light coagulation for retinal detachment
Light Commander xenon illuminator
light cross-slot screwdriver
light electron microscope
light emitter
light exposure
light guide bundle
light microscope
light microscopy (LM)
light monitoring probe
light pen

light pipe
light pipe pick
light pipette
light wire appliance
light-around-wire technique
Lightblade laser
lighted retractor
lighted speculum
lighted stent
lighted stylet
lighted stylet-guided oral
    intubation
light-emitting diode (LED)
lightning cataract
Lightning high-speed vitrectomy
    handpiece
Lightstic 180 (or 360) fiberoptic
    laser
Light-Veley (*also* Dr. Light-
    Veley)
Light-Veley bur
Light-Veley cranial drill
Light-Veley drill
Light-Veley headrest
LightWare micro retractor
LightWear headlight
Ligmajet syringe
ligneous struma
lignocaine anesthetic agent
LIH hook pin
Liks Russian disk rotation heart
    valve
Lilienthal bullet probe
Lilienthal incision
Lilienthal rib guillotine
Lilienthal rib spreader
Lilienthal-Sauerbruch retractor
Lilienthal-Sauerbruch rib
    spreader
Liliequist membrane
Lillehei forceps
Lillehei pacemaker
Lillehei retractor
Lillehei valve forceps
Lillehei valve prosthesis
Lillehei valve-grasping forceps
Lillehei-Cruz-Kaster valve
    prosthesis
Lillehei-Kaster aortic value
    prosthesis
Lillehei-Kaster cardiac valve
    prosthesis

Lillehei-Kaster mitral valve
    prosthesis
Lillehei-Kaster pivoting disk
Lillehei-Kaster pivoting-disk
    prosthetic valve
Lillehei-Warden catheter
Lillie alligator scissors
Lillie antral trocar
Lillie attic cannula
Lillie attic hook
Lillie cannula
Lillie ear hook
Lillie frontal sinus probe
Lillie gouge
Lillie hook
Lillie intestinal forceps
Lillie knife
Lillie nasal speculum
Lillie probe
Lillie rectus tendon clamp
Lillie retractor
Lillie rongeur
Lillie scissors
Lillie sinus bone-nibbling
    rongeur
Lillie speculum
Lillie tissue-holding forceps
Lillie tonsillar knife
Lillie tonsillar scissors
Lillie trocar
Lillie-Killian septal bone forceps
Lillie-Killian septal forceps
Lillie-White tenaculum
Lilliput neonatal oxygenator
LIMA graft (left internal
    mammary artery graft)
limb and elbow protector
limb bud
limb deformity
limb duplication
limb girdle
limb holder
limb hypertrophy
limb lead
limb reduction abnormality
limb reduction anomaly
limb salvage
limb splint
limbal approach
limbal compression
limbal groove
limbal incision

limbal sutures
limbal-based flap
limb-body wall complex
Limberg local transposition flap
Limberg technique
Limberg-type cutaneous flap
limb-girdle dystrophy
limbic lobe
limbic suture
limb-lengthening procedure
limb-salvage procedure
limb-salvage surgery
limb-saving procedure
limb-saving technique
limb-sparing operation
limb-sparing procedure
limb-sparing surgery
limb-threatening problem
limbus (*pl.* limbi)
limbus alveolaris mandibulae
limbus alveolaris maxillae
limbus corneae
limitation of motion (LOM)
limitation of surgery
limited anterior small
    thoracotomy (LAST)
limited examination
limited fasciectomy
limited gastrectomy
limited hemorrhoidectomy
limited hepatectomy
limited joint motion
limited joint movement
limited obturator node
    dissection
limited pancreatectomy
limited prognosis
limited range of motion
limited resection
limited straight-leg raising
limited thoracotomy
limited-contact dynamic
    compression plate
limiting membrane
limiting plate
Lin clamp
Linatrix sutures
Linburg sign
Lincoff design of Storz scleral
    buckling balloon catheter
Lincoff eye implant
Lincoff lens sponge

Lincoff operation
Lincoff scleral sponge implant
Lincoff Silastic sponge
Lincoff sponge implant material
Lincoff sponge rod
Lincoln cardiovascular scissors
Lincoln deep scissors
Lincoln pediatric scissors
Lincoln-Metzenbaum scissors
Lindbergh pump
Lindblom position
Linde cryogenic probe
Linde cryoprobe
Linde walker
Lindegaard ratio
Lindell classification
Lindeman bone cutter
Lindeman bur
Lindeman cannula
Lindeman hysteroflator
Lindeman knee procedure
Lindeman needle
Lindeman procedure
Lindeman self-retaining uterine
    vacuum cannula
Lindeman transfusion needle
Lindeman-Silverstein Arrow tube
Lindeman-Silverstein tube
Lindeman-Silverstein ventilation
    tube
Lindemann bur
Lindesmith operation
Lindholm anatomical tracheal
    tube
Lindholm microlaryngoscope
Lindholm operating laryngoscope
Lindholm operation
Lindholm technique
Lindholm tendo calcaneus
    repair
Lindholm tracheal tube
Lindholm-Stille elevator
Lindley carbide-jaw needle
    holder
Lindley needle holder
Lindley scissors
Lindner anastomosis clamp
Lindner corneoscleral sutures
Lindner cyclodialysis spatula
Lindner cyclodialysis spoon
Lindner operation
Lindner sclerotomy

Lindner spatula
Lindorf lag screw
Lindorf position screw
Lindsay nail
Lindsay operation
Lindsay-Rea forceps
Lindstrom arcuate incision
    marker
Lindstrom Centrex lens
Lindstrom lens-insertion forceps
Lindstrom modified J-loop, 3-
    piece reverse PMMA optic
    intraocular lens
Lindstrom Star nucleus
    manipulator
Lindstrom-Chu aspirating
    speculum
Lindvall meniscectomy knife
Lindvall-Stille meniscal knife
line
    accretion line
    AC-PC line
    action line
    air-fluid line
    alveolar point-basion line
    alveolar point-nasal point line
    alveolar point-nasion line
    alveolobasilar line
    alveolonasal line
    Amberg lateral sinus line
    Amici line
    aneuploid cell line
    angular line
    anocutaneous line
    anorectal line
    anterior axillary line (AAL)
    anterior commissure-posterior
        commissure line
    antitension line (ATL)
    arcuate line
    Arlt line
    arterial line (A-line)
    arterial mean line
    atopic line
    auriculomastoid line
    axillary line
    azygoesophageal line
    B cell line
    basal line
    basinasal line
    Beau line
    biepicondylar line

line (*continued*)
    bimastoid line
    bisector line
    bismuth line
    bite line
    black line
    Blaschko line
    Bloominstadt lines
    blue line
    Bolton-nasion line
    Brodel bloodless line
    bunny scrunch lines
    Burton line
    calcification line
    calciotraumatic line
    Camper line
    canthomeatal line
    Cantlie line
    CaSki cell line
    cell line
    cement line
    cemental line
    cementing line
    central venous line
    central venous pressure line
    cerebral reference line
    cervical line (CL)
    Chamberlain line
    Chaussier line
    Clapton line
    cleavage line
    clivus canal line
    Codman ICP
        monitoring line
    colonic mucosal line
    Conradi line
    contour line
    Converse skin lines
    corneal iron line
    coronal suture lines
    coronoid line
    Correra line
    costoclavicular line
    costophrenic septal line
    Cox skin lines
    Crampton line
    craze line
    crease line
    crinkle line
    cross arch fulcrum line
    curved radiolucent line
    CVP line

line (*continued*)
cyma line
D line
Daubenton line
delay line
demarcation line
Dennie lines
Dennie-Morgan line
dentate line
dependency skin lines
developmental line
digastric line
division line
division skin lines
dominant skin lines
Donders line
dotted line
Douglas line
drool line
dynamic facial skin lines
dynamic line
Ebner line
Egger line
elastic line
elastic skin lines
emission line
epiphyseal line
equipotential line
established cell line
external oblique line
face line
Farre line
Farre white line
fat line
fat-density line
feathered-edged proximal
   finishing line
feather-edged proximal
   finishing line
Feiss line
femoral head line
Ferry line
fine line
fingerprint line
finish line
Fishgold line
Fleischner line
flexion skin lines
flexure line
flexure skin lines
fold line
foramen magnum line

line (*continued*)
force line
fracture line
Fraenkel line
Frankfort horizontal light line
Frankfort horizontal line
Fraunhofer lines
frontal zygomatic suture line
frontozygomatic suture line
frown line
Fraenkel white line
fulcrum line
Futcher line
gallbladder-vena cava line
Gant line
Garrett orientation line
gas density line
gaussian line
George line
germ line
gingival finishing line
gingival line
glabellar frown line
glabellar line
glabelloalveolar line
gluteal line
Granger line
gravitational line
gravitational skin lines
gravity line
gray line
growth arrest line
Gubler line
gum line
Hampton line
Harris growth arrest line
Harris line
Hawkins line
Helmholtz line
hemiclavicular line
hemostatic staple line
Hickman line
Hickman Silastic
   semipermanent central line
high lip line
high smile line
Hilgenreiner horizontal Y line
Hilgenreiner line
Hilgenreiner-Perkins line
Hilton white line
His line
Holdaway line

line (*continued*)

Holden line
hot line
Hudson line
Hudson-Stahli line
Hueter line
human AML cell line
humeral line
Hunter line
Hunter-Schreger line
Hylamer acetabular line
hyperfunctional facial lines
hyperfunctional glabellar line
hyperkinetic facial lines
iliopectinate line
iliopectineal line
imaginary line
incision line
incremental line
infraciliary line
infracostal line
infraorbitomeatal line
innominate line
intercondylar line
intermediate line
internal oblique line
interpupillary line
interspinal line
Intertech Perkin-Elmer gas
    sampling line
intertrochanteric line
intertubercular line
intravenous line
iron line
iron-Hudson-Stahli line
isodose line
isoelectric line
IV line
joint line
Jurkat T-cell line
Koehler line
Kaplan cardinal line
Kaplan oblique line
Keasbey line
Kerley A, B, C lines
Khodadoust line
Kilian line
knife-edged finishing line
labial line
lack of strongness to the jaw
    line
lambda suture line

line (*continued*)

lambdoid suture line
Langer cleavage line
Langer lines
Langhans line
Lanz line
lateral joint line
lead line
Linton line
lip line
load line
long line
Looser lines
lorentzian line
low lip line
lower midclavicular line
lucent line
lumbar gravitational line
lymphoblastoid cell line
M line
Mach line
MacNab line
mamillary line
mammary line
mare's tail line
marionette line
maximal tension skin lines
McGregor basal line
McGregor line
McKee line
McRae foramen magnum line
median line
Medigel Z Line
Mees line
mercurial line
methylene blue line
Meyer line
Meyerding spondylolisthesis
    classification line
midaxillary line
midclavicular line
midcostal line
middle cranial fossa line
Middleton line
midheel line
midhumeral line
midmalleolar line
midpoint to meatal line
midscapular line
midsternal line
milk lines
minimal tension skin lines

line (*continued*)
  Moloney line
  monitoring lines
  Monro line
  Monro-Richter line
  Morgan line
  Morris hepatoma cell line
  mucogingival line
  mucosal line
  Muehrcke line
  murine mesangial cell line
  myelomonocytic cell line
  mylohyoid line
  Nafion dryer line
  nasion-alveolar point line
  nasobasilar line
  nasolabial line
  natural line
  natural skin lines
  neonatal line
  neuronal cell line
  nipple line
  nuchal line
  Nelaton line
  Obersteiner-Redlich line
  oblique line
  obturator line
  occipitomastoid suture lines
  odontoid perpendicular line
  Ohngren line
  omphalospinous line
  orbital line
  orbitomeatal line
  orthostatic lines
  Owen line
  oxygen supply line
  palato-occipital line
  Pall leukogard-6 arterial line
  pararectal line
  paraspinal line
  parasternal line
  paravertebral line
  Pastia line
  pectate line
  pectinate line
  pectineal line
  percutaneous line
  peripheral arterial line
  Perkins vertical line
  physeal line
  PICC line
  Pickerill imbrication line

line (*continued*)
  pigmentary demarcation line
  pleural line
  pleuroesophageal line
  plumb line
  Poirier line
  Poupart line
  preaxillary line
  primary suture line
  principal line
  properitoneal fat line
  protrusive line
  psoas line
  pubic hair line
  pubococcygeal line
  pupillary line
  radio signal line
  radiocapitellar line
  radiolucent crescent line
  radiolucent line
  recessional line
  rectal floor line
  Reid base line
  rejection line
  relaxed skin tension lines
    (RSTLs)
  resonance line
  resting line
  Restylane/Perlane for
    fine/deep lines
  retentive fulcrum line
  reversal line
  Rex-Cantli-Serege line
  Richter-Monro line
  right midinguinal line
  Robson line
  rolandic line
  Roser-Nelaton line
  sacral arcuate line
  sacral horizontal plane line
  sagittal suture line
  Salter incremental lines
  Sampoelesi line
  scapular line
  Schoemaker line
  Schreger lines
  Schwalbe line
  sclerotic line
  scurvy line
  semilunar line
  septal lines
  Seraflo blood line

line (*continued*)

Shenton line
simian line
sinus line
skin lines
smoker's lines
S-N line
Snellen line
soleal line
Sorenson catheter for CVP line
spectral line
sphenofrontal suture line
sphenoparietal suture line
Spieghel line
Spigelius line
spinolamellar line
spinolaminar line
spinous interlaminar line
spiral line
squamous suture lines
stabilizing fulcrum line
sternal line
Stocker line
straight line
stress skin lines
stromal line
Stahli line
Stahli pigment line
subclavian line
subcostal line
subcutaneous fat lines
submammary line
supracondylar line
supracrestal line
survey line
suture line
Sydney line
sylvian line
Tatagiba line
T-cell line
teardrop line
temporal line
tender line
tension skin lines
tentorial line
terminal line
Terry line
Terry skin lines
Thompson line
Thorpe 4-mirror vitreous
    fundus laser line
tibiofibular line

line (*continued*)

Toldt line
TPN line
trapezoid line
triradiate line
trough line
Turk line
Twining line
Tycos pressure infusion line
Ullman line
V line
vena cava-gallbladder line
venous line
vertical corrugator line
vertical glabellar frown lines
Vesling line
vibrating line
visual line
Voigt line
von Ebner line
Wackenheim clivus canal line
water density line
Webster line
Webster skin lines
Wegner line
widening of suture lines
Winberger line
wrinkle line
Zoellner line
Zahn lines
zero line
Z-shaped suture line
zygomatic suture line
zygomaticofrontal suture lines
line angle
line focus principle
line incision
line infection
line of Bechterew
line of demarcation
line of direction
line of fixation
line of fracture
line of Gennari
line of Kaes
line of occlusion
line of Ogston
line of Toldt
line of Zahn
line test
line width
linea alba

linea alba buccalis
linea alba cervicalis
linea aspera
linea corneae senilis
linea glutea
linea semilunaris
linea temporalis
linea terminalis pelvis
linear accelerator unit
linear amputation
linear and whorled nevoid
    hypermelanosis
linear array scanner
linear array transducer
linear array-hydrophone
    assembly
linear atrophy
linear cautery
linear convex array scanner
linear craniectomy
linear defect
linear density
linear depression
linear erosion
linear fracture
linear graft
linear groove
linear incision
linear in-line ligature carrier
Linear KGT tonometer
linear lesion
linear marking
linear opacification
linear osteotomy
linear polyethylene sutures
linear potentiometer
linear raphe
linear scarring
linear scissor punch
linear scleroderma
linear skin incision
linear skin lesion
linear skull fracture
linear stapler
linear stapling device
linear strand
linear telangiectases
linear thermal expansion
linear transverse incision
linear ulcer
linear variable-differential
    transducer

linearly polarized near-infrared
    irradiation
linear-type echoendoscope
Lineback adenoidal punch
lined flap
Linell-Ljungberg classification
linen sutures
linen thread sutures
line-of-pull of the suspensions
    suture
lines of expression
lines of Retzius
lines of von Ebner
Lingeman 3-in-1 procedure drape
Lingeman kit
Lingeman TUR drape
lingua
lingua alba
lingua dissecta
lingua fissurata
lingua frenata
lingua geographica
lingua nigra
lingua plicata
lingua villosa alba
lingua villosa nigra
linguadental (*variant of*
    linguodental)
lingual alveolus
lingual angle
lingual aponeurosis
lingual approach
lingual apron
lingual arch
lingual arch-forming pliers
lingual artery
lingual attachment
lingual bar
lingual block
lingual bone
lingual branch
lingual button
lingual cavity
lingual clasp
lingual corpuscle
lingual cortical plate
lingual crossbite
lingual cyst
lingual development groove
    (LDG)
lingual dovetail
lingual duct

lingual embrasure
lingual flange
lingual flap
lingual folium
lingual follicle
lingual foramen
lingual forceps
lingual fossa (LF)
lingual frenulum
lingual frenum
lingual ganglion
lingual gingiva
lingual gland
lingual groove (LG)
lingual guillotine
lingual gyrus
lingual hemiatrophy
lingual hemorrhoid
lingual hypoplasia
lingual inclination
lingual lisp
lingual lobe
lingual lymph follicle
lingual lymph node
lingual mandibular periosteum
lingual movement
lingual mucoperiosteal flap
lingual mucosa
lingual nerve
lingual occlusion
lingual papilla
lingual papillae
lingual paralysis
lingual peak
lingual periosteum
lingual placement
lingual plate
lingual plexus
lingual quinsy
lingual raphe
lingual root
lingual saliva
lingual salivary gland depression
lingual septum
lingual shield
lingual spatula
lingual splint
lingual split-bone technique
lingual strap
lingual sulcus
lingual surface
lingual surface of tooth

lingual thyroid
lingual thyroid carcinoma
lingual tongue flap
lingual tonsillectome
lingual tonsillectomy
lingual tonsils
lingual trophoneurosis
lingual vein
lingual villi
lingual wire
linguine sign
lingula (*pl.* lingulae)
lingula mandibulae
lingula of mandible
lingular bronchus
lingular segment
lingulectomy
linguoalveolar
linguoalveolar area
linguoangular
linguoaxial
linguoaxiogingival
linguocervical ridge
linguoclination
linguoclusion
linguodental area
linguodistal (LD)
linguofacial trunk
linguogingival fissure
linguogingival groove
linguogingival ridge
linguogingival shoulder
linguoincisal (LI)
linguoincisal edge (LIE)
linguoincisal line angle
linguo-occlusal angle
linguo-occlusal line angle
linguopalatal contact
linguopapillitis
linguoplacement
linguoplasty
linguoplate
linguoplate major connector
linguoproximal
linguopulpal (LP)
lining anesthesia
lining mucosa
lining of organ
linitis plastica
Link anatomical hip
Link approximator
Link boutonnière finger splint

Link cementless hip prosthesis
Link cementless reconstruction
hip prosthesis
Link Endo-Model rotational knee
prosthesis
Link Lubinus SP II hip
prosthesis
Link MP hip noncemented
reconstruction prosthesis
Link stack split splint
Link toe splint
Link total hip
Linkow blade implant
Linkow dental implant
material
Link-Plus retention pin
Linnartz forceps
Linnartz intestinal clamp
Linnartz stomach clamp
Linn-Graefe iris forceps
Linscheid tendon transfer
Linscheid test
Linson electronic cell counter
Linton clamp
Linton elastic hose
Linton esophageal tube
Linton flap
Linton hook
Linton incision
Linton line
Linton operation
Linton procedure
Linton radical vein ligation
Linton retractor
Linton shunt
Linton splanchnic retractor
Linton stocking
Linton subfascial ligation
Linton tourniquet
Linton tourniquet clamp
Linton tube
Linton vein hook
Linton vein stripper
Linton vein stripping
Linton-Blakemore needle
Linton-Nachlas tube
Linton-Talbott operation
Lintro-Scan scanner
Linvatec absorbable screw
Linvatec Advantage shaver
Linvatec arthroscopic infusion
pump

Linvatec bioabsorbable
interference screw
Linvatec cannula
Linvatec driver
Linvatec blade resector
Linvatec meniscal anchor suture
Linx exchange guidewire
Linx extension wire
Linx guidewire extension
Linx guidewire extension
cardiac device
lion forceps
lion jaw tenaculum
lion-head clamp
Lionheart catheter
lion-jaw bone holder
lion-jaw bone-holding forceps
lion-jaw clamp
lion-jaw tenaculum
Lion's Claw grasper
Lion's Paw grasper
Liotta total artificial heart
Liotta-BioImplant LPB prosthetic
valve
Liotta-BioImplant prosthetic
valve
lip adhesion operation
lip and vermilion reconstruction
lip augmentation
lip biting
lip border advancement
lip bumper
lip clamp
lip competency
lip curtain
lip elevator
lip enhancement
lip flap
lip furrow band
lip habit appliance
lip hypertonia
lip incompetence
lip line
lip movements
lip of cervix
lip of mouth
lip paresthesia
lip pit
lip plumper
lip pucker
lip reconstruction
lip reflex

lip region
lip retractor
lip rounding
lip sclerotomy
lip shave
lip sulcus
lip sutures
lip switch flap
lip traction bow
lip tumor
lip vermilion
lipectomy
    abdominal lipectomy
    blunt suction lipectomy
    jowl reduction lipectomy
    orbital lipectomy
    suction lipectomy
    suction-assisted lipectomy
        (SAL)
    transjunctional lipectomy
    Tulip harvesting system for
        suction lipectomy
    ultrasound-assisted lipectomy
        (UAL)
Lipectron ultrasonic lancet
Lipectron ultrasonic scalpel
lipexeresis
lipid infusion
Lipikar balm
Lipikar oil
Lipisorb dressing
lip-lip flap
lip-nose complex
lipo layering technique
lipoaspirate
lipoaspirated material
lipoaspiration
lipoatrophy
lipoblastoma
lipocele
lipocontour
lipocontouring
lipocytic lesion
lipodissector (*see* dissector)
lipodystrophy
lipofilling
lipogenic tumor
lipogranuloma
lipogranulomatosis
lipohypertrophic mass
lipohypertrophy
lipoid granuloma

lipoid histiocytoma
lipoid hyperplasia
lipoid material
lipoid nephrosis
lipoidosis
lipoinfiltration
lipoinjection technique
lipolysis
lipoma (*pl.* lipoma, lipomata)
    atypical lipoma
    conjunctival lipoma
    hypopharyngeal lipoma
    laryngeal lipoma
    posttraumatic lipoma
    salivary lipoma
    spindle cell lipoma
    subcutaneous lipoma
lipoma arborescens
lipoma aspiration
lipomatosis
lipomatous ileocecal value
lipomatous infiltration
lipomatous lesion
lipomatous-like tissue
lipomelanic reticulosis
lipomusculoplasty
lipomyxoma
liponecrosis
liponecrotic pseudocyst
lipophagic granuloma
lipoplasty
    blunt suction-assisted
        lipoplasty
    Fischer aspirative lipoplasty
    full-leg circumferential
        lipoplasty
    Illouz aspirative lipoplasty
    Kesselring aspirative
        lipoplasty
    power-assisted lipoplasty
        (PAL)
    Schrudde aspirative lipoplasty
    Teimourian aspirator
        lipoplasty
    traditional lipoplasty
    ultrasound-assisted lipoplasty
        (UAL)
liporestructure
liposarcoma
liposculpture
liposculpturing
liposhaver

lipostructure
liposuction
    extended liposuction
    massive all layer liposuction
        (MALL)
    submental liposuction
    syringe-assisted liposuction
    tumescent liposuction
    ultrasonic liposuction
    ultrasound liposuction
    ultrasound-assisted CAST
        liposuction
    ultrasound-assisted liposuction
    wet technique liposuction
liposuction cannula
liposuction divot
liposuction fat fillant implant
liposuction technique
liposuction-assisted
liposuctioning
liposurgery
lipotropic agent
Lippes intrauterine loop
Lippes loop intrauterine device
    (Lippes loop IUD)
Lippman hip prosthesis
Lippy incus prosthesis
Lippy modified prosthesis
Lipschiff knife
Lipschwitz needle
Lipscomb orthopedic procedure
Lipscomb technique
Lipscomb-Anderson drill guide
Lipscomb-Anderson procedure
Lipscomb-Henderson-Elkins
    technique
Lipsett operation
Lipsett scissors
Lipshultz epididymovasostomy
    microdissection scissors
lip-splitting incision
lipstick sign
lip-sucking habit crib
liquefaction
liquefaction necrosis
liquefaction of fat
liquefaction of vitreous
liquefactive necrosis
LiquiBand topical wound-
    closure adhesive
liquid biopsy
liquid conductor Bovie

liquid extraction
liquid intake
liquid nitrogen
liquid organic dye laser
liquid vitreous-aspirating
    cannula
Liquiderm dressing
Liquiderm liquid adhesive
Liquiderm liquid healing
    bandage
Lisch nodules
LISCO sponge
Lisfranc amputation
Lisfranc ankle dislocation
Lisfranc articulation
Lisfranc disarticulation
Lisfranc dislocation
Lisfranc foot fracture
Lisfranc fracture
Lisfranc fracture-dislocation
Lisfranc joint
Lisfranc ligament
Lisfranc operation
Lissauer bundle
Lissauer paralysis
Lissauer tract
Lissauer zone
Lister bandage
Lister bandage scissors
Lister conjunctival forceps
Lister dressing
Lister forceps
Lister knife
Lister lens manipulator
Lister mules
Lister technique
Lister tubercle
Lister-Burch eye speculum
Liston amputating knife
Liston amputation knife
Liston bone-cutting forceps
Liston forceps
Liston knife
Liston operation
Liston phalangeal knife
Liston plaster-of-Paris scissors
Liston rongeur
Liston scissors
Liston shears
Liston splint
Liston-Key bone-cutting forceps
Liston-Key-Horsley rib shears

Liston-Key-Horsley forceps
Liston-Littauer bone-cutting
  forceps
Liston-Littauer rongeur
Liston-Luer-Whiting rongeur
Liston-Ruskin bone-cutting
  rongeur
Liston-Ruskin shears
Liston-Stille bone-cutting forceps
Lite blade
Lite hip cast
Liteflex intraocular lens
liter (l or L)
lith II pacemaker
lithiasis
lithium pacemaker
lithium-powered pacemaker
lithocenosis
lithoclast
Lithoclast lithotripter
Lithoclast lithotriptor
lithocystotomy
lithodialysis
Lithognost flashlamp pulsed dye
  laser
litholabe
litholapaxy
    Bigelow litholapaxy
    endoscopic bladder
      litholapaxy
litholysis
litholyte
litholytic
lithometer
lithonephria
lithonephritis
lithonephrotomy
lithoscope
Lithospec lithotriptor
Lithostar lithotripsy unit
Lithostar lithotripter
Lithostar lithotriptor
Lithostar nonimmersion
  lithotriptor
lithotome
lithotomist
lithotomy
    bilateral lithotomy
    celsian lithotomy
    Celsus lithotomy
    dorsal lithotomy
    high lithotomy

lithotomy (*continued*)
  lateral lithotomy
  marian lithotomy
  median lithotomy
  mediolateral lithotomy
  percutaneous
    cholangioscopic lithotomy
  percutaneous transhepatic
    cholangioscopic lithotomy
    (PTCSL)
  perineal lithotomy
  Petersen lithotomy
  prerectal lithotomy
  rectal lithotomy
  rectovesical lithotomy
  suprapubic lithotomy
  Trendelenburg-position
    lithotomy
  vaginal lithotomy
  vesical lithotomy
  vesicovaginal lithotomy
lithotomy forceps
lithotomy legholder
lithotomy position
lithotomy procedure
lithotomy-Trendelenburg
  position
lithotony
lithotresis
lithotripsy
  biliary lithotripsy
  blind lithotripsy
  candela lithotripsy
  cystoscopic electrohydraulic
    lithotripsy
  dry lithotripsy
  (EHL)
  electrohydraulic shock wave
    lithotripsy (ESWL)
  endoscopic electrohydraulic
    lithotripsy
  endoscopic pulsed dye laser
    lithotripsy
  endoscopic-controlled
    lithotripsy
  external shock wave
    lithotripsy
  extracorporeal piezoelectric
    shock wave lithotripsy
  extracorporeal shock wave
    lithotripsy (ESWL)
  intracorporeal laser lithotripsy

lithotriptor (*continued*)
tubeless lithotriptor
ultrasonic lithotriptor
water cushion lithotriptor
Wilson-Cook mechanical
  lithotriptor
lithotriptor machine
lithotriptor probe
lithotriptoscope
lithotriptoscopy
lithotrite
  Alcock lithotrite
  Alcock-Hendrickson
    lithotrite
  Bigelow lithotrite
  Hendrickson lithotrite
  Keyes lithotrite
  Loewenstein lithotrite
  Lowsley lithotrite
  Marmite lithotrite
  Ravich lithotrite
  Reliquet lithotrite
  Teale gorget lithotrite
  Teevan lithotrite
  Thompson lithotrite
  Wolf lithotrite
lithotrity
LITT forceps
Littauer bone-cutting forceps
Littauer cilia forceps
Littauer ciliary forceps
Littauer dissecting scissors
Littauer ear polyp forceps
Littauer ear-dressing forceps
Littauer Junior suture scissors
Littauer nasal-dressing forceps
Littauer rongeur
Littauer scissors
Littauer stitch scissors
Littauer suture scissors
Littauer-Liston bone-cutting
  forceps
Littauer-Liston forceps
Littauer-West cutting forceps
Littauer-West rongeur
Littell cannula
little head of mandible
Little intraocular lens implant
Little Leaguer's elbow
Little Leaguer's shoulder
Little retractor
Little technique

Little-Arnott tripod intraocular
  lens
Littleford introducer
Littleford-Spector introducer
Littler carrying scissors
Littler dissecting scissors
Littler neurovascular island flap
Littler operation
Littler procedure
Littler scissors
Littler suture carrying scissors
Littler technique
Littler-Cooley technique
Littler-Eaton reconstruction
Littlewood amputation
Littlewood operation
Littlewood tissue forceps
Littmann defibrillation pad
Littmann ECG electrode
Litton dental handpiece
Littre glands
Littre hernia
Littre operation
Littre sutures
Littre-Richter hernia
Litvak-Pereyra ligature needle
Litwak aortic bypass
Litwak cannula
Litwak clamp
Litwak left atrial-aortic bypass
Litwak mitral valve scissors
Litwak utility scissors
Litwin dissecting scissors
Lively splint
liver abscess
liver allograft
liver allotransplantation
liver bed
liver biopsy
liver biopsy needle
liver biopsy set
liver cell adenoma
liver coil
liver damage
liver death
liver disease
liver distention
liver donation
liver edge
liver enlargement
liver failure
liver flap

liver flap sign
liver function
liver hanging maneuver
liver injury
liver involvement
liver laceration
liver lobe
liver lobule
liver metastasis
liver nodule
liver operation
liver recipient
liver resection
liver retractor
liver scan
liver scintiphoto
liver shadow
liver shock
liver span
liver spot
liver tender
liver transplant
liver transplantation
liver tumor
liver wire ablation
liver, kidneys, and spleen (LKS)
liver, spleen, and kidneys (LSK)
liver-holding clamp
Livermore trocar
Livernois lens-holding forceps
Livernois pickup and folding
     forceps
Livernois-McDonald forceps
Liverpool elbow implant
Liverpool knee prosthesis
liver-spleen scan
Livewire Duo-Decapolar
     catheter
Livewire TC Compass ablation
     catheter
livid cyanosis
lividity
Livierato reflex
Livierato sign
living donor partial
     hepatectomy
living homograft
living relative donor
living suture
living-related donor
living-related donor
     transplantation

living-related liver
     transplantation (LRLT)
living-related small bowel
     transplant
Livingston bar
Livingston forceps
Livingston intramedullary bar
Livingston triangle
Livingstone therapy
livor mortis
Lizar operation
LKB/Wallach scintillation
     counter
LKS (liver, kidneys, and
     spleen)
LLC (long-leg cast)
LLETZ/LEEP loop electrode
LLL (left lower lobe)
LLL brace
Llobera fixation forceps
Llorente dissecting forceps
Lloyd adapter
Lloyd adapter counterbore
Lloyd bronchial catheter
Lloyd Davis modified lithotomy
     position
Lloyd double catheter
Lloyd esophagoscopic catheter
Lloyd flexion distraction table
Lloyd nail driver
Lloyd nail extractor
Lloyd tube
Lloyd Davies clamp
Lloyd Davies occlusion forceps
Lloyd Davies rectal scissors
Lloyd Davies scissors
Lloyd Davies clamp
Lloyd Davies operation
Lloyd Davies sigmoidoscope
Lloyd Davies stirrups
Lloyd-Roberts clubfoot
     procedure
Lloyd-Roberts fracture
     technique
Lloyd-Roberts osteotomy
Lloyd-Roberts-Lettin technique
LLQ (left lower quadrant)
LMA (laryngeal mask airway)
LMA position (left
     mentoanterior position)
LMA-Unique disposable
     laryngeal mask airway

LMP position (left
  mentoposterior position)
LMT position (left
  mentotransverse position)
L'Nard long opponens hand and
  wrist orthosis
L'Nard Multi-Podus orthosis
L'Nard thoracolumbosacral orthosis
Lo Bak spinal support
Lo Bak spinal support prosthesis
LOA position (left
  occipitoanterior position)
load line
load-bearing graft
load-deflection rate
loading applicator
loading dose
load-sharing
lobar atelectasis
lobar atrophy
lobar emphysema
lobar hemorrhage
lobar hyperplasia
lobar pneumonia
lobar resection
lobar sclerosis
lobe enlargement
lobe of brain
lobe of liver
lobe of lung
lobe of pituitary gland
lobe of prostate
lobe of thyroid gland
lobe resection
lobectomy
  deep lobectomy
  Falconer lobectomy
  hepatic lobectomy
  ipsilateral thyroid lobectomy
  ipsilateral total lobe and
    contralateral subtotal
    lobectomy
  pulmonary lobectomy
  sleeve lobectomy
  temporal lobectomy
  thyroid lobectomy
  total ipsilateral lobectomy
  total lobectomy
  unilateral lobectomy
lobectomy forceps
lobectomy of lung
lobectomy of prostate

lobectomy of thyroid
lobectomy scissors
lobectomy tourniquet
lobed placenta
lobe-grasping forceps
lobe-holding forceps
Lobell splinter forceps
Lobenstein-Tarnier forceps
lobotomy
  frontal lobotomy
  prefrontal lobotomy
  radical prefrontal lobotomy
  transorbital lobotomy
lobotomy electrode
lobotomy needle
lobotomy of brain
Lobstein ganglion
lobster bone-reduction forceps
lobster hand deformity
lobster-claw deformity
lobster-claw foot
lobster-claw hand
lobster-claw operation
lobster-tail catheter
lobster-type clamp
lobular architecture of liver
lobular carcinoma in situ
lobular hyperplasia
lobular patches of atelectasis
lobular pattern
lobulated contour
lobulated kidney
lobulated mass
lobulated tongue
lobulated tumor mass
lobulation
lobule
lobule of epididymis
lobule of Zuckerkandl
lobulette
lobulus (pl. lobuli)
LOC guidewire extension
local abscess
local analgesia
local anaphylaxis
local anesthesia
local anesthetic
local disease
local epineurotomy
local excision
local exhaust ventilation
local field block

local flap
local gradient coil
local hepatectomy
local infection
local infiltration
local infiltrative anesthesia (LIA)
local injection
local instillation
local invasion
local involvement
local irradiation
local leakage
local lesion
local metastasis
local muscle flap
local nerve block
local radiation therapy
local radical resection
local reaction
local recurrence
local recurrence of carcinoma
local rotation flap
local skin flap
local standby anesthesia
    technique
local surgery
local therapy
local tissue infiltration
local tumor extension
local vasodilation
Localio procedure
Localio sacral tumor procedure
Localio-Francis-Rossano resection
localization
localization films
localization of disease
localization signal
localization study
localization technique
localization test
localized abdominal sign
localized abscess
localized adiposity
localized advancement flap
localized cancer
localized defect
localized inflammation
localized lesion
localized leukocyte mobilization
localized mass
localized mucocutaneous
    candidiasis

localized neurological sign
localized nodular tenosynovitis
localized pain
localized plaque formation
localized prostate cancer
localized radiotherapy
localized scleroderma
localized sepsis
localized signs of weakness
localized tenderness
localized vitiligo
localizer
    Berman localizer
    FlashPoint optical localizer
    Risser localizer
    Roper-Hall localizer
    Suetens-Gybels-Vandermeulen
        angiographic localizer
    Urrets-Zavalia localizer
    Wildgen-Reck localizer
localizer cast
localizing electrode
localizing neurological sign
localizing probe
localizing sign
locally advanced condition
locally advanced disease
locally invasive congenital
    cellular blue nevus of scalp
locator (see also metal locator,
    magnet)
    apex locator
    ASIS femoral head locator
    Berman foreign body locator
    Berman metal locator
    Berman-Moorhead metal
        locator
    Bronson-Turner foreign body
        locator
    foreign body locator
    Gill-Thomas locator
    metal locator
    Neosono MC apex locator
    nerve locator
    Odontometer electronic apex
        locator
    Porex nerve locator
    Root ZX spec locator
    Roper-Hall locator
    saddle locator
    Sweet locator
lochia alba

lochia cruenta
lochia purulenta
lochia rubra
lochia sanguinolenta
loci (*sing.* locus)
lock finger
lock knee
lock needle
lock stitch
lock sutures
Locke bone clamp
locked joint
locked knee
locked septal displacement
locked sutures
Lockhart-Mummery probe
Lockhart-Mummery retractor
locking clamp
locking device
locking nut
locking of joint
locking prosthesis
locking reconstruction plate
locking running sutures
locking screw
locking stitch
locking stylet
locking sutures
lockjaw
Locklin stitch scissors
lock-stitch sutures
Lockwood clamp
Lockwood intestinal forceps
Lockwood ligament
Lockwood tendon
Lockwood tissue forceps
Lockwood-Allis intestinal
    forceps
Lockwood-Allis tissue forceps
locomotor ataxia
loculated abscess
loculated effusion
loculated emphysema
loculated empyema
loculated fluid
loculated pleural effusion
loculation syndrome
locus (*pl.* loci)
Loeffler (*also* Löffler)
Loeffler sutures
Loeffler-Ballard incision
Loening stomach tube

Loesche classification
Loetwig ganglion
Loewenthal bundle
Loewi suspension device
Lofberg thyroid retractor
Lofberg vaginal speculum
Löffler (*see* Loeffler)
Lofric disposable urethral
    catheter
Lofstrand brace
Lofstrand crutches
Logan bow support
Logan box
Logan dissector
Logan elevator
Logan lacrimal sac self-retaining
    retractor
Logan lip traction bow
Logan periosteal elevator
Logan retractor
Logan traction bow
loge de Guyon ulnar nerve block
Logol solution
Logracino bunionectomy
logrolling maneuver
Loehlein diameter
Loehlein operation
Loehlein-Baehr lesion
Lok-it screwdriver
Lok-screw double-slot
    screwdriver
Lok-screw screwdriver
lollipop bite-block
LOM (limitation of motion)
Lombard mastoid rongeur
Lombard-Beyer rongeur
Lombard-Beyer rongeur forceps
Lombard-Boies rongeur
Lombart radioscope
Lombart tonometer
Londermann corneal trephine
Londermann operation
London College foil carrier
London elbow hinge
London forceps
London narrow-bladed retractor
London prosthesis
London retractor
London tissue forceps
London total elbow
lone atrial fibrillation
Lone Star retractor

long abductor muscle
long abductor tendon
long above-elbow cast
long ACE fixed-wire balloon
 catheter
long adductor muscle
long- and short-level rotational
 manipulation
long arm navicular cast
long arm splint
long atraumatic retractor
long axis of kidney
long axis scan
long axis view
Long Beach stereotactic robot
long below-elbow cast
long blunt nerve hook
long bone fracture
long bone reconstruction
long bone survey
Long Brite Tip guiding catheter
long ciliary arteries
long ciliary nerves
long coarse bur
long cone technique
long double upright brace
long extensor muscle
long external lateral ligament
long face syndrome
long fibular muscle
long finger
long flexor muscle
long gyrus of insula
Long hysterectomy forceps
long intestinal tube
Long Island College Hospital
 placenta forceps
Long Island forceps
long leg cylinder cast
long leg immobilizer
long leg plaster cast
long leg posterior molded splint
long leg splint
long leg walking cast
long lesion
long levator muscle
long limb gastric bypass
long nail-mounted drill guide
long needle
long nerve of Bell
long oblique incision
long occluder

long palate hook
long palmar muscle
long periosteal elevator
long peroneal muscle
long philtrum
long plantar ligament
long posterior ciliary artery
long posterior ciliary axis
long process of incus
long radial extensor muscle
long rectangular flap
long rotator muscles
long scalpel
long scissors
long segment spinal fusion
Long stitch scissors
long thoracic nerve
long tissue forceps
Longacre graft augmentation
long-arm cast (LAC)
long-armed cast
long-bore collimator
long-cone radiograph
Longdwel catheter
Longdwel catheter needle
Longdwel needle
Longdwel Teflon catheter
longer-segment obstruction
long-face syndromes
long-handle curet
long-handle offset gouge
Longhem prosthesis
longhorn-shaped incision
longissimus muscle
longitudinal aberration
longitudinal arc of skull
longitudinal arch
longitudinal arch supports
longitudinal arteriogram
longitudinal axis
longitudinal bundle
longitudinal cerebral fissure
longitudinal choledochotomy
longitudinal cystotomy
longitudinal diameter
longitudinal enterotomy
longitudinal esophageal stricture
longitudinal fissure of cerebrum
longitudinal fold
longitudinal fold of duodenum
longitudinal fracture
longitudinal incision

longitudinal laceration
longitudinal ligament
longitudinal medial bundle
longitudinal melanonychia
longitudinal midline incision
longitudinal muscle
longitudinal muscle of tongue
longitudinal myotomy
longitudinal nerves
longitudinal plane
longitudinal presentation
longitudinal raphe
longitudinal raphe of tongue
longitudinal ridge of hard palate
longitudinal side-to-side
    anastomosis
longitudinal sinus
longitudinal spinal bar
longitudinal sulcus
longitudinal suture of palate
longitudinal sutures
longitudinalis inferior muscle
longitudinalis superior muscle
long-jaw basket forceps
long-leg brace
long-leg cast (LLC)
long-limb gastric artery bypass
Longmire anastomosis
Longmire operation
Longmire valvulotome
Longmire-Gutgeman gastric
    reconstruction
Longmire-Mueller curved
    valvulotome
Longmire-Storm clamp
long-nose retriever snare
long-nosed sphincterotome
Longo hemorrhoidectomy
long-skin flap blepharoplasty
long-span rigid plate
long-standing condition
long-stretch bandage
long-term ambulatory physiologic
    surveillance monitor
long-term bone-instrumentation
    interface
long-term central venous access
    catheter placement
long-term epidural
    catheterization
long-term internal jugular
    catheter

long-term oxygen therapy
long-term tip graft camouflage
long-tract sign
Longuet incision
Longuet operation
longus capitis muscle
longus colli muscle
long-wave irradiation
long-wearing contact lens
Lonnecken tube
Look capsular polisher
Look coaxial flexible disposable
    cannula
Look cortex extractor
Look cystotome
Look I&A coaxial cannula
Look irrigating lens loupe
Look micropuncture device
Look retrobulbar needle
Look sutures
Loomis ring
loop (*see also* loupe)
    2-angled polypropylene loop
    Adler tripronged lens error
        loop
    afferent loop
    air-filled loop
    alpha loop
    alpha sigmoid loop
    Amenabar lens loop
    angled lens loop
    angled nucleus removal loop
    arterial loop
    Atwood loop
    Aus-Jena-Gullstrand lens loop
    Axenfeld nerve loop
    Beck twisted wire snare loop
    Beebe lens loop
    Berens lens loop
    Berger loop
    Berget lens loop
    Biebl loop
    Billeau ear loop
    Billeau Teflon-coated loop
    Billeau-House ear loop
    bipolar urological loop
    Blair-Ivy loop
    blind loop
    bowel loop
    Bricker loop
    Bunnell finger loop
    Bush stabilized cutting loop

loop (*continued*)

Callahan lens loop
Cannon endarterectomy loop
capillary loop
Castroviejo lens loop
central chemoreflex loop
cerebral-sacral loop
cervical loop
Clayman-Knolle irrigating lens loop
Clayman-Knolle lens loop
closed loop
colonic loop
colostomy loop
contiguous loop
Cordonnier ureteroileal loop
cutting loop
Diaflex retrieval loop
diathermic loop
distended afferent loop
double-reverse alpha sigmoid loop
Duncan loop
duodenal loop
ear loop
efferent loop
electrodes loop
Elschnig-Weber loop
endarterectomy loop
expressor loop
finger loop
Flynn lens loop
foreign body loop
FormFlex lens loop
Gamma transverse colon loop
Gerdy interauricular loop
Gill-Welsh lens loop
Gill-Welsh-Morrison lens loop
Gobin-Weiss loop
Greenwald cutting loop
hairpin loop
haptic loop
Henle loop
House wire loop
House-Billeau ear loop
Hyrtl loop
ileal loop
Ilg lens loop
interauricular loop
intestinal loop
intracapsular lens loop
irrigating lens loop

loop (*continued*)

irrigating vectis loop
Ivy loop
Ivy wire loops
jejunal interposition of Henle loop
jejunal loop
jejunal Roux-en-Y loop
jejunum loop
Kirby intracapsular lens loop
Kirby intraocular lens loop
Kirby lens loop
Kleinsasser lens loop
Knapp lens loop
Knolle-Pearce irrigating lens loop
Knolle-Pearce lens loop
Kraff nucleus lens loop
Lemoine-Searcy fixation anchor loop
Lempert-Storz lens loop
lenticular loop
Lewis lens loop
Lippes intrauterine loop
Look irrigating lens loop
lyodura loop
maxi-vessel loops
McKenzie leukotomy loop
Medevice surgical loop
Meyer temporal loop
nephronic loop
N-shaped sigmoid loop
nuclear removal loop
nuclear delivery loop
nylon loop
Oculus lens loop
Olympus resectoscope loop
open loop
ostomy loop
Pearce-Knolle irrigating lens loop
peduncular loop
peripheral chemoreflex loop
physiologic endometrial ablation/resection loop (PEARL)
platinum loop
pressure length loop
prosthetic loop
puborectalis loop
Ransford loop
re-entrant loop

loop (*continued*)

resectoscope cutting loop
retrieval loop
Roux-en-Y loop
rubber vessel loop
Sarns safety loop
Schroeder tenaculum loop
scoops and loops
sentinel loop
sigmoid loop
Silastic loop
Simcoe double-end lens loop
Simcoe II posterior chamber
    nucleus delivery loop
Simcoe nucleus lens loop
snare loop
Snellen lens loop
soft wire loop
spring wire loop
Stierlen lens loop
Stoerck loop
Storz Universal lens loop
subclavian loop
Surgitite ligating loop
Sut-Fit loop
Teflon Silastic loop
tenaculum hook loop
terminal ileal loop
thyroid loop
toe loop
tonsillar loop
tonsillectome loop
tripronged loop
twisted wire loop
twisted wire snare loop
unipolar cutting loop
Uresil radiopaque silicone-
    band vessel loops
ureteroileal loop
V. Mueller vascular loop
vaginal speculum loop
vascular loop
vectis loop
vector loop
Vedder loop
venous loop
ventricular loop
vessel loop
Vieussens loop
Visitec nucleus removal loop
Ward-Lempert lens loop
Weber-Elschnig lens loop

loop (*continued*)

Wilder lens loop
wire loop
loop & hook strapping
loop ball electrode
loop choledochojejunostomy
loop colostomy
loop colostomy set
loop curet
loop diathermy cervical
    conization
loop distribution
loop diuretics
loop electrocautery excision
    procedure (LEEP)
loop electrode
loop electrosurgical excision
    procedure (LEEP)
loop electrosurgical excision
    procedure conization
loop esophagojejunostomy
loop fixation
loop forearm graft
loop gastric bypass
loop gastric bypass procedure
loop gastric bypass technique
loop gastrojejunostomy
loop ileostomy
loop ileostomy construction
loop jejunostomy
loop of bowel
loop of suture material
loop of Vieussens
loop ostomy bridge
loop retractor
loop scaler
loop scissors
loop shunt
loop stoma
loop sutures
loop transverse colostomy
looped cautery
loop-end ileostomy
loop-fixated intraocular lens
loopogram
loopography
loop-on mucosa suture
    technique
loop-over wrap
loops of redundant colon
loop-tipped electrode
loop-type snare forceps

loop-type stone-crushing forceps
Loopuyt needle
loose bodies
loose body forceps
loose body grasper
loose body suction forceps
loose cartilage
loose connective tissue
loose fracture
loose fragment
loose intra-articular body
loose knee procedure
loose premaxilla
loose shoulder
loosely approximated
loosely closed
loosening of prosthetic joint
Looser lines
Looser zone
Loosett maneuver
LOP position (left occipitoposterior position)
lop-ear deformity
Lopez enteral valve
Lopez-Enriquez operation
Lopez-Reinke tonsillar dissector
Lo-Por arterial prosthesis
Lo-Por tracheal tube
Lo-Por vascular graft
Lo-Por vascular graft prosthesis
LoPresti fiberoptic esophagoscope
LoPresti panendoscope
LoPro right angle ArthroWand
Lo-Pro tracheal tube
Lo-Profile balloon
Lo-Profile balloon catheter
Lo-Profile II balloon catheter
Lo-Profile steerable dilatation catheter
Lo-Profile urostomy pouch
Loptex laser intraocular lens implant
Lord cup
Lord dilation of hemorrhoid
Lord hemorrhoidectomy
Lord hydrocelectomy
Lord operation
Lord press-fit hip prosthesis
Lord total hip
Lord total hip prosthesis
Lordan chalazion forceps

Lordan forceps
Lordan hook
Lordan muscle-splitting hook
Lord-Blakemore tube
lordoscoliosis
lordosis creation
lordotic curve
lordotic projection
lordotic view
Lore subglottic forceps
Lore suction tip-holding forceps
Lore suction tube
Lore suction tube and tip-holding forceps
Lore suction tube-holding forceps
Lore-Lawrence tracheotomy tube
Lore-Lawrence tube
lorentzian line
Lorenz bandage scissors
Lorenz brace
Lorenz chisel
Lorenz gauze packer
Lorenz needle holder
Lorenz operation
Lorenz osteotomy
Lorenz PC/TC scissors
Lorenz position
Lorenz procedure
Lorenz reamer
Lorenz screw
Lorenz sign
Lorenz titanium screws and plate
Lorenz tube
Lorenzo bone fixation screw
Lorenzo reamer
Lorenzo screw
Lorenzo SMO prosthesis
Lorenz-Rees nasal rasp
Loreta operation
Lorez PC/TC ultra-sharp knife
Lorfan anesthesia
Lorfan anesthetic agent
lorgnette occluder
Lorie antral trephine
Lorie cheek retractor
Lorie retractor
Lorie tonsillar suture instrument
Lorie trephine
Loring ophthalmoscope
Lorna nonperforating towel clamp

lorry-driver fracture
Lortat-Jacob approach
Lorus knee orthosis
Losee knee reconstruction
Losee maneuver
Losee modification
Losee modification of MacIntosh
    technique
Losee sling and reef technique
Lossen operation
loss-of-resistance technique
L-osteotomy
LOT position (left
    occipitotransverse position)
Lotheissen femoral hernia repair
Lotheissen hernia repair
Lotheissen herniorrhaphy
Lotheissen operation
Lotheissen-McVay operation
Loth-Kirschner drill
Lothrop dissector
Lothrop frontoethmoidectomy
    procedure
Lothrop hemostat
Lothrop knife
Lothrop ligature forceps
Lothrop retractor
Lothrop tonsillar knife
Lothrop tonsillar retractor
Lothrop uvula retractor
Lo-Trau side-cutting needle
Lottes intramedullary nail
Lottes operation
Lottes pin
Lottes reamer
Lottes reduction technique
Lottes rod
Lottes triflange intramedullary
    nail
lotus position
loud piping rales
loud systolic murmur
Loughnane prostatic hook
Louis angle
Louis instrumentation
Louisville elevator
Lounsbury placenta curet
loupe (see also loop)
    Adler lens loupe
    Arlt lens loupe
    Bausch & Lomb Duoloupe
        lens loupe

loupe (continued)
    Bausch-Lomb loupe
    Beebe binocular loupe
    Beebe lens loupe
    Berens lens loupe
    binocular loupe
    binocular prism loupe
    binocular surgical loupe
    Callahan lens loupe
    Castroviejo lens loupe
    Codman magnifying loupe
    corneal loupe
    corneal monocular loupe
    Daviel lens loupe
    Denlan magnifying loupe
    Duoloupe lens loupe
    ear loupe
    Elschnig-Weber loupe
    eye loupe
    fiberoptic loupe
    Galilean loupe
    Gullstrand lens loupe
    Gullstrand-Zeiss lens loupe
    Ilg lens loupe
    intracapsular lens loupe
    Keeler panoramic loupe
    Keeler spotlight lens loupe
    Keeler wide-angle lens loupe
    Keeler-Galilean surgical loupe
    Kirby intracapsular lens loupe
    Lempert-Storz loupe
    lens loupe
    Lewis loupe
    Magill magnifying loupe
    Magni-Focuser lens loupe
    magnifying loupe
    Mark II Magni-Focuser loupe
    Mark lens loupe
    May hook-on lens loupe
    McKenzie leukotomy loupe
    New Orleans Eye and Ear
        loupe
    New Orleans lens loupe
    nucleus delivery loupe
    nucleus removal loupe
    ocular Gamboscope loupe
    operating loupe
    Opticaid lens loupe
    Opt-Visor loupe
    panoramic loupe
    plastic Berger eye loupe
    prism loupe

loupe (*continued*)
    Simcoe II nucleus delivery
      loupe
    Storz binocular loupe
    Storz binocular prism loupe
    surgical loupe
    Troutman lens loupe
    Weber-Elschnig lens loupe
    Wilder loupe
    Zeiss lens loupe
    Zeiss operating field loupe
    Zeiss-Gullstrand loupe
loupe magnification
Lours leukotome
Lovac fundal contact lens
Lovac fundal contact lens
    implant
Lovac fundus contact lens
    implant
Lovac gonioscopic lens
Lovas 6-mirror gonioscopic
    lens
Love leukotome
Love nasal splint
Love nasopharyngeal retractor
Love nerve retractor
Love nerve root retractor
Love pituitary rongeur
Love splint
Love uvula retractor
Love-Adson periosteal elevator
Love-Gruenwald alligator forceps
Love-Gruenwald cranial rongeur
Love-Gruenwald intervertebral
    disk rongeur
Love-Gruenwald laminectomy
    rongeur
Love-Gruenwald pituitary forceps
Love-Gruenwald pituitary rongeur
Lovejoy retractor
Love-Kerrison rongeur
Love-Kerrison rongeur forceps
Lovelace bladder forceps
Lovelace gallbladder traction
    forceps
Lovelace gallbladder trocar
Lovelace hemostatic forceps
Lovelace lung-grasping forceps
Lovelace thyroid traction
    vulsellum forceps
Lovelace tissue forceps
Lovelace traction lung forceps

Lovelace traction tissue forceps
Loversan infusion set
Lovitt-Uhler modification of
    Jewett post-fusion brace
Lovset maneuver
Low (*see* Low)
Low (*see* Löw, Loew)
Loew (*see* Low)
low anterior resection
low bleed implants
low central venous pressure
    anesthesia
low cervical cesarean section
low cervical spine fusion
low cesarean section
low dose rate (LDR)
low forceps
low frequency
low grade
low incision
low intermittent suction
low level
low ligation
low lip line
low lumbar spine fracture
low median nerve palsy
low median/ulnar nerve palsy
low midline incision
low outlet forceps
Low Profile legholder
Low Profile plastic body jacket
low profile plate
low rectal cancer
low small-bowel obstruction
low spinal anesthesia
low stirrups
low thoracic level epidural
    anesthesia
low threshold
low tracheotomy
low transverse incision
low ulnar nerve palsy
low viscosity cement (LVC)
low voltage
low-attenuation lesion
low-back pain
Loew-Beer forceps
Loew-Beer position
Loew-Beer projection
Loew-Beer view
low-collar incision
low-compliance balloon

low-contact dynamic compression plate
low-contact stress plate
low-current electrocautery
low-current monopolar coagulation
low-dose anesthetic
low-dose irradiation
low-dose therapy
Lowe microtome knife
Lowe ring
Lowe-Breck cartilage knife
Lowe-Breck elbow prosthesis
Lowe-Breck meniscectomy knife
Lowell glaucoma knife
Lowell pleural needle
Lowell reduction
Lowenberg forceps
low-energy collimator
low-energy fracture
low-energy laser
Lowenstein lithotrite
Lowenstein operation
lower abdomen
lower abdominal organ
lower airway obstruction
lower anterior forceps
lower arch
lower back
lower blepharoplasty
lower cervical spine posterior stabilization
lower cervical spine procedure
lower clival region
lower esophageal sphincter (LES)
lower extremity bypass
lower extremity edema
lower extremity nerve block
lower extremity occlusive disease
lower extremity reconstruction
lower extremity surgery
lower eyelid
lower fragment
lower frontal bone fracture
Lower gall duct forceps
lower ganglion of glossopharyngeal nerve
lower gastrointestinal hemorrhage
lower GI procedure

lower GI series
lower GI tract foreign body
lower jaw
lower lateral cartilage
Lower lateral forceps
Lower lateral scissors
lower lid sling procedure
lower limb
lower limb prosthesis
lower lip-splitting incision
lower lobe of lung
lower mantle
lower margin of field
lower midclavicular line
lower midline incision
lower motor neuron lesion
lower nephron syndrome
lower operation for femoral hernia
lower panendoscopy
lower plexus compression
lower pole laceration
lower quadrant abdominal incisional hernia
lower trapezius flap
Lower trocar
lower uterine segment cesarean section
lower uterine segment incision
lower extremity fracture
Lower-Shumway cardiac transplant
lowest splanchnic nerve
lowest thyroid artery
Lowette needle
Lowette-Verner needle
low-flow anesthetic technique
low-flow regulator
low-flux cellulose-based membrane
low-flux cuprophane membrane
low-flux dialysis membrane
low-flying bird incision
low forceps delivery
low forceps operation
low-frequency jet ventilation
low-friction arthroplasty (LFA)
low-grade dysplasia
low-grade MALT lymphoma
low-grade squamous intraepithelial lesion
low-grade suction unit

Lowis intervertebral disk forceps
Lowis IV disk rongeur forceps
Lowis periosteal elevator
low-level echo enhancement
Lowman bone clamp
Lowman bone-holding clamp
Lowman bone-holding forceps
Lowman chisel
Lowman flatfoot procedure
Lowman hand retractor
Lowman rongeur
Lowman sling procedure
Lowman-Gerster bone clamp
Lowman-Hoglund chisel
Lowman-Hoglund clamp
Lown cardioverter
Lown classification
Lown technique
low-pass filter
low-pitched bowel sounds
low-power optics for myopic correction lens
low-pressure voice prosthesis
low-profile angioplasty balloon
low-profile balloon-positioning catheter
low-profile breast implant
low-profile mitral heart valve
low-profile prosthesis
low-profile R-K marker
low-profile valve prosthesis
low-profile, port implantable port
low-resistance fundoplication
low-riding patella
low-risk papillary cancer
low-segment transverse incision
low-set hyoid
Lowsley grasping forceps
Lowsley hemostat
Lowsley lithotrite
Lowsley lobar anatomy
Lowsley needle
Lowsley nephropexy
Lowsley operation
Lowsley prostate retractor
Lowsley prostatic forceps
Lowsley prostatic lobe-holding forceps
Lowsley prostatic traction
Lowsley prostatic tractor

Lowsley retractor with hand-sutured closure
Lowsley ribbon-gut needle
Lowsley stone crusher
Lowsley suprapubic tractor
Lowsley urethroscope
Lowsley-Luc forceps
Lowsley-Peterson cystoscope
Lowsley-Peterson endoscope
Lowsman operation for talipes valgus
low-speed rotation angioplasty catheter
low-speed rotational angioplasty
low-speed tapered carbide bur
low-tension pulse
low-viscosity bone cement
loxotomy
L-plasty repair
L-plate
LPS balloon
LPS catheter
LPS Peel-Away introducer
LR (lateral rectus)
LR needle
LR shunt
L-resection guide
L-rod implant material
L-rod instrumentation
LSA position (left sacroanterior position)
LScA position (left scapuloanterior position)
LScP position (left scapuloposterior position)
L-shaped aneurysm clip
L-shaped capsular incision
L-shaped cautery
L-shaped elevator
L-shaped miniplate
L-shaped skin excision
LSI silver self-adhesive disposable electrode
LSK (liver, spleen, and kidneys)
LSK microkeratome
LSP position (left sacroposterior position)
LSU reciprocation-gait orthosis brace
LTIL (lunotriquetral interosseous ligament)

LTR (laryngotracheal reconstruction)
L-transposition of great arteries (levotransposition of great arteries)
LTTF (lateral transverse thigh flap)
LTX PTCA catheter
L-type capsulotomy
L-type nose-bridge prosthesis
Lu corneal marker
Lubafax dressing
Lubinus acetabular component
Lubinus knee prosthesis
Luebke uterine vacuum cannula
lubricating jelly
Lubri-Flex ureteral stent
Lubri-Flex urologic stent
Lubriglide-coated guidewire
Luc ethmoid forceps
Luc nasal-cutting forceps
Luc operation
Luc septum forceps
Luc septum-cutting forceps
Lucae bayonet
Lucae bayonet dressing forceps
Lucae bayonet ear forceps
Lucae bayonet tissue forceps
Lucae bone hammer
Lucae bone mallet
Lucae dissecting forceps
Lucae dressing forceps
Lucae ear forceps
Lucae ear perforation knife
Lucae ear probe
Lucae ear speculum
Lucae eustachian catheter
Lucae hook
Lucae mastoid mallet
Lucae probe
Lucas alveolar curet
Lucas chisel
Lucas gouge
Lucas groove
Lucas-Cottrell operation
Lucas-Cottrell osteotomy
Lucas-Murray knee arthrodesis
Lucas-Murray operation
lucent calculi
lucent defect
lucent line
lucent lung lesion

Lucite eye implant
Lucite implant
Lucite pessary
Lucite sphere implant
Luck bone drill
Luck bone saw
Luck fasciotome
Luck hallux valgus procedure
Luck operation
Luck procedure for Dupuytren contracture release
Luck saw
Luck-Bishop saw
Luckett operation
Ludloff bunionectomy
Ludloff hallux valgus procedure
Ludloff incision
Ludloff medial approach
Ludloff operation
Ludloff osteotomy
Ludloff sign
Ludloff technique
Ludwig angle
Ludwig applicator
Ludwig ganglion
Ludwig labyrinth
Ludwig middle ear applicator
Ludwig plane
Ludwig sinus applicator
Luedde exophthalmometer
Luedde measurement
Luedde transparent rule
Luer bone curet
Luer bone rongeur
Luer cannula lock
Luer connector
Luer curet forceps
Luer double-ended tracheal retractor
Luer eye speculum
Luer gallstone scoop
Luer hemorrhoidal forceps
Luer mallet
Luer needle
Luer reconstruction plate
Luer rongeur
Luer rongeur forceps
Luer scoop
Luer speaking tube
Luer speculum
Luer S-shaped retractor
Luer suction cannula adapter

Luer thoracic rongeur
Luer tip cap
Luer tip syringe
Luer tracheal cannula
Luer tracheal double-ended
    retractor
Luer tracheal tube
Luer-Friedman bone rongeur
Luer-Hartmann rongeur
Luer-Koerte scoop
Luer-Liston-Wheeling rongeur
Luer-Lok adapter
Luer-Lok B-D syringe
Luer-Lok catheter connection
Luer-Lok jet ventilator connector
Luer-Lok male adapter plug
Luer-Lok needle
Luer-Lok port
Luer-Lok pump
Luer-Stille rongeur
Luer-Whiting mastoid rongeur
Luer-Whiting rongeur forceps
Luethy-Beck needle holder
lugged plate
Lugol iodine preparation
lugolized
Luhr fixation plate
Luhr implant
Luhr implant screw
Luhr mandibular plate
Luhr MCS bone plate
Luhr microbone plate
Luhr microfixation cranial plate
Luhr microfixation system plate
    cutter
Luhr microfixation system plate-
    holding forceps
Luhr microfixation system pliers
Luhr microplate
Luhr minifixation bone plate
Luhr miniplate
Luhr pan plate
Luhr Vitallium micromesh plate
Luhr Vitallium screw
Luikart forceps
Luikart Iconoclast blunt
    dissection instrument
Luikart obstetrical forceps
Luikart-Bill forceps
Luikart-Bill traction handle
Luikart-Kielland obstetrical
    forceps

Luikart-McLane obstetrical
    forceps
Luikart-Simpson obstetrical
    forceps
Luke procedure
Lukens aspirator
Lukens bone wax dressing
Lukens cannula
Lukens catgut sutures
Lukens collecting tube
Lukens collector
Lukens double-channel irrigator
Lukens double-ended tracheal
    retractor
Lukens enterotome
Lukens enterotomy
Lukens epiglottic retractor
Lukens irrigator
Lukens needle
Lukens orthodontic band
Lukens suction tube
Lukens thymus retractor
Lukens tracheal double-ended
    retractor
Lukens trap
Lukes-Butler Hodgkin disease
    classification
Lukes-Collins classification
LUL (left upper lobe)
Lulu clamp
Lumaguide infusion catheter
lumbar accessory movement
    technique
lumbar anesthetic technique
lumbar anterior root stimulator
    implant
lumbar aortogram
lumbar aortography
lumbar aortography needle
lumbar approach
lumbar arcades
lumbar arteries
lumbar colotomy
lumbar corset
lumbar curvature
lumbar curve
lumbar disk herniation
lumbar diskectomy
lumbar drainage
lumbar epidural abscess
lumbar epidural anesthesia
lumbar epidural endoscopy

lumbar extension
lumbar facet injection
lumbar flexure
lumbar ganglion
lumbar gravitational line
lumbar hemangioma
lumbar hemilaminectomy
lumbar hernia
lumbar intersomatic fusion
    expandable cage
lumbar laminectomy
lumbar lordotic curve
lumbar lymph nodes
lumbar musculature
lumbar myelogram
lumbar nephrotomy
lumbar nerve block
lumbar nerve root injection
lumbar nerves
lumbar orthosis
lumbar pedicle fixation
lumbar pedicle screw
lumbar periosteal turnover flap
lumbar peritoneal catheter
lumbar plexus
lumbar plexus block
lumbar port
lumbar puncture
lumbar puncture needle
lumbar reflex
lumbar region
lumbar retractor
lumbar roll
lumbar scoliosis
lumbar spinal cord lesion
lumbar spinal fusion
lumbar spine
lumbar spine biopsy
lumbar spine burst fracture
lumbar spine fusion
lumbar spine kyphotic
    deformity
lumbar spine lesion
lumbar spine segmental fixation
lumbar spine stabilization
lumbar spine transpedicular
    fixation
lumbar splanchnic nerves
lumbar spur
lumbar spurring
lumbar subarachnoid catheter
lumbar sutures

lumbar sympathectomy
lumbar sympathetic block
lumbar veins
lumbar vertebrae
lumbar vertebral interbody fusion
Lumbard airway
lumbarization
lumbocolostomy
lumbocolotomy
lumbocostoabdominal triangle
lumbodorsal fascia
lumboiliac incision
lumboinguinal nerve
lumboperitoneal shunt
lumbosacral angle
lumbosacral back flap
lumbosacral belt
lumbosacral corset
lumbosacral curve
lumbosacral disk protrusion
lumbosacral dislocation
lumbosacral fusion
lumbosacral fusion elevator
lumbosacral joint
lumbosacral junction fracture
lumbosacral orthosis
lumbosacral plexus lesion
lumbosacral projection
lumbosacral root lesion
lumbosacral series
lumbosacral spine
lumbosacral spine transpedicular
    instrumentation
lumbosacral sprain
lumbosacral strain
lumbosacral support
lumbosacral support pelvic
    traction
lumbosacral trunk
lumbotomy retractor
lumbrical bar
lumbrical muscle flap
lumbrical muscles
Lumbrical-Plus finger
Lumelec pacing catheter
lumen (*pl.* lumina)
lumen cannula
lumen finder
lumen of appendix
lumen of artery
lumen of bowel
lumen of bronchial artery

lumen of gut
lumen of vein
Lumenator injectable guidewire
Lumi alloy
lumiform splint
lumina (*sing.* lumen)
Lumina guidewire
Lumina rod lens arthroscope
luminal defect
luminal irregularity
luminal narrowing
luminal stent
lumina-operating telescope
lumina-SL telescope
Luminexx biliary stent
luminous intensity
luminous ophthalmoscope
luminous rays
Lumiwand light
Lumonics YAG laser
lump kidney
lumpectomy
lumpy jaw
Lunar DPX densitometer
Lunar DPX total-body scanner
Lunar Expert densitometer
lunar hymen
lunate bone
lunate dislocation
lunate excision
lunate fracture
lunate implant
lunate prosthesis
lunate sinus of radius
lunate sinus of ulna
Lund operation
Lund-Browder burn chart
Lund-Dodick punch
Lunderquist catheter
Lunderquist coat hanger wire
Lunderquist guide
Lunderquist guidewire
Lunderquist wire
Lunderquist working wire
Lunderquist-Ring torque guide
Lundholm plate
Lundholm screw
Lundia dialyzer holder
Lundquist nephrostomy wire
Lundsgaard blade
Lundsgaard knife
Lundsgaard rasp

Lundsgaard sclerotome
Lundsgaard-Burch corneal rasp
Lundsgaard-Burch corneal
   raspatory
Lundsgaard-Burch knife
Lundsgaard-Burch rasp
Lundsgaard-Burch sclerotome
Lundstrom arcuate incision marker
Lundy fascial needle
Lundy laryngoscope
Lundy tubing hand-roller
Lundy-Irving caudal needle
Luneau retinoscopy rack
lung abscess
lung base
lung biopsy
lung brushings
lung calculus
lung cancer
lung carcinoma
lung cavity
lung clamp
lung disease
lung dissecting scissors
lung elasticity
lung exclusion clamp
lung fields
lung forceps
lung function studies
lung hilus
lung imaging fluorescence
   endoscope
lung infarct
lung infiltrate
lung lingula
lung markings
lung metastasis
lung parenchyma
lung resection
lung retractor
lung scan
lung scissors
lung tissue
lung tissue forceps
lung tourniquet
lung transplantation
lung volume reduction (LVR)
lung volume reduction surgery
lung washings
lung-grasping forceps
lung-imaging fluorescent
   endoscopy

lungs clear to percussion and auscultation
lunotriquetral fusion
lunotriquetral instability
lunotriquetral interosseous ligament (LTIL)
lunotriquetral joint
lunotriquetral ligament
lunotriquetral ligament tear
lunotriquetral motion
lunotriquetral shear test
lunotriquetral tear
Luntz-Dodick punch
Luomanen oral airway
Luongo cannula
Luongo curet
Luongo elevator
Luongo hand retractor
Luongo instruments
Luongo needle
Luongo retractor
Luongo septal elevator
Luongo sphenoid irrigating cannula
lupus anticoagulant
lupus erythematosus
lupus erythematosus-like rash
lupus pernio
lupus verrucosus
lupus vulgaris
lupus-associated valve disease
LUQ (left upper quadrant)
Luque cerclage wire
Luque fixation device
Luque II plate
Luque II screw
Luque II segmental spinal instrumentation
Luque instrumentation
Luque instrumentation concave technique
Luque instrumentation convex technique
Luque loop fixation
Luque L-rod
Luque rod
Luque rod fixation
Luque segmental spinal instrumentation
Luque semirigid segmental spinal instrumentation
Luque sublaminar wire

Luque sublaminar wiring technique
Luque wire
Luque-Galveston fixation
LUS examination
LUS scanning technique
Luschka-Magendie foramen
Luschka bursa
Luschka cartilage
Luschka crypt
Luschka foramen
Luschka ganglion
Luschka gland
Luschka joints
Luschka laryngeal cartilage
Luschka muscles
Luschka nerve
Luschka sinus
Luschka tonsil
Lusk instrument
Lusskin bone drill
Luster investment material
lutein cells
luteinize
Lutembacher syndrome
Luther-Peter lid everter
Luther-Peter retractor
Lutkens sphincter
Lutz automatic reprocessor
Lutz septal forceps
Lutz septal ridge forceps
Lutz septal ridge-cutting forceps
Luxar NovaPulse CO_2 laser
Luxar Silhouette noninvasive body appearance equipment
luxatio erecta shoulder dislocation
luxation
Luxation patellar saw
Luxator extractor
Luxo illuminated magnifier
Luxo surgical illuminator
Luxtec illuminated surgical telescope
Luxtec surgical telescope
luxus heart
Luys body syndrome
Luys segregator
Luys separator
LV apex cannula (left ventricular apex cannula)

LVAD (left ventricular assist device)
LVAS implantable pump
LVC cement (low viscosity cement)
LVEDP (left ventricular end-diastolic pressure)
LVR procedure
LX needle
Lyda-Ivalon-Lucite orbital implant
Lyda-Ivalon-Lucite implant
Lyden technique
Lyden-Lehman technique
Lyman incision
Lyman Smith brace
Lyman Smith traction
Lyman Smith toe drop brace
Lyman Smith tractor
lymph capillary
lymph cells
lymph channel
lymph circulation
lymph dialysis
lymph gland
lymph involvement
lymph node adenopathy
lymph node biopsy
lymph node classification
lymph node disease
lymph node dissection
lymph node enlargement
lymph node involvement
lymph node irradiation
lymph node metastasis
lymph node resection
lymph node-bearing tissue
lymph nodule
lymph space
lymph vessel invasion (LVI)
lymphadenectomy
    3-field lymphadenectomy
    axillary lymphadenectomy
    bilateral lymphadenectomy
    D2 lymphadenectomy
    elective lymphadenectomy
    endocavitary pelvic lymphadenectomy (ECPL)
    extended pelvic lymphadenectomy
    inguinal lymphadenectomy

lymphadenectomy (*continued*)
    Japanese-style lymphadenectomy
    laparoscopic pelvic lymphadenectomy
    mediastinal lymphadenectomy
    Meigs pelvic lymphadenectomy
    para-aortic lymphadenectomy
    pelvic lymphadenectomy
    prophylactic lymphadenectomy
    regional lymphadenectomy
    retroperitoneal lymphadenectomy
    selective lymphadenectomy
    sentinel lymphadenectomy
    staging lymphadenectomy
    thoracoabdominal retroperitoneal lymphadenectomy
lymphadenitis
lymphadenocele
lymphadenoid tissue
lymphadenoma
lymphadenopathy
lymphadenopathy-associated virus (LAV)
lymphadenosis
lymphadenotomy
lymphangiectasis
lymphangiectomy
lymphangioendothelioma
lymphangiogram (LAG)
lymphangiography
lymphangiohemangioma
lymphangioleiomyomatosis
lymphangioma
lymphangioma circumscriptum
lymphangioma superficium simplex
lymphangiomyomatosis
lymphangioplasty
lymphangiorrhaphy
lymphangiosarcoma
lymphangiotomy
lymphangitic metastasis
lymphangitis
lymphatic capillary
lymphatic chain
lymphatic channel
lymphatic dissection

lymphatic drainage
lymphatic duct
lymphatic edema
lymphatic fistula
lymphatic fluid
lymphatic follicle
lymphatic follicle of tongue
lymphatic invasion
lymphatic involvement
lymphatic malformation
lymphatic massage
lymphatic metastasis
lymphatic nodules
lymphatic obstruction
lymphatic sinuses
lymphatic spread
lymphatic tissue
lymphatic trunk
lymphatic vessels
lymphatic vessels of mouth
lymphaticostomy
lymphaticovenous anastomosis
lymphaticovenous bypass
lymphaticovenous malformation
    (LVM)
lymphatics
lymphaticum
lymphaticus
lymphatolysis
lymphedema
lymphoadenoma
lymphoblastoid cell line
lymphocele drainage
lymphocelectomy
lymphocyte
lymphocyte cell
lymphocyte migration
lymphocytic choriomeningitis
lymphocytic infiltration
lymphocytoma
lymphoepithelial carcinoma
lymphoepithelial cyst
lymphoepithelial lesion
lymphoepithelial proliferation
lymphoepithelioma
lymphogenous metastasis
lymphogranuloma
lymphoid hyperplasia
lymphoid infiltration
lymphoid irradiation
lymphoid mass
lymphoid polyp

lymphoid ring
lymphoid tissue
lymphoidectomy
lymphoma
    Burkitt lymphoma
    Castleman lymphoma
    cutaneous T-cell lymphoma
        (CTCL)
    Darmstruck lymphoma
    diffuse large cell lymphoma
    endemic Burkitt lymphoma
    extranodal malignant
        lymphoma
    extranodal non-Hodgkin
        lymphoma
    follicular lymphoma
    gastric MALT lymphoma
    gastric non-Hodgkin lymphoma
    giant follicle lymphoma
    high-grade MALT lymphoma
    Hodgkin lymphoma
    Kiel classification of non-
        Hodgkin lymphoma
    large-cell lymphoma
    low-grade MALT lymphoma
    malignant lymphoma
    MALT lymphoma
    mucosa-associated lymphoid
        tissue lymphoma
    node lymphoma
    non-Hodgkin lymphoma
    primary gastric lymphoma
        (PGL)
    primary gastric non-Hodgkin
        lymphoma
    small bowel lymphoma
    sporadic Burkitt lymphoma
    testicular lymphoma
    undifferentiated lymphoma
lymphoma implant
lymphoma relapse
lymphomatoid granuloma
lymphomatoid papulosis
lymphomatosa
lymphomatosum
lymphomatous infiltrate
lymphomyeloma
lymphonodular pharyngitis
lymphoplasty
lymphoproliferation
lymphoproliferative disorder
lymphoproliferative lesion

lymphorrhea
lymphosarcoma
lymphosarcomatous nodule
LymphoScan nuclear imaging
  system scanner
lymphoscintigraphy
lymphostatic verrucosis
lymphovascular invasion
lymphovenous malformation
Lynch blunt dissector
Lynch cup-shaped curet forceps
Lynch curet
Lynch dissector
Lynch electrode
Lynch frontal sinus exploration
Lynch frontoethmoidectomy
  procedure
Lynch incision
Lynch knife
Lynch laryngeal dissector
Lynch laryngeal forceps
Lynch laryngeal knife handle
Lynch laryngoscope
Lynch mucosa separator plate
Lynch obtuse-angle laryngeal
  knife
Lynch operation
Lynch right-angle knife
Lynch scissors
Lynch septal splint
Lynch sinusectomy
Lynch spatula
Lynch splint
Lynch straight knife
Lynch suspension
  laryngoscope
Lynch syndrome
Lynch tonsillar dissector
Lynch tonsillar knife
Lynco arch support
Lynco foot orthosis
Lynell intraocular lens
Lynn Achilles-tendon
  procedure
Lynn technique
Lynx OTW catheter

Lynx over-the-wire balloon
  catheter
LYOfoam A water-resistant
  dressing
LYOfoam C dressing
LYOfoam T dressing
LYOfoam wound dressing
Lyon forceps
Lyon ring
Lyon tube
Lyon-Horgan operation
Lyon-Horgan procedure
lyophilized bone graft
lyophilized dura graft
lyophilized dural patch
lyophilized extract
lyophilized graft
lyophilized pigskin
lyophilized (freeze dried)
lyre of uterus
lyre of vagina
Lyrelle patch
lyre-shaped finger
lyre-shaped finger hook
lysed adhesions
lysis of adhesions
lysis time
lysogenic induction
LySonix ultrasound device
LySonix aspirator
LySonix irrigator
lysosomal enzyme disorder
lysosomal membrane
lysosomal storage disease
Lyster tube
Lyster water bag
lytic area
lytic blockade
lytic bone lesion
lytic cocktail
lytic defect
lytic disease
lytic lesion
Lytle metacarpal splint
Lytle splint
Lytle sutures

M Beaver blade
M line
Moenckeberg arteriosclerosis
Moenckeberg degeneration
Moenckeberg sclerosis
MA (main arteriole, mental age)
ma (milliamperes)
M-A tube (Miller-Abbott tube)
MAA (mandibular advancement
    appliance)
MAC (monitored anesthesia
    care)
MAC anesthesia
MAC cervical collar
Macaluso stent remover
MacAusland bone hammer
MacAusland bone mallet
MacAusland chisel
MacAusland dissector
MacAusland elbow arthroplasty
MacAusland finishing-ball
    reamer
MacAusland finishing-cup
    reamer
MacAusland mallet
MacAusland muscle retractor
MacAusland operation
MacAusland procedure
MacAusland reamer
MacAusland retractor
MacAusland skid
MacAusland-Kelly retractor
MacCallan classification
MacCallum knife
MacCallum patch
MacCarthy procedure
MacCarty forceps
MacCarty procedure
MacDonald clamp
MacDonald dissector
MacDonald periosteal elevator
macerated
macerated fetus

maceration
    flap maceration
    perianal maceration
    skin maceration
Macewen classification
Macewen drill
Macewen hernia operation
Macewen herniorrhaphy
Macewen operation
Macewen osteotomy
Macewen saw
Macewen sign
Macewen symptom
Macewen triangle
Macewen-Shands osteotomy for
    coxa vara
Macey tendon carrier
MacFee incision
MacFee neck flap
MacGregor conjunctival forceps
MacGregor forceps
MacGregor mules
MacGregor osteotome
Mach line
Machat adjustable aspirating
    wire speculum
Machat double-ended marker
Machat superior flap LASIK
    marker
Machek operation
Machek ptosis operation
Machek-Blaskovics operation
Machek-Brunswick operation
Machek-Gifford operation
Machemer calipers
Machemer cutter
Machemer diamond-dust-coated
    foreign body forceps
Machemer diamond-dusted
    forceps
Machemer flat lens
Machemer infusion contact lens
Machemer lens

Machemer magnifying
vitrectomy lens
Machemer scleral knife
Machemer sclerotomy knife
Machemer VISC (vitreous
infusion suction cutter)
Machemer VISC vitrector
Machemer vitreous cutter
Machemer vitreous infusion
suction cutter (Machemer
VISC)
Machida
Machida fiberoptic
laryngoscope
Machida light source
connector
Machida bronchoscope
Machida FDS
(fiberduodenoscope)
Machida fiber-duodenoscope
Machida fiberduodenoscope
(FDS)
Machida fiberoptic
laryngoscope
Machida flexible endoscope
Machida nasolaryngoscope
machining
computer assisted
design/computer assisted
machining
Machlett collimator
MacIntosh blade
MacIntosh fiberoptic
laryngoscope blade
MacIntosh implant
MacIntosh knee prosthesis
MacIntosh laryngoscope
MacIntosh operation
MacIntosh over-the-top ACL
reconstruction
MacIntosh over-the-top
reconstruction of knee
MacIntosh over-the-top repair
MacIntosh prosthesis
MacIntosh sign
MacIntosh technique
MacIntosh tibial plateau
prosthesis
MacIntosh tibial prosthesis
Mack lingual tonsillar
tonsillectome
Mack tonometer

Mack tonsillectome
MacKay contour retractor
MacKay contour self-retaining
retractor
MacKay nasal splint
MacKay retractor
MacKay-Marg tonometer
Mack-Brunswick operation
Mackenrodt incision
Mackenrodt operation
MacKenty antral tube
MacKenty cleft palate knife
MacKenty elevator
MacKenty forceps
MacKenty knife
MacKenty laryngectomy tube
MacKenty periosteal elevator
MacKenty punch
MacKenty scissors
MacKenty septal elevator
MacKenty sphenoid punch
MacKenty tissue forceps
MacKenty tube
MacKenty-Converse periosteal
elevator
Mackenzie (*see also* McKenzie)
Mackenzie amputation
MacKenzie syndrome
Mackid operation
Mackinnon modification
MacKinnon-Dellon
Diskriminator instrument
Mackler esophageal tube
Mackler intraluminal tube
Mackler intraluminal tube
prosthesis
Mackler tube prosthesis
MacKool capsule retractor
Maclay scissors
Maclay tonsillar scissors
Macmed pediatric
intramedullary nail
MacNab line for facet
imbrication
MacNab operation
MacNab shoulder repair
MacNab-Dall spinal fusion
MacNab-English shoulder
prosthesis
MacNichol-Voutsinas
classification
Macon Hospital speculum

MacRae spatula
macrocalcification
macrocephaly
macrocheilia
macrodactyly
macrodontia
macroelectrode recording
    technique
macrofilled resin
macrofiller
Macrofit hip prosthesis
macrofollicular lesion
macrogingivae
macroglobulin
macroglobulinemia
macroglossia
    amyloid macroglossia
    unilateral macroglossia
macroglossic
macrognathia
    mandibular macrognathia
    maxillary macrognathia
macrognathic
macroinjection of autologous fat
macromastia
macro-mesh
macrophage
    blood-borne macrophage
    chemotactic factor for
        macrophage (CFM)
    pulpal macrophage
    tissue macrophage
    tissue-borne macrophage
macrophage-activating factor
    (MAF)
macrophage-inhibiting factor
    (MIF)
macrophallus
macrophonia
Macroplastique bulking agent
Macroplastique implantable
    device
Macroplastique material
macrorhinia
macroscopic anatomy
macroscopic concavity
macroscopic involvement
macroscopic lesion
macroscopic tumor removal
macrosomia
    fetal macrosomia
macrosomic baby

macrostomia
macrotia
macrotooth
macrotrauma
MacroVac
macrovascular coronary lesion
macula (*pl.* maculae)
macula adherens
macula degeneration
macula flava
macula retinoscope
macula-off retinal detachment
macular atrophy
macular change
macular contact lens
macular degeneration
macular ectopia
macular fan
macular hair cell
macular rash
macular star
macular vascular birthmark
macule
    bruise-like macules
    cafe au lait macule (CALM)
    reddish macule
maculopapillary bundle
maculopapular bundle
maculopapular rash
MacVicar double-end strabismus
    retractor
MAD (maximum accumulated
    dose)
Madayag biopsy needle
Madayag needle
Maddacrawler walker
Madden clamp
Madden dissector
Madden forceps
Madden herniorrhaphy
Madden hook
Madden incisional
    herniorrhaphy
Madden intestinal clamp
Madden ligature carrier
Madden repair of incisional
    hernia
Madden sympathectomy hook
Madden technique
Madden-Potts forceps
Madden-Potts intestinal forceps
Madden-Potts tissue forceps

Maddox caudal needle
Maddox LASIK spatula
Maddox needle
Maddox pliers
Maddox prism
Maddox rod
Maddox rod occluder
Madeira-Stern suture hook
Madelung deformity
Madlener operation
Madlener sterilization
Madoff suction tube
Madonna fingers
madreporic femoral component
madreporic hip prosthesis
Madsen tympanoscope
Madura foot
Maestro bipolar dual-chamber
    pacemaker
Maestro implantable cardiac
    pacemaker
Maestro pacemaker
MAF (macrophage-activating
    factor, master apical file)
Maffucci syndrome
Magellan monitor
Magendie foramen
Magendie space
magenta tongue
Magerl posterior cervical screw
    fixation
Magerl translaminar facet screw
    fixation technique
Maggi disposable biopsy needle
    guide
Magic microcatheter
Magic Torque guidewire
Magic-Wall stent
Magielski bayonet canal knife
Magielski canal knife
Magielski cautery
Magielski chisel
Magielski coagulating forceps
Magielski coagulation cautery
Magielski coagulator
Magielski curet
Magielski electrocoagulator
Magielski elevator
Magielski forceps
Magielski hook
Magielski needle
Magielski stapes chisel

Magielski tonsil forceps
Magielski tonsil-seizing forceps
Magielski-Heermann strut forceps
Magill band
Magill catheter forceps
Magill catheter-introducing
    forceps
Magill endotracheal catheter
Magill endotracheal forceps
Magill laryngoscope
Magill magnifying loupe
Magill orthodontic band
Magill endotracheal tube
Magill tube
Magitot disease
Magitot keratoplasty
Magitot keratoplasty operation
Maglinte catheter
Magna-Finder locating device
MagnaPod pain relief magnet
Magna-SL scanner
Magnathotics orthotic
MAGneedle controller
MAGneedle driver
magneprobe
Magnes imager
Magnes whole-body scanner
Magnes magnetic source imaging
magnesium oxide
magnesium salicylate
magnesium tuning forks
magnet (*see also* locator, metal
    locator)
  air-core magnet
  Alnico magneprobe magnet
  Atlas-Storz eye magnet
  Berman magnet
  Bonaccolto magnet
  bronchoscopic magnet
  Bronson magnet
  Bronson-Magnion eye magnet
  Coronet magnet
  C-shaped resistive magnet
  doughnut magnet
  ear magnet
  Eindhoven magnet
  elbow magnet
  endoscopic magnet
  Equen stomach magnet
  eye magnet
  Firlene eye magnet
  foot magnet

magnet (*continued*)
  foreign body magnet
  GE Signa magnet
  Grafco magnet
  Gruening magnet
  Haab eye magnet
  Hamblin magnet
  hand-held eye magnet
  Hirschberg magnet
  Holinger bronchoscopic
    magnet
  Holinger endoscopic magnet
  Holinger magnet
  horseshoe magnet
  implant magnet
  Lancaster eye magnet
  large-bore magnet
  Magnex magnet
  Mag-Optin eye magnet
  Mellinger magnet
  Mueller giant eye magnet
  needle magnet
  nonenclosed magnet
  Norris tip magnet
  open magnet
  original Sweet eye magnet
  Oxford magnet
  pancake MRI magnet
  passively shimmed
    superconducting magnet
  Patel intraocular magnet
  permanent magnet
  Ralks eye magnet
  rare earth intraocular magnet
  Schumann giant eye magnet
  Scientronics magnet
  shim magnet
  shimmed magnet
  short-bore magnet
  stomach magnet
  Storz magnet
  Storz-Atlas eye magnet
  suction magnet
  superconducting magnet
  surgical power magnet
  Sweet electric magnet
  Sweet eye magnet
  Sweet original magnet
  Szluc eye magnet
  Tectonic magnet
  temporary magnet
  Tesla magnet

magnet (*continued*)
  Thomas magnet
  Trowbridge-Campau eye
    magnet
  tubular magnet
  Walker magnet
  Wildgen-Reck magnet
  Wildgen-Reck metal locator
    magnet
magnet operation
magnet splint
magnet therapy
magnet wire
magnetic cup
magnetic extraction
magnetic extractor
magnetic eye implant
magnetic eye probe
magnetic field
magnetic imaging guidance
magnetic implant
magnetic induction
magnetic induction device
magnetic internal ureteral stent
magnetic jaw tracking device
magnetic mat pad
magnetic microsphere
magnetic motion transducer
magnetic operation
magnetic radiation exposure
magnetic resonance
  angiography (MRA)
magnetic resonance
  cholangiopancreatography
magnetic resonance endoscope
magnetic resonance imaging
  (MRI)
magnetic resonance imaging
  cholangiography
magnetic resonance imaging-
  guided focused ultrasound
  sector transducer
magnetic resonance venography
  (MRV)
magnetic retriever
magnetic source imaging (MSI)
magnetic stimulator
magnetic wrap
magnetization
magnetoencephalography
magnetogyric ratio
Magnetom scanner

Magnetom MRI imager
magnetometer probe
Magnetriever ureteral stent
  retriever
Magnetrode cervical unit
magnet-tipped flexible catheter
Magnex magnet
Magnex MR scanner
magnification
magnifier
  anastigmatic aural magnifier
  aural magnifier
  Bruening Japanese
    anastigmatic aural magnifier
  Bruening-Storz anastigmatic
    aural magnifier
  Circline magnifier
  Coil magnifier
  Japanese Bruening
    anastigmatic aural magnifier
  Luxo illuminated magnifier
  Optelec Passport magnifier
  Storz adjustable magnifier
  Storz-Bruening anastigmatic
    aural magnifier
  Storz-Bruening ear magnifier
  Zeiss binocular head
    magnifier
Magni-Focuser lens loupe
magnifying colonoscope
magnifying loupe
magnitude preparation-rapid
  acquisition gradient echo
  (MP-RAGE)
magnitude shunt
magnum
  foramen magnum
  os magnum
Magnum chisel
Magnum curet
magnum foramen
Magnum guidewire
Magnum knot pusher
Magnus operation
Magnuson abduction humeral
  splint
Magnuson abduction humerus
  splint
Magnuson arthroplasty
Magnuson circular twin saw
Magnuson double counter-
  rotating saw

Magnuson patellar procedure
Magnuson reduction technique
Magnuson saw
Magnuson single circular saw
Magnuson splint
Magnuson strut
Magnuson strut miniplate strut
Magnuson technique
Magnuson transplantation of
  subscapularis tendon
Magnuson twist drill
Magnuson valve prosthesis
Magnuson-Cromie prosthesis
Magnuson-Cromie valve
  prosthesis
Magnuson-Stack arthroplasty
Magnuson-Stack operation
Magnuson-Stack procedure
Magnuson-Stack shoulder
  arthroplasty
Magnuson-Stack shoulder
  arthrotomy
Mag-Optin eye magnet
Magovern ball-valve mallet
Magovern ball-valve prosthesis
Magovern heart valve
Magovern-Cromie ball-cage
  prosthetic value
Magovern-Cromie valve
  prosthesis
MAGPI (meatal advancement
  and glanuloplasty
  procedure)
MAGPI hypospadias repair
MAGPI operation
MAGPI technique
Ma-Griffith technique
Ma-Griffith tendo calcaneus
  repair
Magrina-Bookwalter vaginal
  Deaver blade
Magrina-Bookwalter vaginal
  retractor
Magrina-Bookwalter vaginal
  retractor ring
Maguire-Harvey vitreous cutter
Mahaim bundle in heart
Mahan procedure
Mahler sign
Mahoney dilator
Mahoney intranasal antral
  speculum

Mahoney speculum
Mahorner dilator
Mahorner thyroid retractor
Mahorner-Mead operation
Mahurkar catheter
Mahurkar curved extension
    catheter
Mahurkar dual-lumen catheter
Mahurkar dual-lumen dialysis
    catheter
Mahurkar dual-lumen femoral
    catheter
Mahurkar dual-lumen femoral
    dialysis catheter
Mahurkar fistular needle
Maier dressing forceps
Maier forceps
Maier hemostat
Maier polyp forceps
Maier sinus
Maier sponge forceps
Maier uterine forceps
Maier uterine-dressing forceps
Mailith pacemaker
Mailler colon forceps
Mailler cut-off forceps
Mailler intestinal forceps
Mailler rectal forceps
Mailman coronary guidewire
main arteriole (MA)
main bronchus
main bundle
main pancreatic duct (MPD)
main pancreatic duct stent
main pulmonary artery
main renal vein
main stem bronchus
main venule (MV)
Maine gonioscope
Maingot clamp
Maingot gallbladder tube
Maingot hemostat
Maingot hysterectomy forceps
Maingot operation
Mainstay urologic soft tissue
    anchor
mainstem intubation
Mainster retina laser lens
Mainster Ultra Field laser lens
Mainster wide-field lens
maintainer
    anterior chamber maintainer

maintainer (*continued*)
  Blumenthal anterior chamber
    maintainer
  Fary anterior chamber
    maintainer
  filter maintainer
  Gerber space maintainer
  Lewicky self-retaining
    chamber maintainer
  Mayne space maintainer
  self-retaining chamber
    maintainer
maintainer cast space
maintenance chemotherapy
maintenance dialysis
maintenance dose
maintenance level
maintenance therapy
Mainz pouch
Mainz pouch augmentation
Mainz pouch cutaneous urinary
    diversion
Mainz pouch operation
Mainz pouch urinary resector
Mainz pouch urinary reservoir
Mainz urinary reservoir pouch
Mair operation
Maison retractor
Maisonneuve amputation
Maisonneuve bandage
Maisonneuve fibular fracture
Maisonneuve fracture
Maisonneuve sign
Maisonneuve urethrotome
Maitland technique
Majestro-Ruda-Frost tendon
    technique
Majewski nasal curet
major abdominal surgery
major airway
major amputation
major anchorage
major connector
major connector bar
major fissure
major fracture
major histocompatibility
    complex (MHC)
major liver resection
major motor group
major nonvascular abdominal
    surgery

major operation
major palatine artery
major salivary glands
major surgery
major trauma
major vascular injury
Makar coagulator
Maki pylorus-preserving
    gastrectomy
Maki scissors
Makkas operation
Makler cannula
Makler counting chamber
Makler insemination
Makler sperm counting device
Mako shaver blade
Malacarne space
malacotic teeth
malacotomy
maladaptive response
Maladie de Graeffe operation
maladie-de-Roger
maladjustment
Malaga flap
malaise
malalignment
  vermilion-white line
      malalignment
malar alloplastic augmentation
malar arch
malar area
malar bag
malar bag suctioning
malar bone
malar butterfly rash
malar complex fracture
malar crest of great wing of
    sphenoid bone
malar deficiency
malar elevator
malar eminence
malar facial augmentation
malar fat pad
malar flatness
malar fold
malar foramen
malar fracture
malar glands
malar hypoplasia
malar implant
malar incision
malar ligament complex

malar margin
malar mound
malar pad
malar periosteum-SMAS flap
    fixation suture
malar process
malar prominence
malar prosthesis
malar shell augmentation
malar surface of zygomatic bone
malar tuberosity
malarplasty procedure
malar-zygomatic region
Malassez debris
Malassez epithelial rest
Malawar fibular resection
Malawer excision technique
Malbec operation
Malbran operation
Malcolm-Lynn cervical retractor
    frame
Malcolm-Rand carbon-composite
    headholder
Malcolm-Rand cranial x-ray
    frame
maldevelopment
male abdominoplasty
male castration
male catheter
male catheterization
male compression girdle
male flank
male foreheadplasty
male pattern baldness
male pseudohermaphroditism
male reproductive organs
male soprano voice
Malecot 2-wing catheter
Malecot 2-wing drain
Malecot 4-wing catheter
Malecot 4-wing drain
Malecot catheter
Malecot gastrostomy tube
Malecot nephrostomy catheter
Malecot nephrostomy tube
Malecot reentry catheter
Malecot self-retaining urethral
    catheter
Malecot Silastic catheter
Malecot suprapubic cystostomy
    catheter
Malecot tube

Malecot urethral catheter
maleruption
male-to-female transsexual
Malette-Spencer coronary
  cannula
malformation
  adult Chiari malformation
  angiographically occult
    intracranial vascular
    malformation (AOIVM)
  anorectal malformation
  Arnold-Chiari malformation
  arrhinia malformation
  arteriovenous malformation
    (AVM)
  atrioventricular malformation
    (AVM)
  A-V malformation
  Bing-Siebenmann
    malformation
  bronchopulmonary foregut
    malformation
  capillary malformation
  capillary vascular
    malformation
  cardiac valvular malformation
  cardiovascular malformation
  cavernous malformation
  central nervous system
    malformation
  cerebral arteriovenous
    malformation
  cerebral vascular
    malformation
  cerebrovascular malformation
  Chiari malformation
    (types I, II, III, IV)
  cloacal malformation
  clomiphene fetal
    malformation
  congenital brain malformation
  congenital cystic adenomatoid
    malformation
  congenital heart malformation
  congenital malformation
  congenital vascular
    malformation
  craniofacial malformation
  cutaneous malformation
  cystic adenomatoid
    malformation (CAM)
  Dandy-Walker malformation

malformation (*continued*)
  DeMyer system of cerebral
    malformation
  Dieulafoy vascular
    malformation
  dural arteriovenous
    malformation
  dysraphic malformation
  Ebstein malformation
  extremity malformation
  faciotelencephalic
    malformation
  fast-flow arterial
    malformations
  fetal cystic adenomatoid
    malformation
  flocculonodular arteriovenous
    malformation
  foregut malformation
  frontal arteriovenous
    malformation
  frontoparietal arteriovenous
    malformation
  galenic venous malformation
  gastric arteriovenous
    malformation
  glomus arteriovenous
    malformation
  high-flow arterial
    malformation
  high-flow arteriovenous
    malformation
  holoprosencephalic
    malformation
  infratentorial arteriovenous
    malformation
  intracerebral arteriovenous
    malformation
  intracerebral vascular
    malformation
  intracranial arteriovenous
    malformation
  intracranial vascular
    malformation
  intramedullary arteriovenous
    malformation
  intramuscular venous
    malformation
  lymphatic malformation
  lymphaticovenous
    malformation (LVM)
  lymphovenous malformation

malformation (*continued*)
mermaid malformation
Michel malformation
mixed venous-lymphatic
malformation
Mondini malformation
Mondini pulmonary
arteriovenous malformation
Mondini-Alexander
malformation
multiple glomuvenous
malformation (GVM)
neural axis vascular
malformation
neural crest malformation
occipital malformation
occult cerebrovascular
malformation
occult vascular malformation
orbital arteriovenous
malformation
osseous craniofacial
arteriovenous malformation
pulmonary arterial
malformation
pulmonary arteriovenous
malformation
radiculomeningeal spinal
vascular malformation
retinal arteriovenous
malformation
rugose frontonasal
malformation
Scheibe malformation
sink-trap malformation
spinal vascular malformation
split hand malformation
split foot malformation
split-cord malformation
supratentorial arteriovenous
malformation
Taussig-Bing malformation
telencephalic malformation
teratogen-induced
malformation
thalamocaudate arteriovenous
malformation
Uhl malformation
vaginal malformation
vascular malformation
vein of Galen malformation
venous malformation

malformation sequence
malformed fetus
malfunctional occlusion
Malgaigne amputation
Malgaigne clamp
Malgaigne fossa
Malgaigne fracture
Malgaigne hernia
Malgaigne hook
Malgaigne luxation
Malgaigne patellar hook
Malgaigne pelvic fracture
Malibu cervical orthosis
malic dehydrogenase
malignant adenoma
malignant atrophic papulosis
malignant blue nevus
malignant chondroma
malignant degeneration
malignant disease
malignant dyskeratosis
malignant external otitis
malignant external otitis
syndrome
malignant fibroma
malignant fibrous histiocytoma
malignant granular cell
myoblastoma
malignant granuloma
malignant growth
malignant
hemangioendothelioma
malignant hemangiopericytoma
malignant hyperthermia
malignant lesion
malignant lymphoepithelioma
malignant lymphoma
malignant melanoma
malignant mesenchymal tumor
malignant midline reticulosis
malignant necrotizing otitis
externa (MNOE)
malignant neoplasm
malignant odontogenic tumor
malignant pancreatic disease
malignant papillomatosis
malignant papulosis
malignant pemphigus
malignant pituitary lesion
malignant pleomorphic
adenoma
malignant polyp

malignant process
malignant reticulosis
malignant schwannoma
malignant transformation
malignant tumor
malignant ulcer
malignoma
Maliniac nasal brace
Maliniac nasal rasp
Maliniac nasal raspatory
Maliniac nasal retractor
malinterdigitation
Malis angled bayonet forceps
Malis angled-up bipolar forceps
Malis bipolar coagulation
   forceps
Malis bipolar cutting forceps
Malis bipolar instrument
Malis bipolar irrigating forceps
Malis bipolar microcoagulator
Malis brain retractor kit
Malis cerebellar retractor
Malis cerebral retractor
Malis clip applier
Malis bipolar coagulator
Malis coagulator
Malis cup forceps
Malis curet
Malis dissector
Malis electrocautery
Malis electrocoagulation unit
Malis elevator
Malis hinge clamp
Malis irrigating forceps stylet
Malis irrigation forceps
Malis irrigation tubing set
Malis jeweler bipolar forceps
Malis ligature passer
Malis microcuret
Malis microdissector
Malis needle holder
Malis nerve hook
Malis neurological scissors
Malis neurosurgical scissors
Malis retractor
Malis scissors
Malis solid state coagulator
Malis titanium microsurgical
   forceps
Malis-Frazier suction tube
Malis-Jensen bipolar forceps
Malis-Jensen microbipolar forceps

MALL (massive all layer
   liposuction)
Mallampati oropharyngeal
   classification
Mallampati pharyngeal visibility
   classification
Mallampati score
Mallard incision
malleability
malleable blade
malleable blade retractor
malleable copper retractor
malleable facial implant
malleable metal finger splint
malleable microsurgical suction
   device
malleable multipore suction
   tube
malleable passing needle
malleable plate
malleable probe
malleable prosthesis
malleable retractor
malleable ribbon retractor
malleable rod
malleable scoop
malleable screw
malleable spatula
malleable stainless steel
   retractor
malleable stylet
mallear fold
mallear ligament
malleo-incudal joint
malleolar artery
malleolar folds
malleolar fracture
malleolar gel sleeve
malleolar plexus
Malleoloc anatomic ankle
   orthosis
malleolus (*pl.* malleoli)
   lateral malleolus
   medial malleolus
malleolus muscle
malleostapedial assembly
malleotomy
Malleotrain active ankle
   support
Malleotrain ankle sleeve
Malleotrain ankle support
malleovestibulopexy

mallet
  aluminum mallet
  Bakelite mallet
  Bergman mallet
  Blount mallet
  Blount nylon mallet
  bone mallet
  Boxwood mallet
  brass mallet
  bronze mallet
  Brown mallet
  Carroll aluminum mallet
  cervical mallet
  Chandler mallet
  Children's Hospital mallet
  combination mallet
  Cooper mallet
  copper mallet
  Cottle mallet
  Crane mallet
  Doyen bone mallet
  Gerzog bone mallet
  Gerzog mastoid mallet
  Hajek mallet
  hard mallet
  Heath mallet
  Heister mallet
  Henning mallet
  Hibbs mallet
  Jarit mallet
  Kirk mallet
  lead-filled head mallet
  lead-filled mallet
  Lucae bone mallet
  Lucae mastoid mallet
  Luer mallet
  MacAusland bone mallet
  Magovern ball-valve mallet
  mastoid mallet
  Mead mallet
  Meyerding solid aluminum
    mallet
  nasal mallet
  Newhart mallet
  No Bounce mallet
  nylon face mallet
  nylon head mallet
  Ombredanne mallet
  orthopedic mallet
  polyethylene-faced mallet
  Ralks mallet
  Rica bone mallet

mallet (*continued*)
  Richards combination mallet
  Rissler mallet
  Rush mallet
  slotted mallet
  small brass mallet
  small head mallet
  SMIC surgical mallet
  Smith-Petersen mallet
  solid copper head mallet
  standard-pattern mallet
  steel mallet
  Steinbach mallet
  Stille mallet
  surgical mallet
  Swanson mallet
  White mallet
mallet finger deformity
mallet fracture
Mallet scale shoulder external
    rotation
mallet toe deformity
malleus
  caput malleus
  cog-tooth of malleus
  external ligament of malleus
  fixed malleus
  hallux malleus
  handle of malleus
  head of malleus
  ligament of malleus
  manubrium of malleus
  osteoma of malleus
malleus bone
malleus cutter
malleus forceps
malleus handle
malleus head
malleus nipper
malleus punch
malleus-footplate assembly
malleus-incus prosthesis
malleus-stapes assembly
Mallinckrodt angiographic
    catheter
Mallinckrodt catheter
Mallinckrodt endotracheal tube
Mallinckrodt Laser-Flex tube
Mallinckrodt scanner
Mallinckrodt ultra tag labeling
    kit
Mallinckrodt vertebral catheter

Mallory pacemaker
Mallory technique
Mallory-Head hip component
Mallory-Head hip program
Mallory-Head hip prosthesis
Mallory-Head Interlok primary
   femoral component
Mallory-Head Interlok rasp
Mallory-Head Interlok reamer
Mallory-Head porous primary
   femoral prosthesis
Mallory-Weiss lesion
Mallory-Weiss mucosal rupture
Mallory-Weiss mucosal tear
Mallory-Weiss procedure
Mallory-Weiss syndrome
Mallory-Weiss tear
Malmo hip splint
Malm-Himmelstein pulmonary
   valvulotome
Malmstrom cup
malocclusion
   Ackerman-Proffitt
      classification of
      malocclusion
   class I, II, III, IV malocclusion
   closed-bite malocclusion
   deflective malocclusion
   open bite malocclusion
   Simons classification of
      malocclusion
   teeth malocclusion
malocclusion index
malodorous discharge
malomaxillary sutures
Malone ACE procedure
Malone antegrade continence
   enema procedure
Maloney bougie
Maloney catheter
Maloney esophageal dilator
Maloney mercury bougie
Maloney mercury-filled dilator
Maloney mercury-filled
   esophageal dilator
Maloney no-hole lens
   manipulator
Maloney tapered bougie
Maloney tapered esophageal
   bougie
Maloney tapered-tip dilator
Maloney-Hurst dilator

Maloney-type bougie
Malpighi vesicles
malpighian bodies
malpighian capsule
malpighian cell
malposition
   bilateral malposition
   extension malposition
   functional malposition
   implant malposition
   inferior malposition
   superior malposition
   teeth malposition
malpositioned
malpositioned tooth
malrotation
malsensing pacemaker
Malström cup
Malstrom extraction
Malström vacuum extractor
Malström-Westman cannula
MALT (mucosa-associated
   lymphoid tissue)
Malt technique in liver
   transplantation
Malteno glaucoma artificial valve
Maltese cross lens
Maltese cross-patterned flap
maltreatment
malturned
Maltz angle knife
Maltz bayonet saw
Maltz button-end knife
Maltz cartilage knife
Maltz knife
Maltz nasal rasp
Maltz nasal saw
Maltz needle
Maltz rasp
Maltz raspatory
Maltz retractor
Maltz saw
Maltz-Anderson nasal rasp
Maltz-Lipsett nasal rasp
Maltz-Lipsett rasp
Maltz-Lipsett raspatory
Maltzman needle
malunion of fracture
malunion of zygoma
malunited calcaneus fracture
malunited forearm fracture
malunited fracture

malunited radial fracture
mamilla (*pl.* mamillae)
mamillary body
mamillary duct
mamillary line
mamillary process
mamillary sutures
mammalian cell membrane
Mammalok localization needle
mammaplasty
  Arie reductive mammaplasty
  Arie-Pitanguy mammaplasty
  Arie reductive mammaplasty
  Ashford mammaplasty
  augmentation mammaplasty
  Biesenberger reduction
    mammaplasty
  bilateral McKissock reduction
    mammaplasty
  devil's incision mammaplasty
  endoscopic transaxillary
    submuscular augmentation
    mammaplasty
  Goulian mammaplasty
  Lejour mammaplasty
  McIndoe nipple placement in
    reduction mammaplasty
  McKissock reduction
    mammaplasty
  Mouly reduction
    mammaplasty
  owl reduction mammaplasty
  periareolar mammaplasty
  Pitanguy reduction
    mammaplasty
  reconstructive mammaplasty
  reduction mammaplasty
  reductive mammaplasty
  Schatten mammaplasty
  Skoog mammaplasty
  Strombeck technique for
    reduction mammaplasty
  Toronto two-stage
    mammaplasty
  vertical mammaplasty
  Wyse reduction mammaplasty
mammaplasty procedure
mammaplasty reduction
  technique
mammary abscess
mammary artery
mammary body

mammary branches
mammary calculus
mammary duct ectasia
mammary fistula
mammary fold
mammary gangrene
mammary glands
mammary implant
mammary involvement
mammary line
mammary node biopsy
mammary prosthesis
mammary ptosis procedure
mammary region
mammary ridge
mammary souffle
mammary support
mammary support dressing
mammary vein
mammary vessels
mammary-coronary tissue
  forceps
mammascope
  acute-tipped mammascope
  central blunt-tipped
    mammascope
Mammatech breast prosthesis
mammectomy
mammiform
mammillaplasty
mammillary body
mammillo-accessory ligament
Mammo Mask illuminator
mammogram
mammogram lesion
mammographic abnormality
mammographic evaluation
mammographic lesion
mammography
Mammo-lock needle
Mammopatch gel self-adhesive
  dressing
Mammopatch gel self-adhesive
  scar treatment
mammoplasia
mammoplasty (mammaplasty
  preferred)
Mammotest Plus breast
  aspiration
Mammotome core biopsy device
mammotomy
management of anesthesia

Manan cutting needle
Manan needle
Manashil sialography catheter
Manche LASIK forceps
Manche LASIK speculum
Manchester colporrhaphy
Manchester knee replacement
Manchester nasal osteotome
Manchester operation
Manchester repair
Manchester uterine suspension
Manchester-Donald-Fothergill
    operation
Manchester-Fothergill operation
Manchu cotton dressing
Mancini technique
Mancusi-Ungaro scissors
mandatory laparoscopy
Mandelbaum cannula
Mandelbaum catheter
Mandelbaum ear knife
Mandelbaum-Nartolozzi-Carney
    patellar tendon repair
Mandelkorn suture lysis lens
mandible
    alveolar arch of mandible
    alveolar border of mandible
    alveolar limbus of mandible
    alveolar margin of mandible
    alveolar process of mandible
    alveolar surface of mandible
    alveolar yokes of mandible
    articular fossa of mandible
    ascending ramus of the
        mandible
    backward autorotation of the
        mandible
    body of mandible
    breadth of mandible
    cant of mandible
    cant of occlusal plane of
        mandible
    condyle of mandible
    coronoid process of mandible
    disappearing mandible
    extraoral open reduction of
        mandible
    head of condyloid process of
        mandible
    hypoplastic mandible
    incisive fossa of mandible
    inferior border of mandible

mandible (*continued*)
    jutting mandible
    lateral oblique projection of
        mandible
    length of mandible
    lingula of mandible
    little head of mandible
    median cleft of lower lip and
        mandible
    mental tubercle of mandible
    mylohyoid sulcus of mandible
    neck of mandible
    peripheral osteoma of
        mandible (POM)
    prognathic mandible
    protruding mandible
    pterygoid tuberosity of
        mandible
    ramus of mandible
    retrognathic mandible
    retruded mandible
    sagittal splitting of mandible
    short mandible
    space of body of mandible
    subcondylar fracture of the
        mandible
    subcondylar greenstick
        fracture of the mandible
    symphysial height of
        mandible
    temporal process of mandible
    vertical osteotomy of ramus
        of mandible
    yoke of mandible
mandible panogram
mandible radiography
mandible rim
mandible splint
mandibular advancement
mandibular advancement
    appliance (MAA)
mandibular alveolar mucosa
mandibular alveolus
mandibular angle
mandibular angle fracture
    intraoral open reduction
    microplate
mandibular angle fracture
    intraoral open reduction
    screw
mandibular anteroposterior
    ridge slope

mandibular arch
mandibular arch bar
mandibular artery
mandibular articulation
mandibular axis
mandibular base
mandibular bicuspid
mandibular bicuspid radiograph
mandibular block
mandibular body fracture
mandibular body length
mandibular body retractor
mandibular bone
mandibular border
mandibular branchial arch
mandibular bridging plate
mandibular canal
mandibular cartilage
mandibular centric relation
mandibular condylar hypoplasia
mandibular condyle
mandibular condyle fracture
mandibular condylectomy
mandibular contour
mandibular crest
mandibular cuspid
mandibular cuspid radiograph
mandibular cuspid-first bicuspid
   radiograph
mandibular cyst
mandibular defect
mandibular deficiency
mandibular dentition
mandibular dentitional
   odontectomy
mandibular depth
mandibular deviation
mandibular disk
mandibular dislocation
mandibular distraction
mandibular distraction
   osteogenesis
mandibular distractor
mandibular equilibration
mandibular excess
mandibular fissure
mandibular fixation
mandibular foramen
mandibular forceps
mandibular fossa
mandibular functional
   reconstruction

mandibular gland
mandibular glide
mandibular gliding movement
mandibular guide prosthesis
mandibular guide-plane
   prosthesis
mandibular head
mandibular hemisection
mandibular hinge position
mandibular hypoplasia
mandibular impression
mandibular incisor
mandibular incisor crowding
mandibular incisor radiograph
mandibular joint
mandibular leiomyosarcoma
mandibular lingual flange
mandibular lymph nodes
mandibular macrognathia
mandibular median cyst
mandibular mesh
mandibular micrognathia
mandibular miniplate
mandibular molar
mandibular molar radiograph
mandibular nerve
mandibular nerve block
mandibular neurovascular canal
mandibular notch
mandibular occlusal view
mandibular orthopedic
   repositioning appliance
mandibular osteotomy
   advancement
mandibular osteotomy-
   genioglossus advancement
mandibular overdenture
mandibular plane
mandibular plane angle
mandibular plane to hyoid
mandibular port
mandibular positioning device
mandibular premolar
mandibular process
mandibular prognathism
mandibular prosthesis
mandibular protraction
mandibular protrusion
mandibular ramus
mandibular ramus fracture
mandibular ramus osteotomy
mandibular range of motion

mandibular reconstruction
mandibular recontouring
   alveolectomy
mandibular reflex
mandibular rest position
mandibular restriction
mandibular retraction
mandibular retrognathia
mandibular retrognathism
mandibular retroposition
mandibular retrusion
mandibular ridge
mandibular sagittal deficiency
mandibular sagittal split
   osteotomy
mandibular sieving
mandibular sling
mandibular space
mandibular spine
mandibular splint
mandibular split
mandibular staple bone plate
   (MSBP)
mandibular sulcus
mandibular surgery
mandibular swing approach
mandibular swing operation
mandibular swing technique
mandibular symphysis
mandibular symphysis
   comminution
mandibular symphysis fracture
mandibular teeth
mandibular torus
mandibular trusion
mandibular vestibule
mandibular visceral arch
mandibular wiring
mandibular-sparing technique
mandibulectomy
   anterior mandibulectomy
   lateral mandibulectomy
   marginal mandibulectomy
   right segmental
      mandibulectomy
   segmental mandibulectomy
mandibulofacial dysostosis
mandibulomasseteric
mandibulomaxillary fixation
mandibulo-oculofacial
   dyscephaly
mandibulotomy

mandrel
   disk mandrel
   endosseous implant needle
      mandrel
   Moore mandrel
   Morgan mandrel
   snap-on mandrel
mandrel graft
mandrin
mandrin dilator
mandrin guide
maneuverability
maneuver
   Addison maneuver
   Adson maneuver
   Allen maneuver
   Allis maneuver
   alpha loop maneuver
   Apley maneuver
   avoidance maneuver
   Barlow maneuver
   Barton maneuver
   Bielschowsky maneuver
   Bigelow maneuver
   Bill maneuver
   Bracht maneuver
   Brandt-Andrews maneuver
   Bruhat maneuver
   bunching maneuver
   BURP maneuver
   Buzzard maneuver
   Cairns maneuver
   Carlo Traverso maneuver
   Chassard-Lapine maneuver
   circumduction maneuver
   closed manipulative maneuver
   Colanis maneuver
   cold pressor testing maneuver
   corkscrew maneuver
   costoclavicular maneuver
   Cottle maneuver
   Crede maneuver
   Cushieri maneuver
   Dandy maneuver
   deglutition maneuver
   delay maneuver
   DeLee maneuver
   Dix-Hallpike maneuver
   doll's eye maneuver
   doll's head maneuver
   Engel-Lysholm maneuver
   Epley maneuver

maneuver (*continued*)
  Essex-Lopresti maneuver
  Falconer maneuver
  Finkelstein maneuver
  flexion-extension maneuver
  flexor pollicis longus
    substitution maneuver
  Fog maneuver
  forceps maneuver
  forward-bending maneuver
  Fowler maneuver
  Fowler-Stephens maneuver
  Frenzel maneuver
  Gifford maneuver
  Gowers maneuver
  grunting maneuver
  Hallpike maneuver
  Hallpike-Dix maneuver
  Halsted maneuver
  Hampton maneuver
  heel-to-ear maneuver
  Heiberg-Esmarch maneuver
  Heimlich maneuver
  hemodynamic maneuver
  Hillis-Mueller maneuver
  Hippocratic maneuver
  Hodge maneuver
  Hoguet maneuver
  Hueter maneuver
  hyperabduction maneuver
  hyperventilation maneuver
  Jahss maneuver
  jaw thrust maneuver
  Jendrassik maneuver
  Jonnson maneuver
  J-type maneuver
  jugular compression
    maneuver
  Kappeler maneuver
  key-in-lock maneuver
  Ko-Airan maneuver
  Kocher maneuver
  Krackow maneuver
  Kristeller maneuver
  Lachman maneuver
  Lasegue maneuver
  Leadbetter maneuver
  Lecompte maneuver
  Levret maneuver
  liver hanging maneuver
  logrolling maneuver
  Losee maneuver

maneuver (*continued*)
  Lovset maneuver
  Massini maneuver
  Mattox maneuver
  Mauriceau maneuver
  Mauriceau-Levret maneuver
  Mauriceau-Smellie maneuver
  Mauriceau-Smellie-Veit
    maneuver
  McDonald maneuver
  McKenzie extension
    maneuver
  McMurray circumduction
    maneuver
  McMurray maneuver
  McRoberts maneuver
  Mendelsohn maneuver
  meticulous maneuver
  midforceps maneuver
  military maneuver
  Mueller maneuver
  modified Ritgen maneuver
  Moore head-tilt maneuver
  Mueller maneuver
  Mueller-Hillis maneuver
  Munro Kerr maneuver
  notch-and-roll maneuver
  Nylen-Barany maneuver
  oculocephalic maneuver
  Ortolani maneuver
  osteoclasis maneuver
  Pajot maneuver
  Patrick maneuver
  Pelosi maneuver
  peroral maneuver
  Phalen maneuver
  Phaneuf maneuver
  Pinard maneuver
  positive maneuver
  postural fixation back
    maneuver
  Prague maneuver
  Prentiss maneuver
  Pringle maneuver
  Proetz maneuver
  pull maneuver
  push maneuver
  Queckenstedt maneuver
  recruitment maneuver
  re-expansion maneuver
  relative response attributable
    to the maneuver

maneuver (*continued*)
  reverse Bigelow maneuver
  Ritgen maneuver
  Rivero-Carvallo maneuver
  rotation-compression
    maneuver
  Rubin maneuver
  Saxtorph maneuver
  scalene maneuver
  Scanzoni maneuver
  Scanzoni-Smellie maneuver
  scarf maneuver
  Schartzmann maneuver
  Schatz maneuver
  Schreiber maneuver
  Sellick maneuver
  shoeshine maneuver
  Slocum maneuver
  Smellie maneuver
  Spurling maneuver
  squatting maneuver
  Steel maneuver
  Stimson maneuver
  straightening maneuver
  surgical maneuver
  Thorn maneuver
  tire-iron maneuver
  Tobey-Ayer maneuver
  Toynbee maneuver
  U-turn maneuver
  Valsalva maneuver
  van Hoorn maneuver
  wall push maneuver
  Wigand maneuver
  Woods maneuver
  Woods screw maneuver
  Wright maneuver
  Zavanelli maneuver
Mangat curvilinear chin
    prosthesis
mangled extremity syndrome
Mangoldt epithelial graft
Manhattan Eye and Ear spatula
Manhattan Eye and Ear corneal
    dissector
Manhattan Eye and Ear probe
Manhattan Eye and Ear spat
Manhattan Eye and Ear
Manhattan Eye and Ear suturing
    forceps
ManHood absorbent pouch
Manhurkar catheter

Mani catheter
Mani cerebral catheter
manic reaction
manifest deviation
manifestation
  initial manifestation
man-in-the-barrel syndrome
manipulation
  back manipulation
  bile duct manipulation
  catheter manipulation
  cervical manipulation
  contact manipulation
  cranial nerve manipulation
  digital manipulation
  direct manipulation
  endoscopic manipulation
  fine manipulation
  gamete manipulation
  general thrust manipulation
  gross manipulation
  guidewire manipulation
  Hippocrates manipulation
  indirect manipulation
  interceptive orthodontic
    manipulation
  joint manipulation
  laparoscopic dissection and
    manipulation
  laser manipulation
  Leadbetter hip manipulation
  long- and short-level rotational
    manipulation
  manual manipulation
  myofascial manipulation
  noncontact manipulation
  opening wedge manipulation
  pancreatic duct manipulation
  passive joint manipulation
  percutaneous stone
    manipulation
  pharmacologic manipulation
  physical manipulation
  postureteroscopic
    manipulation
  shunt manipulation
  skin-subcutaneous dissection
    with SMAS manipulation
  SMAS manipulation
  specific thrust manipulation
  spinal manipulation
  thrust manipulation

manipulation of fracture
manipulation of joint
manipulation of muscle
manipulation of prosthetic
  device
manipulative therapy
manipulator
  4-degrees-of-freedom
    manipulator
  Barrett flange lens
    manipulator
  Barrett irrigating lens
    manipulator
  button lip lens manipulator
  button-tip manipulator
  ClearView uterine
    manipulator
  Drysdale nucleus
    manipulator
  Feaster lens manipulator
  Friedman Phaco/IOL
    manipulator
  Gall-Addison uterine
    manipulator
  Grieshaber 2-function
    manipulator
  Grieshaber 3-function
    manipulator
  Grieshaber manipulator
  Guimaraes implantable
    contact lens manipulator
  Hasson uterine manipulator
  Hirschman lens manipulator
  hook manipulator
  Hulka uterine manipulator
  HUMI uterine manipulator
  iris lens manipulator
  irrigating lens manipulator
  Jaffe-Maltzman lens
    manipulator
  Judson-Smith manipulator
  Koch phaco manipulator
  Kuglen angled lens
    manipulator
  Kuglen irrigating lens
    manipulator
  Kuglen lens manipulator
  Kuglen straight lens
    manipulator
  lens manipulator
  Lester lens manipulator
  Levy-Kuglen lens manipulator

manipulator (*continued*)
  Lieberman MicroFinger
    manipulator
  Lindstrom Star nucleus
    manipulator
  Lister lens manipulator
  Maloney no-hole lens
    manipulator
  McIntyre irrigating iris
    manipulator
  Microbeam manipulator
  multi-coordinate manipulator
  Osher nucleus lens
    manipulator
  Pelosi uterine manipulator
  Ramirez manipulator
  Rappazzo intraocular
    manipulator
  RUMI uterine manipulator
  Sargis uterine manipulator
  Sinskey lens manipulator
  Smith-Leiske lens manipulator
  uterine manipulator
  Valtchev uterine manipulator
  Vico angled manipulator
  Visitec Vico manipulator
  ZUMI uterine manipulator
manipulator/injector
  Harris-Kronner uterine
    manipulator/injector
    (HUMI)
  HUMI uterine
    manipulator/injector
  Kronner Manipujector uterine
    manipulator/injector
  Zinnanti uterine
    manipulator/injector
manipulator/splitter
Manketelow transfer procedure
Mankin procedure
Mankin resection
Mankin technique
Mann forceps
Mann procedure
Mann technique
Mann-Bollman fistula
Mann-Coughlin procedure
Mann-Coughlin-DuVries
    cheilectomy
Mann-DuVries arthroplasty
Mann-DuVries technique
Mannerfelt chisel

Mannerfelt gouge
Mannerfelt raspatory
Mannerfelt retractor
Mannerfelt syndrome
Manning forceps
Manning retractor
Mannis sutures
Mannis suture probe
Mannkopf sign
Mann-Williamson operation
Mann-Williamson ulcer
manometer (*see also* sphygmomanometer)
  Capsuel CPAP manometer
  catheter-tipped manometer
  DeVilbiss CPAP manometer
  Dinamap ultrasound blood pressure manometer
  Ethitek automated protection manometer
  Harvard manometer
  Honan manometer
  Riva-Rocci manometer
  spinal manometer
  strain-gauge manometer
  Tycos manometer
  Validyne manometer
  ventilator pressure manometer
manometer stopcock
manometer-tipped catheter
manometric catheter
manometric evaluation
manometric flame
manometric pressure
manometric technique
manometry
  anal manometry
  aneroid manometry
  anorectal manometry
  balloon reflex manometry
  biliary manometry
  ERCP manometry
  esophageal manometry
  laparoscopic transcystic sphincter of Oddi manometry
  rectosigmoid manometry
manoptoscope
Manschot intraocular implant lens
Mansfield catheter

Mansfield balloon
Mansfield balloon catheter
Mansfield balloon dilatation catheter
Mansfield bioptome
Mansfield dilatation balloon catheter
Mansfield forceps
Mansfield orthogonal electrode catheter
Mansfield Polaris electrode
Mansfield Scientific dilatation balloon catheter
Mansfield-Webster deflectable curve catheter
Manske technique
Manske-McCarroll-Swanson centralization
Manske-McCarroll-Swanson incision
Manson double-ended strabismus hook
Manson-Aebli corneal section scissors
Manson-Aebli scissors
Mansson urinary pouch
Mantel laryngoscope
Mantel-Haenszel analysis
Mantis retrograde forceps
Mantisol drain
mantle block
mantle dentin
mantle field
mantle irradiation
mantle radiation treatment
mantle technique
mantle therapy
Mantoux needle
Mantz dilator
Mantz rectal dilator
manual core endarterectomy
manual delivery of placenta
manual dermatome
manual dermatome thickness gauge
manual esthesiometer
manual extraction
manual injection
manual inspection
manual keratometer
manual lithotriptor
manual manipulation

manual osteotome
manual palpation
manual positioning
manual push-pull technique
manual reduction of dislocation
manual reduction of fracture
manual removal of placenta
manual resuscitation bag
manual retractor
manual traction
manual ventilation
manubriogladiolar junction
manubriosternal joint
manubriosternal junction
manubrium (*pl.* manubria)
manubrium of malleus
manudynamometer
many-tailed bandage
many-tailed dressing
Manz gland
MAP (mean arterial pressure;
    motor nerve action
    potential)
MAPcath stylet
map-guided endocardial
    resection surgery
Maple Leaf orthosis
maplike skull
Mapper hemostasis EP mapping
    sheath
mapping
    auditory brain mapping
    body surface Laplacian
      mapping
    brain mapping
    catheter mapping
    electrophysiologic mapping
    gene mapping
    intraoperative lymphatic
      mapping
    nerve mapping
    sentinel lymphatic mapping
mapping catheter
mapping/ablation catheter
MapWire J-tip guidewire
Maquet endoscopy table
Maquet knee operation
Maquet operating table
Maquet procedure
Maquet table
Maquet technique
Maquet tibial procedure

Marafioti-Westin rod
Maragiliano body
marantic clot
Marathon guiding catheter
Marax bronchodilator
Marbach episiotomy scissors
Marbach-Weil technique
marble bone disease
marble bones
marbleized
Marcaine hydrochloride
    anesthetic agent
march foot
march fracture
March laser lens
March laser sclerostomy needle
March technique
Marchant zone
March-Barton forceps
Marchetti operation
Marcks knife
Marcks operation
Marckwald operation
Marco refractor
Marco chart projector
Marco lensometer
Marco manual keratometer
Marco prism exophthalmometer
Marco radius gauge
Marco slit lamp
Marcon colon decompression
    set
Marcove-Lewis-Huvos shoulder
    girdle resection
Marcus-Balourdas-Heiple ankle
    fusion technique
Marcuse forceps
Marcuse tube clamp
Marcy hernia repair
Marcy operation
Mardis soft stent
Mardis-Dangler ureteral stent set
Marena by LySonix compression
    garment
Marfan epigastric puncture
Marfan syndrome
margin
    alveolar margin
    bone margin
    carious restoration margin
    cavity margin
    cavosurface margin

margin (*continued*)
- ceramometal margin
- cervical margin
- ciliary margins
- close margin
- corneal margin
- costal margin
- costochondral margin
- demarcated margin
- dentate margin
- dissection margin
- enamel margin
- eyelid margin
- falciform margin
- free gastric margin
- free gingival margin
- free gum margin
- frontal margin
- gastric margin
- gingival margin
- hepatic margin
- incisal margin
- infraorbital margin
- intercostal margin
- interosseous margin
- lacrimal margin
- lambdoid margin
- lid margin
- malar margin
- mastoid margin
- mesovarian margin
- metal crown margin
- negative margin
- obtuse margin
- occipital margin
- opposing margin
- orbital margin
- parietal margin
- positive resection margin
- positive surgical margin
- psoas margin
- pupillary margin
- resection margin
- revised wound margins
- skin margins
- smooth margin
- squamous margin
- superior margin
- supraorbital margin
- surgical margin
- temporal margin
- tumor-free margin

margin (*continued*)
- vermilion margin
- vermilion-free margin
- well-demarcated margin
- wound margins
- zygomatic margin

margin invasion
margin of field
margin of tongue
margin of wound
margin resection
margin resection involvement
margin trimmer
marginal nevus
marginal tubercle
marginal zone
marginal adaptation
marginal alopecia
marginal artery
marginal bevel
marginal chalazion forceps
marginal clamp
marginal crest
marginal excess
marginal excision
marginal fracture
marginal gingiva
marginal gingivitis
marginal incision
marginal insertion
marginal integrity of amalgam
marginal mandibular branch
marginal mandibular nerve
marginal mandibular resection
marginal mandibulectomy
marginal nevus
marginal periodontitis
marginal portion
marginal process of malar bone
marginal resection
marginal ridge
marginal ridge fracture
marginal sinus
marginal sinus rupture
marginal spinning
marginal traumatic alopecia
marginal tubercle
marginal tubercle of zygomatic
   bone
marginal ulcer
marginal zone
margination

margin-finishing knife
marginoplasty
marginotomy
  inferior marginotomy
  superior marginotomy
  supplementary marginotomy
margo alveolaris
margo incisalis
margo temporalis
Margolis appliance
Margulies coil
Margulies coil intrauterine
  device
Margulies intrauterine device
Margulies spiral intrauterine
  device
marian lithotomy
Marici bronchoscope
Marin bur
Marin operation
Marin reamer
Marino rotatable
  transsphenoidal curet
Marino rotatable
  transsphenoidal enucleator
Marino rotatable
  transsphenoidal horizontal-
  ring curet
Marino rotatable
  transsphenoidal knife
  handle
Marino rotatable
  transsphenoidal right-angle
  hook
Marino rotatable
  transsphenoidal round
  dissector
Marino rotatable
  transsphenoidal spatula
  dissector
Marino rotatable
  transsphenoidal vertical-
  ring curet
Marino transsphenoidal curet
Marinr catheter
Marion disease
Marion drain
Marion screw
marionette groove
marionette line
Marion-Moschcowitz
  culdoplasty

Marion-Reverdin needle
Mario-Stone staple
Marjolin ulcer
mark
  needle marks
  Permark micropigmentation
  mark
  port wine mark
  raspberry mark
  strawberry mark
  stretch marks
Mark II total knee retractor
Mark II knee retractor
Mark II Chandler total knee
  retractor
Mark II concave total knee
  retractor
Mark II distal femur distractor
Mark II femoral component
  extractor
Mark II Kodros radiolucent awl
Mark II lateral collateral
  ligament retractor
Mark II Magni-focuser loupe
Mark II modular weighted
  retractor
Mark II retractor
Mark II Stubbs short-prong
  collateral ligament retractor
Mark II Stulberg hip positioner
Mark II tibial component extractor
Mark II Wixson hip positioner
Mark III halo
Mark IV Moss decompression-
  feeding catheter
Mark IV nasogastric tube
Mark IV repair
Mark IX lens
Mark lens loupe
Mark-7 intrauterine sound
marked falling curve
marked localized reaction
marked narrowing
markedly comminuted
markedly dilated
markedly enlarged
Markel cell
Markel cell cancer (*also* scleral
  marker)
marker
  Accu-line Products skin
  marker

marker (*continued*)
Accu-Line surgical marker
Allskin marker
Amsler chart marker
Amsler scleral marker
Anastomark flexible coronary
  graft marker
Arrowsmith corneal marker
astigmatic marker
biprong muscle marker
Bores radial marker
Brems astigmatism marker
Castroviejo corneal transplant
  marker
Castroviejo scleral marker
Chayet corneal marker
Codman marker
cookie-cutter areolar marker
corneal transplant marker
cytokeratin marker
D'Assumpcao rhytidoplasty
  marker
Dell astigmatism marker
Desmarres marker
diamond green marker
Donahoo marker
Dulaney LASIK marker
ear marker
epithelial marker
E-rosette cell marker
Etch-Master instrument
  marker
facelift flap marker
fecal marker
Feldman radial keratotomy
  marker
fine-line tissue marker
Fink biprong marker
Fink muscle marker
Freeman cookie-cutter areolar
  marker
Friedlander incision marker
Gass scleral marker
genetic markers
Glomark fluorescent skin
  marker
gold ear marker
Gonin marker
Gonin-Amsler scleral marker
Green corneal marker
Green optical crater marker
Green-Kenyon corneal marker

marker (*continued*)
Hoffer corneal marker
Hoopes corneal marker
House-Urban ear marker
House-Urban gold ear marker
House-Urban marker
Hunkeler frown incision
  marker
I marker
instrument marker
intentional marker
interspace width marker
Kremer triple-optical zone
  corneal marker
Landstrom arcuate incision
  marker
Landstrom astigmatic marker
lead pellet marker
low-profile R-K marker
Lu corneal marker
Lundstrom arcuate incision
  marker
Machat double-ended marker
Machat superior flap LASIK
  marker
McDonald optic zone marker
Mendez corneal marker
metallic skin marker
Mickey and Minnie surgical
  marker
MicroMark tissue marker
Neumann double corneal
  marker
Neumann-Shepard corneal
  marker
neuroendocrine marker
neuropeptide marker
nipple marker
Nordan-Ruiz trapezoidal
  marker
O'Brien marker
O'Connor marker
ocular marker
Oshar-Neumann 8-line corneal
  marker
oval optical zone marker
periodontal pocket marker
phenotypic marker
Price radial marker
radial keratotomy marker
radiopaque end marker
retroreflective marker

marker (*continued*)
  Richey condyle marker
  RK marker
  roentgenographic opaque
    marker
  round optical zone marker
  Ruiz adjustable marker
  Ruiz-Shepard marker
  Saunders-Paparella marker
  scleral marker
  Shepard optical center marker
  Simcoe corneal marker
  Sitzmarks radiopaque marker
  skin marker
  Skin Skribe marker
  SklarScribe skin marker
  Soll suture and incision
    marker
  Squeeze-Mark surgical marker
  Storz radial incision marker
  tantalum-ball marker
  tape marker
  Thornton corneal marker
  Thornton 360-degree arcuate
    marker
  Thornton low-profile marker
  T-incision marker
  TLS surgical marker
  trephine marker
  tumor marker
  vein graft ring marker
  Visitec RK zone marker
  Vismark skin marker
  Vismark surgical skin marker
  window rasp marker
  X-act cutaneous x-ray marker
marker catheter
marker transit studies
market stitch
Markham biopsy needle
Markham-Meyerding
    hemilaminectomy retractor
marking pen
marking pencil
marking pocket
markings
  bronchovesicular markings
  convolutional markings
  fibrotic markings
  haustral markings
  interstitial markings
  linear markings

markings (*continued*)
  lung markings
  peribronchial markings
  pulmonary vascular markings
  skin markings
  superficial venous markings
  template markings
  Weise-pattern markings
marking scissors
Markley orthodontic wire
Markley retention pin
Markley retractor
Marks-Bayne technique for
    thumb duplication
Markwalder bone rongeur
Markwalder forceps
Markwalder rib forceps
Markwalder rib rongeur
Marlen airing hook
Marlen belt
Marlen biliary drainage kit
Marlen clamp
Marlen colostomy appliance
Marlen gas relief pouch
Marlen ileostomy bag
Marlen leg bag
Marlen Odor-Ban pouch
Marlen SkinShield adhesive skin
    barrier
Marlen Solo ileostomy pouch
Marlen weightless bag
Marlen zip-closed pouch
Marlen's Ultra one-piece
    pouch
Marlex atraumatic obstetrical
    tenaculum
Marlex atraumatic tenaculum
Marlex band
Marlex bandage
Marlex closure
Marlex graft
Marlex hernial repair
Marlex mesh
Marlex mesh abdominal
    rectopexy
Marlex mesh closure
Marlex mesh graft
Marlex mesh implant
Marlex mesh prosthesis
Marlex mesh rectopexy
Marlex mesh sling
Marlex mesh snare

Marlex methyl methacrylate
    prosthesis
Marlex methyl methacrylate
    sandwich
Marlex Perfix plug
Marlex plug technique
Marlex prosthesis
Marlex screen
Marlex sheet
Marlex sponge
Marlex sutures
Marlex tenaculum
Marlin cervical collar
Marlin cervical orthosis
Marlin thoracic catheter
Marlow disposable cannula
Marlow disposable trocar
Marlow Primus handle
Marlow Primus instrument
Marlow Primus tip
Marmor knee prosthesis
Marmor modular knee
    prosthesis
Marmor procedure
Marmor prosthesis
Marmor tibial prosthesis
Marmor total knee prosthesis
Maroon lip curet
Maroon-Jannetta neurodissector
Marquardt bone rongeur
Marquest Respirgard II nebulizer
Marquette 3-channel laser
    holder
Marquette 8000 Holter monitor
Marquette electrocardiograph
Marquette Holter recorder
Marquette monitor
Marquette Responder 1500
    multifunctional defibrillator
Marquez-Gomez conjunctival
    graft
Marquez-Gomez operation
Marquis probe
Marritt dilator
marrow
    bone marrow
    cancellous cellular marrow
    fat marrow
    fatty marrow
    gelatinous marrow
    incompatible bone marrow
    mismatched marrow

marrow (*continued*)
    particulate cancellous bone
        and marrow (PCBM)
    spinal marrow
    yellow marrow
marrow ablation
marrow cavity
marrow depression
marrow embolism
marrow injection
marrow nailing
marrow space
marrow spoon
marrow-lymph gland
Marrs intrauterine catheter
MARS revision acetabular
    component
Marsan belt
Marseille pancreatitis
    classification
Marshall knee procedure
Marshall ligament repair
    technique
Marshall meniscectomy
Marshall oblique vein
Marshall syndrome
Marshall vein
Marshall V-sutures
Marshall-Marchetti operation
Marshall-Marchetti repair
Marshall-Marchetti-Krantz
    operation
Marshall-Marchetti-Krantz
    uterine suspension
Marshall-McIntosh technique
Marshall-Taylor vacuum
    extraction
Marshik tonsillar forceps
Marshik tonsil-seizing forceps
marsupial flap
marsupial graft
marsupial notch
marsupial pouch
marsupial skin flap
marsupialization of abscess
marsupialization of cyst
marsupialization of lesion
marsupialization technique
Martel conductor
Martel intestinal clamp
Martin abdominal retractor
Martin anoplasty

Martin ballpoint scissors
Martin bandage
Martin bipolar coagulation
    forceps
Martin blade
Martin bur
Martin cartilage chisel
Martin cartilage clamp
Martin cartilage forceps
Martin cartilage scissors
Martin cheek retractor
Martin dermal curet
Martin diamond wire cutter
Martin drainage tube
Martin endarterectomy stripper
Martin gouge
Martin hip gouge
Martin hook
Martin incision
Martin laryngectomy tube
Martin lip retractor
Martin meniscal forceps
Martin modification
Martin muscle clamp
Martin nasopharyngeal biopsy
    forceps
Martin nasopharyngeal forceps
Martin needle
Martin nerve root retractor
Martin operation
Martin palate retractor
Martin patellar wiring technique
Martin pelvimeter
Martin plane
Martin probe
Martin rectal hook
Martin rectal hook retractor
Martin rectal speculum
Martin reduction technique
Martin retractor
Martin rubber dressing
Martin scissors
Martin screw for hip fracture
Martin snare
Martin speculum
Martin stripper
Martin Surefit lens pusher
Martin technique
Martin throat scissors
Martin thumb forceps
Martin tissue forceps
Martin tracheostomy tube

Martin uterine fistula probe
Martin uterine needle
Martin uterine sound
Martin uterine tenaculum
    forceps
Martin vaginal retractor
Martin vaginal speculum
Martin wire cutter
Martin-Davy rectal speculum
Martinez corneal dissector knife
Martinez corneal transplant
    centering ring
Martinez corneal trephine blade
Martinez disposable corneal
    trephine
Martinez double-ended corneal
    dissector
Martinez keratome
Martinez knife-dissector
Martinez-Castro keratome
Martin-Gruber anastomosis
Martini bone curet
Martinotti cells
Martius operation
Martius-Harris operation
Martorell ulcer
Marwedel gastrostomy
Marwedel operation
Marx classification of microtia
Marx needle
Marx protocol for ORN
    treatment
Mary Jane breast pump
Maryan biopsy punch forceps
Maryfield introducer
Maryfield introducer catheter
Maryland bridge
Maryland dissector
Maryland monopolar
    electrosurgical dissector
Marzola hair restoration surgery
Masciulli silicone sponge
Mascot indirect ophthalmoscope
masculinizing genitoplasty
Masera septal organ
Masing needle holder
mask
    AccuroX mask
    AeroChamber facemask
    Aquaplast mask
    Armstrong CPR mask
    bag and mask

mask (*continued*)
  Baker-Lima-Baker mask
    (BLB mask)
  Bili mask
  BLB mask (Baker-Lima-Baker
    mask)
  BLB mask (Boothby-Lovelace-
    Bulbulian mask)
  Boothby-Lovelace-Bulbulian
    mask (BLB mask)
  bridgeless mask
  cataract mask
  cold compress mask
  convolution mask
  CP2 Inflat-A-Mask inflatable
    sinus mask
  double-cataract mask
  EndoShield mask
  face mask
  Finney mask
  high-humidity facemask
  high-humidity tracheostomy
    mask
  Hudson-type oxygen mask
  isolation facemask
  Kuhn mask
  laryngeal mask
  LaserSite facial mask
  meter mask
  mouth mask
  nonrebreathing mask
  Olympic mask
  open face mask
  Orfit mask
  oxygen mask
  partial rebreathing mask
  Patil-Syracuse mask
  PEP mask
  Petit facial mask
  Phantom nasal mask
  Puritan mask
  rebreathing mask
  Rendell-Baker Soucek mask
  reservoir facemask
  Ring cataract mask
  Rudolph mask
  SealEasy resuscitation mask
  surgical mask
  Swiss Therapy eye mask
  Venti mask
  ventilated mask
  Venturi mask

mask leak
mask lift
masked fat
Masket forceps
Masket phaco spatula
masking
  backward masking
  central masking
  effective masking
  forward masking
  initial masking
  maximum masking
  peripheral masking
  upward masking
masking efficiency
masking level difference
masking technique
masklike face
masklike facies
Mason
    abdominotranssphincteric
    resection
Mason clamp
Mason gastroplasty
Mason incision
Mason leg holder
Mason operation
Mason radial head fracture
    classification
Mason splint
Mason suction tube
Mason vascular clamp
Mason vertical-banded
    gastroplasty
Mason-Allen hand splint
Mason-Allen snare
Mason-Allen splint
Mason-Allen Universal hand
    splint
Mason-Allen Universal sling
Mason-Auvard speculum
Mason-Auvard weighted vaginal
    speculum
Mason-Judd bladder retractor
Mason-Judd retractor
Mason-Judd self-retaining
    retractor
Mason-Likar limb lead
    modification
Mason-School aspirating needle
masoseptal deviation
masquerade technique

mass
- abdominal wall mass
- abdominopelvic mass
- achromatic mass
- adnexal mass
- appendiceal mass
- bisected mass
- body cell mass
- calcified mass
- cancerous mass
- cavitary mass
- complex chest mass
- congenital mass
- critical mass
- cystic mass
- definite mass
- discrete mass
- echogenic mass
- electronic mass
- enlarged mass
- esophageal mass
- exophytic mass
- expansile abdominal mass
- extrauterine pelvic mass
- extrinsic mass
- firm cell mass
- flank mass
- freely movable mass
- fungating mass
- hard indurated colon mass
- hilar mass
- hyperintense mass
- incudomalleolar mass
- indurated mass
- inflammatory mass
- infra-auricular mass
- injection mass
- intra-abdominal mass
- intraluminal mass
- intravascular mass
- intrinsic mass
- jelly-like mass
- lateral mass
- lipohypertrophic mass
- lobulated mass
- lobulated tumor mass
- localized mass
- lymphoid mass
- mediastinal mass
- mobile mass
- multilocular mass
- muscle mass

mass (*continued*)
- obstructing mass
- ovarian mass
- palpable mass
- parametrial mass
- paravertebral mass
- pelvic mass
- perihilar mass
- perineal mass
- peripheral mass
- phlegmonous mass
- pleural mass
- polypoid mass
- pulsatile mass
- pulsating mass
- questionable mass
- radiopaque mass
- rectal mass
- retroareolar mass
- retromammilar mass
- ropy mass
- salivary gland mass
- sclerotic cemental mass
- scrotal mass
- soft tissue mass
- solid-appearing mass
- sonolucent mass
- spherical mass
- Stent mass
- subcutaneous mass
- subcutaneous perineal mass
- subpleural mass
- superior perihilar mass
- suprahilar mass
- tender mass
- tissue mass
- umbilicated mass
- vascular mass
- ventrolateral mass

mass concentration
mass defect
mass excision
mass flow controller
mass lesion
mass reflex
mass spectrophotometric detector
MASS syndrome (mitral valve, aorta, skeleton, skin)
Massachusetts General Hospital (*see* MGH)
Massachusetts hemostat

Massachusetts Vision Kit
massage
   cardiac massage
   carotid massage
   chest cardiac massage
   closed chest cardiac massage
   cross-friction massage
   diathermy and massage
   external cardiac massage
   gingival massage
   glandular massage
   gum massage
   heart massage
   hydropneumatic massage
   lymphatic massage
   scar massage
   vibratory massage
Masseran trepan bur
masseter
masseter abscess
masseter muscle
masseter muscle flap
masseter muscle hypertrophy
masseter muscle transfer
masseter reflex
masseter tendon
masseteric area
masseteric artery
masseteric fascia
masseteric hypertrophy
masseteric nerve
masseteric reflex
masseteric space
masseteric vein
masseter-mandibular-pterygoid
   space
Massie driver
Massie extractor
Massie II nail
Massie II plate
Massie inserter
Massie nail
Massie nail assembly
Massie screwdriver
Massie sliding graft
Massie sliding nail
Massie sliding nail tube
Massini maneuver
Massiot polytome
massive all layer liposuction
   (MALL)
massive ascites

massive bleeding
massive bowel resection
massive collapse
massive dose
massive dose technique
massive heart attack
massive hemoptysis
massive hemorrhage
massive incisional hernioplasty
massive infection
massive involvement
massive lower GI bleeding
massive malignant infiltration
massive pulmonary hemorrhagic
   edema
massive radiation
massive resorption
massive sliding graft
massive sliding nail
massive transfusion protocol
massive transfusion
massive tumor
Masson fascial needle
Masson fascial stripper
Masson fasciatome
Masson needle
Masson needle holder
Masson trichrome stain
Masson-Luethy needle holder
Masson-Mayo-Hegar needle
   holder
Masson Vital needle holder
Masson trichrome method
MAST (military antishock
   trousers)
mast cell
MAST pants
MAST suit
MAST technique
mastadenoma
mastalgia
mastectomy
   Auchincloss mastectomy
   breast reconstruction after
     mastectomy
   complete skin-sparing
     mastectomy
   extended radical mastectomy
   Halsted radical mastectomy
   McKissock mastectomy
   McWhirter mastectomy
   Meyer mastectomy

mastectomy (*continued*)
  modified radical mastectomy
  Patey mastectomy
  radical mastectomy
  salvage mastectomy
  simple mastectomy
  simultaneous LATRAM and
    mastectomy (SLAM)
  skin-sparing mastectomy
  subcutaneous mastectomy
  toilet mastectomy
  total mastectomy
  transareolar mastectomy
  Urban mastectomy
  Willy Meyer radical
    mastectomy
mastectomy closure
mastectomy incision
mastectomy knife
mastectomy scar
mastectomy skin flap
mastectomy skin flap retractor
mastectomy support
Mastel trifaceted diamond blade
master apical file (MAF)
master cast
master cement
master cone
master gland
master IG bundle
Master screwdriver
Master step foot prosthesis
Master-Allen syndrome
Masterbrace 3 functional ACL
  knee brace
MasterFlex pump
Masters intestinal clamp
Masterson hysterectomy forceps
Masterson pelvic clamp
Masters-Schwartz intestinal
  clamp
Masters-Schwartz liver clamp
Masterstim interferential
  stimulator
masthelcosis
masticating surface
mastication disorder
mastication muscle
masticator space
  monoplegia masticatoria
masticatory bone
masticatory fat pad

masticatory force
masticatory mandibular
  movement
masticatory movements
masticatory mucosa
masticatory muscle
masticatory space
masticatory spasm
Mastin goiter forceps
Mastin muscle clamp
Mastin muscle forceps
mastitis
  chronic cystic mastitis
  cystic mastitis
  granulomatous mastitis
  silicone mastitis
Mastner median episiotomy and
  repair
mastocarcinoma
mastocele
mastochondroma
mastocytosis
mastodynia
mastogram
mastography
mastoid abscess
mastoid air cells
mastoid angle of parietal bone
mastoid antrotomy
mastoid antrum
mastoid bone
mastoid bone bur
mastoid bowl
mastoid bur
mastoid canaliculi
mastoid catheter
mastoid cavity
mastoid chisel
mastoid cortex
mastoid curet
mastoid dressing
mastoid emissary vein
mastoid empyema
mastoid fascia
mastoid fontanelle
mastoid foramen
mastoid fossa
mastoid gouge
mastoid groove
mastoid incision
mastoid knife
mastoid mallet

mastoid margin
mastoid node
mastoid notch
mastoid obliteration operation
mastoid operation
mastoid packer
mastoid pneumatization
mastoid pressure
mastoid probe
mastoid process
mastoid raspatory
mastoid region
mastoid retractor
mastoid rongeur
mastoid rongeur forceps
mastoid search
mastoid searcher
mastoid self-retaining retractor
mastoid sinus
mastoid suction tube
mastoid sutures
mastoid tip
mastoid tip cell
mastoid wall
mastoid-conchal suture
mastoidectomy
    Bondy mastoidectomy
        (type I, II, III)
    canal wall-down
        mastoidectomy
    canal wall-up mastoidectomy
    cortical mastoidectomy
    modified radical
        mastoidectomy
    radical mastoidectomy
    simple mastoidectomy
    Stacke mastoidectomy
    tympanoplasty mastoidectomy
mastoideum
mastoideus
mastoiditis
    Bezold mastoiditis
    coalescent mastoiditis
    Pneumocystis carinii
        mastoiditis
    sclerosing mastoiditis
    sclerotic mastoiditis
mastoidotomy
mastoidotympanectomy
mastoid-retaining retractor
mastoncus
mastopathia

mastopathy
mastopexy
    Benelli mastopexy
    double-skin mastopexy
    dual-pedicle
        dermoparenchymal
        mastopexy (DPM)
    endoscopic mastopexy
    Goulian mastopexy
    internal mastopexy
    modified Kiel mastopexy
    periareolar mastopexy
    reduction mastopexy
    Wise pattern mastopexy
mastopexy form
mastopexy breast augmentation
mastoplastia
mastoplasty
mastoptosis
mastorrhagia
mastorrhaphy
mastoscirrhus
mastosis
mastostomy
mastotomy
Mast-Spieghel-Pappas
    classification
Masuka modified thymic
    carcinoma classification
Masy angioscope
MAT (multifocal atrial
    tachycardia)
Matas aneurysmectomy
Matas aneurysmoplasty
Matas band
Matas operation
Matas vessel band
Matchett prosthesis
Matchett-Brown femoral head
    replacement
Matchett-Brown hip arthroplasty
Matchett-Brown hip
    endoprosthesis
Matchett-Brown hip prosthesis
Matchett-Brown stem rasp
matching donor
matchstick graft
mater
    arachnoid mater
    dura mater
    lateral lacunae of cranial dura
        mater

mater (*continued*)
  pia mater
  venous sinus of dura mater
materia (*pl.* materiae)
materia alba
materia dentica
material
  2-paste polysulfide rubber
    impression material
  3M Tegapore wound contact
    material
  Absorb-its material
  Accugel impression material
  Accumix impression material
  acrylic implant material
  Acuflex impression material
  Adaptic II dental restorative
    material
  agar hydrocolloid impression
    material
  agar impression material
  agar-alginate impression
    material
  Agarloid impression material
  Algee impression material
  alginate impression material
  Algitec impression material
  allogeneic lyophilized bone
    graft implant material
  allogeneic material
  Alveograf bone-grafting
    material
  Aneuroplast acrylic material
  Apligraf skin graft material
  Apligraf venous ulcer graft
    material
  Aquaplast alloplastic material
  Aquaplast rapid setting splint
    material
  Aquaplast splinting materials
  Audisil silicone ear mold
    material
  Augmen bone-grafting
    material
  Aurovest investment material
  autograft material
  autophagocytosed cellular
    material
  Avitene hemostatic material
  Balnetar graft materials
  base material
  baseplate material

material (*continued*)
  Biobrane graft material
  bioceramic implant material
  biocompatible bone graft
    substitute material
  biocompatible spacing
    material
  Bioglass bone substitute
    material
  Bioglass bone graft substitute
    material
  Biograft bovine heterograft
    material
  BioMend periodontal material
  Bio-Oss corticalis bone graft
    material
  Bio-Oss spongiosa bone graft
    material
  Bioplastique augmentation
    material
  Biovert implant material
  block-out material
  Bonaccolto monoplex orbital
    implant material
  bone graft material
  bone implant material
  bone substitute material
  bovine graft material
  brittle material
  Calcitite bone graft material
  Canals-N root canal filling
    material
  carbonaceous material
  Carboplast sheet orthotic
    material
  Carbo-Seal graft material
  Carbo-Zinc skin barrier
    material
  cast material
  Castorit investment material
  Celestin graft material
  Cellolite material
  celluloid graft material
  celluloid implant material
  CeraMed bone grafting
    material
  chrome-cobalt-molybdenum
    material
  coating material
  Codman cranioplastic
    material
  Coe impression material

material (*continued*)

Coe investment material
collagen hemostatic material
Collagraft bone graft matrix material
Collastat microfibrillar collagen hemostat material
colloid impression material
Coltene impression material
Coltex impression material
Compafill dental restorative material
Compalay dental restorative material
Compamolar dental restorative material
composite materials
contrast material
corundum ceramic implant material
Cranioplastic acrylic cranioplasty material
Cresatin dental material
Cristobalite investment material
Crossfire polyethylene material
Curaderm hydrocolloid dressing material
Cutinova Cavity wound filling material
cyanoacrylate fixed orbital silicone sleds implant material
cyanographic contrast material
Cyano-Dent material
dental material
Dentemp filling material
Dentloid impression material
Dermalogen material
Derma-Sil impression material
DermAssist wound filling material
Dermatell hydrocolloid dressing material
Dermostat eye implant material
devascularized material
Dextran barrier material
Diviplast impression material
double-lumen breast implant material

material (*continued*)

DualMesh material
ductile material
Duplicone silicone dental impression material
Durafill dental restorative material
Durapatite bone replacement material
Dur-A-Sil ear impression material
Duraval Hook & Loop strap material
Dynafabric material
DynaLeap balloon material
Edwards Teflon intracardiac patch implant material
elastic impression material
elastomeric impression material
Elgiloy clip material
Embarc bone repair material
Endo-Avitene collagen hemostatic material
Endur bonding material
eosinophilic proteinaceous material
Epicel skin graft material
epoxy die material
Estilux dental restorative material
Evazote cushioning material
Expander mammary implant material
Fastcure denture repair material
Fastrak traction material
fatty material
fecal material
Fermit N occlusal hole blockage material
fibrinous material
fibrocartilaginous material
filling material
Fletching femoral hernia implant material
Flexicon material
Flexistone impression material
FlowGel barrier material
Fotofil dental restorative material

material (*continued*)
  Frosted Flex earmold material
  G-C Vest investment material
  gelatinous material
  Geristore repair material
  glass ionomer restorative
    material
  glycolide trimethylene
    carbonate material
  gold weight and wire spring
    implant material
  Gore cast liner material
  Gore SAM patch material
  Gore subcutaneous
    augmentation material
    (SAM)
  Gore-Tex alloplastic material
  Gore-Tex augmentation
    material (GTAM)
  Gore-Tex periodontal material
  Gore-Tex regenerative
    material
  Graflex material
  Grafton bone grafting material
  grumose material
  grumous material
  Guttaform dental impression
    material
  Gypsona cast material
  Gypsona rapid-setting cast
    material
  Hand-Aid strapping material
  Hapex bioactive material
  Hapset bone graft plaster
    material
  Healos synthetic bone
    grafting material
  heavy body impression material
  hemostatic material
  Herculon suture material
  heterologous material
  Hircoe denture base material
  homograft implant material
  Hydrocal cast material
  hydrocolloid impression
    material
  hydroxyapatite ceramic
    material
  hydroxyapatite implant
    material
  impacted fecal material
  implant material

material (*continued*)
  Impregum impression
    material
  impression material
  inelastic impression material
  infested material
  injection of radiopaque
    material
  insertion of radioactive
    material
  Insta-Mold silicone ear
    impression material
  Interceed barrier material
  intermediate restoration
    material (IRM)
  Interpore bone replacement
    material
  Interpore ceramic material
  intrathecal contrast material
  intravenous contrast material
  irreversible hydrocolloid
    impression material
  IV bolus injection of contrast
    material
  Ivalon material
  Kaltostat wound packing
    material
  Karaya self-adhesive
    conductive material
  Keolar implant material
  Kerr Permplastic material
  Kerr Traycon material
  Kevlar material
  Lactomer skin staple material
  Langinate impression material
  Lash-Loeffler penile implant
    material
  LEAP balloon material
  light body impression material
  Lincoff sponge implant
    material
  Linkow dental implant
    material
  lipoaspirated material
  lipoid material
  loop of suture material
  L-rod implant material
  Luster investment material
  Macroplastique material
  MediFlex earmold material
  Medpor allograft material
  Medpor alloplastic material

material (*continued*)

Medpor block facial structure building material
methyl methacrylate implant material
mucoid material
Multidex wound-filling material
MycroMesh graft material
nonabsorbent material
Nu Gauze packing material
Omega splinting material
Ommaya reservoir implant material
Omniflex impression material
opaque material
Opotow filling material
Opotow material
Optisson contrast material
OrthoDyn bone substitute material
Orthoglass splint material
Ortho-Jel impression material
osteoconductive bone grafting material
OsteoGen bone grafting material
OsteoGen HA Resorb implant material
Osteogenics BoneSource synthetic bone replacement material
Osteograf bone grafting material
Osteograf/D dense bone grafting material
Osteograf/LD low density bone grafting material
Osteograf/N natural bone grafting material
Pacific Coast demineralized bone grafting material
Paladon implant material
Palfique Estelite tooth shade resin material
Paradentine dental restorative material
paraffin implant material
particulate material
PE Lite material
Pearlon impression material
Pearman penile implant material

material (*continued*)

PerioGlas material
Perma-Cryl denture base material
PermaMesh material
PermaSoft reline material
Permatone denture material
Phynox cobalt alloy clip material
plaster impression material
plastic restoration material
plastic wax material
platinum material
Platorit investment material
Poloxamer 407 barrier material
polyether graft material
polyether implant material
polyether impression material
polyether prosthesis material
polyether rubber impression material
polyethylene implant material
polysulfide impression material
polysulfide rubber impression material
polyurethane elastomer material
polyurethane implant material
polyvinyl alcohol splinting material
polyvinyl implant material
Polyviolene polyester material
Polyviolene polyester suture material
PolyWic wound filling material
Porocoat material
porous materials
porous prosthetic materials
precollagenous filamentous material
ProOsteon implant graft material
Proplast porous implant material
Proplast-Teflon material
Protegen material
Protouch material
provisionally acceptable material

material (*continued*)
  Provit filling material
  purulent material
  radar absorbent material (RAM)
  Ramitec bite material
  regular body impression material
  reline material
  Rema Exakt investment material
  Reprodent acrylic tooth material
  residual contrast material
  restorative dental materials
  restorative material
  reversible hydrocolloid impression material
  rubber impression material
  SAM facial implant material
  sanguineous material
  Scialom dental implant material
  Scutan temporary splint material
  SeamGuard staple line material
  sebaceous material
  semisolid material
  Septosil impression material
  Shearing posterior chamber implant material
  shell implant material
  shiny material
  ShowerSafe protector material
  Silastic material
  silicate restorate material
  silicone impression material
  silicone rubber impression material
  Sili-Gel impression material
  Silon silicone thermoplastic splinting material
  silver material
  Small-Carrion penile implant material
  solid buckling implant material
  solid silicone exoplant implant material
  soupy material
  spacing material

material (*continued*)
  Spicel skin graft material
  Spitz-Holter valve implant material
  splinting material
  sponge silicone implant material
  SR Isosit dental restorative material
  SR Ivocap denture material
  SR Ivolen impression material
  SR Ivoseal impression material
  StaTic impression material
  Stellite ring material
  stimoceiver implant material
  subcutaneous augmentation material (SAM)
  Surgamid polyamide suture material
  Surgical Nu-Knit absorbable hemostatic material
  surrounding graft material
  suture material
  synthetic suture material
  Szulc orbital implant material
  tantalum material
  Teflon material
  temporary endodontic restorative material (TERM)
  temporary material
  thermoplastic impression material
  tissue equivalent material
  tissue mandrel implant material
  titanium implant material
  transcatheter umbrella implant material
  tridodecylmethylammonium chloride graft coating material (TDMAC)
  Tru-Chrome band material
  tubular Gore-Tex SAM material
  tunnel-type implant material
  twisted cotton nonabsorbable surgical suture material
  unacceptable material
  Uroplastique material
  Usher Marlex mesh implant material
  vasodepressor material

material (*continued*)
  Vicryl suture material
  vinyl polysiloxane impression
    material
  Vitallium implant material
  Vitremer glass-ionomer
    restorative material
  wash impression material
  Wheeler graft material
  Wirosol investment material
  Wirovest investment material
  Xantopren impression
    material
  Zenotech graft material
  zinc oxide-eugenol
    impression material
material failure break point
maternal anesthesia
maternal birthing position
maternal bleed
maternal deprivation syndrome
maternal fracture
maternal mercury exposure
maternal placenta
Mathes-Nahai classification
    for muscle circulation
    (types I-IV)
Mathews drill
Mathews drill point
Mathews forceps
Mathews hand drill
Mathews load drill
Mathews olecranon fracture
    classification
Mathews osteotome
Mathews rectal speculum
Mathews speculum
Mathieu double-ended retractor
Mathieu foreign body forceps
Mathieu holder
Mathieu island onlay flap
Mathieu needle
Mathieu needle holder
Mathieu pliers
Mathieu procedure
Mathieu raspatory
Mathieu retractor
Mathieu technique
Mathieu tongue forceps
Mathieu tongue-seizing forceps
Mathieu urethral forceps
Mathieu-Kocher needle holder

Mathieu-Olson needle holder
Mathieu-Ryder needle holder
Mathieu-Stille needle holder
Mathys cementless prosthesis
Mathys prosthesis
matricectomy
matrix (*pl.* matrices)
  ACCOR dental matrix
  amalgam matrix
  bone matrix
  cartilage matrix
  celluloid matrix
  Class V cervical matrix
  Collagraft bone graft matrix
  custom matrix
  demineralized bone matrix
  dentin matrix
  dentinal matrix
  direct porcelain matrix
  distal nail matrix
  DuraGen absorbable dural
    graft matrix
  Dynafill graft biomedium
    mineralized bone matrix
  enamel matrix
  extracellular matrix (ECM)
  germinal matrix
  glomerular extracellular matrix
  groove of nail matrix
  human tissue collagen matrix
  mesangial matrix
  Mylar matrix
  myxochondroid matrix
  nail matrix
  NeoDura matrix
  nuclear matrix (NM)
  organic matrix
  Osteovit bone matrix
  perilacunar mineral matrix
    (PMM)
  PermaMesh hydroxyapatite
    woven sheet matrix
  plastic matrix
  platinum foil matrix
  predentin matrix (PDM)
  proximal nail matrix
  Raven matrix
  resin matrix
  resin shell matrix
  sterile matrix
  T-band matrix
  Walser matrix

matrix band
matrix calculus
matrix cells
matrix metalloproteinase (MMP)
matrix pliers
matrix retainer
matrix sentence
matrix vesicles
Matroc femoral head
Matsen procedure
Matson elevator
Matson operation
Matson periosteal elevator
Matson raspatory
Matson rib elevator
Matson rib spreader
Matson rib stripper
Matson stripper
Matson-Alexander elevator
Matson-Alexander raspatory
Matson-Alexander rib elevator
Matson-Alexander rib stripper
Matson-Mead apicolysis retractor
Matson-Mead periosteal stripper
Matson-Mead stripper
Matson-Plenk raspatory
Matsuda titanium surgical
    instruments
Matsura preparation
Matta-Saucedo fixation
matte black forceps
matted node
Matthew cross-leg clamp
Matthew forceps
Matti-Russe bone graft
Matti-Russe technique
Mattis corneal scissors
Mattis scissors
Mattison-Upshaw retractor
Mattox aortic clamp
Mattox maneuver
Mattox-Potts scissors
mattress stitch
mattress suture otoplasty
mattress sutures
mattressed onlay graft
maturation
maturational lag
maturative stage
mature bite
mature bone
mature cataract

mature cell
mature dentin
mature ovum
mature placenta
mature stump
mature teratoma
maturing temperature
Matzenauer vaginal speculum
Matzner tube
Mauch hydraulic knee
Mauck operation
Mauck procedure
Mauermayer stone punch
Mauksch operation
Mauksch-Maumenee-Goldberg
    operation
Maumenee capsule forceps
Maumenee corneal forceps
Maumenee cross-action capsule
    forceps
Maumenee erysiphake
Maumenee eye knife
Maumenee forceps
Maumenee goniotomy cannula
Maumenee goniotomy knife
Maumenee iris hook
Maumenee straight-action
    capsule forceps
Maumenee Suregrip forceps
Maumenee tissue forceps
Maumenee trephine
Maumenee vitreous sweep
    spatula
Maumenee vitreous-aspirating
    needle
Maumenee-Barraquer vitreous
    sweep spatula
Maumenee-Colibri corneal
    forceps
Maumenee-Colibri forceps
Maumenee-Goldberg operation
Maumenee-Park erysiphake
Maumenee-Park eye speculum
Maumenee-Park lid speculum
Maunder oral screw gag
Maunder oral screw mouth gag
Maunoir hydrocele
Maunoir iris scissors
Maunsell sutures
Maunsell-Weir operation
Mauriceau maneuver
Mauriceau-Levret maneuver

Mauriceau-Smellie maneuver
Mauriceau-Smellie-Veit
  maneuver
Maverick balloon dilatation
  catheter
Max Fine scissors
Max Fine tying forceps
Max Force balloon dilatation
  catheter
Max Force TTS biliary balloon
  dilatation catheter
Max forceps
Max Plus MR scanner
Max ventilator
Maxam sutures
MaxBloc bite block
MaxCast fiberglass casting tape
MaxCast tape
Maxilith pacemaker
Maxilith pacemaker pulse
  generator
maxilla (*pl.* maxillae)
  alveolar arch of maxilla
  alveolar border of maxilla
  alveolar canal of maxilla
  alveolar limbus of maxilla
  alveolar process of maxilla
  alveolar surface of maxilla
  alveolar yokes of maxilla
  anterior nasal spine of maxilla
  anterior surface of maxilla
  body of maxilla
  clothesline evulsion of maxilla
  conchal crest of maxilla
  facial surface of maxilla
  Fergusson excision of maxilla
  frontal process of maxilla
  greater palatine sulcus of
    maxilla
  incisive fossa of maxilla
  inferior maxilla
  inferior turbinal crest of
    maxilla
  infraorbital groove of maxilla
  infraorbital ridge of maxilla
  infraorbital sulcus of maxilla
  infratemporal surface of
    maxilla
  lacrimal groove of maxilla
  lacrimal sulcus of maxilla
  medial surface of maxilla
  nasal crest of maxilla

maxilla (*continued*)
  nasal notch of maxilla
  palatine groove of maxilla
  palatine lamina of maxilla
  palatine process of maxilla
  palatine sulci of maxilla
  palatine sulcus of maxilla
  posterior surface of maxilla
  retroinclined maxilla
  spine of maxilla
  sulcus of nasal process of
    maxilla
  superior maxilla
  superior turbinal crest of
    maxilla
  superolateral surface of
    maxilla
  yoke of maxilla
  zygomatic buttress of maxilla
  zygomatic process of maxilla
maxilla radiograph
maxillary alveolar protrusion
maxillary alveolectomy
maxillary alveoloplasty
maxillary alveolus
maxillary anchorage
maxillary and mandibular
    disharmony
maxillary angle
maxillary anterior tooth
maxillary antrotomy
maxillary antrum
maxillary antrum closure
maxillary arch
maxillary arch bar
maxillary artery
maxillary articulation
maxillary bicuspid
maxillary bite plate
maxillary bone
maxillary buttress
maxillary canal
maxillary canine
maxillary crest
maxillary cuspid
maxillary cyst
maxillary deficiency
maxillary deformity
maxillary dental prosthesis
maxillary dentition
maxillary depth
maxillary disimpaction forceps

maxillary division
maxillary downgrafting
maxillary excess
maxillary excision
maxillary expansion
maxillary first molar alveolus
maxillary fissure
maxillary foramen
maxillary fossa
maxillary fracture
maxillary fracture forceps
maxillary gland
maxillary hiatus
maxillary hypoplasia
maxillary impression
maxillary incisor
maxillary incisor retraction
maxillary intrusion
maxillary ligament
maxillary lymph node
maxillary macrognathia
maxillary malignant
  mesenchymoma
maxillary median anterior cyst
maxillary micrognathia
maxillary molar
maxillary neoplasm
maxillary nerve
maxillary nerve block
maxillary occlusal view
maxillary osteotomy
maxillary ostium
maxillary plane
maxillary posterior tooth
maxillary process of zygomatic
  bone
maxillary prognathism
maxillary prominence
maxillary prosthesis
maxillary protraction
maxillary protrusion
maxillary rampart
maxillary recontouring
  alveolectomy
maxillary removal and
  reinsertion
maxillary restoration
maxillary retardation
maxillary retrognathia
maxillary retroinclination
maxillary retroposition
maxillary retrusion

maxillary ridge
maxillary sinus
maxillary sinus cannula
maxillary sinus carcinoma
maxillary sinus cavity
maxillary sinus cyst
maxillary sinus Foley catheter
  balloon placement
  technique
maxillary sinus mucocele
maxillary sinuses
maxillary sinusitis
maxillary sinusoscopy
maxillary sinusotomy
maxillary stent
maxillary surface
maxillary surface of great wing
maxillary surface of
  perpendicular plate of
  palatine bone
maxillary surgery
maxillary teeth
maxillary torus
maxillary trusion
maxillary tubercles
maxillary tuberosity
maxillary veins
maxillary-zygomatic hypoplasia
maxillectomy
maxillitis
maxilloalveolar breadth
maxilloalveolar index
maxilloalveolar length
maxillodental
maxillofacial abnormality
maxillofacial and facioproximal
  surface toothbrushing
maxillofacial anomaly
maxillofacial bone screw
maxillofacial fracture
maxillofacial injury
maxillofacial osteotome
maxillofacial prosthesis
maxillofacial prosthodontics
maxillofacial reconstruction
maxillofacial region
maxillofacial skeletal
  advancement
maxillofacial surgery
maxillofrontale
maxillojugal
maxillomandibular anchorage

maxillomandibular disharmony
maxillomandibular dysplasia
maxillomandibular elastic
maxillomandibular fixation
  (MMF)
maxillomandibular record
maxillomandibular registration
maxillomandibular relation
maxillomandibular traction
maxillonasal dysostosis
maxillopalatine
maxillotomy
maxillozygomatic complex
Maxima II TENS unit
Maxima II transcutaneous
  electrical nerve stimulator
maximal contrast
maximal drug concentration
maximal expiratory flow rate
maximal intensity
maximal static response assay of
  facial motion
maximal stress
maximal tension skin lines
maximal ventilation rate
maximal voluntary ventilation
maximum accumulated dose
  (MAD)
maximum acoustic output
maximum amplitude
maximum bite force
maximum breathing capacity
maximum dimension
maximum dosage
maximum duration of sustained
  blowing
maximum frequency range
maximum intensity projections
  (MIPs)
maximum intercuspation
maximum interincisal distance
  (MID)
maximum masking
maximum movement
maximum occipital point
maximum permissible
  concentration
maximum permissible dose
  (MPD)
maximum power output (MPO)
maximum pressure
maximum stimulation test (MST)

maximum voluntary ventilation
  (MVV)
Max-I-Probe endodontic
  irrigation syringe
Max-I-Probe irrigation probe
Maxisorb test plate
maxi-vessel loops
Maxon absorbable sutures
Maxorb alginate wound dressing
Maxum Carr-Locke angled
  forceps
Maxum reusable endoscopic
  forceps
Maxxum balloon catheter
Maxxus orthopaedic latex
  surgical glove
May anatomical bone plate
May bone plate
May hook-on lens loupe
May kidney clamp
May ophthalmoscope
Maydl colostomy
Maydl hernia
Maydl operation
Maydl pessary
Maydl procedure
Mayer forceps
Mayer nasal splint
Mayer orthotic
Mayer pessary
Mayer position
Mayer reflex
Mayer speculum
Mayer splint
Mayer trapezius transfer
Mayer vaginal speculum
Mayer view
Mayer-Rokitansky syndrome
Mayer-Rokitansky-Küster-Hauser
  syndrome (MRKHS)
Mayfield 3-pin skull clamp
Mayfield aneurysm clamp
Mayfield aneurysm clip
Mayfield aneurysm forceps
Mayfield aneurysm hemostat
Mayfield applying forceps
Mayfield bayonet osteotome
Mayfield bone rongeur
Mayfield brain spatula
Mayfield CIS-RE aneurysm clamp
Mayfield CIS-RE aneurysm clip
Mayfield clip applicator

Mayfield curet
Mayfield disposable skull pin
Mayfield fixation frame
Mayfield head clamp
Mayfield head holder
Mayfield headrest
Mayfield incision
Mayfield malleable brain spatula
Mayfield miniature clip applier
Mayfield osteotome
Mayfield pediatric horseshoe
    headrest
Mayfield pediatric horseshoe
    pad
Mayfield radiolucent base unit
Mayfield radiolucent head
    holder
Mayfield radiolucent headrest
Mayfield retractor
Mayfield skull clamp
Mayfield skull clamp adapter
Mayfield skull clamp pin
Mayfield skull-pin head holder
Mayfield spatula
Mayfield spinal curet
Mayfield swivel horseshoe
    headrest
Mayfield table
Mayfield temporary aneurysm
    clip applier
Mayfield tic head holder
Mayfield-Kees clip
Mayfield-Kees head holder
Mayfield-Kees headrest
Mayfield-Kees table attachment
May-Harrington forceps
Maylard incision
Mayne muscle control appliance
Mayne space maintainer
Mayo abdominal retractor
Mayo approach
Mayo bone-cutting forceps
Mayo bunion deformity
    procedure
Mayo bunion repair
Mayo bunionectomy
Mayo cannula
Mayo carpal instability
    classification
Mayo carrier
Mayo catgut needle
Mayo clamp

Mayo common duct probe
Mayo common duct scoop
Mayo common duct spoon
Mayo coronary perfusion
    cannula
Mayo coronary perfusion tip
Mayo curved scissors
Mayo cystic duct scoop
Mayo dissecting scissors
Mayo elbow prosthesis
Mayo external vein stripper
Mayo fibroid hook
Mayo forceps
Mayo gallstone scoop
Mayo gastrojejunostomy
Mayo goiter ligature carrier
Mayo hammertoe correction
Mayo hemostat
Mayo herniorrhaphy
Mayo holder
Mayo hook
Mayo hysterectomy
Mayo instrument table
Mayo instrument tray
Mayo intestinal needle
Mayo kidney clamp
Mayo kidney pedicle forceps
Mayo kidney stone probe
Mayo knife
Mayo linen sutures
Mayo long dissecting scissors
Mayo modified total elbow
    arthroplasty
Mayo needle
Mayo needle holder
Mayo operating scissors
Mayo operation
Mayo perfusing O ring
Mayo probe
Mayo pyloric vein
Mayo resection arthroplasty
Mayo retractor
Mayo rheumatoid elbow
    classification
Mayo round blade scissors
Mayo sacroiliac belt
Mayo scissors
Mayo scoop
Mayo semiconstrained elbow
    prosthesis
Mayo stand
Mayo straight scissors

Mayo stripper
Mayo sutures
Mayo tissue forceps
Mayo total ankle prosthesis
Mayo trocar needle
Mayo trocar-point needle
Mayo ureter isolation forceps
Mayo uterine probe
Mayo uterine scissors
Mayo vein stripper
Mayo vessel clamp
Mayo-Adams appendectomy
    retractor
Mayo-Adams retractor
Mayo-Adams self-retaining
    retractor
Mayo-Adson self-retaining
    retractor
Mayo-Blake gallstone forceps
Mayo-Boldt appendix inverter
Mayo-Boldt inverter
Mayo-Collins appendectomy
    retractor
Mayo-Collins double-ended
    retractor
Mayo-Collins mastoid retractor
Mayo-Collins retractor
Mayo-Fueth inversion procedure
Mayo-Fueth operation
Mayo-Gibbon heart-lung
    machine
Mayo-Guyon kidney clamp
Mayo-Guyon vessel clamp
Mayo-Harrington dissecting
    scissors
Mayo-Harrington forceps
Mayo-Harrington scissors
Mayo-Hegar curved-jaw needle
    holder
Mayo-Heuter bunionectomy
Mayo-Kelly appendix inverter
Mayo-Lexer scissors
Mayo-Lovelace abdominal
    retractor
Mayo-Lovelace clamp
Mayo-Lovelace crusher
Mayo-Lovelace spur crusher
Mayo-Lovelace spur crushing
    clamp
Mayo-Myers external vein
    stripper
Mayo-New scissors

Mayo-Noble dissecting scissors
Mayo-Ochsner cannula
Mayo-Ochsner forceps
Mayo-Ochsner hemostat
Mayo-Ochsner suction trocar
    cannula
Mayo-Ochsner trocar
Mayo-Pean forceps
Mayo-Pean hemostat
Mayo-Polya gastric resection
Mayo-Potts dissecting scissors
Mayo-Potts scissors
Mayo-Robson gallstone scoop
Mayo-Robson gastrointestinal
    forceps
Mayo-Robson incision
Mayo-Robson intestinal clamp
Mayo-Robson intestinal forceps
Mayo-Robson operation
Mayo-Robson position
Mayo-Robson scoop
Mayo-Russian gastrointestinal
    forceps
Mayo-Simpson retractor
Mayo-Sims dissecting scissors
Mayo-Sims scissors
Mayo-Stille dissecting scissors
Mayo-Stille operating scissors
Mayo-Ward hysterectomy
Mays operation
Mazas hinge elbow
Maze III procedure
Mazet knee disarticulation
Mazet technique
Mazlin intrauterine device
Mazlin spring intrauterine
    device (spring IUD)
Mazur operation
Mazzariello-Caprini stone
    forceps
Mazzocco flexible lens forceps
Mazzocco silicone intraocular
    lens
MB&J hip drape
MB&J knee positioner
MBD (minimal brain
    dysfunction)
MBD syndrome
MBE cast
M-blade
M-brace corneal trephine
MBS snap-on orthotic

Mc (*see also* Mac)
MC (mesenchymal
    chondrosarcoma)
mc (millicuries)
MCA (middle cerebral artery)
MCA occlusion
McAfee approach
McAllister needle holder
McAllister scissors
McArdle sign
McArdle syndrome
McArthur incision
McArthur operation
McAtee compression screw
    device
McAtee olecranon compression
    screw device
McAtee olecranon device
McAtee screw
McAtee-Tharias-Blazina
    arthroplasty
McBride bunion repair
McBride bunionectomy
McBride cup
McBride femoral prosthesis
McBride operation
McBride pin
McBride plate
McBride procedure
McBride prosthesis
McBride tripod-pin traction
McBride-Akin operation
McBride-Moore prosthesis
McBurney appendectomy
McBurney appendectomy
    incision
McBurney fenestrated retractor
McBurney incision
McBurney operation
McBurney point
McBurney retractor
McBurney sign
McBurney thyroid retractor
McCabe antral retractor
McCabe canal knife
McCabe crurotomy saw
McCabe crus guide fork
McCabe dissector knife
McCabe elevator
McCabe facial nerve dissector
McCabe flap knife dissector
McCabe measuring instrument

McCabe parotidectomy retractor
McCabe perforation rasp
McCabe posterior fossa retractor
McCabe rasp
McCabe-Farrior rasp
McCaffrey positioner
McCain TMJ cannula
McCain TMJ curet
McCain TMJ forceps
McCall culdoplasty
McCall curet
McCall festoon
McCall instrument
McCall operation
McCall scaler
McCall stitch
McCall-Schumann operation
McCall-Schumann procedure
McCannel implant
McCannel intraocular implant
    lens
McCannel lens
McCannel ocular pressure
    reducer
McCannel sutures
McCarroll operation
McCarroll osteotomy hip
McCarroll-Baker procedure
McCarthy bladder evacuator
McCarthy catheter
McCarthy coagulation electrode
McCarthy cystoscope
McCarthy diathermic knife
McCarthy diathermic knife
    electrode
McCarthy electrode
McCarthy electrotome
McCarthy endoscope
McCarthy evacuator
McCarthy forceps
McCarthy Foroblique operating
    telescope
McCarthy fulguration electrode
McCarthy loop operating
    electrode
McCarthy miniature electrotome
McCarthy miniature loop
    electrode
McCarthy miniature
    resectoscope
McCarthy miniature telescope
McCarthy panendoscope

McCarthy resectoscope
McCarthy telescope
McCarthy visual hemostatic
  forceps
McCarthy-Alcock forceps
McCarthy-Alcock hemostatic
  forceps
McCarthy-Campbell miniature
  cystoscope
McCarthy-Peterson cystoscope
McCash procedure for
  Dupuytren contracture
McCash-Randall operation
McCaskey antral catheter
McCaskey antral curet
McCaskey catheter
McCaskey sphenoid cannula
McCaslin keratome
McCaslin knife
McCaslin knife-needle
McCaslin needle
McCaslin needle-knife
McCaslin wave-edge keratome
McCathy Foroblique
  panendoscope cystoscope
McCauley operation for talipes
  equinovarus
McCauley technique
McClamary elevator
McCleery-Miller anastomosis
McCleery-Miller intestinal
  anastomosis clamp
McCleery-Miller intestinal clamp
McCleery-Miller locking device
McClintock placental forceps
McClintock uterine forceps
McClure eye scissors
McClure iris scissors
McClure scissors
McCollough elevator
McCollough internal tibial
  torsion brace
McCollough osteotome
McCollough rasp
McCollough strabismus forceps
McCollough suturing forceps
McCollough tying forceps
McCollum attachment
McCollum tube
McComb procedure
McConnell extensile approach
McConnell knee technique

McConnell medial glide patellar
  taping technique
McConnell median and ulnar
  nerve approach
McConnell orthopedic headrest
McConnell shoulder positioner
McConnell technique
McCool capsule retractor
McCormick-Blount procedure
McCort sign
McCoy septal forceps
McCoy septum-cutting forceps
McCrae cystoscope
McCrae dilator
McCrae infant sound
McCrae sound
McCraw gracilis myocutaneous
  flap
McCraw technique
McCullough externofrontal
  retractor
McCullough forceps
McCullough hysterectomy
  clamp
McCullough retractor
McCullough strabismus forceps
McCullough suture forceps
McCullough suture-tying forceps
McCullough suturing forceps
McCullough utility forceps
McCune-Albright syndrome
McCurdy needle
McCurdy staphylorrhaphy
  needle
McCutchen hip
McCutchen hip implant
McCutchen press-fit titanium
  femoral implant
McCutchen SLT hip prosthesis
McDavid ankle guard
McDavid hinged knee guard
McDavid knee brace
McDermott clip
McDermott extractor
McDonald bone plate
McDonald cerclage
McDonald cervical cerclage
McDonald dissector
McDonald expressor
McDonald gastric clamp
McDonald lens-folding forceps
McDonald maneuver

McDonald operation
McDonald optic zone marker
McDonald pelvimetry
McDonald procedure
McDougal prostatectomy clamp
McDowell mouth gag
McDowell needle
McDowell operation
McDowell reflex
McElroy curet
McElroy instrument
McElveney procedure
McElveney punch
McElvenny technique
McElvenny-Caldwell procedure
McEvedy operation
MCF shoulder orthosis
McFadden aneurysm clip
McFadden clip
McFadden cross-legged clip
McFadden Vari-Angle aneurysm clip
McFadden Vari-Angle clip applier
McFadden-Kees clip
McFarland bone graft
McFarland tibia graft
McFarland-Osborne approach
McFarland-Osborne lateral approach
McFarland-Osborne technique
McFarlane skin flap
McFarlane technique
McGannon eye retractor
McGannon forceps
McGannon iris retractor
McGannon lens forceps
McGannon refractor
McGannon retractor
McGaw skinfold calipers
McGaw volumetric pump
McGee canal elevator
McGee crimper
McGee ear piston prosthesis
McGee footplate pick
McGee forceps
McGee middle ear instrument
McGee operation
McGee oval-window rasp
McGee piston
McGee platinum/stainless steel piston

McGee prosthesis needle
McGee raspatory
McGee splint
McGee stainless piston
McGee tympanoplasty knife
McGee wire crimper
McGee wire-closure forceps
McGee wire-crimper forceps
McGee wire-crimping forceps
McGee-Caparosa wire crimper
McGee-Paparella wire-crimping forceps
McGee-Priest wire crimper
McGee-Priest wire forceps
McGee-Priest wire-closure forceps
McGee-Priest wire-crimping forceps
McGee-Priest-Paparella closure forceps
McGee-Priest-Paparella crimper-forceps
McGehee elbow prosthesis
McGhan breast implant
McGhan breast prosthesis
McGhan eye implant
McGhan facial implant
McGhan fill kit
McGhan implant
McGhan intraocular lens
McGhan lens
McGhan Magna-Site tissue expander
McGhan MicroTorque permanent eyelining machine
McGhan mini-motor rotary bur machine
McGhan plastic surgical needle
McGhan tissue expander
McGhan 3M intraocular lens
McGill forceps
McGill neurological percussor
McGill operation
McGill retractor
McGivney hemorrhoidal forceps
McGivney hemorrhoidal ligator
McGivney ligator
McGlamry elevator
McGlamry-Downey procedure
McGoey Vitallium punch
McGoey-Evans acetabular cup

McGoey-Evans cup
McGoon cannula
McGoon coronary perfusion
    catheter
McGoon technique
McGovern nipple
McGowan needle
McGowan-Keeley tube
McGravey forceps
McGravey tissue forceps
McGraw elastic ligature
McGraw sutures
McGregor basal line
McGregor conjunctival forceps
McGregor forceps
McGregor forehead flap
McGregor line
McGregor needle
McGuire clamp
McGuire corneal scissors
McGuire forceps
McGuire marginal chalazion
    forceps
McGuire operation
McGuire pelvic positioner
McGuire rib spreader
McGuire scissors
McGuire urinal
McHenry scissors
McHenry tonsillar artery forceps
McHenry tonsillar forceps
McHugh facial nerve knife
McHugh flap knife
McHugh oval speculum
McHugh-Farrior canal knife
McIndoe-Reese alar cartilage
    suture fixation
McIndoe bone-cutting forceps
McIndoe cartilage scissors
McIndoe chisel
McIndoe colpocleisis
McIndoe dissecting forceps
McIndoe dressing forceps
McIndoe elevator
McIndoe incision
McIndoe inlay graft
McIndoe nasal chisel
McIndoe nipple placement in
    reduction mammaplasty
McIndoe operation
McIndoe orthopedic procedure
McIndoe osteotome

McIndoe procedure
McIndoe rasp
McIndoe raspatory
McIndoe retractor
McIndoe rongeur forceps
McIndoe scissors
McIndoe skin graft
McIndoe technique
McIndoe vaginal creation
McIndoe vaginal reconstruction
McIndoe-Hayes construction
McIndoe-Hayes procedure
McIntosh double-lumen catheter
McIntosh double-lumen
    hemodialysis catheter
McIntosh suture-holding forceps
McIntyre anterior chamber
    cannula
McIntyre aspirating unit
McIntyre aspiration needle
McIntyre coaxial cannula
McIntyre cystitome
McIntyre fish-hook needle
    holder
McIntyre guarded cystotome
McIntyre guarded irrigating
    cystitome set
McIntyre I&A needle
McIntyre infusion handpiece
McIntyre infusion set
McIntyre intracapsular lens
    extraction
McIntyre intraocular implant
    lens
McIntyre irrigating iris hook
McIntyre irrigating iris
    manipulator
McIntyre irrigating spatula
McIntyre irrigating unit
McIntyre irrigation needle
McIntyre irrigation-aspiration
    needle
McIntyre irrigation
McIntyre lacrimal cannula
McIntyre lens
McIntyre microhook
McIntyre needle
McIntyre nylon cannula
    connector
McIntyre splint
McIntyre-Binkhorst irrigating
    cannula

McIver nephrostomy catheter
McIver nephrostomy tube
McIvor mouth gag
McKay ear forceps
McKay-Simons clubfoot
   operation
McKee brace
McKee femoral prosthesis
McKee hinge elbow
McKee line
McKee prosthesis
McKee speculum
McKee table
McKee totally constrained
   elbow prosthesis
McKee tri-fin nail
McKee-Farrar acetabular cup
McKee-Farrar cup
McKee-Farrar hip prosthesis
McKee-Farrar rasp
McKee-Farrar total hip
   arthroplasty
McKee-Farrar total hip
   prosthesis
McKeever-MacIntosh
   hemiarthroplasty
McKeever arthrodesis
McKeever bunionectomy
McKeever cartilage knife
McKeever clavicle procedure
McKeever foot procedure
McKeever knee prosthesis
McKeever knife
McKeever medullary clavicle
   fixation
McKeever open reduction
McKeever operation
McKeever patella cap prosthesis
McKeever patella prosthesis
McKeever prosthesis
McKeever Vitallium cap
   prosthesis
McKeever-Buck elbow
   technique
McKeever-Buck fragment
   excision
McKenna Tide-Ur-Ator evacuator
McKenna Tide-Ur-Ator irrigator
McKenzie (see also Mackenzie)
McKenzie bone drill
McKenzie brain clip-applying
   forceps

McKenzie bur
McKenzie cervical roll
McKenzie clamp
McKenzie clip
McKenzie clip rack
McKenzie clip-applying forceps
McKenzie cranial drill
McKenzie enlarging bur
McKenzie extension maneuver
McKenzie grasping forceps
McKenzie hemostasis clip
McKenzie leukotome
McKenzie leukotomy loop
McKenzie leukotomy loupe
McKenzie lumbar roll
McKenzie night roll
McKenzie operation
McKenzie perforating twist drill
McKenzie perforator
McKenzie perforator drill
McKenzie silver brain clip
McKenzie sphenoid punch
McKenzie V-clip
McKernan Adson forceps
McKernan-Potts forceps
McKesson mouth gag
McKesson mouth probe
McKesson mouth tube
McKesson restrictor
McKibbin splint
McKinley EpM pump
McKinney eye speculum
McKinney fixation ring
McKinney speculum
McKissock incision
McKissock keyhole areolar
   template
McKissock mammaplasty
McKissock mastectomy
McKissock operation
McKissock pedicle flap
   technique
McKissock reduction
   mammaplasty
McKissock sutures
MCL (medial collateral ligament)
McLane obstetrical forceps
McLane pile forceps
McLane-Luikart obstetrical
   forceps
McLane-Tucker obstetrical
   forceps

McLane-Tucker-Kjelland forceps
McLane-Tucker-Luikart forceps
McLaughlin acromioplasty
McLaughlin approach
McLaughlin carpal scaphoid
    screw
McLaughlin extractor
McLaughlin hip plate
McLaughlin incision
McLaughlin laser mirror
McLaughlin laser vaginal
    measuring rod
McLaughlin nail
McLaughlin operation
McLaughlin osteosynthesis
    device
McLaughlin plate
McLaughlin procedure
McLaughlin quartz rod
McLaughlin screw
McLaughlin speculum
McLaughlin tarsorrhaphy
McLaughlin tendon rupture
    repair
McLaughlin Vitallium nail
McLaughlin-Hay technique
McLaughlin-Ryder incision
McLean capsule forceps
McLean capsulotomy scissors
McLean clamp
McLean corneoscleral sutures
McLean forceps
McLean muscle-recession forceps
McLean operation
McLean ophthalmic forceps
McLean ophthalmological
    forceps
McLean prism contact lens
McLean prismatic fundus laser
    lens
McLean scissors
McLean sutures
McLean technique
McLean tonometer
McLean-Tucker obstetrical
    forceps
McLean-Tucker-Kjelland
    obstetrical forceps
McLean-Tucker-Luikart
    obstetrical forceps
McLeary bone forceps
McLeod padded clavicular splint

MCL-N (midclavicular line to
    nipple)
MCM smart laser
McMahon nephrostomy hook
McMahon-Laird incision
McMaster bone graft
McMaster technique
McMurray circumduction
    maneuver
McMurray femoral neck
    osteotomy
McMurray knife
McMurray maneuver
McMurray sign
McMurray tenotomy knife
McNaught keel
McNaught keel laryngeal
    prosthesis
McNaught prosthesis
McNealey visceral retractor
McNealey-Glassman clamp
McNealey-Glassman visceral
    retainer
McNealey-Glassman-Babcock
    forceps
McNealey-Glassman-Babcock
    viscera-holding forceps
McNealey-Glassman-Babcock
    visceral forceps
McNealey-Glassman-Mixter
    clamp
McNealey-Glassman-Mixter
    forceps
McNealey-Glassman-Mixter
    ligature-carrying aneurysm
    forceps
McNealy-Glassman-Babcock
    forceps
McNeer classification
McNeill-Chamberlain
    sternotomy
McNeill-Goldmann blepharostat
McNeill-Goldmann blepharostat
    ring
McNeill-Goldmann ring
McNeill-Goldmann scleral ring
McNutt driver
McNutt extractor
MCP (metacarpophalangeal)
    total joint
MCP finger joint prosthesis
MCP joint

McPherson angled forceps
McPherson bent forceps
McPherson corneal forceps
McPherson corneal section
  scissors
McPherson eye speculum
McPherson iris spatula
McPherson irrigating forceps
McPherson lens forceps
McPherson microbipolar
  forceps
McPherson microconjunctival
  scissors
McPherson microcorneal
  forceps
McPherson microiris forceps
McPherson microsurgery eye
  needle holder
McPherson microsuture forceps
McPherson microtenotomy
  scissors
McPherson needle holder
McPherson scissors
McPherson spatula
McPherson speculum
McPherson straight bipolar
  forceps
McPherson suture-tying forceps
McPherson suturing forceps
McPherson trabeculotome
McPherson tying forceps
McPherson tying iris forceps
McPherson-Castroviejo corneal
  microscissors
McPherson-Castroviejo corneal
  section scissors
McPherson-Castroviejo
  microcorneal scissors
McPherson-Pierse forceps
McPherson-Pierse microcorneal
  forceps
McPherson-Pierse microsuturing
  forceps
McPherson-Vannas iris
  microscissors
McPherson-Vannas iris scissors
McPherson-Vannas microiris
  scissors
McPherson-Westcott
  conjunctival scissors
McPherson-Westcott stitch
  scissors

McPherson-Wheeler blade
McPherson-Wheeler eye knife
McPherson-Wheeler iris
  microknife
McPherson-Ziegler iris knife
McPherson-Ziegler microiris
  knife
McPherson-Ziegler microknife
McQueen vitreous forceps
McQuigg clamp
McQuigg forceps
McQuigg-Mixter bronchial
  forceps
McRae foramen magnum line
McReynolds calcaneus
  procedure
McReynolds driver
McReynolds driver-extractor
McReynolds extractor
McReynolds eye spatula
McReynolds hook
McReynolds keratome
McReynolds knife
McReynolds open reduction
  technique
McReynolds operation
McReynolds pterygium
  keratome
McReynolds pterygium knife
McReynolds pterygium
  operation
McReynolds pterygium scissors
McReynolds pterygium
  transplant
McReynolds scissors
McReynolds spatula
McReynolds transplant of
  pterygium
McReynolds-Castroviejo
  keratome
McReynolds-Castroviejo
  pterygium knife
McRoberts maneuver
McShirley electromallet
McShirley electromallet
  condenser
McSpadden compactor
McSpadden endodontic
  technique
MCT (motor coordination test,
  mucocilary transport)
M-cup vacuum extraction device

McVay hernia repair
McVay hernioplasty
McVay herniorrhaphy
McVay incision
McVay inguinal hernial repair
McVay operation
McVay procedure
McVay technique
McVay-Cooper ligament repair
MCW cement adhesive
McWhinnie dissector
McWhinnie electrode
McWhinnie tonsillar dissector
McWhirter mastectomy
McWhirter hemostat
McWhirter posterior shoulder
  approach
McWhirter tonsillar forceps
McWhirter tonsillar hemostat
McXim file
MD brace (Medical Design
  brace)
MDA ultrasound-assisted
  lipoplasty machine
MDS adhesive
MDS microdebrider
Meacham-Scoville forceps
Mead bone rongeur
Mead bridge remover
Mead crown remover
Mead dental rongeur
Mead forceps
Mead Johnson tube
Mead lancet knife
Mead mallet
Mead mastoid rongeur
Mead periosteal elevator
Meadox bifurcated graft
Meadox Dacron mesh
Meadox Dardik biograft
Meadox Microvel arterial graft
Meadox Microvel double-velour
  Dacron graft
Meadox Microvel double-velour
  knitted Dacron arterial graft
Meadox Microvel graft
Meadox Surgimed catheter
Meadox Surgimed Doppler
  probe
Meadox Teflon felt pledget
Meadox woven velour
  prosthesis

Meadox-Cooley woven low-
  porosity prosthesis
Meadox-Cooley woven low-
  porosity vascular prosthesis
mean arterial pressure (MAP)
mean circulation time
mean foundation plane
mean normalized systolic
  ejection rate
mean pressure
mean rejection grade (MRG)
mean residual gap (MRG)
Means-Lernan mediastinal
  crunch
Meares-Stamey technique
Mears-Rubash approach
measurement control handle
measurement film
measurer
  Bunnell digital exertion
    measurer
  Pach-Pen corneal thickness
    measurer
measuring gauge
measuring guide
measuring rod
measuring wire
measuring-mounting catheter
Measuroll sutures
meat forceps
meat hook retractor
meatal advancement and
  glanuloplasty procedure
  (MAGPI)
meatal atresia
meatal cartilage
meatal clamp
meatal dilator
meatal incision
meatal sound
meatal spine
meatal stenosis
meat-grasping forceps
meatoantrotomy
meatoplasty
meatoplasty and glanuloplasty
  (MAGPI)
meatorrhaphy
meatoscope
  Hubell meatoscope
  Huegli meatoscope
meatoscopy

meatotome
  Bunge meatotome
  Bunge ureteral meatotome
  Dreisse meatotome
  electric meatotome
  Ellik meatotome
  Huegli meatotome
  Otis meatotome
  Riba electric ureteral
    meatotome
  ureteral meatotome
meatotomy
  Spence urethral meatotomy
  ureteral meatotomy
  urethral meatotomy
meatotomy electrode
meatotomy knife
meatotomy scissors
meatus
  anterior middle meatus
  external acoustic meatus
  external meatus
  inferior meatus
  middle meatus
  nasal meatus
  spina meatus
  superior meatus
  urethral meatus
  urinary meatus
meatus clamp
MEC (mucoepidermoid
  carcinoma)
mechanical anastomosis
mechanical avulsion
mechanical axis
mechanical axis cord
mechanical biliary obstruction
mechanical blepharoptosis
mechanical block
mechanical bowel obstruction
mechanical condenser
mechanical creep of skin
mechanical device
mechanical duct obstruction
mechanical
  esophagojejunostomy
mechanical extrahepatic
  obstruction
mechanical finger
mechanical finger forceps
mechanical heart
mechanical ileus

mechanical insulin pump
mechanical intestinal
  obstruction
mechanical labyrinthectomy
mechanical lithotripsy
mechanical longitudinal/sector
  scanning echoendoscope
mechanical obstruction
mechanical occlusion
mechanical percussor
mechanical perforation
mechanical pulp exposure
mechanical radial-scanning
  instrument
mechanical respirator
mechanical retention
mechanical rotating probe
mechanical scanner
mechanical separator
mechanical small-bowel
  obstruction
mechanical stimulation
mechanical stimulus
mechanical strain
mechanical styptic
mechanical tooth separation
mechanical triturator
mechanical ureteral dilation
mechanical variceal
  compression
mechanical ventilation
mechanical ventilation
  anesthetic technique
mechanical ventilator
mechanical vitrector
mechanically assisted respirator
mechanically balanced
  occlusion
mechanized scissors
mechanoactivation
mechanogastrography
mechanoreceptor
mechanotherapy
Meckel band
Meckel cartilage
Meckel cave
Meckel cavity
Meckel diverticulectomy
Meckel diverticulum
Meckel ganglion
Meckel ganglionectomy
Meckel operation

Meckel rod
Meckel scan
Meckel space
Meckel sphenopalatine
    ganglionectomy
meckelectomy
meconium
meconium aspiration
meconium aspiration
    syndrome
meconium aspirator
meconium discharge
meconium fluid
meconium ileus
meconium plug
meconium plug syndrome
meconium-stained amniotic
    fluid
Mecring acetabular prosthesis
Mecron cannulated cancellous
    screw
Mecron titanium Voorhoeve
    sheath
Medallion intraocular lens
    implant
Medallion lens
Medallion lens expressor
Medarmor puncture-resistant
    gloves
Medasonics transcranial
    Doppler
Med-Co flexible catheter
Medcomp catheter
Medcor pacemaker
MedDev gold eyelid implant
Meadox vascular graft
Medela breast pump
Medela Dominant vacuum
    delivery pump
Medela manual breast pump
Medela membrane regulator
Medena continent ileostomy
    catheter
Mederma topical gel
Medevice surgical loop
Medex syringe infusion pump
Medfusion syringe infusion
    pump
MedGraphics body
    plethysmograph
Medi bandage scissors
Medi vascular stockings

media (sing. medium)
  acute otitis media (AOM)
  adhesive otitis media
  aerotitis media
  auris media
  barotitis media
  catarrhal otitis media
  chronic cholesteatomatous
      otitis media
  chronic granulation otitis
      media
  chronic otitis media
  chronic suppurative otitis
      media (CSOM)
  hydrophilic filter media
  instillation of diagnostic
      media
  mucoid otitis media
  mucoserous otitis media
  necrotizing otitis media
  noncholesteatomatous
      chronic suppurative otitis
      media
  nonsuppurative otitis media
  otitis media
  phalanx media
  purulent otitis media
  reflex otitis media
  refracting media
  scala media
  secretory otitis media (SOM)
  serous otitis media (SOM)
  suppurative otitis media
      (SOM)
  tuberculous otitis media
  tunica media
medial angle
medial angle of eye
medial antebrachial cutaneous
    nerve
medial anterior malleolus artery
medial aperture
medial aspect
medial aspiration
medial bicipital sulcus
medial bicortical screw
medial border
medial brachial cutaneous nerve
medial canthal fissure
medial canthal tendon
medial canthoplasty
medial canthus

medial capsular imbrication
medial capsule
medial capsulorrhaphy
medial circumflex artery of
    thigh
medial circumflex femoral artery
medial clear space
medial cleft of lip
medial cleft of palate
medial collateral ligament (MCL)
medial commissure of eyelids
medial compartment
medial condyle
medial crus
medial crus of lower lateral
    cartilage
medial cutaneous nerve
medial cutaneous thigh flap
medial deviation
medial dissection
medial distally based
    fasciocutaneous flap
medial dog ears
medial dorsal cutaneous nerve
medial elevation
medial eminence
medial epicanthoplasty
medial epicondyle
medial extradural approach
medial flap
medial foramen
medial forearm flap
medial geniculate
medial incision
medial incudal fold
medial inferior genicular artery
medial inguinal fossa
medial joint level
medial ligament
medial lobule
medial longitudinal fasciculus
medial malleolus
medial malleolus fixation
medial malleolus resection
medial meniscectomy
medial meniscus
medial muscle
medial nasal concha
medial nasofrontal process
medial nerve
medial oblique and low lateral
    osteotomy

medial orbital wall fracture
medial osteotomy
medial palpebral arteries
medial palpebral commissure
medial palpebral ligament
medial parapatellar capsular
    approach
medial parapatellar incision
medial plantar artery
medial plantar nerve
medial plantar sensory flap
medial plateau of tibia
medial portion
medial protrusion
medial pterygoid muscle
medial pterygoid nerve
medial pterygoid plate
medial puboprostatic ligaments
medial rectus
medial rectus muscle
medial repair
medial rotation procedure
medial slip
medial superior genicular artery
medial supraclavicular nerves
medial surface
medial surface of maxilla
medial talocalcaneal ligament
medial tarsal arteries
medial tarsal artery
medial turbinate bone
medial umbilical fold
medial unicortical screw
medial upper arm flap
medial vestibular nucleus
medial wall
medialis obliquus imbrication
medialization
    fracture medialization
    greenstick medialization
    incomplete medialization
    vocal cord medialization
medialize
medially reflected
medial-to-lateral tumor removal
median alveolar cyst
median antebrachial vein
median anterior maxillary cyst
median appendectomy incision
median arcuate ligament
median artery
median aspect

median basilic vein
median cephalic vein
median cleft face syndrome
median cleft lip
median cleft of lower lip and
      mandible
median corpectomy
median cubital vein
median episiotomy
median facial cleft
median fissure
median forehead flap
median furrow of prostate
median glossoepiglottic fold
median groove
median groove of tongue
median harelip
median ileostomy catheter
median incision
median jaw relation
median labiomandibular
      glossotomy
median laryngotomy
median line
median lingual sulcus
median lithotomy
median longitudinal raphe
median mandibular cyst
median mandibular point
median maxillary anterior
      alveolar cleft
median nerve
median nerve block
median nerve compression
median nerve compression test
median occlusal position
median palatal cyst
median palatine suture
median parapatellar incision
median plane
median raphe
median raphe plane
median retruded jaw relation
median retruded relation
median rhinoscopy
median rhomboid glossitis
median sacral artery
median sagittal plane
median section
median sternotomy
median sternotomy incision
median sulcus

median thyrohyoid fold
median thyrohyoid ligament
median umbilical fold
median vein
median-sagittal plane
mediastinal cannula
mediastinal catheter
mediastinal cavity
mediastinal dissection
mediastinal drain
mediastinal esophagojejunostomy
mediastinal hemorrhage
mediastinal irradiation
mediastinal lymph node biopsy
mediastinal lymph node
      dissection
mediastinal lymphadenectomy
mediastinal mass
mediastinal node biopsy
mediastinal organ
mediastinal pleura
mediastinal plexus
mediastinal shadow
mediastinal shift
mediastinal space
mediastinal sump connector
mediastinal sump filter
mediastinal thickening
mediastinal tube
mediastinal tumor
mediastinal tumor excision
mediastinal veins
mediastinal widening
mediastinitis
   descending necrotizing
      mediastinitis (DNM)
   fulminant mediastinitis
mediastinoscope
   Carlens fiberoptic
      mediastinoscope
   Freiburg mediastinoscope
   Goldberg MPC
      mediastinoscope
   John A. Tucker
      mediastinoscope
   Tucker mediastinoscope
mediastinoscopic examination
mediastinoscopy
mediastinoscopy aspirating
      needle
mediastinoscopy-assisted
      transhiatal esophagectomy

mediastinotomy
mediastinum
mediate amputation
Medi-Band bandage
medical adhesive remover
medical ankle orthosis
medical care evaluation
medical cyclotron
Medical Design brace (MD brace)
medical diathermy
medical dilation
Medical Dynamics needle arthroscope
medical intervention
Medical Optics eye implant
Medical Optics intraocular lens implant
Medical Resources hydrophilic wound dressing
medical systemic condition
medical therapy
Medical Workshop intraocular lens implant
Medicam insufflator
Medicamat ultrasound device
Medicamat ultrasound-assisted lipoplasty machine
medicated bougie
medication-induced hyperplasia
medication-induced injury
Medici aerosol adhesive tape remover dressing
medicinal leech
medicinal nebulizer
medicinal preparation
medicodental
Medicon contractor
Medicon forceps
Medicon instruments
Medicon rib retractor
Medicon spreader
Medicon ultrasonic liposuction device
Medicon liposuction device
Medicon wire-twister forceps
Medicon-Jackson rectal forceps
Medicon-Packer mosquito forceps
Medicornea Kratz intraocular lens implant
Medicut cannula

Medicut catheter
Medicut intravenous needle
Medifill collagen hemostatic wound dressing
MediFlex earmold material
Mediflex-Booker device
Mediform dural graft
Mediform dural substitute
Medigel Z Line
Medi-graft vascular prosthesis
Medi-Jector adapter
Medi-Jector injector
Medilas fiberTome laser
Medilas Nd:YAG surgical laser
MedImage scanner
Medina ileostomy catheter
Medina ileostomy catheter tube
Meding tonsil enucleator
Meding tonsil enucleator tonometer
Meding tonsil enucleator tonsillectome
Medinol NIRside slotted stent
Medinvent vascular stent
mediocarpal articulation
mediocollateral ligament of knee
mediolateral episiotomy
mediolateral lithotomy
mediolateral projection
mediolateral view
medionasal process
mediotarsal amputation
mediotrusion
Medipatch Gel Z adhesive dressing
Mediplast plaster
Medipore Dress-it dressing
Medipore H soft cloth surgical tape
Medipore H surgical tape
MediPort implanted vascular device
MediPort infusion vascular access device
MediPort machine
MediPort double-lumen catheter
Medi-Quet surgical tourniquet
Medi-Quet tourniquet
Medi-Quick topical ointment
Medi-Rip dressing
Medirule measuring device

Medis off-line quantitative
　　coronary angiogram
Mediscus low-air-loss bed
MediSense Pen 2 blood glucose
　　meter
MediSense Pen 2 self blood
　　glucose monitor
Mediskin hemostatic sponge
Mediskin porcine biological
　　wound dressing
Medison scanner
Medispec Econolith spark plug
　　lithotriptor
Medistat hemostatic sponge
Medi-Stim stimulator
Medi-Strumpf elastic stockings
Medisupra mattress
Meditape
Meditape tape
Meditec laser
Meditech arterial dilatation
　　catheter
Meditech arterial dilatation
　　catheter
Meditech balloon catheter
Meditech bandage contact lens
Meditech bipolar probe
Meditech catheter
Meditech fascial dilator
Meditech flexible stiffening
　　cannula
Meditech guidewire
Meditech IVC filter
Meditech Mansfield dilating
　　catheter
Meditech multipurpose basket
Meditech occlusion balloon
　　catheter
Meditech sheath
Meditech steerable catheter
Meditech stone basket
Meditech wire
Meditron bipolar generator with
　　irrigation
Meditronic coronary stent
medium (*pl.* media)
medium below-elbow cast
medium chromic sutures
medium forceps
medium lesion
medium screwdriver
medium-energy collimator

Medivent self-expanding
　　coronary stent
Medivent vascular stent
MedJet microkeratome
Medline Aero-Flow II air
　　mattress
Medline Alpha subacute care bed
Medline deluxe air mattress
Medline Derma-Gel dressing
Medline gauze sponge
Medline gel/foam wheelchair
　　cushion
Medline Lap-pal safety cushion
Medline positioner
Medline roll
Medline Saf-T-Side mattress
MedLite YAG laser
Med-Logics microkeratome
Med-Neb respirator
Medoc-Celestin endoprosthesis
Medoc-Celestin pulsion tube
Medoc-Celestin tube
Medoff sliding femoral plate
Medoff sliding fracture plate
Medos valve
Medos-Hakim valve
Medox Dacron mesh
Medpor allograft material
Medpor alloplastic material
Medpor biomaterial implants
Medpor biomaterial wedge
Medpor block facial structure
　　building material
Medpor facial implant
Medpor malar implant
Medpor reconstructive implant
Medpor surgical implant
Medrad angiographic injectors
Medrad automated power
　　injector
Medrad catheter
Medrad contrast medium
　　injector
Medrad injector
Medrad angiographic injector
Medrafil sutures
Medrafil wire sutures
Meds eye protector
Medscand cervical spatula
Medscand Cytobrush Plus cell
　　collector
Medscand Pap smear kit

Medspec MR imaging system scanner

Medstone extracorporeal shock wave lithotriptor

Medstone STS lithotripter

Medstone STS shockwave generator

Medtel pacemaker

Medtronic Activitrax pacemaker

Medtronic Activitrax rate-responsive unipolar ventricular pacemaker

Medtronic aortic punch

Medtronic coronary stent

Medtronic balloon catheter

Medtronic bipolar pacemaker

Medtronic Chardack pacemaker

Medtronic corkscrew electrode pacemaker

Medtronic Cyberlith pacemaker

Medtronic defibrillator implant support device

Medtronic demand pacemaker

Medtronic device

Medtronic electrode catheter

Medtronic electrosurgical handpiece

Medtronic external tachyarrhythmia control device

Medtronic external-internal pacemaker

Medtronic GEM III implantable cardioverter defibrillator

Medtronic Hancock aortic punch

Medtronic Hancock valve

Medtronic Hemopump

Medtronic porcine bioprosthesis valve

Medtronic interventional vascular stent

Medtronic device

Medtronic Jewel AF arrhythmia management device

Medtronic Jewel Plus defibrillator

Medtronic Micro Jewel defibrillator

Medtronic Minix pacemaker

Medtronic pacemaker

Medtronic Pacette pacemaker

Medtronic prosthetic valve

Medtronic pulse generator

Medtronic Pulsor Intrasound pain reliever

Medtronic Spirit lead

Medtronic SPO pacemaker

Medtronic Spring lead

Medtronic stent

Medtronic stent graft

Medtronic Symbios pacemaker

Medtronic SynchroMed implantable pump

Medtronic temporary pacemaker

Medtronic Thera i-series cardiac pacemaker

Medtronic tip

Medtronic Transvene endocardial lead

Medtronic tremor control therapy device

Medtronic Zuma guiding catheter

Medtronic-Alcatel pacemaker

Medtronic-Byrel-SX pacemaker

Medtronic-Hall device

Medtronic-Hall heart valve

Medtronic-Hall heart valve prosthesis

Medtronic-Hall monocuspid tilting-disk valve

Medtronic-Hall tilting-disk valve prosthesis

Medtronic-Hancock device

Medtronic-Laurens-Alcatel pacemaker

Medtronic Zyrel pacemaker

medulla (*pl.* medullae)

medulla oblongata

medulla spinalis

medullaris

medullary adenocarcinoma

medullary artery

medullary bone graft

medullary callus

medullary canal

medullary canal reamer

medullary carcinoma

medullary cavity

medullary cells

medullary fixation

medullary fold

medullary graft
medullary nail
medullary nail fixation
medullary nailing
medullary pin
medullary rod
medullary segment
medullary space
medullary sponge kidney
medullary tube
medullated fibers and sheaths
medullated nerve
medullated nerve fiber
medullectomy
medulloblastoma
medulloblastoma metastasis
medullogram
medusa (*pl.* medusae)
  caput medusae
Med-Wick nasal pack
MedX camera
MedX functional testing
  machine
MedX knee machine
MedX Mark II lumbar extension
  machine
MedX physical therapy device
MedX scanner
MedX stretch machine
Meek clavicle sling
Meek island sandwich graft
Meek operation
Meek snare
Meeker deep-surgery forceps
Meeker gallbladder forceps
Meeker gallstone clamp
Meeker hemostatic forceps
Meeker intestinal forceps
Meeker monopolar
  electrosurgical dissector
Meeker right-angle clamp
Meek-Wall dermatome
Meek-Wall microdermatome
meerschaum probe
Mees line
Mefilm dressing
Mefix adhesive tape
MEG (magnetoencephalography)
Mega prosthesis
megacolon
megacystis-megaureter
  syndrome

megacystis-microcolon-intestinal
  hypoperistalsis syndrome
megadolichovertebrobasilar
  anomaly
megadont
megadontia
megadontism
megadontismus
MegaDyne arthroscopic hook
  electrode
MegaDyne cautery
MegaDyne electrocautery pencil
MegaDyne E-Z clean cautery tip
MegaDyne clean laparoscopic
  electrode
megaesophagus
MegaFlo infusion set
megaglossia
megagnathia
MegaLink biliary stent
megalodont
megalodontia
megalogastria
megaloglossia
megalourethra
megapockets
Megarcart electrocardiograph
MegaSonics PTCA catheter
Megasource penile prosthesis
megaureter clamp
megavoltage machine
Mehn-Quigley technique
Mehta intraocular lens
Meibom gland
meibomian cyst
meibomian expressor forceps
meibomian foramen
meibomian forceps
meibomian gland carcinoma
meibomian gland expressor
meibomian gland
Meige disease
Meige syndrome
Meigs curet
Meigs endometrial curet
Meigs hemostat
Meigs operation
Meigs pelvic lymphadenectomy
Meigs radical hysterectomy
Meigs retractor
Meigs suture technique
Meigs sutures

Meigs uterine curet
Meigs-Okabayashi procedure
Meigs-Wertheim hysterectomy
Meissner corpuscles
Meissner ganglion
Meissner plexus
Meissner tactile corpuscle
Meisterschnitt incision
MEL 60 excimer laser
MEL 60 scanning laser
MEL 70 flying spot laser
melanin
melanin-pigmented cells
melanization
melanoameloblastoma
melanocyte
melanocyte-stimulating
    hormone
melanocyte-stimulating
    hormone-inhibiting factor
melanocytic atypia
melanocytic conjunctival lesion
melanocytic lesion
melanocytic nevus
melanocytoma
melanoderma
melanoderma chloasma
melanogenesis
melanoglossia
melanoleukoderma colli
melanoma
    ABCDs of melanoma
        (asymmetry, border, color,
        diameter)
    acral-lentiginous melanoma
    benign juvenile melanoma
    Breslow classification for
        malignant melanoma
    Breslow microstaging system
        for malignant melanoma
    Clark classification of
        malignant melanoma (levels
        I-IV)
    Clark-Elder classification of
        malignant melanoma
    Clark-McGovern classification
        of malignant melanoma
    cutaneous melanoma
    desmoplastic melanoma
    Elder classification of
        malignant melanoma
    halo melanoma

melanoma (*continued*)
    juvenile melanoma
    lentigo maligna melanoma
    malignant melanoma
    neurotropic melanoma
    nodular melanoma
    sinonasal melanoma
    subungual melanoma
    suburethral melanoma
    superficial malignant
        melanoma
    superficial spreading
        melanoma
    uveal melanoma
melanoma in situ (MIS)
melanoma warning sign
melanonychia
melanonychia striata (MS)
melanoplakia
melanosarcoma
melanosis
melanosis diffusa congenita
melanosome
melanotic ameloblastoma
melanotic cancer
melanotic carcinoma
melanotic freckle
melanotic freckle of Hutchinson
melanotic lesion
melanotic neuroectodermal
    tumor
melanotic sarcoma
melanotic whitlow
melanotrichosis
melanotrichosis linguae
melasma
melatonin
Melauskas acrylic orbital implant
Melco suction
melena
Meleney gangrene
Meleney synergistic gangrene
Meleney ulcer
melenic stool
Melgisorb calcium alginate
    dressing
Melkersson syndrome
Melkersson-Rosenthal syndrome
Malleoloc anatomic ankle
    orthosis
Meller cyclodialysis spatula
Meller lacrimal sac retractor

Meller operation
Meller retractor
Meller spatula
Meller speculum
Mellinger eye speculum
Mellinger fenestrated blades
   speculum
Mellinger magnet
Mellinger speculum
Mellinger-Axenfeld eye speculum
Melmed blood freezing bag
melocervicoplasty
melolabial flap
melon seed body
Melone distal radius fracture
   classification
melonoplasty (*variant of*
   meloplasty)
meloplasty
Melt elevator
Meltzer adenoid punch
Meltzer adenoid punch forceps
Meltzer anesthesia
Meltzer nasopharyngoscope
Meltzer sign
Meltzer tonsillar punch
membrana adventitia
membrana eboris
membrana tympani
membrane
   acute inflammatory
      membrane
   acute pyogenic membrane
   adamantine membrane
   adventitious membrane
   allantoic membrane
   alveolocapillary membrane
   alveolodental membrane
   amniotic membrane
   antibasement membrane
   antiglomerular basement
      membrane
   antitubular basement
      membrane
   antral membrane
   arachnoid membrane
   artificial rupture of
      membranes (ARM)
   asymmetric unit membrane
   atlantoccipital membrane
   Barkan membrane
   barrier membrane

membrane (*continued*)
   basal cell membrane
   basement membrane
   basilar membrane
   basolateral membrane
   Bichat membrane
   bilaminar membrane
   BioBarrier membrane
   BioGen nonporous barrier
      membrane
   Bio-Gide resorbable barrier
      membrane
   Bio-Gide resorbable bilayer
      barrier membrane
   BioMend collagen membrane
   Biopore membrane
   bioresorbable guided tissue
      membrane
   Bowman membrane
   Bruch membrane
   Brunn membrane
   Cargile membrane
   cell membrane
   cellulose-based membrane
   chorioallantoic membrane
   chorion membranes
   choroidal neovascular
      membrane
   cloacal membrane
   collodion membrane
   congenital pyloric membrane
   conjunctival membrane
   connective tissue membrane
   cricothyroid membrane
   cricotracheal membrane
   cricovocal membrane
   croupous membrane
   crush-border membrane
   cuprophane membrane
   cuticular membrane
   cyclitic membrane
   cystic membrane
   cytoplasmic membrane
   Debove membrane
   decidual membrane
   Demours membrane
   dentinoenamel membrane
   Descemet membrane
   dialyzer membrane
   diphtheritic membrane
   drum membrane
   dry mucous membrane

membrane (*continued*)

Duddell membrane
dysmenorrheal membrane
egg membrane
elastic membrane
enamel membrane
endothelial cell basement
   membrane
epipapillary membrane
epiretinal membrane
epithelial basement
   membrane
ePTFE augmentation
   membrane
ePTFE membrane
erythrocyte membrane
exocoelomic membrane
false membrane
fenestrated membrane
fetal membranes
fibroelastic membrane
fibroproliferative membrane
fibrous membrane
Fielding membrane
filtration-slit membrane
fold of tympanic membrane
follicular membranes
Fresnel membrane
germinal membrane
glassy membrane
glial membrane
gliotic membrane
glomerular basement
   membrane
Golgi membranes
Gore Resolut regenerative
   tissue membrane
Gore-Tex augmentation
   membrane (GTAM)
Gore-Tex membrane
Gore-Tex surgical membrane
Haller membrane
Hemophan membrane
Henle elastic membrane
Henle fenestrated membrane
Heuser membrane
high-flux dialysis membrane
hourglass membrane
Hovius membrane
Huxley membrane
hyaline basement membrane
hyalitis anterior membrane

membrane (*continued*)

hyaloid membrane
hyaloid posterior membrane
hymenal membrane
hyoglossal membrane
hyperemic membranes
hyperplastic membrane
idiopathic preretinal
   membrane
Imtec BioBarrier membrane
inflammatory membrane
inner limiting membrane
intact membrane
intercostal membrane
intermuscular membrane
internal elastic membrane
interosseous membrane
interposition membrane
invaginated membrane
ivory membrane
Jackson membrane
Jacob membrane
labyrinth membrane
labyrinthine membrane
Liliequist membrane
limiting membrane
low-flux cellulose-based
   membrane
low-flux cuprophane
   membrane
low-flux dialysis membrane
lysosomal membrane
mammalian cell membrane
membrane peeler
microvillus membrane
moist mucous membrane
mucous membranes
NaK-ATPase membrane
Nasmyth membrane
neovascular membrane
neuronal membrane
nictitating membrane
nuclear membrane
obturator membrane
olfactory membrane
onion skin-like membrane
oropharyngeal membrane
otolithic membrane
outer limiting membrane
Payr membrane
peridental membrane
perineal membrane

membrane (*continued*)

periodontal membrane (PM)
periorbital membrane
peritoneal membrane
phrenoesophageal membrane
pial-glial membrane
placental membrane
plasma membrane
plastic membrane
polyacrylonitrile membrane
porous filter membrane
postsynaptic membrane
Preclude pericardial
   membrane
Preclude peritoneal membrane
Preclude spinal membrane
premature rupture of
   membranes (PROM)
preretinal membrane
presynaptic membrane
proper membrane
prophylactic membrane
pseudoserous membrane
pulpodentinal membrane
pupillary membrane
purpurogenous membrane
pyogenic membrane
quadrangular membrane
Ranvier membrane
Reichert membrane
Reissner membrane
renal brush border membrane
resorbable bilayer collagen
   membrane
restrictive membrane
retained placenta and
   membranes
reticular membrane
retrocorneal membrane
Rivinus membrane
rolling membrane
ruptured membranes
Ruysch membrane
ruyschian membrane
salpingopalatine membrane
salpingopharyngeal
   membrane
sarcolemmal membrane
Scarpa membrane
schneiderian membrane
schneiderian respiratory
   membrane

membrane (*continued*)

Schultze membrane
Schwalbe membrane
secondary membrane
semi-impermeable membrane
semipermeable membrane
Seprafilm bioresorbable
   membrane
serous membrane
Shrapnell membrane
Slavianski membrane
small intestinal membrane
spiral membrane
statoconic membrane
stripping membrane
stylomandibular membrane
subepithelial membrane
subimplant membrane
submucous membrane
subretinal neovascular
   membrane
suprapleural membrane
surface membrane
syncytiovascular membrane
synovial membrane
tarsal membrane
tectorial membrane
TelGen-FD guided tissue
   regeneration membrane
TelGen-FD plastic membrane
Tenon membrane
thickened synovial membrane
thin basement membrane
thin plastic membrane
thyrohyoid membrane
Toldt membrane
Tourtual membrane
trabecular membrane
tubular basement membrane
tympanic membrane
undulating membrane
unilaminar membrane
unit membrane
urea-impermeable membrane
urogenital membrane
urorectal membrane
urothelial basement
   membrane
vernix membrane
vestibular membrane
virginal membrane
vitelline membrane

membrane (*continued*)
   vitreal membrane
   vitreous membrane
   Volkmann membrane
   von Brunn membrane
   Wachendorf membrane
   wrinkling membrane
   yolk membrane
   Zinn membrane
membrane artificial lung
membrane bridge
membrane catheter technique
membrane current
membrane expansion theory
membrane forceps
membrane instability
membrane of brain
membrane of cervix uteri
membrane of Demours
membrane of Descemet
membrane of joint
membrane of Liliequist
membrane of meninges
membrane of tympanum
membrane oxygenator
membrane peeler
membrane peeling
membrane perforator
membrane permeability
membrane potential
membrane rupture
membrane trafficking
membrane-coating granule
membranectomy
membrane-puncturing forceps
membranous acute inflammation
membranous adhesion
membranous canal
membranous cataract
membranous gingivostomatitis
membranous labyrinth
membranous laryngitis
membranous lining
membranous obstruction
membranous pharyngitis
membranous septum
membranous stomatitis
membranous tissue
membranous tube
membranous urethra
membranous ventricular septal
   defect

membranous wall
Meme breast prosthesis
Meme implant
Meme mammary implant
Memford-Gurd arthroplasty
Memokath catheter
memory catheter
memory splint
MemoryLens foldable
   intraocular lens
MemoryTrace AT ambulatory
   cardiac monitor
Memotherm colorectal stent
Memotherm endoscopic biliary
   stent
Memotherm Flexx biliary stent
Memotherm nitinol stent
MEN syndrome
Mendel dorsal reflex of foot
Mendel ligature forceps
Mendel-Bekhterev sign
mendelian theory
Mendelsohn maneuver
Mendelson syndrome
Mendez corneal marker
Mendez cystotome
Mendez degree calipers
Mendez degree gauge
Mendez multi-purpose LASIK
   forceps
Mendez ultrasonic cystotome
Mendez-Schubert aorta punch
Menelaus triple arthrodesis
Menetrier disease
Menge operation
Menge pessary
Menge stem pessary
Mengert index
Mengert membrane-puncturing
   forceps
Menghini biopsy technique
Menghini cannula
Menghini liver biopsy needle
Menghini needle
Menghini percutaneous liver
   biopsy
Menghini technique for
   percutaneous liver biopsy
Menghini-Wildhirt laparoscope
Meniere disease
Meniere quadrad
Meniere syndrome

meningeal adhesions
meningeal arteries
meningeal artery
meningeal carcinoma
meningeal groove
meningeal hemorrhage
meningeal hernia
meningeal layer
meningeal nerve
meningeal veins
meningeal vessels
meningeorrhaphy
meninges (*sing.* meninx)
  glistening transparent meninges
  innermost membrane of
    meninges
  membrane of meninges
meningioma
  cutaneous meningioma
  extracranial meningioma
  parasagittal meningioma
  posterior cranial fossa
    meningioma
meningioma en plaque
meningismus
meningitis
  AIDS-related cryptococcal
    meningitis
  bacterial meningitis (BM)
  cryptococcal meningitis
  otitic meningitis
  spinal meningitis
meningocele
meningococci
meningoencephalocele
meningoencephalomyelitis
meningothelial cell
meningovascular syphilis
meninx (*pl.* meninges)
meniscal basket forceps
meniscal bone
meniscal clamp
meniscal curet
meniscal cutter
meniscal excision
meniscal fluid
meniscal hook scissors
meniscal knife
meniscal lens
meniscal mirror
meniscal posterior concave
  intraocular lens

meniscal repair
meniscal repair needle
meniscal retractor
meniscal sign
meniscal staple
meniscal suture grabber
meniscal tear
meniscectomy
  arthroscopic meniscectomy
  Marshall meniscectomy
  medial meniscectomy
  total meniscectomy
meniscectomy blade
meniscectomy knife
meniscectomy probe
meniscectomy scissors
meniscofemoral ligament
meniscoresis
meniscotome
  Bowen-Grover meniscotome
  Dyonics meniscotome
  Grover meniscotome
  Smillie meniscotome
  Storz meniscotome
meniscotome power unit
meniscotome sheath
meniscus (*pl.* menisci)
  bucket-handle tear of
    meniscus
  lateral meniscus
  medial meniscus
  slipped meniscus
  tear of meniscus
  torn lateral meniscus
  torn medial meniscus
  triangular fibrocartilage
    meniscus
Meniscus Arrow implant
meniscus of acromioclavicular
  joint
meniscus of knee
meniscus of temporomaxillary
  joint
Menlo Care catheter
Mennen plate
menogingivitis
menometrorrhagia
menorrhagia
menorrhea
menses
Mensor-Scheck hanging-hip
  procedure

Mensor-Scheck technique
menstrual aspiration
menstrual cycle induction
menstrual extraction
menstruation
menstruation gingivitis
mental age (MA)
mental artery
mental block injection
mental branches
mental canal
mental extraoral radiography
mental foramen
mental height
mental muscle
mental nerve
mental nerve block
mental point
mental process
mental projection
mental protuberance
mental region
mental retardation
mental ridge
mental spine
mental squama
mental status evaluation
mental status examination
mental tubercle of mandible
mental V-Y island advancement
     island flap
mentalis band
mentalis muscle
Mentanium vitreoretinal
     instrument set
mentoanterior position
mentolabial furrow
mentolabial sulcus
mento-occipital diameter
mentoparietal diameter
mentoplasty
mentoplasty augmentation
mentoposterior position
Mentor absorbent pouch
Mentor biliary stent
Mentor bladder pacemaker
Mentor breast implant
Mentor breast prosthesis
Mentor cautery
Mentor coude catheter
Mentor Exeter ophthalmoscope
Mentor fine-focus microscope

Mentor Foley catheter
Mentor Foley catheter with
     comfort sleeve
Mentor GFS penile prosthesis
Mentor implant
Mentor inflatable penile
     prosthesis
Mentor injector gun
Mentor IPP penile prosthesis
Mentor lens
Mentor lipoplasty machine
Mentor malleable penile
     prosthesis
Mentor malleable semirigid
     penile implant
Mentor Mark II penile prosthesis
Mentor monitor
Mentor penile prosthesis with
     rear-tip extender
Mentor prostate biopsy needle
Mentor Resi prosthesis
Mentor Self-Cath penile
     prosthesis
Mentor Self-Cath soft catheter
Mentor Siltex implant
Mentor Spectrum contour
     expander
Mentor straight catheter
Mentor Tele-Cath ileal conduit
     sampling catheter
Mentor tissue expander
Mentor ultrasound device
Mentor ultrasound-assisted
     lipoplasty machine
Mentor wet-field cautery
Mentor wet-field coagulator
Mentor wet-field cordless
     coagulator
Mentor wet-field electrocautery
Mentor wet-field hemostatic
     eraser
Mentor-Maumenee Suregrip
     forceps
Mentor-Urosan external
     catheter
mentotransverse position
mentum anterior position
mentum posterior position
mentum transverse position
meperidine anesthetic agent
mephitic gangrene
Mepiform dressing

Mepiform self-adherent silicone dressing
Mepilex dressing
Mepilex foam dressing
Mepitel contact-layer wound dressing
Mepitel dressing
Mepitel nonadherent silicone dressing
mepivacaine hydrochloride anesthetic agent
Mepore absorptive dressing
mEq (milliequivalents)
Mercator catheter
Mercedes cannula
Mercedes incision
Mercedes tip
Mercedes tip cannula
Mercedes-Benz sign
Mercer cartilage knife
Mercier catheter
Mercier operation
Mercier sound
Merck respirator
mercurial line
mercurial stomatitis
mercuric oxide
Mercurio position
mercurochrome
mercuroscopic expansion
mercury bougie
mercury cell-powered pacemaker
mercury-containing balloon
mercury-filled bougie
mercury-filled dilator
mercury-filled esophageal bougie
mercury-in-rubber strain gauge
mercury-in-Silastic strain gauge
mercury-weighted bougie
mercury-weighted dilator
mercury-weighted rubber bougie
mercury-weighted tube
Merendino technique
Meridian intersegmental table
Meridian pacemaker
Meridian ST femoral implant component
meridional aberration
meridional implant

meridional refractometer
meridional section
Merindino operation
Merit-B periodontal probe
Merkel cell carcinoma
Merkel cell carcinoma of buttock
Merkel corpuscles
Merkel disk
Merkel filtrum ventriculi
Merkel fossa
Merkel muscle
Merlin arthroscopy blade
Merlin bendable blade
Merlin stone forceps
MERmaid kit
mermaid malformation
Mermingas operation
Merocel epistaxis packing
Merocel nasal packing
Merocel sponge
Merocel surgical spear
Merocel tampon
merocrine gland
MeroGel dressing
MeroGel nasal dressing and sinus stent
MeroGel nasal packing
MeroGel nasal stent
MeroGel sinus stent
Merrem IV
Merriam forceps
Merrifield knife
Merrill Supramid suturing technique
Merrill-Levassier retractor
Merrimack laser adapter
Merry Walker ambulation device
Mershon arch
Mershon band pusher
Mersilene band
Mersilene braided nonabsorbable sutures
Mersilene dressing
Mersilene gauze
Mersilene graft
Mersilene implant
Mersilene mesh
Mersilene mesh dressing
Mersilene prosthesis
Mersilene sutures
Mersilene tape

Mersilene tape ligature
Mersilk suture
Merthiolate
Merthiolate dressing
Mertz keratoscopy ring
Mery gland
Merz aortic punch
Merz hysterectomy forceps
Merz-Vienna nasal speculum
Mesalt sodium chloride
   impregnated dressing
mesangial matrix expansion
mesencephalic flexure
mesencephalic hemorrhage
mesencephalic low-density
   lesion
mesencephalic reticular
   formation
mesencephalic tractotomy
mesencephalon
mesencephalotomy
mesenchymal cell
mesenchymal chondrosarcoma
   (MC)
mesenchymal cleft
mesenchymal lesion
mesenchymal mixed tumor
mesenchymal neoplasm
mesenchymal sarcoma
mesenchymal tissue
mesenchymal tumor
mesenchyme
mesenchymoma
mesenterectomy
mesenteric adhesions
mesenteric angiography
mesenteric arcade
mesenteric arteriovenous fistula
mesenteric artery
mesenteric attachments
mesenteric border
mesenteric bypass graft
mesenteric circulation
mesenteric cyst
mesenteric fistula
mesenteric ganglion
mesenteric gland
mesenteric hematoma
mesenteric hernia
mesenteric infarction
mesenteric inferior artery
mesenteric lymph nodes

mesenteric nodal disease
mesenteric node
mesenteric rupture
mesenteric stranding
mesenteric superior artery
mesenteric superior vein
mesenteric thrombosis
mesenteric triangle
mesenteric vascular lesion
mesenteric vasodilator infusion
mesenteric vein
mesentericoparietal fossa
mesentericoportal axis
mesenteriopexy
mesenteriorrhaphy
mesenteriplication
mesentery
   appendiceal mesentery
   leaves of mesentery
mesentery abscess
mesentorrhaphy
mesh
   Auto Suture surgical mesh
   Bard Sperma-Tex preshaped
     mesh
   Bard-Marlex mesh
   Brennen biosynthetic surgical
     mesh
   Composix mesh
   craniomaxillofacial mesh
   Dacron mesh
   Dexon mesh
   Dexon polyglycolic acid mesh
   Dexon surgically knitted
     mesh
   DualMesh hernia mesh
   Dumbach mini mesh
   Dumbach regular mesh
   Dumbach titanium mesh
   Epicon mesh
   Ethicon mesh
   Flared patch mesh
   FortaGen mesh
   Gore-Tex mesh
   Herniamesh surgical mesh
   Hexcelite mesh
   intraperitoneal onlay mesh
   Kugel mesh
   Leibinger Micro Dynamic
     mesh
   macro-mesh mesh
   mandibular mesh

mesh (*continued*)
  Marlex mesh
  Meadox Dacron mesh
  Mersilene mesh
  micro mesh
  mixed mesh
  MycroMesh biomaterial
  Mylar mesh
  Parietex composite mesh
  PerFix Marlex mesh plug
  Permacol mesh
  polyamide mesh
  polyglactin mesh
  polyglycolic acid mesh
  polypropylene mesh
  polytetrafluoroethylene mesh
  Prolene mesh
  Sepramesh biosurgical
    composite
  sintered titanium mesh
  skin graft expander mesh
  skin graft mesh
  skin mesh
  Sperma-Tex preshaped mesh
  stainless steel mesh
  steel mesh
  Supramid polyamide mesh
  surgical metallic mesh
  Surgipro hernia mesh
  SynMesh mesh
  synthetic mesh
  tantalum mesh
  Teflon mesh
  ThermoFX mesh
  TiMesh cranial mesh
  TiMesh orbital mesh
  TiMesh titanium mesh
  titanium mesh
  Trelex natural mesh
  Usher Marlex mesh
  Vicryl mesh
  Visilex polypropylene mesh
  Vitallium mesh
  zippered mesh
mesh graft
mesh graft urethroplasty
mesh herniorrhaphy
mesh implantation
mesh myringotomy tube
mesh plug hernioplasty
mesh prosthesis
mesh removal

mesh repair
mesh skin graft
mesh stent
mesh stent prosthesis
mesh sutures
meshed ball implant
meshed graft
meshed split-thickness skin graft
mesher
  Collin mesher
  skin graft mesher
  Tanner mesher
  Zimmer skin graft mesher
Meshgraft skin expander
meshwork
  coagulation meshwork
  trabecular meshwork
mesial occlusion
mesial surface
mesioangular impaction
mesioangular position
mesioaxial
mesioaxiogingival
mesioaxioincisal
mesiobuccal (MB)
mesiobuccal alveolus
mesiobuccal canal
mesiobuccal developmental
    groove (MBDG)
mesiobuccal line angle
mesiobucco-occlusal (MBO)
mesiobucco-occlusal point angle
mesiobuccopulpal (MBP)
mesiocervical
mesioclination
mesioclusion
mesiodens (*pl.* mesiodentes)
mesiodistal clasp
mesiodistal fracture
mesiodistal plane
mesiodistal width
mesiodistocclusal (MOD)
mesiogingival (MG)
mesioincisal
mesioincisodistal (MID)
mesiolabial (MLA)
mesiolabial bilobed
    transposition flap
mesiolabial line angle
mesiolabioincisal (MLAI)
mesiolabioincisal point angle
mesiolingual (ML)

mesiolingual developmental
groove (MLDG)
mesiolingual fossa (MLF)
mesiolingual groove (MLG)
mesiolingual line angle
mesiolinguoincisal (MLI)
mesiolinguoincisal point angle
mesiolinguo-occlusal (MLO)
mesiolinguo-occlusal point angle
mesiolinguopulpal (MLP)
mesio-occlusal (MO)
mesio-occlusal line angle
mesio-occlusion
mesio-occlusodistal (MOD)
mesiopalatal
mesioplacement
mesiopulpal (MP)
mesiopulpolabial (MPLA)
mesiopulpolingual (MPL)
mesioversion
mesoappendicitis
mesoappendix
meso-bi-ileal shunt
mesobranchial area
Mesocaine anesthetic
mesocaval anastomosis
mesocaval H-graft shunt
mesocaval interposition shunt
mesocecum
mesocolic band
mesocolic hernia
mesocolic involvement
mesocolic lymph nodes
mesocolic shelf
mesocolon
  sigmoid mesocolon
  transverse mesocolon
mesocolopexy
mesocoloplication
mesocuneiform bone
mesoderm
mesodermal core
mesodermal segment
mesodermal somite
mesodermal tumor
mesodont
mesodontia
mesodontic
mesodontism
mesoesophageal dissection
mesogastrium
mesognathic

mesognathous
mesolateral fold
mesonephric adenocarcinoma
mesonephric drain
mesonephric duct
mesonephric fold
mesopexy
mesorectal excision
mesorectum
mesorrhaphy
mesosalpinx
mesosigmoid
mesosigmoidopexy
mesostomia
mesostructure
mesostructure bar
mesostructure conjunction bar
mesostructure implant
mesotaurodontism
mesothelial cell layer
mesothelial cells
mesothelioma
mesothenar muscle
mesotympanum
mesouterine fold
mesovarian margin
mesovarium
Messerklinger endoscope
Messerklinger sinus endoscopy
  set
Messerklinger technique
Messing root canal gun
Messner plate
META (methacryloxyethyl
  trimellitic anhydride)
Meta DDDR pacemaker
Meta II pacemaker
Meta MV cardiac pacemaker
Meta rate-responsive pacemaker
metabolator
metabolic bone disease
metabolic calculus
metabolic complication
metabolic disorder
metabolic disturbance
metabolic evaluation
metabolic heat load stimulator
metabolic rate
metabolic sialadenosis
metabolic stone
metabolism
metacarpal arteries

metacarpal bones
metacarpal broach
metacarpal double-ended
    retractor
metacarpal epiphyseal centers
metacarpal fracture
metacarpal hand
metacarpal head
metacarpal head fracture
metacarpal neck fracture
metacarpal of wrist
metacarpal saw
metacarpal shaft fracture
metacarpal splint
metacarpal veins
metacarpectomy
metacarpocarpal articulations
metacarpophalangeal (MCP)
metacarpophalangeal
    joint arthroplasty
metacarpophalangeal
    articulation
metacarpophalangeal implant
metacarpophalangeal joint
metacarpophalangeal prosthesis
metacarpothenar reflex
metachronous metastasis
metachronous tumor
metaconid
metaconule
metafacial angle
metaidoioplasty (*spelled also*
    metoidioplasty)
metal adapter
metal and rubber block
metal applicator
metal ball-tip catheter
metal band
metal band sutures
metal bar retractor
metal base
metal bracket
metal bucket-handle prosthesis
metal cannula
metal catheter
metal clamp
metal clip
metal connector
metal crown margin
metal electrode
metal femoral head prosthesis
metal Fox shield

metal hemi-toe implant
metal hybrid orthosis
metal interface
metal irrigating tip
metal locator (*see also* locator,
    magnet)
metal nail
metal needle
metal olive
metal opaquer
metal orthopedic implant
metal pin
metal plate
metal prosthesis
metal reconstruction plate
metal rod
metal ruler
metal scleral shield
metal screw
metal sewing ring
metal sound
metal splint
metal suction connector
metal syringe
metal tongue depressor
Metal Z stent
metal-augmented polymer stent
metal-backed acetabular
    component hip implant
metal-backed socket
metal-ball tip cannula
metal-coated stent
Metaline dressing
metallic clamp
metallic clip
metallic cranioplasty
metallic fixation device
metallic foreign body (MFB)
metallic fragment
metallic frontal needle
metallic implant
metallic oxide paste
metallic pointer
metallic restoration
metallic rod fixation
metallic screw
metallic skin marker
metallic sphere introducer
metallic stain
metallic staple
metallic stent
metallic sutures

metallic-dense shadow
metallic-tip cannula
metallic-tip catheter
metalloproteinase
   matrix metalloproteinase
    (MMP)
metal-olive dilator
metal-on-metal articulating
   intervertebral disk
   prosthesis
metal-plated die
metal-tipped cannula
metal-tipped stent pusher
metal-weighted Silastic feeding
   tube
metanephric duct
metaphysial abscess
metaphysial flair
metaphysial tibial fracture
metaphysis
metaplasia
metaplasia of pulp
metaplastic carcinoma
metaplastic polyp
Metaport catheter
metarteriole
metastasis (*pl.* metastases)
   adnexal metastasis
   adrenal metastasis
   aortic node metastasis
   axillary node metastasis
   bilobar liver metastasis
   biochemical metastasis
   biopsy-proven metastasis
   blastic metastasis
   bone metastasis
   bony metastasis
   brain metastasis
   breast metastasis
   calcareous metastasis
   calcified liver metastasis
   calcifying metastasis
   cannonball metastasis
   cardiac metastasis
   cavitating metastasis
   celiac lymph node metastasis
   cerebral metastasis
   cervical metastasis
   chiasmal metastasis
   choroidal metastasis
   clivus metastasis
   colonic metastasis

metastasis (*continued*)
   colorectal metastasis
   contact metastasis
   contralateral axillary
    metastasis
   cutaneous metastasis
   cystic metastasis
   diffuse metastasis
   direct metastasis
   distal metastasis
   distant metastasis
   drop metastasis
   duodenal metastasis
   echopenic liver metastasis
   epidural metastasis
   extracapsular metastasis
   extrahepatic metastasis
   extralymphatic metastasis
   extrathoracic metastasis
   fallopian tube metastasis
   floxuridine in hepatic
    metastasis
   gastric bed metastasis
   gastrointestinal metastasis
   generalized metastasis
   hematogenic metastasis
   hematogenous metastasis
   hematopoietic metastasis
   hemorrhagic metastasis
   hepatic colorectal metastasis
   hernia metastasis
   implantation metastasis
   incisional metastasis
   inguinal lymph node
    metastasis
   intracapsular metastasis
   intracranial metastasis
   intrahepatic metastasis
   intramucosal metastasis
   in-transit metastasis
   intraparotideal metastasis
   intrapulmonary metastasis
    (IPM)
   laparoscopic port site
    metastasis
   lateroaortic metastasis
   leptomeningeal metastasis
   liver metastasis
   local metastasis
   lung metastasis
   lymph node metastasis
   lymphangitic metastasis

metastasis (*continued*)
  lymphatic metastasis
  lymphogenous metastasis
  medulloblastoma metastasis
  metachronous metastasis
  multiple metastases
  necrotic metastasis
  neoplasm metastasis
  nodal metastasis
  noncolorectal liver metastasis
    (NCRLM)
  nonneuroendocrine
    metastasis
  occult metastasis
  ocular metastasis
  omental metastasis
  orbital metastasis
  osseous metastasis
  osteoblastic metastasis
  ovarian cancer metastasis
  paracardiac metastasis
  parasellar metastasis
  parenchymal brain metastasis
  pelvic metastases
  periesophagogastric lymph
    node metastasis
  peritoneal metastasis
  placental metastasis
  pleural metastasis
  port site metastasis
  precocious metastasis
  pulmonary metastasis
  regional metastasis
  remote metastases
  resectable liver metastasis
  retrobulbar orbital metastasis
  satellite metastasis
  septic metastasis
  serosal metastasis
  serosal-peritoneal metastasis
  skeletal metastasis
  skip metastasis
  soft tissue metastasis
  sphenoid sinus metastasis
  spinal metastasis
  stomach cancer metastasis
  subcutaneous metastasis
  synchronous hepatic metastasis
  synchronous metastasis
  testicular metastasis
  transplantation metastasis
  tumor node metastasis (TNM)

metastasis (*continued*)
  tumor-to-tumor metastasis
  unique noncolorectal liver
    metastasis
  unresectable metastasis
  uterine sarcoma metastasis
  uveal metastasis
  vascular metastasis
  Virchow metastasis
metastasis, age, completeness of
    resection, local invasion,
    and tumor size (MACIS)
metastasize
metastatic abscess
metastatic adenocarcinoma
metastatic basal cell carcinoma
metastatic cancer
metastatic carcinoma
metastatic colorectal cancer
metastatic colorectal carcinoma
metastatic disease
metastatic focus
metastatic implant
metastatic implantation
metastatic involvement
metastatic lesion
metastatic neoplasm
metastatic node
metastatic prostatic carcinoma
metastatic renal cell carcinoma
metastatic site
metastatic spread
metastatic tumor
metastatic tumor removal
Metasul hip joint component
Metasul hip prosthesis
Metasul joint
Metasul metal-on-metal hip
    prosthesis
metatarsal artery
metatarsal bone
metatarsal cuneiform exostosis
metatarsal cuneiform joint
metatarsal fracture
metatarsal free vascularized graft
metatarsal head
metatarsal head resection
metatarsal joint
metatarsal osteotomy
metatarsal splint
metatarsal stem broach
metatarsal ulcer

metatarsal veins
metatarsectomy
metatarsocuneiform articulation
metatarsophalangeal
    joint arthroplasty
metatarsophalangeal (MTP)
metatarsophalangeal
    articulations
metatarsophalangeal
    endoprosthesis
metatarsophalangeal joint
metatarsophalangeal joint
    disarticulation
metatarsophalangeal joint
    dislocation
metatarsus abductus
metatarsus adductus
metatarsus equinus
metatarsus primus varus
metatypical carcinoma
Metcalf spring drop brace
Metcher eye speculum
Metcher speculum
Metcoff pediatric biopsy needle
methacrylate
    2-hydroxyethyl methacrylate
        (HEMA)
    bisphenol A-glycidyl
        methacrylate (bis-GMA)
    butyl methacrylate
    dimethyl methacrylate
    ethyl methacrylate
    glyceryl methacrylate
    hydroxyethyl methacrylate
    methyl methacrylate
    poly-1-hydroxyethyl
        methacrylate
    poly-2-hydroxyethyl
        methacrylate (poly-HEMA)
    polymethyl methacrylate
        (PMMA)
    vinyl ethyl methacrylate
methacryloxyethyl trimellitic
    anhydride (META)
methamphetamine exposure
methemoglobinemia
method of Cosman
method of Quinones
Methodist Hospital head holder
Methodist suction tube
Methodist vascular suction
    tube

methohexital sodium anesthetic
    agent
methoxyflurane anesthetic
    agent
methyl cellulose paste
methyl cyanoacrylate glue
methyl ethyl ketone
methyl methacrylate adhesive
methyl methacrylate beads
    implant
methyl methacrylate block
methyl methacrylate bone
    cement
methyl methacrylate cement
methyl methacrylate cement
    adhesive
methyl methacrylate
    cranioplastic plug
methyl methacrylate ear stent
methyl methacrylate eye
    implant
methyl methacrylate glue
methyl methacrylate graft
methyl methacrylate implant
    material
methyl methacrylate polymer
methylene blue dye
methylene blue dye localization
methylene blue insufflation
methylene blue line
methylprednisolone
Metico forceps
meticulous hemostasis
meticulous maneuver
metodontiasis
metoidioplasty (*variant of*
    metaidoioplasty)
metopic craniosynostosis
metopic point
metopic suture
metopic synostosis
metopic synostosis reoperation
metopoplasty
Metra PS procedure kit
MetraGrasp ligament grasper
MetraPass suture passer
Metras bronchial catheter
Metras catheter
MetraTie knot pusher
Metrecom device
Metrecom digitizer
metric ophthalmoscope

metric ophthalmoscopy
metrizamide cisternogram
metrizamide myelography
metrizamide-filled balloon
metro catheter
MetroFlex endoscopic cart
metroperitoneal fistula
metroplasty
metrorrhagia
mets (*slang for* metastases)
Mett tube
Mettelman prejowl chin implant
Mettler Dia-Sonic electrosurgical
  unit
Mettler electrotherapy
metycaine hydrochloride
  anesthetic agent
Metzelder modification activator
Metzel-Wittmoser forceps
Metzenbaum baby tonsillar
  scissors
Metzenbaum chisel
Metzenbaum dissecting scissors
Metzenbaum dressing scissors
Metzenbaum gouge
Metzenbaum knife
Metzenbaum long scissors
Metzenbaum needle holder
Metzenbaum operating scissors
Metzenbaum septal knife
Metzenbaum septum knife
Metzenbaum tonsillar forceps
Metzenbaum tonsillar scissors
Metzenbaum-Lipsett plastic
  scissors
Metzenbaum-Lipsett scissors
Metzenbaum-Tydings forceps
Metzger infant knife
Meuli arthroplasty
Meurig Williams spinal fusion
  plate
Meurmann external ear anomaly
  grade
MEVA probe
Mewissen infusion catheter
Meyenburg disease
Meyenburg-Altherr-Uehlinger
  syndrome
Meyer biliary retractor
Meyer cartilage
Meyer cervical orthosis
Meyer cyclodiathermy needle

Meyer hockey-stick incision
Meyer incision
Meyer light pipe
Meyer line
Meyer loop
Meyer mastectomy
Meyer needle
Meyer olive-tipped vein stripper
Meyer operation
Meyer organ
Meyer sinus
Meyer spiral vein stripper
Meyer Swiss diamond knife
  lancet
Meyer Swiss diamond lancet
  knife
Meyer Swiss diamond wedge
  knife
Meyer temporal loop
Meyerding aluminum hammer
Meyerding bone graft
Meyerding bone skid
Meyerding chisel
Meyerding curet
Meyerding curved gouge
Meyerding double-ended
  retractor with skin hook
Meyerding facet eroder
Meyerding finger retractor
Meyerding gouge
Meyerding laminectomy
  blade
Meyerding laminectomy self-
  retaining retractor
Meyerding mallet
Meyerding nail
Meyerding osteotome
Meyerding prosthesis
Meyerding retractor
Meyerding retractor blade
Meyerding saw-toothed curet
Meyerding self-retaining
  laminectomy retractor
Meyerding skid
Meyerding skin hook
Meyerding skin hook and
  retractor
Meyerding solid aluminum
  mallet
Meyerding spondylolisthesis
  classification line
Meyerding-Deaver retractor

Meyerding-Van Demark
    technique
Meyer-Halsted incision
Meyers hip procedure
Meyers quadratus muscle-
    pedicle bone graft
Meyer-Schwickerath coagulator
Meyer-Schwickerath light
    coagulation
Meyer-Schwickerath operation
Meyers-McKeever avulsion
    fracture classification
Meyers-McKeever tibial fracture
    classification
Meyerson sign
Meyhoeffer bone curet
Meyhoeffer chalazion curet
Meyhoeffer eye knife
Meyhoeffer knife
Meynert retroflex bundle
Meynet bundle
Meynet commissure
Meynet decussation
Meynet nodes
Meynet nodosities
Meynet tract
MF (mitogenic factor)
MF heel protector
MFB (metallic foreign body)
MFH (malignant fibrous
    histiocytoma)
MG (mesiogingival)
MG II knee prosthesis
MGH (Massachusetts General
    Hospital)
MGH elevator
MGH forceps
MGH glenoid punch
MGH knee prosthesis
MGH needle holder
MGH osteotome
MGH periosteal elevator
MGH uterine vulsellum forceps
MGH vulsellum forceps
MGJ (mesiogingival junction)
MGM glenoidal punch
MHC (major histocompatibility
    complex)
MHN (Mohs hardness number)
MI (myocardial infarct;
    myocardial infarction)
Miami J collar cervical traction

Miami cervical collar
Miami cervical traction
Miami cervical fracture brace
Miami fracture brace
Miami J cervical collar
Miami scoliosis brace
Mibelli angiokeratomas
MIC bolus gastrostomy tube
MIC gastroenteric tube
MIC jejunal tube
MIC jejunostomy tube
MICA 3X sleeve
Mich compression arthrodesis
Michael Reese prosthesis
Michael Reese shoulder
    prosthesis
Michaelson operation
Michal I procedure
Michal II procedure
Michel anomaly
Michel aortic clamp
Michel clip
Michel clip hemostat
Michel clip-applying forceps
Michel clip-removing forceps
Michel deformity
Michel malformation
Michel pick
Michel rhinoscopic mirror
Michel scalp clip
Michel suture clip
Michel tissue forceps
Michel trephine
Michel wound clip
Michele trephine
Michele vertebral aspiration
Michelis intraocular implant lens
Michelson bronchoscope
Michelson infant bronchoscope
Michelson-Sequoia air drill
Michel-Wachtenfeldt clip
Michigan forceps
Michigan intestinal forceps
Michigan probe
Michigan University intestinal
    forceps
Mick afterloading needle
Mick applicator
Mick seed applicator
Mickey and Minnie surgical
    marker
Mic-Key gastrostomy tube

Micra knife
Micra needle holder
Micrins forceps
Micrins microsurgical sutures
Micrins needle holder
Micro 100 irrigation kit
Micro catheter
Micro Diamond-Point
  microsurgery instruments
Micro Discoblator
Micro E irrigation kit
Micro FET isometric force
  dynamometer
Micro Link endoscope fiber
micro liquid extraction
micro mesh
Micro Minix pacemaker
Micro oral surgery handpiece
Micro Plus screw
Micro punctum plug
micro round-tip needle
micro scissors
Micro Series wire driver
Micro Stent II
micro Westcott scissors
microabrasion
microabscess
micro-adaption plate
microadenoma
MicroAire bone saw
MicroAire bur
MicroAire cannula
MicroAire drill
MicroAire instruments
MicroAire oscillating bone saw
MicroAire osteotome
MicroAire pneumatic power
  instrument
microAllis forceps
microamperage electrical nerve
  stimulator
microamps TENS unit
microanalyzer
microanastomosis
microanastomosis approximator
microanastomosis clip
microanastomosis clip
  approximator
microaneurysm
microangiopathy
microarterial clamp
microarterial clamp applier

microarterial forceps
microaspirator (*see also*
  aspirator)
  Ergo microaspirator
microball hook
microballoon (*see also* balloon)
  implantable silicone
    microballoon
  Rand microballoon
microballoon probe
microbar
microbayonet forceps
microbayonet rasp
microbayonet scoop
Microbeam manipulator
microbial action
microbial pathogen
microbial plaque
microbiliary inflammation
microbiopsy forceps
microbipolar forceps
MicroBite forceps
microblade (*see also* blade)
  Beaver microblade
  Sharptome microblade
microblade knife
Microblator ArthroWand
Microbond NP
microbone curet
microbore Tygon tube
microbrachycephaly
microbrenner
microbronchoscopic grasping
  forceps
microbronchoscopic tissue
  forceps
microbulldog clamp
microbulldog clip
microcalipers (*see also* calipers)
  Storz microcalipers
MicroCAP ArthroWand
microcap scalpel
Micro-Cast collimator
microcatheter (*see also*
  catheter)
  AngioOPTIC microcatheter
  Cardima Pathfinder
    microcatheter
  Hydrolyser microcatheter
  Magic microcatheter
  Prowler microcatheter
  Renegade microcatheter

microcatheter (*continued*)
    Terumo SP hydrophilic-polymer-coated microcatheter
    Tracker microcatheter
    UltraLite flow-directed microcatheter
microcautery unit
Microcell alternating pressure pad
Microcell chamber
microcellular organism
microcephaly
microcheilia (*also* microchilia)
microchilia (*variant of* microcheilia)
microcirculation
microcirculatory failure
microclamp (*see also* clamp)
    bulldog microclamp
    disposable microclamp
    Kapp microclamp
    Khodadad microclamp
microclamp clip
microclamp forceps
microclip (*see also* clip)
    Heifitz microclip
    Khodadad microclip
    Kleinert-Kutz microclip
    Schwasser microclip
    Williams microclip
    Yasargil microclip
    Zylik microclip
microclip applier
microclip forceps
microcoagulator (*see also* coagulator)
    Malis bipolar microcoagulator
    Polar-Mate bipolar microcoagulator
micrococcus (*pl.* micrococci)
microcoil
micro-Colibri forceps
microcolon
microconjunctival scissors
microconnector
microcorneal forceps
microcorneal scissors
microcrack
microcrimped prosthesis
microcrystalline wax
microcup pituitary forceps

microcuret (*see also* curet)
    Acurette microcuret
    Hardy microcuret
    HemoCue microcuret
    Malis microcuret
    Rhoton microcuret
    Ruggles microcuret
microcurie
microcurrent electrode
microcurrent therapy
microcystic adnexal carcinoma
microcystic disease
microcystitome (*see also* cystitome)
    Lieppman microcystitome
microdebrider (*see also* debrider)
    Hummer microdebrider
    Linvotec microdebrider
    MDS microdebrider
    Radnoid microdebrider
    Stryker microdebrider
    Wizard microdebrider
microdensitometer
    Vickers microdensitometer
microdensitometric
microdermabrader (*see also* abrader, dermabrader)
    Pelle Peel microdermabrader
microdermabrasion crystals
microdermatome (*see also* dermatome)
    Meek-Wall microdermatome
microdirect laryngoscopy
microdiskectomy
microdissecting forceps
microdissection
microdissector (*see also* dissector)
    Crockard microdissector
    Hardy microdissector
    Kurze microdissector
    Malis microdissector
    Rhoton microdissector
    Yasargil microdissector
Microdon dressing
microdont
microdontia
    relative generalized microdontia
    single-tooth microdontia
    true generalized microdontia

microdontism
micro-Doppler instrument
microdressing forceps
microdrill
    high-speed microdrill
    Shea microdrill
    Treace microdrill
microdrilling guide
microdroplet
    silicone microdroplet
microdroplet liquid silicone
    injections
microelectrode
    tungsten microelectrode
microelectrode recording
    technique
microelectrode technique
microembolic disease
microembolization
microendoprobe (see also
    endoprobe)
    Toshiba microendoprobe
microendoscope (see also
    endoscope)
    Omegascope flexible
        microendoscope
    ophthalmic laser
        microendoscope
    Toshiba microendoscope
microendoscopic optical catheter
microetcher
microetching technique
microextractor forceps
microfibrillar collagen
microfibrillar collagen hemostat
Microfil injection
Microfil silicone-rubber injection
    compound
Microfil solution
microfilament bundle
microfilter (see filter)
microfixation
Micro-Flow compactor (MFC)
MicroFlow phacoemulsification
    needle
Microfoam dressing
Microfoam surgical tape
microforceps (see also forceps)
    Adson microforceps
    Anis microforceps
    bipolar microforceps
    Birks-Mathelone microforceps

microforceps (continued)
    Colibri microforceps
    Collis microforceps
    Decker microforceps
    iris microforceps
    iris suture microforceps
    Jako laryngeal microforceps
    Jako-Kleinsasser microforceps
    jeweler's microforceps
    Koslowski microforceps
    Nicola microforceps
    Rhoton microforceps
    Scanlan microforceps
    Sparta microforceps
    V. Mueller laser Rhoton
        microforceps
    Yasargil microforceps
microfracture
MicroFrance minimally invasive
    surgical instruments
MicroFrance pediatric backbiter
Microfuge tube
MicroFuse Infuser
microgastria
Microgel surface-enhanced
    ventilation tube
microgenia
Microglass pH electrode
MicroGlide corneal sutures
MicroGlide exchange wire
MicroGlide reciprocating
    osteotome
microglossia
microglossic
micrognathia
    adult acquired micrognathia
    mandibular micrognathia
    maxillary micrognathia
    Pierre Robin micrognathia
micrognathia with peromelia
micrognathic appearance
micrograft dilator
micrograft punctiform
    technique
micrograph
Micro-Guide catheter
Microgyn II urinary
    incontinence device
Micro-Halogen otoscope
micro-Halsted arterial
    forceps
microhandpiece

microhemostat (*see also* hemostat)
O'Brien-Storz microhemostat
microhook (*see also* hook)
Bonn microhook
McIntyre microhook
Shambaugh-Derlacki microhook
Simcoe microhook
microhysteroscope (*see also* hysteroscope)
Hamou contact microhysteroscope
Micro-Imager high-resolution digital camera
microimpactor (*see also* impactor)
Codman microimpactor
microimplant (*see also* implant)
Artecoll injectable microimplant
Bioplastique injectable microimplant
silicone microimplant
microinstrument
Jako laryngeal microinstrument
Yasargil microinstruments
microinvasive carcinoma classification
microinvasive catheter
microinvasive technique
microiris hook
microiris knife
microiris scissors
microirrigator (*see also* irrigator)
Stryker microirrigator
microischemia
Microjet Quark portable pump
Microjet-based cutting and debriding device
micro-jeweler's monopolar forceps
microkeratome (*see also* keratome)
Barraquer microkeratome
Barraquer-Carriazo microkeratome
Carriazo-Barraquer microkeratome
Chiron ACS microkeratome

microkeratome (*continued*)
Corneal Shaper microkeratome
FlapMaker disposable microkeratome
Hanastome microkeratome
Krumeich-Barraquer microkeratome
LSK microkeratome
MedJet microkeratome
Med-Logics microkeratome
ML microkeratome
One Disposable microkeratome
Ruiz microkeratome
Summit Krumeich-Barraquer microkeratome
microknife (*see also* knife)
Karlin microknife
McPherson-Wheeler iris microknife
McPherson-Ziegler microknife
Microknit arterial prosthesis
Microknit patch graft
Microknit vascular graft
Microknit vascular graft prosthesis
Microlance blood lancet
MicroLap endoscope
MicroLap Gold microlaparoscope
microlaparoscope (*see also* laparoscope)
Imagyn microlaparoscope
microlaparoscopic cholecystectomy
microlaparoscopic Nissen fundoplication
microlaryngeal endotracheal tube
microlaryngeal grasping forceps
microlaryngeal instruments
microlaryngeal laser probe
microlaryngeal scissors
microlaryngeal surgery
microlaryngoscope (*see also* laryngoscope)
Abramson-Dedo microlaryngoscope
anterior commissure microlaryngoscope
Dedo-Jako microlaryngoscope

microlaryngoscope (*continued*)
  Fragen anterior commissure
    microlaryngoscope
  Jako microlaryngoscope
  Lindholm microlaryngoscope
microlaryngoscopy
  direct microlaryngoscopy
  suspension
    microlaryngoscopy
  Thornell microlaryngoscopy
Microlase transpupillary diode
    laser
microleakage
Microlens cystourethroscope
Microlens direct-vision
    telescope
Microlens Foroblique telescope
Microlens hook
Microlet electrode needle
Micro-Line arterial forceps
Micro-Line artery forceps
microlipofilling of the cheeks
    and chin
microlipoinjection
microlipoplasty
Microlith P pacemaker
Microlith pacemaker plus
    generator
microlithiasis
Microloc knee prosthesis
Micro-Lok implant
microlumbar disk excision
microlumbar diskectomy
microlumbar diskectomy
    retractor
micromandible
micromanipulation technique
micromanipulator (*see also*
    manipulator)
  microscope-mounted
    micromanipulator
  MicroSpot micromanipulator
  self-centering
    micromanipulator
  UniMax 2000 laser
    micromanipulator
micromanometer (*see also*
    manometer)
micromanometer catheter
micromanometer-tip catheter
MicroMark clip
MicroMark tissue marker

micromat
MicroMax Speed drill
micromaxilla
micromechanical retention
Micromedics surgical
    instrument
micromembranous stethoscope
micrometastasis
    (*pl.* micrometastases)
micrometastatic peritoneal
    disease
micrometastic disease
micrometer
  diamond micrometer
  Tolman micrometer
  Ultrasonic micrometer
micrometer knife
MicroMewi multiple sidehole
    infusion catheter
MicroMewi multi-sidehole
    infusion catheter
micromirror (*see also* mirror)
  Apfelbaum micromirror
  Silverstein micromirror
MicroMirror gold sensor
Micro-Mist disposable nebulizer
MicroMite anchor sutures
micromoles
micro-mosquito curved scissors
micro-mosquito straight scissors
micromultiplane
    transesophageal
    echocardiographic probe
micromyelia
Micron bobbin ventilation tube
micron needle
micronebulizer (*see also*
    nebulizer)
  Bird micronebulizer
microneedle
microneedle holder
microneedle holder forceps
micronerve hook
microneurolysis
microneurorrhaphy
microneurosurgery
microneurosurgery forceps
microneurosurgical forceps
microneurovascular anastomosis
Microny SR+ single-chamber,
    rate-responsive pulse
    generator

Micro-One dissecting forceps
micro-operative procedure
micro-organism
  gram-negative microorganism
  gram-positive microorganism
  pathogenic microorganism
micropannus
micropapillary carcinoma
microparticle
MicroPeel
Micro-Pen handpiece
micropenis
microphallus
microphonoscope
microphthalmus
micropigmentation handpiece
micropin (*see also* pin)
  Pischel micropin
micropin forceps
micropipette
micropituitary rongeur
micropituitary scissors
microplate (*see also* plate)
  AO-Titanium microplate
  C-shaped microplate
  Luhr microplate
  mandibular angle fracture
    intraoral open reduction
    microplate
microplate fixation
micropoint cautery
micropoint needle
micropoint sutures
Micropore dressing
Micropore hypoallergenic tape
Micropore surgical tape dressing
Micropore tape
microporosity
microporous paper taping
microprobe (*see also* probe)
  laser microprobe
microprobe ophthalmic laser
microprobe surgical tape
microprobe tip
microprocessor
micropuncture
micropuncture guidewire
micropuncture introducer
    needle
Micropuncture Peel-Away
    introducer
microradiograph

microradiography
microrasp (*see also* rasp,
    raspatory, microraspatory)
  Scanlan microrasp
microraspatory (*see* raspatory,
    rasp)
  Yasargil microraspatory
microreciprocating saw
microreconstruction
microretractor (*see also*
    retractor)
  flexible arm microretractor
microroentgenography
microrongeur (*see also* rongeur)
  Davol microrongeur
  Decker microrongeur
  Kerrison microrongeur
microruler (*see* ruler)
microruptor
  LASAG microruptor
microsagittal saw
Microsampler device
microscalpel (*see also* scalpel)
  Oasis feather microscalpel
microscanner (*see also* scanner)
  pQCT microscanner
microscissors (*see also* scissors)
  bayonet microscissors
  Castroviejo corneal
    microscissors
  Castroviejo microscissors
  Collis microscissors
  curved conventional
    microscissors
  DORC microforceps and
    microscissors
  Gill-Welsh-Vannas angled
    microscissors
  iris microscissors
  Jacobson microscissors
  Jako laryngeal microscissors
  Jako-Kleinsasser microscissors
  Kamdar microscissors
  Keeler microscissors
  Kleinsasser laryngeal
    microscissors
  Kurze microscissors
  McPherson-Castroviejo
    corneal microscissors
  McPherson-Vannas iris
    microscissors
  pinch-handle microscissors

microscissors (*continued*)
  Rhoton microscissors
  Rhoton titanium
    microscissors
  round-tip microscissors
  Scanlan microscissors
  Shutt microscissors
  straight microscissors
  Twisk microscissors
  V. Mueller laser Rhoton
    microscissors
  Westcott microscissors
  Yasargil microscissors
microscope
  Accu-Scope microscope
  acoustic microscope
  AFI Micros 5 microscope
  analytical electron
    microscope (AEM)
  aural microscope
  Barraquer-Zeiss microscope
  Beckerscope binocular
    microscope
  beta ray microscope
  BHTU microscope
  binocular microscope
  Bio-Optics specular
    microscope
  Bitumi monobjective
    microscope
  capillary microscope
  centrifuge microscope
  cine microscope
  Codman-Mentor microscope
  Cohan microscope
  Cohan-Barraquer microscope
  color contract microscope
  comparison microscope
  compound microscope
  confocal microscope
  Contraves microscope
  conventional transmission
    electron microscope
  CooperVision microscope
  corneal microscope
  coupling microscope
  Czapski microscope
  darkfield microscope
  Derlacki-Shambaugh
    microscope
  EIE 150F operating
    microscope

microscissors (*continued*)
  electron microscope
  Elmiskop 101 electron
    microscope
  endothelial specular
    microscope
  epic microscope
  Fiberlite microscope
  fiberoptic microscope
  fluorescence microscope
  fluorescent microscope
  Galilean microscope
  Greenough microscope
  Haag-Streit microscope
  Hallpike-Blackmore ear
    microscope
  Heyer-Schulte microscope
  high-voltage electron
    microscope
  Hitachi H-series electron
    microscope
  hypodermic microscope
  infrared microscope
  integrating microscope
  interference microscope
  ion microscope
  JedMed Trigem microscope
  JEM electron microscope
  Joel scanning electron
    microscope
  Kaps operating microscope
  Keeler-Konan Specular
    microscope
  Kelar microscope
  Konan noncontact specular
    microscope
  laser microscope
  Leica microscope
  Leitz microscope
  light electron microscope
  light microscope
  Mentor fine-focus microscope
  Moller microscope
  nailfold capillary microscope
  Neibauer-Kleinert microscope
  Olympus microscope
  Olympus fluorescence
    microscope
  Olympus microscope
  OM 2000 operating
    microscope
  Omni 2 microscope

microscissors (*continued*)
  Omni operating microscope
  opaque microscope
  operating microscope
  OPMI operating microscope
  Opmi surgical microscope
  Opmi microscope
  Opmi-6 operating microscope
  Optiphot microscope
  Optique microscope
  phase microscope
  phase-contrast microscope
  Philips electron microscope
  photon microscope
  pneumatic microscope
  polarizing microscope
  Project Research Ophthalmic
    specular microscope
  projector x-ray microscope
  Pro-Koester wide-field SCM
    microscope
  Protege Plus microscope
  real-time confocal scanning
    laser microscope
  rectified microscope
  rectified polarizing
    microscope
  reflecting microscope
  Rheinberg microscope
  scanning electron microscope
  scanning laser acoustic
    microscope
  scanning slit confocal
    microscope
  scanning transmission
    electron microscope
  scanning tunneling
    microscope
  schlieren microscope
  Seiler surgical microscope
  Shambaugh operating
    microscope
  Shambaugh-Derlacki
    microscope
  simple microscope
  slit-lamp microscope
  SMZ zoom stereo microscope
  specular microscope
  stereoscopic microscope
  Storz microscope
  Storz-Urban surgical
    microscope

microscissors (*continued*)
  stroboscopic microscope
  surgical microscope
  tandem scanning confocal
    microscope
  television microscope
  tonsillectomy with operating
    microscope
  Topcon SP-series non-contact
    specular microscope
  transmission electron
    microscope (TEM)
  trinocular microscope
  ultrasonic microscope
  ultraviolet microscope
  Universal electron
    microscope
  Urban microscope
  Varimic microscope
  video specular microscope
  video-rate 2-photon laser
    scanning microscope
  Weck ceiling-mount operating
    microscope
  Weck operating microscope
  Weck-cel operating
    microscope
  Welch Allyn portable
    binocular microscope
  Wild operating microscope
  Wild surgical microscope
  x-ray microscope
  x-ray tomographic
    microscope
  Yasargil microscope
  Yasargil surgical microscope
  Zeiss Axioskop microscope
  Zeiss phase-contrast
    microscope
  Zeiss operating microscope
  Zeiss Opmi surgical
    microscope
  Zeiss Opmi-6 operating
    microscope
  Zeiss electron
    microscope
  Zeiss-Jena surgical
    microscope
  Zeiss-Barraquer cine
    microscope
  Zeiss-Barraquer surgical
    microscope

microscissors (*continued*)
  Zeiss-Cohan-Barraquer
    microscope
  Zeiss-Contraves operating
    microscope
  Zeiss-Jena surgical
    microscope
microscope eyepiece
microscope-mounted
  micromanipulator
microscopic diagnosis
microscopic disease
microscopic epididymal sperm
  aspiration
microscopic hook
microscopic invasion
microscopic multifocal
  medullary carcinoma
microscopic resection
microscopic scissors
microscopically controlled surgery
microscopy
  binocular microscopy
  cryoelectron microscopy
  double-immunofluorescence
    microscopy
  electron microscopy
  fluorescence microscopy
  immunofluorescent
    microscopy
  light microscopy (LM)
  scanning electron microscopy
    (SEM)
  specular microscopy
  television microscopy
  transmission electron
    microscopy (TEM)
microscrew (*see also* screw)
  Barouk microscrew
  forehead elevation and
    fixation with percutaneous
    microscrews
MicroSeal nebulizer
MicroSeal ophthalmic
  handpiece
microsecond pulsed flashlamp
  pumped dye laser
Microsect curet
microsection
microserrefine (*see also*
  serrefine)
  Storz microserrefine

MicroShape keratome
Micro-Sharp blade
MicroSkin urostomy pouch
MicroSmooth probe
Microsnap hemostatic forceps
Micro-Soft Stream sidehole
  infusion catheter
Microsoftrac catheter
microsomatic
microsomia
  craniofacial microsomia
  hemifacial microsomia
MicroSpan capnometer
MicroSpan hysteroscope
MicroSpan sheath
microspatula (*see also* spatula)
  Osher malleable microspatula
microspectroscope
microspectroscopy
microsphere
  Embosphere microsphere
  magnetic microsphere
  paramagnetic microsphere
  Super-Bright microsphere
Microspike approximator
Microspike approximator clamp
microsponge (*see also* sponge)
  Alcon microsponge
  Schachar-Gills microsponge
  Teardrop microsponge
  Weck-cel microsponge
Microsponge Teardrop sponge
MicroSpot micromanipulator
Micross dilatation catheter
Micross SL balloon
MicroStable liner locking
  mechanism
microstaple (*see also* staple)
  Barouk microstaple
microstaple holder
Microstat handpiece
Microstat ultrasonic nebulizer
MicroStim 100 TENS device
microstomia
microstomia prevention
  appliance
microsurgery
microsurgery biopsy forceps
microsurgery dissector
microsurgery needle holder
microsurgery procedure
microsurgery retractor

microsurgery technique
microsurgical biopsy forceps
microsurgical breast
    reconstruction
microsurgical diskectomy
microsurgical dissector
microsurgical ear hook
microsurgical ear pick
microsurgical ear replantation
microsurgical epididymal sperm
    aspiration
microsurgical free flap
microsurgical grasping
    forceps
microsurgical knife
microsurgical procedure
microsurgical retractor
microsurgical scissors
microsurgical spatula
microsurgical technique
microsurgical tubocornual
    anastomosis
microsurgical tying forceps
microsuture (*see also* sutures)
    Sharpoint microsutures
microsuture forceps
microsuture-tying forceps
microsyringe
Microtek cupped forceps
Microtek Heine otoscope
Microtek scissors
Micro-Temp pad
Micro-Temp pump
microtenotomy scissors
Microthin pacemaker
microtia
microtia reconstruction
microtip bipolar forceps
microtip bipolar jeweler's
    forceps
microtip phaco tip
microtip pressure transducer
microtissue forceps
microtitration plate reader
microtome
    Cryo-Cut microtome
    Leica vibrating knife
        microtome
    Leitz microtome
    rotary microtome
    sliding microtome
    Stadie-Riggs microtome

microtonometer (*see also*
    tonometer)
    Computon microtonometer
Micro-Touch medical gloves
microtrabecular hepatocellular
    carcinoma
Micro-Tracer portable ECG
microtransducer (*see also*
    transducer)
    imbedded microtransducer
    Konigsberg microtransducer
microtransducer catheter
microtransducer technique
microtrauma
microtubule
micro-tubulotomy technique
Micro-Two forceps
microtying eye forceps
microtying forceps
MicroTymp tympanometric
    device
microutility forceps
MicroVac catheter
microvascular abnormalities
microvascular anastomosis
microvascular bone transfer
microvascular clamp
microvascular clamp-applying
    forceps
microvascular clip
microvascular decompression
    (MVD)
microvascular free flap transfer
microvascular free gracilis
    transfer
microvascular free posterior
    interosseous flap
microvascular free tissue
    transfer
microvascular graft
microvascular modified Alm
    retractor
microvascular needle holder
microvascular neurosurgery
microvascular reconstruction
microvascular scissors
microvascular STA-MCA kit
microvascular surgery
microvascular surgical
    anastomosis
microvascular technique
microvascular thrombosis

microvascular toe transfer
microvascular tying forceps
microvascularize
Microvasic Rigiflex balloon
Microvasive minisnare
Microvasive biliary device
Microvasive biliary stent
Microvasive controlled radial
    expansion esophageal
    dilator
Microvasive disposable alligator-
    shaped forceps
Microvasive Geenen Endotorque
    guidewire
Microvasive Glidewire
Microvasive Glidewire
    guidewire
Microvasive instrumentation
Microvasive One Step Button
    gastrostomy
Microvasive papillotome
Microvasive radial jaw biopsy
    forceps
Microvasive retrieval balloon
Microvasive Rigiflex balloon
    catheter
Microvasive Rigiflex balloon
    dilator
Microvasive Rigiflex through-
    the-scope balloon
Microvasive Rigiflex TTS balloon
Microvasive sclerotherapy
    needle
Microvasive Speedband
    Superview ligator
Microvasive stent
Microvasive stiff piano wire
    guidewire
Microvasive ultratome
microvascular free flap
Microvel double velour graft
Microvel graft
Microvel implant
Microvel prosthesis
Microvena Amplatz Goose Neck
    snare
Microvena Das Angel Wings
    occluder
Micro-Vent implant
MicroVent ventilator
Micro-Vent implant
microvesicle

microvessel density (MVD)
microvessel hook
microvessel knife
MicroView sheath-based
    catheter
microvillar cell
microvillus membrane
microvillus (*pl.* microvilli)
Microvit cutter
Microvit probe
Microvit scissors
Microvit vitrector
microvitreoretinal blade (MVR)
microvitreoretinal spatula
microvolt
microwave coagulation
microwave diathermy
microwave fixation
microwave radiation injury
microwave therapy
Microtek scissors
Micro-Z neuromuscular
    stimulator
micturition bag
micturition reflex
MID (maximum interincisal
    distance)
MIDA CoroNet instrumentation
midabdominal transverse
    incision
midabdominal wall
Midas alloy
Midas Rex drill
Midas Rex instrumentation
Midas Rex knife
Midas Rex pneumatic
    instrument
Midas Rex pneumatic tool
Midas Rex bur guard
midaxillary line
midaxillary line incision
midbody
midbrain
    aqueduct of midbrain
    tectum of midbrain
    tegmentum of midbrain
midbrain reticular formation
MID-CAB (minimally invasive
    direct coronary artery
    bypass)
midcarpal arthroscopy
midcarpal capsule

midcarpal disarticulation of
    wrist
midcarpal dislocation
midcarpal joint
midcarpal SLAC
midcavity forceps
midcervical apophyseal joint
midclavicular line
midclavicular line to nipple
    (MCL-N)
midconcha cymba
midcoronal plane
midcostal line
midcycle phase
mid-depth
middle cardiac cervical nerve
middle cardiac vein
middle cerebral artery (MCA)
middle cerebral artery occlusion
middle cerebral peduncle
middle cervical ganglion
middle clunial nerves
middle colic artery
middle colic vein
middle collateral artery
middle constrictor pharyngeal
    muscle
middle cranial fossa
middle cranial fossa line
middle ear arrow-tube
middle ear aspirator
middle ear calipers
middle ear canal knife
middle ear capsule knife
middle ear chisel
middle ear cleft
middle ear curet
middle ear dermoid cyst of
    ovary
middle ear effusion (MEE)
middle ear elevator
middle ear excavator
middle ear forceps
middle ear hoe
middle ear hook
middle ear implant
middle ear infection
middle ear knife
middle ear muscle reflex
middle ear neoplasm
middle ear ring curet
middle ear strut forceps

middle ear suction cannula
middle extrahepatic bile duct
middle finger
middle fossa
middle fossa approach
middle fossa plate
middle fossa retractor
middle fossa syndrome
middle fossa vestibular
    neurectomy
middle frontal gyrus
middle genicular artery
middle gluteal muscle
middle latency response (MLR)
middle lobe bronchus
middle lobe of prostate
middle meatal antrostomy
middle meatus
middle meningeal artery
middle meningeal vein
middle nasal concha
middle nasal vault
middle palatine suture
middle palmar space
middle pharyngeal constrictor
middle portion
middle rectal artery
middle rectal vein
middle scalene muscle
middle sinuses
middle suprarenal artery
middle temporal artery
middle temporal vein
middle thyroid vein
middle turbinate
middle umbilical fold
middle umbilical ligament
middle vault deformity
middle vesical artery
middle zone
Middledorf retractor
Middledorpf splint
middle-ear dermoid cyst of ovary
Middlesex-Pointe retractor
Middleton adenoid curet
Middleton curet
Middleton line
Middleton rongeur
midesophageal diverticulum
midexpiratory flow rate
midface
midface alloplastic augmentation

midface avulsion flap
midface degloving technique
midface fracture
midface hypoplasia
midface lift
midface malar zygomatic
    cheekbone complex
midface suspension face-lift
    surgery
midface trauma
midfacial breadth
midfacial degloving
midfacial fracture
midfacial hypoplasia
midfacial rejuvenation
midfacial retrusion
midfemoral block
midflow rate
midfoot fracture
midforceps delivery
midforceps maneuver
midforceps operation
midfrontal plane
midgastric electrode
midget MRI scanner
midgut ischemia
midheel line
midhumeral line
mid-infrared pulsed laser
midlamellar cicatricial retraction
midlamellar contracture
Midland tilt table
midlateral approach
midline abdominal crease
midline abdominal incision
midline aponeurotic closure
midline cranio-orbital clefting
midline disharmony
midline disk herniation
midline episiotomy
midline exposure
midline forehead flap
midline incision
midline incisional hernia
midline incisional hernioplasty
midline lethal granuloma
midline lower abdominal incision
midline malignant reticulosis
    granuloma
midline medial approach
midline oblique incision
midline of the columella

midline plication of the anterior
    rectus sheath
midline position
midline sagittal glossotomy
midline scar
midline spinal approach
midline sternum-splitting
    incision
midline structures
midline tumor
midline upper abdominal
    incision
midlung field
midmalleolar line
midoccipital electrode
midpalatal opening
midpalatal suture opening
midpalatine raphe
midpalmar abscess
midpalmar space
midpalmar space abscess
midpapillary short axis
midpelvic anteroposterior
    diameter
midpelvic diameter
midpenile hypospadias
midplane
midpoint
midpoint to meatal line
midportion
midroot
midsacral region
midsagittal plane
midscapular line
midsection
midshaft fracture
midshaft of bone
midsigmoid colon
midsternal line
midsternum-splitting incision
midstream aortogram catheter
midsystolic buckling
midsystolic closure of aortic
    valve
midtarsal
midtemporal area
midtemporal focus
midtemporal spiking
midthalamic plane
midthigh
midtibial perforator
mid-to-deep dermal peel

midtransverse colon
midtrimester bleeding
Miescher tube
Miescher tubule
MIF (macrophage inhibiting
    factor, migration inhibiting
    factor)
Mighty Bite Zimmon lateral
    biopsy cup forceps
Mignon cataract extractor
migraine abortive therapy
migraine equivalent
migraine headache
migrated tooth
migrating abscess
migration
    calculus migration
    early implant migration
    electrode migration
    epithelial migration
    gallstone migration
    gap migration
    implant migration
    lymphocyte migration
    physiologic mesial migration
    postoperative migration
    tooth migration
migration abnormality
migration of tooth
migration-inhibiting factor (MIF)
migratory cells
migratory deep vein
    thrombophlebitis
Mik (see Mikulicz)
Mikaelsson catheter
Mikamo double-eyelid operation
Mikhail bone block
Mikros pacemaker
Mikro-Tip micromanometer-
    tipped catheter
Mikro-Tip transducer
Mikulicz abdominal retractor
Mikulicz angle
Mikulicz aphthae
Mikulicz cells
Mikulicz clamp
Mikulicz colostomy
Mikulicz crusher
Mikulicz disease
Mikulicz drain
Mikulicz enterectomy
Mikulicz forceps

Mikulicz gastrectomy
Mikulicz gastrotomy
Mikulicz incision
Mikulicz liver retractor
Mikulicz operation
Mikulicz pack
Mikulicz pad
Mikulicz peritoneal clamp
Mikulicz peritoneal forceps
Mikulicz pharyngoesophageal
    reconstruction
Mikulicz pyloroplasty
Mikulicz retractor
Mikulicz spatula
Mikulicz sponge
Mikulicz syndrome
Mikulicz tarsectomy
Mikulicz tonsillar forceps
Mikulicz-Radecki clamp
Mikulicz-Radecki drain
Mikulicz-Vladimiroff amputation
Mikulicz-Vladimiroff operation
Milan uterine curet
Milch condylar fracture
    classification
Milch cuff resection of ulna
    technique
Milch elbow fracture
    classification
Milch elbow technique
Milch humeral fracture
    classification
Milch operation
Milch resection plate
Milch ulna procedure
mild chromic sutures
mild concussion
mild to moderate pain
mild trabeculation
mild traumatic brain injury
    (mTBI)
Miles abdominoperineal
    resection
Miles antral curet
Miles bone chisel
Miles clamp
Miles clip
Miles nasal punch
Miles operation
Miles proctosigmoidectomy
Miles punch biopsy forceps
Miles rectal clamp

Miles retractor
Miles skin clip
Miles Teflon clip
Miles vacuum infiltration
   processor
Miles vena cava clip
Milewski driver
Milex forceps
Milex Jel-Jector cream
Milex Jel-Jector vaginal
   applicator
Milex pessary
Milex retractor
Milex spatula
Milex vaginal insufflator
Milford mallet finger technique
miliary abscess
miliary acne
miliary aneurysm
miliary carcinosis
miliary embolism
miliary granulomatous
   inflammation
miliary sclerosis
military antishock trousers
   (MAST)
military brace position
military maneuver
military tuck position
milium (*pl.* milia)
milk abscess
milk ducts
milk gland
milk lines
milked out
milked superiorly
milk-ejection reflex
milk-filled cyst
milkmaid's elbow dislocation
milkman's fracture
milkman's syndrome
milky ascites
milky fluid
milky urine
mill
   3M bone mill
   DePuy bone mill
   Lere bone mill
Millar catheter
Millar catheter-tipped
   transducer
Millar Doppler catheter

Millar micromanometer
   catheter
Millar Mikro-Tip catheter
   pressure transducer
Millar catheter
Millar pigtail angiographic
   catheter
Millar urodynamic catheter
Millard advancement rotation
   flap reconstruction
Millard bilateral cleft lip
   repair
Millard cheiloplasty
Millard clamp
Millard creed
Millard double hook
Millard flap
Millard forehead flap
Millard forked flap technique
Millard graft augmentation
Millard island flap
Millard modification of
   Kernahan and Elsahy
   striped Y classification for
   cleft lip and palate
Millard mouth gag
Millard operation
Millard retroauricular and
   medial chondrocutaneous
   flap
Millard rotation-advancement lip
   repair
Millard rotation-advancement
   operation
Millard rotation-advancement
   technique
Millard rotation-advancement
   unilateral cleft lip
   repair
Millard thimble hook
Millard thimble retractor
millardian rotation advancement
   principle
Mille Pattes screw
Mille Pattes technique
Mille Patts screw
Millen retropubic prostatectomy
Millen technique
Millender arthroplasty
Millender-Nalebuff wrist
   arthrodesis
Millenia balloon catheter

Millenia percutaneous
    transluminal coronary
    angioplasty (PTCA)
    catheter
Millen-Read modification
Miller 9-prong small rake
Miller articulating forceps
Miller bayonet forceps
Miller bone file
Miller bougie
Miller bracket positioner
Miller curet
Miller cystoscope
Miller dental elevator
Miller dilator
Miller dissecting scissors
Miller endotracheal tube
Miller fiberoptic laryngoscope
    blade
Miller flatfoot operation
Miller forceps
Miller laryngoscope
Miller operating scissors
Miller operation
Miller operation for talipes
    valgus
Miller position
Miller procedure
Miller raspatory
Miller ratchet injector
Miller rectal forceps
Miller rectal scissors
Miller retractor
Miller scissors
Miller septostomy catheter
Miller speculum
Miller syndrome
Miller technique
Miller tonsillar dissector
Miller tonsillar knife
Miller tube
Miller vaginal speculum
Miller-Abbott catheter
Miller-Abbott double-channel
    intestinal tube
Miller-Abbott double-lumen
    intestinal tube
Miller-Abbott intestinal tube
Miller-Abbott tube (M-A tube)
Miller-Apexo elevator
Miller-Fisher variant of Guillain-
    Barre syndrome

Miller-Galante hip prosthesis
Miller-Galante knee arthroplasty
Miller-Galante total knee implant
Miller-Galante
    unicompartmental knee
Miller-Senn double-ended
    retractor
Miller-Senn retractor
Millesi interfascicular grafts
Millesi modified technique
Millesi nerve graft
Millesi scissors
Millet needle
Millet neurological test
    instrument
Millet test hammer
Millette
Millette tonsil knife
Millette-Tydings knife
mill-house murmur
milliamperes (ma)
millicuries (mc)
milliequivalents (mEq)
Milligan double-ended
    dissection
Milligan double-ended dissector
Milligan self-retaining retractor
Milligan speculum
Milligan-Morgan
    hemorrhoidectomy
milligrams (mg)
millijoules (mJ)
Milliknit arterial prosthesis
Milliknit Dacron prosthesis
Milliknit vascular graft
    prosthesis
milliliters (ml)
millimeter ruler
millimeters (mm)
millimoles (mM)
Millin bladder neck spreader
Millin bladder retractor
Millin bladder spatula
Millin boomerang needle holder
Millin capsule forceps
Millin capsule-grasping forceps
Millin clamp
Millin ligature-guiding forceps
Millin lobe-grasping forceps
Millin operation
Millin prostatectomy forceps
Millin retractor

Millin retropubic bladder retractor
Millin self-retaining retractor
Millin suction tube
Millin T-shaped angled forceps
Millin T-shaped forceps
Millin-Bacon bladder neck spreader
Millin-Bacon bladder self-retaining retractor
Millin-Bacon retropubic prostatectomy retractor
Millin-Bacon spreader
milliner's needle
Millin-Read operation
Millipore filter
Millipore sutures
Millipore ultrafree-CL centrifugal filter
milliseconds (msec)
millivolts (mV)
Mill-Rose biopsy forceps
Mill-Rose cytology brush
Mill-Rose esophageal injector
Mill-Rose instrument cleaner
Mill-Rose RiteBite biopsy forceps
Mill-Rose spiral stone basket
Mill-Rose Surebrite biopsy forceps
Mill-Rose tube
Mills arteriotomy scissors
Mills cautery
Mills circumflex scissors
Mills coronary endarterectomy set
Mills coronary endarterectomy spatula
Mills dressing
Mills forceps
Mills microvascular needle holder
Mills operative peripheral angioplasty catheter
Mills tissue forceps
Mills valvulotome
Milteck scissors
Miltex blepharoplasty scissors
Miltex bone saw
Miltex disposable biopsy punch
Miltex gum
Miltex ligature knife

Miltex nail nipper
Miltex pump
Miltex retractor
Miltex rib spreader
Miltex saberback rhytidectomy scissors
Miltex stitch scissors
Miltex surgical instruments
Miltex tenaculum hook
Miltex undermining scissors
Miltner-Wan calcaneus resection
Milton-Adams suspension
Milwaukee brace
Milwaukee orthosis
Milwaukee scoliosis brace
Milwaukee scoliosis orthosis
Milwaukee shoulder
Milwaukee snare
Mi-Mark disposable endocervical curet
Mi-Mark endocervical curet set
mimetic hyperkinesis
mimetic modulation
mimetic muscle
MindSet toe splint
Miner osteotome
mineral oil aspiration
mineral oil foreign body
mineral salt
mineral trioxide aggregate (MTA)
mineral wax
mineralization
    calcospherite mineralization
    capsular mineralization
    dystrophic mineralization
mineralized tissue
Minerva back jacket
Minerva cast
Minerva collar
Minerva jacket
Minerva orthosis
Minerva plaster collar
Minerva plaster jacket
Minerva plastic jacket
Minerva robot
Ming gastric carcinoma classification
Mingazzini-Foerster operation
Mingograf 6-channel electrocardiograph
Mingograf recorder

Mingograf
    electroencephalograph
mini-applier (*see* applier)
mini Bio-Phase suture anchor
Mini Crown stent
Mini automatic implantable
    cardioverter defibrillator
mini lag screw
Mini Orbita plate
Mini speech processor
Mini Stryker power drill
mini trephine
mini Würzburg screw
miniabdominoplasty
miniature blade
miniature bulldog clamp
miniature carrier
miniature electrotome
miniature intestinal forceps
miniature loop electrode
miniature plugger
miniature probe
miniature scissors
miniature sound
miniature ultrasound suction
    device
miniature uterine cavity
miniaturized ultrasound catheter
    probe
minibasket (*see also* basket)
    Shutt minibasket
    Wilson-Cook minibasket
miniblade
minibladebreaker (*see also*
    minibladebreaker)
    Troutman-Barraquer
        minibladebreaker
minibrachioplasty (axillary
    dermolipectomy)
Minicath catheter
miniclip (*see* clip)
    Stangel fallopian tube miniclip
minidialyzer
mini-dose
minidriver instruments
Minidyne
mini-facelift
Mini-Fibralux pocket otoscope
minifixator (*see also* fixator)
    Pennig minifixator
Mini-Flex flexible Harris uterine
    injector

miniforceps (*see* forceps)
    Kern miniforceps
minigraft dilator
Miniguard adhesive patch
Miniguard stress incontinence
    device
MiniHeart nebulizer
mini-Hoffmann external fixator
mini-Hohmann retractor
mini-keratoplasty scissors
mini-Lambotte osteotome
minilaparoscope (*see also*
    laparoscope)
    Aslan 2-mm minilaparoscope
    Pixie minilaparoscope
minilaparoscopic
    cholecystectomy
minilaparotomy
minilaparotomy Falope-ring
    applicator
minilaparotomy incision
minilaparotomy technique
mini-Lexer osteotome
Minilith pacemaker
Minilith pacemaker plus
    generator
miniloop
    Olympus HX-21L detachable
        miniloop
Minilux headlight
Minilux pocket otoscope
minimal access general surgery
minimal alveolar concentration
minimal anesthetic
    concentration (MAC)
minimal assistance
minimal bactericidal
    concentration
minimal bleeding
minimal blood loss
minimal brain dysfunction
    (MBD)
minimal extensibility
minimal instrumentation
minimal leak technique
minimal rhinoplasty
minimal tension skin lines
minimal transurethral
    resection
minimal access procedure
minimal access technique
minimal-change disease

minimal-change nephrotic
    syndrome
minimal incision pubovaginal
    suspension
minimal lesion nephrotic
    syndrome
minimallet (*see also* mallet)
    Gam-Mer minimallet
minimally displaced fracture
minimally invasive approach
minimally invasive biopsy
minimally invasive direct
    coronary artery bypass
    (MIDCAB)
minimally invasive
    esophagectomy
minimally invasive mitral valve
    repair
minimally invasive procedure
minimally invasive robotic heart
    valve surgery
minimally invasive surgical
    technique
minimastopexy
Mini-Matic implant
MiniMed III infusion pump
mini-meniscus blade
mini-micro forceps
mini-Monoka canalicular
    stent
minimum alveolar anesthetic
    concentration
minimum alveolar concentration
    (MAC)
minimum bactericidal
    concentration
minimum detectable
    concentration
minimum effective analgesic
    concentration
minimum effective
    concentration (MEC)
minimum lethal concentration
minimum local analgesic
    concentration (MLAC)
mini-Mustarde procedure
Mini-Neb nebulizer
mini-ophthalmic drain
mini-Orthofix fixator
MiniOx oxygen monitor
MiniOX pulse oximeter
miniphage

miniplate (*see also* plate)
    2-hole miniplate
    2-holed miniplate
    8-hole miniplate
    Champy miniplate
    L-shaped miniplate
    Luhr miniplate
    mandibular miniplate
    Storz miniplate
    titanium miniplate
    Vitallium miniplate
miniplate fixation
miniplate strut
mini-pouch
    CenterPointLock 2-point
        ostomy system: closed mini-
        pouch
    closed mini-pouch
    Filter Security closed mini-
        pouch
    Guardian 2-piece ostomy
        system: closed mini-pouch
    Premier drainable mini-pouch
    Sur-Fit mini-pouch
miniprobe (*see also* probe)
    high-frequency miniprobe
Mini-Profile dilatation
    catheter
minipump (*see also* pump)
    Alzer osmotic minipump
    osmotic minipump
MiniQuad XL lens
minirazor bladebreaker
miniscope
    Candela miniscope
miniscrew
MiniSite laparoscope
minisnare (*see also* snare)
    Microvasive minisnare
mini Snyder Hemovac
Mini-Space IUI catheter
ministaple (*see also* stable)
    Bio-R-Sorb resorbable
        ministaple
    Richards ministaple
MiniStim TENS unit
mini-Sugita clip
mini-tuck abdominoplasty
mini-Ullrich bone clamp
mini-Wright peak flowmeter
Minix pacemaker
mink encephalopathy

Minkoff-Jaffe-Menendez
    posterior approach
Minkoff-Nicholas procedure
Minneapolis hip prosthesis
Minnesota 4-lumen tube
Minnesota EKG classification
Minnesota Mining and
    Manufacturing Company
    (see 3M)
Minnesota retractor
Minnesota thermal disk
    temperature testing device
Minnesota tube
minor amputation
minor connector
minor connector bar
minor discomfort
minor fissure
minor gland obstruction
minor injury
minor laceration
minor operation
minor procedure
minor rhytids
minor salivary glands
Minor sign
minor splenic injury
minor sublingual duct
minor surgery
minor surgery scissors
minor vessel
minor wound
Minos air drill
Minotaur labyrinth
Minsky circle
Minsky operation
Minuet DDD pacemaker
minute anatomy
minute bleeding mucosal ulcer
minute polypoid lesion
minute ventilation (VE)
Mipron digital computer-assisted
    calipers
Mira cautery
Mira diathermy
Mira drill
Mira electrocautery
Mira endovitreal cryopencil
Mira female trochanteric reamer
Mira femoral head reamer
Mira laser
Mira photocoagulator

Mira reamer
Mira scissors
Mira tip eye cautery
Mira unit
Mira-Charnley reamer
Miracompo filling instrument
Mirage guidewire
Mirage over-the-wire balloon
    catheter
Miragel implant
Miragel sponge
Miralene sutures
Miralva vaginal applicator
Mirasorb sponge
Mirault operation
Mirault-Blair-Brown method of
    cleft lip repair
Mirault-Brown-Blair operation
Mire silicone rod
Mirizzi syndrome
mirror cannula
mirror focus
mirror hand
mirror holder
mirror image
mirror laryngoscope
mirror lift
mirror lift look
mirror-based reflective optics
mirror-image breast biopsy
mirror-image laryngoscopy
mirroring of extremities
MIS (melanoma in situ)
misarticulation
miscarriage
Mischler reservoir
Mischler shunt
Mischler valve
Mischler-Pudenz shunt
microscope
misdirection
Misdom-Frank curet
Miskimon cerebellar self-
    retaining retractor
Miskimon cerebellar self-
    retaining retractor
mismatch negativity (MMN)
mismatched marrow
missed abortion
missed fracture
missile injury
missile track abscess

missile-caused wound
Missouri catheter
Misstique female external
     urinary collector
mist tent
mist therapy
Mistette nasal spray pump
Misti Gold prosthesis
Mistogen nebulizer
Mistogen passover humidifier
Misty-Neb nebulizer
Mital elbow release
Mital elbow release technique
Mitchel aortotomy clamp
Mitchel-Adam clamp
Mitchel-Adam multipurpose
     clamp
Mitchell basket
Mitchell bunionectomy
Mitchell cartilage knife
Mitchell distal osteotomy
Mitchell knife
Mitchell operation
Mitchell osteotome
Mitchell osteotomy
Mitchell stone basket
Mitchell ureteral stone dislodger
Mitchell-Clark hernia repair
Mitchell-Diamond biopsy
     forceps
Mitchell-Diamond forceps
Mitek absorbable bone anchor
Mitek anchor
Mitek anchor appliance
Mitek Fastin threaded anchor
Mitek GII Easy Anchor
Mitek GII suture anchor
Mitek Knotless anchor sutures
Mitek ligament anchor
Mitek Micro anchor
Mitek Micro QuickAnchor
Mitek Mini GII anchor
Mitek Mini GLS anchor
Mitek Panalok anchor
Mitek rotator cuff anchor
Mitek SuperAnchor
     instrument
Mitek sutures
Mitek Tacit threaded anchor
miter technique
mitigated echolalia
Mitner rotary bone rasp

mitochondrion
     (*pl.* mitochondria)
mitogenic factor (MF)
Mitraflex dressing
Mitraflex foam dressing
Mitraflex wound dressing
mitral annuloplasty
mitral balloon commissurotomy
mitral commissurotomy
mitral dilator
mitral forceps
mitral hook
mitral insufficiency
mitral knife
mitral regurgitation
mitral stenosis knife
mitral valve aneurysm
mitral valve commissurotomy
mitral valve dilator
mitral valve disorder
mitral valve echo score
mitral valve fusion
mitral valve gradient
mitral valve homograft graft
mitral valve leaflet tip
mitral valve prolapse syndrome
mitral valve prosthesis
mitral valve repair
mitral valve replacement
mitral valve retractor
mitral valve ring
mitral valve scissors
mitral valve spreader
mitral valve hinging operation
mitral valve holding forceps
mitral valvotomy
mitral valvulotomy
Mitrathane wound dressing
Mitrofanoff
     appendicovesicostomy
Mitrofanoff continent urinary
     diversion technique
Mitrofanoff procedure
Mitroflow pericardial prosthetic
     valve
Mitrothin pacemaker
Mitsubishi angioscope
Mitsubishi angioscopic catheter
Mittelman implant
Mittelman prejowl-chin
     implants
Mittlemeir broach

Mittlemeir ceramic hip prosthesis
Mittlemeir ceramic total hip
Mittlemeir femoral prosthesis
Mity Hedstrom file
Mity Roto rotary instrument
Mityvac extractor
Mityvac obstetric vacuum extractor cup
Mityvac Super M cup
Mityvac vacuum extraction delivery
Mitz procedure
mixed abscess
mixed amputation
mixed anesthesia
mixed cataract
mixed condition
mixed connective tissue disease
mixed dentition
mixed failure
mixed fat-water density lesion
mixed glands
mixed gonadal dysgenesis
mixed hemangioma
mixed hemorrhoids
mixed hypertrophy
mixed joint
mixed laterality
mixed lesion
mixed mesh
mixed nasality
mixed nerve
mixed odontoma
mixed rhythm
mixed sclerotic and lytic bone lesion
mixed sore
mixed spasm
mixed tumor
mixed tumor of salivary gland
mixed type parapharyngeal schwannoma
mixed venous-lymphatic malformation
mixed cholesterol gallstone
MixEvac bone cement mixer
Mixter arterial forceps
Mixter baby hemostatic forceps
Mixter brain biopsy punch
Mixter clamp
Mixter common duct Dilaprobe

Mixter common duct irrigating Dilaprobe dilator
Mixter common duct probe
Mixter Dilaprobe probe
Mixter dilating probe
Mixter dissector
Mixter full-curve forceps
Mixter gall duct forceps
Mixter gall duct probe
Mixter gallbladder forceps
Mixter gallstone forceps
Mixter general operating scissors
Mixter hemostat
Mixter irrigating probe
Mixter ligature-carrier clamp
Mixter mosquito forceps
Mixter needle
Mixter operating scissors
Mixter pediatric forceps
Mixter pediatric hemostatic forceps
Mixter probe
Mixter punch
Mixter right-angle clamp
Mixter scissors
Mixter thoracic clamp
Mixter thoracic forceps
Mixter tube
Mixter ventricular needle
Mixter-McQuigg forceps
Mixter-O'Shaughnessy dissecting forceps
Mixter-O'Shaughnessy hemostatic forceps
Mixter-O'Shaughnessy ligature forceps
Mixter-O'Shaughnessy dissecting and ligature forceps
Mixter-Paul arterial forceps
Mixter-Paul hemostatic forceps
Miya hook
Miya hook ligament carrier
Miya hook ligature carrier
Mize-Bucholz-Grogen approach
Mizuho surgical Doppler
Mizuno technique
Mizuno-Hirohata-Kashiwagi technique
Mizzy needle
mJ (millijoule)
MK ophthalmoscope

MKG knee support
MKII automated scanner
MKS II knee brace
ML (mesiolingual)
MLA (mesiolabial)
Mladick abdominoplasty
Mladick concave cannula
Mladick convex cannula
Mladick ear reconstruction
MLAI (mesiolabioincisal)
MLT tube
MM (malignant melanoma)
mm (millimeters)
mM (millimoles)
mM/L (millimoles per liter)
MM-6000 colposcope
MMC (myelomeningocele)
MMF (maxillomandibular
    fixation)
MMG/O'Neil catheter
mmHg (millimeters of mercury)
MMK procedure
MMM (3M; Minnesota Mining and
    Manufacturing Company)
MMM drape (3M drape)
MMM dressing (3M dressing)
MMM Vi-Drape (3M Vi-Drape)
MMN (mismatch negativity)
M-mode sector transducer
MMS (Mohs micrographic
    surgery)
MMS low-profile acetabular cup
MND (modified neck dissection)
Müller (see Müeller)
Muller duct body
Muller maneuver
Muller tray
Muller-Hillis maneuver
mullerian dimple
mullerian duct
mullerian duct anomaly
mullerian duct aplasia
mullerian duct derivation
    syndrome
mullerian duct fusion
mullerian tumor
MNOE (malignant necrotizing
    otitis externa)
MO (myositis ossificans)
MO needle
Moberg advancement flap
Moberg advancement pedicle

Moberg arthrodesis
Moberg bone plate
Moberg chisel
Moberg forceps
Moberg key-pinch procedure
Moberg osteotome
Moberg pickup test
Moberg procedure
Moberg retractor
Moberg volar advancement flap
Moberg-Gedda fracture
Moberg-Gedda open reduction
Moberg-Stille forceps
Moberg-Stille retractor
mobile air chair
mobile bearing knee implant
mobile cecum
mobile gallbladder
mobile kidney
mobile mass
mobile testicle
mobile wad compartment of
    foramen
Mobilimb CPM device
mobilization
  bony mobilization
  cervical mobilization
  circumferential mobilization
  esophageal mobilization
  joint mobilization
  localized leukocyte
    mobilization
  stapes mobilization
mobilized cecum
mobilized uterus
mobilizer
  Derlacki ear mobilizer
  Derlacki mobilizer
  Derlacki-Hough mobilizer
  ear mobilizer
  Hough-Derlacki mobilizer
  Therabite mobilizer
  Valtchev uterine mobilizer
Mobin-Uddin filter
Mobin-Uddin umbrella filter
Mobin-Uddin umbrella vena
    cava filter
Mobin-Uddin vena caval filter
Mobitz heart block
Mobitz I AV heart block
Mobitz I block
Mobitz II AV heart block

Mobitz II block
Möbius (*see* Moebius)
Moebius syndrome
Mobley-Webster needle holder
Moblvac suction unit
Mochida CO_2 laser
MOD femoral drill guide
model
    bladder-prostate model
    casting model
    corpectomy model
    foot model
    Gail breast cancer risk model
    immunocompetent squamous
        cell cancer model
    implant model
    Westmore model
model plaster
model trimmer
modeling composition
modeling compound
modeling plastic
modeling plastic impression
mode-locked laser
moderate contractions
moderate hyperplasia
moderate narrowing
moderate pain
moderate shift
moderate voltage
moderately differentiated
    adenoma
moderately differentiated
    neuroendocrine carcinoma
modified abdominoplasty
modified anterior hairline
    forehead lift
modified autogenous latissimus
    breast reconstruction
modified Bassini herniorrhaphy
modified Belsey fundoplication
modified Bernard-Burow
    technique
modified birdcage coil
modified brachial technique
modified Cantwell technique
modified cast
modified caulking gun
modified chest lead
modified Child technique
modified Chopart amputation
modified CIF needle

modified C-loop intraocular lens
modified desmosome
modified dorsalis pedis
    myofascial flap
modified electron-beam CT
    scanner
modified Essed-Schroeder
    corporoplasty
modified fishtail excision
modified flap operation
modified Frost sutures
modified Gibson incision
modified Grace plate
modified graft
modified Harrington rod
modified Hassan open
    technique
modified Heller
    esophagomyotomy
modified Hoke-Miller flatfoot
    procedure
modified Irving-type tubal
    ligation
modified J-loop, posterior
    chamber intraocular lens
modified junctional complex
modified Kiel mastopexy
modified Konno procedure
modified Krukenberg procedure
modified lateral pharyngotomy
modified lithotomy position
modified Loeb and de la Plaza
    technique blepharoplasty
modified Mallet scale
modified Mark IV R-wave-
    triggered power injector
modified McVay herniorrhaphy
modified mold and surface
    replacement arthroplasty
modified Moore hip locking
    prosthesis
modified neck dissection (MND)
modified Norfolk procedure
modified operation
modified Oppenheimer splint
modified Peck onlay graft
modified pen grasp
modified piggyback technique
modified polymer
modified Pomeroy technique
modified position
modified procedure

modified prosthesis
modified Pulvertaft classification
for mutilating injuries
(categories 1-5)
modified radical hysterectomy
modified radical mastectomy
modified radical mastoidectomy
modified radical neck dissection
modified Rashkind PDA
occluder
modified reconstruction
modified Risdon approach
modified Ritgen maneuver
modified Robert Jones
dressing
modified Sacks-Vine push-pull
technique
modified sclerectomy punch
modified Seldinger procedure
modified Seldinger technique
modified Shouldice hernioplasty
modified shunt
modified Singapore flap
modified Skoog technique
modified spatula needle
modified submental flared-tip
retractor
modified suction tube
modified Sugiura procedure
modified surgical procedure
modified TAPP hernioplasty
modified technique
modified Toupe procedure
modified Toupe technique
modified Van Lint anesthesia
modified V-Y advancement
technique
modified Weber-Fergusson
incision
modified Weber-Fergusson
procedure
modified Weinhold
abdominoplasty
modified Whitehead
hemorrhoidectomy
modified Wies procedure
modified Younge forceps
modified zinc oxide-eugenol
cement
Modny drill
Modny guide
Modny pin

Modulap cutting and
coagulating probe
Modulap probe
modular Austin Moore hip
prosthesis
modular head remover
modular implant
modular instrumentation
modular Iowa Precoat total hip
prosthesis
modular knee prosthesis
modular prosthesis
modular temPPThotic kit
modular total hip prosthesis
modulation
Modulith SL 20 lithotriptor
Modulock posterior spinal
fixation
Modulock posterior spinal
fixation device
Moe alar hook
Moe bone curet
Moe gouge
Moe impactor
Moe intertrochanteric plate
Moe modified Harrington rod
Moe nail
Moe osteotome
Moe plate
Moe procedure
Moe scoliosis technique
Moe spinal fusion
Moe subcutaneous rod
Moebius (see Möbius)
Moebius anomaly
Moebius cataract knife
Moebius knife
Moebius sign
Moehle cannula
Moehle corneal forceps
Moehle forceps
Moehle scissors
Moeller glossitis
Moeller laser
Moersch bronchoscope
Moersch bronchoscopic forceps
Moersch bronchoscopic
specimen forceps
Moersch cardiospasm dilator
Moersch electrode
Moersch esophagoscope
Moe spinal hook

Moffat-Robinson bone plate
   collector
Mogen circumcision clamp
mogiarthria
mogilalia
Mohn microsurgery
Mohr clamp
Mohr finger splint
Mohr pinchcock clamp
Mohr splint
Mohr syndrome
Mohrenheim fossa
Mohrenheim space
Mohr-Tranebjaerg syndrome
Mohs chemotherapy
Mohs defect
Mohs excision of basal cell
   carcinoma
Mohs fresh tissue chemosurgery
   technique
Mohs hardness number (MHN)
Mohs hardness scale
Mohs hardness test
Mohs index
Mohs micrographic
   chemosurgery
Mohs micrographic surgery
   (MMS)
Mohs micrographic surgery by
   fixed-tissue technique
Mohs microsurgical resection
Mohs procedure
Mohs resection
Mohs surgery
Mohs technique
Mohs wound
Moire topography index
moist compress
moist dressing
moist gangrene
moist heat
moist interactive dressing
moist lap packs
moist mucous membrane
moist rales
moist tape
moistened fine mesh gauze
   dressing
moistened tape
moisture chamber
moisture exchanger
moisture-retentive dressing

molal solution
molar
   impacted molar
   mandibular molar
   maxillary molar
   third molar
molar glands
molar pregnancy
molar tooth fracture
mold
   acrylic mold
   Altchek vaginal mold
   Aquaplast mold
   Biothotic orthotic mold
   casting mold
   cesium mold
   Counsellor vaginal mold
   dental mold
   endolaryngeal brachytherapy
      mold
   filter mold
   Hydro-Cast dental mold
   inlay mold
   occlusal mold
   Silastic mold
   silicone mold
   sodium alginate wool mold
   Teflon mold
mold acetabular arthroplasty
mold arthroplasty
mold guide
molded ankle-foot orthosis
molded splint
molded Teflon
molder's sign
Moldestad vein hook
molding
   border molding
   compression molding
   injection molding
   tissue molding
molding helmet
molding of head
molding temperature
mole
   atypical mole
   B-K moles
   hairy mole
   hydatidiform mole
   pigmented mole
   spider mole
mole melanoma syndrome

molecular external layer
molecular lesion
molecular mimicry
molecular technique
molecule
  cell adhesion molecule (CAM)
  collagen molecule
  neurotransmitter molecule
  polymerized
    mucopolysaccharide
    molecule
  tropocollagen molecule
moleskin and felt scissors
moleskin bandage
moleskin padding
moleskin traction
moleskin traction hitch dressing
Molestick padding
Molesworth elbow procedure
Molesworth-Campbell approach
Molesworth-Campbell elbow
  approach
molilalia
Molina mandibular distractor
Molina needle catheter
Moll glands
Moller disease
Moller microscope
Mollison mastoid rongeur
Mollison self-retaining retractor
Mollo boots
molluscum contagiosum
Molnar disk
Molnlycke dressing
Moloney hernia repair
Moloney line
Molt curet
Molt dissector
Molt elevator
Molt forceps
Molt guillotine
Molt mouth gag
Molt mouth prop
Molt pedicle forceps
Molt periosteal elevator
Molteno double-plate implant
Molteno drainage
Molteno drainage eye implant
Molteno episcleral explant
Molteno implant drain
Molteno implant drainage
  device

Molteno shunt tube
Molt-Storz guillotine
Molt-Storz tonsillectome
molybdenum radiation therapy
molybdenum rotating anode
  x-ray tube
molybdenum target tube
molybdenum-technetium
  generator
Momberg tourniquet
Momberg tube
Momentum pacemaker
Monaghan respirator
Monaghan ventilator
Monakow bundle
Monakow fasciculus aberrans
Monaldi drain
Monaldi operation
monangle hoe
Monarch knee brace
monarticular
monaural hearing
Monckeberg arteriosclerosis
Monckeberg degeneration
Monckeberg sclerosis
Moncorps knife
Moncrieff anterior chamber
  irrigating cannula
Moncrieff anterior chamber
  irrigator
Moncrieff cannula
Moncrieff discission
Moncrieff irrigator
Moncrieff operation
Mondini anomaly
Mondini deafness
Mondini deformity
Mondini dysplasia
Mondini malformation
Mondini pulmonary
  arteriovenous malformation
Mondini-Alexander
  malformation
Mondor disease
Monel metal radium applicator
mongolian spot
mongolism
monitor leads
monitor muscle flap
monitored anesthesia care
  (MAC)
monitored anesthesia control

monitored bed
monitoring
  2-dimensional monitoring
  Accutracker II ambulatory
    blood pressure monitoring
  airway gas monitoring
  anesthetic monitoring
  anticoagulant monitoring
  anticoagulation monitoring
  blood pressure monitoring
  cardiac monitoring
  central venous pressure
    monitoring
  close monitoring
  depth of anesthesia
    monitoring
  Doptone monitoring
  ECOG monitoring
  electronic fetal monitoring
    (EFM)
  electrophysiologic monitoring
  epicardial monitoring
  esophageal pH monitoring
  evoked external urethral
    sphincter potential
    monitoring
  external fetal monitoring
  fetal heart rate monitoring
  hemodynamic monitoring
  hospital monitoring
  intracranial pressure
    monitoring
  intraoperative
    neurophysiologic
    monitoring (IOM)
  intraoperative parathyroid
    hormone monitoring
  intraoperative transcranial
    Doppler monitoring
  invasive hemodynamic
    monitoring
  laboratory monitoring
  neuromuscular blockade
    monitoring
  outcome monitoring
  post-tetanic count monitoring
  pressure monitoring
  radiation monitoring
  screw position perioperative
    monitoring
  standard patient monitoring
  telemetric monitoring

monitoring (*continued*)
  tissue pH monitoring
  transcutaneous oxygen
    monitoring
  vigilance monitoring
  water vapor monitoring
monitoring cannula
monitoring lines
monitoring probe
monitoring technique
MoniTorr lumbar catheter
Moniz sign
Monk hip prosthesis
Monk orthopedic procedure
Monks malar elevator
Monks operation
Monks-Esser flap
Monks-Esser island flap
monangle chisel
monangled
monarticular
monobloc advancement
monobloc appliance
monobloc femoral component
monobloc tibial component
monochromatic aberration
monochromatic radiation
monoclonal adenoma
monoclonal antibody
monoclonal expansion
Monocorps milium knife
monocortical bone
monocortical screw
Monocryl poliglecaprone
    sutures
Monocryl sutures
monocular bandage
monocular dressing
monocular eye dressing
monocular fixation
monocular patch
monocular rotations
monocular vision
monocuspid tilting disk heart
    valve
monocyte
monocytoid cell
monofascicular nerve
monofilament
monofilament absorbable
    sutures
monofilament clear sutures

monofilament green sutures
monofilament nylon sutures
monofilament polypropylene
    sutures
monofilament skin sutures
monofilament snare wire
monofilament stainless steel
    wire
monofilament steel sutures
monofilament sutures
monofilament test
monofilament wire
monofilament wire sutures
Monofixateur external fixator
monofixation syndrome
Monoflex lens
monofoil catheter
Monogram total knee
    instrument
Monoject bone marrow
    aspirator
Monoject laceration irrigation
    tray
Monoject sphygmomanometer
Monoject suction tube
Monojector fingerstick device
Monoka canalicular stent
Monoka tube
MonoLith single-piece
    mechanical lithotriptor
Monolyth oxygenator
monomalleolar ankle fracture
monomanual delivery
monomaxillary
monomer filter
monomer suction biopsy tube
monomorphic adenoma
monomorphic pattern
mononuclear cell infiltration
monocular indirect
    ophthalmoscope
monoplegia masticatoria
monopodal ankylotic stapes
monopolar cautery
monopolar coagulating forceps
monopolar coagulation
monopolar connection cord
monopolar electrocautery
monopolar electrocoagulation
monopolar insulated forceps
monopolar temporary electrode
monopolar tissue forceps

Monopty needle
Monorail angioplasty catheter
Monorail catheter
Monorail guidewire
Monorail imaging catheter
Monorail Piccolino catheter
Monorail Speedy balloon
monorail technique
Monoscopy locking trocar
Monosof sutures
monospherical total shoulder
    arthroplasty
monostotic fibrous dysplasia
monostotic lesion
monostructure implant
monostrut
monostrut Bjork-Shiley valve
monostrut cardiac valve
    prosthesis
monostrut heart valve
monostrut valve
monosynaptic reflex
monotypic lesion
Monro abscess
Monro bursa
Monro foramen
Monro line
Monro sulcus
Monro-Richter line
mons pubis
Monson curve
monster rongeur
montage
    circumferential bipolar
        montage
    coronal bipolar montage
    transverse bipolar montage
    triangular bipolar montage
Montague abrader
Montague lane
Montague plane
Montague proctoscope
Montague sigmoidoscope
Montefiore tracheal tube
Montefiore tube
Monteggia dislocation
Monteggia equivalent lesion
Monteggia forearm fracture
Monteggia fracture
Monteggia fracture-dislocation
Montenovesi cranial forceps
Montenovesi cranial rongeur

Montenovesi cranial rongeur forceps
Montenovesi rongeur
Montercaux ankle fracture
Montercaux fracture
Montevideo units (uterine contractions)
Montgomery esophageal tube
Montgomery glands
Montgomery laryngeal keel
Montgomery laryngeal stent
Montgomery salivary bypass tube
Montgomery speaking valve
Montgomery speculum
Montgomery Stomeasure device
Montgomery strap dressing
Montgomery straps
Montgomery tape
Montgomery thyroplasty implant
Montgomery T-piece tube
Montgomery tracheal cannula
Montgomery tracheal tube
Montgomery T-tube
Montgomery tubercles
Montgomery vaginal speculum
Montgomery-Bernstine speculum
Monticelli-Spinelli distraction technique
Monticelli-Spinelli distractor
Monticelli-Spinelli frame
Montreal positioner
Montrose dressing applicator
Moody fixation forceps
Moolgaoker forceps
Moon boot
Moon boot brace
Moon rectal retractor
Moon-Robinson prosthesis inserter
Moon-Robinson stapes prosthesis
moon-shaped face
moon-shaped facies
Moor monitor
Moore adjustable nail
Moore approach
Moore blade plate
Moore bone drill
Moore bone elevator

Moore bone reamer
Moore bone retractor
Moore button
Moore chisel
Moore direction finder
Moore disk
Moore drill
Moore driver
Moore elevator
Moore extractor
Moore femoral neck prosthesis
Moore fixation pin
Moore forceps
Moore fracture
Moore gallbladder spoon
Moore gallstone scoop
Moore gouge
Moore head-tilt maneuver
Moore hip prosthesis
Moore hip-locking prosthesis
Moore hollow chisel
Moore hooked extractor
Moore humeral head procedure
Moore lens-inserting forceps
Moore mandrel
Moore measuring rod
Moore nail
Moore nail extractor
Moore nail set
Moore operation
Moore osteotome
Moore osteotomy
Moore pin
Moore plate
Moore posterior approach
Moore prosthesis
Moore prosthesis extractor
Moore prosthesis mortising chisel
Moore prosthesis rasp
Moore rasp
Moore raspatory
Moore reamer
Moore retractor
Moore rod
Moore scoop
Moore self-locking prosthesis
Moore shoulder procedure
Moore sliding nail plate
Moore spinal fusion gouge
Moore spoon
Moore stem rasp

Moore technique
Moore template
Moore thoracoscope
Moore tibial plateau fracture
    classification
Moore tracheostomy buttons
Moore tube
Moore-Blount driver
Moore-Blount extractor
Moore-Blount plate
Moore-Blount screwdriver
Moore-Corradi operation
Moorehead cheek retractor
Moorehead clamp
Moorehead dental retractor
Moorehead dissector
Moorehead ear knife
Moorehead elevator
Moorehead knife
Moorehead periosteotome
Moorehead pressure anesthesia
    unit
Moorehead retractor
Moorehead suction anesthesia
Mooren ulcer
Moore-Troutman corneal
    scissors
Moorfields curet
Moorfields cystotome
mooring fibers
mop-end tear
Morand foot
Moran-Karaya disk
Moran-Karaya ring
Morax keratoplasty
Morax operation
morbid obesity
morbidity
morbidly obese
morbilliform basal cell
    carcinoma
morcel
morcellation operation
morcellation technique
morcellator
    Cook tissue morcellator
    Diva laparoscopic morcellator
    electric tissue morcellator
    electromechanical morcellator
    Elmore tissue morcellator
    high-speed electrical tissue
        morcellator

morcellator (*continued*)
    motorized morcellator
    OPERA Star morcellator
    rotating morcellator
    Semm morcellator
    Steiner electromechanical
        morcellator
    tissue morcellator
morcellement nephrectomy
morcellement operation
morcellization
morcellized bone graft
morcellizer
    Rubin septal morcellizer
    Tessier rib morcellizer
    Yarmo morcellizer
Morch respirator
Morch swivel adapter
Morch swivel tracheostomy tube
Morch tracheostomy tube
Morch tube
Morch ventilator
Morel ear
Moreland-Marder-Anspach
    femoral stem removal
Morel-Fatio blepharoplasty
Morel-Fatio-Lalardie operation
Morel-Lavele lesion
Moren-Moretz vena caval clip
Moreno clamp
Moreno gastroenterostomy
    clamp
Morestin operation
Moretsky LASIK hinge protector
    fixation ring
Moretz clip
Moretz prosthesis
Moretz Tab ventilation tube
Moretz Tytan ventilation tube
Morgagni appendix
Morgagni cartilage
Morgagni column
Morgagni concha
Morgagni foramen
Morgagni fossa
Morgagni hernia
Morgagni nodules
Morgagni sphere
Morgagni ventricle
morgagnian cataract
morgagnian cyst
Morgagni-Larrey type hernia

Morgan fold
Morgan lens
Morgan line
Morgan mandrel
Morgan pelvic support
Morgan proctoscope
Morgan therapeutic lens
Morgan vent tube introducer
Morgan-Boehm proctoscope
Morgan-Casscells meniscus
    suturing technique
Morganstern continuous-flow
    operating cystoscope
Morgenstein blunt forceps
Morgenstein gouge
Morgenstein hook
Morgenstein periosteal knife
Morgenstein spatula
Morgenstein-Kerrison rongeur
Mori knife
Moria 1-piece speculum
Moria obturator
Moria trephine
Moria-France
    dacryocystorhinostomy
    clamp
moribund
Morinaga hemorrhoidectomy
Morison incision
Morison pouch
Moritz-Schmidt forceps
Moritz-Schmidt knife
Moritz-Schmidt laryngeal forceps
Morland scanner
Morley peritoneocutaneous
    reflex
morning glory optic disk
    anomaly
Moro reflex
morpheaform basal cell
    carcinoma
morphea-like lesion
morphine anesthetic
    agent
morphine narcotic analgesic
    therapy
morphofunctional vulvar
    reconstruction
morphogenic stage
morphologic classification
morphologic feature
morphological sex

morphology
    Antoni classification of
        schwannoma morphology
    craniofacial morphology
    lesion morphology
morphotype
Morquio sign
Morquio syndrome
Morrell crown remover
Morrey total elbow arthroplasty
Morrey-Bryan total elbow
    arthroplasty
Morris aortic clamp
Morris biphase screw
Morris cannula
Morris catheter
Morris defibrillator
Morris drain
Morris forceps
Morris hepatoma cell line
Morris incision
Morris mitral valve spreader
Morris retractor
Morris Silastic thoracic drain
Morris splint
Morris taper
Morris thoracic catheter
Morrison neurovascular free flap
Morrison skin hook
Morrison technique
Morrison toe flap
Morrison-Hurd dissector
Morrison-Hurd pillar retractor
Morrison-Hurd retractor
Morrison-Hurd tonsillar
    dissector
Morrissey Gigli-saw guide
Morrow-Brown needle
morsal teeth
Morscher anterior cervical plate
Morscher titanium cervical plate
Morse aortic scissors
Morse backward-cutting aortic
    scissors
Morse blade
Morse head
Morse instrument handle
Morse manifold
Morse modified Finochietto
    retractor
Morse retractor
Morse scissors

Morse sternal retractor
Morse sternal spreader
Morse suction tube
Morse tape lock of modular hip
    implant component
Morse taper
Morse taper stem
Morse towel clip
Morse valve
Morse valve retractor
Morse-Andrews suction tube
Morse-Ferguson suction tube
morselized cartilage
morselizer
    Rubin septal morselizer
Morson forceps
Morson trocar
mortality rate
mortar kidney
Mortara 12-lead monitor
mortise
    ankle mortise
    tibiofibular mortise
mortise of joint
mortise x-ray view
mortising chisel
Morton bandage
Morton dislodger
Morton foot
Morton neuroma
Morton ophthalmoscope
Morton plane
Morton stone dislodger
Morton toe
Morton toe support
Mortson V-shaped clip
Morwel cannula
Morwel ultrasound device
Morwel ultrasound-assisted
    lipoplasty machine
mosaic development
mosaic duodenal mucosal
    pattern
mosaicism
    chromosomal mosaicism
mosaicism of cervix
Moschcowitz enterocele repair
Moschcowitz hernia repair
Moschcowitz operation
Moschcowitz procedure
Mose concentric ring
Mose technique

Moseley fasciatome
Moseley glenoid rim prosthesis
Mosher bag
Mosher cardiospasm dilator
Mosher curet
Mosher dilator
Mosher drain
Mosher esophagoscope
Mosher esophagoscope tube
Mosher ethmoid curet
Mosher ethmoid punch
Mosher ethmoid punch forceps
Mosher forceps
Mosher intubation tube
Mosher lifesaver antichoke
        suction device
Mosher lifesaver retractor
Mosher lifesaver tube
Mosher lifesaving tracheal
        suction tube
Mosher lifesaving tube
Mosher nasal speculum
Mosher operation
Mosher punch
Mosher retractor
Mosher speculum
Mosher suction tube
Mosher tube
Mosher urethral speculum
Mosher-Toti operation
Moskowitz procedure
Mosley anterior shoulder repair
Mosley shoulder repair
Mosley stone crusher
mosque-shaped opening
mosquito clamp
mosquito forceps
mosquito hemostat
mosquito hemostatic clamp
mosquito hemostatic forceps
mosquito lid clamp
Moss balloon triple-lumen
        gastrostomy tube
Moss cage
Moss classification
Moss decompression feeding
    catheter
Moss feeding tube
Moss gastric decompression
    tube
Moss gastrostomy tube
Moss G-tube PEG

Moss hook
Moss instrumentation
Moss Mark IV gastrostomy tube
Moss Mark IV nasal tube
Moss Mark IV tube
Moss nasal tube
Moss operation
Moss rod
Moss Suction Buster catheter
Moss Suction Buster tube
Moss T-anchor needle
Moss T-anchor needle introducer
Moss T-anchor needle introducer
  gun
Moss tube
Moss-Harms basket
Moss-Miami spinal
  instrumentation
Motais operation
Moteno shunt tube
moth-eaten bone destruction
mother cell
mother cyst
Mother Jones dressing
mother yaw
mother-baby endoscope
mother-daughter endoscope
mother-to-infant transmission
motile organism
motilin effect
motility
  esophageal motility
motility eye implant
motion
  abdominal respiratory motion
  active range of motion
    (AROM)
  active-assistive range of
    motion
  back-and-forth motion
  brownian motion
  cartwheel motion
  ciliary motion
  cogwheel motion
  extraocular motion (EOM)
  eye motion
  finger motion
  full range of motion
  functional range of motion
  gentle rocking motion
  gliding motion
  helical axis of motion

motion (*continued*)
  JACE continuous passive
    motion (CPM) wrist device
  joint motion
  knee motion
  leg motion
  limitation of motion (LOM)
  limited joint motion
  limited range of motion
  lunotriquetral motion
  mandibular range of motion
  maximal static response assay
    of facial motion
  peristaltic motion
  range of motion (ROM)
  rocking motion
  rolling motion
  rotatory motion
  scapholunate motion
  scapulothoracic motion
  short arc motion (SAM)
    protocol
  subtalar motion
motion barrier
motion-preserving procedure
motokinesthetics
motor activity
motor and sensory function
motor aphasia
motor area
motor axon
motor center
motor control test
motor coordination test
  (MCT)
motor decussation
motor defect
motor development
motor disorder
motor endplate
motor examination
motor fibers
motor function
motor fusion
motor impairment
motor nerve
motor nerve action potential
  (MAP)
motor nerve of tongue
motor neuron
motor oil peritoneal fluid
motor point block

motor point block anesthetic technique

motor power and coordination

motor reflexes

motor root of trigeminal nerve

motor roots of submandibular ganglion

motor skills

motorized cannula

motorized morcellator

Mott body

Mott double-ended retractor

Mott raspatory

Mott retractor

mottled appearance

mottled area

mottled calcification

mottled in appearance

mottling of extremities

Mouchet fracture

mould (*variant of* mold)

Mould arthroplasty

Moult curet

Moult mouth prop

Moulton lacrimal duct tube

Mouly reduction mammaplasty

Mount forceps

Mount intervertebral disk forceps

Mount intervertebral disk rongeur forceps

Mount laminectomy rongeur

Mount-Mayfield aneurysm forceps

Mount-Mayfield forceps

Mount-Olivecrona clip applier

Mount-Olivecrona forceps

Mouradian humeral rod

Moure esophagoscope

Moure-Coryllos rib shears

mouse-tooth clamp

mouse-tooth forceps

Mousseau-Barbin esophageal tube

Mousseau-Barbin prosthetic tube

moustache (*spelled also* mustache)

moustache dressing

moustache-like flap

mouth

   angle of mouth

   by mouth (per os, p.o., po, PO)

   commissure of lips of mouth

   dentulous sore mouth

mouth (*continued*)

   denture sore mouth

   depressor muscle of angle of mouth

   diaphragm of mouth

   dry mouth

   floor of mouth (FOM)

   glands of mouth

   levator muscle of angle of mouth

   lip of mouth

   lymphatic vessels of mouth

   numerary mouth

   orbicular muscle of mouth

   orbicularis muscle of mouth

   orifice of the mouth

   phlegmon of floor of mouth

   putrid sore mouth

   roof of mouth

   trench mouth

   vestibule of mouth

   white mouth

mouth breathing

mouth flora

mouthgag (*see* gag)

   Boettcher-Jennings mouthgag

   Boyle-Davis mouthgag

   Brophy mouthgag

   Brown-Davis mouthgag

   Brown-Fillebrown-Whitehead mouthgag

   Brown-Whitehead mouthgag

   Collis mouthgag

   Crowe-Davis mouthgag

   Dann-Jennings mouthgag

   Davis mouthgag

   Davis ring mouthgag

   Davis-Crowe mouthgag

   Denhardt-Dingman moughgag

   Dilner-Doughty mouthgag

   Dingman mouthgag

   Dingman-Denhardt mouthgag

   Dingman-Millard mouthgag

   Dott mouthgag

   Dott-Kilner mouthgag

   Doyen mouthgag

   Doyen-Jansen mouthgag

   Ferguson mouthgag

   Ferguson-Ackland mouthgag

   Ferguson-Brophy mouthgag

   Ferguson-Gwathmey mouthgag

mouthgag (*continued*)
  Frohm mouthgag
  Fulton mouthgag
  Green mouthgag
  Green-Sewall mouthgag
  Hayton-Williams mouthgag
  Heister mouthgag
  Hibbs mouthgag
  Jansen mouthgag
  Jansen-Sluder mouthgag
  Jennings Loktite mouthgag
  Jennings mouthgag
  Jennings-Skillern mouthgag
  Kilner mouthgag
  Kilner-Dott mouthgag
  Kilner-Doughty mouthgag
  Lane mouthgag
  Lange mouthgag
  Leivers mouthgag
  Lewis mouthgag
  Maunder oral screw
    mouthgag
  McDowell mouthgag
  McIvor mouthgag
  McKesson mouthgag
  Millard mouthgag
  Mithoefer-Jansen mouthgag
  Molt mouthgag
  mouthgag
  Negus mouthgag
  Newkirk mouthgag
  oral screw mouthgag
  oral speculum mouthgag
  palate-type mouthgag
  Proetz mouthgag
  Proetz-Jansen mouthgag
  Pynchon mouthgag
  Rabbit mouthgag
  Ralks-Davis mouthgag
  Rew-Wyly mouthgag
  Roser mouthgag
  Roser-Koenig mouthgag
  Seeman-Seiffert mouthgag
  side mouthgag
  Sluder mouthgag
  Sluder-Ferguson mouthgag
  Sluder-Jansen mouthgag
  Sydenham mouthgag
  Thackray mouthgag
  Trousseau mouthgag
  Wesson mouthgag
  Whitehead mouthgag

mouthgag (*continued*)
  Whitehead-Jennings
    mouthgag
  Wolf Loktite mouthgag
  Wolf mouthgag
mouthgag tooth plate
mouthguard
mouth hygiene
mouth lamp
mouth mask
mouth mirror
mouth preparation
mouth prop
mouth rehabilitation
mouth stick
mouthgag frame
mouthgag tongue depressor
  blade
mouth-to-mouth resuscitation
mouth-to-mouth ventilation
movability
movable
movable joint
movable kidney
movable-arm clasp
move normally
moved and positioned
movement
  ballistic movement
  Bennett movement
  bodily movement
  border tissue movement
  brownian movement
  choreiform movements
  compensatory movement
  conjugate eye movement
  conjugate movement
  contralateral movement
  coordinate muscle
    movement
  cutting movement
  dentogenic movement
  distal movement
  downward movement
  dystonic movement
  empty movement
  eruptive tooth movement
  extraneous movement
  extraocular movement
    (EOM)
  eye movement
  eyeball movement

movement (*continued*)

Facial Grading System
voluntary movement
(FGSM)
fetal movement
forced movement
forward movement
free mandibular movement
functional mandibular
movement
gliding movement
grinding movement
hinge movement
hinge-axis movement
hypoactive movements
incessant movements
incremental movement
intermediary movement
involuntary movement
inward movement
jaw movement
jerking eye movements
jerky movements
joint movement
labial movement
lateral movement
laterotrusive movement
limited joint movement
lingual movement
lip movements
mandibular gliding movement
masticatory mandibular
movement
masticatory movements
maximum movement
nonfunction mandibular
movement
opening mandibular
movement
oral commissure movement
outward movement
passive joint movement
pendular movement
pendulum movement
peristaltic movement
pistoning movement
posterior border movement
protrusive movement
random movement
rapid alternating movements
rapid eye movements (REM)
retrusive movement

movement (*continued*)

rolling movement
rotational movement
sagittal mandibular movement
skilled movements
smooth-pursuit eye
movement
sudden movement
tipping movement
translatory movement
trunk movement
upward movement
volition oral movement
voluntary movement
movement disorder
moving strip x-ray technique
moxibustion
Moynihan bile duct probe
Moynihan clamp
Moynihan clip
Moynihan forceps
Moynihan gall duct forceps
Moynihan gallstone probe
Moynihan gallstone scoop
Moynihan gastrojejunostomy
Moynihan incision
Moynihan intestinal forceps
Moynihan intestinal operation
Moynihan kidney pedicle
forceps
Moynihan operation
Moynihan position
Moynihan probe
Moynihan respirator
Moynihan scoop
Moynihan speculum
Moynihan towel clamp
Moynihan towel forceps
Moynihan-Navratil forceps
Moynihan-Navratil speculum
Mozart ear
MP (metacarpophalangeal)
MP (metatarsophalangeal)
MP joint arthroplasty
MPA1 catheter
MPA2 catheter
M-Pact cast cutter
M-Pact cast spreader
M-Pact flexible orthotic
MPAPC (mucus-producing
adenopapillary
carcinoma)

MPC automated intravitreal
  scissors
MPC coagulation forceps
MPC scissors
MPD (main pancreatic duct,
  maximum permissible dose,
  myofascial pain-
  dysfunction)
MPD stent
MPD syndrome
MPF catheter
MPH (mandibular plane to
  hyoid)
MPL aspirating syringe
MPL dental needle
MPL intraosseous needle
M-plasty
M-plasty excision
M-plasty technique
MPM bandage
MPM conductive hydrogel
  dressing
MPM GelPad dressing
MPM hydrogel dressing
MPM multilayer dressing
MPO (maximum power output)
Mport lens inserter
MPR drain catheter
MP-RAGE technique
MPS (mucopolysaccharidosis,
  myofascial pain syndrome)
MRA (magnetic resonance
  angiography)
MRG (mean rejection grading,
  mean residual gap)
MRI (magnetic resonance
  imaging)
  intraoperative MRI
  spin-echo MRI
  surface-coil MRI
MRI cholangiography
MRI probe head
MRI scan
MRKHS (Mayer-Rokitansky-
  Küster-Hauser syndrome)
MRL blood pressure monitor
MRL oximeter
MRM-2 oxygen consumption
  monitor
MS (melanonychia striata)
MS Classique balloon dilatation
  catheter

MSBP (mandibular staple bone
  plate)
msec (milliseconds)
M-series bur (M-1, M-2, etc.)
MSI (magnetic source imaging)
MSRs (muscles, strength,
  reflexes)
MST (maximum stimulation
  test)
MST cryoprobe
Mt. Clemens Hospital clip
  applier
Mt. Sinai skull clamp pin
MTA brace
MTA headlamp
MTBE (methyl tert-butyl ether)
MTBE therapy
MTC Ventcontrol ventricular
  catheter
MTP (metatarsophalangeal)
MTS electrohydraulic piston
M-type extractor
Mubarak-Hargens
  decompression technique
Mucat cervical sampling device
mucilaginous gland
mucin clot test
mucinase
mucinosis
  cutaneous focal mucinosis
  oral focal mucinosis
mucinous adenocarcinoma
mucinous adenoma
mucinous carcinoma
mucinous cell adenocarcinoma
mucinous cyst
mucinous plaque
mucinous tumor
muciparous gland
Muck forceps
Muck tonsillar forceps
Muck tonsillar hemostat
mucobuccal fold
mucobuccal reflection
mucocele
  frontal sinus mucocele
  maxillary sinus mucocele
  retention mucocele
  sinus mucocele
mucochondrocutaneous flap
mucociliary blanket
mucociliary drainage pathway

mucociliary flow
mucociliary transport (MC)
mucoclasis
mucocutaneous border
mucocutaneous candidiasis
mucocutaneous hemorrhoid
mucocutaneous junction
mucocutaneous leishmaniasis
mucocutaneous lesion
mucocutaneous lymph node
    syndrome
mucocutaneous melanosis
mucocutaneous pigmentation of
    Peutz-Jeghers syndrome
mucocutaneous wart
mucoepidermal carcinoma
mucoepidermoid carcinoma
    (MEC)
mucoepidermoid carcinoma of
    parotid
mucoepidermoid carcinoma of
    the tongue
mucoepidermoid lesion
mucoepidermoid tumor
mucogingival junction
mucogingival line
mucogingival surgery
mucoid discharge
mucoid impaction
mucoid material
mucoid otitis media
mucoid secretion
mucolabial fold
mucolytic
mucoparous gland
mucoperichondrial elevation
mucoperichondrial flap
mucoperichondrial sleeves
mucoperichondrium
mucoperiosteal elevator
mucoperiosteal flap
mucoperiosteal flap operation
mucoperiosteal flap technique
mucoperiosteal flap trimming
mucoperiosteal implant
    placement
mucoperiosteal lining
mucoperiosteal periodontal flap
mucoperiosteal periodontal
    graft
mucoperiosteal pushback
    palatoplasty

mucoperiosteal sliding flap
mucoperiosteum
mucopolysaccharidosis (MPS)
    (*pl.* mucopolysac-
    charidoses)
mucopurulent discharge
mucopurulent exudate
mucopurulent hemorrhagic
    effusion
mucopyelocele
mucopyocele
mucormycosis
    rhinocerebral mucormycosis
    rhino-orbital mucormycosis
    rhino-orbitocerebral
      mucormycosis
mucorrhea
mucosa
    alveolar mucosa
    alveolar ridge mucosa
    antral mucosa
    beefy red mucosa
    bladder mucosa
    buccal mucosa
    burned out mucosa
    cardiac mucosa
    cobblestone mucosa
    cobblestoning of mucosa
    colorectal mucosa
    columnar mucosa
    conchal mucosa
    dorsal lingual mucosa
    duodenal mucosa
    ectopic gastric mucosa
    effacement of mucosa
    endocervical mucosa
    esophageal mucosa
    ethmoidal mucosa
    foveolar gastric mucosa
    free graft from urinary
      bladder mucosa
    friable mucosa
    fundic mucosa
    gastric mucosa
    gastroduodenal mucosa
    gastrointestinal mucosa
    gingival mucosa
    hypermobile mucosa
    hyperplastic mucosa
    intestinal mucosa
    jejunal mucosa
    laryngeal mucosa

mucosa (*continued*)
 ligamental mucosa
 lingual mucosa
 lining mucosa
 mandibular alveolar mucosa
 masticatory mucosa
 nasal mucosa
 normal-appearing mucosa
 oral mucosa
 palatal mucosa
 palatine mucosa
 passed per mucosa
 per mucosa
 pyloric mucosa
 quilting of septal mucosa
 rectal mucosa
 reflecting mucosa
 respiratory mucosa
 retromolar mucosa
 retrotuberosity mucosa
 retrotuberous mucosa
 septal mucosa
 specialized mucosa
 sublingual mucosa
 sulcular gastric mucosa
 swollen mucosa
 tear of mucosa
 throat mucosa
 tracheal mucosa
 vaginal mucosa
 vestibular mucosa
 vomer mucosa
mucosa elevator
mucosa knife
mucosa speculum
mucosa-associated lymphoid
  tissue lymphoma
mucosal ablation
mucosal abnormality
mucosal advancement
mucosal barrier
mucosal biopsy
mucosal blood vessel
mucosal coat
mucosal collar
mucosal cuff
mucosal cyst
mucosal destruction
mucosal excision
mucosal folds
mucosal graft
mucosal grafting

mucosal guideline pattern
mucosal hernia
mucosal horn
mucosal implant
mucosal inflammation
mucosal insert
mucosal invasion
mucosal island
mucosal lesion
mucosal line
mucosal needle aspiration
mucosal neuroma syndrome
mucosal patch replacement
mucosal pattern
mucosal periodontal flap
mucosal periodontal graft
mucosal prelaminated flap
mucosal proctectomy and
  ileoanal pull-through
mucosal relaxing incision
  technique
mucosal rent
mucosal separator plate
mucosal sleeve resection
mucosal suspensory ligament
mucosal tear
mucosal transudate
mucosal vascular dilation
mucosalize
mucosa-to-mucosa anastomosis
mucosa-to-mucosa closure
mucosa-to-mucosa Roux-en-Y
  hepaticojejunostomy
mucosectomy
mucoserous cells
mucoserous otitis media
mucosis otitis
mucositis
 radiation mucositis
 xerostomic mucositis
mucosobuccal fold
mucostatic
mucotome
 Castroviejo-Steinhauser
  mucotome
 Norelco mucotome
mucous (*adjective*)
mucous alveolus
mucous blanket
mucous cell
mucous cyst
mucous desiccation

mucous discharge
mucous fistula
mucous fluid
mucous forceps
mucous glands
mucous lake of stomach
mucous membrane graft
mucous membrane lesion
mucous membrane of lip
mucous membrane of tongue
mucous membranes
mucous otitis
mucous patch
mucous plaque
mucous plug
mucous plug syndrome
mucous polyp
mucous retention cyst
mucous retention phenomenon
mucous stool
mucous thread
mucous tissue
mucous tubule
mucoviscidosis
mucus
  glairy mucus
  nasal mucus
  olfactory mucus
  salivary mucus
  uterine mucus
mucus (*noun*)
mucus forceps
mucus knife
mucus-producing
    adenopapillary carcinoma
    (MPAPC)
mucus-secreting cell
mucus-secreting gland
Muehrcke band
Muehrcke line
Mueller (*also* Müller)
Mueller alkaline battery cautery
Mueller aortic clamp
Mueller bronchial clamp
Mueller bur
Mueller catheter
Mueller catheter guide
Mueller cautery
Mueller cesarean section
Mueller clamp
Mueller coronary perfusion
    cannula

Mueller curet
Mueller Currentrol cautery
Mueller duct
Mueller duct body
Mueller Duo-Lock hip prosthesis
Mueller electric corneal
    trephine
Mueller electric trephine
Mueller electrocautery
Mueller electronic tonometer
Mueller eye shield
Mueller eye speculum
Mueller femoral supracondylar
    fracture classification
Mueller fibers
Mueller fixation device
Mueller forceps
Mueller giant eye magnet
Mueller hip arthroplasty
Mueller hip plate
Mueller hip prosthesis
Mueller lacrimal sac retractor
Mueller laparoscopic
    instrumentation
Mueller maneuver
Mueller micrograin prosthesis
Mueller muscle
Mueller needle
Mueller operation
Mueller osteotomy
Mueller patellar tendon graft
Mueller pediatric clamp
Mueller prosthesis
Mueller refractor
Mueller retractor
Mueller round Gigli saw
Mueller saw
Mueller scissors
Mueller sclerectomy
Mueller shield
Mueller shield eye implant
Mueller sign
Mueller speculum
Mueller suction tube
Mueller technique
Mueller telescope
Mueller test
Mueller tibial fracture
    classification
Mueller tongue blade
Mueller tonometer
Mueller total hip

Mueller total hip prosthesis
Mueller tray
Mueller trephine
Mueller Ultralite brace
Mueller vaginal hysterectomy
Mueller vena cava clamp
Mueller vena caval clamp
Mueller-Balfour retractor
Mueller-Balfour self-retaining
   retractor
Mueller-Charnley hip prosthesis
Mueller-Charnley total hip
   prosthesis
Mueller-Dammann pulmonary
   artery banding
Mueller-Frazier suction tube
Mueller-Frazier tube
Mueller-Hillis maneuver
Mueller-Hinton supplemented
   agar plate
Mueller-LaForce adenotome
Mueller-Markham patent ductus
   forceps
Mueller-Poole suction tube
Mueller-Poole tube
Mueller-Pynchon suction tube
Mueller-Pynchon tube
Mueller-type acetabular cup
Mueller-type femoral head
   replacement
Mueller-Yankauer suction tube
Mueller-Yankauer tube
Muenster cast
Muer anoscope
Muer proctoscope
MUGA (multiple gated
   acquisition)
MUGA cardiac blood pool scan
MUGA scan
MUGA test
Muhlberger implant
Muhlberger orbital implant
Muhlberger orbital implant
   prosthesis
Muhlberger orbital prosthesis
Muhlmann appliance
Mui Scientific 6-channel
   esophageal pressure probe
Muir cautery clamp
Muir hemorrhoidal forceps
Muir rectal cautery clamp
Muir rectal speculum

Muirhead pelvic rest
Muirhead-Little pelvic rest
   tractor
mulberry calculus
mulberry cell
mulberry fat
mulberry gallstone
mulberry lesion
mulberry spot
Mulder angle
Mulder sign
Muldoon dilator
Muldoon lacrimal dilator
Muldoon lacrimal probe
Muldoon lid retractor
Muldoon meibomian forceps
Muldoon retractor
Muldoon tube
mules
   Bishop-Harman mules
   Colibri mules
   Gill-Hess mules
   Graefe mules
   Halsted mules
   Heath mules
   Kulvin-Kalt mules
   Lister mules
   MacGregor mules
   Paton-Berens mules
Mules eye implant
Mules graft
Mules implant
Mules operation
Mules prosthesis
Mules scoop
Mules sphere eye implant
Mules sphere implant
mule-spinner's cancer
Mulholland sphincterotomy
Mullan percutaneous trigeminal
   ganglion microcompression
   set
Mullan trigeminal ganglion
   microcompression set
Mullan wire
Müller (see Mueller)
mullerian dimple
mullerian duct
mullerian duct anomaly
mullerian duct aplasia
mullerian duct derivation
   syndrome

mullerian duct fusion
mullerian tumor
Mulligan anastomosis clamp
Mulligan cervical biopsy
    punch
Mulligan dissector
Mulligan prosthesis
Mulligan Silastic prosthesis
Mullins blade
Mullins blade and balloon
    septostomy
Mullins blade technique
Mullins cardiac device
Mullins catheter introducer
Mullins decompressor
Mullins modification
Mullins sheath
Mullins transseptal atrial
    septostomy
Mullins transseptal catheter
Mullins transseptal
    catheterization sheath
Mullins transseptal introducer
Mullins transseptal sheath
multangular bone
multangular ridge fracture
multangulum majus
MultAport cannula
Multi Dopplex II Doppler
multi-access catheter
multiaxial classification
multiaxial joint
multiaxial screw
multiaxis foot
Multibite biopsy forceps
Multibite multiple sample
    biopsy forceps
multicellular stent
multicentric glomus tumor
multichannel cochlear implant
Multiclip disposable ligating clip
    device
Multicor Gamma pacemaker
Multicor II cardiac pacemaker
Multicor II pacemaker
multicrystal gamma camera
multicuspid teeth
Multidex maltodextrin wound
    dressing
Multidex wound-filling material
multidirectional distractor
multielectrode basket catheter

multielectrode impedance
    catheter
multielectrode probe
multifidus muscle
multifilament steel sutures
multifilament sutures
multifilament wire
multifire clip applicator
Multifire Endo GIA stapler
Multifire Endo GIA stapling
    device
Multifire Endo hernia clip
    applier
Multifire GIA stapler
Multifire GIA-series stapler
Multifire TA-series stapler
Multifire VersaTack stapler
Multi-Fit Luer-Lok control
    tonsillar syringe
multiflanged Portnoy catheter
Multiflex catheter
Multiflex stent
multifocal atrial tachycardia
    (MAT)
multifocal contractions
multifocal enhancing lesion
multifocal heartbeats
multifocal inflammation
multifocal lymphocytic infiltrate
multifocal extensive disease
multiforme
    atypical erythema multiforme
    bullous erythema multiforme
    erythema multiforme
multigland disease
multigland hyperplasia
multiglandular disease
multiglandular parathyroid
    hyperplasia
multihit injury
multiholed tube
multilamellar body
multilaminar
MultiLase D copper vapor laser
MultiLase Nd:YAG surgical laser
multilayer design catheter
multi-layered graft
multilead electrode
multileaf collimator
multilesion angioplasty
multilevel atherosclerotic
    arterial occlusive disease

multilevel fracture
multilevel laminectomy
multilevel spinal fusion
Multi-Link Duet stent
Multi-Link Penta stent
Multi-Link Pixel stent
Multilink stent
Multi-Link Tetra coronary stent
Multilith pacemaker
Multiload Cu-375 intrauterine
    device
multiload occlusive clip
    applicator
multiloaded clip applier
multilobed placenta
multilobular cyst
multilocular cyst
multilocular cystic lesion
multilocular mass
multiloculated
multilumen catheter
multilumen manometric
    catheter
multilumen probe
Multi-Med triple-lumen catheter
Multi-Med triple-lumen infusion
    catheter
multimodal adjuvant therapy
multimodal analgesia
multimodality therapy
multinodular goiter
multinucleated dentinoblastic cell
multinucleated giant cell
multiorgan failure (MOF)
multiorgan hernia
multiorgan system dysfunction
multiorgan system failure
multipara
multiparity
multiparous female
multiplanar endoscopic facial
    rejuvenation technique
multiplanar image
multiplanar mandibular
    distractor
multiplanar reconstructions
multiplanar upper facial
    rejuvenation technique
multiplane intracavitary probe
multiple abutment
multiple abutment support
multiple amputation

multiple anchorage
multiple apertures
multiple benign sarcoma
multiple biopsies
multiple births
multiple clasp
multiple core biopsy
multiple endocrine neoplasia
multiple endocrine neoplasia
    syndrome (type 2a, 2b)
multiple exostoses of jaw
multiple fasciotomies
multiple foci
multiple foramina
multiple fractures
multiple fragmentations
multiple gated acquisition
    (MUGA)
multiple gland hyperplasia
multiple glomuvenous
    malformation (GVM)
multiple hamartoma syndrome
multiple hereditary hemorrhagic
    telangiectases
multiple hydatid disease
multiple idiopathic hemorrhagic
    sarcoma
multiple jointed digitizer
    scanner
multiple line scan imaging
multiple loop archwire
multiple loop wiring
multiple mechanism inhaled
    anesthetic
multiple metastases
multiple mucosal neuroma
    syndrome
multiple myeloma
multiple organ dysfunction
    (MOD)
multiple organ dysfunction
    syndrome (MODS)
multiple organ failure (MOF)
multiple organ failure syndrome
multiple organ system failure
multiple papillomatosis
multiple resectoscope
multiple site inhaled anesthetic
multiple spin-echo imaging
multiple surgical excisions
multiple system organ failure
multiple tenotomies

multiple therapy
multiple trauma
multiple washings
multiple-action rongeur
multiple-echo imaging
multiple-lumen tube
multiple-piece intraocular lens
multiple-pin hole occluder
multiple-plane imaging
multiple-point electrode
multiple-point sacral fixation
multiple-port incision
multiple-port incision procedure
multiple-port incision technique
multiple-punch resection
multiple-stage approach
multiple-stage omphalocele
   repair
multiple-suture synostosis
multiplex catheter
Multi-Ply reusable electrode
multipoint contact plate
Multipoise headrest
multipolar bipolar cup
multipolar coagulation
multipolar electrocautery
multipolar electrocoagulation
multipolar electrode catheter
multipolar impedance catheter
MultiPro biopsy needle
multiprogrammable pacemaker
multiprogrammable pulse
   generator
multiprong rake retractor
Multipulse compression pump
multipurpose ball electrode
multipurpose catheter
multipurpose clamp
multipurpose forceps
multipurpose instruments
multipurpose laryngoscope
multipurpose retractor
multipurpose valve
multiray fracture
multirod collimator
multirooted abutment
multirooted tooth
multiscope
   roaming optical access
      multiscope (ROAM)
multisegmental resection
multisensor catheter

multiseptate gallbladder
multisided Z-plasty closure
multispan fracture hook
Multispatula cervical sampling
   device
multistaged carrier flap
multistaged reconstruction
Multistim electrode catheter
multistrand sutures
multisystem disorder
multisystem failure
multisystem organ failure
   (MSOF)
multisystem trauma
multitoothed cartilage forceps
MultiVac TriStar ArthroWand
MultiVac XL ArthroWand
multivacuolated
multivesicular body
multivisceral graft
multiwire camera
multiwire proportional chamber
Mumford arthroscopy
Mumford clavicle resection
Mumford Gigli-saw guide
Mumford operation
Mumford procedure
Mumford resection
Mumford-Gurd arthroplasty
Mumford-Neer procedure
mummified fetus
mummified pulp
mummylike wrap
Munchen endometrial biopsy
   curet
Mundie placenta forceps
Mundie placental forceps
Munich-Crosstreet anoscope
Munnell operation
Munro abscess
Munro-Parker laparoscopic
   hysterectomy classification
Munro brain scissors
Munro classification of orbital
   hypertelorism (types A-D)
Munro Kerr bladder flap
Munro Kerr cesarean section
Munro Kerr incision
Munro Kerr maneuver
Munro microabscess
Munro point
Munro retractor

Munro scissors
Munro self-retaining retractor
Munson sign
Munster cast
mural ameloblastoma
mural aneurysm
mural kidney
mural pregnancy
Murdock eye speculum
Murdock speculum
Murdock-Wiener eye speculum
Murdock-Wiener speculum
Muldoon eye speculum
murine graft
murine mesangial cell line
Murless fetal head extractor
Murless head extractor
Murless head extractor forceps
Murless head retractor
Murless vector head extractor
murmur
    aortic murmur
    aortic regurgitation murmur
    apical murmur
    Austin Flint murmur
    Bellows murmur
    cardiac murmur
    cardiopulmonary murmur
    cardiorespiratory murmur
    Carey-Coombs murmur
    crescendo murmur
    crescendo-decrescendo
      murmur
    decrescendo early systolic
      murmur
    decrescendo murmur
    diamond-shaped murmur
    diastolic murmur
    ejection murmur
    end-diastolic murmur
    endocardial murmur
    end-systolic murmur
    exit block murmur
    exocardial murmur
    faint diastolic murmur
    functional cardiac murmur
    Gibson murmur
    Graham Steell murmur
    harsh murmur
    heart murmur
    hemic murmur
    holosystolic murmur

murmur (*continued*)
    Hope murmur
    hourglass murmur
    incidental murmur
    innocent murmur
    inorganic murmur
    inspiratory murmur
    Levine gradation of cardiac
      murmurs (grades 1-6)
    loud systolic murmur
    mill-house murmur
    musical murmur
    organic murmur
    pericardial murmur
    pleuropericardial murmur
    prediastolic murmur
    presystolic murmur
    raucous murmur
    respiratory murmur
    rubs or murmurs
    seesaw murmur
    subclavicular murmur
    systolic murmur
    to-and-fro murmur
    Traube murmur
Murphy approach
Murphy ball reamer
Murphy ball-end hook
Murphy bone gouge
Murphy bone lever
Murphy bone skid
Murphy brace
Murphy button
Murphy chisel
Murphy common duct dilator
Murphy dilator
Murphy drip tube
Murphy endotracheal tube
Murphy forceps
Murphy gallbladder retractor
Murphy gouge
Murphy hook
Murphy intestinal needle
Murphy kidney punch
Murphy knife
Murphy light
Murphy needle
Murphy osteotome
Murphy percussion
Murphy plaster knife
Murphy punch
Murphy rake retractor

Murphy reamer
Murphy retractor
Murphy scissors
Murphy sign
Murphy splint
Murphy tonsillar forceps
Murphy treatment
Murphy tube
Murphy-Balfour center blade
Murphy-Balfour retractor
Murphy-Johnson anastomosis
    button
Murphy-Lane bone elevator
Murphy-Lane bone skid
Murphy-Lane lever
Murphy-Lane skid
Murphy-Pean hemostatic forceps
MurphyScope neurologic device
Murray forceps
Murray holder
Murray knee prosthesis
Murray operation
Murray-Jones arm splint
Murray-Thomas arm splint
Murtagh self-retaining infant
    scalp retractor
muscle
    3rd peroneal muscle
    abdominal external oblique
        muscle
    abdominal internal oblique
        muscle
    abductor hallucis muscle
    abductor muscle
    abductor pollicis longus
        muscle
    adductor longus muscle
    adductor magnus muscle
    adductor muscle
    advancement of muscle
    advancement of ocular
        muscle
    advancement of superior
        oblique muscle
    Aeby muscle
    agonistic muscle
    airway smooth muscle (ASM)
    alar muscle
    anconeus muscle
    ansa hypoglossus muscle
    antagonistic muscle
    anterior auricular muscle

muscle (*continued*)
    anterior scalene muscle
    anterior serratus muscle
    anterior superficialis muscle
    anterior tibial muscle
    antitragicus muscle
    antitragus muscle
    aponeurosis of external
        oblique muscle
    articular muscle
    aryepiglottic muscle
    arytenoid muscle
    auricular muscle
    belly of the muscle
    biceps muscle
    bipennate muscle
    Bochdalek muscle
    Bovero muscle
    Bowman ciliary muscle
    Bowman muscle
    brachial muscle
    brachialis muscle
    brachioradial muscle
    brachioradialis muscle
    Brücke muscle
    bronchoesophageal muscle
    buccal muscle
    buccinator muscle
    bulbocavernous muscle
    canine muscle
    capillary muscle
    cardiac muscle
    Casser muscle
    casserian muscle
    ceratocricoid muscle
    ceratopharyngeal muscle
    Chassaignac axillary muscle
    cheek muscle
    chest muscles
    chin muscle
    chondroglossus muscle
    chondropharyngeal muscle
    ciliary muscle
    circular fibers of ciliary
        muscle
    circular muscle
    coccygeal muscle
    congenerous muscles
    constrictor muscle
    contracting and relaxing of
        muscles
    contraction of muscles

muscle (*continued*)

contracture of interosseous muscles
coracobrachial muscle
corrugator muscle
corrugator supercilii muscle
Crampton muscle
cremaster muscle
cremasteric muscle
cricoarytenoid muscle
cricopharyngeal muscle
cricopharyngeus muscle
cricothyroid muscle
crushed muscle
cutaneous muscle
dartos muscle
deep flexor muscle
deep muscle
deltoid muscle
denervated muscle
depressor anguli oris muscle
depressor labii inferioris muscle
depressor labii oris muscle
depressor muscle
depressor septi muscle
diaphragmatic muscle
diastasis of muscle
digastric muscle
dilator naris muscle
dorsal interosseous muscles
dorsal muscle
dorsal sacrococcygeal muscle
drainage of muscle
epicranius muscle
epimeric muscle
epitrochleoanconeus muscle
erector muscle
eustachian muscle
extensor carpi radialis brevis muscle
extensor digiti minimi muscle
extensor digitorum longus muscle
extensor digitorum muscle
extensor hallucis longus muscle
extensor indicis muscle
extensor muscle
extensor pollicis brevis muscle
external anal sphincter muscle

muscle (*continued*)

external intercostal muscles
external oblique muscle
external obturator muscle
external pterygoid muscle
external rectus muscle
extracostal muscle
extralaryngeal muscle
extraocular muscles (EOM)
extrinsic muscle
facial mimetic muscle
facial muscle
fast twitch muscle
fast-twitch fatigable skeletal muscle
FDP muscle
FDS muscle
femoral muscle
fibular muscle
fixator muscles
flexor carpi ulnaris muscle
flexor digitorum brevis muscle
flexor digitorum longus muscle
flexor hallucis longus muscle
flexor muscle
Folius muscle
FPL muscle
free tissue transfer of muscle
frontal belly of the occipitofrontal muscle
frontalis muscle
fusiform muscle
Gantzer muscle
gastric sling muscle
gastrocnemius muscle
gastrosoleus muscle
Gavard muscle
gemellus muscle
genioglossus muscle
geniohyoglossus muscle
geniohyoid muscle
glossopalatine muscle
glossopharyngeal muscle
gluteal muscle
gracilis muscle
great adductor muscle
greater pectoral muscle
greater psoas muscle
greater rhomboid muscle
greater trochanter muscle

muscle (*continued*)

greater zygomatic muscle
greatest gluteal muscle
guarding of muscle
Guthrie muscle
hamstring muscle
heart muscle
herniation of muscle
Hilton muscle
Horner muscle
Houston muscle
hyoglossal muscle
hyoglossus muscle
hypaxial muscle
hyperactive glabellar muscle
hyperactive muscle
hypertonic muscle
hypomeric muscle
hypothenar muscles
hypotonic muscle
iliac muscle
iliococcygeal muscle
iliocostal muscle
iliocostalis dorsi muscle
iliocostalis lumborum muscle
iliopsoas muscle
incisive muscle
inferior constrictor
   pharyngeal muscle
inferior gemellus muscle
inferior oblique muscle
inferior posterior serratus
   muscle
inferior rectus muscle
inferior tarsal muscle
infrahyoid muscles
infrahyoid strap muscle
infraspinatus muscle
infraspinous muscle
innermost intercostal muscles
innervated muscles
inspiratory muscles
interarytenoid muscle
intercostal muscle
intercostalis externus muscle
intercostalis internus muscle
internal intercostal muscles
internal oblique muscle
internal obturator muscle
internal pterygoid muscle
internal thyroarytenoid muscle
interosseous muscle

muscle (*continued*)

interspinal muscles
intertransverse muscles
intra-auricular muscle
intraocular muscles
involuntary muscle
ipsilateral mentalis muscle
iridic muscles
ischiocavernous muscle
Jarjavay muscle
Jung muscle
Koyter muscle
Lancisi muscle
Landstrom muscle
Langer muscle
lateral cricoarytenoid muscle
lateral pterygoid muscle
lateral rectus muscle
latissimus dorsi muscle
left gluteal muscle
left rhomboid muscle
lesser zygomatic muscle
levator anguli oris muscle
levator ani muscle
levator costae muscle
levator glandulae thyroidea
   muscle
levator labii superioris
   alaeque nasi muscle
levator labii superioris muscle
levator muscle
levator palatini muscle
levator veli palatini muscle
long abductor muscle
long adductor muscle
long extensor muscle
long fibular muscle
long flexor muscle
long levator muscle
long muscle
long palmar muscle
long peroneal muscle
long radial extensor muscle
long rotator muscles
longissimus muscle
longitudinal muscle
longitudinalis inferior muscle
longitudinalis superior muscle
longus capitis muscle
longus colli muscle
lumbrical muscles
Luschka muscles

muscle (*continued*)
   malleolus muscle
   manipulation of muscle
   masseter muscle
   mastication muscle
   masticatory muscle
   medial muscle
   medial pterygoid muscle
   medial rectus muscle
   mental muscle
   mentalis muscle
   Merkel muscle
   mesothenar muscle
   middle constrictor pharyngeal
      muscle
   middle gluteal muscle
   middle scalene muscle
   mimetic muscle
   Mueller muscle
   multifidus muscle
   musculus transversus menti
      muscle
   mylohyoid muscle
   mylopharyngeal muscle
   nasal muscle
   nasalis muscle
   nasolabial muscle
   nonstriated muscle
   oblique arytenoid muscle
   oblique muscle
   obliquus abdominis externus
      muscle
   obliquus abdominis internus
      muscle
   obliquus inferior muscle
   obliquus superior muscle
   obturator muscle
   occipital belly of the
      occipitofrontal muscle
   occipital muscle
   occipitofrontal muscle
   occipitofrontalis muscle
   Ochsner muscle
   ocular muscle
   Oddi muscle
   omohyoid muscle
   opposing muscle
   orbicular muscle
   orbicularis muscle
   orbicularis oculi muscle
   orbicularis oris muscle
   orbital muscle

muscle (*continued*)
   palatal muscle
   palatoglossal muscle
   palatoglossus muscle
   palatopharyngeal muscle
   palatopharyngeus muscle
   palmar interosseous muscle
   palmar muscle
   palmaris longus muscle
   papillary muscles
   paraspinal muscles
   paraspinous muscles
   paraverterbral muscle
   pectinate muscles
   pectineal muscle
   pectoral muscles
   pectoralis major muscle
   pectoralis minor muscle
   pennate muscle
   penniform muscle
   perioral muscle
   periorbital orbicularis oculi
      muscle
   peroneal muscle
   peroneus tertius muscle
   pharyngeal constrictor muscle
   pharyngopalatine muscle
   pharyngopalatinus muscle
   Phillips muscle
   piriform muscle
   plantar interosseous muscles
   plantar muscle
   platysma muscle
   pleuroesophageal muscle
   popliteal muscle
   postaxial muscle
   posterior auricular muscle
   posterior cricoarytenoid
      muscle
   posterior scalene muscle
   posterior tibial muscle
   preaxial muscle
   procerus muscle
   profundus muscle
   pronator muscle
   pronator quadratus muscle
   pronator teres muscle
   psoas muscle
   pterygoid muscle
   pubococcygeal muscle
   puboprostatic muscle
   puborectal muscle

muscle (*continued*)

pubovaginal muscle
pubovesical muscle
pulled muscle
pyramidal muscle
quadrate muscle
quadratus labii inferioris muscle
quadratus labii superioris muscle
quadratus lumborum muscle
quadriceps muscle
radial extensor muscle
radial flexor muscle
rectococcygeal muscle
rectourethral muscle
rectouterine muscle
rectovesical muscle
rectus abdominis muscle
rectus capitis muscle
rectus femoris muscle
rectus labii muscle
rectus medialis muscle
rectus muscle
rectus superioris muscle
relaxing of muscles
resection-recession of eye muscles
rhomboid muscle
ribbon muscles
rider's muscle
Riolan muscle
Riordan repair of muscle
risorius muscle
rotator muscles
Rouget muscle
round pronator muscle
Ruysch muscle
Saba classification of shoulder muscles
sacrococcygeal muscle
sacrospinal muscle
salpingopharyngeal muscle
Santorini muscle
sartorius muscle
scalene muscle
scalenus anterior muscle
scalenus medius muscle
scalenus posterior muscle
scalp muscle
semimembranosus muscle
semimembranous muscle

muscle (*continued*)

semispinal muscle
semitendinous muscle
serratus anterior muscle
serratus muscle
serratus posterior inferior muscle
serratus posterior superior muscle
sheath of rectus abdominis muscle
sheath of rectus muscle
short abductor muscle
short adductor muscle
short anconeus muscle
short extensor muscle
short fibular muscle
short flexor muscle
short levator muscles
short palmar muscle
short peroneal muscle
short radial extensor muscle
short rotator muscles
shortening of ocular muscle
skeletal muscle
slow-twitch fatigue-resistant skeletal muscle
smaller pectoral muscle
smaller psoas muscle
smallest adductor muscle
smallest scalene muscle
smooth muscle
Soemmering muscle
soleus muscle
somatic muscles
spastic muscle
sphincter muscle
spinal muscle
splenius muscle
stapedius muscle
sternal muscle
sternoclavicularis muscle
sternocleidomastoid muscle
sternocleidomastoideus muscle
sternocostal muscle
sternohyoid muscle
sternohyoideus muscle
sternomastoid muscle
sternothyroid muscle
sternothyroideus muscle
strap muscles

muscle (*continued*)

stretching of muscle
striated muscle
striped muscle
styloglossus, muscle
stylohyoid muscle
stylopharyngeal muscle
stylopharyngeus muscle
subclavius muscle
subcostal muscles
subcostalis muscle
subscapular muscle
subvertebral muscles
superciliary depressor muscle
superficial flexor muscle
superior auricular muscle
superior constrictor muscle
superior constrictor
  pharyngeal muscle
superior gemellus muscle
superior muscle
superior oblique muscle
superior posterior serratus
  muscle
superior rectus muscle
superior tarsal muscle
supinator muscle
suprahyoid muscles
supraspinous muscle
suspensory muscle
synergic muscles
synergistic muscle
tagged muscles
tarsal muscle
tear of muscle
temporal muscle
temporalis muscle
temporoparietal muscle
tendinous chiasm of flexor
  digitorum sublimis muscle
tensor fasciae latae muscle
tensor muscle
tensor tympani muscle
tensor veli palatini muscle
teres major muscle
teres minor muscle
teres muscle
thenar muscle
thyroarytenoid muscle
thyroepiglottic muscle
thyrohyoid muscle
thyropharyngeal muscle

muscle (*continued*)

tibial muscle
tibialis anterior muscle
tibialis posterior muscle
torn muscle
tracheal muscle
trachealis muscle
trachelomastoid muscle
tragus muscle
transference of muscle
transpalpebral corrugator
  muscle
transplantation of muscle
transplantation of ocular
  muscle
transverse arytenoid muscle
transverse muscle
transverse perineal muscle
transversospinal muscle
transversus abdominis muscle
transversus linguae muscle
transversus perinei profundus
  muscle
transversus thoracis muscle
trapezius muscle
Treitz muscle
triangular muscle
triceps muscle
trunk muscles
tympanic muscle
ulnar extensor muscle
ulnar flexor muscle
underlying chest muscles
unipennate muscle
unstriated muscle
uterine muscle
uvula muscle
uvular muscle
vaginal muscles
Valsalva muscle
vastus lateralis muscle
vastus medialis muscle
vastus medialis obliquus
  muscle
ventral sacrococcygeal muscle
vertical muscle
verticalis linguae muscle
vestigial muscle
visceral muscle
vocal muscle
vocalis muscle
voluntary muscle

muscle (*continued*)
 wasting of muscle
 Wilson muscle
 yoked muscles
 zygomatic muscle
 zygomaticomandibular muscle
 zygomaticus major muscle
 zygomaticus minor muscle
 zygomaticus muscle
muscle advancement technique
muscle and neurological
  stimulation electrotherapy
  device
muscle atrophy
muscle belly
muscle biopsy
muscle biopsy clamp
muscle bleeding points
muscle breakdown
muscle bulk
muscle bundle
muscle clamp
muscle contraction
muscle contraction headache
muscle control
muscle coordination
muscle cramp
muscle dissection
muscle distraction
muscle energy technique
muscle fascicle
muscle fiber
muscle fixation
muscle flap
muscle forceps
muscle function
muscle graft
muscle guarding
muscle hernia
muscle hook
muscle implantation
muscle injuries
muscle lysis
muscle mass
muscle pain
muscle pedicle
muscle prosthesis
muscle re-education
muscle relaxant
muscle repair
muscle repositioning
muscle resection

muscle response
muscle rupture
muscle sense
muscle sliding operation
muscle sling
muscle spindle
muscle stamp
muscle status
muscle stimulation
muscle strain
muscle tension
muscle tension headache
muscle testing
muscle tightness
muscle tissue
muscle tone
muscle tonicity
muscle tonus
muscle transfer
muscle transposition
muscle trimming
muscle tumor
muscle-access abdominoplasty
muscle-balancing procedure
muscle-periosteal flap
muscle-plasty
 V-Y muscle-plasty
muscles, strength, reflexes
 (MSRs)
muscle-splitting incision
muscle-splitting technique
muscle-tendon transplantation
muscular aches
muscular anesthesia
muscular artifact
muscular asthenopia
muscular atrophy
muscular attachment
muscular bolster
muscular contraction
muscular control
muscular defect
muscular disease
muscular dystrophy
muscular graft
muscular layer
muscular pain
muscular paralysis
muscular reflex
muscular relaxation
muscular rheumatism
muscular rigidity

muscular sclerosis
muscular senses
muscular spasm
muscular strabismus
muscular structure
muscular tension
muscular tissues
muscular tone
muscular torticollis
muscular trabeculation
muscular tremors
muscular tube
muscular twitching
muscular veins
muscular ventricular septal
   defect
muscular wall
muscular weakness
muscularis tunnel closure
musculature
   aponeurotic musculature
   cervical musculature
   contralateral musculature
   external musculature
   facial mimetic musculature
   hip musculature
   jerking musculature
   lumbar musculature
   paraspinous musculature
   paravertebral musculature
   pelvic musculature
   thickened musculature
   uvulopalatine musculature
musculoaponeurotic control
musculoaponeurotic layer
musculoaponeurotic plication
musculocartilaginous structure
musculocutaneous amputation
musculocutaneous artery
musculocutaneous flap
musculocutaneous flap skin
   paddle
musculocutaneous free flap
musculocutaneous nerve
musculocutaneous perforator
musculocutaneous vein
musculofascial flap
musculofascial laxity
musculofascial layers
musculofascial plication
musculofascial structures
musculofascial wall

musculofascially
musculomucosal
   facial artery musculomucosal
   (FAMM) flap
musculoperitoneal
musculophrenic artery
musculophrenic veins
musculoplasty
musculoskeletal allograft-
   transmitted infections
musculoskeletal disorder
musculoskeletal evaluation
musculoskeletal tissue
musculospiral groove
musculospiral nerve
musculotendinous aponeurosis
musculotendinous cuff
musculotendinous flap
musculovascular pedicle
musculus antitragicus
musculus helicis major
musculus helicis minor
musculus levator anguli oris
musculus levator labii superioris
musculus risorius
musculus tensor fasciae latae
musculus transversus menti
   muscle
musculus vastus lateralis
musculus zygomaticus major
Museholdt forceps
Museholdt nasal-dressing forceps
Museux forceps
Museux tenaculum
Museux tenaculum forceps
Museux uterine forceps
Museux uterine vulsellum
   forceps
Museux vulsellum forceps
Museux-Collins uterine
   vulsellum forceps
Musgrave-Dupertuis graft
   augmentation
mush clamp
mush heart
mushroom catheter
mushroom corneal graft
mushroom impactor
mushroom overlap of pars
   interarticularis
mushrooming
mushroom-type plate

Musial tissue forceps
musical bowel sounds
musical murmur
muslin dressing
Mussen frame
mustache (*variant of* moustache)
Mustang steerable guidewire
Mustard atrial baffle repair
Mustard flap otoplasty
Mustard iliopsoas transfer
Mustard intra-atrial operation
Mustard intra-atrial procedure
Mustard operation
mustard plaster
mustard poultice
Mustard transposition of great arteries
Mustard transposition of great vessels
Mustarde awl
Mustarde forceps
Mustarde four-flap epicanthal repair
Mustarde graft
Mustarde lateral cheek rotation flap
Mustarde operation
Mustarde otoplasty
Mustarde procedure
Mustarde rotation-advancement flap
Mustarde rotational cheek flap
Mustarde sutures
Mustarde technique
Mustarde-Furnas otoplasty
Mustarde 4-flap epicanthal repair
mutagen
mutagenic
mutilation
mutilization
mutton chop flap
MV (main venule)
mV (millivolts)
MVD (microvascular decompression, microvessel density)
MVR (microvitreoretinal)
MVR blade
MVR plate
MVS cannula

MVS phacoemulsifier
MVV ventilator
myalgia
myasthenia gravis
myasthenia laryngis
myasthenic facies
mycelium (*pl.* mycelia)
mycetoma
mycobacteria (*pl.* of mycobacterium)
mycobacterial infection
mycobacterial lymphadenitis
mycobacterial nodal infection
mycobacterium
mycobacterium (*pl.* of mycobacteria)
mycomyringitis
mycosis
    antral mycosis
    systemic mycosis
mycosis fungoides
mycosis leptothrica
mycotic aneurysm
mycotic disease
mycotic stomatitis
MycroMesh biomaterial
MycroMesh graft material
mydriasis
mydriatic eye drops
mydriatic pupils
mydriatic rigidity
myectomy
myelin globules
myelin kidney
myelin sheath
myelinated axon
myelinated nerve fibers
myelinated sensory nerve fiber
myelination
myelinization
myeloblastoma
myelocytoma
myelogenous callus
myelogenous disease
myelogram
myelography
myelography needle
myeloid cell
myeloid leukemia
myeloid metaplasia
myeloid tissue
myeloid/erythroid ratio

myeloma
myelomeningocele (MMC)
myelomeningocele repair
myelomonocytic cell line
Myelo-Nate needle
Myelo-Nate set
myeloparalysis
myelopathic muscular atrophy
myelopathy
myelosuppressed
myelotomy
   Bischoff myelotomy
   commissural myelotomy
myelotomy knife
myenteric plexus
myenteric reflex
Myers intraluminal stripper
Myers knee retractor
Myers punch
Myers retractor
Myers stripper
Myers vein stripper
Myerson antrum trocar
Myerson biting punch
Myerson biting tip
Myerson bronchial forceps
Myerson electrode
Myerson forceps
Myerson laryngeal forceps
Myerson laryngectomy saw
Myerson miniature laryngeal
   biopsy forceps
Myerson punch
Myerson saw
Myerson sign
Myerson snout
Myerson trocar
Myerson wash tube
Myerson-Moncrieff cannula
myofasciitis
myiasis
Mylar catheter
Mylar matrix
Mylar mesh
Mylar sheeting
Mylar strip
Myles adenotome
Myles antral curet
Myles cannula
Myles clamp
Myles curet
Myles forceps

Myles guillotine
Myles guillotine adenotome
Myles guillotine tonsillectome
Myles hemorrhoidal clamp
Myles hemorrhoidal forceps
Myles nasal forceps
Myles nasal punch
Myles nasal speculum
Myles nasal cutting forceps
Myles punch
Myles sinus antral cannula
Myles sinus cannula
Myles snare
Myles speculum
Myles tonsillectome
Myles tonsillectome snare
Myles-Ray speculum
mylohyoid fossa
mylohyoid groove
mylohyoid groove of inferior
    maxillary bone
mylohyoid line
mylohyoid muscle
mylohyoid nerve
mylohyoid region
mylohyoid ridge
mylohyoid sulcus
mylohyoid sulcus of mandible
mylopharyngeal muscle
Mynol endodontic cement
myoablative therapy
myoblastoma
   granular cell myoblastoma
   malignant granular cell
     myoblastoma
Myobock artificial hand
myocardial clamp
myocardial conduction defect
myocardial contusion
myocardial damage
myocardial dilator
myocardial disease
myocardial electrode
myocardial fibers
myocardial fibrosis
myocardial hypertrophy
myocardial infarct (MI)
myocardial infarction (MI)
myocardial inflammation
myocardial insufficiency
myocardial ischemia
myocardial lead

myocardial necrosis
myocardial perforation
myocardial perfusion
myocardial perfusion imaging
myocardial revascularization
myocardial rupture
myocardial scar
myocardial tumors
myocardiectomy
myocardiopathy
myocardiorrhaphy
myocardiotomy
myocardium
myocardosis
myocervical collar
myochromic
myoclasis
myoclonal antibodies
myoclonic jerk
myoclonic seizure
myoclonus
myocontrol signals
Myocure blade
Myocure blade scalpel
Myocure knife
myocutaneous flap
myocutaneous graft
myodermal flap
myoelectric control prosthesis
myoelectric prosthesis
myoepithelial cell
myoepithelial cell island
myoepithelial cell process
myoepithelial sialadenitis
myoepithelioma
myofascial flap
myofascial manipulation
myofascial pain syndrome (MPS)
myofascial pain-dysfunction
    (MPD)
myofascial trigger point
myofasciitis
myofiber atrophy
myofibroblast cell
myofibroblast contraction
myofibrositis
myofunctional therapy
myogaleal
myogenic blepharoptosis
myoglobin tubular obstruction
myognathus
myograph

myography
myoid cells
myoid cyst
myoma (*pl.* myomas, myomata)
myoma fixation instrument
myoma screw
myomalacia cordis
myomata
myomata uteri
myomatectomy
myomectomy
    abdominal myomectomy
    laparoscopic esophageal
        myomectomy
    uterine myomectomy
myometrial
myometrium
myomotomy
myomucosal flap
myonephropexy
myoneural blockade
myoneural blocking agent
myoneural junction
myoneurectomy
myoneuroma
myoneurosis
myoneurotization
myopathic facies
myopathic paralysis
myopathy
myopectoral inhibition of
    pacemaker
myoplastic muscle stabilization
myoplasty
myopotential
Myopulse muscle stimulator
myorrhaphy
myosarcoma
myositis ossificans (MO)
myositis ossificans progressiva
myospherulosis
myostasis
Myostim unit
Myosynchron muscle stimulator
myotactic
myotasis
myotatic contraction
myotatic irritability
myotatic reflex
myotenontoplasty
myotenotomy
Myotest nerve stimulator

myotome distribution of nerve
myotomy
  circular myotomy
  cricopharyngeal myotomy
  diverticulectomy with
    myotomy
  esophageal myotomy
  Heller myotomy
  hyoid myotomy
  laparoscopic Heller myotomy
  longitudinal myotomy
  procerus muscle myotomy
Myotone EMG monitor
myotonia
  acquired myotonia
  congenital myotonia
  dystrophic myotonia
myotonic cataract
myotonic discharges
myotonic reflexes
myotonic response
myovascular sphincter
Myrhaug procedure
Myriadlase laser
myringeal web
myringectomy
myringitis
myringitis bullosa
myringodectomy
myringodermatitis
myringomycosis
myringoplasty
myringoplasty knife
myringostapediopexy
myringotome
  barbed myringotome
  Buck myringotome

myringotome (*continued*)
  Rica myringotome
  SMIC myringotome
myringotome knife
myringotomy
myringotomy and grommet
  insertion
myringotomy drain tube
myringotomy incision
myringotomy knife
myringotomy knife blade
myringotomy knife handle
myringotomy tube
myringotomy with aspiration
myringotomy with insertion of
  polyethylene collar
  buttons
Myrtle leaf probe
Mystic balloon catheter
myxochondroid matrix
myxochondroid stroma
myxofibroma
myxoid crystal
myxoid cyst
myxoid cystoma
myxoid liposarcoma
myxoid lobule
myxoid neurofibroma
myxoid stroma
myxolipoma
myxoma
myxomatosis
myxomatous degeneration
myxomatous tissue
myxomembranous colitis
myxoneurosis
myxosarcoma

9th cranial nerve (9th)
9th cranial nerve
    (glossopharyngeal)
N₂O cryosurgical unit
Nabatoff vein stripper
Nabers probe
Naboth cysts
Naboth follicles
Naboth glands
Naboth vesicles
nabothian cyst
nabothian follicle
nabothian gland
NAC (nipple-areolar complex)
Nachlas gastrointestinal tube
Nachlas-Linton esophagogastric
    balloon tamponade device
Nachlas-Linton tube
Naclerio diaphragm retractor
Nadbath akinesia
Naden-Rieth femoral prosthetic
    head
Naden-Rieth implant
Naden-Rieth prosthesis
Nadler bipolar coaptation forceps
Nadler superior radial scissors
Naegele obstetrical forceps
Naffziger operation
Naffziger-Poppen-Craig orbital
    decompression
Nagamatsu incision
Nagaraja endoscopic nasal
    biliary drainage set
Nagashima antroscope trocar
Nagashima laryngostroboscope
Nagashima right-angle antroscope
Nagele scissors
Nagele obliquity
Nagele pelvis
Nagele maneuver
Nager acrofacial dysostosis
Nager palatal needle
Nager syndrome

Nager tonsillar needle
Nagielski needle
Nahai tensor fascia lata flap
Nahai tensor fasciae latae flap
Nahai-Mathes classification of fas-
    ciocutaneous flaps (types A-C)
Nahai-Mathes fasciocutaneous
    flap (types A-C)
Nahigian butterfly flap
Nahigian Z-plasty
nail
  3-flanged nail
  4-flanged nails
  adjustable nail
  Albizzia nail
  antegrade/retrograde
    compression nail
  Augustine boat nail
  Boehler hip nail
  Badgley nail
  Barr nail
  Bickel intramedullary nail
  Biomet ankle arthrodesis nail
  blind medullary nail
  boat nail
  bowing of nail
  Brooker double-locking
    unreamed tibial nail
  Brooker-Wills interlocking nail
  Burgess nail
  Calandruccio nail
  cannulated nail
  Capener nail
  Chandler unreamed
    interlocking tibial nail
  clincher nail
  closed Kuntschner nail
  cloverleaf nail
  condylocephalic nail
  Coventry nail
  crutch and belt femoral
    closed nail
  Curry hip nail

nail (*continued*)
  DePuy nail
  Derby nail
  Deyerle nail
  diamond nail
  Dooley nail
  double-ended nail
  eggshell nail
  elastic stable intramedullary nail
  Ender intramedullary nail
  Engel-May nail
  Fenton nail
  flexible intramedullary nail
  fluted Sampson nail
  fluted titanium nail
  fracture nail
  Frosh procedure for ingrown
    nail
  Gamma trochanteric locking nail
  Gissane spike nail
  Grosse-Kempf femoral nail
  Grosse-Kempf interlocking nail
  Grosse-Kempf tibial nail
  Hagie pin nail
  Hahn bone nail
  half-and-half nail
  Hansen-Street intramedullary
    nail
  Hansen-Street self-broaching nail
  Hansen-Street solid
    intramedullary nail
  Harold Crowe drill nail
  Harris condylocephalic nail
  Harris hip nail
  Harris intramedullary nail
  Harris medullary nail
  hexhead nail
  hip nail
  Holt nail
  hooked intramedullary nails
  hooked medullary nail
  Huckstep intramedullary
    compression nail
  I-beam nail
  IM nail
  IMSC 5-hole nail
  ingrown nail
  Inro surgical nail
  insertion of nail
  intramedullary ANK nail
  intramedullary Kuntscher nail
  intramedullary nail

nail (*continued*)
  intramedullary skeletal kinetic
    distractor nail (ISKD)
  intramedullary supracondylar
    multihole nail
  Inyo nail
  Jewett hip nail
  Johannson hip nail
  Kaessmann nail
  Ken sliding nail
  Kirschner interlocking
    intramedullary nail
  Klemme locked
    intramedullary nail
  Knowles pin nail
  Koslowski hip nail
  Kuntscher cloverleaf nail
  Kuntscher intramedullarynail
  Lewis nail
  Lindsay nail
  Lottes intramedullary nail
  Lottes triflange intramedullary
    nail
  Macmed pediatric
    intramedullary nail
  Massie sliding nail
  massive sliding nails
  McKee tri-fin nail
  McLaughlin Vitallium nail
  medullary nail
  metal nail
  Meyerding nail
  Moe nail
  Moore adjustable nails
  nested nails
  Neufeld nail
  noncannulated nail
  Norman tibial nail
  Nylok self-locking nail
  Nystroem hip nail
  Nystroem-Stille hip nail
  Orthofix intramedullary nail
  OrthoSorb pin nail
  osteotomy nail
  Palmer bone nail
  Peterson nail
  Pidcock nail
  Pugh self-adjusting nail
  Recon nail
  Redler nail
  retropulsion of nail
  Revision nail

nail (*continued*)
Richards nail
R-T nail
Rush intramedullary nail
Russell-Taylor delta tibial nail
Russell-Taylor interlocking
    medullary nail
Russell-Taylor interlocking nail
Russell-Taylor tibial
    interlocking nail
Rydell nail
Sampson fluted nail
Schneider intramedullary nail
Schneider medullary nail
Seidel humeral locking nail
self-adjusting nail
self-broaching nail
sinus of nail
sliding nail
Slocum-Smith-Petersen nail
slotted nail
Smillie nail
Smith-Peterson cannulated nail
Smith-Peterson femoral neck
    nail
Smith-Peterson transarticular
    nail
spring-loaded nail
Staples osteotomy nail
Steinmann extension nail
Street diamond-shaped nail
supracondylar nail
Sven Johansson femoral neck
    nail
Synthes titanium elastic nail
Temple University nail
Terry nails
Thatcher nail
Thornton nail
threaded portion of nail
Tiemann nail
titanium elastic nail
triflange intramedullary nail
triflange nail
True/Flex intramedullary nail
Uniflex intramedullary nail
Venable-Stuck nail
Vesely nail
Vesely-Street nail
Vitallium nail
V-medullary nail
Watson-Jones nail

nail (*continued*)
Webb bolt nail
Williams interlocking Y nail
Z-fixation nail
Zickel intramedullary nail
Zimmer intramedullary nail
Zimmer telescoping nail
nail bed
nail cutter
nail disorder
nail drill
nail extension
nail fold
nail groove
nail injury
nail lunula
nail matrix
nail nipper (*see* nipper)
nail plate (*see* plate)
nail scissors
nail-bending device
nail-cutting forceps
nail-driving guidewire
nail-extracting forceps
nail-fold capillaroscopy
nail-fold capillary microscope
nail-fold removal
nailing of bone
nailing of hip
nail-nipper scissors
nail-patella syndrome
nail-patella-elbow syndrome
nail-plate fixation
nail-plate removal
nail-pulling forceps
nail-to-nail bed angle
Nakamura brace
Nakao Ejector biopsy forceps
Nakao snare
Nakayama anastomosis
Nakayama clamp
Nakayama instruments
Nakayama microvascular stapler
Nakayama ring
Nakayama staple
Nalebuff classification
Nalebuff wrist arthrodesis
Nalebuff-Goldman strut
Nalebuff-Millender lateral band
    mobilization technique
NAMI DDV ligator
Namic angiographic syringe

Namic catheter
Namic localization needle
Nance analysis of arch length
Nance leeway space
nanocurie (nCi)
nanogram (ng)
Nanolas Nd:YAG laser
nanoliter (nl)
nanometer (nm)
nanomole
nanopascal
Nanos 1 pacemaker
nape of neck flap
naphthalinic cataract
napkin-ring calcar allograft
napkin-ring annular lesion
napkin-ring carcinoma
napkin-ring compression
napkin-ring defect
napkin-ring lesion
Napoleon Bonaparte sign
Naraghi-DeCoster reduction
      clamp
Narath omentopexy
Narath operation
narcolocal analgesia
Narcomatic flowmeter
narcotic agent
narcotic analgesic
narcotic antagonist
narcotic drug
narcotic effect
nares constriction
naris (pl. nares)
   anterior naris
   compressor muscle of naris
   constrictor naris
   dilator naris
   posterior naris
naris constriction
naris internae
Narkomed anesthesia machine
Naropin anesthetic
narrow AO dynamic
      compression plate
narrow cone
narrow Deaver retractor
narrow duodenal opening
narrow elevator
narrow field
narrow gauze roll
narrow lens

narrow retractor
narrow rim
narrow-angle glaucoma
narrow-bite bone rongeur
narrowed blood vessel
narrowed duct
narrowed valve
narrow-field laryngectomy
NarrowFlex intra-aortic balloon
      catheter
narrowing and lipping
nasal accessory artery
nasal airway obstruction
nasal ala
nasal alligator forceps
nasal antrostomy
nasal aperture
nasal applicator
nasal arch
nasal arteries
nasal aspirator
nasal bistoury
nasal bivalve speculum
nasal bone crusher
nasal bone forceps
nasal border
nasal branches
nasal bridge
nasal calculus
nasal canal
nasal cannula
nasal canthus
nasal capsule
nasal cartilage
nasal cartilage guide
nasal cartilage-cutting board
nasal cartilage-holding forceps
nasal catarrh
nasal catheter
nasal cavity
nasal cavity cancer
nasal chamber
nasal chisel
nasal chisel-osteotome
nasal chondroma
nasal concha
nasal congestion
nasal contour
nasal crest of maxilla
nasal crest of palatine bone
nasal cross-sectional area
nasal culture

nasal curet
nasal cutting forceps
nasal deformity
nasal dilator
nasal discharge
nasal dissection
nasal dissector
nasal dome cartilage
nasal dorsal implant
nasal dorsal-angled scissors
nasal dorsum
nasal douche
nasal drainage
nasal drip pad
nasal duct
nasal dysplasia
nasal elevator
nasal eminence
nasal endoscopic surgery
nasal endoscopic telescope
nasal endoscopy
nasal endoscopy telescope
nasal feeding
nasal flaring
nasal floor
nasal foramen
nasal forceps
nasal fossa
nasal fracture
nasal gavage
nasal glands
nasal glioma
nasal gouge
nasal height
nasal hemorrhage
nasal hook
nasal hump forceps
nasal hump gouge
nasal hump-cutting forceps
nasal incision
nasal insertion forceps
nasal instruments
nasal intubation
nasal irrigator
nasal knife
nasal knife blade
nasal lisp
nasal lower lateral forceps
nasal mallet
nasal meatus
nasal mucosa
nasal mucus

nasal muscle
nasal myiasis
nasal needle
nasal needle holder
nasal needle holder forceps
nasal nerve
nasal notch of maxilla
nasal obstruction
nasal osteotome
nasal pack
nasal packing
nasal pancreatogram
nasal passage
nasal plastic instruments
nasal polyp forceps
nasal polyp hook
nasal polypectomy
nasal polypus forceps
nasal probe
nasal process
nasal prongs
nasal punch
nasal pyramid
nasal rasp
nasal recess
nasal reconstruction
nasal reflex
nasal retractor
nasal ridge
nasal rongeur
nasal root
nasal sac
nasal saw
nasal saw blade
nasal scissors
nasal septal reconstruction
nasal septal abscess
nasal septal forceps
nasal septal perforation
nasal septoplasty
nasal septum
nasal septum reconstruction
   (NSR)
nasal sill
nasal sinus
nasal smear
nasal snare wire
nasal snare wire carrier
nasal speculum
nasal spine of frontal bone
nasal spine of palatine bone
nasal splint

nasal spur
nasal stenosis
nasal stent cutter
nasal strut
nasal suction cup
nasal suction tip
nasal suction tube
nasal suture
nasal suture needle
nasal swivel knife
nasal tampon
nasal tampon sponge
nasal tamponade
nasal tenaculum
nasal tip deformity
nasal tip projection
nasal tip-plasty
nasal trephine
nasal truss
nasal tube
nasal turbinate
nasal valve collapse
nasal valve suspension
nasal vault
nasal vein
nasal venous arch
nasal venule
nasal verge
nasal vestibule
nasal vestibulitis
nasal washings
nasal wing
nasal-cutting forceps
nasal-cutting tip
nasal-dressing forceps
nasal-grasping forceps
nasalis muscle
nasal-labial furrow
nasal-packing forceps
nasal-septal fracture
nasal-tip dressing
Nasa-Spec nasal speculum
nascent vasculature
Nashold biopsy needle
Nashold electrode
nasi
nasion perpendicular
nasion point
nasion soft tissue
nasion-alveolar point line
nasion-pogonion facial axis plane
nasion-pogonion measurement

nasion-point A plane
nasion-point B plane
nasoalveolar cyst
nasoantral window
nasobasilar line
nasobiliary catheter
nasobiliary catheter
    cholangiogram
nasobiliary drainage
nasobiliary pigtail catheter
    placement
nasobiliary tube
nasobregmatic arc
nasociliary branches of
    ophthalmic nerve
nasociliary ganglion
nasociliary nerve
nasocystic catheter
nasocystic drain
nasocystic drainage tube
nasoduodenal feeding tube
nasoendoscope (see endoscope)
    Hirschman nasoendoscope
nasoendotracheal anesthesia
nasoendotracheal intubation
nasoendotracheal tube
nasoenteric feeding tube
nasoesophageal feeding tube
nasoethmoidal fracture
nasoethmoidal-orbital fracture
naso-ethmoid-orbital fracture
nasofacial analysis
nasofacial groove
nasofrontal angle
nasofrontal duct
nasofrontal orifice
nasofrontal osteotome
nasofrontal suture
nasofrontal vein
nasogastric aspirate
nasogastric drainage
nasogastric feeding tube
nasogastric intubation
nasogastric suction
nasogastric tube
nasograph
nasoileal tube
nasojejunal feeding tube
nasojugal fold
nasojugal grove
nasolabial angle
nasolabial crease

nasolabial cyst
nasolabial droop
nasolabial flap
nasolabial fold (NLF)
nasolabial groove
nasolabial junction
nasolabial ligament
nasolabial line
nasolabial muscle
nasolabial reflex
nasolabial rotation flap
nasolabial stigma
nasolabial sulcus
nasolacrimal canal
nasolacrimal duct
nasolacrimal duct probe
nasolacrimal dysfunction
nasolacrimal groove
nasolacrimal sac
nasolacrimal tube
nasolaryngopharyngoscope
nasolaryngoscope (*see*
   laryngoscope)
   Machida nasolaryngoscope
nasomalarmaxillary
nasomandibular fixation
nasomandibular ligament
nasomaxillary balloon
nasomaxillary buttress
nasomaxillary dysplasia
nasomaxillary fracture
nasomaxillary groove
nasomaxillary suture
nasomental reflex
naso-occipital arc
naso-ocular cleft
naso-orbital fracture
naso-orbitoethmoid (NOE)
   fracture
nasopalatine canal
nasopalatine cyst
nasopalatine duct
nasopalatine duct cyst
nasopalatine foramen
nasopalatine groove
nasopalatine injection
nasopalatine nerve
nasopalatine nerve block
nasopalatine plexus of Woodruff
nasopalatine recess
nasopancreatic catheter
nasopancreatic drainage

nasopharyngeal abscess
nasopharyngeal airway
nasopharyngeal angiofibroma
nasopharyngeal applicator
nasopharyngeal area
nasopharyngeal biopsy
nasopharyngeal biopsy forceps
nasopharyngeal bursa
nasopharyngeal carcinoma
   (NPC)
nasopharyngeal cyst
nasopharyngeal fiberscope
nasopharyngeal fibroma
nasopharyngeal groove
nasopharyngeal hematoma
nasopharyngeal hemorrhage
nasopharyngeal pack
nasopharyngeal retractor
nasopharyngeal secretion
nasopharyngeal speculum
nasopharyngeal sponge
nasopharyngeal stenosis
nasopharyngeal tube
nasopharyngectomy
nasopharyngolaryngofiberscope
   (*see* fiberscope)
nasopharyngolaryngoscope
nasopharyngoscope (*see*
   pharyngoscope)
   ACMI nasopharyngoscope
   Broyles nasopharyngoscope
   flexible nasopharyngoscope
   Holmes nasopharyngoscope
   Meltzer nasopharyngoscope
   Yankauer nasopharyngoscope
nasopharynx
nasoplasty
nasoseptal deviation
nasoseptal reconstruction
nasostat
   balloon nasostat
   Gottschalk nasostat
Naso-Tamp nasal packing sponge
nasotracheal catheter
nasotracheal intubation
nasotracheal intubation anesthesia
nasotracheal suctioning
nasotracheal tube
nasoturbinal
nasoturbinal concha
nasovesicular catheter
nasovesicular catheter technique

Nassif parascapular flap
Nataf lateral flap
natal cleft
natatory ligament
Natelson tube
Nathan pacemaker
natiform skull
National cautery
National cautery electrode
National coagulator
National cystoscope
National ear speculum
National general-purpose
    cystoscope
National Graves vaginal speculum
National instruments
National proctoscope
National speculum
National transilluminator
native anatomy
native caudate lobe
native renal biopsy
native valve
natural amputation
natural bypass
natural joint
natural line
natural pacemaker
natural skin lines
natural suture
natural teeth
NaturaLase Er:YAG laser
NaturaLase erbium laser
natural-feel breast prosthesis
Natural-Hip prosthesis
Natural-Loc acetabular cup
    prosthesis
Natural-Loc RM acetabular cup
Natural-Lok acetabular cup
Natural-Lok acetabular cup
    prosthesis
Natural-Y breast prosthesis
Natvig wire-twister forceps
Naugh os calcis apparatus tractor
Naugle orbitometer
    exophthalmometer
Nauth traction device
NavAblator catheter
Navarre interventional radiology
    device
navicular abdomen
navicular arthritis

navicular bone
navicular fat stripe sign
navicular fossa
navicular fossa of male urethra
navicular fracture
navicular pad
navicular projection
navicular screw
naviculocapitate fracture
naviculocuneiform fusion
navigated brain tumor surgery
navigational surgery
Navigator flexible endoscope
Naviport deflectable tip guiding
    catheter
Naviport hollow-lumen guiding
    catheter
Navius stent
Navratil retractor
Navratil stirrups
Nazorcap capnographic
    respiratory monitor
NB (newborn)
NBIH catheter
NC Bandit catheter
NC Big Ranger OTW balloon
    catheter
NC Cobra balloon
NCC Hi-Lo Jet endotracheal tube
nCi (nanocurie)
NC-stat nerve conduction
Nd:YAG (neodymium:yttrium-
    aluminum-garnet) laser
Nd:YAG (neodymium-doped
    yttrium-aluminum-garnet)
    laser
Nd:YAG laser
Nd:YAG laser ablation
Nd:YAG laser irradiation
Nd:YAG laser therapy
Nd:YAG laser with Hexascan
Nd:YLF laser
NDM adhesive wound dressing
NDSB occlusion balloon catheter
Neal cannula
Neal catheter
Neal catheter trocar
Neal fallopian cannula
Neal insufflator
Nealon technique
Neal-Robertson litter
near fixation

near visual point
near-anatomic position
near-and-far suture technique
near-and-far sutures
near-edge of incision
near-far sutures
near-infrared electronic
    endoscope
Nearly Me breast form
near-term gestation
near-total esophagectomy
near-total gastrectomy
near-total laryngectomy
NEB hip arthroplasty
NEB total hip prosthesis
Nebauer ophthalmoendoscope
Nebauer ophthalmoscope
Nebinger-Praun operation
Nebuhaler inhaler
nebulization ventilator
nebulized solution
Nec Loc cervical collar
Necelon surgical gloves
neck
    adenoid cystic carcinoma of
        head and neck (ACCHN)
    anatomic neck
    aortic neck
    bladder neck
    bur neck
    condylar neck
    congenital cartilaginous rest
        of the neck (CCRN)
    femoral neck
    fibular neck
    fiddler neck
    functional assessment of
        cancer therapy-head and
        neck (FACT-HN)
    gallbladder neck
    Girdlestone excision of
        femoral head and neck
    implant neck
    implant superstructure neck
    innervation of head and neck
    osteotomy of condylar neck
    Pauwels fracture of proximal
        femoral neck
    radial neck
    ridge of mandibular neck
    squamous cell carcinoma of
        head and neck (SCCHN)

neck (*continued*)
    stiff neck
    stiffness of neck
    sulcus of mandibular neck
    supple neck
    surgical neck
    transverse artery of neck
    turkey gobbler neck
    V-Y plasty of bladder neck
neck dissection
neck exploration
neck extension position
neck flap
neck flexion
neck fracture
neck implant substructure
neck jowl
neck lift
neck of condyle
neck of femur
neck of mandible
neck of middle turbinate
neck of organ or structure
neck rest
neck roll
neck sign
neck support
neck vein distention
neck veins
neck wound
Neck-Hugger cervical support
    pillow
Neck-Roll aromatherapy hot/
    cold pack
neck-shaft angle
Necktrac traction device
neck-wrap halter
necrobiotic xanthogranuloma
necropsy
necrosectomy
necrosis (*pl.* necroses)
necrotic abscess
necrotic debris
necrotic flap
necrotic hemorrhoid
necrotic inflammation
necrotic metastasis
necrotic pulp
necrotic tissue
necrotic ulcer
necrotic ulceration
necrotic zone

necrotizing external otitis
necrotizing fasciitis (NF)
necrotizing granuloma
necrotizing granulomatous
    inflammation
necrotizing myofascial fungal
    infection
necrotizing myofasciitis
necrotizing otitis media
necrotizing sialometaplasia
necrotizing soft tissue infection
    (NSTI)
necrotizing ulcerative
    gingivostomatitis
necrotizing ulcerative stomatitis
necrotizing vasculitis
necrotomy
NED (no evidence of disease)
needle
    4-seded cutting needle
    abdominal needle
    Abrams biopsy needle
    Abrams needle
    Abscession needle
    abscission needle
    Accucore II biopsy needle
    Accuject dental needle
    Ackerman needle
    Acland needle
    ACS needle
    active length needle
    Acumaster acupuncture
        needle
    Adair-Veress needle
    Addix needle
    Adson aneurysm needle
    Adson scalp needle
    Adson suture needle
    Adson-Murphy trocar point
        needle
    advancement needle
    Agnew tattooing needle
    Agrikola tattooing needle
    Ailee needle
    air aspirator needle
    Albarran-Reverdin needle
    Alcon irrigating needle
    Alcon reverse cutting needle
    Alcon spatula needle
    Alcon taper-cut needle
    Alcon taper-point needle
    Aldrete needle

needle (*continued*)
    Alexander tonsil needle
    Altmann needle
    AMC needle
    Amersham needle
    Amplatz angiography needle
    Amsler aqueous transplant
        needle
    Anchor surgical needle
    anesthesia block needle
    aneurysm needle
    angiography needle
    angular needle
    antral needle
    antral trocar needle
    antrum-exploring needle
    aortic root perfusion needle
    aortogram needle
    aortography needle
    aqueous transplant needle
    arachnophlebectomy needle
    Arkan sharpening-stone
        needle
    Arrow-Fischell needle
    arterial blood needle
    arterial needle
    arteriogram needle
    arteriography needle
    ASAP channel-cut automated
        biopsy needle
    ASAP prostate biopsy needle
    aspirating needle
    aspiration biopsy needle
    aspiration needle
    Atkinson retrobulbar needle
    Atkinson single-bevel blunt-tip
        needle
    Atkinson tip peribulbar needle
    Atraloc surgical needle
    atraumatic needle
    atraumatic suture needle
    Austin needle
    AV fistula needle
    B&D needle
    Babcock needle
    Ballade needle
    Barbara needle
    Bard Biopty cut needle
    Bard biopsy needle
    Barker needle
    Barraquer needle
    Barraquer-Vogt needle

needle (*continued*)

Barrett hebosteotomy needle
Bauer biopsy needle
BD bone marrow biopsy needle
BD SafetyGard needle
BD SafetyGlide needle
BD SafetyGlide shielding hypodermic needle
BD spinal needle
Beath needle
Becton-Dickinson Teflon-sheathed needle
Beeth needle
Bengash needle
bent blunt needle
bent needle
Berbecker needle
Bergeret-Reverdin needle
Berges-Reverdin needle
Bergstrom needle
beveled thin-walled needle
Beyer paracentesis needle
bicurved needle
Biegelseisen needle
Bier lumbar puncture needle
Bierman needle
biopsy needle
Biopty cut biopsy needle
Biopty cut needle
Biosearch needle
bipolar needle
Birtcher electrosurgical needle
Black-Decker needle
Blackmon needle
Blair-Brown needle
bleeding needle
block anesthesia needle
block needle
blunt needle
blunt-end sialogram needle
bone marrow biopsy needle
bone marrow needle
Bonney suture needle
boomerang bladder needle
Bovie needle
Bowman cataract needle
Bowman iris needle
Bowman stop needle
brain biopsy needle
Braun needle
breast localization needle

needle (*continued*)

BRK transseptal needle
Brockenbrough curved needle
Brockenbrough transseptal needle
Brophy needle
Brophy-Deschamps needle
Brown cleft palate needle
Brown staphylorrhaphy needle
Brown-Sanders fascial needle
Brughleman needle
Brunner ligature needle
Buerger prostatic needle
Buncke quartz needle
Bunnell tendon needle
Burr butterfly needle
butterfly IV needle
butterfly needle
BV-2 needle
Caldwell needle
Calhoun needle
Calhoun-Hagler lens needle
Calhoun-Merz needle
Campbell ventricular needle
cardioplegic needle
Cardiopoint cardiac surgery needle
Carlens needle
carotid angiogram needle
Carpule needle
Carroll needle
Castroviejo vitreous-aspirating needle
cataract needle
cataract-aspirating needle
catgut needle
catheter needle
caudal needle
cerebral angiography needle
cervical needle
cervical suture needle
cervix suture needle
cesium needle
Charles flute needle
Charles vacuuming needle
Charlton antral needle
Charlton antrum needle
Chiba biopsy needle
Chiba eye needle
Chiba transhepatic cholangiography needle

needle (*continued*)

- Childs-Phillips intestinal plication needle
- Childs-Phillips plication needle
- Cibis ski needle
- CIF needle
- Clagett needle
- Clas von Eichen needle
- Cleasby spatulated needle
- cleft palate needle
- Cloquet needle
- coaxial sheath cut-biopsy needle
- Cobb-Ragde needle
- Cobe AV fistular needle
- Colapinto transjugular needle
- Colorado microdissection needle
- Colts cutting needle
- Colver tonsil needle
- Colver tonsillar needle
- concentric needle
- Concept Multi-Liner lining needle
- Concept suturing needle
- cone biopsy needle
- Cone ventricular needle
- Conrad-Crosby biopsy needle
- Conrad-Crosby bone marrow biopsy needle
- Continental needle
- Control Release pop-off needle
- conventional needle
- Cook endomyocardial needle
- Cook endoscopic curved needle driver
- Cook Longdwel needle
- Cook percutaneous entry needle
- Cooley aortic vent needle
- Cooley ventricular needle
- Cooper chemopallidectomy needle
- Cooper ligature needle
- Cooper pallidectomy needle
- CooperVision irrigating needle
- CooperVision spatulated needle
- Cope biopsy needle
- Cope pleural biopsy needle
- Cope thoracentesis needle
- copper-clad steel needle

needle (*continued*)

- Core aspiration/injection needle
- Core CO_2 insufflation needle
- corneal needle
- corneal suture needle
- Corson needle
- Coston iris needle
- couching needle
- Cournand arterial needle
- Cournand arteriography needle
- Cournand-Grino angiography needle
- Cournand-Potts needle
- Craig biopsy needle
- Crawford fascial needle
- Crown biopsy needle
- CTX needle
- C-type acupuncture needle
- CU-8 needle
- Culp biopsy needle
- Curran knife needle
- Curry cerebral needle
- curved suture needle
- curved transjugular needle
- CUSALap ultrasonic accessory needle
- Cushing needle
- Cushing ventricular needle
- cut biopsy needle
- cut taper needle
- cutting needle
- cyclodiathermy needle
- dacryocystorhinostomy needle
- Daily cataract needle
- Daiwa dental needle
- Damshek needle
- Dandy ventricular needle
- Dandy-Cairns brain needle
- Dandy-Cairns ventricular needle
- Dattner needle
- Davis knife needle
- Davis tonsillar needle
- Dean antral needle
- Dean iris knife needle
- Dean iris needle
- Dean knife needle
- Dean-Senturia needle
- DeBakey needle
- debridement needle

needle (*continued*)

Dees renal needle
Dees suture needle
Deknatel needle
Delbert-Reverdin needle
Denis Browne cleft palate
    needle
DePuy-Weiss tonsillar needle
D'Errico ventricular needle
Deschamps ligature needle
Deschamps-Navratil ligature
    needle
desiccation needle
desiccation-fulguration needle
Desmarres paracentesis
    needle
Devonshire needle
Diamond SharpPoint needle
diamond-point suture needle
diathermal needle
diathermic needle
diathermic precut needle
Dieckmann intraosseous
    needle
Dingman malleable passing
    needle
Dingman passing needle
discission needle
diskogram needle
diskographic needle
disposable acupuncture
    needle
disposable aspiration needle
disposable biopsy needle
disposable injection needle
disposable suturing needle
Dispos-A-Ture single-use
    surgical needle
Dix needle
DLP cardioplegic needle
DN acupuncture needle
docking needle
Docktor needle
Dorsey needle
Dos Santos aortography needle
Dos Santos lumbar
    aortography needle
double-barreled needle
double-hub emulsifying needle
double-lumen needle
double-tipped center-
    threading needle

needle (*continued*)

double-webbed needle
Douglas suture needle
Doyen needle
dragonhead needle
Drapier needle
Drews cataract needle
Drews lavage needle
D-Tach removable needle
Duff debridement needle
dumbbell needle
Dupuy-Dutemps needle
Dupuy-Weiss tonsillar needle
dural needle
Durham needle
Durrani dorsal vein complex
    ligation needle
DuVries needle
Dyonics needle
Echo-Coat ultrasound biopsy
    needle
echogenic needle
egress needle
EJ bone marrow biopsy needle
electrodes needle
electrosurgical needle
Ellis foreign body needle
Elschnig extrusion needle
Emmet needle
Emmet-Murphy needle
Empire needle
Endopath Ultra Veress needle
Entree disposable CO_2
    insufflation needle
epilation needle
Epstein needle
Erosa disposable hypodermic
    needle
Espocan combined
    spinal/epidural needle
Estridge ventricular needle
Ethalloy TruTaper
    cardiovascular needle
Ethicon needle
Ethicon straight taper-point
    needle
Ethiguard needle
Euro-Med aspiration needle
eXcel-DR disposable/reusable
    Glasser laparoscopic needle
eXcel-DR pneumothorax
    needle

needle (*continued*)
 exploring needle
 extended round needle
 ExtraSafe butterfly infusion
  needle
 extrusion needle
 eye needle
 eyed needle
 eyed suture needle
 eyeless atraumatic suture
  needle
 eyeless needle
 eyeless suture needle
 E-Z-EM Cut biopsy needle
 Falk needle
 Farah cystoscopic needle
 fascia needle
 fascial needle
 fat-injection needles
 Federspiel needle
 Fein needle
 Fergi needle
 Ferguson round-body needle
 Ferguson suture needle
 Ferris disposable bone
  marrow aspiration needle
 Field-Lee biopsy needle
 filiform steel needle
 filter needle
 fine intestinal needle
 fine needle
 Finochietto needle
 Fischer pneumothoracic
  needle
 Fisher eye needle
 fishhook needle
 fistula needle
 fistular needle
 flat spatula needle
 flexible aspiration needle
 flexible biopsy needle
 flexible injection needle
 Floyd pneumothorax needle
 flute needle
 Flynt aortography needle
 Foltz needle
 foreign body needle
 Frackelton fascial needle
 Framer tendon-passing needle
 Francke needle
 Frankfeldt hemorrhoidal needle
 Franklin liver puncture needle

needle (*continued*)
 Franklin-Silverman biopsy
  needle
 Franklin-Silverman prostatic
  biopsy needle
 Franseen liver biopsy needle
 Frazier ventricular needle
 Frederick pneumothoracic
  needle
 Frederick pneumothorax
  needle
 Freenseen liver biopsy needle
 French spring-eye needle
 French-eye needle
 Fritz vitreous transplant needle
 front wall needle
 full-intensity needle
 Gallie fascia needle
 Gallini bone marrow
  aspiration needle
 ganglion injection needle
 Gardner suture needle
 gastrointestinal needle
 GC needle
 general closure needle
 Geuder corneal needle
 Geuder keratoplasty needle
 Gill needle
 Gillmore needle
 Girard anterior chamber
  needle
 Girard cataract-aspirating
  needle
 Girard phacofragmatome
  needle
 Girard-Swan needle
 gold needle
 Goldbacher rectal needle
 Goldenberg Snarecoil bone
  marrow biopsy needle
 Goldmann knife needle
 Gordh needle
 Gorsch needle
 Graefe iris needle
 GraNee needle
 Grantham lobotomy needle
 Greene needle
 Greenfield needle
 Greenwald needle
 Grice suture needle
 Grieshaber corneal needle
 Grieshaber eye needle

needle (*continued*)

Grieshaber iris needle
Grieshaber ophthalmic needle
Gripper needle
Guest needle
Gynex extended-reach needle
Haab knife needle
Hagedorn operation suture needle
Hagedorn suture needle
half-intensity needle
Halle septal needle
Halsey needle
hammer-type acupuncture needle
harelip needle
Harken heart needle
Harvard needle
Haverhill needle
Hawkeye suture needle
Hawkins breast localization needle
Hawkins-Akins needle
Hearn needle
heart needle
Hegar needle
Hegar-Baumgartner needle
Hemoject needle
hemorrhoidal needle
Henton suture needle
Henton tonsillar needle
Henton tonsillar suture needle
heparin needle
heparin-flushing needle
Hessburg lacrimal needle
Hey-Groves needle
Heyner-double needle
high-risk needle (HR needle)
Hingson-Edwards needle
Hingson-Ferguson needle
Hobbs needle
Hoen ventricular needle
Holinger needle
hollow needle
Homer localization needle
Homerlok needle
hooked needle
hookwire needle
Hosford-Hicks needle
Hourin tonsil needle
Hourin tonsillar needle
House stapes needle

needle (*continued*)

House-Barbara shattering needle
House-Rosen needle
Howard Jones needle
Howell biliary aspiration needle
Howell biopsy aspiration needle
HR needle (high-risk needle)
Huber point needle
Hunstad infusion needle
Hurd suture needle
Hustead epidural needle
Hutchins biopsy needle
hypodermic needle
Hypospray jet injection needle
Icofly infusion needle
Ilg needle
Iliff-Wright fascia needle
Illinois needle
illuminated suction needle
Impex aspiration and injection needle
Indian club needle
Infusaid needle
Ingersoll tonsil needle
Ingersoll tonsillar needle
injection needle
Injex disposable needle
insulated electrode needle
internal nucleus hydrodelineation needle
intestinal plication needle
intraosseous needle
intravenous needle
Iocare titanium needle
IOLAB irrigating needle
IOLAB taper-cut needle
IOLAB taper-point needle
IOLAB titanium needle
iridium needle
iris needle
irrigating-positioning needle
Ito needle
IV needle
J needle
Jalaguier-Reverdin needle
Jameson strabismus needle
Jamshidi adult needle
Jamshidi liver biopsy needle
Jamshidi-Kormed bone marrow biopsy needle

needle (*continued*)
- Jelco needle
- JMS injection needle
- Jonesco wire suture needle
- Jordan needle
- Kader fishhook needle
- Kall modification of Silverman needle
- Kalt corneal needle
- Kalt eye needle
- Kalt vein needle
- Kangnian acupuncture needle
- Kaplan tracheostomy needle
- Kara needle
- Karras angiography needle
- Keith abdominal needle
- Kelly intestinal needle
- Kelman needle
- KeyMed disposable variceal injection needle
- kidney suture needle
- kidney suturing needle
- King suture needle
- Klatskin liver biopsy needle
- Klein infiltration needle
- Klima-Rosegger sternal needle
- Knapp iris knife needle
- Knight needle
- Kobak needle
- Koch nucleus hydrolysis needle
- Kohn needle
- Koontz hernia needle
- Kopan breast lesion localization needle
- Kormed disposable liver biopsy needle
- Kratz diamond-dusted needle
- Kronecker aneurysm needle
- lacrimal needle
- Lagleyze needle
- Lahey needle
- Laminex needle
- Lane cleft palate needle
- Lane suture needle
- Lane suturing needle
- Lapides needle
- Laredo-Bard needle
- large-bore needle
- large-bore slotted aspirating needle
- Lee-Westcott needle
- Lee needle

needle (*continued*)
- Leighton needle
- L'Esperance needle
- Lewicky needle
- Lewis Pair-Pak needle
- Lewy Teflon glycerin-mixture injection needle
- Lewy-Holinger Teflon injection needle
- Lewy-Rubin needle
- Lewy-Rubin Teflon glycerin-mixture injection needle
- Lichtwicz antral needle
- Lichtwicz-Bier antral needle
- ligature needle
- Lindeman transfusion needle
- Linton-Blakemore needle
- Lipschwitz needle
- List needle
- Litvak-Pereyra ligature needle
- liver biopsy needle
- lobotomy needle
- lock needle
- long needle
- Longdwel catheter needle
- Look retrobulbar needle
- Lo-Trau side-cutting needle
- Lowell pleural needle
- Lowette needle
- Lowette-Verner needle
- Lowsley ribbon-gut needle
- LR needle
- Luer needle
- Luer-Lok needle
- Lukens needle
- lumbar aortography needle
- lumbar puncture needle
- Lundy fascial needle
- Lundy-Irving caudal needle
- Luongo needle
- LX needle
- Madayag biopsy needle
- Maddox caudal needle
- Magielski needle
- Mahurkar fistular needle
- malleable passing needle
- Maltz needle
- Maltzman needle
- Mammalok localization needle
- Mammo-lock needle
- Manan cutting needle
- Mantoux needle

needle (*continued*)

March laser sclerostomy
  needle
Marion-Reverdin needle
Markham biopsy needle
Martin uterine needle
Marx needle
Mason-School aspirating
  needle
Masson fascial needle
Mathieu needle
Maumenee vitreous-aspirating
  needle
Mayo catgut needle
Mayo intestinal needle
Mayo trocar needle
Mayo trocar-point needle
McCaslin needle
McCurdy staphylorrhaphy
  needle
McDowell needle
McGee prosthesis needle
McGhan plastic surgical
  needle
McGowan needle
McGregor needle
McIntyre aspiration needle
McIntyre I&A needle
McIntyre irrigation needle
McIntyre irrigation/aspiration
  needle
mediastinoscopy aspirating
  needle
Medicut intravenous needle
Medicut needle
Menghini liver biopsy needle
meniscal repair needle
Mentor prostate biopsy
  needle
metal needle
metallic frontal needle
Metcoff pediatric biopsy needle
Meyer cyclodiathermy needle
Mick afterloading needle
micro round-tip needle
MicroFlow phaco-emul-
  sification needle
Microlet electrode needle
micron needle
micropoint needle
micropuncture introducer
  needle

needle (*continued*)

Microvasive sclerotherapy
  needle
Millet needle
milliner's needle
Mixter ventricular needle
Mizzy needle
MO needle
modified CIF needle
modified spatula needle
Monopty needle
Morrow-Brown needle
Moss T-anchor needle
MPL dental needle
MPL intraosseous needle
Mueller needle
Multi-Pro biopsy needle
Murphy intestinal needle
myelography needle
Myelo-Nate needle
Nager palatal needle
Nager tonsillar needle
Nagielski needle
Namic localization needle
nasal needle
nasal suture needle
Nashold biopsy needle
Nelson ligature needle
neurography needle
neurosurgical suture needle
Neville ascending aortic air
  vent needle
New oral needle
Newman rectal injection
  needle
Nichols-Deschamps-Navratil
  ligature needle
Noci stimuli needle
NoKor needle
noncoring Huber needle
noncutting needle
noncutting suture needle
nonferromagnetic needle
Nordenstrom biopsy needle
Nordenstrom Rotex II biopsy
  needle
Nottingham colposuspension
  needle
nucleus hydrolysis needle
Oaks double needle
O'Brien airway needle
obstetrical anesthesia needle

needle (*continued*)
  obstetrical block anesthesia
    needle
  Ochsner needle
  Oldfield needle
  olive-tipped needle
  Olympus sclerotherapy
    needle
  Olympus reusable oval cup
    forceps with needle
  OmniTip side-firing laser
    needle
  Op-Pneu laparoscopy needle
  optical needle
  Optivis Surgalloy needle
  oral needle
  Osgood needle
  Osterballe precision needle
  Ostycut bone biopsy needle
  Overholt rib needle
  Pace ventricular needle
  Page needle
  Pajunk needle
  Palmer-Drapier needle
  palpating needle
  Pannett needle
  Paparella straight needle
  paracentesis needle
  paracervical nerve block
    needle
  paraPRO paracentesis needle
  Parhad needle
  Parhad-Poppen needle
  Parker needle
  Parker-Pearson needle
  Payr vein needle
  pediatric biopsy needle
  Pencan spinal needle
  Penfield biopsy needle
  Pentax prototype needle
  PercuCut biopsy needle
  PercuGuide needle
  percutaneous cutting needle
  percutaneous needle
  Pereyra needle
  peribulbar needle
  pericardiocentesis needle
  permanent needle
  Permark micropigmentation
    needle
  PermaShap suture and needle
  Pharmaseal needle

needle (*continued*)
  pilot needle
  Pischel needle
  Pitkin needle
  plain eye needle
  pleural biopsy needle
  plication needle
  Plum-Blossom acupuncture
    needle
  Pneumo-Matic insufflation
    needle
  Pneumo-Needle needle
  pneumoperitoneum needle
  pneumothoracic injection
    needle
  pneumothorax injection
    needle
  pneumothorax needle
  Politzer paracentesis needle
  polypropylene needle
  polytef-sheathed needle
  pop-off needle
  Poppen ventricular needle
  positioning needle
  postmortem suture needle
  Potocky needle
  Potter needle
  Potts needle
  Potts-Cournand angiography
    needle
  precision lancet cutting
    needle
  PrecisionGlide needle
  Presbyterian Hospital
    ventricular needle
  Pricker needle
  probe needle
  ProBloc insulated regional
    block needle
  Promex biopsy needle
  prostatic biopsy needle
  Protect Point needle
  pudendal block anesthesia
    needle
  pudendal needle
  Pulec needle
  puncture needle
  puncture-tip needle
  Punctur-Guard needle
  Quantico needle
  quartz needle
  Quick-Core biopsy needle

needle (*continued*)

Quincke spinal needle
Quincke-Babcock needle
Quincke-point spinal needle
radium needle
Radpour needle
Ranfac soft-tissue needle
Rashkind septostomy needle
razor-tip needle
RCB biopsy needle
rectal injection needle
rectal needle
renal needle
retrobulbar needle
retrobulbar prosthesis needle
Retter aneurysm needle
Reverdin suturing needle
reverse-cutting needle
Rhoton straight point needle
rib needle
ribbon gut needle
Rica aneurysm needle
Rica cerebral angiography
    puncture needle
Rica suturing needle
Rider-Moeller needle
Riedel corneal needle
Riley arterial needle
Ring drainage catheter needle
Riza-Ribe grasping needle
Robb needle
Roberts needle
Robinson-Smith needle
Rochester aortic vent needle
Rochester-Meeker needle
Rolf lance needle
root needle
Rosen needle
Rosenthal aspiration needle
Roser needle
Ross needle
Rotex II biopsy needle
Rotex needle
round body needle
round needle
Rubin needle
Rubin-Arnold needle
Ruskin antral needle
Ruskin antral trocar needle
Ruskin sphenopalatine
    ganglion needle
Rutner biopsy needle

needle (*continued*)

Rycroft needle
Sabreloc needle
Sachs needle
SafeTap tapered spinal needle
Safety AV fistula needle
Sahli needle
Salah sternal needle
Salah sternal puncture needle
SampleMaster biopsy needle
Sanders-Brown needle
Sanders-Brown-Shaw
    aneurysm needle
Sato cataract needle
Saunders cataract needle
Saunders-Paparella needle
Savariaud-Reverdin needle
Scabbard needle
scalp vein needle
scalpene needle
Schanz needle
Schecter-Bryant aortic vent
    needle
Scheer needle
Scheie cataract needle
Scheie cataract-aspirating
    needle
Schmieden needle
Schmieden-Dick needle
Schuknecht needle
Schutt needle
scleral spatula needle
sclerostomy needle
sclerotherapy needle
Scoville ventricular needle
screw-tipped intraosseous
    needle
Sedan-Nashold needle
Seirin acupuncture needle
Seldinger arterial needle
Seldinger gastrostomy needle
self-aspirating cut-biopsy
    needle
septal needle
Septoject needle
Seraflo AV fistular needle
seton needle
Seven-Star acupuncture
    needle
Shambaugh palpating needle
Sharpoint Ultra-Guide
    ophthalmic needle

needle (*continued*)

  shattering needle
  Sheldon-Spatz vertebral
    arteriogram needle
  Sheldon-Swann needle
  Shirodkar aneurysm needle
  Shirodkar cervical needle
  short needle
  sialography needle
  side-cutting spatulated needle
  side-flattened needle
  sidewall holed needle
  silver needle
  Silverman biopsy needle
  Silverman-Boeker needle
  Simcoe anterior chamber
    receiving needle
  Simcoe aspirating needle
  Simcoe irrigating-positioning
    needle
  Simcoe suture needle
  Simmonds cricothyrotomy
    needle
  Sims abdominal needle
  Singer needle
  SITE I&A needle
  SITE macrobore plus needle
  SITE phaco I&A needle
  ski needle
  skinny Chiba needle
  skinny needle
  Sklar ligature needle
  slotted needle
  Sluder needle
  small-bore needle
  small-caliber needle
  SmallPort needle
  SmartNeedle
  SMIC suture needle
  Smiley-Williams arteriography
    needle
  Solitaire needle
  SonoVu US aspiration needle
  spatula-split needle
  spatulated half-circle needle
  sphenopalatine ganglion
    needle
  sphenopalatine needle
  spinal needle
  Spinelli biopsy needle
  spoon needle
  spring-eye needle

needle (*continued*)

  spring-hook wire needle
  Sprotte epidural needle
  Sprotte spinal needle
  spud needle
  stab needle
  Stallerpointe needle
  Stamey needle
  standard needle
  stapes needle
  staphylorrhaphy needle
  steel-winged butterfly
    needle
  Steis bone marrow transplant
    needle
  StereoGuide needle
  stereotactic breast biopsy
    needle
  sternal needle
  sternal puncture needle
  Stifcore aspiration needle
  Stifcore transbronchial
    aspiration needle
  Stille-Mayo-Hegar needle
  Stille-Seldinger needle
  Stimuplex block needle
  Stocker cyclodiathermy
    puncture needle
  stop needle
  Storz aspiration biopsy needle
  Storz flexible injection needle
  strabismus needle
  straight needle
  straight suture needle
  straight suturing needle
  straight-point needle
  Strasbourg-Fairfax in vitro
    fertilization needle
  Straus curved retrobulbar
    needle
  Strauss needle
  stress on needle
  Sturmdorf cervical needle
  Sturmdorf pedicle needle
  Stylus suture needle
  Subco needle
  subconjunctival needle
  suction biopsy needle
  Sudan needle
  Sulze diamond-point needle
  SuperGlide needle
  Sure-Cut biopsy needle

needle (*continued*)

Suresharp blood collecting needle
Suresharp dental needle
Sur-Fast needle
surgeon's regular needle
surgical needle
Surgicraft suture needle
Surgimedics air aspirator needle
Surgineedle pneumoperitoneum needle
Sutton biopsy needle
suture needle
suture-release needle
suturing needle
swaged arthroscopic needles
swaged needle
swaged-on needle
Swann needle
Swann-Sheldon needle
Swedgeon already-threaded needle
Symmonds needle
Szabo-Berci needle
taper needle
Tapercut needle
tapered needle
taper-point needle
taper-point suture needle
tattooing needle
Tauber needle
tax double needle
Teflon glycerin-mixture injection needle
Teflon needle
Teflon-coated hollow-bore needle
Teflon-covered needle
Tek-Pro needle
TEMNO biopsy needle
tendon needle
Terry-Mayo needle
Terumo AV fistula needle
Terumo dental needle
Terumo hypodermic needle
Tew needle
thermistor needle
THI needle
thin acupuncture needle
thin-walled needle

needle (*continued*)

Thomas needle
thoracentesis needle
Thornton needle
threaded eye needle
through-the-scope injection needle
Ticsay transpubic needle
tie-on needle
tissue desiccation needle
titanium alloy needle
titanium needle
Titus venoclysis needle
Tocantins bone marrow biopsy needle
Todd eye cautery needle
tonsillar needle
tonsillar suture needle
Torrington French spring needle
transaxillary needle
translocation needle
transpubic needle
Travenol biopsy needle
Travert needle
triple-lumen needle
trocar needle
Troutman needle
Tru Taper Ethalloy needle
Tru-Cut biopsy needle
Tru-Cut liver biopsy needle
Trupp ventricular needle
tungsten microdissection needle
Tuohy aortography needle
Tuohy lumbar aortography needle
Tuohy spinal needle
Turkel liver biopsy needle
Turkey sternal needle
Turner biopsy needle
Turner-Warwick urethroplasty needle
Tworek bone marrow-aspirating needle
Ultra-Core biopsy needle
ultrasonic cataract-removal lancet needle
Ultra-vue amniocentesis needle
UMI needle
Unimar J needle

needle (*continued*)
  University of Illinois biopsy needle
  University of Illinois marrow needle
  University of Illinois sternal puncture needle
  Updegraff cleft palate needle
  Updegraff staphylorrhaphy needle
  urethroplasty needle
  uterine needle
  V. Mueller paracervical nerve block needle
  V. Mueller pudendal nerve block needle
  Vacutainer needle
  vacuuming needle
  Variject needle
  Vastack needle
  Veenema-Gusberg prostatic biopsy needle
  Veirs needle
  Venaflo needle
  Venflon needle
  venipuncture needle
  venous needle
  venting aortic Bengash needle
  ventricular needle
  Verbrugge needle
  Veress pneumoperitoneum needle
  Veress spring-loaded laparoscopy needle
  Veress-Frangenheim needle
  Vicat needle
  Vim needle
  Vim-Silverman biopsy needle
  Virginia needle
  Visi-Black surgical needle
  Visitec retrobulbar needle
  vitreous transplant needle
  vitreous-aspirating needle
  Vogt-Barraquer corneal needle
  von Graefe knife needle
  Voorhees needle
  Walker tonsillar needle
  Wang needle
  Wangensteen intestinal needle
  Wannagat injection needle
  Ward French-eye needle
  Ward-French needle

needle (*continued*)
  Waterfield needle
  Watson-Williams needle
  wedge-line needle
  Weeks needle
  Weiss needle
  Welsh olive-tipped needles
  Wergeland double needle
  Wertheim-Navratil needle
  Westcott biopsy needle
  Westerman-Jensen needle
  whirlybird needle
  Whitacre spinal needle
  Wiener eye needle
  Williams cystoscopic needle
  Williamson biopsy needle
  Wilson-Cook electrode needle
  winged steel needle
  Wolf antral needle
  Wolf-Veress needle
  Wood aortography needle
  Wooten eye needle
  Worst needle
  Wright fascia needle
  Wright ophthalmic needle
  Wright ptosis needle
  Wright-Crawford needle
  Yale Luer-Lok needle
  Yang needle
  Yankauer septal needle
  Yankauer suture needle
  Yueh centesis catheter needle
  Zavala lung biopsy needle
  Ziegler iris needle
  Zoellner needle
needle ablation
needle arthroscopy
needle aspiration
needle aspiration biopsy
needle biopsy
needle catheter jejunostomy
needle core biopsy
needle count
needle dissector
needle driver
needle electrode
needle endosseous implant
needle endosteal implant
needle extension
needle forceps
needle guide (*see* guide)
needle holder (*see* holder)

needle holder clamp
needle holder forceps
needle hydrophone
needle laparoscopy
needle localization
needle localization breast
    biopsy
needle magnet
needle marks
needle point suture passer/
    incision closure guide
needle probe
needle puncture
needle site
needle spatula
needle spoon
needle spud
needle stick
needle suspension procedure
needle thermocouple
needle thoracentesis procedure
needle thoracentesis technique
needle tip catheter
needle tract implantation
Needle-Ease device
needle-holder forceps
needle-knife
    McCaslin needle-knife
    Ziegler eye needle-knife
    Ziegler needle-knife
needle-knife fistulotome
needle-knife papillotome
needle-knife sphincterotome
needle-knife technique
needle-knife wire
Needleless Suture
needle-localized open biopsy
    (NLOB)
needle-nose pliers
needle-nose rongeur
needle-nose vise-grip pliers
needle-nosed pliers
needlepoint cautery
needlepoint electrocautery
Needle-Pro needle protection
    device
needles-and-pins sensation
needlescope device
Needlescoper endoscope
needlescopic laparoscopic
    cholecystectomy
needlestick injury

needle-through-needle single
    interspace technique
needle-tipped sphincterotome
needling of cataract
needling of lens
Neef hammer
Neer acromioplasty
Neer capsular shift procedure
Neer classification of shoulder
    fractures
Neer femur fracture
    classification
Neer hemiarthroplasty
Neer I shoulder joint prosthesis
Neer II proximal humerus
    prosthesis
Neer II shoulder joint prosthesis
Neer II shoulder prosthesis
Neer II shoulder replacement
Neer II total shoulder system
    implant
Neer modification
Neer open reduction
Neer posterior shoulder
    reconstruction
Neer resection of acromion
Neer shoulder fracture
    classification
Neer shoulder prosthesis
Neer shoulder replacement
    prosthesis
Neer unconstrained shoulder
    arthroplasty
Neer-Horowitz humeral fracture
    classification
Neff meniscus knife
Neff percutaneous access set
negative appendectomy
negative aspiration
negative biopsy
negative bone scan
negative breast biopsy
negative control enzyme
    induction
negative culture
negative effect
negative eyepiece
negative findings
negative laparotomy
negative margin
negative pressure
negative pressure device

negative pressure therapy
negative reaction
negative results
neglected rupture
negligible blood loss
Negus bronchoscope
Negus laryngoscope
Negus mouth gag
Negus pusher
Negus telescope
Negus tonsillar forceps
Negus-Broyles bronchoscope
Negus-Green forceps
Neher operation
Nehra-Mach operation
Neibauer hand
Neibauer hand prosthesis
Neibauer prosthesis
Neibauer-Cutter operation
Neibauer-Glynn procedure
Neibauer-King open reduction
Neibauer-Kleinert microscope
Neill-Mooser body
Neil-Moore meatotomy
    electrode
Neil-Moore perforator drill
Neiman nasal splint
Neisser syringe
Neitz CT-R cataract camera
Neivert chisel
Neivert dissection
Neivert dissector
Neivert double-ended retractor
Neivert hook
Neivert knife
Neivert knife guide
Neivert knife guide and
    retractor
Neivert nasal polyp hook
Neivert needle holder
Neivert osteotome
Neivert polyp hook
Neivert retractor
Neivert rocking gouge
Neivert snare
Neivert tonsillar knife
Neivert tonsillar snare
Neivert-Anderson osteotome
Neivert-Eves tonsillar snare
Neivert-Eves tonsillar wire
Neivert-Neivert needle holder
Nek-L-O hot & cold pillow

Nek-L-O orthopedic
    support/comfort pillow
Nelaton ankle dislocation
Nelaton bullet probe
Nelaton catheter
Nelaton dislocation
Nelaton dislocation of ankle
Nelaton fold
Nelaton line
Nelaton operation
Nelaton rubber tube drain
Nelaton sphincter
Nelaton urethral catheter
Nellcor N10 ETCO$_2$/SpO$_2$
    monitor
Nellcor N-499 fetal oxygen
    saturation monitor
Nellcor N-series pulse oximeter
Nellcor Symphony blood
    Nellcor Symphony N-3000
    pulse oximeter
Nellcor Symphony N-3100
    noninvasive blood pressure
    monitor
Nelson empyema trocar
Nelson first-rib raspatory
Nelson general operating scissors
Nelson ligature needle
Nelson lobectomy scissors
Nelson lung forceps
Nelson lung-dissecting forceps
Nelson lung-dissecting scissors
Nelson needle
Nelson retractor
Nelson rib self-retaining retractor
Nelson rib spreader
Nelson rib stripper
Nelson rocker knife
Nelson scissors
Nelson self-retaining rib retractor
Nelson thoracic scissors
Nelson thoracic trocar
Nelson tissue forceps
Nelson trocar
Nelson uterine scissors
Nelson-Bethune rib shears
Nelson-Bethune shears
Nelson-Martin forceps
Nelson-Metzenbaum scissors
Nelson-Patterson empyema trocar
Nelson-Roberts stripper
Nelson Vital dissecting scissors

Nembutal anesthetic agent
Nemdi tweezer epilation device
neoadjuvant therapy
neoadjuvant total androgen
    ablation
neocartilage formation
neoclitoris (*pl.* neoclitorides)
neoclitoroplasty
neo-coagulator (*see.* coagulator)
    Codman-Shurtleff neo-
    coagulator
neocystostomy
NeoDerm dressing
neodermis
NeoDura matrix
neodymium laser
neodymium:yttrium-aluminum-
    garnet (Nd:YAG) laser
neodymium:yttrium-lithium-
    fluoride photodisruptive
    laser
neodymium:yytrium-aluminum-
    garnet
neodymium-doped yttrium-
    aluminum-garnet (Nd:YAG)
    laser
Neo-Fit neonatal endotracheal
    tube grip
Neo-Fit neonatal endotracheal
    tube holder
Neoflex bendable knife
Neoflex electrocautery knife
neoglottic reconstruction
Neoguard percussor
neointima formation
NeoKnife cautery
Neoknife electrosurgical
    instrument
Neolens lens
Neolyte laser indirect
    ophthalmoscope
Neomed cautery
Neomed electrocautery
neonatal anesthesia
neonatal death
neonatal internal jugular
    puncture kit
neonatal intracranial hemorrhage
neonatal intraventricular
    hemorrhage
neonatal line
neonatal monitor

neonatal pulmonary
    transplantation
neonatal scissors
neonatal sternal retractor
neonatal vascular clamp
neonatal vascular forceps
neonate examination
neonate ventilation
NeoNaze nasal function
    restoration device
neo-omphaloplasty
neoplasia
neoplasm
neoplasm metastasis
neoplastic disease
neoplastic disorder
neoplastic fracture
neoplastic growth
neoplastic hyperplasia
neoplastic lesion
neoplastic polyp
neoplastic port site implant
neoplasty
Neoplex catheter
Neoplush foam
neoprene ankle support
neoprene back support
neoprene dressing
neoprene elbow sleeve
neoprene glove
neoprene hinged-knee brace
neoprene orthosis
neoprene Osgood-Schlatter knee
    brace
neoprene sleeves
neoprene splint
neoprene support
neoprene wrist brace
neoprene wrist orthosis
NeoProbe gamma detection probe
NeoProbe portable radioisotope
    detector
Neos pacemaker
neosalpingostomy
Neo-Sert umbilical vessel catheter
Neo-Sert umbilical vessel
    catheter insertion set
Neosonic piezo ultrasonic unit
Neosono MC apex locator
Neostar Pheres-Flow triple-
    lumen catheter
neostigmine

neostomy
NeoTect imaging agent
Neo-Therm neonatal skin
    temperature probe
Neo-trak 515A neonatal monitor
Neotrode II neonatal electrode
neo-ureterocystotomy
neovaginal cavity
neovaginal introitus
neovascular bundle
neovascular glaucoma
neovascular membrane
neovascularization
Neovision micro mirror
NeoVO$_2$R volume control
    resuscitator
nephralgia
nephrectomy
    abdominal nephrectomy
    anterior nephrectomy
    hand-assisted laparoscopic
        live-donor nephrectomy
    laparoscopic donor
        nephrectomy (LDN)
    laparoscopic-assisted living
        donor nephrectomy
    laser partial nephrectomy
    morcellement nephrectomy
    paraperitoneal nephrectomy
    posterior nephrectomy
    subcapsular nephrectomy
    transperitoneal nephrectomy
    transplant nephrectomy
nephritic calculus
nephritic syndrome
nephritis
nephroarteriolar sclerosis
nephroblastoma
nephrocapsectomy
nephrocolic ligament
nephrocolopexy
nephrocystanastomosis
nephrogenic ascites
nephrogenic tissue
nephrogram
nephrography
nephrolithiasis
nephrolithotomy
nephrolithotomy forceps
nephrolithotripsy
nephrolumbar ganglion
nephrolysis

nephroma
NephroMax catheter set
nephronic loop
nephron-sparing surgery
nephro-omentopexy
nephropathic cardiopathy
nephropathy
nephropexy
nephrophthisis
nephroplasty
nephroptosis
nephropyelolithotomy
nephropyeloplasty
nephropyeloureterostomy
nephrorrhagia
nephrorrhaphy
nephrosclerosis
nephroscope
nephroscopy
nephrosis
nephrosonephritis
nephrosplenopexy
Nephross dialyzer
nephrostomy
nephrostomy catheter
nephrostomy clamp
nephrostomy drainage
nephrostomy hook
nephrostomy speculum
nephrostomy tube
nephrotic edema
nephrotic syndrome
nephrotome plate
nephrotomic cavity
nephrotomic cavity occlusal cavity
nephrotomogram
nephrotomography
nephrotomy
nephrotoxic
nephrotoxicity
nephroureterectomy
nephroureterocystectomy
NeProbe radioactivity detector
NER (no evidence of recurrence)
NERD (no evidence of recurrent
    disease)
nerve
    3rd cranial nerve
    4th cranial nerve
    5th cranial nerve
    6th cranial nerve (cranial
        nerve 6)

nerve (*continued*)

7th cranial nerve (7)
8th cranial nerve
9th cranial nerve
10th cranial nerve
11th cranial nerve
12th cranial nerve
3rd occipital nerve
abdominopelvic splanchnic
  nerve
abducens nerve
  (cranial nerve 6)
abducent nerve
accessory nerve (cranial
  nerve 11)
accessory nerves
accessory phrenic nerves
accompanying artery of
  sciatic nerve
accompanying vein of
  hypoglossal nerve
acoustic nerve
acousticofacial nerve
afferent nerve
alveolar nerve
ampullary nerve
anastomosis of nerves
anococcygeal nerves
anterior alveolar branch of
  maxillary nerve
anterior ampullary nerve
anterior auricular nerve
anterior ethmoidal branch of
  ophthalmic nerve
anterior ethmoidal nerve
anterior interosseous
  nerve
anterior labial nerve
anterior palatine nerve
anterior scrotal nerves
area of facial nerve
Arnold nerve
auditory nerve
auricular nerve
auriculotemporal nerve
avulsion of nerve
avulsion of optic nerve
axillary nerve
bath for the nerve
blunting of nerve
Bock nerve
brachial plexus nerve

nerve (*continued*)

Brailey stretching of
  supratrochlear nerve
buccal nerve
buccinator nerve
canals for lesser palatine
  nerves
cardiac nerves
caroticotympanic nerves
carotid nerve
carotid sinus nerve
celiac nerves
centripetal nerve
cerebral nerves
cervical branch of facial nerve
cervical nerves
cervical sympathetic nerve
chorda tympani nerve
ciliary nerves
circumflex nerve
clunial nerves
coccygeal nerve
cochlear nerve
common fibular nerve
common palmar digital nerves
common peroneal nerve
common plantar digital nerves
compressed nerves
cranial nerves (1-12, also I-XII)
crushing of nerve
cubital nerve
cupping of nerve
cutaneous nerve
deep nerve
deep peroneal nerve
deep petrosal nerve
deep temporal nerve
dental nerve
depressor nerve
derangement of vasomotor
  nerves
diaphragmatic nerve
digastric nerve
digital nerve
dorsal antebrachial cutaneous
  nerve
dorsal branch of nerve
dorsal digital nerves
dorsal nerve
dorsal scapular nerve
dorsal sensory branch of
  ulnar nerve

nerve (*continued*)
  efferent nerve
  esodic nerve
  ethmoidal nerve
  external carotid nerve
  external genu of facial nerve
  external nasal nerve
  external popliteal nerve
  external pterygoid nerve
  external spermatic nerve
  extrinsic nerve
  facial nerve (cranial nerve 7)
  femoral cutaneous nerve
  femoral nerve
  fibroma of nerve
  fibular nerve
  fold of laryngeal nerve
  foramina for olfactory nerves
  frontal nerve
  frontalis nerve
  gangliated nerve
  ganglion of nerve
  geniculum of facial nerve
  genitofemoral nerve
  glossopharyngeal nerve
    (cranial nerve 9)
  gluteal nerve
  Goldman nerve
  graft of nerve
  great auricular nerve
  greater occipital nerve
  greater palatine nerve
  greater petrosal nerve
  greater splanchnic nerve
  greater superficial nerve
  greater superficial petrosal
    nerve
  groove for nasal nerve
  groove for radial nerve
  hemorrhoidal nerves
  hiatus of canal for greater
    petrosal nerve
  hiatus of canal for lesser
    petrosal nerve
  hypogastric branch of
    iliohypogastric nerve
  hypogastric nerve
  hypoglossal nerve (cranial
    nerve 12)
  Hyrtl nerve
  iliohypogastric nerve
  ilioinguinal nerve

nerve (*continued*)
  inferior alveolar nerve (IAN)
  inferior cardiac cervical nerve
  inferior clunial nerves
  inferior ganglion of
    glossopharyngeal nerve
  inferior gluteal nerve
  inferior laryngeal nerve
  inferior nasal nerve
  inferior nerve
  inferior rectal nerves
  infraoccipital nerve
  infraorbital branch of
    maxillary nerve
  infraorbital nerve
  infratrochlear branch of
    ophthalmic nerve
  infratrochlear nerve
  inguinal nerve
  intercostal nerves
  intercostobrachial nerves
  intermediate dorsal cutaneous
    nerve
  intermediate nerve
  intermediate supraclavicular
    nerves
  internal carotid nerve
  internal rectal nerve
  interosseous anterior nerve
  interosseous cruris nerve
  interosseous dorsalis nerve
  interosseous nerve
  interosseous posterior nerve
  intratrochlear nerve
  ischiadic nerve
  Jacobson nerve
  Jannetta vascular
    decompression of 5th nerve
  jugular ganglion of
    glossopharyngeal nerve
  jugular nerve
  labial nerves
  labioglossopharyngeal nerve
  lacrimal nerve
  Lancisi nerve
  Langley nerves
  laryngeal nerve
  Latarjet nerve
  lateral ampullary nerve
  lateral antebrachial cutaneous
    nerve
  lateral cutaneous nerve

nerve (*continued*)

lateral dorsal cutaneous nerve
lateral femoral cutaneous nerve
lateral plantar nerve
lateral pterygoid nerve
lateral supraclavicular nerves
left hypogastric nerve
lesser occipital nerve
lesser palatine nerves
lesser petrosal nerve
lesser superficial petrosal nerve
levator nerve
lingual nerve
long ciliary nerves
long thoracic nerve
longitudinal nerves
lower ganglion of glossopharyngeal nerve
lowest splanchnic nerve
lumbar nerves
lumbar splanchnic nerves
lumboinguinal nerve
Luschka nerve
mandibular nerve
marginal mandibular nerve
masseteric nerve
maxillary nerve
medial antebrachial cutaneous nerve
medial brachial cutaneous nerve
medial cutaneous nerve
medial dorsal cutaneous nerve
medial nerve
medial plantar nerve
medial pterygoid nerve
medial supraclavicular nerves
median nerve
medullated nerve
meningeal nerve
mental nerve
middle cardiac cervical nerve
middle clunial nerves
mixed nerve
monofascicular nerve
motor nerve
motor root of trigeminal nerve
musculocutaneous nerve
musculospiral nerve
mylohyoid nerve
myotome distribution of nerve
nasal nerve

nerve (*continued*)

nasociliary branches of ophthalmic nerve
nasociliary nerve
nasopalatine nerve
obturator nerve
occipital nerve
ocular nerve
oculomotor nerve (cranial nerve 3)
olfactory nerve (cranial nerve 1)
ophthalmic nerve
ophthalmic recurrent nerve
optic nerve (cranial nerve 2)
palatine nerve
palmar digital nerves
parasympathetic nerve
pectoral nerve
pelvic splanchnic nerves
perineal nerve
peripheral nerves
peroneal nerve
petrosal nerve
phrenic nerve
phrenicoabdominal nerves
pinched nerve
plantar digital nerves
plantar nerve
pneumogastric nerve
popliteal nerve
posterior ampullary nerve
posterior auricular nerve
posterior cutaneous femoral nerve
posterior cutaneous nerve
posterior ethmoidal nerve
posterior interosseous nerve
posterior labial nerves
posterior scrotal nerves
posterior tibial nerve
proper palmar digital nerves
proper plantar digital nerves
pterygoid nerve
pterygopalatine nerves
pudendal nerve
radial nerve
rectal nerves
recurrent laryngeal nerves
recurrent nerve
right hypogastric nerve
saccular nerve

nerve (*continued*)
 sacral nerves
 sacral splanchnic nerves
 saphenous nerve
 Scarpa nerve
 sciatic nerve
 scrotal nerves
 secretory nerve
 sensory branch of radial nerve
  (SBRN)
 sensory nerve
 sensory root of trigeminal
  nerve
 short ciliary nerves
 sinus nerve
 sinu-vertebral nerve
 small sciatic nerve
 somatic nerves
 spermatic nerve
 sphenopalatine nerves
 spinal accessory nerve
 spinal nerves
 splanchnic nerve
 stapedial nerve
 stimulation of peripheral
  nerves
 stretching of nerve
 stylohyoid nerve
 stylopharyngeal nerve
 subclavian nerve
 subcostal nerve
 subcutaneous temporal nerves
 sublingual nerve
 submaxillary nerves
 suboccipital nerve
 subscapular nerves
 sudomotor nerves
 sulcus for greater palatine
  nerve
 superficial fibular nerve
 superficial middle petrosal
  nerve
 superficial nerve
 superficial peroneal nerve
 superficial radial nerve
 superior alveolar nerve
 superior ampullar nerve
 superior cardiac cervical nerve
 superior cervical cardiac nerve
 superior clunial nerves
 superior ganglion of
  glossopharyngeal nerve

nerve (*continued*)
 superior gluteal nerve
 superior laryngeal nerve
 supraclavicular nerves
 supraorbital nerve
 suprascapular nerve
 supratrochlear nerve
 supreme cardiac nerves
 sural nerve
 sympathetic nerve
 temporal facial nerve
 temporal nerves
 tentorial nerve
 terminal nerves
 thoracic cardiac nerve
 thoracic nerve
 thoracodorsal nerve
 tibial nerve
 Tiedemann nerve
 tonsillar nerves
 transverse cervical nerve
 transverse nerve
 trigeminal nerve (cranial
  nerve 5)
 trochlear nerve (cranial
  nerve 4)
 trophic nerve
 tympanic nerve
 ulnar nerve
 uterine nerve
 utricular nerve
 utriculoampullar nerve
 vagal accessory nerve
 vagal nerve
 vaginal nerves
 vagus nerve (cranial nerve 10)
 vascular circle of optic nerve
 vascular nerve
 vasoconstrictor nerve
 vasosensory nerve
 vena comitans of hypoglossal
  nerve
 vertebral nerve
 vestibular nerve
 vestibulocochlear nerve
  (cranial nerve 8)
 vidian nerve
 Wrisberg nerve
 zygomatic nerve
 zygomaticofacial nerve
 zygomaticotemporal nerve
nerve accommodation

nerve action potential
nerve activity
nerve anastomosis
nerve approximator
nerve avulsion
nerve biopsy
nerve block
nerve block anesthesia
nerve block infusion
Nerve Block Infusion Kit
nerve branch
nerve bundle
nerve cable graft
nerve cell body
nerve cell fibers
nerve center
nerve coaptation
nerve compression
nerve compression anesthesia
nerve compression-degeneration
    syndrome
nerve crush injury
nerve cuff
nerve damage
nerve deafness
nerve decompression
nerve deficit
nerve dissection
nerve distribution
nerve endings
nerve entrapment
nerve evulsion
nerve factor
nerve fascicle
Nerve Fiber Analyzer laser
    ophthalmoscope
nerve fiber bundle
nerve fiber bundle layer
nerve fibers
nerve force
nerve gap
nerve graft
nerve growth factor (NGF)
nerve holder
nerve hook
nerve impingement
nerve implantation
nerve impulse
nerve injury
nerve involvement
nerve locator
nerve loss

nerve mapping
nerve monitor
nerve of Grassi
nerve of Latarjet
nerve of pterygoid canal
nerve of Wrisberg
nerve protector
nerve pull hook
nerve receptors
nerve retractor
nerve root compression
nerve root injection
nerve root laminectomy dissector
nerve root retractor
nerve root sleeve injection
nerve rootlet ablation
nerve separator spatula
nerve sheath
nerve sign
nerve signal
nerve stimulant
nerve stimulation
nerve stimulator (*see also*
    stimulator)
nerve stimulator anesthetic
    technique
nerve suture technique
nerve sutures
nerve tabes
nerve tissue
nerve tumor
nerve-approximating clamp
nerve-blocking anesthesia
nerve-integrity monitor
NervePace nerve conduction
    monitor
NervePace nerve conduction
    testing machine
nerve-sparing dissection
nervous damage
nervous system involvement
nervous tissues
Nesacaine-CE anesthetic agent
Nesbit cystoscope
Nesbit electrode
Nesbit electrotome
Nesbit hemostatic bag
Nesbit operation
Nesbit plication
Nesbit resection of prostate
Nesbit snare
Nesbit tonsillar snare

Nesbit tuck procedure
Nesta stitch sutures
nested nails
nested trocar
Nestor guiding catheter
net shunt
Netra intravascular ultrasound
Netterville double-ended
    elevator
Nettleship canaliculus dilator
Nettleship iris repositor
Nettleship-Wilder lacrimal
    dilator
Neubauer artery
Neubauer cannula
Neubauer foreign body forceps
Neubauer lancet cannula
Neubauer scissors
Neubauer vitreous
    microextractor forceps
Neubeiser adjustable forearm
    splint
Neuber bone tube
Neuber drainage tube
Neuber operation
Neubuser tube-seizing forceps
Neufeld cast
Neufeld device
Neufeld driver
Neufeld femoral nail plate
Neufeld nail
Neufeld pin
Neufeld plate
Neufeld rolling traction
Neufeld screw
Neufeld traction
Neufeld tractor
NeuFlex metacarpophalangeal
    joint implant
Neugebauer-LeFort procedure
Neuhann cystotome
Neumann calipers block
Neumann cell
Neumann depth gauge
Neumann double corneal marker
Neumann razor blade fragment
    holder
Neumann scissors
Neumann-Shepard corneal
    marker
Neurain drill
Neurairtome drill

neural apraxia
neural arch
neural arch defect
neural archresection technique
neural atrophy
neural axis vascular malformation
neural canal
neural crest cell
neural crest malformation
neural crest mesenchymal
    connective tissue
    framework
neural deafness
neural discharge
neural dissector
neural element
neural filament
neural fold
neural foramen
neural impulse
neural lesion
neural parenchyma
neural pathway
neural prosthesis
neural retinal layer
neural stimuli
neural transmitter
neural tube defect
neuralgia
neuralgia facialis vera
neurapraxic lesion
neuraxial neurolytic block
neuraxis irradiation
neurectasia
neurectomy
    Abbe neurectomy
    Cotte neurectomy
    cranial neurectomy
    gastric neurectomy
    middle fossa vestibular
        neurectomy
    opticociliary neurectomy
    presacral neurectomy
    Selig intrapelvic obturator
        neurectomy
    spinal neurectomy
    splanchnic neurectomy
neurenteric cyst
neurexeresis
neurilemma
neurilemmatosis
neurinoma

neuritis
Neuro N-50 lesion generator
Neuro Stim 2000 MK1
    stimulator
neuroablative technique
neuroacanthocytosis
Neuro-Aide testing device
neuroanastomosis
NeuroAvitene applicator
neuroblastoma
neurocentral joint
neurocentral suture
neurocirculatory asthenia
NeuroCol neurosurgical sponge
NeuroControl Freehand implant
neurocutaneous flap
neurocutaneous island flap
neurocutaneous syndrome
NeuroCybernetic prosthesis
neurodiagnostic evaluation
neurodiagnostic scanner
neurodissector (*see also* dissector)
    Maroon-Jannetta
        neurodissector
    Penfield neurodissector
    Rhoton neurodissector
    Schmieden-Taylor
        neurodissector
    Tonnis-Adson neurodissector
NeuroDrape surgical drape
neuroectodermal tumor
NeuroEdge neurovascular
    catheter
neuroeffector junction
neuroelectric event
neuroemergency
neuroencephalomyelopathy
neuroendocrine cancer
neuroendocrine carcinoma
neuroendocrine marker
neuroendocrine skin carcinoma
neuroendocrine tumor of larynx
neuroepithelial cells
neuroepithelioma
neurofibrillary tangles
neurofibroma
neurofibroma of larynx
neurofibromatosis
neuroforamina
neurogenic bladder
neurogenic blepharoptosis
neurogenic dysarthria

neurogenic dysphagia
neurogenic factor
neurogenic fracture
neurogenic pulmonary edema
    (NPE)
neuroglia
neurography needle
Neuroguard transcranial Doppler
Neuroguide monitor
Neuroguide optical handpiece
Neuroguide peel-away catheter
    introducer
Neuroguide suction-irrigation
    adapter
Neuroguide Visicath viewing
    catheter
neurohypophysectomy
Neurolase microsurgical CO_2
    laser
neurolemma
neurolemmoma
neuroleptanalgesia anesthesia
neuroleptanalgesia anesthetic
    technique
neuroleptic malignant syndrome
    (NMS)
neuroleptic medication
neurologic complication
neurologic disease
neurologic disorder
neurologic evaluation
neurologic examination
neurologic injury
neurologic surgery
neurological assessment
neurological complications
neurological defect
neurological deficit
neurological disease
neurological disorder
neurological disturbance
neurological dysfunction
neurological emergency
neurological examination
neurological function
neurological impairment
neurological instability
Neurological Institute elevator
Neurological Institute periosteal
    elevator
neurological nerve conduction
    velocity examination

neurological percussion hammer
neurological percussor
neurological scissors
neurological sign
neurological sponge
neurological surgery
neurological survey
neurological sutures
neurological symptoms
neurological syndrome
neurological trauma
neurological tuning fork
neurologically intact
neurolysis
neurolytic celiac plexus block (NCPB)
neuroma excision
neuroma relocation surgery
NeuroMate sterotactic robot
Neuromed Octrode implantable pain management device
Neuromeet nerve approximator
Neuromeet nerve ending approximator
Neuromeet soft tissue approximator
Neuromeet universal soft tissue approximator
neurometer device
neuromotor dysfunction
neuromuscular block
neuromuscular blockade (NMB)
neuromuscular blockade monitoring
neuromuscular blocking agents
neuromuscular choristoma
neuromuscular control
neuromuscular disorder
neuromuscular electrical stimulator (NMES)
neuromuscular firing
neuromuscular stimulator
neuromuscular junction
neuromuscular pedicle graft
neuromuscular system electric induction
neuromyography
neuron
neuronal cell line
neuronal circuit
neuronal membrane

neuro-ophthalmologic examination
Neuropath biofeedback device
neuropathic bladder
neuropathic foot
neuropathic fracture
neuropathic incontinence
neuropathy
Neuropedic multidensity mattress
Neuropedic neurolon mattress
neuropeptide marker
Neuroperfusion pump
neurophysiologic examination
neuroplasty
neuroradiography
neuroradiologic evaluation
neuroretinopathy
neurorrhaphy
neurosarcocleisis
NeuroScan 3D imager
NeuroSector ultrasound
neurosensorial free medial plantar flap
neurosensory cells
neurosensory flap
neurosensory island flap
Neurosign 100 nerve monitor
NeuroStim TENS unit
neurostimulating procedure
neurostimulation
neurosurgery
neurosurgical anesthesia
neurosurgical approach
neurosurgical bur
neurosurgical connector
neurosurgical dissector
neurosurgical dressing forceps
neurosurgical elevator
neurosurgical forceps
neurosurgical head holder
neurosurgical headrest
neurosurgical intervention
neurosurgical knife
neurosurgical ligature forceps
neurosurgical light
neurosurgical needle holder
neurosurgical pledget
neurosurgical procedure
neurosurgical suction forceps
neurosurgical sutures
neurosurgical suture needle

neurosurgical tissue forceps
neurosutures
neurotization
neurotmetic injury
neurotologic examination
neurotome
    Bradford enucleation
        neurotome
    enucleation neurotome
    Hall neurotome
neurotomy
    acoustic neurotomy
    glossopharyngeal neurotomy
    opticociliary neurotomy
    retrogasserian neurotomy
Neurotone biofeedback device
neurotonic reaction
neurotony
neurotoxic drug
Neuro-Trace instrument
neurotransmitters
neurotripsy
neurotropic atrophy
neurotropic environment
neurotropic melanoma
neurotropic virus
neurovascular anatomy
neurovascular bundle
neurovascular complication
neurovascular compression
    syndrome
neurovascular compromise
neurovascular cross
    compression (NVCC)
neurovascular forceps
neurovascular free flap
neurovascular infrahyoid island
    flap for tongue
    reconstruction
neurovascular island flap
neurovascular island graft
neurovascular island pedicle flap
neurovascular lesion
neurovascular scissors
neutral density filter
neutral electrode
neutral hip position
neutral hook
neutral occlusion
neutral point
neutral position
neutral position splint

neutral reaction
neutral spine position
Neutral WEDGE immobilizer
neutralization plate fixation
neutralizing
Neutrocim dental cement
neutron beam therapy
neutron capture therapy
neutron radiation
neutron therapy machine
neutropenic patient
neutrophilic infiltration
neutrophilic inflammation
neutrophilic leukocyte
Neuwirth-Palmer forceps
Nevada gonioscope
Neviaser acromioclavicular
    technique
Neviaser clavicle procedure
Neviaser operation
Neviaser-Wilson-Gardner
    technique
Neville ascending aortic air vent
    needle
Neville stent
Neville tracheal prosthesis
Neville tracheal reconstruction
    prosthesis
Neville tracheobronchial
    prosthesis
Neville-Barnes forceps
Nevins dressing forceps
Nevins tissue forceps
nevoid anomaly
nevoid basal cell carcinoma
nevoid basal cell carcinoma
    syndrome
nevoid hypermelanosis
nevoid lesion
nevoid pigmentation
nevoid telangiectasia
nevus (pl. nevi)
    agminated blue nevus
    atypical nevus
    balloon cell nevus
    basal cell nevus
    Becker nevus
    benign cellular blue nevus
    benign nevus
    blue nevus
    capillary nevus
    cellular blue nevus

nevus (*continued*)
  comedones epidermal nevus
  common blue nevus
  common nevus
  compound nevus
  congenital nevus
  connective tissue nevus
  epidermal nevus
  faun tail nevus
  flammeus nevus
  giant congenital nevus
  giant pigmented nevus
  hairy nevus
  halo blue nevus
  halo nevus
  inflammatory linear verrucous
    epidermal nevus (ILVEN)
  intradermal nevus
  Ito nevus
  junctional nevus
  malignant blue nevus
  marginal nevus
  melanocytic nevus
  pigmented nevus
  spider nevus
  Spitz nevus
  stocking nevus
  vascular nevus
nevus cell
nevus fibrosus
nevus vascularis
nevus verrucosus
Nevyas double sharp cystotome
Nevyas drape retractor
Nevyas lens forceps
New biopsy forceps
new bone formation
new dermis
New electrode
New England Baptist acetabular
    cup
New England Baptist
    arthroplasty
New England scoliosis brace
New forceps
new growth
new happy bur
New hook
New Jersey hemiarthroplasty
    prosthesis
New Jersey-LCS shoulder
    prosthesis

New Jersey-LCS total knee
    prosthesis
New Luer-type speaking tube
New MindSet toe splint
New oral needle
New Orleans corneal cutting
    block
New Orleans endarterectomy
    stripper
New Orleans endarterectomy
    stripper set
New Orleans Eye & Ear Hospital
    fixation forceps
New Orleans Eye & Ear forceps
New Orleans Eye & Ear loupe
New Orleans Eye & Ear fixation
    forceps
New Orleans lens
New Orleans lens loupe
New Orleans loupe
New Orleans needle holder
New Orleans stripper
New scissors
New speaking tube
New suture scissors
New tenaculum
New tissue forceps
New tracheal hook
New tracheal retractor
New tracheostomy hook
New tracheotomy hook
New tube
New ultra-thick powder-free
    latex surgical glove
New Weavenit Dacron
    prosthesis
New York erysiphake
New York Eye and Ear cannula
New York Eye and Ear fixation
    forceps
New York Eye and Ear forceps
New York Eye and Ear Hospital
    fixation forceps
New York glass suction tube
New York Heart Association
    classification of heart
    disease (I-IV)
New York Heart Association
    heart disease classification
New York Hospital electrode
New York Hospital retractor
New York Hospital suction tube

New York Orthopedic front-opening orthosis
New York speculum
New York University insert for orthosis
New Yorker guidewire
newborn (NB)
newborn anesthesia
newborn examination
newborn eyelid retractor
Newell lid retractor
Newell nucleus hook
Newhart incus hook
Newhart mallet
Newhart-Casselberry snare
Newhart-Smith cup
Newington orthosis
Newington plate
Newkirk mouth gag
New-Lambotte osteotome
NewLife oxygen concentrator
NewLife therapeutic mattress
Newman forceps
Newman hook
Newman knife
Newman needle
Newman plate
Newman procedure
Newman proctoscope
Newman radial neck and head fracture classification
Newman rectal injection needle
Newman tenaculum
Newman tenaculum forceps
Newman toenail plate
Newman uterine knife
Newman uterine tenaculum
Newman uterine tenaculum forceps
Newport cartilage gouge
Newport collar
Newport MC hip orthosis
Newport MC hip orthosis brace
Newport medical instrument
Newport total hip orthosis
Newport ventilator
Newton disk
Newton LLT guidewire
newtonian aberration
newtonian body
Newton-Morgan retractor
Newvicon camera tube

Newvicon vacuum chamber pickup tube
Newvicon vacuum tube
NewVues lens
Nexacryl tissue adhesive
NexGen complete knee replacement
NexGen complete knee replacement components
NexGen knee component
NexGen knee implant
NexGen offset stem extension
NexStent carotid stent
Nextep knee brace
Nexus linear ablation catheter
Nexus hip prosthesis
Nexus implant
nexus-type junction
Ney articulator
Nezhat irrigator
Nezhat suction-irrigator
Nezhat-Dorsey Trumpet Valve hydrodissector
ng (nanogram)
NG (nasogastric)
NG aspirate
NG feeding tube
NG strip nasal tube fastener
NG tube
Niagara temporary dialysis catheter
Niamtu video imaging
Nibbler device
Nibbler laparoscopic probe
Nibblit laparoscopic device
Niblitt dissector
N'ice Stretch night splint
Nichamin fixation ring
Nichamin hydrodissection cannula
Nichamin laser-assisted intrastromal keratomileusis (LASIK) irrigating cannula
Niche knife
Nichol clamp
Nichol procedure
Nichol rongeur
Nichol speculum
Nichol vaginal suspension procedure
Nicholas 5-in-1 reconstruction technique

Nicholas ligament technique
Nicholas medial compartment
   reconstruction
Nichols aortic clamp
Nichols infundibulectomy
   rongeur
Nichols procedure
Nichols sacrospinous fixation
Nichols-Deschamps-Navratil
   ligature needle
Nichols-Jehle coronary
   multihead catheter
nickel-and-dime lesion
Nickell cystoscope adapter
Nickel-Perry technique
nickel-titanium file
nicking
Nicks procedure
Nicola clamp
Nicola forceps
Nicola gouge
Nicola incision
Nicola microforceps
Nicola operation for shoulder
   dislocation
Nicola pituitary rongeur
Nicola rasp
Nicola raspatory
Nicola shoulder arthroplasty
Nicola shoulder procedure
Nicola tendon clamp
Nicolet Compass
   electromyography
   instrument
Nicolet Elite obstetrical Doppler
Nicolet Nerve Integrity Monitor
   (NIM-2)
Nicolet Pathfinder I recording
   device
Nicolet SM-300 stimulator
Nicolet/EME Muller and Moll
   probe fixation device
Nicoll bone graft
Nicoll cancellous bone graft
Nicoll cancellous insert graft
Nicoll classification
Nicoll fracture operation
Nicoll fracture repair procedure
Nicoll plate
Nicoll tendon prosthesis
nictitating membrane
Nida nicking operation

Nidek stereodisk camera
Nidek objective automatic
   refractor
Nidek excimer laser
Niebauer finger-joint
   replacement prosthesis
Niebauer implant
Niebauer trapeziometacarpal
   arthroplasty
Niebauer trapezium
   replacement prosthesis
Niebauer-Cutter implant
Niebauer-King technique
Niedner anastomosis clamp
Niedner commissurotomy knife
Niedner dissecting forceps
Niedner knife
Niedner pulmonic clamp
Niedner valvulotome
Niehaber prosthesis
Niemann splenomegaly
Niemeier classification
Niemeier gallbladder perforation
night drainage bag
night splint
Nightimer carpal tunnel support
Nightingale examining lamp
nightstick fracture
NIH cardiomarker catheter
NIH left ventriculography
   catheter
NIH marking catheter
NIH mitral valve forceps
NIH mitral valve-grasping forceps
Nikon aspheric lens
Nikon camera
Nikon microprocessor-
   controlled camera
Nikon fundus camera
Nikon magnifying lens
Nikon zoom photo slit lamp
Nilsson suction tube
Nilsson-Stille abortion suction
   tube
Nimbus Hemopump cardiac
   assist device
Niplette device
nipper
   anterior crurotomy nipper
   crural nipper
   crurotomy nipper
   cuticle nipper

nipper (*continued*)
  Dieter nipper
  Dieter-House nipper
  English anvil nail nipper
  Hough anterior crurotomy
    nipper
  Hough crurotomy nipper
  House malleus nipper
  House-Dieter malleus nipper
  Lempert malleus nipper
  malleus nipper
  Miltex nail nipper
  nail nipper
  Rica malleus head nipper
  SMIC malleus head nipper
  Tabb crural nipper
  Turnbull nail nipper
  Turnbull nipper
  Wister nipper
nipper nail drill
nipping at arteriovenous
    crossings
nipple
  aortic nipple
  areola of nipple
  boxing of nipple
  circumference of the chest at
    the nipple (C-N)
  connecting nipple
  cystoscopic connecting
    nipple
  darkening of nipples
  donor nipple
  everted nipple
  free transplantation of nipple
  invaginated nipple
  Kock nipple
  McGovern nipple
  midclavicular line to nipple
    (MCL-N)
  Nuk nipple
  Paget disease of nipple
nipple discharge
nipple everted
nipple grafting
nipple inversion
nipple line
nipple marker
nipple plasty
nipple reconstruction
nipple retraction
nipple shadow

nipple site
nipple transposition
nipple valve
nipple-areolar amputation
nipple-areola tattoo
nippled stoma
nipple-flat duct resection
nipple-to-inframammary fold
    distance (N-IMF)
NIR Elite over-the-wire stent
NIR ON Ranger balloon
    expandable stent
NIR ON Ranger premounted stent
NIR paclitaxel-coated coronary
    stent
NIR Primo balloon expandable
    stent
NIR Primo Monorail stent
NIR with SOX coronary stent
NIR with SOX over-the-wire
    coronary stent
Niro arch bars
Niro bone-cutting forceps
Niro wire-twister forceps
Niro wire-twisting forceps
Niroyal Advance balloon
    expandable stent
Niroyal Elite Monorail coronary
    stent
Niroyal Monorail stent
NIRS (near infrared spectroscopy)
Nirschl operation
Nirschl fasciotomy
Nirschl procedure
Nirschl technique
NIRstent
Nirvana pressure-reducing
    mattress
Nisbet eye forceps
Nisbet fixation forceps
Nisentil anesthetic agent
Nishimoto Sangyo scanner
Nishizaki-Wakabayashi suction
    tube
Nissen 360-degree
    transabdominal
    fundoplication
Nissen 360-degree wrap
    fundoplication
Nissen antireflux operation
Nissen cystic forceps
Nissen fundoplasty

Nissen fundoplication
Nissen fundoplication operation
Nissen fundoplication procedure
Nissen fundoplication technique
Nissen fundoplication wrap
Nissen gall duct forceps
Nissen gastrectomy
Nissen hallux forceps
Nissen hiatal hernia repair
Nissen operation
Nissen procedure
Nissen repair
Nissen rib spreader
Nissen sutures
Nissenbaum surgical exposure
Nissen-Rosseti fundoplication
    procedure
Nissen-Rosseti fundoplication
    technique
Nissen-Rossetti fundoplication
Nite Train-R enuresis
    conditioning device
Ni-Ti alloy compression stapler
nitinol guidewire
nitinol mesh stent
nitinol mesh-covered frame
nitinol self-expanding coil stent
nitinol shape-memory alloy wire
nitinol subglottic stenosis stent
nitinol thermal memory stent
nitrile glove
nitroglycerin transdermal patch
Nitrospray Plus cryosurgical
    device
nitrous oxide anesthetic agent
nitrous oxide-opioid-barbiturate
    anesthetic technique
nitrous oxide-oxygen-opioid
    anesthetic technique
Nivita lens
Nizetic operation
nl (nanoliter)
NL3 guider
NLite laryngoscope
N-loop
nm (nanometer)
NMR LipoProfile device
no appreciable change
No Bounce mallet
no evidence of disease (NED)
no evidence of recurrence
    (NER)

no evidence of recurrent disease
    (NERD)
no line of demarcation
No Pour Pak suction catheter kit
no significant change
No Sting barrier film
no-absorption anesthesia
Nobel Biocare implant
Nobelpharma gold prosthetic
    retaining screw
Nobelpharma implant
Nobetec dental cement
Nobis aortic occluder
Noble bowel plication
Noble iris forceps
Noble operation
Noble position
Noble procedure for volvulus
Noble scissors
Noble small bowel plication
Noble-Mengert perineal repair
Noblock retractor
no-bone reconstruction
Noci stimuli needle
Nocito eye implant
nocturnal penile tumescence
    monitor
nodal arrhythmia
nodal beat
nodal bigeminy
nodal disease
nodal extirpation
nodal involvement
nodal metastasis
nodal nuchal plane
nodal point
nodal arrhythmia
nodal tachycardia
nodal tissue
node
    accessory node
    aortic lymph node
    Aschoff node
    Aschoff-Tawara node
    atrioventricular node
    AV node (atrioventricular
        node)
    axillary node
    Bouchard nodes
    buccal lymph node
    calcified lymph node
    calcified node

node (*continued*)

Calot node
caval nodes
cecal mesocolic lymph nodes
celiac lymph nodes
cervical lymph node
cervical node
Cloquet node
common iliac lymph nodes
cryosurgical interruption of AV node
cubital lymph nodes
deep cervical jugulodigastric nodes
deep facial lymph node
deep lateral node
deep parotid node
Delphian lymph node
Delphian node
diaphragmatic node
Durck node
external iliac lymph node
facial node
femoral nodes
Flack node
gastroepiploic lymph node
hard subcutaneous node
Heberden nodes
hemal node
hilar lymph nodes
hilar node
His-Tawara node
ileocolic lymph nodes
iliac lymph nodes
inferior deep cervical node
infrarenal node
inguinal lymph node
inguinal nodes
jugular chain lymph node
jugular lymph nodes
jugulodigastric nodes
jugulo-omohyoid node
juxtaregional lymph node
Keith node
Keith-Flack node
Koch node
lingual lymph node
lumbar lymph nodes
lymph nodes
mandibular lymph nodes
mastoid node
matted node

node (*continued*)

maxillary lymph node
mesenteric lymph nodes
mesenteric node
mesocolic lymph nodes
metastatic node
Meynet nodes
Osler nodes
pancreaticosplenic lymph node
parapharyngeal lymph nodes
parasternal lymph nodes
paratracheal nodes
parotid lymph node
Parrot node
pelvic lymph node
pelvic node
periaortic lymph node
periaortic nodes
perigastric lymph nodes
pharyngeal lymph node
phrenic lymph node
popliteal lymph node
positive node
prelaryngeal node
pretracheal node
pyloric lymph node
questionable node
Ranvier nodes
regional node
residual node
retroperitoneal lymph node
retrorectal lymph node
Rotter interpectoral nodes
S-A node (sinoatrial node)
scalene lymph node
scalene node
Schmorl node
sentinel node
shotty lymph node
shotty node
singer's node
sinus node
Sister Mary Joseph lymph node
subcutaneous intraocular node
subdigastric lymph nodes
submandibular lymph nodes
submental lymph nodes
succulent nodes
superficial nodes

node (*continued*)
  superior mesenteric lymph
    nodes
  superior tracheobronchial
    lymph nodes
  supraclavicular lymph nodes
  supraclavicular node
  swollen lymph nodes
  Tawara node
  tibial lymph node
  Troisier node
  Virchow sentinel node
  Virchow-Troisier node
node biopsy
node dissection
node involvement
node lymphoma
node-negative disease
node-positive breast cancer
node-positive disease
nodose ganglion
nodose rheumatism
nodosity
nodoventricular bypass tract
nodular amyloidosis
nodular basal cell carcinoma
nodular density
nodular fasciitis
nodular goiter
nodular granulomatous
    vasculitis
nodular hidradenoma
nodular histiocytosis
nodular lesion
nodular liver
nodular melanoma
nodular scleritis
nodular subepidermal fibrosis
nodular thyroid
nodular tumor
nodular ulcerative basal cell
    carcinoma
nodular vasculitis
nodularity
nodulation
nodule
  Aschoff nodule
  Bohn nodules
  Bouchard nodules
  Busacca nodules
  calcified nodule
  Cherney thyroid nodule

nodule (*continued*)
  chest nodules
  cold nodule
  Cruveilhier nodules
  cutaneous nodule
  cutaneous-subcutaneous
    nodule
  Dalen-Fuchs nodules
  discrete nodule
  fibrocystic nodules
  fibrohyaline nodule
  fibrous nodule
  Gamna nodules
  Gamna-Gandy nodule
  Gandy-Gamna nodule
  hot nodule
  Jeanselme nodule
  juxta-articular nodule
  Kerckring nodule
  Koeppe nodule
  Koester nodule
  Lisch nodules
  liver nodule
  lymph nodule
  lymphatic nodules
  lymphosarcomatous nodule
  Morgagni nodules
  Paterson nodules
  pearly nodule
  pedunculated nodule
  pulmonary nodules
  retrosternal nodule
  rheumatic nodule
  satellite nodule
  Schmorl nodule
  singer's nodule
  solitary nodule
  subcutaneous nodule
  surfer's nodules
  thymic nodule
  ulcerated nodule
  vestigial nodule
nodule-in-nodule lesion
nodulocystic acne
nodulo-vegetating
    keratoacanthoma
Noel-Thompson operation
Nogenol dental cement
Noiles posterior stabilized knee
Noiles posterior stabilized knee
    prosthesis
Noiles rotating hinge knee

Noiles rotating hinge total knee
Noiles rotating hinge total knee
    prosthesis
Noiles rotating hinge knee
    mechanism
Noiles rotating-hinge total knee
    prosthesis
NoKor needle
Nokrome bifocal lens
Nolan needle holder
Noland-Budd cervical curet
no-leak technique
No-Lok compression screw
no-loop gastrojejunostomy
Nomos multiprogrammable
    R-wave inhibited demand
    pacemaker
non sequitur
nonabsorbable surgical sutures
nonabsorbable sutures
nonabsorbent material
nonaddictive painkillers
nonadherent foam
nonadhering dressing
nonadhesive dressing
nonanatomic renal bypass
nonanatomic wedge resection
nonaneurysmal
    perimesencephalic
    subarachnoid hemorrhage
non-Arcon articulator
nonarticular distal radial fracture
nonautologous implant
nonbacterial thrombotic
    endocardial lesion
nonbench surgery
nonbiological signal
nonblanchable, abnormally
    colored lesion
noncalcified stone
noncancer death
noncannulated nail
noncardiac surgery
noncaseating granuloma
noncemented component
noncemented prosthesis
noncemented total hip
    arthroplasty
noncholesteatomatous chronic
    suppurative otitis media
noncircumferential antireflux
    procedure

noncirrhotic liver
noncirrhotic metabolic liver
    disease
noncolorectal liver metastasis
    (NCRLM)
noncomminuted fracture
noncommunicating hydrocele
noncompetitive pacemaker
noncompliant balloon
noncompliant patient
nonconductive guidewire
nonconstrained knee prosthesis
noncontact manipulation
Non-Contact tonometer
noncontiguous fracture
noncontributory history
noncoring Huber needle
noncornified epithelium
noncrosslinked silicones
noncrushing anterior resection
    clamp
noncrushing bowel clamp
noncrushing clamp
noncrushing common duct
    forceps
noncrushing forceps
noncrushing gastroenterostomy
    clamp
noncrushing gastrointestinal
    clamp
noncrushing intestinal clamp
noncrushing intestinal forceps
noncrushing liver-holding clamp
noncrushing pickup forceps
noncrushing tissue-holding
    forceps
noncrushing vascular clamp
noncutting needle
noncutting suture needle
nondeciduous placenta
nondepolarizing block
nondepolarizing blockade
nondermatomal sensory
    abnormality (NDSA)
nondescent of cecum
nondetachable endovascular
    balloon
nondetachable occlusive balloon
nondetachable silicone balloon
    catheter
nondialysis time
nondismembered anastomosis

nondisplaced crack fracture
nondisplaced fracture
nondistended abdomen
nondistinctive features
nondominant gland
nondyskeratotic leukoplakia
nonenclosed magnet
nonepithelial bone cyst
nonepithelial tumor
nonerosive gastric mucosal
　lesion
noneverting sutures
nonfade scope
nonfamilial multiglandular
　disease
nonfatal complication
nonfebrile-associated vesicular
　eruption
nonfenestrated Fontan
　procedure
nonfenestrated forceps
nonferromagnetic clip
nonferromagnetic MR-
　compatible frame
nonferromagnetic needle
nonferromagnetic positioning
　device
nonfiberoptic bronchoscopy
nonfilamented form
nonflotation catheter
non-flow-compensated
　sequences
non-flow-directed catheter
nonfunction mandibular
　movement
nonfunctional
nonfunctioning
nonhealing
non-heart-beating donor
　(NHBD)
nonhinged constrained knee
　prosthesis
nonhinged knee prosthesis
non-Hodgkin lymphoma
nonhornified epithelium
nonimmunologic complication
Nonin Onyx pulse oximeter
noninfective extra-abdominal
　complication
noninfiltrating lobular
　carcinoma
noninflammatory

nonintegrated transvenous
　defibrillation lead
nonintegrated tripolar lead
noninterfering separator
noninvasive assessment
noninvasive continuous cardiac
　output monitor
noninvasive diagnosis
noninvasive evaluation
noninvasive lesion
noninvasive pacemaker
　programming
noninvasive paddle
noninvasive positive-pressure
　ventilation (NPPV)
noninvasive procedure
noninvasive temporary
　pacemaker
noninversion
nonirritating diet
nonisometric graft
nonkeratinized epithelium
nonkeratinizing carcinoma
nonlatex dental dam
nonloadbearing regions of the
　craniofacial skeleton
nonlocalized inflammation
nonmagnetic dressing forceps
nonmagnetic tissue forceps
nonmalignant disease
nonmalignant tissue
nonmarginal syndesmophytes
nonmarital introitus
nonmedullated nerve fiber
nonmeningiomatous malignant
　lesion
nonmucosal hemorrhoidectomy
nonnecrotizing granulomatous
　inflammation
nonneoplastic tumorlike lesion
nonneuroendocrine metastasis
nonoccluding earmold
nonocclusive dressing
nonocclusive mesenteric
　ischemia syndrome
nonocclusive mesenteric
　thrombosis
nonoperative approach
nonoperative closure
nonoperative diagnosis
nonoperative reduction
nonopportunistic infection

nonpalpable invasive breast cancer
nonpalpable mammographic abnormality
nonpenetrating corneal graft
nonpenetrating keratoplasty
nonpenetrating rupture
nonpenetrating wound
nonperforating towel clamp
nonperforating towel forceps
nonperforative lesion
nonphysial fracture
nonphysiologic position
nonpitting edema
nonplicated appendicocystostomy
nonpneumatic tourniquet
nonporous-coated endoprosthesis
nonproductive cough
nonprosthetic closure
nonradiating pain
nonradioactive metal pellets
nonrebreathing anesthesia
nonrebreathing mask
nonrebreathing valve
nonresorbable fixation
nonresorbable hydroxyapatite
non-rib-spreading thoracotomy incision
non-rib-spreading thoracotomy incision procedure
nonrigid endoscope
nonrotational burst fracture
nonsecretory sigmoid cystoplasty
nonseptate cavity
nonsevered injury
nonslipping forceps
nonspecific change
nonspecific gas pattern
nonspecific therapy
nonsterile technique
nonstick gauze
nonstress test (NST)
nonstriated muscle
nonsuppurative otitis media
nonsurgical therapy
nonsynovial joint
nonthoracotomy system antitachycardia device
nontoothed forceps

nontoxic goiter
nontraumatic cardiac tamponade
nontraumatic hernia
nontraumatizing catheter
nontraumatizing forceps
nontraumatizing viscera forceps
nonunion
nonunion fracture
nonunion of fracture
nonunited fracture
nonvalved graft
nonvascular abdominal surgery
nonvascularized bone graft (NVBG)
nonvascularized fibular strut graft
nonviable scar
nonviable tissue
nonvolitional facial expression
nonweightbearing (NWB)
nonweightbearing brace
nonwoven sponge
Noon AV fistula clamp
noose suture technique
noose sutures
NoProfile balloon
NoProfile balloon catheter
Norco ulnar deviation support
Norcross periosteal elevator
Nord appliance
Nord orthodontic plate
Nordan tying forceps
Nordan-Colibri forceps
Nordan-Ruiz trapezoidal marker
Nordenstrom biopsy needle
Nordent amalgam condenser
Nordent bone chisel
Nordent bone curet
Nordent bone file
Nordent excavator
Nordent filling instrument
Nordent hoe
Nordent oral surgery elevator
Nordent periodontic knife
Nordent-Oschsenbein periodontic chisel
Nordin-Ruiz trapezoidal marker
Nordson debrider
Nordt knot tightener
Norelco mucotome
Norfolk intrauterine aspiration catheter

Norfolk technique
Norian skeletal repair system
    cancellous bone cement
Norian SRS cement
Norland digital oscilloscope
Norland bone densitometer
normal anatomic position
normal caliber duct
normal condition
normal occlusion
normal planar MR anatomy
normal saline
normal vital sign
normal-appearing mucosa
Norman tibial bolt
Norman tibial nail
Norman tibial pin
Normigel hydrogel dressing
Normlgel protective wound
    dressing
normoactive bowel sounds
normoactive bowel tones
normoactive reflexes
normoblast
normocephalic
normophysiological reflexes
normothermia
Norport pump
Norrbacka bone elevator
Norrbacka-Stille level
Norris button
Norris sponge forceps
Norris tip magnet
Nortech SLED electrode
Northbent suture scissors
Northgate dual-purpose
    lithotriptor
Northpedic cast cutter
North-South retractor
Northville brace
Norton adjustable cup reamer
Norton ball reamer
Norton endotracheal tube
Norton flow-directed Swan-Ganz
    thermodilution catheter
Norton operation
Norton-Latzko extraperitoneal
    cesarean section
Norwich approach
Norwood forceps
Norwood operation for
    hypoplastic left-sided heart

Norwood rectal snare
Norwood univentricular heart
    procedure
nose anesthesia
nose bridge-lid reflex
nose cleft
nose clip
nose guard splint
nosebleed
nose-bridge prosthesis
nosecone
nose-eye reflex
Nosik transorbital leukotome
nosocomial gangrene
nosocomial infection
nostril elevator
nostril sills
notch
    acetabular notch
    antegonial notch
    aortic notch
    cardiac notch
    Carhart notch
    cerebellar notch
    chin notch
    clavicular notch
    coracoid notch
    cotyloid notch
    craniofacial notch
    dicrotic notch
    ethmoidal notch
    fibular notch
    frontal notch
    gastric notch
    greater ischiatic notch
    greater sacrosciatic notch
    greater sciatic notch
    hamular notch
    Hutchinson crescentic notch
    inferior thyroid notch
    inferior vertebral notch
    interarytenoid notch
    interclavicular notch
    intercondylar notch
    interlobar notch
    intertragic notch
    interventricular notch
    ischiatic notch
    jugular notch
    Kernohan notch
    labial notch
    lesser sciatic notch

notch (*continued*)
  mandibular notch
  marsupial notch
  mastoid notch
  palatine notch
  parotid notch
  popliteal notch
  preoccipital notch
  presternal notch
  pterygoid notch
  pterygomaxillary notch
  radial notch
  rivinian notch
  Rivinus notch
  sacroiliac notch
  sacrosciatic notch
  scapular notch
  sciatic notch
  semicircular trochlear notch
  semilunar notch
  Sibson notch
  sigmoid notch
  sternal notch
  sternoclavicular notch
  superior thyroid notch
  supraorbital notch
  suprascapular notch
  suprasternal notch
  tentorial notch
  thyroid notch
  trochlear notch
  tympanic notch
  ulnar notch
  umbilical notch
  vertebral notch
notch correction
notch filter
notch-and-roll maneuver
notched rotation osteotomy
notched ruler
notched wave
notcher device
notching of pulmonic valve
notchplasty blade
notchplasty procedure
notch-shaped erosion
Noto dressing forceps
Noto ovum forceps
Noto polypus forceps
Noto sponge forceps
Noto sponge-holding forceps
no-touch surgical technique

no-touch technique
Nott vaginal speculum
Nott-Guttmann vaginal
  speculum
Nottingham colposuspension
  needle
Nottingham introducer
Nottingham One-Step tapered
  dilator
Nottingham ureteral dilator
Nounton blade
Nourse bladder syringe
Nova Aid lens
Nova Curve lens
NOVA skin testing instrument
Nova hook
Nova II machine
Nova II pacemaker
Nova MR pacemaker
Nova Soft II lens
Nova thermodilution catheter
NovaCath multilumen infusion
  catheter
Novack special extraction set
Novacor DIASYS left ventricular
  assist device
Novacor left ventricular assist
  device
Novacor LVAD (Novacor left
  ventricular assist device)
Novacor pump
Novafil sutures
Novaflex intraocular lens
NovaGold breast implant
Novagold mammary implant
Novak biopsy curet
Novak fixation forceps
Novak uterine curet
Novak uterine suction curet
Novak-Schoeckaert endometrial
  biopsy curet
Novak-Schoeckaert endometrial
  curet
NovaLine excimer laser
Novametrix pulse oximeter
NovaPulse CO_2 laser
Novar oral illuminator
NovaSaline inflatable breast
  implant
Novascan scanning headpiece
  laser
Novasome microvesicle

Novastent
Novatec LightBlade laser
Novex wedged wheelchair
    cushion
Novo-10a CBF measuring device
Novocain anesthetic agent
Novofil sutures
NovolinPen device
Novoste catheter
Novulase laser
Novus ophthalmoscope
Novus LC threaded interbody
    fusion cage
NOxBOX II monitor
noxious stimulus
Noyes anterior cruciate
    reconstruction
Noyes chalazion punch
Noyes ear forceps
Noyes iridectomy scissors
Noyes iris scissors
Noyes nasal forceps
Noyes nasal-dressing forceps
Noyes punch
Noyes rongeur
Noyes speculum
Noyes-Shambaugh alligator
    scissors
NPO (nothing by mouth)
NSAID analgesic
N-shaped sigmoid loop
NSR (nasal septal
    reconstruction)
NST (nonstress test)
N-Terface contact-layer wound
    dressing
N-Terface graft dressing
Nu Gauze dressing
Nu Gauze packing material
Nu Gauze sponge
Nu-Brede packing and
    debridement sponge
nubular blade
nuchae
nuchal cord
nuchal flexure
nuchal ligament
nuchal line
nuchal region
nuchal ridge
nuchal rigidity
nuchofrontal projection

Nuck canal
Nuck diverticulum
Nuck hydrocele
nuclear bleeding scan
nuclear cataract
nuclear external layer
nuclear imaging
nuclear matrix (NM)
nuclear medicine
nuclear membrane
nuclear pacemaker
nuclear powered pacemaker
nuclear probe
nuclear scanner
nucleic acid
nucleoplasty
nucleotide
Nucleotome diskectomy
    instruments
Nucleotome Endoflex
    instrument
Nucleotome Flex II cutting
    probe
Nucleotome Micro I probe
Nucletron applicator
Nucleus 22 cochlear implant
nucleus ambiguous lesion
nucleus delivery cannula
nucleus delivery loop
nucleus delivery loupe
nucleus erysiphake
nucleus expressor
nucleus hydrolysis needle
Nucleus multichannel cochlear
    implant
nucleus of Gudden
nucleus of Luys
nucleus of Perlia
nucleus of Rose
nucleus pulposus herniation
nucleus removal loop
nucleus removal loupe
nucleus rotator
nucleus spatula
Nu-Comfort colostomy
    appliance
Nu-Derm foam island dressing
Nuform gauze
Nu-Gel clear hydrogel wound
    dressing
Nugent aspirator
Nugent erysiphake

Nugent fixation forceps
Nugent iris hook
Nugent rectus forceps
Nugent soft cataract aspirator
Nugent superior rectus forceps
Nugent utility forceps
Nugent-Gradle stitch scissors
Nugent-Green-Dimitry
    erysiphake
Nugowski forceps
Nuhn glands
Nu-Hope adhesive
Nu-Hope adhesive waterproof
    skin barrier
Nu-Hope drainable one-piece
    pouch
Nu-Hope hole cutter
Nu-Hope ileostomy pouch
Nu-Hope neonatal and preemie
    pouches
Nu-Hope urinary pouch
Nuk nipple
Nu-Knit absorbable hemostat
nulligravida
Nulling pattern on x-ray
nullipara
nulliparous introitus
nulliparous patient
NuMed intracoronary Doppler
    catheter
NuMed single balloon
numerary mouth
numerary renal anomaly
nummular lesion
Nunc cryotube
Nunez sternal approximator
Nunez aortic clamp
Nunez approximator
Nunez auricular clamp
Nunez clamp
Nunez tube
Nunez ventricular ventilation
    tube
Nunez-Nunez knife
Nunez-Nunez mitral stenosis
    knife
Nupercaine hydrochloride
    anesthetic agent
Nuport PEG tube
NURD (nonuniform rotational
    distortion)
Nurolon suture

nursemaid's elbow
Nussbaum intestinal clamp
Nussbaum intestinal forceps
Nussbaum narcosis
nut alignment guide
nutcracker esophagus
nutcracker fracture
nutcracker's syndrome
Nu-Thor thoracostomy device
Nu-Tip disposable scissor tip
Nu-Tip laparoscopic scissors
nutmeg liver
NutraCol hydrocolloid wound
    dressing
NutraDress zinc-saline dressing
NutraFil hydrophilic B dressing
Nutraflex Poole tube
NutraGauze hydrophilic wound
    dressing
Nu-Trake cricothyrotomy device
NutraStat calcium alginate
    wound dressing
NutraVue hydrogel dressing
Nutricath silicone elastomer
    catheter
nutrient arteries of humerus
nutrient canal of bone
nutrient flap
nutrient foramen
nutrient vessel
Nuttall operation
Nuttall retractor
Nuvistor electronic tonometer
NUVO barrier film
Nu-Vois artificial larynx
NuVue lens
Nuwave transcutaneous
    electrical nerve stimulator
Nu-wrap rolls dressing
NWB (nonweightbearing)
Nyboer esophageal electrode
Nycore angiography catheter
Nycore angiography pigtail
    catheter
Nycore cardiac device
Nyhus classification
Nyhus-Nelson gastric
    decompression tube
Nyhus-Nelson jejunal feeding
    tube
Nyhus-Potts intestinal forceps
Nylen-Barany maneuver

Nylok bolt
Nylok self-locking nail
nylon 66 sutures
nylon face mallet
nylon hand scrub brush
nylon head hammer
nylon head mallet
nylon loop
nylon monofilament sutures
nylon nut
nylon retention sutures
nylon scrub brush
nylon sutures
nylon vascular prosthesis

nystagmograph
nystagmus bulb
Nystroem abdominal suction
    tube
Nystroem hip nail
Nystroem nail driver
Nystroem retractor
Nystroem tumor forceps
Nystroem-Stille driver
Nystroem-Stille hip nail
Nystroem-Stille retractor
Nytone enuretic control unit
NYU-Hosmer electric elbow and
    prehension actuator

1-minimum alveolar concentration (1-MAC)
O₂ disposable boot device
OA (occipital artery)
OA knee brace
Oakley-Fulthorpe technique
Oaks double needle
Oaks double straight cannula
Oasis collagen plug
Oasis feather microscalpel
Oasis wound dressing
Oasys brace
oat cell carcinoma
OB-10 Comfort bite block
Obagi sign
O'Beirne sphincter
O'Beirne sphincter tube
Ober incision
Ober operation
Ober sign
Ober tendon passer
Ober tendon technique
Ober-Barr brachioradialis transfer
Ober-Barr transfer technique
Oberhill obstetrical forceps
Oberhill retractor
Oberhill self-retaining retractor
Oberst operation
Obersteiner-Redlich line
Ober-Young operation
obese abdomen
obese support
obesity-hypoventilation syndrome
oblique aberration
oblique amputation
oblique arytenoid muscle
oblique astigmatism
oblique bandage
oblique conus
oblique coronal plane
oblique diameter

oblique facial cleft
oblique fiber
oblique film
oblique fissure
oblique flap
oblique flap in mucogingival surgery
oblique fracture
oblique head
oblique hernia
oblique incision
oblique inguinal hernia
oblique inguinal incision
oblique lateral projection
oblique line
oblique muscle
oblique muscle hook
oblique popliteal ligament
oblique position
oblique presentation
oblique prism
oblique projection
oblique ramus sliding osteotomy
oblique relaxing incision
oblique retinacular ligament
oblique sagittal gradient-echo MR imaging
oblique septum
oblique sinus of pericardium
oblique spot view
oblique study
oblique subcondylar osteotomy
oblique subcondylar ramus osteotomy
oblique tendon
oblique vein
oblique view
oblique-forward-viewing instrument
obliquely contracted pelvis
oblique-viewing echoendoscope
oblique-viewing endoscope
obliquity reflex

obliquus abdominis externus
   muscle
obliquus abdominis internus
   muscle
obliquus inferior muscle
obliquus superior muscle
obliteration
   balloon-occluded retrograde
      transvenous obliteration
      (B-RTO)
   endoscopic extirpation
      cicatricial obliteration
   fibrous obliteration
   percutaneous transhepatic
      obliteration
   posterior sulcus obliteration
   radiographic obliteration
   subdeltoid fat plane
      obliteration
   total ear obliteration
obliterative inflammation
obliterative labyrinthitis
obliterative vascular disease
oblong fovea of arytenoid
   cartilage
O'Brien airway needle
O'Brien akinesia
O'Brien anesthesia
O'Brien block
O'Brien capsular shift procedure
O'Brien cataract
O'Brien fixation forceps
O'Brien foreign body spud
O'Brien hook
O'Brien marker
O'Brien needle holder
O'Brien pelvic halo operation
O'Brien phrenic retractor
O'Brien rib hook
O'Brien rib retractor
O'Brien rongeur
O'Brien spatula
O'Brien stitch scissors
O'Brien suture scissors
O'Brien tissue forceps
O'Brien-Elschnig forceps
O'Brien-Mayo scissors
O'Brien-Storz microhemostat
Obstbaum lens spatula
Obstbaum synechia spatula
obstetric anesthesia
obstetric brachial plexus injury

obstetric position
obstetrical analgesia
obstetrical anesthesia
obstetrical anesthesia needle
obstetrical binder
obstetrical block anesthesia
   needle
obstetrical complication
obstetrical decapitating hook
obstetrical delivery
obstetrical double-armed sutures
obstetrical forceps
obstetrical history
obstetrical hook
obstetrical hysterectomy
obstetrical infection
obstetrical instruments
obstetrical operation
obstetrical position
obstetrical retractor
obstetrical spoon
obstetrical stirrups
obstetrical surgery
obstetrical traction handle
obstetrical traction injury
obstetrical ultrasonography
obstetrics instrument set
obstructed airway
obstructed labor
obstructed nares
obstructed shunt
obstructed shunt tube
obstructed testis
obstructed tube
obstructing adhesions
obstructing airway
obstructing colorectal cancer
obstructing lesion
obstructing mass
obstruction
   acute intestinal obstruction
   adherence obstruction
   adynamic intestinal
      obstruction
   airflow obstruction
   airway obstruction
   anorectal outlet obstruction
   ball-valve obstruction
   biliary obstruction
   biliary tract obstruction
   bowel obstruction
   bronchial obstruction

obstruction (*continued*)
  catheter obstruction
  check-valve obstruction
  closed-loop intestinal
    obstruction
  clot-induced urinary tract
    obstruction
  colon obstruction
  colonic obstruction
  common bile duct
    obstruction
  common duct obstruction
  complete obstruction
  complex left ventricular
    outflow tract obstruction
  ductal obstruction
  duodenal obstruction
  duodenojejunal obstruction
  esophageal obstruction
  extrahepatic bile duct
    obstruction
  extrahepatic biliary
    obstruction
  extrahepatic binary
    obstruction
  extrahepatic obstruction
  extrahepatic portal vein
    obstruction (HPO)
  extrahepatic venous
    obstruction
  extramural upper airway
    obstruction
  extrinsic obstruction
  false colonic obstruction
  fecal obstruction
  fecalith obstruction
  food bolus obstruction
  foreign body obstruction
  free of obstruction
  functional cystic duct
    obstruction
  gall duct obstruction
  gallstone obstruction
  gastric outlet obstruction
  hepatic obstruction
  hepatic venous outflow
    obstruction
  high small-bowel
    obstruction
  high-grade obstruction
  idiopathic obstruction
  impassable obstruction

obstruction (*continued*)
  intermittent subclavian vein
    obstruction
  intestinal obstruction
  ipsilateral portal vein
    obstruction
  junction obstruction
  large-bowel obstruction
  laryngeal obstruction
  left-sided colorectal
    obstruction
  longer-segment obstruction
  low small-bowel obstruction
  lower airway obstruction
  lymphatic obstruction
  mechanical biliary
    obstruction
  mechanical bowel obstruction
  mechanical duct obstruction
  mechanical extrahepatic
    obstruction
  mechanical intestinal
    obstruction
  mechanical obstruction
  mechanical small-bowel
    obstruction
  membranous obstruction
  minor gland obstruction
  myoglobin tubular
    obstruction
  nasal airway obstruction
  nasal obstruction
  ostial obstruction
  outflow tract obstruction
  outlet obstruction
  papillary obstruction
  paralytic colonic obstruction
  paralytic intestinal
    obstruction
  parotid obstruction
  partial bowel obstruction
  partial mechanical
    obstruction
  portal obstruction
  portal vein obstruction
  postoperative airway
    obstruction
  pyloric obstruction
  pyloric outlet obstruction
  pyloroduodenal obstruction
  renal obstruction
  salivary duct obstruction

obstruction (*continued*)
  shunt obstruction
  simple mechanical
    obstruction
  sit of obstruction
  small-bowel obstruction
    (SBO)
  stop-valve airway
    obstruction
  strangulated bowel
    obstruction
  strangulation obstruction
  sublingual obstruction
  submandibular obstruction
  suprahepatic venous
    obstruction
  top-valve airway obstruction
  total obstruction
  tracheal obstruction
  tubal obstruction
  tube obstruction
  upper airway obstruction
  ureteropelvic obstruction
  ureterovesical obstruction
  urinary tract obstruction
  vascular obstruction
  vein obstruction
  vena caval obstruction
  venous obstruction
  ventricular inflow tract
    obstruction
  ventricular outflow tract
    obstruction
obstructive airway defect
obstructive airway disease
obstructive defect
obstructive disease
obstructive esophagogastric
  cancer
obstructive lesion
obstructive problem
obstructive pulmonary
  dysfunction
obstructive sialadenitis
obstructive site
obstructive sleep apnea
obstructive symptoms
obtainer space
obtunded
obtundity
Obtura injectable technique
obturating embolus

obturator
  Alcock obturator
  Alcock-Timberlake obturator
  anoscope with obturator
  atraumatic distending
    obturator
  Beall mitral obturator
  blunt obturator
  blunt-tipped obturator
  cannulated obturator
  coagulating suction cannula
    obturator
  concave obturator
  concave sheath and obturator
  convex obturator
  convex sheath and obturator
  Cripps obturator
  cystoscope obturator
  deflecting obturator
  distending obturator
  double-catheterizing sheath
    and obturator
  Ellik-Shaw obturator
  Endopath Optiview
    laparoscopic obturator
  Endotrac obturator
  eyed obturator
  Fitch obturator
  Frazier suction tube
    obturator
  Hemaflex PTCA sheath with
    obturator
  Hemaquet PTCA sheath with
    obturator
  Hirschman anoscope with
    obturator
  Hirschman proctoscope with
    obturator
  Keene obturator
  Keene self-sealing sleeve and
    obturator
  LaparoSAC obturator
  Leusch atraumatic obturator
  Moria obturator
  Optiview optical surgical
    obturator
  palatal obturator
  Rumel tourniquet eyed
    obturator
  sheath and obturator
  Storz atraumatic distending
    obturator

obturator (*continued*)
  Storz deflecting obturator
  suction tube obturator
  Thal-Mantel obturator
  Thermafil Plus obturator
  Timberlake obturator
  tourniquet-eyed obturator
  tracheal tube with obturator
  ureteral catheter obturator
  visual obturator
obturator appliance
obturator artery
obturator avulsion fracture
obturator bypass
obturator crest
obturator cystoscope
obturator deflecting
  resectoscope
obturator fascia
obturator foramen
obturator fossa
obturator groove
obturator hernia
obturator line
obturator membrane
obturator muscle
obturator nerve
obturator nerve block
obturator nerve damage
obturator nerve injury
obturator resectoscope
obturator shelf
  cystourethropexy
obturator sign
obturator test
obturator urethroscope
obturator veins
obturatoria stapedis fold
obtuse angle
obtuse cervicomandibular angle
obtuse margin
obtuse-angle knife
Obwegeser awl
Obwegeser channel retractor
Obwegeser incision
Obwegeser orthognathic
  surgery instrument
Obwegeser osteotomy
Obwegeser periosteal elevator
Obwegeser periosteal retractor
Obwegeser sagittal mandibular
  osteotomy

Obwegeser splitting chisel
Obwegeser stripper
Obwegeser-Dalpont internal
  screw fixation
OC (occlusocervical)
occipital anchorage
occipital angle
occipital angle of parietal bone
occipital artery
occipital belly of the
  occipitofrontal muscle
occipital bone
occipital border
occipital brachycephaly
occipital cephalocele
occipital condyle fracture
occipital condyle syndrome
occipital crest
occipital diploic vein
occipital emissary vein
occipital foramen
occipital fracture
occipital groove
occipital lobe
occipital malformation
occipital margin
occipital muscle
occipital nerve
occipital plagiocephaly
occipital plane
occipital point
occipital protuberance
occipital region
occipital segment
occipital sinus
occipital spur
occipital squama
occipital suture
occipital triangle
occipital vein
occipitoanterior position
occipitoatlantal articulation
occipitoatlantal dislocation
occipitoatlantoaxial anomaly
occipitocervical fixation
occipitocervical fusion
occipitocervical stabilization
occipitofrontal circumference
occipitofrontal diameter
occipitofrontal muscle
occipitofrontalis muscle
occipitomastoid suture

occipitomastoid suture lines
occipitomeatal view
occipitomental diameter
occipitoparietal suture
occipitoposterior position
occipitosacral position
occipitosphenoidal suture
occipitosphenoidal
    synchondrosis
occipitotemporal convolution
occipitotransverse position
occiput posterior
occluded blood vessel
occluded duct
occluded fistula
occluded intracranial vessel
occluded lisp
occluder
    Amplatzer septal occluder
    aorta occluder
    ASDOS umbrella occluder
    Bard clamshell septal
        occluder
    black-white occluder
    Brockenbrough curved-tip
        occluder
    CardioSeal septal occluder
    catheter tip occluder
    clip-on/tie-on occluder
    eye occluder
    Florester vascular occluder
    Halberg trial clip occluder
    Heifitz carotid occluder
    Heishima balloon occluder
    Kean occluder
    long occluder
    lorgnette occluder
    Maddox rod occluder
    Microvena Das Angel Wings
        occluder
    modified Rashkind PDA
        occluder
    multiple-pin hole occluder
    Nobis aortic occluder
    pinhole occluder
    Pram combination occluder
    radiolucent plastic occluder
    Rashkind double-disk
        umbrella occluder
    red lens occluder
    Rumison side port fixation
        occluder

occluder (*continued*)
    short occluder
    single occluder
    square-shaped occluder
occluding centric relation
    record
occluding clamp
occluding forceps
occluding fracture frame
occluding ligature
occlusal adjustment
occlusal analysis
occlusal balance
occlusal cant
occlusal cavity
occlusal cephalometric analysis
occlusal clearance
occlusal climate
occlusal contact
occlusal contouring
occlusal correction
occlusal cross section
        radiograph
occlusal curvature
occlusal curve
occlusal disharmony
occlusal disturbance
occlusal embrasure
occlusal equilibration
occlusal form
occlusal function
occlusal guide
occlusal harmony
occlusal imbalance
occlusal interference
occlusal jaw relation
occlusal level
occlusal mold
occlusal pattern
occlusal perception
occlusal pivot
occlusal plane
occlusal plane angle
occlusal plane plate
occlusal position
occlusal pressure
occlusal quadrant view
occlusal recontouring
occlusal registration
occlusal rehabilitation
occlusal relation
occlusal relationship

occlusal rest angle
occlusal rest bar
occlusal splint
occlusal stability
occlusal stent
occlusal sulcus
occlusal surface
occlusal therapy
occlusal trauma
occlusal vertical dimension
occlusal wear
occlusal zone
occlusion
　2-plane occlusion
　abnormal occlusion
　acentric occlusion
　adjusted occlusion
　adjustment occlusion
　afunctional occlusion
　anatomic occlusion
　Andrews 6 keys to normal
　　occlusion
　angioplasty-related vessel
　　occlusion
　anterior occlusion
　aortic occlusion
　arterial occlusion
　artery occlusion
　attritional occlusion
　balanced occlusion
　bilateral balanced occlusion
　bimaxillary protrusive
　　occlusion
　branch vein occlusion
　buccal occlusion
　capsular occlusion
　carotid artery occlusion
　central occlusion
　centrally balanced occlusion
　centric occlusion
　centric relation occlusion
　centrically balanced occlusion
　cerebrovascular occlusion
　class I, II, III occlusion
　clip occlusion
　contralateral carotid artery
　　occlusion
　convenience occlusion
　coronary occlusion
　crossbite occlusion
　curve of occlusion
　dental occlusion

occlusion (*continued*)
　distal occlusion
　eccentric occlusion
　edge-to-edge occlusion
　embolic occlusion
　endovascular balloon
　　occlusion
　end-to-end occlusion
　enteromesenteric occlusion
　faulty eccentric occlusion
　graft occlusion
　habitual occlusion
　hemihepatic vascular
　　occlusion
　high occlusion
　ideal occlusion
　inflow occlusion
　intermittent inflow occlusion
　IVC occlusion
　labial occlusion
　laparoscopic total occlusion
　　(LTO)
　lateral occlusion
　line of occlusion
　lingual occlusion
　malfunctional occlusion
　MCA occlusion
　mechanical occlusion
　mechanically balanced
　　occlusion
　mesial occlusion
　middle cerebral artery
　　occlusion
　neutral occlusion
　normal occlusion
　outlet occlusion
　plastic stent occlusion
　posterior occlusion
　postnormal occlusion
　prenormal occlusion
　protrusive occlusion
　rapid occlusion
　retrusive occlusion
　skeletal occlusion
　spherical form of occlusion
　subclavian artery occlusion
　terminal occlusion
　thrombotic occlusion
　tourniquet occlusion
　transfemoral balloon
　　occlusion
　trauma from occlusion

occlusion (*continued*)
  traumatic occlusion
  traumatogenic occlusion
  traumatogenic pulpal
    occlusion
  tubal occlusion
  vascular occlusion
  vein occlusion
  venous occlusion
  working occlusion
occlusion analysis
occlusion balance
occlusion balloon
occlusion catheter
occlusion clamp
occlusion coil
occlusion forceps
occlusion multipurpose clamp
occlusion pressure
occlusion therapy
occlusive balloon
occlusive cant
occlusive carotid artery disease
occlusive collodion dressing
occlusive coronary artery
    disease
occlusive disease
occlusive dressing
occlusive ileus
occlusive moisture-retentive
    dressing
occlusive semipermeable
    dressing
occlusive therapy
occlusive wafer
occlusocervical (OC)
occlusogingival
occlusor
occlusorehabilitation
occult bleeding
occult blood
occult cancer
occult carcinoma
occult cerebrovascular
    malformation
occult cholelithiasis
occult cleft palate
occult compression injury
occult diaphragmatic injury
occult enterotomy
occult extrahepatic disease
occult fracture

occult hepatic disease
occult infection
occult irresectable disease
occult lesion
occult malformation of the skull
    base
occult metastasis
occult scaphoid fracture
occult spina bifida
occult systemic disease
occult talar lesion
occult trauma
occult vascular malformation
occupational abrasion
occupational therapy
occupational toxin exposure
OCG (oral cholecystogram)
ochre hemorrhage
Ochsenbein gingivectomy
Ochsenbein-Luebke flap
Ochsner aortic clamp
Ochsner arterial clamp
Ochsner arterial forceps
Ochsner artery clamp
Ochsner artery forceps
Ochsner ball-tipped scissors
Ochsner cartilage forceps
Ochsner diamond-edged scissors
Ochsner ether inhaler
Ochsner flexible spiral gallstone
    probe
Ochsner gall duct probe
Ochsner gallbladder trocar
Ochsner gallbladder tube
Ochsner gallstone probe
Ochsner hemostat
Ochsner hemostatic forceps
Ochsner hook
Ochsner malleable retractor
Ochsner muscle
Ochsner needle
Ochsner position
Ochsner probe
Ochsner ribbon retractor
Ochsner ring
Ochsner scissors
Ochsner spiral probe
Ochsner thoracic clamp
Ochsner thoracic trocar
Ochsner tissue forceps
Ochsner tissue/cartilage forceps
Ochsner treatment

Ochsner tube
Ochsner vascular retractor
Ochsner wire twister
Ochsner-DeBakey spur crusher
Ochsner-Dixon arterial forceps
Ochsner-Favaloro self-retaining
  retractor
Ochsner-Fenger gallstone probe
Ockerblad forceps
Ockerblad kidney clamp
Ockerblad ureter technique
Ockerblad vessel clamp
Ockerblad-Boari flap
OCL (Orthopedic Casting
  Laboratory)
OCL bowel prep
OCL flexible casting tape
OCL volar splint
o'clock position (1 through 12)
O'Connell sutures
O'Connor abdominal retractor
O'Connor biopsy forceps
O'Connor clamp
O'Connor depressor
O'Connor double-edged curet
O'Connor drape
O'Connor eye forceps
O'Connor finger cup
O'Connor flat tenotomy hook
O'Connor grasping forceps
O'Connor hex probe knife
O'Connor hook
O'Connor hook punch
O'Connor hook scissors
O'Connor iris forceps
O'Connor left-curve knife
O'Connor lid clamp
O'Connor lid forceps
O'Connor lip clamp
O'Connor marker
O'Connor meniscotomy knife
O'Connor muscle hook
O'Connor operating
  arthroscope
O'Connor operating scope
O'Connor operation
O'Connor probe knife
O'Connor retractor
O'Connor retrograde knife
O'Connor right-curve knife
O'Connor scleral depressor
O'Connor sheath

O'Connor sponge forceps
O'Connor straight knife
O'Connor tenotomy hook
O'Connor vaginal retractor
O'Connor-Elschnig fixation
  forceps
O'Connor-O'Sullivan self-
  retaining vaginal retractor
O'Connor-O'Sullivan abdominal
  retractor
O'Connor-O'Sullivan self-
  retaining retractor
O'Connor-O'Sullivan self-
  retaining vaginal retractor
O'Connor-Peter operation
Octa-Hex implant
octapolar catheter
octapolar lead
Octopus holder
Octopus retractor
OCTR (open carpal tunnel
  release)
Oculaid lens
ocular adnexa
ocular adnexal lesion
ocular ballottement
ocular barrier
ocular cautery
ocular cup
ocular dysmetria
ocular dystopia
ocular fundi
ocular Gamboscope lens
ocular Gamboscope loupe
ocular globe
ocular headache
ocular hypotelorism
ocular inflammation
ocular marker
ocular metastasis
ocular motility disorder
ocular muscle
ocular nerve
ocular pressure
ocular pressure reducer
ocular prosthesis
ocular radiation therapy
ocular refraction
ocular region
ocular tendon
ocular tension
ocular torticollis

ocular tremor
ocular vesicle
ocular-mucous membrane
    syndrome
OcuLight ophthalmic laser
oculoauriculovertebral dysplasia
oculobuccogenital syndrome
oculocardiac reflex (OCR)
oculocephalic maneuver
oculocephalic vascular anomaly
oculocutaneous laser
oculocutaneous telangiectasia
oculodento-osseous dysplasia
oculofacial cleft
oculogram
oculogyric stimulator
oculomandibulodyscephaly
oculomandibulofacial syndrome
oculomotor decussation
oculomotor foramen
oculomotor ganglion
oculomotor nerve (cranial
    nerve 3)
oculomotor nerve sign
oculomotor sulcus
oculopharyngeal syndrome
oculoplastic surgery
Oculo-Plastik ePTFE ocular
    implant
oculoplasty corneal protector
oculoplethysmography
oculovertebral syndrome
Oculus lens loupe
ocutome
    Berkeley ocutome
    CooperVision ocutome
    disposable ocutome
    O'Malley ocutome
ocutome probe
ocutome vitrectomy unit
ocutome vitrector
ocutome vitreous blade
ODAM defibrillator
odd facet
Oddi muscle
Oddi sphincter
Odelca camera unit
O'Dell spicule forceps
Odgen plate
Odland ankle prosthesis
Odman-Ledin catheter
O'Donaghue knee splint

O'Donaghue splint
O'Donaghue stirrup splint
O'Donnell operation
O'Donoghue ACL reconstruction
O'Donoghue cotton cast
O'Donoghue cystourethroscope
O'Donoghue dressing
O'Donoghue facetectomy
O'Donoghue operation
O'Donoghue probe
O'Donoghue procedure
O'Donoghue triad
odontalgia
odontalgia dentalis
odontectomy
    dentitional odontectomy
    mandibular dentitional
        odontectomy
odontexesis
odontogenic fibrosarcoma
odontogenic keratocyst
odontogenic myxofibroma
odontogenic myxoma
odontogenic tumor
odontoid condyle fracture
odontoid fracture
odontoid fracture internal
    fixation
odontoid neck fracture
odontoid peg-grasping forceps
odontoid perpendicular line
odontoid process
odontoid screw fixation
odontoid screw placement
odontoma
    composite odontoma
    dens invaginatus gestant
        odontoma
    mixed odontoma
odontoplasty
odontoscopy
odontotomy
odor absorbent dressing
odoriferous gland
O'Dwyer intubation
O'Dwyer intubation tube
OEC forearm splint
OEC hip prosthesis
OEC knee immobilizer
OEC lag screw component with
    keyway
OEC wrist splint

Oehlers type 3 dens invagination
Oertli knife
Oertli lid retractor
Oertli razor bladebreaker knife
Oertli sutures
Oertli wire lid retractor
OES colonoscope
Oesch hook
Oettingen abdominal self-retaining retractor
Oettingen abdominal retractor
  congenital absence of (organ, organ part, tissue, etc.)
  indicative of
  surgical absence of (breast, limb, uterus, etc.)
off-center isoperistaltic technique
off-pump coronary artery bypass (OPCAB)
offset hand retractor
offset hinge prosthesis
offset modified prosthesis
offset operating laparoscope
offset reamer
offset reverse dome bunionectomy (ORD bunionectomy)
offset suspension feeder
O'Gawa cataract-aspirating cannula
O'Gawa irrigating cannula
O'Gawa needle holder
O'Gawa suture forceps
O'Gawa suture-fixation forceps
O'Gawa 2-way I&A cannula
O'Gawa tying forceps
O'Gawa-Castroviejo tying forceps
Ogden Anchor soft tissue device
Ogden classification of fractures
Ogden epiphysial fracture classification
Ogden knee dislocation classification
Ogden soft tissue to bone anchor
Ogden-Senturia eustachian inflator
Ogee acetabular component
Ogilvie femoral herniorrhaphy

Ogilvie operation
Ogsten-Luc operation
Ogston operation
Ogston-Luc operation
Ogura cartilage forceps
Ogura fossa
Ogura nasal saw
Ogura operation
Ogura saw
Ogura technique
Ogura tissue and cartilage forceps
Ogura tissue forceps
Oh femoral component
OH pressurizer (Oxy-Hood pressurizer)
O'Hanlon forceps
O'Hanlon gastrointestinal clamp
O'Hanlon intestinal clamp
O'Hanlon-Poole suction tube
O'Hara forceps
O'Hara operation
O'Harris-Petruso cup
O'Harris-Petruso ring
OHD (organic heart disease)
Ohio bed
Ohio Bubble humidifier
Ohio critical care ventilator
Ohio Hope resuscitator
Ohio Nuclear Delta scanner
Ohio pressure infuser
Ohio resuscitation unit
Ohio Vortex respiration monitor
Ohl periosteal elevator
Ohmeda 5250 respiratory gas monitor
Ohmeda 6200 CO_2 monitor
Ohmeda computer-controlled infusion pump
Ohmeda continuous-vacuum regulator
Ohmeda hand-held oximeter
Ohmeda intermittent suction unit
Ohmeda probe
Ohmeda pulse oximeter
Ohmeda thoracic suction regulator
ohmmeter
Ohngren line
oil glands
oiled silk dressing

oiled silk sutures
OIU cold knife
Ojemann cortical stimulator
Okamura technique
Oklahoma ankle joint orthosis
Oklahoma ankle prosthesis
Oklahoma iris wire retractor
Okmian microneedle holder
Okonek-Yasargil tumor fork
Olair mouth mirror
Olatunbosun cerclage
Olbert balloon
Olbert balloon catheter
Olbert balloon dilatation
    catheter
Olbert balloon dilator
Olbert NoProfile balloon
    dilatation catheter
old posterior cyst
old scarring
old smoothie bur
Oldberg brain retractor
Oldberg dissector
Oldberg elevator
Oldberg intervertebral disk
    forceps
Oldberg intervertebral disk
    rongeur
Oldberg laminectomy rongeur
Oldberg pituitary rongeur
Oldberg pituitary rongeur
    forceps
Oldberg retractor
Oldberg straight retractor
Oldfield needle
O'Leary lesser curvature
    gastroplasty
O'Leary modification
olecranon bursa
olecranon fossa
olecranon fracture
olecranon ligament
olecranon process
olecranon spur
oleoarthrosis
oleothorax
Olerud internal fixator
Olerud PSF rod
Olerud PSF screw
olfactive angle
olfactory anesthesia
olfactory angle

olfactory area
olfactory bulb
olfactory bundle
olfactory cilia
olfactory cleft
olfactory foramen
olfactory ganglion
olfactory glands
olfactory groove
olfactory membrane
olfactory mucus
olfactory nerve (cranial nerve 1)
olfactory nerve sign
olfactory sulcus of nose
olfactory tract
olfactory vesicle
Oliair articulator
oligoclonal band
oligonucleotide probe
oligosegmental correction
olisthetic vertebra
olivary body
olivary catheter
olivary dilator
olive
    expandable olive
    metal olive
    palpable pyloric olive
    Sippy dilating olives
olive dilator
olive ring
olive tip
olive wire
Olivecrona aneurysm clamp
Olivecrona aneurysm clip
Olivecrona aneurysm forceps
Olivecrona angular scissors
Olivecrona brain spatula
Olivecrona clip applier
Olivecrona clip-applying and
    removing forceps
Olivecrona clip-applying forceps
Olivecrona conchotome
Olivecrona double-ended
    dissector
Olivecrona dura scissors
Olivecrona endaural rongeur
Olivecrona guillotine scissors
Olivecrona mastoid rongeur
Olivecrona rongeur forceps
Olivecrona saw
Olivecrona scissors

Olivecrona silver clip
Olivecrona spatula
Olivecrona trigeminus knife
Olivecrona wire saw
Olivecrona-Gigli wire saw
Olivecrona-Stille dissector
Olivecrona-Toennis clip-applying
    forceps
Oliver scalp retractor
olive-tipped monopolar
    electrosurgical dissector
olives passed over guidewire
olive-tipped bougie
olive-tipped cannula
olive-tipped catheter
olive-tipped dilator
olive-tipped irrigator
olive-tipped needle
olive-tipped stripper
Olivier-Bertrand-Tipal frame
olivocerebellar tract
olivocochlear bundle of
    Rasmussen
olivopontocerebellar atrophy
Olk membrane peeler knife
Olk retinal spatula
Olk vitreoretinal pick
Olk vitreoretinal spatula
Ollier arthrodesis approach
Ollier disease
Ollier graft
Ollier incision
Ollier lateral approach
Ollier layer
Ollier operation
Ollier rake retractor
Ollier raspatory
Ollier technique
Ollier thick split free graft
Ollier-Murphy approach in hip
    arthroplasty
Ollier-Thiersch graft
Ollier-Thiersch implant
Ollier-Thiersch operation
Ollier-Thiersch prosthesis
Olliger splint
Olsen bayonet monopolar
    forceps
Olsen cholangiogram clamp
Olsen-Hegar needle holder
Olshausen operation
Olshausen procedure

Olshausen sign
Olshausen suspension
Olshevsky tube
Olyco articulator
Olyco mouth mirror
Olympia articulator
Olympia mouth mirror
Olympia Vacpac support
Olympia Vacpac support device
Olympian forehead
Olympic mask
Olympic needle holder
Olympic Neostraint immobilizer
Olympus alligator-jaw
    endoscopic forceps
Olympus angioscope
Olympus automatic reprocessor
Olympus basket-type
    endoscopic forceps
Olympus biopsy forceps
Olympus bronchoscope
Olympus choledochofiberscope
Olympus cholangioscope
Olympus choledochoscope
Olympus choledochofiberscope
Olympus clip-fixing device
Olympus colonoscope
Olympus colonofiberscope
Olympus cystofiberscope
Olympus cystoscope
Olympus detachable miniloop
Olympus diagnostic laparoscope
Olympus dilatation catheter
Olympus disposable cannula
Olympus disposable trocar
Olympus duodenofiberscope
Olympus duodenoscope
Olympus echoendoscope
Olympus endocamera
Olympus endoscope
Olympus endoscopic biopsy
    forceps
Olympus endoscopic camera
Olympus endoscopic forceps
Olympus endoscopic ultrasound
    scanner
Olympus endosonography
    image processor
Olympus endoscopic suture-
    cutting forceps
Olympus endoscopic
    ultrasound

Olympus Endo-Therapy
  disposable biopsy forceps
Olympus enteroscope
Olympus esophagofiberscope
Olympus esophagoscope
Olympus fibercolonoscope
Olympus flexible
  echocolonoscope
Olympus flexible gastroscope
Olympus flexible laryngoscope
Olympus flexible sigmoidoscope
Olympus fluorescence
  microscope
Olympus fiberoptic
  duodenoscope
Olympus fiberoptic
  bronchoscope
Olympus fiberoptic cystoscope
Olympus fiberoptic
  duodenoscope
Olympus fiberoptic instrument
Olympus fiberoptic
  sigmoidoscope
Olympus fiberscope
Olympus flexible ENT scope
Olympus flexible
  hysterofiberscope
Olympus flexible sigmoidoscope
Olympus forward-viewing
  endoscope
Olympus gastrocamera
Olympus gastroscope
Olympus gastrostomy
Olympus grasping rat-tooth
  forceps
Olympus heater probe
Olympus hot biopsy forceps
Olympus hysteroscope
Olympus injector
Olympus laryngoscope
Olympus light source connector
Olympus lithotriptor
Olympus magnetic extractor
  forceps
Olympus magnifying
  colonoscope
Olympus microscope
Olympus miniature camera
Olympus miniature ultrasonic
  probe
Olympus minisnare forceps
Olympus monopolar cannula

Olympus needle
Olympus needle-knife
  papillotome
Olympus neonatal cystoscope
Olympus oblique-viewing
  flexible fiberscope
Olympus One-Step button
Olympus One-Step Button
  gastrostomy tube
Olympus operating camera
Olympus operating laparoscope
Olympus panendoscope
Olympus pediatric colonoscope
Olympus pelican-type
  endoscopic forceps
Olympus pediatric
  duodenoscope
Olympus pediatric endoscope
Olympus resectoscope loop
Olympus reflex camera
Olympus reusable oval cup
  forceps
Olympus reusable oval cup
  forceps with needle
Olympus rubber-tip endoscopic
  forceps
Olympus sclerotherapy needle
Olympus scope
Olympus semicircular snare
Olympus shark-tooth
  endoscopic forceps
Olympus side-viewing
  endoscope
Olympus sigmoidoscope
Olympus snare cautery device
Olympus sphincterotome
Olympus stone retrieval basket
Olympus translaparoscopic
  choledochofiberscope
Olympus tripod-type
  endoscopic forceps
Olympus twin-channel
  gastroscope
Olympus ultrasonic
  esophagoprobe
Olympus ultrasonic endoscope
Olympus ultrathin balloon-fitted
  ultrasound probe
Olympus ultrathin endoscope
Olympus ureterorenofiberscope
Olympus video endoscope
Olympus video enteroscope

Olympus video duodenoscope
Olympus video duodenoscope
Olympus video push endoscope
Olympus wash catheter
Olympus W-shaped endoscopic
    forceps
O'Malley jaw fracture splint
O'Malley knife
O'Malley ocutome
O'Malley self-adhering lens
    implant
O'Malley vitrector
O'Malley-Heintz infusion
    cannula
O'Malley-Heintz vitreous cutter
O'Malley-Pearce-Luma lens
Ombredanne forceps
Omega 5600 noninvasive blood
    pressure monitor
Omega compression hip screw
Omega screw
Omega splinting material
Omega-NV balloon
OmegaPort access port
Omegascope flexible
    microendoscope
omega-shaped incision
    score
OMENS (orbit, mandible, ear,
    cranial nerves, and soft
    tissue) score
omental adhesions
omental adhesive band
omental appendage
omental band
omental bursa
omental cake
omental cyst
omental enterocleisis
omental filler
omental flap
omental graft
omental hernia
omental metastasis
omental nodal disease
omental patch
omental plug
omental recess
omental skin graft
omental studding
omental transposition
omental transposition flap

omentectomy
omentofixation
omentopexy
    Narath omentopexy
omentoplasty
omentorrhaphy
omentosplenopexy
omentotomy
omentum
    colic omentum
    gastric omentum
    gastrocolic omentum
    gastrohepatic omentum
    gastrosplenic omentum
    greater omentum
    incarcerated omentum
    lesser omentum
    pancreaticosplenic omentum
    splenogastric omentum
    transposed omentum
omentum majus flap procedure
omentum minus
omentumectomy
Omer sternoclavicular
    dislocation
Omer technique
Omer-Capen carpectomy
Omer-Capen technique
Omiderm transparent adhesive
    film dressing
Ommaya cerebrospinal fluid
    reservoir
Ommaya reservoir device
Ommaya reservoir implant
    material
Ommaya reservoir prosthesis
Ommaya reservoir transensor
Ommaya retromastoid reservoir
Ommaya shunt
Ommaya side-port flat-bottomed
    reservoir
Ommaya spinal fluid reservoir
Ommaya suboccipital reservoir
Ommaya ventricular reservoir
Ommaya ventricular tube
Omni 2 microscope
Omni Bloc bite blocks
Omni catheter
Omni knee brace
Omni laser tip
Omni operating microscope
Omni press

Omni pretibial buttress
Omni retractor
Omni SST balloon
Omni-Atricor pacemaker
Omnicarbon heart valve
    prosthesis
Omnicarbon prosthetic valve
OmniCath atherectomy catheter
Omnicor pacemaker
Omnicor programmer
Omni-Ectocor pacemaker
Omnifit acetabular cup
Omnifit HA femoral component
Omnifit HA hip stem
Omnifit HA hip stem prosthesis
Omnifit intraocular lens
Omnifit knee prosthesis
Omniflex balloon
Omniflex balloon catheter
Omniflex head
Omniflex impression material
Omni-Flexor device
OmniLink biliary stent
Omniloc dental implant
OmniMed argon-fluoride
    excimer laser
OmniMedia XRS scanner
Omni-Orthocor pacemaker
Omni-Park eyelid speculum
OmniPhase penile prosthesis
OmniPhase semirigid penile
    prosthesis
OmniPulse holmium laser
Omniscience heart valve
Omniscience prosthetic valve
Omniscience single-leaflet
    cardiac valve prosthesis
Omniscience tilting-disk valve
Omniscience valve device
Omni-Stanicor pacemaker
OmniStent
Omni-Theta pacemaker
OmniTip side-firing laser needle
Omni-Tract vaginal retractor
Omnivac splint
Omni-Ventricor pacemaker
omocervical flap
omoclavicular fossa
omoclavicular triangle
omohyoid muscle
omphalectomy
omphalelcosis

omphalic
omphalocele
omphalomesenteric duct
omphalomesenteric veins
omphalomesenteric vessels
omphalospinous line
omphalotomy
Omron compressor nebulizer
Omron Hem-601 automatic
    digital wrist blood pressure
    monitor
Omron/Marshall 97 automatic
    oscillometric digital blood
    pressure monitor
OMS (oral and maxillofacial
    surgery)
OMU (ostiomeatal unit)
On2 lateral transfer device
oncocytic adenoma
oncocytic epithelial cell
oncocytic schneiderian
    papilloma (OSP)
oncocytoid carcinoid
oncocytoid change
oncocytosis
oncogenic virus
oncologic anatomy
oncologic mandibular resection
On-Command catheter
oncoplastic carcinoma
oncoplastic surgery
Oncor ApopTaq Kit
oncotaxis
oncotic pressure
oncotomy
One-vessel angioplasty
One disposable microkeratome
One Time dressing kit
One Time sharp debridement tray
One Time skin stapler
One Time staple remover
One Touch blood glucose
    monitor
one-buttress defect
on-edge mattress sutures
one-hand speculum
one-handed knot
one-hold angiographic catheter
one-horn bridge
O'Neill cardiac clamp
O'Neill cardiac surgical scissors
O'Neill scissors

one-lung anesthesia
one-lung ventilation (OLV)
one-lung ventilation anesthetic
    technique
one-part fracture
one-phase subperiosteal implant
    technique
one-piece lip retractor
one-piece ostomy pouch
one-piece shunt with reservoir
one-plane deformity
one-plate haptic silicone
    intraocular lens
one-pour technique
one-session removal
one-sheet pack
One-Shot anastomotic instrument
one-sixth molar lactate solution
one-snip punctum operation
one-stage amputation
one-stage esthetic correction
one-stage grafting
one-stage hypospadias repair
one-stage left colectomy
one-stage operation
one-stage
    pancreatoduodenectomy
one-stage posterior mediastinal
    esophagoplasty
one-stage procedure
One-Time disposable skin
    stapler
One-Touch blood glucose meter
One-Touch electrolysis unit
one-vessel angioplasty
Ong capsulotomy scissors
Onik-Cohen percutaneous
    access catheter
onion peel appearance
onion scale lesion
onion skin-like membrane
onion-bulb changes on biopsy
onlay (ON)
onlay bone graft
onlay bone grafting
onlay bone patch
onlay cortical graft
onlay Dacron prosthesis
onlay graft
onlay grafting
onlay implant
onlay island flap

onlay patch anastomosis
onlay splint
onlay technique
onlay tip graft
onlay-tube onlay-urethroplasty
    technique
On-Q pump
onset of blockade
on-table angiogram
on-table irrigation
onychauxis
onychectomy
onychia
onychocryptosis
onychogryphosis
onychomycosis
onychomycosis nigricans
onychoplasty
onychorrhexis
onychotomy
Onyx finger pulse oximeter
Onyx-R NiTi file
oocyte extrusion
oophorectomy
oophoritic cyst
oophorocystectomy
oophorohysterectomy
oophoropexy
oophoroplasty
oophorosalpingectomy
oophorostomy
oophorotomy
oophorrhaphy
oothecectomy
oozing
    shunt-site oozing
OP-1 implant (osteogenic
    protein 1)
Opaca-Garcea ureteral catheter
opacification
    corneal opacification
    coronary opacification
    cortical opacification
    faint opacification
    lens opacification
    linear opacification
    stringy opacification
opacified frontal sinus
opacifying
opacity
    capsular opacities
    Caspar ring opacity

opacity (*continued*)
  corneal opacity
  lens opacity
  subcapsular opacity
  vitreous opacity
Opal tissue ablation device
opaque arthrography
opaque calculus
opaque material
opaque medium
opaque microscope
opaque myringotomy tube
opaque shadows
opaque wire suture
OPCAB (off-pump coronary artery bypass)
open adjustable silicone gastric banding
open adrenalectomy
open airway
open amputation
open anesthesia
open anti-reflux surgery
open apex
open appendectomy (OA)
open biopsy
open bite malocclusion
open brain biopsy
open capsulotomy
open carpal tunnel release (OCTR)
open cavity
open C-D hook
open cholecystectomy
open colectomy
open common bile duct exploration
open coronal brow lift
open disk surgery
open dislocation
open diverticulectomy
open drainage
open dressing
open drop anesthesia
open drop technique
open earmold
open electrocautery snare
open endarterectomy
open endotracheal inhalation anesthesia
open esophagectomy
open esophagomyotomy

open facemask
open facelift
open fistula
open flap technique
open foreheadplasty
open fracture
open fundoplication
open harvesting technique
open Hasson technique
open head injury
open heart surgery
open hemorrhoidectomy
open hernia operation
open herniorrhaphy
open inhalation anesthesia
open laparoscopic approach
open laparoscopic technique
open laparoscopy
open laparotomy
open lens
open liver biopsy
open loop
open lung biopsy
open magnet
open method harvest
open miniabdominoplasty
open mitral commissurotomy
open Nissen fundoplication (ONF)
open Nissen operation
open oblique osteotomy
open operation
open osteotomy
open palm technique
open perineal biopsy
open reconstruction
open reconstructive procedure
open reduction
open reduction and fixation
open reduction and internal fixation (ORIF)
open reduction of dislocation
open reduction of fracture
open reduction of fracture-dislocation
open reduction with internal fixation (ORIF)
open repair
open retroperitoneal high ligation
open rhinoplasty

open skull fracture
open sphincterotome
open stereotactic craniotomy
open surgical biopsy
open surgical cordotomy
open surgical therapy
open technique
open thimble splint
open transaxillary breast
    augmentation (OTBA)
open valvulotomy
open vertical banded
    gastroplasty
open wound
open-angle glaucoma
open-approach nose reshaping
open-book fracture
open-celled foam
open-end aspirating tube
open-end ostomy pouch
open-ended ureteral catheter
open-gloving technique
opening ABD wedge
    bunionectomy
opening axis
opening flap
opening mandibular movement
opening snap
opening wedge
opening wedge manipulation
opening wedge osteotomy
open-look effect
open-loop intraocular lens
open-patch technique
open-pore structure
OpenSail balloon catheter
open-side vaginal speculum
open-sky cryoextraction
    operation
open-sky procedure
open-sky rhinoplasty
open-sky technique
open-sky vitrectomy
open-tube rigid bronchoscope
OPERA Star morcellator
OPERA Star hysteroscope
operable cancer
operable case
opera-glass deformity
opera-glass hand
operant procedure
operated cleft

operating esophagoscope
operating gastroscope
operating knife
operating loupe
operating microscope
operating otoscope
operating platform
operating scissors
operating scope
operating suite
operating table
operating telescope
operating voltage
operation
  1-snip punctum operation
  1-stage operation
  2nd-look operation
  2-stage operation
  3-snip punctum operation
  ab externo filtering operation
  Abbe operation
  Abbott operation
  Abbott-Lucas shoulder
      operation
  Abbe small bowel operation
  Abbe-Estlander operation
  abdominal pull-through
      operation
  Abell operation
  Abernethy operation
  Aburel operation
  accessory feminizing
      operation
  Adams ectropion operation
  Adams hip operation
  Adelmann operation
  Adler operation
  Agee fiberoptic carpal tunnel
      operation
  Agnew operation
  AKC varicose vein operation
  Albee hip operation
  Albee-Delbet operation
  Albert knee operation
  Aldridge operation
  Alexander operation
  Alexander-Adams operation
  Allarton operation
  Allen operation
  Allingham operation
  Allison gastroesophageal
      reflux operation

operation (*continued*)

Allport operation
Almoor operation
Alouette operation
Alsus-Knapp operation
Altemeier operation
Alvis operation
Ambrose operation
Ammon operation
Amsler corneal graft
  operation
Amussat operation
Anagnostakis operation
anal stretch operation
anastomotic operation
Anderson operation
Anderson-Hutchins tibial
  fracture operation
Andrews bottle operation
Anel operation
Angelucci operation
Annandale knee operation
annular corneal graft
  operation
Anson-McVay operation
anterior fusion operation
anterior Polya operation
antimesenteric fat operation
antiperistaltic operation
antireflux operation
antral window operation
aorticopulmonary window
  operation
Appolito operation
Argyll Robertson operation
Arie-Pitanguy mammary ptosis
  operation
Arie-Pitanguy operation
Arion sling operation
Arlt operation
Arlt-Jaesche operation
Armistead ulnar lengthening
  operation
Armsby operation
Arrowhead operation
Arroyo operation
Arruga operation
Arruga-Berens operation
Arslan operation
arterial switch operation
Asai operation
Asch operation

operation (*continued*)

Ashford retracted nipple
  operation
atrial baffle operation
Auchincloss operation
Auclair operation
Avila operation
Axer operation
Aylett operation
Babcock operation
Bacon-Babcock operation
Badal operation
Badgley operation
Baffle operation
Bailey operation
Baker patellar advancement
  operation
Baker translocation operation
Baldwin operation
Baldy operation
Baldy-Webster operation
Ball operation
Ball-Hoffman operation
Bancroft-Plenk operation
Band-Aid operation
Bangerter operation
Bangerter pterygium
  operation
Bankart-Putti-Platt operation
Bardelli operation
bariatric operation
Barkan double cyclodialysis
  operation
Barkan goniotomy operation
Barkan-Cordes linear cataract
  operation
Barker operation
Barnard operation
Barr tendon transfer
  operation
Barraquer enzymatic
  zonulolysis operation
Barrie-Jones
  canaliculodacryorhino-
  stomy operation
Barrio operation
Barsky operation
Barton operation
Barwell operation
Basset operation
Bassini operation
Basterra operation

operation (*continued*)

Bateman modification of
  Mayer transfer operation
Battle operation
Baudelocque operation
Baudet-Fontan operation
Baum operation
Baynton operation
Beard operation
Beard-Cutler operation
Beath operation
Beatson operation
Beck I operation
Beck II operation
Becker operation
Beck-Jianu operation
Beer cataract flap operation
Belfield operation
Bell operation
Belmas operation
Belsey antireflux operation
Belsey Mark IV antireflux
  operation
Belsey Mark IV operation
Benedict operation
Bennett operation
Bent operation
Berens pterygium transplant
  operation
Berens sclerectomy operation
Berens-Smith operation
Berger operation
Berke operation
Berke-Motais operation
Bernard operation
Bernard-Burow operation
Berry operation
Best operation
Bethke operation
Bevan operation
Bevan-Rochet operation
Beyea operation
Bielschowsky operation
Bier operation
Biesenberger operation
Bigelow operation
biliary-enteric anastomosis
  operation
Billroth I operation
Billroth II operation
Binnie operation
Bircher operation

operation (*continued*)

Birch-Hirschfeld entropion
  operation
Bischoff operation
Bissell operation
Björk operation
Blair ptosis correction
  operation
Blair-Brown operation
Blair-Brown-McDowell
  operation
Blair-Byars operation
Blair-Wehrbein operation
Blalock operation
Blalock-Hanlon operation
Blalock-Taussig operation
Blasius lid flap operation
Blasius lid operation
Blaskovics canthoplasty
  operation
Blaskovics dacryostomy
  operation
Blaskovics lid operation
Blatt operation
Bloch-Paul-Mikulicz operation
Blocker operation
Block-Paul-Mixter operation
Bloodgood operation
bloodless operation
Blount operation
Blundell-Jones operation
Boari operation
Bobb operation
Bobroff operation
Boehm operation
Boerema-Crile operation
Bogue operation
bolster operation
Bonaccolto-Flieringa vitreous
  operation
Bondy operation
Bonnet enucleation operation
Bonney operation
Bonzel operation
Bora operation
Borggreve operation
Borthen operation
Bose operation
Bossalino blepharoplasty
  operation
Bosworth operation
Bottini operation

operation (*continued*)
 bottle hernia operation
 bottle operation
 Bouilly operation
 Bowman operation
 Boyd operation
 Boyes operation
 Bozeman operation
 Brackett operation
 Brailey operation
 Brauer operation
 Braun operation
 Braun-Wangensteen operation
 Brenner operation
 Brett operation
 Brewer operation
 Bricker operation
 Bridge operation
 bridge pedicle flap operation
 Briggs strabismus operation
 Bristow operation
 Brittain operation
 Broadbent operation
 Brock operation
 Brockman operation
 Bromley foreign body
  operation
 Bronson foreign body removal
  operation
 Brophy cleft palate
  operation
 Brown operation
 Brown-Blair operation
 Brunschwig operation
 Bryant operation
 buccal pedicle-flap operation
 Buck operation
 buckling operation
 Budinger blepharoplasty
  operation
 Buie operation
 bunion operation
 Bunnell operation
 Burch eye evisceration
  operation
 Burckhardt operation
 Burgess operation
 Burow flap operation
 Butler 5th toe operation
 buttonhole operation
 Buzzi operation
 bypass operation

operation (*continued*)
 Byron Smith ectropion
  operation
 Cairns operation
 Caldwell operation
 Caldwell-Luc window
  operation
 Calhoun-Hagler lens
  extraction operation
 Callahan operation
 Callisen operation
 Calot operation
 Camey I operation
 Camey II operation
 Campbell operation
 Campbell-Goldthwait patella
  dislocation operation
 Campodonico operation
 Canfield operation
 capital operation
 Carmody-Batson operation
 Carnochan operation
 Carpue operation
 Carrel operation
 Carter operation
 Casanellas lacrimal operation
 Casey operation
 Caslick operation
 Cassel operation
 Castroviejo operation
 Castroviejo-Scheie
  cyclodiathermy operation
 cataract extraction operation
 cataract flap operation
 cataract operation
 Cattell operation
 cautery operation
 Cave operation
 Cave-Rowe operation
 Cawthorne operation
 Cecil urethral stricture
  operation
 Cecil-Culp operation
 celsian operation
 Celsus spasmodic entropion
  operation
 Celsus-Hotz operation
 cerclage operation
 cesarean operation
 Chandler vitreous operation
 Chandler-Verhoeff operation
 Chaput anal operation

operation (*continued*)
- Charcot operation
- Charles operation
- Cheatle-Henry operation
- Chevalier Jackson operation
- Cheyne operation
- Chiazzi operation
- Chiene operation
- Child operation
- Childress operation
- Chopart operation
- Cibis operation
- cinch operation
- cinching operation
- Civiale operation
- Clagett operation
- Clark operation
- Clayton operation
- clean operation
- clean-contaminated operation
- Cleasby iridectomy operation
- cleft palate operation
- Cleveland-Bosworth-Thompson operation
- Cloutier operation
- Cloward operation
- cluster operation
- Coakley sinus operation
- Codivilla operation
- Coffey operation
- Cohen operation
- Cole operation
- Colles operation
- Collin-Beard operation
- Collis antireflux operation
- Collis-Nissen operation
- Colonna operation
- Colonna-Ralston operation
- colorectal operation
- Colp-Hofmeister operation
- Coltart talus fracture operation
- Comberg foreign body operation
- combined operation
- commando operation
- comparison operation
- Compere operation
- complete wrap Nissen operation
- composite operation
- computer-assisted operation

operation (*continued*)
- Conn operation
- Connell operation
- Conrad orbital blowout fracture operation
- Continent operation
- conventional operation
- Converse operation
- Conway operation
- Cooley operation
- Cooper operation
- corneal graft operation
- corrective operation
- cosmetic operation
- Cotte operation
- Cotting toenail operation
- Cottle operation
- Counsellor-Davis artificial-vagina operation
- Cozen-Brockway operation
- Crafoord operation
- Crawford sling operation
- Credo operation
- Creevy operation
- Crego operation
- crescent operation
- Crespo operation
- Crile-Matas operation
- Cripps operation
- Critchett operation
- Crock encircling operation
- Cronin operation
- Crutchfield operation
- cryoextraction operation
- cryotherapy operation
- Csapody orbital repair operation
- Culp-Calhoon operation
- Culp-Scardino operation
- Cupper-Faden operation
- curative sphincter-saving operation
- curative-intent operation
- Curtin operation
- Curtis operation
- Cushing operation
- Cusick operation
- Cusick-Sarrail ptosis operation
- Custodis scleral buckle operation
- Cutler operation
- Cutler-Beard operation

operation (*continued*)
 cyclodiathermy operation
 Czermak pterygium operation
 Czerny operation
 dacryoadenectomy operation
 dacryocystectomy operation
 dacryocystorhinotomy
  operation
 dacryocystostomy operation
 Dalgleish operation
 Dallas operation
 Dammann-Muller operation
 Damus-Kaye-Stansel operation
 Dana operation
 Dandy operation
 Danforth fetal operation
 Daviel operation
 Davies-Colley operation
 Davis operation
 day-case operation
 de Grandmont operation
 de Lapersonne operation
 de Vincentiis operation
 Debeyre rotator cuff
  operation
 debulking operation
 Decker operation
 decompression operation
 Dees operation
 Deiter operation
 DeKlair operation
 Del Toro operation
 DeLee operation
 Delorme rectal prolapse
  operation
 Delorme-Fowler operation
 Demel-Ruttin operation
 Denans operation
 Denis Browne operation
 Denker sinus operation
 Dennis operation
 Denonvilliers operation
 Denuse operation
 Derby operation
 Derlacki operation
 Descemet operation
 Desmarres operation
 Devine operation
 Dewar-Harris operation
 DeWecker operation
 Diamond-Gould syndactyly
  operation

operation (*continued*)
 Dianoux trichiasis operation
 diathermy operation
 Dick operation
 Dickey operation
 Dickey-Fox operation
 Dickson shelf operation
 Dickson-Diveley operation
 Dickson-Wright operation
 Dieffenbach operation
 Dieffenbach-Duplay operation
 Dieffenbach-Szymanowski-
  Kuhnt operation
 Dieffenbach-Warren operation
 Dieffenbach-Webster
  operation
 distal Roux-en-Y gastric
  operation
 Dittel operation
 DKS operation
 Doderlein roll-flap operation
 Doderlein-Kronig operation
 Dohlman operation
 Doleris operation
 d'Ombrain operation
 Donald operation
 Donald-Fothergill operation
 Doppler operation
 Dorrance operation
 Dott operation
 Dotter operation
 double eyelid operation
 double-flap operation
 double-needle cataract
  operation
 Douglas operation
 Dourmashkin operation
 Dowell operation
 Doyen operation
 Doyle operation
 Dragstedt operation
 Dragstedt-Tanner operation
 Drummond-Morison
  operation
 Dudley operation
 Duhamel colon operation
 D^{u}hrssen operation
 Duke-Elder operation
 Dunn operation
 Dunn-Brittain operation
 Dunnington operation
 Duplay operation

operation (*continued*)
Dupuy-Dutemps operation
Dupuytren operation
Durham flatfoot operation
Durham-Caldwell operation
Durman operation
Durr operation
Duverger-Velter operation
Dwyer clawfoot operation
Eagleton operation
Eaton-Malerich fracture-
  dislocation operation
Edebohls operation
Eden-Lawson operation
Edlan-Mejchar operation
effector operation
Effler operation
Effler-Groves operation
Eggers operation
Eitner operation
Ekehorn operation
elephantiasis operation
Elliot operation
Ellis operation
Ellis-Jones operation
Elmslie-Cholmeley operation
Eloesser operation
Elschnig canthorrhaphy
  operation
Elschnig operation
Ely operation
emergency operation
emergent operation
Emmet operation
endorectal ileal pull-through
  operation
enterobiliary operation
entropion operation
epithelial inlay operation
epithelial onlay operation
epithelial outlay operation
equilibrating operation
Erbakan inferior fornix
  operation
Erich operation
Escapini cataract operation
Esmarch operation
Esser eyelid operation
Esser inlay operation
Estes operation
Estlander operation
Evans operation

operation (*continued*)
Everett-TeLinde operation
Eversbusch ptosis operation
eversion operation
evisceration operation
Ewing operation
exploratory operation
extra-abdominal operation
extracapsular cataract
  extraction operation
eyelid operation
eyelid ptosis operation
Eyler operation
facelift operation
Faden strabismus operation
Fahey operation
Fairbanks operation
Falk operation
Falk-Shukuris operation
Fansler-Frykman operation
Fanta cataract operation
Farabeuf operation
Farill operation
Farmer hallux valgus
  operation
Fasanella operation
Fasanella-Servat
  blepharoptosis operation
Fasanella-Servat ptosis
  operation
fascia lata sling operation
Federov operation
fenestrated Fontan operation
fenestration operation
Fenton operation
Fergus operation
Fergusson operation
Ferris Smith operation
Fick operation
Filatov operation
filtering operation
Fink cataract operation
Finney operation
Finochietto operation
Finsterer operation
Finsterer-Hofmeister
  operation
Finzi-Harmer operation
Fisher operation
Flajani operation
flap operation
Fleming operation

operation (*continued*)
floating forehead operation
Foerster operation
Foerster-Penfield operation
Foley operation
Fomon operation
Fontan operation
forceps operation
Fothergill operation
Fothergill-Donald operation
Fothergill-Hunter operation
Fothergill-Shaw operation
Fould entropion operation
Fowler operation
Fox entropion operation
Franceschetti coreoplasty
  operation
Franceschetti corepraxy
  operation
Franceschetti deviation
  operation
Franceschetti keratoplasty
  operation
Franceschetti pupil deviation
  operation
Franco operation
Frazier operation
Frazier-Spiller operation
Freckner operation
Fredet-Ramstedt operation
Freeman operation
French skin flap operation
French supracondylar fracture
  operation
Freund operation
Freyer operation
Fricke eyelid operation
Frickman I operation
Frickman II operation
Friede operation
Friedenwald ptosis
  operation
Friedenwald-Guyton
  operation
Friedreich foot operation
Fritsch operation
Frommel operation
frontal sinus operation
Frost operation
Frost-Lang operation
Fuchs canthorrhaphy
  operation

operation (*continued*)
Fuchs iris bombe transfixion
  operation
Fukala operation
Fuller operation
Furlow-Fisher modification of
  Virag 1 operation
fusion operation
Gabarro operation
Gaillard operation
Galeazzi patellar operation
gallbladder operation
Gallie operation
Gallie-LeMesurier operation
Gant operation
Gardner operation
gastric bypass operation
Gatellier operation
Gauderer-Ponsky PEG
  operation
Gavello operation
Gayet operation
Gaza operation
Georgariou operation
Gersuny operation
Ghormley operation
Gibson operation
Gifford delimiting keratotomy
  operation
Gigli operation
Gill operation
Gilles operation
Gillespie operation
Gilliam operation
Gilliam-Doleris operation
Gillies scar correction
  operation
Gillies-Fry operation
Gillies-Kilner operation
Gill-Stein operation
Gil-Vernet operation
Giordano operation
Giralde operation
Girard keratoprosthesis
  operation
Girdlestone operation
Gittes operation
glass hand operation
Glenn operation
Goebel-Frangenheim-Stoeckel
  operation
Goebel-Stoeckel operation

operation (*continued*)
Goffe operation
gold weight and wire spring
operation
Goldmann-Larson foreign
body operation
Goldsmith operation
Goldthwait operation
Gomez-Marquez lacrimal
operation
Gonin cautery operation
Gonin operation
goniopuncture operation
goniotomy operation
Goodall-Power operation
Gottschalk operation
Gradle keratoplasty operation
Graefe operation
Graham operation
Graham-Roscie operation
Grant operation
Grant-Ward operation
Greaves operation
Green operation
Green-Armytage operation
Grice-Green operation
Grimsdale operation
Gritti operation
Grondahl-Finney operation
Gross operation
Grossman operation
Guleke-Stookey operation
Gussenbauer operation
Gutzeit dacryostomy
operation
Guyon operation
Guyton ptosis operation
Haas dislocation operation
Hagedorn operation
Hagedorn-LeMesurier
operation
Hagerty operation
Hagner operation
Hahn operation
Haight operation
Hajek operation
Halpin operation
Halsted operation
Halsted-Ferguson operation
Hammond operation
Hampton small bowel
operation

operation (*continued*)
Hancock operation
Handley operation
hanging hip operation
hanging toe operation
harelip operation
Harman operation
Harmon operation
Harms-Dannheim
trabeculotomy operation
Harrington operation
Harris operation
Hartley-Krause operation
Hartmann operation
Hasner operation
Hassab operation
Hatcher operation
Haultain operation
Hauser operation
Haverhill ear operation
Haynes operation
Heaney operation
Heath operation
Heaton operation
Hegar operation
Heifitz operation
Heile operation
Heimlich operation
Heine operation
Heineke operation
Heineke-Mikulicz hypospadias
operation
Heisrath operation
Heitz-Boyer operation
Heller operation
Heller-Belsey operation
Heller-Dor operation
Heller-Nissen operation
hemi-Fontan operation
Henderson operation
Henry operation
Henry-Geist operation
Herbert operation
Hess eyelid operation
Hess ptosis operation
Heuter operation
Hey operation
Hey-Groves operation
Heyman operation
Heyman-Herndon operation
Hibbs operation
Hiff operation

operation (*continued*)

Higgins operation
high-forceps operation
Hill antireflux operation
Hill hiatus hernia operation
Hill-Allison operation
Hinsberg operation
Hippel operation
Hirst operation
His-Haas operation
Hochenegg operation
Hoffa operation
Hoffa-Lorenz operation
Hofmeister operation
Hofmeister-Finsterer
  operation
Hofmeister-Polya operation
Hogan operation
Hoguet operation
Hohmann operation
Hoke operation
Holmes operation
Holth operation
Hood operation
Hopkins operation
Horay operation
Horgan operation
Horner operation
Horsley operation
Horton-Devine operation
Horvath operation
Horwitz-Adams operation
Hotchkiss operation
Hotz entropion operation
Hotz-Anagnostakis operation
Hough operation
Houston operation
Howorth operation
Hueter-Mayo operation
Hufnagel operation
Huggins operation
Hughes eyelid operation
Humby operation
Hummelsheim operation
Hunt operation
Hunter operation
Huntington operation
Hunt-Transley operation
Hutch operation
Hutch ureteral reflux
  operation
Hyams operation

operation (*continued*)

Hybbinette-Eden operation
hypopyon operation
hypospadias operation
I-beam hip operation
ileal pull-through operation
ileoanal endorectal pull-
  through operation
Iliff ptosis operation
Iliff-Haus operation
Imre flap operation
Imre lateral canthoplasty
  operation
Imre lid operation
indentation operation
Indian skin flap operation
initial operation
intermediate operation
interposition operation
interval operation
intracapsular cataract
  extraction operation
inversion operation
Ionescu operation
iridectomy operation
iridencleisis operation
iridodialysis operation
iridotomy operation
iris inclusion operation
iris stretching operation
Irvine operation
Irving sterilization operation
Irwin operation
Israel operation
Italian operation
Ivalon sponge-wrap operation
Jaboulay operation
Jaboulay-Doyen-Winkleman
  operation
Jackson-Babcock operation
Jacobaeus operation
Jaesche operation
Jaesche-Arlt operation
Jaime lacrimal operation
Jameson operation
Jansen operation
Jantene operation
Japanese standard operation
Japanese-style operation
Jarvis operation
Jay-Monnet acromioclavicular
  operation

operation (*continued*)
Jelks operation
Jensen operation
Jewett operation
Jianu-Beck operation
Jobert de Lamballe operation
Johnson operation
Jones hammertoe operation
Joplin operation
Joseph operation
Judd operation
Judet operation
Kader operation
Kader-Senn operation
Kasai operation
Katzin operation
Kaufman operation
Kaye antihelix operation
Kaye-Damus-Stansel operation
Kazanjian operation
Keegan operation
keel operation
Keen operation
Kehr operation
Keller hallux rigidus
    operation
Keller hallux valgus operation
Keller-Madlener operation
Kellogg-Speed operation
Kelly urinary incontinence
    operation
Kelly-Deming operation
Kelly-Kennedy operation
Kelly-Stoeckel operation
Kelman operation
Kennedy urinary
    incontinence operation
Kennedy-Pacey operation
keratectomy operation
keratocentesis operation
keratomileusis operation
keratoplasty operation
keratotomy operation
Kessler operation
Key operation
Kidner operation
kidney-sparing operation
Kjelland operation
Killian frontal sinus operation
Killian-Freer operation
Kilner operation
King operation

operation (*continued*)
King vocal cord operation
King-Richards operation
Kirby operation
Kirkaldy-Willis operation
Kirmisson operation
Kirschner operation
Kitlowski operation
Kleinert operation
Kling-Richards operation
Knapp flap operation
Knapp lid operation
Knapp pterygium operation
Knapp-Imre lid operation
Knapp-Wheeler-Reese
    operation
Kocher operation
Kochs operation
Kock operation
Koeberle operation
Koenig operation
Koenig-Wittek operation
Koerte-Ballance operation
Koffler operation
Kolle-Lexer operation
Kolomnin operation
Kondoleon operation
Konno operation
Kono operation
Kowalzig operation
Kraske operation
Kraupa operation
Krause operation
Krause-Wolfe operation
Kreibig operation
Kreiker operation
Krempen-Silver-Sotelo
    nonunion operation
Kreuscher operation
Krieberg operation
Krimer operation
Kroener operation
Krönlein operation
Krönlein-Berke operation
Kropp operation
Krukenberg operation
Kuhnt eyelid operation
Kuhnt-Helmbold operation
Kuhnt-Szymanowski eyelid
    operation
Kuhnt-Thorpe operation
Kuster operation

operation (*continued*)

Kustner operation
Kwitko operation
Labbe operation
LaCarrere operation
Ladd operation
Lagleyze eyelid operation
Lagleyze-Trantas operation
Lagrange modification of
    Arruga operation
Lagrange modification of
    Berens operation
Lahey operation
laissez-faire lid operation
Lam operation
Lambrinudi operation
Lancaster operation
Lanchner operation
Landolt operation
Lane operation
Lane-Lannelongue operation
Lange operation
Langenbeck operation
Lannelongue operation
Lanz operation
laparoscopic Hassab
    operation
Laroyenne operation
Larrey operation
laryngeal drop operation
laryngeal keel operation
Lash operation
Latzko operation
Laurens operation
Lawson operation
Leadbetter operation
Leadbetter-Politano operation
Leahey operation
LeFort-Neugebauer operation
LeFort operation
Legg operation
LeMesurier operation
Lempert operation
Lennander operation
Leopold operation
L'Episcopo operation
Leriche operation
Lester Jones operation
Levine dislocation operation
Levine hip dislocation
    operation
Lewis operation

operation (*continued*)

Lexer operation
Lich operation
Lichtenstein operation
lid operation
lid ptosis operation
lid suture operation
Liebolt operation
limb-sparing operation
Lincoff operation
Lindesmith operation
Lindholm operation
Lindner operation
Lindsay operation
Linton operation
Linton-Talbott operation
lip adhesion operation
Lipsett operation
Lisfranc operation
Liston operation
Littler operation
Littlewood operation
Littre operation
liver operation
Lizar operation
Lloyd-Davis operation
lobster-claw operation
logical operation
Lohlein operation
Londermann operation
Longmire operation
Longuet operation
Lopez-Enriquez operation
Lord operation
Lorenz operation
Loreta operation
Lossen operation
Lotheissen operation
Lotheissen-McVay operation
Lottes operation
Lowenstein operation
low-forceps operation
Lowsley operation
Luc operation
Lucas-Cottrell operation
Lucas-Murray operation
Luck operation
Luckett operation
Luco operation
Ludloff operation
Lund operation
Lynch operation

operation (*continued*)

Lyon-Horgan operation
MacAusland operation
Macewen hernia operation
Machek ptosis operation
Machek-Blaskovics operation
Machek-Brunswick operation
Machek-Gifford operation
MacIntosh operation
Mack-Brunswick operation
Mackenrodt operation
Mackid operation
MacNab operation
Madlener operation
Magitot keratoplasty
   operation
magnet operation
magnetic operation
Magnus operation
Magnuson operation
Magnuson-Stack operation
MAGPI operation
Mahorner-Mead operation
Maingot operation
Mainz pouch operation
Mair operation
Majewsky operation
major operation
Makkas operation
Malbec operation
Malbran operation
Manchester operation
Manchester-Donald-Fothergill
   operation
Manchester-Fothergill
   operation
mandibular swing operation
Mann-Williamson operation
Maquet knee operation
Marchetti operation
Marcks operation
Marckwald operation
Marcy operation
Marin operation
Marquez-Gomez operation
Marshall-Marchetti operation
Marshall-Marchetti-Krantz
   operation
Martin operation
Martius operation
Martius-Harris operation
Marwedel operation

operation (*continued*)

Mason operation
mastoid obliteration operation
mastoid operation
Matas operation
Matson operation
Mauck operation
Mauksch operation
Mauksch-Maumenee-Goldberg
   operation
Maumenee-Goldberg
   operation
Maunsell-Weir operation
Maxur operation
Maydl operation
Mayo operation
Mayo-Fueth operation
Mayo-Robson operation
Mays operation
Mazur operation
McArthur operation
McBride operation
McBride-Akin operation
McBurney operation
McCall operation
McCall-Schumann operation
McCarroll operation
McCash-Randall operation
McDonald operation
McDowell operation
McEvedy operation
McGavic operation
McGee operation
McGill operation
McGuire operation
McIndoe operation
McKay-Simons clubfoot
   operation
McKeever operation
McKenzie operation
McKissock operation
McLaughlin operation
McLean operation
McReynolds pterygium
   operation
McVay operation
Meckel operation
Meek operation
Meigs operation
Meller operation
Menge operation
Mercier operation

operation (*continued*)

Merindino operation
Mermingas operation
Meyer operation
Meyer-Schwickerath
 operation
Michaelson operation
midforceps operation
mika operation
Mikamo double-eyelid
 operation
Mikulicz operation
Mikulicz-Vladimiroff operation
Milch operation
Miles operation
Millard rotation-advancement
 operation
Miller flatfoot operation
Millin operation
Millin-Read operation
Mingazzini-Foerster operation
minor operation
Minsky operation
Mirault operation
Mirault-Brown-Blair operation
Mitchell operation
mitral valve-hinging operation
modified flap operation
modified operation
Monaldi operation
Moncrieff operation
Monfort operation
Monks operation
Moore operation
Moore-Corradi operation
Moran operation
Morax operation
morcellation operation
morcellement operation
Morel-Fatio-Lalardie operation
Morestin operation
Moschcowitz operation
Mosher operation
Mosher-Toti operation
Moss operation
Motais operation
motivating operation
Moynihan intestinal operation
Moynihan operation
mucoperiosteal flap operation
Mueller operation
Mules operation

operation (*continued*)

Mumford operation
Munnell operation
Murray operation
muscle sliding operation
Mustard intra-atrial operation
Mustard operation
Mustarde operation
myectomy operation
myelomeningocele operation
myotomy operation
Naffziger operation
Narath operation
Nebinger-Praun operation
Neher operation
Nehra-Mach operation
Neibauer-Cutter operation
Nesbit operation
Neuber operation
Neviaser operation
Nicoll fracture operation
Nida nicking operation
Nirschi operation
Nissen antireflux operation
Nissen fundoplication
 operation
Nizetic operation
Noble operation
Noel-Thompson operation
Norton operation
Norwood operation
Nuttall operation
Nelaton operation
Ober operation
Oberst operation
Ober-Young operation
O'Brien pelvic halo operation
obstetrical operation
O'Connor operation
O'Connor-Peter operation
O'Donnell operation
O'Donoghue operation
Ogilvie operation
Ogston operation
Ogston-Luc operation
Ogura operation
O'Hara operation
Ollier operation
Ollier-Thiersch operation
Olshausen operation
Ombredanne operation
open hernia operation

operation (*continued*)
  open Nissen operation
  open operation
  open-sky cryoextraction
    operation
  optical iridectomy operation
  orbital implant operation
  Ord operation
  orthognathic operation
  orthotopic hemi-Koch
    operation
  Osborne operation
  Osgood operation
  Osmond-Clarke shoulder
    operation
  osteoplastic frontal sinus
    operation
  O'Sullivan operation
  outlay operation
  outpatient thyroid operation
  Overholt operation
  Owen operation
  Oxford operation
  Paci operation
  Pagenstecher operation
  palatal pushback operation
  palatoplasty pushback
    operation
  palliative operation
  Palma operation
  Palmer-Widen operation
  Palomo operation
  Panas operation
  Pancoast operation
  pancreaticobiliary operation
  pantaloon operation
  parallel operation
  parathyroid operation
  Parker-Kerr operation
  Parkes operation
  Parkhill operation
  Partsch operation
  Patey operation
  pattern cut corneal graft
    operation
  Patterson operation
  Paufique detached retina
    operation
  Paul-Mikulicz operation
  Pauwels fracture operation
  Payne operation
  Pean operation

operation (*continued*)
  pedicle flap operation
  Peet operation
  Pemberton operation
  Pereyra operation
  peripheral iridectomy
    operation
  Peter operation
  Petersen operation (GI)
  Peterson operation (gyn)
  Phaneuf-Graves operation
  pharyngeal flap operation
  Pheasant elbow dislocation
    operation
  Phelps operation
  Phemister operation
  Physick operation
  Pico operation
  Pierce-O'Connor operation
  pinning operation
  Pirogoff operation
  plastic operation
  plombage operation
  pocket operation
  Politano-Leadbetter operation
  Politzer operation
  Pollock operation
  Polya operation
  Polyak operation
  Pomeroy operation
  Poncet operation
  Porro operation
  Porro-Veit operation
  portacaval shunt operation
  Portmann interposition
    operation
  Poth operation
  Potts operation
  Potts-Smith operation
  Potts-Smith-Gibson operation
  Poulard operation
  Poulard-Pochissov operation
  Power operation
  Pozzi operation
  Preziosi operation
  Price operation
  probing lacrimonasal duct
    operation
  protective antireflux
    operation
  pterygium operation
  pubovaginal operation

operation (*continued*)
Puestow operation
Puestow-Gillesby operation
pull-through operation
pulsed-mode operation
Puntenney operation
Putti operation
Putti-Platt shoulder
    dislocation operation
Puusepp operation
pyloric occlusion operation
Quaglino operation
Quenu-Mayo operation
radical antrum operation
radical operation
Ragnell operation
Ramadier operation
Ramstedt operation
Randall operation
Randall-Tennison operation
Rankin operation
Ransohoff operation
rapid pull-through operation
Rashkind operation
Rastan operation
Rastelli operation
Raverdino operation
Ray-Brunswick-Mack
    operation
Ray-McLean operation
Read-McIndoe operation
Recamier operation
reconstruction operation
reconstructive operation
rectal pull-through operation
Redmond Smith operation
re-entry operation
Reese ptosis operation
Reese-Cleasby operation
Reese-Jones-Cooper operation
Regnoli operation
Rehne-Delorme operation
Reichenheim operation
Reichenheim-King operation
Reis-Wertheim operation
repeat operation
resectional phase of operation
resurfacing operation
Reverdin operation
Richardson operation
Richet operation
Ridell operation

operation (*continued*)
Ridley operation
Ridlon operation
Rienhoff-Tanner operation
Rigaud operation
Ripstein rectal prolapse
    operation
Rives operation
Rizzoli operation
Rodney Smith biliary stricture
    operation
Rodney Smith operation
Roger Anderson operation
rollflap operation
Rose operation
Rosenburg operation
Rosengren operation
Rose-Thompson operation
Rouge operation
Routier operation
Routte operation
Roux operation
Roux-en-Y operation
Roux-Goldthwait dislocation
    operation
Roveda operation
Rovsing operation
Rowbotham operation
Rowinski operation
Royle operation
RPT operation
Rubbrecht operation
Rubin operation
Ruedemann operation
Russe operation
Rycroft operation
Ryerson operation
saccus operation
sacroabdominoperineal pull-
    through operation
sacrofixation operation
Sade modification of
    Norwood operation
Saemisch operation
Saenger operation
Safar operation
Salter operation
Sanders operation
Saraf toenail operation
Sato operation
Sauer-Bacon operation
Savin operation

operation (*continued*)

Sawar ptosis operation
Sawyer operation
Sayoc operation
Sayre operation
Sbarbaro operation
Scanzoni operation
Scarpa operation
Schanz operation
Schauffler operation
Schauta vaginal operation
Schauta-Amreich vaginal
   operation
Schauta-Wertheim operation
Schede operation
Scheie operation
Schepens operation
Schimek operation
Schirmer operation
Schlatter operation
Schmalz operation
Schoemaker-Wangensteen
   operation
Schoenbein operation
Schreck-Mensor hanging hip
   operation
Schroeder operation
Schuchardt operation
Schuchardt-Pfeifer operation
Schuknecht operation
Schwartze operation
Schwartze-Stacke operation
scleral buckling operation
scleral fistula operation
scleral fistulectomy operation
scleral shortening operation
scleroplasty operation
Scott operation
scrotal pouch operation
Scudder operation
sector iridectomy operation
Seddon operation
Sedillot operation
Selinger operation
Semb operation
semielective operation
Senn operation
Senning transposition
   operation
sensor operation
serial operation
Serre operation

operation (*continued*)

seton operation
Sever operation
Sever-L'Episcopo operation
Sewell-Boyden operation
sex change operation
Shaffer operation
Sharrard operation
Shaw operation
Sheldon-Pudenz operation
shelf operation
shelving operation
Shirodkar operation
Shirodkar-Barter operation
Shugrue operation
shunt operation
Sichi operation
Silva-Costa operation
Silver-Hildreth eyelid
   operation
Simon operation
simple operation
Simpson operation
single-stage operation
sinus operation
Sistrunk operation
Sjoqvist operation
Skoog operation
slant muscle operation
sling operation
Slocum operation
Smith eyelid operation
Smith-Boyce operation
Smith-Gibson operation
Smith-Indian operation
Smith-Kuhnt-Szymanowski
   operation
Smith-Petersen operation
Smith-Robinson operation
Smithwick operation
Snellen entropion operation
Snellen ptosis operation
Soave operation
Socin operation
Sofield operation
Somerset-Mack hand
   operation
Sondergaard operation
Sonneberg operation
Sordille operation
Soria operation
Soriano operation

operation (*continued*)
Sorrin operation
Sotteau operation
Sourdille keratoplasty
operation
Sourdille ptosis operation
Souttar operation
Spaeth cystic bleb operation
Spaeth ptosis operation
Spalding-Richardson operation
spasmodic entropion
operation
Speas strabismus operation
Speed operation
Spencer-Watson Z-plasty
operation
sphincter-saving operation
Spinelli operation
Spivack operation
splenorenal venous operation
splitting lacrimal papilla
operation
Ssabanejew-Frank operation
Stacke operation
staging operation
Staheli shelf operation
Stallard eyelid operation
Stallard flap operation
Stallard-Liegard operation
Stamey operation
Stamm operation
Stamm-Kader operation
Stanischeff operation
stapes mobilization operation
State operation
station pull-through operation
Steele-Stewart operation
Stein operation
Steinach operation
Steindler operation
step graft operation
stereotactic operation
Stetta operation
Stevenson operation
Stock operation
Stocker operation
Stoffel operation
Stokes operation
Stookey-Scarff operation
strabismus operation
Straith eyelid operation
Strampelli-Valvo operation

operation (*continued*)
Strap operation
Strassman operation
Strassman-Jones operation
Streatfield operation
Streatfield-Fox operation
Streatfield-Snellen operation
string operation
Strombeck operation
Stromeyer-Little operation
Sturmdorf operation
Suarez-Villafranca operation
subcutaneous operation
Sugarbaker operation
Sugiura abdominal pull-
through operation
Summerskill operation
suprapubic urethrovesical
suspension operation
suspensory sling operation
Swan operation
Swanson operation
Swenson operation
switch operation
Syme operation
symmetry operation
synchrocyclotron operation
Szymanowski operation
Szymanowski-Kuhnt operation
Taarnhoj operation
tack operation
tagliacotian operation
talc operation
Talma operation
Tanner operation
Tanner-19 anti-bile reflux
operation
Tansini operation
Tansley operation
Tanzer operation
Tasia operation
Taussig operation
Taussig-Morton operation
Teale operation
Teale-Knapp operation
TeLinde operation
TeLinde-Everett operation
Tennison operation
Tennison-Randall operation
tenotomy operation
Terrillon operation
Terson operation

operation (*continued*)

Tessier craniofacial operation
Tessier facial dysostosis operation
Tessier operation
Textor operation
Thal fundic patch operation
Thiersch anal incontinence operation
Thiersch graft operation
Thomas operation
Thomson operation
Thorek operation
Thornell operation
thyroid operation
Tikhoff-Linberg operation
Tillett operation
Tompkins operation
tongue-in-groove operation
tongue-tie operation
Torek operation
Torek-Bevan operation
Torkildsen operation
Torpin operation
total excisional operation
Toti operation
Toti-Mosher operation
Townley-Paton operation
Trainor operation
Trainor-Nida operation
transposition operation
transsphenoidal operation
Trantas operation
trapdoor scleral buckle operation
Trauner operation
Travel operation
Trendelenburg operation
Treves operation
trichiasis operation
Tripier operation
Troutman operation
Truc operation
Tubby-Steindler operation
Tudor operation
Tudor-Thomas operation
Tuffier operation
tumbling technique operation
Turnbull multiple ostomy operation
Turner operation
Twombly operation

operation (*continued*)

Twombly-Ulfelder operation
Tzanck operation
Uchida operation
Ulloa operation
unattended laboratory operation
Urban operation
urologic operation
uterine suspension operation
Uyemura operation
vacuum extraction operation
van Buren operation
Van Gorder operation
van Hook operation
Van Millingen operation
Veau operation
Veau-Axhausen operation
Veau-Wardill-Kilner pushback operation
Vecchietti operation
Veirs operation
Verhoeff operation
Verhoeff-Chandler operation
Vermale operation
Verneuil operation
Vernon-David operation
Verwey eyelid operation
Vidal operation
Viers operation
Vineberg operation
Virag operation
visor flap operation
Vladimiroff operation
Vogel operation
Vogt operation
von Ammon operation
von Bergmann operation
von Blaskovics-Doyen operation
von Burow operation
von Hackler operation
von Kraske operation
von Langenbeck operation
Voronoff operation
Voss hanging-hip operation
Vulpius operation
Vulpius-Compere operation
V-Y operation
Wagner hand operation
Wagoner operation
Waldhauer operation

operation (*continued*)

Walter Reed operation
Walthardt operation
Wangensteen operation
Wardill-Kilner operation
Wardill-Kilner-Veau operation
Ward-Mayo operation
Warner-Farber operation
Warren operation
Waters operation
Waterston operation
Watkins operation
Watkins-Wertheim operation
Watson operation
Watson-Jones operation
Watzke self-holding sleeve
   operation
Waugh operation
Way operation
Webster operation
Weeker operation
Weeks operation
weight-reduction operation
Weinberg operation
Weiner operation
Weir operation
Weis operation
Weisinger operation
Wendell Hughes operation
Werb operation
Wertheim operation
Wertheim-Schauta operation
Wertheim-Taussig operation
West operation
Weve operation
Wharton operation
Wharton-Jones V-Y operation
Wheeler operation
Wheeler-Reese operation
Wheelhouse operation
Whipple operation
Whitacre operation
White operation
Whitehead operation
Whitman operation
Whitnall sling operation
Wicherkiewicz operation
Wiener operation
Wies operation
Wilkinson operation
Williams-Richardson
   operation

operation (*continued*)

Wilmer operation
Wilms operation
Wilson operation
Wilson-Jones patellar operation
window operation
winged V-flap operation
Winiwarter operation
Wise operation
Witzel operation
Woelfer operation
Wolfe ptosis operation
Wolff operation
Wood operation
Woodman operation
Woodward operation
Worst operation
Worth ptosis operation
Wright operation
Wullstein-Zollner operation
Wutzer operation
W-Y operation
Wyeth operation
Wylie operation
Wyllys-Andrews operation
Wynn cleft lip operation
Yankauer operation
Young operation
Young-Dees operation
Young-Dees-Leadbetter
   operation
Yount operation
Zahradnicek operation
Zancolli operation
Zickel subtrochanteric
   fracture operation
Ziegler operation
Zieman operation
Zimaloy operation
Zimmerman operation
Z-plastic relaxing operation
Z-plasty operation
Zylik operation
operation drape
operation microscope drape
operative amputation
operative approach
operative arthroscopy
operative arthrotomy
operative biliary bypass
operative cholangiography (OC)
operative choledochoscopy

operative correction
operative damage
operative delivery
operative diagnosis
operative drainage
operative excision
operative exposure
operative field
operative findings
operative incision
operative intervention
operative mortality flow
operative perforation
operative procedure
operative reconstruction
operative repair
operative scar
operative site
operative site complication
operative suite
operative surgery
operative technique
operative therapy
operative wound
opercular fold
operculectomy
operculum (*pl.* opercula)
   dental operculum
   orbital operculum
OPG-Gee instrument
O'Phelan technique
ophryospinal angle
Ophtec lens
Ophtec occlusion implant
Ophthaine anesthetic agent
Ophthalas argon/krypton laser
Ophthalas krypton laser
Ophthalas laser
ophthalmectomy
ophthalmia
ophthalmic anesthesia
ophthalmic artery
ophthalmic blade
ophthalmic calipers
ophthalmic cautery
ophthalmic cautery electrode
ophthalmic cup
ophthalmic electrocautery
ophthalmic endoscope
ophthalmic examination
ophthalmic hook
ophthalmic irrigator

ophthalmic knife
ophthalmic lamp
ophthalmic laser
   microendoscope
ophthalmic nerve
ophthalmic ointment
ophthalmic pick
ophthalmic plexus
ophthalmic recurrent nerve
ophthalmic sable brush
ophthalmic sponge
ophthalmic tumor
ophthalmic ultrasonography
ophthalmic vein
ophthalmic vesicle
ophthalmodynamometer
   Bailliart
      ophthalmodynamometer
   dial-type
      ophthalmodynamometer
   Dynoptor
      ophthalmodynamometer
   electronic
      ophthalmodynamometer
   Reichert
      ophthalmodynamometer
   suction
      ophthalmodynamometer
ophthalmodynamometry
ophthalmoendoscope
   Nebauer
      ophthalmoendoscope
   Zylik ophthalmoendoscope
ophthalmologic anesthesia
ophthalmomeningeal vein
ophthalmometer
   American Optical
      ophthalmometer
   Haag-Streit ophthalmometer
   Javal ophthalmometer
   OM 4 ophthalmometer
ophthalmoplegia
   basal ophthalmoplegia
   internuclear ophthalmoplegia
   (INO)
ophthalmoscope
   Alcon indirect
      ophthalmoscope
   Bailliart ophthalmoscope
   binocular ophthalmoscope
   confocal scanning laser
      ophthalmoscope

ophthalmoscope (*continued*)
  cordless monocular indirect
    ophthalmoscope
  direct ophthalmoscope
  Doran pattern stimulator
    ophthalmoscope
  Exeter ophthalmoscope
  Fisons indirect binocular
    ophthalmoscope
  Friedenwald
    ophthalmoscope
  Ful-Vue ophthalmoscope
  ghost ophthalmoscope
  Grafco ophthalmoscope
  Gullstrand ophthalmoscope
  Halberg indirect
    ophthalmoscope
  halogen coaxial
    ophthalmoscope
  halogen ophthalmoscope
  Helmholtz ophthalmoscope
  Highlight spectral indirect
    ophthalmoscope
  indirect laser ophthalmoscope
  indirect ophthalmoscope
  Keeler polarizing
    ophthalmoscope
  Loring ophthalmoscope
  luminous ophthalmoscope
  Mascot indirect
    ophthalmoscope
  May ophthalmoscope
  Mentor Exeter
    ophthalmoscope
  metric ophthalmoscope
  MK IV ophthalmoscope
  mono-ocular indirect
    ophthalmoscope
  Morton ophthalmoscope
  Nebauer ophthalmoscope
  Neolyte laser indirect
    ophthalmoscope
  Nerve Fiber Analyzer laser
    ophthalmoscope
  Novus ophthalmoscope
  Panoramic nonmydriatic
    ophthalmoscope
  polarizing ophthalmoscope
  Polle pod attachment for
    ophthalmoscope
  Propper binocular indirect
    ophthalmoscope

ophthalmoscope (*continued*)
  Propper-Heine
    ophthalmoscope
  reflecting ophthalmoscope
  Reichert binocular indirect
    ophthalmoscope
  Reichert Ful-Vue binocular
    ophthalmoscope
  Rodenstock scanning laser
    ophthalmoscope
  scanner laser
    ophthalmoscope
  scanning laser
    ophthalmoscope
  Schepens binocular indirect
    ophthalmoscope
  Schepens indirect
    ophthalmoscope
  Schepens ophthalmoscope
  Schepens-Pomerantzeff
    ophthalmoscope
  Schultz-Crock binocular
    ophthalmoscope
  TopSS scanning laser
    ophthalmoscope
  visuscope ophthalmoscope
  Welch Allyn ophthalmoscope
  Zeiss ophthalmoscope
ophthalmoscope camera
ophthalmoscopic examination
ophthalmoscopy
  direct ophthalmoscopy
  indirect ophthalmoscopy
  metric ophthalmoscopy
ophthalmotomy
Ophthalon sutures
ophthalsonic pachymeter
Opiela brace
opioid analgesia
opioid analgesic
opioid anesthesia
opioid anesthetic
opisthocheilia
opisthogenia
opisthognathism
opisthotonos position
OpMi colposcope
OpMi microscopic drape
OpMi operating microscope
OpMi PRO magis surgical
  microscope
OpMi VISU microscope

OPMI-6 operating microscope
Opmilas surgical laser
Opmilas CO_2 laser
Opmilas CO_2 multipurpose laser
Opotow filling material
Opotow Jelset material
Oppenheim brace
Oppenheim spring wire splint
Oppenheimer knuckle-bender
   splint
Oppenheimer spring wire splint
Op-Pneu insufflator
Op-Pneu laparoscopy needle
opponens splint
opponensplasty
  Bran opponensplasty
  Brand opponensplasty
  Camitz opponensplasty
  Ring sublimis opponensplasty
  Royle-Thompson
    opponensplasty
opportunistic complication
opportunistic infection
opposed loop-pair quadrature
   magnetic resonance coil
opposing margin
opposing muscle
opposing portal
opposing vocal cord
opposite side
oppressive pain
Opraflex dressing
Opraflex incise drape
OpSite drape
OpSite dressing
OpSite Flexifix transparent film
   dressing
OpSite Flexigrid adhesive film
   dressing
OpSite Flexigrid dressing
OpSite Flexigrid transparent
   adhesive film dressing
OpSite occlusive dressing
OpSite PLUS dressing
OpSite wound dressing
Opta 5 catheter
Optelec Passport magnifier
Op-Temp cautery
Op-Temp disposable
   electrocautery
Opthascan Mini-A scanner
optic axis

optic canal
optic center
optic chiasm
optic chiasm compression
optic commissure
optic cup
optic decussation
optic disk
optic evagination
optic foramen
optic ganglion
optic implant
optic iridectomy
optic keratoplasty
optic nerve (cranial nerve 2)
optic papilla
optic papilla cavity
optic radiation
optic recess
optic tract
optic tract compression
optic tract syndrome
optic vesicle
Opticaid lens loupe
optical aberration
optical aspirating curet
optical biopsy
optical biopsy forceps
Optical catheter
optical cavity
optical coherence reflectometry
   (OCR)
optical correction
optical density
optical digitizer
optical esophagoscope
optical iridectomy
optical iridectomy operation
optical keratoplasty
optical laryngoscope
optical needle
optical nodal point
optical pachymeter
Optical Radiation intraocular lens
optical stylet
optically transparent electrode
Opticath oximeter catheter
OptiChamber drug holding
   device
opticociliary neurectomy
opticociliary neurotomy
opticociliary vessels

opticomalacia
Opticon catheter
opticostriate region
Opti-Fix acetabular component
Opti-Fix acetabular cup
Opti-Fix femoral component
Optiflex intraocular lens
Optiflex lens
Opti-Flow permanent dialysis
  catheter
Opti-Gard eye protector
Optilume prostate balloon
  dilator
Optima bipolar pulse generator
Optima contact lens
Optima diamond knife
Optima pacemaker
Optima pulse generator
optimal diastolic pressure
optimal dose
optimal technique
optimal therapy
OptiMax Supreme pressure-
  reduction mattress
Optimed glaucoma pressure
  regulator
Optimum blade
Optiphot-2UD microscope
Optiplanimat automated unit
Opti-Plast XT balloon catheter
Optipore scrub sponge
Optipore wound-cleaning
  sponge
Optique microscope
OptiQue sensing catheter
Optiscope angioscope
Optiscope catheter
Optison echocardiography
  agent
Optiva catheter
Optiview optical surgical
  obturator
Optiview trocar
Optivis Surgalloy needle
Opti-Vu lens
Optokinetic stimulator
optometer
Opt-Visor lens
Opt-Visor loupe
Opus pacemaker
ora serrata
Oracle Focus PTCA catheter

Oracle Focus ultrasound
  imaging catheter
Oracle intravascular ultrasound
  catheter
Oracle Megasonics catheter
Oracle MegaSonics coronary
  balloon/imaging catheter
Oracle Micro catheter
Oracle Micro intravascular
  ultrasound catheter
Oracle Micro Plus PTCA
  catheter
Ora-Gard disposable intraoral
  bite block
O'Rahilly limb deficiency
  classification
oral administration
oral agent
oral analgesic
oral and maxillofacial surgery
  (OMS)
oral anesthesia
oral anesthetic
oral anesthetic technique
oral anomaly
oral antibiotic
oral anticoagulant
oral anticoagulation
oral antimicrobial prophylaxis
oral arch
oral atresia
oral cancer
oral candidiasis
oral cavity abnormality
oral cavity cancer
oral cephalocele
oral cholecystogram
oral cleft
oral commissure movement
oral commissuroplasty
oral complication
oral contents
oral contraceptive
oral corticosteroid
oral diaphragm
oral dose
oral drug
oral endotracheal intubation
oral endotracheal tube
oral esophageal tube
oral feeding
oral fissure

oral fistula
oral focal mucinosis
oral forceps
oral fossa
oral gangrene
oral hairy leukoplakia
oral implant
oral implantology
oral intubation
oral irrigation
oral leukoplakia
oral lighted-stylet intubation
oral Mondini
oral mucosa graft
oral myiasis
oral needle
oral panendoscope
oral passages
oral peripheral examination
oral pharyngeal airway
oral plate
oral reconstruction
oral restorative surgery
oral rongeur forceps
oral route
oral screw
oral screw mouth gag
oral screw tongue depressor
oral secretions
oral speculum mouth gag
oral squamous cell carcinoma
    (oral SCC)
oral surface
oral surgery rongeur
oral temperature
oral temperature device
oral tissues
oral trauma
oral urogram
oral urography
oral vestibular depth
Oral-Cath catheter
Orandi blade
Orandi knife
Orandi technique
orange dye laser
Orascoptic fiberoptic headlight
Orascoptic loupe extension
OraSure HIV-1 oral specimen
    collection device
OraSure HIVG-1 collection
    device

OraSure salivary collection
    device
Oratek chisel
Oratek device
Oratek thermal shrinking
    probe
Orban curet
Orban knife
orbicular alignment
orbicular incision
orbicular muscle
orbicular muscle of mouth
orbicular retractor
orbicular ring
orbicularis block
orbicularis laxity
orbicularis muscle of mouth
orbicularis oculi muscle
orbicularis oculi reflex
orbicularis oris muscle
orbiculociliary fiber
Orbis-Sigma cerebrospinal fluid
    shunt valve
Orbis-Sigma cerebrospinal fluid
    valve
Orbis-Sigma shunt
Orbit blade
orbital abscess
orbital akinesia
orbital anesthesia
orbital aperture
orbital apex syndrome
orbital arteriovenous
    malformation
orbital axis
orbital blow-in fracture
orbital blow-out fracture
orbital bone
orbital border of sphenoid
    bone
orbital branches
orbital canal
orbital cavity
orbital cellulitis
orbital compartment syndrome
orbital contents
orbital decompression
orbital depressor
orbital dysmorphology
orbital eminence
orbital enucleation compressor
orbital exenteration

orbital exenteration
  gastroscopic access
  technique
orbital extension
orbital fasciae
orbital fat
orbital fat was grasped and
  swept
orbital fissure
orbital fistula
orbital floor fracture
orbital floor implant
orbital floor prosthesis
orbital fracture
orbital fracture reduction
orbital height
orbital hematoma
orbital hernia
orbital hypertelorism
orbital hypotelorism
orbital implant
orbital implant operation
orbital infection
orbital layer
orbital lesion
orbital line
orbital lipectomy
orbital margin
orbital metastasis
orbital muscle
orbital neurovascular bundle
orbital operculum
orbital plane
orbital plate
orbital process
orbital projections
orbital prosthesis
orbital region
orbital retractor
orbital ridge
orbital rim fracture
orbital rim reconstruction
orbital roof fracture
orbital septum
Orbital shoulder stabilizer brace
orbital support
orbital surgery
orbital wall fracture
orbitale nasion
orbital-palpebral furrow
orbitomaxillary defect
orbitomaxillectomy

orbitomeatal line
orbitomeatal plane
orbitonasomaxillary defect
orbitopalpebral mutilization
orbitopathy
orbitosphenoidal bone
orbito-temple distance
orbitotomy
  Kronlein orbitotomy
  lateral orbitotomy
orbitozygomatic temporopolar
  approach
orbitozygomaticomalar bone
  ridge
Orbix x-ray unit
Orbscan pachymeter
ORC anterior chamber
  intraocular lens
ORC posterior chamber
  intraocular lens
ORC posterior chamber
  intraocular lens implant
Orca surgical blade
ORC-B Ranfac cholangiographic
  catheter
orchectomy (variant of
  orchiectomy)
orchidectomy
orchidoepididymectomy
orchidopexy
orchidoplasty
orchidorrhaphy
orchidotomy
orchiectomy
orchiopexy
  eversion orchiopexy
  Fowler-Stephens orchiopexy
  laparoscopic orchiopexy
  Torek orchiopexy
  transscrotal orchiopexy
orchioplasty
orchiorrhaphy
orchiotomy
orchipexy
orchiplasty
orchotomy
ORD bunionectomy (offset
  reverse dome
  bunionectomy)
Ord operation
ordinal classification
Oregon prosthesis

Oregon tunneler
O'Reilly esophageal retractor
Orentreich punch
Oreopoulos-Zellerman catheter
Oretorp meniscectomy knife
Oretorp retractable knife
Orfit mask
Orfit splint
Orfizip body jacket
Orfizip knee cast
organ
  cadaveric organ
  calcified organ
  conjoined organs
  contralateral organ
  dilatation of organ
  dilated organ
  diseased organ
  distal portion of organ
  donated organ
  drainage of organ
  duplication of organ
  enlarged organ
  enlargement of organ
  eversion of organ
  excision of organ
  exenteration of pelvic organs
  exposed organ
  female reproductive organs
  fibrous organ
  foreign body in organ
  gangrenous organ
  graft of organ
  harvest organ
  harvesting an organ
  healthy appearing organ
  hollow organ
  infantile organ
  infected organ
  inflamed organ
  inflammation of organ
  injured organ
  internal female genital organ
  internal male genital organ
  Jacobson organ
  laceration of organ
  lardaceous organ
  left organ
  lesion of organ
  lining of organ
  lower abdominal organ
  male reproductive organs

organ (*continued*)
  Masera septal organ
  mediastinal organ
  Meyer organ
  palpable organ
  palpably enlarged organ
  pelvic organs
  rejected organ
  rejection of organ
  removal of organ
  reproductive organs
  solid organ
  supernumerary organ
  transplanted organ
  upper abdominal organs
  vital organs
  vomeronasal organ (VNO)
organ ablation
organ allograft
organ bank
organ donation
organ donor
organ dysfunction
organ exenteration
organ failure
organ graft
organ of Corti
organ of Zuckerkandl
organ perfusion
organ rejection
organ sharing
organ source
organ transplant
organ transplantation
organ viability
Organdi blade
organic dental cement
organic disease
organic disorder
organic dysfunction
organic heart disease (OHD)
organic lesion
organic matrix
organic murmur
organic origin
organic pain
organic short bowel syndrome
organic stricture
organically impaired brain
  function
organized clot
organized hematoma

organizing hemorrhagic cyst
organizing inflammation
organizing thrombus
organoid
organomegaly
Organon percutaneous
    implant
organoscopy
organ-specific antigen
organ-specific pattern of injury
Orgen spinal bone growth
    stimulator
Oriental VY flap
ORIF (open reduction and
    internal fixation)
orifacial angle
orifice
    anal orifice
    anorectal orifice
    aortic orifice
    atrioventricular orifice
    auriculoventricular orifice
    cardiac orifice
    external orifice
    external urethral orifice
    floor of orifice
    heart orifices
    hymenal orifice
    internal acoustic orifice
    internal urethral orifice
    nasofrontal orifice
    patent orifice
    pharyngeal orifice
    pulmonary trunk orifice
    pyloric orifice
    segmental orifices
    stadium-type of ureteral
        orifice
    tricuspid orifice
    tympanic orifice
    ureteral orifice
    urethral orifice
    uterine orifice
    vaginal orifice
    vesical orifice
    vesicourethral orifice
    widely patent orifice
orifice of the mouth
Origin balloon
Origin tacker
Origin trocar
original incision

Original Jacknobber II muscle-
    massage device
original Sweet eye magnet
original tumor site
originating infection
O-ring attachments
Orion anterior cervical plate
Orion balloon
Orion device
Orion inhaler
Orion lumbar support
Orion pacemaker
Orion plate and screw
Oris pin
Orlando hip-knee-ankle-foot
    orthosis
Orley retractor
Orlon vascular prosthesis
Orlowski stent
Ormco appliance
Ormco band scissors
Ormco ligature director
Ormco orthodontic arch-
    expander
Ormco orthodontic hemostat
Ormco orthodontic pliers
Ormco pin
Ormco preformed band
Ormond disease
oroantral fistula
orocutaneous fistula
orodigitofacial dysostosis
oroendotracheal tube
orofacial carcinoma
orofacial clefting
orofacial dysfunction syndrome
orofacial fistula
orofacial muscle imbalance
orofacial reconstruction
orofaciodigital syndrome
orogastric Ewald tube
oromandibular defect
oromandibular dystonia
oromandibular lesion
oromandibular reconstruction
oromandibular rehabilitation
oromaxillary
oronasal fistula
oronaso-ocular cleft
oro-ocular cleft
oropharyngeal airway
oropharyngeal anesthesia

oropharyngeal approach
oropharyngeal candidiasis
oropharyngeal carcinoma
oropharyngeal defect
oropharyngeal hemorrhage
oropharyngeal membrane
oropharyngeal pack
oropharyngeal reconstruction
oropharyngeal ulcer
oropharynx pack
orotracheal intubation
orotracheal tube
Orozco plate
Orr automatic reprocessor
Orr forceps
Orr gall duct forceps
Orr incision
Orr rectal prolapse repair
Orr technique
Orr treatment
Orr-Buck extension tractor
Orr-Loygue proctopexy
Orr-Loygue transabdominal
    proctopexy
Orthair bunionectomy
    instruments
Orthair orthopedic instruments
Orthair oscillating saw
Orthairtome II drill
Orthex cannulated titanium
    bone screw
Orthicon camera
Ortho Cytofluorograf
    cytometer
Ortho diaphragm kit
ortho disk
Ortho Dx electromedical
    stimulator
Ortho System cytometer
Ortho Tech cock-up wrist splint
Ortho Tech performer knee
    brace
Ortho-Arch II orthotic
Ortho-Athrex instrument
Orthoband traction band
Ortho-Biotic recliner
OrthoBone pillow
orthocardiac reflex
Ortho-Cel pad
Orthoceph x-ray unit
Orthocomp cement
Orthocor II pacemaker

Orthoderm consummate air
    therapy bed
Orthoderm convertible mattress
orthodontic appliance
orthodontic band
orthodontic band driver
orthodontic base plate
orthodontic cement
orthodontic impression tray
orthodontic ligature
orthodontic procedure
orthodontic therapy
orthodontics
    corrective orthodontics
    cosmetic orthodontics
    interceptive orthodontics
    preventive orthodontics
    prophylactic orthodontics
    surgical orthodontics
orthodox procedure
OrthoDyn bone substitute
    material
Orthofix Cervical-Stim cervical
    bone growth stimulator
Orthofix external fixation
    device
Orthofix external fixator
Orthofix intramedullary nail
Orthofix lengthening device
Orthofix distractor
Orthofix monolateral femoral
    external fixator
Orthofix pin
Orthofix prosthesis
Orthofix screw
Orthoflex dressing
Orthoflex elastic plaster
    bandage
Ortho-Foam elbow/heel pad
OrthoFrame external fixation
Orthofuse implantable growth
    stimulator
OrthoGel liner
Ortho-Gen bone growth
    stimulator
Ortho-Glass cast material
Ortho-Glass splint material
orthognathia
orthognathic occlusal relator
orthognathic operation
orthognathic surgery
orthognathism

orthognathous
orthognathus
orthogonal film
orthogonal laser
orthogonal plane
orthogonal radiofrequency coil
Ortho-Grip silicone rubber
    handle
Ortho-Ice Multipaks pack
Ortho-Jel impression material
orthokeratinized variant
Ortho-last splint
Ortholav irrigation and suction
    device
Ortholav pulsed irrigator
Ortholav suction
Ortholoc IM instrumentation
Ortholoc prosthesis
OrthoLogic bone growth
    stimulator
Orthomatrix binder
Orthomedics brace
Orthomedics Stretch and Heel
    splint
Orthomite adhesive
Ortho-Mold spinal brace
Ortho-Mold splint
OrthoNail intramedullary
    fixation device
orthopaedic (*variant of*
    orthopedic)
Orthopaedic Trauma Association
    classification
orthopaedics (*variant of*
    orthopedics)
OrthoPak bone growth
    stimulator
OrthoPak II bone growth
    stimulator
Orthopantomograph-series
    panoramic x-ray machine
orthopedic (*spelled also*
    orthopaedic)
orthopedic anesthesia
orthopedic anomaly
orthopedic bone file
orthopedic broach
orthopedic bur
orthopedic chisel
orthopedic curet
orthopedic cutting instrument
orthopedic depth gauge

orthopedic drill
orthopedic dynamometer
orthopedic elevator
orthopedic fixation device
orthopedic forceps
orthopedic goniometer
orthopedic gouge
orthopedic hammer
orthopedic hardware
orthopedic hemostat
orthopedic impactor
orthopedic knife
orthopedic mallet
orthopedic osteotome
orthopedic pin
orthopedic plate
orthopedic rasp
orthopedic reamer
orthopedic rod
orthopedic rongeur
orthopedic scissors
orthopedic screw
orthopedic staple
orthopedic strap clavicle splint
orthopedic surgery
orthopedic surgical pliers
orthopedic surgical procedure
orthopedic surgical stripper
orthopedic table
orthopedic Universal drill
orthopedic wrench
orthopedics (*spelled also*
    orthopaedics)
orthopelvimetry
Orthoplast dressing
Orthoplast fracture brace
Orthoplast isoprene splint
Orthoplast jacket
Orthoplast slipper cast
orthoplastic rhinoplasty
orthopnea
orthopnea position
OrthoPro ankle support
Orthoptic eye patch
orthorhythmic pacemaker
orthoroentgenogram
orthoroentgenography
orthoscopic lens
Orthoset cement
Orthoset radiopaque bone
    cement adhesive
orthosis

Orthosleep pillow
OrthoSorb absorbable pin
OrthoSorb pin fixation
OrthoSorb pin nail
Orthostar surgical table
orthostatic drainage
orthostatic dyspnea
orthostatic hypotension
orthostatic lines
orthostatic tachycardia
orthotic attachment implant
orthotic coiled spring twister
orthotic device
orthotic plate
orthotonos position
orthotopic
   appendicocystostomy
orthotopic biventricular
   artificial heart
orthotopic bladder
orthotopic bone graft
orthotopic cardiac transplant
orthotopic graft
orthotopic heart transplantation
orthotopic hemi-Koch operation
orthotopic liver transplant
   (OLT)
orthotopic transplant
orthotopic transplantation
orthotopic univentricular
   artificial heart
orthotopic urinary diversion
Ortho-Trac adhesive skin
   traction bandage
orthotripsy
Orthotron machine
Ortho-Vent bandage
OrthoVise orthopedic
   instrument
OrthoVise orthotic
Orticochea flap
Orticochea pharyngoplasty
Orticochea procedure
Orticochea scalping technique
Ortolani click
Ortolani maneuver
Orton enamel cleaver
Ortved stone dislodger
os (*Pl.* ossa)
   cervical os
   endocervical os
   external os

os (*continued*)
   internal os
   per os (p.o., PO, or po)
   pinpoint os
os calcis
os cuboideum
os epitympanicum
os ethmoidale
os frontale
os hyoideum
os interparietale
os lacrimale
os lunatum
os magnum
os mastoideum
os nasale
os occipitale
os odentoideum
os orbiculare
os palatinum
os parietale
os penis
os pubis
os pubis spline
os sphenoidale
os temporale
os trigonum
os triquetrum
os unguis
os uteri
os vesalianum pedis
os zygomaticum
Osada 2-stage palatoplasty
Osada saw
Osbon pressure-point tension
   ring
Osbon technique for impotence
Osborne goniometer
Osborne lesion of elbow
Osborne ligament
Osborne operation
Osborne osteotomy plate
Osborne posterior approach
Osborne punch
Osborne-Cotterill elbow
   procedure
Osborne-Cotterill elbow
   technique
Osborne-Cotterill procedure
oscheoplasty
Osciflator balloon inflation
   syringe

oscillating cannula
oscillating grid
oscillating nystagmus
oscillating saw
oscillating sternotomy saw
oscillation
oscillator
   Hayek oscillator
   Zimmer Orthair oscillator
oscillatory saw
oscillatory ventilation
oscillometric blood pressure
   cuff
oscillometrics
oscillometry
oscilloscope
   cathode ray oscilloscope
   Norland digital oscilloscope
   Sanborn oscilloscope
   single-channel
      electromyograph
      oscilloscope
   single-channel nonfade
      oscilloscope
   Tektronix digital oscilloscope
Oscor atrial lead
Oscor pacemaker
Oscor pacing leads
Osgood modified technique
Osgood needle
Osgood operation
Osgood supracondylar
   osteotomy of femur
Osgood-Schlatter disease
Osgood-Schlatter lesion
Oshar-Neumann 8-line corneal
   marker
O'Shaughnessy arterial forceps
O'Shaughnessy clamp
O'Shea lens
Osher air-bubble removal
   cannula
Osher bipolar coaptation
   forceps
Osher capsular forceps
Osher conjunctival forceps
Osher corneal scissors
Osher diamond knife
Osher foreign body forceps
Osher globe rotator
Osher haptic forceps
Osher internal calipers

Osher iris retractor
Osher irrigating implant hook
Osher lens
Osher lens-vacuuming cannula
Osher lid retractor
Osher malleable microspatula
Osher micrometer cataract knife
Osher needle holder
Osher nucleus lens manipulator
Osher nucleus stab expressor
Osher pan-fundus lens
Osher superior rectus forceps
Osher surgical keratometer
Osher surgical posterior pole
   lens
Osher-Fenzel hook
Osher-Fresnel intraocular lens
Oshukova collapsible bougie
   guide
OSI arthroscopic well-leg holder
OSI extremity elevator
Osler hemangiomatosis
Osler nodes
Osler triad
Osler-Weber-Rendu syndrome
Osmette osmometer
OSMO reverse-osmosis unit
OsmoCyte island wound care
   dressing
OsmoCyte PCA pillow wound
   dressing
OsmoCyte pillow
OsmoCyte pillow dressing
osmolarity of blood
osmometer
Osmond-Clarke shoulder
   operation
Osmond-Clarke technique
osmosis
osmostat
osmotic minipump
osmotic pressure
Osoff-Karlen laryngoscope
OSP (oncocytic schneiderian
   papilloma)
OssaTron orthotripsy
OsseoCare drill
OsseoCare drilling equipment
OsseoCare machine
osseocartilaginous craniofacial
   skeleton
Osseodent dental implant

Osseodent surgical drill
osseointegrated cylinder implant
osseointegrated implant
    rehabilitation
osseointegrated oral implant
osseointegration process
osseoprosthesis
osseotendinous
Osseotite 2-stage procedure
    implant
Osseotite dental implant
osseous abnormality
osseous anomaly
osseous cleft
osseous craniofacial
    arteriovenous malformation
osseous dysplasia
osseous fixation
osseous flap
osseous genioplasty
osseous graft
osseous grafting
osseous heteroplasia
osseous implant
osseous labyrinth
osseous lesion
osseous metastasis
osseous pin
osseous portion
osseous spiral lamina
osseous structures
osseous surgery
osseous tissue
osseus rheumatism
ossicle-holding clamp
ossicle-holding forceps
ossicular chain reconstruction
ossicular chain replacement
    prosthesis
ossicular replacement prosthesis
ossiculectomy
ossiculotomy
ossification
    ectopic ossification
    heterotopic ossification
    labyrinthine ossification
    reaction ossification
    reactive ossification
    vitreous ossification
ossification centers
ossified edge
ossifying cartilage

ossifying fibroma
ossifying inflammation
Ossloff-Karlan laser
    laryngoscope
Ossloff-Karlan-Dedo
    laryngoscope
Ossloff-Karlan-Jako laryngoscope
Ossoff-Karlan laser forceps
Ossoff-Karlan laser laryngoscope
Ossoff-Karlan laser suction tube
Ossoff-Karlan microlaryngeal
    laser probe
Ossoff-Karlan-Dedo
    laryngoscope
Ossoff-Karlan-Jako laryngoscope
Ossoff-Karlen laryngoscope
Ossof-Sisson surgical stent
Ostby dam frame
ostectomy
    Dingman ostectomy
    wedge ostectomy
ostectomy plate
Osteo implant
OsteoAnalyzer densitometer
OsteoAnalyzer device
osteoarthritic changes
osteoarthritic knee brace
osteoarthritic lipping
osteoarthritis (OA)
    generalized osteoarthritis
        (GOA)
    rheumatoid osteoarthritis
    temporomandibular joint
        osteoarthritis (TMJ-OA)
osteoarthritis disease
osteoarthropathy
    hypertrophic
        osteoarthropathy
osteoarthrotomy
osteoarticular allograft
osteoarticular allograft
    transplantation
osteoarticular defect
osteoarticular graft
osteoblastic lesion
osteoblastic metastasis
osteoblastic sinusitis
Osteobond copolymer bone
    cement
OsteoCap hip prosthesis
osteocartilaginous body
osteocartilaginous excision

osteocartilaginous exostosis
osteocartilaginous framework
osteocartilaginous graft
osteocartilaginous growth
osteocartilaginous loose body
osteochondral allograft
osteochondral defect
osteochondral exostosis
osteochondral fragment
osteochondral graft
osteochondral injury
osteochondral junction
osteochondral lesion
osteochondral loose body
osteochondral reconstruction
osteochondral slice fracture
osteochondrodystrophy
osteochondroma
osteochondromatosis
osteochondrosis
osteoclasia
osteoclasis
osteoclasis maneuver
osteoclast
  Collin osteoclast
  Phelps-Gocht osteoclast
  Rizzoli osteoclast
osteoclast-activating factor
osteoclasty
osteocollagenous fibers
osteoconductive bone grafting
  material
osteocutaneous fillet flap
osteocutaneous scapular flap
osteodensitometry
osteodistractor
osteodystrophy
osteofibroma
osteofibrosis
Osteofil allograft paste
OsteoGen bone graft
OsteoGen bone grafting material
OsteoGen bone growth
  stimulator
OsteoGen HA dental implant
OsteoGen HA Resorb implant
  material
OsteoGen implantable
  stimulator
Osteogen resorbable osteogenic
  bone-filling implant
osteogenesis

osteogenesis imperfecta
  congenita syndrome
osteogenetic fibers
osteogenic fibroma
osteogenic myxoma
osteogenic sarcoma
osteogenic tissue
Osteogenics BoneSource
  synthetic bone replacement
Osteogenics BoneSource
  synthetic bone replacement
  material
Osteograf binder
Osteograf bone grafting material
Osteograf/D dense bone grafting
  material
Osteograf/LD low-density bone
  grafting material
Osteograf/N natural bone
  grafting material
osteoid sarcoma
osteointegrated dental implant
Osteo-Lock endodontic
  stabilization kit
Osteolock HA femoral
  component
Osteolock hip prosthesis
Osteolock acetabular component
osteolysis
osteolytic bone lesion
osteolytic calvarial lesion
osteoma
osteoma of malleus
osteomalacia
Osteomatrix bone filler
osteomeatal sinus tract
Osteomed screw
osteomicrotome
Osteomin freeze-dried bone
osteomusculocutaneous flap
osteomyelitis
osteomyelofibrotic syndrome
osteomyocutaneous flap
Osteon bur
Osteon drill
osteonecrosis
osteonic bone
Osteonics acetabular dome hole
  plug
Osteonics femoral component
Osteonics hip prosthesis
Osteonics jig

Osteonics Omnifit-HA
  component
Osteonics Omnifit-HA hip
  stem
Osteonics prosthesis
Osteonics reamer
Osteonics Scorpio insert
Osteonics-HA coated implant
osteopathia striata syndrome
osteopathic lesion
osteoperiosteal bone graft
osteoperiosteal flap
osteoperiostitis
osteopetrosis
osteopetrotic scar
osteophyte
osteophyte elevator
osteophyte formation
osteoplastic amputation
osteoplastic bone flap
osteoplastic craniotomy
osteoplastic flap
osteoplastic flap clamp
osteoplastic frontal sinus
  operation
osteoplastic frontal sinus
  procedure
osteoplastic necrotomy
osteoplastic reconstruction
osteoplastic rhinoplasty
osteoplasty
Osteoplate implant
osteoporosis
osteoporosis circumscripta
osteoporosis pseudoglioma
  syndrome
osteoporotic compression
  fracture
osteoporotic fracture
osteoporotic lesion
osteoporotic marrow defect
OsteoPower drilling and cutting
  machine
osteopulmonary arthropathy
osteorrhaphy
osteosarcoma
osteosclerotic lesion
OsteoSet bone filler
Osteoset bone graft substitute
osteospongioma
osteostat
  Riordan osteostat

OsteoStat single-use power
  surgical equipment
Osteostim electrical bone
  growth stimulator
OsteoStim implantable bone
  growth stimulator
Osteostim prosthesis
osteosutures
osteosynthesis
  distraction osteosynthesis
  wire osteosynthesis
osteotome (*see also*
  periosteotome)
alar osteotome
Albee osteotome
Alexander perforating
  osteotome
Amico osteotome
Anderson-Neivert osteotome
Andrews osteotome
A-O osteotome
API osteotome
Army pattern osteotome
articular osteotome
articulation osteotome
Bakelite-handled osteotome
Barsky nasal osteotome
bayonet osteotome
beat-up osteotome
Blount scoliosis osteotome
Bowen osteotome
Box osteotome
Buck osteotome
Burton osteotome
Campbell osteotome
Carroll osteotome
Carroll-Legg osteotome
Carroll-Smith-Petersen
  osteotome
Cavin osteotome
Chermel osteotome
Cherry osteotome
Cinelli guarded osteotome
Clayton osteotome
Cloward spinal fusion
  osteotome
Cobb osteotome
Codman osteotome
Compere osteotome
Converse guarded osteotome
Cook osteotome
Cottle chisel osteotome

osteotome (*continued*)

Cottle crossbar chisel osteotome
Cottle-Medicon osteotome
Crane osteotome
Cross osteotome
curved osteotome
Dautrey osteotome
Dautrey-Munro osteotome
Dawson-Yuhl osteotome
Dileant osteotome
Dingman osteotome
Duray-Read osteotome
Duray-Ward osteotome
Epstein osteotome
flexible blade osteotome
Fomon osteotome
Frazier osteotome
French-pattern osteotome
Furnas bayonet osteotome
guarded osteotome
hand surgery osteotome
Hardt-Delima osteotome
Hendel guided osteotome
hexagonal handle osteotome
Hibbs osteotome
Hohmann osteotome
Hoke osteotome
Hough osteotome
Houston nasal osteotome
Howorth osteotome
Jarit hand surgery osteotome
Kazanjian action-type osteotome
Kezerian osteotome
lacrimal osteotome
Lahey Clinic osteotome
Lahey Clinic thin osteotome
Lahey osteotome
Lambotte osteotome
Lambotte-Henderson osteotome
lateral osteotome
Legg osteotome
Leinbach osteotome
Lexer osteotome
MacGregor osteotome
Manchester nasal osteotome
manual osteotome
Mathews osteotome
maxillofacial osteotome
Mayfield bayonet osteotome

osteotome (*continued*)

McCollough osteotome
McIndoe osteotome
Meyerding osteotome
MGH osteotome
Micro-Aire osteotome
Miner osteotome
mini-Lambotte osteotome
mini-Lexer osteotome
Mitchell osteotome
Moberg osteotome
Moe osteotome
Moore osteotome
Murphy osteotome
nasal osteotome
nasofrontal osteotome
Neivert osteotome
Neivert-Anderson osteotome
New-Lambotte osteotome
orthopedic osteotome
osteotomy osteotome
Padgett osteotome
Parkes lateral osteotomy osteotome
Parkes-Quisling osteotome
Peck osteotome
perforating osteotome
Quisling-Parkes osteotome
Read osteotome
Rhoton osteotome
Richards-Hibbs osteotome
Rish osteotome
Ristow osteotome
Roos osteotome
Rowland osteotome
Rubin nasofrontal osteotome
scoliosis osteotome
Sheehan osteotome
Shepard osteotome
Silver nasal osteotome
Simmons osteotome
single-guarded osteotome
sinus lift osteotome
slotting-bur osteotome
Smith-Petersen curved osteotome
Smith-Petersen straight osteotome
spinal fusion osteotome
Stille osteotome
Stille-pattern osteotome
Stille-Stiwer osteotome

osteotome (*continued*)
  straight osteotome
  Stryker impact osteotome
  Swanson osteotome
  Swiss-pattern osteotome
  Tardy osteotome
  Tessier osteotome
  U.S. Army osteotome
  U.S. Army-pattern osteotome
  Ultra-Cut Hoke osteotome
  Ultra-Cut Smith-Petersen
    osteotome
  vomer osteotome
  Ward nasal osteotome
  West osteotome
  Wood osteotome
osteotomized
osteotomy
  abductory wedge osteotomy
  Albee osteotomy
  Amstutz-Wilson osteotomy
  Anderson-Fowler osteotomy
  angulation osteotomy
  Baker-Hill osteotomy
  ball-and-socket osteotomy
  Bardach modification of
    Obwegeser mandibular
    osteotomy
  bifurcation osteotomy
  bijaw osteotomy
  bijaw segmental dentoalveolar
    setback osteotomy
  bilateral mandibular sagittal
    split osteotomy
  bilateral sagittal split
    advancement osteotomy
  bilateral sagittal split
    osteotomy (BSSO)
  blind osteotomy
  block osteotomy
  Blount displacement
    osteotomy
  Blundell-Jones osteotomy
  Borden-Spencer-Herndon
    osteotomy
  Brackett hip osteotomy
  Brett osteotomy
  Brett-Campbell tibial
    osteotomy
  buccal osteotomy
  bunion osteotomy
  C sliding osteotomy

osteotomy (*continued*)
  C-form osteotomy
  chevron osteotomy
  Chiari osteotomy
  Chuinard femoral osteotomy
  closed osteotomy
  closed subcondylar osteotomy
  closed wedge osteotomy
  closing base wedge
    osteotomy
  Cole osteotomy
  Cotton osteotomy
  Coventry osteotomy
  Crego osteotomy
  cuneiform osteotomy
  cup-and-ball osteotomy
  Dautrey osteotomy
  derotation osteotomy
  dial osteotomy
  Dickson osteotomy
  displacement osteotomy
  dorsiflexor wedge osteotomy
  Dunn-Hess osteotomy
  DuVries osteotomy
  Dwyer osteotomy
  Eppright osteotomy
  eversion osteotomy
  extension osteotomy
  external osteotomy
  femoral shortening osteotomy
  Ferguson-Thompson-King
    osteotomy
  Fernandez osteotomy
  French elbow osteotomy
  Fulkerson osteotomy
  Gant hip osteotomy
  Hass hip osteotomy
  high tibial osteotomy
  hinge osteotomy
  horizontal osteotomy
  horseshoe LeFort I osteotomy
  Houston osteotomy
  innominate osteotomy
  inverted-L osteotomy
  Irwin pelvic osteotomy
  Jahss osteotomy
  Keller bunion osteotomy
  Kessel-Bonney extension
    osteotomy
  Kramer-Craig-Noel osteotomy
  Langenskiold hip osteotomy
  lateral osteotomy

osteotomy (*continued*)
LeFort I osteotomy
LeFort II osteotomy
Leach-Igou step-cut medial
    osteotomy
LeFort III advancement
    osteotomy
LeFort II-type midface
    osteotomy
LeFort I-type osteotomy
LeFort maxillary osteotomy
LeFort osteotomy
L-form osteotomy
linear osteotomy
Lloyd-Roberts osteotomy
Lorenz osteotomy
Lucas-Cottrell osteotomy
Ludloff osteotomy
Macewen osteotomy
mandibular ramus osteotomy
mandibular sagittal split
    osteotomy
maxillary osteotomy
McMurray femoral neck
    osteotomy
medial oblique and low lateral
    osteotomy
medial osteotomy
metatarsal osteotomy
Mitchell distal osteotomy
Moore osteotomy
Mueller osteotomy
notched rotation osteotomy
oblique ramus sliding
    osteotomy
oblique subcondylar
    osteotomy
oblique subcondylar ramus
    osteotomy
Obwegeser sagittal
    mandibular osteotomy
open oblique osteotomy
open osteotomy
opening wedge osteotomy
Pauwels adduction osteotomy
pelvic osteotomy
Pemberton osteotomy
perforation osteotomy
periodontal osteotomy
Plateau osteotomy
posterior maxillary segmental
    osteotomy

osteotomy (*continued*)
Pott eversion osteotomy
Pott tibial osteotomy
proximal osteotomy
radial wedge osteotomy
reduction osteotomy
Reverdin osteotomy
reverse facial osteotomy
rotation osteotomy
rotational advancement
    osteotomy
Rubin osteotomy
sagittal ramus osteotomy
sagittal split mandibular
    osteotomy
sagittal split osteotomy (SSO)
sagittal split ramus osteotomy
    (SSRO)
sagittal split osteotomy
Salter innominate osteotomy
Salyer modification of
    Obwegeser mandibular
    osteotomy
Samilson calcaneal osteotomy
Schanz osteotomy
Schede rotation osteotomy
segmental alveolar osteotomy
Shantz osteotomy
shelf osteotomy
sliding oblique osteotomy
Smith-Petersen osteotomy
Sofield osteotomy
Southwick osteotomy
Speed osteotomy
Sponsel osteotomy
Stamm osteotomy
Steele osteotomy
step-cut osteotomy
step-down osteotomy
subapical osteotomy
subcondylar osteotomy
subtrochanteric osteotomy
Sutherland-Greenfield
    osteotomy
tarsal wedge osteotomy
Tessier osteotomy
thin osteotomy
total midface osteotomy
transtrochanteric osteotomy
transverse osteotomy
triple innominate osteotomy
truncated osteotomy

osteotomy (*continued*)
 varus osteotomy
 vertical osteotomy
 vertical ramus mandibular
  osteotomy
 vestibular osteotomy
 visor osteotomy
 Wagoner osteotomy
 wedge osteotomy
 Whitman osteotomy
 Winter anterior osteotomy
 Z-cut osteotomy
 zygomaticomaxillary
  osteotomy
osteotomy nail
osteotomy of condylar neck
osteotomy osteotome
osteotomy pin
osteotomy plate
osteotribe (*see* rasp)
osteotripsy
osteotrite
OsteoView device
OsteoView digital bone
  densitometer
Osteovit bone matrix
Osterballe precision needle
osteum internum
ostial lesion
ostial obstruction
ostial sphincter
Ostic plaster dressing
ostiomeatal complex
ostiomeatal stent
ostiomeatal unit (OMU)
ostium (*pl.* ostia)
 abdominal ostium
 accessory maxillary ostium
 accessory maxillary sinus
  ostium
 accessory ostium
 anterior ostium
 ethmoidal ostium
 frontal ostium
 maxillary ostium
 pharyngeal ostium
 sphenoidal ostium
ostomy appliance
ostomy bag
ostomy loop
Ostrom antral punch
Ostrom antrum punch-tip forceps

Ostrom nose punch
Ostrom punch forceps
Ostrum-Furst syndrome
Ostrup harvesting technique
Ostrup vascularized rib graft
Ostycut bone biopsy needle
O'Sullivan operation
O'Sullivan self-retaining
  abdominal retractor
O'Sullivan vaginal retractor
O'Sullivan-O'Connor self-
  retaining abdominal
  retractor
O'Sullivan-O'Connor abdominal
  retractor
O'Sullivan-O'Connor self-
  retaining abdominal
  retractor
O'Sullivan-O'Connor self-
  retaining retractor
O'Sullivan-O'Connor vaginal
  retractor
O'Sullivan-O'Connor vaginal
  speculum
Oswestry staples
Oswestry-O'Brien spinal
  stapler
Osypka atrial lead
Osypka Cereblate electrode
Osypka rotational angioplasty
Oti Vac lighted suction unit
otic depression
otic ganglion
otic labyrinth
otic periotic shunt procedure
otic shunt
Otis anoscope
Otis bougie à boule
Otis bougie à boule dilator
Otis bulb cystoscope
Otis meatotome
Otis proctoscope
Otis prostatic urethral sound
Otis urethral sound
Otis urethrotome
Otis urological bougie
Otis-Brown cystoscope
otitic meningitis
otitis
 furuncular otitis
 malignant external otitis
 mucosis otitis

otitis (*continued*)
  mucous otitis
  necrotizing external otitis
otitis externa
otitis interna
otitis media
Otlinger technique
Otocap myringotomy blade
Otocap myringotomy scalpel
otogenous pyemia
OtoLam laser
otolithic membrane
otologic cup forceps
otologic scissors
otomandibular dysostosis
otomandibular syndrome
Oto-Microscope
otomicrosurgical transtemporal
    approach
Oto-mid permanent ventilation
    tube
otonecrectomy
otopexy
otopharyngeal tube
otoplasty
  Adams otoplasty
  Alexander otoplasty
  anterior-posterior otoplasty
  Crikelair otoplasty
  Davis-Kitlowski otoplasty
  Dieffenbach otoplasty
  flap otoplasty
  Furniss otoplasty
  incisionless otoplasty
  mattress suture otoplasty
  Mustard flap otoplasty
  Mustarde otoplasty
  Mustarde-Furnas otoplasty
  Peled knifeless otoplasty
  Stenstrom otoplasty
  Straith otoplasty
  Tan otoplasty
  Vogel otoplasty
otorrhea
OtoScan device
otosclerectomy
otoscleronectomy
otosclerosis
otosclerotic fixation
otosclerotic process
otoscope
  acoustic otoscope

otoscope (*continued*)
  Advanced beta otoscope
  Alpha fiberoptic pocket
    otoscope
  Bruening pneumatic
    otoscope
  Brunton otoscope
  diagnostic otoscope
  fiberoptic otoscope
  Grafco otoscope
  halogen otoscope
  Jako suspension otoscope
  micro-halogen otoscope
  Microtek Heine otoscope
  Mini-Fibralux pocket
    otoscope
  Minilux pocket otoscope
  operating otoscope
  pneumatic otoscope
  Politzer air-bag otoscope
  Rica pneumatic otoscope
  Riester otoscope
  Siegel pneumatic otoscope
  SMIC pneumatic otoscope
  StarMed video otoscope
  surgical otoscope
  Toynbee otoscope
  video otoscope
  Welch Allyn dual-purpose
    otoscope
  Welch Allyn operating
    otoscope
  Wullstein ototympanoscope
    otoscope
otoscopic examination
otoscopy
ototome drill
ototome irrigation kit
ototome otologic drill
ototomy
Otovent autoinflation kit
Oto-Wick ear sponge
Ottenheimer common duct
    dilator
Ott-Mayo channel sampling kit
Otto Barkan Bident retractor
Otto Bock Greissinger Plus foot
    prosthesis
Otto Bock modular rotary
    hydraulic knee
Otto Bock Safety constant-
    friction knee

Otto Bock system electric hands prosthesis
Otto forceps
Otto pelvis
Otto pelvis dislocation
Otto tissue forceps
Ottoback modular knee joint
Ottoback children's hydraulic knee joint
Ottoback knee prosthesis
Ouchterlony gel diffusion technique
Ouchterlony technique
Oudard procedure
Oudin resonator
Oughterson forceps
OutBound syringe
outcome monitoring
outcropping of lesions
outer aspect
outer border
outer canthus
outer convexity
outer ear
outer fibrous layer
outer interrupted silk sutures
outer layer
outer limiting membrane
outer rim
outer surface
outer table bones of skull
outer table graft
outer table of frontal bone
outer table of skull
Outerbridge classification
Outerbridge ridge
Outerbridge scale
Outerbridge uterine dilator
outermost covering
outermost layer
outflow cannula
outflow cardiac patch
outflow control
outflow tract
outflow tract obstruction
outfolding
outfracture
outgoing
outgrowth
   bagpipe vertebral outgrowth
   comma-shaped vertebral outgrowth

outgrowth (*continued*)
   teardrop vertebral outgrowth
   vertebral outgrowth
outlay operation
outlet
   gastric outlet
   overflow outlet
   pelvic outlet
   relaxed vaginal outlet
   Roos test for thoracic outlet
   transverse diameter of pelvic outlet
   vaginal outlet
outlet cannula
outlet forceps
outlet forceps delivery
outlet narrowing
outlet obstruction
outlet occlusion
outlet strut fracture
outlining
out-of-body surgery
out-of-phase endometrial biopsy
outpatient anesthesia
outpatient biopsy
outpatient endoscopy
output
   cardiac output
   Fick measurement of cardiac output
   fluid output
   inadequate cardiac output
   insensible fluid output
   intake and output (I&O)
   intraoperative urine output
   maximum acoustic output
   maximum power output (MPO)
   urinary output
output device
output signal processor
outrigger splint
outrigger wire
outrigger wrist splint
outside diameter
outside-to-outside arthroscopy technique
outward movement
outward rotation
OV-1 surgical keratometer
ova (*sing.* ovum)
oval amputation

oval cup erysiphake
oval cup forceps
oval cutting bur
oval esophagoscope
oval incision
oval knife
oval niche
oval optical zone marker
oval piston gauge
oval speculum
oval window
Oval-8 finger splint
oval-form colonic groove
oval-open esophagoscope
oval-shaped
oval-window curet
oval-window excavator
oval-window hook
oval-window pick
oval-window piston evacuator
ovarian ablation
ovarian abscess
ovarian artery
ovarian calculus
ovarian cancer
ovarian cancer metastasis
ovarian carcinoma debulking
ovarian clear cell
    adenocarcinoma
ovarian cycle
ovarian cyst
ovarian cystectomy
ovarian dermoid cyst
ovarian duct
ovarian fimbria
ovarian follicle
ovarian fossa
ovarian hernia
ovarian hyperstimulation
    syndrome
ovarian incision
ovarian ligament
ovarian mass
ovarian overstimulation
    syndrome
ovarian plexus
ovarian pregnancy
ovarian stroma
ovarian trocar
ovarian tube
ovarian tumor
ovarian vein

ovarian vein syndrome
ovarian wedge resection
ovariectomy
ovarioabdominal pregnancy
ovariocentesis
ovariosalpingectomy
ovariotomy
    Beatson ovariotomy
ovary
    accessory ovary
    hilus of ovary
    middle-ear dermoid cyst of
        ovary
    polycystic ovary (PCO)
    wandering ovary
ovary forceps
over-and-out cheek flap
over-and-over suture technique
over-and-over sutures
over-and-over whip sutures
overbite
    deep overbite
    excessive overbite
    vertical overbite
overbite/overjet relationship
overcorrected position
overcorrection
overcouch tube
overdenture
    mandibular overdenture
overdevelopment
overdistention
overdosage
overdrive atrial pacing
overflow outlet
overgrafting
overgrowth
overhang
    excess overhang
Overhauser effect on x-ray
Overhauser technique
overhead fracture frame
Overhold-Jackson bronchoscope
Overholt clip-applying forceps
Overholt dissecting forceps
Overholt double-ended elevator
Overholt elevator
Overholt needle
Overholt operation
Overholt periosteal elevator
Overholt procedure
Overholt raspatory

Overholt retractor
Overholt rib needle
Overholt rib raspatory
Overholt rib spreader
Overholt thoracic forceps
Overholt-Finochietto rib
  spreader
Overholt-Geissendoerfer
  dissecting forceps
Overholt-Geissendoerfer arterial
  forceps
Overholt-Jackson bronchoscope
Overholt-Mixter dissecting
  forceps
overlap midline incisional
  hernioplasty
overlapping closure
overlapping incision
overlapping pincer
overlapping suture technique
overlapping sutures
overlay cantilever bone graft
overlay mattress
overlying skin
overprojecting nasal tip
overriding aorta
overripe cataract
overrotation
oversensing pacemaker
Overstreet endometrial polyp
  forceps
Overstreet polyp forceps
over-the-door traction unit
over-the-endoscope Witzel
  dilator
over-the-guidewire esophageal
  dilator
over-the-needle infusion catheter
over-the-top cruciate repair
over-the-top position
over-the-wire pacing lead
over-the-wire (OTW)
OTW (over-the-wire)
over-the-wire probe
over-the-wire PTCA balloon
  catheter
over-the-wire technique
Overton dowel graft
Overton shunt
Overton spinal fusion
overtransfusion
overtube (*see* tube)

over-tying wire
overzealous flaring
Oves cervical cup
oviduct
  fimbriated oviduct
  pavilion of oviduct
oviductal pregnancy
ovoid
  Delclos ovoid
  Henschke ovoid
ovoid outline
ovoid packing
ovoid radium application
ovulation cycle
ovulation induction
ovulation rate
ovulatory menstruation
ovum (*pl.* ova)
ovum curet
ovum forceps
Owatusi double catheter
Owen balloon
Owen catheter
Owen cloth dressing
Owen gauze dressing
Owen hemostatic bag
Owen line
Owen Lo-Profile dilation catheter
Owen nonadherent surgical
  dressing
Owen operation
Owen position
Owen rayon gauze
Owen sutures
owl eye inclusion body
owl reduction mammaplasty
Oxaine anesthetic agent
oxalate calculus
oxethazaine anesthetic agent
Oxford large-bore imaging
  system scanner
Oxford fixator
Oxford magnet
Oxford Medilog frequency-
  modulated recorder
Oxford miniature vaporizer
  inhaler
Oxford nonkinking cuffed tube
Oxford operation
Oxford prosthesis
Oxford technique
Oxford total knee prosthesis

Oxford tube
Oxford uncompartmental device
OxiFlow meter
oximetric catheter
Oximetrix oximeter
oximetry
oximetry catheter
Oxinium femoral head
Oxiplex adhesive barrier
Oxiport blade
OxiScan pulse oximeter
Oxisensor fetal oxygen
    saturation monitor
Oxisensor oxygen transducer
Oxycel cautery
Oxycel cotton
Oxycel dressing
Oxycel gauze
Oxycel hemostat
Oxycel pack
Oxycyte perfluorocarbon-based
    blood substitute
oxygen
  ambient oxygen
  blow-by oxygen
  hyperbaric oxygen (HBO)
  inspired oxygen
  triflow oxygen
oxygen administration
oxygen cisternography
oxygen effect
oxygen extraction rate
oxygen mask
oxygen saturation meter
oxygen supply line
oxygen therapy
oxygenated blood
oxygenated hemoglobin
oxygenation
  disk oxygenation
  extracorporeal membrane
    oxygenation (ECMO)
oxygenator
  Bentley oxygenator
  bubble oxygenator
  Capiox hollow flow
    oxygenator
  Capiox-E bypass system
    oxygenator
  Cobe oxygenator
  Cobe Optima hollow-fiber
    membrane oxygenator

oxygenator (*continued*)
  DeBakey heart pump
    oxygenator
  Digi-Dyne cardiopulmonary
    bypass oxygenator
  disk oxygenator
  extracorporeal membrane
    oxygenator (ECMO)
  extracorporeal pump
    oxygenator
  film oxygenator
  Gambro oxygenator
  High Flex bubble
    oxygenator
  Kay-Cross oxygenator
  Lilliput neonatal oxygenator
  Maxima Plus plasma resistant
    fiber oxygenator
  membrane oxygenator
  Monolyth oxygenator
  Oxy-Hood oxygenator
  pump oxygenator
  rotating disk oxygenator
  Sarns membrane oxygenator
  Sci-Med oxygenator
  screen oxygenator
  Shiley oxygenator
  SpiralGold oxygenator
oxygenator pump
oxygen-starved tissue
Oxyguard mouth block
Oxyguard oxygenating
    mouthguard
Oxy-Hood oxygenator
Oxy-Hood pressurizer
Oxylator emergency
    resuscitation device
OxyLead interconnect cable
Oxymizer device
Oxy-Quik Mark IV oxygen
    inhalator
oxyquinoline dressing
Oxyrak pulse oximeter
OxyShuttle pulse oximeter
OxyTemp hand-held pulse
    oximeter
oxytocin
Oxytrak pulse oximeter
Oxy-Ultra-Lite ambulator oxygen
    systems
Oyloidin sutures
oyster splint

P&A (percussion and auscultation)
PAS Port catheter
PAS Port Fluoro-Free catheter
PD Access with peel-away needle introducer
P.R. heat moldable insert
PA (posteroanterior; pulmonary artery)
PA radiofrequency probe
PA and lateral projections (posteroanterior)
PA banding (pulmonary artery banding)
PA film (posteroanterior film)
PA lordotic projection (posteroanterior lordotic projection)
PA position (posteroanterior position)
PA projection (posteroanterior projection)
PA view (posteroanterior view)
PA position-monitoring catheter
PABP (pulmonary artery balloon pump)
PAC (premature atrial contraction)
pacchionian foramen
pacchionian glands
pacchionian granulation
Pace hysterectomy knife
Pace periosteal elevator
Pace Plus System scanner
Pace ventricular needle
Pacel bipolar pacing catheter
pacemaker
   AA1 single-chamber pacemaker
   AAT pacemaker
   Accufix pacemaker
   Acculith pacemaker

pacemaker (*continued*)
   Activitrax single-chamber responsive pacemaker
   Activitrax variable rate pacemaker
   activity-guided pacemaker
   activity-sensing pacemaker
   Actros pacemaker
   AddVent atrial-ventricular pacemaker
   adjustment of cardiac pacemaker
   AEC pacemaker
   Aequitron pacemaker
   Affinity pacemaker
   AFP pacemaker
   AICD pacemaker
   AID-B pacemaker
   Alcatel pacemaker
   American Optical Cardiocare pacemaker
   American Optical R-inhibited pacemaker
   Amtech-Killeen pacemaker
   antitachycardia pacemaker
   AOO pacemaker (atrial asynchronous)
   Arco atomic pacemaker
   Arco lithium pacemaker
   artificial pacemaker
   Arzco pacemaker
   Astra pacemaker
   ASVIP pacemaker
   asynchronous mode pacemaker
   asynchronous ventricular VOO pacemaker
   atrial demand-inhibited pacemaker
   atrial demand-triggered pacemaker
   atrial synchronous ventricular-inhibited pacemaker
   atrial tracking pacemaker

pacemaker (*continued*)

  atrial triggered ventricular-inhibited pacemaker

  Atricor Cordis pacemaker

  Atricor pacemaker

  atrioventricular junctional pacemaker (AV junctional pacemaker)

  atrioventricular sequential pacemaker (AV sequential pacemaker)

  atrioventricular synchronous pacemaker (AV synchronous pacemaker)

  Aurora dual-chamber pacemaker

  Autima II dual-chamber cardiac pacemaker

  automated external defibrillator pacemaker (AEDP)

  AV junctional pacemaker (atrioventricular junctional pacemaker)

  AV sequential pacemaker (atrioventricular sequential pacemaker)

  AV synchronous pacemaker (atrioventricular synchronous pacemaker)

  Avius sequential pacemaker

  Axios pacemaker

  Basix pacemaker

  Betacel-Biotronik pacemaker

  bifocal demand pacemaker

  Biorate pacemaker

  Biotronik demand pacemaker

  bipolar Medtronic pacemaker

  bipolar pacemaker

  bladder pacemaker

  breathing pacemaker

  burst pacemaker

  Byrel pacemaker

  cardiac pacemaker

  Cardio-Control pacemaker

  Cardio-Pace Medical Durapulse pacemaker

  Chardack Medtronic pacemaker

  Chardack-Greatbatch pacemaker

pacemaker (*continued*)

  Chorus rate-responsive dual-chamber pacemaker

  Chronocor external pacemaker

  Chronos pacemaker

  cilium pacemaker

  Circadia dual-chamber rate-adaptive pacemaker

  Classix pacemaker

  Command pacemaker

  committed mode pacemaker

  Cook pacemaker

  cor pacemaker

  Coratomic pacemaker

  Coratomic R-wave inhibited pacemaker

  Cordis Atricor pacemaker

  Cordis Chronocor pacemaker

  Cordis Ectocor pacemaker

  Cordis fixed-rate pacemaker

  Cordis Gemini pacemaker

  Cordis Multicor pacemaker

  Cordis Omni Stanicor Theta transvenous pacemaker

  Cordis Omnicor Stanicor pacemaker

  Cordis Sequicor pacemaker

  Cordis Stanicor unipolar ventricular pacemaker

  Cordis Synchrocor pacemaker

  Cordis Ventricor pacemaker

  Cortomic pacemaker

  Cosmos pulse-generator pacemaker

  CPI Astra pacemaker

  CPI Maxilith pacemaker

  CPI Microthin lithium-powered programmable pacemaker

  CPI Microthin pacemaker

  CPI Minilith pacemaker

  CPI Ultra pacemaker

  CPI Vigor pacemaker

  CPI Vista-T pacemaker

  cross-talk pacemaker

  Cyberlith demand pacemaker

  Cybertach automatic-burst atrial pacemaker

  Daig pacemaker

  Dart pacemaker

pacemaker (*continued*)

Dash single-chamber rate-adaptic pacemaker

DDD pacemaker (dual-sensing, -pacing, -mode)

DDI mode pacemaker

Delta pacemaker

demand cardiac pacemaker

demand pacemaker

Devices, Ltd. pacemaker

Diag screw-in lead pacemaker

Dialog pacemaker

Diamond pacemaker

Diplos pacemaker

Discovery pacemaker

Dromos pacemaker

dual-chamber AV sequential pacemaker

dual-chamber Medtronic Kappa pacemaker

dual-chamber pacemaker

dual-pass pacemaker

Durapulse pacemaker

DVI pacemaker

ECT pacemaker

Ectocor pacemaker

ectopic atrial pacemaker

ectopic pacemaker

Ela Chorus pacemaker

Elecath pacemaker

electric cardiac pacemaker

Electrodyne pacemaker

electronic pacemaker

Elema pacemaker

Elema-Schonander pacemaker

Elevath pacemaker

Elgiloy lead-tip pacemaker

Elite dual-chamber rate-responsive pacemaker

Encor pacemaker

endocardial bipolar pacemaker

endocardial pacemaker

Enertrax pacemaker

Enterra pacemaker

Entity pacemaker

epicardial pacemaker

Ergos O_2 dual-chamber rate-responsive pacemaker

escape pacemaker

external asynchronous pacemaker

pacemaker (*continued*)

external demand pacemaker

external pacemaker

external transthoracic pacemaker

external-internal pacemaker

externally controlled noninvasive programmed stimulation pacemaker

Fast-Pass lead pacemaker

fixed-rate asynchronous atrial pacemaker

fixed-rate asynchronous ventricular pacemaker

fixed-rate pacemaker

fully automatic pacemaker

fully automatic, atrioventricular universal dual-channel pacemaker

Galaxy pacemaker

GE pacemaker

Gemini pacemaker

General Electric pacemaker

Genisis dual-chamber pacemaker

Guardian pacemaker

Guidant pacemaker

heart pacemaker

hermetically sealed pacemaker

hysteresis of pacemaker

hysteresis rate of pacemaker

Identity pacemaker

implantable pacemaker

implantation of pacemaker

implanted pacemaker

insertion of pacemaker

Integrity pacemaker

Intermedics atrial antitachycardia pacemaker

Intermedics Cyberlith multiprogrammable pacemaker

Intermedics lithium-powered pacemaker

Intermedics Marathon dual-chamber rate-responsive pacemaker

Intermedics Quantum pacemaker

Intermedics Quantum unipolar pacemaker

pacemaker (*continued*)
    Intermedics Stride pacemaker
    Intermedics Thinlith
        pacemaker
    Intertach pacemaker
    intraperitoneal migration of
        pacemaker
    isotopic pulse generator
        pacemaker
    Jade pacemaker
    junctional pacemaker
    Kairos pacemaker
    Kalos pacemaker
    Kantrowitz pacemaker
    Kappa pacemaker
    Kelvin pacemaker
    Kelvin Sensor pacemaker
    Lambda Omni Stanicor
        pacemaker
    Lambda pacemaker
    latent pacemaker
    Laurens-Alcatel nuclear
        powered pacemaker
    Legend pacemaker
    Leios pacemaker
    Leptos pacemaker
    Leukos pacemaker
    Lillehei pacemaker
    lith II pacemaker
    lithium pacemaker
    lithium-powered pacemaker
    Maestro implantable cardiac
        pacemaker
    Mailith pacemaker
    malsensing pacemaker
    Maxilith pacemaker
    Medcor pacemaker
    Medtel pacemaker
    Medtronic Activitrax rate-
        responsive unipolar
        ventricular pacemaker
    Medtronic bipolar pacemaker
    Medtronic Byrel-SX
        pacemaker
    Medtronic Chardack
        pacemaker
    Medtronic corkscrew
        electrode pacemaker
    Medtronic Cyberlith
        pacemaker
    Medtronic demand
        pacemaker

pacemaker (*continued*)
    Medtronic Elite pacemaker
    Medtronic external/internal
        pacemaker
    Medtronic Minix pacemaker
    Medtronic pacemaker
    Medtronic Pacette pacemaker
    Medtronic Symbios
        pacemaker
    Medtronic temporary
        pacemaker
    Medtronic Thera i-series
        cardiac pacemaker
    Medtronic Kappa pacemaker
    Medtronic-Alcatel pacemaker
    Medtronic-Laurens-Alcatel
        pacemaker
    Medtronic-Zyrel pacemaker
    Mentor bladder pacemaker
    mercury cell-powered
        pacemaker
    Meridian pacemaker
    Meta pacemaker
    Meta rate-responsive
        pacemaker
    Micro Minix pacemaker
    Microlith pacemaker
    Microthin pacemaker
    Mikros pacemaker
    Minilith pacemaker
    Minix pacemaker
    Minuet pacemaker
    Mitrothin pacemaker
    Momentum pacemaker
    Multicor Gamma pacemaker
    Multicor cardiac pacemaker
    Multicor pacemaker
    Multilith pacemaker
    multiprogrammable
        pacemaker
    myopectoral inhibition of
        pacemaker
    Nanos pacemaker
    Nathan pacemaker
    natural pacemaker
    Neos pacemaker
    Nomos multiprogrammable
        R-wave inhibited demand
        pacemaker
    noncompetitive pacemaker
    noninvasive temporary
        pacemaker

pacemaker (*continued*)
- Nova pacemaker
- nuclear pacemaker
- nuclear powered pacemaker
- Omni-Atricor pacemaker
- Omnicor pacemaker
- Omni-Ectocor pacemaker
- Omni-Orthocor pacemaker
- Omni-Stanicor pacemaker
- Omni-Theta pacemaker
- Omni-Ventricor pacemaker
- Optima pacemaker
- Opus pacemaker
- Orion pacemaker
- Orthocor pacemaker
- orthorhythmic pacemaker
- Oscor pacemaker
- oversensing pacemaker
- Pacesetter Affinity pacemaker
- Pacesetter Regency pacemaker
- Pacesetter Synchrony pacemaker
- Pacette pacemaker
- Paragon pacemaker
- Pasar tachycardia reversion pacemaker
- Pasys pacemaker
- PDx pacing and diagnostic pacemaker
- permanent myocardial pacemaker
- permanent pacemaker
- permanent rate-responsive pacemaker
- permanent transvenous demand pacemaker (PTDP)
- permanent transvenous pacemaker
- permanent ventricular pacemaker
- Permathane Pacesetter lead pacemaker
- Philos pacemaker
- Phoenix single-chamber pacemaker
- Phymos pacemaker
- physiologic pacemaker
- Pinnacle pacemaker
- PolyFlex implantable pacing lead pacemaker
- PolyFlex lead pacemaker

pacemaker (*continued*)
- Precept pacemaker
- Prima pacemaker
- Prism-CL pacemaker
- Programalith AV pacemaker
- Programalith pacemaker
- programmable pacemaker
- Programmer pacemaker
- Prolith pacemaker
- Prolog pacemaker
- Pulsar pacemaker
- Pulsar implantable pacemaker
- P-wave-triggered ventricular pacemaker
- Q-T interval sensing pacemaker
- Quantum pacemaker
- radiofrequency pacemaker
- rate-modulated pacemaker
- rate-responsive pacemaker
- Reflex pacemaker
- Relay cardiac pacemaker
- rescuing pacemaker
- respiratory-dependent pacemaker
- reversion pacemaker
- RS4 pacemaker
- R-synchronous pacemaker
- Ruby pacemaker
- SAVVI synchronous pacemaker
- Schaldach electrode pacemaker
- Schultz pacemaker
- screw-in-lead pacemaker
- Seecor pacemaker
- Sensolog pacemaker
- Sensor Kelvin pacemaker
- sensor-based single-chamber pacemaker
- Sequicor pacemaker
- Shaldach pacemaker
- shifting pacemaker
- Siemens-Elema multiprogrammable pacemaker
- Siemens-Pacesetter pacemaker
- single-chamber pacemaker
- single-pass pacemaker
- sinus node pacemaker
- sinus pacemaker
- Solar pacemaker

pacemaker (*continued*)
Solis pacemaker
Solus pacemaker
Sorin pacemaker
Spectraflex pacemaker
Spectrax bipolar pacemaker
Spectrax programmable
  Medtronic pacemaker
standby pacemaker
Stanicor Gamma pacemaker
Stanicor Lambda demand
  pacemaker
Starr-Edwards hermetically
  sealed pacemaker
Stride cardiac pacemaker
Swing pacemaker
Symbios dual-chamber
  pacemaker
synchronous burst pacemaker
synchronous mode
  pacemaker
Synchrony pacemaker
Synergyst pacemaker
Syticon bipolar demand
  pacemaker
tachycardia-terminating
  pacemaker
Tachylog pacemaker
Telectronics pacemaker
temperature-sensing
  pacemaker
temporary pacemaker
temporary transvenous
  pacemaker
Thera-SR pacemaker
Thermos pacemaker
Thinlith pacemaker
tined lead pacemaker
Topaz pacemaker
transcutaneous pacemaker
transmural antitachycardia
  pacemaker
transpericardial pacemaker
transthoracic pacemaker
transvenous catheter
  pacemaker
transvenous pacemaker
transvenous ventricular
  demand pacemaker
Trilogy pacemaker
Trios M pacemaker
Triumph VR pacemaker

pacemaker (*continued*)
Ultra pacemaker
undersensing malfunction of
  pacemaker
Unilith pacemaker
unipolar atrial pacemaker
unipolar atrioventricular
  pacemaker
unipolar pacemaker
unipolar sequential
  pacemaker
Unity pacemaker
Unity-C cardiac pacemaker
USCI Vario permanent
  pacemaker
variable rate pacemaker
VAT pacemaker
VDD pacemaker
Ventak pacemaker
Ventricor pacemaker
ventricular asynchronous
  pacemaker
ventricular demand
  pacemaker
ventricular demand-inhibited
  pacemaker
ventricular demand-triggered
  pacemaker
ventricular pacemaker
ventricular-suppressed
  pacemaker
ventricular-triggered
  pacemaker
Versatrax cardiac pacemaker
Versatrax pacemaker
Vicor pacemaker
Vigor pacemaker
Vista pacemaker
Vitatrax pacemaker
Vitatron Diamond pacemaker
Vitatron pacemaker
Vivalith-10 pacemaker
Vivatron pacemaker
VVD mode pacemaker
VVI bipolar Programalith
  pacemaker
VVI pacemaker
VVI single-chamber
  pacemaker
VVI/AAI pacemaker
VVIR single-chamber rate-
  adaptive pacemaker

pacemaker (*continued*)
 VVT pacemaker
 wandering atrial pacemaker (WAP)
 wandering pacemaker
 Xyrel pacemaker
 Xyticon bipolar demand pacemaker
 Zitron pacemaker
 Zoll pacemaker
pacemaker adaptive rate
pacemaker battery
pacemaker catheter
pacemaker electrode
pacemaker failure
pacemaker generator
pacemaker lead
pacemaker lead attachment
pacemaker lead fracture
pacemaker pocket
pacemaker pouch
pacemaker programmer
pacemaker rhythm
pacemaker syndrome
Paceport catheter
Pace-Potts forceps
pacer-cardioverter defibrillator (PCD)
Pacesetter pacemaker
Pacesetter Affinity pacemaker
Pacesetter pacemaker programmer
Pacesetter knee brace
Pacesetter pacemaker
Pacesetter programmable pulse generator
Pacesetter Regency pacemaker
Pacesetter Synchrony pulse generator
Pacesetter Synchrony pacemaker
Pacesetter Tendril pacing lead
Pacesetter Tendril steroid-eluting active-fixation pacing lead
Pacesetter Trilogy pulse generator
Pacette pacemaker
Pacewedge dual-pressure bipolar pacing catheter
Pacey technique
pachometer

Pach-Pen corneal thickness measurer
Pach-Pen tonometer
Pach-Pen pachymeter
pachyblepharon
pachyblepharosis
pachycephaly
pachycheilia
pachydactyly
pachyderma circumscripta
pachyderma laryngis
pachyderma lymphangiectatica
pachydermatous
pachydermoperiostosis
pachyglossia
pachygnathous
pachymeter
 Advent pachymeter
 Compuscan-P pachymeter
 corneal pachymeter
 ophthalsonic pachymeter
 optical pachymeter
 Orbscan pachymeter
 Pach-Pen XL pachymeter
 Packo pars plana cannula pachymeter
 Sonogage ultrasound pachymeter
 Villasensor ultrasonic pachymeter
pachymeter, pachometer
pachymucosa
pachynsis
pachyonychia
pachyonychia congenita
pachyotia
pachyperiosteoderma
Pachysomia
Paci operation
Pacific Coast demineralized bone grafting material
Pacific Coast demineralized cortical bone powder
Pacific Coast flexible laminar bone strip
Pacifico cannula
Pacifico catheter
pacing
 Baim-Turi pacing
 cardiac pacing
 electronic diaphragm pacing

pacing (*continued*)
  implantable cardioverter-
    defibrillator/atrial
    tachycardia pacing
  incremental pacing
  overdrive atrial pacing
pacing and sensing
pacing catheter
pacing electrode
pacing electrode wire
pacing wire
pacing impulse
pacing technique
pacing wire
pacing wire electrode
Pacini corpuscles
pacinian corpuscles
pack
Pack technique
Packard intraocular lens
packed cell volume
packed red blood cells
packed with gauze
Pack-Ehrlich deep iliac
    dissection
packer
  Allport gauze packer
  Allport packer
  Angell gauze packer
  August automatic gauze
    packer
  Balshi packer
  Bernay gauze packer
  Bernay uterine gauze packer
  Bernay uterine packer
  dental amalgam packer
  gauze packer (*see* packer)
  iodoform gauze packer
  Jewett bone chip packer
  Kitchen postpartum gauze
    packer
  Kreiselman packer
  Lorenz gauze packer
  mastoid packer
  Ralks nasal gauze packer
  Torpin automatic uterine
    gauze packer
  Woodson dural separator and
    packer
  Woodson gauze packer
Packer mosquito forceps
Packer tunnel silicone sponge

packing
  Adaptic gauze packing
  Algiderm wound packing
  Brodhead uterine gauze
    packing
  dry packing
  gauze packing (*see* packing)
  Gelfoam packing
  ice packing
  incision and packing
  intranasal packing
  iodoform gauze packing
  Kaltostat hydrofiber wound
    packing
  Merocel epistaxis packing
  Merocel nasal packing
  Merogel nasal packing
  nasal packing
  ovoid packing
  polyurethane packing
  Pope Merocel ear packing
  removal of packing
  Rhino Rocket nasal packing
  SinuSeal nasal packing
  transvenous packing
  vaginal packing
  Vaseline petrolatum packing
  Weimert epistaxis packing
  wet packing
packing forceps
packing strip
Pac-Kit Army-type tourniquet
Packo pars plana cannula
Packo pars plana cannula
    pachymeter
paclitaxel-coated coronary stent
Pac-Man flap for closure of
    pressure sores
pad
PAD (percutaneous automated
    diskectomy)
pad electrode
pad sign
padded aluminum splint
padded board splint
padded clamp
padded knee supports
padded plywood splint
padded splint
paddle
  boomerang-shaped skin paddle
  cardioversion paddles

paddle (*continued*)
  compression paddle
  crescentic-shaped skin paddle
  cutaneous paddle
  defibrillation paddle
  defibrillator paddle
  elliptical transverse skin
    paddle
  fleur-de-lis-shaped skin paddle
  horizontal-shaped skin paddle
  musculocutaneous flap skin
    paddle
  noninvasive paddle
  Rosen nucleus paddle
  sentinel skin paddle
  skin paddle
  spot-compression paddle
  thin-skin paddle
  Y-shaped skin paddle
Padgett baseline pinch gauge
Padgett dermatome
Padgett dermatome blade
Padgett endoscope
Padgett graft
Padgett hydraulic hand
  dynamometer
Padgett implant
Padgett manual dermatome
Padgett mesh skin graft
Padgett osteotome
Padgett prosthesis
Padgett shark-mouth cannula
Padgett-Concorde suction
  cannula
Padgett-Hood dermatome
Padgett-Hood electrodermatome
Padua bladder urinary pouch
PAF (platelet-activating factor,
  platelet-aggregating factor)
PAFD (percutaneous abscess
  and fluid drainage)
Page knife
Page needle
Page procedure
Page tonsillar forceps
Page tonsillar knife
Pagenstecher linen thread sutures
Pagenstecher operation
Pagenstecher scoop
Pagenstecher suture technique
Pagenstecher sutures
Paget carcinoma

Paget cells
Paget disease of bone
Paget disease of nipple
Paget extramammary disease
Paget I syndrome
Paget II syndrome
Paget-von Schrotter syndrome
PAIC (procedures, alternatives,
  indications, complications)
pain induction
pain syndrome
pain threshold gauge
pain threshold reduction
Paine carpal tunnel
  retinaculotome
Paine syndrome
paint-gun injury
paired vertebral arches
Pairolero classification of
  sternotomy wound
  infection (types I-III)
Pais fracture
Pajot decapitating hook
Pajot maneuver
Pajunk needle
Palacos bone cement
Palacos cement adhesive
Palacos radiopaque bone
  cement
Paladon graft
Paladon implant material
Paladon prosthesis
palatal access
palatal alveolar fracture
palatal aponeurosis
palatal arch
palatal area
palatal bar
palatal bone
palatal cleft
palatal closure
palatal connector
palatal dimple
palatal distraction
palatal edema
palatal expansion
palatal expansion appliance
palatal fistula
palatal flap
palatal fronting
palatal gland
palatal height index

palatal incompetence
palatal index
palatal insufficiency
palatal island flap
palatal length
palatal lengthening procedure
palatal lift
palatal lifting device
palatal linguoplate
palatal mucoperiosteal flap
palatal mucosa
palatal muscle
palatal obturator
palatal papillomatosis
palatal paralysis
palatal plane
palatal plate
palatal prosthesis
palatal pushback
palatal pushback operation
palatal ramping
palatal reflex
palatal root
palatal seal
palatal shelf
palatal shelves
palatal split
palatal strap
palate
  arched palate
  artificial palate
  bilateral cleft lip and palate
    (BCLP)
  bilateral cleft palate
  bony hard palate
  bony palate
  breadth of palate
  Byzantine arch palate
  cleft lip and palate (CLP)
  cleft of primary palate
  cleft palate
  complete cleft palate
  cutaneous suture of palate
  falling palate
  gothic palate
  hard cleft palate
  hard palate
  height of palate
  incomplete cleft palate
  Kernahan-Elsahy striped Y
    classification for cleft lip
    and palate

palate (*continued*)
  length of palate
  longitudinal ridge of hard
    palate
  longitudinal suture of palate
  medial cleft of palate
  occult cleft palate
  partial cleft palate
  pendulous palate
  pillar of soft palate
  posterior nasal spine to soft
    palate (PNSP)
  premaxillary palate
  primary palate
  secondary palate
  smoker's palate
  soft cleft palate
  soft palate
  submucosal cleft palate
  submucous cleft palate
  subtotal cleft palate
  total cleft palate
  unilateral cleft of lip and palate
palate bone
palate elevator
palate fracture
palate hook
palate lengthening
palate myograph
palate plate
palate pusher hook
palate reconstruction
palate retractor
palate-free activator
palate-splitting appliance
plate-type mouth gag
palatine aponeurosis
palatine arch
palatine artery
palatine block anesthesia
palatine bone fissure
palatine bones
palatine canal
palatine durum
palatine folds
palatine foramen
palatine glands
palatine groove of maxilla
palatine groove of palatine bone
palatine index
palatine lamina of maxilla
palatine mucosa

palatine nerve
palatine notch
palatine papilla cyst
palatine process of maxilla
palatine protuberance
palatine raphe
palatine recess
palatine reflex
palatine ridge
palatine root
palatine ruga
palatine shelf
palatine spine
palatine sulci of maxilla
palatine sulcus of maxilla
palatine surface
palatine suture
palatine tonsil
palatine torus
palatine uvula
palatine vein
palatine velum
palatine vertical plate of palatine
palatine vessel
palatoalveolar fistula
palatoethmoid suture
palatoglossal
palatoglossal band
palatoglossal fold
palatoglossal muscle
palatoglossus muscle
palatognathous
palatography
palatomaxillary arch
palatomaxillary canal
palatomaxillary cleft
palatomaxillary groove of
    palatine bone
palatomaxillary index
palatomaxillary suture
palatonasal
palato-occipital line
palatopharyngeal arch
palatopharyngeal closure
palatopharyngeal fold
palatopharyngeal mechanism
palatopharyngeal muscle
palatopharyngeal ring
palatopharyngeal sphincter
palatopharyngeus muscle
palatopharyngoplasty
palatopharyngorrhaphy

palatoplasty
    4-flap palatoplasty
    alveolar extension
        palatoplasty
    Brown push-back palatoplasty
    Delaire palatoplasty
    diathermy palatoplasty
    Frolova primary palatoplasty
    Furlow double-opposing
        Z-plasty palatoplasty
    laser palatoplasty
    mucoperiosteal pushback
        palatoplasty
    Osada 2-stage palatoplasty
    pharyngeal flap palatoplasty
    posterior palatoplasty
    push-back palatoplasty
    Samonara palatoplasty
    Veau palatoplasty
    Veau-Wardill palatoplasty
    Veau-Wardill-Kilner
        palatoplasty
    V-Y palatoplasty
    Wardill palatoplasty
    W-Y palatoplasty
palatoplasty pushback
        operation
palatoplegia
palatoproximal
palatorrhaphy
    functional palatorrhaphy
    Langenbeck palatorrhaphy
    Langenbeck with pharyngeal
        flap palatorrhaphy
    primary palatorrhaphy
    V-Y pushback palatorrhaphy
palatorrhaphy elevator
palatoschisis
palatovaginal canal
palatovaginal groove
palatovaginal sulcus
palatum (pl. palata)
palatum durum
palatum durum osseum
palatum fissum
palatum molle
palatum ogivale
palatum osseum
Palek colostomy irrigation
        starter set
Palex expansion screw
Paley classification

Palfique Estelite tooth shade
  resin material
Palfyn sinus
Palfyn suture technique
Palfyn sutures
palindromic rheumatism
palisaded
Pall leukocyte removal filter
Pall leukogard arterial line
Pall transfusion filter
Pallab finger splint
palliative bypass
palliative cerebrospinal shunt
  procedure
palliative esophagostomy
palliative gastrostomy
palliative hepatojejunostomy
palliative operation
palliative procedure
palliative resection
palliative surgery
palliative surgical procedure
palliative technique
palliative therapy
palliative total gastrectomy
pallidectomy
  chemical pallidectomy
pallidoansection
pallidoansotomy
pallidotomy
Pallin lens spatula
Pallin spring-assisted syringe
palm guard
palm space
palma manus
Palma operation
palmar advancement flap
palmar aponeurosis
palmar aponeurosis pulley
palmar approach
palmar arch
palmar beak ligament
palmar clip
palmar contraction
palmar crease
palmar cross-finger flap
palmar digital arteries
palmar digital nerves
palmar digital veins
palmar dysesthesia
palmar erythema
palmar fascia

palmar fasciitis
palmar fibromatosis
palmar flap
palmar flexion
palmar incision
palmar interosseous arteries
palmar interosseous muscle
palmar ligaments
palmar metacarpal arteries
palmar metacarpal veins
palmar muscle
palmar plate
palmar pulley
palmar pulp
palmar radial arch
palmar radioulnar ligament
palmar reflex
palmar skin bridge
palmar space
palmar splint
palmar swab kit
palmaris longus composite
  flap
palmaris longus muscle
palmaris longus tendon
palmate folds
Palmaz arterial stent
Palmaz balloon-expandable iliac
  stent
Palmaz balloon-expandable stent
Palmaz biliary stent
Palmaz Corinthian transhepatic
  biliary stent
Palmaz vascular stent
Palmaz-Schatz balloon-
  expandable stent
Palmaz-Schatz biliary stent
Palmaz-Schatz coronary stent
Palmaz-Schatz Crown balloon-
  expandable stent
Palmaz-Schatz Mini Crown stent
PalmCups percussor
Palmer biopsy drill forceps
Palmer biopsy forceps
Palmer bone nail
Palmer cruciate ligament guide
Palmer cutting forceps
Palmer dilator
Palmer grasping forceps
Palmer lens
Palmer ovarian biopsy
  forceps

Palmer technique
Palmer transscaphoid perilunar
    dislocation
Palmer uterine dilator
Palmer-Buono contact lens
Palmer-Dobyns-Linscheid
    ligament repair
Palmer-Drapier forceps
Palmer-Drapier needle
Palmer-Widen operation
Palmer-Widen shoulder
    technique
palmomental reflex
Palomar E200 laser
Palomo operation
Palomo procedure
Palomo technique
palpability of pulses
palpable adenopathy
palpable mass
palpable organ
palpable pulse
palpable pyloric olive
palpable rib diastasis
palpable thrill
palpably enlarged organ
palpating finger
palpating needle
palpation
palpation probe
palpator
    Farrior blunt palpator
palpatory examination
palpatory percussion
palpebra (*pl.* palpebrae)
palpebra inferior
palpebra superior
palpebrae
    coloboma palpebrae
    tarsus inferior palpebrae
    tarsus superior palpebrae
palpebral arteries
palpebral cartilage
palpebral commissure
palpebral fascia
palpebral fissure
palpebral fold
palpebral furrow
palpebral glands
palpebral raphe
palpebral region
palpebral veins

palpebral-malar sulcus (tear
    trough)
palpebromalar sulci
palpebronasal fold
palpitations
palsy
    Bell palsy
    cerebral palsy
    Erb palsy
    Erb-Duchenne palsy
    facial nerve palsy
    facial palsy
    high median nerve palsy
    high ulnar nerve palsy
    His-Haas procedure for long
        thoracic nerve palsy
    House grade facial palsy
    Klumpke palsy
    low median nerve palsy
    low median/ulnar nerve palsy
    low ulnar nerve palsy
    posterior interosseous nerve
        palsy
    radial nerve palsy
    tardy median palsy
    tardy palsy
    ulnar nerve palsy
    Whitman procedure for long
        thoracic nerve palsy
    Zeir procedure for long
        thoracic nerve palsy
Palumbo dynamic patellar brace
Palumbo knee brace
Palumbo sleeve
Palumbo stabilizing knee brace
PAM (potential acuity meter)
pampiniform body
pampiniform plexus
pampiniform vein
PAN (posterior ampullary nerve)
pan splint
Panacryl absorbable sutures
Panalok absorbable anchor
Panalok absorbable soft tissue
    anchor
Panalok absorbable sutures
Panalok QuickAnchor Plus
    suture anchor
Panalok RC absorbable soft
    tissue anchor
Panalok RC QuickAnchor Plus
    suture anchor

Panas ptosis correction
    technique
pancake MRI magnet
panchamber UV lens
panclavicular dislocation
Pancoast operation
Pancoast suture technique
Pancoast sutures
Pancoast tumor
pancolectomy
pancraniomaxillofacial
    fracture
pancreas
   aberrant pancreas
   accessory pancreas
   acinarization of pancreas
   artificial endocrine pancreas
   Aselli pancreas
   ectopic pancreas
   head of pancreas
   heterotopic pancreas
   lesser pancreas
   tail of pancreas
   Willis pancreas
   Winslow pancreas
pancreas cancer
pancreas divisum
pancreas transplant (PTX)
pancreas transplantation
pancreas-kidney transplantation
pancreatectomy
   Child pancreatectomy
   complete laparoscopic distal
     pancreatectomy (C-LDP)
   conventional distal
     pancreatectomy
   distal pancreatectomy
   donor pancreatectomy
   en bloc distal pancreatectomy
   laparoscopic distal
     pancreatectomy
   left-to-right subtotal
     pancreatectomy
   limited pancreatectomy
   subtotal pancreatectomy
   total pancreatectomy
   Whipple pancreatectomy
pancreatic abscess
pancreatic adenocarcinoma
pancreatic anastomosis
pancreatic ascites
pancreatic autotransplantation

pancreatic biopsy
pancreatic body
pancreatic bypass
pancreatic calculus
pancreatic carcinoma
pancreatic complication
pancreatic cutaneous fistula
pancreatic cyst
pancreatic cystoduodenostomy
pancreatic disease
pancreatic duct dilatation
pancreatic duct manipulation
pancreatic duct stent
pancreatic endoprosthesis
pancreatic endoscopy
pancreatic extract
pancreatic fluid collection
pancreatic hamartoma
pancreatic head cancer
pancreatic imaging
pancreatic intraluminal radiation
    therapy
pancreatic islet cell tumor
pancreatic pseudocyst
pancreatic ranula
pancreatic stump closure
pancreatic stump leak
pancreatic surgery
pancreatic tail resection
pancreatic tissue
pancreatic transplantation
pancreatic tumor localization
pancreatic veins
pancreaticobiliary ductal
    junction
pancreaticobiliary ductography
pancreaticobiliary endoscopy
pancreaticobiliary operation
pancreaticobiliary sphincter
pancreaticobiliary tract
pancreaticocystoduodenostomy
pancreaticocystoenterostomy
pancreaticocystogastrostomy
pancreaticocystojejunostomy
pancreaticocystostomy
pancreaticoduodenal allograft
pancreaticoduodenal arterial
    arcade
pancreaticoduodenal arteries
pancreaticoduodenal
    transplantation
pancreaticoduodenal veins

pancreaticoduodenectomy
  Whipple
    pancreaticoduodenectomy
pancreaticoduodenostomy
  Child
    pancreaticoduodenostomy
  Dennis-Varco
    pancreaticoduodenostomy
  Waugh-Clagett
    pancreaticoduodenostomy
  Whipple
    pancreaticoduodenostomy
pancreaticoenterostomy
pancreaticogastric anastomosis
pancreaticogastric folds
pancreaticogastrointestinal
    anastomosis
pancreaticogastrostomy
pancreaticogastrostomy
    anastomosis (PGA)
pancreaticogastrostomy
    reconstruction
pancreaticoileostomy
pancreaticojejunal anastomosis
pancreaticojejunostomy
  caudal
    pancreaticojejunostomy
  distal pancreaticojejunostomy
  DuVal
    pancreaticojejunostomy
  DuVal-Puestow
    pancreaticojejunostomy
  end-to-end intussuscepted
    pancreaticojejunostomy
  end-to-end inverting
    pancreaticojejunostomy
  lateral
    pancreaticojejunostomy
  Puestow
    pancreaticojejunostomy
  Roux-en-Y
    pancreaticojejunostomy
pancreaticojejunostomy
    anastomosis (PJA)
pancreaticopleural fistula
pancreaticosplenic ligament
pancreaticosplenic lymph
    node
pancreaticosplenic
    omentum
pancreatic-preserving total
    gastrectomy

pancreatitis
  calcareous pancreatitis
  perilobar pancreatitis
pancreatitis dysfunction
pancreatitis-related hemorrhage
pancreatoduodenectomy
  1-stage
    pancreatoduodenectomy
  2-stage
    pancreatoduodenectomy
  Brunschwig
    pancreatoduodenectomy
  conventional
    pancreatoduodenectomy
  Whipple
    pancreatoduodenectomy
pancreatoduodenectomy bypass
pancreatoduodenostomy
pancreatoenterostomy
pancreatogram
  nasal pancreatogram
pancreatography
pancreatojejunostomy
  Puestow
    pancreatojejunostomy
pancreatolithectomy
pancreatolithotomy
pancreatomy
pancreatotomy
pancreectomy
pancreolithotomy
pancreoprivic
Pancretec pump
pan-culture
Panda gastrostomy tube
Panda nasoenteric feeding tube
Panda NCJ kit
Panelipse panoramic radiograph
Panelipse panoramic x-ray
    machine
panendography
panendoscope
  cap-fitted panendoscope
  fiberoptic panendoscope
  flexible forward-viewing
    panendoscope
  Foroblique panendoscope
  French-McCarthy
    panendoscope
  Kelly panendoscope
  LoPresti panendoscope
  McCarthy panendoscope

panendoscope (*continued*)
  Olympus panendoscope
  oral panendoscope
  Stern-McCarthy
    panendoscope
  Storz panendoscope
  Wolf rigid panendoscope
panendoscope electrode
panendoscopy
  fiberoptic panendoscopy
  lower panendoscopy
  upper panendoscopy
Panex panoramic radiograph
Panex-E (panoral) panoramic
    x-ray machine
panfacial fracture
panfundoscope
  Rodenstock panfundoscope
Pang biopsy forceps
Pang nasopharyngeal forceps
Pang technique
panhysterectomy
panhystero-oophorectomy
panhysterosalpingectomy
panhysterosalpingo-
    oophorectomy
Panje implant
Panje prosthesis
Panje tube
Panje voice box
Panje voice button laryngeal
    prosthesis
Panje voice prosthesis
Panje voice valve
Panje-Shagets tracheoesophageal
    fistula forceps
panmetatarsal head resection
panmucosal inflammatory cell
    infiltration
panmural
Pannett needle
pannicular hernia
panniculectomy
panniculitis
  histiocytic cytophagic
    panniculitis
  septal panniculitis
panniculotomy
panniculus (*pl.* panniculi)
  abdominal panniculus
  hanging panniculus
panniculus adiposus

panniculus carnosus
Pannu intraocular lens
Pannu-Kratz-Barraquer speculum
pannus
  abdominal pannus
  redundant pannus
  rheumatoid pannus
pannus formation
PanoGauge hydrogel-
    impregnated gauze
PanoGauze dressing
PanoGauze hydrogel-
    impregnated gauze
PanoGauze hydrogel-
    impregnated gauze dressing
panogram
  mandible panogram
Panoplex hydrogel dressing
pan-oral radiography
Panoramic nonmydriatic
    ophthalmoscope
Panoramic Ultra-Widefield
    ophthalmic imaging device
panoramic loupe
panoramic radiograph
panoramic roentgenogram
panoramic series
panoramic view
panoramic x-ray machine
Panorex films
Panorex panoramic x-ray
    machine
Panorex radiograph
Panorex view
Panorex x-ray
PanoView Optics lens
PanoView rod-lens ureteroscope
panproctocolectomy
panretinal ablation
Pansch fissure
pan-sensitive
pantalar fusion
pantaloon brace
pantaloon embolism
pantaloon hernia
pantaloon inguinal hernia
pantaloon operation
pantaloon patch
Panther catheter
pantomographic view
pantomography
  concentric pantomography

pantoscope
pants-over-vest capsulorrhaphy
pants-over-vest hernia repair
pants-over-vest herniorrhaphy
pants-over-vest repair
pants-over-vest sutures
pants-over-vest technique
panty cast
Panvue scope
Panzer gallbladder scissors
Pap smear
Papanicolaou smear
Papanicolaou smear tray
Paparella angled-ring curet
Paparella calipers
Paparella canal knife
Paparella catheter
Paparella curet
Paparella duckbill elevator
Paparella elevator
Paparella fenestrometer
Paparella footplate pick
Paparella incudostapedial joint
    knife
Paparella knife
Paparella mastoid curet
Paparella middle ear instrument
Paparella monkey-head holder
Paparella myringotomy tube
Paparella needle
Paparella otologic surgery
    elevator
Paparella pick
Paparella polyethylene tube
Paparella probe
Paparella rasp calipers
Paparella retractor
Paparella scissors
Paparella self-retaining retractor
Paparella sickle knife
Paparella stapes curet
Paparella straight needle
Paparella tissue press
Paparella tube
Paparella type II ventilation tube
Paparella wire-cutting scissors
Paparella-Frazier suction tube
Paparella-Hough excavator
Paparella-House curet
Paparella-House knife
Paparella-McCabe crurotomy saw
Paparella-Weitlaner retractor

Papavasiliou olecranon fracture
    classification
papaverine hydrochloride
paper drape
paper point
paper tape
Papercuff disposable blood
    pressure cuff
paper-doll fetus
Papette cervical collector
papilla (*pl.* papillae)
    atrophied papilla
    anal papilla
    calciform papilla
    capitate papillae
    circumvallate papilla
    clavate papilla
    conic papillae
    dermal papillae
    filiform papilla
    filiform papillae
    foliate papillae
    fungiform papillae
    hair papilla
    hypertrophied papilla
    incisive papilla
    lacrimal papilla
    lingual papilla
    lingual papillae
    optic papilla
    palatine papilla
    parotid papilla
    renal papillae
    retrocuspid papilla
    sublingual papilla
    tactile papilla
    vallate papilla
    Vater papilla
    vestibular papilla
papilla (*pl.* papillae)
papilla drain
papilla graft
papilla mammae
papilla of Santorini
papilla of Vater
papilla pili
papillae (*sing.* papilla; *see* papilla)
papillae linguales
papillae of corium
papillary adenocarcinoma
papillary adenoma
papillary cancer

papillary carcinoma
papillary cyst
papillary cystadenoma
  lymphomatosum
papillary cystic adenoma
papillary dermal peel
papillary duct
papillary ectasia
papillary foramen
papillary gastric carcinoma
papillary hidradenoma
papillary hyperplasia
papillary keratosis
papillary lesion
papillary muscle rupture
papillary muscles
papillary obstruction
papillary pedicle graft
papillary reconstruction
papillary squamous
  carcinoma
papillary stenosis
papillary thyroid carcinoma
papillary tumor
papillary varices
papillectomy
papilloma (*pl.* papillomas,
  papillomata)
  basal cell papilloma
  cutaneous papilloma
  fibroepithelial papilloma
  intracanalicular papilloma
  intracystic papilloma
  inverted ductal papilloma
  inverted schneiderian
    papilloma
  inverting papilloma
  keratotic papilloma
  oncocytic schneiderian
    papilloma (OSP)
  sinonasal papilloma
  soft papilloma
  squamous cell papilloma
  squamous papilloma
  tracheal papilloma
  villous papilloma
papilloma forceps
papillomacular nerve fiber
  bundle
papillomatosis
  confluent and reticulated
    papillomatosis

papillomatosis (*continued*)
  florid cutaneous
    papillomatosis
  inflammatory papillomatosis
  laryngeal papillomatosis
  malignant papillomatosis
  multiple papillomatosis
  palatal papillomatosis
papillomatous goiter
Papillon-Leage and Psaume
  syndrome
Papillon-Lefevre syndrome
papillosphincterectomy
papillotome
  30-30 papillotome
  Accuratome precurved
    papillotome
  Apollo 3 triple-lumen
    papillotome
  Bard Companion papillotome
  Bilisystem wire-guided
    papillotome
  Classen-Demling papillotome
  Cremer-Ikeda papillotome
  double-lumen tapered-tip
    papillotome
  dual-lumen papillotome
  Erlangen papillotome
  Frimberger-Karpiel 12 o'clock
    papillotome
  Howell rotatable papillotome
  Huibregtse-Katon papillotome
  Microvasive papillotome
  needle-knife papillotome
  Olympus needle-knife
    papillotome
  Piggyback needle-knife
    papillotome
  precut papillotome
  ProForma double-lumen
    papillotome
  shark fin papillotome
  Swenson papillotome
  Wilson-Cook papillotome
  Wiltek papillotome
  wire-guided papillotome
  Zimmon papillotome
papillotome/sphincterotome
  Soehendra
    papillotome/sphincterotome
  Soehendra Precut
    papillotome/sphincterotome

papillotome/sphincterotome
(*continued*)
Swenson wire-guided
papillotome/sphincterotome
papillotomy
endoscopic papillotomy
laparoscopic transcystic
papillotomy
Papineau bone graft staging
(stages I-III)
Papineau cancellous graft
Papineau sequestrectomy and
curettage
Papineau technique
papular acne
papular acrodermatitis
papular fibroplasia
papule
indurated papule
keratotic papule
red papule
split papule
papulopustular lesion
papulosis
atrophic papulosis
bowenoid papulosis
lymphomatoid papulosis
malignant atrophic papulosis
malignant papulosis
papulosquamous
papulosquamous dermatitis
papulosquamous lesion
papulous vaginitis
papulovesicular
papulovesicular lesion
papulovesicular rash
papyraceous fetus
papyraceous layer
papyraceous scar
Paquelin cautery
PAR (procedures, alternatives,
risks)
par glissement hernia
PAR room (postanesthesia
recovery room)
Par scissors
para (1, 2, 3, etc.)
para-aortic hematoma
para-aortic lymph node
dissection
para-aortic lymphadenectomy
para-aortic node irradiation

parabiotic flap
parabola of urinary stream
paracardiac metastasis
paracentesis (*pl.* paracenteses)
paracentesis abdominis
paracentesis capitis
paracentesis cordis
paracentesis knife
paracentesis needle
paracentesis pericardii
paracentesis pulmonis
paracentesis thoracis
paracentesis vesicae
paracentetic
paracentral lobe
paracentral lobule
paracentral nerve fiber bundle
paracervical anesthetic
paracervical block anesthesia
paracervical injection
paracervical nerve block needle
paracervix
Parachute Corkscrew suture
anchor
parachute deformity
parachute jumper's dislocation
parachute mitral valve
Parachute stone retrieval device
parachute valve
Paracine dressing
paraclavicular thoracic outlet
decompression
paracolic abscess
paracolic gutter
paracollicular biopsy
paracolon
paracorporeal heart
paracostal incision
paradental pyorrhea
Paradentine dental restorative
material
Paradigm insulin pump
Paradigm Link blood glucose
monitor
paradoxical contraction
paradoxical effect
paradoxical embolism
paradoxical extensor reflex
paradoxical pulse
paradoxical reflex
paradoxical technique
paraduodenal fold

paraduodenal fossa
paraduodenal hernia
paraesophageal diaphragmatic
  hernia
paraesophageal hiatal hernia
paraesophageal varices
paraextrophy skin flap
parafascicular thalamotomy
  (PFT)
paraffin block
paraffin dressing
paraffin gauze
paraffin graft
paraffin implant
paraffin implant material
paraffin prosthesis
paraffin-impregnated gauze
paraganglioma
  laryngeal paraganglioma
ParaGard intrauterine device
paraglenoid groove
paraglenoid sulcus
paraglossia
paraglottic space
paragnathus
Paragon ambulatory pump
Paragon Champion stent
Paragon Complete implant
Paragon coronary stent
Paragon implant
Paragon infuser
Paragon laser
Paragon nitinol stent
Paragon pacemaker
parahiatal hernia
parahippocampal gyrus
Parahisian catheter
paraileostomal hernia
parainguinal incision
parajejunal fossa
parakeratinized cyst
parakeratinized epithelium
parakeratosis
parakeratotic layer
paralaryngeal space
paraldehyde
paralingual sulcus
parallel flow dialyzer
parallel incision
parallel jaw clip
parallel loop electrode
parallel operation

parallel opposing tangential
  fields
parallel pin kit
parallel plate dialyzer
parallel plate hemodialyzer
parallel technique
parallel to wound edges
parallel-hole medium sensitivity
  collimator
paralleling cone position
paralleling technique
parallel-jaw spring clip
parallel-plate flow chamber
parallel-transverse incision
paralunate dislocation
paralysis
  abductor paralysis
  adductor paralysis
  Basedow paralysis
  bilateral abductor paralysis
  bilateral adductor paralysis
  bilateral facial paralysis
  Brown-Sequard paralysis
  central facial paralysis
  compression paralysis
  conjugate paralysis
  cricothyroid paralysis
  Duchenne-Erb paralysis
  facial nerve paralysis
  facial paralysis
  fascial sling for facial paralysis
  faucial paralysis
  frontalis muscle paralysis
  hernia paralysis
  hypesthesia and paralysis
  hypoglossal paralysis
  idiopathic facial paralysis
  incomplete facial paralysis
  incomplete paralysis
  Klumpke paralysis
  labioglossolaryngeal paralysis
  laryngeal motor paralysis
  laryngeal sensory paralysis
  lingual paralysis
  Lissauer paralysis
  muscular paralysis
  myopathic paralysis
  palatal paralysis
  partial paralysis
  Peabody classification of foot
    and ankle paralysis
  permanent paralysis

paralysis (*continued*)
  progressive paralysis
  Ramsay Hunt facial paralysis
  residual paralysis
  respiratory paralysis
  sensory paralysis
  soft palate paralysis
  spinal paralysis
  sudden paralysis
  trigeminal nerve paralysis
  unilateral adductor paralysis
  unilateral vocal cord paralysis
    (UVCP)
  Volkmann ischemic paralysis
  X paralysis
paralytic agent
paralytic colonic obstruction
paralytic ileus
paralytic intestinal obstruction
paralyzed limb
Parama pulse wave generator
paramagnetic contrast injection
paramagnetic enhancement
    accentuation by chemical
    shift imaging
paramagnetic microsphere
ParaMax angled driver
paramedial sulcus
paramedian appendectomy
    incision
paramedian approach
paramedian forehead flap
paramedian incision
paramedian pontine reticular
    formation
paramedian sagittal plane
paramediastinal shadow
paramesonephric duct
parameter
  baseline parameters
  conventional parameter
  effect parameter
  fetal growth parameters
  hemologic parameters
parametrial curettage
parametrial fixation
parametrial mass
parametrial thickening
parametric hematocele
parametrium clamp
parametrium forceps
paramuscular incision

paranasal sinuses
paraneoplastic acrokeratosis
paranephric abscess
paranephric body
paranephric fat body
paraneural anesthesia
paraneural block
paraneural infiltration
paraoperative
paraorbital lesion
paraovarian cyst
parapatellar arthrotomy
parapatellar incision
paraperitoneal hernia
paraperitoneal nephrectomy
parapharyngeal fat
parapharyngeal lymph nodes
parapharyngeal space
parapharyngeal space abscess
parapharyngeal tumor
paraphimosis
paraplegia
paraplegia in extension
Parapost bur
paraPRO paracentesis needle
parapubic hernia
pararectal abscess
pararectal fistula
pararectal fossa
pararectal line
pararectus approach
pararectus incision
pararenal fat
pararenal space
PARAS (postauricular and
    retroauricular scalping)
parasaccular hernia
parasacral anesthesia
parasacral block
parasagittal incision
parasagittal lesion
parasagittal meningioma
parasagittal plane
Parascan scanning device
parascapular flap
parascapular incision
parasellar metastasis
parasellar syndrome
paraseptal cartilage
parasitic cyst
Parasmillie double-bladed knife
parasol tube

paraspinal approach
paraspinal line
paraspinal muscles
paraspinal thrust
paraspinous aspect
paraspinous fascia
paraspinous muscles
paraspinous musculature
parasternal examination
parasternal line
parasternal lymph nodes
parasternal tissue
parastomal hernia
parasympathetic ganglion
parasympathetic nerve
parasymphyseal fracture
parasymphyseal region
parasymphysis area
parasystole
paraterminal body
parathyroid adenoma
parathyroid autograft
parathyroid biopsy
parathyroid carcinoma
parathyroid extract
parathyroid gland
parathyroid hyperplasia
parathyroid operation
parathyroid surgery
parathyroid tetany
parathyroid tumor ablation
parathyroidectomy
    2-1/2 gland
        parathyroidectomy
    endoscopic
        parathyroidectomy
paratracheal nodes
Paratrend 7 continuous blood
    gas monitor
paratrigeminal syndrome
paratrooper fracture
paratubular adhesions
paraumbilical hernia
paraumbilical incision
paraumbilical perforator
paraumbilical veins
paraurethral duct
paraurethral glands
paraurethral suspension
parauterine adhesions
paravaginal abscess
paravaginal defect repair

paravaginal hysterectomy
paravaginal incision
paravariceal injection
paraventricular veins
paravertebral anesthesia
paravertebral block
paravertebral ganglion
paravertebral line
paravertebral lumbar
    sympathetic block
paravertebral mass
paravertebral muscle spasm
paravertebral musculature
paravertebral thoracoplasty
paravesical fossa
paravesical pouch
paravesical space
ParCA catheter
parchment heart
parchment induration
Pardos scissors
Pare reduction
Pare suture technique
Pare sutures
pared with motor saw
Parel-Crock vitreous cutter
parenchyma
    breast parenchyma
    lung parenchyma
    neural parenchyma
    renal parenchyma
parenchyma infiltration
parenchyma testis
parenchymal brain metastasis
parenchymal density
parenchymal dissection
parenchymal hematoma
parenchymal infiltrate
parenchymal laceration
parenchymal route of injection
parenchymal scarring
parenchymal softening
parenchymal sparing surgery
parenchymal tissue
parenchymatous carcinoma
parenchymatous change
parenchymatous goiter
parenchymatous implantation
parenchymatous injection
parenchymatous intracerebral
    hemorrhage
parenchymatous tissue

parenteral administration
parenteral alimentation
parenteral analgesia
parenteral analgesic
parenteral anesthesia
parenteral hyperalimentation
parenteral therapy
parenthesis tip
paresis
paresthesia
paresthesia anesthetic technique
paretic analgesia
paretic lagophthalmos
parfocal defraction lens
Parhad needle
Parhad-Poppen needle
Parham band
Parham support
Parham-Martin band
Parham-Martin bone clamp
Parham-Martin bone-holding
    clamp
Parham-Martin fracture device
Parham-Martin rongeur
paries (*pl.* parietes)
parietal angle
parietal angle of the sphenoid
    bone
parietal area
parietal bone
parietal border
parietal cephalocele
parietal defect
parietal diameter
parietal eminence
parietal emissary vein
parietal fistula
parietal foramen
parietal hernia
parietal lamina
parietal layer
parietal lobe
parietal margin
parietal peritoneum
parietal pleura
parietal pregnancy
parietal presentation
parietal shunt
parietal suture
parietes (*sing.* paries)
Parietex composite mesh
parietocolic fold

parietography
parietomastoid suture
parieto-occipital approach
parieto-occipital fissure
parieto-occipital flap
parieto-occipital region
parieto-occipital suture
parieto-orbital projection
parietoperitoneal fold
parietotemporal region
Paris classification
Paris manual therapy table
Parisian peel
Paritene mesh graft
Park aneurysm
Park blade septostomy
Park blade septostomy catheter
Park eye speculum
Park irrigating cannula
Park lens implantation forceps
Park Medical Systems scanner
Park rectal spreader
park-bench position
Parke-Davis splint
Parker clamp
Parker double-ended retractor
Parker fixation forceps
Parker incision
Parker knife
Parker knife-needle
Parker micropump insulin
    infuser
Parker needle
Parker retractor
Parker serrated discission knife
Parker tenotomy knife
Parker thumb retractor
Parker tube
Parker-Bard blade
Parker-Bard handle
Parker-Glassman intestinal clamp
    set
Parker-Heath anterior chamber
    syringe
Parker-Heath cautery
Parker-Heath electrocautery
Parker-Heath eye syringe
Parker-Heath piggyback probe
Parker-Kerr basting stitch
Parker-Kerr basting sutures
Parker-Kerr end-to-end
    enteroenterostomy

Parker-Kerr enteroenterostomy
Parker-Kerr forceps
Parker-Kerr intestinal clamp
Parker-Kerr operation
Parker-Kerr suture technique
Parker-Kerr sutures
Parker-Mott double-ended
 retractor
Parker-Pearson needle
Parkes hump gouge
Parkes lateral osteotomy
 osteotome
Parkes nasal raspatory
Parkes nasal retractor
Parkes operation
Parkes osteotome
Parkes rasp
Parkes-Quisling osteotome
Parkes-Weber hemangiomatosis
Parkes-Weber syndrome
Park-Guyton eye speculum
Park-Guyton-Callahan eye
 speculum
Park-Guyton-Maumenee
 speculum
Parkhill operation
Parkinson disease
Parkinson head holder
Parkland fluid requirement
 formula for burn patients
Parkland resuscitation
Parkland tubal ligation
Park-Maumanee eye speculum
Park-Maumanee lid speculum
Parks anal retractor
Parks anal speculum
Parks bidirectional Doppler
 flowmeter
Parks fistulotomy
Parks hemorrhoidectomy
Parks ileoanal anastomosis
Parks ileoanal reservoir
Parks ileostomy pouch
Parks method of anal
 fistulotomy
Parks partial sphincterotomy
Parks retractor
Parks sphincterotomy
Parks staged fistulotomy
Parks transanal anastomosis
Parma band
Parodi catheter

Parona space
paronychia bur
paro-oophoritic cyst
parosteal osteosarcoma
parotic recess
parotid body
parotid capsule
parotid carcinoma
parotid cyst
parotid dissection
parotid duct ligation
parotid duct transposition
parotid fascia
parotid gland abscess
parotid ligation
parotid lobe
parotid lymph node
parotid lymph node hyperplasia
parotid notch
parotid obstruction
parotid papilla
parotid plexus
parotid resection
parotid saliva
parotid sialodochoplasty
parotid space
parotid tumor
parotid veins
parotidectomy
 Aveline Gutierrez
  parotidectomy
 facial nerve-preserving
  parotidectomy
 lateral parotidectomy
 radical parotidectomy
 superficial parotidectomy
 total parotidectomy
parotidectomy procedure
parotidectomy retractor
parotideomasseteric region
parotiditis
parotid-masseteric area
parotidoscirrhus
parotitis
parous cervix
parous introitus
parovarian cyst
paroxysmal atrial fibrillation
 (PAF)
Parrish procedure
Parrish-Mann hammertoe
 technique

Parrot atrophy of newborn
Parrot-beak deformity
parrot jaw
Parrot sign
parrot-beak basket
parrot-beak basket biter
parrot-beak flap
parrot-beak meniscus tear
parrot-beak shape of distal
   esophagus
parry fracture
pars (*pl.* partes)
pars defect
pars flaccida defect
pars plana
pars pylorica
pars superior duodeni
Parsonage-Turner syndrome
Parsonnet aortic clamp
Parsonnet coronary probe
Parsonnet dilator
Parsonnet epicardial retractor
Parsonnet pouch
Parsonnet probe
Parsonnet pulse generator
   pouch
Par-Style needle holder
partes (*sing.* pars)
partial alveolectomy
partial amputation
partial anesthesia
partial anodontia
partial bowel obstruction
partial breech delivery
partial breech extraction
partial bypass
partial central hypophysectomy
partial cleft palate
partial colectomy
partial cricotracheal resection
partial cystectomy
partial diskectomy
partial dislocation
partial duplication
partial ethmoidectomy
partial excision
partial facetectomy
partial gastrectomy (PG)
partial gastric resection
partial glossectomy
partial hemilaminectomy
partial hepatectomy

partial hepatic vascular
   exclusion (PHVE)
partial ileal bypass
partial impairment
partial inferior retrocolic end-to-
   side gastrojejunostomy
partial internal hemipelvectomy
partial keratoplasty
partial laryngectomy
partial laryngopharyngectomy
   (PLP)
partial liquid ventilation
partial mechanical obstruction
partial mesh excision
partial occlusion clamp
partial occlusion forceps
partial ossicular
   reconstructive/replacement
   prosthesis (PORP)
partial ossicular replacement
   prosthesis (PORP)
partial pack
partial paralysis
partial plate
partial pressure
partial rebreathing anesthesia
partial rebreathing mask
partial resection
partial subfascial abdominoplasty
partial superior retrocolic end-
   to-side gastrojejunostomy
partial syndactyly
partial union of fracture
partial weightbearing (PWB)
partial zonal dissection
partial-breast irradiation
partially occluding clamp
partially-implantable catheter
partially-threaded pin
partial-occlusion clamp
partial-occlusion forceps
partial-occlusion inferior vena
   cava clip
partial-thickness burn
partial-thickness craniectomy
partial-thickness flap
partial-thickness graft
partial-throw surgeon knot
particle beam radiation therapy
particulate cancellous bone and
   marrow (PCBM)
particulate cancellous bone graft

particulate contaminants
particulate material
particulate matter
Partipilo clamp
Partipilo gastrostomy
Partnership implant
Partnership instrument
Partsch bone chisel
Partsch bone gouge
Partsch gouge
Partsch operation
parumbilical hernia
parumbilical incision
Parvin gravity technique
Parvin reduction
PAS technique
PASA (proximal articular set angle)
Pasar tachycardia reversion pacemaker
PASG (pneumatic antishock garment)
Pasqualini implant
Passage balloon dilation catheter
Passage exchange balloon
passage of blood
passage of catheter
passage of clots
passage of flatus
passage of instrument
passage of meconium
passage of sound
passage of stone
passage of tissue
Passager device
Passager endoprosthesis
Passager introducing sheath
Passager stent
passageway
Passarelli one-pass capsulorrhexis forceps
Passavant bar
Passavant cushion
Passavant fold
Passavant pad
Passavant ridge
passed per mucosa
passed with difficulty
passed with ease
passed without difficulty

passer
  Arans pulley passer
  Batzdorf cervical wire passer
  Brand tendon passer
  Bunnell tendon passer
  Cappio suture passer
  Carroll tendon passer
  Carter-Thomason suture passer
  Charnley wire passer
  Concept 2-pin passer
  Concept graft passer
  Crile wire passer
  DeMayo suture passer
  dermis-fat passer
  Dingman wire passer
  Ferszt ligature passer
  Framer tendon passer
  Furlow cylinder passer
  Gallie tendon passer
  Garrett vein passer
  Gore suture passer
  Hewson ligature passer
  Hewson suture passer
  Hoefflin suture passer
  Holter distal catheter passer
  Incavo wire passer
  Joplin tendon passer
  Kleinert tendon passer
  Lahey ligature passer
  ligature passer
  Malis ligature passer
  MetraPass suture passer
  Ober tendon passer
  O'Donahue ligature passer
  O'Donahue suture passer
  Protect-a-Pass suture passer
  pulley passer
  Schnidt passer
  Shuttle-Relay suture passer
  SpeedPass suture passer
  suture passer
  tendon passer
  Uni-Shunt catheter passer
  Wedeen wire passer
  wire passer
  Withers tendon passer
  Yankauer ligature passer
passer
passing forceps
passive clot
passive contraction

passive exercise
passive flexion
passive gliding technique
passive immunity
passive joint manipulation
passive joint movement
passive motion device
passive placement
passive relaxation
passive stretching
passive track detector
passive tremor
passive vasodilation
passively flexed
passively shimmed
    superconducting magnet
Passow chisel
Passport Balloon-on-a-Wire
    dilatation catheter
Passport bedside monitor
Passport instrumentation
Passy-Muir tracheostomy and
    ventilator speaking valves
Passy-Muir tracheostomy
    speaking valve
paste
    Abbot paste
    aluminum paste
    Ethicon paste
    metallic oxide paste
    methyl cellulose paste
    Multi-Form dual purpose
        impression paste
    Osteofil allograft paste
    Regenafil allograft paste
    Replicare paste
    Teflon paste
    Unna paste
paste filler
paste plate
Pastia line
Pastia sign
Pasys pacemaker
patch (*see also* graft, implant,
    prosthesis)
    achromic patch
    aortic patch
    ash-leaf patch
    autologous pericardial patch
    Bard Composix Kugel patch
    BioGlue surgical patch
    blood patch

patch (*continued*)
    butterfly patch
    cardiac patch
    Cardiofix pericardium patch
    Carrel patch
    colic patch
    colonic patch
    cotton-wool patch
    Dacron intracardiac patch
    Dacron Sauvage patch
    defibrillation patch
    Donaldson eye patch
    Dura-Guard patch
    eczematous patch
    Edwards patch
    electrodispersive skin patch
    epicardial defibrillator patch
    epidural blood patch
    eye patch
    felt patch
    Fluoropassiv thin-wall carotid
        patch
    Fluoropassiv thin-wall carotid
        patches
    FTO eye patch
    full-time occlusion eye patch
    Gelseal vascular patch
    glue patch
    Gore-Tex cardiovascular patch
    Gore-Tex soft-tissue patch
    Graham omental patch
    gray patch
    Grillo patch
    gusset-type patch
    Hemarrest patch
    herald patch
    Hutchinson patch
    intracardiac patch
    Ionescu-Shiley pericardial
        patch
    Ivalon patch
    Kugel hernia patch
    lyophilized dural patch
    Lyrelle patch
    MacCallum patch
    Miniguard adhesive patch
    monocular patch
    moth patch
    mucous patch
    nitroglycerin transdermal
        patch
    omental patch

patch (*continued*)
  onlay bone patch
  Orthoptic eye patch
  outflow cardiac patch
  pantaloon patch
  pericardial patch
  peritoneal patch
  Permacol patch
  Peyer patch
  pigskin patch
  polypropylene intracardiac
    patch
  polytef soft-tissue patch
  Prolene hernia system onlay
    patch
  Prolene hernia system
    underlay patch
  Pro-Ophtha eye patch
  prosthetic patch
  RapiSeal patch
  Rutkow sutureless plug and
    patch
  salmon patch
  sandwich patch
  sclerotic calvarial patch
  shagreen patch
  Silastic patch
  smoker's patches
  Snugfit eye patch
  soldier patch
  Stat-padz defibrillator patch
  Syvek patch
  Tanne corneal patch
  Teflon felt patch
  Teflon intracardiac patch
  Testoderm patch
  Thal gastric patch
  Tissue-Guard bovine
    pericardial patch
  Torpedo eye patch
  transannular patch
  Vascu-Guard peripheral
    vascular patch
  vascularized fascial patch
  vein patch
  velour patch
  venous sheath patch
  white patch
  wicking glue patch
patch amnesia
patch angioplasty
patch aortoplasty

patch booster
patch clamp electrophysiology
patch closure of defect
patch dressing
patch esophagoplasty
patch eye
patch graft
patch implant
patch lesion
patch procedure for Peyronie
    disease
patch prosthesis
patch stage
patch technique
patch test scarring
patch testing
patch-graft angioplasty
patchplasty
    profunda Dacron patchplasty
patch-reinforced mattress sutures
patchy area
patchy infiltrate
patchy infiltration
patchy ulceration
Patel intraocular magnet
patella
  ballotable patella
  bipartite patella
  floating patella
  high-riding patella
  low-riding patella
  release of patella
  retinacular release of patella
  skyline view of patella
  slipping patella
  squinting patella
  tripartite patella
  winking patella
patella alta
patella apprehension test
patella baja
patella bone saw
patella cap prosthesis
patella compression
patella disease
patella dislocation
patella turndown approach
patellapexy
patellaplasty
patellar aligner
patellar band
Patellar Band knee protector

patellar button
patellar cement clamp
patellar chondromalacia
patellar clamp
patellar dome
patellar drill guide
patellar facet cartilage
patellar fold
patellar hook
patellar intra-articular dislocation
patellar ligament
patellar prosthesis
patellar reamer guide
patellar reflex
patellar resection guide
patellar retinaculum
patellar sleeve fracture
patellar synovial fold
patellar tendon repair
patellar tendon weightbearing
    brace orthosis
patellar tendon-bearing below-
    knee prosthesis
patellar tendon-bearing cast
    (PTB)
patellar tendon-bearing walking
    cast (PTB walker)
patellar tracking
patella-resurfacing implant
patellectomy
    Soto-Hall patellectomy
    Soto-Hall-West patellectomy
    West patellectomy
patelloadductor reflex
patellofemoral articulation
patellofemoral prosthesis
patency of veins
patent canal of Nuck
patent duct
patent ductus arteriosus (PDA)
patent ductus arteriosus ligation
patent ductus clamp
patent ductus forceps
patent ductus retractor
patent fallopian tube
patent graft
patent iridectomy
patent lumen
patent opening
patent orifice
patent stent
patent tube

Paterson brain clip forceps
Paterson cannula
Paterson laryngeal cannula
Paterson laryngeal forceps
Paterson long-shank brain clip
Paterson nodules
Paterson procedure
Paterson pseudarthrosis of
    tibia
Paterson technique
Patey axillary node dissection
Patey fracture
Patey mastectomy
Patey operation
path of insertion
path of removal
Pathfinder catheter
Pathfinder exchange guidewire
Pathfinder irrigation device
Pathfinder mini microcatheter
Pathfinder wire
pathogenic micro-organism
pathognomonic phleboliths
pathognomonic symptom
pathologic amputation
pathologic atrophy
pathologic barrier
pathologic change
pathologic classification
pathologic compression
    fracture
pathologic condition
pathologic diagnosis
pathologic disease
pathologic dislocation
pathologic examination
pathologic fracture
pathologic pedicle fracture
pathologic histology
pathologic lesion
pathologic organism
pathologic perforation
pathologic process
pathologic reflex
pathologic rigidity
pathologic specimen
pathologic stool
pathologic tissue examination
pathological anatomy
pathology and staging
pathology examination
pathometer attachment

pathway
  afferent-efferent pathway
  atrio-His pathway
  coagulation pathway
  extrinsic pathway
  mucociliary drainage
    pathway
  neural pathway
  sensory pathway
  subarachnoid pathways
patient dose monitor
patient electrode
patient plate
patient self-administration
  device
patient-controlled analgesia
  (PCA)
patient-controlled analgesia
  administered epidurally
  (PCAE)
patient-controlled anesthesia
  pump
patient-controlled epidural
  analgesia (PCEA, PEA)
patient-controlled intranasal
  analgesia (PCINA)
patient-controlled intravenous
  anesthesia
patient-matched implant
patient-operated selector
  mechanism
Patil stereotactic system I, II
Patil-Syracuse mask
Paton anterior chamber lens
  implant forceps
Paton capsular forceps
Paton corneal dissector
Paton corneal forceps
Paton corneal knife
Paton corneal transplant forceps
Paton corneal trephine
Paton double spatula
Paton extra-delicate forceps
Paton eye needle holder
Paton eye shield
Paton knife
Paton needle holder
Paton see-through corneal
  trephine
Paton single spatula
Paton suturing forceps
Paton transplant spatula

Paton tying/stitch removal
  forceps
Paton-Berens mules
Patrick drill
Patrick maneuver
Patrick sign
Patrick test
Patrick trigger area
pattern
  abdominal wall venous
    pattern
  acanthomatous pattern
  acinar pattern
  airway pattern
  anhaustral colonic gas pattern
  arborization pattern
  bowel pattern
  caliceal pattern
  class III ring avulsion injury
    pattern
  coarsened mucosal fold
    pattern
  Collimator plugging pattern
  contraction pattern
  crescendo pattern
  cribriform pattern
  detrusor pattern
  diffraction pattern
  dominant pattern
  drainage pattern
  echo pattern
  echogenic pattern
  electrocautery pattern
  fishnet pattern
  fleur-de-lis breast
    reconstruction pattern
  fold pattern
  gas pattern
  genetic pattern
  ground-glass pattern
  gull-wing pattern
  haustral pattern
  honeycomb pattern
  hyperdivergent facial pattern
  hyperdivergent skeletal
    pattern
  identical pattern
  inconclusive pattern
  incremental appositional
    pattern
  irregular amputated mucosal
    pattern

pattern (*continued*)
  lobular pattern
  mitten pattern
  monomorphic pattern
  mosaic duodenal mucosal
    pattern
  mucosal guideline pattern
  mucosal pattern
  nonspecific gas pattern
  occlusal pattern
  recorded pattern
  reticular pattern
  rugal pattern
  signet-ring pattern
  soap-bubble pattern
  speckled pattern
  spike pattern
  spindling patterns
  spread pattern
  stellate pattern
  strain pattern
  submucosal vascular pattern
  vascular pattern
  wear pattern
  Wise pattern
  Wolfe mammographic
    parenchymal patterns
pattern arborization
pattern-cut corneal graft
  operation
pattern of degenerative change
pattern of drainage
pattern trephine
pattern umbilical scissors
pattern-cut corneal graft
Patterson bronchoscopic
  forceps
Patterson empyema trocar
Patterson operation
Patterson specimen forceps
Patterson trocar
Patterson-Nelson empyema trocar
Pattey modified radical
  mastectomy
Patton bur
Patton cannula
Patton esophageal dilator
Patton nasal speculum
Patton septal speculum
patty
  Cellolite patty
  Codman patty

patty (*continued*)
  Cottonoid patty
  sponge patties
patulent
patulous abdomen
Pauchet gastrectomy
Pauchet procedure
paucity of findings
Paufique blade
Paufique corneal knife
Paufique corneal trephine
Paufique detached retina
  operation
Paufique graft knife
Paufique keratoplasty
Paufique keratoplasty knife
Paufique lamellar knife
Paufique operation
Paufique suturing forceps
Paufique synechotomy
Paufique trephine
Paufique-Duredge knife
Paul condom bag
Paul drainage tube
Paul hemostatic bag
Paul intestinal drainage tube
Paul lacrimal sac retractor
Paul retractor
Paul tendon hook
Paul-Mikulicz operation
Paul-Mikulicz resection
Paul-Mixter tube
Paulos ligament technique
Paulson infertility microtissue
  forceps
Paulson infertility microtying
  forceps
Paulson knee retractor
Paulus chin plate
Paulus midfacial plate
Pauly point
Pautler infusion cannula
Pautrier abscess
Pauwels adduction osteotomy
Pauwels angle
Pauwels femoral neck fracture
  classification
Pauwels fracture
Pauwels fracture forceps
Pauwels fracture of proximal
  femoral neck
Pauwels fracture operation

Pauwels osteotomy
Pauwels technique
Pauwels Y-osteotomy
pavement cells
Pavenik monodisk device
pavilion of oviduct
paving-stone degeneration
Pavlik harness
Pavlik harness splint
Pavlik hip harness
Pavlo-Colibri corneal forceps
Pavulon anesthesia
paw pigmentation
Pawlik triangle
pawlike hand
Payman intraocular forceps
Payne jejunoileostomy
Payne operation
Payne retractor
Payne-DeWind jejunoileal bypass
Payne-Ochsner arterial forceps
Payne-Pean arterial forceps
Payne-Pean arterial forceps
Payne-Pean forceps
Payne-Rankin arterial forceps
Payr abdominal retractor
Payr clamp
Payr forceps
Payr gastrectomy
Payr gastrointestinal clamp
Payr grooved director
Payr membrane
Payr probe
Payr pylorus clamp
Payr pylorus forceps
Payr resection clamp
Payr retractor
Payr sign
Payr stomach clamp
Payr vein needle
Payr-Schmieden probe
PB-FOxS pediatric femoral
    sensor kit
PBI (penile pressure/brachial
    pressure index)
PBI Medical copper vapor laser
PBI MultiLase D copper vapor
    laser
PBII blue loop lens
PBN hysterosalpingography
    catheter
PC EDO ophthalmic office laser

PC EEA stapler
PC shunt
PC-1000 panoramic x-ray
    machine
PC-7 needle
PCA (porous coated
    anatomic)
PCA acetabular cup
PCA E-series hip replacement
PCA hip
PCA hip component
PCA infuser
PCA knee
PCA knee prosthesis
PCA modular total knee
PCA periodontal pack
PCA pump
PCA revision total knee
PCA total hip
PCA total knee replacement
PCA unicompartmental knee
PCAE (patient-controlled
    analgesia administered
    epidurally)
PCA-plus infusion device
PCBM (particulate cancellous
    bone and marrow)
PC-IOL lens
PCL-oriented placement
    marking hook
PCNL (percutaneous
    nephrostolithotomy)
PCO (polycystic ovary)
PCR (progressive condylar
    resorption)
PCW (pulmonary capillary
    wedge)
PD (probing depth)
PD defibrillator
PD copper band
PD excavator
PD orthodontic wire
PD preformed crown
PD reamer
PD SS matrix band
PDA (patent ductus arteriosus)
PDA (posterior descending
    artery)
PDB preperitoneal distention
    balloon
pDEXA x-ray peripheral bone
    densitometer

PDFG (platelet-derived growth factor)
PDL (periodontal ligament)
PDL intraligamentary syringe
PDS (polydioxanone)
PDS Endoloop sutures
PDS sutures (polydioxanone sutures)
PDS Vicryl sutures
PDT guidewire
PDT guiding catheter
PDx pacing and diagnostic pacemaker
PE (pharyngoesophageal)
PE LITE material
PE Plus II balloon dilatation catheter
PE Plus II peripheral balloon catheter
PE tube (polyethylene tube; pressure equalization tube)
Peabody bunionectomy
Peabody classification of foot and ankle paralysis
Peabody foot procedure
Peabody splint
Peabody tibialis tendon transfer
Peabody-Mitchell bunionectomy
Peacekeeper cannula
peacock dressing
Peacock rhizotomy hook
Peacock transposing technique
peak expiratory flow
peak expiratory flow rate
peak flow meter
peak lidocaine concentration (Cmax)
peak systolic gradient
peak transaortic valve gradient
peak-and-trough levels
peaked pupil
Peakometer urinary flow-rate meter
peak-to-peak deflection
peak-to-peak systolic gradient
Pean amputation
Pean arterial forceps
Pean GI forceps
Pean hemostatic clamp
Pean hemostatic forceps
Pean hysterectomy
Pean hysterectomy clamp
Pean hysterectomy forceps
Pean incision
Pean intestinal clamp
Pean intestinal forceps
Pean operation
Pean position
Pean sponge forceps
Pean vessel clamp
Pean-Billroth I gastrectomy
peanut dissector
peanut eye implant
peanut forceps
peanut sponge
peanut sponge-holding forceps
peanut-fenestrated forceps
peanut-grasping forceps
PEAP (positive end-airway pressure)
peapod bead-type forceps
peapod chisel
peapod intervertebral disk forceps
peapod intervertebral disk rongeur
Pearce coaxial I&A cannula
Pearce eye speculum
Pearce intraocular glide
Pearce nucleus hydrodissector
Pearce posterior chamber intraocular lens
Pearce posterior chamber intraocular lens implant
Pearce Tripod cataract lens
Pearce Tripod intraocular lens
Pearce Tripod lens
Pearce vaulted-Y lens implant
Pearce-Keates bifocal intraocular lens
Pearce-Knolle irrigating lens loop
Pearlcast polymer plaster bandage
Pearlon impression material
pearly nodule
Pearman penile implant material
Pearman penile prosthesis
Pearman penile Silastic prosthesis
Pearman transurethral hemostatic bag
Pearsall Chinese twisted sutures
Pearsall silk sutures
pear-shaped bur

pear-shaped extension tube
pear-shaped fluted bag
pear-shaped heart
pear-shaped nerve hook
Pearson attachment to Thomas
    frame
Pearson attachment to Thomas
    splint
Pearson clavicle attachment
    splint
Pearson position
Pease bone drill
Pease reamer
Pease-Thomson traction bow
Peat hemostat
peau d'orange
PeBA anchor
Pedicle finder
Peck chisel
Peck osteotome
Peck rake retractor
Peck scissors
Peck-Joseph scissors
Peck-Vienna nasal speculum
Pecquet duct
pectate line
pectenotomy
pectinate body
pectinate ligament
pectinate line
pectinate muscles
pectineal crural hernia
pectineal fascia
pectineal hernia
pectineal ligament
pectineal line
pectineal muscle
pectoral catheter
pectoral fascia
pectoral fremitus
pectoral girdle
pectoral glands
pectoral groove
pectoral muscles
pectoral nerve
pectoral reflex
pectoral regions
pectoralis major (PM)
pectoralis major flap
pectoralis major muscle
pectoralis major myocutaneous
    flap

pectoralis minor
pectoralis minor flap
pectoralis minor muscle
pectoralis minor muscle transfer
pectoralis muscle implant
pectoralis myocutaneous
    esophagoplasty
pectoralis myocutaneous flap
pectoralis myofascial flap
pectus carinatum deformity
pectus deformity
pectus excavatum deformity
pectus gallinatum
pectus recurvatum
Peczon I&A cannula
Peczon I&A unit
pedal edema
pedal pulse
Pederson speculum
Pederson vaginal speculum
pedestal massage table
Pediastrol self-irrigating bladder
    irrigator
Pedia-Trake tube
pediatric abdominal retractor
pediatric airway
pediatric analgesic
pediatric anesthetic
pediatric balloon catheter
pediatric biopsy needle
pediatric biplane TEE probe
pediatric bone rongeur
pediatric bridge
pediatric bronchoscope
pediatric bulldog clamp
pediatric cardiovascular
    surgery
pediatric catheter
pediatric C-D hook
pediatric colonoscopy
pediatric Cotrel-Dubousset rod
pediatric drainable pouch
pediatric endoscope
pediatric endoscopy
pediatric esophagogastro-
    duodenoscopy
pediatric esophagoplasty
pediatric esophagoscope
pediatric feeding tube
pediatric Foley catheter
pediatric forceps
pediatric gastroscope

pediatric Hendren retractor blade
pediatric hepatojejunostomy
pediatric hernia
pediatric injury
pediatric intussusception
pediatric Karickhoff laser lens
pediatric laparoscopic surgical
    procedure
pediatric lid speculum
pediatric mastoid retractor blade
pediatric nasogastric tube
pediatric ophthalmic surgery
pediatric perineal retractor ring
pediatric pigtail catheter
pediatric PRAFO brace
pediatric pressure relief ankle-
    foot orthosis
pediatric Racine adapter
pediatric radiotherapy anesthesia
pediatric rectal dilator
pediatric scissors
pediatric self-retaining retractor
pediatric speculum
pediatric surgery
pediatric telescope
pediatric 3-mirror laser lens
pediatric transfer pouch
pediatric TSRH hook
pediatric urostomy pouch
pediatric vascular clamp
Pedic sponge
Pedicath catheter
pedicle
   circumflex scapular pedicle
   dermal pedicle
   dermal vascularized pedicle
   dominant pedicle
   fasciovascular pedicle
   Filatov-Gillies tubed pedicle
   inferior pedicle
   latissimus dorsi segmental
     musculovascular pedicle
   Moberg advancement
     pedicle
   muscle pedicle
   musculovascular pedicle
   Ponten-type tubed pedicle
   renal pedicle
   stump of pedicle
   superior dermal pedicle
   thoracoacromial pedicle
   vascular pedicle

pedicle anatomy
pedicle C-D hook
pedicle clamp
pedicle connector
pedicle entrance point
pedicle evaluation
pedicle fat graft
pedicle flap
pedicle flap donor site
pedicle flap operation
pedicle forceps
pedicle graft
pedicle groin flap
pedicle hook
pedicle implant
pedicle intact
pedicle kinking
pedicle ligation
pedicle localization
pedicle mucoperiosteal flap
pedicle of lung
pedicle of spleen
pedicle plate
pedicle prosthesis
pedicle screw
pedicle screw-rod fixation
pedicle stump
pedicled
pedicled cartilage graft
pedicled cyst
pedicled enteric donor site
pedicled galeal frontalis flap
pedicled jejunal reconstruction
pedicled latissimus flap
pedicled mucosa flap
pedicled myocutaneous flap
pedicled pericranial flap
pedicled skin graft
pedicled tibial bone flap
pedicolaminar fracture-
    dislocation
pedicular fixation
pediculated cells
Pedi-Cushions cushion
Pedifix hammertoe pad
PediKair pediatric low-air-loss bed
Pedilen polyurethane foam
Pediplast cushion
pedography
peduncle
   cerebellar peduncle
   cerebral peduncle

peduncle (*continued*)
   middle cerebral peduncle
   superior cerebellar peduncle
peduncular loop
pedunculated adenoma
pedunculated fibroid
pedunculated growth
pedunculated lesion
pedunculated loose body
pedunculated nodule
pedunculated polyp
pedunculotomy
peel off
Peel Pak bag
peel-away banana catheter
peel-away catheter
peel-away introducer
Peel-Away introducer set
peel-away sheath
Peeler-Cutter vitrector
peeling
   chemical face peeling
   chemical peeling
   glycolic acid peeling
   membrane peeling
   phenol peeling
peel-off catheter
PEEP (positive end-expiratory
      phase/pressure)
Peep ventilator
Peers towel clamp
Peet forceps
Peet lighted splanchnic retractor
Peet mosquito forceps
Peet nasal rasp
Peet operation
Peet splanchnic resection
Peet splinter forceps
Peet technique for leg
      constricture
PEG (percutaneous endoscopic
      gastrostomy; polyethylene
      glycol)
peg board lateral positioning
      device
peg bone graft
peg cells
peg flap
peg graft
PEG insertion
peg latissimus dorsi flap breast
      reconstruction

PEG lavage (polyethylene glycol
      lavage)
PEG procedure (percutaneous
      endoscopic gastrostomy
      procedure)
PEG self-adhesive elastic
      dressing (polyethylene
      glycol self-adhesive elastic
      dressing)
PEG tube, percutaneous
      endoscopic gastrostomy tube
peg-and-socket articulation
peg-and-socket hammertoe repair
peg-and-socket joint
peg-and-socket technique
Pegasus Nd:YAG surgical laser
pegged tibial prosthesis
peg-top prosthesis
      parallel-transverse incision
Pehr abduction splint
Peiper-Beyer bone rongeur
Peiper-Beyer laminectomy rongeur
PELCA (percutaneous excimer
      laser coronary angioplasty)
Pelco prosthetic valve
Peled knifeless otoplasty
Pelger-Huet anomaly
pelican biopsy forceps
Pelikan Sun lancing device
Pelkmann foreign body forceps
Pelkmann gallstone forceps
Pelkmann sponge forceps
Pelkmann uterine forceps
Pelkmann uterine-dressing
      forceps
Pell-Gregory classification
Pelle Peel microdermabrader
pellucidum septum
Pelorus stereotactic frame
Pelosi illuminator
Pelosi maneuver
Pelosi technique
Pelosi uterine manipulator
pelvectomy
pelvic abscess
pelvic adhesions
pelvic adhesive disease
pelvic aneurysm
pelvic aspiration biopsy
pelvic avulsion fracture
pelvic axis
pelvic block

pelvic bone
pelvic canal
pelvic cavity
pelvic clamp
pelvic colon
pelvic colon of Waldeyer
pelvic colonic surgery
pelvic deformities
pelvic diameter
pelvic diaphragm
pelvic direction
pelvic drainage
pelvic endometriosis
pelvic examination
pelvic exenteration
pelvic fixation
pelvic floor
pelvic floor dysfunction
pelvic fossa
pelvic fracture
pelvic ganglion
pelvic girdle
pelvic gutter
pelvic ileal reservoir
    construction
pelvic inflammation
pelvic inflammatory disease (PID)
pelvic inlet
pelvic irradiation
pelvic kidney
pelvic laparoscopy
pelvic laparotomy
pelvic lymph node dissection
    (PLND)
pelvic lymphadenectomy
pelvic lymphocelectomy
pelvic malignancy
pelvic mass
pelvic measurements
pelvic metastases
pelvic muscular support
pelvic musculature
pelvic node dissection
pelvic obliquity
pelvic organ exenteration
pelvic organs
pelvic osteotomy
pelvic outlet
pelvic peritoneal cavity
pelvic peritoneal graft
pelvic peritoneum
pelvic peritonitis

pelvic phased-array coil
pelvic plane
pelvic plexus
pelvic pouch procedure
pelvic presentation
pelvic reconstruction kit
pelvic reduction forceps
pelvic relaxation
pelvic ring fractures
pelvic scanography
pelvic sling
pelvic snare
pelvic splanchnic nerves
pelvic splint
pelvic stabilization orthosis
pelvic steal test
pelvic straddle fracture
pelvic strait
pelvic support
pelvic tilt
pelvic tissue forceps
pelvic traction
pelvic ultrasound
pelvic version
pelvic viscera
pelvic wall
pelvic washings
pelvic-femoral angle
pelvifemoral
pelvifixation
pelvilithotomy
pelvimeter
    Barbara pelvimeter
    Baudelocque pelvimeter
    Breisky pelvimeter
    Collin pelvimeter
    Collyer pelvimeter
    DeLee pelvimeter
    DeLee-Breisky pelvimeter
    Douglas measuring plate
        pelvimeter
    Douglas pelvimeter
    Hanely-McDermott pelvimeter
    Martin pelvimeter
    Pilling-Douglas pelvimeter
    Rica pelvimeter
    Schneider pelvimeter
    Thole pelvimeter
    Thomas pelvimeter
    Thoms pelvimeter
    Williams internal pelvimeter
    Williams pelvimeter

pelvimetry
  McDonald pelvimetry
  x-ray pelvimetry
pelvimetry study
pelvioileoneocystostomy
pelviolithotomy
pelvioneostomy
pelvioplasty
pelvioprostatic capsule
pelvioscopy
pelviostomy
pelviotomy
pelviradiography
pelvirectal anesthesia
pelvis (*pl.* pelves)
  android pelvis
  assimilation pelvis
  axis pelvis
  beaked pelvis
  bifid pelvis
  bifurcation of renal pelvis
  brim of pelvis
  contracted pelvis
  Deventer pelvis
  dolichopellic pelvis
  flat pelvis
  funnel-shaped pelvis
  greater pelvis
  gynecoid pelvis
  inadequate pelvis
  intrapelvic kidney pelvis
  kidney pelvis
  kyphotic pelvis
  linea terminalis pelvis
  Nagele pelvis
  obliquely contracted pelvis
  Otto pelvis
  rachitic pelvis
  redundant pelvis
  renal pelvis
  Robert pelvis
  rostrate pelvis
  rotation of pelvis
  small pelvis
  Techmedica total pelvis
  true pelvis
pelvisacral
pelviscope
pelviscopic clip ligation
    technique
pelviscopic intrafascial
    hysterectomy

pelvisection
pelviureteroplasty
pelvivertebral angle
pelvoscopy
Pemberton clamp
Pemberton forceps
Pemberton operation
Pemberton osteotomy
Pemberton retractor
Pemberton sigmoid anastomosis
Pemberton sigmoid clamp
Pemberton spur crusher
Pemberton spur-crushing clamp
Pemco cannula
Pemco prosthetic valve
Pemco pump
Pemco retractor
Pemco valve prosthesis
pemphigus vegetans
pen pump insulin infuser
Penberthy double-action
    aspirator
Pencan spinal needle
pencil
  Blaisdell skin pencil
  cataract pencil
  caustic pencil
  cautery pencil
  Cheshire electrosurgical
    pencil
  disposable electrosurgical
    pencil
  electrosurgical pencil
  glaucoma pencil
  hand-switching electrocautery
    pencil
  Handtrol electrosurgical
    pencil
  marking pencil
  MegaDyne electrocautery
    pencil
  retinal detachment pencil
  skin pencil
  straight bipolar pencil
  Valleylab pencil
  vitreous pencil
  Wallach cryosurgical pencil
  Wallach pencil
  Weck electrosurgery pencil
pencil cautery
pencil Doppler probe
pencil dosimeter

pencil drain
pencil-grip instrument
pencil-handled laryngoscope
pencil-in-cup deformity
pencil-probe Doppler
pencil-shaped stools
pencil-tip cautery
pencil-tip drill
pencil-tipped drill
pencil-tipped electrode
Pendoppler ultrasonic fetal
   heart detector
Pendula cast cutter
pendular movement
Penduloff incision
pendulous abdomen
pendulous breasts
pendulous palate
pendulous urethra
pendulous uvula
pendulum movement
pendulum rhythm
pendulum scalpel
penectomy
penetrating abdominal trauma
penetrating corneal graft
penetrating corneal transplant
penetrating drill
penetrating fracture
penetrating graft
penetrating keratoplasty
penetrating liver injury
penetrating rupture
penetrating thoracoabdominal
   injury
penetrating trauma
penetrating ulcer
penetrating wound
penetration fracture
penetrator
Penfield biopsy needle
Penfield clip
Penfield dissector
Penfield elevator
Penfield forceps
Penfield needle
Penfield neurodissector
Penfield retractor
Penfield silver clip
Penfield suture forceps
Penfield watchmaker suture
   forceps

penile agenesis
penile amputation
penile block
penile brachial pressure index
penile cancer
penile carcinoma
penile clamp
penile deformity
penile discharge
penile Doppler
penile epispadias
penile erection
penile flap
penile girth enhancement
penile hypospadias
penile implant
penile induration
penile injection therapy
penile injury
penile island flap
penile lengthening
penile lesion
penile plethysmography
penile pneumoplethysmography
penile pressure/brachial
   pressure index (PBI)
penile prosthesis
penile prosthesis cylinders
penile reconstruction
penile reflex
penile rupture
penile shaft
penile sheath
penile skin
penile skin inversion
penile skin inversion
   vaginoplasty
penile vein occlusion therapy
penile venous ligation surgery
penile wart
penile-scrotal incision
Peninject injector
penis
   artery of bulb of penis
   bulb of penis
   buried penis
   cavernous nerves of penis
   cavernous veins of penis
   clubbed penis
   corpora cavernosa penis
   corpus cavernosum penis
   corpus spongiosum penis

penis (*continued*)
  crus penis
  deep artery of penis
  deep veins of penis
  dorsal artery of penis
  dorsal nerve of penis
  dorsal veins of penis
  erectile elements of the penis
  frenulum of penis
  glans of penis
  glans penis
  helicine arteries of penis
  os penis
  prepuce of penis
penis clamp
penlight cautery
Penlon infant resuscitator
Penn finger drill
Penn pouch
Penn scissors
Penn State artificial heart
Penn State total artificial heart
Penn State ventricular assist
  device
Penn swivel hook
Penn trocar
Penn tuning fork
Penn umbilical scissors
Pennal classification
Penn-Anderson scleral fixation
  forceps
pennate muscle
pennate suction catheter
penniform muscle
Pennig dynamic wrist fixator
Pennig minifixator device
Pennine leg bag
Pennine Nelaton catheter
Pennine-O'Neil urinary catheter
  introducer
Pennington clamp
Pennington elevator
Pennington hemorrhoidal
  forceps
Pennington hemostatic forceps
Pennington rectal speculum
Pennington septal dissector
Pennington septal elevator
Pennington tissue forceps
Pennington tissue-grasping
  forceps
Pennybacker rongeur

penoplasty
penoscrotal edema
penoscrotal hypospadias
penoscrotal incision
Penrose drain
Penrose seton
Penrose sump drain
Penrose tourniquet
Penrose tube
PENSIL catheter (Penn State
  Intravascular Lung catheter)
PentaCath catheter
pentagon lobule graft
pentagonal block excision
pentalogy of Fallot
Pentalumen catheter
PentaPace QRS catheter
Pentax ultrasound
  gastrofiberscope
Pentax bronchoscope
Pentax choledochocystonephro-
  fiberscope
Pentax colonofiberscope
Pentax duodenoscope
Pentax video endoscope
Pentax EndoNet digital
  endoscope
Pentax ultrasound gastroscope
Pentax EUP-EC-series ultrasound
  gastroscope
Pentax colonoscope
Pentax duodenofiberscope
Pentax echoendoscope
Pentax linear scanning
  echoendoscope
Pentax ultrasound endoscope
Pentax fiberoptic sigmoidoscope
Pentax fiberscope
Pentax flexible endoscope
Pentax flexible sigmoidoscope
Pentax gastroscope
Pentax light source connector
Pentax lithotripter
Pentax lithotriptor
Pentax nasopharyngolaryngo-
  fiberscope
Pentax prototype needle
Pentax side-viewing endoscope
Pentax pediatric colonoscope
Penthrane anesthetic agent
pentobarbital anesthetic agent
pentose phosphate shunt

Pentothal anesthetic agent
Pneumotachometer
peptic gland
peptic stricture
peptic ulcer disease (PUD)
per contiguum
PER fracture (pronation, external rotation fracture)
perforating osteotome
per high power field
per mucosa
per os (p.o., PO, or po)
per primam healing
per primam intentionem
per rectum
per secundam healing
per secundam intentionem
per urethram
per vaginam
perambulating ulcer
Percaine anesthetic agent
Per-C-Cath catheter
Perception scanner
perceptual expansion
perceptual-motor match
Percival gastric balloon
Perclose closure device
Perclose PVS device
Perclose suture device
Perclose technique
Perclose vascular closure device
Perclose/Prostar device
percolator irrigator
Percoll filter
Percoll technique
Percor dilator
Percor dual-lumen intra-aortic balloon catheter
Percor intra-aortic balloon catheter
Percor-DL catheter (dual-lumen catheter)
Percor-Stat intra-aortic balloon
Percor-Stat-DL catheter (dual-lumen catheter)
perc-q-cath
PercuCut biopsy needle
PercuCut cut-biopsy needle
Percufix catheter cuff kit
Percuflex Amsterdam stent
Percuflex biliary stent
Percuflex endopyelotomy stent

Percuflex flexible biliary stent
Percuflex nephrostomy catheter
Percuflex Plus ureteral stent
PercuGuide needle
percussible
percussion
    auscultatory percussion
    bimanual percussion
    chest percussion
    clear to percussion
    dullness to percussion
    fist percussion
    hyperresonance to percussion
    Koranyi percussion
    Kronig percussion
    Murphy percussion
    palpatory percussion
    resonant on percussion
    resonant to percussion
    shifting dullness on percussion
    tenderness to percussion
percussion and auscultation (P&A)
percussion hammer
percussion note
percussion of bone
percussion sound
percussion therapy
percussion wave
percussive ventilation
Percu-Stay catheter fastener
PercuSurge recovery system device
percutaneous abscess and fluid drainage (PAFD)
percutaneous abscess drainage (PAD)
percutaneous access kit
percutaneous alcohol injection
percutaneous antegrade biliary drainage
percutaneous antegrade pyelography
percutaneous antegrade urography
percutaneous anterior gastropexy
percutaneous aortic valvuloplasty (PAV)
percutaneous appendectomy

percutaneous arterial
cannulation
percutaneous arteriogram
percutaneous arteriography
percutaneous aspiration
percutaneous atherectomy
device
percutaneous automated
diskectomy (PAD)
percutaneous balloon
angioplasty
percutaneous balloon aortic
valvuloplasty
percutaneous balloon aspiration
percutaneous balloon dilation
percutaneous balloon
valvuloplasty
percutaneous biopsy
percutaneous brachial sheath
percutaneous cardiopulmonary
bypass support
percutaneous carotid
arteriography (PCA)
percutaneous catheter
percutaneous catheter
cecostomy
percutaneous catheter
commissurotomy
percutaneous catheter drainage
percutaneous catheter insertion
percutaneous catheter
introducer kit
percutaneous catheterization
percutaneous central venous
catheter
percutaneous cholangiogram
percutaneous cholangiography
percutaneous cholangioscopic
lithotomy
percutaneous cholecystectomy
percutaneous
cholecystolithotomy
percutaneous cholecystostomy
percutaneous cordotomy
percutaneous coronary
rotational atherectomy
percutaneous CT-guided
aspiration
percutaneous cutting needle
percutaneous diskectomy
percutaneous dorsal column
stimulator implant

percutaneous drainage catheter
percutaneous embolization
therapy
percutaneous endoscope
percutaneous endoscopic
gastrojejunostomy
percutaneous endoscopic
gastrostomy (PEG)
percutaneous endoscopic
gastrostomy insertion
percutaneous endoscopic
removal
percutaneous endoscopy
percutaneous enterostomy
percutaneous epididymal sperm
aspiration
percutaneous epidural electrode
percutaneous epidural nerve
stimulator
percutaneous ethanol ablation
percutaneous ethanol injection
percutaneous ethanol injection
therapy
percutaneous excisional breast
biopsy (PEBB)
percutaneous exposure
percutaneous external drainage
(PED)
percutaneous femoral
arteriogram
percutaneous femoral-femoral
cardiopulmonary bypass
percutaneous fetal cystoscopy
percutaneous fine-needle
aspiration
percutaneous fine-needle
aspiration biopsy
percutaneous fine-needle
pancreatic biopsy
percutaneous fixation
percutaneous gastroenterostomy
percutaneous gastrostomy
percutaneous hepatobiliary
cholangiography
percutaneous injury (PI)
percutaneous insertion
technique
percutaneous interventional
technique
percutaneous intra-aortic
balloon counterpulsation
catheter (PIBC catheter)

percutaneous Judkins technique
percutaneous laser angioplasty
percutaneous lead introducer
percutaneous line
percutaneous liver biopsy
percutaneous localization
percutaneous low-stress
 angioplasty
percutaneous lumbar
 diskectomy
percutaneous microwave
 coagulation therapy
percutaneous mitral balloon
 commissurotomy
percutaneous mitral balloon
 valvotomy (PMV)
percutaneous mitral balloon
 valvuloplasty
percutaneous mitral valvotomy
percutaneous native renal
 biopsy
percutaneous needle
percutaneous needle liver
 biopsy
percutaneous nephroscope
percutaneous
 nephrostolithotomy (PCNL)
percutaneous nephrostomy
percutaneous nephrostomy
 Malecot catheter
percutaneous nephrostomy tube
percutaneous nephrostomy tube
 placement
percutaneous pancreas biopsy
percutaneous patent ductus
 arteriosus closure
percutaneous pencil Doppler
 probe
percutaneous pin
percutaneous pin insertion
percutaneous pinning
percutaneous plantar fasciotomy
percutaneous portocaval
 anastomosis
percutaneous puncture
percutaneous radical
 cryosurgical ablation
percutaneous radiofrequency
 catheter ablation
percutaneous reduction
percutaneous rotational
 thrombectomy catheter

percutaneous route
percutaneous splenoportal
 venography
percutaneous stent
percutaneous stone
 manipulation
percutaneous stone removal
percutaneous stricture dilatation
 (PSD)
percutaneous subclavian-
 subclavian bypass
percutaneous thecoperitoneal
 shunt
percutaneous transatrial mitral
 commissurotomy
percutaneous transcatheter
 therapy
percutaneous transfemoral
 arteriography
percutaneous transfemoral
 technique
percutaneous transhepatic
 approach
percutaneous transhepatic
 biliary drainage (PTBD)
percutaneous transhepatic
 biliary drainage catheter
percutaneous transhepatic
 biliary procedure
percutaneous transhepatic
 cardiac catheterization
percutaneous transhepatic
 cholangiogram
percutaneous transhepatic
 cholangiography (PTC)
percutaneous transhepatic
 cholangioscopic lithotomy
 (PTCSL)
percutaneous transhepatic
 cholangioscopy
percutaneous transhepatic
 cholecystoscopy
percutaneous transhepatic
 decompression (PTD)
percutaneous transhepatic
 drainage (PTD)
percutaneous transhepatic
 obliteration
percutaneous transhepatic
 pigtail catheter
percutaneous transhepatic
 portography

percutaneous transjugular approach
percutaneous translumbar aortography
percutaneous transluminal angioplasty (PTA, PTLA)
percutaneous transluminal angioscopy
percutaneous transluminal atherectomy
percutaneous transluminal balloon dilatation (PTBD)
percutaneous transluminal coronary angioplasty (PTCA)
percutaneous transluminal coronary angioplasty catheter
percutaneous transluminal renal angioplasty (PTRA)
percutaneous transtracheal bronchography
percutaneous transtracheal jet ventilation (PTV)
percutaneous transvenous mitral commissurotomy
percutaneous tumor ablation
percutaneous ultrasonic lithotripsy
percutaneous ultrasonic lithotriptor
percutaneous ureteral stent
percutaneous vasectomy
percutaneously
Percy amputating saw
Percy amputation retractor
Percy bone retractor
Percy cautery
Percy clamp
Percy hemostat
Percy intestinal forceps
Percy plate
Percy retractor
Percy tissue forceps
Percy-Wolfson gallbladder forceps
Percy-Wolfson gallbladder retractor
PerDUCER Pericardial access device
Perdue tonsillar hemostat

Perdue tonsillar hemostat forceps
Perell fetoscope
Pereyra bladder neck suspension
Pereyra bladder suspension
Pereyra ligature cannula
Pereyra needle
Pereyra needle driver
Pereyra needle suspension
Pereyra operation
Pereyra paraurethral suspension
Pereyra procedure
Pereyra vesicourethral suspension
Pereyra-Lebhertz modification of Frangenheim-Stoeckel procedure
Pereyra-Raz cystourethropexy
Perez-Castro forceps
Perfecta hip prosthesis
Per-fit percutaneous tracheostomy kit
PerFix hernia plug
PerFix Marlex mesh plug
PerFixation screw
Perflex stainless steel stent
Perflex stainless steel stent and delivery system biliary stent
perforated acid peptic ulcer
perforated appendix
perforated cancer
perforated diverticulum
perforated eardrum
perforated gallbladder
perforated space
perforated ulcer
perforated viscus
perforating abscess
perforating alveolar artery
perforating appendicitis
perforating arteries
perforating arteries of foot
perforating arteries of hand
perforating arteries of internal mammary
perforating branches
perforating bur
perforating drill
perforating forceps
perforating fracture
perforating keratoplasty

perforating osteotome
perforating twist drill
perforating ulcer
perforating ulcer of foot
perforating vein
perforating wound
perforation
  advanced tumor perforation
  amebic perforation
  appendiceal perforation
  Bezold perforation
  bladder perforation
  bowel perforation
  cardiac perforation
  colon perforation
  colonic perforation
  corneal perforation
  cortical perforation
  diaphragm perforation
  ductal system perforation
  duodenal system perforation
  esophageal perforation
  frank perforation
  gallbladder perforation
  gastric perforation
  gastrointestinal perforation
  guidewire perforation
  iatrogenic perforation
  ileal perforation
  inflammatory perforation
  instrumental perforation
  intestinal perforation
  intraperitoneal perforation
  lateral perforation
  mechanical perforation
  myocardial perforation
  nasal septal perforation
  Niemeier gallbladder
    perforation
  operative perforation
  pathologic perforation
  peritoneal perforation
  prepyloric perforation
  pyloroduodenal perforation
  retroduodenal perforation
  retroperitoneal perforation
  root perforation
  sealing perforation
  septal perforation
  strip perforation
  sublabial perforation
  tooth perforation

perforation (*continued*)
  traumatic perforation
  ureteral perforation
  uterine perforation
  vascular perforation
  ventricular perforation
  viscus perforation
perforation osteotomy
perforation peritonitis
perforation rasp
perforation risk
perforative appendicitis
perforative lesion
perforator
  Acra-Cut cranial perforator
  Aesculap skull perforator
  Amnihook amniotic
    membrane perforator
  amniotic membrane
    perforator
  Anspach cranial perforator
  antral perforator
  Baylor amniotic perforator
  Bishop antral perforator
  Bishop antrum perforator
  Blot perforator
  Boyd perforator
  Chapman-Dintenfass
    perforator
  Codman disposable perforator
  cranial perforator
  cranial twist drill perforator
  Cushing cranial perforator
  DeLee-Pierce membrane
    perforator
  D'Errico perforator
  Dodd perforator
  fascial perforator
  fasciocutaneous perforator
  Friesner ear perforator
  hand ear perforator
  hand perforator
  Heifitz skull perforator
  Hillis perforator
  hunterian perforator
  incompetent perforator
  Joseph antral perforator
  Kalinowski perforator
  Lasette laser finger perforator
  Lempert perforator
  McKenzie perforator
  membrane perforator

perforator (*continued*)
  midtibial perforator
  musculocutaneous perforator
  periumbilical perforator
  Politzer ear perforator
  powered automatic skull
    perforator
  Royce tympanum perforator
  segmental perforators
  septocutaneous perforator
  septomuscular perforator
  Smellie obstetrical perforator
  Smith perforator
  spondylophyte annular
    dissector perforator
  Stein membrane perforator
  Stryker perforator
  Thornwald antral perforator
  tibial perforator
  tributaries and perforators
  tympanum perforator
  Wellaminski antral perforator
  Williams ear perforator
  Wilson amniotic perforator
perforator and tributaries
perforator drill
perforator vessel
perforator-based flap
perforators tied
Performa ultrasound
performance
Performance knee prosthesis
performance status
Performance surgical
  instruments
performed in routine fashion
performer ultralight knee brace
Perf-Plate cranial plate
perfusate
perfusion
  aortic perfusion
  blood perfusion
  cardiac perfusion
  cerebral perfusion
  continuous hyperthermic
    peritoneal perfusion
  continuous sanguineous
    perfusion
  coronary artery perfusion
  coronary perfusion
  distal aortic perfusion
  distal visceral perfusion

perfusion (*continued*)
  ex vivo perfusion
  extracorporeal liver perfusion
  extracorporeal perfusion
  extremity perfusion
  Hancock coronary perfusion
  hepatic perfusion
  hyperthermic isolated limb
    perfusion (HILP)
  hypothermic hepatic
    perfusion
  in situ hypothermic perfusion
  in-line perfusion
  intramural blood perfusion
  intraperitoneal hyperthermic
    perfusion
  isolated heat perfusion
  isolated hepatic perfusion
  isolated limb perfusion (ILP)
  isolated perfusion
  Langendorff perfusion
  myocardial perfusion
  organ perfusion
  peripheral perfusion
  Pulmopak pump for arterial
    perfusion
  pulsatile perfusion
  regional perfusion
  retrograde cardiac perfusion
  sanguineous perfusion
  splanchnic perfusion
  superficial renal cortical
    perfusion (SRCP)
  systemic perfusion
  tissue perfusion
  visceral perfusion
perfusion cannula
perfusion catheter
perfusion defect
perfusion flow rate
perfusion hypothermia
  technique
perfusion lung scan
perfusion measurement
  technique
perfusion monitor
perfusion of coronary artery
perfusion pressure
perfusion rate
perfusion scan
perfusion study
perfusion technique

perfusion therapy
perfusor
 Belsey perfusor
perialveolar wiring
periampullary cancer
periampullary carcinoma
periampullary diverticulum
periampullary tumor
perianal abscess
perianal anorectal space
perianal fistula abscess
perianal hematoma
perianal incision
perianal maceration
perianal reflex
perianal skin
perianal skin tag
perianal wart
perianeurysmal hemorrhage
periaortic chain
periaortic irradiation
periaortic lymph node
periaortic mediastinal
 hematoma
periaortic nodes
periapical abscess
periapical curet
periapical curettage
periapical lesion
periapical osteofibrosis
periapical surgery
periapical tooth repair
periappendiceal abscess
periaqueductal gray electrode
periareolar area
periareolar de-epithelialization
periareolar incision
periareolar mammaplasty
periareolar mastopexy
periareolar retractor
periareolar scar
periareolar technique
periarterial pad
periarterial sympathectomy
periarticular calcification
periarticular fluid collection
periarticular fracture
periarticular osteoporosis
periarticular soft tissue swelling
periarticular soft tissues
periauricular
peribronchial cuffing

peribronchial markings
peribronchiolar lymphocyte
 infiltration
peribulbar anesthesia
peribulbar anesthetic technique
peribulbar injection
peribulbar needle
pericallosal artery
pericallosal veins
pericanalicular fibroadenoma
pericapillary cells
pericapsular fat infiltration
pericardectomy
pericardiac veins
pericardiacophrenic artery
pericardiacophrenic veins
pericardial baffle
pericardial biopsy
pericardial cavity
pericardial decompression
pericardial effusion
pericardial fat pad
pericardial flap
pericardial fluid
pericardial fluid examination
pericardial fusion
pericardial hematoma
pericardial murmur
pericardial patch
pericardial peel
pericardial pleura
pericardial puncture
pericardial raspatory
pericardial recess
pericardial reflex
pericardial rub
pericardial rupture
pericardial sac
pericardial sling
pericardial snare
pericardial space
pericardial tumor
pericardial xenograft
pericardicentesis
pericardiectomy
pericardiocentesis needle
pericardiolysis
pericardiomediastinitis
pericardioplasty in pectus
 excavatum repair
pericardiorrhaphy
pericardiostomy

pericardiotomy scissors
pericardiotomy syndrome
pericarditis
pericardium
pericardotomy
pericaval
pericecal abscess
pericholecystic abscess
pericholecystic adhesions
pericholecystic edema
pericholecystic fluid collection
Pericranial
perichondral arthroplasty
perichondral circulation
perichondrial elevator
perichondrial flap
perichondrial graft
perichondrial-periosteal tissue
perichondritis
    arytenoid perichondritis
    laryngeal perichondritis
perichondrium on the cranial
    aspect
perichondrocutaneous graft
perichoroidal space
pericolic abscess
pericolic membrane syndrome
pericolonic abscess
pericolonic penetration
pericolostomy hernia
Peri-Comfort seating cushion
periconchal sulcus
pericoronal abscess
pericoronal flap
pericortical clamp
pericostal suture
pericostal suture technique
pericranial temporalis flap
pericyte
pericytic venules
peridectomy
peridental ligament
peridental membrane
peridental space
peridentinoblastic space
peridiaphragmatic hematoma
peridural anesthesia
Peries medicated hygienic wire
    dressing
periesophageal abscess
periesophageal lymph node
    dissection

periesophagogastric lymph
    node metastasis
Periflow peripheral balloon
    angioplasty-infusion
    catheter
Periflow peripheral balloon
    catheter
perifollicular mesenchyme
perigastric adhesions
perigastric lymph nodes
Peri-Gel pack
perigenicular vascular injury
perigingival implant
perigraft hematoma
Peri-Guard vascular graft guard
perihepatic abscess
perihepatic space
perihernial
perihilar area
perihilar mass
perihilar scarring
peri-implant ligament
peri-implant space
peri-infarction block
peri-infarction conduction
    defect
perilacunar mineral matrix
    (PMM)
perilenticular space
perilimbal incision
perilimbal suction
perilobar pancreatitis
perilobular duct
perilunar instability (PLI)
perilunar transscaphoid
    dislocation
perilunate carpal dislocation
perilunate dislocation
perilunate fracture
perilunate fracture-dislocation
perilymph fistula
perilymph fluid
perilymphatic cavity
perilymphatic duct
perilymphatic fistula (PLF)
perilymphatic space
perimeter earmold
perimetry
perinatal injury
perinatal morbidity
perinatal mortality
perinatal support sutures

perineal abscess
perineal analgesia
perineal anesthesia
perineal area
perineal artery
perineal artery axial flap
perineal bandage
perineal biopsy
perineal body
perineal defect
perineal dissection
perineal fascia
perineal flap
perineal hernia
perineal hypospadias
perineal incision
perineal laceration
perineal lithotomy
perineal mass
perineal membrane
perineal needle biopsy
perineal nerve
perineal pad
perineal prostatectomy
perineal prostatectomy retractor
perineal reconstruction
perineal reflection
perineal region
perineal repair
perineal retractor
perineal section
perineal self-retaining
    retractor
perineal sheet
perineal sinus
perineal skin tag
perineal space
perineal support
perineal support sutures
perineal tear
perineal tissue
perineal urinary fistula
perineocele
perineometer
  Gynos perineometer
  Kegel perineometer
  Peritron perineometer
perineoplasty
  Hierst perineoplasty
  single-stage castration, vaginal
    construction perineoplasty
  Tait perineoplasty

perineorrhaphy
  Clark perineorrhaphy
  Simon perineorrhaphy
perineotomy
perineovaginal fistula
perinephric abscess
perinephric air injection
perinephric capsule
perinephric fascia
perinephric fat
perinephric fluid collection
perinephric hematoma
perinephric space hemorrhage
perineum
perineural anesthesia
perineural block
perineural channels
perineural fibroblastoma
perineural infiltration
perineural invasion
perineurial suture
perineurium
perinuclear contact
perinuclear space
Perio Pik irrigator
Perio Temp dental probe
periocular bulge
periocular festooning
periocular injection
periocular pigmentation
periocular rhytids
periodic dilatation
periodic slowing
periodic transitory
    menogingivitis
periodontal anesthesia
periodontal bony defect
periodontal defect
periodontal disease
periodontal flap
periodontal inflammation
periodontal intrabony defect
periodontal knife
periodontal lesion
periodontal ligament (PDL)
periodontal ligament anesthesia
periodontal membrane (PM)
periodontal osteotomy
periodontal pocket marker
periodontal probe
periodontal prosthesis
periodontal therapy

periodontitis
PerioGlas material
PerioGlas synthetic bone graft
perioneorrhaphy
    Emmet-Studdiford
        perioneorrhaphy
perioperative analgesia
perioperative antibiotic therapy
perioperative complication
perioperative death
perioperative reduction
perioportal cirrhosis
perioptic subarachnoid space
perioral dermatitis
perioral flaw
perioral muscle
periorbital cellulitis
periorbital ecchymosis
periorbital edema
periorbital fat
periorbital hematoma
periorbital infection
periorbital lipoinfiltration
periorbital membrane
periorbital orbicularis oculi
        muscle
periorbital soft tissue
periorbital swelling
periorbital wrinkle
periosteal adherence to the
        calvarium
periosteal band
periosteal bone
periosteal cyst
periosteal elevation
periosteal elevator (see elevator)
periosteal fibroma
periosteal flap
periosteal flaps raised
periosteal ganglion
periosteal graft
periosteal implantation
periosteal level
periosteal membranous lining
periosteal new bone formation
periosteal raspatory
periosteal release
periosteal stripping
periosteal thickening
periosteal vessel
periosteoplastic amputation
periosteorrhaphy

periosteotome
    Alexander costal
        periosteotome
    Alexander-Farabeuf costal
        periosteotome
    baby costal periosteotome
    Ballenger periosteotome
    Brophy periosteotome
    Brown periosteotome
    costal periosteotome
    Dean periosteotome
    Ferris Smith-Lyman
        periosteotome
    Fomon periosteotome
    Freer periosteotome
    Jansen periosteotome
    Joseph periosteotome
    Moorehead periosteotome
    Potts periosteotome
    Speer periosteotome
    Vaughan periosteotome
    West-Beck periosteotome
periosteotomy
periosteum (pl. periostea)
periosteum elevator
periosteum sheath
periosteum stripper
periostitis
Periotest implant
Periotest gold screw
periotic duct
periotic space
PerioWise probe
peripad
peripalpebral
peripancreatic abdominal
        drainage
peripancreatic fat plane
peripapillary retinal edema
peripapillary scotoma
peripartum endoscopy
Peri-Patch peritoneal catheter
        extension set
peripatellar incision
peripatellar pain
peripelvic cyst
peripharyngeal space
peripheral ameloblastoma
peripheral aneurysm
peripheral apnea
peripheral arterial aneurysmal
        disease

peripheral arterial line
peripheral artery bypass
peripheral atherectomy
    catheter
peripheral balloon angioplasty
peripheral blood
peripheral blood vessel forceps
peripheral blood vessels
peripheral cataract
peripheral chemoreflex loop
peripheral circulation
peripheral extremity edema
peripheral fields
peripheral fusion
peripheral glioma
peripheral hepatojejunostomy
peripheral indwelling
    intermediate infusion
    device
peripheral interface adapter
peripheral iridectomy
peripheral iridectomy forceps
peripheral iridotomy
peripheral laceration
peripheral laser angioplasty
    (PLA)
peripheral long-line catheter
peripheral masking
peripheral mass
peripheral mesh dissection
peripheral microcirculation
peripheral nerve block
peripheral nerve block
    anesthesia
peripheral nerve block
    anesthetic technique
peripheral nerve glove
peripheral nerve injury
peripheral nerve lesion
peripheral nerve repair
peripheral nerve stimulation
peripheral nerves
peripheral neuropathy
peripheral ossifying fibroma
peripheral osteoma of mandible
    (POM)
peripheral panretinal ablation
peripheral perfusion
peripheral pulses
peripheral reflex
peripheral temporomandibular
    joint remodeling

peripheral triangular
    fibrocartilage complex
peripheral vascular clamp
peripheral vascular disease
peripheral vascular forceps
peripheral vascular retractor
peripheral vascular surgery
peripheral venous cannulation
peripheral vessel
peripheral vision
peripherally inserted central
    catheter (PICC)
peripherally inserted central
    venous catheter (PICVC)
periportal carcinoma
periportal cirrhosis
periportal sinusoidal dilatation
periportal sinusoidal dilation
periprosthetic breast abscess
periprosthetic fibrous capsule
periprosthetic fracture
periprosthetic leak
periprosthetic space infection
perirectal abscess
perirectal incision
perirectal incision and drainage
perirectal inflammation
perirectal pelvic dissection
perirenal fascia
perirenal fat
perirenal hematoma
perirenal insufflation
perirenal space
perirenal tissues
periscapular incision
periscapularly
periscleral space
periscopic lens
perisellar vascular lesion
perisinusoidal space
perispinal area
perispondylitis
    Gibney perispondylitis
peristalsis
    absent peristalsis
    decreased peristalsis
    retrograde peristalsis
    reversed peristalsis
peristaltic activity
peristaltic anastomosis
peristaltic motion
peristaltic movement

peristaltic rushes
peristaltic sounds
peristaltic unrest
peristaltic valve
peristaltic wave
perisylvian
peritectomy
Peritest perimeter
perithelium
peritomist
peritomy
peritoneal abscess
peritoneal adenocarcinoma
peritoneal adhesion
peritoneal anatomy
peritoneal aspiration
peritoneal attachments
peritoneal autoplasty
peritoneal band
peritoneal biopsy
peritoneal button
peritoneal cancer
peritoneal catheter
peritoneal cavity
peritoneal cavity abscess
peritoneal clamp
peritoneal closure
peritoneal cytological
    assessment
peritoneal defect
peritoneal dialysis
peritoneal dialysis catheter
peritoneal disease
peritoneal drainage
peritoneal encapsulation
peritoneal floor
peritoneal fluid
peritoneal fluid examination
peritoneal forceps
peritoneal hernia
peritoneal incision
peritoneal insertion of shunt
peritoneal insufflation
peritoneal lavage
peritoneal membrane
peritoneal metastasis
peritoneal mouse
peritoneal patch
peritoneal perforation
peritoneal puncture
peritoneal reconstruction
peritoneal reflection

peritoneal reflux control
    catheter
peritoneal sac
peritoneal shunt
peritoneal sign
peritoneal space
peritoneal studding
peritoneal surface
peritoneal tap
peritoneal-atrial shunt
peritonealization
peritonealize
peritoneal-venous shunt
peritoneocaval shunt
peritoneocentesis
peritoneoclysis
peritoneocutaneous reflex
peritoneography
peritoneointestinal reflex
peritoneojugular shunt
peritoneopericardial
    diaphragmatic hernia
peritoneopericardial hernia
peritoneoplasty
peritoneoscope
    Photo-Flash peritoneoscope
    Storz peritoneoscope
peritoneoscopy
peritoneotomy
peritoneovenous shunt
peritoneum
    abdominal peritoneum
    exposing peritoneum
    fold of peritoneum
    intestinal peritoneum
    parietal peritoneum
    pelvic peritoneum
    vesicouterine peritoneum
    visceral peritoneum
peritonitis
    pelvic peritonitis
    perforation peritonitis
peritonization
peritonize
peritonsillar abscess
peritonsillar cellulitis
peritonsillar space
peritonsillar tags
peritrochanteric fracture
Peritron perineometer
peritubal syndrome
periumbilical abscess

periumbilical incision
periumbilical perforator
periumbilical port
periungual desquamation
periungual telangiectasia
periungual wart
periureteral abscess
periurethral abscess
periurethral duct carcinoma
periurethral tissues
perivascular cells
perivascular lymph spaces
perivascular space
peri-Vaterian duodenum
peri-Vaterian therapeutic
    endoscopic procedure
periventricular hyperintense
    lesion
periventricular white matter
    lesion
periventricular-intraventricular
    hemorrhage
perivesical abscess
perivesical fascia
perivesical hernia
Peri-Warm pack
PERK protocol (prospective
    evaluation of radial
    keratotomy protocol)
Perkins applanation tonometer
Perkins elevator
Perkins otologic retractor
Perkins split-weight tractor
Perkins tonometer
Perkins traction
Perkins vertical line
Per-Lee equalizing tube
Per-Lee middle ear tubes
Per-Lee myringotomy tube
Per-Lee ventilation tube
Perlmann tumor of kidney
Perlon sutures
Perlstein brace
Perlstein orthosis
Perma-Cath catheter
Perma-Cath drain
Permacol mesh
Permacol patch
Perma-Cryl denture base
    material
Perma-Flow coronary bypass
    graft

Perma-Hand braided silk sutures
Perma-Hand silk sutures
Permalens lens
PermaMesh hydroxyapatite
    woven sheet matrix
PermaMesh material
Perman cartilage forceps
permanent anticoagulant
    therapy
permanent bipolar magnet
    placement
permanent callus
permanent cardiac pacing
    lead
permanent cartilage
permanent colostomy
permanent damage
permanent deformation
permanent end colostomy
permanent ileostomy
permanent implant
permanent lead introducer
permanent lip augmentation
permanent loop ileostomy
permanent magnet
permanent myocardial
    pacemaker
permanent needle
permanent pacemaker
permanent paralysis
permanent pedicle flap
permanent rate-responsive
    pacemaker
permanent remission
permanent silicone catheter
permanent stoma
permanent stricture
permanent transvenous demand
    pacemaker (PTDP)
permanent transvenous
    pacemaker
permanent ventricular
    pacemaker
Perman-Stille abdominal
    retractor
PermaRidge alveolar ridge
    augmentation
PermaRidge delivery syringe
Permark Enhancer III
    pigmenting unit
Permark micropigmentation
    mark

Permark micropigmentation needle
PermaSeal dialysis access graft
PermaSharp suture and needle
PermaSharp PGA sutures
PermaSoft reline material
Permathane lead
Permathane Pacesetter lead pacemaker
Permatone denture material
PermCath dual-lumen catheter
permeability
permeation analgesia
permeation anesthesia
permucosal endosteal implant
permucosal needle aspiration
Perneczky aneurysm clip
peromelia
Perone laser-assisted intrastromal keratomileusis (LASIK) marker
Perone LASIK flap forceps
peroneal artery
peroneal compartment syndrome
peroneal dislocation
peroneal groove
peroneal injury
Peroneal island flap
peroneal muscle
peroneal nerve
peroneal nerve entrapment
peroneal retinaculum
peroneal sheath
peroneal sign
peroneal sulcus
peroneal tendon
peroneal tendon sheath
peroneal tubercle
peroneal veins
peroneal vessels
peroneus brevis flap
peroneus longus flap
peroneus tertius muscle
peroral approach
peroral cholangiopancreatoscopy
peroral cholangioscopy
peroral endoscopy
peroral esophageal dilation
peroral esophageal prosthesis
peroral gastroscope

peroral intestinal biopsy
peroral maneuver
peroral pneumocolon double-contrast follow-through
peroral retrograde pancreaticobiliary ductography
perpendicular
nasion perpendicular
perpendicular plane
perpendicular plate of ethmoid
perpendicular squama
perpetual arrhythmia
Per-Q-Cath CVP catheter
Perras mammary prosthesis
Perras-Papillon breast prosthesis
Perritt fixation forceps
Perritt lens forceps
PERRLA (pupils equal, round, react to light and accommodation)
Perry extensile anterior approach
Perry forceps
Perry ileostomy bag
Perry Noz-Stop kit
Perry ostomy irrigator
Perry pediatric Foley latex catheter
Perry procedure for genu recurvatum
Perry technique
Perry-Foley catheter
Perry-Nickel technique
Perry-O'Brien-Hodgson technique
Perry-Robinson cervical technique
persistent breast abnormality
persistent fetal circulation
persistent generalized lymphadenopathy
persistent lop ear
persistent muellerian duct syndrome
persistent occiput posterior position
Persona monitoring kit
Personal Best peak flowmeter
Personal Catheter 100% silicone intermittent catheter

Personna Plus disposable Teflon scalpel
Personna Plus MicroCoat surgeon's blade
Personna prep blades
Personna surgical blade
Perspex button
Perspex CQ intraocular lens
Perspex CQ-Shearing-Simcoe-Sinskey lens
Perspex rod
Perspex tube
perspiratory gland
Per-Stat-DL catheter
Perstein joint
Perthes incision
Perthes lesion
Perthes procedure
Perthes reamer
pertinent findings
Pertrach percutaneous tracheostomy tube
pertrochanteric fracture
pertubation
pervasive
pervenous catheter
pes abductus
pes anserinus
pes cavus
pes equinus
pes planus
pes valgus
pes varus
PE-series implantable pronged unipolar electrode
Pess lid everter
pessary
    Albert-Smith pessary
    Biswas Silastic vaginal pessary
    bladder neck support pessary
    Blair modification of Gellhorn pessary
    blue ring pessary
    Chambers doughnut pessary
    Chambers intrauterine pessary
    cube pessary
    cup pessary
    diaphragm pessary
    doughnut pessary
    Dumas pessary
    Dumontpallier pessary

pessary (*continued*)
    Dutch pessary
    Emmet-Gellhorn pessary
    Findley folding pessary
    Gariel pessary
    Gehrung pessary
    Gellhorn pessary
    globe prolapsus pessary
    Gold pessary
    Gynefold prolapse pessary
    Gynefold retrodisplacement pessary
    Hodge pessary
    hollow Lucite pessary
    intrauterine pessary
    lever pessary
    Lucite pessary
    Maydl pessary
    Mayer pessary
    Menge pessary
    Menge stem pessary
    Milex pessary
    Plexiglas Gellhorn pessary
    Plexiglas pessary
    Prentif pessary
    Prochownik pessary
    prolapse ring pessary
    prolapsus pessary
    red pessary
    retrodisplaced pessary
    retroversion pessary
    ring pessary
    safety pessary
    Smith retroversion pessary
    Smith-Hodge pessary
    stem pessary
    Thomas pessary
    Vimule pessary
    White foam pessary
    Wylie stem pessary
    Zwanck radium pessary
pessary doughnut
Pesso reamer
PET (positron emission tomography)
PET balloon
PET balloon Simpson atherectomy device
PET scanning
petaling the cast
petechia (*pl.* petechiae)
petechial hemorrhage

Peter operation
Peter-Bishop forceps
Peters anomaly
Peters tissue forceps
Petersen bag
Petersen lithotomy
Petersen operation (GI)
Petersen rectal bag
Peterson cervical collar
Peterson nail
Peterson operation (gyn)
PET-guided biopsy
Petit aponeurosis
Petit canal
Petit facial mask
Petit hernia
Petit herniotomy
Petit ligament
petit mal
Petit suture technique
Petit sutures
Petit tourniquet
PETite scanner
Petralit dental cement
Petrie spica cast
petrobasilar suture
petroclinoid ligament
petroclival suture
petrolatum dressing
petrolatum gauze
petrolatum gauze dressing
petrolatum-impregnated gauze
petro-occipital fissure
petro-occipital joint
petro-occipital synchondrosis
petrosal approach
petrosal artery
petrosal foramen
petrosal fossa
petrosal ganglion
petrosal nerve
petrosal ridge
petrosal sinuses
petrosal sulcus
petrosphenobasilar suture
petrosphenoid
petrosphenoidal syndrome
petrospheno-occipital suture of
    Gruber
petrosquamosal
petrosquamous fissure
petrosquamous sutures

petrotympanic fissure
petrotympanic suture
petrous apices
petrous bone
petrous pyramid
petrous pyramid air cell
    exploration
petrous pyramid air cells
petrous pyramid exenteration
petrous pyramid fracture
petrous ridge
petrous tips
petrous-to-supraclinoid bypass
PETT (positron emission
    transaxial/transverse
    tomography)
Pettigrove laser-assisted
    intrastromal keratomileusis
    set
Pettigrove LASIK set
Petz clamp
Petz clip
Peutz-Jeghers syndrome
Peyer glands
Peyer patch
Peyer plaque
    Peyman wide-field lens
Peyman full-thickness eyewall
    resection
Peyman intraocular forceps
Peyman special optics for low
    vision lens
Peyman vitrectomy unit
Peyman vitrector
Peyman vitreophage unit
Peyman vitreous scissors
Peyman vitreous-grasping
    forceps
Peyman wide-field lens
Peyman-Green vitrectomy lens
Peyman-Green vitreous forceps
Peyman-Tennant-Green lens
Peyronie disease
Peyronie-like plaque
Peyrot thorax
Peyton brain spatula
Pezzer (see de Pezzer)
PF Lee pediatric goniolens
PF night splint
Pfannenstiel incision
Pfannenstiel transverse
    approach

Pfau atticus punch
Pfau atticus sphenoidal punch
Pfau polyp forceps
PFC component (Press-Fit
    condylar component)
Pfeiffer mechanical dosing pump
Pfeiffer procedure
Pfeiffer syndrome
Pfeiffer-Grobety activator
PFFD (proximal focal femoral
    deficiency)
Pfister stone basket
Pfister-Schwartz basket forceps
Pfister-Schwartz sheath
Pfister-Schwartz stone basket
Pfister-Schwartz stone dislodger
Pfister-Schwartz stone retriever
Pfizer scan
Pfluger tube
PFO-Star occluder
PFT (parafascicular thalamotomy)
PFTE shunt
    (polyfluorotetraethylene
    shunt)
PGIA instrument
PGK (Panos G. Koutrouvelis,
    M.D. stereotactic device
PGK (Panos G. Koutrouvelis, M.D.)
pH electrode placement
pH probe
Phaco Emulsifier Cavitron unit
Phaco-4 diamond step knife
phacocystectomy
phacoemulsification
    Cavitron-Kelman
        phacoemulsification
    Kelman phacoemulsification
        (KPE)
phacoemulsification cautery
phacoemulsifier
    Cavitron Phacoemulsifier
    KCP phacoemulsifier
    Kelman Phacoemulsifier
    MVS Phacoemulsifier
phacoemulsifier-aspirator
phacoemulsifier-extractor
phacoerysis
PhacoFlex foldable intraocular
    lens implant
PhacoFlex intraocular lens
PhacoFlex lens
phacolysis

phagedenic ulcer
Phakic lens
phakodialysis spatula
phakofragmatome
    Girard phakofragmatome
phalangeal articulation
phalangeal bone
phalangeal broach
phalangeal clamp
phalangeal diaphysial fracture
phalangeal dislocation
phalangeal forceps
phalangeal fracture
phalangeal fracture fixation
phalangeal knife
phalangeal malunion correction
phalangeal set
phalangeal tuft
phalangectomy
phalanges (*sing.* phalanx)
phalangization
phalangophalangeal amputation
phalanx (*pl.* phalanges)
    BIOPRO implant for the
        proximal phalanx
    buckle fracture of phalanx
    buckling fracture of the phalanx
    clubbing of distal phalanges
    cutaneous ligaments of
        phalanges
    delta phalanx
    distal phalanx
    floating distal phalanx
    shaft of phalanx
    terminal phalanx
phalanx distalis
phalanx media
phalanx proximalis
Phalen maneuver
Phalen position
Phalen sign for carpal tunnel
Phalen test
phallectomy
phallic reconstruction
phalloplasty
phallotomy
phallourethroplasty
phallus
Phaneuf arterial forceps
Phaneuf artery forceps
Phaneuf clamp
Phaneuf hysterectomy forceps

Phaneuf maneuver
Phaneuf peritoneal forceps
Phaneuf uterine artery forceps
Phaneuf uterine artery scissors
Phaneuf vaginal forceps
Phaneuf-Graves operation
Phaneuf-Graves repair
phantom aneurysm
Phantom cardiac guidewire
phantom clamp
phantom frame
phantom hand
Phantom interference screw
phantom limb pain
Phantom nasal mask
phantom pain
phantom pregnancy
Phantom V Plus balloon
  dilatation catheter
Pharmacia corneal trephine
Pharmacia Intermedics
  ophthalmic intraocular lens
Pharmacia intraocular lens
Pharmacia lancet
Pharmacia Visco J-loop lens
pharmacologic manipulation
Pharmaseal catheter
Pharmaseal closed drain
Pharmaseal disposable cervical
  dilator
Pharmaseal disposable uterine
  sound
Pharmaseal drain
Pharmaseal needle
Pharmex disposable catheter
pharmacologically induced
  erection
pharyngeal airway
pharyngeal anesthesia
pharyngeal aperture
pharyngeal arches
pharyngeal artery
pharyngeal branch of internal
  maxillary artery
pharyngeal branch of
  pterygopalatine ganglion
pharyngeal bursa
pharyngeal calculus
pharyngeal canal
pharyngeal cavity
pharyngeal cleft
pharyngeal constrictor muscle

pharyngeal exudate
pharyngeal fascia
pharyngeal fistula
pharyngeal flap operation
pharyngeal flap palatoplasty
pharyngeal glands
pharyngeal grooves
pharyngeal hemisphincter
pharyngeal hypophysis
pharyngeal insufflation anesthesia
pharyngeal lymph node
pharyngeal mirror
pharyngeal orifice
pharyngeal ostium
pharyngeal pack
pharyngeal plexus
pharyngeal pouch syndrome
pharyngeal raphe
pharyngeal recess
pharyngeal reflex
pharyngeal retractor
pharyngeal septum
pharyngeal space
pharyngeal speculum
pharyngeal spine
pharyngeal tonsil
pharyngeal tube
pharyngeal tubercle
pharyngeal veins
pharyngeal wall
pharyngeal wall augmentation
pharyngeal wall carcinoma
pharyngectomy
pharyngitis
  atrophic pharyngitis
  lymphonodular pharyngitis
  membranous pharyngitis
  pustular pharyngitis
pharyngitis sicca
pharyngobasilar fascia
pharyngocutaneous fistula
pharyngoepiglottic fold
pharyngoesophageal (PE)
pharyngoesophageal defect
pharyngoesophageal
  diverticulectomy
pharyngoesophageal
  diverticulum
pharyngoesophageal pads
pharyngoesophageal
  reconstruction
pharyngoesophageal sphincter

pharyngoesophagoplasty
pharyngogram
pharyngoinfraglottic duct
pharyngolaryngectomy
pharyngomaxillary fissure
pharyngomaxillary space
pharyngonasal cavity
pharyngopalatine arch
pharyngopalatine muscle
pharyngopalatinus muscle
pharyngoplasty
  Barsky pharyngoplasty
  Hynes pharyngoplasty
  Orticochea pharyngoplasty
  sphincter pharyngoplasty
  Wardill pharyngoplasty
pharyngorrhaphy
pharyngoscope
pharyngoscopy
pharyngotomy
  lateral pharyngotomy
  modified lateral pharyngotomy
pharyngotympanic cephalalgia
pharyngotympanic groove
pharyngotympanic tube
pharynx
  constrictor muscle of pharynx
  vault of pharynx
  vestibule of pharynx
phase I block
phase II block
phase microscope
phase-contrast microscope
phased array sector transducer
phased array ultrasonographic
  device
phased-array body-coil MR
  imaging
phase-encoding direction
phase-sensitive detector
phase-sensitive gradient-echo
  MR imaging
phasic activity
Phazet lancet
Pheasant elbow dislocation
  operation
Pheasant elbow technique
Pheasant technique
Pheifer-Young retractor
Phelan vein stripper
Phelps brace
Phelps gracilis test

Phelps operation for talipes
  equinovarus
Phelps orthosis
Phelps partial resection
Phelps splint
Phelps-Baker gracilis test
Phelps-Gocht osteoclast
Phemister acromioclavicular pin
  fixation
Phemister approach
Phemister biopsy trephine
Phemister brace
Phemister elevator
Phemister graft
Phemister incision
Phemister medial approach
Phemister onlay bone graft
Phemister operation
Phemister punch
Phemister rasp
Phemister raspatory
Phemister raspatory elevator
Phemister reamer
Phemister splint
Phemister-Bonfiglio technique
phenol neurolysis
phenol peeling
phenolized gelatin compound
phenol-preserved extract
phenomenon
  Ashman phenomenon
  Austin Flint phenomenon
  autoimmune phenomenon
  Beevor phenomenon
  Bell phenomenon
  cavitation phenomenon
  cellulite phenomenon
  coronary steal phenomenon
  declamping phenomenon
  extravasation phenomenon
  jaw-winking phenomenon
  Kasabach-Merritt phenomenon
  lateral constriction
    phenomenon
  mattress phenomenon
  mucous retention phenomenon
phenomenon of cellulite
phenomenon of compression
  atelectasis
phenopeel
phenotypic lymphocyte
phenotypic marker

phenylalanine mustard
pheochromocytoma
pheresis
 CFC pheresis (continuous-flow centrifugation pheresis)
 FL pheresis (filtration leukapheresis)
 IFC pheresis (intermittent-flow centrifugation pheresis)
Philadelphia cervical collar
Philadelphia cocktail
Philadelphia collar
Philadelphia collar cervical support
Philadelphia collar cervical traction
Philadelphia tonsil knife
Philips electron microscope
Philips endorectal transducer
Philips endovaginal transducer
Philips Gyroscan scanner
Philips small-bore system scanner
Philips spiral CT scanner
Philips toe force gauge
Philips Tomoscan CT scanner
Philips ultrasound machine
Phillips bougie
Phillips catheter
Phillips clamp
Phillips dilator
Phillips fixation forceps
Phillips forceps
Phillips muscle
Phillips recessed-head screw
Phillips rectal clamp
Phillips screw
Phillips screwdriver
Phillips swan neck forceps
Phillips urethral catheter
Phillips urethral whip bougie
Phillips urologic catheter
Philly bolt
Philos DR pacemaker
philtral column elevation
philtral dimple
philtral flap de-epithelization centering and reconstruction
philtral height
philtral malrotation

philtral roll
philtral symmetry
philtral tubercle
philtral tunnel dissection
philtral unit
philtral vermilion
philtrum (pl. philtra)
 long philtrum
 rotation of philtrum
 two-ridge philtrum
phimosis forceps
phimosis vaginalis
Phipps forceps
pHisoDerm
pHisoHex
phlebectomy
phlebitic induration
phlebitis
phleboclysis
phlebogram
phlebography
phlebolith
phlebolithiasis
phleboplasty
phleborrhagia
phleborrhaphy
phleborrheogram (PRG)
 Cranley-Graff phleborrheogram
 Grass-Cranley phleborrheogram
phleborrheograph
phleborrheography
phlebosclerosis
phlebothrombosis
phlebotome
phlebotomy
phlegm
phlegmon of floor of mouth
phlegmonous abscess
phlegmonous mass
phlegmonous ulcer
Phocas syndrome
Phoenix pacemaker
Phoenix Anti-Blok ventricular catheter
Phoenix outrigger splint
Phoenix single-chamber pacemaker
Phoenix total artificial heart
Phoenix total hip prosthesis
phonating edge

phonating structure
phonoangiography
phonocardiogram
phonocardiogram study
phonocardiography
phonocatheterization
Phoropter (*also* Phorotor)
phoropter retractor
Phoroptor (*also* Phoropter)
phosphatase
phosphate scan
phosphotungstic acid-
    magnesium chloride
    precipitation
photic stimulation
photic-evoked response
    stimulator
photoablation
photoabsorptiometry
photoallergic reaction
photochemotherapy
photocoagulation
    hemorrhoid infrared
        photocoagulation
    Ialo photocoagulation
    infrared photocoagulation
    intralesional laser
        photocoagulation (ILP)
    laser photocoagulation
    proliferative retinopathy
        photocoagulation (PRP)
photocoagulator (*see also*
    coagulator)
    American Optical
        photocoagulator
    argon laser photocoagulator
    Coherent argon laser
        photocoagulator
    Mira photocoagulator
    xenon arc photocoagulator
    xenon photocoagulator
    Zeiss photocoagulator
photoculdoscope
PhotoDerm PL laser
PhotoDerm PL, VL pulsed light
    device
PhotoDerm laser
PhotoDerm pulsed dye laser
photodisrupting laser
photodynamic therapy (PDT)
photoelectric multiplier tube
Photo-Flash peritoneoscope

photofluorographic examination
photogastroscope
    Krentz photogastroscope
PhotoGenica laser
PhotoGenica pulsed dye laser
photographic radiometer
photoionization detector
photo-kerato attachment
photokeratoscope
photolaparoscope
    Lent photolaparoscope
photometer
    Foerster photometer
    HemoCue photometer
photomultiplier tube
photon beam densitometry
Photon laser
Photon LaserPhaco probe
Photon LaserPhacolysis Probe
Photon micro implantable
    cardioverter defibrillator
photon microscope
photon-deficient bone lesion
photon-deficient lesion
photo-ophthalmia
PhotoPoint laser
photoradiation therapy
photorefractive keratectomy
    (PRK)
photorefractive keratoplasty
photo-strobe
phototherapeutic keratectomy
phototherapy
photothermal laser ablation
photothermolysis
photovaporization
photovaporizing laser
photovolt pH meter
phrenemphraxis
phrenic arteries
phrenic avulsion
phrenic evulsion
phrenic ganglion
phrenic lymph node
phrenic nerve block
phrenic nerve block anesthetic
    technique
phrenic nerve stimulation
phrenic retractor
phrenic surface of spleen
phrenic veins
phrenicectomized

phrenicectomy forceps
phreniclasia
phreniclasis
phrenicoabdominal nerves
phrenicocolic ligament
phrenicoesophageal ligament
phrenicoexeresis
phrenicolienal ligament
phreniconeurectomy
phrenicosplenic ligament
phrenicostomy
phrenicotomy
phrenicotripsy
phrenoesophageal ligament
phrenoesophageal membrane
phrenopericardial angle
phrenoplegia
phrygian cap deformity
phrygian cap of gallbladder
phthisis
Phylax implantable cardioverter
    defibrillator
Phylax AV dual chamber
    implantable cardioverter
    defibrillator
phylloides
Phymos 3D pacemaker
Phynox clip
Phynox cobalt alloy clip
Phynox cobalt alloy clip
    material
physeal fracture
physeal line
physeal plate
physial (see physeal)
physical barrier
physical capacity evaluation
physical examination
physical manipulation
physician-applied resurfacing
physician's pickup forceps
physician's splinter forceps
Physick operation
Physick pouch
physiognomic length
physiologic aspect
physiologic atrophy
physiologic barrier
physiologic curettement
physiologic endometrial
    ablation/resection loop
    (PEARL)

physiologic excavation
physiologic mesial migration
physiologic pacemaker
physiologic rest position
physiologic, physiological
physiological dead space
Physio-Stim Lite bone growth
    stimulator
Phystan implant
phytobezoar
PI disposable stapler
PI surgical stapler
pia mater
PIAC test for heart disease
pial-glial membrane
piano-style guidewire stent
piano-wire adhesion
piano-wire dorsiflexion brace
PIBC catheter (percutaneous
    intra-aortic balloon
    counterpulsation catheter)
PICA (posterior inferior
    cerebellar artery,
    posterior inferior
    communicating artery)
PICC (peripherally inserted
    central catheter)
PICC line
Piccolino Monorail balloon device
Piccolino Monorail catheter
Pichlmayer procedure
Pichlmayer technique
pick
    anterior footplate pick
    Austin pick
    Bellucci pick
    Burch fixation pick
    Burch ophthalmic pick
    Cooley pick
    Crabtree dissector pick
    Crane dental pick
    dental pick
    Desmarres fixation pick
    double-ended root tip dental
        pick
    Drews pick
    Farrior anterior footplate pick
    Farrior footplate pick
    Farrior oval-window pick
    Farrior posterior footplate
        pick
    fiberoptic pick

pick (*continued*)
  fixation pick
  footplate pick
  Guilford-Wright footplate pick
  Guilford-Wright stapes pick
  Hayden footplate pick
  Hoffmann scleral fixation pick
  Hough footplate pick
  Hough stapedectomy
    footplate pick
  House obtuse pick
  House oval-window pick
  House strut pick
  House-Barbara pick
  House-Crabtree dissector pick
  Kos pick
  light pipe pick
  McGee footplate pick
  Michel pick
  microsurgical ear pick
  Olk vitreoretinal pick
  ophthalmic pick
  oval-window pick
  Paparella footplate pick
  posterior footplate pick
  Rhein pick
  Rice pick
  right-angle pick
  Rosen pick
  Saunders-Paparella pick
  Scheer pick
  Schuknecht pick
  scleral pick
  Shea pick
  Sinskey pick
  slightly curved ear pick
  slightly curved pick
  small pick
  stapedectomy footplate pick
  stapes pick
  strut pick
  Tabb knife pick
  Trent eye pick
  Wells scleral suture pick
  Wilder pick
  Wright-Guilford footplate pick
  Wright-Guilford stapes pick
Pick and Go monitor
Pick bundle
pick chisel
pick knife
Picker camera

Picker scanner
Picker collimator
Picker helical CT scanner
Picker spiral CT scanner
Picker Synerview scanner
Picker Vanguard deep therapy
  unit
Picker Vista MRI scanner
Picker Vista MagnaScanner
  scanner
Pickerill imbrication line
picket fence guide
Pickett scissors
Pickrell hook
Pickrell retractor
pickup forceps
pickup noncrushing forceps
pickup screw
pickup spatula suture
pickup tube
Pico operation
Pico-ST low-profile balloon
  catheter
Pico-T II PTCA balloon catheter
Picot incision
Picot vaginal retractor
Picot vaginal speculum
Picot weighted speculum
Picotip steroid-eluting lead
picture-in-picture monitor
PID (pelvic inflammatory
  disease)
Pidcock nail
Pidcock pin
Pie Medical ultrasound
piebald skin
piecemeal removal
pie-crusting skin graft
Piedmont all-cotton elastic
  dressing
Piedmont fracture of radius
Pier abduction splint
Pierce antral trocar
Pierce antral wash tube
Pierce antrum wash tube
Pierce attic cannula
Pierce cheek retractor
Pierce coaxial I&A cannula
Pierce cryptotome
Pierce dissector
Pierce double-ended elevator
Pierce elevator

Pierce I&A unit
Pierce mastoid rongeur
Pierce nasal cup
Pierce raspatory
Pierce rongeur
Pierce saccade
Pierce submucous dissector
Pierce syringe
Pierce trocar
Pierce tube
Pierce washing tube
Pierce-Donachy Thoratec
    ventricular assist device
Pierce-Donachy ventricular
    assist device
Pierce-Kyle trocar
Pierce-O'Connor operation
piercing instrument
Pierre Robin micrognathia
Pierre Robin sequence
Pierrot-Murphy advancement
    insertion
Pierrot-Murphy ankle procedure
Pierrot-Murphy tendon
    technique
Pierse Colibri forceps
Pierse corneal Colibri-type
    forceps
Pierse corneal forceps
Pierse eye speculum
Pierse fixation forceps
Pierse tip forceps
Pierse-Colibri corneal utility
    forceps
Pierse-Hoskins forceps
Piersol point
Pierson attachment
Pierson traction
piesimeter
piezoelectric lithotripsy
piezoelectric shock wave
    lithotriptor
piezoelectric stimulator
piezoelectric transducer
Piezolith
    lithotriptor
Piezolith-EPL lithotripter
piezo-resistive transducer
Piffard dermal curet
Piffard placental curet
pigeon breast deformity
pigeon chest

pigeon toe
Pigg-O-Stat immobilization
    device
Pigg-O-Stat x-ray chair
piggyback contact lens
piggyback heart transplant
piggyback implant
piggyback IV fluid
piggyback liver transplantation
piggyback mammary prosthesis
piggyback needle-knife
    papillotome
piggyback probe
piggybacking
pigment cell transplantation
pigment epithelial lesion
pigmentary atrophy
pigmentary changes
pigmentary demarcation line
pigmentary dyschromia
pigmentation
    bear-track pigmentation
    bismuth pigmentation
    brown/black pigmentation
    nevoid pigmentation
    paw pigmentation
    periocular pigmentation
pigmentation mismatch
pigmented ameloblastoma
pigmented basal cell carcinoma
pigmented gallstone
pigmented lesion
pigmented linear streak
pigmented mole
pigmented nevus
pigmented villonodular synovitis
    (PVNS)
pigment-laden
pigmentosus
Pigott forceps
pigskin graft
pigskin patch
pigtail biliary stent
pigtail catheter
pigtail endoprosthesis
pigtail nephrostomy drain
pigtail nephrostomy tube
pigtail probe
pigtail stent
pigtail tendon stripper
Pike jawed forceps
pilar tumor of scalp

Pilcher bag catheter
Pilcher hemostatic bag
Pilcher hemostatic suprapubic
   bag
Pilcher suprapubic hemostatic
   bag
pile clamp
pile forceps
pileous gland
pillar
   anterior pillar
   bladder pillars
   dissector and pillar
   external pillar
   Herring lateral pillar
   inner pillar
   internal pillars
   iris pillars
   posterior pillar
   tonsillar pillar
   Uskow pillar
pillar and dissector
pillar cells
pillar forceps
pillar of diaphragm
pillar of fauces
pillar of fornix
pillar of soft palate
pillar projection
pillar retractor
pillar-and-post microsurgical
   retractor
pillar-grasping forceps
Pillet hand prosthesis
Pilliar total hip replacement
Pilling bronchoscope
Pilling clamp
Pilling collector
Pilling dilator
Pilling Duralite tracheal tube
Pilling Duralite tube
Pilling Excalibur gauge
Pilling fiberoptic illuminator
Pilling forceps
Pilling gouge
Pilling laryngofissure shears
Pilling microanastomosis clamp
Pilling needle holder
Pilling pediatric clamp
Pilling retractor
Pilling shears
Pilling stethoscope

Pilling sutures
Pilling tracheostomy tube
Pilling tube
Pilling vascular needle holder
Pilling Weck Y-stent forceps
Pilling Wolvek sternal
   approximator
Pilling-Douglas pelvimeter
Pilling-Favaloro retractor
Pilling-Hartmann speculum
Pilling-Liston bone utility
   forceps
Pilling-Negus clamp-on aspirator
Pilling-Ruskin rongeur
pillion fracture
Pillo Pro dressing
Pillo-Boot Lower leg positioning
   device
Pillo-Pedic cervical traction
   pillow
pillow fracture
pillow sign
pillow splint
pillow-shaped balloon
pilocarpine
pilojection
pilomatrixoma carcinoma
pilon ankle fracture
pilon fracture
pilonidal abscess
pilonidal cyst
pilonidal cystectomy
pilonidal cystectomy and
   sinusectomy
pilonidal dimple
pilonidal fistula
pilonidal sinus
pilosebaceous opening
pilosebaceous unit
Pil-O-Splint wrist splint
pilot bur
pilot drill
pilot needle
Pilot point screw
Pilot suturing guide
piloting trocar
Pilotip catheter
Pilotip catheter guide
pin (*see also* guide pin)
   Ace pin
   apex pin
   Arthrex zebra pin

pin (*continued*)

ARUM Colles fixation pin
ASIF screw pin
Asnis pin
Austin Moore pin
Barr pin
beaded hip pin
Beath pin
Belos compression pin
bevel-point Rush pin
Biofix system pin
biphasic pin
Boehler pin
Boehler-Knowles hip pin
Boehler-Steinmann pin
Böhler-Steinmann pin
Bohlman pin
breakaway pin
Breck pin
calibrated guide pin
calibrated pin
calibrated-tip threaded guide pin
Canakis beaded hip pin
cancellous pin
Caspar distraction pin
Charnley pin
cloverleaf pin
Co-Cr-Mo pin
Compere threaded pin
Conley pin
cortical pin
Craig pin
Crowe pilot point on Steinmann pin
Crowe-tip pin
Crutchfield skull-tip pin
Davis pin
Delitala T-pin
deluxe FIN pin
Denham pin
DePuy pin
derotational pin
Deyerle pin
distraction pin
distractor pin
duodenal pin
Ender pin
endodontic pin
Fahey hip pin
Fahey-Compere pin
femoral guide pin

pin (*continued*)

Fisher half pin
fixation pin
friction lock pin
Furniss-Clute pin
Getz root canal pin
Gingrass-Messer pin
Gouffon hip pin
guide pin
guidepin
Hagie hip pin
Hahnenkratt root canal pin
Hansen-Street pin
Hatcher pin
Haynes pin
Hegge pin
Hessel-Nystrom pin
Hewson breakaway pin
hexhead pin
hip pin
Hoffmann apex fixation pin
Hoffmann transfixion pin
hook-end intramedullary pin
insertion of pin
Intraflex intramedullary pin
intramedullary pin
Jones pin
Jurgan pin
Kirschner wire pin
Knowles hip pin
Kronendonk pin
Kronfeld pin
Kuntscher femur guide pin
lateral guide pin
LIH hook pin
Link-Plus retention pin
Lottes pin
Marble bone pin
Markley retention pin
Mayfield disposable skull pin
Mayfield skull clamp pin
McBride pin
mechanic's pin
medullary pin
metal pin
Modny pin
Moore fixation pin
Moule screw pin
Mt. Sinai skull clamp pin
Neufeld pin
Norman tibial pin
Oris pin

pin (*continued*)
Ormco pin
Orthofix pin
orthopedic pin
OrthoSorb absorbable pin
osseous pin
osteotomy pin
partially-threaded pin
percutaneous pin
Pidcock pin
pinion pin
Pischel pin
Pugh hip pin
rasp pin
removal of pin
resorbable polydioxanone pin
restorative pin
ReUnite orthopedic pin
revolving Ge-68 pin
Rhinelander pin
Rica wire guide pin
Riordan pin
Rissler pin
Rissler-Stille pin
Roger Anderson pin
Rush intramedullary fixation
  pin
Rush intramedullary pin
Rush safety pin
safety pin
Safir pin
Sage pin
sail of pin
Scand pin
Schanz pin
Schneider self-broaching pin
Schweitzer pin
self-broaching pin
self-tapering pin
Shantz pin
Shriners Hospital pin
Shriners pin
skeletal pin
Smillie pin
Smith-Petersen fracture pin
SMo Moore pin
smooth pin
Snap fixation pin
spring pin
sprue pin
stabilizing guide pin
Stader pin

pin (*continued*)
Steinmann calibrated pin
Steinmann calibration pin
Steinmann fixation pin
Street medullary pin
strut-type pin
Surgin hemorrhage occluder
  pin
Synthes guide pin
tapered pin
threaded guide pin
threaded pin
tibial guide pin
tibial pin
titanium half pin
torlone fixation pin
trochanteric pin
Turner hip pin
tutoFix cortical pin
union broach retention pin
Venable-Stuck fracture pin
von Saal medullary pin
Walker hollow quill pin
Watanabe pin
Watson-Jones guide pin
Webb pin
Zimfoam pin
Zimmer pin
pin chuck
pin crimper
pin cutter
pin endosseous implant
pin guard
pin guide
pin head holder
pin headrest
pin holder
pin implant
pin suture technique
pin sutures
pin tract sinus
pin vise
pin wheel
pin-and-plaster fixation
Pinard fetoscope
Pinard maneuver
Pinard sign
pin-bending forceps
pin-bone interface
pincers
pinch biopsy
pinch forceps

pinch gauge
pinch graft
pinch nose strut
pinch skin graft
pinch tree
pinchcock clamp
pinchcock mechanism
pinched nerve
pinch-grasp injection technique
pinch-handle microscissors
pinching pain
pin-cushion distortion
pin-deburring die
pineal body
pineal calcification
pineal gland
pinealectomy
pinealoma
pinealotomy
pineapple bur
pineapple contouring burr
ping-pong ball deformity
ping-pong fracture
pinhole camera
pinhole collimator
pinhole occluder
pinion head holder
pinion headrest
pinion pin
pink dressing
pink twisted cotton sutures
Pinkerton balloon catheter
pinky compression procedure
    (lens implant surgery)
Pinnacle contact Nd:YAG fiber
Pinnacle introducer sheath
Pinnacle pacemaker
pinnectomy
pinning operation
Pinocchio tip deformity
pinpoint electrocoagulation
pinpoint gastric mucosal
    defect
pinpoint gastric mucosal defect
    bleeding
pinpoint os
pinpoint pupils
pinprick analgesia
pins-and-needles sensation
pin-seating forceps
Pinto dissector tip
Pinto distractor

Pinto superficial dissection
    cannula
pin-to-bar clamp
pin-tract infection
pinwheel exam
pinwheel hypesthesia
pinwheel sensation gauge
PIP (pressure inversion point,
    proximal interphalangeal)
PIP (proximal interphalangeal)
    total joint
PIP Hydrogel breast implants
PIP joint
Pipe check kit PAD device
Pipelle biopsy
Pipelle endometrial curet
Pipelle endometrial suction
    catheter
Pipelle endometrial suction
    curet
Pipelle-deCornier endometrial
    curet
Piper lateral wall retractor
Piper obstetrical forceps
piperocaine hydrochloride
    anesthetic agent
pipestem artery
pipette
PIPIDA hepatobiliary scanning
    agent
piping rales
Pipkin femoral fracture
    classification
Pipkin fracture
Pipkin posterior hip dislocation
    classification
Pipkin subclassification of
    Epstein-Thomas
    classification
Piranha uteroscopic biopsy
    forceps
Pirie bone
piriform angle
piriform aperture access
piriform aperture stenosis
piriform aperture wiring
piriform crest
piriform fossa
piriform muscle
piriform opening
piriform process
piriform recess

piriform rim
piriform sills
piriform sinus
piriformis syndrome
Pirogoff amputation
Pirogoff angle
Pirogoff operation
Pirquet decompressor
Pirquet tongue depressor
Pisces device
Pisces electrode
Pisces implant
Pisces spinal cord stimulation
    device
Pischel electrode
Pischel elevator
Pischel forceps
Pischel micropin
Pischel micropin forceps
Pischel needle
Pischel pin
Pischel scleral ruler
pisiform bone
pisiform fracture
pisihamate ligament
pisitriquetral joint
pisometacarpal ligament
pisotriquetral joint
Pistofidis cervical biopsy forceps
pistol-grip hand drill
pistol-grip instrument
pistol-shot pulse
piston
    Austin piston
    Causse piston
    Guilford-Wright Teflon wire
        piston
    House piston
    House stapes piston
    McGee piston
    McGee platinum/stainless
        steel piston
    McGee stainless piston
    MTS electrohydraulic piston
    Schuknecht Teflon piston
    stainless steel piston
    stapes piston
    Teflon piston
    Teflon-wire piston
piston prosthesis
    Schuknecht Teflon wire
        priston prosthesis

piston sign
piston stapes prosthesis
piston strut
piston wire
pistoning movement
piston-type prosthesis
pit
    anal pit
    colonic pit
    commissural pit
    gastric pit
    herniation pit
    labial pit
    lip pit
    postanal pit
pit and fissure cavity
Pitanguy abdominoplasty
Pitanguy clamp
Pitanguy fat
Pitanguy flap demarcator
Pitanguy forceps
Pitanguy-McIndoe gouge
Pitanguy mammaplasty
Pitanguy reduction
    mammaplasty
Pitanguy-type breast reduction
pitch-workers' cancer
Pitha foreign body forceps
Pitha urethral forceps
Pitie-Salpetriere saphenous vein
    hook
Pitkin dermatome
Pitkin needle
Pitkin syringe
Pitocin augmentation of labor
Pitocin drip
Pitt tracheostomy tube
pitting defect
pitting edema
Pittman needle holder
Pittsburgh triangular frame
pituitary ablation
pituitary adenoma
pituitary body
pituitary capsulectomy
pituitary capsulectomy knife
pituitary curet
pituitary disorder
pituitary elevator
pituitary endocrine disorder
pituitary forceps
pituitary fossa

pituitary gland
pituitary gland transplantation
pituitary growth hormone
pituitary lesion
pituitary rongeur
pituitary rongeur forceps
pituitary stalk
pituitary tumor
pituitectomy
Pituitrin uterine injection
pivot aneurysm clip
pivot aneurysm clip applier
Pivot balloon
pivot clip applier
Pivot fixed-wire balloon catheter
pivot joint
pivot lock
pivot microanastomosis
     approximator
pivot microanastomosis clip
     applier
pivot point
pivotal disk heart valve
pivoting table
Pixsys FlashPoint camera
Pixsys FlashPoint digitizer
PKS-25 apparatus stapler
PLA (peripheral laser
     angioplasty)
place of articulation
placebo therapy
placed in position
placed in traction
placement
     4-point diamond placement
     5-port fan placement
     aortic graft placement
     band placement
     biliary sphincterotomy and
        stent placement
     bone graft placement
     bur-hole placement
     catheter placement
     catheter tip placement
     clip placement
     dilator placement
     electrode placement
     endoscopic biliary stent
        placement
     endotracheal tube placement
     esophageal prosthetic
        placement

placement (*continued*)
     eyelid sulcus placement
     feeding tube placement
     filter placement
     fluoroscopic placement
     graft placement
     implant placement
     infrarenal endograft
        placement
     intrapleural catheter
        placement
     Kirschner wire placement
     K-wire placement
     lead placement
     lingual placement
     long-term central venous
        access catheter placement
     mucoperiosteal implant
        placement
     nasobiliary pigtail catheter
        placement
     odontoid screw placement
     passive placement
     percutaneous nephrostomy
        tube placement
     permanent bipolar magnet
        placement
     permanent pacemaker
        placement
     pH electrode placement
     plate placement
     posterolateral bone graft
        placement
     postfistula placement
     radiologic biliary stent
        placement
     retropectoral placement
     retropubic placement
     rod placement
     sacral screw placement
     screw placement
     shunt placement
     Spetzler technique for shunt
        placement
     stent placement
     suprarenal filter placement
     surgical placement
     Surgicel implant placement
     temporary pacemaker
        placement
     T-tube placement
     tube placement

placement (*continued*)
  ureteral stent placement
  variable screw placement
  ventriculoperitoneal shunt
    placement
  wire-guided placement
placement forceps
placenta
  accessory placenta
  adherent placenta
  battledore placenta
  bidiscoidal placenta
  bilobate placenta
  bilobed placenta
  bipartite placenta
  choriovitelline placenta
  deciduous placenta
  dichorionic placenta
  duplex placenta
  endotheliochorial placenta
  expelled placenta
  fetal placenta
  fragment of placenta
  fundal placenta
  furcate placenta
  hemoendothelial placenta
  horseshoe placenta
  incarcerated placenta
  lobed placenta
  manual delivery of placenta
  manual removal of placenta
  maternal placenta
  mature placenta
  multilobed placenta
  nondeciduous placenta
  premature separation of
    placenta
  removal of placenta
  retained placenta
  Schultze placenta
  Stallworthy placenta
  stone placenta
  succenturiate placenta
  syndesmochorial placenta
  trilobate placenta
  tripartite placenta
  uterine placenta
  zonary placenta
  zonular placenta
placenta accreta
placenta bipartita
placenta clamp

placenta curet
placenta delivered
placenta expelled
placenta extracted
placenta forceps
placenta intact
placenta previa
placenta previa forceps
placenta reflexa
placenta removed
placenta retained
placenta scan
placental band
placental barrier
placental bruit
placental circulation
placental clamp
placental curet
placental dysfunction
placental dystocia
placental extrusion
placental forceps
placental fragment
placental growth hormone
placental hemangioma syndrome
placental hemorrhage
placental implantation
placental index
placental insufficiency
placental localization
placental membrane
placental metastasis
placental presentation
placental septum
placental site
placental tissue
placental tissue transplant
placental transfusion
placental villi
placentogram
placentography
Placer guidewire
Placido da Costa disk
Placido disk
Placido keratoscope
placing of clamp
plafond fracture
plagiocephaly
  compensational frontal
    plagiocephaly
  deformational frontal
    plagiocephaly

plagiocephaly (*continued*)
  frontal plagiocephaly
  lambdoid synostotic
    plagiocephaly
  occipital plagiocephaly
  synostotic frontal
    plagiocephaly (SFP)
  unilateral plagiocephaly
plagiocephaly headband
plagiocephaly without
  synostosis
plain catgut sutures
plain collagen suture
plain ear hook
plain eye needle
plain films
plain films of abdomen
plain forceps
plain gauze
plain gauze ABD
plain gut sutures
plain interrupted sutures
plain pattern plate
plain rib shears
plain rotary scissors
plain screwdriver
plain sutures
plain thumb forceps
plain tie
plain tissue forceps
plain vesical trocar
plain view
plain wire speculum
plain x-ray
plain-end grooved director
plain-line articulator
plain-pattern plate
planar circular coil
planar mesh implant
planar image
planar incision
Planas approach
plane
  1st parallel pelvic plane
  2nd parallel pelvic plane
  3rd parallel pelvic plane
  4th parallel pelvic plane
  Addison plane
  Aeby plane
  alveolar point-meatus plane
  anatomic plane
  angel hair plane

plane (*continued*)
  auriculoinfraorbital plane
  axial plane
  axiobuccolingual plane
  axiolabiolingual plane
  axiomesiodistal plane
  Ba-N plane (basion-nasion
    plane)
  base plane
  biplane intracavitary plane
  Bolton nasion plane
  Bolton-Broadbent plane
  Broca visual plane
  buccolingual plane
  Camper plane
  cephalometric plane
  cleavage plane
  coronal plane
  cove plane
  cranial base plane
  cross-sectional plane
  cusp plane
  datum plane
  Daubenton plane
  diffuse plane
  equatorial plane
  equivalent retracting plane
  extended supraplatysmal
    plane (ESP)
  extended supraplatysmal
    plane (ESP) dissection
  extended supraplatysmal plane
    (ESP) face-lift technique
  eye-ear plane
  facet plane
  facial plane
  fascial plane
  fat plane
  flexion-extension plane
  focal plane
  Frankfort horizontal plane
  Frankfort mandibular plane
  French plane
  frontal plane
  guide plane
  guiding plane
  Hensen plane
  His plane
  Hodge plane
  horizontal plane
  interspinal plane
  intertubercular plane

plane (*continued*)
   ischiorectal fossa plane
   labiolingual plane
   Listing plane
   longitudinal plane
   Ludwig plane
   mandibular plane
   Martin plane
   maxillary plane
   mean foundation plane
   median plane
   median raphe plane
   median sagittal plane
   mesiodistal plane
   midcoronal plane
   midfrontal plane
   midsagittal plane
   midthalamic plane
   Montague plane
   Morton plane
   nasion-pogonion facial axis
     plane
   nasion-point A plane
   nasion-point B plane
   nodal nuchal plane
   oblique coronal plane
   occipital plane
   occlusal plane
   orbital plane
   orbitomeatal plane
   orthogonal plane
   palatal plane
   paramedian sagittal plane
   parasagittal plane
   pelvic plane
   peripancreatic fat plane
   perpendicular plane
   pocket plane
   preglenoid plane
   preseptal-suborbicularis
     dissection plane
   primary movement plane
   principal plane
   reinforced the immediately
     subcutaneous plane
   sagittal plane
   scan plane
   sella-nasion plane
   sensitive plane
   short-axis plane
   slant of occlusal plane
   sliding plane

plane (*continued*)
   SN plane
   spectacle plane
   spinous plane
   sternal plane
   sternoxiphoid plane
   subcostal plane
   subcutaneous plane
   subgaleal plane
   subpectoral plane
   subperiosteal vomerine-
     ethmoidal plane
   subplatysmal plane
   sub-SMAS plane
   supracrestal plane
   supracristal plane
   suprasternal plane
   symmetry plane
   tangential plane
   temporal plane
   tension planes
   terminal plane
   thalamic plane
   thoracic plane
   tissue plane
   tooth plane
   transaxial scan plane
   transection plane
   transpyloric plane
   transtubercular plane
   transverse plane
   umbilical plane
   varus-valgus plane
   vertical plane
   visual plane
   von Ihring plane
   wide plane
   wire osteotomy plane
plane configuration
plane joint
plane of dissection
Plange spud
planigram
planimetry
plano lens
plano T-bandage
planoconcave
planoconcave lens
planoconvex eye implant
planoconvex lens
planoconvex nonridge lens
planoconvex-shaped disk

planographic examination
planovalgus deformity
planovalgus feet
plantar approach
plantar arch
plantar artery
plantar aspect
plantar aspect of foot
plantar axial x-ray
plantar calcaneal spur
plantar calcaneocuboid
   ligament
plantar compartmental anatomy
plantar condylectomy
plantar digital arteries
plantar digital nerves
plantar digital veins
plantar fascia
plantar fasciitis
plantar fasciitis night splint
plantar fasciotomy
plantar flexion
plantar flexion-inversion
   deformity
plantar flexors
plantar foot defect
plantar forefoot ulcer
plantar interosseous muscles
plantar ligaments
plantar longitudinal incision
plantar metatarsal arteries
plantar metatarsal vein
plantar muscle
plantar nerve
plantar reflex
plantar response
plantar space
plantar surface
plantar verruca
plantar view
plantar wart
plantar-flexed metatarsal
plantaris tendon
plaque
   atheromatous plaque
   augmentation plaque
   chorionic plaque
   cobblestone-like plaques
   dental plaque
   fibromyelinic plaques
   Hollenhorst plaque
   meningioma en plaque

plaque (*continued*)
   microbial plaque
   mucinous plaque
   mucous plaque
   Peyer plaque
   Peyronie-like plaque
   Randall plaque
   Redlich-Fisher miliary plaque
   talc plaque
plaque fracture
plaque incision
plaque radiotherapy
plaque retriever
plaque rupture
plaque technique
plaque-like lesion
plaquing
plasma cell portal infiltration
plasma clot diffusion chamber
plasma concentration
plasma endotoxin concentration
plasma exchange
plasma exchange therapy
plasma expander
plasma gastrin concentration
plasma iron concentration
plasma membrane
plasma norepinephrine
   concentration
plasma protein fraction
plasma renin concentration
plasma scalpel
plasma separation rate
plasma TFE vascular graft
plasma transfusion
plasma urea concentration
plasma volume expander
plasma volume expansion
Plasmalyte
plasmapheresis
plasmid-carrying cell
plasmin coagulation
plasmin-inhibitor complex (PIC)
Plastalume bulb-ended splint
Plastalume straight splint
plaster bandage
plaster boot
plaster cast
plaster cast application burn
plaster cast cutter
plaster cast knife
plaster dressing

plaster impression material
plaster knife
plaster pants dressing
plaster pants prosthesis
plaster saw
plaster shears
plaster spatula
plaster spline
plaster splint
plaster spreader
plaster-of-Paris bandage (POP
    bandage)
plaster-of-Paris cast
plaster-of-Paris dressing
plaster-of-Paris jacket
plaster-of-Paris scissors
plaster-of-Paris splint
Plastibell circumcision
Plastibell circumcision clamp
Plastibell circumcision device
Plastibell clamp
Plastibell compression
    instrument
plastic achillotenotomy
plastic Adzef sheet
plastic and reconstructive
    surgery
plastic ball
plastic ball eye implant
plastic Berger eye loupe
plastic bowing fracture
plastic bridge colostomy pouch
plastic cannula
plastic catheter
plastic closure
plastic clot
plastic collar
plastic conformer
plastic connector
plastic construction
plastic corneal protector
plastic crown
plastic curet
plastic drape
plastic dressing
plastic endoprosthesis
plastic eye knife box
plastic eye shield
plastic femoral plug
plastic floor reaction orthosis
plastic forceps
plastic implant

plastic induration
plastic lens
plastic ligature
plastic matrix
plastic membrane
plastic motor
plastic mouth guard
plastic needle holder
plastic operation
plastic orthosis
plastic prism
plastic reconstruction
plastic repair
plastic restoration material
plastic revision
plastic scalp clip
plastic scissors
plastic sewing ring
plastic Silastic
plastic sphere eye implant
plastic sphere implant
plastic splint
plastic stent
plastic stent occlusion
plastic suction tip
plastic surgery
plastic surgery elevator
plastic surgery scissors
plastic suture technique
plastic sutures
plastic syringe
plastic Tiemann catheter
plastic tube
plastic utility scissors
plastic wax material
plastic-cuffed tracheostomy tube
Plasticor torque-type prosthesis
Plasti-Pore ossicular replacement
    prosthesis
Plasti-Pore strut
Plasti-Pore TORP (Plasti-Pore
    total ossicular replacement
    prosthesis)
Plasti-Pore total ossicular
    replacement prosthesis
    (Plasti-Pore TORP)
Plastizote arch support
Plastizote cervical collar
Plastizote collar
Plastizote foot bed
Plastizote neck collar
Plastizote orthotic

Plastizote orthotic device
Plastizote plate
Plastodent dental impression
   adhesive
Plast-O-Fit thermoplastic
   bandage
Plastogel
plasty
   Bradford-Young Y-V plasty
   double-eyelid plasty
   Kleinert volar V-Y plasty
   lid plasty
   nipple plasty
   V-Y plasty
   Y-V plasty
   Y-Z plasty
plastyma muscle tightening
plastyma muscle
plate (*see also* nail plate)
   3D-flat Lactosorb plate
   2-hole plate
   3-hole plate
   4-hole anteromedial Alta
     straight plate
   4-hole side plate
   6-hole stainless steel plate
   6-hole mandibular plate
   7-hole plate
   absorbable plate
   acetabular reconstruction
     plate
   AIO compression plate
   Alta channel bone plate
   Alta condylar buttress plate
   Alta femoral plate
   Alta supracondylar bone plate
   anal plate
   anchor plate
   AO compression plate
   AO dynamic compression
     plate
   AO reconstruction plate
   AOI compression plate
   ASIF broad dynamic
     compression bone plate
   atresia plate
   Babcock plate
   Badgley plate
   Bagby compression plate
   Balser hook plate
   base plate
   Batchelor plate

plate (*continued*)
   bent blade plate
   Berke-Jaeger lid plate
   Bimler elastic plate
   biodegradable plate
   Blackstone anterior cervical
     plate
   blade plate
   Blair talar body fusion blade
     plate
   Blair tibiotalar arthrodesis
     blade plate
   Blanchard traction device
     blade plate
   blood agar plate
   Blount blade plate
   bone flap fixation plate
   bone plate
   bony atretic plate
   bony plate
   Bosworth spline plate
   breast plate
   broad AO dynamic
     compression plate
   Brophy plate
   buccal alveolar plate
   buccal cortical plate
   Burns plate
   butterfly-shaped monoblock
     vertebral plate
   buttress plate
   Capener nail plate
   CAPIS compression plate
   CAPIS reconstruction plate
   Caspar anterior cervical plate
   Caspar trapezoidal plate
   cervical plate
   Champy bone plate
   CHS supracondylar bone
     plate
   cloverleaf plate
   coaptation plate
   cobra plate
   cobra-head plate
   Coffin split plate
   Collison plate
   compression plate
   compression screw plate
   Concise side plate
   condylar blade plate
   condylar lag screw plate
   connecting plate

plate (*continued*)

contoured anterior spinal
  plate
cortical bone plate
cortical oral plate
craniocervical plate
craniomaxillofacial plate
cribriform plate
Crockard midfacial osteotomy
  retractor plate
C-shaped plate
Danek cervical fusion plate
Davis tooth plate
DC plate
DCFAO plate
deck plate
dental plate
depth plate
DePuy plate
Deyerle bone graft plate
disposable ground plate
dorsal plate
double-angled blade plate
double-H plate
Doughty tongue plate
Driessen hinged plate
Dupont distal humeral plate
dural plate
Dwyer-Hall plate
Dynamic Bridging plate
dynamic compression plate
  (DCP)
eccentric dynamic
  compression plate
Eggers bone plate
Elliot femoral condyle blade
  plate
Elliot femoral condyle plate
Elliot knee plate
Elliott blade plate
Ellis buttress plate
epiphyseal plate
ethmoid plate
ethmoidomaxillary plate
femoral condyle plate
femoral plate
fenestrated compression plate
finger plate
flat plate
Foley plate
Fresnel zone plate
fusion plate

plate (*continued*)

gait plate
Gallannaugh bone plate
gallbladder plate
Galveston plate
Gambro Liendia plate
Geibel blade plate
Gelfilm plate
genial advancement plate
graft blade plate
ground plate
Haid cervical plate
Haid Universal bone plate
half-circle plate
Hansen-Street anchor plate
Hardy-Rand-Rittler plate
Harlow plate
Harm posterior cervical plate
Harris plate
Hawley bite plate
Hicks lugged plate
hilar plate
Hoen skull plate
Holt nail plate
Hospidex microtiter plate
Hotz-type alveolar molding
  plate
Howmedica plate
H-shaped plate
Hubbard plate
ICS plate
impactor plate
infraorbital plate
inner lip plate
insertion of metal plate
interfragmentary plate
intertrochanteric plate
Ishihara pseudoisochromatic
  plate
isochromatic plate
Jaeger bone plate
Jaeger lid plate
Jaeger metal lid plate
Jewett double-angle
  osteotomy plate
Jewett nail overlay plate
Jewett nail plate
Jewett slotted plate
Ken plate
Kessel osteotomy plate
keyed supracondylar plate
Kilner-Doughty plate

plate (*continued*)

Kingsley orthodontic plate
Kirschner TOD plate
Kleer base plate
knee plate
Laing osteotomy plate
Lane fracture plate
Langenskiold fusion of growth plate
lateral pterygoid plate
Lawson-Thornton plate
L-buttress plate
lead plate
Leibinger 3-D bone plate
Leibinger Micro Plus plate
Leibinger Wurzberg plate
Letournel acetabular fracture bone plate
Letournel fracture plate
lid plate
limited-contact dynamic compression plate
limiting plate
lingual cortical plate
lingual plate
locking reconstruction plate
long-span rigid plate
Lorenz titanium screws and plate
low profile plate
low-contact dynamic compression plate
low-contact stress plate
Luer reconstruction plate
lugged plate
Luhr fixation plate
Luhr mandibular plate
Luhr bone plate
Luhr microbone plate
Luhr microfixation cranial plate
Luhr minifixation bone plate
Luhr pan plate
Luhr Vitallium micromesh plate
Lundholm plate
Luque II plate
Lynch mucosa separator plate
malleable plate
mandibular bridging plate
mandibular staple bone plate (MSBP)

plate (*continued*)

Massie plate
maxillary bite plate
Maxisorb test plate
May anatomical bone plate
McBride plate
McDonald bone plate
McLaughlin hip plate
medial pterygoid plate
Medoff sliding femoral plate
Medoff sliding fracture plate
Mennen plate
Messner plate
metal plate
metal reconstruction plate
Meurig Williams spinal fusion plate
micro-adaption plate
middle fossa plate
Milch resection plate
Mini Orbita plate
Moberg bone plate
modified Grace plate
Moe intertrochanteric plate
Moore blade plate
Moore sliding nail plate
Moore-Blount plate
Morscher anterior cervical plate
Morscher titanium cervical plate
mouth gag tooth plate
mucosal separator plate
Mueller hip plate
Mueller-Hinton-supplemented agar plate
multipoint contact plate
mushroom-type plate
MVR plate
nail plate
narrow AO dynamic compression plate
nephrotome plate
Neufeld femoral nail plate
Newington plate
Newman toenail plate
Nicoll plate
Nord orthodontic plate
occlusal plane plate
Odgen plate
oral plate
orbital plate

plate (*continued*)

   Orion anterior cervical plate
   Orozco plate
   orthodontic base plate
   orthopedic plate
   orthotic plate
   Osborne osteotomy plate
   ostectomy plate
   osteotomy plate
   palatal plate
   palate plate
   palmar plate
   partial plate
   paste plate
   patient plate
   Paulus chin plate
   Paulus midfacial plate
   pedicle plate
   Percy plate
   Perf-Plate cranial plate
   physeal plate
   plain pattern plate
   Plastizote plate
   polydioxanone plate
   polyethylene plate
   PolyMedics plate
   Profil-O-Plastic preshaped
     chin plate
   Profil-O-Plastic preshaped
     midfacial plate
   pseudoisochromatic plate
   pterygoid plate
   Pugh plate
   Pyramid anterior lumbar plate
   reconstruction plates
   resorbable plate
   Rhinelander plate
   Richards hip screw plate
   Richards side plate
   Richards-Hirschhorn plate
   Robin orthodontic plate
   Rohadur gait plate
   round hole plate
   Roy-Camille plate
   safety plate
   Schwartz plate
   Schweitzer spring plate
   screw plate
   self-compressing plate
   semitubular blade plate
   semitubular plate
   Senn bone plate

plate (*continued*)

   serpentine bone plate
   serpentine plate
   Shelton plate
   Sherman bone plate
   side plate
   Silastic plate
   Skirrow agar plate
   skull plate
   slide plate
   slotted bone plate
   slotted plate
   Smith-Petersen bone plate
   Smith-Petersen
     intertrochanteric plate
   SMO plate
   snap-on inserter plate
   spinal fusion plate
   spring plate
   stabilization plate
   Stahl calipers plate
   stainless steel AO plate
   staple bone plate
   steel plate
   Steffee pedicle plate
   Steffee screw plate
   Steinhauser plate
   Storz plate
   suction plate
   supracondylar plate
   supraorbital plate
   symmetrical sacral plate
   symmetrical thoracic
     vertebral plate
   Synthes AO reconstruction
     plate
   Synthes dorsal distal plate
   Synthes maxillofacial locking
     reconstruction plate
   Synthes maxillofacial titanium
     plate
   Synthes metallic plate
   Synthes stainless steel
     minifragment plate
   Synthes titanium
     minifragment plate
   Tacoma sacral plate
   tantalum plate
   tarsal plate
   T-buttress plate
   Teflon plate
   Temple University plate

plate (*continued*)
　tendon plate
　thoracolumbosacral plate
　Thornton side plate
　THORP-type mandibular
　　reconstruction plate
　tibial fixation plate
　tibial plate
　tibial relocation plate
　TiMesh orthognathic strap
　　plate
　titanium hollow-screw
　　osseointegrating
　　reconstruction plate
　　(THORP)
　titanium optimized design
　　plate (TOD plate)
　TOD plate (titanium
　　optimized design plate)
　toe plate
　tongue plate
　Townsend-Gilfillan plate
　transverse widening of
　　cribriform plate
　trochanteric plate
　T-shaped AO plate
　tubular plate
　Tupman osteotomy plate
　Universal bone plate
　urethral plate
　V-blade plate
　Venable bone plate
　vestibular oral plate
　Vitallium Elliott knee plate
　Vitallium Hicks radius plate
　Vitallium Wainwright blade
　　plate
　Vitallium Walldius mechanical
　　knee plate
　volar plate
　VSP plates
　V-type intertrochanteric plate
　vulcanite dental plate
　Wainwright osteotomy plate
　Wenger slotted plate
　Whitman plate
　Wiener gold plate
　Wilson spinal fusion plate
　wing plate
　Wright knee plate
　Wurzburg plate
　Yaeger lid plate

plate (*continued*)
　Y-bone plate
　Zimmer femoral condyle
　　blade plate
　Zimmer hip plate
　Zuelzer hook plate
plate and screw fixation
plate bender
plate cutter
plate fixation
plate placement
plateau fracture
plateau joint surface
plate-holding clamp
plate-holding forceps
platelet factor
platelet gel
platelet tissue factor
platelet trapping
platelet-activating factor (PAF)
platelet-aggregating factor (PAF)
platelet-derived growth factor
　　(PDGF)
plateletpheresis
platelet-rich plasma gel (PRPG)
platelet-shaped knife
plates and screws
plate-screw fixation
platform forceps
platform lift
platform walker
Platina clip implant cataract lens
Platina clip lens
Platina intraocular lens implant
plating
　compression instruments for
　　bone plating
　compression plating
　Leibinger plating
platinum blade electrode
platinum blade meatotomy
　　electrode
platinum conjunctival smear
　　spatula
platinum embolization coil
platinum eyelid implant
platinum filter
platinum foil matrix
platinum iridium capsule
platinum loop
platinum material
platinum microcoil

platinum oxygen electrode
Platinum Plus guidewire
platinum probe spatula
Platinum stationary table
platinum wire
platinum-Dacron microcoil
Platou osteotomy
platysma deep-tissue facelift
platysma facelift
platysma flap
platysma muscle
platysma myocutaneous flap
platysma plication
platysma reflex
platysma resection
platysma rhytidectomy
platysmal band
platysmal imbrication
platysmal transection
platysmaplasty
Playfair uterine caustic
    applicator
Pleatman pouch
Pleatman sac
pledget
    cotton pledget
    cottonoid pledget
    Dacron pledget
    felt pledget
    Gelfoam pledget
    Gelfoam-soaked pledget
    Meadox Teflon felt pledget
    neurosurgical pledget
    polypropylene pledget
    prethreaded Teflon pledget
    Teflon felt pledget
pledget dressing
pledget sponge
pledget sutures
pledgeted Ethibond sutures
pledgeted mattress sutures
pledgeted sutures
PlegiaGuard safety device
Plenk-Matson rasp
Plenk-Matson raspatory
pleomorphic adenocarcinoma
pleomorphic adenoma
pleomorphic liposarcoma
pleomorphism
plesiosectional tomography
Plester retractor
plethoric dysmenorrhea

plethysmogram
plethysmograph
plethysmography
pleura
    cervical pleura
    costal pleura
    cupula of pleura
    diaphragmatic pleura
    discission of pleura
    hydrops of pleura
    lavage of pleura
    mediastinal pleura
    parietal pleura
    pericardial pleura
    thickened pleura
    visceral pleura
pleuracentesis
pleuracotomy
pleural abrasion
pleural adhesion
pleural biopsy needle
pleural biopsy needle shears
pleural biopsy punch
pleural bleb
pleural calculus
pleural cavity
pleural cupola
pleural dissector
pleural effusion
pleural fibrosis
pleural fluid aspiration
pleural fluid collection
pleural fluid examination
pleural fremitus
pleural friction rub
pleural lavage
pleural line
pleural mass
pleural metastasis
pleural peel
pleural plaquing
pleural pleurisy
pleural poudrage
pleural rale
pleural reaction
pleural rub
pleural sac
pleural scarring
pleural shock
pleural space
pleural suction tube
pleural surface

pleural symphysis
pleural thickening
pleural tube
pleural villi
pleuralized
pleurectomy forceps
Pleur-evac chest catheter
Pleur-evac device
Pleur-evac suction
Pleur-evac suction tube
pleurisy
pleurobiliary fistula
pleurocentesis
pleurodesis
pleuroesophageal fistula
pleuroesophageal line
pleuroesophageal muscle
pleurolysis
pleuroparietopexy
pleuropericardial incision
pleuropericardial murmur
pleuropericardial window
pleuroperitoneal canal
pleuroperitoneal fold
pleuroperitoneal foramen
pleuroperitoneal hernia
pleuroperitoneal space
pleuropexy
pleuropneumonolysis
pleuropulmonary congestion
pleurotomy
Pleurovac chest catheter
Pleurx pleural catheter
plexectomy
plexiform angioma
plexiform external layer
plexiform lesion
plexiform neuroma
Plexiglas eye implant
Plexiglas Gellhorn pessary
Plexiglas graft
Plexiglas jig
Plexiglas pessary
Plexiglas prosthesis
Plexiglas radiographic ruler
Plexiglas splint
Plexiglas tissue equivalency
    block
PlexiPulse compression device
plexus (*pl.* plexus, plexuses)
    abdominal aortic plexus
    aortic plexus

plexus (*continued*)
  areolar venous plexus
  arterial plexus
  Auerbach mesenteric plexus
  basilar plexus
  Batson plexus
  biliary plexus
  brachial plexus
  capillary plexus
  cardiac plexus
  carotid plexus
  celiac plexus
  cervical plexus
  choroid plexus
  coccygeal plexus
  colonic myenteric plexus
  common carotid plexus
  cystic plexus
  dermal vascular plexus
  esophageal plexus
  Exner plexus
  gastric plexus
  gastroesophageal variceal
      plexus
  Haller plexus
  hemorrhoidal plexus
  hepatic plexus
  Hovius plexus
  hypogastric plexus
  hypoglossal plexus
  ileocolic plexus
  intermediate plexus
  internal carotid venous plexus
  internal mammary plexus
  internal plexus
  internal thoracic lymphatic
      plexus
  Jacobson plexus
  Kiesselbach plexus
  laryngeal plexus
  lingual plexus
  lumbar plexus
  malleolar plexus
  mediastinal plexus
  Meissner plexus
  myenteric plexus
  ophthalmic plexus
  ovarian plexus
  pampiniform plexus
  parotid plexus
  pelvic plexus
  pharyngeal plexus

plexus (*continued*)
  porta hepatis plexus
  prostatic plexus
  prostaticovesical plexus
  pterygoid plexus
  ranine vein plexus
  rectal plexus
  renal plexus
  rete plexus
  sacral plexus
  Santorini plexus
  Sappey plexus
  Stensen plexus
  subepithelial nerve plexus
  subepithelial plexus
  submucosal venous plexus
  suboccipital plexus
  subpleural mediastinal plexus
  suprarenal plexus
  sympathetic carotid plexus
  testicular plexus
  thyroid plexus
  tympanic plexus
  ureteric plexus
  uterine plexus
  uterovaginal plexus
  vaginal plexus
  venous plexus
  venous vertebral plexus
  vertebral plexus
  vesicoprostatic plexus
  Woodruff nasopalatine plexus
plexus anesthesia
plexus of Santorini
plexus pampiniformis
Pley capsular forceps
Pley extracapsular forceps
Pley forceps
PLF (perilymphatic fistula)
PLI (perilunar instability)
plica (*pl.* picae)
plica duodenalis
plica duodenojejunalis
plica duodenomesocolica
plica epigastrica
plica gastropancreatica
plica ileocecalis
plica nasi
plica paraduodenalis
plica semilunaris
plica sublingualis
plica umbilicalis

plicae (*sing.* plica)
plicated appendicocystostomy
plicated tongue
plicating suture technique
plicating sutures
plication
  buccinator plication
  Childs-Phillips bowel plication
  disk plication
  endoscopic muscle plication
  fascial plication
  fundal plication
  fusiform plication
  galea aponeurosis plication
  Graham plication
  Kelly plication
  Kelly-Kennedy vaginal
    plication
  musculoaponeurotic plication
  musculofascial plication
  Nesbit plication
  Noble bowel plication
  Noble small bowel plication
  platysma plication
  Rehne-Delorme plication
  renal plication
  retractor plication
  soft-tissue plication
  suture plication
  tongue plication
  transgastric plication
  transmesenteric plication
  vertical rectus plication
plication face-lift
plication needle
plication of bowel
plication procedure
plication sutures
Plicator endoscopic device
plicecotomy
plicotomy
pliers
  Allen pliers
  Allen root pliers
  Bailey pliers
  Beck pliers
  Becker-Parkin pliers
  bending pliers
  Berbecker pliers
  College pliers
  crown-crimping pliers
  debonding pliers (DP)

pliers (*continued*)
  dental pliers
  extraction pliers
  fisherman's pliers
  Jacob-Swan goniotomy pliers
  Jelenko pliers
  K-Y pliers
  ligature-locking pliers
  ligature-tying pliers
  lingual arch-forming pliers
  Luhr Microfixation System
    pliers
  Maddox pliers
  Mathieu pliers
  matrix pliers
  needle-nose pliers
  needle-nose vise-grip pliers
  Ormco orthodontic pliers
  orthopedic surgical pliers
  Power Grip pliers
  Reill wire-cutting pliers
  Risley pliers
  root pliers
  Schwarz arrow-forming pliers
  slip-joint pliers
  SMIC pliers
  Sontec pliers
  square-end pliers
  Stille flat pliers
  Swan-Jacob goniotomy pliers
  threader rod holder pliers
  vice-grip pliers
PLIF procedure (posterior
    lumbar interbody fusion
    procedure)
PLM (precise lesion measuring)
plombage operation
Plondke uterine forceps
Plondke uterine-elevating
    forceps
P-loop
plop
  cardiac tumor plop
  tumor plop
PLP (partial
    laryngopharyngectomy)
plug
  Air-Lon decannulation plug
  Air-Lon plug
  Alcock catheter plug
  Alcock plug
  Avina female urethral plug

plug (*continued*)
  Bard mesh PerFix hernia plug
  Berkeley brass scleral plug
  bile plug
  Biomet plug
  Bio-Plug canal plug
  bone femoral plug
  bone plug
  brass scleral plug
  Buck plug
  Catamaran swim plug
  catheter plug
  choanal plug
  collagen plug
  Coloplast 1-piece conseal
    plug
  Coloplast 2-piece conseal
    plug
  Concept bone tunnel plug
  Corner plug
  cotton plug
  Counsellor plug
  decannulation plug
  Diomet plug
  Dittrich plug
  Doc's earplug
  Dohlman plug
  dome hole plug
  EaglePlug tapered-shaft
    punctum plug
  EagleVision Freeman punctum
    plug
  Exeter intramedullary bone
    plug
  femoral plug
  fibrin plug
  Freeman punctum plug
  gastrostomy plug
  glass vaginal plug
  Herniamesh surgical plug
  Herrick lacrimal plug
  Insta-Putty silicone earplug
  intramedullary canal plug
  Isberg scleral plug
  Johnston gastrostomy plug
  Johnston plug
  Kirschner femoral canal plug
  Luer-Lok male adapter plug
  Mack ear plugs
  meconium plug
  methyl methacrylate
    cranioplastic plug

plug (*continued*)
  Micro punctum plug
  mucous plug
  Oasis collagen plug
  omental plug
  Osteonics acetabular dome hole plug
  PerFix hernia plug
  PerFix Marlex mesh plug
  plastic femoral plug
  polypropylene plug
  punctum plug
  Reich-Nechtow plug
  R-Med plug
  scleral plug
  sealing window plug
  Seidel plug
  self-seating plug
  Shiley decannulation plug
  Sims vaginal plug
  Super punctum plug
  tapered-shaft punctum plug
  TearSaver punctum plug
  Teflon Bardic plug
  Umbrella punctum plug
  Woodson plug
plug cutter
plug prosthetic mesh repair
plug-finishing bur
plugger
  amalgam plugger
  Bredall amalgam plugger
  Dower bone plugger
  endodontic plugger
  miniature plugger
  Mity plugger
  Schilder plugger
  serrated amalgam plugger
  SMIC root canal plugger
plugging
  stent plugging
plugging instrument
plumb line sign
plumb line test
plumbeous zirconate titanate tip
Plum-Blossom acupuncture needle
Plum-Blossom needle
Plume-Away evacuator
Plumicon camera tube
Plummer bag
Plummer esophageal dilator

Plummer modified bougie
Plummer water-filled pneumatic esophageal dilator
Plummer-Vinson applicator
Plummer-Vinson dilator
Plummer-Vinson esophageal dilator
Plummer-Vinson radium applicator
Plummer-Vinson radium esophageal applicator
Plummer-Wilson syndrome
plumping graft
plural pregnancy
plus power lens
Plystan graft
Plystan implant
Plystan prosthesis
PM (pectoralis major, Periodontal membrane)
PMH scissors
PMI (point of maximal impulse)
PMI implant
PMMA (polymethyl methacrylate)
PMMA bone cement
PMMA centering sleeve
PMMA contact lens
PMMA hard contact lens
PMMA intraocular lens
PMT AccuSpan tissue expander
PMT Cortac cortical electrode
PMT Depthalon depth electrode
PMT halo brace
PMT InVac in-line suction control device
PMT MicroVac suction device
PMT tissue expander
Pnetax Spotmatic camera
Pneu Care ICU dynamic low-air-loss bed
Pneu Care Pedibed dynamic pediatric low-air-loss bed
Pneu Knee brace
pneumatic 4-bar linkage knee
pneumatic ankle tourniquet
pneumatic antishock garment (PASG)
pneumatic antishock trousers
pneumatic artificial larynx
pneumatic bag

pneumatic bag esophageal
    dilatation
pneumatic bag esophageal
    dilation
pneumatic balloon catheter
pneumatic balloon catheter
    dilation
pneumatic balloon dilator
pneumatic chair lift
pneumatic compression
pneumatic compression
    stockings
pneumatic cuff
pneumatic dilatation
pneumatic dilator
pneumatic garment
pneumatic microscope
pneumatic otoscope
pneumatic reduction
pneumatic retinopexy
pneumatic space
pneumatic splint
pneumatic tonometer
pneumatic tourniquet
pneumatization
pneumatonographer
pneumatonography
pneumatonometer
pneumectomy
pneumo sleeve
pneumoarthrogram
pneumoballistic lithotriptor
pneumocentesis
pneumocisternogram
pneumocisternography
pneumococcal infection
pneumocystis carinii
    mastoiditis
pneumodissection
pneumoencephalogram
pneumoencephalography
pneumogastric nerve
pneumogram
pneumography
pneumogynogram
pneumogynography
pneumolysis
Pneumomat laparoscopic
    insufflator
Pneumo-Matic insufflation
    needle
pneumomediastinogram

pneumomediastinography
pneumonectomy
Pneumo-Needle needle
pneumonocentesis
pneumonolysis
    extraperiosteal pneumonolysis
    extrapleural pneumonolysis
    intrapleural pneumonolysis
pneumonopexy
pneumonoresection
pneumonorrhaphy
pneumonotomy
pneumoperitoneum needle
pneumopexy
pneumoplethysmography
pneumoresection
pneumostatic dilation
pneumostatic dilator
pneumotach
pneumotachometer
pneumothoracic injection
    needle
pneumothorax
    closed pneumothorax
    extrapleural pneumothorax
    iatrogenic tension
        pneumothorax
    induced pneumothorax
    induced tension
        pneumothorax
    spontaneous pneumothorax
pneumothorax apparatus (*see*
    apparatus)
pneumothorax injection needle
pneumothorax needle
Pneumotron ventilator
pneumoventriculogram
pneumoventriculography
pneupac resuscitator
pneupac ventilator
PNSP (posterior nasal spine to
    soft palate)
POC (presurgical orthopedic
    correction)
POC balloon
POC Bandit catheter
pocket chamber
pocket depth
pocket epithelium
pocket infection
pocket of pus
pocket operation

pocket plane
pocket probe
Pocket-Dop blood-flow detector
Pocket-Dop fetal heart rate
    monitor
pocketed calculus
Pocketpeak peak flowmeter
podalic extraction
podalic version
Pogon chair
Pogrund lateral approach
Poh mouth mirror
point
    abrasive point
    absorbent paper point
    absorbent point
    Addison point
    alveolar point
    anchoring point
    anterior focal point
    APACHE-II point
    apophysary point
    apophysial point
    associated myofascial trigger
        point
    auricular point
    axial point
    B point
    Barker point
    bifurcation point
    bleeding point
    blur point
    Boas point
    Bolton point
    bounce point
    Boyd point
    break point
    Brinell hardness indenter
        point
    Broadbent registration point
    Capp point
    Capuron point
    cardinal point
    Castellani point
    central-bearing point
    change point
    Chauffard point
    chin point
    choroid point
    Clado point
    cleft high points
    coagulated bleeding points

point (*continued*)
    condenser point
    conjugate point
    contact area point
    convenience point
    convergence point
    copular point
    corresponding point
    craniometric point
    Crowe pilot point
    Crutchfield-Raney drill point
    cut point
    D point
    de Mussy point
    Desjardins point
    disparate point
    dorsal point
    drill point
    E point
    electrodesiccated bleeding
        point
    end point
    entry point
    equivalence point
    Erb point
    ethmoid registration point
    Excell polishing point
    exit point
    eye point
    F2 focal point
    far point
    faulty contact point
    fibromyalgia trigger point
    fixation point
    fixed point
    focal bleeding point
    focal image point
    focal point
    forceps point
    freezing point
    fulguration of bleeding points
    fusing point
    gingival point
    glenoid point
    growing point
    gutta-percha point
    Gueneau de Mussy point
    Halle point
    Hartmann point
    hinge-axis point
    Hoku point
    ice point

point (*continued*)
  identical point
  ignition point
  image point
  impaction point
  incident point
  incisal point
  incisor point
  insertion point
  isoelectric point
  isometric point
  isosbestic point
  jugal point
  jugomaxillary point
  justrous central yellow point
  Keen point
  key point
  Knoop hardness indenter
    point
  Kocher point
  Krackow point
  lacrimal point
  Lanz point
  Larrey point
  Legat point
  Mackenzie point
  material failure break point
  Mathews drill point
  maximum occipital point
  McBurney point
  median mandibular point
  melting point
  mental point
  metopic point
  motor point
  multiple sensitive point
  Munro point
  muscle bleeding points
  myofascial trigger point
  nasion point
  near visual point
  neutral point
  nodal point
  null point
  occipital point
  optical nodal point
  painful point
  paper point
  Pauly point
  pedicle entrance point
  Piersol point
  pivot point

point (*continued*)
  posterior focal point
  power point
  powered automatic stopping
    drill point
  preauricular point
  pressure inversion point (PIP)
  pressure point
  primary myofascial trigger
    point
  principal point
  purchase point
  radix point
  Ramond point
  Raney-Crutchfield drill point
  referred point
  respiratory inversion point
  restoration point
  retention point
  retrograde insertion point
  retromandibular point
  Robson point
  root canal point
  rotary mounted point
  sacral brim target point
  satellite myofascial trigger
    point
  secondary focal point
  secondary myofascial trigger
    point
  self-stopping drill point
  sella-nasion-B point
  sensitive point
  separation point
  set point
  Sippy point
  spinal point
  Starlite point
  Steinmann pin with Crowe
    pilot point
  stereo-identical point
  Sudeck critical point
  sulfur and silver point
  supra-auricular point
  supraorbital point
  sylvian point
  tender point
  tender trigger points
  thermal death point
  trial point
  trigger point
  triple point

point (*continued*)
  Trousseau point
  twist drill points
  Universal drill point
  Valleix point
  virtual point
  visual point
  Vogt point
  Vogt-Hueter point
  Weber point
  white point
  William Dixon Cratex point
  wood point
  yellow point
  Z point
  zygomaxillary point
point angle
point centric
point electrode
point forceps
point imaging
point of abscess
point of election
point of inflection
point of maximal impulse (PMI)
point of proximal contact
point resolved spectroscopy
point scanning
point source
point tenderness
point-counting image
pointed awl
pointed cone bur
pointed head
pointed pinna
pointed scissors
pointed-tip electrode
pointer
  Baton laser pointer
  hip pointer
  LaserMed laser pointer
  metallic pointer
  shoulder pointer
Pointer 1-piece all-PMMA
    intraocular lens
point-in-space stereotactic
    biopsy
point-of-reduction clamp
point-search instrument
Poirier glands
Poirier line
Poiseuille space

poker spine
Polack keratoscope
Poland anomaly
Poland classification of fractures
Poland epiphysial fracture
    classification
Poland physical injury
    classification
Poland syndrome
Polar Bair forced-air active
    cooling device
cryotherapy device
polar cataract
polar presentation
Polar Vantage XL heart rate
    monitor
Polar wrist monitor
polarimeter
  confocal scanning laser
      polarimeter
  scanning laser polarimeter
Polaris adjustable spinal cage
    implant
Polaris cage
Polaris electrode
Polaris 1.32 Nd:YAG laser
Polaris laparoscope
Polaris catheter
Polaris Mansfield/Webster
    deflectable tip
Polaris reusable cutter
Polaris reusable dissector
Polaris reusable forceps
Polaris reusable grasper
Polaris reusable laparoscopic
    instrument
Polaris steerable diagnostic
    catheter
polarizing microscope
polarizing ophthalmoscope
Polar-Mate bipolar coagulator
Polar-Mate bipolar
    microcoagulator
polarographic needle electrode
Polaroid camera
Polaroid instant endocamera
Polarus humeral rod
Polavision Land camera for
    endoscopy
Polcyn elevator
pole ligation
pole of kidney

pole of the breast
pole of the hamate
Polhemus digitizer scanner
Polhemus digitizer
policeman's heel
poliglecaprone 25 sutures
polio laryngoscope
Polisar-Lyons adapted tracheal
  tube
Polisar-Lyons tracheal tube
polisher
  Anis ball reverse-curvature
    capsular polisher
  Anis disk capsular polisher
  Bechert capsular polisher
  Buedding squeegee cortex
    extractor and polisher
  capsular polisher
  Carborundum polisher
  Drews capsular polisher
  Freeman capsular polisher
  Gill-Welsh capsular polisher
  Holladay posterior capsular
    polisher
  Jensen capsular polisher
  Jensen diamond polisher
  Knolle capsular polisher
  Knolle polisher
  Knolle posterior capsule
    polisher
  Kraff capsular polisher
  Kratz polisher
  Kratz-Jensen polisher
  Look capsular polisher
  Tennessee capsular polisher
  Terry silicone capsular
    polisher
  Torchia capsular polisher
  Yaghouti LASIK Polisher
polishing brush
polishing bur
polishing disk
Politano-Leadbetter anastomosis
Politano-Leadbetter operation
Politano-Leadbetter tunnel
  creation
Politzer air bag
Politzer air syringe
Politzer air-bag otoscope
Politzer angular ear knife
Politzer bag
Politzer ear knife

Politzer ear perforator
Politzer ear speculum
Politzer knife
Politzer operation
Politzer otoscope
Politzer paracentesis needle
Politzer speculum
politzerization
Politzer-Ralks knife
Polk finger goniometer
Polk goniometer
Polk placental forceps
Polk sponge forceps
Pollack ureteral catheter
Polle pod attachment for
  ophthalmoscope
Polley-Bickel trephine
pollicization
  Buck-Gramcko pollicization
  index finger pollicization
pollicization procedure
Pollock amputation
Pollock atraumatic grasper
Pollock catheter
Pollock double corneal forceps
Pollock operation
Pollock punch
Pollock sweetheart periosteal
  elevator
Pollock wimp wire impactor
Pollock zygoma elevator
Pollock-Dingman elevator
polly beak deformity
polly beak nasal deformity
polly-beak deformity of nose
Polmedco endotracheal tube
  cuff
Polmenus digitizer
Polokoff rasp
Poloxamer 407 barrier material
POLY balloon catheter
Poly CS device
Poly Surgiclip absorbable clip
poly-1-hydroxyethyl
  methacrylate
poly-2-hydroxyethyl
  methacrylate (poly-HEMA)
Polya anastomosis
Polya gastrectomy
Polya gastroenterostomy
Polya gastrojejunostomy
Polya operation

Polya procedure
Polya technique
Polyak eye retractor
Polyak operation
polyamide mesh
polyamide sutures
polyaxial cervical screw
polyaxial joint
polybutester sutures
polycarboxylate cement
Poly-Cath catheter
polycationic histochemical
    probe
Polycel bone composite
    prosthesis
polycentric knee prosthesis
polycentric prosthesis
polyclonal hyperplasia
polycycloidal tomography
polycystic disease
polycystic kidney disease (PKD)
polycystic liver
polycystic ovary (PCO)
polycystic renal disease
polydactylism
polydactyly
    index finger polydactyly
    thumb polydactyly
    Wassel classification of thumb
        polydactyly
Polydek sutures
Polyderm foam wound dressing
polydioxanone plate
polydioxanone sutures (PDS)
Polydor Preforms orthotic
polyester fiber sutures
polyester sutures
polyester-reinforced Dacron
    tape
polyether graft material
polyether implant material
polyether impression material
polyether prosthesis material
polyether rubber impression
    material
polyethylene ball
polyethylene cannula
polyethylene catheter
polyethylene cement
polyethylene collar button
polyethylene drain
polyethylene drainage tube

polyethylene eye implant
polyethylene foam
polyethylene glycol lavage
polyethylene graft
polyethylene implant
polyethylene implant material
polyethylene intravenous
    catheter
polyethylene linear implant
    component
polyethylene liner
polyethylene plate
polyethylene prosthesis
polyethylene retractor tape
polyethylene snare
polyethylene socket
polyethylene sphere implant
polyethylene stent
polyethylene strut
polyethylene sutures
polyethylene talar prosthesis
polyethylene terephthalate
    balloon
polyethylene tube
polyethylene vein stripper
polyethylene-faced driver
polyethylene-faced mallet
polyfilament sutures
PolyFlex implantable pacing
    lead pacemaker
PolyFlex lead
PolyFlex lead pacemaker
PolyFlex traction dressing
PolyFlo peripherally inserted
    central catheter
polyfluorotetraethylene shunt
    (PFTE shunt)
Polyform splint
polygalactic acid sutures
PolyGIA stapler
PolyGIA stapling device
polyglactic acid sutures
polyglactin 910 sutures
polyglactin mesh
polyglecaprone 25 sutures
polyglycolate sutures
polyglycolic acid
polyglycolic acid mesh
polyglycolic acid sutures
polyglycolic mesh
polyglycolic sutures
polyglycolide implant

polyglyconate sutures
poly-HEMA (poly-2-hydroxyethyl
  methacrylate)
polylactide absorbable screw
polylactide implant
polylobar liver
Polymed splint
PolyMedics plate
PolyMem adhesive surgical
  wound dressing
PolyMem foam wound dressing
PolyMem wound care dressing
polymer
  Bioplastique polymer
  fibrin glue polymer
  human tissue polymer
  methyl methacrylate polymer
  modified polymer
  thermoplastic polymer
  thermosetting polymer
polymer anesthetic
polymer tooth replica implant
polymer-coated, drug-eluting
  stent
PolymerFriction total knee
polymeric carbon
polymeric endoluminal paving
  stent
polymerization
polymethyl methacrylate
  (PMMA)
polymethyl methacrylate bone
  cement
polymethyl methacrylate ear
  splint
polymethyl methacrylate implant
polymorphonuclear cell
polymorphonuclear leukocyte
polymorphous
polymyxin
polyneuritis
polyneuropathy
polyolefin copolymer balloon
polyolefin elastomer
polyp
  adenomatous polyp
  benign adenomatous polyp
  broad-based polyp
  cervical polyp
  choanal polyp
  colonic polyp
  colorectal polyp

polyp (*continued*)
  duodenal polyp
  endocervical polyp
  endometrial polyp
  fibroepithelial polyp
  fibrovascular polyp
  hamartomatous gastric polyp
  Hopmann polyp
  hyperplastic gastric polyp
  hyperplastic polyp
  inflammatory fibroid polyp
  intestinal polyp
  juvenile polyps
  laryngeal polyp
  lymphoid polyp
  malignant polyp
  metaplastic polyp
  mucous polyp
  nasal polyp
  neoplastic polyp
  pedunculated polyp
  polypoid polyp
  postinflammatory polyp
  precancerous polyp
  rectal polyp
  retention polyp
  sentinel polyp
  sessile polyp
  stalk of polyp
  tubular polyp
  tubulovillous polyp
  villoglandular polyp
  villous polyp
polyp forceps
polyp grasper
polyp snare
polyp stalk
polypectomy
  colonoscopic polypectomy
  electrosurgical snare
    polypectomy
  endocervical polypectomy
  endoscopic polypectomy
  endoscopic sessile
    polypectomy
  Hirano polypectomy
  incomplete polypectomy
  nasal polypectomy
  sigmoidoscopy with rectal
    polypectomy
polypectomy snare
Poly-Plus Dacron vascular graft

polypoid adenoma
polypoid lesion
polypoid mass
polypoid polyp
polypoid superficial gastric
    carcinoma
polypoid tissue
polyposis coli
polyposis gastrica
polyposis intestinalis
polyposis ventriculi
polypotome
polypotrite
polypous endocarditis
polypous gastritis
polypropylene braid
polypropylene button
polypropylene button sutures
polypropylene glycol ankle-foot
    orthosis
polypropylene glycol
    thoracolumbosacral
    orthosis
polypropylene intracardiac
    patch
polypropylene intraocular lens
polypropylene mesh
polypropylene needle
polypropylene pledget
polypropylene plug
polypropylene sutures
polypus forceps
polyradicular joint disease
Polyrox Fractal active fixation
    lead
polyscope
Polysil-Foley catheter
Polyskin II dressing
Polysorb 55 stapler
Polysorb absorbable staple
Polysorb heel cub
Polysorb liner
Polysorb suture
Polysporin ointment
Polystan cardiotomy reservoir
Polystan catheter
Polystan implant
Polystan perfusion cannula
Polystan shunt
Polystan venous return catheter
Polystim electrode
polystyrene foam

polysulfide impression material
polysulfide rubber impression
    material
polysyndactyly
Polytec LaseAway Q-switched
    ruby laser
PolyTech nonlatex self-adhering
    urinary external catheter
polytef soft tissue patch
polytef-sheathed needle
polytetrafluoroethylene-covered
    stent
polytetrafluoroethylene (PTFE)
    prosthesis
polytetrafluoroethylene (PTFE)
    stent graft
polytetrafluoroethylene graft
    (PTFE graft)
polytetrafluoroethylene implant
polytetrafluoroethylene
    membrane graft
polytetrafluoroethylene mesh
polytome
polytome instrument
Polytrac Gomez retractor
Polytrac retractor
PolyTrach dressing
polyunguia
polyurethane bandage
polyurethane elastomer material
polyurethane foam dressing
polyurethane foam embolus
polyurethane graft
polyurethane implant
polyurethane implant material
polyurethane nasoenteric
    catheter
polyurethane packing
polyurethane prosthesis
polyurethane stent
polyurethane-coated silicone
    breast implant
polyuria
polyvinyl alcohol
polyvinyl alcohol foam
polyvinyl alcohol splint
polyvinyl alcohol splinting
    material
polyvinyl alcohol sponge
polyvinyl bougie
polyvinyl catheter
polyvinyl chloride balloon

polyvinyl chloride endotracheal tube
polyvinyl curet
polyvinyl dilator
polyvinyl drain
polyvinyl graft
polyvinyl implant
polyvinyl implant material
polyvinyl prosthesis
polyvinyl sponge
polyvinyl sponge implant
polyvinyl tube
polyvinyl tubing
Polyviolene polyester material
Polyviolene polyester sutures
PolyWic dressing
PolyWic wound filling material
POM (peripheral osteoma of the mandible)
Pomeranz aortic clamp
Pomeranz hiatal hernia retractor
Pomeranz retractor
Pomeroy ear syringe
Pomeroy manner
Pomeroy operation
Pomeroy salpingectomy
Pomeroy sterilization
Pomeroy syringe
Pomeroy tubal ligation
pommel cushion
POMS 20/50 oxygen conservation device
Poncet operation
Ponka anesthetic technique
Ponka herniorrhaphy
Ponka local anesthesia technique
Ponka technique for local anesthesia
pons (*pl.* pontes)
pons cerebelli
pons hepatis
pons oblongata
pons tarini
pons varolii
Ponseti splint
Ponsky Endo Sock retrieval bag
Ponsky Endo-Sock specimen retrieval bag
Ponsky PEG tube
Ponsky guidewire insertion technique

Ponsky-Gauderer PEG procedure
Ponsky-Gauderer PEG tube
pont of Arrhigi
Ponten fasciocutaneous flap
Ponten-type tubed pedicle
pontes (*sing.* pons)
pontile hemianesthesia
pontine angle
pontine flexure
pontine hemorrhage
pontine lesions
pontine paramedian reticular formation
pontine tumor
Pontocaine anesthetic agent
pontomedullary junction
pontoon spica cast
Ponten fasciocutaneous flap
Pool Pfeiffer self-locking clip
pool sucker
Poole abdominal suction tube
Poole suction tip
Poole suction tube
Poole trocar
poorly defined
poorly differentiated
poorly visualized
POP bandage (plaster-of-Paris bandage)
pop scar
Pope halo dressing
Pope Merocel ear packing
Pope Merocel ear wick
Pope rectal knife
Pope wick
popliteal aneurysm
popliteal artery
popliteal artery occlusive disease (PAOD)
popliteal bypass
popliteal cyst
popliteal entrapment
popliteal fossa
popliteal groove
popliteal incision
popliteal lymph node
popliteal muscle
popliteal nerve
popliteal notch
popliteal pulse
popliteal retractor
popliteal space

popliteal vein
popliteal web syndrome
pop-off needle
pop-off sutures
pop-on self-adhering male external catheter
Poppen aortic clamp
Poppen coagulator
Poppen electrosurgical coagulator
Poppen elevator
Poppen fashion
Poppen forceps
Poppen Gigli-saw guide
Poppen intervertebral disk forceps
Poppen intervertebral disk rongeur
Poppen laminectomy rongeur
Poppen needle
Poppen periosteal elevator
Poppen pituitary rongeur
Poppen rongeur
Poppen scissors
Poppen suction tube
Poppen sympathectomy scissors
Poppen ventricular needle
Poppen-Blalock carotid artery clamp
Poppen-Gelpi laminectomy self-retaining retractor
Poppers tonsillar guillotine
poppet
    ball poppet
    barium-impregnated poppet
    disk poppet
    prosthetic poppet
    prosthetic valve poppet
poppet valve
porcelain aorta
porcelain cervical ditching technique
porcelain fracture
porcelain gallbladder
porcelain inlay
porcine graft
porcine heart valve
porcine heterograft
porcine heterograft prosthesis
porcine valve
porcine xenograft
porcupine skin

porencephalic cyst
Porex implant
Porex Medpor implant
Porex nerve locator
Porex PHA implant
Porex tissue expander
Porges Neoflex dilator
Porges stone dislodger
Porites coral material
Porocoat coating
Porocoat material
Porocool prosthesis
porokeratosis
Porolon sponge
poroplastic splint
porotomy
porous bones
porous coat cup for Richards hip prosthesis
porous coated anatomic knee prosthesis (PCA knee prosthesis)
porous coating
porous filter membrane
porous hydroxyapatite
porous ingrowth fixation
porous materials
porous metallic stent
porous polyethylene implant
porous prosthetic materials
porous-coated anatomic
poorly compliant bladder
Porro cesarean hysterectomy
Porro cesarean section
Porro hysterectomy
Porro operation
Porro-Veit operation
Porstmann technique
port
    A-Port implantable port
    Berkeley infusion terminal port
    butterfly needle infusion port
    CathLink 20 implanted port
    Celsite brachial port
    Celsite implanted port
    Celsite pediatric port
    chest port
    Cordis multipurpose access port
    Dialock access port
    endoscopic access port (EAP)

port (*continued*)
  endoscopic threaded imaging
    port
  EndoTIP imaging port
  Gill-Welsh guillotine port
  Hassan-type port
  Hasson blunt port
  implantable infusion port
  Infuse-A-Port port
  infusion port
  injection port
  low-profile, port implantable
    port
  Luer-Lok port
  lumbar port
  mandibular port
  OmegaPort access port
  periumbilical port
  Quinton Q-Port vascular
    access port
  single port
  supraclavicular port
  tangential port
  Thora-Port port
  Titanium VasPort port
  treatment port
  Universal catheter access port
  Vasport access port
  venous access port
  Visiport port
  Vortex Clear-Flow port
port displacement
port incision
port of entry
port protector
port site hernia
port site metastasis
port wine mark
porta hepatis
porta hepatis plexus
porta lienis
Porta Pulse 3 portable
    defibrillator
portable aspirator
portable C-arm image intensifier
    fluoroscopy
portable cephalostat
portable dialysis unit
portable insulin infusion
    pump
portable respirator
portable suction aspirator

portable topical hyperbaric
    oxygen extremity chamber
Port-A-Cath device
Port-A-Cath implantable catheter
portacaval anastomosis
portacaval H graft
portacaval shunt
portacaval shunt operation
portacaval transposition
port-access technique for
    coronary bypass surgery
portal bifurcation
portal block
portal cannula
portal catheter
portal circulation
portal decompression
portal decompression surgery
portal drainage
portal eosinophilic
    inflammation
portal fissure
portal hypertension
portal hypertensive bleeding
portal infusion
portal lymphadenopathy
portal nodal involvement
portal obstruction
Portal Pro 2 treatment chair
portal shunt
portal sinus
portal space
portal systemic anastomosis
portal to systemic venous shunt
portal tract inflammation
portal triad clamping
portal vascular bed
portal vein catheterization
portal vein obstruction
portal vein reconstruction
portal vein resection
portal vein thrombosis
portal venography
portal-collateral circulation
portal-hypophysial circulation
portal-systemic encephalopathy
    (PSE)
portal-systemic shunt
portal-systemic shunt surgery
Porta-Lung noninvasive
    extrathoracic ventilator
Portaray dental x-ray unit

portarenal shunt
Porta-Resp monitor
Porta-Stat cephalostat
Portazam portable exam chair
Portdial kidney machine
Porter duodenal forceps
Porterfield catheter
Porter-Kolpe biliary biopsy set
Porter-O-Surgical cutter
Porter-Richardson-Vainio elbow
　　synovectomy
Porter-Richardson-Vainio
　　technique
Portex bacterial filter
Portex Blue Line tracheostomy
　　tube
Portex cannula
Portex chorionic villus sampling
　　catheter
Portex nasopharyngeal airway
Portex Neo-Vac meconium
　　suction device
Portex nylon cannula
Portex Per-fit tracheostomy kit
Portex Per-Fit tracheostomy tube
Portex preformed blue line
　　tracheal tube
Portex speaking tube
Portex SS endotracheal tube cuff
Portex Thermo-Vent heat and
　　moisture device
Portex ThermoVent heat and
　　moisture exchanger
Portex tracheostomy
Portex tracheostomy tube
Portex endotracheal tube
　　cuff
Portex-Gibbon catheter
portligature
Portmann drill
Portmann interposition
　　operation
Portmann retractor
Portmann speculum
Portmann speculum holder
portmanteau procedure
Portnoy catheter
Portnoy DPV device
Portnoy multiflanged catheter
Portnoy ventricular cannula
Portnoy ventricular catheter
Portnoy ventricular-end shunt

portoenterostomy
　　Anderson portoenterostomy
　　Kasai portoenterostomy
portogram
portograph
portography
　　percutaneous transhepatic
　　　portography
　　splenic portography
　　transhepatic portography
portoportal anastomosis
portopulmonary shunt
portopulmonary venous
　　anastomosis
portorenal shunt
portosystemic anastomosis
portosystemic collateral
　　circulation
portosystemic encephalopathy
portosystemic shunt
portosystemic vascular shunt
Porto-vac catheter
Porto-vac suction tube
PortSaver PercLoop device
port-wine hemangioma
port-wine macrocheilia
port-wine stain
port-wine stain birthmark
Porzett splint
Posada fracture
Posada-Vasco orbital retractor
Posey bar kit
Posey belt
Posey grip
Posey restraint
Posey sling
Posey snare
Posey support
Posican scanner
Posilok instrument holder
Posi-Stop drill
position
　　abdominal brace position
　　Adams position
　　adduction position
　　airplane position
　　Albers-Schoenberg position
　　Albert position
　　anatomic position
　　anatomical position
　　angular position
　　anomalous position

position (*continued*)
  antecolic position
  anterior oblique position
  antero-oblique position
  anteverted position
  antiembolic position
  anti-Trendelenburg position
  arch-and-slouch position
  arm extension position
  arm position
  arm-extension position
  asynclitic position
  back-up position
  backward position
  barber chair position
  batrachian position
  bayonet fracture position
  beach chair position
  Bertel x-ray position
  birthing position
  bisecting angle cone position
  Blackett-Healy position
  body position
  Bonner position
  Boyce position
  Bozeman position
  Brickner position
  brow position
  brow-anterior position
  brow-down position
  brow-posterior position
  brow-up position
  Buie position
  calcaneal stance position
  calibrated position
  Camp-Coventry position
  cardiac position
  cardinal position
  Casselberry position
  catheter position
  centric position
  cervical position
  chest position
  chin position
  claw-toe position
  Cleaves position
  coiled position
  condylar hinge position
  consonant position
  convergence position
  conversion of position
  corrected sternal position

position (*continued*)
  cottonloader position
  craniocaudad position
  cross-table lateral position
  curved flank position
  cuspid-molar position
  decortical position
  decubitus position
  Depage position
  dissociated position
  distoangular position
  dorsal decubitus position
  dorsal elevated position
  dorsal inertia position
  dorsal lithotomy position
  dorsal position
  dorsal recumbent position
  dorsal rigid position
  dorsal supine position
  dorsodecubitus position
  dorsorecumbent position
  dorsosacral position
  dorsosupine position
  Duncan position
  eccentric jaw position
  Edebohls position
  electrical heart position
  elevated position
  Elliot position
  emprosthotonos position
  en face position
  English position
  equinus position
  erect position
  eversion position
  exaggerated sniffing position
  extended position
  extra-abdominal position
  extrathoracic position
  extreme Trendelenburg position
  face-down position
  face-to-pubes position
  Feist-Mankin position
  fetal head position
  fetal position
  Fick position
  figure-4 position
  final cone position
  final consonant position
  first cone position
  flank position
  flexed position

position (*continued*)
  flexion position
  forehead-nose position
  Fowler position
  fracture position
  French position
  frogleg position
  frog-legged position
  froglike position
  frontoanterior position
  frontoposterior position
  frontotransverse position
  Fuchs position
  functional position
  fusion-free position
  Gaynor-Hart position
  genucubital position
  genufacial position
  genupectoral position
  gingival position
  Grashey position
  gravity-free position
  greater curve position
  head and neck in extended
    position
  head dependent position
  head-up tilt position
  heart position
  heterophoric position
  high stirrups position
  hinge position
  hook-lying position
  horizontal position
  hornpipe position
  incomplete breech position
  infraumbilical position
  initial consonant position
  intercuspal position
  intraperitoneal position
  intrathoracic position
  intrinsic minus position
  inversion position
  inverted jackknife position
  Isherwood position
  jackknife position
  Jahss position
  James position
  jaw-to-jaw position
  jet pilot position
  Johnson position
  joint position
  Jones position

position (*continued*)
  Jonge position
  jumper-knee position
  kidney position
  knee-chest position
  knee-elbow position
  kneeling position
  kneeling-squatting position
  Kraske position
  Kurzbauer position
  Low-Beer position
  Lange position
  LAO position
  Larkin position
  lateral anterior position
  lateral anterior x-ray position
  lateral decubitus position
  lateral position
  lateral prone position
  lateral rectus position
  lateral recumbent position
  Law position
  Lawrence position
  leapfrog position
  left anterior oblique position
  left decubitus position
  left lateral decubitus position
  left lateral position
  left mentoanterior position
    (LMA position)
  left mentoposterior position
    (LMP position)
  left mentotransverse position
    (LMT position)
  left occipitoanterior position
    (LOA position)
  left occipitoposterior position
    (LOP position)
  left occipitotransverse
    position (LOT position)
  left sacroanterior position
    (LSA position)
  left sacroposterior position
    (LSP position)
  left scapuloanterior position
    (LScA position)
  left scapuloposterior position
    (LScP position)
  left-side-down position
  Leonard-George position
  levo-transposed position
  Lewis position

position (*continued*)
Lindblom position
lithotomy position
lithotomy-Trendelenburg
  position
Lloyd Davis modified
  lithotomy position
LMA position (left
  mentoanterior position)
LMP position (left
  mentoposterior position)
LMT position (left
  mentotransverse position)
LOA position (left
  occipitoanterior position)
LOP position (left
  occipitoposterior position)
Lorenz position
LOT position (left
  occipitotransverse position)
lotus position
LSA position (left
  sacroanterior position)
LScA position (left
  scapuloanterior position)
LScP position (left
  scapuloposterior position)
LSP position (left
  sacroposterior position)
Low-Beer position
mandibular hinge position
mandibular rest position
maternal birthing position
Mayer position
Mayo-Robson position
median occlusal position
mentoanterior position
mentoposterior position
mentotransverse position
mentum anterior position
mentum posterior position
mentum transverse position
Mercurio position
mesioangular position
midline position
military brace position
military tuck position
Miller position
missionary position
modified lithotomy position
modified position
Moynihan position

position (*continued*)
near-anatomic position
neck extension position
neutral hip position
neutral position
neutral spine position
Noble position
nonphysiologic position
normal anatomic position
oblique position
obstetric position
obstetrical position
occipitoanterior position
occipitoposterior position
occipitosacral position
occipitotransverse position
occlusal position
Ochsner position
o'clock position (1 through
  12)
opisthotonos position
orthopnea position
orthotonos position
overcorrected position
over-the-top position
Owen position
PA position (posteroanterior
  position)
paralleling cone position
park-bench position
Pean position
Pearson position
persistent occiput posterior
  position
Phalen position
physiologic rest position
placed in position
posterior border position
posteroanterior position
postreduction position
postural resting position
prayer position
premuscular position
primary position
Proetz position
prone jackknife position
prone position
prone split-leg position
protrusive occlusal position
proximal bow position
pterygoid position
pulmonary position

position (*continued*)

quasistatic stressed position
RAO position
reclining position
rectus position
recumbent position
rest position
retrocolic position
retromuscular position
retruded position
reverse Trendelenburg position
reverse Waters x-ray position
reverted to normal position
Rhese position
right acromiodorsoposterior position
right anterior oblique position
right antero-oblique position
right decubitus position
right lateral position
right mentoanterior position (RMA position)
right mentoposterior position (RMP position)
right mentotransverse position (RMT position)
right occipitoanterior position (ROA position)
right occipitoposterior position (ROP position)
right occipitotranverse position (ROT position)
right sacroanterior position (RSA position)
right sacroposterior position (RSP position)
right scapuloanterior position (RScA position)
right scapuloposterior position (RScP position)
right-side-down position
RMA position (right mentoanterior position)
RMP position (right mentoposterior position)
RMT position (right mentotransverse position)
ROA position (right occipitoanterior position)
Robson position

position (*continued*)

ROP position (right occipitoposterior position)
Rose head-extension position
ROT position (right occipitotransverse position)
RScA position (right scapuloanterior position)
RScP position (right scapuloposterior position)
RSP position (right sacroposterior position)
SA position (sacroanterior position)
sacroanterior position (SA position)
sacrodextra anterior position
sacrodextra posterior position
sacroposterior position (SP position)
sacrotransverse position
Samuel position
scapuloanterior position
scapuloposterior position
Schuller position
scissor-leg position
scultetus position
semierect position
semi-Fowler position
semilateral position
semioblique position
semiprone position
semireclining position
semirecumbent position
semiupright position
series II acetabular cup position
Settegast position
shock position
shoe-and-stocking position
Simon position
Sims position
sitting position
ski position
sniffing position
SP position (sacroposterior position)
spinal fusion position
static position
Staunig position
Stecher position
steep Trendelenburg position

position (*continued*)
Stenver position
Stern position
sternal position
subcostal position
sulcus fixated position
supine position
Tarrant position
Taylor position
terminal hinge position
tonsil position
tooth position
tooth-to-tooth position
Towne position
translational position
Trendelenburg position
tricuspid position
tuck position
Twining position
unbuckled flat position
upright position
usual anatomic position
Valentine position
vertex position
vertical divergence position
Walcher position
Waters x-ray position
Waters-Waldron position
Wigby-Taylor position
Williams position
Wolfenden position
W-sitting position
Zanelli position
position ametropia
position in space
positional release therapy
positioned and draped
positioner
acetabular cup positioner
acetabular positioner
Assistant Free Stulberg leg
positioner
Bareskin knee positioner
beach chair positioner
body positioner
Body Wrap foam positioner
BodyCushion positioner
Cook stent positioner
Craniad cup positioner
cup positioner
eggcrate positioner
Foot Waffle positioner

positioner (*continued*)
forehead positioner
Grasshopper positioner
Hold-and-Hold positioner
IMP Universal lateral
positioner
Kirschenbaum foot positioner
knee positioner
lateral positioner
leg positioner
Mark II Stulberg hip
positioner
Mark II Wixson hip positioner
MB&J knee positioner
McCaffrey positioner
McConnell shoulder
positioner
McGuire pelvic positioner
Medline positioner
Miller bracket positioner
Montreal positioner
Picket Fence leg positioner
Prep-Assist positioner
Profex arthroscopic leg
positioner
ProForm positioner
Schlein shoulder positioner
shoulder abduction
positioner
Stulberg hip positioner
Stulberg Mark II leg
positioner
SurgAssist leg positioner
Ther-A-Shapes positioner
TMJ head positioner
Vac-Pac positioner
Wixson hip positioner
Zimfoam pad and patient
positioner
positioning needle
positioning of patient
positioning pillow
positioning platform
position-sensing catheter
positive airway pressure
positive bowel sounds
positive charge
positive control enzyme
induction
positive culture
positive end-airway pressure
(PEAP)

positive end-expiratory phase (PEEP)
positive end-expiratory pressure (PEEP)
positive eyepiece
positive finding
positive maneuver
positive node
positive pressure
positive reaction
positive resection margin
positive result
positive shear test (excessive skin laxity)
positive surgical margin
positive torsion
positive x-ray finding
positive-pressure ventilation (PPV)
Positran technique
Positrap mini-retrieval basket
Positrap retriever
positrocephalogram
positrocephalography
Positrol cardiac device
Positrol catheter
Positrol Bernstein catheter
Positrol USCI catheter
positron computed tomography
positron emission tomography (PET)
positron emission tomography balloon (PET balloon)
positron emission tomography-guided biopsy
positron scintillation camera
Posner diagnostic gonioprism
Posner diagnostic lens
Posner procedure
Posner slit lamp
Posner surgical gonioprism
post C-section
post dam
Post forceps
post implant
post laser balm
Post total shoulder arthroplasty
Post trocar and washing cannula
Post washing cannula
postablation defect
postabortal infection
postacute phase

postadrenalectomy syndrome
postage-stamp skin graft
postalveolar cleft palate fistulation (CPF)
postanal gut
postanal pit
postanal repair
postanesthesia
postanesthesia recovery room (PAR room)
postanesthetic central nervous system dysfunction
postangioplasty angiogram
postangioplasty intimal flap
postaural approach
postauricular and retroauricular scalping (PARAS)
postauricular approach
postauricular area
postauricular artery
postauricular ear dressing
postauricular graft
postauricular incision
postauricular retractor
postauricular sulcus
postaxial duplication of the 5th ray (types I-III)
postaxial muscle
postbiopsy renal AV fistula
postbiopsy vascular complication
postbulbar diverticula
postbulbar duodenal ulcer
postbulbar ulcer
postburn bone marrow failure
postcannulation
postcapillary venules
postcardinal veins
postcardiotomy intra-aortic balloon pumping
postcardiotomy syndrome
postcaval shunt
postcaval ureter
postcentral gyrus
postcentral vein
postcerebrovascular accident
postcesarean anesthesia
postcesarean section
postcholecystectomy syndrome
postcoital bleeding
postcolonoscopy distention syndrome

postcommissurotomy syndrome
postcoronary angioplasty
postcricoid region
postcricoid space
postcricoid web
postcystoscopy
postductal coarctation
postembolization syndrome
posterior fossa circulation
posterior abdominal wall
posterior alveolar artery
posterior ampullary nerve
posterior annular ligament
posterior approach
posterior arch fracture
posterior articular aorta
posterior aspect
posterior auricular artery
posterior auricular branch of
    external carotid artery
posterior auricular flap
posterior auricular groove
posterior auricular muscle
posterior auricular nerve
posterior auricular vein
posterior belly
posterior bone block
posterior border jaw relation
posterior border movement
posterior border of petrous
    portion of temporal bone
posterior border position
posterior bow femoral fracture
posterior canal separator
posterior capsular zonular
    barrier
posterior capsule
posterior capsulorrhaphy
posterior capsulotomy
posterior cecal artery
posterior cerebral artery
posterior cervical fixation
posterior cervical fusion
posterior cervical lip
posterior cervical space
posterior chamber intraocular
    lens
posterior chamber lens implant
posterior circulation aneurysm
posterior circumflex humeral
    artery
posterior colporrhaphy

posterior column cordotomy
posterior column fracture
posterior commissure
posterior communicating artery
posterior condyloid foramen
posterior conjunctival arteries
posterior convex intraocular
    lens
posterior costotransversectomy
    approach
posterior cranial fossa
    meningioma
posterior cricoarytenoid muscle
posterior crossbite
posterior cruciate ligament
posterior crus
posterior cutaneous femoral
    nerve
posterior cutaneous nerve
posterior cyst
posterior descending artery
    (PDA)
posterior diaphragmatic
    gastropexy
posterior distraction
    instrumentation
posterior element fracture
posterior ethmoid
posterior ethmoidal artery
posterior ethmoidal branch of
    ophthalmic artery
posterior ethmoidal foramen
posterior ethmoidal nerve
posterior exenteration
posterior explant
posterior facial height
posterior facial vein
posterior false ligament
posterior flap technique
posterior focal point
posterior footplate pick
posterior forceps
posterior fossa
posterior fossa craniotomy
posterior fossa decompression
posterior fossa retractor
posterior fracture
posterior fracture-dislocation
posterior fundoplasty
posterior ghosting artifacts
posterior hemicircular incision
posterior hip dislocation

posterior hook-rod spinal instrumentation
posterior horn
posterior impaction
posterior incision
posterior incudal ligament
posterior infarction
posterior inferior cerebellar artery (PICA)
posterior inferior communicating artery (PICA)
posterior intercostal arteries
posterior intercostal veins
posterior internal orbital canal
posterior interosseous artery
posterior interosseous nerve
posterior interosseous nerve compression syndrome
posterior interosseous nerve palsy
posterior interventricular
posterior intraoccipital joint
posterior intraoccipital synchondrosis
posterior inverted-U approach
posterior iridodialysis
posterior jejunostomy
posterior labial artery
posterior labial hernia
posterior labial nerves
posterior labial veins
posterior lacrimal crest
posterior lamina
posterior laparoscopic approach
posterior lateral nasal arteries
posterior layer
posterior leaf of broad ligament
posterior leaf-spring ankle-foot orthosis
posterior ligament
posterior lobule
posterior longitudinal bundle
posterior lower cervical spine surgery
posterior lumbar approach
posterior lumbar interbody fusion (PLIF)
posterior lumbar interbody fusion procedure
posterior lumbar interbody fusion surgery

posterior lumbar spine and sacrum surgery
posterior maxillary segmental osteotomy
posterior median fissure
posterior median sulcus
posterior meningeal artery
posterior midline approach
posterior naris
posterior nasal spine
posterior nasal spine to soft palate (PNSP)
posterior neck surface coil
posterior nephrectomy
posterior nerve root
posterior occipital fontanelle
posterior occipitocervical approach
posterior occlusal discrepancy
posterior occlusion
posterior palatal seal area
posterior palate hook
posterior palatine arch
posterior palatine artery
posterior palatine sutures
posterior palatoplasty
posterior pelvic exenteration
posterior pillar
posterior Polya procedure
posterior rectopexy
posterior rectus sheath
posterior reduction device
posterior repair
posterior rhizotomy
posterior ring fracture
posterior scalene muscle
posterior screw fixation
posterior scrotal nerves
posterior scrotal veins
posterior segment
posterior segmental fixation
posterior septal artery
posterior septal artery of nose
posterior septal space
posterior shoulder dislocation
posterior sinuses
posterior skin flap
posterior spinal artery
posterior spinal fusion
posterior splint
posterior stab incision

posterior subcapsular cataract (PSC)
posterior sulcus obliteration
posterior superior alveolar artery
posterior surface of maxilla
posterior suspensory ligament
posterior symblepharon
posterior synechia formation
posterior table
posterior talocalcaneal ligament
posterior temporal diploic vein
posterior thigh bar
posterior tibial artery
posterior tibial muscle
posterior tibial nerve
posterior tibial recurrent artery
posterior tibial tendon
posterior tibial vein
posterior transolecranon approach
posterior transthoracic incision
posterior tympanic artery
posterior upper cervical spine surgery
posterior urethral retractor
posterior urethroscope
posterior vagal trunk
posterior vaginal hernia
posterior vein of left ventricle
posterior view
posterior vitrectomy
posterior wall fracture
posterior-interbody lumbar spinal fusion
posterior-lateral lobule
posterior-lateral lumbar spinal fusion
posteriorly
posteroanterior (PA)
posteroanterior film
posteroanterior lordotic projection
posteroanterior mandible radiograph
posteroanterior position
posteroanterior sinus radiograph
posteroanterior skull radiograph
posteroanterior study
posteroanterior view
posteroanterior x-ray view
posteroinferior aspect

posterointermediate sulcus
posterolateral approach
posterolateral aspect
posterolateral bone graft placement
posterolateral bundle
posterolateral costotransversectomy incision
posterolateral costotransversectomy technique
posterolateral flap
posterolateral fontanelle
posterolateral herniation
posterolateral incision
posterolateral infarction
posterolateral interbody fusion
posterolateral lumbosacral fusion
posterolateral nasal artery
posterolateral sclerosis
posterolateral sulcus
posteromedial approach
posteromedial aspect
posteromedial dislocation
posteromedian lobule
posterosuperior iliac spine
posterotemporal fontanelle
posterotemporal region
posterotransverse diameter
postevacuation film
postexchange bilirubin
postexcision cavity
postexcitation wave
postextraction bleeding
postextraction hemorrhage
postextubation laryngospasm
postfistula placement
postfracture lesion
postfundoplication syndrome
postganglionic neuron
postgastrectomy bleed
postgastrectomy cancer
postgastrectomy dysfunction
postgastrectomy hemorrhage
postgastrectomy syndrome
postglenoid foramen
postglomerular arteriole
Post-Harrington erysiphake
postinfarction ventriculoseptal defect

postinflammatory
hypopigmentation
postinflammatory polyp
postinjury immunologic defect
postirradiation fracture
postirradiation sialadenitis
postirradiation syndrome
postischemic administration
postischemic stenosis
postlaminectomy syndrome
postlaryngectomy
postlaser conization
postlaser edema
postligation
postlumbar puncture
postlymphangiography
abdomen
postmastectomy
postmastectomy reconstruction
postmaxillectomy collapsed
cheek
postmaxillectomy deformity
postmembrane rupture
postmenopausal bleeding
postmenopausal breasts
postmortem clot
postmortem examination
postmortem suture needle
postmyocardial infarction
postnasal applicator
postnasal balloon
postnasal bleeding
postnasal catarrh
postnasal discharge
postnasal dressing
postnasal drip
postnasal sponge forceps
postnasal tube
postnatal therapy
postnecrotic tissue
postnormal occlusion
postoperative abscess
postoperative adhesions
postoperative airway
obstruction
postoperative analgesia
postoperative analgesic
postoperative anastomotic leak
postoperative anesthesia
postoperative anticoagulation
therapy
postoperative bleeding

postoperative care
postoperative change
postoperative chemotherapy
postoperative choledochoscopy
postoperative complication
postoperative condition
postoperative course
postoperative death
postoperative diagnosis
postoperative discomfort
postoperative ductal dilation
postoperative dysphagia
postoperative flexor tendon
traction brace
postoperative followup
postoperative followup
evaluation
postoperative forehead descent
postoperative fracture
postoperative hematoma
postoperative hemorrhage
postoperative hepatic failure
postoperative hypertension
postoperative ileus
postoperative immobilization
postoperative infection
postoperative irradiation
postoperative irrigation-suction
drainage
postoperative liver failure
postoperative mammary
support
postoperative migration
postoperative pain
postoperative pleurobiliary
fistula
postoperative progress
postoperative puckers
postoperative reaction
postoperative recovery
postoperative regimen for oral
early feeding (PROEF)
postoperative relief
postoperative renal dysfunction
postoperative repair
postoperative respiratory
complication
postoperative shock
postoperative status
postoperative systemic
chemotherapy
postoperative tetany

postoperative ventilation
postoperative vomiting
postoperative withdrawal
postoperative wound infection
postoral arches
postorbital pain
postpalatal seal area
postpartum hemorrhage
postpartum sterilization
postpeel hyperpigmentation
postpeel hypopigmentation
postpeel pigmentary changes
postperfusion syndrome
postpericardiotomy syndrome
postpharyngeal abscess
postpharyngeal space
postphlebitic syndrome
postplaced sutures
postpoliomyelitic contracture
postpolypectomy bleed
postpolypectomy coagulation
    syndrome
postpolypectomy hemorrhage
postponed labor
postprandial distention
postprandial pain
postpyloric feeding tube
postradiation fistula
postradiation therapy
postradiation xerostomia
postradical neck dissection
postreduction films
postreduction position
postreduction status
postrenal
postresection defect
postresection filling technique
postsclerotherapy
    hyperpigmentation
postseizure
postsphenoid bone
postsphincterotomy ERCP
    cannulation
postsplenectomy
postsplenectomy complication
postsplenic
poststenotic dilatation
poststenotic dilation
poststyloid space
postsurgery exercises
postsurgical abdomen
postsurgical anomaly

postsurgical course
postsurgical endoscopy
postsurgical followup
postsurgical nervous damage
postsurgical recurrent ulcer
postsynaptic membrane
post-term birth
posttetanic count monitoring
posttransfusion
posttranslation modification
posttransplant
    immunosuppression
    therapy
posttransplant
    lymphoproliferative disease
    (PTLD)
posttransplant
    lymphoproliferative
    disorder (PTLD)
posttrauma
posttraumatic
    autotransplantation
posttraumatic hemorrhage
posttraumatic lipoma
posttraumatic pancreatic-
    cutaneous fistula
posttraumatic renal failure
posttraumatic rhinoplasty
posttraumatic spinal deformity
posttraumatic spondylitis
posttraumatic stress disorder
posttraumatic subcapsular
    hepatic fluid collection
posttreatment hemorrhage
posttubal ligation syndrome
post-TUR clamp
post-TUR irrigation clamp
post-TUR irrigation control
    clamp
Post-T-Vac vacuum erection
    device
postural changes
postural deformity
postural drainage
postural fixation back maneuver
postural fixation test
postural hypertension
postural hypotension
postural reduction
postural resting position
postural therapy
postural tone

postural version
Posture Curve lumbar cushion
Posture Wedge seat cushion
postureteral ligation
postureteroscopic manipulation
posturethroplasty review
    speculum
postvagotomy dysphagia
postvagotomy gastroparesis
postvagotomy syndrome
postvoiding cystogram
postvoiding cystography
postvoiding film
postvoiding residual (PVR)
postzygomatic space
Potain aspirating trocar
Potain aspirator
Potain sign
Potain trocar
potassium space
potassium titanyl phosphate
    laser
potential
    compound muscle action
        potential (CMAP)
    demarcation potential
    denervation potential
    electric potential
    electrode potential
    evoked action potential
    evoked potential
    extraneous electrode
        potential
    fasciculation potential
    fibrillating action potentials
    fibrillation potential
    His potential
    laser-evoked potential
    membrane potential
    motor nerve action potential
        (MAP)
    nerve action potential
    reduction potential
    risk potential
    somatosensory evoked
        potential (SEP)
    teratogenic potential
    visual evoked potential
        (VEP)
potential acuity meter (PAM)
potential cautery
potentially curative procedure

potentially lethal x-ray damage
    repair
potentially resectable lesion
potentiometer
Potenza finger arthrodesis
Poth operation
Potocky needle
Pott abscess
Pott aneurysm
Pott ankle fracture
Pott eversion osteotomy
Pott fracture
Pott gangrene
Pott paraplegia
Pott puffy tumor
Pott splint
Pott tibial osteotomy
Potter coarctation forceps
Potter classification of
    polycystic kidney
Potter facies
Potter knee arthrodesis
Potter modified knife
Potter needle
Potter sickle knife
Potter sponge forceps
Potter tonsillar forceps
Potter version
Potter-Bucky diaphragm
Potts 60-degree angled scissors
Potts anastomosis
Potts aortic clamp
Potts aortic-pulmonary artery
    anastomosis
Potts bronchial forceps
Potts bulldog forceps
Potts cardiovascular clamp
Potts coarctation clamp
Potts coarctation forceps
Potts dental elevator
Potts dilator
Potts dissector
Potts divisional clamp
Potts ductus clamp
Potts elevator
Potts expansile dilator
Potts expansile knife
Potts expansile valvulotome
Potts fixation forceps
Potts infant rib shears
Potts intestinal forceps
Potts knife

Potts ligature
Potts needle
Potts operation
Potts patent ductus clamp
Potts patent ductus forceps
Potts periosteotome
Potts procedure
Potts pulmonic clamp
Potts rib shears
Potts scissors
Potts shears
Potts shunt
Potts splint
Potts tenaculum
Potts tenotomy scissors
Potts thumb forceps
Potts tie sutures
Potts valvulotome
Potts vascular scissors
Potts-Cournand angiography
    needle
Potts-DeBakey clamp
Potts-DeMartel gall duct scissors
Potts-Nevins dressing forceps
Potts-Niedner aorta clamp
Potts-Riker dilator
Potts-Riker valvulotome
Potts-Satinsky clamp
Potts-Smith anastomosis
Potts-Smith aortic clamp
Potts-Smith aortic occlusion
    clamp
Potts-Smith arterial scissors
Potts-Smith bipolar forceps
Potts-Smith cardiovascular
    scissors
Potts-Smith dissecting
    scissors
Potts-Smith dressing forceps
Potts-Smith monopolar
    forceps
Potts-Smith needle holder
Potts-Smith operation
Potts-Smith pulmonic clamp
Potts-Smith reverse scissors
Potts-Smith side-to-side
    anastomosis
Potts-Smith tenaculum
Potts-Smith tissue forceps
Potts-Smith vascular scissors
Potts-Smith-Gibson operation
Potts-Yasargil scissors

pouch
1-piece ostomy pouch
2-piece ostomy pouch
3-loop ileal pouch
Bard closed-end adhesive
    pouch
Bard drainage adhesive pouch
Bard ostomy pouch
Bard security pouch
bladder replacement urinary
    pouch
blind rectal pouch
blind upper esophageal
    pouch
Bongort 1-piece drainable
    pouch
Bongort 1-piece ostomy
    pouch
Bongort ostomy pouch
Bongort urinary diversion
    pouch
branchial pouch
Broca pouch
Cardio-Cool myocardial pouch
Cardio-Cool myocardial
    protection pouch
CenterPointLock 2-piece
    ostomy system: closed
    pouch
CenterPointLock 2-piece
    ostomy system: drainable
    pouch
cheek pouch
closed-end ostomy pouch
Coloplast colostomy pouch
Coloplast flange pouch
Coloplast 1-piece post-op
    drainable pouch
Coloplast 1-piece small
    drainable pouch
Coloplast 1-piece standard
    drainable pouch
Coloplast pouch
Coloplast 2-piece small
    drainable pouch
Coloplast 2-piece small
    urostomy pouch
coloplasty pouch
Coloset ostomy pouch
colostomy pouch
continent ileal pouch
ConvaTec ostomy pouch

pouch (*continued*)

ConvaTec urostomy pouch
Cymed Micro skin pouch
Dansac 1-piece pouch
Dansac mini 1-piece pouch
Dansac oval 1-piece pouch
Dansac ileal pouch
Dansac Karaya seal pouch
Dansac ostomy pouch
Dansac standard 1-piece
  pouch
dartos pouch
Dennis Brown pouch
dermal pouch
double-loop pouch
Douglas pouch
drainable ostomy pouch
Durahesive Wafer pouch
female urinary pouch
FirstChoice closed pouch
FirstChoice postoperative
  drainable pouch
FirstChoice urostomy pouch
Florida urinary pouch
Fobi pouch
gastric pouch
Guardian 2-piece ostomy
  system: closed pouch
Guardian 2-piece ostomy
  system: drainable pouch
Guardian 2-piece ostomy
  system: urostomy pouch
Hartmann pouch
hepatorenal pouch
hernia pouch
HolliGard seal closed stoma
  pouch
Hollister First Choice pouch
Hollister HolliGard pouch
Hollister Karaya ostomy
  pouch
Hollister Karaya seal pouch
Hollister ostomy pouch
Hollister Premium pouch
H-shaped ileal pouch
Hunt-Lawrence pouch
ileoanal pouch
ileocecal pouch
ileostomy pouch
jejunal pouch
J-shaped ileal pouch
Karaya seal pouch

pouch (*continued*)

Karaya seal closed stoma
  pouch
Kock pouch
laryngeal pouch
lateral-lateral pouch
Le Bag urinary pouch
Lo-Profile urostomy pouch
Mainz urinary reservoir pouch
ManHood absorbent pouch
Mansson urinary pouch
Marlen gas relief pouch
Marlen Odor-Ban pouch
Marlen Solo ileostomy pouch
Marlen zip-closed pouch
Marlen's Ultra 1-piece pouch
Marsupial pouch
Mentor absorbent pouch
MicroSkin urostomy pouch
Morison pouch
Nu-Hope drainable 1-piece
  pouch
Nu-Hope ileostomy pouch
Nu-Hope urinary pouch
open-end ostomy pouch
pacemaker pouch
Padua bladder urinary
  pouch
paravesical pouch
Parks ileostomy pouch
Parsonnet pouch
Parsonnet pulse generator
  pouch
pediatric drainable pouch
pediatric transfer pouch
pediatric urostomy pouch
Penn pouch
pharyngeal pouch
Physick pouch
plastic bridge colostomy
  pouch
Pleatman pouch
Preemie pouch
Premier drainable pouch
Premier urostomy pouch
Premium closed pouch
Premium drainable pouch
Prussak pouch
QT pouch
Rathke pouch
Reality vaginal pouch
rectal pouch

pouch (*continued*)
  rectouterine pouch
  rectovaginal pouch
  rectovesical pouch
  renal pouch
  retracted penis pouch
  Rowland pouch
  Sheet Plus pouch
  side-to-side jejunal pouch
  Squibb Sur-Fit ostomy pouch
  Squibb urostomy pouch
  S-shaped ileal pouch
  S-shaped pouch
  Studer pouch
  suprapatellar pouch
  Sur-Fit flexible and drainable
    pouch
  Sur-Fit Mini pouch
  Sur-Fit Natura pouch
  Sur-Fit urostomy pouch
  Sur-Fit wafer and drainable
    pouch
  Tena pouch
  Tenador male pouch
  terminal ileal pouch
  Torbot plastic pouch
  Torbot rubber pouch
  United Max-E pouch
  United Surgical Bongort
    Lifestyle pouch
  United Surgical Featherlite
    ileostomy pouch
  United Surgical Shear Plus
    pouch
  United Surgical Soft & Secure
    pouch
  urostomy pouch
  vallecular pouch
  vesicouterine pouch
  VPI nonadhesive pouch
  Willis pouch
  W-shaped ileal pouch
  Zenker pouch
pouch biopsy
pouch dilatation
pouch failure
pouch of Douglas
pouch of Hartmann
pouch of Morison
pouch of Munro
pouch reconstruction
pouched ileostomy

pouchitis
pouchography
pouch-type sling
poudrage
  Beck poudrage
  pleural poudrage
  talc poudrage
Poulard entropion
Poulard operation
Poulard-Pochissov operation
pounds of traction
Poupart inguinal ligament
Poupart ligament shelving edge
Poupart line
Pousson pigtail catheter
Poutasse renal artery clamp
Poutasse renal artery forceps
powder blower
powder board
powder burn
powdered bone graft
power cannula
power Doppler
power Doppler imaging
power Doppler ultrasound
power drill
Power Grip pliers
power injection
power injector
power peak filter
power point
power rasp
power router
power thrombectomy
power-assisted lipoplasty (PAL)
PowerCut drill blade
powered automatic skull
  perforator
powered automatic stopping
  drill point
Powerflex balloon catheter
Powerflex tape
Powerforma surgical drill
PowerGrip stent
Powermatic table
PowerStar bipolar scissors
PowerVision ultrasound
Pozzi operation
Pozzi procedure
Pozzi tenaculum
Pozzi tenaculum forceps
PPD dialyzer

PPG (polypropylene glycol)
PPG probe
PPG-AFO brace (ankle-foot orthosis brace)
PPG-TLSO brace (thoracolumbar standing orthosis brace)
PPT orthotic device
Praeger iris hook
PRAFO adjustable orthotic
PRAFO KAFO attachment
pragmatic anomaly
Prague maneuver
Prall urethral sound
Pram combination occluder
pramoxine hydrochloride anesthetic agent
Pratt anoscope
Pratt antrum curet
Pratt bivalve retractor
Pratt bivalve speculum
Pratt crypt hook
Pratt curet
Pratt cystic hook
Pratt dilator
Pratt director
Pratt ethmoid curet
Pratt hemostatic forceps
Pratt hook
Pratt nasal curet
Pratt open reduction
Pratt probe
Pratt proctoscope
Pratt rectal dilator
Pratt rectal director
Pratt rectal hook
Pratt rectal probe
Pratt rectal scissors
Pratt rectal speculum
Pratt scissors
Pratt sigmoid speculum
Pratt sound
Pratt technique
Pratt tenaculum
Pratt tissue forceps
Pratt T-shaped hemostatic forceps
Pratt urethral sound
Pratt uterine dilator
Pratt vulsellum forceps
Pratt-Sims closure
Pratt-Smith hemostatic forceps
Pratt-Smith tissue-grasping forceps

Pravay syringe
prayer position
preadventitial dissection
prealveolar cleft
preampullary portion of bile duct
preaponeurotic fat
preauricular area
preauricular crease
preauricular cyst
preauricular fistula
preauricular fossa
preauricular groove
preauricular incision
preauricular pain
preauricular point
preauricular radiation therapy
preauricular scar
preauricular sinus
preauricular sulcus
preaxial muscle
preaxial thumb duplication (types I-IV)
preaxillary line
precancerous erythroplakia
precancerous lesion
precancerous polyp
precannulation antibiotic
precapillary anastomosis
precapillary sphincter
precardinal veins
precatheterization
Preceder interventional guidewire
precentral gyrus
Precept DR pacemaker
prechiasmal compression
prechiasmal optic nerve lesion
precipitating cause
precipitating lesion
precipitating noxious event
precipitin tube
Precise anastomotic coupler
Precise disposable skin stapler
precise dissection
precise lesion measuring (PLM)
precise lesion measuring device
Precision Cosmet lens
Precision eye implant
precision lancet cutting needle
Precision miniature and microminiature scalpel

Precision Osteolock femoral
   component
Precision Osteolock femoral
   prosthesis
Precision Osteolock hip
   prosthesis
Precision refractor
Precision Tack instrument
Precision-Cosmet intraocular
   lens implant
PrecisionGlide needle
Preci-Slot dental attachment
Precisor direct-bite biopsy
   forceps
Preci-Vertix kit
preclotted graft
Preclude dura substitute
   prosthesis
Preclude pericardial membrane
Preclude peritoneal membrane
Preclude spinal membrane
Precoat Plus femoral prosthesis
Precoat Plus total hip
precocious metastasis
precollagenous filamentous
   material
precommissural bundle
precompression jig
precontoured unit rod
precordial region
precornified cell
precostal anastomosis
precursor
precursor lesion
precut incision
precut papillotome
precut sphincterotome
precut sutures
Predator balloon catheter
predental space
predentin matrix (PDM)
predialysis plasma phosphate
   concentration
prediastolic murmur
predorsal bundle
pre-eclampsia of pregnancy
pre-eclamptic liver disease
pre-eclamptic toxemia
Preefer eye speculum
pre-ejection time
pre-emptive analgesia
pre-emptive anesthesia

pre-epiglottic space
pre-evacuation film
pre-excitation syndrome
preexisting lesion
prefollicle cells
preformed catheter
preformed clasp
preformed Cordis catheter
preformed polyvinyl chloride
   endotracheal tube
prefrontal bone
prefrontal bone of von
   Bardeleben
prefrontal lobotomy
prefrontal region
preganglionic cardiac
   sympathetic blockade
preganglionic cells
preganglionic neurons
preganglionic sympathetic block
preganglionic sympathetic
   denervation
preglenoid plane
preglomerular arteriole
pregnancy
   1st trimester of pregnancy
   2nd trimester of pregnancy
   3rd trimester of pregnancy
   abdominal pregnancy
   Baudelocque operation for
     extrauterine pregnancy
   bigeminal pregnancy
   cervical pregnancy
   cornual pregnancy
   ectopic pregnancy
   extrauterine pregnancy
   fallopian pregnancy
   false pregnancy
   gemellary pregnancy
   heterotopic pregnancy
   horseshoe pregnancy
   hydatid pregnancy
   incomplete pregnancy
   intraligamentous ectopic
     pregnancy
   intraligamentous pregnancy
   intramural pregnancy
   intraperitoneal pregnancy
   molar pregnancy
   mural pregnancy
   ovarian pregnancy
   ovarioabdominal pregnancy

pregnancy (*continued*)
oviductal pregnancy
parietal pregnancy
phantom pregnancy
plural pregnancy
pre-eclampsia of
pregnancy
sacrofetal pregnancy
sacrohysteric pregnancy
spurious pregnancy
striae of pregnancy
term pregnancy
termination of pregnancy
tubal pregnancy
tubo-ovarian pregnancy
tubouterine pregnancy
unruptured ectopic
pregnancy
uterine pregnancy
uteroabdominal pregnancy
utero-ovarian pregnancy
uterotubal pregnancy
pregnancy-induced anesthesia
prehepatic coma
prehepatic edema
prehyoid gland
preinsular gyri
preinvasive carcinoma
preischemic administration
Preiser disease
prejowl anterior mandibular
sulcus
prejowl depression
prejowl sulcus
prelabor membrane rupture
prelacrimal area
prelaryngeal node
preliminary film
preliminary impression
preliminary iridectomy
preliminary studies
premalignant fibroepithelioma
premalignant lesion
premammary abscess
premandible alloplastic
augmentation
premandible implant
premandibular arch
premandibular augmentation
premasseteric space abscess
premature airway closure
premature amnion rupture

premature atrial contraction
(PAC)
premature beat
premature birth
premature closure of valve
premature contact
premature contraction
premature delivery
premature ductus arteriosus
closure
premature labor
premature membrane rupture
premature rupture of
membranes (PROM)
premature separation of
placenta
premature ventricular
contraction (PVC)
premaxilla peripyriform
deficiency
premaxillary palate
premaxillary suture
premembrane rupture
premenarche
premenopausal
premenstrual
Premier drainable mini-pouch
Premier drainable pouch
Premier I&A unit
Premier urostomy pouch
Premiere vitreous cutter
Premium circular stapler
Premium CEEA circular stapling
device
Premium closed pouch
Premium drainable pouch
Premium Plus disposable stapler
Premium Poly stapler
Premo guidewire
premolar teeth
premolars
premonitory contraction
premonitory pain
premotor area
premotor neuron
premounted stent
premuscular mesh technique
premuscular position
premuscular prosthetic repair
prenatal course
prenatal development
prenatal diagnosis

prenatal diethylstilbestrol
   exposure
prenatal dislocation
prenatal therapy
prenormal occlusion
Prentif pessary
Prentiss forceps
Prentiss maneuver
preoccipital notch
preoperative analgesia
preoperative anesthetic
preoperative biopsy
preoperative care
preoperative cast
preoperative checklist
preoperative diagnosis
preoperative evaluation
preoperative hair clippers
preoperative imaging
preoperative induction
   chemotherapy
preoperative lesion
preoperative localization
preoperative
   lymphoscintigraphy
preoperative orders
preoperative percutaneous
   aspiration
preoperative retrograde
   cholangiogram
preoperative sedation
preoperative staging evaluation
preoperative systemic
   chemotherapy
preoperative therapy
preoral gut
prep
   Colonlite bowel prep
   Condon antibiotic prep
   Dulcolax bowel prep
   Fleet bowel prep
   GoLytely bowel prep
   inadequate bowel prep
   iodo prep
   OCL bowel prep
   scrub prep
   Septisol prep
   surgical prep
prep and drape
prep for delivery
prepalatal cleft
prepancreatic arch

prepapillary bile duct
prepared and draped in routine
   manner
prepared cavity impression
preparotid access
preparotid fascia
Prep-Assist legholder
Prep-Assist positioner
prepatellar bursa
prepatellar bursa inflammation
preperitoneal anesthesia
preperitoneal approach
preperitoneal bleeder
preperitoneal distention balloon
preperitoneal fat
preperitoneal space
Prep-IM hip bone preparation
   kit
preplaced sutures
preplacental hemorrhage
preplatysmal fat
Prepodyne scrub
Prepodyne solution
prepped and draped in routine
   manner
preprosthetic augmentation
preprosthetic surgery
Preptic dressing
prepubic fascia
prepuce forceps
prepuce of penis
preputial calculus
preputial gland
preputial island graft
preputial space
preputiotomy
prepyloric atresia
prepyloric gastric ulcer
prepyloric perforation
prepyloric sphincter
prepyloric ulcer
prepyloric vein
prerectal lithotomy
prereduction film
preretinal hemorrhage
preretinal membrane
presacral anesthesia
presacral anomaly
presacral block
presacral cystic lesion
presacral fascia
presacral insufflation

presacral neurectomy
presacral rectopexy
presacral resection
presacral space
presaturation technique
Presbyterian Hospital forceps
Presbyterian Hospital occluding
    clamp
Presbyterian Hospital
    staphylorrhaphy elevator
Presbyterian Hospital T-clamp
Presbyterian Hospital tubing
    clamp
Presbyterian Hospital
    ventricular needle
presection sutures
presence of infection
presenile sclerosis
present breast width (PBW)
present illness
presentation
    breech presentation
    brow presentation
    brow-up presentation
    cephalic presentation
    compound presentation
    face presentation
    footling breech presentation
    footling presentation
    frank breech presentation
    full breech presentation
    head down presentation
    lateral presentation
    longitudinal presentation
    oblique presentation
    parietal presentation
    pelvic presentation
    placental presentation
    polar presentation
    torso presentation
    transverse lie presentation
    transverse presentation
    vertex presentation
preseptal cellulitis
preseptal space
preseptal-suborbicularis
    dissection plane
preservation technique
preshaped catheter
Preshaw clamp
presigmoid-transtransversarium
    intradural approach

presphenoethmoid suture
presplenic fold
press
    Cali-Press graft press
    CamStar power leg press
    fascial press
    House Gelfoam press
    Omni press
    Paparella tissue press
    Sheehy fascial press
    tissue graft press
    tissue press
press plate needle holder
press-button chuck
Press-Fit condylar component
    (PFC component)
Press-Fit condylar total knee
Press-Fit femoral component
press-fit implant
press-fit prosthesis
Press-Mate model 8800T blood
    pressure monitor
Presso cardiac device
Presso-Elastic dressing
press-on prism
Pressoplast compression
    dressing
Pressore wrapping pressure
    monitor
Presso-Superior dressing
pressure
    abdominal pressure
    airway pressure
    aortic blood pressure
    aortic dicrotic notch pressure
    aortic pressure
    aortic pullback pressure
    arterial pressure
    back pressure
    bladder pressure
    bleeding controlled with
        direct pressure
    blood pressure
    bone marrow pressure
    capillary pressure
    capillary wedge pressure
    carbon dioxide pressure
    central venous pressure (CVP)
    cerebrospinal pressure
    closing pressure
    closure pressure
    compartment pressure

pressure (*continued*)

continuous distending airway pressure
continuous negative airway pressure
continuous positive airway pressure (CPAP)
cuff pressure
depressed systolic pressure
diastolic blood pressure
diastolic pressure
disk pressure
elevated pressure
end-diastolic pressure
endocardial pressure
end-systolic pressure
esophageal peristaltic pressure
esophageal sphincter pressure
expiratory pressure
extrinsic pressure
fluid pressure
gastric pressure
Gould Statham pressure
high blood pressure
high intraluminal pressure
hydrostatic pressure
hypogastric pressure
inspiratory pressure
instantaneous pressure
insufflation pressure
intracardiac pressure
intracranial pressure (ICP)
intraluminal pressure
intraocular pressure (IOP)
intrauterine pressure
intravascular pressure
intraventricular pressure
intrinsic pressure
leak point pressure
left ventricular end-diastolic pressure
manometric pressure
mastoid pressure
maximum pressure
mean arterial pressure (MAP)
mean pressure
negative pressure
occlusal pressure
occlusion pressure
ocular pressure
oncotic pressure

pressure (*continued*)

optimal diastolic pressure
osmotic pressure
partial pressure
perfusion pressure
positive airway pressure
positive end-airway pressure (PEAP)
positive end-expiratory pressure (PEEP)
positive pressure
pulmonary capillary wedge pressure
pulmonary pressure
pulmonary wedge pressure
rectal pressure
relieve pressure
stump pressure
systemic pressure
systolic pressure
tenderness on pressure
torr units of pressure
transmembrane pressure (TMP)
venous pressure
ventilation peak pressure
ventricular end-diastolic pressure
ventricular pressure
wedge pressure
pressure alopecia
pressure anesthesia
pressure applied
pressure atrophy
pressure bandage
pressure changes
pressure control inverse ratio ventilation (PCIRV)
pressure control ventilation (PCV)
pressure cuff
pressure dressing
pressure elevator
pressure equalization tube
pressure equalizing tube
pressure forceps
pressure fracture
pressure gangrene
pressure gauge
pressure glove
pressure gradient
Pressure Guard guidewire
pressure half-time technique

pressure increment rate
pressure injector
pressure inversion point (PIP)
pressure length loop
pressure maintained
pressure monitoring
pressure pack
pressure patch dressing
pressure phosphene tonometer
pressure point
pressure pump
pressure regulated
electrohydraulic lithotripsy
pressure relief ankle-foot
orthosis
pressure relief padding
pressure ring
pressure sensation
Pressure Sense monitor
Pressure Sentinel reamer
pressure shield
pressure support ventilation
(PSV)
pressure transducer
pressure urgency
pressure velocity (PV)
pressure ventilator
pressure wound
pressure-controlled inverse ratio
ventilation
pressure-cycled ventilator
PressureEasy cuff inflation
device
Pressurefuse automatic constant
pressure device
PressureGuard IV alternating
pressure mattress
pressure-point tension ring
pressure-preset ventilator
pressure-regulated volume
control ventilation
pressure-relief cushion
Pressure-Specified Sensory
Device
pressurizer
Pressurometer blood pressure
monitor
prestenotic dilatation
presternal notch
presternal space
Presto cardiac device
Preston dynamometer

Preston ligamentum flavum
forceps
Preston pinch gauge
prestyloid recess
prestyloid space
presumptive diagnosis
presurgical medical evaluation
presurgical orthopedic
correction (POC)
presurgical orthopedic
correction (POC) device
presurgical orthopedics,
gingivoperiosteoplasty, and
lip adhesion (POPLA)
presynaptic membrane
presystolic murmur
pretapped synthes lag screw
pretarsal fold
pretarsal space
pretemporal space
preternatural anus
prethreaded Teflon pledget
pretibial edema
pretibial fever
pretracheal fascia
pretracheal layer
pretracheal node
pretracheal space
pretransplant evaluation
pretransplant surgery
pretreatment evaluation
prevacuum sterilizer
Pre-Vent boot style stirrup pad
Pre-Vent elbow protector
Pre-Vent heel protector
Pre-Vent knee crutch pad
Pre-Vent OR table pad
Pre-Vent Pneumotach flowmeter
Pre-Vent ulnar nerve protector
preventive intravesical therapy
preventive orthodontics
preventricular artery
preventricular stenosis
prevertebral fascia level
prevertebral ganglia
prevertebral ganglion
prevertebral layer
prevertebral space
prevertebral space abscess
prevesical space of Retzius
Preziosi operation
prezonular space

PRG (phleborheogram)
Pribram suction tube
Price corneal punch
Price muscle biopsy clamp
Price muscle clamp
Price operation
Price radial marker
Price-Thomas bronchial clamp
Price-Thomas bronchial forceps
Price-Thomas clamp
Price-Thomas forceps
Price-Thomas rib stripper
Pricker needle
prickle-cell carcinoma
prick-test concentration
Pridie incision
Pridie-Koutsogiannis procedure
Priessnitz bandage
Priessnitz compress
Priessnitz dressing
Priest wasp-waist laryngostat
Priestley-Smith retinoscope
Priestly catheter
prilocaine hydrochloride
    anesthetic agent
Prima laser
Prima Laser catheter
Prima laser guidewire
Prima pacemaker
Prima Series speculum
Prima Total Occlusion device
Primaderm foam dressing
Primalloy alloy
Primapore absorptive wound
    dressing
Primapore tape and gauze
    wound dressing
primarily vascularized organ
    transplant
primary abscess
primary adenocarcinoma
primary adhesion
primary amputation
primary anastomosis
primary anesthetic
primary antecubital jump
    bypass (PAJB)
primary arteriovenous fistula
primary bile duct carcinoma
primary bone graft
primary brain tumor
primary cancer

primary carcinoma
primary choana
primary cleft
primary clip
primary closure
primary colostomy
primary contraction of skin graft
primary diagnostic endoscopy
primary end-to-end anastomosis
primary ganglion
primary gangrene
primary gastric lymphoma
    (PGL)
primary gastric non-Hodgkin
    lymphoma
primary hemorrhage
primary hyperparathyroidism
primary indirect inguinal hernia
primary inguinal herniorrhaphy
primary intra-axial brain tumor
primary intraosseous carcinoma
primary lesion
primary macular atrophy of skin
primary movement plane
primary myofascial trigger point
primary nerve repair
primary neuroendocrine
    carcinoma of the skin
primary palate
primary palatorrhaphy
primary perineal hypospadias
    surgery
primary position
primary procedure
primary renal calculus
primary repair
primary resection
primary sequestrum
primary skin graft
primary suture line
primary suture technique
primary sutures
primary trimming bur
primary union
primary wound closure
primary access incisions
Primbs suturing forceps
Prime balloon
Primer compression dressing
Primer compression wrap
priming of artificial kidney
priming of pump

priming solution
primip (primipara)
primip
primiparous patient
primitive dislocation
primitive gut
primitive knot
primordial catheter tube
primordial cyst
Primus prostate machine
Prince advancement forceps
Prince clamp
Prince dissecting scissors
Prince electrocautery
Prince eye cautery
Prince knife
Prince muscle clamp
Prince muscle forceps
Prince rongeur
Prince scissors
Prince tonsillar scissors
Prince trachoma forceps
Prince ureteropelvioplasty
Prince-Potts tonsillar scissors
principal artery of thumb
principal fiber bundle
principal visual direction
Pringle clamp
Pringle incision
Pringle maneuver
Pringle vascular control
Pringle vascular control
    procedure
Pringle vascular control
    technique
Printz anesthesia unit
Printz aspirator
Printz suction
Prinzmetal angina
prion-associated spongiform
    encephalopathies
prism
    Allen-Thorpe gonioscopic
        prism
    bar prism
    base-down prism
    Becker gonioscopic prism
    Berens prism
    binocular prism
    DermaGard prism
    diopter prism
    Drews inclined prism

prism (*continued*)
    Fresnel prism
    Goldmann contact lens prism
    gonioscopic prism
    hand-held rotary prism
    Jacob-Swan gonioscopic
        prism
    Keeler prism
    lens prism
    Maddox prism
    oblique prism
    plastic prism
    press-on prism
    Risley rotary prism
    scanning prism
    square prism
    Storz binocular prism
Prism gamma camera
prism diopters
prism loupe
prismatic contact lens
prismatic gonioscopic lens
prismatic goniotomy lens
Prism-CL pacemaker
Pritchard arthroplasty
Pritchard cannula
Pritchard elevator
Pritchard speculum
Pritchard syringe
Pritchard total elbow prosthesis
Pritchard-Walker elbow hinge
Pritikin scleral punch
prizefighter's ear
Prizm defibrillator
Prizm Electro-Mesh Sock
    electrode
Prizm Electro-Mesh Z-Stim-II
    stimulator
Pro Peak decubitus pad
Pro Pulse irrigator
Pro Relief gel/foam wheelchair
    cushion
PRO traction table
PRO/Covers ultrasound probe
    sheath
Pro/Pel cannulated interference
    screw
Pro/Pel coating
Pro/Pel coating cardiac device
Pro-8 ankle brace
proactive hemostasis
ProAdvantage knee prosthesis

Pro-Bal protected balloon-tipped catheter
probang
probe (*see also* cryoprobe)
  4-beam laser Doppler Probe
  8-channel cross-sectional anal sphincter probe
  24-hour esophageal probe
  Acolysis coronary probe
  acoustic impedance probe
  ADD side-directed probe
  Alcon vitrectomy probe
  Aloka MP-PN ultrasound probe
  Amoils probe
  Amussat probe
  Ando motor-driven probe
  AnEber probe
  Anel lacrimal probe
  angled probe
  Arbuckle sinus probe
  Arndorfer esophageal motility probe
  Aspir-Vac probe
  back-stop laser probe
  Bakes probe
  Balectrode pacing probe
  Bard probe
  Barr fistula probe
  Barr rectal probe
  Becker probe
  Beckman probe
  Benger probe
  Berman-Werner probe
  Beyer pigtail probe
  BiCAP bipolar hemostatic probe
  BiCAP bipolar laparoscopic probe
  biliary balloon probe
  biometry probe
  biopsy probe
  biplane sector probe
  bipolar circumactive probe
  bipolar endostasis probe
  bipolar hemostasis probe
  bipolar probe
  Birtcher electrocautery probe
  blind endosonography probe
  blood-flow probe
  blunt lacrimal probe
  blunt probe
  blunt-tip probe

probe (*continued*)
  Bodian lacrimal pigtail probe
  Bodian minilacrimal probe
  Bowman lacrimal probe
  Brackett dental probe
  brain probe
  Brenner rectal probe
  Bresgen frontal sinus probe
  Bresgen sinus probe
  Brock probe
  Brodie fistula probe
  bronchoscopic probe
  Bruel-Kjaer transvaginal ultrasound probe
  Brunner probe
  Brymill cryosurgical probe
  Buck ear probe
  Buie fistula probe
  bullet probe
  Bunnell dissecting probe
  Bunnell forwarding probe
  calibrated probe
  canaliculus probe
  cardiac probe
  Castroviejo lacrimal sac probe
  cataract probe
  catheter ultrasound probe
  catheter-based ultrasound probe
  Chandler V-pacing probe
  Cherry brain probe
  Cherry probe
  Circon-ACMI electrohydraulic lithotriptor probe
  Clinitex Charles endophotocoagulator probe
  CO_2 laser probe
  coagulation probe
  Coakley nasal probe
  Cody magnetic probe
  common duct probe
  conical probe
  Contact Laser bullet probe
  Contact Laser chisel probe
  Contact Laser conical probe
  Contact Laser convex probe
  Contact Laser flat probe
  Contact Laser interstitial probe
  Contact Laser round probe
  continuously perfused probe

probe (*continued*)

convex probe
coronary artery probe
Corson needle electrosurgical probe
Crawford canaliculus probe
Criticare sensor probe
cross-sectional anal sphincter probe
cryogenic probe
cryopexy probe
cryotherapy probe
C-Trak handheld gamma probe
curved retinal probe
Dandy probe
Desjardins gallstone probe
dilating probe
dilator probe
disposable probe
dissecting probe
dissection probe
Dix spud probe
Dobbhoff bipolar coagulation probe
Dodick photolysis probe
Doppler flow echocardiographic probe
Doppler flow probe
Doppler 4-beam laser probe
Doppler ultrasonic probe
dot-plotted probe
double-ended chrome probe
double-ended nickelene probe
double-ended probe
double-ended silver probe
drum probe
Dymer excimer delivery probe
ear probe
Earle rectal probe
echocardiographic probe
electric probe
electrohydraulic lithotripsy probe
electrohydraulic lithotriptor probe
electromagnetic flow probe
electromagnetic focusing field probe

probe (*continued*)

electrosurgical monopolar spatula probe
Ellis foreign body spud needle probe
Ellis foreign body spud probe
Emmet uterine probe
end-fire transrectal probe
endocavitary probe
Endocavity probe
endocervical probe
endolaser probe
Endopath needle tip electrosurgery probe
Endo-P-Probe endorectal probe
endoscopic BiCAP probe
endoscopic heat probe
EndoSound ultrasound probe
EndoStasis probe
Endotrac probe
Envision endocavity probe
Esmarch tin bullet probe
esophageal temperature probe
eustachian probe
extended sector ultrasonic probe
eye probe
eyed probe
Fenger gall duct probe
Fenger gallbladder probe
Fenger gallstone probe
Fenger spiral gallstone probe
Ferguson esophageal probe
fiberoptic probe
FIDUS probe
filiform bougie probe
Fish antral probe
Fish sinus probe
fistula probe
flexible endosonography probe
flexible probe
flow probe
Fluhrer bullet probe
Fluhrer rectal probe
fluorescent probe
fluoroptic thermometry probe
Fogarty biliary balloon probe
Fogarty biliary probe

probe (*continued*)

foreign body probe
forwarding probe
Fraenkel sinus probe
fragmentation probe
free-spinning probe
French lacrimal probe
French-pattern lacrimal probe
Fresgen frontal sinus probe
Frigitronics freeze-thaw
cryopexy probe
frontal sinus probe
Gabor probe
gall duct probe
Gallagher bipolar mapping
probe
gallstone probe
galvanic probe
gamma probe
gamma-detecting probe
Gant rectal probe
gear shift pedicle probe
Geldmacher tendon-passing
probe
general probe
Gillquist-Oretorp-Stille probe
Gilmore probe
Girard Fragmatome probe
Girdner probe
Gold probe
Goldman-Fox probe
Gross probe
Hagar probe
hand-held exploring electrode
probe
hand-held mapping probe
Harms trabeculotomy probe
Hayden probe
heater probe
Heller probe
Henning-Keinkel stomach
probe
Hertzog pliable probe
Hewlett-Packard biplane probe
Hewlett-Packard omniplane
probe
high-density endocavity probe
high-frequency miniature
probe
high-resolution probe
Hitachi convex ultrasound
probe

probe (*continued*)

Hitachi convex-convex
biplane probe
Hitachi fingertip ultrasound
probe
Hitachi linear ultrasound probe
Hitachi transrectal ultrasound
probe
Hitachi transvaginal
ultrasound probe
Hoffrel transesophageal probe
Hotz ear probe
Huber probe
Ilg probe
Iliff lacrimal probe
illuminated probe
illuminated ureter probe
illumination probe
Injectate probe
injection gold probe
IntraDop probe
intraductal ultrasound probe
intraluminal probe
intraoperative ultrasonic probe
intrauterine probe
irrigating probe
Jackson probe
Jacobson blood vessel probe
Jacobson vas deferens probe
Jako laryngeal probe
Jannetta probe
Jansen-Newhart mastoid
probe
J-hook electrosurgical probe
Jobson-Horne probe
Josephberg probe
Kalk palpitation probe
Kartch pigtail probe
Keeler-Amoils curved cataract
probe
Keeler-Amoils glaucoma
probe
Keeler-Amoils long-shank
retinal probe
Keeler-Amoils microcurved
cataract probe
Keeler-Amoils ophthalmic
long-shank probe
Keeler-Amoils ophthalmic
Machemer retinal probe
Keeler-Amoils ophthalmic
straight cataract probe

probe (*continued*)

    Keeler-Amoils ophthalmic
      vitreous probe
    Keeler-Amoils-Machemer
      retinal probe
    Kennerdell-Maroon probe
    Killian probe
    Kirschner guiding probe
    Kistner probe
    Kleinsasser probe
    Knapp iris probe
    Kocher probe
    Koenig probe
    Kron bile duct probe
    Kron gall duct probe
    KTP laser probe
    lacrimal duct probe
    lacrimal intubation probe
    laparoscopic Doppler probe
    large-bore heat probe
    Larry rectal probe
    laryngeal probe
    laser probe
    laser-Doppler flowmetry
      probe
    laser-Doppler Periflux probe
    Laserflow Doppler probe
    Lente silver nitrate probe
    L-hook electrosurgical probe
    Liebreich probe
    light monitoring probe
    Lilienthal bullet probe
    Lillie frontal sinus probe
    Linde cryogenic probe
    lithotriptor probe
    localizing probe
    Lockhart-Mummery probe
    Lucae ear probe
    magnetic eye probe
    magnetometer probe
    malleable probe
    Manhattan Eye and Ear
      probe
    Mannis suture probe
    Marquis probe
    Martin uterine fistula probe
    mastoid probe
    Max-I-Probe irrigation probe
    Mayo common duct probe
    Mayo kidney stone probe
    Mayo uterine probe
    McKesson mouth probe

probe (*continued*)

    Meadox Surgimed Doppler
      probe
    mechanical rotating probe
    Meditech bipolar probe
    meerschaum probe
    meniscectomy probe
    Merit-B periodontal probe
    Michigan probe
    microballoon probe
    microlaryngeal laser probe
    micromultiplane
      transesophageal
      echocardiographic probe
    MicroSmooth probe
    Microvit probe
    miniature probe
    miniaturized ultrasound
      catheter probe
    Mixter common duct probe
    Mixter Dilaprobe probe
    Mixter dilating probe
    Mixter gall duct probe
    Mixter irrigating probe
    Modulap probe
    monitoring probe
    Moynihan bile duct probe
    Moynihan gallstone probe
    Mui Scientific 6-channel
      esophageal pressure probe
    Muldoon lacrimal probe
    multielectrode probe
    multilumen probe
    multiplane intracavitary probe
    Myrtle leaf probe
    Nabers probe
    nasal probe
    nasolacrimal duct probe
    needle probe
    NeoProbe gamma detection
      probe
    NeoTherm neonatal skin
      temperature probe
    Nibbler laparoscopic probe
    nuclear probe
    Nucleotome cutting probe
    Nucleotome Micro probe
    Nelaton bullet probe
    Ochsner flexible spiral
      gallstone probe
    Ochsner gall duct probe
    Ochsner gallstone probe

probe (*continued*)
  Ochsner spiral probe
  Ochsner-Fenger gallstone
    probe
  ocutome probe
  O'Donoghue probe
  Ohmeda probe
  oligonucleotide probe
  Olympus heater probe
  Olympus heat probe
  Olympus ultrathin balloon-
    fitted ultrasound probe
  Olympus transendoscopic
    probe
  Olympus miniature ultrasonic
    probe
  Olympus endoscopic probe
  Oratek thermal shrinking
    probe
  Ossoff-Karlan microlaryngeal
    laser probe
  over-the-wire probe
  Osypka radiofrequency probe
  palpation probe
  Paparella probe
  Parker-Heath piggyback probe
  Parsonnet coronary probe
  Parsonnet probe
  Payr probe
  Payr-Schmieden probe
  pediatric biplane TEE probe
  pencil Doppler probe
  percutaneous pencil Doppler
    probe
  Perio Temp dental probe
  periodontal probe
  PerioWise probe
  pH probe
  Photon LaserPhacolysis Probe
  piggyback probe
  pigtail probe
  pocket probe
  polycationic histochemical
    probe
  Pratt rectal probe
  Probex probe
  pulpal microdialysis probe
  quartz fiberoptic probe
  Quickert lacrimal probe
  Quickert-Dryden lacrimal
    probe
  Quickert-Dryden probe

probe (*continued*)
  radiometer probe
  rectal probe
  Reddick-Saye Lav-1 I&A probe
  Reddick-Saye Lav-1 irrigating
    and aspirating probe
  reflectance
    spectrophotometric probe
  reverse-cutting meniscal
    probe
  reverse-cutting probe
  Rica ear probe
  Richards probe
  right-angle blunt probe
  rigid endosonography probe
  Ritleng probe
  RNA probe
  Robicsek vascular probe
  Rockey dilating probe
  Rohrschneider probe
  Rolf lacrimal probe
  Rollet lacrimal probe
  Rosen ear probe
  Rosen endaural probe
  salpingeal probe
  Sandhill probe
  Sarns temperature probe
  Schmieden probe
  scissors probe
  Sheer probe
  Shirodkar probe
  side-hole cannulated probe
  Siemens linear probe
  Siemens vaginal probe
  silver probe
  Silverstein stimulator probe
  Simpson lacrimal probe
  Simpson sterling lacrimal
    probe
  Sims uterine probe
  simultaneous thermal
    diffusion blood flow and
    pressure probe
  sinus probe
  Skillern sinus probe
  Skillern sphenoid probe
  Skillern sphenoidal probe
  SMIC periodontal abscess
    probe
  SmokEvac electrosurgical
    probe
  Softflo fiberoptic probe

probe (*continued*)
Somnus probe
Sonablate transrectal probe
Sonocath ultrasound probe
spatula electrosurgical probe
spear-ended chrome probe
spear-pointed nickelene
    probe
Spectraprobe-Max probe
Spencer labyrinth exploration
    probe
sphenoidal probe
Spiesman fistula probe
SpineStat side-directed
    diskectomy probe
spinning probe
spiral probe
Stacke probe
standard hook electrosurgical
    probe
Storz pigtail probe
Storz-Bowman lacrimal probe
straight retinal probe
suction probe
Surgiflex suction/irrigation
    probe
Swiss Lithoclast pneumatic
    lithotripsy probe
tactile probe
Teflon probe
telephone probe
temperature probe
Theobald sinus probe
thermistor probe
through-the-scope catheter
    probe
tin-bullet probe
trabeculotomy probe
transcranial Doppler probe
transesophageal
    echocardiography probe
transesophageal probe
Transonic flow probe
transrectal probe
TrueVision transvaginal probe
truncated probe
Tufcote epilation probe
tulip probe
tumor probe
ultrasonic probe
ultrasound catheter probe
Universal vaginal probe

probe (*continued*)
Urrets-Zavalia probe
USCI probe
uterine probe
vacuum intrauterine probe
Valliex uterine probe
Vasamedics implantable prism
    laser probe
Versadopp Doppler probe
vertebrated probe
Vibrodilator probe
ViraType probe
vitrector probe
Vygantas-Wilder retinal
    drainage probe
Wasko common duct probe
water probe
Weaver sinus probe
Welch Allyn rectal probe
Werb right-angle probe
whalebone eustachian probe
whirlybird probe
Williams lacrimal probe
wire probe
Woodson probe
Worst double-ended pigtail
    probe
Worst pigtail probe
Xomed rectal probe
Yankauer salpingeal probe
Yellow Springs probe
Yeoman probe
YSI Foley probe
YSI neonatal temperature
    probe
Ziegler lacrimal probe
Ziegler needle probe
probe balloon catheter
probe catheter
probe catheterization
probe dilator
probe needle
probe point scissors
probe shield
probe spatula
probe-ended grooved director
probe-point scissors
Probex probe
probing catheter
probing depth (PD)
probing lacrimonasal duct
    operation

probing of lacrimonasal duct
probing of wound
probing sheath exchange
  catheter
problematic wound
ProBloc insulated regional block
  needle
procaine hydrochloride
  anesthetic agent
procallus formation
Procath electrophysiology
  catheter
procedure (*see also* operation,
  technique)
  1st-stage procedure
  2-stage procedure
  2-step procedure
  2nd-look procedure
  3-stage procedure
  4-flap procedure
  4-incision procedure
  4-port procedure
  5-incision procedure
  Abbe-McIndoe procedure
  Abbe-McIndoe-Williams
    procedure
  Abbe-Wharton-McIndoe
    procedure
  abdominal procedure
  abdominoplasty procedure
  ablative procedure
  Adair procedure
  Adams procedure
  Adasoy procedure
  adipofascial sural flap
    procedure
  adjunctive procedure
  advancement procedure
  aesthetic procedure
  Akin procedure
  Akiyama procedure
  Albee shelf procedure
  Albee-Delbert procedure
  Albert-Chase procedure
  Aldridge sling procedure
  Al-Ghorab procedure
  Aliston procedure
  Allan calcaneus procedure
  Allport ptosis correction
    procedure
  Altemeier rectal prolapse
    procedure

procedure (*continued*)
  Alvis ptosis correction
    procedure
  anchorage procedure
  anchovy procedure
  Anderson procedure
  Anderson-Fowler procedure
  Angelucci ptosis correction
    procedure
  antegrade continence enema
    procedure
  antenna procedure
  anterior Polya procedure
  anterior stabilization procedure
  anti-incontinence procedure
  antireflux procedure
  AO procedure
  apron flap procedure
  Armistead procedure
  arterial reconstructive
    procedure
  arterial switch procedure
  articulatory procedure
  Atosoy procedure
  augmentation procedure
  autogenous fascia lata sling
    procedure
  Axer-Clark procedure
  B.H. Moore procedure
  Badgley combination
    procedure
  Bailey-Dubow femoral shaft
    procedure
  Baiter modification of
    Shirodkar procedure
  Baker patellar tendon
    procedure
  Baldy-Webster procedure
  balloon fenestration
    procedure
  Bandi procedure
  Bankart procedure
  Barr procedure
  Barsky procedure
  Bartlett procedure
  baseline procedure
  Bassini procedure
  Batista procedure
  Baxter-D'Astous procedure
  Bell-Tawse procedure
  Belsey fundoplication
    procedure

procedure (*continued*)

Bentall procedure
Bergenhem procedure
Berman-Gartland procedure
Bernard lip reconstruction procedure
Bick procedure
Bickel-Moe procedure
bilateral inguinal hernia repair procedure
bilateral procedures
Bilhaut-Cloquet procedure
biliary procedure
Billroth I procedure
Billroth II procedure
Bing-Taussig heart procedure
Bjork method of Fontan procedure
bladder chimney procedure
Blair-Brown procedure
Blalock procedure
Blalock-Hanlon procedure
Blalock-Taussig procedure
Blatt procedure
Blatt-Ashworth procedure
Blazina procedure
blocking procedure
Boari bladder flap procedure
bone block procedure
Bonferroni-Holm procedure
bony procedure
Bora procedure
Bose procedure
Bosworth procedure
bowel refashioning procedure
Boyce-Vest procedure
Boyd-Anderson biceps procedure
Boyd-Bosworth procedure
Boyd-McLeod tennis elbow procedure
Boyd-Sisk shoulder procedure
Boytchev procedure
Brackett-Osgood knee procedure
Brahms mallet toe procedure
Brantigan procedure
Brantigan-Voshell procedure
Braun shoulder procedure
breast-conserving procedure
Bricker procedure
Bridle procedure

procedure (*continued*)

Bristow-Helfet procedure
Bristow-Latarjet procedure
Bristow-May procedure
Brock procedure
Brockman clubfoot procedure
Brostrom procedure
Brostrom-Gould foot procedure
Brown-McDowell procedure
Bryan procedure
Bucknall procedure
Bugg-Boyd procedure
Bunnell procedure
Bunnell-Williams procedure
Burch bladder suspension procedure
Burkhalter procedure
burn-out procedure
bypass procedure
Byron Smith lazy-T procedure
Calandriello procedure
Caldwell-Durham procedure
Caldwell-Luc window procedure
Callia floating umbilicus procedure
CAM procedure (coblation-assisted microdisc)
Camey procedure
Campbell-Akbarnia procedure
Campbell-Goldthwait procedure
canalith repositioning procedure
capsular shift procedure
Carolinas Laparoscopic Advanced Surgery Program procedure
carotid ablative procedure
Castaneda procedure
Castle procedure
cataract procedure
catheter-directed interventional procedure
Cave-Rowe patellar procedure
Cawthorne-Day procedure
cecal imbrication procedure
Cecil procedure
Celestin procedure
cervical spine stabilization procedure

procedure (*continued*)
  cervicofacial rhytidectomy
    procedure
  cervicomandibular angle
    correction through
    Guyuron's procedure
  Chamberlain procedure
  Chambers procedure
  Charles procedure
  Chassar Moir sling procedure
  Chassar Moir-Sims procedure
  Chaves procedure
  checkrein procedure
  Cherry-Crandall procedure
  cherry-picking procedure
  Chester-Winter procedure
  chin-contouring procedure
  Chrisman-Snook ankle
    procedure
  Cibis liquid silicone procedure
  ciliary procedure
  cineplastic procedure
  circulatory arrest procedure
  Clancy-Zoellner procedure
  CLASP procedure
  Clayton procedure
  Cleveland procedure
  Cloward procedure
  coblation-assisted microdisc
    procedure
  cocked hat procedure
  Cockett procedure
  Cody tack procedure
  Cohen antireflux procedure
  Cole intubation procedure
  Collin-Beard procedure
  Collis gastroplasty procedure
  Collis-Nissen esophageal
    lengthening procedure
  Collis-Nissen fundoplication
    procedure
  colon procedure
  colpoplasty procedure
  combined contour procedure
  commando procedure
  compartment procedure
  Compere femoral lengthening
    procedure
  complete procedure
  composite pelvic resection
    procedure
  concentration procedure

procedure (*continued*)
  Connolly procedure
  controlled procedure
  conventional procedure
  core drilling procedure
  coronary artery
    revascularization procedure
  coronary bypass procedure
  corporeal rotation procedure
  corrective procedure
  corridor procedure
  Couch-DeRosa-Throop hip
    procedure
  Cox Maze procedure
  Crohnlein procedure
  Cracchiolo procedure
  Crowel-Beard ptosis
    procedure
  curative procedure
  curative-intent procedure
  Custodis nondraining
    procedure
  Cutler-Beard bridge flap
    procedure
  cyclodestructive procedure
  Cyclops procedure
  dacryocystorhinostomy
    procedure
  Daggett procedure
  Damian graft procedure
  Damus-Kaye-Stansel
    procedure
  Damus-Stansel-Kaye
    procedure
  Danus-Fontan procedure
  Darrach procedure
  dartos pouch procedure
  Das Gupta scapula procedure
  Datta procedure
  Davis-Kitlowski procedure
  Davydov procedure
  de-airing procedure
  DeBakey-Creech procedure
  debubbling procedure
  debulking procedure
  Dees-Young procedure
  degloving procedure
  Denis Browne procedure
  dental procedure
  dental prosthetic laboratory
    procedure
  dermoplasty procedure

procedure (*continued*)
Devine-Devine procedure
Dewar posterior cervical fixation procedure
Dewar-Barrington procedure
Deyerle procedure
diagnostic procedure
dialysis procedure
Dickson-Diveley procedure
Dillwyn Evans procedure
dislocation procedure
distal procedure
DKS procedure
domino procedure
Donald procedure
Donders procedure
Donoghue knee procedure
Dor fundoplication procedure
Dorrance procedure
dorsal root entry zone procedure
dot-blot procedure
double-blind procedure
double-stapled ileoanal reservoir procedure
Douglas procedure
Downey-McGlamery procedure
DREZ procedure
drop-back procedure
drop-foot procedure
Duckett procedure
Duhamel procedure
Dukes procedure
duToit rotator cuff procedure
duToit-Roux shoulder procedure
Duval procedure
DuVries procedure
Dwyer clubfoot procedure
Dwyer scoliosis procedure
Ebbehoj procedure
Eberbusch ptosis correction procedure
Eden-Hybbinette procedure
Eden-Lange procedure
Edwards procedure
Effler-Groves mode of Allison procedure
elective surgical procedure
elimination procedure

procedure (*continued*)
Ellis-Jones peroneal tendon procedure
Ellison knee procedure
Elmslie procedure
Elmslie-Trillat patellar procedure
Ely procedure
emergency procedure
endolacrimal procedure
endorectal ileoanal pull-through procedure
endorectal pull-through procedure
endoscopic mucosal procedure
endoscopic mucosal resection procedure
endoscopic procedure
endoscopy procedure
end-to-end reconstruction procedure
enucleation procedure
Eriksson knee procedure
esophageal sling procedure
Estes procedure
evacuation procedure
Evans foot procedure
Evans-Steptoe procedure
Everard Williams procedure
ex situ in vivo procedure
excisional biopsy procedure
exploratory procedure
extended Ross procedure
extra-anatomic bypass procedure
extra-articular procedure
extracorporeal procedure
Eyler elbow procedure
face-neck rejuvenation procedure
Faden procedure
Fahey-O'Brien procedure
failed procedure
Fairbanks-Sever shoulder procedure
Fasanella-Servat ptosis correction procedure
fascial sling procedure
fenestration procedure
fiberoptic intubation procedure

procedure (*continued*)

Ficat procedure
fillet flap procedure
filtering procedure
Fired-Hendel procedure
flap advancement procedure
flip-flap procedure
floating umbilicus procedure
floppy Nissen fundoplication
    procedure
followup procedure
Fontan modification of
    Norwood procedure
Fontan-Baudet procedure
Fontan-Kreutzer procedure
forage procedure
Fowler-Stephens procedure
Fox-Blazina knee procedure
Frank procedure
Fredet-Ramstedt procedure
free flap procedure
Fried-Green foot procedure
Froimson biceps procedure
frontalis sling procedure
Frost procedure
Fulford procedure
Furlow procedure
fusion procedure
Gaenslen procedure
Galeazzi procedure
Gallie procedure
Garceau clubfoot procedure
Garceau-Brahms clubfoot
    procedure
Garden procedure
Gartland procedure
gaseous laparoscopy
    procedure
gasless laparoscopy
    procedure
gastric bypass procedure
    (GBP)
gastric emptying procedure
    (GEP)
gastric procedure
gastric pull-through
    procedure
gastric pull-up procedure
gastric stapling procedure
gastric valve tightening
    procedure
gauntlet flap procedure

procedure (*continued*)

Gelman procedure
general laparoscopic surgical
    procedure
genioplasty procedure
Gerard resurfacing procedure
Giannestras metatarsal
    procedure
Giannestras step-down
    procedure
Gilchrist procedure
Gill dropfoot procedure
Gillies cocked hat procedure
Gillies elevation procedure
Gill-Jonas modification of
    Norwood procedure
Gilquist procedure
Gil-Vernet procedure
Girard procedure
Girdlestone hip procedure
Girdlestone-Taylor procedure
Gittes procedure
Gittes-Loughlin procedure
Glenn procedure
Goebel procedure
Goebel-Stoeckel-Frangenheim
    procedure
Goldner-Hayes procedure
Goldthwait procedure
Goldthwait-Hauser procedure
Gould procedure
Goulding procedure
Graber-Duvernay hip
    procedure
gracilis procedure
Green scapular procedure
Green-Banks procedure
Gregoir-Lich procedure
Gurd procedure
Guyuron procedure
gynecological procedure
Halban procedure
hallux valgus procedure
Hambly procedure
Hammon procedure
hamular procedure
Hancock procedure
Hanley rectal bladder
    procedure
Harada-Ito procedure
Harewood suspension
    procedure

procedure (*continued*)
Hark procedure
Harmon deltoid procedure
Harris-Beath flatfoot procedure
Harris-Mueller procedure
Hartmann procedure
Hass procedure
Hastings procedure
Hauser heel cord procedure
Hauser knee procedure
Hauser patellar tendon procedure
Hawkins procedure
Hedley procedure
Heifitz ingrown nail procedure
Heinig procedure
hemi-Fontan procedure
hemi-Koch procedure
heparinization procedure
Hepp-Couinaud biliary tract procedure
Herndon procedure
Herndon-Heyman procedure
hex procedure
Heyman clubfoot procedure
Heyman-Herndon clubfoot procedure
Hibbs foot procedure
high-risk procedure
Hill procedure
Hinman procedure
Hitchcock biceps procedure
Hodor-Dobbs procedure
Hoffer procedure
Hoffman and Mohr procedure
Hoffmann-Clayton procedure
Hoffmann-Keller-Lapidus procedure
Hofmeister procedure
Hohmann tennis elbow procedure
Hoke flatfoot procedure
Hoke-Miller procedure
Holz procedure
Hood procedure
Hotz procedure
Hovanian procedure
Howorth procedure
Howorth-Keillor procedure
Huber procedure

procedure (*continued*)
Hueston flap procedure
Hughston patellar procedure
Hughston-Hauser procedure
Hui-Linscheid procedure
Hummelsheim procedure
hyperventilation procedure
hypoglossal facial transfer procedure
hypothermic procedure
IDET procedure
ileal pull-through procedure
ileoanal pouch procedure
ileoanal pull-through procedure
iliac buttressing procedure
Ilizarov leg-lengthening procedure
Illouz procedure
imaging procedure
in situ procedure
Inclan-Ober scapula procedure
inferior pedicle inverted-T procedures
infrarenal template procedure
Inge procedure
Ingelman-Sundberg gracilis muscle procedure
Ingram procedure
initial screening procedure
inner ear tack procedure
Insall procedure
installation procedure
intercalary allograft procedure
interlaminar procedure
interventional procedure
intestinal bypass procedure
intra-abdominal laser procedure
intra-abdominal procedure
intra-articular procedure
intraoperative procedure
intraparavariceal procedure
intraperitoneal procedure
invasive procedure
Ionescu tri-leaflet valve procedure
island-flap procedure
isolated procedure
Ito procedure
J.R. Moore procedure

procedure (*continued*)
Jacobaeus procedure
Jaeger-Hamby procedure
Jaffe procedure
Jahss procedure
Jannetta microvascular
   decompression procedure
Jansey procedure
Japas foot procedure
Jatene arterial switch
   procedure
jejunoileal bypass reversal
   procedure
Jensen transposition
   procedure
Jobe-Glousman capsular shift
   procedure
Johnson procedure
Johnson-Spiegel procedure
Johnston buttonhole
   procedure
Jonas modification of
   Norwood procedure
Jones ankle procedure
Jones knee procedure
Jones toe procedure
Jones tube procedure
Junod procedure
Juvara procedure
Kaliscinski ureteral procedure
Kapel elbow procedure
Karakousis-Vezeridis
   procedure
Karhunen-Loeve procedure
Karlsson procedure
Kasai procedure
Kaufman incontinence
   procedure
Kawaii-Yamamoto procedure
Kelikian tendon transfer
   procedure
Kelikian-McFarland
   procedure
Keller procedure
Kelling-Madlener procedure
Kelly plication procedure
Kendrick procedure
Kennedy procedure
Kessel-Bonney procedure
Kestenbach-Anderson
   procedure
Kestenbaum eye procedure

procedure (*continued*)
keyhole coronary bypass
   procedure
Kidner foot procedure
Kidner podiatric procedure
Kiehn-Earle-DesPrez
   procedure
Killian frontoethmoidectomy
   procedure
King hip fusion procedure
Kleinert volar pedicle
   procedure
Knapp procedure
Knobby-Clark procedure
Ko-Airan bleeding control
   procedure
Kocher ureterosigmoidostomy
   procedure
Kock pouch modified
   procedure
Kole procedure
Kolmogorov-Smirnov
   procedure
Kondoleon-Sistrunk
   elephantiasis procedure
Konno procedure
Kortzeborn hand procedure
Koutsogiannis procedure
Kraske procedure
Kronlein procedure
Kropp procedure
Krukenberg procedure
Kuhnt-Szymanowski
   ectropion repair
   procedure
Ladd procedure
Lairmonth procedure
Lam modification of Jones
   procedure
Lane procedure
Lange metatarsus varus
   procedure
Langenskiold procedure
Langevin updating procedure
laparoscopic bladder neck
   suture suspension
   procedure
laparoscopic Burch procedure
laparoscopic bypass
   procedure
laparoscopic lymph node
   dissection procedure

procedure (*continued*)

laparoscopic Nissen fundoplication procedure

laparoscopic para-aortic lymph node sampling procedure

laparoscopic surgical procedure

laparoscopic tubal banding procedure

laparoscopically-assisted endorectal pull-through procedure

laparoscopic-assisted procedure

Lapides urological procedure

Larmon forefoot procedure

laryngopharyngoeso-phagectomy procedure

laser coagulation vaporization procedure (LCVP)

laser-balloon procedure

Lash procedure

LAST coronary bypass procedure

Latarget procedure

lateral tarsal strip procedure

lathing procedure

latissimus dorsi procedure

Latram mastectomy procedure

Lauenstein procedure

Lauenstein wrist procedure

Leadbetter procedure

Leadbetter-Politano procedure

Lee procedure

LeFort osteotomy procedure

LeFort procedure (I, II, III)

left atrial isolation procedure

Lempert procedure

lens delivered by tumbling procedure

Leone eye procedure

Lepird procedure

L'Episcopo-Zachary shoulder procedure

Lester Martin modification of Duhamel procedure

Lewis-Tanner procedure

Lich procedure

life-sustaining procedure

limb-lengthening procedure

procedure (*continued*)

limb-salvage procedure

limb-saving procedure

limb-sparing procedure

Lindeman knee procedure

Linton procedure

Lipscomb orthopedic procedure

Lipscomb-Anderson procedure

lithotomy procedure

Littler procedure

Lloyd-Roberts clubfoot procedure

Localio sacral tumor procedure

loop electrocautery excision procedure (LEEP)

loop electrosurgical excision procedure (LEEP)

loop gastric bypass procedure

loose knee procedure

Lorenz procedure

Lothrop frontoethmoidectomy procedure

lower cervical spine procedure

lower GI procedure

lower lid sling procedure

Lowman flatfoot procedure

Lowman sling procedure

Luck hallux valgus procedure

Ludloff hallux valgus procedure

Luke procedure

LVR procedure

Lynch frontoethmoidectomy procedure

Lynn Achilles-tendon procedure

Lyon-Horgan procedure

MacAusland procedure

Magnuson patellar procedure

Magnuson-Stack procedure

Mahan procedure

malarplasty procedure

Mallory-Weiss procedure

Malone ACE procedure

Malone antegrade continence enema procedure

mammaplasty procedure

procedure (*continued*)

mammary ptosis procedure
Manketelow transfer procedure
Mankin procedure
Mann procedure
Mann-Coughlin procedure
Maquet tibial procedure
Marmor procedure
Marshall knee procedure
Marshall-Marchetti procedure
Marshall-Marchetti-Krantz procedure
Martius procedure
Mathieu procedure
Matsen procedure
Mauck procedure
Maydl procedure
Mayo bunion deformity procedure
Mayo-Fueth inversion procedure
Maze III procedure
McBride procedure
McCall-Schumann procedure
McCarroll-Baker procedure
McComb procedure
McCormick-Blount procedure
McDonald procedure
McElveney procedure
McElvenny-Caldwell procedure
McGlamry-Downey procedure
McIndoe orthopedic procedure
McIndoe-Hayes procedure
McKeever clavicle procedure
McKeever foot procedure
McLaughlin procedure
McReynolds calcaneus procedure
McVay procedure
meatal advancement and glanuloplasty procedure (MAGPI)
medial rotation procedure
Meigs-Okabayashi procedure
meloplasty procedure
Menson-Scheck hanging-hip procedure
Meyers hip procedure
Michal I procedure

procedure (*continued*)

Michal II procedure
micro-operative procedure
microsurgery procedure
microsurgical epididymal sperm aspiration procedure
microsurgical procedure
Milch ulna procedure
Miller flatfoot procedure
Miller procedure
minimal access procedure
minimally invasive procedure
mini-Mustarde procedure
Minkoff-Nicholas procedure
minor procedure
Mitrofanoff procedure
Mitz procedure
MMK procedure
Moberg key-pinch procedure
modified Belsey fundoplication procedure
modified Hoke-Miller flatfoot procedure
modified Konno procedure
modified Krukenberg procedure
modified Norfolk procedure
modified procedure
modified Seldinger procedure
modified Sugiura procedure
modified surgical procedure
modified Toupe procedure
modified Weber-Fergusson procedure
modified Wies procedure
Moe procedure
Mogensen procedure
Mohs procedure
Molesworth elbow procedure
Monk orthopedic procedure
Moore humeral head procedure
Moore shoulder procedure
Moschcowitz laparoscopic procedure
Moskowitz heat procedure
motion-preserving procedure
multiple-port incision procedure
Mumford procedure
Mumford-Neer procedure
muscle-balancing procedure

procedure (*continued*)

Mustard intraatrial procedure
Mustarde otoplasty procedure
Myrhaug procedure
needle suspension procedure
needle thoracentesis
  procedure
Neer capsular shift procedure
Neibauer-Glynn procedure
Nesbit tuck procedure
Neugebauer-LeFort procedure
neurostimulating procedure
neurosurgical procedure
Neviaser clavicle procedure
Newman procedure
Nichol vaginal suspension
  procedure
Nichols procedure
Nicks procedure
Nicola shoulder procedure
Nicoll fracture repair
  procedure
Nirschl procedure
Nissen fundoplication
  procedure
Nissen-Rosseti fundoplication
  procedure
noncircumferential antireflux
  procedure
nonfenestrated Fontan
  procedure
noninvasive procedure
non-rib-spreading
  thoracotomy incision
  procedure
Norwood univentricular heart
  procedure
notchplasty procedure
nursing procedure
O'Brien capsular shift
  procedure
O'Donoghue procedure
Olshausen procedure
omentum majus flap
  procedure
open reconstructive
  procedure
open-sky procedure
operant procedure
operative procedure
orthodontic procedure
orthodox procedure

procedure (*continued*)

orthopedic surgical
  procedure
Orticochea procedure
Osborne-Cotterill elbow
  procedure
Osmond-Clarke foot
  procedure
osteoplastic frontal sinus
  procedure
otic periotic shunt procedure
Oudard procedure
Overholt procedure
Page procedure
palatal lengthening
  procedure
palliative cerebrospinal shunt
  procedure
palliative procedure
Palomo procedure
parotidectomy procedure
Parrish procedure
Paterson procedure
Pauchet procedure
Peabody foot procedure
pediatric laparoscopic
  surgical procedure
PEG procedure (percutaneous
  endoscopic gastrostomy
  procedure)
pelvic pouch procedure
percutaneous transhepatic
  biliary procedure
Pereyra procedure
Pereyra-Lebhertz modification
  of Frangenheim-Stoeckel
  procedure
peri-vaterian therapeutic
  endoscopic procedure
Perthes procedure
Pfeiffer procedure
phalloplasty procedure
Pichlmayer procedure
Pierrot-Murphy ankle
  procedure
pinky compression procedure
  (lens implant surgery)
PLIF procedure (posterior
  lumbar interbody fusion
  procedure)
pollicization procedure
Polya procedure

procedure (*continued*)
  Ponsky-Gauderer PEG
    procedure
  portmanteau procedure
  Posner procedure
  posterior lumbar interbody
    fusion procedure
  posterior Polya procedure
  potentially curative procedure
  Potts procedure
  Pozzi procedure
  Pridie-Koutsogiannis
    procedure
  primary procedure
  Pringle vascular control
    procedure
  proper sterilization procedure
  psoas hitch procedure
  Puestow biliary tract procedure
  Puestow-Gillesby procedure
  pull-through procedure
  push-back procedure
  Putti-Platt shoulder procedure
  Putti-Scaglietti procedure
  Quaegebeur procedure
  Quickert procedure
  radical procedure
  radiologic procedure
  Ramstedt procedure
  Ransley procedure
  Rashkind cardiac procedure
  Rastan-Konno procedure
  Rastelli procedure
  Raz procedure
  Raz-Leach procedure
  realignment procedure
  recess-resect procedure
  reconstruction procedure
  reconstructive plastic
    procedure
  reconstructive procedure
  reduction-augmentation
    procedure
  reefing procedure
  Rehbein procedure
  Reichel-Polya procedure
  Recamier procedure
  Reichenheim-King procedure
  Reid-Baker procedure
  repeat procedure
  restorative procedure
  resurfacing procedure

procedure (*continued*)
  retrogasserian procedure
  revascularization procedure
  Reverdin-Green bunion
    procedure
  reverse filling procedure
  reverse Mauck procedure
  reverse Putti-Platt procedure
  reversed extensor digitorum
    muscle island flap
    procedure
  revision procedure
  Richardson procedure
  Richter-Albrich procedure
  Ridlon procedure
  Riedel frontoethmoidectomy
    procedure
  Righini procedure
  Riordan procedure
  Ripstein procedure
  Robinson procedure
  Robinson-Smith procedure
  Rochet procedure
  Rockwood shoulder
    procedure
  Rockwood-Matsen capsular
    shift procedure
  rolled tendon anchovy
    procedure
  Rose procedure
  Ross procedure
  rotation-transposition cleft lip
    procedure
  Rotozyme diagnostic
    procedure
  routine procedure
  Roux-en-Y procedure
  Roux-Goldthwait procedure
  Ruiz procedure
  Ruiz-Mora procedure
  Ruiz-Morgan procedure
  Ryerson procedure
  sacroiliac buttressing
    procedure
  Sade modification of
    Norwood procedure
  Saha shoulder procedure
  Salle procedure
  salting-out procedure
  salvage procedure
  Samilson procedure
  sartorial slide procedure

procedure (*continued*)

Sato procedure
Sauve-Kapandji procedure
Savin procedure
Sayoc procedure
Scaglietti procedure
Schauffler procedure
Schenk-Eichelter vena cava plastic filter procedure
Schoemaker procedure
Schonander procedure
Schrock procedure
scleral buckling procedure
Scottish Rite procedure
screening procedure
Scudder procedure
Scuderi procedure
secondary procedure
second-look procedure
segment-oriented procedure
Segura procedure
Selakovich procedure
Seldinger procedure
semitendinosus procedure
Senning transposition procedure
septation procedure
Shauta-Aumreich procedure
Shea procedure
shelf hip procedure
Shirodkar procedure
short lever specific contact procedure
Siffert-Forster-Nachamie clubfoot procedure
Silfverskiold knee procedure
Silovi procedure
Silver procedure
Simplate procedure
single-stage procedure
Sistrunk procedure
sling procedure
Smith-Robinson procedure
Snow procedure
Soave abdominal pull-through procedure
Soave endorectal pull-through procedure
Soave pull-through procedure
Somerville procedure
Sondergaard procedure
Southwick slide procedure

procedure (*continued*)

spatial localization procedure
Speed sternoclavicular procedure
Spence procedure
sphincter-saving procedure
sphincter-sparing procedure
spinal-locking procedure
Spira procedure
Spittler procedure
split anterior tibial tendon procedure
Stack shoulder procedure
staged procedure
Stagnera procedure
Staheli shelf procedure
STA-MCA bypass procedure
Stamey modification of Pereyra procedure
Stamey procedure
Stamey-Martius procedure
Stamm procedure
standard gastric resection Whipple procedure
standard procedure
standard stripping procedure
standard surgical procedure
Stanley Way procedure
Stansel procedure
STA-peg procedure
staple procedure
stapled reconstruction procedure
Staples-Black-Brostrom ankle procedure
stapling procedure
steal procedure
Steindler procedure
stereotactic needle core biopsy procedure
stereotaxic procedure
sterile procedure
sternum turnover procedure
sternum-splitting procedure
Stewart-Harley ankle procedure
Steytler-Van Der Walt procedure
Stone procedure
Stoppa procedure
strategy procedure
Strayer procedure

procedure (*continued*)
Stretta procedure
strip procedure
Studer pouch procedure
suburethral rectus fascial sling
   procedure
suburethral sling procedure
Sugiura procedure
supramesocolic surgical
   procedure
surgical enucleation
   procedure
surgical procedure
surveillance procedure
Sutherland hip procedure
Sutherland thigh procedure
Sutro procedure
Swenson pull-through
   procedure
switch procedure
Syme procedure
Tachdjian procedure
takedown procedure
Tanagho modification of
   Burch procedure
tarsal strip procedure
Taylor procedure
Temple procedure
terminal Syme procedure
termination of procedure
Thal fundoplication
   procedure
Thiersch procedure
Thiersch-Duplay proximal
   tube procedure
ThinPrep procedure
Thomas procedure
Thomas-Thompson-Straub
   gluteus medius procedure
Thompson procedure
Thompson-Terwilliger
   procedure
Tikhoff-Linberg procedure
TIPS procedure
toe fillet flap procedure
Torkildsen shunt procedure
total fundoplication
   procedure
Toti procedure
touch-up procedure
Toupe procedure
TRAM flap procedure

procedure (*continued*)
TRAM procedure (transverse
   rectus abdominis
   myocutaneous procedure)
transblepharoplasty
   procedure
transendoscopic procedure
transhepatic antegrade biliary
   drainage procedure
transvaginal Burch procedure
transverse rectus abdominis
   muscle flap procedure
transverse rectus abdominis
   myocutaneous procedure
   (TRAM procedure)
Trillat procedure
triple-wire procedure
TriVex procedure
Tsai-Stillwell procedure
tuck procedure
tumbling procedure
uncinate procedure
uncut Collis-Nissen
   fundoplication procedure
unilateral inguinal hernia
   repair procedure
unilateral procedure
untethering procedure
up-and-down staircases
   procedure
upper cervical spine
   procedure
ureteral patch procedure
urethral vesicle suspension
   procedure
urinary diversion procedure
urologic laparoscopic surgical
   procedure
urologic surgical procedure
uvulopalatoplasty procedure
vaginal needle suspension
   procedure
vaginal suspension
   procedure
vaginal wall sling procedure
vaginoplasty procedure
valvulotomy procedure
Van de Kramer fecal fat
   procedure
Van Nes procedure
vascular procedure
VATS procedure

procedure (*continued*)
 Veleanu-Rosianu-Ionescu
  procedure
 ventriculoperitoneal shunting
  procedure
 Verdan hand procedure
 video-assisted thoracic
  surgical procedure
 Vineberg procedure
 Vulpius procedure
 Vulpius-Stoffel procedure
 V-Y pushback procedure
 W procedure
 Wagner tibial lengthening
  procedure
 Waldhausen procedure
 Walsh procedure
 Wardill-Kilner procedure
 Wassmund procedure
 Waterhouse transpubic
  procedure
 Waterston-Cooley procedure
 Watson-Cheyne-Burghard
  procedure
 Watson-Jones ankle procedure
 Weaver-Dunn procedure
 Weber procedure
 Weber-Fergusson procedure
 Weiss procedure
 West-Soto-Hall knee
  procedure
 Wheeler halving procedure
 Whipple procedure
 White slide procedure
 Whitman talectomy
  procedure
 Whitman-Thompson
  procedure
 Wiberg shelf procedure
 Wies procedure
 Williams procedure
 Williams-Haddad procedure
 Wilson procedure
 Wilson-Jacobs procedure
 Wilson-Jones procedure
 Wilson-McKeever shoulder
  procedure
 Winograd ingrown nail
  procedure
 Winter procedure
 Wolf procedure
 Womack procedure

procedure (*continued*)
 Woodward scapula procedure
 yoke transposition procedure
 York-Mason procedure
 Young flatfoot procedure
 Young-Dees procedure
 Yount procedure
 Y-plasty procedure
 Z procedure
 Zadik ingrown nail procedure
 Zancolli static lock procedure
 Zancolli-Lasso procedure
 Zarins-Rowe procedure
 Zoellner-Clancy procedure
 Z-plasty procedure
procedure drape
procedure time
procedures, alternatives,
  indications, complications
  (PAIC)
procedures, alternatives, risks
  (PAR)
Proceed hemostatic sealant
Proceed hemostatic surgical
  sealant
Procel Cast Liner
procerus and corrugator
  ablation
procerus muscle
procerus muscle myotomy
process
 acromial process
 acromion process
 alveolar process
 anterior clinoid process
 anterior process
 arytenoid process
 basilar process
 Burlar process
 burn process
 capitular process
 caudate process
 clinoid process
 cochleariform process
 condyloid process
 conoid process
 coracoid process
 coronoid process
 cortical process
 cribriform plate of alveolar
  process
 cribriform process

process (*continued*)
  cylinder process
  destructive process
  diskiform process
  ensiform process
  ethmoidal process
  external mastoid process
  falciform process
  fibro-osseous process
  fibrous process
  fovea of condyloid process
  fragmentation process
  frontal process
  frontonasal process
  glenoid process
  hamular process
  implant-layering process
  infectious process
  infiltrative process
  inflammatory process
  intercellular matrix process
  intercondylar process
  irradiation process
  knobby process
  lacrimal process
  laser stereolithography
    process
  lateral process
  lenticular process
  malar process
  malignant process
  mamillary process
  mandibular process
  mastoid process
  maxillary process
  medial nasofrontal process
  medionasal process
  mental process
  myoepithelial cell process
  nasal process
  odontoid process
  olecranon process
  orbital process
  osseointegration process
  otosclerotic process
  palatine process
  pathologic process
  piriform process
  pterygoid process
  radial styloid process
  secondary process
  septic process

process (*continued*)
  sphenoid process
  sphenoidal process
  spinous process
  styloid process
  superior articulating process
  tissue process
  transverse process
  trochlear process
  uncinate process
  ungual process
  vermiform process
  vocal process
  xiphoid process
  zygomatic process
processed carbon implant
processus vaginalis
Prochownik pessary
procidentia of uterus
ProClude transparent adhesive
    film dressing
Pro-Clude transparent wound
    dressing
Procomat small-tank
    semiautomatic processor
Procomp pelvic muscle
    reeducation equipment
ProCross Rely balloon
ProCross Rely over-the-wire
    balloon catheter
proctalgia fugax
proctectasia
proctectomy
  abdominoperineal
    proctectomy
  laparoscopic proctectomy
  pull-through proctectomy
Procter-Livingston
    endoprosthesis
Procter-Livingston tube
procteurynter
procteurysis
proctoclysis
proctococcypexy
proctocolectomy
  abdominal proctocolectomy
  laparoscopic total
    proctocolectomy
proctocolonoscopy
proctocystoplasty
proctocystotomy
proctoelytroplasty

proctogram
proctography
proctologic ball electrode
proctologic biopsy forceps
proctologic cotton carrier
proctological biopsy forceps
proctological grasping forceps
proctological polyp forceps
proctolysis
proctoperineoplasty
proctoperineorrhaphy
proctopexy
   Orr-Loygue proctopexy
   Orr-Loygue transabdominal
     proctopexy
   Ripstein proctopexy
proctoplasty
proctoptosis
Proctor cheek retractor
Proctor elevator
Proctor laryngopharyngoscope
Proctor laryngostat
Proctor mucosal elevator
Proctor phrenectomy forceps
Proctor phrenicectomy forceps
Proctor retractor
Proctor suction tube
Proctor-Hellens laryngostat
proctorrhaphy
proctoscope
   ACMI proctoscope
   Bacon proctoscope
   Bodenheimer proctoscope
   Boehm proctoscope
   Brinkerhoff proctoscope
   Buie-Hirschman proctoscope
   Fansler proctoscope
   Gabriel proctoscope
   Goldbacher proctoscope
   Hirschman proctoscope
   Hirschman-Martin
     proctoscope
   Ives proctoscope
   Kelly proctoscope
   Lieberman proctoscope
   Montague proctoscope
   Morgan proctoscope
   Morgan-Boehm proctoscope
   Muer proctoscope
   National proctoscope
   Newman proctoscope
   Otis proctoscope

proctoscope (*continued*)
   Pratt proctoscope
   Pruitt proctoscope
   rotating speculum
     proctoscope
   Salvati proctoscope
   Sims proctoscope
   Sklar proctoscope
   Strauss proctoscope
   Turrell proctoscope
   Tuttle proctoscope
   Vernon-David proctoscope
   Welch Allyn proctoscope
   Yeoman proctoscope
proctoscopic air
proctoscopic examination
proctoscopic fulguration
    electrode
proctoscopic speculum
proctoscopy
proctosigmoidectomy
proctosigmoiditis
proctosigmoidopexy
proctosigmoidoscope
   ACMI fiberoptic
     proctosigmoidoscope
   ACMI proctosigmoidoscope
   fiberoptic
     proctosigmoidoscope
proctosigmoidoscopic
   evaluation
proctosigmoidoscopic
   examination
proctosigmoidoscopy
proctostenosis
proctostomy
proctotome
proctotomy
   external proctotomy
   internal proctotomy
proctovalvotomy
ProCyte transparent adhesive
    film dressing
Prodigy lens inserter
prodromal labor
prodromal symptom
prodromic sign
production inflammation
products of conception
ProDynamic monitor
Proetz atomizer
Proetz decompressor

Proetz displacement syringe
Proetz displacement technique
Proetz maneuver
Proetz mouth gag
Proetz position
Proetz syringe
Proetz tongue depressor
Proetz-Jansen mouth gag
Profex arthroscopic leg
    positioner
Profex arthroscopic tourniquet
Profex cast padding
profile
    aortic valve velocity profile
    biometric profile
    biophysical profile (BPP)
    cardiac profile
    coagulation profile
    dose profile
    facial profile
    retrognathic profile
    ultra low profile (ULP)
    urethral pressure profile
        (UPP)
Profile hip prosthesis
Profile pediatric polypectomy
    snare
Profile Plus balloon dilatation
    catheter
Profile Plus dilatation catheter
ProFile variable taper rotary
    instrument
profilometer
    Bartlett-Edwards profilometer
    Cottle profilometer
    laryngofissure profilometer
    laryngoscope profilometer
    Straith profilometer
Profil-O-Plastic preshaped chin
    plate
Profil-O-Plastic preshaped
    midfacial plate
Profix confirming tibial insert
Profix porous femoral
    component
proflavin wool dressing
Proflex dilatation catheter
ProFlex wrist support
Pro-Flo XT catheter
Profore 4-layer bandage
Profore 4-layer wound
    dressing

ProForm maxim pressure
    reduction mattress
ProForm maxim-VE pressure
    reduction mattress
ProForm positioner
ProForma cannula
ProForma double-lumen
    papillotome
profunda Dacron patchplasty
profunda endarterectomy
profunda femoris artery
profundaplasty
profundus artery fracture
profundus function
profundus muscle
profundus tendon
profuse bleeding
profuse hemorrhage
profuse menstruation
profuse sweating
Progestasert intrauterine device
Pro-glide orthosis
Pro-glide splint
prognathia
prognathic mandible
prognathism
    basilar prognathism
    bimaxillary prognathism
    mandibular prognathism
    retromaxillary prognathism
prognostic block
prognostic factors
prognostic indicators
progonoma of jaw
prograde technique
Programalith AV pacemaker
Programalith pulse generator
Programalith pacemaker
programmable pacemaker
programmable pulse generator
programmable pump
Programmer pacemaker
programmer wand
progressive abdominal
    distention
Progressive ankle orthosis
progressive bacterial synergistic
    gangrene
progressive compression
progressive condition
progressive condylar resorption
    (PCR)

progressive dilation
progressive dilators
progressive disease
progressive enlargement
progressive extraction
progressive failure
progressive gangrene
progressive hemifacial atrophy
progressive idiopathic
  atrophoderma
progressive lingual hemiatrophy
progressive liver failure
progressive paralysis
progressive parenchymal
  destruction
progressive perilunar instability
  (stages I-IV)
progressive respiratory failure
progressive symptoms
progressive systemic sclerosis
progressive temporomandibular
  joint remodeling
progressive tension suture
  technique in
  abdominoplasty
Project research ophthalmic
  specular microscope
projection
  axial projection
  basilar projection
  basovertical projection
  biplane projection
  blow-out view projection
  bony projection
  Caldwell projection
  carpal tunnel projection
  cone projection
  coned AP projection
  cone-down projection
  cross-sectional projection
  dorsoplantar projection
  filtered-back projection
  flexion-extension projection
  frog-leg projection
  frontal projection
  half-axial projection
  horizontal projection
  inferosuperior axial
    projection
  inferosuperior projection
  inferosuperior tangential
    projection

projection (*continued*)
  intraoral projection
  lateral jaw projection
  lateral projection
  lateromedial oblique
    projection
  Lauenstein x-ray projection
  Low-Beer projection
  left lateral projection
  lordotic projection
  lumbosacral projection
  maximum intensity
    projections (MIPs)
  mediolateral projection
  mental projection
  nasal tip projection
  navicular projection
  nuchofrontal projection
  oblique lateral projection
  oblique projection
  orbital projections
  PA and lateral projections
    (posteroanterior)
  PA lordotic projection
    (posteroanterior lordotic
    projection)
  PA projection
    (posteroanterior
    projection)
  parieto-orbital projection
  pillar projection
  posteroanterior lordotic
    projection
  recumbent lateral
    projection
  sagittal projection
  scaphoid projection
  semiaxial anteroposterior
    projection
  semiaxial projection
  semiaxial transcranial
    projection
  skyline projection
  spider projection
  spiny projection
  submentovertical axial
    projection
  sunrise projection
  superoinferior projection
  superoinferior tangential
    projection
  tangential projection

projection (*continued*)
  Templeton-Zim carpal tunnel
    projection
  tip projection
  Towne projection
  transcranial projection
  transoral projection
  transverse projection
  tunnel projection
  verticosubmental projection
  Zim carpal tunnel projection
projection fiber damage
projection tract imaging
projection-reconstruction
    imaging
projection-reconstruction
    technique
projective technique
projector x-ray microscope
Pro-Koester wide-field
    microscope
Prokop intraocular lens
prolabium
prolapse
  anal prolapse
  Birnbaum procedure for
    vaginal prolapse
  frank prolapse
  hemorrhoidal prolapse
  intestinal prolapse
  iris prolapse
  Kocks operation for uterine
    prolapse
  leaflet prolapse
  rectal prolapse
  reduction of rectal prolapse
  Ripstein operation for rectal
    prolapse
  Thiersch procedure for rectal
    prolapse
  uterine prolapse
  vaginal prolapse
  Watkins transposition operation
    for uterine prolapse
Prolapse coil
prolapse of Morgagni
prolapse ring pessary
prolapsed fibroid
prolapsed hemorrhoid
prolapsed mitral valve syndrome
prolapsed rectum
prolapsed stoma

prolapsed vaginal wall
prolapsed valve
prolapser
prolapsing internal hemorrhoid
prolapsus ani
prolapsus pessary
prolapsus recti
Prolase lateral firing Nd:YAG
    laser
Prolene hernia system
    connector
Prolene hernia system onlay
    patch
Prolene hernia system underlay
    patch
Prolene mesh
Prolene mesh sheet
Prolene mesh silo
Prolene polypropylene sutures
Prolene stitch
Prolene sutures
proliferating pilar cyst
  lymphoepithelial proliferation
  synovial proliferation
  vascular proliferation
proliferative endometrium
proliferative fasciitis
proliferative inflammation
proliferative lesion
proliferative phase of wound
    healing
proliferative retinopathy
    photocoagulation (PRP)
ProLine endoscopic instrument
Prolith pacemaker
Prolog pacemaker
prolonged postoperative
    ventilation
prolonged rupture
PROloop electrosurgical device
PROloop instrument
prolotherapy
PROM (premature rupture of
    membranes)
Promex biopsy needle
prominence
  Ammon scleral prominence
  bony prominence
  canine prominence
  forehead prominence
  hilar prominence
  laryngeal prominence

prominence (*continued*)
  malar prominence
  maxillary prominence
  pulmonary prominence
  sacral prominence
  vertebral prominence
promontory of tympanum
prompt emptying
prompt excretion of dye
prompt surgical closure
Pron pillow
pronation and supination
pronation control
pronation injury
pronation sign
pronation spring-control device
pronation, external rotation
    fracture (PER fracture)
pronation-abduction fracture
pronation-abduction injury
pronation-eversion fracture
pronation-eversion injury
pronation-eversion-external
    rotation injury
pronator drift
pronator drill
pronator muscle
pronator quadratus muscle
pronator reflex
pronator syndrome
pronator teres muscle
pronator teres syndrome
prone cranial support device
prone jackknife position
prone position
prone rectus test
prone reduction
prone split-leg position
pronephric duct
Pronex pneumatic device
Proneze pad
Proneze pillow
pronged retractor
pronglike excementosis
Pronova sutures
Pron-Pillo head positioning
    device
Pronto cement
Pro-Ophtha absorbent stick
    sponge
Pro-Ophtha drape
Pro-Ophtha dressing

Pro-Ophtha eye pad
Pro-Ophtha eye patch
ProOsteon bone implant
ProOsteon bone implant graft
ProOsteon implant coralline
    hydroxyapatite bone void
    filler
ProOsteon Implant granule
ProOsteon implant graft
    material
ProOsteon synthetic bone
    implant
prop graft
Propaq Encore vital signs
    monitor
proparacaine hydrochloride
    anesthetic agent
proper alignment and
    apposition of fracture
proper hepatic artery
proper lamina
proper ligament
proper membrane
proper palmar digital arteries
proper palmar digital nerves
proper plantar digital arteries
proper plantar digital nerves
proper sterilization procedure
properitoneal fat
properitoneal fat line
properitoneal hernia
properitoneal inguinal hernia
properitoneal space
prophy angles (prophylactic)
prophylactic angiographic
    intervention
prophylactic angles
prophylactic antibiotic therapy
prophylactic anticoagulation
prophylactic bone graft
prophylactic cholecystectomy
prophylactic colectomy
prophylactic course
prophylactic fasciotomy
prophylactic gastroenterostomy
prophylactic gastrojejunostomy
prophylactic irradiation
prophylactic lymphadenectomy
prophylactic membrane
prophylactic operative
    stabilization
prophylactic orthodontics

prophylactic resection
prophylactic skeletal fixation
prophylactic surgery
prophylactic therapy
prophylaxis
Proplast allograft
Proplast facial implant
Proplast graft
Proplast porous implant material
Proplast nasal implant
Proplast pad
Proplast preformed facial
   implant
Proplast preformed implant
Proplast prosthesis
Proplast staples
Proplast-Teflon disk implant
Proplast-Teflon material
propofol infusion
proportional assist ventilation
proportional facial analysis
propoxycaine hydrochloride
   anesthetic agent
Propper binocular indirect
   ophthalmoscope
Propper retinoscope
Propper-Heine ophthalmoscope
proprioception
proprioceptive head-turning
   reflex
proprioceptive neuromuscular
   facilitation approach
proprius tendon
proptosed
proptosis
proptotic globe
propylene dressing
Proscope anoscope
prosopoanoschisis
prosopodiplegia
prosopodysmorphia
prosoponeuralgia
prosopoplegia
prosopoplegic
prosoposchisis
prosopospasm
Prospec disposable speculum
prospective evaluation of radial
   keratotomy protocol (PERK
   protocol)
ProSpeed CT scanner
ProstaCoil self-expanding stent

prostaglandin suppository
Prostakath urethral stent
Prostalac total hip prosthesis
Prostalase laser
Prostaprobe catheter
Prostar Plus percutaneous
   closure device
Prostar XL hemostatic puncture
   closure device
Prostar XL percutaneous closure
   device
ProstaScint diagnostic imaging
   agent
prostate
   base of prostate
   boggy prostate
   Cecil transurethral resection
     of prostate
   fibroadenomatous hyperplasia
     of prostate
   lateral lobes of prostate
   lobe of prostate
   lobectomy of prostate
   median furrow of prostate
   middle lobe of prostate
   Nesbit resection of
     prostate
   suprapubic excision of
     prostate
   transurethral resection of
     prostate (TURP)
prostate cancer
prostate gland
prostatectomy
   Alexander prostatectomy
   Belt prostatectomy
   laparoscopic radical
     prostatectomy
   Millen retropubic
     prostatectomy
   perineal prostatectomy
   retropubic prevesical
     prostatectomy
   retropubic prostatectomy
   suprapubic prostatectomy
   suprapubic transvesical
     prostatectomy
   transurethral prostatectomy
   transvesical prostatectomy
   Young prostatectomy
prostatectomy bag
prostatectomy forceps

prostatic adenocarcinoma
prostatic adenoma
prostatic aluminum
    electrode
prostatic biopsy needle
prostatic biopsy set
prostatic bridge catheter
prostatic calculus
prostatic cancer
prostatic capsule
prostatic carcinoma
prostatic catheter
prostatic cavity
prostatic dissector
prostatic diverticulum
prostatic driver
prostatic duct
prostatic enlargement
prostatic enucleator
prostatic forceps
prostatic fossa
prostatic fraction
prostatic ganglion
prostatic hook
prostatic hypertrophy
prostatic lobe forceps
prostatic lobe-holding forceps
prostatic needle holder
prostatic plexus
prostatic punch
prostatic retractor
prostatic scissors
prostatic sinus
prostatic stent
prostatic tissue
prostatic tractor
prostatic trocar
prostatic urethra
prostatic utricle
prostatic vesicle
prostaticovesical plexus
prostaticovesiculectomy
prostatism
prostatitis
prostatocystotomy
prostatolithotomy
prostatoseminovesiculectomy
prostatotomy
prostatovesicular junction
prostatovesiculectomy
Prostatron transurethral
    thermotherapy device

prosthesis (*pl.* prosthesis) (*see also* graft, implant, patch, valve)
2-prong stem finger prosthesis
2-pronged stem finger
    prosthesis
4-A Magovern prosthesis
4-A Magovern valve prosthesis
4-bar polycentric knee
    prosthesis
Accolade hip prosthesis
accordion prosthesis
Ace Kyle prosthesis
Acrax prosthesis
acrylic bar prosthesis
acrylic prosthesis
Acticon neosphincter
    prosthesis
AcuMatch M series modular
    femoral hip prosthesis
Adrian-Flat prosthesis
Airprene hinged knee
    prosthesis
Akiyama prosthesis
Alivium prosthesis
Aljan prosthesis
Allen-Brown prosthesis
Allo-Pro prosthesis
Allurion foot prosthesis
Alumina cemented total hip
    prosthesis
Alvarez valve prosthesis
Ambicor inflatable prosthesis
Ambicor penile prosthesis
AMC wrist prosthesis
American Heyer-Schulte chin
    prosthesis
American Heyer-Schulte
    mammary prosthesis
American Heyer-Schulte
    rhinoplasty prosthesis
American Heyer-Schulte
    testicular prosthesis
American Heyer-Schulte-
    Hinderer malar prosthesis
American Heyer-Schulte-
    Radovan tissue expander
    prosthesis
American Medical Systems
    inflatable penile prosthesis
American Medical Systems
    penile prosthesis

prosthesis (*continued*)

AML orthopedic prosthesis
AML total hip prosthesis
AMS penile prosthesis
AMS Ambicore penile prosthesis
AMS Hydroflex penile prosthesis
AMS inflatable penile prosthesis
AMS malleable penile prosthesis
AMS semirigid penile prosthesis
AMS Ultrex penile prosthesis
Amsterdam-type prosthesis
Anametric knee prosthesis
Anatomic Precoat hip prosthesis
Anatomique osteal prosthesis
Anderson columella prosthesis
Angelchik antireflux prosthesis
ankle prosthesis
antibiotic-loaded acrylic cement total joint prosthesis
anti-incontinence penile prosthesis
antireflux prosthesis
aortic valve prosthesis
aortofemoral prosthesis
Apollo hip prosthesis
Apollo knee prosthesis
Arion rod eye prosthesis
Arizona condylar tibial plateau prosthesis
Armstrong-Schuknecht stapes prosthesis
arterial graft prosthesis
arterial prosthesis
articulated chin prosthesis
Ashley breast prosthesis
Ashworth Dow Corning prosthesis
Atkinson endoprosthesis
Atkinson prosthesis
attachment of prosthesis
Attenborough total knee prosthesis
A-Turner prosthesis
Aufranc hip prosthesis

prosthesis (*continued*)

Aufranc-Turner cemented hip prosthesis
auricular prosthesis
Austin Moore hip prosthesis
Autophor femoral prosthesis
Balance hip prosthesis
ball valve prosthesis
ball-and-cage prosthesis
ball-and-cage valve prosthesis
ball-and-socket ankle prosthesis
ball-cage prosthesis
ball-type prosthesis
ball-valve prosthesis
Balnetar prosthesis
Bankart shoulder prosthesis
Bard prosthesis
Barnard mitral valve prosthesis
Bateman bipolar cup hip prosthesis
Bateman finger joint prosthesis
Bateman finger prosthesis
Bateman Universal proximal femur prosthesis (UPF prosthesis)
Bateman UPF shoulder prosthesis
Bateman UPF prosthesis (Universal proximal femur prosthesis)
Baxter mechanical valve prosthesis
BDH hip prosthesis
Beall disk valve prosthesis
Beall mitral valve prosthesis
Bechtol cemented hip prosthesis
Bechtol glenohumeral joint prosthesis
Becker breast prosthesis
Becker hand prosthesis
Becker mammary prosthesis
Becker tissue expander prosthesis
Beck-Stefee total ankle prosthesis
below-knee prosthesis
Bentall cardiovascular prosthesis
Berens prosthesis

prosthesis (*continued*)
Bi-Angular shoulder prosthesis
bicondylar ankle prosthesis
bifurcated aortofemoral prosthesis
bifurcated seamless prosthesis
bifurcation prosthesis
bileaflet prosthesis
biliary duct prosthesis
bilioduodenal prosthesis
Bi-Metric hip prosthesis
Bi-Metric Interlok femoral prosthesis
Bi-Metric porous primary femoral prosthesis
Bingham knee prosthesis
Bio-Chromatic hand prosthesis
Bioclad with pegs reinforced acetabular prosthesis
Bioglass prosthesis
biograft umbilical prosthesis
Bio-Groove acetabular prosthesis
Bio-Groove Macrobond femoral prosthesis
Bio-Groove total hip prosthesis
Biolox ball head prosthesis
Biomet AGC knee prosthesis
Biomet hip prosthesis
Biomet total toe prosthesis
biometric prosthesis
Bionic ear prosthesis
Bionit vascular prosthesis
bipolar cup hip prosthesis
bipolar prosthesis
bisque-baked prosthesis
Bivona Duckbill voice prosthesis
Bivona low-resistance voice prosthesis
Bivona Ultra Low voice prosthesis
Bivona-Colorado dummy prosthesis
Bivona-Colorado voice prosthesis
Bjork prosthesis
Bjork-Shiley aortic valve prosthesis

prosthesis (*continued*)
Bjork-Shiley convexoconcave 60-degree valve prosthesis
Bjork-Shiley floating disk prosthesis
Bjork-Shiley mitral valve prosthesis
BK prosthesis, (below-knee prosthesis)
bladder-neck support prosthesis
Blair-Brown prosthesis
Blauth knee prosthesis
Blazina prosthesis
Blom-Singer indwelling low-pressure voice prosthesis
Blom-Singer tracheoesophageal prosthesis
Bock knee prosthesis
Bograb Universal offset ossicular prosthesis
bone prosthesis
bone-anchored prosthesis
bovine collagen material prosthesis
bovine pericardial prosthesis
Boyne dental prosthesis
Braun prosthesis
Braunwald prosthesis
Braunwald-Cutter ball-valve prosthesis
Braun-Wangensteen prosthesis
breast prosthesis
Bridge prosthesis
Brigham total knee prosthesis
Buchholz hip prosthesis
Buchholz knee prosthesis
Buchholz total hip prosthesis
Buechel-Pappas total ankle prosthesis
Byars mandibular prosthesis
Byers prosthesis
bypass prosthesis
cable-operated hand prosthesis
CAD hip prosthesis
CAD prosthesis
Caffiniere prosthesis
caged-ball valve prosthesis
calcar replacement femoral prosthesis

prosthesis (*continued*)

Callender technique hip prosthesis
Calnan-Nicole prosthesis
Calnan-Nicoll synthetic joint prosthesis
Calnan-Nicolle synthetic joint prosthesis
camouflage prosthesis
Canadian hip disarticulation prosthesis
Capetown aortic valve prosthesis
Capetown prosthesis
CarboMedics cardiac valve prosthesis
Carbon Copy foot prosthesis
Carbon Copy lightweight prosthesis
Carbo-Seal ascending aortic prosthesis
CardioFix pericardium patch
Cardona eye prosthesis
carpal prosthesis
Carpentier annuloplasty ring prosthesis
Carpentier-Edwards aortic valve prosthesis
Carpentier-Edwards valve prosthesis
Carpentier-Rhone-Poulenc mitral rings prosthesis
Carrion penile prosthesis
cartilage prosthesis
Cartwright heart prosthesis
Cartwright valve prosthesis
Cartwright vascular prosthesis
Cathcart orthocentric hip prosthesis
Catterall prosthesis
Causse-Shea prosthesis
CDH Precoat Plus hip prosthesis
Celestin endoesophageal prosthesis
celluloid prosthesis
Centralign Precoat hip prosthesis
ceramic hip prosthesis
ceramic ossicular prosthesis
Ceramion prosthesis

prosthesis (*continued*)

Ceravital incus replacement prosthesis
Ceravital partial ossicular replacement prosthesis (PORP)
Ceravital total ossicular replacement prosthesis (TORP)
CFE Taperloc hip prosthesis
CFS hip prosthesis
Charcot prosthesis
Charnley acetabular cup prosthesis
Charnley cemented hip prosthesis
Charnley hip prosthesis
Charnley knee prosthesis
Charnley total hip prosthesis
Charnley-cobra total hip prosthesis
Charnley-Hastings prosthesis
Charnley-Moore hip prosthesis
Charnley-Mueller cemented hip prosthesis
chessboard prosthesis
chin prosthesis
Chopart partial foot prosthesis
Cintor knee prosthesis
Cirrus foot prosthesis
clamshell prosthesis
cleft palate prosthesis
Cloutier unconstrained knee prosthesis
cobalt-chromium alloy prosthesis
cochlear prosthesis
Co-Cr-Mo prosthesis
Co-Cr-W-Ni alloy prosthesis
collagen prosthesis
collagen tape prosthesis
collar prosthesis
College Park TruStep foot prosthesis
combination gel and inflatable mammary prosthesis
compartmental total knee prosthesis

prosthesis (*continued*)

computerized assisted design prosthesis
condylar prosthesis
Conley mandibular prosthesis
constrained hinged knee prosthesis
constrained nonhinged knee prosthesis
constrained total knee prosthesis
contoured Dow Corning Silastic prosthesis
convexoconcave valve prosthesis
Cooley Dacron prosthesis
Cooley-Bloodwell mitral valve prosthesis
Cooley-Bloodwell-Cutter prosthesis
Cooley-Cutter prosthesis
Coonrad prosthesis
Coonrad wrist prosthesis
Coonrad-Morrey total elbow prosthesis
Cox-Uphoff double-lumen breast prosthesis
cranial prosthesis
Creench insertion of vascular prosthesis
crimped Dacron prosthesis
crimped woven prosthesis
crimped wire prosthesis
Cronin Silastic mammary prosthesis
crook measuring prosthesis
CROS hearing aid prosthesis
Cross-Jones disk valve prosthesis
Cross-Jones valve prosthesis
cruciate-retaining prosthesis
cruciate-sacrificing prosthesis
Crutchfield tongs prosthesis
CSF prosthesis
CUI artificial breast prosthesis
CUI chin prosthesis
CUI eye sphere prosthesis
CUI gel mammary prosthesis
CUI nasal prosthesis
CUI saline mammary prosthesis
CUI tendon prosthesis

prosthesis (*continued*)

CUI testicular prosthesis
cup hip prosthesis
custom pectus excavatum per moulange prosthesis
custom total alloplastic TMJ reconstruction prosthesis
Cutter aortic valve prosthesis
Cutter SCDK prosthesis
Cutter-Smeloff aortic valve prosthesis
Cutter-Smeloff cardiac valve prosthesis
cylinder penile distendible prosthesis
cylinder penile nondistendible prosthesis
Dacomed Omni Phase penile prosthesis
Dacron arterial prosthesis
Dacron bifurcation prosthesis
Dacron valve prosthesis
Dacron vascular prosthesis
Dacron vessel prosthesis
Dallop-type fascial prosthesis
DANA shoulder prosthesis
Dardik umbilical prosthesis
d'Aubigne prosthesis
Davis prosthesis
de la Caffiniere trapeziometacarpal prosthesis
De Paco prosthesis
Deane unconstrained knee prosthesis
DeBakey prosthesis
DeBakey valve prosthesis
DeBakey vascular prosthesis
DeBakey Vasculour-II vascular prosthesis
Dee elbow prosthesis
definitive prosthesis
DeLaura knee prosthesis
DeLaura-Verner knee prosthesis
Delrin biomaterial joint replacement prosthesis
Delrin frame of valve prosthesis
dental prosthesis
Deon hip prosthesis
DePalma hip prosthesis

prosthesis (*continued*)
 DePuy dual-lock hip
  prosthesis
 Deune knee prosthesis
 DeVega prosthesis
 Dilamezinsert penile
  prosthesis
 Dimension hip prosthesis
 Dimension-C femoral stem
  prosthesis
 discoid valve prosthesis
 disk valve prosthesis
 distal radioulnar joint
  prosthesis (DRUJ
  prosthesis)
 Doherty prosthesis
 double-pigtail prosthesis
 double-rod penile prosthesis
 DoubleStent biliary
  endoprosthesis
 Dow Corning contoured
  Silastic prosthesis
 Dow Corning mammary
  prosthesis
 Dow Corning Silastic
  prosthesis
 Dragstedt prosthesis
 DRUJ prosthesis
 dual-chambered prosthesis
 dual-lock Depuy hip
  prosthesis
 dual-lock hip prosthesis
 dual-lock total hip prosthesis
 Dubinet prosthesis
 duckbill voice prosthesis
 Duocondylar knee
  prosthesis
 Duo-Lock hip prosthesis
 Duo-Patella knee prosthesis
 Duracon prosthesis
 Dura-II positionable penile
  prosthesis
 DuraPhase inflatable penile
  prosthesis
 DuraPhase semirigid penile
  prosthesis
 Duromedics valve prosthesis
 DynaFlex penile prosthesis
 dynamic penile prosthesis
 E2 foot prosthesis
 ear pinna prosthesis
 ear piston prosthesis

prosthesis (*continued*)
 Eaton trapezium finger joint
  replacement prosthesis
 Eaton upper limb prosthesis
 Edwards seamless prosthesis
 Edwards Teflon intracardiac
  patch prosthesis
 Edwards Teflon intracardiac
  prosthesis
 Efteklar-Charnley hip
  prosthesis
 Ehmke ear prosthesis
 Ehmke platinum Teflon
  prosthesis
 Eicher hip prosthesis
 elbow prosthesis
 ELP femoral prosthesis
 Endo hinged knee prosthesis
 Endo rotating knee joint
  prosthesis
 Endo sled prosthesis
 endoesophageal prosthesis
 endoskeletal prosthesis
 Engh porous metal hip
  prosthesis
 Englehardt femoral prosthesis
 English-McNab shoulder
  prosthesis
 Entegra prosthesis
 EPTFE graft prosthesis
 ERCP conventional prosthesis
 Eriksson knee prosthesis
 ESKA-Jonas penile prosthesis
 EsophaCoil prosthesis
 esophageal prosthesis
 Esser prosthesis
 Estecar prosthesis
 Ethicon Polytef paste
  prosthesis
 Ethrone prosthesis
 Evolution hip prosthesis
 Ewald elbow prosthesis
 expandable prosthesis
 external prosthesis
 F.R. Thompson hip
  prosthesis
 facial prosthesis
 fallopian tube repair
  prosthesis
 fascia lata prosthesis
 femoral head prosthesis
 femoral prosthesis

prosthesis (*continued*)

femorofemoral crossover prosthesis
fenestra prosthesis
Fett carpal prosthesis
finger prosthesis
Finn hinged knee replacement
Finn knee revision prosthesis
Finney penile prosthesis
Finney-flexirod penile prosthesis
fixed expansion prosthesis
fixed femoral head prosthesis
Flatt finger prosthesis
Flatt thumb prosthesis
FLEX H/A total ossicular prosthesis
Flex-Foot prosthesis
flexible penile prosthesis
Flexi-Flate penile prosthesis
Flexi-Flate inflatable penile prosthesis
Flexi-rod penile prosthesis
Flexi-rod semirigid penile prosthesis
Fountain design prosthesis
Fox prosthesis
Fox-Blazina prosthesis
Fredricks mammary prosthesis
free prosthesis
Free-Flow system prosthesis
Freeman modular total hip prosthesis
Freeman-Samuelson knee prosthesis
Freeman-Swanson knee prosthesis
Freestyle aortic root bioprosthesis
full-thickness prosthesis
fully constrained tricompartmental knee prosthesis
Gaffney ankle prosthesis
Galante hip prosthesis
gel-filled prosthesis
gel-saline Surgitek prosthesis
Gemini hip system prosthesis
Genesis knee prosthesis

prosthesis (*continued*)

Geomedic femoral condyle prosthesis
Geomedic knee prosthesis
Geomedic total knee prosthesis
Geometric knee prosthesis
Geometric total knee prosthesis
Georgiade breast prosthesis
GFS Mark II inflatable penile prosthesis
Gianturco expandable metallic biliary stent
Gilbert prosthesis
Gilfillan humeral prosthesis
Giliberty acetabular prosthesis
Giliberty cup hip prosthesis
Giliberty total hip prosthesis
Gillette joint prosthesis
Gillies prosthesis
glass penile prosthesis
gliding prosthesis
glottic prosthesis
Golaski-UMI vascular prosthesis
golf tee-shaped polyvinyl prosthesis
Goodhill prosthesis
Gore-Tex knee prosthesis
Gore-Tex vascular prosthesis
Gott low-profile prosthesis
Gott mitral valve prosthesis
Gott-Daggett heart valve prosthesis
Greissinger foot prosthesis
Gripper acetabular cup prosthesis
Groningen voice prosthesis
Gruppe wire prosthesis
GSB elbow prosthesis
GSB knee prosthesis
Guepar hinged knee prosthesis
Guepar knee prosthesis
Guepar total knee prosthesis
Guilford-Wright prosthesis
Gunston knee prosthesis
Gunston polycentric knee prosthesis
Gunston-Hult knee prosthesis

prosthesis (*continued*)

Gustilo knee prosthesis
Haering esophageal prosthesis
Hall-Kaster mitral valve prosthesis
Hall-Kaster tilting disk valve prosthesis
Hamas upper limb prosthesis
Hammersmith mitral prosthesis
Hammersmith mitral valve prosthesis
Hancock aortic valve prosthesis
Hancock mitral valve prosthesis
Hancock porcine valve prosthesis
Hanger prosthesis
Hanslik patellar prosthesis
Harken prosthesis
Harris cemented hip prosthesis
Harris hip prosthesis
Harris Micromini prosthesis
Harris precoat cemented hip prosthesis
Harris precoat prosthesis
Harris total hip prosthesis
Harris-Galante hip prosthesis
Harris-Galante porous hip prosthesis
Harris-Galante porous metal hip prosthesis
Harrison interlocking mesh prosthesis
Hartley mammary prosthesis
Haynes-Stellite implant metal prosthesis
HD2 total hip prosthesis
heart prosthesis
heart valve prosthesis
Helanca seamless tube prosthesis
Henschke-Mauch lower limb prosthesis
Herbert knee prosthesis
heterograft prosthesis
Hexcel total condylar knee system prosthesis
Hexcel total condylar prosthesis

prosthesis (*continued*)

Heyer-Schulte breast prosthesis
Heyer-Schulte chin prosthesis
Heyer-Schulte malar prosthesis
Heyer-Schulte mammary prosthesis
Heyer-Schulte testicular prosthesis
HG Multilock hip prosthesis
Hinderer malar prosthesis
hinged constrained knee prosthesis
hinged great toe replacement prosthesis
hinged implant prosthesis
hinged total knee prosthesis
hinged-leaflet vascular prosthesis
hinge-knee prosthesis
hingeless heart valve prosthesis
hip cup prosthesis
hip disarticulation prosthesis
Hittenberger prosthesis
HKAFO prosthesis
hollow sphere prosthesis
homograft prosthesis
Hosmer elbow prosthesis
Hosmer WALK prosthesis
Hosmer weight-activated locking knee prosthesis
House incus replacement prosthesis
House piston prosthesis
House stainless steel mesh prosthesis
House stapes wire prosthesis
House tantalum prosthesis
House wire stapes prosthesis
House wire-fat prosthesis
Howmedica Kinematic II knee prosthesis
Howmedica orthopedic prosthesis
Howmedica Universal total knee prosthesis
Howorth prosthesis
Howse-Coventry hip prosthesis
HPS II total hip prosthesis

prosthesis (*continued*)

HSS knee prosthesis
HSS total condylar knee prosthesis
Hufnagel disk heart valve prosthesis
Hufnagel low-profile heart prosthesis
Hufnagel valve prosthesis
Hunter tendon prosthesis
hybrid prosthesis
hydraulic incontinent prosthesis
hydraulic knee unit prosthesis
Hydroflex inflatable penile prosthesis
Hydroflex penile prosthesis
Hydroxial hip prosthesis
hydroxyapatite ossicular prosthesis
I-beam hemiarthroplasty hip prosthesis
Identifit hip prosthesis
Image custom external breast prosthesis
immediate fit prosthesis
immediate postoperative prosthesis (IPOP)
Impact modular porous prosthesis
implant-borne prosthesis
implant-supported fixed prosthesis
Impra collagen-impregnated Dacron prosthesis
incontinence prosthesis
incus replacement prosthesis
Indong Oh prosthesis
Infinity modular hip prosthesis
inflatable mammary prosthesis
inflatable Mentor penile prosthesis
inflatable penile prosthesis
inflatable prosthesis
inflatable urinary incontinence prosthesis
Inro fingernail prosthesis
Inro toenail prosthesis
Insall-Burstein knee prosthesis

prosthesis (*continued*)

Insall-Burstein total knee prosthesis
insertion of prosthesis
Integral Interlok femoral prosthesis
Integrity acetabular cup prosthesis
interlocked mesh prosthesis
Intermedics Natural-Knee knee prosthesis
internal ear prosthesis
Inter-Op acetabular prosthesis
intracardiac patch prosthesis
intraluminal tube prosthesis
IntraStent DoubleStrut biliary endoprosthesis
Introl bladder neck support prosthesis
Ionescu-Shiley aortic valve prosthesis
Iowa total hip prosthesis
iridium prosthesis
ischial weightbearing prosthesis
isoelastic pelvic prosthesis
Ivalon prosthesis
Jenny mammary prosthesis
Jewett prosthesis
Jobst stocking prosthesis
Jonas penile prosthesis
Jonas silicone-silver penile prosthesis
Jonas silver penile prosthesis
Joplin toe prosthesis
JSCI-DeBakey vascular prosthesis
Judet hip prosthesis
Judet press-fit hip prosthesis
KAFO prosthesis
Kastec mitral valve prosthesis
Kaster mitral valve prosthesis
Kaufman anti-incontinence prosthesis
Kaufman incontinence prosthesis
Kaufman male urinary incontinence prosthesis
Kaufman penile prosthesis
Kaufman urinary incontinence prosthesis

prosthesis (*continued*)

Kay-Shiley disk valve prosthesis
Kay-Shiley valve prosthesis
Kay-Suzuki disk prosthesis
Kay-Suzuki disk valve prosthesis
Kay-Suzuki valve prosthesis
KD chin prosthesis
Keeler prosthesis
Kessler upper limb prosthesis
Kinematic rotating-hinge total knee prosthesis
Kinematic total knee prosthesis
Kinematic rotating-hinge knee prosthesis
Kinemax Plus knee prosthesis
Kirschner total shoulder prosthesis
KMC femoral stem prosthesis
KMP femoral stem prosthesis
KMW/PC femoral prosthesis
knee prosthesis
knee-bearing prosthesis
knitted prosthesis
knitted Teflon prosthesis
knitted vascular prosthesis
Koenig MPJ prosthesis
Krause-Wolfe prosthesis
Lacey prosthesis
Lagrange-Letoumel hip prosthesis
Lagrange-Letoumel hip socket prosthesis
LAI knee prosthesis
Lanceford porous metal hip prosthesis
Landers-Foulks prosthesis
laryngeal prosthesis
Lash-Loeffler penile prosthesis
Lash-Masler penile prosthesis
Lash-Moser prosthesis
latex prosthesis
Lattimer Silastic testicular prosthesis
Leadbetter-Politano ureteral implant prosthesis
Leake Dacron mandible prosthesis
Leeds-Keio ligament prosthesis

prosthesis (*continued*)

Leinbach hip prosthesis
Lewis expandable adjustable prosthesis
Lezinski Flex-HA PORP ossicular chain prosthesis
Lillehei valve prosthesis
Lillehei-Cruz-Kaster valve prosthesis
Lillehei-Kaster aortic value prosthesis
Lillehei-Kaster cardiac valve prosthesis
Lillehei-Kaster mitral valve prosthesis
Link cementless reconstruction hip prosthesis
Link MP hip noncemented reconstruction prosthesis
Lippman hip prosthesis
Lippy incus prosthesis
Lippy modified prosthesis
Liverpool knee prosthesis
Lo Bak spinal support prosthesis
locking prosthesis
London prosthesis
Longevity V-line hip prosthesis
Longhem prosthesis
Lo-Por arterial prosthesis
Lo-Por vascular graft prosthesis
Lord press-fit hip prosthesis
Lord total hip prosthesis
Lorenzo SMO prosthesis
Lowe-Breck elbow prosthesis
lower limb prosthesis
low-pressure voice prosthesis
low-profile prosthesis
low-profile valve prosthesis
L-type nose-bridge prosthesis
Lubinus knee prosthesis
lunate prosthesis
MacIntosh knee prosthesis
MacIntosh tibial plateau prosthesis
MacIntosh tibial prosthesis
Mackler intraluminal tube prosthesis
Mackler tube prosthesis

prosthesis (*continued*)

MacNab-English shoulder prosthesis
Macrofit hip prosthesis
madreporic hip prosthesis
Magnuson valve prosthesis
Magnuson-Cromie valve prosthesis
Magovern ball-valve prosthesis
Magovern-Cromie valve prosthesis
malar prosthesis
malleable prosthesis
malleus-incus prosthesis
Mallory-Head hip prosthesis
Mallory-Head porous primary femoral prosthesis
mammary prosthesis
Mammatech breast prosthesis
mandibular guide prosthesis
mandibular guide-plane prosthesis
mandibular prosthesis
Mangat curvilinear chin prosthesis
MAPF femoral stem prosthesis
Marlex mesh prosthesis
Marlex methyl methacrylate prosthesis
Marmor knee prosthesis
Marmor modular knee prosthesis
Marmor tibial prosthesis
Marmor total knee prosthesis
Master step foot prosthesis
Matchett prosthesis
Matchett-Brown hip prosthesis
Matchett-Brown prosthesis
Mathys cementless prosthesis
Matrol femoral head prosthesis
maxillary dental prosthesis
maxillary prosthesis
maxillofacial prosthesis
Mayo elbow prosthesis
Mayo semiconstrained elbow prosthesis
Mayo total ankle prosthesis
M-C prosthesis
McBride femoral prosthesis
McBride-Moore prosthesis

prosthesis (*continued*)

McCutchen SLT hip prosthesis
McGee ear piston prosthesis
McGehee elbow prosthesis
McGhan breast prosthesis
McKee femoral prosthesis
McKee totally constrained elbow prosthesis
McKee-Farrar hip prosthesis
McKee-Farrar total hip prosthesis
McKeever knee prosthesis
McKeever patella cap prosthesis
McKeever patella prosthesis
McKeever Vitallium cap prosthesis
McNaught keel laryngeal prosthesis
MCP finger joint prosthesis
Meadox woven velour prosthesis
Meadox-Cooley woven low-porosity prosthesis
Meadox-Cooley woven low-porosity vascular prosthesis
Mecring acetabular prosthesis
Medi-graft vascular prosthesis
Medtronic-Hall heart valve prosthesis
Medtronic-Hall tilting-disk valve prosthesis
Mega prosthesis
Megasource penile prosthesis
Meme breast prosthesis
Mentor Alpha 1 inflatable penile prosthesis
Mentor breast prosthesis
Mentor inflatable penile prosthesis
Mentor malleable penile prosthesis
Mentor Mark penile prosthesis
Mentor Resi prosthesis
Mentor Self-Cath penile prosthesis
Mersilene prosthesis
mesh prosthesis
mesh stent prosthesis
metacarpophalangeal prosthesis

prosthesis (*continued*)

metal bucket-handle prosthesis
metal femoral head prosthesis
metal-on-metal articulating intervertebral disk prosthesis
metal prosthesis
Metasul hip prosthesis
Metasul metal-on-metal hip prosthesis
Meyerding prosthesis
MGH knee prosthesis
Michael Reese shoulder prosthesis
microcrimped prosthesis
Microknit arterial prosthesis
Microknit vascular graft prosthesis
Microloc knee prosthesis
Microvel prosthesis
Miller-Galante hip prosthesis
Milliknit arterial prosthesis
Milliknit Dacron prosthesis
Milliknit vascular graft prosthesis
Minneapolis hip prosthesis
Misti Gold prosthesis
mitral valve prosthesis
Mittlemeir ceramic hip prosthesis
Mittlemeir femoral prosthesis
modified Moore hip locking prosthesis
modified prosthesis
modular Austin Moore hip prosthesis
modular Iowa Precoat total hip prosthesis
modular knee prosthesis
modular prosthesis
modular total hip prosthesis
Monk hip prosthesis
monostrut cardiac valve prosthesis
Moon-Robinson stapes prosthesis
Moore femoral neck prosthesis
Moore hip prosthesis
Moore hip-locking prosthesis
Moore self-locking prosthesis

prosthesis (*continued*)

Moretz prosthesis
Moseley glenoid rim prosthesis
Mueller Duo-Lock hip prosthesis
Mueller hip prosthesis
Mueller micrograin prosthesis
Mueller total hip prosthesis
Mueller-Charnley hip prosthesis
Mueller-Charnley total hip prosthesis
Muhlberger orbital implant prosthesis
Muhlberger orbital prosthesis
Mules prosthesis
Mulligan prosthesis
Mulligan Silastic prosthesis
Murray knee prosthesis
muscle prosthesis
myoelectric control prosthesis
myoelectric prosthesis
Naden-Rieth prosthesis
natural-feel breast prosthesis
Natural-Hip prosthesis
Natural-Y breast prosthesis
NEB total hip prosthesis
Neer shoulder joint prosthesis
Neer proximal humerus prosthesis
Neer shoulder joint prosthesis
Neer shoulder prosthesis
Neer shoulder replacement prosthesis
Neibauer hand prosthesis
neural prosthesis
NeuroCybernetic prosthesis
Neville tracheal prosthesis
Neville tracheal reconstruction prosthesis
Neville tracheobronchial prosthesis
New Jersey hemiarthroplasty prosthesis
New Jersey-LCS shoulder prosthesis
New Jersey-LCS total knee prosthesis
New Weavenit Dacron prosthesis
Nexus hip prosthesis

prosthesis (*continued*)

Nicoll tendon prosthesis
Niebauer finger-joint replacement prosthesis
Niebauer trapezium replacement prosthesis
Noiles posterior stabilized knee prosthesis
Noiles rotating-hinge total knee prosthesis
noncemented prosthesis
nonconstrained knee prosthesis
nonhinged constrained knee prosthesis
nonhinged knee prosthesis
nose-bridge prosthesis
nylon vascular prosthesis
ocular prosthesis
Odland ankle prosthesis
OEC hip prosthesis
offset hinge prosthesis
offset modified prosthesis
Oklahoma ankle prosthesis
Ollier-Thiersch prosthesis
Ommaya reservoir prosthesis
Omnicarbon heart valve prosthesis
Omnifit HA hip stem prosthesis
OmniPhase penile prosthesis
OmniPhase semirigid penile prosthesis
Omniscience single-leaflet cardiac valve prosthesis
onlay Dacron prosthesis
orbital floor prosthesis
orbital prosthesis
Oregon prosthesis
Orlon vascular prosthesis
Orthofix prosthesis
Ortholoc prosthesis
ossicular chain replacement prosthesis
ossicular replacement prosthesis
OsteoCap hip prosthesis
Osteolock hip prosthesis
Osteonics hip prosthesis
Osteostim prosthesis
Otto Bock Greissinger foot prosthesis

prosthesis (*continued*)

Otto Bock system electric hands prosthesis
Ottoback knee prosthesis
Oxford total knee prosthesis
Padgett prosthesis
Paladon prosthesis
palatal prosthesis
Panje voice button laryngeal prosthesis
Panje voice prosthesis
paraffin prosthesis
partial ossicular reconstructive/replacement prosthesis (PORP)
Passy-Muir tracheostomy speaking valve
patch prosthesis
patella cap prosthesis
patellar prosthesis
patellar tendon-bearing below-knee prosthesis
patellofemoral prosthesis
PC Performer knee prosthesis
PCA knee prosthesis
Pearman penile prosthesis
Pearman penile Silastic prosthesis
pedicle prosthesis
pegged tibial prosthesis
peg-top prosthesis
Pemco valve prosthesis
penile prosthesis
Perfecta hip prosthesis
Performance knee prosthesis
periodontal prosthesis
peroral esophageal prosthesis
Perras mammary prosthesis
Perras-Papillon breast prosthesis
Phoenix total hip prosthesis
piggyback mammary prosthesis
Pillet hand prosthesis
piston prosthesis
piston stapes prosthesis
piston-type prosthesis
Pitt talking tracheostomy tube
plaster pants prosthesis
Plasticor torque-type prosthesis

prosthesis (*continued*)

Plasti-Pore ossicular replacement prosthesis
Plasti-Pore total ossicular replacement prosthesis (Plasti-Pore TORP)
Plexiglas prosthesis
Plystan prosthesis
Polycel bone composite prosthesis
polycentric knee prosthesis
polycentric prosthesis
polyethylene prosthesis
polyethylene talar prosthesis
polyurethane prosthesis
polyvinyl prosthesis
porcine heterograft prosthesis
porcine prosthesis
Porocool prosthesis
porous coat cup for Richards hip prosthesis
porous coated anatomic knee prosthesis (PCA knee prosthesis)
Precision Osteolock femoral prosthesis
Precision Osteolock hip prosthesis
Preclude dura substitute prosthesis
Precoat Plus femoral prosthesis
press-fit prosthesis
Pritchard total elbow prosthesis
ProAdvantage knee prosthesis
Profile hip prosthesis
Proplast prosthesis
Prostalac hip prosthesis
Prostalac total hip prosthesis
prosthetic antibiotic-loaded acrylic cement total joint prosthesis
Protasul femoral prosthesis
Protek hip prosthesis
Protek Protasul vanadium-free titanium alloy prosthesis
Proud septal prosthesis
Provox voice prosthesis
PTB cast prosthesis
PTS prosthesis
Quantum foot prosthesis

prosthesis (*continued*)

RAM knee prosthesis
Ranawat-Burstein hip prosthesis
Rancho external fixation prosthesis
Randelli shoulder prosthesis
Rashkind double-disk occluder prosthesis
Rastelli prosthesis
Reese prosthesis
removable expansion prosthesis
replacement of prosthesis
replacement prosthesis
Reverdin prosthesis
Revive system penile prosthesis
R-HAB lighter weight ankle prosthesis
Richards hydroxyapatite PORP prosthesis
Richards hydroxyapatite TORP prosthesis
Richards maximum contact cruciate-sparing prosthesis
Richards Zirconia femoral head prosthesis
Ring hip prosthesis
Ring knee prosthesis
Ring total hip prosthesis
Robert Bent Brigham total knee prosthesis
Robert Brigham knee prosthesis
Robinson incus replacement prosthesis
Robinson middle ear prosthesis
Robinson piston prosthesis
Robinson stapes prosthesis
Robinson-Moon stapes prosthesis
Robinson-Moon-Lippy stapes prosthesis
Rochester HKAFO prosthesis
Rock-Mulligan prosthesis
Rose L-type nose bridge prosthesis
Rosen inflatable urinary incontinence prosthesis
Rosen urinary prosthesis

prosthesis (*continued*)

Rosenfeld hip prosthesis
Rosenfeld total hip prosthesis
Rosi bridge prosthesis
rotating-hinge knee prosthesis
Rothman Institute femoral
  prosthesis
Ruddy stapes prosthesis
SACH prosthesis
sacral segmental nerve
  stimulation implantable
  neural prosthesis
saddle prosthesis
Safian design prosthesis
Safian rhinoplasty prosthesis
Saint George knee prosthesis
Saint Jude prosthesis
Sampson prosthesis
Sauerbruch limb prosthesis
Sauvage Bionit femoral
  prosthesis
Sauvage fabric graft prosthesis
Sauvage filamentous
  prosthesis
Savastano hemi-knee
  prosthesis
Savastano total knee
  prosthesis
Sbarbaro tibial prosthesis
Scarborough prosthesis
SCDK heart valve prosthesis
SCDT heart valve prosthesis
Scheer Teflon prosthesis
Scheer Tef-wire prosthesis
Schlein total elbow prosthesis
Schlein trisurface ankle
  prosthesis
Schuknecht Gelfoam wire
  prosthesis
Schuknecht piston prosthesis
Schuknecht stapes prosthesis
Schuknecht Teflon wire
  piston prosthesis
Schuknecht Tef-Wire
  prosthesis
Schurring ossicle cup
  prosthesis
Scott inflatable penile
  prosthesis
screw-retained prosthesis
scrotal-perineal incontinence
  prosthesis

prosthesis (*continued*)

Scuderi prosthesis
Scurasil device prosthesis
SE prosthesis
seamless prosthesis
seamless tube prosthesis
Seattle Foot prosthesis
Select ankle prosthesis
Select shoulder prosthesis
self-articulating femoral
  prosthesis
self-centering Universal hip
  prosthesis
self-locking prosthesis
semiconstrained prosthesis
semirigid penile prosthesis
Sense-of-Feel prosthesis
Servital prosthesis
Sevastano knee prosthesis
shaft prosthesis
Shea bail-hook prosthesis
Shea malleus gripper
  prosthesis
Shea polyethylene prosthesis
Shea Teflon piston prosthesis
Sheehan knee prosthesis
Sheehan total knee prosthesis
Sheehy incus replacement
  prosthesis
Sheehy-House incus
  replacement prosthesis
shell prosthesis
Shier knee prosthesis
shoulder prosthesis
Silastic ball spacer prosthesis
Silastic chin prosthesis
Silastic fimbrial prosthesis
Silastic mammary prosthesis
Silastic otoplasty prosthesis
Silastic penile prosthesis
Silastic sheeting keel
  prosthesis
Silastic standard elastometer
  prosthesis
Silastic testicular prosthesis
Silflex intramedullary
  prosthesis
silicone doughnut prosthesis
silicone elastomer prosthesis
silicone gel prosthesis
silicone trapezium prosthesis
Silima breast prosthesis

prosthesis (*continued*)

Siloxane prosthesis
Siltex Becker breast prosthesis
Singer-Blom electrolarynx prosthesis
Singer-Blom ossicular prosthesis
Singh speech system voice rehabilitation prosthesis
single-axis ankle prosthesis
single-rod penile prosthesis
Sinterlock implant metal prosthesis
Sivash hip prosthesis
SKI knee prosthesis
Small-Carrion penile prosthesis
Small-Carrion semirigid penile prosthesis
Smeloff-Cutter aortic valve prosthesis
Smeloff-Cutter ball-valve prosthesis
Smeloff-Cutter heart valve prosthesis
Smith Silastic prosthesis
Smith total ankle prosthesis
Smith-Petersen hip cup prosthesis
SMo prosthesis
Snyder breast prosthesis
solid silicone orbital prosthesis
solid-ankle, cushioned-heel foot prosthesis
Sorin mitral valve prosthesis
Sparks mandrel prosthesis
Spectron cemented hip prosthesis
Spectron hip prosthesis
Spectron metal-backed cup for Richards hip prosthesis
Speed radial cap prosthesis
sphere prosthesis
spherocentric knee prosthesis
split-thickness prosthesis
Springlite lower limb prosthesis
S-ROM femoral stem prosthesis
S-ROM hip prosthesis

prosthesis (*continued*)

S-ROM system prosthesis
St. George total elbow prosthesis
St. George total hip prosthesis
St. George total knee prosthesis
St. Jude Medical aortic valve prosthesis
St. Jude Medical valve prosthesis
St. Jude mitral valve prosthesis
St. Jude valve prosthesis
stabilocondylar knee prosthesis
stainless steel mesh prosthesis
stainless steel prosthesis
stainless steel wire prosthesis
standard neck Universal for Richards hip prosthesis
Stanmore shoulder prosthesis
stapedectomy prosthesis
stapes prosthesis
Starr ball heart prosthesis
Starr-Edwards aortic valve prosthesis
Starr-Edwards ball valve prosthesis
Starr-Edwards mitral prosthesis
Starr-Edwards valve prosthesis
STD+ titanium total hip prosthesis
steel wire prosthesis
Steffee prosthesis
stem prosthesis
stemmed tibial prosthesis
stentless porcine aortic valve prosthesis
Stenzel rod prosthesis
Stevens-Street elbow prosthesis
STH-2 total hip prosthesis
straight-stem prosthesis
subdermal prosthesis
Subrini penile prosthesis
Sulzer prosthesis
SuperCup acetabular cup prosthesis
Supramid prosthesis
surgical prosthesis

prosthesis (*continued*)
Surgitek Flexi-Flate penile prosthesis
Surgitek Flexi-rod penile prosthesis
Surgitek inflatable penile prosthesis
Surgitek mammary prosthesis
Surgitek penile prosthesis
Sutter double-stem silicone implant prosthesis
Sutter MCP finger joint prosthesis
Sutter-Smeloff heart valve prosthesis
sutureless valve prosthesis
Swanson finger joint prosthesis
Swanson flexible hallux valgus prosthesis
Swanson great toe prosthesis
Swanson metacarpal prosthesis
Swanson metatarsal prosthesis
Swanson Silastic elbow prosthesis
Swanson Silastic prosthesis
Swanson wrist prosthesis
Syme amputation prosthesis
Syme foot prosthesis
Synatomic knee prosthesis
Synatomic total knee prosthesis
Synergist Erection penile prosthesis
T-28 hip prosthesis
tantalum mesh prosthesis
tantalum prosthesis
tantalum stapes prosthesis
Taperloc femoral prosthesis
TARA total hip prosthesis
TCCK unconstrained knee prosthesis
Techmedica prosthesis
Teflon intracardiac patch prosthesis
Teflon mesh prosthesis
Teflon sheeting prosthesis
Teflon trileaflet prosthesis
Teflon wire piston prosthesis
Teflon woven prosthesis
Tef-wire prosthesis

prosthesis (*continued*)
temporary prosthesis
tendon prosthesis
testicular prosthesis
Tevdek prosthesis
Thackray hip prosthesis
Tharies hip replacement prosthesis
Thiersch prosthesis
Thompson femoral head prosthesis
Thompson femoral neck prosthesis
Thompson hemiarthroplasty hip prosthesis
threaded titanium acetabular prosthesis (TTAP)
Thrust femoral prosthesis
Ti CoCr hip prosthesis
Ti-BAC hip prosthesis
tibial plateau prosthesis
tibial prosthesis
tibiofemoral prosthesis
Tilastin hip prosthesis
tilting-disk aortic valve prosthesis
titanium ball prosthesis
titanium prosthesis
Tivanium hip prosthesis
TK Optimizer knee prosthesis
TMJ fossa-eminence prosthesis
toe prosthesis
toe-to-thumb prosthesis
TORP ossicular prosthesis
torque-type prosthesis
total alloplastic TMJ reconstruction prosthesis
total condylar knee prosthesis
total hip prosthesis
total knee prosthesis
total ossicular prosthesis
total ossicular reconstruction/replacement prosthesis (TORP)
Townley knee prosthesis
Townley TARA prosthesis
Townley total knee prosthesis
TR-28 hip prosthesis
trapeziometacarpal joint replacement prosthesis

prosthesis (*continued*)

Trapezoidal-28 total hip prosthesis
Trautman Locktite prosthesis
Triad prosthesis
trial prosthesis
triaxial elbow prosthesis
triaxial semiconstrained elbow prosthesis
Tricon-M cruciate-sparing prosthesis
Tricon-M patellar prosthesis
Tricon-M total knee prosthesis
trileaflet aortic prosthesis
trileaflet prosthesis
Trilicon external breast prosthesis
Tronzo prosthesis
trunnion-bearing hip prosthesis
TruStep foot prosthesis
TTAP-ST acetabular prosthesis
tube prosthesis
Turner prosthesis
Tygon esophageal prosthesis
UCBL prosthesis
UCI knee prosthesis
UCI prosthesis
UHI Universal head system hip prosthesis
Ultra Low resistance voice prosthesis
Ultraflex esophageal prosthesis
Ultrec Plus penile prosthesis
umbrella-type prosthesis
unconstrained knee prosthesis
unconstrained prosthesis
undersized prosthesis
unicondylar prosthesis
Uni-Flate penile prosthesis
Universal femoral head prosthesis
Universal prosthesis
UPF prosthesis (Universal proximal femur prosthesis)
upper extremity myoelectric prosthesis
urinary incontinence prosthesis

prosthesis (*continued*)

UroLume endourethral Wallstent prosthesis
USCI bifurcated Vasculour prosthesis
USCI Sauvage Bionit bifurcated vascular prosthesis
USCI Sauvage side-limb prosthesis
Usher Marlex mesh prosthesis
Utah arm electronic prosthesis
vaginal prolapse prosthesis
Valls prosthesis
valve prosthesis
valved voice prosthesis
Vanghetti limb prosthesis
vascular prosthesis
Vascutek vascular prosthesis
vessel prosthesis
Viscoheel prosthesis
Viscoheel SofSpot prosthesis
Vitallium alloy cobalt-chrome prosthesis
Vitallium hip prosthesis
Vitallium Moore self-locking prosthesis
Vivosil prosthesis
voice prosthesis
Voltz wrist joint prosthesis
Wada hingeless heart valve prosthesis
Wada valve prosthesis
Wagner resurface prosthesis
Walldius knee prosthesis
Walldius total knee prosthesis
Walldius Vitallium mechanical knee prosthesis
Wallstent esophageal prosthesis
Wallstent iliac endoprosthesis
Warsaw hip prosthesis
Waugh ankle prosthesis
Waugh knee prosthesis
Wayfarer prosthesis
Weavenit valve prosthesis
Weavenit vascular prosthesis
Weck-cel prosthesis
Wehrs incus prosthesis
Weller total hip joint prosthesis

prosthesis (*continued*)
Wesolowski vascular prosthesis
Wesolowski Weavenit vascular prosthesis
Wheeler prosthesis
Whiteside total hip prosthesis
Wiles prosthesis
Wilke boot prosthesis
Wilson-Cook esophageal balloon prosthesis
Wilson-Cook plastic prosthesis
wire mesh prosthesis
wire stapes prosthesis
wire-fat ear prosthesis
wire-Gelfoam prosthesis
Wolfe prosthesis
woven-tube vascular graft prosthesis
woven-tube vascular prosthesis
Wright knee prosthesis
wrist prosthesis
Xenophor femoral prosthesis
Zimaloy femoral head prosthesis
Zimaloy hip prosthesis
Zimaloy knee prosthesis
Zimmer Centralign Precoat hip prosthesis
Zimmer shoulder prosthesis
Zimmer tibial prosthesis
Zimmer total hip prosthesis
Ziramic femoral head prosthesis
Zirconia orthopedic prosthesis
Zweymuller hip prosthesis
Zweymuller-Alloclassic prosthesis
prosthesis extractor with hand grip
prosthesis fin
prosthesis fixation
prosthesis interface
prosthesis sizing set
prosthesis smooth wire
prosthesis-cement interface
prosthetic antibiotic-loaded acrylic cement
prosthetic antibiotic-loaded acrylic cement total joint prosthesis

prosthetic appliance
prosthetic arterial graft
prosthetic arthroplasty
prosthetic ball valve
prosthetic cup
prosthetic device
prosthetic dislocation
prosthetic foam
prosthetic fracture
prosthetic graft
prosthetic heart
prosthetic heart valve
prosthetic hemiarthroplasty
prosthetic implant
prosthetic incisional hernioplasty
prosthetic integration
prosthetic lens
prosthetic loop
prosthetic mesh repair
prosthetic patch
prosthetic patch graft
prosthetic poppet
prosthetic reconstruction
prosthetic replacement arthroplasty
prosthetic ring annuloplasty
prosthetic sizer
prosthetic socket
prosthetic valve
prosthetic valve holder
prosthetic valve poppet
prosthetic valve sewing ring
prosthetic valve suture ring
Prosthex sponge
prosthodontics
ProSys silicone sterile 2-way, Foley catheter
ProSys silicone sterile 3-way, Foley catheter
Protasul femoral prosthesis
Protasul prosthetic hip
ProTech instrument protection tray
Protect-Point needle
Protectaid contraceptive sponge
Protect-a-Pass suture passer
protected bronchoscopic brush
protected knife handle
protective antireflux operation
protective bandage
protective dressing

protective eye pad
protective eye shield
protective goggles
protective recovery balm
Protecto splint
protector plus wire
Protector suturing device
Protege syringe infusion pump
Protege Plus microscope
Protegen material
proteinaceous aqueous
    exudation
Protek hip prosthesis
Protek joint
Protek joint implant
Protek Protasul vanadium-free
    titanium alloy prosthesis
ProTon portable tonometer
proton pump inhibition therapy
prototype cholangioscope
Protouch material
Protouch orthopedic padding
Protouch pad
Protouch synthetic orthopedic
    padding
ProTrac ACL tibial guide
ProTrac cruciate reconstruction
    measurement device
protractor
protruded disk
protruding ear
protruding fat
protruding mandible
protrusio acetabulum
protrusio cage
protrusio deformity
protrusion
    anal protrusion
    bimaxillary dentoalveolar
        protrusion
    bimaxillary protrusion
    disk protrusion
    double protrusion
    hernial protrusion
    intrapelvic protrusion
    iris protrusion
    jaw protrusion
    lumbosacral disk protrusion
    mandibular protrusion
    maxillary alveolar protrusion
    maxillary protrusion
    medial protrusion

protrusion lisp
protrusive condyle
protrusive excursion
protrusive incisal guide angle
protrusive jaw relation
protrusive line
protrusive movement
protrusive occlusal position
protrusive occlusion
protuberance
    Bichat protuberance
    bony protuberance
    chin protuberance
    external occipital
        protuberance
    mental protuberance
    occipital protuberance
    palatine protuberance
    transverse occipital
        protuberance
protuberant abdomen
Proud adenoidectomy forceps
Proud fascia crusher
proud flesh
proud graft
Proud infant turbinate speculum
Proud septal prosthesis
Proust space
Pro-Vent ABG kit
Pro-Vent arterial blood sampling
    kit
Providence Hospital artery
    forceps
Providence Hospital clamp
Providence Hospital classic
    forceps
Providence Hospital hemostat
Providence Hospital hemostatic
    forceps
Provider 5500 patient-controlled
    analgesia device
Provider ambulatory dual-
    channel infusion pump
provisional canthoplasty
provisional fixation
provisional ligature
provisional liner
provisional stabilization
provisionally acceptable
    material
Provit filling material
Provocative sensitivity balloon

provoked response
Provox speaking valve
Provox voice prosthesis
Prowler microcatheter
Proxi-Floss cleaning appliance
proximal aorta
proximal articular set angle (PASA)
proximal bowel distention
proximal carpal row
proximal cavity
proximal clot
proximal colon
proximal electrode
proximal femoral fracture
proximal femoral resection
proximal focal femoral deficiency (PFFD)
proximal gastrectomy
proximal gastric cancer
proximal gastric resection
proximal humeral fracture
proximal incision
proximal interphalangeal (PIP)
proximal interphalangeal joint
proximal interphalangeal joint approach
proximal jejunum
proximal ligatures
proximal loop syndrome
proximal myofascial dysfunction
proximal nail matrix
proximal osteotomy
proximal radioulnar articulation
proximal row carpectomy
proximal shaft
proximal space
proximal splenorenal shunt
proximal subclavian injury
proximal tendon rupture
proximal tibia
proximal tibial metaphysial fracture
proximal tibiofibular joint dislocation
proximal ureter
proximal vascular control
proximally retracted
proximate cause
proximate disposable skin stapler
Proximate flexible linear stapler
Proximate intraluminal stapler

Proximate linear cutter
Proximate linear cutter stapler
Proximate linear stapler
Proximate skin staples
proximate space
Proximate curved intraluminal stapler
Proxi-Strip sutures
Proxi-Strip wound closures
PRP (proliferative retinopathy photocoagulation)
Pruitt anoscope
Pruitt irrigation catheter
Pruitt occlusion catheter
Pruitt proctoscope
Pruitt rectal speculum
Pruitt vascular shunt
Pruitt-Inahara autoperfusion shunt
Pruitt-Inahara balloon-tipped perfusion catheter
Pruitt-Inahara carotid shunt
Pruitt-Inahara vascular shunt
prune belly syndrome
prune belly abdomen
pruned-tree appearance
pruned-tree arteriogram
prune juice peritoneal fluid
pruritus erythematous patch
pruritus lesion
pruritus senilis
Prussak fibers
Prussak pouch
Prussak space
Pryor-Pean retractor
Pryor-Pean vaginal retractor
PS-2 needle
PSA thermoplastic orthosis
PSA-1 monitor
psammoma bodies
PSC (posterior subcapsular cataract)
PSCE (presurgical clotting evaluation)
pseudarthrosis repair
pseudoaneurysm formation
pseudoarthrosis repair
pseudobiopsy technique
pseudoblind loop syndrome
pseudoboutonniere deformity
pseudocancerous lesion
pseudocapsule
pseudocarcinomatous hyperplasia

pseudochylous ascites
pseudocoarctation of aorta
pseudocyst formation
pseudocystobiliary fistula
pseudoepithelioma
pseudoepitheliomatous
    hyperplasia
pseudoexfoliation syndrome
pseudofollicular salpingitis
pseudohermaphroditism
  female
      pseudohermaphroditism
  male pseudohermaphroditism
pseudocyst drainage
pseudohernia
pseudohypoparathyroidism
pseudoisochromatic plate
pseudojoint formation
pseudo-Kaposi sarcoma
pseudoligamentous
pseudolymphoma syndrome
pseudomallet deformity
pseudomedial longitudinal
    fasciculus lesion
pseudomelanoma
pseudomelia
pseudomembrane
pseudomembranous acute
    inflammation
pseudomotor cerebri
pseudoneurogenic bladder
pseudo-obstruction
pseudo-orbital hypertelorism
pseudoparalysis
pseudophake
pseudophakia
pseudophakos
pseudopod formation
pseudopolypoid changes
pseudosarcomatous fasciitis
pseudoscar
pseudoserous membrane
pseudotabes
pseudotumor cerebri
pseudotumor cerebrimeningeal
    biopsy
pseudovaginal hypospadias
pseudoxanthoma elasticum
    syndrome
PSIS (posterosuperior iliac spine)
psoas abscess
psoas bladder hitch

psoas hitch procedure
psoas line
psoas margin
psoas muscle
psoas retractor
psoas sheath block
psoas sign
psoas test
psoriatic spondylitis
psoriatic-type scale
PSS powered disposable skin
    stapler
PSVT (paroxysmal
    supraventricular
    tachycardia)
psychocardiac reflex
PTA (percutaneous transluminal
    angioplasty)
PTB (patellar tendon-bearing)
PTB brace
PTB cast
PTB cast prosthesis
PTBD catheter (percutaneous
    transhepatic biliary
    drainage catheter)
PTC (percutaneous transhepatic
    cholangiography)
PTCA (percutaneous
    transluminal coronary
    angioplasty)
PTCA catheter
PTD (percutaneous transhepatic
    decompression/drainage)
pterional approach
pterional craniotomy
pterygium colli
pterygium keratome
pterygium knife
pterygium operation
pterygium scissors
pterygium transplant
pterygoid bone
pterygoid canal
pterygoid chisel
pterygoid fissure
pterygoid fossa
pterygoid fovea
pterygoid hamulus
pterygoid lamina
pterygoid muscle
pterygoid nerve
pterygoid notch

pterygoid plate
pterygoid plexus
pterygoid position
pterygoid process
pterygoid ridge of sphenoid
    bone
pterygoid tuberosity of
    mandible
pterygomandibular fold
pterygomandibular raphe
pterygomandibular space
pterygomandibular space
    abscess
pterygomasseteric sling
pterygomaxillary buttress
pterygomaxillary fissure
pterygomaxillary fossa
pterygomaxillary notch
pterygomaxillary region
pterygomaxillary separation
pterygomaxillary space
pterygopalatine canal
pterygopalatine fissure
pterygopalatine fossa
pterygopalatine fossa
    syndrome
pterygopalatine ganglion
pterygopalatine groove
pterygopalatine nerves
pterygopalatine space
pterygopharyngeal space
PTFE (polytetrafluoroethylene)
    prosthesis
PTFE (polytetrafluoroethylene;
    Teflon)
PTFE endovascular graft
PTFE Gore-Tex graft
PTFE graft
PTFE shunt
PTFE-containing implant
PTFE-covered Palmaz stent
PTLA (percutaneous
    transluminal angioplasty)
ptosis clamp
ptosis correction
ptosis forceps
ptosis knife
ptosis of lacrimal glands
ptosis of submandibular glands
ptosis of the chin
ptosis scissors
ptosis sling

ptosis snare
ptosis surgery
ptotic breast
ptotic brow
ptotic earlobe
ptotic eyebrow
ptotic kidney
ptotic malar fat pad
PTRA (percutaneous
    transluminal renal
    angioplasty)
PTS prosthesis
PTVA (percutaneous transseptal
    ventricular assist)
ptyalectasis
ptyalolithiasis
ptyalolithotomy
pubic angle
pubic arch
pubic body
pubic bone
pubic crest
pubic diastasis
pubic fixation
pubic hair
pubic hair line
pubic ramus
pubic region
pubic symphysis
pubic tubercle
pubioplasty
pubiotomy
    Gigli pubiotomy
    Siebold pubiotomy
    Stoltz pubiotomy
pubis (*pl.* pubes)
pubocapsular ligament
pubocervical fascia
pubocervical ligament
pubococcygeal line
pubococcygeal muscle
pubococcygeoplasty
pubofemoral ligament
puboprostatic ligament
puboprostatic muscle
puborectal muscle
puborectalis loop
pubosacral diameter
pubotuberous diameter
pubovaginal muscle
pubovaginal operation
pubovesical ligament

pubovesical muscle
pubovesicocervical fascia
puboxyphoid incision
Pucci Air orthotic
Pucci pediatrics hand orthosis
Pucci rehab knee orthosis
Pucci splint
Pucci-Seed hook
Pucci-Seed spatula
PUD (peptic ulcer disease)
puddler's cataract
Puddu drill guide
Puddu reconstruction
Puddu tendon technique
pudenda
pudendal anesthesia
pudendal arteriography
pudendal artery
pudendal artery angiography
pudendal block
pudendal block anesthesia
pudendal block anesthesia
    needle
pudendal canal
pudendal hernia
pudendal needle
pudendal needle guide
pudendal nerve
pudendal vein
pudendal vessels
Pudenz barium cardiac catheter
Pudenz connector
Pudenz flushing chamber
Pudenz infant cardiac catheter
Pudenz peritoneal catheter
Pudenz reservoir
Pudenz shunt
Pudenz tube
Pudenz valve
Pudenz valve-flushing shunt
Pudenz ventricular catheter
Pudenz ventriculoatrial shunt
Pudenz-Heyer clamp
Pudenz-Heyer shunt
Pudenz-Heyer vascular catheter
Pudenz-Heyer-Schulte valve
Pudenz-Schulte thecoperitoneal
    shunt
pudic vessel
puerperal eclampsia
puerperal hematoma
puerperal sterilization

Puestow anatomosis
Puestow biliary tract procedure
Puestow dilator
Puestow guidewire
Puestow operation
Puestow
    pancreaticojejunostomy
Puestow pancreatojejunostomy
Puestow wires
Puestow-Gillesby operation
Puestow-Gillesby procedure
Puestow-Olander
    gastrointestinal tube
Puestow-Olander GI tube
puffy tumor
Pugh barrel component
Pugh classification
Pugh driver
Pugh hip pin
Pugh plate
Pugh self-adjusting nail
Pugh tractor
Pugh-Child bleeding esophageal
    varices grading scale
    classification
Puig Massana-Shiley
    annuloplasty ring
Puig Massana-Shiley
    annuloplasty valve
puka chisel
Pulec-Freedman classification of
    congenital aural atresia
Pulec needle
pull knife
pull maneuver
pull rasp
pull screw
pull-apart introducer
pullback pressure gradient
pulled muscle
pulled taut
pulled tendon
pulley passer
pulley reconstruction
pulley suture technique
pulley sutures
pulley tendon
pulleys
pull-out button
pull-out sutures
pull-out wire
pull-out wire suture technique

pull-out wire sutures
pull-through abdominoperineal
	resection
pull-through operation
pull-through procedure
pull-through proctectomy
pull-through technique
Pulmo-Aide ventilator
Pulmonair 40 bed
pulmonary abscess
pulmonary acid aspiration
	syndrome
pulmonary aneurysm
pulmonary angiogram
pulmonary aortic anastomosis
pulmonary apex
pulmonary arborization
pulmonary arterial catheter
pulmonary arterial clamp
pulmonary arterial forceps
pulmonary arterial malformation
pulmonary arterial snare
pulmonary arterial vent
pulmonary arteriography
pulmonary arteriole
pulmonary arteriovenous fistula
	(PAF)
pulmonary arteriovenous
	malformation
pulmonary artery (PA)
pulmonary artery arteriogram
pulmonary artery balloon pump
	(PABP)
pulmonary artery banding
pulmonary artery catheter
pulmonary artery
	catheterization
pulmonary artery clamp
pulmonary artery forceps
pulmonary artery sling
pulmonary artery wedge
	angiogram
pulmonary aspiration
pulmonary autograft (PA)
pulmonary balloon
pulmonary balloon valvuloplasty
pulmonary bed
pulmonary bypass
pulmonary capillary wedge
	(PCW)
pulmonary capillary wedge
	pressure

pulmonary cavity
pulmonary circulation
pulmonary clamp
pulmonary complication
pulmonary conduit outflow
	tract
pulmonary disease
pulmonary dysfunction
pulmonary edema
pulmonary effect
pulmonary embolectomy
pulmonary embolism
pulmonary embolism clamp
pulmonary embolization
pulmonary embolus
pulmonary fibrosis
pulmonary fields
pulmonary flotation catheter
pulmonary flow
pulmonary function
pulmonary hemorrhage
pulmonary hilus
pulmonary homograft
pulmonary hypertension
pulmonary infiltration
pulmonary innominate
	anastomosis
pulmonary involvement
pulmonary lesion
pulmonary ligament
pulmonary lobectomy
pulmonary lobule
pulmonary
	lymphangioleiomyomatosis
pulmonary
	lymphangiomyomatosis
pulmonary metastasis
pulmonary nodulectomy clamp
pulmonary nodules
pulmonary outflow tract
pulmonary perfusion scanning
pulmonary position
pulmonary pressure
pulmonary prominence
pulmonary pulse
pulmonary resection
pulmonary resistance
pulmonary retractor
pulmonary segment
pulmonary stenosis repair
pulmonary subclavian
	anastomosis

pulmonary sulcus syndrome
pulmonary sympathetic
    blockade
pulmonary toilet
pulmonary transplantation
pulmonary triple-lumen catheter
pulmonary trunk orifice
pulmonary valve anomaly
pulmonary valve disease
pulmonary valve gradient
pulmonary valve knife
pulmonary valve replacement
pulmonary valvotomy
pulmonary valvuloplasty
pulmonary valvulotome
pulmonary valvulotomy
pulmonary vascular abnormality
pulmonary vascular markings
pulmonary vasculature
pulmonary vein
pulmonary venous connection
    anomaly
pulmonary venous return anomaly
pulmonary ventilation
pulmonary vesicles
pulmonary vessel clamp
pulmonary vessel forceps
pulmonary wedge pressure
pulmonary-gas exchange
Pulmonex dynamic air therapy
    unit
pulmonic clamp
pulmonic closure
pulmonic insufficiency
pulmonic stenosis
pulmonic stenosis clamp
pulmonic valve
pulmonocoronary reflex
Pulmopak pump
Pulmosonic ultrasonic nebulizer
pulp
    dental pulp
    finger pulp
    metaplasia of pulp
    mummified pulp
    necrotic pulp
    palmar pulp
    splenic pulp
pulp amputation
pulp approach
pulp canal file
pulp canal therapy

pulp cavity
pulp chamber
pulp extirpation
pulp flap
pulpa dentis
pulpa lienis
pulpal devitalization
pulpal excavations
pulpal macrophage
pulpal microdialysis probe
pulpar cells
Pulpdent cavity liner
pulpectomy
pulped muscle dressing
pulpless tooth
pulpodentinal membrane
pulpoperiapical lesion
pulpotomy
pulpy testis
Pulsair tonometer
Pulsair.5 oxygen portable unit
Pulsar DDD pacemaker
Pulsar implantable pacemaker
pulsatile assist device
pulsatile cardiopulmonary
    bypass
pulsatile hematoma
pulsatile mass
pulsatile perfusion
pulsatile pressure lavage
pulsating aneurysm
pulsating aorta
pulsating low-air-loss bed
pulsating mass
pulsating pain
pulsation
pulsator
Pulsator anaerobic syringe
Pulsator dry heparin arterial
    blood gas kit
Pulsatron hand-held nerve
    stimulator
pulse
    abdominal pulse
    biferious pulse
    bigeminal pulse
    bounding pulse
    cannonball pulse
    carotid pulse
    centripetal venous pulse
    cordy pulse
    coupled pulse

pulse (*continued*)
    dicrotic pulse
    digitalate pulse
    dorsalis pedis pulse
    elastic pulse
    entoptic pulse
    feeble pulse
    femoral pulse
    filiform pulse
    guttural pulse
    imperceptible pulse
    infrequent pulse
    irradiation pulse
    jugular pulse
    Kussmaul pulse
    low-tension pulse
    palpability of pulses
    palpable pulse
    paradoxical pulse
    pedal pulse
    peripheral pulses
    pistol-shot pulse
    popliteal pulse
    pulmonary pulse
    quick pulse
    radial pulse
    rising pulse
    saphenous pulse
    short pulse
    strong and equal pulses
    strong and regular pulses
    strong pulse
    thready pulse
    tibial pulse
    tricrotic pulse
    trigeminal pulse
    trip-hammer pulse
    venous pulse
    wiry pulse
pulse generator
pulse lavage irrigation
pulse monitor
pulse oximeter
pulse oximetry device
pulse spray catheter
pulse wave Doppler
pulse width
pulsed angiolaser
pulsed Doppler
pulsed Doppler images
pulsed Doppler spectral
    analysis
pulsed Doppler ultrasonic
    flowmeter
pulsed Doppler ultrasound
pulsed dye laser
pulsed echo methods
pulsed galvanic stimulator
pulsed irrigation
pulsed laser ablation
pulsed light
pulsed metal vapor laser
pulsed sonogram
pulsed tunable dye laser
pulsed ultrasonic velocity
    detector
pulsed yellow dye laser
pulsed-mode operation
pulsed-range gated Doppler
    instrument
pulsed-wave ultrasound
PulseMaster laser
Pulse-Pak infusion kit
PulseSpray injector
pulse-wave configurations
pulsion hernia
Pulsolith pulsed-dye laser
Pulsolith laser lithotripter
pulsus alternans
pulsus tardus
pulverize
Pulvertaft fishmouth incision
Pulvertaft interweaving method
    for hand surgery
Pulvertaft sutures
Pulvertaft weave technique
pump bump
pump failure
pump oxygenator
pump primed
Pump Vac III
pumped dye laser
pump-reservoir
punch
    Abrams biopsy punch
    Abrams pleural biopsy punch
    Accuflex punch
    Acufex duckbill punch
    Acufex linear punch
    Acufex rotary punch
    adenoid punch
    Adler attic ear punch
    Ainsworth punch
    Alexander antrostomy punch

punch (*continued*)
- Alexander biopsy punch
- Anderson antrum punch
- angular oval punch
- antral punch
- antrostomy punch
- aorta punch
- aortic punch
- attic ear punch
- atticus punch
- baby Tischler biopsy punch
- backbiting bone punch
- backward-biting ostrum punch
- Bailey punch
- Baker punch
- Barron donor corneal punch
- Baumgartner punch
- Berens corneoscleral punch
- Beyer atticus punch
- biopsy punch
- biting punch
- bone hole punch
- Braasch-Bumpus prostatic punch
- Brewster sinus punch
- Brock infundibular punch
- Brooks adenoid punch
- Bruening punch
- Buerger punch
- canaliculus punch
- cartilage punch
- Caspari suture punch
- Casselberry suture punch
- Casteyer prostatic punch
- Castroviejo corneoscleral punch
- Cault punch
- cervical foraminal punch
- cervical laminectomy punch
- cervical punch
- chalazion punch
- Charnley femoral prosthesis neck punch
- cigar handle basket punch
- circular punch
- Citelli laminectomy punch
- Citelli-Meltzer atticus punch
- Cloward bone punch
- Cloward intervertebral punch
- Cloward square punch
- Cloward-Dowel punch

punch (*continued*)
- Cloward-English punch
- Cloward-Harper cervical punch
- Cloward-Harper punch
- cone biopsy punch
- cone bone punch
- cone skull punch
- Cordes circular punch
- Cordes ethmoidal punch
- Cordes semicircular punch
- Cordes sphenoid punch
- Cordes square punch
- Cordes-New laryngeal punch
- Corgill bone punch
- corneal punch
- corneoscleral punch
- Cottingham punch
- cruciate punch
- cup-biting punch
- cutaneous punch
- Davol canal wall punch
- Derlacki punch
- dermal punch
- Descemet membrane punch
- Deyerle punch
- disposable aortic rotating punch
- Dorsey cervical foraminal punch
- Dyonics suction punch
- DyoVac suction punch
- ear punch
- Ellison glenoid rim punch
- endocervical biopsy punch
- Entrease variable depth punch
- Eppendorfer biopsy punch
- ethmoidal punch
- Ewald-Hensler arthroscopic punch
- Faraci punch
- Faraci-Skillern sphenoid punch
- Fehling TOP ejector punch
- Ferris Smith punch
- Ferris Smith-Gruenwald sphenoid punch
- Ferris Smith-Kerrison punch
- finned-stem punch
- Flateau oval punch
- fluted stem punch

punch (*continued*)
foraminal punch
Frangenheim hook punch
Frenckner-Stille punch
Gass cervical punch
Gass corneoscleral punch
Gass scleral punch
Gass sclerotomy punch
Gaylor punch
Gaylor-Alexander punch
Gelfoam punch
Gellhorn uterine biopsy punch
Gendelach sphenoid punch
Gibbs eye punch
glenoid punch
Goldman cartilage punch
Goosen vascular punch
Gosteyer punch
Graham-Kerrison punch
grasping punch
Gruenwald nasal punch
Gundelach punch
Gusberg endocervical biopsy punch
hair transplant punch
Haitz canaliculus punch
Hajek antral punch
Hajek-Koffler bone punch
Hajek-Koffler sphenoidal punch
Hajek-Skillern sphenoidal punch
Hancock aortic punch
Hardy sellar punch
Harper cervical laminectomy punch
Harris punch
Hartmann biopsy punch
Hartmann ear punch
Hartmann nasal punch
Hartmann tonsillar punch
Hartmann-Citelli ear punch
Hirsch hypophyseal punch
Hoffmann biopsy punch
Hoffmann ear punch
Holth corneoscleral punch
Holth scleral punch
Holth sclerectomy punch
Holth-Rubin punch
Holtz corneoscleral punch
Housepian sellar punch

punch (*continued*)
I-beam cement punch
I-beam Press-Fit punch
infundibular punch
Ingraham infant skull punch
Ingraham skull punch
intervertebral punch
intranasal punch
Jackson punch
Jacobson vessel punch
Jansen-Middleton septal punch
Johnson tonsillar punch
Johnson-Kerrison punch
Joseph punch
Karolinska-Stille punch
Karp aortic punch
Kelly punch
Kelly-Descemet membrane punch
Kennan cervical punch
Kerrison bone punch
Kerrison laminectomy punch
Kerrison-Jacoby punch
Kerrison-Rhoton sella punch
Kevorkian biopsy punch
Keyes cutaneous biopsy punch
Keyes cutaneous punch
Keyes dermal punch
Keyes dermatologic punch
Keyes skin punch
Keyes vulvar punch
keyhole punch
kidney punch
King adenoidal punch
Klause antrum punch
Klause-Carmody antrum punch
Klein punch
Knighton-Kerrison punch
Koffler-Hajek sphenoidal punch
Krause angular oval punch
laminectomy punch
Lange antrum punch
laryngeal punch
Lebsche sternal punch
Leksell punch
Lempert malleus punch
Lermoyez nasal punch
Lewis-Resnik punch

punch (*continued*)

linear scissor punch
Lineback adenoidal punch
Luntz-Dodick punch
MacKenty sphenoid punch
malleus punch
Mauermayer stone punch
McElveney punch
McGoey Vitallium punch
McKenzie sphenoid punch
Medtronic aortic punch
Medtronic Hancock aortic
  punch
Meltzer adenoid punch
Meltzer tonsillar punch
Mendez-Schubert aorta punch
Merz aortic punch
MGH glenoid punch
MGM glenoid punch
Miles nasal punch
Miltex disposable biopsy
  punch
Mixter brain biopsy punch
modified sclerectomy punch
Mosher ethmoid punch
Mulligan cervical biopsy
  punch
Murphy kidney punch
Myers punch
Myerson biting punch
Myles nasal punch
nasal punch
Noyes chalazion punch
O'Connor hook punch
Orentreich punch
Osborne punch
Ostrom antral punch
Ostrom nose punch
Pfau atticus punch
Pfau atticus sphenoidal punch
Phemister punch
pleural biopsy punch
Pollock punch
Price corneal punch
Pritikin scleral punch
prostatic punch
Raney laminectomy punch
Rathke punch
Reaves antral punch
Rhoton sellar punch
Richter laminectomy punch
ring punch

punch (*continued*)

Ronis adenoid punch
Ronis tonsillar punch
Rothman-Gilbard corneal
  punch
Rowe glenoid punch
Rubin-Holth corneoscleral
  punch
Rubin-Holth sclerectomy
  punch
Sachs cervical punch
Scheicker laminectomy punch
Scheinmann biting punch
Schlesinger cervical punch
Schmeden nasal punch
Schmeden tonsillar punch
Schmithhuisen ethmoid
  punch
Schmithhuisen sphenoid
  punch
Schnaudigel sclerotomy
  punch
Schubert biopsy punch
Schubert uterine biopsy
  punch
scleral punch
sclerectomy by punch
sclerectomy punch
sclerectomy with punch
sclerotomy punch
Seiffert grasping punch
Seletz punch
Seletz Universal Kerrison
  punch
sellar punch
semicircular punch
septal punch
Shastid punch
Shutt punch
side-biting ostrum punch
sinus punch
Skillern punch
skin punch
skull cone punch
skull punch
Smeden tonsillar punch
Smillie nail punch
Smithuysen ethmoidal punch
Smithuysen sphenoidal punch
Sokolowski antral punch
Sparks atrioseptal punch
Spencer oval punch

punch (*continued*)

Spencer triangular adenoid punch
sphenoidal bone punch
sphenoidal punch
Spies ethmoidal punch
Spurling-Kerrison laminectomy punch
square punch
Stammberger antrum punch
sternal punch
Stevenson capsule punch
Storz antrum punch
Storz corneoscleral punch
Storz intranasal antral punch
Stough punch
Struempel ear punch
Struyken punch
suction punch
Swan corneoscleral punch
Sweet sternal punch
Takahashi ethmoid punch
Takahashi nasal punch
Tanne corneal punch
Thompson adenoid punch
Thoms-Gaylor biopsy punch
Thomson adenoidal punch
Tischler cervical biopsy punch
Tischler-Morgan biopsy punch
Tomey trabeculectomy punch
tonsillar punch
TOP ejector punch
Townsend biopsy punch
Troutman corneal punch
Turkel prostatic punch
Turrell angular rotating punch
Turrell biopsy punch
Universal antral punch
Universal punch
up-biting punch
uterine biopsy punch
Van Struyken nasal punch
Veenema-Gusberg prostatic biopsy punch
Veenema-Gusberg prostatic punch
vessel punch
Wagner antrum punch
Walser corneoscleral punch
Walton corneoscleral punch
Walton-Schubert punch

punch (*continued*)

Watson-Williams ethmoidal punch
Watson-Williams nasal punch
Weck endoscopic suture punch
Whitcomb-Kerrison laminectomy punch
Wilde ethmoidal punch
Wilde nasal punch
Williams-Watson ethmoidal punch
Wittner biopsy punch
Wittner cervical biopsy punch
Wittner cervical punch
Woolley tibia punch
Yankauer antral punch
Yeoman biopsy punch
punch biopsy
punch block
punch forceps
punch forceps tip
punch graft
punch guide
punch resection
punch resection of vocal cords
punch rongeur
punch tip
punch trephine
punched-out lesions
punched-out ulcer
Pynchon ear snare
puncta calcific stone
punctal dilator
punctal lens
punctate cataract
punctate electrode
punctate electrotome
punctate epithelial keratoplasty
punctate hemorrhage
punctate lesion
punctate ulcer
punctate wound
punctiform lesion
punctum dilator
punctum lacrimale
punctum plug
punctum snip
puncture
    arterial puncture
    cardiac puncture
    carotid puncture

puncture (*continued*)
  cisternal puncture
  Corning puncture
  cranial puncture
  cricothyroid needle puncture
  diabetic puncture
  diathermy puncture
  endoscopic fine-needle
    puncture
  epigastric puncture
  exploratory puncture
  groin puncture
  intracisternal puncture
  lumbar puncture
  Marfan epigastric puncture
  needle puncture
  percutaneous puncture
  pericardial puncture
  peritoneal puncture
  postlumbar puncture
  Quincke puncture
  spinal puncture
  splenic puncture
  sternal puncture
  subdural puncture
  suboccipital puncture
  thecal puncture
  transanal puncture
  transvaginal puncture
  venous puncture
  ventricular puncture
  Ziegler puncture
puncture incision
puncture needle
puncture site
puncture transducer
puncture wound
puncture-tip needle
Punctur-Guard needle
Punctur-Guard Revolution safety
  needle holder
Punctur-Guard Winged Set
puncturing of skin
punktal lens
Puntenney operation
Puntenney tying forceps
Puntowicz arterial forceps
pupil
  Adie pupil
  Argyll Robertson pupil
  blown pupil
  bounding pupil

pupil (*continued*)
  Bumke pupil
  constriction of pupil
  contraction of pupil
  dilated pupil
  dilator muscle of pupil
  exit pupil
  hammock pupil
  Horner pupil
  keyhole pupil
  mydriatic pupils
  peaked pupil
  pinpoint pupils
  sphincter of pupil
  stiff pupil
  updrawn pupil
pupil dilation
pupil dilator
pupil spreader/retractor forceps
pupillary aperture
pupillary block
pupillary border
pupillary change
pupillary dilatation
pupillary line
pupillary margin
pupillary membrane scissors
pupillary reflex
pupillotomy
pupil-to-root iridectomy
PuraPly wound dressing
Pura-Vario stent
Purcell self-retaining abdominal
  retractor
pure blow-out fracture
pure cutting cautery
pure gonadal dysgenesis
pure insular carcinoma
pure refractive surgery
pure ultrafiltration (PUF)
purified bovine collagen
purified cotton
puriform aspect
Puritan-Bennett 7250 metabolic
  monitor
Puritan-Bennett BiLevel Knight
  Star 335 machine
Puritan-Bennett ventilator
Purkinje cells
Purkinje fibers
Purkinje images
Purlon sutures

puromucous
purpuric lesion
purpuric violaceous lesions
purpurogenous membrane
pursestring cervical closure
pursestring ligature
pursestring of black silk
pursestring suture technique
pursestring sutures
Pursuit catheter
purulence
purulent discharge
purulent drainage
purulent edema
purulent exudate
purulent exudation
purulent inflammation
purulent material
purulent otitis media
purulent sputum
pus accumulation
pus at incision site
pus basin
pus cells
pus collection
pus tube
PUSH (Pressure Ulcer Scale for
    Healing)
push cuff
push enteroscopy
push maneuver
push plus refraction technique
pushback
    Dorrance palatal pushback
    palatal pushback
pushback
    Veau-Wardill palatal pushback
pushback palatoplasty
pushback procedure
pushback technique
pusher
    Aker lens pusher
    Arrequi laparoscopic knot
        pusher
    Charnley femoral prosthesis
        pusher
    chorda tympani pusher
    Clark-Reich knot pusher
    component pusher
    De La Vega lens pusher
    Endo-Assist endoscopic knot
        pusher

pusher (*continued*)
    femoral component pusher
    femoral prosthetic pusher
    femoral pusher
    Fresnel lens pusher
    Gazayerli knot pusher
    Geomedic femoral pusher
    heliX knot pusher
    hemispherical pusher
    hook pusher
    Jacobson suture pusher
    Jako knot pusher
    knot pusher
    lens pusher
    Magnum knot pusher
    Martin Surefit lens pusher
    Mershon band pusher
    metal-tipped stent pusher
    MetraTie knot pusher
    Negus pusher
    Ranfac laparoscopic knot
        pusher
    Revo loop handle knot pusher
    Shuletz pusher
    suture pusher
    Visitec lens pusher
pusher catheter
pusher wire
pusher-tier
push-pull catheter
push-pull T technique
push-type enteroscopy
push-up block
Pusto dilatation
pustular acne
pustular inflammation
pustular lesion
pustular pharyngitis
pustular tonsillitis
pustule
Putenney operation
Putnam evacuator catheter
putrefaction
Putterman levator resection
    clamp
Putterman ptosis clamp
Putterman-Chaflin ocular
    asymmetry device
Putti approach
Putti arthrodesis
Putti arthroplasty gouge
Putti bone file

Putti bone rasp
Putti bone raspatory
Putti frame
Putti gouge
Putti knee arthrodesis
Putti operation
Putti posterior approach
Putti rasp
Putti raspatory
Putti shoulder arthrodesis
Putti splint
Putti technique
Putti-Abbott approach
Putti-Platt arthroplasty
Putti-Platt director
Putti-Platt instrumentation
Putti-Platt operation
Putti-Platt shoulder dislocation
    operation
Putti-Platt shoulder procedure
Putti-Scaglietti procedure
putty kidney
Puusepp operation
Puusepp reflex
PV (pressure velocity)
PVB sutures
PVC (premature ventricular
    contraction)
PVC drain
PVFR (postvoiding residual)
P-wave-triggered ventricular
    pacemaker
PWB (partial weightbearing)
Pye cannula
pyelectasia
pyelectasis
pyelitic
pyelitis
pyelocaliectasis
pyelogram
    air pyelogram
    ascending pyelogram
    drip pyelogram
    excretion pyelogram
    excretory pyelogram
    hydrated pyelogram
    infusion pyelogram
    intravenous pyelogram (IVP)
    IV pyelogram
    respiration pyelogram
    retrograde pyelogram
pyelographic study

pyelography
    antegrade pyelography
    ascending pyelography
    drip pyelography
    excretion pyelography
    infusion pyelography
    intravenous pyelography
    IV pyelography
    percutaneous antegrade
        pyelography
    respiration pyelography
    washout pyelography
pyeloileocutaneous anastomosis
pyeloileostomy
pyelolithotomy
pyelolymphatic
pyelonephritic kidney
pyelophlebitis
pyeloplasty
    Anderson-Hynes pyeloplasty
    capsular flap pyeloplasty
    dismembered pyeloplasty
    Foley pyeloplasty
    Foley Y-V pyeloplasty
    Hellstrom pyeloplasty
    Hynes-Anderson
        dismembered pyeloplasty
    laparoscopic dismembered
        pyeloplasty
    Scardino pyeloplasty
    vertical flap pyeloplasty
    Y-V pyeloplasty
pyelorrhaphy
pyeloscopy
pyelostomy
pyelotomy incision
pyelotomy wound
pyeloureteral catheter
pyeloureterogram
pyeloureterography
pyeloureterolysis
pyeloureteroplasty
pyelovenous backflow
pyknotic body
Pyle-Greulich bone age scale
pylon (variant of pilon)
pylon fracture
pylorectomy
pyloric antrum
pyloric autotransplantation
pyloric cap
pyloric channel ulcer

pyloric constriction
pyloric dilation
pyloric gland
pyloric intubation
pyloric lymph node
pyloric mucosa
pyloric obstruction
pyloric occlusion operation
pyloric orifice
pyloric outlet obstruction
pyloric region
pyloric ring
pyloric sphincter
pyloric stenosis dilator
pyloric stricture
pyloric string sign
pyloric vein
pyloric vein of Mayo
pyloric vestibule
pyloristenosis
pylorodilator
pyloroduodenal junction
pyloroduodenal obstruction
pyloroduodenal perforation
pyloroduodenotomy
pylorogastrectomy
pyloromyotomy
    Fredet-Ramstedt
        pyloromyotomy
    laparoscopic pyloromyotomy
    Ramstedt pyloromyotomy
    Ramstedt-Fredet
        pyloromyotomy
pyloroplasty
    Devine pyloroplasty
    double pyloroplasty
    Finney pyloroplasty
    Heineke-Mikulicz pyloroplasty
    Horsley pyloroplasty
    Jaboulay pyloroplasty
    Judd pyloroplasty
    Mikulicz pyloroplasty
    Ramstedt pyloroplasty
    vagotomy and pyloroplasty
    Weinberg modification of
        pyloroplasty
    Weinberg pyloroplasty
pyloroptosis
pyloroscopy
pylorospasm
pylorostenosis
pylorostomy

pylorotomy
pylorus clamp
pylorus of stomach
pylorus separator
pylorus-preserving gastrectomy
    (PPG)
pylorus-preserving surgery
Pynchon applicator
Pynchon cannula
Pynchon decompressor
Pynchon mouth gag
Pynchon nasal speculum
Pynchon suction tube
Pynchon tongue depressor
Pynchon-Lillie tongue depressor
pyocele
pyoderma
pyodermatous skin lesion
pyogenic abscess
pyogenic granuloma
pyogenic membrane
pyoktanin catgut sutures
pyoktanin sutures
pyorrhea
pyosalpinx
pyoureter
PYP scan (pyrophosphate
    scan)
pyramid
    bony pyramid
    cartilaginous pyramid
    nasal pyramid
    petrous pyramid
    renal pyramid
Pyramid anterior lumbar plate
pyramid cannula
pyramid of kidney
pyramid of thyroid
pyramid Toomey tip
pyramidal cataract
pyramidal decussation
pyramidal electrode
pyramidal eminence
pyramidal eye implant
pyramidal fracture
pyramidal function
pyramidal lobe of thyroid
pyramidal muscle
pyramidal tip trocar
pyramidal tract
pyramidal trocar
pyramidal tube

pyramidal tuberosity of palatine
   bone
pyramidotomy
Pyrex tube
pyriform (*see* piriform)
pyriform aperture wiring

pyriform thorax
pyroglycolic acid sutures
Pyrolite heart valve
pyrophosphate scan (PYP scan)
Pyrost bone replacement
pyxigraphic device

Q

Q-angle
Q-band
Q-cath catheter
QCT (quantitative computed tomography)
Q-disk
QIAmp tissue kit
Q-LAS 10 YAG laser
Q-Maxx side-firing laser device
QS (Q-switched)
QS alexandrite laser
QS Nd:YAG laser
QS neodymium:yttrium-aluminum-garnet (Nd:YAG) laser
QS ruby laser
QS ruby/YAG laser
QSA dressing forceps
Q-Star IV pressure-relief mattress
Q-Star Voyager pressure-reduction mattress
Q-switched (QS)
Q-switched alexandrite laser
Q-switched Er:YAG laser
Q-switched Nd:YAG laser
Q-switched neodymium:YAG laser
Q-switched neodymium:yttrium-aluminum-garnet (Nd:YAG) laser
Q-switched ruby laser
Q-switched ruby/YAG laser
Q-T interval sensing pacemaker
QT pouch
Quad cutting tip
Quadcat wire
Quad-Lumen drain
QuadPediatric fundus lens
QuadPolar electrode
quad-ported laser-assisted intrastromal keratomileusis (LASIK) irrigating cannula
Quadracoil ureteral stent

Quadra-Flo infusion catheter
quadrangular cartilage
quadrangular fontanelle
quadrangular lobule of cerebellum
quadrangular membrane
quadrangular space
quadrangular therapy
quadrant
    anterosuperior quadrant
    inner quadrant
    left lower quadrant (LLQ)
    left upper quadrant (LUQ)
    right lower quadrant (RLQ)
    right upper quadrant (RUQ)
Quadrant advanced shoulder brace
quadrant field
quadrant sampling technique
quadrantal cephalalgia
quadrantectomy, axillary dissection, radiation therapy (QUART)
quadrantectomy, axillary dissection, radiotherapy (QUART)
quadriplegic standing frame
quadrapod flap
quadrate gyrus
quadrate lobe
quadrate muscle of upper lip
quadrature cervical spine coil
quadrature phase detector
quadrature radiofrequency receiver coil
quadrature T/L surface coil
quadratus labii inferioris muscle
quadratus labii superioris muscle
quadratus lumborum muscle
quadriceps atrophy
quadriceps jerk
quadriceps muscle

quadriceps reflex
quadriceps tendon
quadricepsplasty
quadricuspid pulmonary valve
quadriga syndrome
quadrilateral brim
quadrilateral cartilage
quadrilateral septum
quadrilateral space
quadrilateral space syndrome
Quadrilite 6000 fiberoptic
    headlight
quadrilobed flap
quadripedal extensor reflex
quadriplegia
quadriplegic
quadripolar 6-French diagnostic
    electrophysiology catheter
quadripolar catheter
quadripolar cutting forceps
quadripolar electrode catheter
quadripolar pacing catheter
quadripolar steerable electrode
    catheter
quadripolar steerable
    mapping/ablation catheter
quadrisected graft dilator
quadrisected minigraft dilator
Quadro dressing
quadruple amputation
quadruple therapy
Quadtro cushion
Quaegebeur procedure
Quaglino operation
QualCare knee brace
QualCraft ankle support
QualCraft short elastic wrist
    support
QualCraft splint
qualitative analysis
qualitative melanin test
Qualtex surgical drape
Quantec endodontic instrument
Quantico needle
Quanticor catheter
quantitative analysis
quantitative computed
    tomography (QCT)
quantitative hepatobiliary
    scintigraphy
Quantum biliary inflation device
Quantum enhancement knife

Quantum enteral pump
Quantum foot prosthesis
Quantum pacemaker
Quantum Ranger OTW balloon
    catheter
Quantum TTC biliary balloon
Quantum TTC biliary balloon
    dilator
quarantine drain
QUART (quadrantectomy,
    axillary dissection,
    radiotherapy)
QUART procedure for breast
    cancer
Quartey technique
quartz abrasive
quartz fiberoptic probe
quartz lamp
quartz mercury ultraviolet lamp
quartz needle
quartz rod
quartz transducer
Quartzo device
quasistatic stressed position
quaternary ammonium chloride
    skin cleanser
Quattro mitral valve
Queckenstedt maneuver
Queckenstedt sign
Queckenstedt test
Queen Anne collar
Queen Anne dressing
quelling reaction
Quengel device
Quenu nail plate removal
    technique
Quenu-Kuss tarsometatarsal
    injury classification
Quenu-Mayo operation
Quenu-Muret sign
quenuthoracoplasty
Quervain (*also* de Quervain)
Quervain abdominal retractor
Quervain cranial forceps
Quervain cranial rongeur forceps
Quervain elevator
Quervain forceps
Quervain fracture
Quervain incision
Quervain release
Quervain rib spreader
Quervain rongeur

Quervain tenolysis
Quervain-Sauerbruch retractor
Questek laser tube
question mark ear
questionable mass
questionable node
questionable sign
questionable significance
Questus Leading Edge
    arthroscopic grasper-cutter
Questus Leading Edge grasper-
    cutter
Questus Leading Edge sheathed
    arthroscopy knife
Questus sheathed knife
Quevedo conjunctival forceps
Quevedo fixation forceps
Quevedo suturing forceps
quick angulation technique
Quick Bend flex clamp
quick catheter
quick connector
Quick scanner
quick pulse
QuickCast splint
QuickCast wrist immobilizer
Quick-cath
Quickcoff device
Quick-Core biopsy needle
QuickDop probe
QuickDraw bone harvester
QuickDraw venous cannula
Quickert grooved director
Quickert grooved director and
    tongue tie
Quickert lacrimal probe
Quickert probe
Quickert procedure
Quickert sutures
Quickert 3-suture technique
Quickert tube
Quickert-Dryden lacrimal probe
Quickert-Dryden tube
Quicket tourniquet
QuickFlash arterial catheter
QuickFurl double-lumen balloon
QuickFurl single-lumen balloon
quick-mount face-bow
    articulator
Quick-Sil starter kit
QuickSilver hydrophilic-coated
    guidewire

QuickSilver hydrophilic-coated
    guidewire
QuickStick padding
Quickswitch
    irrigation/aspiration
    ophthalmic device
quiet bowel sounds
Quiet interference screw
Quik Connect fetal monitor
Quik splint
quill sheath
quilt suture technique
quilt sutures
quilt the septal mucosa
quilted sutures
quilting stitch
Quimby gum scissors
Quinby pelvic fracture
    classification
Quincke puncture
Quincke sign
Quincke spinal needle
Quincke tube
Quincke-Babcock needle
Quincke-point spinal needle
Quinn holder
Quinn needle holder
Quinones uterine-grasping
    forceps
Quinones-Neubuser uterine-
    grasping forceps
quinsy
    lingual quinsy
quinsy tonsillectomy
Quinton biopsy catheter
Quinton central venous catheter
Quinton dual-lumen catheter
Quinton Mahurkar double-
    lumen catheter
Quinton Mahurkar dual-lumen
    catheter
Quinton Mahurkar dual-lumen
    peritoneal catheter
Quinton peritoneal catheter
Quinton Q-Port catheter
Quinton Q-Port vascular access
    port
Quinton Quik-Prep electrode
Quinton suction biopsy
    instrument
Quinton tube
Quinton-Scribner shunt

Quire finger forceps
Quire foreign body forceps
Quire mechanical finger forceps
Quire mechanical finger snare

Quisling intranasal hammer
Quisling-Parkes osteotome
Qwik-Clean dressing
QwikStrip adhesive bandage

R double umbrella device
R&R (recess-resect)
R0, R1, R2 resection
R1 rapid exchange balloon
   catheter
RA (rheumatoid arthritis)
Raaf vascular catheter
Raaf double-lumen catheter
Raaf dual-lumen catheter
Raaf flexible lighted spatula
Raaf forceps
Raaf rongeur
Raaf spatula
Raaf-Oldberg intervertebral disk
   forceps
Raaf-Oldberg rongeur
RAB (remote afterloading
   brachytherapy)
Rabbit mouth gag
Rabiner neurological hammer
Rabinov cannula
racemic modification
racemose gland
Racestyptine retraction ring
rachicentesis
rachigraph
rachilysis
rachiocentesis
rachiometer
rachiotome
  Ralks rachiotome
rachiotomy
rachischisis
rachitic beads
rachitic pelvis
rachitic scoliosis
rachitome
rachitomy
rack
  Austin sterilizing storage rack
  DeVilbiss rack
  ear instrument rack
  eye bottle rack

rack (*continued*)
  Hausmann weight rack
  instrument rack
  Jannetta sterilizing rack
  Jannetta storage rack
  Luneau retinoscopy rack
  McKenzie clip rack
RackBeta scintillation counter
racket amputation
racket incision
racket, racquet
racket-shaped flap
raclage
racquet incision
racquet-shaped incision
Racz catheter
Racz epidural catheter
Racz epidurolysis
rad (radiation absorbed dose)
RAD Airway laryngeal blade
RAD40 sinus blade
radar absorbent material (RAM)
Radcliff perineal retractor
Radcliff retractor
RADenoid adenoidectomy blade
radial
radial abduction
radial artery
radial artery catheter
radial artery of index finger
radial artery reconstruction
radial aspect
radial bone
radial bursa
radial collateral artery
radial collateral ligament
radial column
radial depression
radial deviation
radial drift
radial drift of metacarpal
radial extensor muscle
radial flexor muscle

radial forearm flap
radial forearm free flap
   reconstruction
radial forearm osteocutaneous
   flap
radial fossa
radial foveola
radial fracture reduction
radial fracture site
radial groove
radial head
radial head dislocation
radial head fracture
radial incision
radial index artery
radial iridotomy
radial iridotomy scissors
Radial Jaw biopsy forceps
Radial Jaw bladder biopsy
   forceps
Radial Jaw hot biopsy forceps
Radial Jaw single-use biopsy
   forceps
radial keratotomy (RK)
radial keratotomy knife
radial keratotomy marker
radial laminectomy
radial mutilation injury
radial neck
radial neck fracture
radial nerve block
radial nerve glove
radial nerve palsy
radial nerve splint
radial notch
radial pulse
radial recurrent artery
radial reflex
radial scar
radial sclerosing lesion
radial sector scanning
   echoendoscope
radial sensory compression
radial shaft
radial shortening
radial skin incision
radial sponge
radial styloid fracture
radial styloid process
radial sutures
radial tuberosity
radial tunnel

radial tunnel syndrome
radial veins
radial wedge osteotomy
radial wrinkle
radial wrist examination
radial-based flap
radialis sign
radial-ulnar deviation axis
radiate arteries of kidney
radiating pain
radiation
   accumulative radiation
   biopsy after radiation
   cesium radiation
   cesium tube radiation
   contralateral radiation
   course of radiation
   diagnostic radiation
   dose of radiation
   heat radiation
   interstitial radiation
   intracavitary radiation
   intraoperative radiation
   ionizing radiation
   laser radiation
   massive radiation
   monochromatic radiation
   neutron radiation
   optic radiation
   whole pelvis radiation
radiation absorbed dose (rad)
radiation alopecia
radiation and chemotherapy
radiation beam monitor
radiation burn
radiation damage
radiation dermatitis
radiation dermatosis
radiation exposure
radiation injury
radiation lung disease
radiation monitoring
radiation mucositis
radiation necrosis
radiation of pain
radiation oncology
radiation surgery
radiation therapy
radiation treatment
radiation wound
radiational effect
radiation-induced carcinogenesis

radiation-induced carcinoma
radiation-induced disease
radiation-induced ulceration
radiative hyperthermia device
radical abdominal hysterectomy
radical antrum operation
radical axillary dissection
radical compartmental excision
radical curative surgery
radical cystectomy
radical en bloc removal
radical excision
radical gastrectomy
radical gastric resection
radical hemimaxillectomy
radical hemorrhoidectomy
radical lymph node dissection
radical mastectomy
radical mastoidectomy
radical mediastinal dissection
radical neck dissection
radical operation for hernia
radical parotidectomy
radical prefrontal lobotomy
radical procedure
radical subtotal resection
radical surgery
radical therapy
radical total gastrectomy
radical vaginal hysterectomy
radicle
    biliary radicle
    hepatic radicles
    intrahepatic radicle
    tertiary radicle
radicotomy
radicular abscess
radicular artery
radicular cyst
radicular dentinogenesis
radicular pain
radiculectomy
radiculomedullary fistula
radiculomeningeal spinal
    vascular malformation
RadiMedical fiberoptic pressure-
    monitoring wire
Radin-Rosenthal implant
radioactive applicator
radioactive cobalt
radioactive concentration
radioactive iodine

radioactive rod
radioactive seed implantation
radioactive seeds
radioactive stent
radioactive tag
radioactive tracer
radioactive uptake
radiocapitellar articulation
radiocapitellar line
radiocarpal arch
radiocarpal arthroscopy
radiocarpal articulation
radiocarpal disarticulation
radiocarpal dislocation
radiocarpal fusion
radiocarpal implant
radiocarpal joint
radiocarpal joint capsule
radiocarpal ligament
radiocarpus
radiocurable tumor
radiodense lesion
radiodensity
radiodermatitis
radioencephalogram study
radioepidermatitis
Radiofocus catheter guidewire
Radiofocus Glidewire
    angiography catheter
Radiofocus introducer B kit
radiofrequency ablator
radiofrequency catheter ablation
    (RFCA)
radiofrequency coil
radiofrequency hot balloon
radiofrequency lesion
radiofrequency pacemaker
radiofrequency thermal ablation
    (RFTA)
radiofrequency-generated
    thermal balloon catheter
radiofrequency-generated
    thermal lesion
radiographic apex
radiographic cephalometer
radiographic density
radiographic effect
radiographic evaluation
radiographic evidence
radiographic grid
radiographic image
radiographic lesion

radiographic obliteration
radiographic studies
radiographic technique
radiographic tooth repair
radioguided technique
radiohumeral joint
radioimmunoassay (RIA)
radioimmunoassay kit
radioimmunoglobulin therapy
radioimmunoguided surgery
radioimmunotherapy
radioiodinated
radioiodine ablation
radioisotope applicator
radioisotope camera
radioisotope localization
radioisotope scanning
radioisotope scintigraphy
radioisotope stent
radiologic anatomy
radiologic biliary stent
    placement
radiologic diagnosis
radiologic evaluation
radiologic examination
radiologic magnification study
radiologic portacaval shunt
radiologic procedure
radiologic studies
radiologic technique
radiologic, radiological
radiological examination
radiolucency
radiolucent calculus
radiolucent cranial pin head
    holder
radiolucent crescent line
radiolucent density
radiolucent gallstone
radiolucent lesion
radiolucent line
radiolucent plastic occluder
radiolucent sound
radiolucent spine frame
radiolucent splint
radiolucent stone
radiolunate angle
radiolunate arthrodesis
radiolunate fusion
radiolunate joint
radiometer probe
radionecrosis

radionecrotic tissue
Radionics bipolar coagulation
    unit
Radionics bipolar instrument
Radionics stereotactic head
    frame
Radionics lesion generator
Radionics radiofrequency lesion
    generator
Radionics stimulus generator
radiononopaque stone
radionuclear dynamics
radionucleotide imaging
radionuclide angiogram
radionuclide cineangiogram
radionuclide imaging
radionuclide scanning
radionuclide technique
radiopacity
radiopaque bone cement
radiopaque bougie
radiopaque calibrated catheter
radiopaque contrast medium
radiopaque density
radiopaque dye
radiopaque end marker
radiopaque ERCP catheter
radiopaque foreign body
radiopaque intestinal tube
radiopaque lesion
radiopaque mass
radiopaque medium
radiopaque nitinol stent
radiopaque Silastic catheter
radiopaque skull
radiopaque substance
radiopaque table
radiopaque tantalum stent
radiopharmaceutical
radioresistant tumor
radioscaphoid fusion
radioscapholunate ligament
radiotherapy
radiotranslucent rod
radiotransparent
radioulnar articulation
radioulnar joint
radioulnar subluxation
radioulnar synostosis
radium application
radium applicator
radium capsule

radium implant
radium insertion
radium necrosis
radium needle
radium seeds
radium therapy
radius enteral feeding tube
radius fossa
Radius self-expanding stent
radix (*pl.* radices)
Radix anchor
radix arcus vertebrae
radix dentis
radix facialis
radix linguae
radix longa ganglii ciliaris
radix nasi
radix nasociliaris
radix nervi facialis
radix point
radix Raney jacket
radix unguis
Radley-Liebig-Brown resection
Radley-Liebig-Brown technique
Radnoid microdebrider
radon contamination
radon seed implantation
Radovan breast implant
Radovan subcutaneous tissue
   expander
Radovan tissue expander
Radovan tissue expander tip
Radpour irrigator
Radpour needle
Radpour-House suction tube
Radpour-House suction irrigator
Radstat wrist splint
RAE endotracheal tube
Raeder syndrome
RAE Flex tracheal tube
RAFF (rectus abdominis free
   flap)
Ragnault incision
Ragnell dissecting scissors
Ragnell double-ended retractor
Ragnell drain
Ragnell operation
Ragnell retractor
Ragnell undermining scissors
Ragnell-Davis double-ended
   retractor
Ragnell-Kilner scissors

Rai chronic lymphocytic
   leukemia classification
railway catheter
Raimondi catheter
Raimondi forceps
Raimondi hemostat
Raimondi low-pressure shunt
Raimondi peritoneal catheter
Raimondi scalp hemostatic
   forceps
Raimondi spring peritoneal
   catheter
Raimondi spring peritoneal
   valve
Raimondi tube
Raimondi ventricular catheter
Rainbow cast shoe
Rainbow drill
Rainbow envelope arm sling
Rainbow envelope arm snare
Rainbow fracture frame
Raindrop medication nebulizer
Rainin iris hook
Rainin lens hook
Rainin lens spatula
Rains stent
raised border
raised edge
raised skin flap
raised-arm method to reduce
   dislocated shoulder
rake
   amputation rake
   Blake rake
   Miller 9-prong small rake
   Volkmann rake
rake teeth
rake ulcer
Ralks applicator
Ralks bone drill
Ralks clamp
Ralks drill
Ralks ear forceps
Ralks ear knife
Ralks ear retractor
Ralks elevator
Ralks eye magnet
Ralks fingernail drill
Ralks hammer
Ralks knife
Ralks magnet
Ralks mallet

Ralks nasal gauze packer
Ralks rachiotome
Ralks retractor
Ralks reversible
Ralks sinus applicator
Ralks splinter forceps
Ralks stitch scissors
Ralks suction pressure
    anesthesia unit
Ralks thoracic clamp
Ralks tuning fork
Ralks wire-cutting forceps
Ralks-Davis mouth gag
Ralston-Thompson
    pseudoarthrosis technique
RAM (radar absorbent material)
RAM (rectus abdominis
    musculocutaneous) flap
RAM (rectus abdominis
    myocutaneous) flap
RAM knee prosthesis
Ramadier operation
Rambo endaural incision
Ramdohr sutures
rami (*sing.* ramus)
ramicotomy
Ramirez arteriovenous shunt
Ramirez manipulator
Ramirez periosteal elevator
Ramirez shunt
Ramirez Silastic cannula
Ramirez straight Silastic tube
Ramirez tube
Ramirez winged catheter
ramisection
ramisectomy
Ramitec bite material
Ramond point
Ramond sign
Rampley sponge forceps
ram's horn toenail
Ramsay Hunt facial paralysis
Ramsay Hunt syndrome
Ramsbotham decapitating hook
Ramsbotham knife
Ramsbotham sickle
Ramsden eyepiece
Ramses diaphragm
Ramses diaphragm introducer
Ramsey County pyoktanin
    catgut sutures
Ramsey Hunt syndrome

Ramstedt clamp
Ramstedt operation
Ramstedt procedure
Ramstedt pyloric stenosis dilator
Ramstedt pyloromyotomy
Ramstedt pyloroplasty
Ramstedt-Fredet pyloromyotomy
ramus (*pl.* rami)
ramus blade
ramus blade implant
ramus bone
ramus endosteal implant
ramus of jaw
ramus of mandible
ramus stripper
Ranawat neurologic impairment
    classification
Ranawat-Burstein hip prosthesis
Rancho ankle foot control
    device
Rancho cube
Rancho external fixation
    instrument
Rancho external fixation
    prosthesis
Rancho Los Amigos feeder
Rancho Los Amigos orthosis
Rancho Los Amigos splint
Rancho swivel hinge
Rand bayonet ring curet
Rand forceps
Rand microballoon
Rand retractor for brain surgery
Randall biopsy curet
Randall endometrial biopsy
    curet
Randall kidney stone forceps
Randall lip adhesion
Randall operation
Randall plaque
Randall sign
Randall stone forceps
Randall triangular flap repair
Randall uterine curet
Randall-Brown needle holder
Randall-Tennison operation
Randelli shoulder prosthesis
Rand-House suction tube
Rand-Malcolm cranial x-ray
    frame
Randolph cyclodialysis cannula
Randolph irrigator

random bladder biopsy
random cutaneous flap
random fasciocutaneous flap
random movement
random pattern blood supply
random pattern flap
random temporoparietal fascial
    flap
random-pattern, palmar-based
    flap
Rand-Radpour suction tube
Rand-Wells pallidothalamectomy
    guide
Raney bone drill
Raney clip
Raney clip forceps
Raney cranial drill
Raney curet
Raney dissector
Raney drill
Raney flexion jacket brace
Raney forceps
Raney Gigli-saw guide
Raney jacket
Raney laminectomy punch
Raney laminectomy retractor
Raney laminectomy rongeur
Raney perforator drill
Raney periosteal elevator
Raney punch
Raney retractor
Raney rongeur
Raney rongeur forceps
Raney scalp clip
Raney scalp clip applier
Raney scalp clip-applying
    forceps
Raney spinal fusion curet
Raney spring steel clip
Raney stainless steel scalp clip
Raney stirrup-loop curet
Raney straight coagulating
    forceps
Raney tube
Raney-Crutchfield drill point
Raney-Crutchfield skull traction
    tongs
Ranfac cannula
Ranfac cholangiographic
    catheter
Ranfac laparoscopic knot
    pusher

Ranfac soft-tissue needle
range of excursion
range of motion (ROM)
range of motion of the wrist
range-of-motion brace
Ranger OTW balloon catheter
Ranieri clamp
ranine artery
ranine vein
ranine vein plexus
Ranke angle
Ranke complex
Ranke space
Rankin anastomosis clamp
Rankin arterial forceps
Rankin hemostat
Rankin hemostatic forceps
Rankin intestinal clamp
Rankin operation
Rankin prostatic retractor
Rankin prostatic tractor
Rankin stomach clamp
Rankin sutures
Rankin tractor
Rankin-Crile hemostat
Rankin-Crile hemostatic forceps
Rankin-Kelly hemostat
Rankin-Kelly hemostatic forceps
Rankow forceps
Ransford loop
Ransley procedure
Ransley-Cantwell repair
Ransohoff operation
Ranson acute pancreatitis
    classification
Ranson criteria
Ranvier membrane
Ranvier nodes
Ranvier segments
Ranvier tactile disk
Ranzewski intestinal clamp
RAO position
RAO ventriculogram
RAP cannula
raphe
    lateral canthal raphe
    lateral palpebral raphe
    linear raphe
    lingual raphe
    longitudinal raphe
    median longitudinal raphe
    median raphe

raphe (*continued*)
  midpalatine raphe
  palatine raphe
  palpebral raphe
  pharyngeal raphe
  pterygomandibular raphe
  septal raphe
  supraumbilical raphe
  vertical raphe
rapid alternating movements
rapid bedside imaging
rapid cuff inflator
rapid emptying of dye
rapid exchange balloon
    catheter
rapid exchange Flowtrack
    catheter
rapid eye movements (REM)
rapid filling
rapid infusion pump
rapid maxillary expansion
rapid occlusion
rapid palatal expansion device
rapid pull-through (RPT)
rapid pull-through esophageal
    manometry technique
rapid pull-through operation
rapid scan fluoroscopy
rapid scan technique
rapid sequence filming
rapid sequence induction
    intubation
rapid slide test
rapid tumor lysis syndrome
rapid Y descent
Rapide sutures
RapidFire multiple band ligator
RapidFlap
Rapidgraft arterial vessel
    substitute
rapid-sequence induction (RSI)
rapid-sequence induction of
    anesthesia
rapid-volume approach
RapiSeal patch
Raplon anesthesia
Raplon anesthetic
Rapp forceps
Rapp technique
Rappaport classification
Rappazzo foreign body scissors
Rappazzo haptic scissors

Rappazzo intraocular foreign
    body forceps
Rappazzo intraocular lens
Rappazzo intraocular
    manipulator
Rappazzo iris hook
Rappazzo speculum
Rapp-Hodgkin syndrome
Raptorail catheter
rarefied area
Rascal II anesthetic gas monitor
Rashkind balloon
Rashkind balloon atrial
    septostomy
Rashkind balloon catheter
Rashkind balloon septostomy
Rashkind balloon technique
Rashkind cardiac device
Rashkind cardiac procedure
Rashkind double-disk occluder
    prosthesis
Rashkind double-disk umbrella
    occluder
Rashkind double-umbrella
    device
Rashkind hooked device
Rashkind operation
Rashkind procedure
Rashkind septostomy balloon
    catheter
Rashkind septostomy needle
Rashkind-Miller atrial
    septostomy
Rasmussen aneurysm
rasp (*see also* raspatory)
  Aagesen disposable rasp
  Agris rasp
  Alexander rib rasp
  Alexander-Farabeuf rib rasp
  AMS rasp
  antrum rasp
  Arthrofile orthopedic rasp
  Aufricht glabellar rasp
  Aufricht nasal rasp
  Aufricht-Lipsett nasal rasp
  Austin Moore prosthesis rasps
  Bardeleben rasp
  Barsky nasal rasp
  Bartholdson-Stenstrom rasp
  Beck rasp
  Berne nasal rasp
  Bio-Modular humeral rasp

rasp (*continued*)

Black bone and skin rasp
bone rasp
Bowen rasp
Brawley antrum rasp
Brawley frontal sinus rasp
Brawley sinus rasp
Bristow rasp
Brown rasp
Charnley rasp
Charnley-Mueller rasp
Christmas-tree rasp
circular rasp
Cohen sinus rasp
compound curved rasp
Concept arthroscopy rasp
Converse rasp
convex rasp
corneal rasp
Coryllos rasp
Cottle nasal rasp
Cottle-MacKenty elevator rasp
Davidson-Mathieu-Alexander
    elevator rasp
Davidson-Sauerbruch rasp
Dean antral rasp
diamond nasal rasp
diamond rasp
down-curved rasp
Doyen costal rasp
Doyen rib rasp
ear rasp
Eicher rasp
Endotrac rasp
Epstein bone rasp
F.R. Thompson rasp
facet rasp
Farabeuf bone rasp
Farabeuf-Collen rasp
FeatherTouch automated rasp
femoral rasp
femoral shaft rasp
Filtzer interbody rasp
Fischer nasal rasp
Fomon nasal rasp
Friedman rasp
frontal sinus rasp
Gallagher antral rasp
Gam-Mer rasp
Georgiade rasp
glabellar rasp
Gleason rasp

rasp (*continued*)

Good antral rasp
hand surgery rasp
Hylin rasp
interbody circular rasp
interbody fusion rasp
interbody rasp
Israel nasal rasp
Joseph nasal rasp
Kalinowski rasp
Kalinowski-Verner rasp
Kessler podiatry rasp
Key rasp
Kleinert-Kutz rasp
Lambotte rasp
Lamont nasal rasp
Leurs nasal rasp
Lewis rasp
Lorenz-Rees nasal rasp
Lundsgaard rasp
Lundsgaard-Burch corneal
    rasp
Maliniac nasal rasp
Mallory-Head Interlok rasp
Maltz nasal rasp
Maltz-Anderson nasal rasp
Maltz-Lipsett nasal rasp
Matchett-Brown stem rasp
McCabe perforation rasp
McCabe-Farrior rasp
McCollough rasp
McGee oval-window rasp
McIndoe rasp
McKee-Farrar rasp
McKinty rasp
microbayonet rasp
Mitner rotary bone rasp
Moore prosthesis rasp
Moore stem rasp
nasal rasp
Nicola rasp
orthopedic rasp
Parkes rasp
Peet nasal rasp
perforation rasp
Phemister rasp
Plenk-Matson rasp
Polokoff rasp
power rasp
pull rasp
push rasp
Putti bone rasp

rasp (*continued*)
rat-tail rasp
Reidy rasp
Ringenberg rasp
Riordan rasp
Ritter rasp
Robb-Roberts rotary rasp
Rubin oblique rasp
Saunders-Paparella window
rasp
Schantz sinus rasp
Scheer oval window rasp
Schmidt rasp
side-cutting rasp
sinus rasp
snow plow rasp
Southworth rasp
Spratt nasofrontal rasp
stem rasp
Stenstrom rasp
Stille-Doyen rasp
Stille-Edwards rasp
straight rasp
Sullivan sinus rasp
surgical general rasp
Thompson antral rasp
Thompson sinus rasp
Thompson stem rasp
triangular rasp
trochanteric rasp
ulnar rasp
V. Mueller diamond rasp
Watson-Williams frontal sinus
rasp
Watson-Williams sinus rasp
Wiener antral rasp
Wiener nasal rasp
Wiener Universal frontal sinus
rasp
Wiener-Pierce antral rasp
window rasp
Woodward rasp
rasp pin
raspatory (*see also* rasp)
Alexander rib raspatory
Artmann raspatory
Aufricht raspatory
Aufricht-Lipsett raspatory
Babcock raspatory
Bacon periosteal raspatory
Ballenger raspatory
Barsky cleft palate raspatory

raspatory (*continued*)
Bastow laminectomy
raspatory
Beck pericardial raspatory
Bennett raspatory
Berne nasal raspatory
Berry rib raspatory
Brawley antrum raspatory
bronchocele sound raspatory
Brown raspatory
Brunner raspatory
cleft palate raspatory
Cohen sinus raspatory
Collin raspatory
Converse raspatory
Coryllos rib raspatory
Cottle raspatory
Cushing raspatory
Davidson-Mathieu raspatory
Davidson-Sauerbruch rib
raspatory
Davis raspatory
Dean raspatory
Dolley raspatory
Doyen rib raspatory
Edwards raspatory
Edwards-Verner raspatory
Eicher raspatory
elevator and raspatory
facet raspatory
Farabeuf raspatory
Farabeuf-Collin raspatory
Farabeuf-Lambotte raspatory
Farrior mushroom raspatory
fishtail raspatory
fishtail spatula raspatory
Fomon raspatory
French-pattern raspatory
Friedrich raspatory
Gallagher antral frontal
raspatory
Gam-Mer oblique raspatory
Gleason raspatory
Good frontal raspatory
Hedblom raspatory
Hein raspatory
Herczel rib raspatory
Hill nasal raspatory
Hoen periosteal raspatory
Hopkins Hospital periosteal
raspatory
Hopkins periosteal raspatory

raspatory (*continued*)
Howarth nasal raspatory
Israel raspatory
Jansen mastoid raspatory
Joseph nasal raspatory
Joseph periosteal raspatory
Joseph-Verner raspatory
Kirmisson periosteal
  raspatory
Kleesattel raspatory
Kocher raspatory
Koenig raspatory
Kokowicz raspatory
Ladd raspatory
Lambert-Berry rib raspatory
Lambotte rib raspatory
laminectomy raspatory
Lamont nasal raspatory
Lane periosteal raspatory
Langenbeck periosteal
  raspatory
Langenbeck-O'Brien raspatory
Lebsche raspatory
Lewis nasal raspatory
Lewis periosteal raspatory
Lundsgaard-Burch corneal
  raspatory
Maliniac nasal raspatory
Maltz raspatory
Maltz-Lipsett raspatory
Mannerfelt raspatory
mastoid raspatory
Mathieu raspatory
Matson raspatory
Matson-Alexander raspatory
Matson-Plenk raspatory
McGee raspatory
McIndoe raspatory
Miller raspatory
Moore raspatory
Mott raspatory
Nelson first-rib raspatory
Nicola raspatory
Ollier raspatory
Overholt rib raspatory
Parkes nasal raspatory
pericardial raspatory
periosteal raspatory
Phemister raspatory
Pierce raspatory
Plenk-Matson raspatory
Putti bone raspatory

raspatory (*continued*)
rib elevator and raspatory
rib raspatory
Ritter raspatory
Sauerbruch raspatory
Sauerbruch-Frey raspatory
Sayre periosteal raspatory
Schantz sinus raspatory
Scheuerlen raspatory
Schmidt raspatory
Schneider raspatory
Schneider-Sauerbruch
  raspatory
Sedillot raspatory
Semb rib raspatory
Sewall raspatory
Shuletz raspatory
Shuletz-Damian raspatory
skull raspatory
Spratt raspatory
Stenstrom raspatory
Stille-Crafoord raspatory
Stille-Doyen raspatory
Stille-Edwards raspatory
Stillenberg raspatory
Sullivan raspatory
sympathetic raspatory
Thompson frontal sinus
  raspatory
Trelat palate raspatory
Watson-Williams sinus
  raspatory
Wiberg raspatory
Wiener antral raspatory
Wiener Universal frontal sinus
  raspatory
Willauer raspatory
Williger raspatory
Woodward antral raspatory
xyster raspatory
Yasargil raspatory
Zenker raspatory
Zoellner raspatory
raspberry mark
raspberry tongue
rasping action
Rastan operation
Rastan-Konno procedure
Rastelli graft
Rastelli implant
Rastelli operation
Rastelli procedure

Rastelli prosthesis
Rastelli repair
Rastelli type A, B, C classification
    of atrioventricular septal
    defect
ratchet applicator
ratchet clamp
ratchet tourniquet
ratchet-type brace
rate of cerebral blood flow
    (rCBF)
rate of fluid filtration
rate of maturation
rate-adaptive device
rate-modulated pacemaker
rate-responsive pacemaker
Rath treatment table
Rathke bundle
Rathke folds
Rathke pocket
Rathke pouch
Rathke pouch cyst
Rathke punch
Rathke tumor
Ratliff-Blake gallstone forceps
Ratliff-Mayo gallstone forceps
rat-tail catheter
rat-tail deformity
rat-tail rasp
rat-tail sign
rat-tooth forceps
rat-tooth pickup
rat-tooth rongeur
Rauchfuss sling
Rauchfuss sling splint
Rauchfuss snare
Raulerson introducer syringe
Raven matrix
Ravenna syndrome
Raverdino operation
Ravich bougie
Ravich clamp
Ravich convertible
    cystoscope
Ravich cystoscope
Ravich dilator
Ravich lithotriptoscope
Ravich lithotriptoscope with
    Luer lock
Ravich lithotrite
Ravich needle holder
Ravich ureteral dilator

Ravitch technique for
    reconstruction
rawhide bone hammer
ray
    Bucky rays
    canal rays
    convergent ray
    Dorno rays
    fluorescent ray
    gamma ray
    grenz ray
    luminous rays
    postaxial duplication of the
        5th ray (types I-III)
    roentgen ray
    stiff ray
ray amputation
Ray brain spatula
Ray brain spoon
Ray curet
Ray kidney stone forceps
Ray nasal speculum
Ray pituitary curet
ray resection
Ray rhizotomy electrode
Ray thermistor electrode
Ray screw
Ray speculum
Ray spoon
Ray TFC device
Ray tube
Ray-Brunswick-Mack operation
Ray-Clancy-Lemon technique
Rayhack technique
Raylor bone impactor
Raylor malleable retractor
Ray-McLean operation
Raynaud syndrome
Rayner lens
Rayner-Choyce eye implant
Rayner-Choyce intraocular lens
rayon gauze
rayon strip
Ray-Parsons-Sunday
    staphylorrhaphy elevator
Rayport dural dissector
Rayport dural knife
Rayport knife
Rayport muscle clamp
Ray-Tec band
Ray-Tec dressing
Ray-Tec gauze

Ray-Tec surgical sponge
Ray-Tec x-ray detectable lap pad
Ray-Tec x-ray detectable surgical
    sponge
Raz bladder neck suspension
Raz double-prong ligature
    carrier
Raz 4-quadrant suspension
Raz modification
Raz needle suspension
Raz procedure for stress
    incontinence
Raz urethral suspension
Raz urethropexy
Razel pump
Razi cannula introducer
Raz-Leach procedure
razor
    Bard-Parker razor
    Castroviejo oscillating razor
    Castroviejo razor
    Credo razor
    Detroit Receiving Hospital
        razor
    Emir razor
    Weck-Prep orderly razor
razor blade
razor blade holder
razor blade knife
razor bladebreaker
razor scalpel
razor-blade trephine
razor-tip needle
RB1 sutures
RC1 catheter
RC2 fundus camera
RCB biopsy needle
rCBF (rate of cerebral blood
    flow)
RD (retinal detachment)
Re/Flex filter
reabsorbable sutures
reaccumulation of fluid
reach-and-pin forceps
ReAct NMES device
reaction
    allergic reaction (type I-IV)
    allograft reaction
    anaphylactic reaction
    anaphylactoid reaction
    antigen-antibody reaction
    Arthus reaction

reaction (*continued*)
    autoimmune reaction
    blanching reaction
    cadaveric reaction
    Cupraphane dialyzer reaction
    cutaneous reaction
    delayed reaction
    drug reaction
    dyskinetic and dystonic
        reactions
    dyskinetic reaction
    dystonic reactions
    epicutaneous reaction
    febrile reaction
    fibroblastic reaction
    foreign body reaction
    graft-versus-host reaction
    granulomatous inflammatory
        reaction
    granulomatous reaction
    homograft reaction
    Hunt reaction
    idiosyncratic allergic reaction
    immunity reaction
    implant reaction
    inflammation reaction
    inflammatory reaction
    intracutaneous reaction
    intradermal reaction
    irritative reaction
    late phase reaction
    local reaction
    marked localized reaction
    negative reaction
    neurotonic reaction
    neutral reaction
    photoallergic reaction
    pleural reaction
    positive reaction
    postoperative reaction
    quelling reaction
    reflex-like reaction
    reversible reaction
    skin reaction
    sluggish reaction
    somatization reactions
    suspected transfusion
        reaction
    sympathetic reaction
    systemic reaction
    tibial stress reaction
    trigger reaction

reaction (*continued*)
  untoward reaction
  vascular reaction
  vasomotor reaction
  wheal-and-flare reaction
  white-graft reaction
reaction formation
reaction ossification
reactive angioendotheliomatosis
reactive dilation
reactive hyperemia
reactive hyperostosis
reactive lymphoid lesion
reactive ossification
reactive perforating collagenosis
Read chisel
Read facial curet
Read forceps
Read gouge
Read oral curet
Read osteotome
Read periosteal elevator
Read-McIndoe operation
real reconstruction
realigned fracture
realignment of fracture
    fragments
realignment procedure
realignment rhinoplasty
Reality vaginal pouch
real-time 3-D biplanar
    transperineal prostate
    implantation
real-time B scanner
real-time colonoscopy
real-time confocal scanning laser
    microscope
real-time echo-planar image
real-time endoscopic ultrasound-
    guided fine-needle
    aspiration
real-time imaging
real-time multiplanar image
real-time ultrasonography
real-time ultrasound
real-time video processor
reamer
  acetabular reamer
  acorn reamer
  adjustable cup reamer
  AMBI reamer
  Anatomic/Intracone reamer

reamer (*continued*)
  Aufranc finishing ball reamer
  Aufranc finishing cup reamer
  Aufranc offset reamer
  Austin Moore bone reamer
  ball reamer
  ball-tip reamer
  burred Wright reamer
  CAD reamer
  calcar reamer
  canal reamer
  cannulated 4-flute reamer
  cannulated reamer
  Chamfer reamer
  Charnley deepening reamer
  Charnley expanding reamer
  Charnley taper reamer
  Charnley trochanter reamer
  core reamer
  cylindrical reamer
  debris-retaining acetabular
    reamer
  deepened reamer
  Dentatus reamer
  DePuy reamer
  drill reamer
  Duthie reamer
  end-cutting reamer
  endodontic reamer
  engine reamer
  expanding reamer
  femoral head reamer
  femoral neck reamer
  femoral shaft reamer
  final-cut acetabular reamer
  finishing ball reamer
  finishing cup reamer
  flexible reamer
  flexible-wire bundle reamer
  fluted reamer
  Gray flexible intramedullary
    reamer
  Green-Armytage reamer
  grooving reamer
  Gruca hip reamer
  Hall Versipower reamer
  Harris brace-type reamer
  Harris center-cutting
    acetabular reamer
  Harris-Norton hip reamer
  Henderson reamer
  Hewson-Richards reamer

reamer (*continued*)
  humeral reamer
  Indiana reamer
  Intracone intramedullary
    reamer
  intramedullary reamer
  Jergesen-Trinkle reamer
  Jergesen reamer
  Jewett socket reamer
  K reamer
  Kuntscher shaft reamer
  Lorenz reamer
  Lottes reamer
  MacAusland finishing-ball
    reamer
  MacAusland finishing-cup
    reamer
  Mallory-Head Interlok reamer
  Marin reamer
  medullary canal reamer
  Mira female trochanteric
    reamer
  Mira femoral head reamer
  Mira-Charnley reamer
  Moore bone reamer
  Murphy ball reamer
  Norton adjustable cup reamer
  Norton ball reamer
  offset reamer
  orthopedic reamer
  Osteonics reamer
  PD reamer
  Pease reamer
  Perthes reamer
  Pesso reamer
  Phemister reamer
  Pressure Sentinel reamer
  Reiswig reamer
  revision conical reamer
  Richards barrel reamer
  Richards calibrated reamer
  Rispi reamer
  Rowe glenoidal reamer
  Rush awl reamer
  Schneider nail shaft reamer
  shaft reamer
  shelf reamer
  Smith-Petersen hip reamer
  Sovak reamer
  spherical reamer
  spiral reamer
  spiral trochanteric reamer

reamer (*continued*)
  spot face reamer
  step-cut reamer
  straight reamer
  Sturmdorf cervical reamer
  Swanson reamer
  tapered reamer
  T-handle reamer
  Tinel tapered reamer
  trochanteric reamer
reamer awl
reamer bushing
reamer clamp
reaming awl
reamputation
reanastomosis
renal ectopia
reapplication of cast
reapproximated skin edges
rear-entry ACL drill guide
rear-tip extender
reattached extremity
reattached surgically
reattribution technique
Reaves antral punch
REB rubber-reinforced bandage
Rebar microcatheter
Rebar microvascular catheter
Rebel knee orthosis
rebleeding risk
rebound hyperemia
rebound tenderness
rebreathing anesthesia
rebreathing bag
rebreathing mask
rebreathing technique
Rebuck skin window
    technique
recalcification
recalcitrant ulcer
recalcitrant verruca
Recamier curet
Recamier operation
Recamier procedure
Recamier uterine curet
recanalization
recanalization of artery
recanalization technique
recanalizing thrombosis
recannulization
receding lower jaw
receiver coil

receptor
  epidermal growth factor
    receptor
  E-rosette receptor
  high threshold receptor
  juxtacapillary receptor
  nerve receptors
recess
  Arlt recess
  bony sphenoethmoidal recess
  costodiaphragmatic recess
  costomediastinal recess
  duodenal recess
  epitympanic recess
  facial recess
  frontal recess
  inferior duodenal recess
  inferior omental recess
  infundibuliform recess
  intersigmoid recess
  laryngopharyngeal recess
  nasal recess
  nasopalatine recess
  omental recess
  optic recess
  palatine recess
  parotic recess
  pericardial recess
  pharyngeal recess
  piriform recess
  prestyloid recess
  Rosenmueller recess
  sphenoethmoidal recess
  superior duodenal recess
  superior omental recess
  zygomatic recess
recess of nasopharynx
recessed balloon septostomy
    catheter
recessed-head screw
recessing of tendon
recession forceps
recess-resect procedure
recipient
  designated recipient
  donor recipient
  kidney recipient
  liver recipient
  universal recipient
recipient bed
recipient hepatectomy
recipient of organ transplant

recipient site
recipient vessel
reciprocal innervation
reciprocal ohm meter
reciprocal planing instrument
reciprocal rhythm
reciprocal transfusion
reciprocating cannula
reciprocating gait orthosis
reciprocating saw
reciprocator
recirculation
Recklinghausen disease
Recklinghausen tonometer
recliner air chair
reclining chair
Reclus syndrome
recoarctation of aorta
recombinant DNA technique
recombinant human bone
    morphogenetic protein
    (rhBMP-2)
recombinant human growth
    hormone (rhGH)
recombinant human insulin-like
    growth factor (rhIGF)
Recon nail
reconstruction
  2-stage tendon graft
    reconstruction
  3-D computer reconstruction
  3-dimensional reconstruction
  4-bone SLAC wrist
    reconstruction
  5-1 reconstruction
  Abbe-McIndoe vaginal
    reconstruction
  abdominal wall
    reconstruction
  ACL reconstruction
  AL reconstruction
  alar reconstruction
  Albee hip reconstruction
  Allman ankle reconstruction
  alloplastic reconstruction
  anal sphincter reconstruction
  analytic reconstruction
  Andrews iliotibial band
    reconstruction
  Andrews knee reconstruction
  anterior capsulolabral
    reconstruction

reconstruction (*continued*)

anterior cruciate ligament reconstruction
aortic root reconstruction
aortorenal reconstruction
areolar reconstruction
artery reconstruction
arthroscopic anterior cruciate ligament reconstruction (AACLR)
auricular reconstruction
autogenous reconstruction
Bankart reconstruction
bell flap nipple reconstruction
biliary reconstruction
Billroth I, II reconstruction
BIMA reconstruction
bladder outlet reconstruction
Blom-Singer vocal reconstruction
bone reconstruction
bony reconstruction
box top technique of nipple reconstruction
breast mound reconstruction
breast reconstruction
Brent eyebrow reconstruction
Brown knee joint reconstruction
Browne urethral reconstruction
buccal mucosa graft for urethra reconstruction
Bucknall urethral reconstruction
burn reconstruction
Cabral coronary reconstruction
chest wall reconstruction
Cho anterior cruciate ligament reconstruction
Chrisman-Snook reconstruction
circumferential esophageal reconstruction
Clancy cruciate ligament reconstruction
cleft lip nasal reconstruction
Colonna reconstruction
columellar reconstruction
composite mandibular reconstruction

reconstruction (*continued*)

conjunctival cul-de-sac reconstruction
constrained reconstruction
coronal reconstruction
corporeal reconstruction
cosmetic reconstruction
costochondral graft mandibular ramus reconstruction
costochondral graft reconstruction
craniofacial reconstruction
cruciate ligament reconstruction
Cutler-Beard reconstruction
d'Aubigne femoral reconstruction
d'Aubigne resection reconstruction
dermal pouch reconstruction
Dibbell cleft lip-nasal reconstruction
digital nerve reconstruction
distal vertebral artery reconstruction
double-paddle peroneal tissue transfer reconstruction
dural patch reconstruction
DuVries lateral ankle reconstruction
ear reconstruction
Eaton-Littler ligament reconstruction
Ellison lateral knee reconstruction
Elmslie ankle reconstruction
Elmslie modification of ankle reconstruction
endoscopic anterior cruciate ligament reconstruction
end-to-end reconstruction
epiglottic reconstruction
Eriksson cruciate reconstruction
esthetic breast reconstruction
Eva-Hewes reconstruction
Evans reconstruction
exogenous reconstruction
expanded 2-flap method for microtia reconstruction

reconstruction (*continued*)
exstrophy reconstruction
extended lateral arm free flap for head/neck reconstruction
extensor tendon reconstruction
external genitalia reconstruction
extra-articular reconstruction
eyelid reconstruction
facial artery musculomucosal flap reconstruction
facial reconstruction
finger reconstruction
forehead reconstruction
free bone reconstruction
free fillet extremity flap for reconstruction
free flap reconstruction
free gracilis muscle reconstruction
free tissue transfer reconstruction
functional reconstruction
genital reconstruction
Goldman nasal tip reconstruction
Goldner reconstruction
gracilis myocutaneous vaginal reconstruction
hair-bearing reconstruction
hand reconstruction
Harmon hip reconstruction
head and neck reconstruction
hemimandible reconstruction
House reconstruction
Hughes eye reconstruction
Hughston quadriceps reconstruction
Hughston-Degenhardt reconstruction
Hughston-Jacobson lateral compartment reconstruction
immediate breast reconstruction
implant/flap reconstruction
in situ reconstruction
index metacarpophalangeal joint reconstruction

reconstruction (*continued*)
inferior vena cava reconstruction
infrarenal aortic reconstruction
Inglis reconstruction
innominate artery reconstruction
Insall anterior cruciate ligament reconstruction
Insall-Hood posterior cruciate reconstruction
intra-articular reconstruction
Istanbul flap for phallic reconstruction
iterative reconstruction
IVC reconstruction
joint reconstruction
juxtacubital reconstruction
Krukenberg hand reconstruction
Kugelberg reconstruction
Landolt eyelid reconstruction
Larson ligament reconstruction
laryngeal reconstruction
laryngotracheal reconstruction (LTR)
lateral compartment reconstruction
latissimus dorsi breast reconstruction
Lee reconstruction
LeFort I maxillary reconstruction
L'Episcopo hip reconstruction
Lewis-Tanner subtotal esophagectomy and reconstruction
ligament reconstruction
lip and vermilion reconstruction
lip reconstruction
Littler-Eaton reconstruction
long bone reconstruction
Longmire-Gutgeman gastric reconstruction
Losee knee reconstruction
lower extremity reconstruction
MacIntosh over-the-top ACL reconstruction

reconstruction (*continued*)

mandibular functional
reconstruction
mandibular reconstruction
maxillofacial reconstruction
McIndoe vaginal
reconstruction
microsurgical breast
reconstruction
microtia reconstruction
microvascular reconstruction
Mikulicz pharyngoesophageal
reconstruction
Millard advancement rotation
flap reconstruction
Mladick ear reconstruction
modified autogenous
latissimus breast
reconstruction
modified reconstruction
morphofunctional vulvar
reconstruction
multiplanar reconstruction
multistaged reconstruction
nasal reconstruction
nasal septum reconstruction
(NSR)
nasoseptal reconstruction
Nathan-Trung modification of
Kurkenberg hand
reconstruction
Neer posterior shoulder
reconstruction
neoglottic reconstruction
neurovascular infrahyoid
island flap for tongue
reconstruction
Nicholas medial compartment
reconstruction
nipple reconstruction
no-bone reconstruction
Noyes anterior cruciate
reconstruction
O'Donoghue ACL
reconstruction
open reconstruction
operative reconstruction
oral reconstruction
orbital rim reconstruction
orofacial reconstruction
oromandibular reconstruction
oropharyngeal reconstruction

reconstruction (*continued*)

ossicular chain reconstruction
osteochondral reconstruction
osteoplastic reconstruction
palate reconstruction
pancreaticogastrostomy
reconstruction
papillary reconstruction
pedicled jejunal
reconstruction
peg latissimus dorsi flap
breast reconstruction
penile reconstruction
perineal reconstruction
peritoneal reconstruction
phallic reconstruction
pharyngoesophageal
reconstruction
philtral flap deepithelization
centering and
reconstruction
plastic reconstruction
portal vein reconstruction
postmastectomy
reconstruction
pouch reconstruction
prosthetic reconstruction
Puddu reconstruction
pulley reconstruction
radial artery reconstruction
radial forearm free flap
reconstruction
Ravitch technique for
reconstruction
real reconstruction
renal artery reconstruction
reverse ulnar hypothenar flap
finger reconstruction
reversed island flaps for
forefoot reconstruction
Rosenberg endoscopic
anterior cruciate ligament
reconstruction
Roux gastric reconstruction
Roux-en-Y reconstruction
Rubens free flap for breast
reconstruction
sagittal reconstruction
scalp reconstruction
secondary ear
reconstruction
secondary reconstruction

reconstruction (*continued*)

segmental bone and cartilage reconstruction

sensitive free flap reconstruction

septal reconstruction

sequential bilateral breast reconstruction

Sheen airway reconstruction

single-stage reconstruction

sliding osteotomy in mandibular reconstruction

socket reconstruction

soft tissue expansion reconstruction

soft tissue reconstruction

sphincter reconstruction

S-pouch reconstruction

staged breast reconstruction

staged reconstruction

staircase technique for lip reconstruction

stapled reconstruction

Steffanoff ear reconstruction

stepladder technique for lip reconstruction

sternoclavicular joint reconstruction

subpectoral reconstruction

sural island flap for foot and ankle reconstruction

Swanson reconstruction

synchronous bladder reconstruction

Tagliacozzi nasal reconstruction

TAL breast reconstruction

Tanagho bladder neck reconstruction

Tanzer auricle reconstruction

tenoplastic reconstruction

Thom flap laryngeal reconstruction

thumb reconstruction

Torg knee reconstruction

total autogenous latissimus breast reconstruction

total penile reconstruction

tracheal reconstruction

TRAM flap breast reconstruction

reconstruction (*continued*)

transmandibular reconstruction

tubular reconstruction

tubularized bladder neck reconstruction

Turbinger gastric reconstruction

urethral reconstruction

urinary tract reconstruction

vaginal reconstruction

vaginoperineal reconstruction

vascular reconstruction

Verdan osteoplastic thumb reconstruction

vertebral artery reconstruction

Victor-Gomel microsurgical tubal reconstruction

vulvovaginal reconstruction

Watson-Jones ligament reconstruction

Whitman femoral neck reconstruction

Wirth-Jager posterior cruciate reconstruction

Wookey pharyngoesophageal reconstruction

Young-Dees bladder neck reconstruction

Young-Dees-Leadbetter bladder neck reconstruction

Zancolli reconstruction

Zisser-Madden method of upper lip reconstruction

reconstruction occlusal surface (RecOS)

reconstruction of heel and plantar area

reconstruction of maxillectomy and midfacial defects

reconstruction operation

reconstruction plates

reconstruction procedure

reconstruction technique

reconstructive mammaplasty

reconstructive microsurgery

reconstructive operation

reconstructive plastic procedure

reconstructive preprosthetic surgery

reconstructive procedure

reconstructive rhinoplasty
reconstructive surgery
reconstructive surgical
    procedure
reconstructive sutures
reconstructive technique
recontouring
recontouring alveolectomy
recording cystometer
recording electrode
Recovercare System 3 low-air,
    loss-alternating pressure
    mattress
recovery room (RR)
recovery technique
recrudescent abscess
recruitment maneuver
rectal abscess
rectal ampulla
rectal anesthesia
rectal anesthetic
rectal anesthetic technique
rectal artery
rectal balloon
rectal biopsy forceps
rectal bleeding
rectal bougie
rectal canal
rectal cancer
rectal carcinoma
rectal catheter
rectal cautery snare
rectal cautery wire
rectal clamp
rectal column
rectal crypt hook
rectal curet
rectal cutter
rectal dilation
rectal dilator
rectal director
rectal distention
rectal enema
rectal evacuation
rectal examination
rectal excision
rectal expander
rectal finger cot
rectal fissure
rectal fistula
rectal fistulectomy
rectal floor line

rectal fold
rectal forceps
rectal foreign body
rectal gargle
rectal hemorrhoid
rectal hernia
rectal hook
rectal hook retractor
rectal incontinence
rectal injection cannula
rectal injection needle
rectal irrigator
rectal laceration
rectal lesion
rectal lithotomy
rectal mass
rectal mucosa
rectal multiplane transducer
rectal muscle cuff
rectal needle
rectal nerves
rectal plexus
rectal polyp
rectal pouch
rectal pressure
rectal probe
rectal probe electroejaculation
rectal prolapse
rectal pull-through operation
rectal pulsed irrigation
rectal reflex
rectal retinaculum
rectal retractor
rectal scissors
rectal shelf
rectal sinuses
rectal site
rectal skin tag
rectal snare
rectal speculum
rectal sphincter
rectal stalks
rectal stenosis
rectal stricture
rectal stump
rectal suction biopsy
rectal suppository
rectal surgery
rectal swab
rectal tags
rectal tear
rectal temperature

rectal tenesmus
rectal trauma
rectal trocar
rectal tube
rectal valve
rectal vein
rectal verge
rectal warts
rectangular amputation
rectangular awl
rectangular blade
rectangular brain spatula
rectangular cartilage graft
rectangular flap
rectangular wire
rectectomy
rectified microscope
rectified polarizing microscope
rectilinear scan
rectilinear scanner
rectoanal inhibitory reflex
rectocele
   A&P repair of cystocele and
     rectocele
   anterior and posterior repair
     of cystocele and rectocele
     (A&P repair)
rectocele repair
rectoclysis
rectococcygeal muscle
rectococcypexy
rectocutaneous fistula
rectocystotomy
rectolabial fistula
rectoperineorrhaphy
rectopexy
  abdominal rectopexy
  anterior rectopexy
  Ivalon sponge rectopexy
  Marlex mesh abdominal
    rectopexy
  posterior rectopexy
  presacral rectopexy
  Ripstein anterior sling
    rectopexy
  Ripstein presacral rectopexy
  Teflon sling rectopexy
  Wells posterior rectopexy
rectoplasty
rectorectal intussusception
rectorectostomy
rectoromanoscope

rectoromanoscopy
rectorrhaphy
rectoscope
rectoscopic endometrial ablation
rectoscopy
rectosigmoid anastomosis
rectosigmoid carcinoma
rectosigmoid junction
rectosigmoid manometry
rectosigmoidectomy
rectosigmoidoscope
rectosigmoidoscopy
rectosigmoidostomy
rectosphincteric reflex
rectostomy
rectotome
rectotomy
rectourethral fistula
rectourethral muscle
rectourinary fistula
rectouterine fold
rectouterine ligament
rectouterine muscle
rectouterine pouch
rectovaginal dose
rectovaginal examination
rectovaginal fascia
rectovaginal fistula
rectovaginal fold
rectovaginal pouch
rectovaginal septum
rectovaginal space
rectovaginal surgery
rectovesical center
rectovesical fascia
rectovesical fistula
rectovesical fold
rectovesical lithotomy
rectovesical muscle
rectovesical pouch
rectovesical septum
rectovesical space
rectovestibular fistula
rectovulvar fistula
rectum
  abdominoperineal resection
    of rectum
  Allingham excision of
    rectum
  anastomosis of rectum
  anterior resection of sigmoid
    and rectum

rectum (*continued*)
  Bergenhem implantation of
    ureter into rectum
  colonoscopy per rectum
  decompression of rectum
  exteriorization of rectum
  flexure of rectum
  fold of rectum
  implantation of ureter into
    rectum
  per rectum
  prolapsed rectum
  redundant prolapsed rectum
  transverse folds of rectum
rectum cancer
rectum irrigation
rectus
  gyrus rectus
  inferior rectus (IR)
  lateral rectus (LR)
  medial rectus
  superior rectus
rectus abdominis flap
rectus abdominis free flap (RAFF)
rectus abdominis muscle
rectus abdominis muscle flap
rectus abdominis muscle sheath
rectus abdominis muscle transfer
rectus abdominis
    musculocutaneous (RAM)
    flap
rectus abdominis myocutaneous
    flap (RAM flap)
rectus abdominis sheath
rectus capitis muscle
rectus diastasis
rectus fascia
rectus femoris fasciocutaneous
    flap
rectus femoris flap
rectus femoris muscle
rectus femoris
    musculocutaneous flap
rectus incision
rectus labii muscle
rectus medialis muscle
rectus muscle
rectus muscle hook
rectus muscle-splitting incision
rectus position
rectus sheath hematoma
rectus sheath incision

rectus superioris muscle
rectus traction suture
rectus turnover flap
rectus turnover repair
recumbent incision
recumbent lateral projection
recumbent position
recurrent abdominal pain
    syndrome (RAPS)
recurrent aphthous ulcer
recurrent artery
recurrent aspiration
recurrent bandage
recurrent basal cell carcinoma
recurrent canal
recurrent carcinoma
recurrent cutaneous abscess
recurrent disease
recurrent dislocation
recurrent dysphagia
recurrent episode
recurrent ganglion
recurrent hemorrhage
recurrent hernia
recurrent incisional hernia
recurrent infection
recurrent inflammation
recurrent interosseous artery
recurrent laryngeal nerves
recurrent lesion
recurrent nerve
recurrent nerve injury
recurrent nerve lesion
recurrent patellar dislocation
recurrent pleomorphic adenoma
recurrent squamous cell
    carcinoma
recurrent stricture
recurrent thromboembolic
    complication
recurrent thromboembolic
    disease
recurrent tumor
recurrent ulcer
recurrent vaginal bleeding
recurrent vomiting
recurring hemorrhage
recurvatum
  genu recurvatum
  Heyman procedure for genu
    recurvatum
  pectus recurvatum

recurvatum (*continued*)
　Perry procedure for genu recurvatum
recurvatum angulation deformity
RED (rigid external distraction)
Red Cross adhesive dressing
red ear syndrome
red flare
red granulation
red induration
red laser
red lens occluder
red papule
red pessary
red reflex
Red Reflex lens
red Robinson catheter
red rubber arch
red rubber catheter
red rubber endotracheal tube
RED system rigid external distractor
red wale sign
Red Witch bur
red zone of lip
red-beam laser
Reddick cystic duct cholangiogram catheter
Reddick-Saye cannula
Reddick-Saye Lav-1 I&A probe
Reddick-Saye Lav-1 irrigating and aspirating probe
Reddick-Saye screw
Reddick-Saye screw catheter
Reddick-Saye suture grasper
Reddick-Saye trocar
red-eyed shunt syndrome
Redfield infrared coagulator
Redi-Around finger splint
Redifocus guidewire
Rediform orthotic
RediFurl catheter
RediFurl double-lumen balloon
RediFurl single-lumen balloon
RediFurl Taperseal catheter
RediFurl TaperSeal IAB catheter
RediGuard IAB catheter
Redi-Spec disposable vaginal speculum
Reditron refractometer
Redivac drain

Redivac drainage
Redivac suction drain
Redivac suction tube
Redler nail
Redlich-Fisher miliary plaque
Redman approach
Redmond Smith operation
redness along incision site
Redo intestinal clamp
Redon drain
redressed wound
red-tip aspirator
red-top tube
reduced fracture
reduced liver transplant (RLT)
reduced-height implants
reduced-size graft
reduced-size transplant
reducer
　Cloward cervical dislocation reducer
　Honan eye-pressure reducer
　McCannel ocular pressure reducer
　Norelco allergen reducer
　ocular pressure reducer
　Salinger nasal reducer
reducible hernia
reducing fracture frame
reducing technique
reducing valve
reduction
　afterload reduction
　Agee force-couple splint reduction
　Agnew-Hunt reduction
　alar base reduction
　Allen reduction
　anterior displacement no reduction (ADNR)
　Arie-Pitanguy breast reduction
　axillary endoscopic reduction
　Barsky macrodactyly reduction
　Batista procedure for left ventricular reduction
　Becton open reduction
　Boitzy open reduction
　breast reduction
　Calandriello open hip reduction
　calcaneal fracture reduction

reduction (*continued*)
calf reduction
caudal septal reduction
central cone technique
reduction
closed reduction
cluster reduction
concentric reduction
conchal reduction
Cooper reduction
Cotton reduction
Crego closed reduction
Crosby reduction
Cubbins open reduction
delayed open reduction
Deyerle hip fracture
reduction
Dias-Giegerich open
reduction
dorsal reduction
Eaton closed reduction
Eaton-Malerich reduction
embryo reduction
Essex-Lopresti fracture
reduction
Essex-Lopresti open reduction
femoral neck fracture
reduction
fetal reduction
Flynn femoral neck fracture
reduction
force-couple splint reduction
Fowles open reduction
fracture reduction
fracture-dislocation reduction
Frechet extended scalp
reduction
funic reduction
gravity lumbar reduction
(GLR)
Greeley technique for
gynecomastia reduction
Hankin reduction
Hastings open reduction
hip reduction
Houghton-Akroyd open
reduction
incomplete reduction
indirect reduction
internal fixation, closed
reduction
interproximal reduction

reduction (*continued*)
Ivar Parlmar reduction
Kaplan open reduction
Kinast indirect reduction
King open reduction
Koch shoulder reduction
Kocher shoulder reduction
laser festoon reduction
Lavne reduction
Lejour breast reduction
limb reduction
Lowell reduction
lung volume reduction (LVR)
McKeever open reduction
Meyn reduction
Moberg-Gedda open
reduction
multifetal pregnancy
reduction
Neer open reduction
Neibauer-King open
reduction
nonoperative reduction
open reduction
orbital fracture reduction
pain threshold reduction
Pare reduction
Parvin reduction
percutaneous reduction
perioperative reduction
Pitanguy-type breast
reduction
pneumatic reduction
postural reduction
Pratt open reduction
preload reduction
prone reduction
radial fracture reduction
risk reduction
scalp reduction
septal reduction
short-scar technique breast
reduction
shoulder reduction
side posture reduction
sigmoid loop reduction
Somerville open reduction
Speed open reduction
Speed-Boyd fracture reduction
Speed-Boyd open reduction
spondylolisthesis reduction
stable reduction

reduction (*continued*)
  stapled lung reduction
  sternoclavicular joint
    reduction
  stress reduction
  Strombeck breast reduction
  surgical reduction
  swan-neck deformity
    reduction
  T-breast reduction
  trial reduction
  tuberosity reduction
  tumescent technique breast
    reduction
  vertical pedicle technique
    breast reduction
  volumetric fat reduction
  volvulus reduction
  Wagner fracture reduction
  Wayne County reduction
  Weber-Brunner-Freuler open
    reduction
  weight reduction
  wet technique with
    liposuction breast
    reduction
  Wiener breast reduction
  Wise pattern in breast
    reduction
reduction and internal
  fixation
reduction before resection
reduction division
reduction en masse
reduction genioplasty
reduction instrument
reduction mammaplasty
reduction mastopexy
reduction of fracture
reduction of hernia
reduction of intussusception
reduction of lower palpebral
  bulge
reduction of rectal prolapse
reduction of torsion
reduction of volvulus
reduction osteotomy
reduction potential
reduction ring
reduction syndactyly
reduction technique
reduction ventriculoplasty

reduction-advancement
  genioplasty
reduction-augmentation
  procedure
reductive mammaplasty
redundant abdominal apron
redundant foreskin
redundant pannus
redundant pelvis
redundant prepuce
redundant prolapsed rectum
redundant skin
redundant tissue
redundant upper lid skinfolds
Redy hemodialyzer
Reece osteotomy guide
Reed ventriculorrhaphy
reef knot sutures
reefed vaginal cuff
reefing of joint capsule
reefing of vastus medialis
reefing procedure
Reeh stitch scissors
reel aspiration cannula
re-entrant loop
re-entrant well chamber
Re-Entry Malecot catheter set
re-entry operation
re-epithelialization
Rees dermatome
Rees face-lift scissors
Rees facelift serrated scissors
Rees lighted retractor
Reese advancement forceps
Reese dermatome
Reese dermatome blade
Reese muscle forceps
Reese operation
Reese prosthesis
Reese ptosis knife
Reese ptosis operation
Reese saw
Reese stimulator
Reese-Cleasby operation
Reese-Drum dermatome
Reese-Jones-Cooper operation
re-expansion maneuver
re-expansion of lung
re-exploration
re-exposure
reference catheter
reference electrode

referred pain
referred point
referred sensation
Reflec UV instant camera
reflectance spectrophotometric
    probe
reflected from insertion
reflected laterally
reflected medially
reflected skin flap
reflected upward
reflecting microscope
reflecting mucosa
reflecting ophthalmoscope
reflection
   angle of reflection
   bladder reflection
   diaphragmatic reflection
   hepatoduodenal reflection
   mucobuccal reflection
   perineal reflection
   peritoneal reflection
   serosal reflection
   uterine reflection
Reflection acetabular cup
reflection of scalp
reflection of sternum
reflection site
reflectometer tuning unit
reflectometry
reflex
   abdominal cardiac reflex
   abdominal reflex
   abdominocardiac reflex
   Abrams reflex
   absent gag reflex
   accommodation reflex
   Achilles reflex
   acousticopalpebral reflex
   anal reflex
   Aschner reflex
   atriopressor reflex
   auricular reflex
   auriculopalpebral reflex
   auropalpebral reflex (APR)
   Babinski reflex
   Bainbridge reflex
   Barkman reflex
   basal joint reflex
   Bekhterev-Mendel reflex
   Bezold reflex
   Bezold-Jarisch reflex

reflex (*continued*)
   biceps reflex
   blink reflex
   body righting reflex
   brachioradial reflex
   bregmocardiac reflex
   Breuer-Hering inflation reflex
   bulbocavernosus reflex
   bulbocavernous reflex
   bulbomimic reflex
   cardiopressor reflex
   carotid sinus reflex
   celiac plexus reflex
   cephalopalpebral reflex
   chin reflex
   ciliary reflex
   clasp-knife reflex
   cochleo-orbicular reflex
   cochleopalpebral reflex
   cochleopapillary reflex
   cochleostapedial reflex
   compression reflex
   consensual reflex
   contraction reflex
   copper-wire reflex
   corneal light reflex
   corneal reflex
   corneomandibular reflex
   corneomental reflex
   corneopterygoid reflex
   coronary reflex
   cortex reflex
   cranial reflex
   cremasteric reflex
   crossed extensor reflex
   crossed reflex
   Cushing reflex
   Dagnini reflex
   deglutition reflex
   delayed reflex
   depressor reflex
   doll's eye reflex
   domino reflex
   dorsal reflex
   dorsocuboidal reflex
   dorsum pedis reflex
   elbow reflex
   embrace reflex
   enterogastric reflex
   epigastric reflex
   Erben reflex
   erector-spinal reflex

reflex (*continued*)

esophagosalivary reflex
extensor thrust reflex
external oblique reflex
eyeball compression reflex
eye-closure reflex
eyelash reflex
eyelid-closure reflex
facile reflex
faucial reflex
femoral reflex
finger flexion reflex
finger-thumb reflex
fixation reflex
flexion reflex
flexion-extension reflex
foveolar reflex
front-tap reflex
fusion reflex
gag reflex
Galant abdominal reflex
gastrocnemius reflex
gastrocolic reflex
gastroileal reflex
gastropancreatic reflex
gastropancreatic vagovagal
   reflex
Gault cochleopalpebral reflex
Gifford reflex
Gifford-Galassie reflex
gluteal reflex
Gonda reflex
Gordon reflex
grasp reflex
grasping reflex
Haab reflex
Head paradoxical reflex
head-turning reflex
Hennebert reflex
Hering-Breuer reflex
Hirschberg reflex
hyperactive carotid sinus
   reflex
hyperactive reflex
hypoactive reflex
ileogastric reflex
indirect reflex
inflation reflex
infraspinatus reflex
inguinal reflex
interscapular reflex
intestinointestinal reflex

reflex (*continued*)

ipsilateral reflex
ischemic reflex
Jacobson reflex
jaw jerk reflex
jaw reflex
juvenile reflex
Kehrer reflex
Kisch reflex
knee-jerk reflex
Kocher reflex
labyrinthine righting reflex
lacrimation reflex
laryngeal reflex
laryngopharyngeal reflex
laryngospastic reflex
lash reflex
latent reflex
lid reflex
lip reflex
Livierato reflex
lumbar reflex
mandibular reflex
mass reflex
masseter reflex
masseteric reflex
Mayer reflex
McDowell reflex
metacarpothenar reflex
micturition reflex
middle ear muscle reflex
milk-ejection reflex
monosynaptic reflex
Morley peritoneocutaneous
   reflex
Moro reflex
muscular reflex
myenteric reflex
myotatic reflex
nasal reflex
nasolabial reflex
nasomental reflex
nose bridge-lid reflex
nose-eye reflex
obliquity reflex
oculocardiac reflex (OCR)
orbicularis oculi reflex
orthocardiac reflex
palatal reflex
palatine reflex
palmar reflex
palmomental reflex

reflex (*continued*)

  paradoxical extensor reflex
  paradoxical reflex
  patellar reflex
  patelloadductor reflex
  pathologic reflex
  pectoral reflex
  penile reflex
  perianal reflex
  pericardial reflex
  peripheral reflex
  peritoneocutaneous reflex
  peritoneointestinal reflex
  pharyngeal reflex
  plantar reflex
  platysma reflex
  pronator reflex
  proprioceptive head-turning
    reflex
  psychocardiac reflex
  pulmonocoronary reflex
  pupillary reflex
  Puusepp reflex
  quadriceps reflex
  quadripedal extensor reflex
  radial reflex
  rectal reflex
  rectoanal inhibitory reflex
  rectosphincteric reflex
  red reflex
  relax reflex
  Remak reflex
  renal reflex
  renointestinal reflex
  renorenal reflex
  retrobulbar pupillary reflex
  righting reflex
  Roger reflex
  rooting reflex
  Saenger reflex
  scapular reflex
  scapulohumeral reflex
  silver-wire reflex
  simple reflex
  sole reflex
  Somagyi reflex
  somatointestinal reflex
  spinal reflex
  Starling reflex
  Stookey reflex
  stretch reflex
  styloradial reflex

reflex (*continued*)

  superficial reflex
  supination reflex
  supinator longus reflex
  supraorbital reflex
  suprapatellar reflex
  suprapubic reflex
  supraumbilical reflex
  sympathoexcitation reflex
  tarsophalangeal reflex
  threat reflex
  Throckmorton reflex
  thumb reflex
  tibioadductor reflex
  tracheal reflex
  triceps reflex
  triceps surae reflex
  trigeminal-facial nerve
    reflex
  trigeminofacial reflex
  trigeminus reflex
  Tromner reflex
  ulnar reflex
  vagovagal reflex
  vascular reflex
  vasopressor reflex
  vertical suspension reflex
  vesicointestinal reflex
  vestibulo-ocular reflex
  visceral traction reflex
  viscerocardiac reflex
  visceromotor reflex
  viscerosensory reflex
  viscerotrophic reflex
  withdrawal reflex
  zygomatic reflex
Reflex articulating endoscopic
    cutter
reflex erection
reflex examination
reflex hammer
reflex ileus
reflex incontinence
reflex ligament
reflex neurogenic bladder
reflex otitis media
Reflex pacemaker
reflex response
Reflex skin stapler
reflex stimulation
Reflex SuperSoft steerable
    guidewire

reflex sympathetic dystrophy
   (RSD)
reflex venoconstriction
reflexes
   asymmetric reflexes
   brisk reflexes
   cephalic reflexes
   coordinated reflexes
   deep abdominal reflexes
   deep tendon reflexes (DTRs)
   diminished reflexes
   equal and brisk reflexes
   hypoactive deep tendon
      reflexes
   motor reflexes
   muscles, strength, reflexes
      (MSRs)
   myotonic reflexes
   normoactive reflexes
   normophysiological reflexes
   sacral reflexes
reflexes absent
reflexes equal
reflexive ileus
reflex-like reaction
reflexogenic erection
reflex-type ileus
reflux
   abdominal reflux
   extraesophageal reflux
   gastroesophageal reflux
   hepatojugular reflux
   intrarenal reflux
   ureteral reflux
   urethrovesicular differential
      reflux
   urinary reflux
   venous reflux
   vesicoureteral reflux
reflux esophagitis
reflux filling
reflux from stomach
reflux of barium
reflux of gastric contents
reflux symptoms
reform eye implant
reform implant
reformation of chamber
refracted x-ray
refractibility
refractile body
refracting media

refraction of eye
refraction of lens
refraction test
refractionometer
refractive error
refractive keratoplasty
refractive keratotomy
refractive operative technique
refractive surgery
refractometer
   Abbe refractometer
   AMO refractometer
   Canyon auto refractometer
   Hoya HDR objective
      refractometer
   Hoya MRM objective
      refractometer
   meridional refractometer
   Reditron refractometer
   Speedy-1 Auto refractometer
   Topcon auto refractometer
refractor
   Agrikola refractor
   Amoils refractor
   AR 1000 refractor
   ARK-Juno refractor
   automated refractor
   Barraquer-Krumeich-Swinger
      refractor
   Berens refractor
   Brawley refractor
   Bronson-Turtz refractor
   Campbell refractor
   Canon refractor
   Castallo refractor
   Castroviejo refractor
   Coburn refractor
   CooperVision diagnostic
      imaging refractor
   Desmarres refractor
   Elschnig refractor
   Ferris Smith-Sewall refractor
   Fink refractor
   Goldstein refractor
   Gradle refractor
   Graether refractor
   Green refractor
   Groenholm refractor
   Hartstein refractor
   Hillis refractor
   Humphrey automatic refractor
   Kirby refractor

refractor (*continued*)
  Knapp refractor
  Kronfeld refractor
  Kuglen refractor
  Leland refractor
  Marco refractor
  McGannon refractor
  Mueller refractor
  Nidek objective automatic
    refractor
  Precision refractor
  Reichert refractor
  Remote Vision electronic
    refractor
  Retinomax auto refractor
  Rizzuti refractor
  Rollet refractor
  Schepens refractor
  SR-IV programmed subjective
    refractor
  Stevenson refractor
  Topcon refractor
  Ultramatic Rx Master
    phoroptor refractor
  Wilmer refractor
refractory ascites
refractory encephalopathy
refractory period
refractory variceal hemorrhage
refracture following fracture
refracture of bone
refractured bone
refrigeration anesthesia
Ref-Star catheter
refusion of blood
regained consciousness
Regaud radium colpostat
Regency pulse generator
regeneration
  aberrant regeneration
  axonal regeneration
  bony regeneration
  controlled bone regeneration
  guided bone regeneration
  guided tissue regeneration
  incomplete regeneration
  tissue regeneration
regeneration aberration
regenerative activity
regio (*pl.* regiones)
regio buccalis
regio carpalis anterior

regio carpalis posterior
regio frontalis capitis
regio inframammaria
regio infraorbitalis
regio mammaria
regio mentalis
regio nasalis
regio oralis
regio orbitalis
regio submaxillaris
regio submentalis
regio zygomatica
region
  abdominal region
  adnexal region
  antebrachial region
  anterolateral region
  auricular region
  axillary region
  basilar region
  Broca region
  brow-tail region
  buccal region
  calcaneal region
  cancerous region
  centroparietal regions
  cervical region
  ciliary region
  clavicular region
  crural region
  cubital region
  deltoid region
  dorsal region
  encephalic region
  extrapolar region
  facial regions
  falcine region
  femoral artery-saphenous bulb
    region
  frontal region
  frontocentral region
  frontoparietal region
  genitourinary region
  glabellar region
  hilar region
  hyoid region
  hypochondriac region
  hypogastric region
  iliac region
  infraclavicular region
  inframammary region
  infraorbital region

region (*continued*)
  infrascapular region
  infratemporal region
  inguinal region
  interscapular region
  jugulodigastric region
  labial region
  laryngeal region
  lateral abdominal region
  lateral region
  left lateral region
  lip region
  lower clival region
  lumbar region
  malar-zygomatic region
  mammary region
  mastoid region
  maxillofacial region
  mental region
  midsacral region
  mylohyoid region
  nuchal region
  occipital region
  ocular region
  opticostriate region
  orbital region
  palpebral region
  parasymphyseal region
  parieto-occipital region
  parietotemporal region
  parotideomasseteric region
  pectoral regions
  perineal region
  postcricoid region
  posterotemporal region
  precordial region
  prefrontal region
  pterygomaxillary region
  pubic region
  pyloric region
  retrocardiac region
  rolandic region
  sacral region
  sacrococcygeal region
  scapular region
  sphenopetroclival region
  sternocleidomastoid region
  subareolar region
  subauricular region
  subhyoid region
  submaxillary region
  submental region

region (*continued*)
  superior labial region
  superior palpebral region
  supraclavicular region
  supraorbital region
  suprapubic region
  suprasternal region
  tegmental region
  temporal region
  thoracic region
  thyroid region
  trabecular region
  umbilical region
  upper cervical region
  urogenital region
  vertebral region
  vestibular region
  volar region
  wattled submental region
  ZF region
  zygomatic region
  zygomaticofrontal region
  zygomaticomaxillary region
regional adenopathy
regional anesthesia (RA)
regional anesthetic
regional anesthetic technique
regional block anesthesia
regional cerebral blood flow
regional excision
regional flap
regional free
regional hepatectomy
regional hypoperfusion
regional ileitis
regional involvement
regional lymphadenectomy
regional metastasis
regional muscle transfer
regional node
regional node involvement
regional perfusion
regional recurrence
regional spread
regional vasodilation
regional wall motion
    abnormality (RWMA)
regiones abdominis
regiones fasciales
regiones volares digitorum
    manus
Register needle holder

regloving and regowning
Regnault abdominoplasty
Regnoli operation
regression of symptoms
regressive reconstructive
    approach
regular body impression
    material
regular contractions
regular eye spatula
regular rate and rhythm
regular sinus rhythm
regular Trimshield pad
regurgitant lesion
regurgitation
    aortic regurgitation
    mitral regurgitation
Regu-Vac regulator
Rehbein infant abdominal
    retractor
Rehbein internal steel strut
Rehbein procedure
Rehbein rib spreader
Rehfuss duodenal tube
Rehfuss stomach tube
Rehfuss tube
Rehne abdominal retractor
Rehne skin graft knife
Rehne-Delorme operation
Rehne-Delorme plication
Reich curet
Reichel chondromatosis
Reichel cloacal duct
Reichel-Polya stomach resection
Reichenheim operation
Reichenheim-King operation
Reichenheim-King syndrome
Reichert antroscope
Reichert binocular indirect
    ophthalmoscope
Reichert camera
Reichert cartilage
Reichert fiberoptic
    sigmoidoscope
Reichert flexible sigmoidoscope
Reichert Ful-Vue binocular
    ophthalmoscope
Reichert Ful-Vue spot
    retinoscope
Reichert lensometer
Reichert membrane
Reichert noncontact tonometer

Reichert
    ophthalmodynamometer
Reichert radius gauge
Reichert refractor
Reichert retinoscope
Reichert scar
Reichert sigmoidoscope
Reichert slit lamp
Reichert tonometer
Reichert-Lenschek advanced
    logic lensometer
Reichert-Mundinger stereotactic
    device
Reichert-Mundinger-Fischer
    stereotactic head frame
Reichling corneal scissors
Reichmann ivory rod
Reich-Nechtow arterial clamp
Reich-Nechtow cervical biopsy
    curet
Reich-Nechtow clamp
Reich-Nechtow dilator
Reich-Nechtow hypogastric
    artery forceps
Reich-Nechtow hysterectomy
    forceps
Reich-Nechtow plug
Reicker pillow
Reid classification for mutilating
    injuries (groups 1-6)
Reid retinoscope
Reid-Baker procedure
Reidy rasp
Reif catheter
Reifenstein syndrome
Reil island
Reill forceps
Reill needle holder
Reill wire-cutting pliers
Reilly body
Reilly granulations
reimplantation
    Boari-Ockerblad flap
        reimplantation
    Cohen reimplantation
    end-to-side reimplantation
    Leadbetter-Politano ureteral
        reimplantation
    Leadbetter-Politano
        ureterovesical
        reimplantation
reimplantation of extremity

reimplantation of fingertip
reimplantation of ureter
reimplanted electrode
Reinecke-Carroll lacrimal tube
Reiner bone rongeur
Reiner curet
Reiner ear knife
Reiner ear syringe
Reiner plaster knife
Reiner repair
Reiner rongeur
Reiner-Alexander ear syringe
Reiner-Beck tonsil snare
Reiner-Knight ethmoid-cutting
    forceps
Reinert acetabular extensile
    approach
reinforced anchorage
reinforced tracheostomy tube
reinforcing sutures
reinfusate
reinfusion
Reinhart retractor
Reinhoff arterial forceps
Reinhoff dissector
Reinhoff swan neck clamp
Reinhoff thoracic scissors
Reinke crystals
Reinke edema
Reinke space
reinnervate
reinnervation
reintubation
Reipen cannula
Reipen speculum
Reisinger lens-extracting forceps
Reisseisen muscle
Reissner canal
Reissner membrane
Reis-Wertheim operation
Reis-Wertheim vaginal
    hysterectomy
Reiswig reamer
Reitan CatheterPump
Reiter disease
Reiter syndrome
rejected graft
rejected organ
rejected transplant
rejection
    allograft corneal rejection
    allograft rejection

rejection (*continued*)
    bout of rejection
    chronic allograft rejection
    classical sign of rejection
    graft rejection
    grafted kidney rejection
    homograft rejection
    organ rejection
    threatened transplant
        rejection
    tissue rejection
    transplant rejection
    white graft rejection
rejection cardiomyopathy
    transplant
rejection line
rejection of graft
rejection of organ
rejection of transplant
rejuvenation
    complete facial rejuvenation
    facial rejuvenation
    midfacial rejuvenation
    spectrum concept to skin
        rejuvenation
    upper face rejuvenation
rejuvenation surgery
Relat vaginal speculum
relation
    acentric relation
    acquired eccentric jaw relation
    abnormal occlusal relation
    alar-columella relation
    bimaxillary relation
    buccolingual relation
    centric jaw relation
    centric occluding relation
    centric relation
    cephalometric relation
    dynamic relation
    eccentric jaw relation
    intermaxillary relation
    jaw relation
    lateral relation
    mandibular centric relation
    maxillomandibular relation
    median jaw relation
    median retruded jaw relation
    median retruded relation
    occlusal jaw relation
    occlusal relation
    overbite/overjet relation

relation (*continued*)
  posterior border jaw relation
  protrusive jaw relation
  rest jaw relation
  retruded jaw relation
  ridge relation
  statis relation
  SPC relation
  unstrained jaw relation
  upper tooth to upper lip
    relation
  working bite relation
relational coil
relationship (*see* relation)
relative curative resection
relative generalized microdontia
relative noncurative resection
relative response attributable to
  the maneuver
relaxant effect
relaxation
  complete sphincter relaxation
  esophageal sphincter
    relaxation
  incomplete relaxation
  intraoperative stress
    relaxation
  muscular relaxation
  passive relaxation
  pelvic relaxation
  progressive relaxation
  skin relaxation
  T2 relaxation
relaxation sutures
relaxed anterior wall
relaxed introitus
relaxed pelvic floor
relaxed perineal body
relaxed skin tension lines
  (RSTLs)
relaxed vaginal outlet
relaxing incision
relaxing of muscles
Relay cardiac pacemaker
release
  Agee carpal tunnel release
  Agee fiberoptic carpal tunnel
    release
  carpal tunnel release
  chordee release
  de Quervain release
  depressor septi release

release(*continued*)
  Eberle release
  endoscopic carpal tunnel
    release (ECTR)
  galea-frontalis-occipitalis
    release
  Guyon canal release
  Heyman-Herndon release
  laryngeal release
  Luck procedure for
    Dupuytren contracture
    release
  Mital elbow release
  open carpal tunnel release
    (OCTR)
  periosteal release
  Quervain release
  retro-orbicularis fat pad
    release
  Roos hip flexor release
  single-portal endocarpal
    tunnel release
  syndactylism release
  syndactyly release
  tendon release
  trigger finger release
  Turco clubfoot release
Release nonadhering dressing
release of carpal tunnel
release of patella
release of plantar fascia
release of pus
release of tendo Achillis
release of trigger finger
release sleeve
released compartment
Release-NF camera
Release-NF catheter
releasing incision
Reliance CM femoral
  component
Reliance device
Reliance urinary control insert
Reliance urinary control insert
  catheter
Reliance urinary control stent
Reliavac drain
Relief Band device
relief incision
relief of symptoms
relief space
relieve pressure

relieving incision
reline material
Reliquet lithotrite
relocation of anterior septum to midline
Relton frame pad
Relton-Hall spinal frame
Rely balloon catheter
REM (rapid eye movement)
Rema-Exakt investment material
Remak band
Remak fibers
Remak ganglion
Remak reflex
Remak sign
Remaloy wire
Remanium alloy
Remanium wire
remedial inguinal exploration
remedial surgery
Remedy colostomy appliance
Remedy ileostomy appliance
Remine mastectomy skin flap retractor
remineralization
remission induction
remission of disease
remission of symptoms
remittent fever
remnant gland
remobilization
remodeling
   adaptive temporomandibular joint remodeling
   bilateral forehead remodeling
   bilateral fronto-orbital remodeling
   bone remodeling
   frontocranial remodeling
   fronto-orbital remodeling
   peripheral temporomandibular joint remodeling
   progressive temporomandibular joint remodeling
   supraorbital remodeling
   temporomandibular joint remodeling
   tissue remodeling
remodeling of collagen

remodeling phase of wound healing
remote afterloading brachytherapy (RAB)
remote control afterloading machine
remote metastases
remote pedicle flap
Remote Vision electronic refractor
remottling fracture site
removable appliance
removable expansion prosthesis
removable implant
removable maintainer space
removal
   1-session removal
   arthrotomy with removal
   Bose nail fold removal
   bronchoscopy with removal
   bronchotomy with removal
   Cameron femoral component removal
   cast removal
   cement removal
   Collis-Dubrul femoral stem removal
   colonoscopic removal
   corrugator removal
   en bloc removal
   endoscopic removal
   excisional removal
   extracorporeal CO_2 removal (ECOR)
   forceps removal
   foreign body removal
   gastric coin removal
   gland removal
   Harris femoral component removal
   hump removal
   implant removal
   intracapsular tumor removal
   Jancey nail fold removal
   laparoscopic gallbladder removal
   laser hair removal
   lens removal
   macroscopic tumor removal
   medial-to-lateral tumor removal
   mesh removal

removal (*continued*)
  metastatic tumor removal
  Moreland-Marder-Anspach
    femoral stem removal
  nail-fold removal
  nail-plate removal
  path of removal
  percutaneous endoscopic
    removal
  percutaneous stone removal
  piecemeal removal
  radical en bloc removal
  rib removal
  small polyp removal
  stem removal
  stone removal
  surgical removal (of organ,
    tissue, etc.)
  tattoo removal
  through-the-scope balloon
    removal
  total surgical removal
  transsphenoidal removal
  tube removal
  tumor removal
  ureteral stoma removal
  Winograd nail plate removal
removal of calculus
removal of drain
removal of dressing
removal of emboli
removal of embryo
removal of fetal structure
removal of foreign body
removal of life support
removal of organ
removal of pack
removal of packing
removal of pin
removal of placenta
removal of placental fragments
removal of screw
removal of sutures
Removatron epilator
removed in part
removed in toto
removed manually
remover
  adhesive tape remover
  anterior band remover (ABR)
  Atwood bridge remover
  Atwood crown remover

remover (*continued*)
  Austin Moore corkscrew
    femoral head remover
  Autoclip remover
  Bailey foreign body remover
  Bard adhesive and barrier film
    remover
  Biomet Ultra-Drive cement
    remover
  Braithwaite clip remover
  clip remover
  corkscrew femoral head
    remover
  corneal rust ring remover
  Crown-A-Matic crown and
    bridge remover
  Damon-Julian ring remover
  DMV contact lens remover
  Ferrolite crown remover
  foreign body remover
  frog cortex remover
  Macaluso stent remover
  Mead bridge remover
  Mead crown remover
  medical adhesive remover
  modular head remover
  Morrell crown remover
  One Time staple remover
  Richwil bridge remover
  Richwil crown remover
  ring remover
  Schuknecht foreign body
    remover
  Tott ring remover
  Universal clip remover
  Watanabe pin remover
  Wolfe-Bohler cast remover
Remy separator
renal abnormality
renal adenocarcinoma
renal adenoma
renal allograft
renal allograft rupture
renal angiography
renal angioplasty
renal anomaly
renal arterial embolization
renal arteriogram
renal arteriography
renal artery clamp
renal artery forceps
renal artery occlusive disease

renal artery reconstruction
renal artery stenotic disease
renal artery-reverse saphenous
   vein bypass
renal autotransplantation
renal ballottement
renal biopsy
renal brush border membrane
renal calculus
renal capsulectomy
renal capsulotomy
renal cell carcinoma
renal clamp
renal colic
renal complication
renal cortical lobule
renal crush syndrome
renal cyst ablation
renal cyst decortication
renal cyst hemorrhage
renal decortication
renal disease
renal duplication
renal dysfunction
renal failure
renal fascia
renal fistula
renal fossa
renal function
renal ganglia
renal ganglion
renal hematoma
renal hyperfiltration
renal impression
renal infarction
renal infusion therapy
renal injury
renal labyrinth
renal lobe
renal needle
renal obstruction
renal papillae
renal parenchyma
renal pedicle
renal pelvis
renal plexus
renal plication
renal pouch
renal ptosis
renal pyramid
renal reflex
renal replacement therapy

renal scan
renal shadow
renal sinus
renal sinus retractor
renal sparing surgery
renal sympathetic nerve activity
   recording electrode
renal transplant
renal transplantation
renal tubule
renal tumor
renal ultrasound
renal vascular disease
renal vein renin concentration
renal veins
renal venography
Renalflo hollow fiber dialyzer
Renalin dialyzer
Renard technique
Renatron dialyzer
Rendu-Osler-Weber syndrome
Renegade microcatheter
Re-New laparoscopic
   instruments
renewed tumor activity
Rennig dynamic wrist fixator
renogastric fistula
renogram
renointestinal reflex
renorenal reflex
renovascular hypertension
renovascular stent
Renovist II injector
rent in uterus
rent of intestine
Rentrop catheter
Rentrop classification
Rentrop infusion catheter
Reo Macrodex sutures
reoperative aesthetic surgery
reoperative bariatric surgery
reoperative carotid surgery
reoperative coronary artery
   bypass graft (rCABG)
reoperative pelvic surgery
repair
   1-stage hypospadias repair
   1st-stage repair
   1st-toe Jones repair
   2-flap palatoplasty repair
   2-stage repair
   4-flap cleft palate repair

repair (*continued*)
- 5-in-1 repair
- 5-1 knee ligament repair
- A&P repair
- Abbe repair
- Abraham-Pankovich tendo calcaneus repair
- ACL repair
- Acland repair
- acromioclavicular joint repair
- all-inside repair
- Allison gastroesophageal reflux repair
- Allison hiatal hernia repair
- Alsus-Knapp eyelid repair
- Ammon eyelid repair
- anal sphincter repair
- anatomic repair
- aneurysm repair
- Anson-McVay hernia repair
- anterior and posterior repair
- aortic aneurysm repair
- aortic valve repair
- apertognathia repair
- Arlt epicanthus repair
- Arlt eyelid repair
- Armstrong repair
- Ashley repair
- Atasoy-type repair
- AV repair (aortic valve repair)
- Axhausen cleft lip repair
- Ballen eye repair
- Bankart shoulder repair
- Bankart-Magnuson shoulder repair
- Barsky cleft lip repair
- Bassini inguinal hernia repair
- Bassini-Stetten hernia repair
- Bauer-Tondra-Trusler cleft lip repair
- Bauer-Trusler-Tondra cleft lip repair
- Becker tendon repair
- Belsey hiatal hernia repair
- Belsey Mark IV repair
- Belt hypospadias repair
- Belt-Fugua hypospadias repair
- Bergmann hydrocele repair
- Bick ectropion repair
- bilateral inguinal hernia repair
- bilayer patch hernia repair
- Black repair

repair (*continued*)
- Blackwood meniscal repair
- Blair epicanthus repair
- Blazina patellofemoral repair
- blepharochalasis repair
- blepharoptosis repair
- Block entropion repair
- Boari ureteral flap repair
- Boerema hernia repair
- bone graft repair
- Bosworth tendo calcaneus repair
- bottle repair
- boutonniere repair
- Boyd-Anderson biceps tendon repair
- brachial plexus repair
- Brand tendon repair
- Brom repair
- bronchoplasty repair
- Browne hypospadias repair
- Bunnell ligament repair
- Bunnell tendon repair
- Byers repair
- calvarial repair
- Camille Bernard lip repair
- Campbell-Young incontinence repair
- Cantwell-Ransley epispadias repair
- Caspari repair
- Cecil hypospadias repair
- Cecil-Culp hypospadias repair
- cemental repair
- cleft lip repair
- cleft palate repair
- coarctation repair
- Collis repair
- Collis-Belsey repair
- columellar repair
- commissure repair
- Cooper ligament repair
- cross-trigonal repair
- crural repair
- Cutler repair
- cystocele repair
- Danus-Stanzel repair
- DeBakey-Creech aneurysm repair
- delayed primary repair
- density-dependent repair
- dental repair

repair (*continued*)

Devine hypospadias repair
diaphragmatic crural repair
diaphragmatic hernia repair
Dickey ptosis repair
dog-ear repair
Dowell hernia repair
Duckett procedure for
 hypospadias repair
Duplay hypospadias repair
dural repair
DuVries hammertoe repair
dynamic repair
early thoracoscopic repair
Ecker-Lotke-Glazer patellar
 tendon repair
ectropion repair
Effler hiatal hernia repair
elective hernia repair
elective repair
Elmslie ligament repair
endoluminal repair
endoscopic mitral valve repair
endovascular repair
end-to-end tendon repair
end-to-side repair
entropion repair
epicanthal repair
epineural repair
epineurial repair
episiotomy repair
esophageal repair
Evans ankle ligament repair
exploration and repair
extensor tendon repair
exteriorized uterine repair
extracorporeal repair
extraperitoneal endoscopic
 hernia repair
fascicular repair
femoral hernia repair
fibrous repair
flap valve after hiatal hernia
 repair
flexor tendon repair
Foimson biceps tendon repair
Fontan repair
Fontan-Kreutzer repair
fracture repair
Froimson-Oh repair
functional repair
funicular repair

repair (*continued*)

Gardner meningocele repair
glenohumeral dislocation
 repair
group fascicular repair
Hagedorn-Le Mesurier method
 of cleft lip repair
Halsted-Bassini hernia repair
hammertoe repair
Harrington hernia repair
Harrington-Allison repair
Hatafuku fundus onlay patch
 esophageal repair
hernia repair
Hill hiatus hernia repair
Hill median arcuate repair
histologic tooth repair
Hodgson hypospadias repair
Hodgson-Tuksu tumble flap
 hypospadias repair
Hoguet hernia repair
Hoguet pantaloon hernia
 repair
Hughston button for meniscal
 repair
Husen button for meniscal
 repair
hydrocele repair
hypoplastic left heart repair
hypospadias repair
Iliff eyelid repair
in situ uterine repair
in utero repair
inguinal hernia repair
Jalaguier cleft lip repair
John Wobig entropion repair
joint repair
Jones 1st-toe repair
Jones toe repair
Judd hernia repair
Kelikian-Riashi-Gleason
 patellar tendon repair
Kessler repair
Kleinert repair
Konno repair
Kugel hernia repair
Kuhnt-Junius repair
lacrimal gland repair
Lange tendon lengthening and
 repair
Lange tendon repair
Langenbeck repair

repair (*continued*)

laparoscopic IPOM repair
laparoscopic paraesophageal hernia repair (LPHR)
laparoscopic prosthetic mesh repair
laparoscopic varicocele repair
laparoscopic ventral hernia repair
LaRoque hernia repair
LaRoque-Branson hernia repair
laryngeal repair
Latzko fistula repair
Latzko vesicovaginal fistula repair
LeFort I apertognathia repair
LeFort uterine prolapse repair
LeFort-Wehrbein-Duplay hypospadias repair
LeMesurier repair
levator aponeurosis repair
Lich-Gregoir repair
Lichtenstein hernial repair
Lichtenstein inguinal hernia repair
Lichtenstein mesh repair
Lindholm tendo calcaneus repair
Lotheissen femoral hernia repair
Lotheissen hernia repair
L-plasty repair
MacIntosh over-the-top repair
MacNab shoulder repair
Madden repair
MAGPI hypospadias repair
Ma-Griffith tendo calcaneus repair
Manchester repair
Mandelbaum-Nartolozzi-Carney patellar tendon repair
Marcy hernia repair
Mark IV repair
Marlex hernial repair
Marshall-Marchetti repair
Matsner median episiotomy repair
Mayo bunion repair
McBride bunion repair
McLaughlin tendon rupture repair

repair (*continued*)

McVay hernia repair
McVay inguinal hernial repair
McVay-Cooper ligament repair
medial repair
meniscal repair
mesh repair
Millard bilateral cleft lip repair
Millard rotation-advancement lip repair
Millard rotation-advancement unilateral cleft lip repair
minimally invasive mitral valve repair
Mirault-Blair-Brown method of cleft lip repair
Mitchell-Clark hernia repair
mitral valve repair
Moloney hernia repair
Moschcowitz enterocele repair
Moschcowitz hernia repair
Mosley anterior shoulder repair
Mosley shoulder repair
multiple-stage omphalocele repair
muscle repair
Mustard atrial baffle repair
Mustarde 4-flap epicanthal repair
myelomeningocele repair
Nissen hiatal hernia repair
Noble-Mengert perineal repair
open repair
operative repair
Orr rectal prolapse repair
over-the-top cruciate repair
Palmer-Dobyns-Linscheid ligament repair
pants-over-vest hernia repair
paravaginal defect repair
patellar tendon repair
peg-and-socket hammertoe repair
periapical tooth repair
pericardioplasty in pectus excavatum repair
perineal repair
peripheral nerve repair
Phaneuf-Graves repair
plastic repair

repair (*continued*)
  plug prosthetic mesh repair
  postanal repair
  posterior repair
  postoperative repair
  potentially lethal x-ray
    damage repair
  premuscular prosthetic
    repair
  primary nerve repair
  primary repair
  prosthetic mesh repair
  pseudarthrosis repair
  pseudoarthrosis repair
  pulmonary stenosis repair
  radiographic tooth repair
  Randall triangular flap repair
  Ransley-Cantwell repair
  Rastelli repair
  rectocele repair
  rectus turnover repair
  Reiner repair
  renal injury repair
  retinal detachment repair
  reverse sigma penoscrotal
    transposition repair
  rod fracture repair
  Rodney Smith biliary stricture
    repair
  Rose cleft lip repair
  Rose-Thompson cleft lip
    repair
  rotation-advancement cleft lip
    repair
  rotator cuff repair
  Roux-Goldthwait patella
    repair
  Schepens-Okamura-
    Brockhurst retinal
    detachment repair
  Scuderi tendon repair
  secondary repair
  Senning atrial baffle repair
  Sever-L'Episcopo shoulder
    repair
  Shirodkar-McDonald cervical
    repair
  shoelace-type repair
  shoulder repair
  Shouldice hernia repair
  Shouldice inguinal hernia
    repair

repair (*continued*)
  Shouldice-Bassini hernia
    repair
  single-stage omphalocele
    repair
  Skoog cleft lip repair
  slipped Nissen repair
  Slocum knee repair
  Speed sternoclavicular repair
  Spence-Allen hypospadias
    repair
  sphincter repair
  staged abdominal repair
    (STAR)
  Staples repair
  Staples-Black-Brostrom
    ligament repair
  Stoppa hernia repair
  Stoppa-type laparoscopic
    repair
  Strickland tendon repair
  sublethal x-ray damage repair
  surgical repair
  suture repair
  Symmonds enterocele repair
  Symmonds vaginal prolapse
    repair
  syndactyly repair
  Talesnick scapholunate repair
  Tashiro repair
  Teflon sling repair
  tendon repair
  Tennison-Randall cleft lip
    repair
  Tennison-Randall triangular
    flap repair
  tension repair
  tension-free mesh repair
  tension-free prosthetic mesh
    repair
  tension-free repair
  TEP repair
  Teuffer tendo calcaneus
    repair
  Thal esophageal stricture
    repair
  Thal hiatal hernia repair
  Theirsch-Duplay repair
  thoracic aortic aneurysm
    repair
  thoracoabdominal aortic
    aneurysm repair

repair (*continued*)

  thoracoscopic repair
  tight Nissen repair
  tissue repair
  total extraperitoneal repair
  tracheal repair
  transabdominal preperitoneal
    repair
  transabdominal repair
  triad knee repair
  trichiasis repair
  tricuspid valve repair
  triple ligamentous repair
  triple-A repair (AAA;
    abdominal aortic aneurysm)
  Tsuge tendon repair
  tumble-flap hypospadias
    repair
  Turco-Spinella tendo
    calcaneus repair
  ultrasound-guided
    compression repair (UGCR)
  umbilical hernia repair
  unilateral inguinal hernia
    repair
  unilateral Millard repair
  Usher-Bellis hernia repair
  uterine prolapse repair
  vaginal repair
  vaginal vault repair
  vaginal wall repair
  vascular laceration repair
  Veau cleft lip repair
  Veau-Wardill-Kilner cleft
    palate repair
  Veirs canaliculus repair
  ventral hernia repair
  Verdan tendon repair
  vesicovaginal repair
  vest-over-pants hernia repair
  videoscopic repair
  volar plate repair
  von Langenbeck cleft lip
    repair
  von Langenbeck method
    repair
  von Langenbeck periosteal
    repair
  V-Y push-back cleft palate
    repair
  V-Y retroposition cleft palate
    repair

repair (*continued*)

  Wardill-Kilner cleft palate
    repair
  Wardill-Kilner V-Y palatal
    repair
  Watson-Jones fracture repair
  Wehrbein hypospadias repair
  Wehrbein-Smith hypospadias
    repair
  Wheeler halving repair
  Wicherkiewicz eyelid repair
  Wiener eyelid repair
  Winkelman hydrocele repair
  Wobig entropion repair
  Wynn cleft lip repair
  Y-mesh hernia repair
  York-Mason repair
  Young epispadias repair
  Zancolli claw-hand deformity
    repair
  Z-cleft palate repair
  Ziegler ectropion repair
  Zieman hernia repair
  zigzag bilateral cleft lip repair
  zigzag repair
repair of alveolar ridge defect
repair of defect
reparative cardiac surgery
reparative closure
Repel bioresorbable barrier film
Repela surgical glove
reperfusion catheter
reperfusion injury
reperfusion-induced
    hemorrhage
reperitonealization
reperitonealize
Replace system tapered
    implant
replacement
  allograft joint replacement
  anatomic porous replacement
    (APR)
  aortic root replacement
  aortic valve replacement
  atrioventricular valve
    replacement
  Biolox ceramic ball head for
    hip replacement
  Calcitite bone replacement
  Cosgrove mitral valve
    replacement

replacement (*continued*)
  Coventry total hip
    replacement
  double-compartment knee
    replacement
  endoprosthetic femoral head
    replacement
  Ewald total elbow
    replacement
  fluid replacement
  Freeman total hip
    replacement
  geopatellar-type knee
    replacement
  hard tissue replacement
    (HTR)
  heart valve replacement
  hip replacement
  homograft aortic valve
    replacement
  Howmedica Centrax head
    replacement
  Howmedica total condylar
    knee replacement
  Insall-Burstein total knee
    replacement
  joint replacement
  Kirschner in hi replacement
  hip replacement
  Kirschner total hip
    replacement
  knee replacement
  Konon aortic valve
    replacement
  laparoscopic feeding tube
    replacement
  M2A-38 system for hip
    replacement
  Manchester knee replacement
  Matchett-Brown femoral head
    replacement
  mitral valve replacement
  mucosal patch replacement
  Mueller-type femoral head
    replacement
  Neer II shoulder replacement
  NexGen complete knee
    replacement
  Osteogenics BoneSource
    synthetic bone replacement
  PCA hip replacement
  PCA total knee replacement

replacement (*continued*)
  Pilliar total hip replacement
  pulmonary valve replacement
  Pyrost bone replacement
  SAF hip replacement (self-
    articular femoral hip
    replacement)
  self-articulating femoral hip
    replacement (SAF hip
    replacement)
  Sivash hip replacement
  St. Urban Berlin hip joint
    surface replacement
  Stephee joint replacement
  Street-Stevens humeral
    replacement
  supra-annular mitral valve
    replacement
  temporary skin replacement
  Tharies surface hip
    replacement
  Ti-28 total hip replacement
  tile plate facet replacement
  total hip replacement (THR)
  total knee replacement (TKR)
  Townley anatomic knee
    replacement
  tricompartmental knee
    replacement
  tube replacement
  UCI total knee replacement
  unicompartmental knee
    replacement
  valve replacement
  Wesolowski bifurcation
    replacement
replacement bone
replacement collection bag
replacement fibrosis
replacement graft
replacement joint
replacement prosthesis
replacement surgery
replacement therapy
replacement transfusion
replacer
  iris replacer
  Smith-Fisher iris replacer
replant splint
replantation
  digital replantation
  ear replantation

replantation (*continued*)
  finger replantation
  hand replantation
  heterotopic replantation
  intentional replantation
  microsurgical ear replantation
  scalp replantation
  transmetacarpal replantation
replantation of amputated digit
RepliCare hydrocolloid dressing
Repliderm dressing
Repliform graft
Replogle catheter
Replogle tube
reposited iris
reposition
repositioned
repositioning
  auricular repositioning
  bony repositioning
  incus repositioning
  jaw repositioning
  muscle repositioning
  W-V palatal repositioning
  W-Y palatal repositioning
repositor
  iris repositor
  Knapp iris repositor
  Koman-Nair iris repositor
  Nettleship iris repositor
re-prepped and re-draped
Repro head halter
reprocessor
Reprodent acrylic tooth material
reproduction
reproductive organs
reproductive tract abnormality
rerouting insertion
Resano dissecting scissors
Resano sigmoid forceps
Resano thoracic scissors
rescue analgesia
rescue angioplasty
rescuing pacemaker
Research Medical straight
    multiple-holed aortic
    cannula
resectable carcinoma
resectable hepatic disease
resectable lesion
resectable liver metastasis
resectable periampullary cancer

resectable tumor
resected aneurysm
resected tonsil
resecting fracture
resecting sheath
resection
  abdominal-perineal resection
    (APR)
  abdominoperineal resection
    (APR)
  abdominosacral resection
  absolute curative resection
  absolute noncurative
    resection
  activation map-guided surgical
    resection
  anterior colon resection
  anterior resection
  antral resection
  atrial septal resection
  Badgley iliac wing resection
  Balfour gastric resection
  bar resection
  bilateral resection
  Bilhaut-Cloquet wedge
    resection
  bilobar resection
  bleb resection
  bone resection
  bony bridge resection
  bowel resection
  breast resection
  bronchial sleeve resection
  calcaneonavicular bar
    resection
  Carrell resection
  caudal lamina resection
  cesarean resection
  classical subtotal resection
  Clayton procedure with
    panmetatarsal head
    resection
  cold-cup resection
  coloanal resection
  colon resection
  colonic resection
  colorectal cancer resection
  colosigmoid resection
  combined gastrointestinal
    resection
  combined organ resection
  Commando resection

resection (*continued*)
  complete resection
  composite pelvic resection
  composite resection
  condyle resection
  conservative resection
  corrugator muscle resection
  craniofacial resection
  CRC resection
  cricotracheal resection
  cryo-assisted resection
  cuff resection
  curative resection
  D2 resection
  Darrach ulnar resection
  definitive resection
  diathermic resection
  Dillwyn-Evans resection
  Dwar-Barrington resection
  elective sigmoid resection
  electrocautery resection
  en bloc resection
  endocardial resection
  endocardial-to-epicardial
    resection
  endometrial resection
  endoscopic mucosal resection
    (EMR)
  endoscopic snare resection
  end-to-end ileo-anal
    anastomosis without
    mucosal resection
  epidermoid resection
  epiphysial bar resection
  esophageal resection
  esophagogastric resection
  ex situ-in situ liver resection
  extended resection
  extensive resection
  extra-articular resection
  eyelid resection
  facial nerve resection
  femoral resection
  formal hepatic resection
  gastric leiomyoma resection
  gastric resection
  gastrointestinal resection
  Girdlestone hip resection
  Girdlestone joint resection
  Guller resection
  gum resection
  Gurd resection

resection (*continued*)
  Hartmann resection
  Heineke colon resection
  Henry resection
  hepatic resection
  Hoffmann panmetatarsal head
    resection
  hyoid bone resection
  ileal resection
  ileocolic resection
  ileocolonic resection
  iliac crest resection
  iliac wing resection
  incomplete tumor resection
  infundibular resection
  infundibular wedge resection
  Ingram bony bridge resection
  initial resection
  innominate bone resection
  intercalary resection
  interdental resection
  intestinal resection
  Ivor-Lewis resection
  Janecki-Nelson shoulder girdle
    resection
  jaw-neck resection
  Karakousis-Vezeridis resection
  Kashiwagi calcaneal resection
  kyphos resection
  Langenskiold bony bridge
    resection
  laparoscopic bowel resection
  laparoscopic-assisted small
    bowel resection
  Lartat-Jacob hepatic resection
  lateral rectus resection
  LCVP-aided hepatic resection
  LCVP-assisted major liver
    resection
  lesser resection
  levator resection
  Lewis intercalary resection
  limited resection
  liver resection
  lobar resection
  lobe resection
  local radical resection
  Localio-Francis-Rossano
    resection
  low anterior resection
  lung resection
  lymph node resection

resection (*continued*)

major liver resection
Malawar fibular resection
Mankin resection
Marcove-Lewis-Huvos
   shoulder girdle resection
margin resection
marginal mandibular
   resection
marginal resection
Mason
   abdominotranssphincteric
   resection
massive bowel resection
Mayo-Polya gastric resection
medial malleolus resection
metatarsal head resection
microscopic resection
Miles abdominoperineal
   resection
Miltner-Wan calcaneus
   resection
minimal transurethral
   resection
Mohs microsurgical resection
mucosal sleeve resection
multiple-punch resection
multisegmental resection
Mumford clavicle resection
muscle resection
myotomy-myectomy-septal
   resection
nipple-flat duct resection
nonanatomic wedge resection
oncologic mandibular
   resection
ovarian wedge resection
palliative resection
pancreatic tail resection
panmetatarsal head resection
parotid resection
partial cricotracheal resection
partial gastric resection
partial resection
Paul-Mikulicz resection
Peet splanchnic resection
Peyman full-thickness eyewall
   resection
Phelps partial resection
platysma resection
portal vein resection
presacral resection

resection (*continued*)

primary resection
prophylactic resection
proximal femoral resection
proximal gastric resection
pull-through
   abdominoperineal resection
pulmonary resection
punch resection
R0, R1, R2 resection
radical gastric resection
radical subtotal resection
Radley-Liebig-Brown resection
ray resection
reduction before resection
Reichel-Polya stomach
   resection
relative curative resection
relative noncurative resection
rhinoplasty and submucous
   resection
rim resection
Rockwood resection
root end resection
Schnute wedge resection
scleral resection
sectorial resection
segmental colon resection
segmental colonic resection
segmental lung resection
segmental pulmonary
   resection
segmental resection
segment-oriented hepatic
   resection
segment-oriented liver
   resection
segment-oriented resection
selective subendocardial
   resection
septal resection
skull base tumor resection
sleeve resection
small-bowel resection
soft tissue resection
sphincter-sparing resection
spleen-preserving pancreatic
   resection
standard gastric resection
Stener-Gunterberg sacrum
   resection
strip resection

resection (*continued*)
  subcomplete resection
  submucous resection (SMR)
  subperiosteal resection
  subsegmental resection
  subtotal gastric resection
  subtotal resection
  surgical resection
  synchronous resection
  Tansini gastric resection
  terminal ileal resection
  Thompson resection
  thyroid resection
  Tikhoff-Linberg shoulder
    girdle resection
  Titanium Wedge
    electrosurgical resection
  Torek resection
  Torpin cul-de-sac resection
  total bladder resection
  total upper lip resection
  transanal endoscopic
    microsurgical resection
  transcervical resection
  transmural resection
  transoral odontoid resection
  transsphenoidal microsurgical
    resection
  transsphenoidal pituitary
    resection (TPR)
  transsphenoidal resection
  transthoracic vertebral body
    resection
  transurethral resection (TUR)
  transverse resection
  tumor resection
  ulnar resection
  ultralow anterior resection
  unilateral resection
  VATS wedge resection
  vertebral resection
  Wagner skull resection
  Watson-Cheyne wedge
    resection
  Weaver-Dunn resection
  wedge colon resection
  wedge resection
  wedge-shaped sleeve
    aneurysmal resection
  Whipple resection
resection arthrodesis
resection arthroplasty

resection clamp
resection dermodesis
resection intestinal forceps
resection margin
resection of colon
resectional phase of operation
resectional technique
resection-recession of eye
    muscles
resective colostomy
resective surgery
resectoscope
resector
  Accu-Line distal femoral
    resector
  Accu-Line tibial resector
  distal femoral resector
  Dyonics full-radius resector
  femoral resector
  Friedrich-Petz machine
    resector
  full-radius resector
  full-radius synovial resector
  Gator resector
  Linvatec Lightning blade
    resector
  Mainz pouch urinary resector
  Stryker resector
  Tiger blade resector
  UltraCut blade resector
  XPS Straightshot micro tissue
    resector
resectoscope
  ACMI pediatric resectoscope
  Bard resectoscope
  Baumrucker resectoscope
  Bumpus resectoscope
  cold-punch resectoscope
  continuous irrigation-suction
    resectoscope
  continuous-flow
    resectoscope
  Foroblique resectoscope
  French-Iglesias resectoscope
  Gray resectoscope
  Green resectoscope
  Iglesias continuous-flow
    resectoscope
  Iglesias fiberoptic
    resectoscope
  Kaplan cold-punch
    resectoscope

resectoscope (*continued*)
McCarthy miniature resectoscope
multiple resectoscope
obturator deflecting resectoscope
obturator resectoscope
rotating resectoscope
Scott resectoscope
Stern-McCarthy electrotome resectoscope
Storz cold-punch resectoscope
Storz continuous irrigation-suction resectoscope
Storz-Iglesias resectoscope
Thompson direct full-vision resectoscope
Timberlake resectoscope
Winter-Eber resectoscope
working element resectoscope
resectoscope adapter
resectoscope cable
resectoscope curet
resectoscope cutting loop
resectoscope sheath
resectoscopy
reserve cell carcinoma
reserve fat of Illouz
reserve intraocular lens
reservoir
1-piece shunt with reservoir
abdominal reservoir
Accu-Flo CSF reservoir
Braden flushing reservoir
Braden-CSF flushing reservoir
Camey reservoir
Cardiometrics cardiotomy reservoir
cardiotomy reservoir
Cobe cardiotomy reservoir
contiguous spinal fluid reservoir
continent ileal reservoir
CSF flushing reservoir
Denver reservoir
double J-shaped reservoir
double-barreled reservoir
double-bubble flushing reservoir
double-dome reservoir
fecal reservoir

reservoir (*continued*)
flat bottom reservoir
fluid reservoir
flushing reservoir
Foltz CSF-flushing reservoir
Foltz flushing reservoir
Hakim reservoir
Heyer-Schulte Jackson-Pratt wound-drainage reservoir
Heyer-Schulte wedge-suction reservoir
Heyer-Schulte-Ommaya CSF reservoir
H-H Rickham cerebrospinal fluid reservoir
Holter ventriculostomy reservoir
Holter-Rickham ventriculostomy reservoir
Holter-Salmon-Rickham ventriculostomy reservoir
Holter-Selker ventriculostomy reservoir
ICV reservoir
ileal reservoir
ileoanal reservoir
inflatable penile prosthesis with reservoir
Intersept cardiotomy reservoir
intra-abdominal ileal reservoir
inverted U-pouch ileal reservoir
Jackson-Pratt large-volume suction reservoir
Jackson-Pratt suction reservoir
Jostra cardiotomy reservoir
J-shaped reservoir
J-Vac bulb suction reservoir
J-Vac suction reservoir
Kock ileal reservoir
large-volume suction reservoir
lateral internal pelvic reservoir
LeBag reservoir
Mainz pouch urinary reservoir
Mischler reservoir
Molded Bulb closed wound drainage reservoir
Ommaya cerebrospinal fluid reservoir

reservoir (*continued*)
  Ommaya retromastoid
    reservoir
  Ommaya side-port flat-
    bottomed reservoir
  Ommaya spinal fluid reservoir
  Ommaya suboccipital
    reservoir
  Ommaya ventricular reservoir
  Parks ileoanal reservoir
  Polystan cardiotomy reservoir
  Pudenz reservoir
  retromastoid Ommaya
    reservoir
  Rickham reservoir
  Salmon-Rickham
    ventriculostomy reservoir
  Sci-Med extracorporeal
    silicone rubber reservoir
  Selker ventriculostomy
    reservoir
  Shiley cardiotomy reservoir
  side-port flat-bottomed
    Ommaya reservoir
  S-shaped reservoir
  suboccipital Ommaya
    reservoir
  suction reservoir
  UNI reservoir
  Uni-Shunt with elliptical
    reservoir
  urinary reservoir
  William Harvey cardiotomy
    reservoir
  wound drainage reservoir
residual abscess
residual air
residual barium
residual body
residual contrast material
residual cyst
residual cystic cavity
residual deformity
residual disease
residual dye
residual fragment
residual lesion
residual node
residual pain
residual paralysis
residual ridge
residual scarring

residual skin
residual stone
residual stool
residual tissue
residual tumor
residual urine
residual volume
residual weakness
resin cement
resin matrix
resin shell matrix
resin uptake
resin-uptake ratio
Resipump pump-reservoir
resistance
  abrasion resistance
  airflow resistance
  airway resistance
  aortic valve resistance
  cerebrovascular resistance
  inductive resistance
  pulmonary resistance
  vascular resistance
ResMed CPAP Sullivan III
    machine
Resnick Button bipolar
    coagulator
Resnick Tone Emitter I intraoral
    electrolarynx device
resonance generator
resonance line
resonant abdomen
resonant on percussion
resonant to percussion
resonator
  birdcage resonator
  bridged loop-gap resonator
  Faraday shielded resonator
  flexible surface-coil-type
    resonator
  multicoupled loop-gap
    resonator
  Oudin resonator
resorbable bilayer collagen
    membrane
resorbable fixation
resorbable plate
resorbable plate and screw
resorbable polydioxanone pin
resorbable rigid fixation
resorbable thread clip
    applicator

resorption
  bone resorption
  central resorption
  compensatory bone
    resorption
  frontal bone resorption
  frontal resorption
  graft resorption
  horizontal resorption
  massive resorption
  progressive condylar
    resorption (PCR)
  subchondral bony resorption
  undermining resorption
  vertical resorption
resorption atelectasis
resorption of bone
resorptive defect
ReSound Digital 5000 hearing
    device
respiration
  abdominal respiration
  abdominal-diaphragmatic
    respiration
  absent respiration
  agonal respirations
  apneustic respirations
  artificial respiration
  assisted respiration
  Austin Flint respiration
  bronchovesicular respiration
  cogwheel respiration
  controlled respiration
  deep and regular respirations
  diaphragmatic respiration
  divided respiration
  embarrassed respiration
  fetal respiration
  forced respiration
  grunting respirations
  harsh respiration
  inspiratory respiration
  internal respiration
  interrupted respiration
  irradiation respirations
  Kussmaul respirations
  labored respiration
  laryngeal respiration
  puerile respiration
  spontaneous respiration
  unassisted respiration
respiration assisted anesthesia

respiration bronchoscope
respiration pyelogram
respiration pyelography
respiration unassisted anesthesia
respirator (*see also* ventilator)
  Ambu respirator
  BABYbird respirator
  Bath respirator
  Bear respirator
  Bennett respirator
  Bird respirator
  Bourns electronic adult
    respirator
  Bourns infant respirator
  Bragg-Paul respirator
  Breeze respirator
  cabinet respirator
  Clevedan positive pressure
    respirator
  cuirass respirator
  Dann respirator
  Drinker tank respirator
  Emerson cuirass respirator
  Engstrom respirator
  Gill respirator
  Huxley respirator
  Kirmisson respirator
  MA-1 respirator
  mechanical respirator
  mechanically assisted
    respirator
  Med-Neb respirator
  Merck respirator
  Monaghan respirator
  Morch respirator
  Moynihan respirator
  portable respirator
  Sanders jet ventilation device
    respirator
respiratory activity
respiratory arrest
respiratory assistance
respiratory collapse
respiratory complication
respiratory depression
respiratory distress syndrome
respiratory effort
respiratory exchange
respiratory excursion
respiratory failure
respiratory function
respiratory function monitor

respiratory inversion point
respiratory kinetic therapy
respiratory mucosa
respiratory murmur
respiratory paralysis
respiratory rales
respiratory secretions
respiratory syncytial virus
respiratory therapy
respiratory tract
respiratory tube
respiratory wave
respiratory-dependent
   pacemaker
respiratory-esophageal fistula
respirometer
   Drager respirometer
   Fraser Harlake respirometer
   Haloscale respirometer
   hot-wire respirometer
   Wright respirometer
Respironics BiPAP machine
Respironics CPAP machine
Respond wire
response
   autoimmune response
   biphasic response
   cardiovascular response
   cell-mediated immune
     response
   cortical evoked responses
   detrusor response
   dose response
   electrodermal response
   electroencephalic response
   electronically provoked
     response
   equivocal response
   evoked response
   eye response
   Galant abdominal response
   galvanic response
   grasp response
   histiocytic response
   immune response
   implantation response
   index of response
   inflammatory response
   maladaptive response
   middle latency response
     (MLR)
   muscle response

response (*continued*)
   myotonic response
   plantar response
   provoked response
   reflex response
   rooting response
   skin response
   somatosensory response
   stimulus response
   stress responses
   successive responses
   ventricular response
   visual evoked response (VER)
Response catheter
Response cushion
Response external suction
   device for impotence
Res-Q arrhythmia control device
Res-Q ICD generator
Res-Q Micron implantable
   cardioverter-defibrillator
rest and exercise gated nuclear
   angiogram
Restcue bed
Restcue CC dynamic air therapy
   unit
re-stenosis lesion
resting pan splint
Reston dressing
Reston foam dressing
Reston foam rubber padding
Reston foam wound dressing
Reston hydrocolloid dressing
Reston padding
Reston polyurethane foam
Reston sponge
Restoration GAP acetabular cup
restoration point
restorative colectomy
restorative dental materials
restorative dentistry
restorative fixation
restorative material
restorative pin
restorative procedure
restorative proctocolectomy
   technique
Restore alginate wound dressing
Restore bone implant
Restore CalciCare dressing
Restore dental implant
Restore extra-thin dressing

Restore hydrocolloid dressing
Restore hydrogel dressing
Restore orthobiologic soft-tissue
    implant
Restore Plus wound care
    dressing
Restore threaded implant
restrictive airway defect
restrictive heart disease
restrictive membrane
restrictor
    Biostop G cement restrictor
    Buck femoral cement
        restrictor
    Buck restrictor
    cement restrictor
    Charnley cement restrictor
    E&J restrictor
    Emerson restrictor
    femoral canal restrictor
    McKesson restrictor
    Sahlin restrictor
    Thunberg restrictor
restructuring
Resume electrode
Resurface laser resurfacing
    imaging
resurfacing
    Achilles tendon resurfacing
    bipolar radiofrequency
        resurfacing
    island adipofascial flap in
        Achilles tendon resurfacing
    laser resurfacing
    laser skin resurfacing
    physician-applied resurfacing
    skin resurfacing
resurfacing laser
resurfacing operation
resurfacing procedure
Resuscitaire neonatal
    resuscitation unit
resuscitation
    cardiac resuscitation
    cardiopulmonary resuscitation
    mouth-to-mouth resuscitation
    Parkland resuscitation
resuscitation cart
resuscitation-induced
    pulmonary apoptosis
resuscitative efforts
resuspension of the malar fat pad

re-suture
retained barium
retained contents
retained foreign body
retained gallstone
retained papilla technique
retained placenta
retained placenta and
    membranes
retained placental fragment
retained root
retained stool
retained sutures
retained urine
retainer
    continuous bar retainer
    direct retainer
    extracoronal retainer
    Hahnenkratt retainer
    Hawley retainer
    HygiNet elastic dressing
        retainer
    indirect retainer
    intracoronal retainer
    matrix retainer
    McNealey-Glassman visceral
        retainer
    Mectra Tissue Sample Retainer
    multiple retainer
    series II cup retainer
    space retainer
    SurgiFish visceral retainer
    Thermoskin heat retainer
    Tofflemire retainer
    viscera retainer
retainer arch bar
retainer closure
retainer insert
retainer ring
retaining device
retaining retractor
retardant
Retcam 120 digital camera
rete pegs
rete plexus
rete ridges
rete testis
Retec machine
retention
    excessive fluid retention
    fluid retention
    mechanical retention

retention (*continued*)
  micromechanical retention
  semipermanent retention
  urinary retention
retention bar
retention catheter
retention cyst
retention drill
retention form
retention mucocele
retention point
retention polyp
retention ring
retention suture bolster
retention suture bridge
retention suture technique
retention sutures
retentive fulcrum line
retentive stabilization
Rethi incision
reticular cells
reticular collagen fibers
reticular dermis
reticular formation
reticular lesion
reticular membrane
reticular pattern
reticulate pigmented anomaly
reticulated tissue
reticulocyte
reticuloendothelial cells
reticuloendotheliosis
reticuloendothelioma
reticulogranuloma
reticulohistiocytic granuloma
reticuloid
reticulopathy
reticulosis
  disseminated pagetoid
    reticulosis
  lipomelanic reticulosis
  malignant midline reticulosis
  malignant reticulosis
reticulum
  endoplasmic reticulum
  granular reticulum
  sarcoplasmic reticulum
  striated reticulum
reticulum cell sarcoma
retina
  angiomatosis of retina
  angiopathy of retina

retina (*continued*)
  central artery of retina
  central vein of retina
  coarctate retina
  detached retina
  detachment of retina
  inferior nasal venule of retina
  inferior temporal venule of
    retina
  shot-silk retina
  superior nasal venule of retina
  superior temporal venule of
    retina
  temporal arteriole of retina
  temporal retina
retinacula cutis
retinacular release of patella
retinaculotome
retinaculotomy
retinaculum (*pl.* retinacula)
  dorsal retinaculum
  extensor retinaculum
  flexor retinaculum
  inferior extensor retinaculum
  patellar retinaculum
  peroneal retinaculum
  rectal retinaculum
  vesical retinaculum
retinaculum tendinum
retinal arteriovenous
    malformation
retinal artery
retinal circulation
retinal cones
retinal cryopexy
retinal detachment (RD)
retinal detachment hook
retinal detachment pencil
retinal detachment repair
retinal detachment syringe
retinal diathermy electrode
retinal examination
retinal excavation
retinal exudate
retinal flap
retinal fold
retinal Gelfilm implant
retinal hemorrhage
retinal imbrication
retinal involvement
retinal probe sleeve
retinal puncture cautery

retinal reattachment
retinal rods
retinal surgery
retinal tear
retinal thinning
retinal vein
retinoblastoma-mental
    retardation syndrome
retinocerebral angiomatosis
retinogram
retinoic acid
retinoid dermatitis
Retinopan 45 camera
retinopathy
retinopathy hemorrhage
retinopexy
retinoscope
   Boilo retinoscope
   Copeland streak retinoscope
   electric retinoscope
   Ful-Vue spot retinoscope
   Ful-Vue streak retinoscope
   Keeler retinoscope
   macula retinoscope
   Priestley-Smith retinoscope
   Propper retinoscope
   Reichert Ful-Vue spot
     retinoscope
   Reid retinoscope
   spot retinoscope
   streak retinoscope
   Welch Allyn standard
     retinoscope
   Welch Allyn streak retinoscope
retinoscopy
retractable fiberoptic tube
retractable stylet
retracted columella
retracted penis pouch
retracted stoma
retracting rod
retraction
   intercostal retraction
   lid retraction
   mandibular retraction
   maxillary incisor retraction
   midlamellar cicatricial
     retraction
   nipple retraction
   stimulating skin retraction
   subcostal retractions
   suprasternal retraction

retraction of clot
retraction ring
retraction space
retractor (*see also* rake
    retractor)
   1-piece lip retractor
   2-prong rake retractor
   2-pronged rake retractor
   3-prong retractor
   3-prong rake blade retractor
   4-prong retractor
   4-prong rake retractor
   5-prong rake blade retractor
   6-prong rake retractor
   Abadie self-retaining retractor
   abdominal retractor
   abdominal ring retractor
   abdominal-vascular retractor
   Ablaza aortic wall retractor
   Ablaza-Blanco cardiac valve
     retractor
   Abramson retractor
   Adams retractor
   Adamson retractor
   Adson brain retractor
   Adson cerebellar retractor
   Adson splanchnic retractor
   Adson-Beckman retractor
   Agrikola lacrimal sac retractor
   Aim retractor
   airgun retractor
   Airlift balloon retractor
   alar retractor
   Alden retractor
   Alexander retractor
   Alexander-Ballen orbital
     retractor
   Alexander-Matson retractor
   Alexian Hospital model
     retractor
   Alfreck retractor
   Allen retractor
   Allis lung retractor
   Allison lung retractor
   Allport mastoid bayonet
     retractor
   Allport-Babcock retractor
   Allport-Gifford retractor
   Alm microsurgery retractor
   Alm minor surgery retractor
   Alm self-retaining retractor
   Alter lip retractor

retractor (*continued*)

aluminum cortex retractor
Amenabar iris retractor
American Heyer-Schulte brain
    retractor
Amoils iris retractor
amputation retractor
anal retractor
Anderson double-end retractor
Anderson-Adson self-retaining
    retractor
Andrews tracheal retractor
angled decompression
    retractor
angled iris retractor
angled vein retractor
Ankeney sternal retractor
Ann Arbor phrenic retractor
anterior prostatic retractor
anterior retractor
Anthony pillar retractor
antral retractor
AOR collateral ligament
    retractor
aorta retractor
aorta valve retractor
aortic retractor
aortic valve retractor
Apfelbaum cerebellar retractor
apicolysis retractor
appendectomy retractor
appendiceal retractor
arch rake retractor
Arem retractor
Arem-Madden retractor
arm retractor
Army-Navy retractor
Aronson esophageal
    retractor
Aronson lateral sternomastoid
    retractor
Aronson medial esophageal
    retractor
Arruga eye retractor
Arruga globe retractor
Ashley retractor
Assistant Free retractor
Aston nasal retractor
Aston submental retractor
atrial retractor
atrial septal retractor
Aufranc Cobra retractor

retractor (*continued*)

Aufranc femoral neck
    retractor
Aufranc hip retractor
Aufranc psoas retractor
Aufranc push retractor
Aufricht retractor speculum
Aufricht fiberoptic light
    retractor
Aufricht nasal retractor
Aufricht retractor speculum
Aufricht-Britetrac nasal
    retractor
Austin dental retractor
automated retractor
automatic skin retractor
Auvard weighted vaginal
    retractor
Azar iris retractor
B.E. glass abdominal retractor
Babcock retractor
baby Adson brain retractor
baby Balfour retractor
baby Collin abdominal
    retractor
baby retractor
baby Roux retractor
baby Senn-Miller retractor
baby Weitlaner self-retaining
    retractor
Backmann thyroid retractor
Bacon cranial retractor
Badgley laminectomy
    retractor
Bahnson sternal retractor
Bakelite retractor
Balfour abdominal retractor
Balfour center-blade
    abdominal retractor
Balfour pediatric abdominal
    retractor
Balfour pediatric retractor
Balfour retractor with
    fenestrated blade
Balfour self-retaining retractor
Ballantine hemilaminectomy
    retractor
Ballen-Alexander orbital
    retractor
ball-type retractor
Bankart rectal retractor
Bankart shoulder retractor

retractor (*continued*)

Barkan bident retractor
Baron retractor
Barr rectal retractor
Barr self-retaining rectal
    retractor
Barr self-retaining retractor
Barraquer lid retractor
Barraquer-Krumeich-Swinger
    retractor
Barrett-Adson cerebellum
    retractor
Barron retractor
Barsky nasal retractor
Bauer retractor
Beardsley esophageal
    retractor
Beatty pillar retractor
Beaver retractor
beaver-tail retractor
Bechert-Kratz cannulated
    nucleus retractor
Becker retractor
Beckman goiter retractor
Beckman laminectomy
    retractor
Beckman self-retaining
    retractor
Beckman thyroid retractor
Beckman-Adson laminectomy
    retractor
Beckman-Eaton laminectomy
    retractor
Beckman-Weitlaner
    laminectomy retractor
Bellfield wire retractor
Bellman retractor
Bellucci-Wullstein retractor
Benedict retractor
Beneventi self-retaining
    retractor
Bennett bone retractor
Bennett tibia retractor
bent malleable retractor
Berens esophageal retractor
Berens eye retractor
Berens lid retractor
Berens mastectomy retractor
Berens mastectomy skin flap
    retractor
Berens skin flap retractor
Berens thyroid retractor

retractor (*continued*)

Bergen retractor
Bergman tracheal retractor
Bergman wound retractor
Berkeley retractor
Berkeley-Bonney self-retaining
    abdominal retractor
Berlind-Auvard retractor
Berna infant abdominal
    retractor
Bernay tracheal retractor
Bernstein nasal retractor
Bertin hip retractor
Bethune phrenic retractor
Bicek vaginal retractor
bident retractor
Biestek thyroid retractor
bifid gallbladder retractor
bifid retractor
bifurcated retractor
Biggs mammaplasty retractor
biliary retractor
Billroth ovarian retractor
Billroth-Stille retractor
Bishop retractor
bivalved retractor
Black retractor
bladder retractor
blade retractor
Blair 4-prong retractor
Blair-Brown vacuum retractor
Blakesley uvula retractor
Blanco retractor
Bland perineal retractor
Blount bone retractor
Blount double-prong retractor
Blount hip retractor
Blount knee retractor
Blount single-prong retractor
blunt rake retractor
blunt retractor
boardlike retractor
Bodnar knee retractor
Boley retractor
bone retractor
Bookwalter ring retractor
Bookwalter-Balfour retractor
Bookwalter-Goulet retractor
Bookwalter-Harrington
    retractor
Bookwalter-Hill-Ferguson
    rectal retractor

retractor (*continued*)

Bookwalter-Kelly retractor
Bookwalter-Magrina vaginal retractor
Bookwalter-ring retractor
Bookwalter-St. Mark deep pelvic retractor
Bose retractor
Bosworth nerve root retractor
bowel retractor
Boyd retractor
Boyes-Goodfellow hook retractor
Braastad costal arch retractor
brain retractor
brain silicone-coated retractor
Brantley-Turner vaginal retractor
Brawley scleral wound retractor
Breen retractor
Breisky-Navritrol retractor
Breisky vaginal retractor
Breisky-Navratil straight retractor
Brewster phrenic retractor
Briggs retractor
Brinker hygienic tissue retractor
Brinker tissue retractor
Bristow-Bankart humeral retractor
Bristow-Bankart soft tissue retractor
Brompton Hospital retractor
Bronson-Turtz iris retractor
Brophy tenaculum retractor
Brown uvula retractor
Brown-Burr modified Gillies retractor
Bruch mastoid retractor
Bruening retractor
Brunner retractor
Brunschwig visceral retractor
Buchwalter retractor
Bucy retractor
Bucy spinal cord retractor
Budde halo neurosurgical retractor
Budde halo ring retractor
Buie retractor
Buie-Smith anal retractor

retractor (*continued*)

Buie-Smith retractor
bulb retractor
Bulnes-Sanchez retractor
Burford rib retractor
Burford-Finochietto rib retractor
Busenkell posterior hip retractor
Butler dental retractor
Butler pillar retractor
buttonhook nerve retractor
buttonhook retractor
Bycroft-Brunswick thyroid retractor
Byford retractor
Byrd EndoPlastic retractor
Cairns scalp retractor
Callahan retractor
Campbell lacrimal sac retractor
Campbell nerve root retractor
Campbell self-retaining retractor
Campbell suprapubic retractor
Canadian chest retractor
Cardillo retractor
cardiovascular retractor
Carlens tracheotomy retractor
Carlens-Stille tracheal retractor
Caroline finger retractor
Carroll offset hand retractor
Carroll self-retaining spring retractor
Carroll-Bennett finger retractor
Carten mitral valve retractor
Carter retractor
Caspar cervical retractor
Castallo eyelid retractor
Castallo lid retractor
Castaneda infant sternal retractor
Castroviejo adjustable retractor
Castroviejo lid retractor
cat's paw retractor
Cave knee retractor
cecostomy retractor
cerebellar retractor

retractor (*continued*)
   cerebellum retractor
   cerebral retractor
   cervical disk retractor
   cervical retractor
   Cer-View lateral vaginal
     retractor
   chalazion retractor
   Chamberlain-Fries atraumatic
     retractor
   Chandler knee retractor
   Chandler laminectomy
     retractor
   channel retractor
   Charnley horizontal retractor
   Charnley initial incision
     retractor
   Charnley knee retractor
   Charnley pin retractor
   Charnley self-retaining
     retractor
   Charnley standard stem
     retractor
   Cheanvechai-Favaloro
     retractor
   cheek and tongue retractor
   cheek retractor
   Cherry laminectomy self-
     retaining retractor
   Cherry S-shaped brain
     retractor
   Cheyne retractor
   Children's Hospital pediatric
     retractor
   Chitten-Hill retractor
   Christie gallbladder retractor
   Cibis-Vaiser muscle retractor
   claw retractor
   Clayman lid retractor
   Clevedent retractor
   Cleveland IMA retractor
   Cloward blade retractor
   Cloward brain retractor
   Cloward cervical retractor
   Cloward dural retractor
   Cloward nerve root retractor
   Cloward self-retaining
     retractor
   Cloward tissue retractor
   Cloward-Cushing vein
     retractor
   Cloward-Hoen retractor

retractor (*continued*)
   Cobb retractor
   cobra retractor
   cobra-head retractor
   Cocke large flap retractor
   Cohen retractor
   Cole duodenal retractor
   Coleman retractor
   collapsible tissue retractor
   collar-button iris retractor
   Collin abdominal retractor
   Collin sternal self-retaining
     retractor
   Collin-Hartmann retractor
   Collins-Mayo mastoid
     retractor
   Collis anterior cervical
     retractor
   Collis posterior lumbar
     retractor
   Collis-Taylor retractor
   Colonial retractor
   Colver tonsil retractor
   Comyns-Berkeley retractor
   condylar neck retractor
   Cone laminectomy retractor
   Cone scalp retractor
   Cone self-retaining retractor
   contour retractor
   contour scalp retractor
   Converse alar retractor
   Converse blade retractor
   Converse double-ended alar
     retractor
   Converse double-ended
     retractor
   Converse nasal retractor
   Conway eye retractor
   Conway lid retractor
   Cook rectal retractor
   Cooley aorta retractor
   Cooley atrial retractor
   Cooley atrial valve retractor
   Cooley carotid retractor
   Cooley femoral retractor
   Cooley mitral valve retractor
   Cooley MPC cardiovascular
     retractor
   Cooley neonatal retractor
   Cooley neonatal sternal
     retractor
   Cooley rib retractor

retractor (*continued*)

Cooley sternotomy retractor
Cooley-Merz sternum retractor
Cope double-ended retractor
corner retractor
corrugated forehead retractor
cortex retractor
Coryllos retractor
Cosgrove mitral valve retractor
costal arch retractor
Costenbader retractor
Coston-Trent iris retractor
Cottle alar retractor
Cottle 4-prong retractor
Cottle hook retractor
Cottle knife guide and retractor
Cottle nasal retractor
Cottle pillar retractor
Cottle pronged retractor
Cottle sharp-prong retractor
Cottle single-blade retractor
Cottle soft palate retractor
Cottle thumb hook retractor
Cottle upper lateral exposing retractor
Cottle upper lateral retractor
Cottle weighted retractor
Cottle-Joseph retractor
Cottle-Neivert retractor
Crafoord retractor
Craig-Sheehan retractor
cranial retractor
crank frame retractor
Crawford aortic retractor
Crawford retractor
Crego periosteal retractor
Crile thyroid double-ended retractor
Crockard hard palate retractor
Crockard pharyngeal retractor
Crotti goiter retractor
Crotti thyroid retractor
Crowe-Davis mouth retractor
Cushing aluminum retractor
Cushing angled decompression retractor
Cushing angled retractor
Cushing bivalve retractor
Cushing brain retractor

retractor (*continued*)

Cushing decompression retractor
Cushing nerve retractor
Cushing self-retaining retractor
Cushing S-shaped retractor
Cushing straight retractor
Cushing subtemporal retractor
Cushing vein retractor
Cushing-Kocher retractor
dacryocystorhinostomy retractor
Dallas retractor
Danek self-retaining retractor
Danis retractor
Darling popliteal retractor
Darrach retractor
Dautrey retractor
David-Baker eyelid retractor
Davidoff trigeminal retractor
Davidson erector spinae retractor
Davidson scapular retractor
Davis brain retractor
Davis double-ended retractor
Davis pillar retractor
Davis self-retaining scalp retractor
de la Plaza transconjunctival retractor
Deaver pediatric retractor
DeBakey chest retractor
DeBakey-Balfour retractor
DeBakey-Cooley Deaver-type retractor
DeBakey-Cooley retractor
Decker retractor
decompressive retractor
Dedo laser retractor
deep abdominal retractor
deep blunt rake retractor
deep Deaver retractor
deep rake retractor
deep retractor
DeLaginiere abdominal retractor
Delaney phrenic retractor
DeLee corner retractor
DeLee Universal retractor
DeLee vaginal retractor

retractor (*continued*)
DeLee vesical retractor
DeMartel self-retaining brain
   retractor
Denis Browne pediatric
   retractor
Denis Browne ring retractor
dental retractor
Denver-Wells atrial retractor
Denver-Wells sternal retractor
DePuy retractor
D'Errico nerve retractor
D'Errico nerve root retractor
D'Errico-Adson retractor
Desmarres cardiovascular
   retractor
Desmarres lid retractor
Desmarres valve retractor
Desmarres vein retractor
Deucher abdominal retractor
Devine-Millard-Aufricht
   retractor
Di-Main retractor
Dingman flexible retractor
Dingman Flexsteel retractor
Dingman zygoma hook
   retractor
Dingman-Senn retractor
disposable iris retractor
disposable retractor
Dixon center-blade retractor
Doane knee retractor
Dockhorn retractor
dog chain retractor
Dohn-Carton brain retractor
Dorsey nerve root retractor
Dorton self-retaining retractor
Dott retractor
double-angled retractor
double-bent Hohmann
   acetabular retractor
double-cobra retractor
double-crank retractor
double-ended breast
   retractors
double-ended retractor
double-fishhook retractor
Downing II laminectomy
   retractor
Doyen abdominal retractor
Doyen child abdominal
   retractor

retractor (*continued*)
Doyen vaginal retractor
Dozier radiolucent Bennett
   retractor
Drews iris retractor
Drews-Rosenbaum iris
   retractor
dual nerve root suction
   retractor
Duane retractor
dull retractor
dull-pronged retractor
Dumont retractor
duodenal retractor
dural retractor
dural suction retractor
Duryea retractor
Eastman vaginal retractor
East-West soft tissue retractor
easy-out retractor
Eccentric Y adjustable finger
   retractor
Echols retractor
Eddey parotid retractor
Edinburgh brain retractor
Effenberger retractor
Elias lid retractor
Elite Farley retractor
Emmet obstetrical retractor
Emory EndoPlastic retractor
endaural retractor
Endoflex endoscopic retractor
EndoPlastic retractor
EndoRetract retractor
Endotrac retractor
Enker brain retractor
Enker self-retaining brain
   retractor
epicardial retractor
epiglottis retractor
erector spinae retractor
ESI long, narrow
   mammaplasty retractor
ESI narrow mammaplasty
   retractor
esophageal retractor
examination retractor
eXpose retractor
externofrontal retractor
extraoral sigmoid notch
   retractor
eye retractor

retractor (*continued*)
eyelid retractor
facelift retractor
Falk vaginal retractor
fan elevator retractor
fan liver retractor
Farabeuf double-ended
  retractor
Farley Elite spinal retractor
Farmingdale retractor
Farr self-retaining retractor
Farr spring retractor
Farr wire retractor
Fasanella double-ended iris
  retractor
Fasanella iris retractor
fat pad retractor
Favaloro atrial retractor
Favaloro sternal retractor
Favaloro self-retaining sternal
  retractor
Favaloro retractor
Federspiel cheek retractor
Feldman lip retractor
femoral neck retractor
Ferguson retractor
Ferguson-Moon rectal
  retractor
Fernstroem bladder retractor
Fernstroem-Stille retractor
Ferris Smith orbital retractor
Ferris Smith-Sewall orbital
  retractor
fiberoptic retractor
fiberoptic smoke evacuating
  retractors
finger rake retractor
finger retractor
Fink lacrimal retractor
Finochietto hand retractor
Finochietto infant rib
  retractor
Finochietto laminectomy
  retractor
Finochietto rib retractor
Finochietto-Geissendorfer rib
  retractor
Finsen retractor
Fisch dural retractor
Fisher double-ended retractor
Fisher fenestrated lid retractor
Fisher lid retractor

retractor (*continued*)
Fisher tonsil retractor
Fisher-Nugent retractor
fixed ring retractor
flexible neck rake retractor
flexible shaft retractor
flexible translimbal iris
  retractor
FlexPosure endoscopic
  retractor
Flexsteel ribbon retractor
Foerster abdominal retractor
Foerster abdominal ring
  retractor
Fomon hook retractor
Fomon nasal retractor
Fomon nostril retractor
force fulcrum retractor
Ford-Deaver retractor
Forker retractor
Foss bifid gallbladder
  retractor
Foss bifid retractor
Foss biliary retractor
Foss gallbladder retractor
Fowler self-retaining retractor
Franklin retractor
Franklin malleable retractor
Franz abdominal retractor
Franz retractor
Frater intracardiac retractor
Frazier cerebral retractor
Frazier laminectomy retractor
Frazier lighted retractor
Frazier-Fay retractor
Freeman facelift retractor
Freer dural retractor
Freer skin retractor
Freer submucous retractor
Freiberg hip retractor
Freiberg nerve root retractor
Freidrich-Ferguson retractor
French brain retractor
French S-shaped brain
  retractor
French-Stern-McCarthy
  retractor
Friedman perineal retractor
Friedman vaginal retractor
Friedrich-Ferguson retractor
Fritsch abdominal retractor
Fujita snake retractor

retractor (*continued*)

Fukuda humeral head retractor
Fukushima retractor
Fullerview flexible iris retractor
Fulton retractor
Gabarro retractor
gallbladder retractor
gallows-type retractor
Gam-Mer medial esophageal retractor
Gam-Mer occipital retractor
Gant gallbladder retractor
Garrett peripheral vascular retractor
Garrigue vaginal retractor
gastric resection retractor
Gaubatz rib retractor
Gauthier retractor
Gazayerli endoscopic retractor
Gazayerli-Mediflex retractor
Geissendorfer rib retractor
Gelpi abdominal retractor
Gelpi perineal retractor
Gelpi self-retaining retractor
Gelpi vaginal retractor
Gelpi-Lowrie retractor
general retractor
Gerbode sternal retractor
Gerow-Harrington heart-shaped distal end retractor
Ghazi rib retractor
Gibson-Balfour abdominal retractor
Gifford mastoid retractor
Gifford scalp retractor
Gifford-Jansen mastoid retractor
Gillies single-hook skin retractor
Gil-Vernet lumbotomy retractor
Gil-Vernet renal sinus retractor
Givner eye retractor
Givner lid retractor
Glaser laminectomy retractor
Glass abdominal retractor
Glenner vaginal retractor
Goelet double-ended retractor

retractor (*continued*)

goiter retractor
Goldstein lacrimal sac retractor
Goligher modification of the Berkeley-Bonney retractor
Goligher sternal-lifting retractor
Gomez gastric retractor
Gooch mastoid retractor
Good retractor
Goodhill retractor
Goodyear tonsillar retractor
Goodyear uvula retractor
Gosset abdominal retractor
Gosset appendectomy retractor
Gosset self-retaining retractor
Gott malleable retractor
Goulet retractor
Gradle eyelid retractor
Graether retractor
Grant gallbladder retractor
Gray surgical retractor
Green goiter retractor
Green thyroid retractor
Greenberg Universal retractor
Greenberg-Sugita retractor
Greene retractor
Greenwald retractor
Grice retractor
Grieshaber flexible iris retractor
Grieshaber self-retaining retractor
Grieshaber spring wire retractor
Grieshaber wire retractor
Grieshaber-Balfour retractor
Groenholm lid retractor
Gross iris retractor
Gross patent ductus retractor
Gross-Pomeranz-Watkins atrial retractor
Gross-Pomeranz-Watkins retractor
Gruenwald retractor
Guilford-Wright meatal retractor
Guthrie retractor
Guttmann obstetrical retractor

retractor (*continued*)
  Guttmann vaginal retractor
  Guzman-Blanco epiglottis retractor
  Haight baby retractor
  Haight pulmonary retractor
  Haight rib retractor
  Haight-Finochietto rib retractor
  Hajek antral retractor
  Hajek lip retractor
  half-moon retractor
  halo retractor
  Hamburger-Brennan-Mahorner thyroid retractor
  Hamby brain retractor
  Hamby-Hibbs retractor
  hand retractor
  hand-held retractor
  hard palate retractor
  Hardy lip retractor
  Hardy retractor
  Hardy-Duddy vaginal retractor
  Harken rib retractor
  Harrington bladder retractor
  Harrington Britetrac retractor
  Harrington splanchnic retractor
  Harrington sympathectomy retractor
  Harrington-Deaver retractor
  Harrington-Pemberton sympathectomy retractor
  Harrison chalazion retractor
  Hartstein irrigating iris retractor
  Hartzler rib retractor
  Haslinger palate retractor
  Haslinger uvula retractor
  Hasson retractor
  Haverfield hemilaminectomy retractor
  Haverfield-Scoville hemilaminectomy retractor
  Haynes retractor
  Hays finger retractor
  Hays hand retractor
  Heaney hysterectomy retractor
  Heaney vaginal retractor
  Heaney-Simon hysterectomy retractor

retractor (*continued*)
  Heaney-Simon vaginal retractor
  Hedblom rib retractor
  Heifitz retractor
  Heiss mastoid retractor
  Heiss soft tissue retractor
  Helfrick anal retractor
  Helfrick anal ring retractor
  Helveston Great Big Barbie retractor
  hemilaminectomy retractor
  Henderson self-retaining retractor
  Henley carotid retractor
  Henner endaural retractor
  Henner T-model endaural retractor
  Henning meniscal retractor
  Henrotin retractor
  hernia retractor
  Hertzler baby retractor
  Hertzler baby rib retractor
  Hertzler rib retractor
  Hess nerve root retractor
  Heyer-Schulte brain retractor
  Hibbs laminectomy retractor
  Hibbs self-retaining laminectomy retractor
  Hibbs self-retaining retractor
  Hill rectal retractor
  Hill-Ferguson rectal retractor
  Hill-Ferguson retractor
  Hillis eyelid retractor
  Hillis lid retractor
  Himmelstein retractor
  Himmelstein sternal retractor
  hip retractor
  Hirschman retractor
  Hoen hemilaminectomy retractor
  Hoen scalp retractor
  Hohmann retractor
  Holman lung retractor
  Holscher nerve retractor
  Holscher nerve root retractor
  Holscher root retractor
  Holzbach abdominal retractor
  Holzheimer mastoid retractor
  Holzheimer skin retractor
  Homan retractor
  hook retractor

retractor (*continued*)
Horgan retractor
horizontal flexible bar retractor
horizontal retractor
Hosel retractor
House hand-held double-end retractor
House hand-held retractor
House-Urban middle fossa retractor
Howorth toothed retractor
Huang Universal arm retractor
Hubbard retractor
Hudson bone retractor
humeral retractor
Hunt bladder retractor
Hupp tracheal retractor
Hurd pillar retractor
Hurd tonsillar pillar retractor
Hurson flexible retractor
Hutchinson iris retractor
hysterectomy retractor
IMA retractor
incision retractor
infant abdominal retractor
infant eyelid retractor
infant rib retractor
Inge laminectomy retractor
initial incision retractor
intestinal occlusion retractor
intracardiac retractor
intradural retractor
iris disposable retractor
Iron Intern retractor
irrigating mushroom retractor
Israel blunt rake retractor
Israel rake retractor
Jackson double-ended retractor
Jackson goiter retractor
Jackson self-retaining goiter retractor
Jackson tracheal retractor
Jackson vaginal retractor
Jacobson bladder retractor
Jacobson goiter retractor
Jaeger lid plate retractor
Jaeger lid retractor
Jaffe lid retractor
Jaffe wire lid retractor
Jaffe-Givner lid retractor

retractor (*continued*)
Jako laser retractor
Jannetta posterior fossa retractor
Jansen mastoid retractor
Jansen scalp retractor
Jansen-Gifford mastoid retractor
Jansen-Wagner mastoid retractor
Jari renal sinus retractor
Jarit cross-action retractor
Jarit PEER retractor
Jarit renal sinus retractor
Jarit spring-wire retractor
Jarit-Deaver retractor
Jefferson self-retaining retractor
Joe's hoe retractor
Johns Hopkins gallbladder retractor
Johnson cheek retractor
Johnson hook retractor
Johnson ventriculogram retractor
Jones IMA epicardial retractor
Jorgenson retractor
Joseph skin hook retractor
Joseph wound retractor
Joystick retractor
Judd-Allis intestinal retractor
Judd-Mason bladder retractor
Judd-Mason prostatic retractor
Kalamarides dural retractor
Kanavel-Senn retractor
Kapp total knee retractor
Karmody vascular spring retractor
Kartush insulated retractor
Kasdan retractor
Kaufer type II retractor
Kaufman type II retractor
Keeler-Fison tissue retractor
Keeler-Lancaster lid retractor
Keeler-Rodger iris retractor
Keizer eye retractor
Keizer lid retractor
Keizer-Lancaster lid retractor
Kel retractor
Kelly abdominal retractor
Kelly-Sims vaginal retractor
Kelman iris retractor

retractor (*continued*)
 Kennerdell medial orbital
  retractor
 Kennerdell-Maroon orbital
  retractor
 Kerrison retractor
 kidney retractor
 Killey molar retractor
 Killian-King goiter retractor
 Kilner nasal retractor
 Kilner skin hook retractor
 Kilpatrick retractor
 King goiter retractor
 King goiter self-retaining
  retractor
 King self-retaining goiter
  retractor
 King-Hurd retractor
 Kirby lid retractor
 Kirchner retractor
 Kirkland retractor
 Kirklin atrial retractor
 Kirschenbaum retractor
 Kirschner abdominal retractor
 Kirschner abdominal self-
  retaining retractor
 Kirschner-Balfour abdominal
  retractor
 Kitner retractor
 Kleinert-Kutz hook retractor
 Kleinert-Ragnell retractor
 Kleinsasser retractor
 Klemme appendectomy
  retractor
 Klemme gasserian ganglion
  retractor
 Klemme laminectomy
  retractor
 Kliners alar retractor
 Knapp lacrimal sac retractor
 knee retractor
 Knighton hemilaminectomy
  self-retaining retractor
 Kobayashi retractor
 Kocher bladder retractor
 Kocher blade retractor
 Kocher bone retractor
 Kocher gallbladder retractor
 Kocher goiter self-retaining
  retractor
 Kocher self-retaining goiter
  retractor

retractor (*continued*)
 Kocher-Crotti goiter retractor
 Kocher-Crotti goiter self-
  retaining retractor
 Kocher-Crotti self-retaining
  goiter retractor
 Kocher-Langenbeck retractor
 Kocher-Wagner retractor
 Koenig vein retractor
 Koerte retractor
 Konig retractor
 Korte retractor
 Korte-Wagner retractor
 Kozlinski retractor
 Krasky retractor
 Kretschmer retractor
 Kristeller retractor
 Kristeller vaginal retractor
 Kronfeld eyelid retractor
 Kronlein-Berke retractor
 Kuda retractor
 Kuglen lens retractor
 Kuyper-Murphy sternal
  retractor
 Kwapis subcondylar retractor
 Lack tongue retractor
 lacrimal retractor
 lacrimal sac retractor
 Lahey retractor
 Lahey Clinic nerve root
  retractor
 Lahey goiter retractor
 Lahey thyroid retractor
 laminectomy retractor
 laminectomy self-retaining
  retractor
 Landau vaginal retractor
 Landon narrow-bladed
  retractor
 Lane retractor
 Lange bone retractor
 Lange-Hohmann bone
  retractor
 Langenbeck periosteal
  retractor
 Langenbeck-Cushing vein
  retractor
 Langenbeck-Green retractor
 Langenbeck-Mannerfelt
  retractor
 Laplace liver retractor
 Large self-retaining retractor

retractor (*continued*)
 laryngeal retractor
 laryngofissure retractor
 lateral retractor
 lateral wall retractor
 Latrobe soft palate retractor
 Laufe retractor
 Lawton-Balfour self-retaining
   retractor
 leaflet retractor
 Leasure tracheal retractor
 Leatherman trochanteric
   retractor
 Lee double-ended retractor
 Legen self-retaining retractor
 Legueu bladder retractor
 Legueu kidney retractor
 Lemmon self-retaining sternal
   retractor
 Lemmon sternal retractor
 Lemole atrial valve self-
   retaining retractor
 Lemole mitral valve retractor
 Lempert retractor
 Lempert-Colver retractor
 LeVasseur-Merrill retractor
 Levinthal surgery retractor
 Levy articulating retractor
 Levy perineal retractor
 Lewis uvula retractor
 Leyla self-retaining brain
   retractor
 Leyla-Yasargil retractor
 Leyla-Yasargil self-retaining
   retractor
 lid retractor
 Liddicoat aortic valve
   retractor
 lighted retractor
 LightWare micro retractor
 Lilienthal-Sauerbruch
   retractor
 Lillehei retractor
 Lillie retractor
 Linton splanchnic retractor
 lip retractor
 Little retractor
 liver retractor
 Lockhart-Mummery retractor
 Lofberg thyroid retractor
 Logan lacrimal sac self-
   retaining retractor

retractor (*continued*)
 London narrow-bladed
   retractor
 Lone Star retractor
 long atraumatic retractor
 loop retractor
 Lorie cheek retractor
 Lothrop tonsillar retractor
 Lothrop uvula retractor
 Love nasopharyngeal retractor
 Love nerve retractor
 Love nerve root retractor
 Love uvula retractor
 Lovejoy retractor
 Lowman hand retractor
 Lowsley prostate retractor
 Luer double-ended tracheal
   retractor
 Luer S-shaped retractor
 Luer tracheal double-ended
   retractor
 Lukens double-ended tracheal
   retractor
 Lukens epiglottic retractor
 Lukens thymus retractor
 Lukens tracheal double-ended
   retractor
 lumbar retractor
 lumbotomy retractor
 lung retractor
 Luongo hand retractor
 Luther-Peter retractor
 MacAusland muscle retractor
 MacAusland-Kelly retractor
 MacKay contour retractor
 MacKay contour self-retaining
   retractor
 MacKool capsule retractor
 MacVicar double-end
   strabismus retractor
 Magrina-Bookwalter vaginal
   retractor
 Mahorner thyroid retractor
 Maison retractor
 Maliniac nasal retractor
 Malis cerebral retractor
 malleable blade retractor
 malleable copper retractor
 malleable ribbon retractor
 malleable stainless steel
   retractor
 Maltz retractor

retractor (*continued*)
  mandibular body retractor
  Mannerfelt retractor
  Manning retractor
  manual retractor
  Mark II S total knee retractor
  Mark II Z knee retractor
  Mark II Chandler total knee
    retractor
  Mark II concave total knee
    retractor
  Mark II lateral collateral
    ligament retractor
  Mark II modular weighted
    retractor
  Mark II PCL retractor
  Mark II Stubbs short-prong
    collateral ligament retractor
  Mark II wide PCL knee
    retractor
  Markham-Meyerding
    hemilaminectomy retractor
  Markley retractor
  Martin abdominal retractor
  Martin cheek retractor
  Martin lip retractor
  Martin nerve root retractor
  Martin palate retractor
  Martin rectal hook retractor
  Martin vaginal retractor
  Mason-Judd bladder retractor
  Mason-Judd self-retaining
    retractor
  mastectomy skin flap
    retractor
  mastoid retractor
  mastoid self-retaining
    retractor
  mastoid-retaining retractor
  Mathieu double-ended
    retractor
  Matson-Mead apicolysis
    retractor
  Mattison-Upshaw retractor
  Mayfield retractor
  Mayo abdominal retractor
  Mayo-Adams appendectomy
    retractor
  Mayo-Adson self-retaining
    retractor
  Mayo-Collins appendectomy
    retractor

retractor (*continued*)
  Mayo-Collins double-ended
    retractor
  Mayo-Collins mastoid
    retractor
  Mayo-Lovelace abdominal
    retractor
  Mayo-Simpson retractor
  McBurney fenestrated
    retractor
  McBurney thyroid retractor
  McCabe antral retractor
  McCabe parotidectomy
    retractor
  McCabe posterior fossa
    retractor
  McCool capsule retractor
  McCullough externofrontal
    retractor
  McGannon eye retractor
  McGannon iris retractor
  McGill retractor
  McIndoe retractor
  McNealey visceral retractor
  meat hook retractor
  Medicon rib retractor
  Mediflex Gazayerli retractor
  Meigs retractor
  Meller lacrimal sac retractor
  meniscal retractor
  Merrill-Levassier retractor
  metacarpal double-ended
    retractor
  metal bar retractor
  Meyer biliary retractor
  Meyerding finger retractor
  Meyerding laminectomy self-
    retaining retractor
  Meyerding self-retaining
    laminectomy retractor
  Meyerding skin hook and
    retractor
  Meyerding-Deaver retractor
  microlumbar diskectomy
    retractor
  microsurgery retractor
  microsurgical retractor
  microvascular modified Alm
    retractor
  middle fossa retractor
  Middledorf retractor
  Middlesex-Pointe retractor

retractor (*continued*)
Mikulicz abdominal retractor
Mikulicz liver retractor
Miles retractor
Milex retractor
Millard thimble retractor
Miller retractor
Miller-Senn double-ended
   retractor
Milligan self-retaining
   retractor
Millin bladder retractor
Millin retropublic bladder
   retractor
Millin self-retaining retractor
Millin-Bacon bladder self-
   retaining retractor
Millin-Bacon retropubic
   prostatectomy retractor
Miltex retractor
mini-Hohmann retractor
Minnesota retractor
Miskimon cerebellar self-
   retaining retractor
mitral valve retractor
Moberg retractor
Moberg-Stille retractor
Mollison self-retaining
   retractor
Moon rectal retractor
Moore bone retractor
Moorehead cheek retractor
Moorehead dental retractor
Morris retractor
Morrison-Hurd pillar retractor
Morse modified Finochietto
   retractor
Morse sternal retractor
Morse valve retractor
Mosher lifesaver retractor
Mott double-ended retractor
Mueller lacrimal sac retractor
Mueller-Balfour self-retaining
   retractor
Mufson-Cushing retractor
Muldoon lid retractor
multiprong rake retractor
multipurpose retractor
Munro self-retaining retractor
Murless head retractor
Murphy gallbladder retractor
Murphy rake retractor

retractor (*continued*)
Murphy-Balfour retractor
Murtagh self-retaining infant
   scalp retractor
Myers knee retractor
Naclerio diaphragm retractor
narrow Deaver retractor
narrow retractor
nasal retractor
nasopharyngeal retractor
Navratil retractor
Neivert double-ended
   retractor
Neivert knife guide and
   retractor
Nelson self-retaining rib
   retractor
neonatal sternal retractor
nerve retractor
nerve root retractor
Nevyas drape retractor
New tracheal retractor
New York Hospital retractor
newborn eyelid retractor
Newell lid retractor
Newton-Morgan retractor
Noblock retractor
North-South retractor
Nuttall retractor
Nystroem retractor
Nystroem-Stille retractor
Oberhill self-retaining
   retractor
O'Brien phrenic retractor
O'Brien rib retractor
obstetrical retractor
Obwegeser channel retractor
Obwegeser periosteal
   retractor
Ochsner malleable retractor
Ochsner ribbon retractor
Ochsner vascular retractor
Ochsner-Favaloro self-
   retaining retractor
O'Connor abdominal retractor
O'Connor vaginal retractor
O'Connor-O'Sullivan
   abdominal retractor
O'Connor-O'Sullivan self-
   retaining retractor
Octopus retractor
Oertli lid retractor

retractor (*continued*)
Oertli wire lid retractor
Oettingen abdominal retractor
Oettingen abdominal self-
retaining retractor
offset hand retractor
Oklahoma iris wire retractor
Oldberg brain retractor
Oldberg straight retractor
Oliver scalp retractor
Ollier rake retractor
Omni retractor
Omni-Tract vaginal retractor
orbicular retractor
orbital retractor
O'Reilly esophageal retractor
Orley retractor
Osher iris retractor
Osher lid retractor
O'Sullivan self-retaining
abdominal retractor
O'Sullivan vaginal retractor
O'Sullivan-O'Connor
abdominal retractor
O'Sullivan-O'Connor self-
retaining abdominal
retractor
O'Sullivan-O'Connor self-
retaining retractor
O'Sullivan-O'Connor vaginal
retractor
Otto Barkan Bident retractor
Overholt retractor
Packiam retractor
palate retractor
Paparella self-retaining
retractor
Paparella-Weitlaner retractor
Parker double-ended retractor
Parker thumb retractor
Parker-Mott double-ended
retractor
Parkes nasal retractor
Parks anal retractor
parotidectomy retractor
Parsonnet epicardial retractor
patent ductus retractor
Paul lacrimal sac retractor
Paulson knee retractor
Payne retractor
Payr abdominal retractor
Peck rake retractor

retractor (*continued*)
pediatric abdominal retractor
pediatric self-retaining
retractor
Peet lighted splanchnic
retractor
Pemberton retractor
Pemco retractor
Penfield retractor
Percy amputation retractor
Percy bone retractor
Percy-Wolfson gallbladder
retractor
periareolar retractor
perineal prostatectomy
retractor
perineal retractor
perineal self-retaining
retractor
peripheral vascular retractor
Perkins otologic retractor
Perman-Stille abdominal
retractor
pharyngeal retractor
Pheifer-Young retractor
Phoropter retractor
phrenic retractor
Pickrell retractor
Picot vaginal retractor
Pierce cheek retractor
pillar retractor
pillar-and-post microsurgical
retractor
Pilling retractor
Pilling-Favaloro retractor
Piper lateral wall retractor
Plester retractor
Polyak eye retractor
Polytrac Gomez retractor
Polytrac retractor
Pomeranz hiatal hernia
retractor
popliteal retractor
Poppen-Gelpi laminectomy
self-retaining retractor
Portmann retractor
Posada-Vasco orbital retractor
postauricular retractor
posterior fossa retractor
posterior urethral retractor
Pratt bivalve retractor
Proctor cheek retractor

retractor (*continued*)

pronged retractor
prostatic retractor
Proud-White uvula retractor
Pryor-Pean vaginal retractor
psoas retractor
pulmonary retractor
Purcell self-retaining
abdominal retractor
Quervain abdominal retractor
Quervain-Sauerbruch retractor
Radcliff perineal retractor
Ragnell double-ended
retractor
Ragnell-Davis double-ended
retractor
rake retractor
Ralks ear retractor
Raney laminectomy
retractor
Rankin prostatic retractor
Raylor malleable retractor
rectal hook retractor
rectal retractor
Rees lighted retractor
Rehbein infant abdominal
retractor
Rehne abdominal retractor
Reinhart retractor
Remine mastectomy skin flap
retractor
renal sinus retractor
retaining retractor
retropubic prostatectomy
retractor
retropubic retractor
rib retractor
ribbon malleable retractor
ribbon retractor
Rica bone retractor
Rica brain retractor
Rica mastoid retractor
Rica multipurpose retractor
Rica posterior cranial fossa
retractor
Rica scalp retractor
Ricard abdominal retractor
Richards abdominal retractor
Richardson abdominal
retractor
Richardson appendectomy
retractor

retractor (*continued*)

Richardson-Eastman double-
ended retractor
Richter vaginal retractor
Rigby abdominal retractor
Rigby appendectomy
retractor
Rigby bivalve retractor
Rigby rectal retractor
Rigby vaginal retractor
right-angle retractor
rigid neck rake retractor
ring abdominal retractor
Rissler kidney retractor
Rizzo retractor
Rizzuti iris retractor
Roberts thumb retractor
Robin-Masse abdominal
retractor
Robinson lung retractor
Rochard retractor
Rochester atrial retractor
Rochester atrial septal defect
retractor
Rochester atrial septal
retractor
Rochester colonial retractor
Rochester rake retractor
Rochester-Ferguson double-
ended retractor
Rollet eye retractor
Rollet lacrimal sac retractor
Rollet rake retractor
Rollet skin retractor
Roos brachial plexus root
retractor
Rose double-ended retractor
Rose tracheal retractor
Rosenbaum iris retractor
Rosenbaum-Drews iris
retractor
Rosenbaum-Drews plastic
retractor
Rosenberg full-radius blade
synovial retractor
Rosenberg-Sampson retractor
Ross aortic retractor
Ross aortic valve retractor
Rotalok skin retractor
Rothon retractor
Roux double-ended retractor
Rowe boathook retractor

retractor (*continued*)

Rowe humeral head retractor
Rowe orbital floor retractor
Rowe scapular neck retractor
Rudolph trowel retractor
Rultract internal mammary
  artery retractor
Rumel retractor
Ryecroft retractor
Ryerson bone retractor
Sachs angled vein retractor
Sachs vein retractor
Sachs-Cushing retractor
Samb retractor
Sanchez-Bulnes lacrimal sac
  self-retaining retractor
Sato lid retractor
Sauerbruch retractor
Sauerbruch-Zukschwerdt rib
  retractor
Sawyer rectal retractor
Sayre retractor
scalp retractor
scalp self-retaining retractor
Scanlan pediatric retractor
scapular retractor
Schepens eye retractor
Schepens orbital retractor
Schindler retractor
Schink metatarsal retractor
Schnitker scalp retractor
Schoenborn retractor
Scholten sternal retractor
Schuknecht postauricular self-
  retaining retractor
Schuknecht-Wullstein
  retractor
Schultz iris retractor
Schultz irrigating iris retractor
Schwartz laminectomy
  retractor
Schwartz laminectomy self-
  retaining retractor
scleral wound retractor
Scoville Britetrac retractor
Scoville cervical disk self-
  retaining retractor
Scoville hemilaminectomy
  retractor
Scoville hemilaminectomy
  self-retaining retractor
Scoville laminectomy retractor

retractor (*continued*)

Scoville nerve retractor
Scoville nerve root retractor
Scoville psoas muscle
  retractor
Scoville self-retaining retractor
Scoville-Haverfield
  laminectomy retractor
Scoville-Richter self-retaining
  retractor
Seen retractor
Segond abdominal retractor
Seldin dental retractor
Seletz-Gelpi self-retaining
  retractor
self-adhering lid retractor
self-retaining abdominal
  retractor
self-retaining brain retractor
self-retaining retractor
self-retaining ring retractor
self-retaining skin retractor
self-retaining spring retractor
Sellor rib retractor
Semb lung retractor
Semb self-retaining retractor
Senn double-ended retractor
Senn mastoid retractor
Senn self-retaining retractor
Senn-Dingman double-ended
  retractor
Senn-Green retractor
Senn-Kanavel double-ended
  retractor
Senn-Kanavel retractor
Senn-Miller retractor
Senturia retractor
serrated retractor
serrefine retractor
Sewall orbital retractor
Shambaugh endaural self-
  retaining retractor
Shambaugh endaural retractor
Shambaugh endaural self-
  retaining retractor
sharp-pronged retractor
Shearer lip retractor
Sheehan retractor
Sheldon hemilaminectomy
  retractor
Sheldon hemilaminectomy
  self-retaining retractor

retractor (*continued*)

Sheldon retractor
Sheldon-Gosset self-retaining retractor
Sherwin self-retaining retractor
Sherwood retractor
short Heaney retractor
Shriners Hospital interlocking retractor
Shuletz-Paul rib retractor
Shurly tracheal retractor
sigmoid notch retractor
Silverstein lateral venous sinus retractor
Simon vaginal retractor
Sims double-ended retractor
Sims rectal retractor
Sims vaginal retractor
Sims-Kelly vaginal retractor
single-blade retractor
single-hook retractor
single-prong broad acetabular retractor
Sisson spring retractor
Sisson-Love retractor
Sistrunk band retractor
Sistrunk double-ended retractor
skin flap retractor
skin hook retractor
skin retractor
skin self-retaining retractor
Sloan goiter retractor
Sloan goiter self-retaining retractor
Sluder palate retractor
small rake retractors
Small tissue retractor
SMIC cheek retractor
Smillie knee joint retractor
Smith anal retractor
Smith nerve root suction retractor
Smith rectal retractor
Smith rectal self-retaining retractor
Smith vaginal self-retaining retractor
Smith-Buie anal retractor
Smith-Buie rectal retractor

retractor (*continued*)

Smith-Buie rectal self-retaining retractor
Smith-Buie self-retaining rectal retractor
Smith-Petersen capsular retractor
Smith-Petersen retractor
Smithwick retractor
Snitman endaural retractor
Snitman endaural self-retaining retractor
Sofield retractor
soft palate retractor
soft tissue blade retractor
Spacekeeper retractor
Space-OR retractor
spike retractor
spinal cord retractor
spinal retractor
Spivey iris retractor
splanchnic retractor
spoon retractor
spring retractor
spring-loaded self-retaining retractor
spring-wire retractor
Spurling retractor
S-shaped brain retractor
S-shaped retractor
St. Luke's retractor
St. Mark's Hospital retractor
St. Mark's lipped retractor
St. Mark's pelvis retractor
Stack retractor
Stamey dorsal vein apical retractor
stay suture retractor
Steiner-Auvard vaginal retractor
stereotactic retractor
sternal retractor
sternotomy retractor
Stevens lacrimal retractor
Stevens muscle hook retractor
Stevenson lacrimal retractor
Stevenson lacrimal sac retractor
Stille cheek retractor
Stille heart retractor
Stille-Broback knee retractor
Stiwer retractor

retractor (*continued*)
  Stookey retractor
  Storer thoracoabdominal
    retractor
  Storz retractor
  straight retractor
  Strandell retractor
  Strandell-Stille retractor
  Strully nerve root retractor
  Stuck self-retaining
    laminectomy retractor
  Suarez retractor
  submucous retractor
  Sugita retractor
  suprapubic retractor
  suprapubic self-retaining
    retractor
  surgical retractor
  Sweeney posterior vaginal
    retractor
  Sweet amputation retractor
  sweetheart retractor
  Symmonds hysterectomy
    retractor
  sympathectomy retractor
  table-fixed retractor
  Tang retractor
  Tara retropublic retractor
  Taylor Britetrac retractor
  Taylor fiberoptic retractor
  Taylor spinal retractor
  T-bar retractor
  Tebbetts ribbon retractor
  Teflon iris retractor
  Temple-Fay laminectomy
    retractor
  Tepas retractor
  Terino facial implant retractor
  Tew cranial retractor
  Tew spinal retractor
  Theis self-retaining retractor
  Theis self-retaining rib
    retractor
  Theis vein retractor
  Thoma tissue retractor
  Thomas retractor
  Thompson retractor
  Thorlakson deep abdominal
    retractor
  Thorlakson multipurpose
    retractor
  Thornton iris retractor

retractor (*continued*)
  thumb retractor
  Thurmond iris retractor
  thymus retractor
  thyroid retractor
  tibial retractor
  Tiko pliable iris retractor
  Tiko rake retractor
  Tillary double-ended retractor
  tissue retractor
  titanium wound retractor
  T-malleable retractor
  T-model endaural retractor
  Toennis retractor
  tongue retractor
  tonsillar pillar retractor
  tonsillar retractor
  toothed retractor
  Tower interchangeable
    retractor
  Tower rib retractor
  Tower spinal retractor
  tracheal retractor
  transconjunctival retractor
  transoral retractor
  Trent eye retractor
  trigeminal retractor
  trigeminal self-retaining
    retractor
  Tubinger self-retaining
    retractor
  Tucker-Levine vocal cord
    retractor
  Tuffier abdominal retractor
  Tuffier rib retractor
  Tuffier-Raney laminectomy
    retractor
  Tupper hand-holder and
    retractor
  Turner-Doyen retractor
  Turner-Warwick posterior
    urethral retractor
  Turner-Warwick prostate
    retractor
  Tyrer nerve root retractor
  Tyrrell hook retractor
  U.S. Army double-ended
    retractor
  U.S. Army pattern retractor
  Ullrich laminectomy retractor
  Ullrich self-retaining
    laminectomy retractor

retractor (*continued*)
Ullrich self-retaining retractor
Ullrich-St. Gallen self-retaining
retractor
umbrella retractor
Universal retractor
Upper Hands self-retaining
retractor
upper-lateral exposing
retractor
Urban retractor
USA retractor
U-shaped retractor
uvula retractor
V. Mueller fiberoptic retractor
V. Mueller-Balfour abdominal
retractor
Vacher self-retaining retractor
vacuum retractor
vaginal retractor
vagotomy retractor
Vail lid retractor
Valin hemilaminectomy self-
retaining retractor
Vasco-Posada orbital retractor
vascular retractor
vascular spring retractor
Veenema retropubic retractor
Veenema retropubic self-
retaining retractor
vein hook retractor
vein retractor
ventriculogram retractor
Verbrugge retractor
vertical bone self-retaining
retractor
vertical retractor
vertical self-retaining bone
retractor
vesical retractor
vessel retractor
Viboch graft retractor
Viboch iliac graft retractor
Villalta retractor
Vinke retractor
Visitec iris retractor
Volkmann finger retractor
Volkmann hand retractor
Volkmann pocket retractor
Volkmann rake retractor
W.D. Johnson epicardial
retractor

retractor (*continued*)
Wachtenfeldt-Stille retractor
Walden-Aufricht nasal
retractor
Walker gallbladder retractor
Walker lid retractor
Walter nasal retractor
Walter-Deaver retractor
Wangensteen retractor
Weary nerve hook retractor
Weary nerve root retractor
Webb retractor
Webb-Balfour abdominal
retractor
Webb-Balfour retractor
Webb-Balfour self-retaining
abdominal retractor
Webb-Balfour self-retaining
retractor
Weber retractor
Webster abdominal retractor
Weder retractor
Weder-Solenberger pillar
retractor
Weder-Solenberger tonsil
pillar retractor
Weder-Solenberger tonsillar
retractor
weighted posterior retractor
weighted retractor
Weinberg Joe's hoe double-
ended retractor
Weinberg vagotomy retractor
Weinstein horizontal
retractor
Weinstein intestinal retractor
Weitlaner brain retractor
Weitlaner hinged retractor
Weitlaner microsurgery
retractor
Weitlaner self-retaining
retractor
Wellington Hospital vaginal
retractor
Welsh iris retractor
Wesson perineal retractor
Wesson perineal self-retaining
retractor
Wesson vaginal retractor
Wexler abdominal retractor
Wexler Bantam self-retaining
retractor

retractor (*continued*)
  Wexler deep-spreader blade abdominal retractor
  Wexler large-frame abdominal retractor
  Wexler lateral side-blade abdominal retractor
  Wexler malleable-blade abdominal retractor
  Wexler self-retaining retractor
  Wexler Universal joint abdominal retractor
  Wexler vaginal retractor
  Wexler X-P large abdominal retractor
  Wexler-Balfour retractor
  Wexler-Bantam retractor
  White-Lillie retractor
  White-Proud uvular retractor
  Wichman retractor
  Wieder dental retractor
  Wieder pillar retractor
  Wieder-Solenberger pillar retractor
  Wiet retractor
  Wigderson ribbon retractor
  Wilder scleral self-retaining retractor
  Wilkes self-retaining retractor
  Wilkinson abdominal retractor
  Wilkinson abdominal self-retaining retractor
  Wilkinson ring-frame abdominal retractor
  Wilkinson self-retaining abdominal retractor
  Wilkinson-Deaver blade abdominal retractor
  Willauer-Deaver retractor
  Williams microlumbar retractor
  Williams rod self-retaining retractor
  Willis retractor
  Wills eye lacrimal retractor
  Wilmer cryosurgical iris retractor
  Wilmer iris retractor
  Wilmer-Bagley retractor
  Wilson retractor
  Wiltse iliac retractor

retractor (*continued*)
  Wiltse-Bankart retractor
  Wiltse-Gelpi self-retaining retractor
  Winsburg-White retractor
  wiring retractor
  Wise orbital retractor
  Wolf meniscal retractor
  Wolfson gallbladder retractor
  Woodward retractor
  Worrall deep retractor
  Wort antral retractor
  Wullstein ear self-retaining retractor
  Wullstein self-retaining ear retractor
  Wullstein-Weitlaner self-retaining retractor
  Wylie renal vein retractor
  Wylie splanchnic retractor
  Yasargil retractor
  Yasargil-Leyla brain retractor
  Young anterior prostatic retractor
  Young bifid retractor
  Young bladder retractor
  Young bulb retractor
  Young lateral prostatic retractor
  Young lateral retractor
  Young prostatic retractor
  Yu-Holtgrewe prostatic retractor
  Z retractor
  Zalkind lung retractor
  Zalkind-Balfour center-blade retractor
  Zalkind-Balfour self-retaining retractor
  Zenker retractor
  Zimberg esophageal hiatal retractor
  Zylik-Michaels retractor
retractor blade
retractor clip
retractor hook
retractor oval sprocket frame
retractor plication
retractor-speculum (*see* retractor, speculum)
  Aufricht retractor-speculum
retrieval balloon

retrieval device
retrieval forceps
retrieval loop
retriever
  3-pronged polyp retriever
  basket retriever
  Brimfield magnetic retriever
  Carroll tendon retriever
  Entract stone retriever
  Kleinert-Kutz tendon retriever
  magnetic retriever
  Magnetriever ureteral stent
    retriever
  Pfister-Schwartz stone
    retriever
  plaque retriever
  Positrap retriever
  snail-headed catheter retriever
  Soehendra stent retriever
  stone retriever
  ureteral stone retriever
  Vantec loop retriever
  Warren-Wilder retriever
  Wilson-Cook ministent
    retriever
retroacetabular lesion
retroadductor space
retroareolar mass
retroauricular artery
retroauricular free flap
retroauricular incision
retroauricular sulcus
retroauricular vein
retrobulbar abscess
retrobulbar anesthesia
retrobulbar anesthetic
  technique
retrobulbar block
retrobulbar hematoma
retrobulbar hemorrhage
retrobulbar injection
retrobulbar needle
retrobulbar nerve block
retrobulbar neuralgia
retrobulbar orbital metastasis
retrobulbar prosthesis needle
retrobulbar pupillary reflex
retrobulbar space
retrocalcaneal
retrocardiac region
retrocardiac space
retrocaval ureter

retrocecal abscess
retrocecal appendix
retrocecal hernia
retrocentral sulcus
retrocession
retrochiasmal lesion
retroclavicular injury
retroclusion
retrococcygeal air study
retrocochlear
retrocolic anastomosis
retrocolic
  choledochojejunostomy
retrocolic end-to-side
  choledochojejunostomy
retrocolic end-to-side
  gastrojejunostomy
retrocolic hernia
retrocolic position
retrocorneal membrane
retrocrural celiac plexus block
retrocrural space
retrocuspid papilla
retrodiskal temporomandibular
  joint pad inflammation
retrodisplaced maxilla
retrodisplaced pessary
retrodisplacement
retroduodenal fossa
retroduodenal perforation
retroesophageal aorta
retroesophageal space
retroflexed cystoscopy sheath
retroflexed uterus
retroflexion
retrogasserian neurotomy
retrogasserian procedure
retrogasserian rhizotomy
retrogastric space
retrogenia
retrogeniculate lesion
retroglandular megapockets
retroglandular sulcus
retrognathia
  inferior retrognathia
  mandibular retrognathia
  maxillary retrognathia
  superior maxillary
    retrognathia
retrognathic mandible
retrognathic profile
retrognathism

retrograde aortogram
retrograde arteriogram
retrograde atherectomy
retrograde balloon rupture
retrograde Beaver blade
retrograde bougie
retrograde cannulation
retrograde cardiac perfusion
retrograde catheter insertion
retrograde catheterization
retrograde cholangiogram
retrograde cholecystectomy
retrograde curet
retrograde cystogram
retrograde direction
retrograde dissection
retrograde electrode
retrograde endoscopic approach
retrograde fashion
retrograde femoral approach
retrograde femoral catheter
retrograde filling
retrograde flow
retrograde hernia
retrograde injection
retrograde insertion point
retrograde intrarenal surgery
retrograde intussusception
retrograde knife
retrograde meniscal blade
retrograde occlusion balloon
     catheter
retrograde perfused
     fasciocutaneous flap
retrograde peristalsis
retrograde pyelogram
retrograde tracheal intubation
     anesthetic technique
retrograde ureterogram
retrograde urogram
retrograde valve
retrograde valvuloplasty
retrograde venous drainage
retrograde-cutting hook-shaped
     knife
retrograde-flow flap
Retrografin dye
retrohyoid bursa
retroiliac ureter
retroinclination
retroinclined maxilla
retroinguinal space

retrojection
retrolabyrinthine presigmoid
     approach
retrolental space
retrolenticular
retrolingual
retrolisthesis
retromammary abscess
retromammary bursa
retromammary space
retromammary view
retromammilar mass
retromandibular fossa
retromandibular point
retromandibular triangle
retromandibular vein
retromanubrial
retromastoid craniotomy
retromastoid Ommaya reservoir
retromastoid suboccipital
     craniectomy
Retromax endopyelotomy stent
retromaxillary prognathism
retromolar fossa
retromolar mucosa
retromolar pad
retromolar triangle
retromolar trigone
retromuscular position
retromuscular prosthetic
     technique
retromuscular space
retromylohyoid eminence
retromylohyoid space
retronasal
retro-ocular space
retro-orbicularis fat pad (ROOF)
retro-orbicularis fat pad release
retro-orbicularis ocular fat
     (ROOF)
retro-orbicularis ocular fat pad
     excision
retropapillary apex
retroparotid space
retropatellar fat pad
retropectoral placement
retroperfusion
retroperfusion catheter
retroperfusion pump
retroperitoneal abscess
retroperitoneal adenopathy
retroperitoneal anastomosis

retroperitoneal approach
retroperitoneal bleeding
retroperitoneal cavity
retroperitoneal decompression
retroperitoneal fistula
retroperitoneal gas insufflation
retroperitoneal hematoma
retroperitoneal hemorrhage
retroperitoneal hernia
retroperitoneal injection of air
retroperitoneal lymph node
retroperitoneal
    lymphadenectomy
retroperitoneal pelvic lymph
    node dissection (RPLND)
retroperitoneal perforation
retroperitoneal space
retroperitoneal tumor
retroperitoneal-iliopsoas
    abscess
retroperitoneum
retropexy
retropharyngeal abscess
retropharyngeal approach
retropharyngeal edema
retropharyngeal hematoma
retropharyngeal hemorrhage
retropharyngeal space
retroplacental hematoma
retroplacental lucencies
retroposition
retropubic
    colpourethrocystopexy
retropubic hernia
retropubic Lapides-Ball bladder
    neck suspension
retropubic placement
retropubic prevesical
    prostatectomy
retropubic prostatectomy
retropubic prostatectomy
    retractor
retropubic retractor
retropubic space
retropulsed bone excision
retropulsion
retropulsion of nail
retrorectal abscess
retrorectal lymph node
retroreflective marker
retroscopic lens
retroseptal space

retroseptal transconjunctival
    approach
retrosigmoid approach
retrosinus
retrospective bronchoscopic
    telescope
retrosphenoidal syndrome
retrosternal abnormality
retrosternal air space
retrosternal dislocation
retrosternal fat pad
retrosternal gland
retrosternal hernia
retrosternal nodule
retrosternal pain
retrosternal thyroid
retrotarsal fold
retrotorsion
retrotracheal space
retrotragal incision
retrotuberosity mucosa
retrotuberous mucosa
retrourethral catheterization
retrouterine hematocele
retrouterine hematoma
retrovaginal hernia
retrovaginal septum
retroversion pessary
retroverted uterus
retrovesical space
retrovisceral space
retrozygomatic space
retruded angle of the forehead
retruded centric
retruded contact
retruded jaw relation
retruded mandible
retruded position
retrusion
    bony retrusion
    mandibular retrusion
    maxillary retrusion
    midfacial retrusion
retrusion of the base of the
    columella
retrusive excursion
retrusive movement
retrusive occlusion
Retter aneurysm needle
return-flow cannula
return-flow catheter
return-flow hemostatic catheter

return-flow retention catheter
returning cartilage
Retzius cavity
Retzius space
Retzius veins
Reuben insufflator
Reul aortic clamp
Reul coronary artery scissors
Reul coronary forceps
reuniens duct
ReUnite hand fixation
ReUnite orthopedic pin
ReUnite orthopedic screw
reusable incontinence pant
reusable laparoscopic electrode
reusable vein stripper
Reuse Expanda-graft
    dermatotome
Reuss table
Reuter bobbin
Reuter bobbin collar button
Reuter bobbin implant
Reuter bobbin stainless steel
    drain tube
Reuter bobbin tube
Reuter bobbin ventilation tube
Reuter button
Reuter stainless steel bobbin
Reuter suprabubic trocar
Reuter suprapubic cannula
Reuter tube
Reuter-Wolfe trocar
revascularization
    cardiac revascularization
    myocardial revascularization
    Vineberg cardiac
        revascularization
revascularized bone graft
Reveal camera
Reveal single lens reflex camera
Revelation endocardial
    microcatheter
Revelation Tx microcatheter
reverberation
Reverdin abdominal spatula
Reverdin bunionectomy
Reverdin epidermal free graft
Reverdin graft
Reverdin holder
Reverdin implant
Reverdin operation
Reverdin osteotomy

Reverdin prosthesis
Reverdin skin graft
Reverdin suturing needle
Reverdin-Green bunion
    procedure
Reverdin-Laird bunionectomy
Reverdin-McBride
    bunionectomy
reversal jejunoileal bypass
    surgery
reversal of cervical curve
reversal of lumbar curve
reversal pedicle flap
reverse adenotome
reverse anaphylaxis
reverse augmentation
reverse bandage
reverse Barton fracture
reverse Bennett fracture
reverse bevel incision
reverse Bigelow maneuver
reverse Cole arthrodesis
reverse Colles fracture
reverse crossfinger flap
reverse digital artery flap
reverse digital artery island flap
reverse dorsal digital island flap
reverse Eck fistula
reverse facial osteotomy
reverse filling procedure
reverse flaring
reverse flow
reverse flow island flap
reverse flow vascularization
reverse forearm island flap
reverse gastrectomy
reverse gastric tube
    esophagoplasty
reverse Hill-Sachs lesion
reverse Karapandzic flap
reverse Kingsley splint
reverse knuckle-bender splint
reverse Mauck procedure
reverse medial arm flap
reverse Monteggia fracture
reverse muscle flap
reverse Putti-Platt procedure
reverse Robert view radiograph
reverse scissors
reverse sigma penoscrotal
    transposition repair
reverse sphincterotome

reverse Trendelenburg position
reverse U-flap
reverse ulnar hypothenar flap
    finger reconstruction
reverse Waters x-ray position
reverse wedge technique
reverse-action hypophysectomy
    forceps
reverse-angle skid curet
reverse-bevel laryngoscope
reverse-curve adenoid curet
reverse-curve clamp
reverse-cutting meniscal probe
reverse-cutting needle
reverse-cutting probe
reverse-cutting scissors
reverse-cutting sutures
reversed arm leads
reversed bandage
reversed bypass
reversed digital artery flap
reversed dorsal digital flap
reversed extensor digitorum
    muscle island flap
reversed extensor digitorum
    muscle island flap
    procedure
reversed fasciosubcutaneous
    flap
reversed island flaps for forefoot
    reconstruction
reversed left saphenous vein
    bypass graft
reversed pedicle flap
reversed peristalsis
reversed reimplanted
    appendicocystostomy
reversed rhythm
reversed shunt (right-to-left)
reversed-3 sign
reverse-flow vascularized bone
    graft
reverse-shape eye implant
reverse-shape implant
reverse-threaded screw
reverse-type mastoid
    fasciocutaneous flap
reverse-Y incision
reversible decortication
reversible hydrocolloid
    impression material
reversible ischemic defect

reversible ischemic neurological
    defect (RIND)
reversible knife
reversible lid speculum
reversible perfusion defect
reversible reaction
reversion pacemaker
reverted to normal position
reverting scope
revised wound margins
revision
    debridement and revision
    Dibbell cleft lip-nasal revision
    free flap for burn scar
        revision
    fusiform skin revision
    plastic revision
    scar revision
    W-plasty in scar revision
    W-plasty revision
    Z-plasty revision
revision and closure
revision and debridement
revision conical reamer
revision hip arthroplasty
revision laparoscopy
ReVision nail
revision of amputation stump
revision of graft
revision of scar
revision procedure
revision rhinoplasty
revision tip rhinoplasty
RevitaLase erbium cosmetic laser
Revivac catheter
Revive system penile prosthesis
revivification
Revo loop handle knot pusher
Revo retrievable cancellous
    screw
Revo suture anchor
Revolution lens
revolutions per minute (rpm)
revolving pin
revolving-door island flap
Revots vulsellum tenaculum
Rew-Wyly blade
Rew-Wyly mouth gag
Rex-Cantli-Serege line
Reynolds-Horton alar cartilage
    technique
Reynolds dissecting clamp

Reynolds dissecting scissors
Reynolds infusion catheter
Reynolds resection clamp
Reynolds tongs
Reynolds tube
Reynolds vascular clamp
Reynolds-Jameson vessel scissors
Reynold-Southwick H-graft
    portacaval shunt
Rezaian interbody external
    fixation device
Rezek forceps
Rezifilm dressing
Rezi-last spray-on dressing
Rezinian spinal fixator
Reziplast spray-on dressing
RF (rheumatoid factor)
RF Ablatr ablation catheter
RF balloon catheter
RF Marinr catheter
RF Performer catheter
RFAC-assisted microdisc
    decompression
R-HAB lighter weight ankle
    prosthesis
rhabdoid suture
rhabdomyolysis
rhabdomyoma
rhabdomyosarcoma
rhachotomy
rhagades
rhagadiform
rhegmatogenous retinal
    detachment
Rhein 3-D trapezoid diamond
    blade
Rhein Advantage diamond knife
Rhein capsulorrhexis cystitome
    forceps
Rhein clear corneal diamond
    knife
Rhein fine foldable lens-
    insertion forceps
Rhein pick
Rhein reusable cautery pen
Rheinberg microscope
Rheinstaedter flushing curet
Rheinstaedter uterine curet
rheologic therapy
rheolytic catheter
rheostosis
Rhese position

rheumatic mitral valve
rheumatic nodule
rheumatic scoliosis
rheumatic valvular disease
rheumatoid arthritis (RA)
rheumatoid clawing
rheumatoid factor (RF)
rheumatoid osteoarthritis
rheumatoid pannus
rheumatoid sialadenitis
rheumatoid vasculitis
rhGH (recombinant human
    growth hormone)
rhIGF (recombinant human
    insulin-like growth factor)
Rhinelander clamp
Rhinelander guide
Rhinelander pin
Rhinelander plate
rhinion
    fracture at the rhinion
rhinitis medicamentosa
rhinitis sicca
Rhino Rocket dressing
Rhino Rocket injector
Rhino Rocket nasal packing
Rhino Triangle brace
Rhino Triangle hip abduction
    brace
rhinocanthectomy
rhinocephaly
rhinocerebral mucormycosis
rhinocheiloplasty
rhinocleisis
rhinodacryolith
rhinodymia
rhinofacial
    entomophthoramycosis
rhinokyphectomy
rhinokyphosis
rhinolaryngoscope
rhinolith
rhinolithiasis
rhinomanometer
rhinomanometry
rhinometer
rhinometry
rhinomyomectomy
rhinonecrosis
rhino-orbital mucormycosis
rhino-orbitocerebral
    mucormycosis

rhinophycomycosis
rhinophyma
rhinoplastic correction
rhinoplasty
  adjunctive rhinoplasty
  Bardach cleft rhinoplasty
  Carpue rhinoplasty
  cleft rhinoplasty
  closed rhinoplasty
  conservative subtraction-
    addition rhinoplasty (CSAR)
  cosmetic rhinoplasty
  Cottle rhinoplasty
  dactylocostal rhinoplasty
  endonasal rhinoplasty
  English rhinoplasty
  esthetic rhinoplasty
  extended open-tip
    rhinoplasty
  functional rhinoplasty
  Indian rhinoplasty
  Italian rhinoplasty
  Joseph rhinoplasty
  minimal rhinoplasty
  open rhinoplasty
  open-sky rhinoplasty
  orthoplastic rhinoplasty
  osteoplastic rhinoplasty
  posttraumatic rhinoplasty
  realignment rhinoplasty
  reconstructive rhinoplasty
  revision tip rhinoplasty
  secondary rhinoplasty
  strut rhinoplasty
  submucous resection and
    rhinoplasty
  tagliacotian rhinoplasty
  tension-control suture
    technique in open
    rhinoplasty
  tip rhinoplasty
rhinoplasty and submucous
  resection
rhinoplasty diamond bur
rhinoplasty implant
rhinoplasty saw
rhinoplasty scissors
rhinorrhagia
rhinorrhaphy
rhinorrhea
  cerebrospinal fluid
    rhinorrhea

rhinorrhea (*continued*)
  cerebrospinal rhinorrhea
  CFS rhinorrhea
  gustatory rhinorrhea
  halo test for CSF rhinorrhea
  ipsilateral rhinorrhea
rhinoscleroma
rhinoscope
  Wolf-Post rhinoscope
  Wylie-Post rhinoscope
rhinoscopic mirror
rhinoscopy
  anterior rhinoscopy
  median rhinoscopy
rhinoseptal approach
rhinoseptoplasty
rhinosinusitis
rhinostomy
rhinotomy
rhinovirus
rhizodontropy
rhizolysis
rhizotomy
  anterior rhizotomy
  Dana rhizotomy
  Dandy rhizotomy
  dorsal rhizotomy
  facet rhizotomy
  Fasano test during rhizotomy
  posterior rhizotomy
  retrogasserian rhizotomy
  suboccipital trigeminal
    rhizotomy
  trigeminal rhizotomy
  ventral nerve root rhizotomy
rhodamine laser
Rhode Island dissector
rhodium filter
rhomboid aponeurosis
rhomboid flap
rhomboid fossa
rhomboid glossitis
rhomboid ligament
rhomboid muscle
rhomboid of Michaelis
rhomboid swelling
rhomboid transposition flap
rhonchi (*sing.* rhonchus)
rhonchi and rales
Rhoton 3-prong fork
Rhoton ball dissector
Rhoton bayonet needle holder

Rhoton bayonet scissors
Rhoton bipolar forceps
Rhoton blunt-ring curet
Rhoton cup forceps
Rhoton dissection
Rhoton dural forceps
Rhoton elevator
Rhoton enucleator
Rhoton grasping forceps
Rhoton horizontal-ring curet
Rhoton loop curet
Rhoton microcup forceps
Rhoton microcuret
Rhoton microdissecting forceps
Rhoton microdissector
Rhoton microforceps
Rhoton microneedle holder
Rhoton microscissors
Rhoton microsurgical scissors
Rhoton microtying forceps
Rhoton microvascular forceps
Rhoton nerve hook
Rhoton neurodissector
Rhoton osteotome
Rhoton pituitary curet
Rhoton punch
Rhoton ring tumor forceps
Rhoton round dissector
Rhoton sellar punch
Rhoton spatula dissector
Rhoton spoon curet
Rhoton straight point needle
Rhoton tissue forceps
Rhoton titanium microscissors
Rhoton transsphenoidal bipolar
   forceps
Rhoton tying forceps
Rhoton vertical ring curet
Rhoton-Adson dressing forceps
Rhoton-Adson tissue forceps
Rhoton-Cushing tissue forceps
Rhoton-Merz rotatable coupling
   head
Rhoton-Merz suction tube
Rhoton-Tew bipolar forceps
Rhyder diagnostic catheter
rhythm
   analogous rhythm
   bigeminal rhythm
   cantering rhythm
   cardiac rhythm
   converted rhythm

rhythm (*continued*)
   coupled rhythm
   ectopic rhythm
   erratic heart rhythm
   escape rhythm
   fetal rhythm
   fibrillation rhythm
   force and rhythm (F&R)
   gallop rhythm
   heart rhythm
   idionodal rhythm
   idioventricular rhythm
   irregular heart rhythm
   irregularly irregular rhythm
   junctional rhythm
   mixed rhythm
   pacemaker rhythm
   pendulum rhythm
   reciprocal rhythm
   regular rate and rhythm
   regular sinus rhythm
   reversed rhythm
   sensorimotor rhythm
   sinus rhythm
   spike rhythm
rhythm strip
rhythmia
rhythmic activity
rhythmic breathing
rhythmic initiation technique
rhythmic stabilization
rhythmic wave
rhythmic waxing and waning
rhythmic, rhythmical
rhytid
   forehead rhytids
   glabellar rhytids
   horizontal rhytids
   minor rhytids
   periocular rhytids
   shoulder of rhytid
   superficial rhytids
   transverse rhytids
   vertical lateral glabellar
      rhytids
rhytidectomy
   bidirectional rhytidectomy
   cervicofacial rhytidectomy
   complex superficial
      musculoaponeurotic system
      rhytidectomy
   composite rhytidectomy

rhytidectomy (*continued*)
  deep-plane rhytidectomy
  extended posterior
    rhytidectomy
  full-thickness skin
    rhytidectomy
  platysma rhytidectomy
  SASMAS suspension
    rhytidectomy
  Skoog rhytidectomy
  subcutaneous rhytidectomy
  sub-SMAS rhytidectomy
  superficial plane rhytidectomy
  superficial SMAS
    rhytidectomy
rhytidectomy scissors
rhytidoplasty
RIA (radioimmunoassay)
Riahl coronary compressor
rib
  asternal rib
  bicipital rib
  cervical rib
  component ribs
  contiguous rib
  double-exposed rib
  extrapleural resection of rib
  false ribs
  floating ribs
  rudimentary ribs
  Sauerbruch elevator for first
    rib
  slipping ribs
  true ribs
  vertebral ribs
  vertebrocostal ribs
  vertebrosternal ribs
  Zahn ribs
rib approximator
rib belt
rib brad awl
rib cage
rib cartilage
rib contractor (*see* contractor)
rib costochondral dorsal onlay
    graft
rib cutter
rib drill
rib elevator
rib elevator and raspatory
rib elevator and stripper
rib field treatment

rib graft
rib guillotine
rib involvement
rib lesion
rib needle
rib notches
rib raspatory
rib removal
rib retractor
rib rongeur
rib rongeur forceps
rib shears (*see* shears)
rib spreader (*see* spreader)
rib stripper (*see* stripper)
rib tip syndrome
Riba electric ureteral meatotome
Riba electrourethrotome
    electrode
Riba urethrotome
Riba-Valeira forceps
ribbed hook
Ribble bandage
Ribble dressing
ribbon arch appliance
ribbon arch technique
ribbon blade
ribbon gauze dressing
ribbon gut needle
ribbon gut sutures
ribbon malleable retractor
ribbon muscles
ribbon retractor
ribbon stools
ribbonlike keratitis
ribbon-shaped stools
rib-edge stripper
Ribes ganglion
rib-vertebral angle
Rica anesthetic laryngoscope
Rica aneurysm needle
Rica anterior commissure
    laryngoscope
Rica arterial clamp
Rica bone drill
Rica bone hammer
Rica bone mallet
Rica bone retractor
Rica bone rongeur
Rica brain retractor
Rica brain spatula
Rica cerebral angiography
    puncture needle

Rica cerumen hook
Rica clip-applying forceps
Rica cotton carrier
Rica cranial rongeur
Rica cranioclast
Rica cross-action towel clip
Rica dermatome
Rica ear curet
Rica ear polypus scissors
Rica ear probe
Rica ear speculum
Rica esophagoscopy set
Rica eustachian catheter
Rica forceps holder
Rica hemostatic forceps
Rica infant laryngoscope
Rica laminectomy rongeur
Rica lipoma curet
Rica malleus head nipper
Rica mastoid chisel
Rica mastoid curet
Rica mastoid gouge
Rica mastoid retractor
Rica mastoid rongeur
Rica mastoid suction tube
Rica microarterial clamp
Rica multipurpose retractor
Rica myringotome
Rica nasal septal speculum
Rica pelvimeter
Rica pneumatic otoscope
Rica posterior cranial fossa
    retractor
Rica rongeur
Rica scalp retractor
Rica silver clip
Rica skull perforator set
Rica spinal rongeur
Rica stem clamp
Rica surgical catgut
Rica suture clip
Rica suturing needle
Rica tracheostomy cannula
Rica trigeminal knife
Rica tuning fork
Rica Universal trocar
Rica uterine curet
Rica uterine sound
Rica vaginal speculum
Rica vessel clamp
Rica wire guide pin
Rica wire saw

Rica-Adson forceps
Ricard abdominal retractor
Ricard amputation
Rich forceps
Richard Gruber speculum
Richard Wolf arthroscope
Richard Wolf laparoscopic
    trocar
Richard Wolf diagnostic
    laparoscope
Richard Wolf operating
    laparoscope
Richard-Allan surgical ruler
Richards abdominal retractor
Richards adjustable hip screw
Richards adjustable-angle guide
Richards barrel guide
Richards barrel reamer
Richards bone clamp
Richards bone curet
Richards bone hook
Richards calibrated reamer
Richards calibrated-tip threaded
    guide
Richards chisel
Richards clamp
Richards classic compression
    hip screw
Richards Colles fracture frame
Richards combination mallet
Richards compression device
Richards compression screw
Richards curet
Richards drape
Richards drill guide
Richards ethmoid curet
Richards external fixation
    device for fractures
Richards fixation staple
Richards forceps
Richards headrest
Richards hip screw plate
Richards hydroxyapatite PORP
    prosthesis
Richards hydroxyapatite TORP
    prosthesis
Richards lag screw
Richards lag screw compression
    device
Richards locking rod
Richards mastoid curet
Richards mastoid ethmoid curet

Richards maximum contact cruciate-sparing prosthesis
Richards maximum contact total knee prosthesis (RMC total knee prosthesis)
Richards ministaple
Richards nail
Richards Phillips screwdriver
Richards pillow
Richards pistol-grip drill
Richards probe
Richards prosthesis
Richards screw
Richards side plate
Richards stationary-angle guide
Richards tonsil-grasping forceps
Richards tonsillar forceps
Richards tonsil-seizing forceps
Richards Zirconia femoral head prosthesis
Richards-Andrews forceps
Richards-Cobb spinal elevator
Richards-Cobb spinal gouge
Richards-Hibbs chisel
Richards-Hibbs gouge
Richards-Hibbs osteotome
Richards-Hirschhorn plate
Richards-Lovejoy bone drill
Richards-Moeller pneumatic air-filled dilator
Richardson abdominal retractor
Richardson angle sutures
Richardson appendectomy retractor
Richardson hemostat
Richardson operation
Richardson periosteal elevator
Richardson polyethylene tube introducer
Richardson procedure
Richardson retractor
Richardson right-angle ear knife
Richardson right-angle knife
Richardson rod
Richardson suture technique
Richardson sutures
Richardson technique
Richardson-Eastman double-ended retractor
Richards-Saltzman-Flynn technique
Richards-Schaefer gonioscope

Riche-Cannieu anastomosis
Riches artery forceps
Riches bladder syringe
Riches diathermy forceps
Richet aneurysm
Richet bandage
Richet dressing
Richet operation
Richey condyle marker
Richie brace
Rich-Mar 510 external ultrasound
Richmond bolt
Richmond forceps
Richmond screw
Richmond subarachnoid screw
Richmond subarachnoid twist drill
Richter bone drill
Richter episiotomy scissors
Richter hernia
Richter laminectomy punch
Richter retractor
Richter scissors
Richter screwdriver
Richter suture clip-removing forceps
Richter suture technique
Richter sutures
Richter vaginal retractor
Richter-Heath clip-removing forceps
Richter-Monro line
Richwil bridge remover
Richwil crown remover
Ricketts-Abrams technique
Rickham cup
Rickham reservoir
Rickham reservoir shunt
Riddle coagulator
Rideau technique
Ridell operation
Rider-Moeller cardiac dilator
Rider-Moeller needle
Rider-Moeller pneumatic dilator
rider's bone
rider's muscle
rider's sprain
rider's tendon
ridge
    alveolar ridge
    anatomic ridge

ridge (*continued*)
  bicoronal ridge
  bladder neck ridge
  bony ridge
  buccal cervical ridge
  buccal ridge
  buccal triangular ridge (BTR)
  center of ridge
  crest of alveolar ridge
  crest of ridge
  digastric ridge
  epidermal ridges
  epithelial ridge
  external oblique ridge
  healing ridge
  internal occipital ridge
  interpapillary ridges
  intertrochanteric ridge
  interureteric ridge
  Irv ridge
  key ridge
  linguocervical ridge
  linguogingival ridge
  mammary ridge
  mandibular ridge
  marginal ridge
  maxillary ridge
  mental ridge
  mylohyoid ridge
  nasal ridge
  nuchal ridge
  orbital ridge
  orbitozygomaticomalar bone
    ridge
  Outerbridge ridge
  palatine ridge
  Passavant ridge
  petrosal ridge
  petrous ridge
  residual ridge
  rete ridges
  sphenoidal ridge
  sublingual ridge
  superior petrosal ridge
  support ridge
  supraorbital ridge
  transverse palatine ridge
  trochlear ridge
  ureteric ridge
  vomerine ridge
  zygomaxillare ridge
ridge augmentation

ridge extension
ridge forceps
ridge of mandibular neck
ridge relation
ridged-convoluted villi
ridging
riding embolus
riding-pants deformity
Ridley anterior chamber implant
Ridley anterior chamber lens
    implant
Ridley forceps
Ridley implant cataract lens
Ridley lens
Ridley Mark II lens implant
Ridley operation
Ridley sinus
Ridlon hip dislocation
Ridlon knife
Ridlon operation
Ridlon plaster knife
Ridlon procedure
Ridlon spreader
Ridpath ethmoid curet
Riecker bronchoscope
Riecker respiration
    bronchoscope
Riecker-Kleinsasser
    laryngoscope
Riedel corneal needle
Riedel frontal ethmoidectomy
Riedel frontoethmoidectomy
    procedure
Riedel lobe of liver
Riedel needle
Riedel struma
Rieger stethoscope
Rieger syndrome
Riehl melanoderma
Riehl melanosis
Rienhoff arterial clamp
Rienhoff arterial forceps
Rienhoff clamp
Rienhoff dissector
Rienhoff forceps
Rienhoff general operating
    scissors
Rienhoff needle holder
Rienhoff rib spreader
Rienhoff thoracic scissors
Rienhoff-Finochietto rib
    contractor

Rienhoff-Finochietto rib
  spreader
Rienhoff-Tanner operation
Rienke space
Riepe gastric bubble
Riepe-Bard gastric balloon
Riester otoscope
Ries-Wertheim hysterectomy
Rieux hernia
RIF (rigid internal fixation)
Rife machine
Rifkind sign
Rigal sutures
Rigaud operation
Rigby abdominal retractor
Rigby appendectomy retractor
Rigby bivalve retractor
Rigby rectal retractor
Rigby vaginal retractor
Rigg cannula
Righini procedure
right acromiodorsoposterior
  position
right anterior oblique position
right anterior pararenal space
right antero-oblique position
right aortic arch
right atrial cuff
right bronchus
right bundle-branch block
right caudate lobe
Right Clip applier
right colic artery
right colic vein
right colon
right colonic flexure
right coronary artery
right coronary catheter
right decubitus position
right ear (AD)
right frontal sinus
right gastric artery
right gastric vein
right gastroepiploic artery
right gastroepiploic vein
right gutter
right heart bypass
right heart catheterization
right hemicolectomy
right hemodiaphragm
right hepatic duct
right hilum

right hypogastric nerve
right inferior pulmonary vein
right inguinal hernia (RIH)
right Judkins catheter
right lateral excursion
right lateral position
right lobe hepatectomy
right lower lobe (RLL)
right lower quadrant (RLQ)
right lymphatic duct
right mentoanterior position
  (RMA position)
right mentoposterior position
  (RMP position)
right mentotransverse position
  (RMT position)
right midinguinal line
right occipitoanterior position
  (ROA position)
right occipitoposterior position
  (ROP position)
right occipitotranverse position
  (ROT position)
right ovarian vein
right pulmonary artery
right rectus incision
right sacroanterior position
  (RSA position)
right sacroposterior position
  (RSP position)
right sagittal fissure
right scapuloanterior position
  (RScA position)
right scapuloposterior position
  (RScP position)
right segmental
  mandibulectomy
right superior pulmonary vein
right suprarenal vein
right temporoparietal
  craniotomy
right testicular vein
right umbilical fold
right upper lobe (RUL)
right upper paramedian incision
right upper quadrant (RUQ)
right venous angle
right ventricle
right ventricle-pulmonary artery
  conduit surgery
right ventricular assist device
right ventricular coil

right ventricular inflow tract
right ventricular outflow tract
right ventricular wall device
right-angle bipolar cautery
right-angle blunt probe
right-angle booster clip
right-angle chest catheter
right-angle chest tube
right-angle clamp
right-angle colon clamp
right-angle curet
right-angle drill
right-angle electrode
right-angle elevator
right-angle examining telescope
right-angle forceps
right-angle hook
right-angle knife
right-angle lens
right-angle mattress sutures
right-angle pick
right-angle retractor
right-angle scissors
right-angle technique
right-angle telescope
right-angled bone cutter
right-angled end-to-side
    anastomosis
right-angled erysiphake
right-angled telescopic lens
right-curved scissors
right-handed
right-handed corneal scissors
right-sided injury
right-sided lesion
right-sided submandibular
    transverse incision
right-side-down position
right-to-left shunt
rigid abdomen
rigid ball-shaped alar cartilages
rigid biopsy forceps
rigid cervical immobilization
rigid curet
rigid endoscope
rigid endoscopic surgery
rigid endosonography probe
rigid external distraction (RED)
rigid fixation
rigid gas-permeable contact lens
rigid graft
rigid holding rod

rigid hymen
rigid internal fixation (RIF)
rigid internal fixation device
rigid intranasal endoscope
rigid intraocular lens
rigid kidney stone forceps
rigid lag screw fixation
rigid neck rake retractor
rigid orthosis
rigid pedicle screw
rigid plate fixation
rigid postoperative brace
rigid posture
rigid scoop
rigid sigmoidoscope
rigid sigmoidoscopy
rigid sound
rigidity
    abdominal rigidity
    cerebellar rigidity
    clasp-knife rigidity
    cogwheel rigidity
    decerebrate rigidity
    decorticate rigidity
    guarding and/or rigidity
    hemiplegic rigidity
    muscular rigidity
    mydriatic rigidity
    nuchal rigidity
    pathologic rigidity
    torsional rigidity
    waxlike rigidity
Rigiflator hand-held
    inflation/deflation device
Rigiflex ABD balloon dilatation
    catheter
Rigiflex achalasia balloon
Rigiflex achalasia balloon
    dilator
Rigiflex balloon
Rigiflex balloon dilator
Rigiflex biliary balloon dilatation
    catheter
Rigiflex dilator
Rigiflex OTW balloon dilatation
    catheter
Rigiflex TTS balloon
Rigiflex TTS balloon catheter
Rigiflex TTS balloon dilatation
    catheter
Rigiflex TTS balloon dilator
RigiScan device

RigiScan penile tumescence and
   rigidity monitor
Rigler sign
RIJ catheter
RIK Defender prevention
   mattress
RIK fluid mattress
Riley arterial needle
Riley-Day syndrome
Riley-Smith syndrome
rim
   acetabular rim
   alar rim
   fronto-orbital rim
   helical rim
   infraorbital rim
   intercartilaginous rim
   mandible rim
   narrow rim
   orbital rim
   outer rim
   piriform rim
   scleral rim
   superior orbital rim
   supraorbital rim
   veiling of the alar rim
rim incision
rim necrosis
rim resection
rim sign
rima (*pl.* rimae)
rima glottidis
rima oris
rima palpebrarum
rima vocalis
rim-enhancing lesion
RIND (reversible ischemic
   neurological deficit)
Rindfleisch folds
ring
   Abbe ring
   abdominal ring
   abscess ring
   Ace-Colles half ring
   Airy rings
   AnnuloFlex flexible
      annuloplasty ring
   anorectal ring
   aortic ring
   apex of external ring
   atrioventricular ring
   Bandl obstetric ring

ring (*continued*)
   Bickel ring
   biofragmentable anastomotic
      ring
   blepharostat ring
   Bloomberg SuperNumb
      anesthetic ring
   Bonaccolto scleral ring
   Bonaccolto-Flieringa scleral
      ring
   Bookwalter retractor ring
   Bookwalter segmented ring
   Bookwalter vaginal retractor
      ring
   Bores twist fixation ring
   Brown-Roberts-Wells base ring
   Budde halo ring
   Burr corneal ring
   Buzard-Thornton fixation ring
   Cannon ring
   Carpentier ring
   Carpentier-Edwards
      annuloplasty ring
   cartilage ring
   cartilaginous ring
   cataract mask ring
   CBI stereotactic ring
   centering ring
   Charnley centering ring
   Coats ring
   common tendinous ring
   confidence ring
   constriction ring
   constrictive ring
   contact ring
   Cook continence ring
   corneal ring
   corneal transplant centering
      ring
   Cosman-Roberts-Wells
      stereotactic ring
   Crawford suture ring
   cricoid ring
   deep inguinal ring
   distal esophageal ring
   double-flanged valve-sewing
      ring
   drop-lock ring
   Duran annuloplasty ring
   elastic O ring
   esophageal A ring
   esophageal B ring

ring (*continued*)
- esophageal contractile ring
- esophageal contraction ring
- esophageal mucosal ring
- esophageal muscular ring
- Estring estradiol vaginal ring
- Estring silicone vaginal ring
- external inguinal ring
- external ring
- Falope tubal sterilization ring
- Fine crescent fixation ring
- Fine-Thornton scleral fixation ring
- fixation ring
- Fleisher corneal ring
- Flieringa fixation ring
- Flieringa scleral ring
- Flieringa-Kayser fixation ring
- Flieringa-LeGrand fixation ring
- foam ring
- Gimbel stabilizing ring
- Girard scleral ring
- gold ring
- Graefenberg ring (*also* Gräfenberg)
- half ring
- halo ring
- head ring
- hymenal ring
- Ilizarov ring
- inguinal ring
- Intacs intrastromal corneal ring
- internal abdominal ring
- internal inguinal ring
- intrahaustral contraction ring
- intravaginal ring
- invalid ring
- Japanese erection ring
- Katena ring
- Kayser-Fleischer ring
- KeraVision Intacs intracorneal ring
- KF ring
- Klein-Tolentino ring
- knitted sewing ring
- Landers irrigating vitrectomy ring
- Landers vitrectomy ring
- Landolt C ring
- Landolt ring

ring (*continued*)
- laparotomy sponge ring
- Loomis ring
- Lowe ring
- lymphoid ring
- Lyon ring
- Magrina-Bookwalter vaginal retractor ring
- Martinez corneal transplant centering ring
- Mayo perfusing O ring
- McKinney fixation ring
- McNeill-Goldmann blepharostat ring
- McNeill-Goldmann scleral ring
- Mertz keratoscopy ring
- metal sewing ring
- mitral valve ring
- Moran-Karaya ring
- Moretsky LASIK hinge protector fixation ring
- Mose concentric ring
- Nakayama ring
- Nichamin fixation ring
- Ochsner ring
- O'Harris-Petruso ring
- olive ring
- orbicular ring
- Osbon pressure-point tension ring
- palatopharyngeal ring
- pediatric perineal retractor ring
- plastic sewing ring
- pressure ring
- pressure-point tension ring
- prosthetic valve sewing ring
- prosthetic valve suture ring
- Puig Massana-Shiley annuloplasty ring
- pyloric ring
- Racestyptine retraction ring
- reduction ring
- retainer ring
- retention ring
- retraction ring
- Schatzki esophageal ring
- scleral expander ring
- scleral ring
- Sculptor annuloplasty ring
- Sculptor flexible annuloplasty ring

ring (*continued*)
- semicircular rings
- sewing ring
- Silastic ring
- silicone elastomer ring
- silicone ring
- sizing ring
- SJM Sequin annuloplasty ring
- SJM Tailor annuloplasty ring
- Soemmering ring
- sphincter contraction ring
- sponge ring
- St. Jude annuloplasty ring
- Suarz continence ring
- suction ring
- superficial inguinal ring
- supra-annular suture ring
- suture ring
- symblepharon ring
- Tano ring
- tantalum O ring
- tantalum ring
- tendinous ring
- Thiersch ring
- third cartilaginous ring
- Thornton fixating ring
- Thornton-Fine ring
- titanium ring
- Tolentino ring
- tracheal rings
- Tru-Arc blood vessel ring
- tubal ring
- Turner-Warwick adult retractor ring
- Turner-Warwick pediatric perineal retractor ring
- umbilical ring
- Universal valve prosthesis sewing ring
- V1 halo ring
- vacuum fixation ring
- Valtrac absorbable biofragmentable anastomosis ring
- Valtrac anastomosis ring
- valve ring
- vascular ring
- Villasenor-Navarro fixation ring
- Vossius lenticular ring
- Waldeyer throat ring
- Waldeyer tonsillar ring

ring (*continued*)
- Walsh pressure ring
- Wolf-Yoon ring
- Yoon tubal sterilization ring
- zipper ring

ring abdominal retractor
ring abscess
ring applicator
ring avulsion injury
ring bayonet Rand curet
Ring biliary drainage catheter
ring biliary stent
ring block
ring block digital anesthetic
ring cataract mask
ring cataract mask eye shield
ring cataract mask shield
ring catheter
ring clamp
ring clip
ring curet
ring cushion
ring cutter
Ring drainage catheter needle
ring electrode
ring epiphyses
ring finger
ring forceps
ring fracture
ring graft
ring hip prosthesis
ring knee prosthesis
ring lens expressor
ring lesion
ring man shoulder
ring of bone
ring pessary
ring punch
ring remover
ring shadow
ring stripper
ring sublimis opponensplasty
ring tongue blade
ring total hip prosthesis
ring ulcer
ring ulcer of cornea
ring-cutting saw
ring-disrupting fracture
ringed formed forceps
Ringenberg electrode
Ringenberg rasp

Ringenberg stapedectomy
   forceps
ring-enhancing lesion
Ringer arthroscopy
Ringer's lactate solution
Ringer's solution
ring-handled bulldog clamp
ringing in ears
ring-jawed holding clamp
RingLoc instrument
Ring-McLean catheter
Ring-McLean sump tube
Ring-Moore total hip
ring-rotation forceps
ring-tip forceps
ring-toothed tenaculum
ring-type rigidity measuring
   device
ring-wall lesion
Rinman sign
Rinn XCP radiographic
   paralleling device
Rinne sign
Riolan anastomosis
Riolan arc
Riolan arcade
Riolan arch
Riolan bones
Riolan bouquet
Riolan muscle
Riordan flexible silver cannula
Riordan osteostat
Riordan pin
Riordan procedure
Riordan rasp
Riordan repair of muscle
Riordan tendon transfer
   technique
RIP plethysmograph
rip-cord suture
ripe cataract
ripe cervix
ripple deformity
ripple voltage
rippling
  implant rippling
  superior pole traction
    rippling
  underfill rippling
Ripstein anterior sling
   rectopexy
Ripstein arterial forceps

Ripstein operation for rectal
   prolapse
Ripstein presacral rectopexy
Ripstein procedure
Ripstein proctopexy
Ripstein rectal prolapse
   operation
Ripstein rectopexy
Ripstein tissue forceps
RIS orotracheal intubation
RISA cisternography
Risdon approach
Risdon extraoral incision
Risdon pretragal incision
Risdon wire
Riseborough-Radin classification
   of humeral fractures
Riseborough-Radin intercondylar
   fracture classification
Rish cartilage knife
Rish chisel
Rish osteotome
rising sun appearance of
   olecranon on x-ray
risk
  anesthetic risk
  bleeding risk
  genetic risk
  genetically at risk
  Goldman score of
   cardiovascular risk
  inherent risk
  low risk
  perforation risk
  procedures, alternatives, risks
   (PAR)
  rebleeding risk
  stroke risk
  surgical risk
Risley pliers
Risley rotary prism
risorius muscle
Rispi Micromega reamer
Risser cast
Risser cast table
Risser frame
Risser jacket
Risser localizer
Risser localizer scoliosis cast
Risser sign
Risser technique
Risser turnbuckle cast

Risser wedging jacket
Risser-Cotrel body cast
Rissler kidney retractor
Rissler mallet
Rissler periosteal elevator
Rissler pin
Rissler vein sound
Rissler-Stille pin
Ristow osteotome
RITA ablation catheter
Ritch contact lens
Ritch nylon suture laser lens
Ritch trabeculoplasty laser lens
Ritchie articular pain scale
Ritchie catheter
Ritchie cleft palate tenaculum
Ritchie tenaculum
Ritch-Krupin-Denver eye valve
    insertion forceps
RiteBite biopsy forceps
Ritgen maneuver
Ritisch sutures
Ritleng probe
Ritter bougie
Ritter Bovie
Ritter coagulator
Ritter coagulator electrosurgical
    unit
Ritter dilator
Ritter double-orifice tip
Ritter drain
Ritter fibers
Ritter forceps
Ritter meatal dilator
Ritter rasp
Ritter raspatory
Ritter single-orifice tip
Ritter sound
Ritter suprapubic suction drain
Ritter suprapubic suction tube
Ritter table
Ritter-Bantam Bovie coagulator
Ritter-Bantam Bovie
    electrosurgical unit
Ritter-Oleson technique
ritual circumcision
Riva-Rocci manometer
Riva-Rocci sphygmomanometer
Rivas vascular catheter
Riverbank Laboratories tuning
    fork
Rivero-Carvallo maneuver

Rivero-Carvallo sign
Rives operation
Rives splenectomy
rivet gun
Rivetti-Levinson intraluminal
    shunt
Riviere sign
rivinian foramen
rivinian notch
rivinian segment
Rivinus canals
Rivinus duct
Rivinus gland
Rivinus membrane
Rivinus notch
Rivinus segment
rivus lacrimalis
Riza-Ribe grasper needle
Riza-Ribe grasping needle
Riza-Ribe needle
Rizzo dorsal implant
Rizzo retractor
Rizzoli operation
Rizzoli osteoclast
Rizzuti double-prong forceps
Rizzuti eye expressor
Rizzuti fixation forceps
Rizzuti forceps
Rizzuti graft carrier spatula
Rizzuti iris expressor
Rizzuti iris retractor
Rizzuti keratoplasty scissors
Rizzuti lens expressor
Rizzuti lens hook
Rizzuti retractor
Rizzuti scissors
Rizzuti scleral forceps
Rizzuti scleral knife
Rizzuti superior rectus forceps
Rizzuti-Bonaccolto instruments
Rizzuti-Fleischer instruments
Rizzuti-Furness cornea-holding
    forceps
Rizzuti-Kayser-Fleischer
    instruments
Rizzuti-Lowe instruments
Rizzuti-Maxwell instruments
Rizzuti-McGuire corneal-section
    scissors
Rizzuti-McGuire scissors
Rizzuti-Soemmering instrument
Rizzuti-Spizziri cannula knife

Rizzuti-Verhoeff forceps
RK (radial keratotomy)
RK marker
RL shunt
RLL (right lower lobe)
RLQ (right lower quadrant)
RMA position (right
    mentoanterior position)
RMC total knee prosthesis
    (Richards maximum
    contact total knee
    prosthesis)
RMP position (right
    mentoposterior position)
RMT position (right
    mentotransverse position)
RN clamp
RNA probe
Reutter classification
ROA position (right
    occipitoanterior position)
Roach ball precision attachment
Roach clasp
Roadrunner PC guidewire
Roadrunner wire
Roaf approach
Roaf syndrome
ROAM (roaming optical access
    multiscope)
ROAM right-angled endoscope
roaming optical access
    multiscope (ROAM)
Roane bullet tip
Robb antral cannula
Robb knife
Robb needle
Robb syringe
Robb tonsillar forceps
Robb tonsillar knife
Robb tonsillar sponge forceps
Robbins automatic tourniquet
Robb-Roberts rotary rasp
Robert Bent Brigham total knee
    prosthesis
Robert Brigham knee prosthesis
Robert Brigham prosthesis
Robert Jones bandage
Robert Jones bulky soft
    compressive dressing
Robert Jones compressive
    dressing
Robert Jones splint

Robert ligament
Robert nasal snare
Robert pelvis
Robert view radiograph
Robertazzi nasopharyngeal
    airway
Roberts abdominal trocar
Roberts applicator
Roberts approach
Roberts arterial forceps
Roberts bronchial forceps
Roberts chisel
Roberts dental implant
Roberts episiotomy scissors
Roberts esophageal speculum
Roberts esophagoscope
Roberts folding esophagoscope
Roberts headrest
Roberts hemostatic forceps
Roberts hip dissecting chisel
Roberts laryngoscope
Roberts nasal snare
Roberts needle
Roberts oval esophagoscope
Roberts oval speculum
Roberts self-retaining
    laryngoscope
Roberts shears
Roberts snare
Roberts speculum
Roberts syndrome
Roberts technique
Roberts thumb retractor
Roberts trocar
Roberts-Gill periosteal elevator
Robertshaw bag resuscitator
Robertshaw double-lumen
    endotracheal tube
Robertshaw tube
Roberts-Jesberg esophagoscope
Roberts-Nelson lobectomy
    tourniquet
Roberts-Nelson rib shears
Roberts-Nelson rib stripper
Roberts-Nelson tourniquet
Robertson corneal trephine
Robertson incision
Robertson knife
Robertson sign
Robertson suprapubic drain
Robertson suprapubic trocar
Robertson tonsillar forceps

Robertson tonsillar knife
Robertson tonsil-seizing forceps
Roberts-Singley dressing forceps
Roberts-Singley thumb forceps
Robicheck wire
Robicsek technique
Robicsek vascular probe
Robin chalazion clamp
Robin orthodontic plate
Robin sequence
Robin syndrome
Robinject needle injector
Robin-Masse abdominal
    retractor
Robinow dwarfism
Robinow mesomelic dysplasia
Robinow syndrome
Robinson anterior cervical
    diskectomy
Robinson bag
Robinson belt
Robinson catheter
Robinson cervical spine fusion
Robinson dislodger
Robinson equalizing tube
Robinson flap knife
Robinson hook
Robinson incus replacement
    prosthesis
Robinson lung retractor
Robinson middle ear prosthesis
Robinson piston prosthesis
Robinson pocket arthrometer
Robinson procedure
Robinson retractor
Robinson stapes prosthesis
Robinson stone basket
Robinson stone dislodger
Robinson strut
Robinson tonsillar suction
Robinson urethral catheter
Robinson vein graft
Robinson-Brauer trocar
Robinson-Moon prosthesis
    inserter
Robinson-Moon stapes
    prosthesis
Robinson-Moon-Lippy stapes
    prosthesis
Robinson-Riley cervical
    arthrodesis
Robinson-Smith needle

Robinson-Smith procedure
Robinson-Southwick fusion
    technique
Robinson-Southwick spinal
    fusion
Robles cutting point cannula
Robodoc robot
Roboprep G instrument
Robot Starr II camera
robotic surgery
robotic-automated assist device
robotics-controlled stereotactic
    frame
Robson intestinal forceps
Robson line
Robson point
Robson position
Robson staging of renal cancer
    (I-IV)
ROC suture fastener
ROC XS suture anchor
ROC XS suture fastener
Rocabado posture gauge
Rochard retractor
Rochester aortic vent needle
Rochester atrial retractor
Rochester atrial septal defect
    retractor
Rochester atrial septal retractor
Rochester awl
Rochester bone trephine
Rochester bone trephine device
Rochester clamp
Rochester colonial retractor
Rochester dissector
Rochester dressing
Rochester elevator
Rochester gallstone forceps
Rochester harvest bone cutter
Rochester hip-knee-ankle-foot
    orthosis
Rochester HKAFO prosthesis
Rochester hook clamp
Rochester knife
Rochester laminar dissector
Rochester laminar elevator
Rochester silicone Foley
    catheter
Rochester self-adhering male
    external catheter
Rochester mitral stenosis knife
Rochester needle

Rochester needle holder
Rochester oral tissue forceps
Rochester rake retractor
Rochester recipient bone cutter
Rochester retractor
Rochester Russian tissue forceps
Rochester scissors
Rochester sigmoid clamp
Rochester spinal elevator
Rochester suction tube
Rochester syringe
Rochester tissue forceps
Rochester tracheal tube
Rochester tube
Rochester-Carmalt forceps
Rochester-Carmalt hemostat
Rochester-Carmalt hemostatic
  forceps
Rochester-Carmalt hysterectomy
  forceps
Rochester-Davis forceps
Rochester-Ewald tissue forceps
Rochester-Ferguson double-
  ended retractor
Rochester-Ferguson retractor
Rochester-Ferguson scissors
Rochester-Harrington forceps
Rochester-Kocher clamp
Rochester-Meeker needle
Rochester-Mixter artery forceps
Rochester-Mixter gall duct
  forceps
Rochester-Mueller forceps
Rochester-Ochsner forceps
Rochester-Ochsner hemostat
Rochester-Ochsner hemostat
  forceps
Rochester-Pean clamp
Rochester-Pean forceps
Rochester-Pean hemostat
Rochester-Pean hysterectomy
  forceps
Rochester-Rankin arterial
  forceps
Rochester-Rankin hemostatic
  forceps
Rochester-Russian forceps
Rochet procedure
Rochette bridge
Rock endometrial suction curet
rock-candy lesion
rocker board

rocker boot
rocker knife
rocker-bottom foot
Rockert dilator
Rockey clamp
Rockey dilating probe
Rockey endoscope
Rockey forceps
Rockey mediastinal cannula
Rockey probe
Rockey scoop
Rockey trachea cannula
Rockey vascular clamp
Rockey-Davis appendectomy
  incision
Rockey-Davis incision
Rockey-Thompson catheter
rocking motion
rocking-leg splint
Rock-Mulligan hood
Rock-Mulligan prosthesis
Rockwood acromioclavicular
  injury classification
Rockwood classification
Rockwood clavicular fracture
  classification
Rockwood posterior
  capsulorrhaphy
Rockwood procedure
Rockwood resection
Rockwood shoulder procedure
Rockwood shoulder screw
Rockwood-Green technique
Rockwood-Matsen capsular shift
  procedure
rod
  Acufex rod
  Alta reconstruction rod
  Alta femoral intramedullary rod
  Alta intramedullary rod
  Alta reconstruction rod
  Alta tibial rod
  Auer rod
  Baden Silastic rod
  Bailey rod
  Bickel intramedullary rod
  Biethium ostomy rod
  Biofix absorbable rod
  Biofix fixation rod
  Bobechko rod
  cloverleaf rod
  cold rolled rod

rod (*continued*)
  colostomy rod
  compression rod
  condyle rod
  Cortel insertion of steel rods
  Corti rods
  Cotrel-Dubousset rod
  Danek rod
  degradable polyglycolide rod
  Delrin push rod
  Delta rod
  distraction rod
  double-L spinal rod
  dual square-ended Harrington
    rod
  Dwyer rod
  Edwards Universal rod
  Edwards-Levine rod
  enamel rod
  Ender rod
  Enneking rod
  Fixateur Interne rod
  fixation rod
  flared spinal rod
  flexible round silicone rod
  germinal rod
  glass retracting rod
  glass rod
  Green-Armytage polythene
    rod
  Hamby rod
  Hansen-Street intramedullary
    rod
  Harrington dual square-ended
    rod
  Harris condylocephalic rod
  Heidenhain rods
  Hopkins rod
  House measuring rod
  Hunter rod
  Hunter Silastic rod
  Hunter tendon rod
  Hydroflex penile implant rod
  impactor rod
  impingement rod
  intramedullary rod
  intramedullary alignment rod
  intramedullary Rush rod
  Isola spinal implant system
    eye rod
  Jackson rod
  Jacobs distraction rod

rod (*continued*)
  Jacobs locking hook spinal
    rod
  Kaneda rod
  Kuntscher rod
  Knodt distraction rod
  knurled CD rod (Cotrel-
    Dubousset rod)
  knurled Cotrel-Dubousset rod
  Koenig rod
  Kostuik rod
  laser rod
  Lincoff sponge rod
  Lottes rod
  Luque rod
  Maddox rod
  malleable rod
  Marafioti-Westin rod
  McLaughlin laser vaginal
    measuring rod
  McLaughlin quartz rod
  measuring rod
  Meckel rod
  medullary rod
  metal rod
  Mire silicone rod
  modified Harrington rod
  Moe modified Harrington rod
  Moe subcutaneous rod
  Moore measuring rod
  Moss rod
  Mouradian humeral rod
  Olerud rod
  orthopedic rod
  pediatric Cotrel-Dubousset rod
  Perspex rod
  Polarus humeral rod
  precontoured unit rod
  quartz rod
  radioactive rod
  radiotranslucent rod
  Reichmann ivory rod
  retinal rods
  retracting rod
  Richards locking rod
  Richardson rod
  rigid holding rod
  Rogozinski rod
  round extension rod
  round-ended distraction rod
  Rush rod
  Russell-Taylor delta rod

rod (*continued*)
  Sage forearm rod
  Sage intramedullary rod
  Samson rod
  Schneider rod
  scleral sponge rod
  screw alignment rod
  short rod
  Silastic rod
  silicone flexor rod
  silicone rods
  SinuScope rigid rod
  slotted intramedullary rod
  Sofield rod
  spinal rod
  square-ended distraction rod
  Stader connecting rod
  Stenzel fracture rod
  sterile transverse rod
  Street rod
  telescoping medullary rod
  telescoping rod
  thermoluminescent dosimeter
    rod
  threaded rod
  unit spinal rod
  vaginal laser measuring rod
  Veirs canaliculus rod
  Veirs malleable rod
  Williams rod
  Wiltse system spinal rod
  Wissinger rod
  Y-glass rod
  Zickel II subtrochanteric rod
  Zickel supracondylar rod
  Zielke rod
rod bender
rod cutter
rod electrode
rod fixation
rod fracture repair
rod holder
rod placement
rod sleeve fixation
rod template
Rodenstock panfundoscope
Rodenstock panfundus lens
Rodenstock scanning laser
    ophthalmoscope
Rodenstock slit lamp
rodent ulcer
rodeo thumb

Rodin orbital implant
rodlike structure
Rodman mastectomy incision
Rodney Smith biliary stricture
    operation
Rodney Smith biliary stricture
    repair
Rodney Smith drainage
Rodriguez aneurysm
Rodriguez catheter
Rodriguez-Alvarez catheter
rods and cones
Roe aortic clamp
Roe aortic tourniquet clamp
Roe solution
Roeder clamp
Roeder loop
Roeder loop knot
Roeder manipulative aptitude
    test device
Roeder towel clamp
Roeder towel forceps
Roeltsch forceps
roentgen absorbed dose (rad)
roentgen dosage
roentgen equivalent
roentgen knife
Roentgen knife stereotaxic
    radiosurgical device
roentgen meter
roentgen ray
roentgen therapy
roentgenogram
  cephalometric roentgenogram
  jughandle roentgenogram
  lateral oblique jaw
    roentgenogram
  lateral ramus roentgenogram
  lateral skull roentgenogram
  maxillary sinus
    roentgenogram
  panoramic roentgenogram
  scout roentgenogram
  stress roentgenogram
  submental vertex
    roentgenogram
  thoracic roentgenogram
  Towne projection
    roentgenogram
  transcranial roentgenogram
  Waters view roentgenogram
roentgenograph

roentgenographic evaluation
roentgenographic opaque
    marker
roentgenographic view
roentgenography
Roger amputation
Roger Anderson external fixator
Roger Anderson external
    skeletal fixation device
Roger Anderson facial fracture
    appliance
Roger Anderson fixation bar
Roger Anderson operation
Roger Anderson pin
Roger Anderson pin fixation
    appliance
Roger Anderson splint
Roger Anderson table
Roger Anderson well-leg splint
Roger cervical spine fusion
Roger dissector
Roger forceps
Roger needle holder
Roger reflex
Roger scissors
Roger septal elevator
Roger septal knife
Roger sign
Roger spinal fusion
Roger submucous dissector
Roger syndrome
Roger vascular-toothed
    hysterectomy forceps
Roger wire-cutting scissors
Rogers cervical fusion technique
Rogers sphygmomanometer
Rogers wire cutter
Rogge sterilizing forceps
Rogozinski hook
Rogozinski rod
Rohadur gait plate
Rohadur-Polydor orthotic
Rohadur-Schaefer orthotic
Rohadur-Whitman orthotic
Rohm-Haas PMMA intraocular
    lens
Roho bed
ROHO cushion
Roho Dry Flotation wheelchair
    pad
Roho heel pad
Roho heel protector

Roho high-profile cushion
Roho mattress
Roho Pack-It cushion
Roho solid seat insert
Rohrschneider cannula
Rohrschneider probe
Rokitansky diverticulum
Rokitansky hernia
Rokitansky kidney
Rokitansky tumor
Rokitansky-Aschoff sinus
Rokitansky-Cushing ulcer
Roland dilator
rolandic cortex
rolandic line
rolandic region
Rolando fissure
Rolando fracture
Rolf dilator
Rolf jeweler's forceps
Rolf lacrimal probe
Rolf lance
Rolf lance needle
Rolf muscle hook
Rolf punctum dilator
Rolf utility forceps
Rolf-Jackson cannula
roll
    3M Reston self-adhering foam
        pad and roll
    ACCO cotton roll
    Akton positioning roll
    Celluron dental roll
    cervical roll
    dorsal back roll
    Dutchman's roll
    Fluftex gauze roll
    gluteal banana roll
    instrument roll
    Kerlix bandage roll
    Kerlix gauze roll
    Kling fluff roll
    Krinkle gauze roll
    Lakeside cotton roll
    leg roll
    lumbar roll
    McKenzie cervical roll
    McKenzie lumbar roll
    McKenzie night roll
    Medline roll
    narrow gauze roll
    neck roll

roll (*continued*)
  octagon roll
  philtral roll
  silver Mylar roll
  Skillbuilder half roll
  Stretch gauze roll
  Tensor elastic bandage roll
  Tumble Forms roll
  Veratex cotton roll
roll control bolster
roll stitch
roll tube
Roll-A-Bout mobility device
rolled Colles splint
rolled graft
rolled Instat stent
rolled shoulder lesion
rolled tendon anchovy
    procedure
roller
  Devonshire roller
  hand tubing roller
  intravenous tubing roller
  Spence cranioplastic roller
  Toledo roller
  tubing hand roller
  Unger adenoid pressure roller
roller bandage
roller dressing
roller electrode
roller forceps
roller head perfusion pump
roller knife
roller pump
Roller pump suction tube
RollerBack self-massage device
rollerball endometrial ablation
rollerball technique
rollerbar electrode
rollerbar rel electrode
Rollet anterior chamber irrigator
Rollet chisel
Rollet eye retractor
Rollet incision
Rollet irrigator
Rollet lacrimal probe
Rollet lacrimal sac retractor
Rollet lake retractor
Rollet rake retractor
Rollet retractor
Rollet skin retractor
Rolley I&A unit

rollflap operation
rolling hernia
rolling hiatal hernia
rolling membrane
rolling motion
rolling movement
rolling of conjunctiva
roll-tube technique
Rolnel catheter
Rolodermatome
Rolon spatula
Rolyan arm elevator
Rolyan brace
Rolyan Firm D-Ring wrist
    support
Rolyan foot support
Rolyan Gel Shell splint
Rolyan tibial fracture brace
ROM (range of motion)
ROM exercises (range-of-motion
    exercises)
ROM knee brace
Roman laryngostat
Romana sign
Romano curved surgical drill
romanoscope
Romberg disease
Romberg facial deformity
Romberg hemiatrophy
Romberg hemifacial atrophy
Romberg sign
Romberg spasm
Romberg syndrome
Romberg test
Romberg trophoneurosis
ROMI (rule out myocardial
    infarction)
Rommel cautery
Rommel electrocautery
Rommel-Hildreth cautery
Rommel-Hildreth electrocautery
Rondic sponge dressing
Rondo inhaler
rongeur (*see also* microrongeur)
  Adson bone rongeur
  Adson cranial rongeur
  Adson rongeur
  Andrews-Hartmann ear
    rongeur
  angular rongeur
  antral rongeur
  aortic valve rongeur

rongeur (*continued*)

Bohler rongeur
backbiting rongeur
Bacon bone rongeur
Bacon cranial bone rongeur
Bacon cranial rongeur
Baer bone rongeur
Bailey aortic valve rongeur
bane bone rongeur
Bane mastoid rongeur
Bane-Hartmann bone rongeur
bayonet rongeur
Belz lacrimal sac rongeur
Bethune rib rongeur
Beyer bone rongeur
Beyer endaural rongeur
Beyer laminectomy rongeur
Beyer-Lempert rongeur
Beyer-Stille bone rongeur
biting rongeur
Blakesley laminectomy
   rongeur
Blumenthal bone rongeur
Boehler bone rongeur
Bogle rongeur
Boies-Lombard mastoid
   rongeur
bone punch rongeur
bone rongeur
bone-biting rongeur
bone-cutting rongeur
bony rongeur
Brock cardiac dilator
   rongeur
Bruening-Citelli rongeur
Bucy laminectomy rongeur
Cairns rongeur
Callahan lacrimal rongeur
Campbell laminectomy
   rongeur
Campbell nerve rongeur
Carroll rongeur
Caspar rongeur
cervical rongeur
Cherry-Kerrison laminectomy
   rongeur
chicken-bill rongeur
Cicherelli bone rongeur
Citelli sphenoid rongeur
Cleveland bone rongeur
Cloward intervertebral disk
   rongeur

rongeur (*continued*)

Cloward laminectomy
   rongeur
Cloward pituitary rongeur
Cloward-English laminectomy
   rongeur
Cloward-English rongeur
Cloward-Harper laminectomy
   rongeur
Codman cervical rongeur
Codman laminectomy rongeur
Codman-Kerrison
   laminectomy rongeur
Codman-Leksell laminectomy
   rongeur
Codman-Schlesinger cervical
   laminectomy rongeur
Codman-Schlesinger cervical
   rongeur
Cohen rongeur
Colclough laminectomy
   rongeur
Colclough-Love-Kerrison
   laminectomy rongeur
Converse nasal rongeur
Converse nasal root rongeur
Converse-Lange rongeur
Corbett bone rongeur
Corbett bone-cutting rongeur
Costen rongeur
Costen-Kerrison rongeur
Cottle nasal-biting rongeur
Cottle-Jansen bone rongeur
Cottle-Kazanjian bone rongeur
cranial bone rongeur
Cushing bone rongeur
Cushing intervertebral disk
   rongeur
Cushing laminectomy rongeur
Cushing pituitary rongeur
cystoscopic rongeur
Dahlgren rongeur
Dale first rib rongeur
Dale thoracic rongeur
Davol rongeur
Dawson-Yuhl-Leksell rongeur
Dean bone rongeur
Dean mastoid rongeur
Decker microsurgical rongeur
Decker pituitary rongeur
Defourmental bone rongeur
Defourmental nasal rongeur

rongeur (*continued*)

delicate intervertebral disk rongeur
Dench rongeur
dental rongeur
DePuy rongeur
DeVilbiss cranial rongeur
disk rongeur
double-action rongeur
double-biting rongeur
down-cutting rongeur
duckbill rongeur
Duggan rongeur
DuPuy pituitary rongeur
ear rongeur
Echlin bone rongeur
Echlin duckbill rongeur
Echlin laminectomy rongeur
Echlin-Luer rongeur
endaural rongeur
end-biting blunt-nosed rongeur
end-biting rongeur
Falconer rongeur
Ferris Smith disk rongeur
Ferris Smith intervertebral disk rongeur
Ferris Smith pituitary rongeur
Ferris Smith-Gruenwald rongeur
Ferris Smith-Kerrison disk rongeur
Ferris Smith-Kerrison laminectomy rongeur
Ferris Smith-Kerrison neurosurgical rongeur
Ferris Smith-Spurling disk rongeur
Ferris Smith-Takahashi rongeur
flat-bottomed Kerrison rongeur
FlexTip intervertebral rongeur
Friedman bone rongeur
Frykholm bone rongeur
Fukushima rongeur
Fulton laminectomy rongeur
Gam-Mer rongeur
Garrison rongeur
Giertz rongeur
Glover rongeur
Goldman-Kazanjian rongeur

rongeur (*continued*)

gooseneck rongeur
Gruenwald neurosurgical rongeur
Gruenwald pituitary rongeur
Gruenwald-Love intervertebral disk rongeur
Guleke bone rongeur
Hajek antral rongeur
Hajek downbiting rongeur
Hajek upbiting rongeur
Hajek-Claus rongeur
Hajek-Koffler laminectomy rongeur
Hajek-Koffler sphenoidal rongeur
Hakansson bone rongeur
Hakansson-Olivecrona rongeur
Hardy rongeur
Harper rongeur
Hartmann bone rongeur
Hartmann ear rongeur
Hartmann mastoid rongeur
Hartmann-Herzfeld ear rongeur
Hein rongeur
Henny laminectomy rongeur
Heyman septum-cutting rongeur
Hoen intervertebral disk rongeur
Hoen laminectomy rongeur
Hoen pituitary rongeur
Hoffmann ear rongeur
Horsley bone rongeur
Horsley cranial bone rongeur
Horsley cranial rongeur
Horsley rongeur
Houghton rongeur
Hudson cranial rongeur
Hudson rongeur
Husk mastoid rongeur
Husks bone rongeur
Husks mastoid rongeur
infundibular rongeur
infundibulectomy rongeur
intervertebral disk rongeur
IV disk rongeur (intravertebral disk rongeur)
Ivy mastoid rongeur
Ivy rongeur

rongeur (*continued*)

Jackson intervertebral disk rongeur
Jansen bayonet rongeur
Jansen ear rongeur
Jansen mastoid rongeur
Jansen-Cottle rongeur
Jansen-Middleton rongeur
Jansen-Zaufel bone rongeur
Jarit-Kerrison laminectomy rongeur
Jarit-Ruskin bone rongeur
jaw rongeur
Juers-Lempert endaural rongeur
Juers-Lempert rongeur
Kazanjian-Goldman rongeur
Kerr rongeur
Kerrison cervical rongeur
Kerrison laminectomy rongeur
Kerrison lumbar rongeur
Kerrison mastoid rongeur
Kerrison-Costen ear rongeur
Kerrison-Ferris Smith rongeur
Kerrison-Morgenstein rongeur
Kerrison-Schwartz rongeur
Kerrison-Spurling rongeur
Killian rongeur
Kleinert-Kutz synovectomy rongeur
Koffler-Hajek laminectomy rongeur
lacrimal sac rongeur
laminectomy rongeur
Lane rongeur
Lange-Converse nasal root rongeur
Lebsche rongeur
Leksell bone rongeur
Leksell cardiovascular rongeur
Leksell laminectomy rongeur
Leksell-Stille thoracic rongeur
Leksell-Stille thoracic-cardiovascular rongeur
Lempert bone rongeur
Lempert endaural rongeur
Lempert-Juers rongeur
Lillie sinus bone-nibbling rongeur
Liston rongeur
Liston-Littauer rongeur

rongeur (*continued*)

Liston-Luer-Whiting rongeur
Liston-Ruskin bone-cutting rongeur
Littauer rongeur
Littauer-West rongeur
Lombard mastoid rongeur
Lombard-Beyer rongeur
Lombard-Boies rongeur
Love pituitary rongeur
Love-Gruenwald cranial rongeur
Love-Gruenwald intervertebral disk rongeur
Love-Gruenwald laminectomy rongeur
Love-Gruenwald pituitary rongeur
Love-Kerrison rongeur
Lowman rongeur
Luer bone rongeur
Luer thoracic rongeur
Luer-Friedman bone rongeur
Luer-Liston-Wheeling rongeur
Luer-Stille rongeur
Luer-Whiting mastoid rongeur
Markwalder bone rongeur
Markwalder rib rongeur
Marquardt bone rongeur
mastoid rongeur
Mayfield bone rongeur
Mead bone rongeur
Mead dental rongeur
Mead mastoid rongeur
micropituitary rongeur
Middleton rongeur
Mollison mastoid rongeur
monster rongeur
Montenovesi cranial rongeur
Morgenstein-Kerrison rongeur
Mount laminectomy rongeur
multiple-action rongeur
narrow-bite bone rongeur
nasal rongeur
needle-nose rongeur
Nichol rongeur
Nichols infundibulectomy rongeur
Nicola pituitary rongeur
Noyes rongeur
O'Brien rongeur

rongeur (*continued*)
  Oldberg intervertebral disk
    rongeur
  Oldberg laminectomy rongeur
  Oldberg pituitary rongeur
  Olivecrona endaural rongeur
  Olivecrona mastoid rongeur
  orthopedic rongeur
  Parham-Martin rongeur
  peapod intervertebral disk
    rongeur
  peapod rongeur
  Peiper-Beyer bone rongeur
  Pennybacker rongeur
  Pierce mastoid rongeur
  Pilling-Ruskin rongeur
  pituitary rongeur
  Poppen intervertebral disk
    rongeur
  Poppen laminectomy rongeur
  Poppen pituitary rongeur
  Prince rongeur
  punch rongeur
  Quervain rongeur
  Ruskin bone rongeur
  Raaf rongeur
  Raaf-Oldberg rongeur
  Raney laminectomy rongeur
  rat-tooth rongeur
  Reiner bone rongeur
  rib rongeur
  Rica bone rongeur
  Rica cranial rongeur
  Rica laminectomy rongeur
  Rica mastoid rongeur
  Rica spinal rongeur
  Ronjair air-powered rongeur
  round-nosed rongeur
  Rowland nasal rongeur
  Rottgen-Ruskin bone rongeur
  Ruskin bone rongeur
  Ruskin cranial rongeur
  Ruskin duckbill rongeur
  Ruskin mastoid rongeur
  Ruskin multiple-action rongeur
  Ruskin-Jansen bone rongeur
  Ruskin-Jay heavy-duty rongeur
  Ruskin-Liston bone-cutting
    rongeur
  Ruskin-Rowland bone rongeur
  Ruskin-Storz rongeur
  Sauerbruch rib rongeur

rongeur (*continued*)
  Sauerbruch-Coryllos bone
    rongeur
  Sauerbruch-Coryllos rib
    rongeur
  Sauerbruch-Lebsche rongeur
  Sauerbruch-Stille bone
    rongeur
  Sauer-Lebsche rongeur
  Scaglietti rongeur
  Schlesinger cervical rongeur
  Schlesinger intervertebral disk
    rongeur
  Schlesinger laminectomy
    rongeur
  Schwartz-Kerrison rongeur
  Selverstone intervertebral disk
    rongeur
  Selverstone laminectomy
    rongeur
  Semb gouging rongeur
  Semb-Sauerbruch rongeur
  Semb-Stille bone rongeur
  Shearer bone rongeur
  Shearer chicken-bill rongeur
  Shoemaker rongeur
  side-curved rongeur
  side-cutting rongeur
  Simplex mastoid rongeur
  single-action rongeur
  skinny-nose rongeur
  slender-nose rongeur
  SMIC bone rongeur
  SMIC cranial rongeur
  SMIC laminectomy rongeur
  SMIC mastoid rongeur
  Smith-Petersen laminectomy
    rongeur
  Smith-Petersen rongeur
  Smolik curved rongeur
  Spence intervertebral disk
    rongeur
  Spurling intervertebral disk
    rongeur
  Spurling laminectomy rongeur
  Spurling pituitary rongeur
  Spurling-Kerrison down-biting
    rongeur
  Spurling-Kerrison
    laminectomy rongeur
  Spurling-Kerrison up-biting
    rongeur

rongeur (*continued*)
- Spurling-Love-Gruenwald-Cushing rongeur
- St. Luke's double-action rongeur
- Stellbring synovectomy rongeur
- Stille bone rongeur
- Stille-Beyer rongeur
- Stille-Horsley rongeur
- Stille-Lauer bone rongeur
- Stille-Leksell rongeur
- Stille-Liston double-action rongeur
- Stille-Luer angular duckbill rongeur
- Stille-Luer bone rongeur
- Stille-Luer multiple-action rongeur
- Stille-Luer-Echlin bone rongeur
- Stille-Ruskin rongeur
- Stille-Zaufal-Jansen rongeur
- Stookey cranial rongeur
- Storz cystoscopic rongeur
- Storz duckbill rongeur
- straight rongeur
- Struempel rongeur
- Strully-Kerrison rongeur
- Super Cut laminectomy rongeur
- synovectomy rongeur
- Takahashi rongeur
- taper-jaw rongeur
- Tiedmann rongeur
- Tobey ear rongeur
- Universal Kerrison rongeur
- up-biting rongeur
- Urschel first rib rongeur
- Urschel-Leksell rongeur
- von Seemen rongeur
- Voris intervertebral disk rongeur
- Voris IV disk rongeur
- Wagner rongeur
- Walton rongeur
- Walton-Liston bone rongeur
- Walton-Ruskin bone rongeur
- Watson-Williams intervertebral disk rongeur
- Weil pituitary rongeur
- Weil rongeur

rongeur (*continued*)
- Weil-Blakesley intervertebral disk rongeur
- Weingartner rongeur
- Whitcomb-Kerrison laminectomy rongeur
- Whitcomb-Kerrison rongeur
- White mastoid rongeur
- Whiting mastoid rongeur
- Wilde intervertebral disk rongeur
- Yasargil pituitary rongeur
- Young cystoscopic rongeur
- Zaufel bone rongeur
- Zaufel-Jansen bone rongeur

Ronis adenoid punch
Ronis adenoidal punch
Ronis cutting forceps
Ronis tonsillar punch
Ronjair air-powered rongeur
Rood technique
ROOF (retro-orbicularis ocular fat)
roof disk
roof fracture
roof of mouth
roof of skull
roof of the nail fold
roofing
roof-patch graft
roof-reinforcement ring hip arthroplasty component
PAR room (postanesthesia recovery room)
postanesthesia recovery room (PAR room)
recovery room (RR)
Roos brachial plexus root retractor
Roos first-rib shears
Roos hip flexor release
Roos osteotome
Roos procedure for thoracic outlet syndrome
Roos retractor
Roos rib cutter
Roos rib shears
Roos test for thoracic outlet
Roos transaxillary approach
Roosen clamp
Roosevelt gastroenterostomy clamp

Roosevelt gastrointestinal clamp
root
  anterior nerve roots
  aortic root
  bifurcation of root
  conjoined nerve root
  dorsal nerve root
  facial nerve root
  facial root
  intra-alveolar root
  lingual root
  nasal root
  nerve root
  palatal root
  palatine root
  posterior nerve root
  retained root
  transection of nerve roots
  ventral nerve root
  ventral root
root amputation
root anomaly
root canal broach
root canal drill
root canal file
root canal filling
root canal point
root canal spreader
root canal therapy
root cap
root compression
root dehiscence
root elevator
root end resection
root formation
root fracture
root fusion
root infiltration
root injection
root needle
root of lung
root of tongue
root perforation
root pliers
root rubber dam clamp
root sheath
root sleeve
root z-epicanthoplasty
Rooter splint
root-form dental implant
root-form device
rooting reflex

rooting response
rootlet
ROP position (right
    occipitoposterior position)
rope flap
rope graft
Roper alpha-chymotrypsin
    cannula
Roper cannula
Roper scissors
Roper-Hall localizer
Roper-Hall locator
Roper-Rumel tourniquet
ropivacaine anesthetic
ropy mass
ropy saliva
ropy tumor
Rorabeck fasciotomy
Ros XS suture anchor
Rosa-Berens orbital implant
rosary bougie
rosary-bead esophagus
Rosch catheter
Rosch modification
Roschke dropper sponge
Rosch-Thurmond fallopian tube
    catheterization set
Roscoe-Graham anterior
    gastrojejunostomy
Roscoe-Graham jejunostomy
Rose bed dressing
rose bengal scan
rose bengal sodium I-131 biliary
    scan
Rose cleft lip repair
Rose disimpaction forceps
Rose double-ended retractor
Rose head-extension position
Rose L-type nose bridge
    prosthesis
Rose operation
Rose position
Rose procedure
Rose tamponade
Rose tracheal retractor
Rose-Bradford kidney
rosebud stoma
rosehead bur
Rosen angular elevator
Rosen bayonet separator
Rosen bur
Rosen cartilage knife

Rosen curet
Rosen dissector
Rosen ear incision knife
Rosen ear probe
Rosen elevator
Rosen endaural probe
Rosen fenestrator
Rosen guidewire
Rosen incision
Rosen incision knife
Rosen incontinence device
Rosen inflatable urinary
    incontinence prosthesis
Rosen J-guide guidewire
Rosen knife
Rosen knife curet
Rosen middle ear instrument
Rosen needle
Rosen nucleus paddle
Rosen pick
Rosen probe
Rosen prosthesis
Rosen separator
Rosen splint
Rosen suction
Rosen suction tube
Rosen tube
Rosen urinary prosthesis
Rosen wire
Rosenbach sign
Rosenbaum iris retractor
Rosenbaum-Drews iris retractor
Rosenbaum-Drews plastic
    retractor
Rosenberg dissecting cannula
Rosenberg dissector tip
Rosenberg endoscopic anterior
    cruciate ligament
    reconstruction
Rosenberg full-radius blade
    synovial retractor
Rosenberg gynecomastia
    dissection instrument
Rosenberg meniscal repair kit
Rosenberg retractor
Rosenberg-Sampson retractor
Rosenblatt scissors
Rosenblum rotating adapter
Rosenburg drill guide
Rosenburg operation
Rosenfeld hip prosthesis
Rosengren operation

Rosenmueller body
Rosenmueller cavity
Rosenmueller recess
Rosenmueller valve
Rosenmueller curet
Rosenmueller fossa
Rosenmueller gland
Rosenmüeller (*see* Rosenmueller)
Rosenmueller (*see* Rosenmüeller)
Rosenmüller (*see* Rosenmueller)
Rosenthal ascending vein
Rosenthal aspiration needle
Rosenthal fibers
Rosenthal nail injury classification
Rosenthal needle
Rosenthal urethral speculum
Rosenthal vein
Rosenthal-French nebulization
    dosimeter
Roser mouth gag
Roser needle
Roser-Braun sign
Roser-Koenig mouth gag
Roser-Nelaton line
Rose-Thompson cleft lip repair
Rose-Thompson operation
rose-thorn ulcer
rosette blade
rosette cataract
Rosette strain gauge
Rosi bridge prosthesis
Rosner tonometer
Rosomoff percutaneous
    cordotomy
Ross aortic retractor
Ross aortic valve retractor
Ross body
Ross catheter
Ross needle
Ross procedure
Ross pulmonary porcine valve
Ross technique
Rosser crypt hook
Rossetti modification of Nissen
    fundoplication
Rossmax automatic wristwatch
    blood pressure monitor
Rostan shunt
rostral aspect
rostral pole
rostral transtentorial herniation
rostrally

rostrate pelvis
rostrocaudal extent signal
    abnormality
rostrum (*pl.* rostra)
rostrum of sinus
rostrum of sphenoid
rosy apple cheeks
ROT position (right
    occipitotransverse position)
Rotablator atherectomy device
Rotablator RotaLink Plus
    rotational atherectomy
    device
Rotablator RotaLink rotational
    atherectomy device
Rotablator rotating bur
Rotablator wire
Rotacs guidewire
Rotacs motorized catheter
Rotacs rotational atherectomy
    device
Rotafloppy wire
Rotalink flexible shaft
Rotalok acetabular cup
Rotalok cup
Rotalok cup cementless
    acetabular component
Rotalok skin retractor
rotary basket
rotary bur
rotary cutting instrument
rotary cutting tip
rotary dissector
rotary hub saw
rotary joint
rotary microtome
rotary mounted point
rotary scissors with cigar handle
rotary scissors with loop handle
rotary subluxation
rotatable coupling head
rotatable polypectomy snare
rotatable transsphenoidal
    enucleator
rotatable transsphenoidal
    horizontal ring curet
rotatable transsphenoidal knife
    handle
rotatable transsphenoidal right-
    angle hook
rotatable transsphenoidal round
    dissector

rotatable transsphenoidal
    spatula dissector
rotatable transsphenoidal
    vertical ring curet
rotated down
rotated kidney
rotated to left
rotated to right
rotated upward
rotating adapter
rotating air impactor
rotating anode tube
rotating anoscope
rotating arm impactor
rotating disk oxygenator
rotating forceps
rotating frame imaging
rotating gamma camera
rotating hinge
rotating joint
rotating laryngoscope
rotating mechanism
rotating morcellator
rotating resectoscope
rotating speculum anoscope
rotating speculum proctoscope
rotating sphincterotome
rotating tourniquet
rotating transilluminator
rotating-hinge knee prosthesis
rotating-type cutter
rotation
    axis of rotation
    caudal rotation
    center of rotation
    external rotation
    flap rotation
    flexion, abduction, internal
        rotation (fadir)
    hip rotation
    instantaneous axis of rotation
    internal rotation
    inward rotation
    key-in-lock rotation
    Kjelland rotation
    left rotation
    Mallet scale shoulder external
        rotation
    monocular rotations
    outward rotation
    sagittal rotation
    skin flap rotation

rotation (*continued*)
tip rotation
van Ness rotation
rotation advancement flap
rotation flap
rotation flap cut-back
rotation forceps
rotation fracture
rotation joint
rotation of colon
rotation of flap
rotation of pelvis
rotation of philtrum
rotation operative delivery
rotation osteotomy
rotation skin flap
rotation skin flap technique
rotation therapy
rotation-advancement
continuous rotation-advancement
rotation-advancement cleft lip repair
rotation-advancement flap
rotational ablation
rotational ablation laser
rotational advancement osteotomy
rotational atherectomy device
rotational burst fracture
rotational contact lithotripsy
rotational coronary atherectomy
rotational correction
rotational deformity
rotational deformity of finger
rotational dislocation
rotational dynamic air therapy bed
rotational flap
rotational flap graft
rotational instability
rotational irradiation therapy
rotational movement
rotational x-ray beam dosimetry
rotationally induced shear-strain lesion
rotation-compression maneuver
rotationplasty
rotation-transposition cleft lip procedure

rotator
Bechert nucleus rotator
Bechert-Hoffer nucleus rotator
external rotator
Hosmer above-knee rotator
Howmedica monotube external rotator
internal rotator
Jaffe-Bechert nucleus rotator
Jarit rotator
nucleus rotator
Osher globe rotator
Tennant nuclear ball rotator
rotator cuff arthropathy
rotator cuff injury
rotator cuff lesion
rotator cuff repair
rotator cuff tear
rotator cuff tear arthroplasty
rotator cuff tendinitis
rotator flap
rotator muscles
rotatory hammer
rotatory instability
rotatory motion
rotatory spasm
rotatory subluxation of scaphoid (RSS)
rotatory-variable-differential transducer
RotaWire guidewire
Rotch sign
Rotex II biopsy needle
Rotex needle
Roth arch form
Roth dental cement
Roth endoscopy retrieval net
Roth Grip-Tip suture guide
Roth polyp retrieval net
Roth urethral suture guide
Rothene catheter
Rothman Institute femoral prosthesis
Rothman Institute porous femoral component
Rothman-Gilbard corneal punch
Rothmund syndrome
Rothmund-Thomson syndrome
Rothon retractor
Roticulator clamp stapler
Roto Kinetic bed

Roto Rest delta kinetic therapy
     treatment table
rotoextraction
rotoextractor
Roto-Rest bed
rotoscoliosis
Rotosnare device
rotosteotome
Rotozyme diagnostic procedure
Rotter interpectoral nodes
Rotter node
Rottgen-Ruskin bone rongeur
Roubaix forceps
Roubin-Gianturco flexible coil
     stent
Rouge operation
Rouget muscle
Roughton-Scholander syringe
rouleaux formation
round back deformity
round block suture
round body
round body needle
round bur
round cell
round cell sarcoma
round chuck-end Kirschner wire
round counterbore
round cutting bur
round diamond bur
round dissector
round extension rod
round foramen
round Gigli saw
round hemorrhage
round hole plate
round ligament
round ligament of femur
round ligament of liver
round ligament of uterus
round needle
round nucleus
round optical zone marker
round pronator muscle
round punch forceps
round ruby knife
round shoulder deformity
round speculum
round ulcer
round window
round-blade scissors
round-cell liposarcoma

rounded edge
round-end cutter
round-ended distraction rod
round-handled forceps
round-loop electrode
round-nosed rongeur
round-tip catheter
round-tip microscissors
round-tipped periosteal elevator
round-wire electrode
Rousek extender
Roush tonometer
Roussel-Frankhauser contact lens
route of administration
route of injection
route of insertion
Routier operation
routine bilateral neck exploration
routine laparotomy
routine procedure
routine unilateral exploration
routine urinalysis (RUA)
routine workup
Routte operation
Roux double-ended retractor
Roux gastric reconstruction
Roux gastroenterostomy
Roux limb stump dehiscence
Roux limb stump leak
Roux operation
Roux retractor
Roux sign
Roux spatula
Roux stasis syndrome
Roux-DuToit staple
     capsulorrhaphy
Roux-en-Y (*also* Roux-Y)
Roux-en-Y anastomosis
Roux-en-Y biliary bypass
Roux-en-Y
     choledochojejunostomy
Roux-en-Y esophagojejunostomy
Roux-en-Y gastrectomy
Roux-en-Y gastric bypass
Roux-en-Y gastroenterostomy
Roux-en-Y gastrojejunostomy
Roux-en-Y hepaticojejunal
     anastomosis
Roux-en-Y hepaticojejunostomy
Roux-en-Y hepatojejunostomy
Roux-en-Y incision
Roux-en-Y jejunal limb

Roux-en-Y jejunal loop incision
Roux-en-Y jejunoileostomy
Roux-en-Y limb enteroscopy
Roux-en-Y loop
Roux-en-Y operation
Roux-en-Y pancreaticojejunostomy
Roux-en-Y procedure
Roux-en-Y reconstruction
Roux-Goldthwait dislocation operation
Roux-Goldthwait patella repair
Roux-Goldthwait patellar tendon transfer
Roux-Goldthwait procedure
rove magnetic catheter
Roveda operation
Roveda technique
Rovenstine catheter-introducing forceps
Rovighi sign
Rovsing operation
Rovsing sign
Rovsing-Blumberg sign
row of sutures
Rowbatham orbital decompression
Rowbotham operation
Rowden uterine manipulator injector (RUMI)
Rowe approach
Rowe boathook retractor
Rowe bone elevator
Rowe bone-drilling forceps
Rowe calcaneal fracture classification
Rowe disimpacting forceps
Rowe disimpaction forceps
Rowe elevator
Rowe glenoid punch
Rowe glenoid reamer
Rowe glenoid-reaming forceps
Rowe humeral head retractor
Rowe maxillary forceps
Rowe modified-Harrison forceps
Rowe orbital floor retractor
Rowe posterior approach
Rowe posterior shoulder approach
Rowe punch
Rowe reamer
Rowe retractor

Rowe scapular neck retractor
Rowe-Harrison bone-holding forceps
Rowe-Killey forceps
Rowe-Lowell hip dislocation classification
Rowe-Lowell system for fracture-dislocation classification
Rowen spatula
Rowen spinal fusion gouge
Rowe-Zarins shoulder immobilization
Rowinski dacryostomy
Rowinski operation
Rowland double-action forceps
Rowland double-action hump forceps
Rowland eye knife
Rowland hump forceps
Rowland keratome
Rowland nasal hump forceps
Rowland nasal rongeur
Rowland osteotome
Rowland pouch
Rowsey cannula
Rowsey fixation cannula
Royal crown
Royal disposable skin stapler
Royal Flush angiographic flush catheter
Royal Hospital dilator
Royal Moore opponens pollicis transfer
Royal spoon
Royalite body jacket
Royalite splint
Royalt-Street bougie
Roy-Camille plate
Royce bayonet ear knife
Royce ear knife
Royce forceps
Royce perforator
Royce tympanum perforator
Roylan Gel Shell spica splint
Royl-Derm protectant powder
Royl-Derm wound hydrogel nonadherent dressing
Royle operation
Royle-Thompson FDS transfer
Royle-Thompson opponensplasty
Royle-Thompson transfer technique

RPT (rapid pull-through)
RPT operation
RPT technique
RR (recovery room)
RS4 pacemaker
RScA position (right
    scapuloanterior position)
Rusch-Uchida transjugular liver
    access needle-catheter
RScP position (right
    scapuloposterior position)
RSD (reflex sympathetic
    dystrophy)
RSDCP plate
RSP position (right
    sacroposterior position)
RSS (rotatory subluxation of
    scaphoid)
RSTL (relaxed skin tension
    lines)
R-synchronous VVT pacemaker
RT Advantage ultrasound
RT nail
RTV total artificial heart
RUA (routine urinalysis)
rubber acorn
rubber acorn tip
rubber airway
rubber arch
rubber band hemorrhoidectomy
rubber band ligator
rubber bite liner
rubber bolster
rubber catheter
rubber dam
rubber drain
rubber endoscopic tube
rubber glove
rubber impression material
rubber padding
rubber pegs
rubber punch dam
rubber Scan spray dressing
rubber shod clamp
rubber sponge
rubber sutures
rubber tip
rubber tissue
rubber tube
rubber vessel loop
rubber walking heel
rubber-band extraction

rubber-band hemorrhoid
    ligation
rubber-band ligation
rubber-bulb syringe
rubber-dam clamp
rubber-dam clamp forceps
rubber-dam drain
rubber-reinforced bandage
rubber-shod catheter
rubber-shod clamp
rubber-shod forceps
rubber-shod hook
rubber-tip, rubber-tipped
Rubbrecht extirpation
Rubbrecht operation
Rubbs aortic dilator
Rubens breast flap
Rubens free flap for breast
    reconstruction
Rubens pillow
Rubicon embolic filter
Rubin blade
Rubin bone planer
Rubin Brandborg biopsy tube
Rubin bronchus clamp
Rubin cannula
Rubin cartilage planer
Rubin fallopian tube cannula
Rubin gouge
Rubin hydraulic biopsy tube
Rubin maneuver
Rubin nasal chisel
Rubin nasofrontal osteotome
Rubin needle
Rubin oblique rasp
Rubin operation
Rubin osteotome
Rubin osteotomy
Rubin rasp
Rubin septal morsellizer
Rubin tubal insufflation
Rubin tube
Rubin-Arnold needle
Rubin-Holth corneoscleral
    punch
Rubin-Holth sclerectomy punch
Rubin-Lewis periosteal elevator
Rubin-Quinton small-bowel
    biopsy tube
Rubinstein cryoextractor
Rubinstein cryophake
Rubinstein cryoprobe

Rubinstein-Taybi syndrome
Rubin-Wright forceps
Rubio needle holder
Rubio scissors
Rubio wire-holding clamp
Rubovits clamp
rubrospinal decussation
ruby diamond knife
Ruby II DDD pacemaker
ruby knife
ruby knife scalpel
ruby laser
ruby laser operation for retinal
    detachment
ruby spot
Rucker body
Rudd Clinic hemorrhoidal
    forceps
Rudd Clinic hemorrhoidal
    ligator
Rudd ligator
Ruddock laparoscope
Ruddy dissector
Ruddy incision
Ruddy stapes calipers
Ruddy stapes prosthesis
Rudich treatment unit
rudimentary bone
rudimentary disk space
rudimentary eye
rudimentary metacarpal
rudimentary ribs
rudimentary uterus
rudimentary vagina
Rudolf-Buck suturing device
Rudolph calibrated super
    syringe
Rudolph mask
Rudolph trowel retractor
Ruedemann eye evisceration
Ruedemann eye implant
Ruedemann lacrimal dilator
Ruedemann operation
Ruedemann tonometer
Ruedemann-Todd tendon tucker
Ruedi-Allgower classification
Ruel aorta clamp
Ruel forceps
Ruese bone graft
ruffed canal
Ruffini corpuscles
Ruffini papillary endings

ruga (*pl.* rugae)
rugae gastricae
rugae of stomach
rugae of vagina
rugae vaginales
rugal coarsening
rugal folds
rugal pattern
rugal pattern of stomach
Rugby deep-surgery forceps
rugby knee
Rugelski arterial forceps
rugger jersey spine
Ruggles microcuret
Ruggles surgical instrument
rugose frontonasal malformation
Ruiz adjustable marker
Ruiz fundal contact lens
Ruiz fundal laser lens
Ruiz microkeratome
Ruiz plano fundal lens
Ruiz plano fundus lens implant
Ruiz procedure
Ruiz trapezoidal keratotomy
Ruiz-Cohen round expander
Ruiz-Mora correction
Ruiz-Mora operation for claw
    toe
Ruiz-Mora procedure
Ruiz-Morgan procedure
Ruiz-Shepard marker
RUL (right upper lobe)
rule of nines formula for
    percentage of body surface
    burned
rule out myocardial infarction
    (ROMI)
ruler
  Berndt hip ruler
  Bio-Pen biometric ruler
  bronchoscopic ruler
  centimeter subtraction ruler
  Chernov notched ruler
  Helveston scleral marking
    ruler
  hip ruler
  Hyde astigmatism ruler
  Hyde-Osher keratometric
    ruler
  Joseph measuring ruler
  Krinsky-Prince
    accommodation ruler

ruler (*continued*)
  metal ruler
  millimeter ruler
  notched ruler
  Pischel scleral ruler
  Plexiglas radiographic ruler
  Richard-Allan surgical ruler
  scleral ruler
  Scott No. 2 curved ruler
  Scott ruler
  stainless steel flexible ruler
  Stecher microruler
  steel ruler
  Tabb ruler
  Thornton corneal press-on
    ruler
  Thornton double corneal
    ruler
  ulnar ruler
  V. Mueller ruler
  Walker scleral ruler
  Webster ruler
  Weck astigmatism ruler
ruler calipers
Rultract internal mammary
    artery retractor
rumbling bowel sounds
Rumel aluminum bridge splint
Rumel bronchial hemostat
Rumel cardiac tourniquet
Rumel cardiovascular tourniquet
Rumel catheter
Rumel clamp
Rumel dissecting forceps
Rumel lobectomy forceps
Rumel myocardial clamp
Rumel myocardial tourniquet
Rumel ratchet tourniquet
Rumel ratchet tourniquet eyed
    stylet
Rumel retractor
Rumel rubber clamp
Rumel rubber forceps
Rumel splint
Rumel technique
Rumel thoracic clamp
Rumel thoracic forceps
Rumel thoracic-dissecting
    forceps
Rumel tourniquet
Rumel tourniquet eyed
    obturator

Rumel-Belmont tourniquet
Rumex titanium instruments
RUMI uterine manipulator
Rumison side-port fixation
    occluder
Rumpel-Leede sign
Rumpuffet vessel tourniquet
run-around abscess
run-around infection
running chromic sutures
running continuous sutures
    technique
running continuous sutures
running imbricating sutures
running nylon penetrating
    keratoplasty sutures
running subcuticular sutures
running sutures
running technique
running vascular technique
running W-plasty technique
running-locked stitch
running-locked sutures
rupture
  Achilles tendon rupture
  acute hepatic rupture
  adductor longus muscle
    rupture
  amnion rupture
  aneurysmal rupture
  anterior talofibular ligament
    rupture
  aortic rupture
  balloon rupture
  cardiac rupture
  chamber rupture
  chordae tendineae rupture
  chordal rupture
  choroidal rupture
  collateral ligament rupture
  complete rupture
  crescentic rupture
  diaphragmatic rupture
  distal biceps brachii tendon
    rupture
  ERCP-induced splenic rupture
  esophageal rupture
  flexor tendon rupture
  Frank intrabiliary rupture
  gastric rupture
  hemidiaphragm rupture
  hepatic rupture

rupture (*continued*)
  hernia rupture
  hydatid cyst intrahepatic
    rupture
  incidental rupture
  inflammatory rupture
  infrapatellar tendon rupture
  interventricular septal rupture
  intracapsular rupture
  intramural esophageal rupture
  intraoperative rupture
  intraperitoneal viscus rupture
  intrapleural rupture
  longitudinal ligament rupture
  Mallory-Weiss mucosal rupture
  marginal sinus rupture
  membrane rupture
  mesenteric rupture
  muscle rupture
  myocardial rupture
  neglected rupture
  nonpenetrating rupture
  papillary muscle rupture
  penetrating rupture
  penile rupture
  pericardial rupture
  plaque rupture
  postmembrane rupture
  prelabor membrane rupture
  premature amnion rupture
  premature membrane rupture
  premembrane rupture
  prolonged rupture
  proximal tendon rupture
  renal allograft rupture
  retrograde balloon rupture
  scar rupture
  scleral rupture
  splenic rupture
  spontaneous rupture
  stress rupture
  tendon rupture
  testicular rupture
  total perineal rupture
  traumatic rupture
ruptured abdominal aortic
    aneurysm
ruptured aneurysm
ruptured appendix
ruptured bag of waters
ruptured bladder
ruptured diaphragm

ruptured disk
ruptured disk curet
ruptured disk excision
ruptured episiotomy
ruptured flexor tendon
ruptured ligament
ruptured membranes
ruptured peliotic lesion
ruptured spleen
ruptured uterus
RUQ (right upper quadrant)
Rusch bougie
Rusch bronchial catheter
Rusch coude catheter
Rusch endotracheal tube cuff
Rusch external catheter
Rusch filiform
Rusch follower
Rusch laryngectomy tube
Rusch laryngoscope
Rusch laryngoscope blade
Rusch laryngoscope handle
Rusch laryngoscope lamp
Rusch leg bag
Rusch nephrostomy instrument
Rusch perineal drape
Rusch red rubber rectal tube
Rusch rube
Rusch stent
Ruschelit bougie
Ruschelit catheter
Ruschelit polyvinyl chloride
    endotracheal tube
Ruschelit urethral bougie
Rusch-Foley catheter
Rush awl reamer
Rush bone clamp
Rush driver
Rush driver-bender-extractor
Rush extractor
Rush hammer
Rush incision
Rush intramedullary fixation pin
Rush intramedullary nail
Rush mallet
Rush nail
Rush pin
Rush pin bender
Rush pin driver-bender extractor
Rush pin instrument
Rush pin lead-filled head mallet
    with extractor

Rush pin prosthesis extractor with hand grip
Rush pin reamer awl
Rush pin round bevel-point pin set
Rush reamer
Rush rod
Rush rod insertion
Rush rod instrument
Rush safety pin
Rushkin balloon
Ruskin antral needle
Ruskin antral trocar
Ruskin antral trocar needle
Ruskin bone rongeur
Ruskin bone-cutting forceps
Ruskin bone-splitting forceps
Ruskin cranial rongeur
Ruskin duckbill rongeur
Ruskin mastoid rongeur
Ruskin multiple-action rongeur
Ruskin needle
Ruskin rongeur
Ruskin rongeur forceps
Ruskin sphenopalatine ganglion needle
Ruskin trocar
Ruskin-Jansen bone rongeur
Ruskin-Jay heavy-duty rongeur
Ruskin-Jay rongeur
Ruskin-Liston bone-cutting forceps
Ruskin-Liston bone-cutting rongeur
Ruskin-Liston forceps
Ruskin-Rowland bone rongeur
Ruskin-Rowland bone-cutting forceps
Ruskin-Storz rongeur
Russ tumor forceps
Russ vascular forceps
Russe bone graft
Russe classification
Russe incision
Russe inlay bone graft
Russe operation
Russe technique
Russell dilator
Russell fibular head autograft
Russell forceps
Russell frame
Russell gastrostomy

Russell gastrostomy kit
Russell gastrostomy tray
Russell hydrostatic dilator
Russell hysterectomy forceps
Russell peel-away sheath dilator
Russell percutaneous endoscopic gastrostomy
Russell pin traction
Russell skeletal cervical traction
Russell splint
Russell suction tube
Russell technique
Russell traction
Russell traction device
Russell tractor
Russell traction
Russell-Taylor classification
Russell-Taylor delta rod
Russell-Taylor delta tibial nail
Russell-Taylor interlocking medullary nail
Russell-Taylor interlocking nail
Russell-Taylor interlocking nail instrumentation
Russell-Taylor nail
Russell-Taylor screw
Russell-Taylor tibial interlocking nail
Russian bath
Russian fixation hook
Russian forceps
Russian 4-pronged fixation hook
Russian Pean forceps
Russian thumb forceps
Russian tissue forceps
Rust amputation saw
Rutkow sutureless patch
Rutkow sutureless plug
Rutkow sutureless plug and patch
Rutkow-Robbins-Gilbert classification
Rutledge extended hysterectomy classification
Rutner biopsy needle
Rutner nephrostomy balloon catheter
Rutner stone basket
Rutner stone extractor
Rutner wedge catheter
Reuttner classification
Rutzen ileostomy bag

Ruuska meniscotome
Ruysch membrane
Ruysch muscle
Ruysch tube
Ruysch veins
Ruysch-Armor tube
ruyschian membrane
RVAD centrifugal right
   ventricular assist device
RX Herculink Plus biliary stent
RX perfusion catheter
RX Streak balloon catheter
RX balloon catheter
Rychener-Weve electrode
Rycroft cannula
Rycroft lamp
Rycroft needle
Rycroft operation

Rycroft tying forceps
Rydell nail
Rydel-Seiffert tuning fork
Ryder needle holder
Ryder scissors
Rye Hodgkin disease
   classification
Ryecroft retractor
Ryerson bone graft
Ryerson bone retractor
Ryerson operation
Ryerson procedure
Ryerson retractor
Ryerson technique
Ryerson tenotome
Ryerson tenotome knife
Ryerson triple arthrodesis
Ryle duodenal tube

2nd areola
2nd cranial nerve (optic)
2nd-degree burn
2nd-degree hemorrhoid
2nd-degree operation
2nd-degree radiation injury
2nd-degree sprain
2nd-echo image
2nd-grade fusion
2nd generation lithotriptor
2nd intention wound closure
2nd-line chemotherapy
2nd-line drug
2nd-look biopsy
2nd-look laparoscopy
2nd-look laparotomy
2nd-look procedure
2nd-look surgery
2nd parallel pelvic plane
2nd skin pad
2nd toe wraparound flap
6-eye catheter
6-hole mandibular plate
6-hole stainless steel plate
6-point knee brace
6-prong rake retractor
6th cranial nerve (abducens)
6-wire spiral-tip Segura basket
710 Acuspot
7F Hydrolyser thrombectomy
    catheter
7th cranial nerve (facial)
7-hole plate
7-pin staple
S incision
S root canal file
S stylet
S&C (sclerae and conjunctivae)
SS White surgical
    handpiece bur
SS White clamp
SS White J-Notch surgical
    handpiece bur

SAM (subcutaneous
    augmentation material)
SAM facial implant
SMART (shape memory alloy
    recoverable technology)
    stent
SMART bile duct stent
SMART biliary stent
SA node (sinoatrial node)
SA position (sacroanterior
    position)
Saalfeld comedo extractor
SAB (spontaneous abortion;
    subarachnoid block)
SAB anesthesia (subarachnoid
    block anesthesia)
Saba classification of shoulder
    muscles
Sabbatsberg septum elevator
Saber ArthroWand trocar
Saber blunt-tip surgical trocar
saber incision
saber saw
saber tibia
saber-back scissors
saber-cut approach
saber-cut incision
Saberloc spatula needle
saber-slash incision
Sable balloon catheter
Sable PTCA balloon catheter
sabot heart
Sabra OMS 45 dental handpiece
Sabreloc spatula needle
Sabreloc sutures
sabre-shin deformity
sac
    abdominal sac
    air sacs
    amniotic sac
    aortic sac
    caudal sac
    dural sac

sac (*continued*)
  embryonic sac
  endolymphatic sac
  enterocele sac
  fibrous sac
  fluid-filled sac
  fossa of lacrimal sac
  gestational sac
  greater peritoneal sac
  hernia sac
  hernial sac
  Hilton sac
  ileostomy sac
  indirect hernia sac
  lacrimal sac
  lesser peritoneal sac
  nasal sac
  nasolacrimal sac
  pericardial sac
  peritoneal sac
  pleural sac
  scrotal sac
  subarachnoid sac
  synovial sac
  tear sac
  wide-mouth sac
SAC (short arm cast)
sac cushion
sac extirpation
sac formation
saccade
sacciform kidney
saccular aneurysm
saccular bronchiectasis
saccular collection
saccular colon
saccular cyst
saccular duct
saccular fossa
saccular nerve
saccular spot
sacculation
saccule
  air saccule
  vestibular saccule
saccule of larynx
sacculoutricular duct
sacculus (*pl.* sacculi)
sacculus endolymphaticus
sacculus lacrimalis
sacculus laryngis
saccus (*pl.* sacci)

saccus operation
SACH (solid ankle cushioned
     heel)
SACH foot
SACH foot adapter
SACH heel
SACH implant
SACH orthopedic appliance
SACH prosthesis
Sachs angled vein retractor
Sachs brain suction tube
Sachs brain-exploring cannula
Sachs bur
Sachs catheter
Sachs cervical punch
Sachs dural hook
Sachs dural separator
Sachs elevator
Sachs forceps
Sachs hook
Sachs needle
Sachs nerve separator
Sachs nerve spatula
Sachs punch
Sachs separator
Sachs skull bur
Sachs spatula
Sachs suction tube
Sachs tissue forceps
Sachs urethrotome
Sachs vein retractor
Sachs-Cushing retractor
Sachs-Freer dissector
Sachs-Vine feeding gastrostomy
Sachs-Vine PEG tube
     (percutaneous endoscopic
     gastrostomy tube)
Sachs biliary drain
saclike cavity
sacrococcygeal junction
sacral ala
sacral alar screw
sacral anesthesia
sacral arcuate line
sacral arteries
sacral bar technique
sacral block anesthesia
sacral bone
sacral brim target point
sacral canal
sacral crest
sacral cul-de-sac

Sacral DISH pressure relief back cushion
sacral flexure
sacral foramen
sacral fracture
sacral ganglia
sacral horizontal plane line
sacral nerves
sacral pedicle screw fixation
sacral plexus
sacral prominence
sacral reflexes
sacral region
sacral screw placement
sacral semental nerve stimulation implanatable neural prosthesis
sacral spine fixation
sacral spine fusion
sacral spine modular instrumentation
sacral spine stabilization
sacral spine Universal instrumentation
sacral splanchnic nerves
sacral spot
sacral support
sacral tuberosity
sacral veins
sacral vertebrae
sacral wound
sacrales laterales, arterieae
sacral-foraminal approach
sacralization
sacrectomy
sacroabdominoperineal pull-through operation
sacroanterior position (SA position)
sacrococcygeal articulation
sacrococcygeal cyst
sacrococcygeal defect
sacrococcygeal disk
sacrococcygeal joint
sacrococcygeal muscle
sacrococcygeal region
sacrococcygeal sinus
sacrodextra anterior position
sacrodextra posterior position
sacrofetal pregnancy
sacrofixation operation
sacrogenital fold

sacrogenital ligament
sacrohorizontal angle
sacrohysteric pregnancy
sacroiliac articulation
sacroiliac belt
sacroiliac buttressing procedure
sacroiliac disarticulation
sacroiliac dislocation
Sacroiliac extension fixation
sacroiliac flexion fixation
sacroiliac fracture
sacroiliac joint
sacroiliac notch
sacroiliac strain
sacroma
sacroperineal approach
sacropexy
sacroposterior position (SP position)
sacropubic diameter
sacrosciatic notch
sacrospinal muscle
sacrospinous ligament
sacrospinous ligament suspension
sacrospinous ligament vaginal fixation
sacrotomy
sacrotransverse position
sacrotuberous ligament
sacrouterine fold
sacrouterine ligament
sacrovaginal fold
sacrovesical fold
sacrum fracture
sacrum fusion screw fixation
sac-vein decompression
saddle arch
saddle area
saddle block anesthesia
saddle block spinal anesthesia
saddle coil
saddle curve
saddle defect
saddle deformity of nose
saddle embolism
saddle head
saddle joint
saddle lesion
saddle locator
saddle nose defect
saddle nose deformity

saddle prosthesis
saddle-back nose
saddlebag hernia
saddle-shaped arch
Sade modification of Norwood
    operation
Sadler bone hook
Sadler cartilage scissors
Sadler tissue scissors
Sadowsky hook wire
Saeed Six-Shooter multi-band
    ligator
Saeed technique
Saeed variceal ligator
Saemisch operation
Saemisch ulcer
Saenger macula
Saenger operation
Saenger ovum forceps
Saenger placental forceps
Saenger reflex
Saenger sign
Saenger suture technique
Saenger sutures
Saethre-Chotzen craniosynostosis
Saethre-Chotzen syndrome
SAF hip replacement (self-
    articular femoral hip
    replacement)
Safar bronchoscope
Safar operation
Safar tube
Safar ventilation bronchoscope
Safar-S airway
SAF-Clens wound cleanser
Safco alloy
Safco diamond instrument
Safco polycarbonate crown
Safe Response manual
    resuscitator
Safe spine thoracic-lumbar-sacral
    support
Safe-Cuff blood pressure cuff
Safe-Dwel Plus catheter
SafeTap tapered spinal needle
Safe-T-Coat heparin-coated
    thermodilution catheter
Safetex cervical spatula
SafeTrak epidural catheter
safety AV fistula needle
Safety Clear Plus endotracheal
    tube

safety goggles
safety handle
safety pessary
safety pin
safety pin closer
safety pin finger orthosis
safety pin orthosis
safety pin splint
safety plate
safety strap
safety technique
safety tube
safety-bolt sutures
Safe-Wrap gauze
Saf-Gel hydrogel dressing
SAFHS ultrasound device
Safian design prosthesis
Safian nasal splint
Safian rhinoplasty prosthesis
Safil synthetic absorbable
    surgical sutures
Safir pin
Saf-T E-Z set
Saf-T guidewire
Saf-T shield
Saf-T-Cath
Saf-T-Coil intrauterine device
Saf-T-Sound uterine sound
sag foot
Sage forearm rod
Sage syringe pump
Sage intramedullary rod
Sage pin
Sage snare
Sage technique
Sage tonsil snare
Sage wire
Sage-Clark cheilectomy
Sage-Clark technique
Sage-Salvatore
    acromioclavicular joint
    injury classification
sagittal area
sagittal axis
sagittal cartilage graft
sagittal craniectomy
sagittal crest
sagittal deformity
sagittal diameter
sagittal fissure
sagittal fontanelle
sagittal furrow

sagittal incisure
sagittal linear transducer
sagittal mandibular movement
sagittal orientation
sagittal oscillating saw
sagittal plane
sagittal projection
sagittal ramus osteotomy
sagittal reconstruction
sagittal rotation
sagittal section
sagittal sector transducer
sagittal sinus
sagittal slice fracture
sagittal spin-echo image
sagittal split mandibular
  osteotomy
sagittal split osteotomy (SSO)
sagittal split ramus osteotomy
  (SSRO)
sagittal splitting of mandible
sagittal suture
sagittal suture line
sagittal suture synostosis
sagittal synostosis
sagittal synostosis reoperation
sagittalis inferior, sinus
sagittalis superior, sinus
sagittal-plane imaging
sagittal-split osteotomy
Saha shoulder muscle
  classification
Saha shoulder procedure
Saha transfer technique
Sahara portable bone
  densitometer
Sahli needle
Sahli whistle
sail of cartilage
sail of pin
sail sign
sailor's knot
sailor's skin
Saint (see also St.)
Saint George knee prosthesis
Saint Jude prosthesis
Saint Mark dilator
Saint triad
Sajou laryngeal forceps
Sakati-Nyhan syndrome
Sakellarides calcaneal fracture
  classification

Sakellarides technique for
  forearm contracture
Sakellarides-DeWeese technique
Sakler erysiphake
SAL (suction-assisted lipectomy)
salabrasion
Salah sternal needle
Salah sternal puncture needle
Salem duodenal sump tube
Salem nasogastric tube
Salem pump
Salem sump
Salem sump action nasogastric
  tube
Salem sump drain
Salem sump pump
Salem sump tube
Salenius meniscal knife
Salibi carotid artery clamp
salicylated cotton
saline
  flush with saline
  heparinized saline
  iced saline
  lavaged with sterile saline
  normal saline
  Siltex saline
  sterile saline
saline breast implant
saline compress
saline dressing
saline implant exchange
saline infusion
saline injection
saline irrigation
saline lavage
saline solution
saline technique
saline-filled anatomical breast
  implant
saline-filled expander
saline-filled round breast
  implant
saline-moistened sponge
saline-saturated wool dressing
Saling amnioscope
Salinger nasal reducer
Salinger reducer
Salinger reduction instrument
saliva
  artifical saliva
  chorda saliva

saliva (*continued*)
  ganglionic saliva
  lingual saliva
  parotid saliva
  ropy saliva
  sublingual saliva
  submandibular saliva
  submaxillary saliva
  sympathetic saliva
salivary bypass tube
salivary calculus
salivary duct carcinoma (SDC)
salivary duct obstruction
salivary fistula
salivary gland
salivary gland alveolus
salivary gland aplasia
salivary gland capsule
salivary gland carcinoma
    (SGC)
salivary gland cyst
salivary gland enlargement
salivary gland mass
salivary gland pleomorphic
    adenoma
salivary gland retention cyst
salivary gland tumor
salivary gland virus
salivary gland virus disease
salivary immunoglobulin
salivary lipoma
salivary lithiasis
salivary mucus
salivary stone
salivary tube
salivary duct cyst
salivolithiasis
Salman FES stent
salmon backcut incision
Salmon catheter
salmon patch
salmon-patch hemorrhage
Salmon-Rickham
    ventriculostomy reservoir
Salonpas plaster
salpingeal curet
salpingeal probe
salpingectomy
salpingemphraxis
salpingitis
salpingography
salpingolysis

salpingo-oophorectomy (S-O)
  abdominal salpingo-
    oophorectomy
  unilateral salpingo-
    oophorectomy
salpingo-oophoroplasty
salpingo-oophorostomy
salpingo-oophorotomy
salpingo-oophorrhapy
salpingo-ovarian salpingolysis
salpingo-ovariolysis
salpingopalatine fold
salpingopalatine membrane
salpingopexy
salpingopharyngeal fold
salpingopharyngeal membrane
salpingopharyngeal muscle
salpingoplasty
salpingorrhaphy
salpingoscopy
salpingostomy
salpingotomy
salpingo-ureteroscopy
salt and pepper duodenal
    erosion
Salter epiphysial fracture
    classification
Salter fracture (I-VI)
Salter incremental lines
Salter innominate osteotomy
Salter operation
Salter osteotomy
Salter technique
Salter-Harris epiphysial fracture
    classification
Salter-Harris fracture (I-VI)
salting-out procedure
Salus arch
Salus incision
salvage balloon angioplasty
Salvage catheter
salvage cystectomy
salvage laryngectomy
salvage mastectomy
salvage procedure
salvage surgery
salvage technique
salvage therapy
salvarsan throat irrigation tube
salvatella vein
Salvati proctoscope
Salvatore ligator

Salvatore umbilical cord ligator
Salvatore-Maloney tracheotome
Salyer modification of
    Obwegeser mandibular
    osteotomy
SAM (short arm motion)
SAM facial implant material
SAM protocol
Sam Roberts bronchial biopsy
    forceps
Sam Roberts esophagoscope
Sam Roberts headrest
Sam Roberts self-retaining
    laryngoscope
Samadhi cushion
Samco tube
Samilson calcaneal osteotomy
Samilson procedure
Sammons biplane goniometer
Sampoelesi line
Sampson cyst
Sampson fluted nail
Sampson prosthesis
Samson rod
Samson-Davis infant suction
    tube
Samuels hemoclip-applying
    forceps
Samuels valve
Samuels vein stripper
Samuelson total knee
Sanborn metabolator
Sanborn oscilloscope
Sandalthotics postural support
    orthotic
Sanders bed
Sanders forceps
Sanders incision
Sanders intubation laryngoscope
Sanders jet ventilation device
    respirator
Sanders operation
Sanders oscillating bed
Sanders valve
Sanders vasectomy forceps
Sanders ventilation adapter
Sanders-Brown needle
Sanders-Brown-Shaw aneurysm
    needle
Sanders-Castroviejo suturing
    forceps
Sand-Eze EGD pillow

Sandhill probe
Sandoz balloon replacement
    tube
Sandoz Caluso PEG gastrostomy
    tube
Sandoz feeding suction tube
Sandoz nasogastric feeding
    tube
Sandoz suction feeding tube
sandpaper dermabrader
sandpaper disk
Sandstrom body
Sandström (see Sandstrom)
Sandstrom (also Sandström,
    Sandstroem)
Sandstroem (see Sandstrom)
Sandt suture forceps
Sandt utility forceps
sandwich epicranial flap
sandwich patch
sandwich patch closure
sandwich staghorn calculus
    therapy
sandwiched iliac bone graft
sandwich-type splint
Sanfilippo syndrome
Sanford ligator
Sanger incision
sanguineous
sanguineous cataract
sanguineous drainage
sanguineous exudate
sanguineous fluid
sanguineous infiltration
sanguineous inflammation
sanguineous material
sanguineous perfusion
sanguinopurulent
Sani-Spec vaginal speculum
Sano clip applier
Santiani-Stone classification
Santorini canal
Santorini cartilage
Santorini concha
Santorini duct
Santorini labyrinth
Santorini muscle
Santorini parietal vein
Santorini plexus
Santorini tubercle
Santorini vein
Santorini fissure

Santulli clamp
Santy dissecting forceps
Santy ring-end forceps
saphenectomy
saphenofemoral
saphenofemoral juncture
saphenous artery
saphenous bulb
saphenous flap
saphenous graft
saphenous hiatus
saphenous ICA bypass
saphenous nerve
saphenous pulse
saphenous vein
saphenous vein bypass
saphenous vein bypass graft
    (SVBG)
saphenous vein cannula
saphenous vein interposition
    graft
saphenous vein ligation and
    stripping
saphenous vein patch graft
SAPHfinder balloon dissector
SaphFinder surgical balloon
    dissector
SAPHO (synovitis, acne,
    pustulosis, hyperostosis,
    osteitis)
SAPHO syndrome
SAPHtrak balloon dissector
Sappey fibers
Sappey ligament
Sappey plexus
Sappey vein
sapphire knife
sapphire lens
Sapphire View arthroscope
Sapporo shunt
Saqalain dressing forceps
Saraf toenail operation
Saratoga sump
Saratoga sump catheter
sarcogenic cells
sarcoid
sarcoidosis
sarcolemmal membrane
sarcoma (*pl.* sarcomas,
    sarcomata)
    Abernethy sarcoma
    adipose sarcoma

sarcoma (*continued*)
    alveolar soft part sarcoma
        (ASPS)
    ameloblastic sarcoma
    antral sarcoma
    chondroblastic sarcoma
    chondrogenic sarcoma
    clear cell sarcoma
    craniofacial osteogenic
        sarcoma
    endothelial sarcoma
    epithelial sarcoma (ES)
    epithelioid sarcoma
    Ewing sarcoma
    fascial sarcoma
    fibroblastic sarcoma
    fibrogenic sarcoma
    idiopathic multiple pigmented
        hemorrhagic sarcoma
    intraoral Kaposi sarcoma
    juxtacortical osteogenic
        sarcoma
    Kaposi sarcoma
    melanotic sarcoma
    mesenchymal sarcoma
    multiple benign sarcoma
    osteogenic sarcoma
    osteoid sarcoma
    pseudo-Kaposi sarcoma
    reticulum cell sarcoma
    round cell sarcoma
    serocystic sarcoma
    somatic sarcoma
    synovial sarcoma
    telangiectatic osteogenic
        sarcoma
    tendosynovial tissue sarcoma
    uterine sarcoma
sarcomatoid carcinoma
sarcomatosis cutis
sarcomatous
sarcoplasmic reticulum
Sargis uterine manipulator
Sargis uterine tenaculum
Sargon implant
Sarmiento brace
Sarmiento cast
Sarmiento osteotomy for
        intertrochanteric fracture
Sarmiento osteotomy of hip
Sarmiento trochanteric fracture
        technique

Sarnoff aortic clamp
Sarns pump
Sarns aortic arch cannula
Sarns electric saw
Sarns intracardiac suction
    tube
Sarns membrane oxygenator
Sarns safety loop
Sarns saw
Sarns blood pump
Sarns soft-flow aortic cannula
Sarns temperature probe
Sarns 2-stage cannula
Sarns venous drainage cannula
Sarns vent
Sarns ventricular assist device
Sarns wire-reinforced catheter
Sarot arterial clamp
Sarot arterial forceps
Sarot bold sutures
Sarot bronchial clamp
Sarot cardiovascular needle
    holder
Sarot intrathoracic forceps
Sarot knife
Sarot needle
Sarot needle holder
Sarot petit point needle
    holder
Sarot pleurectomy forceps
Sarot thoracic needle holder
Sarot thoracoscope
Sarot Vital needle holder
SARPE (surgical-assisted rapid
    palatal expansion)
sartorial slide procedure
Sartorius pump
sartorius flap
sartorius muscle
SAS (synthetic absorbable
    suture)
SAS II brace
SASMAS face-lift
SASMAS suspension
    rhytidectomy
Sassouni classification
Sat-A-Lite contoured wedge seat
    cushion
Satchmo syndrome
satellite abscess
satellite cells
satellite ear endoscope

satellite lesion
satellite metastasis
satellite myofascial trigger
    point
satellite nodule
Satellite Plus pulse oximeter
Saticon vacuum chamber
    pickup tube
Saticon vacuum tube
Satin Plus glove
SatinCrescent implant knife
SatinCrescent tunneler
SatinShortCut implant knife
SatinShortcut ophthalmic knife
Satinsky anastomosis clamp
Satinsky aortic clamp
Satinsky cardiac scissors
Satinsky double-curve scissors
Satinsky forceps
Satinsky pediatric clamp
Satinsky thoracic scissors
Satinsky tourniquet
Satinsky vascular clamp
Satinsky vena cava clamp
Satinsky vena caval scissors
SatinSlit implant knife
SatinSlit keratome
Sato cataract needle
Sato corneal knife
Sato eye knife
Sato lid retractor
Sato operation
Sato procedure
Sato speculum
Satterlee advancement forceps
Satterlee amputating saw
Satterlee aseptic saw
Satterlee bone saw
Satterlee bone saw blade
Satterlee capital saw
Satterlee muscle forceps
Satterlee saw
Sattler layer
Sattler veil
saturated solution
saturation index
SaturEyes contact lens
Saturn Splint
saturnine nephritis
Satvioni cryptoscope
saucerization
saucerized biopsy

saucerized cyst
saucer-shaped erosion
Sauer debrider
Sauer eye speculum
Sauer guillotine
Sauer hemostatic tonsillectome
Sauer infant eye speculum
Sauer outer ring forceps
Sauer speculum
Sauer suture forceps
Sauer suturing forceps
Sauer tonometer
Sauer tonsillectome
Sauer-Bacon operation
Sauerbruch elevator for first rib
Sauerbruch implant
Sauerbruch limb prosthesis
Sauerbruch pickup forceps
Sauerbruch prosthesis
Sauerbruch raspatory
Sauerbruch retractor
Sauerbruch rib elevator
Sauerbruch rib forceps
Sauerbruch rib guillotine
Sauerbruch rib rongeur
Sauerbruch rib shears
Sauerbruch rongeur
Sauerbruch-Britsch rib shears
Sauerbruch-Coryllos bone
    rongeur
Sauerbruch-Coryllos rib rongeur
Sauerbruch-Coryllos rib shears
Sauerbruch-Frey raspatory
Sauerbruch-Frey rib elevator
Sauerbruch-Frey rib shears
Sauerbruch-Lebsche rib shears
Sauerbruch-Lebsche rongeur
Sauerbruch-Lilienthal rib
    spreader
Sauerbruch-Stille bone rongeur
Sauerbruch-Zukschwerdt rib
    retractor
Sauer-Lebsche rongeur
Sauer-Sluder tonsillectome
Sauer-Storz tonometer
Sauer-Storz tonsillectome
Sauer-Wiener intranasal
    instruments
Sauflon contact lens
Saunders cataract needle
Saunders cervical traction
Saunders eye speculum

Saunders needle
Saunders-Paparella hook
Saunders-Paparella marker
Saunders-Paparella needle
Saunders-Paparella pick
Saunders-Paparella rasp
Saunders-Paparella stapes hook
Saunders-Paparella window
    rasp
sausage digit
sausage finger
sausage toe
sausaging of vein
Sauvage arterial graft
Sauvage Bionit femoral
    prosthesis
Sauvage Bionit graft
Sauvage Dacron graft
Sauvage fabric graft prosthesis
Sauvage filamentous prosthesis
Sauvage filamentous velour
    graft
Sauvage vein graft
Sauvage-Bionit graft
Sauve-Kapandji procedure
Savage intestinal decompressor
Savage perineal body
Savary bougie
Savary bronchoscope
Savary esophageal dilator
Savary gastrointestinal
    endoscopy
Savary tapered thermoplastic
    dilator
Savary-Gilliard esophageal
    dilator
Savary-Gilliard over-the-wire
    dilator
Savary-Gilliard Silastic flexible
    bougie
Savary-Gilliard tip
Savary-Gilliard wire guide
Savary-Gilliard wire-guided
    bougie
Savary-Miller grading scale
    classification
Savastano hemi-knee prosthesis
Savastano total knee prosthesis
Savin operation
Savin procedure
Savlon splint
SAVVI synchronous pacemaker

saw

- Accutome low-speed diamond saw
- Adams saw
- Adson Gigli saw
- Aesculap saw
- air saw
- air-driven saw
- Albee bone saw
- Allen saw
- amputating saw
- amputation saw
- angular saw
- antral saw
- Arbuckle antral saw
- Arruga saw
- aseptic saw
- Bailey wire saw
- bayonet saw
- Beaver finger ring saw
- Becker-Joseph saw
- Bergman plaster saw
- Bier amputation saw
- Bishop oscillatory electric bone saw
- Bodenham saw
- bone saw
- Bosworth nasal saw
- Bosworth-Joseph nasal saw
- Brown saw
- Brown-Joseph saw
- bur saw
- Butcher saw
- Cayo saw
- chain saw
- Chamfer saw
- Charnley saw
- Charriere amputation saw
- Charriere aseptic metacarpal saw
- Charriere bone saw
- circular saw
- circular twin saw
- Clerf laryngeal saw
- Codman sternal saw
- Converse nasal saw
- Cottle nasal saw
- Cottle Universal nasal saw
- Cottle-Joseph saw
- counterrotating saw
- crosscut saw
- crown saw

saw (*continued*)

- crurotomy saw
- Delrin-handle bone saw
- DeMartel conductor saw
- DeMartel T-wire saw
- diamond saw
- diamond wafering saw
- double-concave rotating saw
- electric laryngofissure saw
- electric saw
- Engle plaster saw
- Farabeuf saw
- Farrior-Joseph bayonet saw
- Farrior-Joseph nasal saw
- femoral head saw
- fenestration saw
- finger ring saw
- fragment pared with motor saw
- Galt saw
- Gigli solid-handle saw
- Gigli wire saw
- Gigli-Strully saw
- gold saw
- Goldman saw
- Gottschalk transverse saw
- Guilford-Wright bur saw
- Guilford-Wullstein bur saw
- Hall sagittal saw
- Hall sternal saw
- Hall Versipower oscillating saw
- Hall Versipower reciprocating saw
- Hall-Zimmer saw
- hand saw
- helical tube saw
- Hetherington circular saw
- Hey skull saw
- Hill-Bosworth saw
- Hough crurotomy saw
- Hough-Wullstein bur saw
- hub saw
- humeral saw
- Iliff dacryoattachment for Stryker saw
- intranasal saw
- Isomet low speed saw
- Isomet precision saw
- Jesse-Stryker saw
- Joseph bayonet saw
- Joseph nasal saw
- Joseph-Farrior saw

saw (*continued*)

Joseph-Maltz angular nasal saw
Joseph-Maltz nasal saw
Joseph-Stille saw
Joseph-Verner saw
Lamont nasal saw
Langenbeck metacarpal amputation saw
Langenbeck metacarpal saw
laryngeal saw
laryngectomy saw
laryngofissure saw
Lebsche wire saw
Lell laryngofissure saw
Luck bone saw
Luck-Bishop saw
luxation saw
Macewen saw
Magnuson circular twin saw
Magnuson double counter-rotating saw
Magnuson single circular saw
Maltz bayonet saw
Maltz nasal saw
McCabe crurotomy saw
metacarpal saw
Micro-Aire bone saw
Micro-Aire oscillating bone saw
microreciprocating saw
microsagittal saw
Miltex bone saw
Mueller round Gigli saw
Myerson laryngectomy saw
nasal saw
Ogura nasal saw
Olivecrona wire saw
Olivecrona-Gigli wire saw
Orthair oscillating saw
Osada saw
oscillating saw
oscillating sternotomy saw
oscillatory saw
Paparella-McCabe crurotomy saw
pared with motor saw
patella bone saw
Percy amputating saw
plaster saw
reciprocating saw

saw (*continued*)

Reese saw
rhinoplasty saw
Rica wire saw
ring-cutting saw
rotary hub saw
round Gigli saw
Rust amputation saw
saber saw
sagittal oscillating saw
Sarns electric saw
Satterlee amputating saw
Satterlee amputation saw
Satterlee aseptic saw
Satterlee bone saw
Satterlee capital saw
Schwartz antral trocar saw
Seltzer saw
separating saw
Shrady saw
silver saw
single circular saw
single-sided bone saw
Skil Saw
Sklar bone saw
skull saw
Slaughter nasal saw
spinal saw
Stedman saw
sternal saw
sternotomy saw
sternum saw
Stille Gigli saw
Stille saw
Stille Gigli wire saw
Stille-Joseph saw
Stiwer finger-ring saw
Stryker autopsy saw
Stryker oscillating saw
subcutaneous saw
surgical saw
transverse saw
Tuke bone saw
Tyler Gigli saw
Tyler spiral Gigli saw
Universal nasal saw
Universal saw
V. Mueller amputating saw
V. Mueller-Gigli saw
Wigmore plaster saw
Williams microsurgery saw
wire saw

saw (*continued*)
 Woakes nasal saw
 Xomed micro-oscillating
  saw
 Zimmer saw
saw guide (*see* guide)
saw handle
saw incision
Sawar ptosis operation
sawdust bed
Sawtell applicator
Sawtell arterial forceps
Sawtell gallbladder forceps
Sawtell hemostat
Sawtell hemostatic forceps
Sawtell laryngeal applicator
Sawtell nasal applicator
Sawtell tonsillar forceps
Sawtell-Davis forceps
Sawtell-Davis hemostat
Sawtell-Davis tonsillar hemostat
  forceps
saw-tooth appearance sign
saw-toothed curet
Sawyer operation
Sawyer rectal retractor
Sawyer rectal speculum
Saxtorph maneuver
SAXX renal stent
Sayoc operation
Sayoc procedure
Sayre bandage
Sayre cast application
Sayre double-end periosteal
  elevator
Sayre double-ended elevator
Sayre dressing
Sayre elevator
Sayre head sling
Sayre head snare
Sayre jacket
Sayre operation
Sayre periosteal elevator
Sayre periosteal raspatory
Sayre raspatory
Sayre retractor
Sayre splint
Sayre suspension traction
Sayre traction
SB tube (Sengstaken-Blakemore
  tube)
Sbarbaro operation

Sbarbaro tibial prosthesis
SBE (subacute bacterial
  endocarditis)
SBE cast
SBMI (silicone gel-filled
  mammary implant)
SBO (small-bowel
  obstruction)
SBRN (sensory branch of radial
  nerve)
SC (supracondylar)
SC suspension
SC-1 needle
SC-5A fiberscope
Scabbard needle
scabbard trachea
scabiform
SCA-EX ShortCutter catheter
Scaglietti closed reduction
  technique
Scaglietti procedure
Scaglietti rongeur
scalar classification
scalar leads
scalar time
scalded-skin syndrome
scale
 Abbreviated Injury Scale
 Bayley infant scale
 Benoist scale
 Binet scale
 Brazelton neonatal assessment
  scale
 Charriere scale
 EMV grading of Glasgow
  coma scale
 Fahrenheit scale
 French catheter scale
 Gardner-Pearson growth grid
  scale
 Glasgow coma scale
 Hachinski ischemic scale
 Hetzel-Dent grading scale
 House-Brackmann facial
  weakness scale
 Kelvin scale
 modified Mallet scale
 Mohs hardness scale
 Outerbridge scale
 Pyle-Greulich bone age scale
 Ritchie articular pain scale
 Schnur scale

scale (*continued*)

  Sessing pressure ulcer
    assessment scale

  Shea pressure ulcer
    assessment scale

scalene adenopathy

scalene biopsy

scalene elevator

scalene fat pad biopsy

scalene lesion

scalene lymph node biopsy

scalene maneuver

scalene muscle

scalene node biopsy (SNB)

scalenectomy

scalenotomy

scalenoverterbral triangle

scalenus anterior muscle

scalenus anterior syndrome

scalenus anticus syndrome

scalenus medius muscle

scalenus posterior muscle

scaling lesion

scaling skin-colored lesion

scallop sign

scalloped closure

scalloping of lower lid

scalloping of vertebrae

scalp clip

scalp clip forceps

scalp clip-applying forceps

scalp closure

scalp contusion

scalp electrode

scalp expansion

scalp extension

scalp forceps

scalp hemostasis clip

scalp hemostat

scalp incision

scalp laceration

scalp lift

scalp muscle

scalp reconstruction

scalp reduction

scalp replantation

scalp retractor

scalp self-retaining retractor

scalp sickle flap

scalp sutures

scalp tissue expansion

scalp tourniquet

scalp vein needle

scalpel (*see also* blade, knife)

  ASR scalpel

  Bard-Parker disposable scalpel

  Bergman scalpel

  blade scalpel

  bone scalpel

  Bowen double-bladed scalpel

  Cavitron scalpel

  Contact Laser scalpel

  Dieffenbach scalpel

  disposable scalpel

  disposable sterile scalpel

  Downing cartilage scalpel

  electrodes scalpel

  electrosurgical scalpel

  Endo-Assist retractable scalpel

  Endotron-Lipectron scalpel

  Epitome scalpel

  feather scalpel

  Green pendulum scalpel

  Guyton-Lundsgaard scalpel

  Hamer scalpel

  Harmonic scalpel

  Hemostatix scalpel

  Jackson tracheal scalpel

  John Green pendulum scalpel

  laser scalpel

  LaserSonics Nd:YAG
    LaserBlade scalpel

  lid scalpel

  Lipectron scalpel

  long scalpel

  Microcap scalpel

  Otocap myringotomy scalpel

  pendulum scalpel

  Personna Plus disposable
    Teflon scalpel

  plasma scalpel

  razor scalpel

  ruby knife scalpel

  sculpturing scalpel

  Shaw scalpel

  Smart scalpel

  stone-age scalpel

  tracheal scalpel

  ultrasonic harmonic scalpel

  ultrasonic scalpel

  ultrasonically activated scalpel

  water scalpel

scalpel blade

scalpel electrode

scalpel guard
scalpel handle
scalpel vulvectomy
scalpene needle
scalping flap
scalping flap of Converse
scan
  3-dimensional computed
    tomography scans
  axial computed tomography
    scan
  bone scan
  brain scan
  CAT scan (computerized axial
    tomography scan)
  cold bone scan
  contrast CT scan
  contrast-enhanced scan
  coronal computed
    tomography scan
  CT scan
  DISIDA scan
  echo scan
  EMI scan
  enhanced scan
  fluorescent scan
  gallbladder scan
  gastric emptying scan
  gated blood pool scan
  gated pool scan
  hepatobiliary scan
  HIDA scan
  indium scan
  indium-111 scan
  indium-64 scan
  iohexol CT scan
  isotope bone scan
  kidney scan
  liver scan
  liver-spleen scan
  long axis scan
  lung scan
  Meckel scan
  MRI scan
  MUGA cardiac blood pool
    scan
  negative bone scan
  nuclear bleeding scan
  perfusion lung scan
  perfusion scan
  Pfizer scan
  phosphate scan

scan (*continued*)
  placenta scan
  PYP scan (pyrophosphate
    scan)
  pyrophosphate scan (PYP
    scan)
  rectilinear scan
  renal scan
  rose bengal scan
  rose bengal sodium I-131
    biliary scan
  SPECT scan
  SPECT Bullseye scans
  sulfur colloid liver scan
  sulfur colloid scan
  TcHIDA scan
  technetium bone scan
  technetium pertechnetate
    scan
  technetium scan
  technetium-99m scan
  thyroid scan
  ultrasound scan
  V/Q lung scan (ventilation-
    perfusion lung scan)
  ventilation lung scan
  ventilation perfusion scan
  ventilation-perfusion lung
    scan (V/Q lung scan)
  xenon ventilation scan
Scan Pattern generator
scan plane
Scand pin
scan-directed biopsy
Scanditronix PET scanner
Scanlan aneurysm clip
Scanlan bipolar coagulator
Scanlan laparoscopic forceps
Scanlan ligator
Scanlan ligature guide
Scanlan microforceps
Scanlan microneedle holder
Scanlan micronerve hook
Scanlan microrasp
Scanlan microscissors
Scanlan microvessel hook
Scanlan pediatric retractor
Scanlan plaster shears
Scanlan rib shears
Scanlan scissors
Scanlan vessel dilator
Scanlan-Crafoord contractor

ScanLite scanner
Scanmate stethoscope
scanner laser ophthalmoscope
scanning
  B-mode scanning
  body scanning
  confocal laser scanning
  duplex scanning
  isotope scanning
  PET scanning
  point scanning
  pulmonary perfusion
    scanning
  radioisotope scanning
  radionuclide scanning
  scintillation scanning
scanning electron microscope
scanning electron microscopy
    (SEM)
scanning excimer laser
scanning fluorometer
scanning laser acoustic
    microscope
scanning laser ophthalmoscope
scanning laser polarimeter
scanning prism
scanning slit confocal
    microscope
scanning technique
scanning transmission electron
    microscope
scanning tunneling microscope
S-cannula
scanography
Scanpor acrylate adhesive
Scanpor surgical tape
Scanpore hypoallergenic tape
Scanzoni forceps
Scanzoni maneuver
Scanzoni operation
Scanzoni-Smellie maneuver
scapha-concha mattress sutures
scapha-helix
scaphocapitate articulations
scaphocapitate fusion
scaphocapitate syndrome
scaphocephalic deformity
scaphocephalous
scaphocephaly
scaphoconchal angle
scaphohydrocephaly
scaphoid abdomen

scaphoid bone
scaphoid fat pad
scaphoid fossa
scaphoid fracture
scaphoid gouge
scaphoid nonunion
scaphoid projection
scaphoid scapula
scaphoid screw guide
scaphoid shift
scaphoid spatula
scaphoid spoon handle
scaphoid tubercle
scaphoid-capitate arthrodesis
scaphoid-capitate fusion
scaphoid-trapezium-trapezoid
    (STT) joint
scapholunate advanced collapse
    (SLAC)
scapholunate angle
scapholunate articulation
scapholunate dislocation
scapholunate disruption
scapholunate dissociation (S-L
    dissociation)
scapholunate gap
scapholunate instability
scapholunate interosseous
    ligament
scapholunate joint space
scapholunate ligament
scapholunate motion
scaphopisocapitate (SPC)
    relationship
scaphotrapeziotrapezoid joint
    (STT joint)
scaphotrapezoid
scapula (pl. scapulae)
  acromion scapulae
  alar scapula
  circumflex artery of scapula
  elevated scapula
  Graves scapula
  scaphoid scapula
  transverse artery of scapula
  wing of scapula
  winged scapula
  Woodward elevation of
    scapula
scapula crest pedicled bone
    graft
scapula free flap

scapular area
scapular artery
scapular blade
scapular elevation
scapular flap transfer
scapular island flap
scapular island flap technique
scapular line
scapular notch
scapular osteocutaneous flap
scapular reflex
scapular region
scapular retractor
scapulectomy
scapuloanterior position
scapuloclavicular articulation
scapuloclavicular joint
scapulohumeral reflex
scapulohumeral type
scapuloperoneal syndrome
scapulopexy
scapuloposterior position
scapulothoracic bursa
scapulothoracic fusion
scapulothoracic motion
scar
    areolar scar
    argon laser-induced scars
    atrophic acne scar
    atrophic facial acne scar
    atrophic scar
    atrophic white scar
    cigarette-paper scars
    circumareolar scar
    contracting scar
    episiotomy scar
    excisional scar
    fusiform scar
    gel-treated scars
    healed scar
    hypertrophic burn scar
    hypertrophic scar
    icepick-type scar
    immature scar
    incisional scar
    infarcted scar
    inferior longitudinal scar
    infra-areolar scar
    infrabrow scar
    inframammary scar
    inverted-T scar
    iridectomy scar

scar (*continued*)
    keloid scar
    lateral scar
    mastectomy scar
    midline scar
    myocardial scar
    nonviable scar
    operative scar
    osteopetrotic scar
    papyraceous scar
    periareolar scar
    pop scar
    preauricular scar
    radial scar
    Reichert scar
    revision of scar
    S-shaped scar
    surgical scar
    thickened scar
    T-shaped scar
    U-shaped scar
    vertical scar
    V-shaped scar
    well-demarcated scar
    well-healed scar
    wrist scar
    Y-shaped scar
    zipper scar
    Z-plasty scar
    Z-shaped scar
scar carcinoma
scar contracture
scar dehiscence
scar elevation index (SEI)
scar fibroblast
scar formation
Scar Fx lightweight silicone
        sheeting
scar massage
scar revision
scar rupture
scar tissue
scarabrasion
Scardino flap
Scardino pyeloplasty
Scardino ureteropelvioplasty
scarf bandage
scarf maneuver
scarf sign
scarification
scarified duodenum
scarifier

scarifier knife
scarifying curet
scarless fetal wound healing
scarlet red gauze dressing
Scarpa adipofascial flap
Scarpa fascia
Scarpa foramen
Scarpa ganglion
Scarpa ligament
Scarpa membrane
Scarpa nerve
Scarpa operation
Scarpa sheath
Scarpa shoe
Scarpa triangle
scarring
   cigarette-paper scarring
   corneal scarring
   fibrocalcareous scarring
   fibrotic scarring
   gastrostomy scarring
   hypertrophic scarring
   keloidal scarring
   linear scarring
   old scarring
   parenchymal scarring
   patch test scarring
   perihilar scarring
   pleural scarring
   residual scarring
scarring alopecia
scatoma
scavenger cell
scavenging tube
SCC (squamous cell carcinoma)
SCCHN (squamous cell carcinoma of head and neck)
SCD (sequential compression device)
SCDK heart valve prosthesis
SCDK-Cutter valve
SCDT heart valve prosthesis
Schaaf foreign body forceps
Schachar blepharostat
Schachar implant cataract lens
Schachar lens
Schachar-Gills microsponge
Schacher ganglion
Schachowa tube
Schacht colostomy appliance
Schaedel clip

Schaedel cross-action towel clamp
Schaedel towel forceps
Schaefer ethmoid curet
Schaefer fixation forceps
Schaefer mastoid curet
Schaefer sponge holder
Schaeffer ethmoid curet
Schaeffer mastoid curet
Schaeffer orthosis
Schaldach electrode pacemaker
Schall laryngectomy tube
Schamberg comedo extractor
Schamberg dermatitis
Schamberg extractor
Schamberg progressive pigmented purpuric dermatosis
Schantz sinus rasp
Schantz sinus raspatory
Schanz brace
Schanz cannula
Schanz cautery
Schanz collar
Schanz collar brace
Schanz electrocautery
Schanz knife
Schanz needle
Schanz operation
Schanz osteotomy
Schanz pin
Schanz Scheie blade
Schanz screw
Schanz trephine
Scharf implant cataract lens
Scharff bipolar forceps
Scharff lens
Schatten mammaplasty
Schatz laser technique
Schatz maneuver
Schatz utility forceps
Schatzker fracture
Schatzker tibial plateau fracture classification
Schatzki esophageal ring
Schatzki syndrome
Schatz-Palmaz tubular mesh stent
Schauffler operation
Schauffler procedure
Schaumann bodies
Schaumann syndrome

Schauta operation
Schauta radical vaginal
    hysterectomy
Schauta vaginal operation
Schauta-Amreich operation
Schauta-Amreich vaginal
    operation
Schaut-Wertheim operation
Schauwecker compression
    wiring
Schauwecker patellar wiring
    technique
Schede bone curet
Schede clot
Schede operation
Schede osteotomy
Schede rotation osteotomy
Schede sequestrectomy
Schede thoracoplasty
Scheer crimper forceps
Scheer elevator
Scheer elevator knife
Scheer hook
Scheer knife
Scheer knife elevator
Scheer middle ear instrument
Scheer needle
Scheer oval window rasp
Scheer pick
Scheer rasp
Scheer Teflon prosthesis
Scheer Tef-wire prosthesis
Scheer-Wullstein cutting bur
Scheibe malformation
Scheicker laminectomy punch
Scheie anterior chamber
    cannula
Scheie blade
Scheie cataract aspiration
Scheie cataract needle
Scheie cataract-aspirating
    cannula
Scheie cataract-aspirating needle
Scheie cautery
Scheie classification
Scheie electrocautery
Scheie goniopuncture knife
Scheie goniotomy knife
Scheie needle
Scheie operation
Scheie ophthalmic cautery
Scheie syndrome

Scheie technique
Scheie trephine
Scheie-Graefe fixation forceps
Scheier hinge
Scheie-Westcott corneal section
    scissors
Scheie-Westcott eye scissors
Scheimpflug camera
Schein syringe
Scheinmann biting punch
Scheinmann biting tip
Scheinmann esophagoscopy
    forceps
Scheinmann laryngeal forceps
schema (pl. schemata)
schematic eye
schematic representation
Schepens binocular indirect
    camera
Schepens binocular indirect
    ophthalmoscope
Schepens clip
Schepens depressor
Schepens electrode
Schepens eye cautery
Schepens eye decompressor
Schepens eye retractor
Schepens forceps
Schepens hollow hemisphere
    implant
Schepens indirect
    ophthalmoscope
Schepens operation
Schepens ophthalmoscope
Schepens orbital retractor
Schepens retinal detachment
    unit
Schepens scleral depressor
Schepens surface electrode
Schepens tantalum clip
Schepens technique
Schepens-Okamura-Brockhurst
    retinal detachment repair
Schepens-Pomerantzeff
    ophthalmoscope
Schepsis-Leach technique
Scher nail biopsy
Scherback speculum
Scherback-Porges vaginal
    speculum
Scherback-Porges vaginal
    speculum set

Scheuermann kyphosis
Schick back support
Schick forceps
Schilder plugger
Schiller D&C technique
Schiller iodine
Schiller test
Schiller-Duvall body
Schillinger suture support
Schimek operation
Schimmelbusch disease
Schindler esophagoscope
Schindler gastroscope
Schindler optical
  esophagoscope
Schindler peritoneal forceps
Schindler retractor
Schindler syndrome
Schink dermatome
Schink metatarsal retractor
Schinzel acrocallosal syndrome
Schiotz tonometer
Schiotz tonometry
Schiotz (*see* Schiøtz)
Schiotz (*also* Schiøtz)
Schirmer operation
Schirmer tear test
Schirmer test
schistosomal bladder carcinoma
Schlosser treatment
Schlösser (*see* Schloesser)
Schloesser (*also* Schlösser)
Schlosser treatment
Schlatter disease
Schlatter gastrectomy technique
Schlatter operation
Schlein arthroplasty
Schlein clamp
Schlein elbow arthroplasty
Schlein shoulder holder
Schlein shoulder positioner
Schlein total elbow prosthesis
Schlein trisurface ankle
  prosthesis
Schlemm canal
Schlesinger cervical punch
Schlesinger cervical punch
  forceps
Schlesinger cervical rongeur
Schlesinger clamp
Schlesinger forceps
Schlesinger Gigli-saw guide

Schlesinger instrument
Schlesinger intervertebral disk
  forceps
Schlesinger intervertebral disk
  rongeur
Schlesinger laminectomy
  rongeur
Schlesinger meniscus-grasping
  forceps
Schlesinger punch
Schlesinger rongeur
Schlesinger rongeur forceps
Schlesinger sign
schlieren microscope
Schmalz operation
Schmeden dural scissors
Schmeden nasal punch
Schmeden punch
Schmeden tonsillar punch
Schmid vascular spatula
Schmidel anastomosis
Schmidt rasp
Schmidt raspatory
Schmidt rod holder
Schmidt syndrome
Schmiedel ganglion
Schmieden needle
Schmieden probe
Schmieden-Dick needle
Schmieden-Taylor dural scissors
Schmieden-Taylor
  neurodissector
Schmieden-Taylor scissors
Schmiedt tube
Schmincke-Regaud
  lymphoepithelial
  carcinoma
Schmorl body
Schmorl furrow
Schmorl groove
Schmorl node
Schmorl nodule
Schmuth modification activator
Schneider arthrodesis
Schneider catheter
Schneider driver-extractor
Schneider extractor
Schneider fixation
Schneider hip fusion
Schneider intramedullary
  fixation of femur
Schneider intramedullary nail

Schneider Magic Wallstent prosthesis
Schneider medullary nail
Schneider nail driver
Schneider nail extractor
Schneider nail shaft reamer
Schneider pelvimeter
Schneider pin
Schneider PTCA instruments
Schneider raspatory
Schneider rod
Schneider self-broaching pin
Schneider stent
Schneider technique
Schneider Wallstent biliary endoprosthesis
schneiderian carcinoma
schneiderian membrane
schneiderian respiratory membrane
Schneider-Sauerbruch raspatory
Schneider-Shiley balloon
Schneider-Shiley catheter
Schneider-Shiley dilatation catheter
Schnidt clamp
Schnidt gall duct forceps
Schnidt hemostat
Schnidt passer
Schnidt thoracic forceps
Schnidt tonsillar forceps
Schnidt tonsillar hemostat
Schnidt tonsillar hemostatic forceps
Schnidt-Rumpler forceps
Schnitker scalp retractor
Schnitman skin hook
Schnur scale
Schnute wedge resection
Schnute wedge resection technique
Schober technique
Schobinger incision
Schocket scleral depressor
Schocket tube implant
Schoemaker (*see also* Schumacher, Schumaker, Shoemaker)
Schoemaker anastomosis
Schoemaker gastrectomy
Schoemaker gastroenterostomy
Schoemaker goiter scissors

Schoemaker intestinal clamp
Schoemaker line
Schoemaker modification
Schoemaker procedure
Schoemaker scissors
Schoemaker thyroid scissors
Schoemaker-Billroth I anastomosis
Schoemaker-Billroth II gastrectomy
Schoemaker-Billroth II intestinal anastomosis
Schoemaker-Loth ligature scssisors
Schoemaker-Wangensteen operation
Schoenberg forceps
Schoenberg intestinal forceps
Schoenberg uterine forceps
Schoenberg uterine-elevating forceps
Schoenborn retractor
Schoenborn (*also* Schonbörn)
Schonbörn (*see* Schoenborn)
Schoenrock laser instrument set
Scholar II vital sign monitor
Scholl knife
Scholl meniscal knife
Scholl meniscus knife
Scholl pad
Scholl solution
Scholten endomyocardial biopsy forceps
Scholten endomyocardial bioptome
Scholten sternal retractor
Schonander procedure
Schonander technique
Schonbein operation
Schönbein (*see* Schonbein)
Schonbein (*also* Schönbein, Schoenbein)
Schoenbein (*see* Schonbein)
SchonCath catheter
Schoonmaker femoral catheter
Schoonmaker multipurpose catheter
Schoonmaker-King single-catheter technique
Schott bath
Schreger lines
Schreger striae

Schreiber maneuver
Schrock procedure
Schröder (*see* Shroeder)
Schroeder (*also* Schröder, Schroder)
Schroder (*see* Schroeder)
Schroeder curet
Schroeder episiotomy scissors
Schroeder forceps
Schroeder forceps tenaculum
Schroeder interlocking sound
Schroeder interlocking uterine sound
Schroeder operating scissors
Schroeder operation
Schroeder scissors
Schroeder tenaculum
Schroeder tenaculum loop
Schroeder tissue forceps
Schroeder uterine curet
Schroeder uterine tenaculum
Schroeder uterine tenaculum forceps
Schroeder uterine vulsellum forceps
Schroeder vulsellum forceps
Schroeder-Braun forceps
Schroeder-Braun uterine forceps
Schroeder-Braun uterine tenaculum forceps
Schroeder-Van Doren tenaculum forceps
Schrotter catheter
Schrötter (*see* Schrotter)
Schrotter (*also* Schrötter, Schroetter)
Schrudde aspirative lipoplasty
Schrudde curet technique
Schrudde rotational flap
Schrudde aspirator lipoplasty
Schubert biopsy punch
Schubert cervical biopsy forceps
Schubert uterine biopsy forceps
Schubert uterine biopsy punch
Schubert uterine biopsy punch forceps
Schubert uterine tenaculum forceps
Schuchardt incision
Schuchardt operation
Schuchardt relaxing incision
Schuchardt-Pfeifer operation

Schuchardt shears
Schuco 2000 nebulizer
Schuknecht chisel
Schuknecht classification of congenital aural atresia
Schuknecht crimper
Schuknecht cutter
Schuknecht elevator
Schuknecht excavator
Schuknecht footplate hook
Schuknecht foreign body remover
Schuknecht Gelfoam wire prosthesis
Schuknecht gouge
Schuknecht hook
Schuknecht knife
Schuknecht middle ear instrument
Schuknecht needle
Schuknecht operation
Schuknecht pick
Schuknecht piston prosthesis
Schuknecht postauricular self-retaining retractor
Schuknecht retractor
Schuknecht roller knife
Schuknecht scissors
Schuknecht sickle knife
Schuknecht spatula
Schuknecht speculum
Schuknecht stapedectomy
Schuknecht stapes hook
Schuknecht stapes prosthesis
Schuknecht suction tip
Schuknecht suction tube
Schuknecht Teflon crimper
Schuknecht Teflon piston
Schuknecht Teflon wire piston prosthesis
Schuknecht Tef-wire prosthesis
Schuknecht temporal trephine
Schuknecht whirlybird excavator
Schuknecht wire
Schuknecht wire crimper
Schuknecht wire-cutting scissors
Schuknecht-Paparella wire-bending die
Schuknecht-Wullstein retractor
Schuletz antral curet
Schuletz pacemaker

Schuletz-Simmons ethmoidal
curet
Schuller duct
Schüller (see Schuller)
Schuller (also Schüller)
Schuller position
Schulte valve
Schultz iris retractor
Schultz irrigating iris retractor
Schultz-Crock binocular
ophthalmoscope
Schultze bundle
Schultze cells
Schultze embryotomy knife
Schultze fold
Schultze knife
Schultze membrane
Schultze placenta
Schumacher (see also
Schoemaker, Schumaker,
Shoemaker)
Schumacher aortic clamp
Schumacher biopsy forceps
Schumacher sternal shears
Schumaker (see also
Schoemaker, Schumacher,
Shoemaker)
Schumaker gynecologic
scissors
Schumaker umbilical cord
scissors
Schutz bundle
Schütz (see Schutz)
Schutz (also Schütz)
Schutz clamp
Schutz clip
Schutz forceps
Schwalbe corpuscle
Schwalbe fissure
Schwalbe foramen
Schwalbe line
Schwalbe membrane
Schwalbe sheath
Schwalbe spaces
Schwann cell
Schwann sheath
Schwann tumor
schwannoma
granular cell schwannoma
malignant schwannoma
mixed type parapharyngeal
schwannoma

Schwarten balloon dilatation
catheter
Schwarten guidewire
Schwarten balloon
Schwartz antral trocar saw
Schwartz arterial aneurysm
clamp
Schwartz bulldog clamp
Schwartz cervical tenaculum
hook
Schwartz clamp
Schwartz clip
Schwartz clip applier
Schwartz clip-applying forceps
Schwartz cordotomy knife
Schwartz endocervical curet
Schwartz expression hook
Schwartz hook
Schwartz intracranial clamp
Schwartz knife
Schwartz laminectomy
retractor
Schwartz laminectomy self-
retaining retractor
Schwartz multipurpose forceps
Schwartz obstetrical forceps
Schwartz plate
Schwartz retractor
Schwartz saw
Schwartz syndrome
Schwartz temporary clamp-
applying forceps
Schwartz tenaculum
Schwartz test
Schwartz trephine
Schwartz trocar
Schwartz vascular clamp
Schwartz-Baumgard technique
Schwartze chisel
Schwartze operation
Schwartze-Stacke operation
Schwartz-Kerrison rongeur
Schwarz arrow-forming pliers
Schwarz bow-type activator
Schwed Flexicut file
Schweigger capsular forceps
Schweigger capsule
Schweigger extracapsular
forceps
Schweigger hand perimeter
Schweitzer pin
Schweitzer spring plate

Schweizer cervix-holding
  forceps
Schweizer speculum
Schweizer uterine forceps
Schweninger-Buzzi anetoderma
Schäfer (*see* Schafer)
Schafer (*also* Schäfer)
Scialom dental implant material
sciatic artery
sciatic foramen
sciatic function index
sciatic hernia
sciatic nerve
sciatic nerve block
sciatic nerve palsy hematoma
sciatic notch
sciatic pain
sciatic scoliosis
sciatica
SCID (severe combined
  immunodeficiency)
Science-Med balloon catheter
Sci-Med angioplasty catheter
Sci-Med Express Monorail
  balloon
Sci-Med extracorporeal silicone
  rubber reservoir
SciMed guiding catheter
SciMed oxygenator
Scimed guiding catheter
SciMed skinny catheter
SciMed Choice floppy wire
scimitar blade
scimitar syndrome
scimitar-blade knife
scintigram
scintigraphic balloon
scintigraphic perfusion defect
scintigraphy
  1-pass scintigraphy
  AMA-Fab scintigraphy
  hepatobiliary scintigraphy
  infarct-avid scintigraphy
  quantitative hepatobiliary
    scintigraphy
  radioisotope scintigraphy
  subtraction scintigraphy
scintillating sesamoids sign
scintillation camera
scintillation counter
scintillation scanner
scintillation scanning

scintimammography (SMM)
scintimammography prone
  breast cushion
scintiphoto
scintiphotography
scintiscan
scintiscanner
scirrhous adenocarcinoma
scirrhous cancer
scirrhous carcinoma
scirrhous lesion
scirrhus
scissor dissection
scissor-leg position
scissors (*see also* shears)
  abdominal scissors
  Abeli tenotomy scissors
  Acufex scissors
  Ada dissecting scissors
  Adson dural scissors
  Adson ganglion scissors
  Adson-Toennis scissors
  Aebli corneal scissors
  Aebli corneal suction scissors
  Aebli tenotomy scissors
  Aebli-Manson scissors
  alligator MacCarty scissors
  alligator scissors
  aloe stitch scissors
  American pattern scissors
  American pattern umbilical
    scissors
  American umbilical scissors
  Anderson converse iris
    scissors
  angled scissors
  angular scissors
  Anis corneal scissors
  anterior chamber synechia
    scissors
  aortic scissors
  AROSupercut scissors
  arterial scissors
  arteriotomy scissors
  Arthro-Force hook scissors
  Aslan endoscopic scissors
  ASSI Supercut scissors
  Asta ligature scissors
  Aston face-lift scissors
  Atkinson corneal scissors
  Atkinson-Walker scissors
  Aufricht scissors

scissors (*continued*)
  automated intravitreal scissors
  Azar corneal scissors
  Babcock wire-cutting scissors
  baby Metzenbaum scissors
  backward-cutting scissors
  Bahama suture scissors
  Bakst cardiac scissors
  ballpoint scissors
  ball-tipped scissors
  Baltimore nasal scissors
  bandage scissors
  Bantam wire scissors
  Bantam wire-cutting scissors
  Bard-Parker scissors
  Barkan scissors
  Barnes vessel scissors
  Barraquer corneal section
    scissors
  Barraquer iris scissors
  Barraquer section scissors
  Barraquer vitreous strand
    scissors
  Barraquer-DeWecker iris
    scissors
  Barraquer-Karakashian
    scissors
  Barsky nasal scissors
  Baruch circumcision scissors
  Baum scissors
  bayonet scissors
  beaded-tip scissors
  Beall circumflex artery
    scissors
  Bechert intraocular scissors
  Becker corneal section
    spatulated scissors
  Becker corneal suture
    scissors
  Becker septal scissors
  Becker spatulated corneal
    section scissors
  Beckman nasal scissors
  Beebe collar scissors
  Beebe wire-cutting scissors
  Bell scissors
  Bellucci alligator scissors
  Bellucci ear scissors
  Bellucci otolaryngology
    scissors
  Bellucci-Paparella scissors
  Berbridge scissors

scissors (*continued*)
  Berens corneal transplant
    scissors
  Berens iridocapsulotomy
    scissors
  Bergman bandage scissors
  Bergman plaster scissors
  Berkeley mechanized scissors
  Berridge gauze scissors
  bipolar cautery scissors
  Birks trabeculectomy scissors
  Biro dermal nevus scissors
  Blanco scissors
  Blot scissors
  Blum arterial scissors
  blunt scissors
  Bodian scissors
  Boettcher tonsil scissors
  Boettcher tonsillar scissors
  Bonn iris scissors
  Bonn miniature iris scissors
  Boochai scissors
  Bowman iris scissors
  Bowman strabismus scissors
  Boyd dissecting scissors
  Boyd tonsillar scissors
  Boyd-Stille tonsillar scissors
  Bozeman scissors
  brain scissors
  Braun episiotomy scissors
  Braun-Stadler bandage scissors
  Braun-Stadler episiotomy
    scissors
  Brooks gallbladder scissors
  Brophy plastic surgery
    scissors
  Brown dissecting scissors
  Brun plastic surgery scissors
  Brun-Stadler episiotomy
    scissors
  Buerger-McCarthy scissors
  Buie operating scissors
  Buie rectal scissors
  bulldog nasal scissors
  bulldog scissors
  Bunge scissors
  Burnham bandage scissors
  Burnham finger bandage
    scissors
  Busch umbilical cord scissors
  Busch umbilical scissors
  calcified tissue scissors

scissors (*continued*)

canalicular scissors
cannula scissors
Caplan angular scissors
Caplan dorsal scissors
Caplan double-action scissors
Caplan nasal bone scissors
Caplan nasal scissors
capsulotomy scissors
Carb-Edge scissors
carbide-jaw scissors
cardiac scissors
cardiovascular scissors
cartilage scissors
Castanares facelift scissors
Castroviejo anterior synechia scissors
Castroviejo corneal scissors
Castroviejo corneal section scissors
Castroviejo corneal transplant scissors
Castroviejo iridocapsulotomy scissors
Castroviejo iris scissors
Castroviejo keratoplasty scissors
Castroviejo microcorneal scissors
Castroviejo section scissors
Castroviejo synechia scissors
Castroviejo tenotomy scissors
Castroviejo-McPherson keratectomy scissors
Castroviejo-Troutman scissors
Castroviejo-Vannas capsulotomy scissors
cataract scissors
Caylor scissors
Chadwick scissors
Charnley cup-trimming scissors
chemopallidectomy scissors
Cherry S-shaped scissors
Chevalier Jackson scissors
Church cardiovascular scissors
Church deep surgery scissors
Church pediatric scissors
Cinelli scissors
Cinelli-Fomon scissors
circumcisional scissors

scissors (*continued*)

circumflex artery scissors
circumflex scissors
Classon deep surgery scissors
Classon pediatric scissors
Clayman-Troutman corneal scissors
Clayman-Westcott scissors
clip-removing scissors
cloth scissors
Codman scissors
Cohan-Vannas iris scissors
Cohan-Westcott scissors
Cohney scissors
cold scissors
collar scissors
Collis scissors
combined needle holder and scissors
conjunctival scissors
Converse nasal tip scissors
Converse plastic surgery scissors
Converse-Wilmer conjunctival scissors
Cooley arteriotomy scissors
Cooley cardiovascular scissors
Cooley probe-point scissors
Cooley reverse-cut scissors
Cooper scissors
cornea scissors
corneal scissors
corneal section scissors
corneal section spatulated scissors
corneal section-enlarging scissors
corneal spatulated scissors
corneal transplant scissors
corneoscleral scissors
coronary artery scissors
coronary scissors
Costa wire suture scissors
Cottle angular scissors
Cottle bulldog nasal scissors
Cottle bulldog scissors
Cottle dorsal scissors
Cottle dressing scissors
Cottle heavy septal scissors
Cottle heavy septum scissors
Cottle nasal scissors
Cottle spring scissors

scissors (*continued*)
Cottle stent scissors
Cottle Vital dorsal angled
scissors
Crafoord lobectomy scissors
Crafoord lung scissors
Crafoord thoracic scissors
Craig angular scissors
craniotomy scissors
crown and bridge scissors
crown scissors
crown-collar scissors
curved iris scissors
curved Mayo scissors
curved operating scissors
curved scissors
curved tenotomy scissors
curved turbinate scissors
curved turbinectomy scissors
curved-on-flat scissors
cuticle scissors
cystoscopic scissors
Dahlgren iris scissors
Dandy neurosurgical scissors
Dandy trigeminal scissors
Davis rhytidectomy scissors
Dean tonsillar scissors
Dean-Trusler scissors
Deaver operating scissors
DeBakey endarterectomy
scissors
DeBakey stitch scissors
DeBakey valve scissors
DeBakey vascular scissors
DeBakey-Metzenbaum
dissecting scissors
DeBakey-Potts scissors
decapitation scissors
Decker microsurgical scissors
deep-surgery scissors
delicate operating scissors
delicate scissors
DeMartel neurosurgical
scissors
DeMartel vascular scissors
Derf scissors
DeWecker eye scissors
DeWecker iridectomy scissors
DeWecker iris scissors
DeWecker-Pritikin iris scissors
Diamond-Edge Supercut
scissors

scissors (*continued*)
diamond-edged scissors
diathermic scissors
diathermy scissors
Diethrich circumflex artery
scissors
Diethrich coronary scissors
Diethrich valve scissors
Diethrich-Hegemann scissors
dissecting scissors
dissecting tonsillar scissors
dissecting vital scissors
dissection scissors
Dixon collar scissors
dorsal scissors
dorsal-angled scissors
Douglas nasal scissors
Doyen abdominal scissors
Doyen dissecting scissors
Doyen-Ferguson scissors
dressing scissors
Dubois decapitation scissors
Duffield cardiovascular
scissors
Dumont angular scissors
Dumont thoracic scissors
dural scissors
Durotip scissors
ear scissors
East-Grinstead scissors
Edelstein scissors
Eiselberg uterine scissors
Eiselberg ligature scissors
Electroscope disposable
scissors
electrosurgical curved
scissors
Emmet uterine scissors
endarterectomy scissors
endoscopic scissors
enterotomy scissors
enucleation scissors
episiotomy scissors
E-series scissors
Esmarch bandage scissors
Esmarch plaster scissors
esophageal scissors
Essrig dissecting scissors
Evershears bipolar curved
scissors
Evershears bipolar
laparoscopic scissors

scissors (*continued*)

Evershears II bipolar curved
scissors
eye scissors
eye stitch scissors
eye suture scissors
F. L. Fischer bayonet scissors
F. L. Fischer microsurgical
neurectomy bayonet
scissors
face-lift scissors
facial plastic surgery scissors
Favaloro coronary scissors
Federspiel scissors
Ferguson abdominal scissors
Ferguson-Metzenbaum
scissors
fine scissors
fine-dissecting scissors
fine-stitch scissors
fine-suture scissors
Finochietto thoracic scissors
Fisch microcrurotomy
scissors
Fiskars scissors
fistula scissors
flap scissors
Fomon angular scissors
Fomon dorsal scissors
Fomon face-lift scissors
Fomon lower lateral scissors
Fomon saber-back scissors
Fomon upper lateral scissors
Fomon Vital dorsal scissors
Foster scissors
Fox scissors
Frahur scissors
Frazier dural scissors
Freeman rhytidectomy
scissors
Freeman-Schepens scissors
Frost scissors
Fulton deep-surgery scissors
Fulton pediatric scissors
gallbladder scissors
ganglion scissors
gauze scissors
Gellquist scissors
gene scissors
general operating scissors
general utility scissors
Giertz-Stille scissors

scissors (*continued*)

Gill scissors
Gill-Hess scissors
Gillies suture scissors
Gill-Welsh scissors
Gill-Welsh-Vannas
capsulotomy scissors
Girard corneoscleral scissors
Glasscock scissors
Glassman scissors
goiter scissors
Goldman septal scissors
Goldman-Fox gum scissors
Goldman-Fox wound
debridement scissors
gold-plated bandage scissors
Gonin-Amsler scleral marker
scissors
Good tonsillar scissors
Good-Reiner tonsil scissors
Gorney face-lift scissors
Gorney rhytidectomy scissors
Gorney septal scissors
Gorney turbinate scissors
Gradle stitch scissors
Graefe scissors
Graham cardiovascular
scissors
Graham pediatric scissors
Grieshaber vertical cutting
scissors
Grieshaber vitreous scissors
Griffon tonsil scissors
Guggenheim scissors
Guggenheim-Schuknecht
scissors
Guilford ear scissors
Guilford-Schuknecht scissors
Guilford-Schuknecht wire-
cutting scissors
Guilford-Wright scissors
guillotine scissors
Guist enucleation scissors
gum scissors
Guyton scissors
Haenig irrigating scissors
Haglund plaster scissors
Haimovici arteriotomy
scissors
Halsey nail scissors
Halsted strabismus scissors
harmonic scissors

scissors (*continued*)

Harrington deep surgical scissors
Harrington-Mayo thoracic scissors
Harrison suture-removing scissors
Harvester bipolar scissors
Harvey wire-cutting scissors
Haynes scissors
Heath clip-removing scissors
Heath suture scissors
Heath suture-cutting scissors
Heath wire-cutting scissors
heavy septal scissors
heavy-angled scissors
Hegemann scissors
Hercules scissors
Heyman nasal scissors
Heyman-Paparella angular scissors
Hi-level bandage scissors
Hill stitch scissors
Hoen laminectomy scissors
Holinger curved scissors
Holmes scissors
hook rotary scissors
hook scissors
Hooper deep surgery scissors
Hooper pediatric scissors
Hoskins-Castroviejo corneal scissors
Hoskins-Westcott tenotomy scissors
Hough scissors
House alligator scissors
House dissecting scissors
House-Metzenbaum scissors
House-Bellucci alligator scissors
House-Bellucci-Shambaugh alligator scissors
Howell coronary scissors
Huey suture scissors
Huger diamond-back nasal scissors
Hunt chalazion scissors
hysterectomy scissors
IMA scissors
in situ valve scissors
incision scissors
insulated curved scissors

scissors (*continued*)

insulated straight scissors
intestinal scissors
intraocular scissors
iridectomy scissors
iridocapsulotomy scissors
iridotomy scissors
iris miniature scissors
iris scissors
Irvine corneal scissors
Irvine probe-point scissors
Jabaley Super-cut scissors
Jabaley-Stille Supercut scissors
Jackson esophageal scissors
Jackson laryngeal scissors
Jackson turbinate scissors
Jacobson bayonet-shaped scissors
Jacobson spring-handled scissors
Jaffe scissors
Jako microlaryngeal scissors
Jameson dissecting scissors
Jameson facelift scissors
Jameson-Werber scissors
Jamison-Metzenbaum scissors
Jannetta bayonet scissors
Jannetta bayonet-shaped scissors
Jannetta-Kurze dissecting scissors
Jansen scissors
Jansen-Middleton scissors
Jarit dissecting scissors
Jarit endarterectomy scissors
Jarit flat-top scissors
Jarit lower lateral scissors
Jarit microstitch scissors
Jarit microsurgery scissors
Jarit peripheral vascular scissors
Jarit stitch scissors
Jesco scissors
Jolly prostatic scissors
Jones dissecting scissors
Jones IMA scissors
Jorgenson dissecting scissors
Jorgenson gallbladder scissors
Jorgenson thoracic scissors
Joseph nasal scissors
Joseph serrated scissors
Joseph-Maltz scissors

scissors (*continued*)
Kahn dissecting scissors
Kantrowitz vascular dissecting scissors
Kantrowitz vascular scissors
Karakashian-Barraquer scissors
Karmody venous scissors
Katena Vannas scissors
Katzeff cartilage scissors
Katzin corneal scissors
Katzin corneal transplant scissors
Katzin transplant scissors
Katzin-Troutman scissors
Kaye blepharoplasty scissors
Kaye face-lift scissors
Kaye fine-dissecting scissors
Kayess bandage scissors
Kazanjian nasal cutting scissors
Keeler intravitreal scissors
Keith scissors
Kelly fistular scissors
Kelly uterine scissors
Kelly-Littauer stitch scissors
keratectomy scissors
keratoplasty scissors
Kilner scissors
Kirby scissors
Kitner dissecting scissors
Kleinert-Kutz tenotomy scissors
Kleinsasser microlaryngeal scissors
Klinkenberg-Loth scissors
Knapp iris scissors
Knapp strabismus scissors
Knight nasal scissors
Knowles bandage scissors
Kocher scissors
Koenig nail-splitting scissors
Koenig-Stille scissors
Koros EndoMax scissors
Kramp scissors
Kreiger-Spitznas vibrating scissors
Kreuscher semilunar cartilage scissors
Kurze dissecting scissors
Lagrange eye scissors
Lagrange sclerectomy scissors

scissors (*continued*)
Lahey Carb-Edge scissors
Lahey Clinic rectal scissors
Lahey delicate scissors
Lahey dissecting scissors
Lahey operating scissors
Lahey thyroid scissors
Lahey-Metzenbaum dissecting scissors
Lakeside nasal scissors
Lambert-Heiman scissors
laminectomy scissors
Landolt enucleation scissors
laparoscopic scissors
laryngeal scissors
laryngofissure scissors
Laschal suture scissors
laser tubal scissors
Lawrie modified circumflex scissors
Lawton corneal scissors
Leather-Karmody in-site valve scissors
left-curved scissors
left-handed cornea scissors
Lejeune scissors
Lexer dissecting scissors
Lexer-Durotip dissecting scissors
ligature scissors
Lillie alligator scissors
Lillie tonsillar scissors
Lincoln cardiovascular scissors
Lincoln deep scissors
Lincoln pediatric scissors
Lincoln-Metzenbaum scissors
Lindley scissors
Lipsett scissors
Lipshultz epididymovasostomy microdissection scissors
Lister bandage scissors
Liston plaster-of-Paris scissors
Littauer dissecting scissors
Littauer Junior suture scissors
Littauer stitch scissors
Littauer suture scissors
Littler carrying scissors
Littler dissecting scissors
Littler suture carrying scissors
Litwak mitral valve scissors

scissors (*continued*)
Litwak utility scissors
Litwin dissecting scissors
Lloyd-Davies rectal scissors
lobectomy scissors
Locklin stitch scissors
long scissors
long stitch scissors
loop scissors
Lorenz bandage scissors
Lorenz PC/TC scissors
Lower lateral scissors
lung dissecting scissors
lung scissors
Lynch scissors
MacKenty scissors
Maclay tonsillar scissors
Maki scissors
Malis neurological scissors
Mancusi-Ungaro scissors
Manson-Aebli corneal section
scissors
Marbach episiotomy scissors
marking scissors
Martin ballpoint scissors
Martin cartilage scissors
Martin throat scissors
Mattis corneal scissors
Mattox-Potts scissors
Maunoir iris scissors
Max Fine scissors
Mayo curved scissors
Mayo dissecting scissors
Mayo long dissecting scissors
Mayo operating scissors
Mayo round blade scissors
Mayo straight scissors
Mayo uterine scissors
Mayo-Harrington dissecting
scissors
Mayo-Lexer scissors
Mayo-New scissors
Mayo-Noble dissecting
scissors
Mayo-Potts dissecting scissors
Mayo-Sims dissecting scissors
Mayo-Stille dissecting scissors
Mayo-Stille operating scissors
McAllister scissors
McClure eye scissors
McClure iris scissors
McGuire corneal scissors

scissors (*continued*)
McHenry scissors
McIndoe cartilage scissors
McLean capsulotomy scissors
McPherson corneal section
scissors
McPherson microconjunctival
scissors
McPherson microtenotomy
scissors
McPherson-Castroviejo
corneal section scissors
McPherson-Castroviejo
microcorneal scissors
McPherson-Vannas iris
scissors
McPherson-Vannas microiris
scissors
McPherson-Westcott
conjunctival scissors
McPherson-Westcott stitch
scissors
McReynolds pterygium
scissors
meatotomy scissors
mechanized scissors
Medi bandage scissors
meniscal hook scissors
meniscectomy scissors
Metzenbaum baby tonsillar
scissors
Metzenbaum dissecting
scissors
Metzenbaum dressing scissors
Metzenbaum long scissors
Metzenbaum operating
scissors
Metzenbaum tonsillar scissors
Metzenbaum-Lipsett plastic
scissors
micro scissors
micro Westcott scissors
microconjunctival scissors
microcorneal scissors
microiris scissors
microlaryngeal scissors
micro-mosquito curved
scissors
micro-mosquito straight
scissors
micropituitary scissors
microscopic scissors

scissors (*continued*)
microsurgical scissors
Microtek scissors
microtenotomy scissors
microvascular scissors
microvit scissors
Microwec scissors
Miller dissecting scissors
Miller operating scissors
Miller rectal scissors
Millesi scissors
Mills arteriotomy scissors
Mills circumflex scissors
Miltex blepharoplasty scissors
Miltex saber-back
  rhytidectomy scissors
Miltex stitch scissors
Miltex undermining scissors
miniature scissors
mini-keratoplasty scissors
minor surgery scissors
Mira scissors
mitral valve scissors
Mixter general operating
  scissors
Mixter operating scissors
Moehle scissors
moleskin and felt scissors
Moore-Troutman corneal
  scissors
Morse aortic scissors
Morse backward-cutting
  aortic scissors
MPC automated intravitreal
  scissors
Mueller scissors
Munro brain scissors
Murphy scissors
Nadler superior radial scissors
Nagel scissors
nail scissors
nail-nipper scissors
nasal dorsal-angled scissors
nasal scissors
Nelson general operating
  scissors
Nelson lobectomy scissors
Nelson lung-dissecting
  scissors
Nelson thoracic scissors
Nelson uterine scissors
Nelson-Metzenbaum scissors

scissors (*continued*)
Nelson Vital dissecting
  scissors
neonatal scissors
Neubauer scissors
Neumann scissors
neurological scissors
neurovascular scissors
New suture scissors
Noble scissors
Northbent suture scissors
Noyes iridectomy scissors
Noyes iris scissors
Noyes-Shambaugh alligator
  scissors
Nugent-Gradle stitch scissors
Nu-Tip laparoscopic scissors
O'Brien stitch scissors
O'Brien suture scissors
O'Brien-Mayo scissors
Ochsner ball-tipped scissors
Ochsner diamond-edged
  scissors
O'Connor hook scissors
Olivecrona angular scissors
Olivecrona dura scissors
Olivecrona dural scissors
Olivecrona guillotine scissors
O'Neill cardiac surgical
  scissors
Ong capsulotomy scissors
operating scissors
Ormco band scissors
orthopedic scissors
Osher corneal scissors
otologic scissors
Panzer gallbladder scissors
Paparella wire-cutting scissors
Par scissors
Pardos scissors
pattern umbilical scissors
Pean scissors
Peck scissors
Peck-Joseph scissors
pediatric scissors
Penn umbilical scissors
pericardiotomy scissors
Peyman vitreous scissors
Phaneuf uterine artery
  scissors
Pickett scissors
plain rotary scissors

scissors (*continued*)

plaster-of-Paris scissors
plastic scissors
plastic surgery scissors
plastic utility scissors
PMH scissors
pointed scissors
Poppen sympathectomy scissors
Potts 60-degree angled scissors
Potts tenotomy scissors
Potts vascular scissors
Potts-De Martel scissors
Potts-DeMartel gall duct scissors
Potts-Smith arterial scissors
Potts-Smith cardiovascular scissors
Potts-Smith dissecting scissors
Potts-Smith reverse scissors
Potts-Smith vascular scissors
Potts-Yasargil scissors
PowerStar bipolar scissors
Pratt rectal scissors
Prince dissecting scissors
Prince tonsillar scissors
Prince-Potts tonsillar scissors
probe-point scissors
prostatic scissors
pterygium scissors
ptosis scissors
pupillary membrane scissors
Pean Scissors
Péan (*see* Pean)
Pean (*also* Péan)
Quimby gum scissors
radial iridotomy scissors
Ragnell dissecting scissors
Ragnell undermining scissors
Ragnell-Kilner scissors
Ralks stitch scissors
Rappazzo foreign body scissors
Rappazzo haptic scissors
Real coronary artery scissors
rectal scissors
Reeh stitch scissors
Rees face-lift scissors
Rees facelift serrated scissors
Reichling corneal scissors
Reinhoff thoracic scissors

scissors (*continued*)

Resano dissecting scissors
Resano thoracic scissors
Reul coronary artery scissors
reverse scissors
reverse-cutting scissors
Reynolds dissecting scissors
Reynolds-Jameson vessel scissors
rhinoplasty scissors
Rhoton bayonet scissors
Rhoton microsurgical scissors
rhytidectomy scissors
Rica ear polypus scissors
Richter episiotomy scissors
Rienhoff general operating scissors
Rienhoff thoracic scissors
right-angle scissors
right-curved scissors
right-handed corneal scissors
Ring ribbon scissors
Rizzuti keratoplasty scissors
Rizzuti-McGuire corneal-section scissors
Roberts episiotomy scissors
Rochester scissors
Rochester-Ferguson scissors
Roger wire-cutting scissors
Roper scissors
Rosenblatt scissors
round-blade scissors
Rubio scissors
Ryder scissors
saber-back scissors
Sadler cartilage scissors
Sadler tissue scissors
Satinsky cardiac scissors
Satinsky double-curve scissors
Satinsky thoracic scissors
Satinsky vena caval scissors
Scanlan scissors
Scheie-Westcott corneal section scissors
Scheie-Westcott eye scissors
Schmieden-Taylor dural scissors
Schoemaker goiter scissors
Schoemaker thyroid scissors
Schoemaker-Loth scissors
Schroeder episiotomy scissors
Schroeder operating scissors

scissors (*continued*)

Schuknecht wire-cutting scissors
Schumaker gynecologic scissors
Schumaker umbilical cord scissors
sclerectomy by scissors
sclerectomy scissors
sclerectomy with scissors
Scott dissecting scissors
Scott right-angle scissors
Scoville scissors
Sealy dissecting scissors
Seiler turbinate scissors
Semb dissecting scissors
semilunar cartilage scissors
septal scissors
serrated iris scissors
Serratex-Mayo dissecting scissors
Serratex scissors
Seutin plaster scissors
Shapshay-Healy laryngeal scissors
Shea vein graft scissors
Shea-Bellucci scissors
Shepard scissors
Shield iridotomy scissors
Shortbent stitch scissors
Shortbent suture scissors
Shutt scissors
sickle scissors
Siebold uterine scissors
Sims general operating scissors
Sims uterine scissors
Sims-Siebold uterine scissors
Sistron scissors
Sistrunk dissecting scissors
slender-tip scissors
Slip-N-Snip scissors
small spring scissors
Smart enucleation scissors
Smellie obstetrical scissors
SMIC collar scissors
SMIC ear polypus scissors
Smith bandage scissors
Smith suture wire scissors
Smith wire-cutting scissors
Smith-Potts scissors
Snowden-Pencer Super-Cut scissors

scissors (*continued*)

Southbent scissors
Spencer eye suture scissors
Spencer stitch scissors
Spetzler scissors
spring iris scissors
spring-handled scissors
Stalzner rectal scissors
StaySharp facelift Supercut scissors
StaySharp Super-cut scissors
Stevens eye scissors
Stevens stitch scissors
Stevens tenotomy scissors
Stevenson alligator scissors
Stille dissecting scissors
Stille Super Cut scissors
Stille-Mayo dissecting scissors
stitch scissors
Stiwer scissors
Storz cystoscopic scissors
Storz delicate iris scissors
Storz intraocular scissors
Storz iris scissors
Storz stitch scissors
Storz wire-cutting scissors
Storz-Westcott conjunctival scissors
strabismus scissors
straight scissors
straight tenotomy scissors
Strully cardiovascular scissors
Strully dissecting scissors
Strully dural scissors
Strully hook scissors
Strully neurological scissors
Strully neurosurgical scissors
Sullivan gum scissors
Super-Cut scissors
superior radial tenotomy scissors
surgical scissors
Sutherland eye scissors
Sutherland-Grieshaber scissors
suture scissors
suture wire-cutting scissors
suture-removing scissors
Sweet delicate pituitary scissors
Sweet esophageal scissors
sympathectomy scissors
Take-apart scissors

scissors (*continued*)
  Tamsco wire-cutting scissors
  Taylor brain scissors
  Taylor craniotomy scissors
  Taylor dural scissors
  Taylor neurosurgical scissors
  tenotomy scissors
  thin-shaft nasal scissors
  Thomas scissors
  Thompson-Walker scissors
  thoracic scissors
  Thorek gallbladder scissors
  Thorek thoracic scissors
  Thorek-Feldman gallbladder
    scissors
  Thorpe pupillary membrane
    scissors
  Thorpe-Castroviejo cataract
    scissors
  Thorpe-Westcott cataract
    scissors
  Thorpe-Westcott scissors
  throat scissors
  Tindall scissors
  tissue scissors
  Toennis anastomosis scissors
  Toennis dissecting scissors
  Toennis-Adson dural scissors
  Toennis-Adson utility scissors
  tonsil-dissecting scissors
  tonsillar scissors
  Torchia conjunctival scissors
  Torchia microcorneal scissors
  Torchia-Vannas micro-iris
    scissors
  tracheal scissors
  tracheostomy scissors
  trigeminal scissors
  Troutman conjunctival scissors
  Troutman corneal scissors
  Troutman corneal section
    scissors
  Troutman microsurgical
    scissors
  Troutman suture scissors
  Troutman-Castroviejo corneal
    section scissors
  Troutman-Katzin corneal
    transplant scissors
  Trusler-Dean scissors
  tubal scissors
  turbinate scissors

scissors (*continued*)
  turbinectomy scissors
  Turner-Warwick diathermy
    scissors
  Twisk scissors
  U.S. Army gauze scissors
  U.S. Army umbilical scissors
  U.S. Army-pattern gauze
    scissors
  umbilical scissors
  Universal wire scissors
  upper lateral scissors
  uterine scissors
  utility bandage scissors
  utility scissors
  V. Mueller curved operating
    scissors
  V. Mueller laser tubal scissors
  V. Mueller operating scissors
  V. Mueller Vital laser Mayo
    dissecting scissors
  valve leaflet excision scissors
  valve scissors
  Vannas capsulotomy scissors
  Vannas corneal scissors
  Vannas iridocapsulotomy
    scissors
  Vannas microcapsulotomy
    scissors
  vascular scissors
  vena caval scissors
  Verdi scissors
  Verhoeff dissecting scissors
  Verner-Joseph scissors
  Vernon wire-cutting scissors
  Vezien abdominal scissors
  vibrating scissors
  Vital iris scissors
  Vital wire-cutting scissors
  Vital Cooley operating
    scissors
  Vital Cooley wire-cutting
    scissors
  Vital-Cottle dorsal angled
    scissors
  Vital-Fomon angular scissors
  Vital-Knapp iris scissors
  Vital-Knapp strabismus
    scissors
  Vital-Mayo dissecting scissors
  Vital-Metzenbaum dissecting
    scissors

scissors (*continued*)
Vital-Nelson dissecting scissors
vitreous strand scissors
Wadsworth scissors
Waldem-Marshall curved dissecting scissors
Walker scissors
Walker-Apple corneal scissors
Walker-Atkinson corneal scissors
Walkmann episiotomy scissors
Walton scissors
Watzke scissors
Weber tissue scissors
Webster meniscectomy scissors
Weck iris scissors
Weck suture scissors
Weck suture-removal scissors
Weck wire-cutting scissors
Weck-Spencer suture scissors
Weller cartilage scissors
Weller dissecting scissors
Wells enucleation scissors
Werb rhinostomy scissors
Wertheim deep-surgery scissors
Wescott stitch scissors
Westcott conjunctival scissors
Westcott double-end scissors
Westcott spring-action scissors
Westcott stitch scissors
Westcott tenotomy scissors
Westcott utility scissors
Westcott-Scheie scissors
Wester meniscectomy scissors
Wexteel scissors
White scissors
Wiechel scissors
Wiechel-Stille bile duct scissors
Wiet otologic scissors
Wilde-Blakesley scissors
Willauer thoracic scissors
Williamson-Noble scissors
Wilmer conjunctival and utility scissors
Wilmer conjunctival scissors
Wilmer iris scissors

scissors (*continued*)
Wilmer-Converse conjunctival scissors
Wilson intraocular scissors
Wincor enucleation scissors
wire carbide-jaw suture scissors
wire scissors
wire-cutting scissors
wire-cutting suture scissors
Wolf curved scissors
Wong-Staal scissors
Woods tonsillar scissors
Wullstein ear scissors
Wutzler circumcision scissors
Yankauer tonsillar scissors
Yasargil bayonet scissors
Yasargil microvascular bayonet scissors
Zoellner scissors
Zylik-Michaels scissors
scissors dissection
scissors forceps
scissors nail drill
scissors plaster shears
scissors probe
scissors-bite crossbite
scissors-excision hemorrhoidectomy
sclera (*pl.* sclerae)
blanching of sclera
blue sclera
buckling of sclera
ectasia of sclera
foramen of sclera
superficial sclera
sclerae and conjunctivae (S&C)
scleral bed
scleral blade
scleral buckle eye implant
scleral buckle procedure for retinal detachment
scleral buckler implant
scleral buckling catheter
scleral buckling operation
scleral buckling procedure
scleral canal
scleral cauterization
scleral depressor
scleral ectasia
scleral expander ring
scleral eye implant

scleral fistula operation
scleral fistulectomy operation
scleral flap
scleral hemorrhage
scleral hook
scleral implant
scleral marker (*see* marker)
scleral pick
scleral plug
scleral punch
scleral resection
scleral resection knife
scleral rim
scleral ring
scleral ruler
scleral rupture
scleral search coil technique
scleral shield
scleral shortening
scleral shortening clip
scleral shortening operation
scleral show
scleral spatula needle
scleral sponge rod
scleral spur
scleral trephine
scleral twist fixation hook
scleral twist-grip forceps
scleral wound retractor
sclerectoiridectomy
sclerectoiridodialysis
sclerectomy
  Berens sclerectomy
  Holth punch sclerectomy
  Lagrange sclerectomy
  Mueller sclerectomy
sclerectomy by punch
sclerectomy by scissors
sclerectomy by trephining
sclerectomy punch
sclerectomy punch forceps
sclerectomy scissors
sclerectomy with punch
sclerectomy with scissors
sclerectomy with trephine
scleriritomy
sclerocorneal junction
sclerodactyly
scleroderma
scleroderma-like eruption
scleroderma-like skin
  thickening

sclerodermatous
sclerodermoid
sclerodermoid graft-versus-host
  disease
sclerolimbal junction
scleronyxis
scleroplasty
scleroplasty operation
sclerosed lens
sclerosing agent
sclerosing basal cell carcinoma
sclerosing hemangioma
sclerosing inflammation
sclerosing injection
sclerosing lesion
sclerosing lipogranulomatosis
sclerosing lymphangitis
sclerosing mastoiditis
sclerosing osteitis
sclerosing substance
sclerosing therapy
sclerosis
  amyotrophic lateral sclerosis
   (ALS)
  cerebellar sclerosis
  diffuse systemic sclerosis
  dorsal sclerosis
  endocardial sclerosis
  gastric sclerosis
  insular sclerosis
  lobar sclerosis
  Mönckeberg (*see*
   Monckeberg)
  Mönckenberg (*also*
   Mönckeberg)
  Monckeberg sclerosis
  miliary sclerosis
  multiple sclerosis
  muscular sclerosis
  nephroarteriolar sclerosis
  posterolateral sclerosis
  presenile sclerosis
  progressive systemic sclerosis
  valvular sclerosis
  venous sclerosis
sclerostenosis
sclerostomy needle
sclerotherapy
  endoscopic injection
   sclerotherapy (EIS)
  endoscopic retrograde
   sclerotherapy

sclerotherapy (*continued*)
  endoscopic variceal
    sclerotherapy (EVS)
  esophageal variceal
    sclerotherapy
  fiberoptic injection
    sclerotherapy
  hemorrhoid sclerotherapy
  injection sclerotherapy
  tetracycline hydrochloride
    sclerotherapy
sclerotherapy complication
sclerotherapy failure
sclerotherapy needle
sclerotic bone lesion
sclerotic calvarial patch
sclerotic cemental mass
sclerotic kidney
sclerotic line
sclerotic mastoiditis
sclerotic rind
sclerotic thickening
scleroticectomy
scleroticochoroidal canal
scleroticonyxis
scleroticopuncture
sclerotome (*see also* knife)
  Alvis-Lancaster sclerotome
  Atkinson sclerotome
  Castroviejo sclerotome
  Curdy sclerotome
  Guyton-Lundsgaard
    sclerotome
  Lancaster sclerotome
  Lundsgaard sclerotome
  Lundsgaard-Burch sclerotome
  Walker-Lee sclerotome
sclerotome blade
sclerotomy
  DeWecker anterior
    sclerotomy
  DeWecker sclerotomy
  Lindner sclerotomy
  lip sclerotomy
  Verhoeff sclerotomy
sclerotomy knife
sclerotomy punch
sclerotomy with drainage
sclerotomy with exploration
sclerotomy with removal of
    foreign body
sclerous tissues

SCM (sternocleidomastoid)
SCM (sternocleidomastoid)
    tumor of infancy
Scobee muscle hook
Scobee oblique muscle hook
Scobee-Allis forceps
SCOI brace
scoliosis
  dextrorotatory scoliosis
  empyematic scoliosis
  ischiatic scoliosis
  levorotatory scoliosis
  lumbar scoliosis
  rachitic scoliosis
  rheumatic scoliosis
  sciatic scoliosis
  S-shaped scoliosis
scoliosis brace
scoliosis correction
scoliosis osteotome
scoliosis surgery
scoliotic curve fixation
Scolitron screw
scoop
  Abbott scoop
  abdominal scoop
  Arlt fenestrated lens scoop
  Arlt lens scoop
  Beck abdominal scoop
  Beck gastrostomy scoop
  Berens lens scoop
  Berens scoop
  common duct scoop
  Councill stone scoop
  cystic duct scoop
  Daviel scoop
  Desjardins gall duct scoop
  Desjardins gallbladder scoop
  Desjardins gallstone scoop
  Elschnig lens scoop
  enucleation scoop
  fenestrated lens scoop
  Ferguson gallstone scoop
  Ferris common duct scoop
  gall duct scoop
  gallbladder scoop
  gallstone scoop
  gastrostomy scoop
  Green lens scoop
  Hess lens scoop
  Kirby intracapsular scoop
  Klebanoff gallstone scoop

scoop (*continued*)
  Knapp lens scoop
  Lang scoop
  lens enucleation scoop
  lens scoop
  Lewis lens scoop
  Luer gallstone scoop
  Luer-Koerte scoop
  malleable scoop
  Mayo common duct scoop
  Mayo cystic duct scoop
  Mayo gallstone scoop
  Mayo-Robson gallstone
    scoop
  microbayonet scoop
  Moore gallstone scoop
  Moynihan gallstone scoop
  Mules scoop
  Pagenstecher scoop
  rigid scoop
  Rockey scoop
  Sellet common duct scoop
  Wells enucleation scoop
  Wilder lens scoop
  Yasargil scoop
Scoop transtracheal catheter
scoops and loops
scope
  baby scope
  colonofiberoptic scope
  Doppler scope
  forward-viewing scope
  Fragen scope
  front-viewing scope
  Fujinon flexible ENT scope
  Hirschowitz gastroduodenal
    scope
  Jesberg scope
  nonfade scope
  O'Connor operating scope
  Olympus flexible ENT scope
  Olympus scope
  operating scope
  Panvue scope
  reverting scope
  rotate scope
  side channel of scope
  side-viewing scope
  Storz scope
  stricture scope
  video image gastrointestinal
    scope

Scopemaster contact
    hysteroscope
scope-straightening twists and
    fold-gathering (on
    colonoscopy)
ScopeTrac support device
Scopette device
Scopinaro pancreaticobiliary
    bypass
score
  airway score
  Apgar score
  cosmetic score
  digital image score
  echo score
  evacuation score
  Gleason prostatic carcinoma
    score
  Gustilo fracture score
  Injury Severity Score (ISS)
  Japan Facial Score
  Mallampati score
  mitral valve echo score (Echo-
    Sc)
  OMENS score
  T-score
scored alar mucocartilaginous
    flap
scoring incision
Scotchcast casting tape
Scotchflex casting tape
scotoma
  Bjerrum scotoma
  centrocecal scotoma
  insular scotoma
  peripapillary scotoma
scotoma junction
scotometer
scotometry
scotopic vision
Scott inflatable penile prosthesis
Scott attic cannula
Scott dissecting scissors
Scott ear speculum
Scott glenoplasty technique
Scott humeral splint
Scott inflatable penile prosthesis
Scott jejunoileal bypass
Scott lens-insertion forceps
Scott nasal suction tube
Scott operation
Scott resectoscope

Scott right-angle scissors
Scott rubber ventricular cannula
Scott ruler
Scott speculum
Scott splint
Scott suction tube
Scott ventricular cannula
Scott-Craig orthosis
Scott-Harden tube
Scottish Rite brace
Scottish Rite hip orthosis
Scottish Rite procedure
Scottish Rite splint
Scott-McCracken elevator
Scott-McCracken periosteal
    elevator
Scott-RCE osteotomy guide
Scotty stainless ankle joint
scotty-dog fracture
scotty-dog graft
scout film
scout negative
scout positive
scout roentgenogram
Scoville blunt hook
Scoville brain forceps
Scoville brain spatula
Scoville brain spatula forceps
Scoville Britetrac retractor
Scoville cervical disk self-
    retaining retractor
Scoville clip
Scoville clip applier
Scoville clip-applying forceps
Scoville curet
Scoville curved hook
Scoville curved nerve hook
Scoville dural hook
Scoville flat brain spatula
Scoville forceps
Scoville hemilaminectomy
Scoville hemilaminectomy
    retractor
Scoville hemilaminectomy self-
    retaining retractor
Scoville laminectomy retractor
Scoville needle
Scoville nerve hook
Scoville nerve retractor
Scoville nerve root retractor
Scoville psoas muscle retractor
Scoville retractor blade

Scoville retractor hook
Scoville ruptured disk curet
Scoville scissors
Scoville self-retaining retractor
Scoville skull trephine
Scoville spatula
Scoville trephine
Scoville ventricular needle
Scoville-Drew clip applier
Scoville-Greenwood bayonet
    neurosurgical bipolar
    forceps
Scoville-Greenwood forceps
Scoville-Haverfield laminectomy
    retractor
Scoville-Hurteau forceps
Scoville-Lewis aneurysm clip
Scoville-Lewis clamp
Scoville-Richter self-retaining
    retractor
scraper
    amalgam scraper
    drum scraper
    Hough drum scraper
scratch incision
scratcher
    Jensen scratcher
    Kratz scratcher
    Kratz-Jensen scratcher
scratch-type incision
screen
    Bjerrum screen
    coagulation screen
    intensifying screen
    Marlex screen
screen oxygenator
screen pneumotach
screw (see also microscrew)
    4-tap screw
    Absolute absorbable screw
    ACE bone screw
    Ace cannulated cancellous
        hip screw
    Ace cannulated cancellous
        screw
    Ace captured hip screw
    Ace cortical bone screw
    Ace hip screw
    Acutrak screw
    adjustable screw
    afterloading screw
    alar screw

screw (*continued*)

Allen screw
Alta cancellous screw
Alta cortical screw
Alta cross-locking screw
Alta lag screw
Alta supracondylar screw
Alta transverse screw
Ambi compression hip screw
Ambi hip screw
amputation screw
anchor screw
anchoring screw
A-O screw
Arthrex sheathed interference
    screw
arthrodesis screw
ASIF screw
Asner screw
Asnis guided screw
Asnis cannulated screw
Asnis guided screw
Aten olecranon screw
axial anchor screw
Barouk cannulated bone
    screw
Basile hip screw
Bechtol screw
bicortical superior border
    screw
bioabsorbable interference
    screw
Biofix absorbable screw
biointerference screw
Biologically Quiet
    interference screw
Biologically Quiet
    reconstruction screw
Bionix self-reinforced smart
    screw
BioRCI bioabsorbable screw
BioSorb endoscopic browlift
    screw
Bone Mulch screw
bone screw
Bosworth coracoclavicular
    screw
Bristow screw
brow lift suspension screw
buttress thread screw
Calcitek retaining screw
Camino subdural screw

screw (*continued*)

cancellous bone screw
cancellous screw
cannulated cancellous lag
    screw
carpal scaphoid screw
Carroll-Girard screw
Caspar cervical screw
Clearfix meniscal screw
Cohort bone screw
Collison screw
compression hip screw (CHS)
compression screw
Concept screw
Concise compression hip
    screw
coracoclavicular screw
cortex screw
cortical anchoring screw
cortical screw
Cotrel pedicle screw
cotton screw
cover screw
craniomaxillofacial screw
Crites laryngeal cotton screw
crown drill screw
cruciate head bone screw
cruciate head screw
cruciform head bone screw
cruciform head-bone screw
Cubbins screw
Demuth hip screw
dental implant cover screw
Dentatus screw
DePuy interference screw
Deyerle screw
distal locking screw
distraction screw
double-threaded Herbert
    screw
Doyen myoma screw
Doyen tumor screw
Druck-Schrauben screw
Duo-Drive cortical bone
    screw
Duo-Drive cortical screw
DuPuy interference screw
Dwyer cancellous screw
Dwyer spinal screw
dynamic condylar screw
    (DCS)
dynamic hip screw

screw (*continued*)

ECT internal fracture fixation
and bone screw
Edwards sacral screw
Eggers screw
encased screw
endocardial screw
EndoFix absorbable
interference screw
expansion screw
eyelet lag screw
Fabian screw
fixateur interne screw
fixation screw
fixing screw
foreign body screw
Geckeler screw
Gentle Threads interference
screw
Gentle Threads resorbable
interference screws
German A-O hip compression
screw
Glasser fixation screw
glenoid fixation screw
Guardsman femoral
interference screw
Hahn screw
Hall spinal screw
Hall-Morris biphase screw
Harris hip screw
healing screw
Heck screw
Henderson lag screw
Herbert bone screw
Herbert scaphoid bone screw
Herbert scaphoid screw
Herbert-Whipple bone screw
hex screw (hexagon)
hexagon screw
hexhead screw
hip screw
Hi-Torque screw
Hoffmann screw
Howmedica lag screw
Howmedica Luer screw
Howmedica Universal
compression screw
Howse-Coventry screw
iliac screw
iliosacral screw
Ilizarov screw

screw (*continued*)

ImplaMed screw
Implant Innovations titanium
screw
implant screw
implant support titanium
screw
insertion of screw
Instrument Makar
biodegradable screw
Integrity acetabular cup
screw
interference screw
interfragmentary lag screw
intracranial pressure monitor
screw
Isola spinal implant system
iliac screw
Isola vertebral screw
Jeter lag screw
Jeter position screw
Jewett pickup screw
Johannson lag screw
Johannson-Stille lag screw
key-free compression screw
KLS-Martin Centre-Drive
screw
Kostuik screw
Kristiansen eyelet lag screw
Kurosaka bone screw
Kurosaka cannulated screw
Kurosaka extremity screw
Kurosaka interference fixation
screw
Kurosaka interference-fit
screw
lag screw
Lane bone screw
lateral screw
Leibinger Micro Plus screw
Leibinger mini Wurzburg
screw
Leinbach olecranon screw
Leone expansion screw
Lewin tonsil screw
Lewis tonsillar screw
Lindorf lag screw
Lindorf position screw
Linvatec absorbable screw
Linvatec bioabsorbable
interference screw
locking screw

screw (*continued*)
Lorenz screw
Lorenzo bone fixation screw
Luhr implant screw
Luhr Vitallium screw
lumbar pedicle screw
Lundholm screw
Luque screw
malleable screw
mandibular angle fracture
intraoral open reduction
screw
Marion screw
Martin screw
maxillofacial bone screw
McAtee screw
McLaughlin carpal scaphoid
screw
Mecron cannulated
cancellous screw
medial bicortical screw
medial unicortical screw
metal screw
metallic screw
Micro Plus screw
Mille Pattes screw
mini lag screw
mini Wurzburg screw
monocortical screw
Morris biphase screw
multiaxial screw
myoma screw
navicular screw
Neufeld screw
Nobelpharma prosthetic
retaining screw
No-Lok compression screw
Olerud screw
Omega compression hip screw
oral screw
Orion plate and screw
Orthex cannulated titanium
bone screw
Orthofix screw
orthopedic screw
Osteomed screw
Palex expansion screw
pedicle screw
PerFixation screw
Periotest Implant Innovations
gold screw
Phantom interference screw

screw (*continued*)
Phillips recessed-head screw
pickup screw
Pilot point screw
plates and screws
polyaxial cervical screw
polylactide absorbable screw
pretapped synthes lag screw
pull screw
quiet interference screw
Ray screw
recessed-head screw
Reddick-Saye screw
removal of screw
resorbable plate and screw
ReUnite orthopedic screw
reverse-threaded screw
Revo retrievable cancellous
screw
Richards adjustable hip screw
Richards classic compression
hip screw
Richards compression screw
Richards lag screw
Richmond subarachnoid
screw
rigid pedicle screw
Rockwood shoulder screw
Russell-Taylor screw
sacral alar screw
sacral pedicle screw
Salzburg screw
Schanz screw
Scolitron screw
screw alignment bar
screw alignment rod
screw compressor
screw depth calibrator
screw depth gauge
screw grip
screw occlusive clamp
screw tap
Scuderi screw
self-tapping bone screw
self-tapping Leibinger lag
screw
set screw
Sharpey screw
Sherman bone screw
Sherman molybdenum screw
Sherman plate and screws
Sherman Vitallium screw

screw (*continued*)

silk screw
Simmons double-hole spinal screw
Simmons-Martin screw
slotted screw
SmartScrew screw
Smith & Nephew screw
Spiessel lag screw
Spiessel position screw
spongiosa screw
stainless steel screw
Steffee screw
Steinhauser lag screw
Steinhauser position screw
step screw
Stryker lag screw
subarachnoid screw
superior thoracic pedicle screw
superlag screw
syndesmosis screw
syndesmotic screw
Syntex screw
Synthes compression hip screw
Texas Scottish Rite Hospital pedicle screw
Thatcher screw
thoracolumbar pedicle screw
Thornton screw
ThreadLoc driver mount screw
ThreadLoc retaining screw
Ti alloy screw
TiMesh emergency screw
titanium mesh screw
titanium screw
tonsillar screw
Townley bone graft screw
Townsend-Gilfillan screw
TPS-coated screw
traction tongs screw
transarticular screw
transfixion screw
transpedicular screw
transsyndesmotic screw
triangulated pedicle screw
Tronzo screw
tulip pedicle screw
tumor screw
TunneLoc interference screw

screw (*continued*)

Venable hip screw
Vilex cannulated screw
Virgin hip screw
Vitallium screw
Weise jack screw
Wood screw
Woodruff screw
Wurzberg screw
Yuan screw
Zielke screw
Zimmer compression hip screw
screw alignment bar
screw alignment rod
screw compressor
screw depth calibrator
screw depth gauge
screw elevator
screw fixation
screw grip
screw home mechanism
screw implantation
screw insertion
screw insertion technique
screw joint
screw occlusive clamp
screw placement
screw plate
screw position perioperative monitoring
screw site
screw stabilization
screw tap
screw tenaculum
screw-and-plate fixation
screw-and-wire fixation
screwdriver
Allen-headed screwdriver
automatic screwdriver
Becker screwdriver
Children's Hospital screwdriver
Collison screwdriver
cross-slot screwdriver
cruciform screwdriver
Cubbins screwdriver
DePuy screwdriver
Dorsey screwdriver
heavy cross-slot screwdriver
hexhead screwdriver
Johnson screwdriver

screwdriver (*continued*)
  Ken screwdriver
  Lane screwdriver
  lever-type screwdriver
  light cross-slot screwdriver
  Lok-it screwdriver
  Lok-screw double-slot
    screwdriver
  Massie screwdriver
  Master screwdriver
  medium screwdriver
  Moore-Blount screwdriver
  Phillips screwdriver
  plain screwdriver
  Richards Phillips screwdriver
  Richter screwdriver
  Shallcross screwdriver
  Sherman screwdriver
  Sherman-Pierce screwdriver
  single cross-slot screwdriver
  Stryker screwdriver
  Trenkle screwdriver
  V. Mueller screwdriver
  White screwdriver
  Williams screwdriver
  Woodruff screwdriver
  Zimmer screwdriver
screwdriver instrument
screwdriver teeth
screw-holding forceps
screw-in epicardial electrode
screw-in lead
screw-in sutureless myocardial
    electrode
screw-in-lead pacemaker
screw-on lead
screw-plate approach
screw-retained prosthesis
screw-tipped intraosseous
    needle
screw-type implant
Screw-Vent implant
Scribner arteriovenous shunt
scroll bones
scroll ear
scrotal area
scrotal compartment
scrotal dressing
scrotal elephantiasis
scrotal hemangioma
scrotal hernia
scrotal hydrocele

scrotal incision
scrotal mass
scrotal nerves
scrotal pouch operation
scrotal sac
scrotal septum
scrotal suspensory support
scrotal swelling
scrotal tongue
scrotal veins
scrotal-perineal incontinence
    prosthesis
scrotectomy
scrotocele
scrotoplasty
Scrotter catheter
scrotum
  shawl scrotum
  testes in scrotum
  watering-can scrotum
scrub file
scrub preparation
scrubbed, prepped, and draped
Scudder intestinal clamp
Scudder intestinal forceps
Scudder operation
Scudder procedure
Scudder skid
Scudder stomach clamp
Scudder technique
Scuderi bipolar coagulating
    forceps
Scuderi forceps
Scuderi procedure
Scuderi prosthesis
Scuderi repair
Scuderi screw
Scuderi technique
Scuderi tendon repair
Scuderi-Callahan flange
SCUF therapy (slow continuous
    ultrafiltration therapy)
Scully functional hip support
Sculptor annuloplasty ring
Sculptor flexible annuloplasty
    ring
sculpturing scalpel
scultetus bandage
scultetus binder
scultetus binder band
scultetus binder dressing
scultetus dressing

scultetus position
Scurasil device prosthesis
Scutan temporary splint material
scutum
scybalous feces
scybalous stool
scybalum (*pl.* scybala)
Scypleth pulse oximeter
SDC (salivary duct carcinoma)
SDC anesthesia
SD Sorb E-Z-Tac implant
SD Sorb meniscal stapler
SE Prosthesis
SE-100 smoke aspiration tip
sea anemone ulcer
Sea-Clens wound cleanser
seal
   cavity seal
   palatal seal
   tight seal
   underwater seal
   velopharyngeal seal
   watertight seal
SealEasy resuscitation mask
sealed applicator
sealed envelope technique
sealed vacuum bottle
sealer extrusion
sealing perforation
Seal-Tight cast protector
Sealy dissecting scissors
Sealy-Laragh technique
SeamGuard staple line material
seamless arterial graft
seamless graft
seamless prosthesis
seamless tube prosthesis
seam-sealer gun
searcher (*see also* bougie, sound)
   Allport mastoid searcher
   Allport-Babcock mastoid
     searcher
   mastoid searcher
Searcy capsular forceps
Searcy chalazion trephine
Searcy erysiphake
Searcy fixation
Searcy fixation anchor
Searcy fixation hook
Searcy forceps
Searcy hook
Searcy oval cup erysiphake

Searcy tonsillectome
Searcy trephine
Searle volume ventilator
SeaSorb alginate wound dressing
seatbelt injury
seatbelt sign
seatbelt fracture
Seated Hamstring Curl exercise
   chair
Seattle classification
Seattle orthosis
sebaceous adenocarcinoma
sebaceous adenoma
sebaceous carcinoma
sebaceous cyst
sebaceous glands
sebaceous horn
sebaceous hyperplasia
sebaceous lymphadenoma
sebaceous material
sebaceous metaplasia
sebaceous skin
Sebbin ultrasound device
Sebbin ultrasound-assisted
    lipoplasty machine
Sebileau hollow
Sebileau periosteal elevator
seborrheic blepharitis
seborrheic dermatitis
seborrheic keratosis
seborrheic verruca
Sebra arm tourniquet
Sechrist infant ventilator
Sechrist hyperbaric chamber
Sechrist neonatal ventilator
Seckel syndrome
secobarbital anesthetic agent
Seconal anesthetic agent
secondary abscess
secondary adhesion
secondary amputation
secondary anesthetic
secondary arrest of dilatation
secondary articulation
secondary branch
secondary carcinoma
secondary cataract
secondary cause
secondary choana
secondary cleft
secondary closure of wound
secondary condition

secondary constriction
secondary contraction of skin
    graft
secondary craniosynostosis
secondary debulking
secondary diagnostic biopsy
secondary ear reconstruction
secondary expansion
secondary fixation
secondary focal point
secondary fracture
secondary gangrene
secondary hemorrhage
secondary hernia
secondary infection
secondary lesion
secondary membrane
secondary myofascial trigger point
secondary occlusal traumatism
secondary palate
secondary procedure
secondary process
secondary ptosis correction
secondary pulmonary lobule
secondary reconstruction
secondary renal calculus
secondary repair
secondary rhinoplasty
secondary site
secondary skin-only face-lift
secondary stage
secondary surgery
secondary suture technique
secondary sutures
secondary telangiectasia
secondary wound closure
Secretan disease
secretion
    excretion and secretion
    external secretion
    gastric secretion
    intestinal secretions
    mucoid secretion
    nasopharyngeal secretion
    oral secretions
    respiratory secretions
    tenacious mucoid secretion
    tracheal secretions
    tracheopulmonary secretions
    viscid secretion
    viscous secretion
    waxlike secretion

secretory activity
secretory adenocarcinoma
secretory canaliculus
secretory carcinoma
secretory duct
secretory immunoglobulin
secretory nerve
secretory otitis media (SOM)
section
    2-step corneal section
    abdominal section
    attached cranial section
    cervical cesarean section
    cesarean section
    classical cesarean section
    corneal section
    corporeal cesarean section
    crash cesarean section
    cross-section
    cryostat section
    cut section
    detached cranial section
    extraperitoneal cesarean
        section
    frozen section
    intraoperative frozen section
    Kerr cesarean section
    Kronig cesarean section
    Krönig (see Kronig)
    Kronig (also Krönig,
        Kroenig)
    Kroenig (see Kronig)
    Latzko cesarean section
    low cervical cesarean section
    low cesarean section
    lower uterine segment
        cesarean section
    median section
    meridional section
    Mueller cesarean section
    Müller (see Mueller)
    Mueller (also Müller)
    Munro Kerr cesarean section
    Norton-Latzko extraperitoneal
        cesarean section
    perineal section
    Porro cesarean section
    postcesarean section
    sagittal section
    serial section
    submitted for frozen section
    tangential section

section (*continued*)
  transperitoneal cesarean
    section
  transverse cesarean section
  transverse section
  vaginal birth after cesarean
    section (VBAC)
  vaginal cesarean section
  Water cesarean section
sectional roentgenography
sectional technique
sector iridectomy
sector iridectomy operation
sector scan echocardiography
sector scanner
sectorial resection
Secu clip
Secund fracture
secundigravida
secundines
secundum atrial septal defect
secundum foramen
Securat suction tube
secure intracorporeal knot
SeCure therapeutic mattress
secured hemostasis
secured with tape
secured with ties
SecureStrand cable
Secur-Its silicone cushion mat
Security+ self-sealing Urisheath
  external catheter
Sedan cannula
Sedan goniometer
Sedan-Nashold needle
sedative effect
sedative therapy
Seddon arthrodesis
Seddon classification for nerve
  injuries (types 1-3)
Seddon costotransversectomy
Seddon modification
Seddon nerve graft
Seddon operation
Seddon technique
Seddon wrist arthrodesis
Sedillot elevator
Sedillot elevator-raspatory
Sedillot operation
Sedillot periosteal elevator
Sedillot raspatory
sedimentary cataract

Seeburger implant
Seecor pacemaker
seed graft
seed implant
Seeker guidewire
Seeligmuller sign
Seeligmüller (*see* Seeligmuller)
Seeligmuller (*also* Seeligmüller)
Seeman-Seiffert mouth gag
Seen retractor
Seep-Pruf ileostomy appliance
SeeQuence disposable lens
Seer cardiac monitor
seesaw murmur
segment
  attenuated lower uterine
    segment
  basilar segment
  bronchopulmonary segments
  bypass occluded segment
  cleft maxillary segment
  cranial segment
  frontal segment
  hepatic segments
  interannular segment
  labyrinthine segment
  lingular segment
  lower uterine segment
  medullary segment
  mesodermal segment
  occipital segment
  posterior segment
  pulmonary segment
  Ranvier segments
  rivinian segment
  Rivinus segment
  stenotic segment
  terminal ileal segment
  uterine segment
segmental alveolar osteotomy
segmental arteries
segmental atelectasis
segmental bone and cartilage
  reconstruction
segmental bone defect
segmental bronchus
segmental buckle
segmental colon resection
segmental colonic resection
segmental compression
  construct
segmental continuity defect

segmental demyelination
segmental dilatation
segmental duct
segmental epidural anesthesia
segmental explant
segmental fixation
segmental fracture
segmental gastrectomy
segmental gracilis muscle
    transplantation
segmental graft
segmental hepatectomy
segmental hyalinizing vasculitis
segmental innervation
segmental involvement
segmental loss of helix
segmental lung resection
segmental mandibulectomy
segmental microvascular
    transfers
segmental orifices
segmental perforators
segmental pulmonary resection
segmental resection
segmental resection of lung
segmental spinal
    instrumentation
segmental stripping
segmental surgery
segmental tendon graft
segmental wall motion
    abnormality (SWMA)
segmental washings
segmentation anomaly
segmentectomy
segmented flap
segmented forms
segmented fracture
segmented ring tripolar lead
segment-oriented hepatic
    resection
segment-oriented liver
    resection
segment-oriented procedure
segment-oriented resection
segment-oriented technique
Segond abdominal retractor
Segond fracture
Segond hysterectomy forceps
Segond spatula
Segond tumor forceps
Segond vaginal spatula

Segond-Landau hysterectomy
    forceps
segregator
    Cathelin segregator
    Harris segregator
    Luys segregator
Segura procedure
Segura stone basket
Segura surgery for esophageal
    varices
Segura-Dretler stone basket
Sehrt clamp
Sehrt compressor
Seidel bone-holding clamp
Seidel catheter
Seidel humeral locking nail
Seidel intramedullary fixation
Seidel plug
Seidel sign
Seidel test for aqueous fluid leak
Seidelin body
Seiff frontalis suspension set
Seiffert esophagoscopy forceps
Seiffert grasping punch
Seiffert laryngeal forceps
Seiffert tip
Seiffert tonsillectome
Seiler cartilage
Seiler conization knife
Seiler surgical microscope
Seiler scissors
Seiler tonsillar knife
Seiler turbinate scissors
Seinsheimer classification of
    subtrochanteric fractures
Seinsheimer femoral fracture
    classification
Seirin acupuncture needle
Seitzinger tripolar cutting
    forceps
seizing forceps
Selakovich procedure
Selby hook
Seldin dental retractor
Seldin elevator
Seldinger arterial needle
Seldinger cardiac catheter
Seldinger cardiac catheterization
Seldinger catheter
Seldinger cystic duct
    catheterization
Seldinger gastrostomy needle

Seldinger needle
Seldinger percutaneous
    technique
Seldinger procedure
Seldinger retrograde wire
Seldinger retrograde
    wire/intubation technique
Seldinger technique
Seldinger-Desilet technique
Selecon coronary angiography
    catheter
Select ankle prosthesis
Select joint orthosis
Select shoulder prosthesis
selective anesthesia
selective angiography
selective arterial embolization
selective bronchial
    catheterization anesthetic
    technique
selective cannulation
selective catheterization
selective coronary arteriogram
selective coronary
    cineangiogram
selective ductal cannulation
selective excitation projection
    reconstruction imaging
selective inguinal node
    dissection
selective injection
selective irradiation
selective lectin-triggered
    apoptosis
selective lymphadenectomy
selective neck dissection (SND)
selective photothermolysis
selective portal decompression
selective subendocardial
    resection
selective thoracic spine fusion
selective vagolysis
selective vagotomy
selective vascular clamping
    (SVC)
Selector ultrasonic aspirator
Seletz cannula
Seletz catheter
Seletz foramen-plugging forceps
Seletz punch
Seletz Universal Kerrison punch
Seletz ventricular cannula

Seletz-Gelpi self-retaining
    retractor
self-adhering lid retractor
self-adjusting nail
self-aligning knee
self-articulating femoral hip
    replacement (SAF hip
    replacement)
self-articulating femoral
    prosthesis
self-aspirating cut-biopsy needle
Selfast dental cement
self-broaching nail
self-broaching pin
Self-Cath coude-tipped catheter
Self-Cath soft catheter
Self-Cath straight-tipped female
    catheter
Self-Cath straight-tipped
    pediatric catheter
Self-Cath straight-tipped soft
    catheter
self-centering micromanipulator
self-centering Universal hip
    prosthesis
self-compressing plate
self-expanding metallic
    endoprosthesis
self-expandable metallic stent
self-expandable stainless steel
    braided endoprosthesis
self-expanding coil stent
self-expanding metallic stent
self-expanding stainless steel
    stent
self-expanding tulip sheath
self-expanding Wallstent
    endoprosthesis
self-guiding catheter
self-inflating bulb
self-inflating tissue expander
self-locking prosthesis
self-locking stitch
self-opening forceps
self-opening rigid snare
self-retaining abdominal
    retractor
self-retaining bone forceps
self-retaining brain retractor
self-retaining brain retractor
    frame
self-retaining catheter

self-retaining chamber maintainer
self-retaining coil stent
self-retaining infusion cannula
self-retaining irrigating cannula
self-retaining laryngoscope
self-retaining retractor
self-retaining retractor blade
self-retaining ring retractor
self-retaining skin retractor
self-retaining speculum
self-retaining spring retractor
self-sealing cannula
self-seating plug
self-stabilizing vitrectomy lens
self-stopping drill point
self-suspension
self-tapering pin
self-tapping bone screw
self-tapping Leibinger lag screw
self-tapping screw-type implant
self-tightening slip knot
Selker ventriculostomy reservoir
Selkin speculum
sella turcica
sella-nasion (S-N) plane
sella-nasion plane
sella-nasion-B point
sella-nasion-subspinale angle
sella-nasion-supramentale angle
sellar punch
Sellheim incision
Sellheim obstetrical level
Sellheim uterine catheter
Sellick maneuver
Sellor clamp
Sellor contractor
Sellor mitral valve knife
Sellor rib contractor
Sellor rib retractor
Sellor valvulotome
Selman clamp
Selman clip
Selman nonslip tissue forceps
Selman peripheral blood vessel forceps
Selman tissue forceps
Selman vessel forceps
Selofix dressing
Selopor dressing
Selrodo bulb
Selrodo nebulizer

Seltzer saw
Selute steroid-eluting lead
Selverstone carotid artery clamp
Selverstone carotid clamp
Selverstone cordotomy hook
Selverstone embolus forceps
Selverstone hook
Selverstone intervertebral disk forceps
Selverstone intervertebral disk rongeur
Selverstone laminectomy rongeur
Selverstone rongeur forceps
SEM (systolic ejection murmur)
Semb bone forceps
Semb bone-cutting forceps
Semb bone-holding clamp
Semb bone-holding forceps
Semb bronchus clamp
Semb dissecting forceps
Semb dissecting scissors
Semb gouging rongeur
Semb ligature forceps
Semb ligature-carrying forceps
Semb lung retractor
Semb nephrectomy technique
Semb operation
Semb raspatory
Semb retractor
Semb rib forceps
Semb rib raspatory
Semb rib shears
Semb rongeur
Semb rongeur forceps
Semb self-retaining retractor
Semb shears
Semb vaginal speculum
Semb-Ghazi dissecting forceps
Semb-Sauerbruch rongeur
Semb-Stille bone rongeur
SEMI (subendocardial myocardial infarction)
semi-adjustable articulator
semiaxial anteroposterior projection
semiaxial projection
semiaxial transcranial projection
semibarber position
semicanal for tensor tympani
semicanal of auditory tube
semicartilaginous

semicircular canals
semicircular ducts (anterior, lateral, posterior, superior)
semicircular gouge
semicircular incision
semicircular punch
semicircular rings
semicircular trochlear notch
semiclosed anesthesia
semiclosed endotracheal anesthesia
semicomatose
semicompressive dressing
semiconductor
semiconscious
semiconstrained prosthesis
semiconstrained total elbow arthroplasty
semicircular line of Douglas
semidecussation
semielective operation
semierect position
semiflat tip electrode
semiflexed incision
semiflexible endoscope
semiflexible intraocular lens
semi-Fowler position
semi-impermeable membrane
semilateral position
semilunar bone
semilunar cartilage
semilunar cartilage knife
semilunar cartilage scissors
semilunar conjunctival fold
semilunar fibrocartilage
semilunar flap
semilunar fold
semilunar ganglion
semilunar hiatus
semilunar incision
semilunar line
semilunar lobule
semilunar notch
semilunar valve
semilunar-tip blade
semimembranosus muscle
semimembranous muscle
seminal ducts
seminal fluid
seminal gland
seminal sutures
seminal vesicle aspiration

seminal vesicles
seminiferous tubules
seminoma
semioblique position
semiocclusive dressing
semiocclusive moisture-retentive dressing
semiopen anesthesia
semiopen dressing
semiopen endotracheal inhalation anesthesia
semiopen hemorrhoidectomy
semioval center
semipedunculated lesion
semipermanent retention
semipermeable dressing
semipermeable membrane
semipermeable membrane dressing
semipressure dressing
semiprone position
semireclining position
semirecumbent position
semirigid catheter
semirigid endoscope
semirigid fiberglass cast
semirigid fixation
semirigid intraocular lens
semirigid penile prosthesis
semirigid polypropylene ankle-foot orthosis
semirigid sigmoidoscope
semishell eye implant
semishell implant
semishelving incision
semisolid material
semispinal muscle
semistuporous patient
semitendinosus procedure
semitendinosus technique
semitendinous muscle
semitubular blade plate
semitubular plate
semiupright film
semiupright position
Semken bipolar forceps
Semken dressing forceps
Semken infant forceps
Semken microbipolar neurosurgical forceps
Semken thumb forceps
Semken tissue forceps

Semken-Taylor forceps
Semm cannula
Semm morcellator
Semm Pelvi-Pneu insufflator
Semm uterine catheter
Semm uterine vacuum cannula
Semm uterine vacuum catheter
Semm Z technique
Semmes curet
Semmes dural forceps
Semmes spinal fusion curet
Semmes-Weinstein
   monofilament test
Semmes-Weinstein pressure
   esthesiometer filament
Semmonds disease
Senear-Usher disease
Senear-Usher syndrome
senescent changes
Sengstaken balloon
Sengstaken nasogastric tube
Sengstaken-Blakemore balloon
Sengstaken-Blakemore device
Sengstaken-Blakemore
   esophageal balloon
Sengstaken-Blakemore
   esophagogastric tamponade
   tube
Sengstaken-Blakemore tube
senile angioma
senile atrophoderma
senile atrophy
senile blepharoptosis
senile cataract
senile chin
senile ectasia
senile elastosis
senile fibroma
senile gangrene
senile hemangioma
senile keratoderma
senile keratoma
senile keratosis
senile lentigo
senile melanoderma
senile sebaceous hyperplasia
senile skin
senile wart
senilis
   alopecia senilis
   arcus senilis
   atrophia cutis senilis

senilis (*continued*)
   atrophoderma senilis
   keratosis senilis
   lentigo senilis
   linea corneae senilis
   pruritus senilis
   verruca plana senilis
   verruca senilis
Senn bone plate
Senn double-ended retractor
Senn forceps
Senn mastoid retractor
Senn operation
Senn self-retaining retractor
Senn speculum
Senn-Dingman double-ended
   retractor
Senn-Green retractor
Senning atrial baffle repair
Senning baffle
Senning bulldog clamp
Senning cardiovascular forceps
Senning correction of
   transposition of great
   vessels
Senning featherweight bulldog
   clamp
Senning intra-arterial baffle
Senning intra-atrial baffle
Senning operation
Senning repair
Senning suction tube
Senning transposition operation
Senning transposition procedure
Senning-Stille clamp
Senn-Kanavel double-ended
   retractor
Senn-Kanavel retractor
Senn-Miller retractor
Senographe breast imaging
Sens dissector
sensate cutaneous flap
sensate flap
sensate medial plantar free flap
sensate pedicled
   neoclitoroplasty
Sensatec forceps
Sensatec scissors
Sensation intra-aortic balloon
   catheter
Sensation snare
Sense-of-Feel prosthesis

Sensimatic electrosurgical unit
sensing catheter
sensing coil
sensitive free flap
    reconstruction
sensitive plane
sensitizing injection
Sensiv endotracheal tube
Senso listening device
Sensolog pacemaker
Sensonic plaque removal
    instrument
Sensor Kelvin pacemaker
sensor operation
sensor-based single-chamber
    pacemaker
sensorimotor arc
sensorimotor cortex
sensorimotor neuropathy
sensorimotor rhythm
sensorimotor stimulation
    approach
sensorimuscular
sensorineural acuity level
    technique
sensorineural deafness
sensorineural hearing loss
sensorium
SensorMedics pressure
    transducer
sensory block
sensory blockade
sensory branch of radial nerve
    (SBRN)
sensory deficit
sensory examination
sensory functions
sensory fusion
sensory hyperesthesia
sensory impairment
sensory loss
sensory nerve
sensory nerve fiber bundle
sensory paralysis
sensory pathway
sensory root of trigeminal nerve
sensory stimulation kit
sensory tract
Sentalloy digital calipers
SentiLite neurological monitor
sentinel bleed
sentinel blood clot

sentinel cells
sentinel fold
sentinel gland
sentinel loop
sentinel lymph node biopsy
sentinel lymphadenectomy
sentinel lymphatic mapping
sentinel node biopsy (SNB)
sentinel node excision
sentinel node localization
sentinel pile
sentinel polyp
sentinel skin paddle
sentinel skin paddle graft
sentinel spinous process
    fracture
sentinel tag
Sentinel-4 neurological monitor
Sentron pigtail angiographic
    micromanometer catheter
Sentron pigtail microtip
    manometer catheter
Senturia forceps
Senturia pharyngeal speculum
Senturia retractor
Senturia speculum
Senturia-Alden specimen
    collector
SEP (somatosensory evoked
    potential)
separating saw
separating wire
separation
    AC separation
    acromioclavicular separation
    E-point septal separation (EPSS)
    incomplete separation
    jaw separation
    mechanical tooth separation
    pterygomaxillary separation
    septal separation
    Weaver-Dunn repair of
        acromioclavicular
        separation
separation point
separator
    Allen stereo separator
    Amicus blood collection
        separator
    Asahi Plasmaflo plasma
        separator
    bayonet separator

separator (*continued*)
- Benson baby pyloric separator
- Benson pylorus separator
- blood cell separator
- Cobe blood cell separator
- curved zonule separator
- cylindrical zonule separator
- Davis nerve separator
- Dorsey dural separator
- double-ball separator
- dural separator
- Elast-O-Chain separator
- Ferrier separator
- finger separator
- flat zonule separator
- Frazier dural separator
- Grant dural separator
- Harris separator
- head spoon separator
- Hoen dural separator
- Horsley dural separator
- House ear separator
- Hunter dural separator
- iliac graft separator
- Kirby curved zonular separator
- Kirby cylindrical zonular separator
- Kirby double-ball separator
- Kirby flat zonular separator
- Kirby intracapsular expressor with curved zonular separator
- Kirby intracapsular lens separator
- Lig-A-Ring separator
- Luys separator
- mechanical separator
- noninterfering separator
- posterior canal separator
- pylorus separator
- Remy separator
- Rosen bayonet separator
- Rosen separator
- Sachs dural separator
- Sachs nerve separator
- Sep-A-Ring separator
- Silverstein nerve separator
- stem spoon separator
- synovial separator
- tonsillar separator
- True separator

separator (*continued*)
- Williger separator
- Woodson dural separator
- zonule separator

separator tube
Sep-A-Ring separator
Seprafilm bioresorbable membrane
Sepramesh biosurgical composite
sepsis syndrome
sepsis-induced disseminated intravascular coagulation
sepsis-induced muscle breakdown
septa (*sing.* septum)
septal annuloplasty
septal artery
septal bone forceps
septal bones
septal branch
septal cartilage
septal cartilage graft
septal chisel
septal chondromucosal graft
septal clamp
septal compression forceps
septal defect
septal deformity
septal deviation
septal displacement
septal dissector
septal elevator
septal forceps
septal fracture
septal gouge
septal hematoma
septal intranasal lining flap
septal knife
septal lines
septal mucoperichondrium
septal mucosa
septal necrosis
septal needle
septal overlap
septal panniculitis
septal perforation
septal posterior nasal arteries
septal punch
septal raphe
septal reconstruction
septal reduction

septal relocation
septal resection
septal ridge forceps
septal scissors
septal separation
septal space
septal speculum
septal splint
septal straightener
septal trephine
septate hymen
septate uterus
septation procedure
septectomy
  Blalock-Hanlon atrial
    septectomy
  Edwards septectomy
septic abortion
septic arthritis
septic complication
septic dactylitis
septic fever
septic joint
septic metastasis
septic process
septic shock
septic wound
Septicare wound cleanser
septicemia
  bacterial septicemia
  cryptogenic septicemia
  streptococcal septicemia
Septisol prep
Septisol soap dressing
septoaponeurotic union
Septocaine anesthetic
septocutaneous island
septocutaneous perforator
septodermoplasty
septofasciocutaneous island
Septoject needle
septomarginal
septomuscular perforator
septonasal
Septopack periodontal dressing
Septopal implant
septoplasty
  endoscopic
    sphenoethmoidectomy
    with septoplasty
  frontal sinus septoplasty
  nasal septoplasty

septorhinoplasty
Septosil impression material
septostomy
  atrial balloon septostomy
  balloon septostomy
  blade and balloon atrial
    septostomy
  Mullins blade and balloon
    septostomy
  Mullins transseptal atrial
    septostomy
  Park blade septostomy
  Rashkind balloon atrial
    septostomy
  Rashkind balloon septostomy
  Rashkind-Miller atrial
    septostomy
septostomy balloon catheter
Septotome septum trimmer
septotomy
septum (pl. septa)
  Adams crushing of nasal
    septum
  alveolar septum
  anterior septum
  bony nasal septum
  bony septum
  cartilage of nasal septum
  cartilaginous septum
  caudal septum
  collagen septum
  deviated nasal septum
  deviated septum
  femoral intermuscular septum
  femoral septum
  fenestrated septum
  hypothenar septum
  interalveolar septum
  interatrial septum
  interauricular septum
  intermuscular septum
  interradicular septum
  interventricular septum
  Korner septum
  lingual septum
  membranous septum
  nasal septum
  oblique septum
  orbital septum
  pellucidum septum
  pharyngeal septum
  placental septum

septum (*continued*)
  quadrilateral septum
  rectovaginal septum
  rectovesical septum
  retrovaginal septum
  scrotal septum
  sinus septum
  sphenoidal sinus septum
  subarachnoid septum
  supravaginal septum
  tarsus orbital septum
septum alveoli
septum femorale
septum interalveolaria maxillae
septum mobile nasi
septum nasi
septum nasi osseum
septum of frontal sinuses
septum of sphenoidal sinuses
septum of tongue
septum orbitale
septum spur
septum-cutting forceps
septum-straightening forceps
Sequeira-Khanuja modification
sequela (*pl.* sequelae)
sequencer
sequencing bead patterns set
sequential administration
sequential bilateral breast
    reconstruction
sequential compression device
sequential extremity pump
sequential free flaps
sequential graft
sequential line imaging
sequential plane imaging
sequential point imaging
sequestration cyst
sequestration dermoid
sequestrectomy
sequestrotomy
sequestrum (*pl.* sequestra)
  bone sequestrum
  primary sequestrum
  tertiary sequestrum
sequestrum forceps
sequestrum formation
Sequicor pacemaker
SER fracture (supination,
    external rotation fracture)
Serafin technique

Serafini hernia
Seraflo AV fistular needle
Seraflo blood line
Seraflo transducer protector
Seraphim clip
Serature clip
Serature spur clip
Serdarevic speculum
Serena Mx hand-held apnea
    detection device
serial angiogram
serial cephalometric x-rays
serial chest x-rays
serial cholangiogram
serial debridement
serial dilation
serial EKGs
serial examinations
serial excisions of skin lesion
serial expansion
serial extraction
serial films
serial imaging
serial injection
serial operation
serial percutaneous liver biopsy
serial radiographic evaluation
serial roentgenography
serial scar excisions
serial scar injections
serial section
serial sonography
serial studies
serial wedged cast
series
  angiographic series
  cardiac series
  diagnostic small bowel series
  gallbladder series
  gastrointestinal series
  lower GI series
  lumbosacral series
  panoramic series
  skeletal series
  small-bowel series
  upper GI series
series II acetabular cup position
series II cup retainer
series II femoral broach
series II humeral head
seriscission
SER IV fracture

serocystadenoma
serocystic sarcoma
serofibrinous inflammation
serologic adhesion
serologic examination
seroma
seroma cavity
seroma formation
Seroma-Cath drainage tube
Seroma-Cath feeding tube
Seroma-Cath wound drainage
    catheter
seromembranous
seromucous glands
seromuscular coat
seromuscular
    enterocystoplasty
seromuscular layer
seromuscular stitch
seromuscular suture
    technique
seromuscular sutures
seromuscular-to-edge sutures
seromyotomy
seropositive
seropurulent discharge
seropurulent sputum
serosa invasion
serosal fibroids
serosal fold
serosal involvement
serosal layer
serosal metastasis
serosal reflection
serosal surface
serosal-peritoneal metastasis
serosanguineous
serosanguineous drainage
serosanguineous fluid
seroserosal silk
seroserosal silk sutures
seroserosal sutures
seroserous suture technique
serous acinus
serous acute inflammation
serous adenocarcinoma
serous alveolus
serous canal
serous cystadenoma
serous exudate
serous fluid
serous glands

serous inflammation
serous layer
serous membrane
serous otitis media (SOM)
serous tumor
serpentine aneurysm
serpentine bone plate
serpentine incision
serpentine plate
serpiginous chancroid
serpiginous ulcer
serpiginous ulceration
serrated amalgam plugger
serrated blade
serrated conjunctival forceps
serrated curet
serrated fine-cutting knife
serrated forceps
serrated grasping tip
serrated iris scissors
serrated knife
serrated retractor
serrated scissors
serrated suture
serrated sutures
serrated T-spatula
Serratex scissors
Serratex-Mayo dissecting
    scissors
serration
serratus anterior
serratus anterior flap
serratus anterior muscle
serratus anterior muscle flap
serratus muscle
serratus posterior inferior
    muscle
serratus posterior superior
    muscle
Serre operation
serrefine (*see also* forceps)
    Blair serrefine
    Dieffenbach serrefine
serrefine clamp
serrefine forceps
serrefine implant
serrefine retractor
Serres angle
Serres glands
serratus anterior muscle
serratus posterior inferior
    muscle

serratus posterior superior
    muscle
Sertoli cells
Sertoli-cell-only syndrome
serum (*pl.* sera)
serum bactericidal
    concentration
serum bilirubin concentration
serum calcium concentration
serum complement (C1-C9)
serum complement level
serum hepatitis (SH)
serum lithium concentration
serum thrombotic accelerator
serum transfusion
Servitel prosthesis
Servo pump
Servo ventilator
sesamatic bone
sesamoid bones
sesamoid cartilage of larynx
sesamoid cartilage of nose
sesamoid cartilages
sesamoidectomy dissector
sesamoiditis
sessile adenoma
sessile hydatid
sessile lesion
sessile polyp
sessile swelling
Sessing pressure ulcer
    assessment scale
Setacure denture repair acrylic
seton
seton drain
seton hip brace
seton needle
seton operation
seton sutures
seton tube
seton wound
Set-Op myringotomy kit
Setopress dressing
Setopress high-compression
    bandage
Settegast position
setting expansion
setting sun sign
Seutin bandage
Seutin plaster scissors
Seutin plaster shears
Sevastano knee prosthesis

Seven-Star acupuncture needle
Sever modification of Fairbank
    technique
Sever operation
severance transurethral bag
severe combined
    immunodeficiency (SCID)
severe traumatic brain injury
severed digit
severed limb
severed surface
severed tendon
Severin classification
Severin implant
Severin intraocular lens
Severin multiple closed-loop
    intraocular lens
Severinghaus electrode
severity of injury
Sever-L'Episcopo operation
Sever-L'Episcopo shoulder repair
Sewall antral cannula
Sewall antral trocar
Sewall brain clip-applying
    forceps
Sewall ethmoidal chisel
Sewall ethmoidal elevator
Sewall mucoperiosteal elevator
Sewall orbital retractor
Sewall raspatory
Sewall retractor
Sewall technique
Sewall trocar
Sewell internal mammary
    implantation
Sewell retractor
Sewell-Boyden flap
Sewell-Boyden operation
SEWHO (shoulder-elbow-wrist-
    hand orthosis)
sewing-machine stitch sutures
sewn-in waterproof drape
sew-on electrode
sex change operation
sex conversion
SEX fracture (supination,
    external rotation fracture)
sex reassignment surgery
sextant technique
Sexton bayonet ear knife
Sexton ear knife
Sexton knife

sexual aberration
sexual evaluation
sexual gland
Seyfert forceps
Seyfert vaginal speculum
Sezary erythroderma
Sezary syndrome
S-flap
S-flap incision
SFP (synostotic frontal
    plagiocephaly)
SFS (superficial fascial system)
SG catheter
SGA (small for gestational age)
Sgarlato hammertoe implant
SGBI (silicone gel-filled breast
    implant)
SGC (salivary gland carcinoma)
SGIA disposable stapler
SGIA stapling device
SH (serum hepatitis)
SH popoff suture
Shaaf eye forceps
Shaaf foreign body forceps
Shaberg-Harper-Allen technique
Shack-Hartmann aberrometer
shadow
    acoustic shadow
    breast shadow
    calcific shadow
    cardiac shadow
    confluent shadows
    gallbladder shadow
    hilar shadow
    kidney shadow
    liver shadow
    mediastinal shadow
    metallic-dense shadow
    nipple shadow
    opaque shadows
    paramediastinal shadow
    renal shadow
    ring shadow
    splenic shadow
    uterine shadow
shadow density
shadow over-the-wire balloon
    catheter
shadow shield
shadow-free laryngoscope
shadow-stripe catheter
Shaeffer rigid orthosis

Shaffer eye knife
Shaffer modification of Barkan
    knife
Shaffer operation
Shaffer-Weiss classification
Shaffner orthopedic inserter
shaft
    cup pusher shaft
    femoral shaft
    fibular shaft
    hair shaft
    humeral shaft
    penile shaft
    proximal shaft
    radial shaft
    Rotalink flexible shaft
    tibial shaft
    ulnar shaft
shaft fracture
shaft of bone
shaft of femur
shaft of fibula
shaft of humerus
shaft of phalanx
shaft prosthesis
shaft reamer
shaggy pericardium
shagreen lesions of lens
shagreen patch
shagreen skin
Shah aural dressing
Shah grommet
Shah myringotomy tube
Shah nasal splint
Shah permanent ventilating tube
Shah permanent ventilation tube
Shahan ophthalmic lamp
Shahan thermophore
Shaher-Puddu classification
Shahinian lacrimal cannula
Shah-Shah intraocular lens
Shaldach pacemaker
Shaldon catheter
Shaldon tube
Shallcross bone shears
Shallcross cystic duct forceps
Shallcross gallbladder forceps
Shallcross hemostat
Shallcross hemostatic forceps
Shallcross nasal forceps
Shallcross nasal-packing forceps
Shallcross plaster shears

Shallcross rib shears
Shallcross screwdriver
Shallcross tonsillar hemostat
Shallcross-Dean gall duct forceps
Shambaugh adenoidal curet
Shambaugh adenotome
Shambaugh elevator
Shambaugh endaural self-
    retaining retractor
Shambaugh endaural elevator
Shambaugh endaural hook
Shambaugh endaural incision
Shambaugh endaural retractor
Shambaugh endaural self-
    retaining retractor
Shambaugh fistula hook
Shambaugh hook
Shambaugh incision
Shambaugh irrigator
Shambaugh knife
Shambaugh microscopic hook
Shambaugh narrow elevator
Shambaugh needle
Shambaugh operating
    microscope
Shambaugh palpating needle
Shambaugh retractor
Shambaugh reverse adenotome
Shambaugh technique
Shambaugh-Derlacki chisel
Shambaugh-Derlacki duckbill
    elevator
Shambaugh-Derlacki endaural
    elevator
Shambaugh-Derlacki knife
Shambaugh-Derlacki microhook
Shambaugh-Derlacki microscope
Shambaugh-Lempert knife
Shampaine headholder
Shampaine orthopaedic table
Shandon cytospin chamber
Shank electrode
Shannon bur
Shantz dressing
Shantz osteotomy
Shantz pin
shape
    ear shape
    echo-signal shape
    fleur-de-lis shape
    keyhole shape
    spherical shape

shape (*continued*)
    uterus normal in size and
        shape
shape memory alloy stent
shape memory clamp
shaped glandular flap
shaped random pattern flap
shaping of breast
Shapiro sign
Shapleigh ear curet
Shapleigh ear wax curet
Shapshay laser bronchoscope
Shapshay-Healy laryngeal
        alligator forceps
Shapshay-Healy laryngeal
        scissors
Shapshay-Healy operating
        laryngoscope
Shapshay-Healy phonatory
        laryngoscope
shark fin papillotome
Shark Fin sphincterotome
Shark forceps
shark-mouth cannula
shark-tip cannula
shark-tooth forceps
Sharley tracheostomy tube
Sharman curet
sharp and blunt dissection
sharp angle
sharp blow
sharp curet
Sharp derma curet
sharp dermal curet
sharp disk
sharp dissection
sharp dissection technique
sharp elevator
sharp hook
sharp incision
sharp knife
sharp loop curet
sharp pain
Sharp point cystotome
sharp spoon
sharp trocar
sharp-and-slow wave
Sharpey fibers
Sharpey screw
Sharplan argon laser
Sharplan CO_2 laser
Sharplan ultrasonic aspirator

SharpLase Nd:YAG laser
Sharpley hook
sharply demarcated
Sharpoint crescent blade
Sharpoint cutting instrument
Sharpoint microsurgical knife
Sharpoint microsutures
Sharpoint ophthalmic
    microsurgical sutures
Sharpoint slit knife
Sharpoint spoon blade
Sharpoint Ultra-Guide
    ophthalmic needle
Sharpoint V-lance blade
sharp-pointed forceps
sharp-pronged retractor
sharps
Sharptome crescent blade
Sharptome microblade
sharp-toothed tenaculum
Sharpy fibers
Sharrard iliopsoas transfer
Sharrard kyphectomy
Sharrard operation
Sharrard transfer
Sharrard transfer technique
shatter hammer
shattering needle
shave biopsy
shave excision
shave excision biopsy
shave excision technique
shaver
    Acufex power shaver
    Dyonics motorized meniscal
        shaver
    Dyonics shaver
shaver catheter
Shaw carotid artery clot stripper
Shaw carotid clot stripper
Shaw catheter
Shaw clot stripper
Shaw knife
Shaw operation
Shaw scalpel
Shaw tube
shawl scrotum
Shea bail-hook prosthesis
Shea bur
Shea curet
Shea ear drill
Shea elevator

Shea fenestration hook
Shea fistular hook
Shea footplate hook
Shea headrest
Shea incision
Shea incision knife
Shea irrigator
Shea knife
Shea malleus gripper prosthesis
Shea microdrill
Shea middle ear instrument
Shea oblique hook
Shea pick
Shea polyethylene drainage tube
Shea polyethylene prosthesis
Shea pressure ulcer assessment
    scale
Shea procedure
Shea prosthesis
Shea speculum
Shea speculum holder
Shea stapedectomy
Shea stapes hook
Shea Teflon piston prosthesis
Shea tube
Shea vein graft scissors
Shea-Anthony bag
Shea-Anthony balloon
Shea-Bellucci scissors
Shea-Hough incision
Shealy facet rhizotomy electrode
shear fracture
shear strain
shear stress
shear test
Shearer bone rongeur
Shearer chicken-bill forceps
Shearer chicken-bill rongeur
Shearer lip retractor
Shearer rongeur
shearing edge
Shearing intraocular implant
    lens
Shearing J-Loop intraocular lens
Shearing posterior chamber
    implant material
Shearing posterior chamber
    intraocular lens
Shearing posterior chamber
    intraocular lens implant
Shearing anterior chamber
    intraocular lens

Shearing suction kit
shears (*see also* scissors)
  ADC Medicut shears
  Bacon rib shears
  Bacon thoracic shears
  Baer rib shears
  bandage plaster shears
  bandage shears
  Bethune rib shears
  Bethune-Coryllos rib shears
  bone shears
  Bortone shears
  Braun-Stadler sternal shears
  Brun plaster shears
  Brunner rib shears
  Clayton laminectomy shears
  Collin rib shears
  Cooley first-rib shears
  Cooley rib shears
  Cooley-Pontius sternal shears
  Cooley-Pontius sternum
    shears
  Coryllos rib shears
  Coryllos-Bethune rib shears
  Coryllos-Moure rib shears
  Coryllos-Shoemaker rib shears
  Diertz shears
  Doyen rib shears
  Dubois shears
  Duval-Coryllos rib shears
  Eccentric locked rib shears
  Endo Shears
  Esmarch plaster shears
  esophageal shears
  Exner rib shears
  Felt shears
  first rib shears
  Frey-Sauerbruch rib shears
  Giertz rib shears
  Giertz-Shoemaker rib shears
  Giertz-Stille rib shears
  Gluck rib shears
  Harrington-Mayo rib shears
  Hercules plaster shears
  Horgan-Coryllos-Moure rib
    shears
  Horgan-Wells rib shears
  Horsley-Stille rib shears
  infant rib shears
  Jackson esophageal shears
  Jackson-Moore shears
  Jarit plaster shears

shears (*continued*)
  Jarit utility shears
  Kazanjian shears
  laminectomy shears
  LaparoSonic coagulating
    shears
  laryngofissure shears
  Lebsche sternal shears
  Lefferst rib shears
  Liston shears
  Liston-Key Horsley rib shears
  Liston-Ruskin shears
  Moure-Coryllos rib shears
  Nelson-Bethune rib shears
  Pilling laryngofissure shears
  plain rib shears
  plaster shears
  pleural biopsy needle shears
  Potts infant rib shears
  Potts rib shears
  rib shears
  Roberts shears
  Roberts-Nelson rib shears
  Roos first-rib shears
  Roos rib shears
  Sauerbruch rib shears
  Sauerbruch-Britsch rib shears
  Sauerbruch-Coryllos rib
    shears
  Sauerbruch-Frey rib shears
  Sauerbruch-Lebsche rib shears
  Scanlan plaster shears
  Scanlan rib shears
  Schuchart pediatric rib shears
  Schumacher sternal shears
  scissors plaster shears
  Semb rib shears
  Seutin plaster shears
  Shallcross bone shears
  Shallcross plaster shears
  Shallcross rib shears
  Shoemaker rib shears
  Shuletz rib shears
  sternal shears
  Stille plaster shears
  Stille rib shears
  Stille-Aesculap plaster shears
  Stille-Ericksson rib shears
  Stille-Giertz rib shears
  Stille-Horsley rib shears
  Stille-pattern rib shears
  Stille-Stiwer plaster shears

shears (*continued*)
Thompson rib shears
Tudor-Edwards rib shears
UltraCision harmonic
laparoscopic cutting shears
utility shears
Walton rib shears
Weck shears
sheath
adventitial sheath
Amplatz sheath
angioplasty sheath
anterior rectus sheath
anterior sheath
Appel-Bercie sheath
Arrow sheath
ArrowFlex sheath
arterial sheath
Bakelite cystoscopy sheath
Bakelite resectoscope sheath
Banana peel sheath
beaked sheath
Berry rotating sheath
biceps tendon sheath
blue Cook sheath
carotid sheath
catheter sheath
check-valve sheath
Colapinto sheath
concave sheath
connective tissue sheath
convex sheath
Cook transseptal sheath
Cordis Bioptone sheath
Cordis sheath
cystoscope sheath
Desilets-Hoffman sheath
documentation sheath
double-channel operating
sheath
Electroshield reusable sheath
enamel rod sheath
epithelial sheath
ERA resectoscope sheath
external rectus sheath
fascial sheath
femoral artery sheath
femoral introducer sheath
femoral sheath
fenestrated sheath
fiberoptic photographic
sheath

sheath (*continued*)
fiberoptic sheath
fibrous sheath
flexor sheath
flexor tendon sheath
French sheath
Futura resectoscope sheath
glial sheath
guiding sheath
Hemaflex sheath
Hemaquet sheath
Huxley sheath
hysteroscope sheath
incandescent sheath
Insul-Sheath vaginal speculum
sheath
integral fiberoptic sheath
Introducer II sheath
introducer sheath
irrigating sheath
IVT percutaneous catheter
introducer sheath
Klein transseptal introducer
sheath
Mapper hemostasis sheath
Mecron titanium Voorhoeve
sheath
Medi-Tech sheath
medullated fibers and sheaths
meniscotome sheath
MicroSpan sheath
midline plication of the
anterior rectus sheath
Mullins transseptal
catheterization sheath
Mullins transseptal sheath
myelin sheath
nerve sheath
O'Connor sheath
Passager introducing sheath
peel-away sheath
penile sheath
percutaneous brachial sheath
periosteum sheath
peroneal sheath
peroneal tendon sheath
Pfister-Schwartz sheath
Pinnacle introducer sheath
posterior rectus sheath
quill sheath
rectus abdominis muscle
sheath

sheath (*continued*)
 rectus abdominis sheath
 rectus sheath
 resecting sheath
 resectoscope sheath
 retroflexed cystoscopy sheath
 root sheath
 Scarpa sheath
 Schwalbe sheath
 Schwann sheath
 self-expanding tulip sheath
 short monorail polyethylene
  imaging sheath
 sigmoidoscope
  documentation sheath
 Silipos Distal Dip prosthetic
  sheath
 single-channel operating
  sheath
 Spectranetics laser sheath
 Storz sheath
 subclavian peel-away sheath
 Super Arrow-Flex
  catheterization sheath
 synovial sheath
 tear-away introducer sheath
 tearaway sheath
 Teflon sheath
 tendinous sheath
 tendon sheath
 Terumo Radiofocus sheath
 transseptal sheath
 trocar sheath
 tulip sheath
 UMI Cath-Seal sheath
 Universal sheath
 ureterorenoscope procedure
  sheath
 USCI angioplasty guiding
  sheath
 vascular sheath
 venous sheath
 Warne penile sheath
 water-filled balloon sheath
sheath and obturator
sheath and side-arm
sheath cystoscope
sheath of rectus abdominis
  muscle
sheath of rectus muscle
sheath of Schwann
sheath with side-arm adapter

sheath-dilator
sheathed flexible gastric forceps
sheathed flexible gastroscopic
  forceps
Shea-TORP shunt
Shea-type parasol myringotomy
  tube
Sheehan chisel
Sheehan gouge
Sheehan knee prosthesis
Sheehan nasal chisel
Sheehan osteotome
Sheehan retractor
Sheehan total knee prosthesis
Sheehan-Gillies needle holder
Sheehy button
Sheehy canal knife
Sheehy collar button
Sheehy collar-button tube
Sheehy collar-button ventilating
  tube
Sheehy collar-button ventilation
  tube
Sheehy fascial press
Sheehy forceps
Sheehy incus replacement
  prosthesis
Sheehy myringotomy knife
Sheehy ossicle-holding clamp
Sheehy ossicle-holding forceps
Sheehy pate collector
Sheehy round knife
Sheehy tube
Sheehy Tytan ventilation tube
Sheehy-House chisel
Sheehy-House curet
Sheehy-House incus
  replacement prosthesis
Sheehy-House knife
Sheehy-House prosthesis
Sheehy-Urban sliding lens
  adapter
Sheen airway reconstruction
Sheen tip graft
sheepskin dressing
Sheer probe
sheer spot Band-Aid dressing
sheet
 barrier sheet
 Biobrane sheet
 cuffed sheet
 fenestrated sheet

sheet (*continued*)
foil sheet
in vitro-growth palatal mucosa sheet
keratinous sheet
lap sheet
lift sheet
Marlex sheet
perineal sheet
plastic Adzef sheet
Prolene mesh sheet
rolled sheet
Silastic sheet
Sil-K silicone sheet
split sheet
tantalum sheet
thyroid sheet
transverse sheet
sheet graft
sheet holder
sheet mesh excision
sheeting
Cica-Care silicone gel sheeting
dural film sheeting
Epi-Derm silicone gel sheeting
Heyer-Schulte dural film sheeting
Mylar sheeting
Scar Fx lightweight silicone sheeting
Sheets cannula
Sheets closed-loop posterior chamber intraocular lens
Sheets cyclodialysis
Sheets glide
Sheets intraocular glide
Sheets intraocular lens
Sheets iris hook
Sheets irrigating vectis
Sheets irrigating vectis cannula
Sheets lens
Sheets lens cutter
Sheets lens forceps
Sheets lens glide
Sheets lens guide
Sheets lens spatula
sheets of nevus cells
Sheets-Hirsch spatula
Sheets-McPherson angled forceps
Sheets-McPherson tying forceps
sheet-wadding dressing

Sheffield gamma unit
Sheffield splint
Sheffield treadmill test
Sheinmann laryngeal forceps
Sheldon catheter
Sheldon clamp
Sheldon hemilaminectomy retractor
Sheldon hemilaminectomy self-retaining retractor
Sheldon retractor
Sheldon spreader
Sheldon-Gosset self-retaining retractor
Sheldon-Pudenz dissector
Sheldon-Pudenz operation
Sheldon-Pudenz tube
Sheldon-Pudenz valve
Sheldon-Spatz vertebral arteriogram needle
Sheldon-Swann needle
shelf
Blumer rectal shelf
buccal shelf
dental shelf
implant shelf
mesocolic shelf
palatal shelf
palatine shelf
rectal shelf
shelf hip procedure
shelf operation
shelf osteotomy
shelf reamer
shelf reconstruction of acetabulum
shelf-type implant
shell ear
shell earmold
shell eye implant
shell fragment
shell graft
shell impactor
shell implant
shell implant material
shell prosthesis
shell wrinkles
shellac-covered catheter
shell-type eye implant
shell-type implant
Shelton femoral fracture classification

Shelton plate
shelving edge of Poupart
    ligament
shelving incision
shelving operation
shelving portion of ligament
Shenstone tourniquet
Shenton arch
Shenton line
Shepard bipolar forceps
Shepard calipers block
Shepard cannula
Shepard curved intraocular lens
    forceps
Shepard drain tube
Shepard flexible anterior
    chamber intraocular lens
Shepard forceps
Shepard grommet
Shepard grommet tube
Shepard grommet ventilation
    tube
Shepard incision depth gauge
Shepard incision irrigating
    cannula
Shepard intraocular lens forceps
Shepard intraocular lens implant
Shepard intraocular lens-
    inserting forceps
Shepard lens
Shepard lens forceps
Shepard optical center marker
Shepard osteotome
Shepard radial keratotomy
    irrigating cannula
Shepard reversed iris hook
Shepard scissors
Shepard Teflon tube
Shepard tying forceps
Shepard ventilation tube
Shepherd fracture
Shepherd hook catheter
shepherd's crook deformity of
    proximal femur
shepherd's hook catheter
Sheridan endotracheal tube cuff
Sheridan tube
Sherlock threaded suture
    anchor
Sherman bone plates
Sherman bone screw
Sherman knife

Sherman molybdenum screw
Sherman plate
Sherman screw
Sherman screwdriver
Sherman suction tube
Sherman Vitallium screw
Sherman-Pierce screwdriver
Sherman-Stille drill
Sherpa guiding catheter
Sherwin self-retaining retractor
Sherwood retractor
shield incision
Shield iridotomy scissors
shielding block
Shields forceps
shield-type graft
Shier knee prosthesis
Shiffrin bone wire
Shiffrin wire crimper
shift to the left
shift to the right
shifting border
shifting dullness
shifting dullness on percussion
shifting pacemaker
Shikani middle meatal
    antrostomy stent
Shiley cardiotomy reservoir
Shiley catheter
Shiley cuffless fenestrated tube
Shiley cuffless tracheostomy
    tube
Shiley decannulation plug
Shiley disposable cannula low
    pressure cuffed
    tracheostomy tube
Shiley distention kit
Shiley endotracheal tube
Shiley extra-length single
    cannula tracheostomy tube
Shiley fenestrated low pressure
    cuffed tracheostomy tube
Shiley French sump tube
Shiley guiding catheter
Shiley heart valve
Shiley Infusaid pump
Shiley irrigation catheter
Shiley JL-4 guiding catheter
Shiley JR-4 guiding catheter
Shiley laryngectomy tube
Shiley low-pressure cuffed
    tracheostomy tube

Shiley neonatal tracheostomy
  tube
Shiley oxygenator
Shiley pediatric tracheostomy
  tube
Shiley pressure-relief adapter
Shiley saphenous vein irrigation
  and pressurization device
Shiley shunt
Shiley single cannula cuffed
  tracheostomy tube
Shiley soft-tip guiding catheter
Shiley sump tube
Shiley Tetraflex vascular graft
Shiley tracheostomy tube
Shiley tube
Shiley valve
Shiley-Bjork tube
Shiley-Ionescu catheter
Shiller solution
shim coil
shim magnet
Shimada classification
Shimadzu cardiac ultrasound
Shimadzu scanner
Shimadzu ultrasound
shimmed magnet
Shimstock occlusion foil
Shinobi wire
SHIP hammertoe implant
SHIP-Shaw rod hammertoe
  implant
Shirley sump wound drain
Shirley wound drain
Shirodkar aneurysm needle
Shirodkar cerclage
Shirodkar cervical needle
Shirodkar operation
Shirodkar probe
Shirodkar procedure
Shirodkar suture technique
Shirodkar sutures
Shirodkar-Barter cervical cerclage
Shirodkar-Barter operation
Shirodkar-McDonald cervical
  repair
Shirodkar-Page cerclage
Shober index for spondylitis
Shoch sutures
shock
  allergic shock
  anaphylactic shock

anaphylactoid shock
anesthetic shock
break shock
burn shock
cardiac shock
cardiogenic shock
declamping shock
deferred shock
electric shock
endotoxic shock
gravitational shock
heart shock
hematogenic shock
hemorrhagic shock
hypovolemic shock
liver shock
pleural shock
postoperative shock
septic shock
surgical shock
systemic shock
testicular shock
traumatic shock
shock block
shock liver
shock position
shock wave lithotripsy (SWL)
shock wave lithotriptor
shocky
shoe-and-stocking position
shoehorn speculum
shoelace fasciotomy closure
shoelace stitch
shoelace suture
shoelace technique
shoelace-type repair
Shoemaker (*see also*
  Schoemaker, Schumacher,
  Schumaker)
Shoemaker intestinal clamp
Shoemaker intraocular lens
  forceps
Shoemaker rib shears
Shoemaker rongeur
Shoemaker shears
Shoepinger incision
Shofu dental cement
Shofu porcelain stain kit
Shone anomaly
Shone catheter
Shooter Saeed multiband
  irrigator

shooting pains
short abductor muscle
short above-elbow cast
short adductor muscle
short anconeus muscle
short arc motion (SAM)
    protocol
short arm cast (SAC)
short arm cylinder cast
short arm navicular cast
short arm plaster splint
short arm posterior molded
    splint
short arm thumb spica cast
short axis
short below-elbow cast
short bundle colonoscope
short calcaneocuboid ligament
short ciliary arteries
short ciliary nerves
short intraocular lens
short coarse bur
short course
short crus of incus
short esophagus type hiatal
    hernia
short extensor muscle
short face syndrome
short fibular muscle
short fine bur
short flexor muscle
short gastric arteries
short gastric branch of lienal
    artery
short gastric veins
short gut syndrome
short Heaney retractor
short increment sensitivity
    index (SISI)
short leg caliper brace
short leg cylinder cast
short leg non-walking cast
short leg non-weightbearing
    cast
short leg plaster cast
short leg splint
short levator muscles
short lever accessory movement
    technique
short lever specific contact
    procedure
short mandible

short monorail polyethylene
    imaging sheath
short needle
short oblique fracture
short occluder
short of breath (SOB)
short palmar muscle
short peroneal muscle
short plantar ligament
short posterior ciliary artery
short posterior ciliary axis
short pulse
short QRS complex
short radial extensor muscle
short rectangular flap
short rod
short rotator muscles
short scar technique
short segment spinal fusion
short tooth forceps
short-acting barbiturate
short-arm Grollman catheter
short-axis plane
Shortbent stitch scissors
Shortbent suture scissors
short-bore magnet
short-bowel syndrome
short-cone technique
ShortCut small-incision knife
ShortCutter catheter
shortening
    esophageal shortening
    Hoffa tendon shortening
    radial shortening
    scleral shortening
    tendon shortening
shortening of bone
shortening of eyeball
shortening of ocular muscle
shortening of round ligament
shortening of sacrouterine
    ligament
shortening of tendon
short-face syndromes
short-gut syndrome
shorthand vertical mattress
    stitch suture technique
short-inversion recovery
    imaging
short-leg brace
short-leg cast (SLC)
short-leg walking cast (SLWC)

short-length tracheal tube
short-limb Roux-en-Y
    gastroenterostomy
shortness of breath (SOB)
short-pulse repetition time/echo
    time image
short-scar technique breast
    reduction
short-scar techniques
short-segment disease
short-segment lesion
short-stretch bandage
short-tip bag
short-tip hemostatic bag
short-tooth forceps
short-wave diathermy
shot compressor
shot-gun approach
shot-perforated
shot-silk retina
shotted sutures
shotty breast
shotty lymph node
shotty node
shoulder
    Bio-Modular shoulder
    Charlotte shoulder
    contracted shoulder
    drop shoulder
    frozen shoulder
    hanging-weight method for
      reducing dislocated
      shoulder
    heel-in-armpit method to
      reduce dislocated shoulder
    knocked-down shoulder
    linguogingival shoulder
    Little Leaguer's shoulder
    loose shoulder
    Milwaukee shoulder
    raised-arm method to reduce
      dislocated shoulder
    ring man shoulder
    square-off sign of shoulder
    subluxed shoulder
shoulder abduction immobilizer
shoulder abduction pillow
shoulder abduction positioner
shoulder amputation
shoulder arthrodesis
shoulder arthroplasty
shoulder blade

shoulder brace
shoulder controller
shoulder cuff
shoulder disarticulation
shoulder dislocation
shoulder drop
Shoulder Ease abduction
    support
shoulder flap
shoulder girdle
shoulder impingement
    syndrome
shoulder joint
shoulder of furrow
shoulder of rhytid
shoulder orthosis
shoulder pointer
shoulder prosthesis
shoulder reduction
shoulder repair
shoulder subluxation inhibitor
    (SSI) brace
shoulder surface coil
shoulder-elbow-wrist-hand
    orthosis (SEWHO)
shoulderRAP wrap
shoulder-strap incision
Shouldice hernia repair
Shouldice hernioplasty
Shouldice herniorrhaphy
Shouldice inguinal hernia repair
Shouldice inguinal
    herniorrhaphy
Shouldice-Bassini hernia repair
shoveller's fracture
shovel-shaped incisor
ShowerSafe cast and bandage
    protector
ShowerSafe protector material
Shprintzen syndrome
Shrady saw
shrapnel fragment
Shrapnell membrane
Shriners Hospital instruments
Shriners Hospital interlocking
    retractor
Shriners Hospital pin
Shriners Hospital retractor
Shriners pin
Shrinker
    Juzo shrinker
    stump shrinker

shriveled skin envelope
shrunken liver
Shug device for male
    contraception
Shuletz pusher
Shuletz raspatory
Shuletz rib shears
Shuletz-Damian raspatory
Shuletz-Paul rib retractor
Shulitz catheter
Shunn gun
Shunn gun transilluminator
shunt
  Accura hydrocephalus shunt
  Allen-Brown vascular access
      shunt
  Ames ventriculoperitoneal
      shunt
  Anastaflo intravascular shunt
  angiographic portacaval shunt
  aorta to pulmonary artery
      shunt
  aorticopulmonary shunt
  aortopulmonary shunt
  aqueous tube shunt
  arteriovenous shunt
  ascending aorta-to-pulmonary
      artery shunt
  ascites shunt
  Assal-Javid cerebrospinal
      shunt
  Austin endolymph
      dispersement shunt
  AV shunt (arteriovenous shunt)
  Baerveldt shunt
  balloon shunt
  Beck shunt
  bidirectional shunt
  biliopancreatic shunt
  Blalock shunt
  Blalock-Taussig shunt
  Brenner carotid bypass shunt
  Brescia-Cimino shunt
  Brisman-Nova carotid
      endarterectomy shunt
  Buselmeier shunt
  capillary bed shunt
  cardiac shunt
  cardiovascular shunt
  carotid bypass shunt
  carotid endarterectomy shunt
  carotid shunt

shunt (*continued*)
  cavamesenteric shunt
  cavernospongiosum shunt
  Cavin shunt
  central nervous system shunt
  cerebrospinal fluid shunt
  Cimino arteriovenous shunt
  Cimino dialysis shunt
  Cobe AV shunt
  Codman Accu-Flow shunt
  conventional shunt
  Cordis-Hakim shunt
  coronary anastomotic shunt
  CSF T-tube shunt
  Denver ascites shunt
  Denver hydrocephalus shunt
  Denver peritoneal-venous
      shunt
  Denver peritoneovenous
      shunt
  Denver pleuroperitoneal
      shunt
  Denver valve shunt
  descending thoracic aorta to
      pulmonary artery shunt
  dialysis shunt
  distal splenorenal shunt
  Dow Corning shunt
  Drapanas mesocaval shunt
  Edwards-Barbaro T-shaped
      syringeal shunt
  endolymphatic subarachnoid
      shunt
  end-to-side portacaval shunt
  end-to-side splenorenal shunt
  esophageal shunt
  extracardiac right-to-left shunt
  extracardiac shunt
  extrahepatic shunt
  Fischer shunt
  Flo-Thru intraluminal shunt
  Foltz shunt
  Foltz-Overton shunt
  Garner balloon shunt
  gastric vena caval shunt
  Gibson inner ear shunt
  Glenn shunt
  Gore-Tex shunt
  Gott shunt
  Gott-Daggett shunt
  Groshong shunt
  Hakim shunt

shunt (*continued*)

Hallin carotid endarterectomy shunt
Hashmat shunt
Hashmat-Waterhouse shunt
Hepacon shunt
hepatofugal porto-systemic venous shunt
Heyer-Schulte hydrocephalus shunt
Heyer-Schulte-Spetzler lumbar peritoneal shunt
H-H neonatal shunt
Holter shunt
House and Pulec otic-periotic shunt
House endolymphatic shunt
Hyde shunt
hydrocephalus shunt
Inahara shunt
Inahara-Pruitt vascular shunt
indwelling nonvascular shunt
initial venous shunt
input shunt
interposition mesocaval shunt
intracardiac shunt
intracardial shunt
intrapericardial aorticopulmonary shunt
intrapulmonary shunt
Javid bypass shunt
Javid carotid shunt
Javid endarterectomy shunt
Javid internal carotid shunt
Kasai peritoneal venous shunt
LaRivetti-Levinson intraluminal shunt
LaVeen ascites shunt
left-to-right shunt
LeVeen dialysis shunt
LeVeen peritoneal shunt
LeVeen peritoneovenous shunt
Levine shunt
Linton shunt
loop shunt
L-R shunt
lumboperitoneal shunt
magnitude shunt
mesobi-ileal shunt
mesocaval H-graft shunt
mesocaval interposition shunt

shunt (*continued*)

mesocaval shunt
Mischler shunt
Mischler-Pudenz shunt
modified shunt
net shunt
obstructed shunt
Ommaya shunt
Orbis-Sigma shunt
otic shunt
Overton shunt
parietal shunt
PC shunt
pentose phosphate shunt
percutaneous thecoperitoneal shunt
peritoneal insertion of shunt
peritoneal shunt
peritoneal-atrial shunt
peritoneal-venous shunt
peritoneocaval shunt
peritoneojugular shunt
peritoneovenous shunt
PFTE shunt (polyfluorotetraethylene shunt)
polyfluorotetraethylene shunt (PFTE shunt)
Polystan shunt
portacaval shunt
portal shunt
portal to systemic venous shunt
portal-systemic shunt
portarenal shunt
Portnoy ventricular-end shunt
portopulmonary shunt
portorenal shunt
portosystemic shunt
portosystemic vascular shunt
postcaval shunt
Potts shunt
proximal splenorenal shunt
Pruitt vascular shunt
Pruitt-Inahara autoperfusion shunt
Pruitt-Inahara carotid shunt
Pruitt-Inahara vascular shunt
PTFE shunt
Pudenz valve-flushing shunt
Pudenz ventriculoatrial shunt
Pudenz-Heyer shunt

shunt (*continued*)
Pudenz-Schulte thecoperitoneal shunt
Quinton-Scribner shunt
radiologic portacaval shunt
Raimondi low-pressure shunt
Ramirez arteriovenous shunt
reversed shunt (right-to-left)
Reynold-Southwick H-graft portacaval shunt
Rickham reservoir shunt
right-to-left shunt
Rivetti-Levinson intraluminal shunt
R-L shunt
Rostan shunt
Scribner arteriovenous shunt
Shea-TORP shunt
Shiley shunt
side-to-side portacaval shunt
Silastic Ames shunt
Silastic ventriculoperitoneal shunt
small-bowel shunt
Spetzler lumbar-peritoneal shunt
Spetzler lumboperitoneal shunt
Spitz-Holter VA shunt
splenorenal bypass shunt
splenorenal shunt
spongiosa shunt
subarachnoid shunt
subduroperitoneal shunt
Sundt carotid endarterectomy shunt
syrinx shunt
systemic-pulmonary artery shunt
T-AnastaFlo shunt
TDMAC heparin shunt
thecoperitoneal Pudenz-Schulte shunt
Thomas femoral shunt
Thomas vascular access shunt
TIPSS shunt
Torkildsen shunt
tracheoesophageal shunt
tracheopharyngeal shunt
transhepatic portacaval shunt
transjugular intrahepatic portal systemic shunt

shunt (*continued*)
T-shaped Edwards-Barbaro syringeal shunt
Uni-Shunt hydrocephalus shunt
Uresil carotid shunt
USCI shunt
Vascu-Flo carotid shunt
Vascushunt shunt
vena cava to pulmonary artery shunt
venous shunt
ventriculoatrial shunt
ventriculocaval shunt
ventriculocisternal shunt
ventriculoperitoneal shunt (VP shunt)
vesicoamniotic shunt
Vitagraft arteriovenous shunt
VP shunt (ventriculoperitoneal shunt)
VS shunt
Warren splenorenal shunt
Waterston shunt
Waterston-Cooley shunt
White glaucoma pump shunt
winged shunt
Winters shunt
shunt cyanosis
shunt filter
shunt for aortic aneurysm
shunt function
shunt infection
shunt kit
shunt manipulation
shunt obstruction
shunt operation
shunt placement
shunt site
shunt surgery
shunt tube
shunt tubing
shunt-site drainage
shunt-site leaking
shunt-site oozing
shunt-tube introducer
Shupe forceps
Shur-Band self-closure elastic bandage
Shur-Clens wound cleanser
Shurly tracheal retractor

Shur-Strip sterile wound closure tape
Shur-Strip wound closure tape
Shuster suture forceps
Shuster tonsillar forceps
shutoff clamp
Shutt Aggressor forceps
Shutt alligator forceps
Shutt basket forceps
Shutt B-scoop forceps
Shutt grasper
Shutt grasping forceps
Shutt hook
Shutt Mantis retrograde forceps
Shutt microscissors
Shutt Mini-Aggressor forceps
Shutt minibasket
Shutt punch
Shutt retrograde forceps
Shutt scissors
Shutt shovel-nosed forceps
Shutt suction forceps
shutter flap
shuttle forceps
Shuttle-Relay suture passer
Shutt-Mantis retrograde forceps
SI joint
sialadenectomy
sialadenography
sialadenoncus
sialadenosis
sialadenotomy
sialoadenectomy
sialoadenolithotomy
sialoadenotomy
sialodochoplasty
sialogenic pain
sialogram
sialographic catheter
sialography needle
sialolith
sialolithotomy
sialometaplasia
sialorrhea
sialoschesis
sialostenosis
sialosyrinx
sibilant rales
Sibson fascia
Sibson groove
Sibson notch
Sibson vestibule

Sichel implant
Sichel iris knife
Sichel movable orbital implant
Sichel orbital implant
Sichi implant
Sichi operation
sick dermatome
sick sinus syndrome
sickle blade
sickle cell anemia
sickle cell ulcer
sickle flap
sickle knife
sickle middle-ear knife
sickle scissors
sickle tonsillar knife
sickle-shape blade
sickle-shaped Beaver blade
sickle-shaped blade
sickle-shaped House knife
sickle-shaped knife
side blade
side channel of scope
side mouth gag
side plate
side posture reduction
side view
side-arm
    sheath and side-arm
side-arm adapter
side-arm nebulizer
side-bending barrier
side-biting clamp
side-biting ostrum punch
side-biting spatula
side-biting Stammberger punch
    forceps
side-curved forceps
side-curved rongeur
side-cut pin cutter
side-cutter
side-cutting basket forceps
side-cutting blade
side-cutting cannula
side-cutting irrigating cystotome
side-cutting rasp
side-cutting rongeur
side-cutting spatula
side-cutting spatulated needle
side-cutting Swanson bur
sidefire laser
side-flattened needle

side-grasping forceps
side-hole cannulated probe
side-hole catheter
side-hole pigtail catheter
side-lip forceps
side-opening laminar hook
side-port airway connector
side-port cannula
side-port flat-bottomed Ommaya
  reservoir
Sideris adjustable buttoned
  device
sideswipe elbow fracture
sideswipe fracture
side-to-end anastomosis
side-to-side anastomosis
side-to-side gastroenterostomy
side-to-side hepatojejunostomy
side-to-side jejunal pouch
side-to-side portacaval shunt
side-to-vein bypass
side-viewing duodenoscope
side-viewing endoscope
side-viewing fiberscope
side-viewing scope
sidewall holed needle
sidewall infusion cannula
sidewinder aortic clamp
sidewinder catheter
sidewinder percutaneous intra-
  aortic balloon catheter
Sidney Stephenson corneal
  trephine
Siebold pubiotomy
Siegel pneumatic otoscope
Siegel stent
Siegel technique
Siegel-Cohen dilating catheter
Sieger insufflator
Siegle ear speculum
Siegle otoscope
Siegler biopsy forceps
Siegler-Hellman clamp
Sielaff gastroscope
Siemens cyclographic tomogram
Siemens scanner
Siemens endorectal transducer
Siemens linear probe
Siemens MRI unit
Siemens open-heart table
Siemens gamma camera
Siemens head unit

Siemens image intensifier
Siemens PTCA open-heart
  sutures
Siemens Doppler
Siemens ventilator
Siemens ultrasound
Siemens whole-body scanner
Siemens Somatom DRB CT
  analyzer unit
Siemens ultrasound
Siemens ultrasound scanner
Siemens echocardiograph
Siemens vaginal probe
Siemens pulse transducer
Siemens multiprogrammable
  pacemaker
Siemens ventilator
Siemens-Pacesetter pacemaker
Siepser intraocular lens
Sierra alloy
Sierra-Sheldon trabeculotome
Sierra-Sheldon tracheotome
SieScape ultrasound
SieScape ultrasound scanner
sieve bone
sieve graft
sievelike pores
Sievert unit
Olympus enteroscope
Siffert-Forster-Nachamie
  clubfoot procedure
Sifoam padding
Sigma infusion pump
Sigma TMB assay kit
sigmoid anastomosis
sigmoid anastomosis clamp
sigmoid arteries
sigmoid bladder
sigmoid clamp
sigmoid colon
sigmoid colon carcinoma
sigmoid colostomy
sigmoid cutaneous fistula
sigmoid cystoplasty
sigmoid enterocystoplasty
sigmoid flexure
sigmoid folds
sigmoid fossa
sigmoid kidney
sigmoid loop
sigmoid loop colostomy
sigmoid loop reduction

sigmoid mesocolon
sigmoid notch
sigmoid notch retractor
sigmoid sinus
sigmoid sinus ligation
sigmoid speculum
sigmoid sulcus
sigmoid veins
sigmoid volvulus
sigmoidal branch of inferior
    mesenteric artery
sigmoidectomy
sigmoid-end colostomy
sigmoid-loop rod colostomy
sigmoidocutaneous fistula
sigmoidopexy
sigmoidoproctectomy
sigmoidoproctostomy
sigmoidorectostomy
sigmoidorrhaphy
sigmoidoscope
    ACMI flexible sigmoidoscope
    adult sigmoidoscope
    Boehm sigmoidoscope
    Buie sigmoidoscope
    disposable sigmoidoscope
    Eder sigmoidoscope
    ESI sigmoidoscope
    fiberoptic sigmoidoscope
    flexible sigmoidoscope
    Frankfeldt sigmoidoscope
    Fujinon flexible
        sigmoidoscope
    Gorsch sigmoidoscope
    Heinkel sigmoidoscope
    Hopkins sigmoidoscope
    Kelly sigmoidoscope
    KleenSpec disposable
        sigmoidoscope
    Lieberman sigmoidoscope
    Lloyd-Davis sigmoidoscope
    Montague sigmoidoscope
    Olympus fiberoptic
        sigmoidoscope
    Olympus flexible
        sigmoidoscope
    Pentax fiberoptic
        sigmoidoscope
    Pentax flexible
        sigmoidoscope
    Reichert fiberoptic
        sigmoidoscope

sigmoidoscope (*continued*)
    Reichert flexible
        sigmoidoscope
    rigid sigmoidoscope
    semirigid sigmoidoscope
    Solow sigmoidoscope
    Strauss sigmoidoscope
    Turrell sigmoidoscope
    Tuttle sigmoidoscope
    Welch Allyn flexible
        sigmoidoscope
    Yeoman sigmoidoscope
sigmoidoscope biopsy forceps
sigmoidoscope documentation
    sheath
sigmoidoscope inflation bulb
sigmoidoscope insulated suction
    tube
sigmoidoscope light carrier
sigmoidoscope replacement
    lamp
sigmoidoscope suction tube
sigmoidoscope with swinging
    window
sigmoidoscopy
    fiberoptic sigmoidoscopy
    flexible fiberoptic
        sigmoidoscopy
    rigid sigmoidoscopy
sigmoidoscopy table
sigmoidoscopy with rectal
    polypectomy
sigmoidosigmoidostomy
sigmoidostomy
sigmoidotomy
sigmoidovesical
sigmoidovesical fistula
sigmoid-rectal intussusception
sign
    Aaron sign
    Abadie sign
    abducens nerve sign
    accessory nerve sign
    accessory sign
    ace of spades sign
    acoustic nerve sign
    acute warning sign
    Adson sign
    Agee sign
    Ahlfeld sign
    air bronchogram sign
    air dome sign

sign (*continued*)
- antecedent sign
- anterior drawer sign
- anterior tibial sign
- Apley sign
- Arnoux sign
- Auenbrugger sign
- Aufrecht sign
- Auspitz sign
- Babinski sign
- Ballance sign
- ballet sign
- Bamberger sign
- barber pole sign
- Barre pyramidal sign
- Battle sign
- beading sign
- Beccaria sign
- Béclard sign
- Beevor sign
- Bekhterev sign
- Berger sign
- Bethea sign
- Bezold sign
- Biermer sign
- Biot sign
- Bjerrum sign
- Blumberg sign
- Boas sign
- Bolt sign
- Bonnet sign
- Bouillaud sign
- bowler hat sign
- bowstring sign
- Boyce sign
- Bozzolo sign
- Bragard sign
- Braun-Fernwald sign
- Braxton Hicks sign
- Brickner sign
- Broadbent inverted sign
- Brockenbrough sign
- Bryant sign
- Barany sign
- Bunnell sign
- Burton sign
- Buschke-Ollendorf sign
- camelback sign
- Cantelli sign
- Cardarelli sign
- cardiorespiratory sign
- Castellino sign

sign (*continued*)
- chain-of-lakes sign
- Charcot sign
- Cheyne-Stokes sign
- chin retraction sign
- choppy sea sign
- Chvostek sign
- Chvostek-Trousseau sign
- Chvostek-Weiss sign
- Claude hyperkinesis sign
- Cleeman sign
- clenched fist sign
- clinical sign
- cobblestoning sign
- Codman sign
- cogwheel sign
- Cole sign
- colon cut-off sign
- comblike redness sign
- Comby sign
- contralateral sign
- Coopernail sign
- Corrigan sign
- cranial nerve sign
- Cruveilhier sign
- cuff sign
- Cullen sign
- Dalrymple sign
- D'Amato sign
- Darier sign
- de la Camp sign
- de Musset sign
- Dejerine sign
- Delmege sign
- Demarquay sign
- Desault hip sign
- dimple sign
- dog-ear sign
- doll's eye sign
- Dorendorf sign
- dorsiflexion sign
- double decidual sac sign
- double-bubble sign
- double-camelback sign
- doughnut sign
- drive-through sign
- Dupuytren sign
- Duroziez sign
- Ellis sign
- empty delta sign
- Erb sign
- Erichsen sign

sign (*continued*)
- Ewart sign
- Ewing sign
- extrapyramidal signs
- fabere sign
- facial nerve sign
- Fajersztajn sign
- fat-pad sign
- Federici sign
- Felson silhouette sign
- Finkelstein sign
- Fischer sign
- flapping tremor sign
- fluid/fluid sign
- focal and lateralizing neurologic signs
- focal motor sign
- focalizing signs
- Fraenkel sign
- Frank sign
- Friedreich sign
- Froment sign
- frontal release sign
- Gaenslen sign
- Gage sign
- Galeazzi sign
- Gauss sign
- Gerhardt sign
- Gifford sign
- Gilbert sign
- Glasgow sign
- glossopharyngeal nerve sign
- Golden sign
- Goldthwait sign
- Goodell sign
- gooseneck sign
- Gowers sign
- Graefe sign
- Granger sign
- great toe sign
- Greene sign
- Grey Turner sign
- Griesinger sign
- Grossman sign
- guarding sign
- Guilland sign
- Gunn closing sign
- hair collar sign
- Hall sign
- Hamman sign
- Hawkins sign
- head-at-risk signs

sign (*continued*)
- Hefke-Turner sign
- Hegar sign
- Henning sign
- Heyring sign
- Hicks sign
- Hill sign
- Hitselberger sign
- Hoaglund sign
- Hoehne sign
- Hoffmann sign
- Homans sign
- Hope sign
- Horn sign
- hot heel sign
- hot patella sign
- Howship-Romberg sign
- Huchard sign
- Hueter sign
- Hutchinson sign
- hypoglossal nerve sign
- iliopsoas sign
- impingement sign
- inhibition sign
- Jacquemier sign
- Jakob reverse pivot shift sign
- Jeanne sign
- Jobe sign
- jugular sign
- Kanavel sign
- Kantor sign
- Kauffman sign
- Keen sign
- Kehr sign
- Kerr sign
- Kimberly sign
- Klemm sign
- Kustner sign
- Koplik sign
- Koranyi sign
- Kussmaul sign
- Kustner sign
- Laennec sign
- Lancisi sign
- Lasegue sign
- lemon sign
- Lennhoff sign
- Leri sign
- Leser-Trelat sign
- Levine sign
- Linburg sign
- Linder sign

sign (*continued*)
   linguine sign
   lipstick sign
   liver flap sign
   Livierato sign
   localized abdominal sign
   localized neurological sign
   localizing neurological sign
   localizing sign
   long-tract sign
   Lorenz sign
   Ludloff sign
   Macewen sign
   MacIntosh sign
   Mahler sign
   Maisonneuve sign
   Mannkopf sign
   May sign
   McArdle sign
   McBurney sign
   McCort sign
   McMurray sign
   melanoma warning sign
   Meltzer sign
   Mendel-Bekhterev sign
   meniscal sign
   Mercedes-Benz sign
   Meyerson sign
   Minor sign
   Moebius sign
   molder's sign
   Moniz sign
   Morquio sign
   Mueller sign
   Mulder sign
   Munson sign
   Murphy sign
   Musset sign
   Myerson sign
   Napoleon Bonaparte sign
   navicular fat stripe sign
   neck sign
   nerve sign
   neurological sign
   normal vital sign
   Obagi sign
   Ober sign
   obturator sign
   oculomotor nerve sign
   oil drop change sign
   olfactory nerve sign
   Olshausen sign

sign (*continued*)
   pad sign
   Parrot sign
   Pastia sign
   Patrick sign
   Payr sign
   peritoneal sign
   peroneal sign
   Phalen sign
   physical sign
   pillow sign
   Pinard sign
   piston sign
   plumb line sign
   Potain sign
   prodromic sign
   pronation sign
   psoas sign
   pyloric string sign
   Quant sign
   Queckenstedt sign
   questionable sign
   Quincke sign
   Quenu-Muret sign
   rabbit-ear sign
   radialis sign
   Ramond sign
   Randall sign
   Rasch sign
   rat-tail sign
   red wale sign
   Remak sign
   Reusner sign
   reversed-3 sign
   Rifkind sign
   Rigler sign
   rim sign
   Rinman sign
   Rinne sign
   Risser sign
   Rivero-Carvallo sign
   Riviere sign
   Robertson sign
   Roger sign
   Romana sign
   Romberg sign
   Rookey sign
   Rosenbach sign
   Roser-Braun sign
   Rotch sign
   Roux sign
   Rovighi sign

sign (*continued*)
Rovsing sign
Rovsing-Blumberg sign
Rumpel-Leede sign
Saenger sign
sail sign
Salmon sign
saw-tooth appearance sign
scallop sign
scarf sign
Schick sign
Schlange sign
Schlesinger sign
scintillating sesamoids sign
seat belt sign
Seeligmueller sign
Seidel sign
setting sun sign
Shapiro sign
Shaver sign
signet ring sign
silhouette sign
silk glove sign
silk sign
Simon sign
Skoda sign
Soto-Hall sign
spilled teacup sign
Spurling sign
squeeze sign
stable vital sign
steeple sign
Steinberg thumb sign
stepladder sign
Sterles sign
Sternberg sign
Stiller sign
Stokes sign
Strauss sign
Strunksy sign
Sumner sign
tail sign
Tansini sign
target sign
tenting sign
Terry fingernail sign
Terry nail sign
Terry-Thomas sign
tethered-bowel sign
Thomayer sign
thumb sign
tibial sign

sign (*continued*)
tibialis sign
Tinel sign
toe sign
Toma sign
trapezius ridge sign
Traube sign
trigeminal nerve sign
trochlear nerve sign
Turner sign
Unschuld sign
vein sign
vital sign
Woelfer sign
Wachenheim-Reder sign
Wahl sign
Walker-Murdock wrist sign
warning sign
Wartenberg sign
Warthin sign
Weber sign
Wernicke sign
Westphal sign
wet leather sign
Wilder sign
Williams sign
wind sock sign
windshield wiper sign
Wolkowitsch sign
Wreden sign
Zaufel sign
sign mechanism for ventilator
    breathing
Signa 1.5 Tesla unit
Signa scanner
Signa imager
SignaDress hydrocolloid
    dressing material
signal attenuation
signal hemorrhage
Signet disposable skin stapler
Signet lens
signet ring shape of scaphoid
signet ring sign on x-ray
signet-ring adenocarcinoma
signet-ring carcinoma
signet-ring cell carcinoma
signet-ring pattern
Signorini tourniquet
Sigualt symphysiotomy
Sigvaris compression stockings
Sigvaris support stockings

Siker mirror laryngoscope
SIL ASCUS lesion
Silastic adhesive
Silastic allograft
Silastic Ames shunt
Silastic ball
Silastic ball spacer prosthesis
Silastic band
Silastic bead embolization
Silastic sterile Foley catheter
Silastic cannula
Silastic catheter
Silastic chin implant
Silastic chin prosthesis
Silastic collar-reinforced stoma
Silastic corneal eye implant
Silastic corneal implant
Silastic coronary artery cannula
Silastic Cronin implant
Silastic Cronin medical adhesive
    silicone
Silastic cup extractor
Silastic Cystocath
Silastic disk heart valve
Silastic drain
Silastic dressing
Silastic elastomer infusion
    catheter
Silastic eustachian tube
Silastic eye implant
Silastic fimbrial prosthesis
Silastic finger implant
Silastic foam dressing
Silastic gel dressing
Silastic graft
Silastic grommet
Silastic Swanson flexible toe
    hinge
Silastic tissue expander
Silastic ileal reservoir catheter
Silastic implant
Silastic indwelling ureteral stent
Silastic injection
Silastic intestinal tube
Silastic keel of vomer
Silastic loop
Silastic lunate arthroplasty
Silastic mammary prosthesis
Silastic material
Silastic medical adhesive
Silastic midfacial malar implant
Silastic mold

Silastic mushroom catheter
Silastic obstetrical vacuum cup
Silastic otoplasty prosthesis
Silastic patch
Silastic penile implant
Silastic penile prosthesis
Silastic plate
Silastic prosthesis
Silastic prosthetic sizer
Silastic rhinoplasty implant
Silastic ring
Silastic ring vertical-banded
    gastric bypass (SRVGB)
Silastic rod
Silastic scleral buckler eye
    implant
Silastic scleral buckler implant
Silastic sheet
Silastic sheeting keel prosthesis
Silastic shunt
Silastic silicone rubber implants
Silastic silo
Silastic silo reduction of
    gastroschisis
Silastic sphere
Silastic sponge
Silastic standard elastometer
    prosthesis
Silastic stent
Silastic strain gauge
Silastic strap
Silastic subdermal implant
Silastic sucker suction tube
Silastic suture button
Silastic tape
Silastic testicular implant
Silastic testicular prosthesis
Silastic thoracic drain
Silastic thyroid drain
Silastic toe implant
Silastic tracheostomy tube
Silastic ventriculoperitoneal
    shunt
Silber microneedle holder
Silber microvascular clamp
Silber technique
Silber vasovasostomy clamp
Silc extractor
Silcath subclavian catheter
Silcock dissection forceps
silent abdomen
silent aspiration

silent attack
silent chest
silent gallstone
silent infection
Silesian bandage
Silesian belt
Silesian belt suspension
Silflex intramedullary prosthesis
Silfverskiold knee procedure
Silfverskiold lengthening
    technique
Silfverskiold procedure
silhouette
    cardiac silhouette
    cardiothymic silhouette
    cardiovascular silhouette
    diaphragmatic silhouette
    heart silhouette
    supracardiac silhouette
Silhouette endoscopic laser
silhouette sign
Silhouette therapeutic mattress
silica contact lens
silica granuloma
silicate filling
silicate restorate material
silicon carbide abrasive
silicon dioxide abrasive
silicon ion therapy
silicon-controlled rectifier
silicone
    Biocell textured silicone
    Corning silicone
    Dow Corning silicone
    ferromagnetic silicone
    noncrosslinked silicones
    Silastic Cronin medical
        adhesive silicone
    small square-groove silicone
    tire-grooved silicone
silicone adhesive
silicone ball heart valve
silicone bleed
silicone block
silicone buckling implant
silicone button
silicone button eye implant
silicone cannula
silicone copolymer
silicone deposition
silicone diode dosimeter
silicone doughnut prosthesis

silicone drain
silicone dressing
silicone elastomer
silicone elastomer arthroplasty
silicone elastomer band
silicone elastomer catheter
silicone elastomer infusion
    catheter
silicone elastomer lens
silicone elastomer prosthesis
silicone elastomer ring
silicone elastomer ring vertical
    gastroplasty
silicone elastomer rubber ball
    implant
silicone epistaxis catheter
silicone eye implant
silicone flexor rod
silicone gel bleed
silicone gel breast implant
silicone gel implant
silicone gel prosthesis
silicone gel-filled breast implant
    (SGBI)
silicone gel-filled mammary
    implant (SGMI)
silicone granuloma
silicone hubless flat drain
silicone implant
silicone implant arthroplasty
silicone implant leakage
silicone impression material
silicone injection
silicone introducer
silicone intubation
silicone leakage
silicone lip augmentation
silicone lubricant
silicone mastitis
silicone meshed motility implant
silicone microdroplet
silicone microdroplet injection
    therapy
silicone microimplant
silicone mold
silicone MP implant
silicone nasal strut implant
silicone pad eye implant
silicone prosthesis
silicone ring
silicone Robinson catheter
silicone rod and sleeve forceps

silicone rod implant
silicone rods
silicone round drain
silicone rubber
silicone rubber arthroplasty
silicone rubber Dacron-cuffed
    catheter
silicone rubber impression
    material
silicone rubber joint
silicone sleeve
silicone sleeve eye implant
silicone sponge
silicone sponge forceps
silicone sponge implant
silicone strip eye implant
silicone sump drain
silicone synovitis
silicone textured mammary
    implant
silicone thoracic drain
silicone tire eye implant
silicone trapezium prosthesis
silicone tube
silicone wrist arthroplasty
silicone-coated, metallic self-
    expanding stent
silicone-filled anatomical breast
    implant
silicone-filled breast implant
silicone-filled implant
silicone-filled mammary implant
silicone-filled round breast
    implant
silicone-lubricated endotracheal
    tube
silicone-treated surgical silk
    suture
silicone-treated sutures
silicone-treated wound
Silicore catheter
Sili-Gel impression material
Silima breast prosthesis
Silipos digital pad
Silipos prosthetic sheath
Silipos silicone wonder cup
Silipos suspension sleeve
Silitek catheter
Silitek ureteral stent
Silitek Uropass stent
silk braided suture
silk glove sign

silk guidewire
silk implantation
silk interrupted mattress
    sutures
silk Mersilene sutures
silk nonabsorbable sutures
silk pop-off sutures
silk screw
silk seton
silk sign
Sil-K silicone sheet
silk stay sutures
silk sutures
silk ties
Silk Touch Flash Scanner laser
silk traction sutures
silk-and-wax catheter
silk-braided sutures
SilkLaser aesthetic CO_2 laser
SilkTouch CO_2 laser scanner
Silktouch laser
Silkworm gut sutures
Silky Polydek sutures
sill length
Sil-Med catheter
Silon pouch chimney
Silon silicone thermoplastic
    splinting material
Silon tent
Silon wound dressing
Silopad body sleeve
Silopad toe sleeve
Silosheath gel liner
Siloskin dressing
Silovi incision
Silovi procedure
Silovi saphenous vein bypass
    graft
Silovi saphenous vein graft
Siloxane graft
Siloxane implant
Siloxane prosthesis
Siltex Becker breast prosthesis
Siltex mammary implant
Siltex saline
Silva-Costa operation
silver bead electrode
Silver bunionectomy
silver cannula
silver catheter
Silver chisel
silver clip

Silver endaural forceps
Silver forceps
Silver knife
silver Mylar roll
Silver nasal osteotome
silver needle
silver nitrate cautery
Silver osteotome
silver probe
Silver procedure
silver saw
silver suture wire
silver sutures
silver-coated stent
silvered contact lens
silver-fork deformity
silver-fork fracture
Silver-Hildreth eyelid operation
silverized catgut sutures
Silverlon wound packing strips
Silverman biopsy needle
Silverman-Boeker cannula
Silverman-Boeker needle
Silver-Skin bunionectomy
SilverSpeed hydrophilic
    guidewire
Silverstein arachnoid dissector
Silverstein auditory canal
    dissector
Silverstein dressing
Silverstein dural elevator
Silverstein facial nerve monitor
Silverstein lateral venous sinus
    retractor
Silverstein malleus clip wire
Silverstein micromirror
Silverstein nerve separator
Silverstein permanent aeration
    tube
Silverstein round knife
Silverstein sickle knife
Silverstein stimulator probe
Silverstein tube
silver-wire appearance of retinal
    arteries
silver-wire reflex
silver-wiring of retinal arteries
SIMA reconstruction (single
    internal mammary artery
    reconstruction)
Simaplast mammary implants
Simcoe anterior chamber lens

Simcoe anterior chamber
    receiving needle
Simcoe anterior chamber
    retaining wire
Simcoe cannula tip
Simcoe C-loop intraocular lens
Simcoe corneal marker
Simcoe cortex cannula
Simcoe cortex extractor
Simcoe double-barreled cannula
Simcoe double-end lens loop
Simcoe eye implant
Simcoe eye speculum
Simcoe handpiece
Simcoe I&A unit
Simcoe aspirating needle
Simcoe double cannula
Simcoe nucleus delivery loupe
Simcoe posterior chamber
    nucleus delivery loop
Simcoe implant
Simcoe implantation forceps
Simcoe interchangeable tip
Simcoe intraocular implant lens
Simcoe intraocular lens implant
Simcoe irrigating-positioning
    needle
Simcoe lens
Simcoe lens-inserting forceps
Simcoe lens-positioning set
Simcoe microhook
Simcoe needle
Simcoe notched irrigating
    spatula
Simcoe nucleus delivery cannula
Simcoe nucleus erysiphake
Simcoe nucleus forceps
Simcoe nucleus lens loop
Simcoe nucleus spatula
Simcoe posterior chamber
    forceps
Simcoe posterior chamber lens
Simcoe reverse I&A cannula
Simcoe reverse-aperture cannula
Simcoe superior rectus forceps
Simcoe suture needle
Simcoe wire speculum
Simcoe-Barraquer eye speculum
Simeone-Erlik side-to-end
    portorenal shunt
simian crease
simian line

Simmonds cricothyrotomy
  needle
Simmonds disease
Simmonds syndrome
Simmonds vaginal speculum
Simmons catheter
Simmons cervical spine fusion
Simmons chisel
Simmons double-hole spinal
  screw
Simmons eye shield
Simmons osteotome
Simmons screw
Simmons sidewinder catheter
Simmons technique
Simmons-Martin screw
Simon bone curet
Simon cheiloplasty
Simon colpocleisis
Simon cup uterine curet
Simon dermatome
Simon expansion arch
Simon fistula hook
Simon fistula knife
Simon incision
Simon nitinol inferior vena cava
  (IVC) filter
Simon operation
Simon perineorrhaphy
Simon position
Simon retractor
Simon sign
Simon speculum
Simon spinal curet
Simon suture technique
Simon sutures
Simon vaginal retractor
Simon vaginal speculum
Simonart band
Simonart bar
Simons classification of
  malocclusion
Simons cleft palate knife
Simons stone-removing forceps
Simplastic catheter
Simplate procedure
simple anchorage
simple angioma
simple apertognathia
simple bone cyst
simple bypass
simple comminuted fracture

simple dislocation
simple excision
simple external drainage
simple flaring suture
simple fracture
simple ganglion
simple hepatojejunostomy
simple interrupted fashion
simple iridectomy
simple joint
simple lentigo
simple mandibular distraction
simple mastectomy
simple mastoidectomy
simple mechanical obstruction
simple microscope
simple operation
simple periodontal flap
simple reflex
simple running sutures
simple sinusotomy
simple skull fracture
simple suture technique
simple sutures
simple syndactyly
simple vesicle
Simplex adhesive
Simplex cement
Simplex cement adhesive
Simplex mastoid rongeur
Simplex premixed bone cement
Simplex bone cement
Simplus dilatation catheter
Simply Wet table
Simpson antral curet
Simpson atherectomy
Simpson atherectomy catheter
Simpson AtheroCath catheter
Simpson coronary AtheroCath
Simpson coronary AtheroCath
  catheter
Simpson curet
Simpson directional coronary
  atherectomy device
Simpson endoscope
Simpson epistaxis balloon
Simpson forceps
Simpson hysteropexy
Simpson lacrimal dilator
Simpson lacrimal probe
Simpson light
Simpson obstetrical forceps

Simpson operation
Simpson peripheral AtheroCath
Simpson PET balloon
    atherectomy device
Simpson sound
Simpson splint
Simpson sterling lacrimal probe
Simpson suction catheter
Simpson sugar-tong splint
Simpson tampon
Simpson balloon catheter
Simpson uterine dilator
Simpson uterine sound
Simpson-Braun obstetrical
    forceps
Simpson-Luikart obstetrical
    forceps
Simpson-Robert dilatation
    catheter
Simpson-Robert guidewire
Simpson-Robert catheter
Simrock speculum
Sims abdominal needle
Sims anoscope
Sims cannula
Sims curet
Sims dilator
Sims double-ended retractor
Sims double-ended speculum
Sims double-ended vaginal
    speculum
Sims general operating scissors
Sims irrigating uterine curet
Sims knife
Sims needle
Sims Per-fit percutaneous
    tracheostomy kit
Sims plug
Sims position
Sims probe
Sims proctoscope
Sims rectal retractor
Sims rectal speculum
Sims retractor
Sims scissors
Sims sound
Sims speculum
Sims sponge holder
Sims suction tip
Sims suture technique
Sims sutures
Sims tenaculum

Sims uterine curet
Sims uterine depressor
Sims uterine dilator
Sims uterine probe
Sims uterine scissors
Sims uterine sound
Sims vaginal decompressor
Sims vaginal plug
Sims vaginal retractor
Sims vaginal speculum
Sims-Kelly vaginal retractor
Sims-Maier clamp
Sims-Maier sponge and dressing
    forceps
Sims-Siebold uterine scissors
simultaneous areolar mastopexy
    and breast augmentation
    (SAMBA)
simultaneous free flaps
simultaneous grafting
simultaneous kidney-pancreas
    transplantation
simultaneous LATRAM and
    mastectomy (SLAM)
simultaneous pancreas and
    kidney (SPK)
simultaneous pancreas-kidney
    transplantation
simultaneous segmental
    hepatectomy
simultaneous thermal diffusion
    blood flow and pressure
    probe
sincipital cephalocele
S-incision
Sinclair spatula
Sinding-Larsen-Johansson lesion
Sine-U-View nasal endoscope
Sinexon dilator
Singer needle
Singer-Blom electrolarynx
    prosthesis
Singer-Blom endoscopic
    tracheoesophageal
    puncture technique
Singer-Blom ossicular prosthesis
Singer-Blom tube
Singer-Blom valve
singer's node
singer's nodule
Singh osteoporosis
    classification

Singh speech system voice rehabilitation prosthesis
single adenoma
single biopsy
single circular saw
single cortical bone onlay
single cross-slot screwdriver
single denture construction
single dynamic graciloplasty
single fracture
single harelip
single hook
single internal mammary artery (SIMA) reconstruction
single injection anesthesia
single lung ventilation
single mechanism inhaled anesthetic
single midline extraperitoneal incision
single need catheter
single occluder
single onlay cortical bone graft
single pedicle TRAM flap
single pigtail stent
single port
single proximal portal technique
single safe-sided chisel
single site inhaled anesthetic
single sleeve bar joint
single space technique
single syndactyly
single-action rongeur
single-armed suture technique
single-armed sutures
single-averaged electrocardiograph
single-axis ankle prosthesis
single-axis friction knee
single-axis locking knee
single-axis Syme foot
single-balloon valvotomy
single-balloon valvuloplasty
single-beveled cutting instrument
single-blade retractor
single-breath induction of anesthesia
single-chamber pacemaker
single-chambered saline implant
single-channel cochlear implant
single-channel electromyograph oscilloscope

single-channel fiberoptic bronchoscope
single-channel in vivo light dosimeter
single-channel nonfade oscilloscope
single-channel operating sheath
single-channel wire-guided sphincterotome
single-contrast study
single-crystal gamma camera
single-echo diffusion imaging
single-fiber EMG electrode
single-field hyperthermia combined with radiation therapy and ultrasound scanner
single-fraction total body irradiation
single-guarded osteotome
single-handed knot sutures
single-hatching undermining
single-head rotating gamma camera
single-holed suction cannula
single-hook retractor
single-hydatid disease
single-incision fasciotomy
single-J urinary diversion stent
single-layer continuous closure
single-level spinal fusion
single-loop tourniquet
single-lumen balloon stone extractor catheter
single-lumen cannula
single-lumen infusion catheter
single-mirror goniolens
single-needle device
single-pass lead
single-pass pacemaker
single-pedicle flap
single-phase current
single-photon densitometer
single-photon electrospinal orthosis
single-plane angiogram
single-plane instrument
single-port laparoscopy
single-port technique
single-portal endocarpal tunnel release

single-prong broad acetabular retractor
single-puncture laparoscopy
single-reference-point instrument
single-rod penile prosthesis
single-running suture
single-shot imaging technique
single-sided bone saw
single-slice gradient-echo image
single-stage castration, vaginal construction perineoplasty
single-stage catheter
single-stage debridement
single-stage omphalocele repair
single-stage operation
single-stage procedure
single-stage reconstruction
single-stage screw implant
single-step esophagoplasty
SingleStitch Phacoflex lens
single-suture craniosynostosis
single-suture synostosis
Singleton empyema trocar
Singleton incision
single-tooth forceps
single-tooth microdontia
single-tooth subperiosteal implant
single-toothed tenaculum
single-use dermatome
single-use electrode
single-wire electrode
Singley clamp
Singley intestinal clamp
Singley intestinal forceps
Singley intestinal tissue forceps
Singley tissue forceps
Singley-Tuttle dressing forceps
Singley-Tuttle intestinal forceps
Singley-Tuttle tissue forceps
Siniscal eyelid clamp
Siniscal-Smith lid everter
sink-trap malformation
sinoaortic denervation
sinoatrial exit block
sinoauricular
sinodural angle
sinogram
sinography
sinonasal carcinoma
sinonasal cavity

sinonasal disease
sinonasal lesion
sinonasal melanoma
sinonasal papilloma
sinonasal tract
sinoscopy trocar
sinospiral muscle bundle
sinotubular junction
sinoventricular
Sinskey blue loop intraocular lenses
Sinskey forceps
Sinskey hook
Sinskey intraocular lens
Sinskey intraocular lens forceps
Sinskey iris hook
Sinskey J-loop intraocular lens
Sinskey lens implant
Sinskey lens manipulator
Sinskey lens-manipulating hook
Sinskey microlens hook
Sinskey microtying forceps
Sinskey needle holder
Sinskey nucleus spatula
Sinskey pick
Sinskey posterior chamber intraocular lens
Sinskey posterior chamber lens
Sinskey-McPherson forceps
Sinskey-Wilson forceps
Sinskey-Wilson foreign body forceps
sintered titanium mesh
Sinterlock implant
Sinterlock implant metal prosthesis
sinuous incision
sinus (*pl.* sinuses)
  1st branchial cleft sinus
  air sinus
  aspiration of sinuses
  confluence of sinuses
  dural confluence of sinuses
  irrigation of sinuses
  lymphatic sinuses
  maxillary sinuses
  middle sinuses
  paranasal sinuses
  petrosal sinuses
  posterior sinuses
  rectal sinuses
  septum of frontal sinuses

sinus (*continued*)

    septum of sphenoidal sinuses
    Waters view of sinuses
    alveolar sinus
    aperture of sphenoid sinus
    Arlt sinus
    Arlt-Jaesche sinus
    barber's pilonidal sinus
    Bascom procedure for repair
      of pilonidal sinus
    basilar sinus
    bony frontal sinus
    bony maxillary sinus
    bony sphenoidal sinus
    branchial cleft sinus
    Breschet sinus
    carotid cavernous sinus
    cavernous sinus
    coronary sinus
    costophrenic sinus
    cranial sinus
    cribriform sinus
    cutaneous sinus
    dermal sinus
    drainage of sinus
    ductal sinus
    dural sinus
    endodermal sinus
    ethmoidal sinus
    excision of sinus
    exenteration of sinus
    frontal paranasal sinus
    frontal sinus
    Huguier sinus
    inferior petrosal sinus
    inferior sagittal sinus
    intercavernous sinus
    lacteal sinus
    lactiferous sinus
    laryngeal sinus
    lateral sinus
    lavage of sinus
    longitudinal sinus
    Luschka sinus
    Maier sinus
    marginal sinus
    mastoid sinus
    maxillary sinus
    Meyer sinus
    nasal sinus
    occipital sinus
    opacified frontal sinus

sinus (*continued*)

    Palfyn sinus
    perineal sinus
    pilonidal sinus
    pin tract sinus
    piriform sinus
    portal sinus
    preauricular sinus
    prostatic sinus
    renal sinus
    Ridley sinus
    right frontal sinus
    Rokitansky-Aschoff sinus
    rostrum of sinus
    sacrococcygeal sinus
    sagittal sinus
    sagittalis inferior, sinus
    sagittalis superior, sinus
    sigmoid sinus
    sphenoidal paranasal sinus
    sphenoidal sinus
    sphenoparietal sinus
    straight sinus
    subarachnoidal sinus
    subperiosteal abscess of
      frontal sinus
    superior longitudinal sinus
    superior petrosal sinus
    superior sagittal sinus
    suprapubic sinus
    tarsal sinus
    thyroglossal sinus
    transverse sinus
    tympanic sinus
    Valsalva sinus
    wide sigmoid sinus
sinus antral cannula
sinus arrest
sinus arrhythmia
sinus balloon
sinus biopsy forceps
sinus block
sinus bradycardia
sinus bur
sinus cannula
sinus cavity
sinus chisel
sinus closure
sinus cranialization
sinus curet
sinus defect
sinus dilator

sinus drainage
sinus elevation
sinus endoscopy
sinus exit block
sinus groove
sinus in the tentorium
sinus irrigation
sinus irrigator
sinus lift osteotome
sinus line
sinus mucocele
sinus nerve
sinus node
sinus node pacemaker
sinus of Morgagni
sinus of nail
sinus operation
sinus pacemaker
sinus probe
sinus punch
sinus rasp
sinus rhythm
sinus septum
sinus suction syringe
sinus surgery
sinus tachycardia
sinus tarsi syndrome
sinus thrombophlebitis
sinus thrombosis
sinus tract
sinus tract cyst
sinus trephine
sinus tympani excavator
sinus unguis
sinus wash bottle
sinus wash tube
SinuScope rigid rod
sinuscopy cannula
SinuSeal resorbable nasal packing
sinusectomy
    branchial cleft sinusectomy
    Lynch sinusectomy
    pilonidal cystectomy and
        sinusectomy
sinuses
sinus-irrigating cannula
sinusitis
    acute frontal sinusitis
    acute maxillary sinusitis
    chronic frontal sinusitis
    chronic maxillary sinusitis
    chronic paranasal sinusitis

sinusitis (*continued*)
    ethmoidal sinusitis
    frontal sinusitis
    isolated sphenoid sinusitis
    maxillary sinusitis
    osteoblastic sinusitis
    sphenoidal sinusitis
    vacuum sinusitis
sinusography
sinusoid
sinusoidal circulation
sinusoidal lesion
sinusoidal spaces
sinusoscopy
sinusotomy
    combined frontal-
        ethmoid-sphenoid
        sinusotomy
    endoscopic intranasal frontal
        sinusotomy
    external frontal sinusotomy
    external sinusotomy
    external sphenoid sinusotomy
    frontal sinusotomy
    intranasal sinusotomy
    maxillary sinusotomy
    simple sinusotomy
    sphenoid sinusotomy
SinuSpacer turbinate stent
sinu-vertebral nerve
Sinvision ultrasound scanner
silicate cement
siphon suction tube
siphonage
Sipple syndrome
Sippy dilating olives
Sippy dilator
Sippy esophageal dilating set
Sippy esophageal dilator
Sippy esophageal dilator pusher
    wire
Sippy point
SIPS (sympathically independent
    pain syndrome)
Siremobil C-arm unit
sireniform fetus
sirenomelia
SIS wound dressing
Sisler lacrimal trephine
Sisson forceps
Sisson fracture-reducing elevator
Sisson spring hook

Sisson spring retractor
Sisson-Cottle septal speculum
Sisson-Love retractor
Sisson-Vienna nasal speculum
Sister Helen Mustard ENT table
Sister Mary Joseph lymph node
sister-hook forceps
Sistron scissors
Sistrunk band retractor
Sistrunk dissecting scissors
Sistrunk double-ended retractor
Sistrunk operation
Sistrunk procedure
Sistrunk retractor
Sistrunk scissors
site
    anastomotic site
    arteriovenous shunt site
    biopsy site
    bleeding site
    carcinoma of uncertain
        primary site
    catheter site
    coaptation site
    colostomy site
    crepitus at fracture site
    curvature site
    donor site
    drain site
    draining incisional site
    endoscopic biopsy site
    excisional biopsy site
    exit site
    extraction site
    fibula donor site
    fracture site
    graft donor site
    graft site
    healing incision site
    immunocompetent site
    implantation site
    incision site
    infected incisional site
    infusion site
    injection site
    injury site
    involved site
    leaking about shunt site
    metastatic site
    needle site
    nipple site
    obstructive site

site (*continued*)
    operative site
    original tumor site
    pedicle flap donor site
    pedicled enteric donor site
    placental site
    pooling site
    prime site
    puncture site
    pus at incision site
    radial fracture site
    recipient site
    rectal site
    redness along incision site
    reflection site
    remottling fracture site
    sanctuary site
    screw site
    secondary site
    shunt site
    sterile site
    stoma site
    surgical site
    tracheotomy site
SiteGuard transparent adhesive
        film dressing
Site-Rite ultrasound scanner
site-specific surgery
Sit-Straight wheelchair cushion
sitting-up view angiogram
situs inversus
situs inversus viscerum
situs perversus
situs solitus
situs tranversus
Sitzmarks radiopaque marker
Siurala classification
Sivash hip prosthesis
Sivash hip replacement
Sivash prosthesis
size
    cardiac size
    chamber size
    clot size
    configuration and size
    donor size
    field size
    generous in size
    gestational size
    gland size
    heart size
    lesion size

size (*continued*)
  overall size
  suture sizes (1-0, 2-0, 3-0, 4-0 [or
    0, 00, 000, 0000], 5-0, etc.)
size and condition normal
sizer
  AP femoral sizer
  AP sizer
  breast sizer
  Dow Corning Silastic
    prosthetic sizer
  femoral sizer
  prosthetic sizer
  Silastic prosthetic sizer
  Whitaker malar sizer
sizing balloon
sizing implants
sizing ring
SJM Sequin annuloplasty ring
SJM Tailor annuloplasty ring
Sjögren syndrome
Sjoqvist operation
SkareKare silicon gel-filled
    cushion
skate flap
skate graft
Skeele chalazion curet
Skeele corneal curet
Skeele eye curet
Skeeter otologic drill
Skeggs-Leonard dialyzer
skeletal abnormalities
skeletal abnormality
skeletal biopsy
skeletal correction
skeletal deformity
skeletal disproportion
skeletal distraction
skeletal fixation
skeletal hypertrophy
skeletal lesion
skeletal maturation
skeletal metastasis
skeletal muscle
skeletal muscle fibers
skeletal occlusion
skeletal open bite
skeletal overgrowth
skeletal pin
skeletal pin fixation
skeletal series
skeletal stabilization

skeletal structure
skeletal tissue
skeletal traction
skeletalization
skeleton
  axial skeleton
  cephalic skeleton
  extralaryngeal skeleton
  non-loadbearing regions of
    the craniofacial skeleton
  osseocartilaginous craniofacial
    skeleton
skeleton earmold
skeleton fine forceps
skeleton hand
skeletonize
Skene catheter
Skene duct
Skene forceps
Skene glands
Skene spoon
Skene tenaculum
Skene tenaculum forceps
Skene uterine curet
Skene uterine forceps
Skene uterine spoon
Skene uterine spoon curet
Skene uterine tenaculum
Skene uterine vulsellum
Skene vulsellum forceps
skenoscope
skew flap
skewer technique
skewfoot
SKI knee prosthesis
ski needle
ski position
skiagram study
skiametry
skiascopy bar
skid
  acetabular skid
  Austin Moore-Murphy bone
    skid
  bone skid
  Davis bone skid
  hip skid
  MacAusland skid
  Meyerding bone skid
  Murphy bone skid
  Murphy-Lane bone skid
  Scudder skid

skid curet
skier's fracture
skier's tear
skier's thumb
Skil-CARE Alarm cushion
Skillern cannula
Skillern curet
Skillern fracture
Skillern phimosis forceps
Skillern probe
Skillern punch
Skillern sinus curet
Skillern sinus probe
Skillern sphenoid cannula
Skillern sphenoid probe
Skillern sphenoidal probe
Skillman arterial forceps
Skillman hemostatic forceps
Skillman mosquito forceps
Skillman prepuce forceps
Skimmer blade
Skimmer laryngeal blade tip
Skimmer RRP laryngeal shaver
skin
   ablated skin
   alligator skin
   appendages of the skin
   biologic creep of skin
   blanched skin
   buttonholing of skin
   chemical peel of skin
   circumferential tearing of skin
   combination skin
   composite cultured skin
      (CCS)
   deciduous skin
   defatting of skin
   degrease the skin
   depigmenting skin
   devitalized skin
   dimpling of breast skin
   dimpling of skin
   elasticity of skin
   farmer's skin
   fish skin
   flaccid skin
   flaking skin
   fold of skin
   glabrous skin
   golfer's skin
   grafted skin
   granulomatous slack skin

skin (*continued*)
   hanging skin
   harvesting skin
   heavy skin
   hooding of the upper lid skin
   India rubber skin
   inherent extensibility of skin
   Integra artificial skin
   juxtabrow skin
   lax skin
   loose skin
   mechanical creep of skin
   overlying skin
   penile skin
   perianal skin
   piebald skin
   porcupine skin
   primary macular atrophy of
      skin
   primary neuroendocrine
      carcinoma of the skin
   puncturing of skin
   redundant skin
   residual skin
   sailor's skin
   sebaceous skin
   senile skin
   shagreen skin
   slack skin
   sloughing of skin
   striate atrophy of skin
   suborbicularis skin
   thickened skin
   tissue-cultured skin
   ultradelicate split-thickness
      scalp skin (UDSTS)
   underlying skin
   viscoelastic property of skin
   wedge of skin
skin approximation
skin atrophy
skin barrier
skin biopsy
skin brassiere
skin breakdown
skin cancer
skin care product
skin clip
skin closure
skin closure strips
skin crease
skin creep

skin depigmentation
skin edge necrosis
skin edges approximated
skin elevator
skin envelope
skin envelope invagination
skin eruption
skin exfoliation
skin expansion
skin expansion technique
skin flap
skin flap retractor
skin flap rotation
skin flap rotation technique
skin forceps
skin graft
skin graft expander mesh
skin graft hook
skin graft knife
skin graft mesh
skin graft mesher
skin grafting
skin grooves
skin gun
skin hook
skin hook retractor
skin incision
skin integrity
skin involvement
skin island
skin knife
skin laxity
skin layers
skin lesion
skin lesion artifact
skin lines
skin loss
skin lubrication therapy
skin maceration
skin margins
skin marker
skin marking pen
skin markings
skin mesh
skin moist
skin necrosis
skin numbness
skin paddle
skin pale
skin pallor
skin paradigm
skin peel

skin pencil
skin planing
skin preparation
skin punch
skin rash
skin reaction
skin relaxation
skin response
skin resurfacing
skin retractor
skin rubor
skin self-retaining retractor
Skin Skribe marker
Skin Skribe pen
Skin Skribe skin marker
skin slough
skin splint
skin spots
skin staple
skin staples
skin stitch
skin stones
skin substitute
skin surface
skin sutures
skin tag
skin test
skin towels
skin traction
skin tumor
skin turgor
skin wheal
skin window
skin window technique
skin/muscle flap blepharoplasty
skin-adipose superficial
    musculoaponeurotic system
    (SASMAS)
skin-adipose unit (SA unit)
Skin Bond skin cement
skin-colored lesion
skin-crease incision
skin-envelope adjustments
skin-equivalent tissue
skin-flap dissection
skinfold calipers
skinfold incision
skin-knife incision
Skinlight Er:YAG laser
Skinlight erbium:YAG (yttrium-
    aluminum-garnet) laser
Skinlight YAG laser

skin-limited histiocytosis
skinline incision
skin-muscle blepharoplasty
Skinner classification
skinning colpectomy
skinning vaginectomy
skinning vulvectomy
skinning vulvovaginectomy
skinny balloon catheter
skinny Chiba needle
skinny dilatation catheter
skinny needle
skinny needle cholangiography
skinny over-the-wire balloon
    catheter
skinny-needle biopsy
skinny-nose rongeur
skin-only periareolar-approach
    mastopexy technique
Skin-Prep protective dressing
Skinscan scanner
Skinsense glove
skin-sparing mastectomy
skin-subcutaneous dissection
    with SMAS manipulation
skin-surfacing technique
SkinTech medical tattooing
    device
Skintegrity hydrogel dressing
SkinTemp biosynthetic collagen
    dressing
skip graft
skip lesion
skip metastasis
skipped beat
skived incision
skiving knife
Sklar anoscope
Sklar bone drill
Sklar bone pin cutter
Sklar bone saw
Sklar cleansers
Sklar cutter
Sklar evacuator
Sklar ligature needle
Sklar pin cutter
Sklar proctoscope
Sklar tonometer
Sklar-Kleen
Sklar-Schiotz jewel tonometer
Sklar-Schiotz tonometer
SklarScribe skin marker

Skoda rale
Skoda sign
Skoda tympany
skodaic resonance
skodaic tympany
Skoog cleft lip repair
Skoog fasciectomy
Skoog fasciotomy
Skoog incision in palmar
    fasciectomy
Skoog mammaplasty
Skoog nasal chisel
Skoog operation
Skoog procedure for Dupuytren
    contracture
Skoog release of Dupuytren
    contracture
Skoog rhytidectomy
Skoog technique
skull
    base of skull
    cloverleaf skull
    hot-cross-bun skull
    inner table bones of skull
    inner table of skull
    lacuna skull
    longitudinal arc of skull
    maplike skull
    natiform skull
    outer table bones of skull
    outer table of skull
    radiopaque skull
    roof of skull
    steeple skull
    suture line of skull
    synchondroses of skull
    table bones of skull
    table of skull
    tower skull
    trilobed cloverleaf skull
    trilobed skull
    West lacuna skull
    West-Engstler skull
skull base chordoma
skull base suture
skull base tumor resection
skull block
skull bur
skull cap
skull clamp
skull closure
skull cone punch

skull elevator
skull film
skull fracture
skull plate
skull punch
skull radiography
skull raspatory
skull saw
skull survey
skull tantalum
skull tongs
skull traction
skull traction drill
skull tractor
skull trephine
skull, occiput, mandibular immobilization (SOMI) brace
skull, occiput, mandibular immobilization (SOMI) orthosis
skull-base approach
Skylark surface electrode
Skylight gamma camera
skyline projection
skyline view of patella
S-L dissociation (scapholunate dissociation)
SLAC (scapholunate advanced collapse)
SLAC pattern of degenerative change
SLAC reconstruction
SLAC sequence
SLAC wrist
SLAC wrist reconstruction
SLAC pattern of degenerative change
SLAC wrist
slack skin
Slade cannula
Slalom balloon
SLAM (simultaneous LATRAM and mastectomy)
Slant haptic intraocular lens
slant hole collimator
Slant lens
slant muscle operation
slant of occlusal plane
SLAP lesion
Slatis frame
slatted plinth table
Slaughter nasal saw

Slavianski membrane
SLC (short leg cast)
sleek catheter
sleep apnea monitor
sleeper sutures
sleeve
  Bard irrigation sleeve
  biocompression pneumatic sleeve
  Charles anterior segment sleeve
  Charles infusion sleeve
  Charles vitrector with sleeve
  Coloplast transparent irrigation sleeve
  Cunningham-Cotton sleeve
  delivery assistance sleeve
  Dent sleeve
  Dexterity Pneumo Sleeve
  drug infusion sleeve
  Dunlop sleeve
  Easy Sleeve
  Edwards-Levine sleeve
  elbow sleeve
  Electro-Mesh sleeve
  EPX suspension sleeve
  gel suspension sleeve
  heel sleeve
  Hemmer connection sleeve
  Iceflex Endurance suction suspension sleeve
  ICEROSS sleeve
  implant sleeve
  Jobst sleeve
  Ken Drive sleeve
  Knit-Rite suspension sleeve
  laparoscopic sleeve
  laparoscopic trocar sleeve
  LocalMed catheter infusion sleeve
  malleolar gel sleeve
  MalleoTrain ankle sleeve
  Mentor Foley catheter with comfort sleeve
  MICA 3× sleeve
  mucoperichondrial sleeves
  neoprene elbow sleeve
  neoprene sleeves
  Palumbo sleeve
  PMMA centering sleeve
  pneumo sleeve
  Preclude IMA sleeve
  release sleeve

sleeve (*continued*)
  retinal probe sleeve
  root sleeve
  silicone sleeve
  Silipos suspension sleeve
  Silopad body sleeve
  Silopad toe sleeve
  Steri-Sleeve sleeve
  Stevens-Charles sleeve
  Super Grip sleeve
  Supramid eye muscle sleeve
  Supramid ptosis sleeve
  Sur-Fit colostomy irrigation
    sleeve
  Surgiport trocar and sleeve
  tri-point K-wire sleeve
  Ultra Duet colostomy
    irrigating sleeve
  Watzke silicone sleeve
  Williams overtube sleeve
sleeve adapter
sleeve bag
sleeve clot
sleeve fracture
sleeve graft
sleeve implant
sleeve lobectomy
sleeve resection
sleeve selector
sleeve technique
sleeve-resection circumcision
sleeve-spreading dilating forceps
sleeve-spreading forceps
slender-nose rongeur
slender-tip scissors
slice fracture
slice graft
Slick stylette endotracheal tube
    guide
slide hammer
slide plate
slide specimen
Slide-On EndoSheath
Slider balloon
Slider catheter
Slidewire extension guide
sliding abdominal hernia
sliding barrel hook
sliding capsular forceps
sliding esophageal hiatal hernia
sliding fat pad technique
sliding flap

sliding genioplasty
sliding hammer
sliding hiatal hernia
sliding horizontal genioplasties
sliding inguinal hernia
sliding inlay bone graft
sliding laryngoscope
sliding lock
sliding microtome
sliding nail
sliding oblique osteotomy
sliding osteotomy in mandibular
    reconstruction
sliding plane
sliding skin flap technique
sliding technique
sliding-rail catheter
sliding-type hiatal hernia
slightly curved ear pick
slightly curved pick
Slik Pak non-stick nasal pack
Slim Fit flex clamp
slimcut blade
Slimfit lens
SlimStem metal scleral shield
Slimthetics orthotic
sling
  acromioclavicular dislocation
    harness sling
  adjustable strap arm sling
  Bobath sling
  cervicofacial sling
  CircOlectric sling
  clavicle strap sling
  Colles sling
  cradle arm sling
  facial sling
  fascial sling
  Freidenwald-Guyton sling
  frontalis sling
  Glisson sling
  Goebel-Stoeckel sling
  hand cock-up sling
  Harris sling
  head sling
  Hoyer lift sling
  levator sling
  mandibular sling
  Marlex mesh sling
  Mason-Allen Universal sling
  Meek clavicle sling
  muscle sling

sling (*continued*)
  pelvic sling
  pericardial sling
  Posey sling
  pouch-type sling
  pterygomasseteric sling
  ptosis sling
  pulmonary artery sling
  Rainbow envelope arm sling
  Rauchfuss sling
  Sayre head sling
  Snoopy arm sling
  static sling
  Straight-In male sling
  strap sling
  Stratasis urethral sling
  sublimis sling
  Supramid ptosis sling
  SurgiSis sling
  Suspend sling
  suspension sling
  Teare arm sling
  temporalis sling
  triangular vaginal patch sling
  UltraSling sling
  Veeder tip sling
  Velpeau sling
  Weil pelvic sling
  Zimmer arm sling
  Zimmer clavicular cross sling
sling and blanket technique
sling and reef technique
sling dressing
sling frame
sling immobilization
sling ligation
sling operation
sling procedure
sling suture technique
sling sutures
sling wrapping technique
sling-and-swathe bandage
sling-dressing
sling-like taping around the
    implant
sling-ring complex
Slinky balloon catheter
Slinky PTCA catheter
slip hernia
Slip-Coat tip
slip-joint pliers
slip-knot ties

Slip-N-Snip scissors
slipped capital femoral
    epiphysis
slipped disk
slipped epiphysis
slipped hernia
slipped meniscus
slipped Nissen fundoplication
slipped Nissen repair
slipped rib cartilage syndrome
slipped strut
slipper cast
slipper-tipped guidewire
slipping epiphysis
slipping patella
slipping rib syndrome
slipping ribs
slip-ring camera
Slip-Sheen catheter
slit blade
slit blade knife
slit catheter technique
slit hemorrhage
slit illuminator
slit lamp
slit scanography
slit ventricle syndrome
slit-lamp camera attachment
slit-lamp cup
slit-lamp examination
slit-lamp fluorophotometer
slit-lamp instrument table
slit-lamp microscope
slitlike defect
slitting of canaliculus
sliver bone graft
SLN (superior laryngeal nerve)
SLN biopsy
SLN localization
Sloan abdominal incision
Sloan dissector
Sloan goiter flap dissector
Sloan goiter retractor
Sloan goiter self-retaining
    retractor
Sloan incision
Sloan retractor
Slocum amputation technique
Slocum anterior rotary drawer
    test
Slocum elevator
Slocum fusion technique

Slocum knee repair
Slocum maneuver
Slocum meniscal clamp
Slocum operation
Slocum pes transfer
Slocum splint
Slocum test
Slocum-Smith-Petersen nail
slope-shouldered lesion
sloping surface
Slot distraction device
slot fracture
slot incision
slot table
slot-blot technique
slotted acetabular
    augmentation
slotted anoscope
slotted bone plate
slotted bronchoscope
slotted handle
slotted instrument
slotted intramedullary rod
slotted laryngoscope
slotted mallet
slotted nail
slotted needle
slotted needle vent
slotted nerve clamp
slotted plate
slotted screw
slotted speculum
slotted sutures
slotted tendon stripper
slotted tube articulated stent
slotted wrench
slotting bur
slotting-bur osteotome
slot-type rim incision
sloughed area
sloughed face-lift
sloughing of skin
sloughing ulcer
slow continuous ultrafiltration
    therapy (SCUF therapy)
slow infusion IV drip
slow maxillary expansion
slow palatal expander
slow phleboclysis
slow spike and wave
slow-flow lesions
slow-pathway ablation

slow-twitch fatigue-resistant
    skeletal muscle
slow-twitch fibers
SLR test (straight leg-raising test)
SLT laser
Sluder adenotome
Sluder cautery electrode
Sluder guillotine
Sluder headband
Sluder hook
Sluder knife
Sluder mouth gag
Sluder needle
Sluder palate retractor
Sluder retractor
Sluder speculum
Sluder sphenoidal hook
Sluder sphenoidal speculum
Sluder tonometer
Sluder tonsillar guillotine
Sluder tonsillar knife
Sluder tonsillar tonsillectome
Sluder tonsillectome
Sluder tonsillectomy
Sluder Universal handle
Sluder-Ballenger tonsillar punch
    forceps
Sluder-Ballenger tonsillectome
Sluder-Demarest tonometer
Sluder-Demarest tonsillectome
Sluder-Ferguson mouth gag
Sluder-Jansen mouth gag
Sluder-Mehta electrode
Sluder-Sauer guillotine
Sluder-Sauer tonometer
Sluder-Sauer tonsillar guillotine
Sluder-Sauer tonsillectome
sludged blood
sludging of circulation
Sluijter-Mehta cannula
SLWC (short leg walking cast)
SMA (superior mesenteric
    artery)
small aperture Steri-Drape drape
small arteries
small blood vessel
small bone chisel
small bone-cutting forceps
small bowel congenital
    abnormality
small bowel diverticular disease
small bowel enteroscopy

small bowel enterotomy
small bowel idiopathic
    intussusception
small bowel lesion
small bowel lymphoma
small bowel surgery
small bowel transplant
small bowel-biopsy
small brass mallet
small caliber
small cardiac vein
small cell carcinoma
small cell lung carcinoma
small cell neuroendocrine
    carcinoma
small cup biopsy forceps
small for gestational age (SGA)
small head mallet
small incisional biopsy
small intestinal endoscopy
small intestinal membrane
small intestine
small joint arthrodesis
small joint arthroplasty
small joint fusion
small loop electrode
small nail spicule bur
small pelvis
small pick
small polyp removal
small rake retractor
small round cell carcinoma
small saphenous vein
small sciatic nerve
small spring scissors
small square-groove silicone
Small tissue retractor
small uterus
small vessel anastomosis
small vessel vasculitis
small volume nebulizer
small-bore cannula
small-bore needle
small bowel enema
small bowel followthrough
small bowel meal
small bowel obstruction (SBO)
small bowel resection
small bowel series
small bowel shunt
small bowel tube
small-caliber needle

Small-Carrion penile implant
    material
Small-Carrion penile prosthesis
Small-Carrion semirigid penile
    prosthesis
Small-Carrion Silastic rod for
    penile implant
small-cell carcinoma
small-cell tumor
small-diameter endosonographic
    instrument
small-droplet fatty liver
smaller pectoral muscle
smaller psoas muscle
smallest adductor muscle
smallest cardiac veins
smallest scalene muscle
small-loop electrode
Smart chalazion forceps
Smart enucleation scissors
Smart laser
Smart nonslipping chalazion
    forceps
Smart position-sensing catheter
Smart scalpel
Smart scissors
Smart splint
Smart Trigger Bear 1000
    ventilator
SmartAnchor suture anchor
SmartBrace brace
Smartdop Doppler
SmartNeedle needle
SmartPins fastener
SmartPrep scanner
SmartScrew bioabsorbable
    implant
SmartScrew screw
SmartWrap elbow brace
SMAS complex
SMAS deep-plane face-lift
SMAS face-lift technique
SMAS fascia
SMAS imbrication face-lift
SMAS lift
SMAS platysma deep-tissue face-
    lift
SMAS platysma face-lift
SMAS plication face-lift
SMAS plication procedure
SMAS rhytidectomy
SMAS facelift technique

SMAS fascia
SMAS layer
SMAS level
SMAS manipulation
SMAS tissue
smasectomy
SMAS-platysma flap
Smead closure
Smead-Jones closure
Smead-Jones stitches
Smead-Jones sutures
smear
   cervical Pap smear
   cervical smear
   endocervical smear
   nasal smear
   Pap smear
   Papanicolaou smear
   stained smear
   throat smear
   vaginal, cervical, endocervical smears (VCE smears)
   VCE smears (vaginal, cervical, endocervical smears)
   wet smear
Smedberg brace
Smedberg dilator
Smedberg hand drill
Smedberg hemostat
Smedberg twist drill
Smeden tonsillar punch
Smedley dynamometer
SMEI ultrasound device
SMEI ultrasound-assisted lipoplasty machine
Smei-sculpture ultrasound device
Smellie crochet hook
Smellie maneuver
Smellie obstetrical forceps
Smellie obstetrical hook
Smellie obstetrical perforator
Smellie obstetrical scissors
Smellie perforator
Smellie scissors
Smeloff prosthetic valve
Smeloff-Cutter aortic valve prosthesis
Smeloff-Cutter ball-cage prosthetic valve
Smeloff-Cutter ball-valve prosthesis

Smeloff-Cutter heart valve prosthesis
SMI cannula
SMI Surgi-Med CPM device
SMIC abdominal spatula
SMIC anterior commissure laryngoscope
SMIC auricular tourniquet
SMIC bone chisel
SMIC bone file
SMIC bone hammer
SMIC bone rongeur
SMIC brain spatula
SMIC cerumen hook
SMIC cheek retractor
SMIC collar scissors
SMIC cranial rongeur
SMIC dermatome
SMIC ear curet
SMIC ear polypus scissors
SMIC ear speculum
SMIC eustachian catheter
SMIC intestinal clamp
SMIC laminectomy rongeur
SMIC malleus head nipper
SMIC mastoid chisel
SMIC mastoid curet
SMIC mastoid gouge
SMIC mastoid rongeur
SMIC mastoid suction tube
SMIC mouth mirror
SMIC myringotome
SMIC nasal septal speculum
SMIC nasal speculum
SMIC periodontal abscess probe
SMIC periodontal file
SMIC periosteal elevator
SMIC pituitary curet
SMIC pliers
SMIC pneumatic otoscope
SMIC rongeur
SMIC root canal plugger
SMIC sternal chisel
SMIC sternal drill
SMIC sternal knife
SMIC surgical catgut
SMIC surgical mallet
SMIC suture needle
SMIC tonsillar guillotine
SMIC tuning fork
SMILE (subperiosteal minimally invasive laser endoscopic)

SMILE facelift
SMILE rhytidectomy
smile incision
smiley-face knotting technique
Smiley-Williams arteriography
	needle
Smiley-Williams needle
smiling incision
Smillie cartilage chisel
Smillie cartilage knife
Smillie chisel
Smillie knee joint retractor
Smillie knife
Smillie meniscal cartilage knife
Smillie meniscectomy chisel
Smillie meniscotome
Smillie meniscus knife
Smillie nail
Smillie nail punch
Smillie pin
Smillie retractor
Smirmaul eyelid speculum
Smirmaul nucleus extractor
Smith anal retractor
Smith anal speculum
Smith and Nephew acetabular
	cup implant
Smith and Nephew barbed
	staple
Smith and Nephew Richards
	forceps
Smith and Nephew screw
Smith and Nephew small barbed
	staple
Smith aneurysmal clip
Smith anoscope
Smith bandage scissors
Smith bone clamp
Smith cartilage stripper
Smith cataract extraction
Smith cataract knife
Smith clamp
Smith cordotomy clamp
Smith cordotomy knife
Smith dislocation
Smith dissector
Smith drill
Smith electrode
Smith endoscopic electrode
Smith expressor
Smith expressor hook
Smith eye speculum

Smith eyelid operation
Smith flexor pollicis longus
	abductorplasty
Smith forceps
Smith fracture
Smith grasping forceps
Smith headlamp
Smith hook
Smith Indian technique
Smith intraocular implant lens
Smith knife
Smith lens expressor
Smith lid expressor
Smith lid hook
Smith lid-retracting hook
Smith lion-jaw forceps
Smith marginal clamp
Smith modification
Smith nerve root suction
	retractor
Smith obstetrical forceps
Smith operation
Smith orbital floor implant
Smith perforator
Smith pessary
Smith posterior cartilage stripper
Smith prosthesis
Smith rectal retractor
Smith rectal self-retaining
	retractor
Smith retractor
Smith retroversion pessary
Smith scissors
Smith Silastic prosthesis
Smith speculum
Smith suture wire scissors
Smith technique
Smith tonsillar dissector
Smith total ankle prosthesis
Smith trabeculotomy
Smith tube
Smith vaginal self-retaining
	retractor
Smith wire-cutting scissors
Smith-Boyce operation
Smith-Buie anal retractor
Smith-Buie rectal retractor
Smith-Buie rectal self-retaining
	retractor
Smith-Buie rectal speculum
Smith-Buie self-retaining rectal
	retractor

Smith-Fisher cataract knife
Smith-Fisher cataract lamp
Smith-Fisher cataract spatula
Smith-Fisher iris replacer
Smith-Fisher iris spatula
Smith-Gibson operation
Smith-Green cataract knife
Smith-Green double-end spatula
Smith-Hodge pessary
Smith-Indian operation
Smith-Kuhnt-Szymanowski
  operation
Smith-Leiske cross-action
  intraocular lens forceps
Smith-Leiske lens manipulator
Smith-Lemli-Opitz syndrome
Smith-Magenis syndrome
Smith-Miller-Patch cryosurgical
  instrument
Smith-Petersen acromioplasty
Smith-Petersen approach
Smith-Petersen arthrodesis
Smith-Petersen arthroplasty
  gouge
Smith-Petersen bone plate
Smith-Petersen cannulated nail
Smith-Petersen capsular
  retractor
Smith-Petersen capsule retractor
Smith-Petersen chisel
Smith-Petersen cup
Smith-Petersen cup arthroplasty
Smith-Petersen curet
Smith-Petersen curved
  osteotome
Smith-Petersen elevator
Smith-Petersen extractor
Smith-Petersen forceps
Smith-Petersen fracture pin
Smith-Petersen gouge
Smith-Petersen hammer
Smith-Petersen hemiarthroplasty
Smith-Petersen hip cup
  prosthesis
Smith-Petersen hip reamer
Smith-Petersen impactor
Smith-Petersen incision
Smith-Petersen intertrochanteric
  plate
Smith-Petersen laminectomy
  rongeur
Smith-Petersen mallet

Smith-Petersen nail
Smith-Petersen nail extractor
Smith-Petersen nailing
Smith-Petersen operation
Smith-Petersen osteotome
Smith-Petersen osteotomy
Smith-Petersen pin
Smith-Petersen plate
Smith-Petersen prosthesis
Smith-Petersen reamer
Smith-Petersen retractor
Smith-Petersen rongeur
Smith-Petersen spatula
Smith-Petersen straight
  osteotome
Smith-Petersen technique
Smith-Petersen tucker
Smith-Petersen wrist arthrodesis
Smith-Petersen bone gouge
Smith-Potts scissors
Smith-Richards instrumentation
Smith-Riley syndrome
Smith-Robinson anterior
  approach
Smith-Robinson anterior cervical
  diskectomy
Smith-Robinson anterior fusion
Smith-Robinson cervical disk
  approach
Smith-Robinson cervical fusion
Smith-Robinson interbody
  fusion
Smith-Robinson operation
Smith-Robinson procedure
Smith-Robinson technique
Smithuysen ethmoidal punch
Smithuysen sphenoidal punch
Smithwick anastomotic clamp
Smithwick blunt nerve hook
Smithwick buttonhook
Smithwick buttonhook button
Smithwick clamp
Smithwick clip
Smithwick clip-applying forceps
Smithwick dissector
Smithwick dissector hook
Smithwick forceps
Smithwick ganglion hook
Smithwick hook
Smithwick nerve dissector
Smithwick nerve hook
Smithwick operation

Smithwick retractor
Smithwick silk buttonhook
Smithwick silver clip
Smithwick sympathectomy
Smithwick sympathectomy
   hook
Smithwick-Hartmann forceps
SMM (scintimammography)
SMo (stainless steel with
   molybdenum)
SMo Moore pin
SMo plate
SMo prosthesis
Smoke Controller device
smoke evacuator suction tube
smoke removal tube
Smokeeter tube
smoker's cancer
smoker's heart
smoker's lines
smoker's palate
smoker's patches
smoker's tongue
SmokEvac electrosurgical probe
SmokEvac smoke evacuator
SmokEvac trumpet valve
Smolik curved rongeur
Smolinski endaural rongeur
smooth broach
smooth cannula
smooth dressing forceps
smooth endoprosthesis
smooth lesion
smooth liver edge
smooth margin
smooth muscle
smooth pin
smooth skin-colored lesion
smooth staple implant
smooth surface cavity
smooth tissue forceps
smooth transfixion wire
Smoothbeam laser
Smoothie Junior bur
smooth-pursuit eye movement
smooth-tipped jeweler's forceps
smooth-tooth forceps
smooth-walled uterus
SMPS (sympathetically
   maintained pain syndrome)
SMR (submucous resection)
SMR speculum

Smuckler tucker
SMZ zoom stereomicroscope
SN (sella nasion)
SN line
SN plane
SNAC (scaphoid nonunion
   advanced collapse)
SNAC wrist
snaggle tooth
snail-headed catheter retriever
SNAP (sensory nerve action
   potential)
snap fixation pin
snap gauge band
Snap Lock wire/pin extractor
snap-frozen biopsy
Snap-Gauge gauge
snap-lock brace
snap-on inserter plate
snap-on mandrel
snapping tendon
snare
   AcuSnare snare
   Alfred snare
   Amplatz retinal snare
   automatic ratchet snare
   Banner enucleation snare
   barbed snare
   Beck-Schenck tonsillar snare
   Beck-Storz tonsillar snare
   BiSNARE bipolar polypectomy
      snare
   Boettcher-Fralow snare
   Bosworth nasal snare
   Brown tonsillar snare
   Bruening ear snare
   Bruening nasal snare
   Bruening tonsillar snare
   Buerger snare
   Captiflex polypectomy snare
   Captivator polypectomy snare
   Castroviejo enucleation snare
   cautery snare
   caval snare
   coaxial snare
   cold snare
   Colles snare
   Cox polypectomy snare
   Crapeau nasal snare
   crescent snare
   cystoscopic snare
   Dean ear snare

snare (*continued*)
  diathermal snare
  diathermic snare
  dissection and snare
  dissection snare
  Douglas mucosal snare
  Douglas nasal snare
  Douglas rectal snare
  Douglas tonsillar snare
  Douglas-Roberts snare
  ear polyp snare
  ear snare
  electrosurgical snare
  endoscopic snare
  enucleation snare
  enucleation wire snare
  Eves tonsillar snare
  Eves-Neivert tonsillar snare
  eye enucleation snare
  Foerster enucleation snare
  Foerster snare
  Farlow tonsil snare
  Farlow tonsillar snare
  Farlow-Boettcher tonsil snare
  fascial snare
  Foerster enucleation snare
  Frankfeldt diathermy snare
  Frankfeldt rectal snare
  Freidenwald-Guyton snare
  frontalis snare
  galvanocaustic snare
  Glegg nasal polyp snare
  Glisson snare
  Goebel-Stoeckel snare
  gooseneck snare
  hand cock-up snare
  Harris snare
  hexagon snare
  Hobbs polypectomy snare
  hot snare
  Hoyer snare
  Jarvis snare
  Krause ear polyp snare
  Krause ear snare
  Krause laryngeal snare
  Krause nasal polyp snare
  Krause nasal snare
  Lange-Wilde snare
  laryngeal snare
  lasso snare
  Layman-Storz snare
  levator snare

snare (*continued*)
  Lewis tonsillar snare
  long-nose retriever snare
  Marlex mesh snare
  Martin snare
  Mason-Allen snare
  Meek snare
  Microvena Amplatz goose
    neck snare
  Milwaukee snare
  Myles tonsillectome snare
  nasal snare
  Neivert tonsillar snare
  Neivert-Eves tonsillar snare
  Nesbit tonsillar snare
  Newhart-Casselberry snare
  Norwood rectal snare
  Olympus semicircular snare
  open electrocautery snare
  pelvic snare
  pericardial snare
  polyethylene snare
  polyp snare
  polypectomy snare
  Posey snare
  Profile pediatric polypectomy
    snare
  ptosis snare
  pulmonary arterial snare
  Pynchon ear snare
  Quire mechanical finger snare
  Rainbow envelope arm snare
  Rauchfuss snare
  rectal cautery snare
  rectal snare
  Reiner-Beck tonsillar snare
  Roberts nasal snare
  rotatable polypectomy snare
  Sage tonsillar snare
  Sayre head snare
  self-opening rigid snare
  Sensation snare
  Singular oval polypectomy
    snare
  SmallHand polypectomy snare
  standard endoscopy
    polypectomy snare
  Stewart lenticular nuclear
    snare
  Stiegler unipolar nasal snare
  Storz snare
  Storz-Beck tonsillar snare

snare (*continued*)
Storz-Beck-Schenck snare
Stutsman nasal snare
Supramid snare
surgical snare
Teare snare
tonsillar snare
Tydings automatic ratchet
    snare
Tydings tonsillar snare
UroSnare cystoscopic tumor
    snare
Veeder tip snare
Wappler polypectomy snare
Weil pelvic snare
Weston rectal snare
Wilde ear polyp snare
Wilde nasal snare
Wilde-Bruening ear snare
Wilde-Bruening nasal snare
Wilson-Cook polypectomy
    snare
wire snare
Wright nasal snare
Wright tonsillar snare
Zimmer snare
snare catheter
snare cautery
snare electrocoagulation
snare enucleator
snare excision biopsy
snare loop biopsy
snare technique
snare tonsillectomy
snare wire
snarl-tip appearance
SND (selective neck dissection)
Sneddon-Wilkinson disease
Snellen conventional reform eye
    implant
Snellen entropion forceps
Snellen entropion operation
Snellen eye chart
Snellen eye implant
Snellen forceps
Snellen lens loop
Snellen line
Snellen operation
Snellen ptosis operation
Snellen reform eye
Snellen soft contact lens
Snellen suture technique

Snellen sutures
Snellen vectis
Sniper Elite guidewire
Snitman endaural retractor
Snitman endaural self-retaining
    retractor
SN-N (sternal notch to nipple)
Snoopy arm sling
Snoopy breast
snoopy deformity
Snornomor device
snow plow rasp
Snow procedure
Snowden-Pencer forceps
Snowden-Pencer insufflator
Snowden-Pencer laparoscopic
    cholecystectomy
    instrument
Snowden-Pencer Super-Cut
    scissors
snowflake cataract
snow-plow injury
snowstorm cataract
Snug denture cushion
Snugfit eye patch
Snugs dressing
Snyder breast prosthesis
Snyder classification
Snyder corneal spring forceps
Snyder deep-surgery forceps
Snyder hemostat
Snyder Hemovac drain
Snyder Hemovac evacuator
Snyder Hemovac silicone sump
    drain
Snyder Hemovac suction tube
Snyder Hemovac tube
Snyder mini-Hemovac drain
Snyder suction device
Snyder Surgivac drainage
Snyder Surgivac suction tube
Snyder trocar
Snyder tube
S-O (salpingo-oophorectomy)
Soaker catheter
SOA-MCA (superficial occipital
    artery-middle cerebral
    artery)
soap-bubble pattern
soapsuds enema
Soave abdominal pull-through
    procedure

Soave endorectal pull-through
procedure
Soave operation
Soave procedure for megacolon
Soave pull-through procedure
Sobel-Kaplitt-Sawyer gas
endarterectomy set
Sober ureterostomy
Socin operation
sock
cast sock
electrode sock
stump sock
TED socks
thromboembolic disease
socks
socket
APOPPS, transtibial prosthetic
socket
concave loading socket
dry socket
flexible socket
Flo-Tech prosthetic socket
hard socket
HD Canadian-type socket
Iceross silicone socket
ICES socket
ischial containment socket
ischial-gluteal weightbearing
socket
joint socket
metal-backed socket
polyethylene socket
prosthetic socket
Pump-It-Up pneumatic socket
standard socket
supracondylar socket
suspension-type socket
tooth socket
socket joint
socket reconstruction
socket wrench
Soderstrom-Corson electrode
sodium chloride-impregnated
gauze
sodium pentothal anesthetic
agent
sodium-potassium aluminum
silicate abrasive
Soehendra
papillotome/sphincterotome
Soehendra catheter dilator

Soehendra dilating catheter
Soehendra dilator
Soehendra lithotripsy set
Soehendra stent extractor
Soehendra stent retrieval device
Soehendra stent retriever
Soehendra Universal catheter
Soemmering area
Soemmering arterial vein
Soemmering external radial
vein
Soemmering foramen
Soemmering ligament
Soemmering muscle
Soemmering ring
Soemmering ring cataract
Soemmering spot
Sof Gel HeelCup orthosis
Sof.Care mattress
Sofamor spinal instrument
Sofamore spinal instrumentation
device
Sof-Band bulky bandage
Sof-Care chair cushion
Sof-Care Plus cushion
Sofflex mattress
Sof-Foam dressing
Sof-Form conforming gauze
Sof-Gel palm shield
Sof-Gel palm shield splint
Sofield femoral deficiency
technique
Sofield operation
Sofield osteotomy
Sofield pseudarthrosis of tibia
Sofield retractor
Sofield retractor blade
Sofield retractor clip
Sofield rod
Sof-Kling conforming bandage
Soflens contact lens
SoFlex lens
Sof-Matt pressure reducing
mattress
Sofomor-Danek component
SofPulse electrotherapy device
Sof-Rol cast pad
Sof-Rol cast padding
Sof-Rol dressing
SOFS (superior orbital fissure
syndrome)
SofSeat pressure relief pad

Sofsilk coated and braided
  sutures
Sofsilk nonabsorbable silk
  sutures
SofSorb absorptive dressing
Soft & Silent diaper pant
soft ankle, cushioned heel
soft ankle, cushioned heel
  orthopaedic appliance
soft cartilage
soft cataract aspirator
soft catheter
soft cleft palate
soft contact lens
soft disk
soft event
soft exudate
soft fold
Soft Guard XL fecal
  incontinence bag
SOF-T guidewire
SOF-T guiding catheter
soft intraocular lens
soft lens
soft lesion
Soft N Dry Merocel sponge
soft palate
soft palate cleft
soft palate paralysis
soft palate retractor
soft palate tip
soft papilloma
soft rubber curet
soft rubber drain
Soft Seal cervical catheter
Soft Shield collagen corneal
  shield
soft silicone sphere implant
soft silicone sponge
soft structure injury
Soft Super Sport orthotic
Soft Support Preforms orthotic
soft tissue abnormality
soft tissue abscess
soft tissue augmentation
soft tissue blade retractor
soft tissue calcification
soft tissue contracture
soft tissue curettage
soft tissue cyst
soft tissue deformity
soft tissue dehiscence

soft tissue elevator
soft tissue expander
soft tissue expansion
  reconstruction
soft tissue gonion
soft tissue hypoplasia
soft tissue mass
soft tissue pinch-thickness at the
  inframammary fold
  (STPTIMF)
soft tissue pinch-thickness
  upper pole (STPTUP)
soft tissue reconstruction
soft tissue resection
soft tissue shaving cannula
soft tissue stranding
soft tissue thickness
soft tissue tumor
soft tissue undercut
soft tissue window
soft tissue windowing
Soft Torque uterine catheter
Soft Touch cup
Soft Touch lancet device
soft triangle of the nose
soft ulcer
soft wart
soft wire loop
soft x-ray examination
soft x-ray film
Soft-Cell permanent dual-lumen
  catheter
SoftCloth absorptive dressing
Softcon contact lens
Softcon lens
SofTec OA knee orthosis
Softech endotracheal tube
Softepil tweezer epilation
  device
Softexe non-adherent sub-
  bandage padding
Soft-EZ reusable electrode
Softeze self-adhering foam pad
Softeze water pillow
Softflo fiberoptic probe
SoftForm facial implant
SoftForm implant
SoftForm tube
Softgut chromic sutures
Softgut surgical chromic catgut
  sutures
Softgut sutures

Softies wrist and forearm splint
Softip arteriography catheter
Softip diagnostic catheter
Softjaw handless clamp
Softjaw insert
SoftLight laser
Softopac intraoral film
Softouch catheter
Softouch Cold/Hot Pack
Softouch guiding catheter
Softouch Headhunter catheter
Softouch multipurpose catheter
Softouch Simmons catheter
Softouch spinal angiography
    catheter
Softouch cardiac pigtail catheter
SofTouch vacuum erection
    device
soft-palate cancer
Softrace gel electrode
Softrac-PTA catheter
Softscan laser scanner
SoftSite multifocal contact lens
Softsplint foot splint
soft-tipped cannula
soft-tipped extrusion handpiece
soft-tipped guidewire
soft-tissue damage
soft-tissue dissection
soft-tissue extremity injury
soft-tissue flap
soft-tissue interface
soft-tissue interposition
soft-tissue lesion
soft-tissue metastasis
soft-tissue plication
soft-tissue Super Sport orthotic
Soft-Touch A-Probe
Soft-Vu angiographic catheter
Soft-Vu Omni flush catheter
Soft-Wand atraumatic tissue
    manipulator balloon
Sof-Wick drain
Sof-Wick drain sponges
Sof-Wick dressing
Sof-Wick lap pad
Sof-Wick sponge
SOF'WIRE spinal fixation
Sohes pacemaker
Soileau Tytan ventilation tube
Soilleau tube
Sokolec elevator

Sokolowski antral punch
Sola Optical Spectralite high-
    index lens
Sola VIP lens
SolAiris oxygen concentrator
solar cautery
solar cheilitis
solar dermatitis
solar elastosis
solar ganglion
solar keratosis
solar lentigo
Solar pacemaker
solar urticaria
Solcia classification
Solcotrans autotransfusion unit
Solcotrans closed vacuum drain
sole laser therapy
sole reflex
sole wedge
Solera thrombectomy catheter
soleus flap
soleus muscle
soleus-fibula free transfer
    reconstruction of lower
    limb
SOLEutions custom orthosis
SOLEutions custom orthotic
    device
SOLEutions orthotic
SOLEutions Prefab orthotic
    device
Solfy ZX ultrasonic unit
solid ankle cushioned heel
    (SACH)
solid buckling implant material
solid copper head mallet
solid hex bolt
solid hidradenoma
solid hyperplasia
solid organ
solid phase extraction
solid silicone buttock implant
solid silicone exoplant implant
    material
solid silicone orbital prosthesis
solid silicone with Supramid
    mesh implant
solid tumor
solid visceral hematoma
solid-ankle, cushioned-heel foot
    prosthesis

solid-appearing mass
solid-phase extraction tube
solid-rod rigid telescope
solid-state coagulator
solid-state esophageal
    manometry catheter
solid-state nuclear track
    detector
solid-state silk sutures
solid-tip catheter
Solis pacemaker
Solitaire needle
solitary bone cyst
solitary bundle
solitary foramen
solitary gland
solitary keratoacanthoma
solitary lesion
solitary nodule
solitary pulmonary
    arteriovenous fistula
solitary rectal ulcer syndrome
solitary simple lymphangioma
Solitens TENS unit
Solitens transcutaneous
    electrical nerve stimulation
    unit
Soll suture and incision marker
Solo catheter
Sol-O-Pake barium
SoloPass catheter
SoloPass biliary stent
SoloPass stent catheter
Solos disposable cannula
Solos disposable trocar
Solos endoscopy diagnostic
    laparoscope
SoloSite hydrogel dressing
SoloSite nonsterile hydrogel
    wound dressing
SoloSite wound gel
Solow sigmoidoscope
soluble bougie
soluble gas technique
soluble ligature
Solus pacemaker
Soluset device
Soluset IV set
solution
    1/6-molar lactate solution
    100th-normal solution
    AF solution (antifog solution)

solution (continued)
    antifogging solution (AF
        solution)
    Anti-Sept bactericidal scrub
        solution
    AstrinGYN solution
    bacitracin solution
    balanced salt solution (BSS)
    Betadine Helafoam solution
    Brompton solution
    Burow solution
    cardioplegic solution
    Cidex solution
    cold cardioplegic solution
    Collins solution
    collodion solution
    Dakin solution
    extravasation irrigation
        solution
    fixative solution
    Hartmann solution
    Hollande solution
    hydrolysis of solution
    hyperalimentation solution
    hypertonic solution
    Hyskon irrigation solution
    iced saline solution
    infusing solutions
    iodophor solution
    irrigated with normal saline
        solution
    irrigated with saline solution
    irrigating solution
    irrigation solution
    Jessner solution
    kanamycin solution
    Kantrex solution
    Klein formula tumescent
        solution
    lactate solution
    lactated Ringer's solution
    lavage solution
    Logol solution
    McCarey-Kaufman solution
    Microfil solution
    molal solution
    nebulized solution
    packaged irrigating solution
    priming solution
    PSKA antibiotic Hank solution
    Ringer's lactate solution
    Ringer's solution

solution (*continued*)
Roe solution
saline solution
saturated solution
Scholl solution
Shiller solution
sodium hyaluronate solution
Storz anti-fog solution
suspended in saline solution
Ultrastop anti-fogging solution
volumetric solution
Zamboni biopsy solution
Zephiran solution
Solvang graft
SOM (serous otitis media, secretory otitis media)
Somagyi reflex
Somanetics INVOS 3100 cerebral oximeter
SomaSensor device
SomaSensor pad
somatic gene-transfer approach
somatic muscles
somatic nerves
somatic sarcoma
Somatics monitoring electrode
Somatics mouth guard
Somatom DR CT scanner
Somatom Plus S whole-body scanner
somatosensory evoked potential (SEP)
somatosensory response
somatostatinoma syndrome
Somers clamp
Somers forceps
Somers tonsillar knife
Somers uterine clamp
Somers uterine elevator
Somers uterine forceps
Somers uterine-elevating forceps
Somerset bur
Somerset-Mack hand operation
Somerville anterior approach
Somerville open reduction
Somerville procedure
Somerville technique
SOMI (skull, occiput, mandibular immobilization)
SOMI brace
SOMI Jr. brace
SOMI orthosis

Somjee-Crabtree temporal bone support clamp
Somnoplasty
SomnoStar apnea testing device
Somnus probe
SON anesthetic agent
Sonablate transrectal probe
sonde coude
Sonde enteroscope
Sondergaard cleft
Sondergaard groove
Sondergaard operation
Sondergaard procedure
Sondermann canal
Sondermann suction tip
Sones arteriography
Sones brachial cutdown technique
Sones cardiac catheterization
Sones Cardio-Marker catheter
Sones cineangiography technique
Sones coronary arteriography
Sones coronary catheter
Sones guidewire
Sones hemostatic bag
Sones Hi-Flow catheter
Sones Positrol catheter
Sones selective coronary arteriogram
Sones technique
Sones vent catheter
Sones Dacron catheter
Songer cable
Songer tonsillar forceps
Sonic Air 1500 device
sonic applicator
sonic curet
sonic surgery
Sonicaid Axis monitor
Sonicaid system 8000 fetal monitor
Sonicath endoluminal ultrasound catheter
Sonicath imaging catheter
Sonicath intravascular ultrasound catheter
Sonicator portable ultrasound
Sonneberg operation
Sonnenberg classification
Sonnenberg sump drain
Sonnenschein nasal speculum

Sonoblate ablation device
Sonocath ultrasound probe
Sonocut ultrasonic aspirator
sonoencephalographic study
Sonogage System Corneo-Gage
 20-MHz center frequency
 transducer
Sonogage ultrasound
 pachymeter
sonography-guided aspiration
sonoguided biopsy
Sonoline Prima ultrasound
Sonoline Siemens ultrasound
 scanner
Sonolith lithotriptor
sonolucent area
sonolucent mass
Sonop handpiece
Sonop ultrasonic aspirator
Sonos cardiovascular ultrasound
Sonos scanner
Sonos ultrasonographic
 transducer
Sonos ultrasound imager
Sono-stat Plus EMG machine
Sono-Stat Plus sound device
Sonotrode lithotriptor
SonoVu aspiration needle
Sontec pliers
Sony color video camera
Sony Promavica still capture
 device
SOOF (suborbicularis oculi fat)
Soonawalla uterine elevator
Soonawalla vasectomy forceps
Soper cone hard contact lens
Soper modification
Sopha Medical gamma camera
Sopher ovum forceps
Sophie mammography unit
Sophy high-resolution collimator
Sophy pressure valve
Soprano cryotherapy unit
SorbaView composite wound
 dressing
Sorbex Thin hydrocolloid
 dressing
Sorbiclear dialyzer
Sorbie calcaneal fracture
 classification
Sorb-It dressing
Sorborthane heel cup

sorbose cushion
Sorbsan alginate dressing
Sorbsan dressing
Sorbsan gel block topical wound
 dressing
Sorbsan topical wound dressing
Sordille operation
Soren ankle fusion
Sorensen aspirator
Sorensen reusable canister
Sorenson catheter for CVP line
Sorenson sinus cleanser
Sorenson thermodilution
 catheter
Sorenson-Yankauer combination
 pump
Soresi cannula
Soria operation
Soriano operation
Sorin cardiac prosthetic valve
Sorin mitral valve prosthesis
Sorin pacemaker
Sorin prosthetic valve
Sorondo hindquarter
 amputation
Sorondo-Ferre amputation
Sorondo-Ferre hindquarter
 amputation
Sorrin operation
SOS guidewire
SOS Omni catheter
Soto USCI balloon
Soto-Hall bone graft
Soto-Hall bone graft technique
Soto-Hall patellectomy
Soto-Hall sign
Soto-Hall-West patellectomy
Sotteau operation
Soules intrauterine insemination
 catheter
Souligoux-Morestin lavage
sound (see also bougie,
 searcher)
 absent breath sounds
 absolute bowel sounds
 active bowel sounds
 adventitious breath sounds
 adventitious sounds
 Allport mastoid sound
 Allport-Babcock sound
 aortic second sound (A2)
 aortic sound

sound (*continued*)

- auscultatory sound
- Bellocq sound
- Bellows sound
- Benique sound
- bladder sound
- bowel sounds
- bronchial breath sounds
- bronchocele sound
- Campbell miniature sound
- Campbell miniature urethral sound
- Campbell urethral sound
- Campbell-French sound
- cardiac sounds
- clicking sound
- coarse breath sounds
- Collin sound
- common duct sound
- cracked-pot sound
- crunching sound
- Davis sound
- dilation with metal sound
- diminished bowel sounds
- diminished breath sounds
- Dittel urethral sound
- Dittel uterine sound
- Ellik sound
- esophageal sound
- eustachian sound
- expiratory sounds
- female sound
- fetal heart sounds (FHS)
- flapping sound
- flexible sound
- Fowler urethral sound
- French steel sound
- French-following metal sound
- fricative sounds
- friction sound
- full-curve sound
- Gouley tunneled urethral sound
- Gouley urethral sound
- graduated sound
- grating sound
- Greenwald sound
- gurgling bowel sounds
- guttural sound
- Guyon dilating sound
- Guyon urethral sound

sound (*continued*)

- Guyon-Benique urethral sound
- heart sounds
- high-pitched bowel sounds
- Hishida pine-needle sound
- Hunt metal sound
- hyperactive bowel sounds
- hypoactive bowel sounds
- infant sound
- infant urethral sound
- inspiratory sounds
- interlocking sound
- Jewett urethral sound
- Jewett uterine sound
- Klebanoff common duct sound
- Kocher bronchocele sound
- Korotkoff sound
- lacrimal sound
- LeFort urethral sound
- LeFort uterine sound
- low-pitched bowel sounds
- Mark-7 intrauterine sound
- Martin uterine sound
- McCrae infant sound
- meatal sound
- Mercier sound
- metal sound
- miniature sound
- musical bowel sounds
- normoactive bowel sounds
- Otis prostatic urethral sound
- Otis urethral sound
- passage of sound
- percussion sound
- peristaltic sounds
- Pharmaseal disposable uterine sound
- positive bowel sounds
- Prall urethral sound
- Pratt urethral sound
- quiet bowel sounds
- radiolucent sound
- Rica uterine sound
- rigid sound
- Rissler vein sound
- Ritter sound
- rumbling bowel sounds
- Saf-T-Sound uterine sound
- Schroeder interlocking uterine sound

sound (*continued*)
   shaking sound
   Simpson uterine sound
   Sims uterine sound
   splitting of heart sounds
   succussion sounds
   tinkling bowel sounds
   to-and-fro friction sounds
   urethral sound
   uterine sound
   Van Buren canvas roll sound
   Van Buren dilating sound
   van Buren urethral sound
   Walther urethral sound
   Winternitz sound
   Woodward sound
   xiphisternal crunching sound
sound level meter
sounds and bougies (*see* bougie, sound)
soupy material
source
   ACMI fiberoptic light source
   cesium sources
   cryogen source
   dual-beam fiberoptic light source
   endoscopic light source
   fiberoptic cold light source
   fiberoptic light source
   implanting radioactive sources
   organ source
   point source
   Storz fiberoptic light source
sourcil fracture
Sourdille forceps
Sourdille keratoplasty
Sourdille keratoplasty operation
Sourdille operation
Sourdille ptosis operation
Souter hinge
Southbent scissors
Southern blot technique
Southern Eye Bank corneal cutting block
Southey anasarca trocar
Southey cannula
Southey capillary drainage tube
Southey trocar
Southey tube
Southey-Leech trocar

Southey-Leech tube
Southwick clamp
Southwick osteotomy
Southwick procedure
Southwick screw extractor
Southwick slide procedure
Southwick-Robinson anterior cervical approach
Southworth rasp
Souttar cautery
Souttar craniotomy incision
Souttar esophageal conductor
Souttar iliac crest fasciotomy
Souttar incision
Souttar operation
Souttar skin incision
Souttar tube
Souttar-Campbell slide
Sovak reamer
Sovally suprapubic suction cup drain
Sovereign bifocal lens
Soviet mechanical bronchial stapler
SP (status post; suprapatellar; sacroposterior)
SP Dynamic Range of Motion Elbow Orthosis
SP Dynamic Range of Motion Knee Orthosis
SP needle holder
SP position (sacroposterior position)
SP6 camera
Spa Bed
space
   5th intercostal space
   abdominal space
   acromioclavicular space
   air space
   alveolar dead space
   anatomic dead space
   anatomical dead space
   anorectal space
   antecubital space
   anterior clear space
   apical space
   arachnoid space
   Aries space
   avascular space
   axillary space
   Bottcher space

space (*continued*)
Berger space
Bogros space
Bowman space
Broca space
buccal space
buccinator space
buccopharyngeal space
Burns space
capsular space
carotid space
cartilage space
central palmar space
cerebral epidural space
Chassaignac space
circumlental space
Colles space
constricted web space
coracoclavicular space
corneal space
costoclavicular space
Cotunnius space
cranial epidural space
craniospinal space
Czermak spaces
danger space
dead space
deep perineal space
deep postanal anorectal
   space
deep space
Denonvilliers space
denture space
digastric space
disk space
Disse space
dorsal subaponeurotic space
echo-free space
edentulous space
embrasure space
endolymphatic space
epicardial space
epicerebral space
epidural space
episcleral space
extracellular space
extraction space
extradural space
extraperitoneal space
extrapleural space
extravascular space
fascial space

space (*continued*)
fat cell space
first web space
fixed maintainer space
Fontana space
Forel space
freeway space
geniohyoid space
gingival space
H-space
haversian space
Henke space
His perivascular space
Holzknecht space
hypothenar space
iliocostal space
incisural space
increased lateral joint space
infraglottic space
inframesocolic space
infraorbital space
infratemporal space
interalveolar space
interarytenoid space
intercellular space
intercellular tissue space
intercondylar space
intercostal space
intercristal space
interdental space
interdigital spaces
interfascial space
interlamellar space
interocclusal rest space
interorbital space
interpedicular joint space
interpleural space
interprismatic space
interproximal space
interradicular space
intersheath space
intersphincteric anorectal
   space
interstitial spaces
intervaginal space
interventricular space
intracristal space
intrafascial space
intramembranous space
intrapharyngeal space
intrathecal space
intravaginal space

space (*continued*)

intravesical space
ischiorectal anorectal space
joint space
K-space
Kiernan space
Larrey space
lateral central palmar space
lateral joint space
lateral pharyngeal space
lateropharyngeal space
lattice space
leeway space
left 5th intercostal space
left intercostal space
leptomeningeal space
Lesgaft space
life space
lymph space
Magendie space
maintainer cast space
Malacarne space
mandibular space
marrow space
masseteric space
masseter-mandibular-
    pterygoid space
masseter-mandibulopterygoid
    space
masticator space
masticatory space
Meckel space
medial clear space
mediastinal space
medullary space
middle palmar space
midpalmar space
Mohrenheim space
Nance leeway space
object space
obtainer space
palm space
palmar space
paraglottic space
paralaryngeal space
parapharyngeal space
pararenal space
paravesical space
Parona space
parotid space
perforated space
perianal anorectal space

space (*continued*)

pericardial space
perichoroidal space
peridental space
peridentinoblastic space
perihepatic space
peri-implant space
perilenticular space
perilymphatic space
perineal space
perinuclear space
perioptic subarachnoid space
periotic space
peripharyngeal space
perirenal space
periscleral space
perisinusoidal space
peritoneal space
peritonsillar space
perivascular lymph spaces
perivascular space
perivitelline space
pharyngeal space
pharyngomaxillary space
physiological dead space
plantar space
pleural space
pleuroperitoneal space
pneumatic space
Poiseuille space
popliteal space
portal space
position in space
postcricoid space
posterior cervical space
posterior septal space
postpharyngeal space
poststyloid space
postzygomatic space
potassium space
predental space
pre-epiglottic space
premasseteric space
preperitoneal space
preputial space
presacral space
preseptal space
presternal space
prestyloid space
pretarsal space
pretemporal space
pretracheal space

space (*continued*)
  prevertebral space
  prevesical space
  prevesicle space
  prezonular space
  properitoneal space
  Proust space
  proximal space
  proximate space
  Prussak space
  pterygomandibular space
  pterygomaxillary space
  pterygopalatine space
  pterygopharyngeal space
  quadrangular space
  quadrilateral space
  rectovaginal space
  rectovesical space
  regainer space
  relief space
  removable maintainer space
  retraction space
  retroadductor space
  retrobulbar space
  retrocardiac space
  retrocrural space
  retroesophageal space
  retrogastric space
  retroinguinal space
  retrolental space
  retromammary space
  retromuscular space
  retromylohyoid space
  retro-ocular space
  retroparotid space
  retroperitoneal space
  retropharyngeal space
  retropubic space
  retroseptal space
  retrosternal air space
  retrotracheal space
  retrovesical space
  retrovisceral space
  retrozygomatic space
  Retzius space
  Rienke space
  right anterior pararenal
    space
  rudimentary disk space
  scapholunate joint space
  Schwalbe spaces
  septal space

space (*continued*)
  sinusoidal spaces
  sphenomaxillary space
  sphenopalatine space
  spinal epidural space
  subacromial space
  subaponeurotic space
  subarachnoid space
  subchorial space
  subcoracoid space
  subdiaphragmatic space
  subdural space
  subepicranial space
  subfascial palmar space
  subfascial web space
  subgaleal space
  subgingival space
  subhepatic space
  sublingual space
  submandibular space
  submasseteric space
  submaxillary space
  submental space
  submucosal space
  subperitoneal space
  subphrenic space
  subpulmonic pleural space
  subretinal space
  subumbilical space
  superficial perineal space
  superior joint space
  supracolic space
  suprahepatic space
  suprahyoid space
  supralevator anorectal space
  supralevator space
  supraomental space
  suprasternal space
  supratentorial space
  Tarin space
  temporal space
  Tenon space
  thenar space
  thenar web space
  thumb-index web space
  thyrohyal space
  tibiofibular clear space
  tissue spaces
  Traube semilunar space
  Trautmann triangular space
  triangular space
  urethrovaginal space

space (*continued*)
  vascular space
  vertebral epidural space
  vesicocervical space
  Virchow space
  Virchow-Robin space
  visceral space
  vitreous space
  Waldeyer space
  web space
  Westberg space
  widened retrogastric space
  yolk space
  Zang space
  zonular space
  zygomaticotemporal space
space myopia
space of body of mandible
space of Donders
space of Fontana
space of Forel
space of Poirier
space of Retzius
space of Retzius abscess
space of Smith
space of Tenon
space of Traube
space-age wire
Spacekeeper retractor
SpaceLabs Holter monitor
SpaceLabs pulse oximeter
Spacemaker balloon dissector
Spacemaker hernia balloon
    dissector
Spacemaker balloon
space-occupying brain lesion
space-occupying disease
space-occupying lesion
Space-OR flexible internal
    retractor
spacer inserter
SpaceSEAL balloon tip cannula
spacing material
spade fingers
spade hand
Spaeth cystic bleb operation
Spaeth facial nerve block
Spaeth ptosis operation
spaghetti drain
spaghetti fat grafting technique
spaghetti wrist
Spaide scleral depressor

Spalding-Richardson
    hysterectomy
Spalding-Richardson operation
Spaleck forceps
Span-aid abduction pillow
Span-aid bed supports
Spandage bandage
Spanish blue virgin silk sutures
Spanish tourniquet
spanner gauge
spanning external fixator
SPARC procedure
spare parts surgery
Spark handheld dynamometer
Sparks atrioseptal punch
Sparks mandrel graft
Sparks mandrel prosthesis
Sparks mandrel technique
sparsity of bone formation
Sparta micro iris forceps
Sparta microforceps
Sparta micro-iris forceps
Spartan jaw wire cutter
spasm
  Bell spasm
  carpopedal spasm
  cerebral spasm
  clinic spasm
  clonic spasm
  diffuse esophageal spasm
  duodenal spasm
  esophageal spasm
  facial spasm
  fixed spasm
  gastrointestinal spasm
  glottic spasm
  hemifacial spasm
  inspiratory spasm
  intention spasm
  laryngeal spasm
  masticatory spasm
  mixed spasm
  muscular spasm
  paravertebral muscle spasm
  Romberg spasm
  rotatory spasm
  stomach spasms
  tonoclonic spasm
  vascular spasm
  vasomotor spasm
  winking spasm
spasmodic entropion operation

spasmodic laryngitis
spasmodic stricture
spasmoid talipes
spastic gait
spastic stricture
spastic thumb-in-palm deformity
spatial localization procedure
spatial resolution
spatial vectorcardiogram
spatially separated foci
spatula
   T-spatula
   Allison lung spatula
   angled iris spatula
   angulated iris spatula
   Ayes spatula
   Aylesbury cervical spatula
   Ayre cervical spatula
   Bakelite spatula
   Banaji spatula
   Bangerter angled iris spatula
   Barraquer cyclodialysis
     spatula
   Barraquer iris spatula
   Barraquer irrigator spatula
   Bechert irrigating spatula
   Berens plastic spatula
   Birks micro push/pull spatula
   brain spatula
   capsule fragment spatula
   Castroviejo cyclodialysis
     spatula
   Castroviejo double-end
     spatula
   Castroviejo synechia spatula
   Cave scaphoid spatula
   cement spatula
   Children's Hospital brain
     spatula
   Clayman spatula
   Cleasby iris spatula
   corneal fascia lata spatula
   corneal graft spatula
   coronary endarterectomy
     spatula
   Crile spatula
   Culler iris spatula
   curved-tipped spatula
   Cushing brain spatula
   Cushing S-shaped brain
     spatula
   cyclodialysis spatula

spatula (*continued*)
   Cytobrush spatula
   Davis brain spatula
   D'Errico brain spatula
   DeWecker iris spatula
   Dixey spatula
   Dorsey spatula
   double spatula
   double-ended spatula
   double-vector brain spatula
   Doyen spatula
   Drews suture pickup spatula
   Drews-Sato capsular fragment
     spatula
   Drews-Sato suture-pickup
     spatula
   duck-billed anodized spatula
   electrosurgical spatula
   Elschnig cyclodialysis spatula
   endarterectomy spatula
   Fisher-Smith spatula
   fishtail spatula
   flat spatula
   Fragmatome tip with
     ultrasound spatula
   Freer nasal spatula
   French hook spatula
   French lacrimal spatula
   French-pattern eye spatula
   French-pattern spatula
   Fukasaku spatula
   Galin lens spatula
   Garron spatula
   Gass endarterectomy spatula
   Gill-Welsh spatula
   Girard synechia spatula
   Green double spatula
   Green eye spatula
   Green lens spatula
   Green replacer spatula
   Gross brain spatula
   Guimaraes ophthalmic flap
     spatula
   Haberer abdominal spatula
   Halle vascular spatula
   Heifitz spatula
   Hersh LASIK retreatment
     spatula
   Hertzog lens spatula
   Hirschman iris spatula
   Hirschman lens spatula
   hook spatula

spatula (*continued*)

hook with spatula
Hough spatula
iridodialysis spatula
iris spatula
irrigating eye spatula
irrigating notched spatula
Jacobson endarterectomy
    spatula
Jaffe intraocular spatula
Jaffe lens spatula
Johnson spatula
Kader intestinal spatula
Kallmorgen vaginal spatula
Katena iris spatula
Kellman-Elschnig cyclodialysis
    spatula
Kennerdell spatula
Killian laryngeal spatula
Kimura platinum spatula
Kirby angulated iris spatula
Kirby iris spatula
Knapp cyclodialysis spatula
Knapp iris spatula
Knolle lens cortex spatula
Knolle lens nucleus spatula
Kocher bladder spatula
Korte abdominal spatula
Krause-Davis spatula
Kummel intestinal spatula
Kwitko lens spatula
Laird cyclodialysis spatula
Legueu spatula
lens spatula
Leriche spatula
Lewicky IOL spatula
Lieppman spatula
Lindner cyclodialysis spatula
lingual spatula
Lynch spatula
Maddox LASIK spatula
malleable spatula
Manhattan Eye & Ear spatula
Masket phaco spatula
Maumenee vitreous sweep
    spatula
Maumenee-Barraquer vitreous
    sweep spatula
Mayfield brain spatula
Mayfield malleable brain
    spatula
McIntyre irrigating spatula

spatula (*continued*)

McPherson iris spatula
McReynolds eye spatula
Medscand cervical spatula
Meller cyclodialysis spatula
microsurgical spatula
microvitreoretinal spatula
Mikulicz spatula
Milex spatula
Millin bladder spatula
Mills coronary
    endarterectomy spatula
Morgenstein spatula
needle spatula
nerve separator spatula
nucleus spatula
O'Brien spatula
Obstbaum lens spatula
Obstbaum synechia spatula
Olivecrona brain spatula
Olk retinal spatula
Olk vitreoretinal spatula
Pallin lens spatula
Paton double spatula
Paton single spatula
Peyton brain spatula
phakodialysis spatula
plaster spatula
platinum conjunctival smear
    spatula
platinum probe spatula
platinum spatula
probe spatula
Raaf flexible lighted spatula
Rainin lens spatula
Ray brain spatula
rectangular brain spatula
regular eye spatula
Reverdin abdominal spatula
Rica brain spatula
Rizzuti graft carrier spatula
Rolon spatula
Roux spatula
Rowen spatula
Sachs nerve spatula
scaphoid spatula
Schmid vascular spatula
Schuknecht spatula
Scoville brain spatula
Scoville flat brain spatula
Segond vaginal spatula
Sheets lens spatula

spatula (*continued*)
  Sheets-Hirsch spatula
  side-biting spatula
  side-cutting spatula
  Simcoe notched irrigating
    spatula
  Simcoe nucleus spatula
  Simmons-Kimbrough
    glaucoma spatula
  Sinclair spatula
  Sinskey nucleus spatula
  SMIC abdominal spatula
  SMIC brain spatula
  Smith-Fisher cataract spatula
  Smith-Fisher iris spatula
  Smith-Green double-end
    spatula
  Smith-Petersen spatula
  spoon and spatula
  spoon spatula
  S-shaped brain spatula
  stainless spatula
  Sterling iris spatula
  Suker cyclodialysis spatula
  surgical spatula
  suture pickup spatula
  synechia spatula
  Tan spatula
  tapered brain spatula
  Tauber vaginal spatula
  Tennant eye spatula
  Thomas spatula
  Thornton malleable spatula
  Tooke spatula
  transplant spatula
  Troutman iris spatula
  Troutman lens spatula
  Troutman-Barraquer iris
    spatula
  Tuffier abdominal spatula
  ultrasound spatula
  University of Kansas eye
    spatula
  vaginal spatula
  vitreous sweep spatula
  wax-removing spatula
  Weary brain spatula
  Wecker iris spatula
  Wecker silver spatula
  Wells eye spatula
  Wheeler cyclodialysis spatula
  Wheeler iris spatula

spatula (*continued*)
  Woodson spatula
  Wullstein transplant spatula
  Wurmuth spatula
  Wylie endarterectomy spatula
spatula and spoon
spatula cannula
spatula cannula tip
spatula dissector
spatula electrosurgical probe
spatula foot
spatula forceps
spatula hook
spatula needle sutures
spatula spoon
spatula tip cannula
spatula-split needle
spatulated half-circle needle
Spaulding classification
Spaulding-Richardson
    hysterectomy
SPC (scaphopisocapitate)
spear blade
spear dural hook
spear-ended chrome probe
Spears USCI laser balloon
Speas strabismus operation
special Colles splint
special wound care
specimen
  biohazard specimen
  biopsy specimen
  catheterized specimen
  cone specimen
  gastrectomy specimen
  pathologic specimen
  slide specimen
  sterile specimen
specimen container
specimen forceps
specimen jar
Speck introducer
Speck-Ange cutter
speckled leukoplakia
speckled pattern of myocardium
SPECT (single photon emission
    computed tomography)
SPECT single-headed camera
SPECT dual-headed camera
SPECT imaging
SPECT scan
spectacle hematoma

spectacle plane
SPECT Bullseye scans
Spectra pad
Spectra-Cath catheter
Spectra-Diasonics ultrasound
Spectraflex pacemaker
spectral analysis
spectral Doppler
Spectralite Transitions lens
Spectramed transducer
Spectranetics laser
Spectranetics laser sheath
Spectranetics P23 Statham
    transducer
Spectranetics support catheter
Spectra-Physics argon laser
Spectra-Physics microsurgical
    laser
Spectraprobe-Max probe
Spectraprobe-PLS laser
    angioplasty catheter
Spectra-System implant
Spectrax bipolar pacemaker
Spectrax programmable
    Medtronic pacemaker
Spectrax SXT pulse generator
Spectron cemented hip
    prosthesis
Spectron femoral component
Spectron hip prosthesis
Spectron metal-backed cup for
    Richards hip prosthesis
Spectron prosthesis
Spectron total hip
Spectron total hip stem
spectrophotometer
spectrophotometry
spectroscopy
spectroscopy-directed laser
spectrum (*pl.* spectra,
    spectrums)
spectrum concept to skin
    rejuvenation
Spectrum Designs facial implant
Spectrum K1 laser
Spectrum ruby laser
Spectrum silicone Foley
    catheter
SPECTurn chair
specular attachment
specular microscope
specular microscopy

Specular reflex slit lamp
speculum
    4-prong finger speculum
    adolescent vaginal speculum
    Adson speculum
    Agrikola eye speculum
    Alfonso eyelid speculum
    Allen-Heffernan nasal speculum
    Allingham rectal speculum
    Amko vaginal speculum
    anal speculum
    anoscope speculum
    Arruga eye speculum
    Arruga globe speculum
    Artisan wide-angle vaginal
        speculum
    Aufricht septal speculum
    Aufricht septum speculum
    Aumence eyelid speculum
    aural speculum
    Auvard Britetrac speculum
    Auvard weighted vaginal
        speculum
    Auvard-Remine vaginal
        speculum
    Auvard-Remine weighted
        speculum
    Azar lid speculum
    Barany speculum
    Barnes speculum
    Barr anal speculum
    Barr rectal speculum
    Barraquer eye speculum
    Barraquer solid speculum
    Barraquer wire lid speculum
    Barraquer wire speculum
    Barraquer-Colibri eye
        speculum
    Barraquer-Douvas eye
        speculum
    Barraquer-Floyd speculum
    Barraquer-Kratz speculum
    Barr-Shuford rectal speculum
    basket-style scleral supporter
        speculum
    Beard eye speculum
    Becker-Park eye speculum
    Beckman nasal speculum
    Beckman-Colver nasal
        speculum
    Bedrossian eye speculum
    Bercovici wire lid speculum

speculum (*continued*)
  Berens eye speculum
  Berlind-Auvard vaginal speculum
  beveled speculum
  Bionix disposable nasal speculum
  Bionix nasal speculum
  bivalved anal speculum
  bivalved ear speculum
  bivalved speculum
  blackened speculum
  Bodenheimer rectal speculum
  Bosworth nasal speculum
  Bosworth nasal wire speculum
  Boucheron ear speculum
  Bovin vaginal speculum
  Bovin-Stille vaginal speculum
  Bowman eye speculum
  Bozeman speculum
  brain speculum
  Braun speculum
  Breisky vaginal speculum
  Breisky-Navratil vaginal speculum
  Breisky-Stille speculum
  Brescio-Breisky-Navratil speculum
  Brewer vaginal speculum
  Brinkerhoff rectal speculum
  Britetrac speculum
  Bronson speculum
  Bronson-Park speculum
  Bronson-Turtz speculum
  Brown ear speculum
  Bruening speculum
  Bruner vaginal speculum
  Barany speculum
  Buie-Hirschman speculum
  Buie-Smith rectal speculum
  Burnett Sani-Spec disposable speculum
  Callahan modification speculum
  Carpel speculum
  Carter septal speculum
  Caspar speculum
  Castallo eye speculum
  Castroviejo eye speculum
  Castroviejo-Barraquer speculum

speculum (*continued*)
  Chelsea-Eaton anal speculum
  Chevalier Jackson laryngeal speculum
  child-size eye speculum
  Clark eye speculum
  Coakley nasal speculum
  Coldlite vaginal speculum
  Coldlite-Graves vaginal speculum
  Colibri speculum
  Collin vaginal speculum
  Converse nasal speculum
  Conway lid speculum
  Cook eye speculum
  Cook rectal speculum
  Cottle nasal speculum
  Cottle septal speculum
  Cottle septum speculum
  Critchett eye speculum
  Culler iris speculum
  Cusco vaginal speculum
  Cushing-Landolt transsphenoidal speculum
  Czerny rectal speculum
  David rectal speculum
  Davy speculum
  DeLee speculum
  DeRoaldes nasal speculum
  Desmarres eye speculum
  Desmarres lid speculum
  DeVilbiss vaginal speculum
  disposable speculum
  disposable vaginal speculum
  Disposo-Spec disposable speculum
  Docherty cheek speculum
  Douglas mucosal speculum
  Douvas-Barraquer speculum
  Downes nasal speculum
  Doyen vaginal speculum
  duckbill speculum
  Dudley-Smith rectal speculum
  Duplay nasal speculum
  Duplay-Lynch nasal speculum
  Dynacor vaginal speculum
  ear speculum
  Eaton nasal speculum
  Eisenhammer speculum
  endaural speculum
  ENT speculum
  Erhardt ear speculum

speculum (*continued*)

Erosa-Spec vaginal speculum
esophageal speculum
eye speculum
eyelid speculum
Fansler rectal speculum
Fanta eye speculum
Farkas urethral speculum
Farrior ear speculum
Farrior oval ear speculum
Farrior oval speculum
Fergusson tubular vaginal
   speculum
fiberoptic vaginal speculum
fine-wire speculum
Flannery ear speculum
flat-bladed nasal speculum
Flint glass speculum
Floyd-Barraquer wire
   speculum
Forbes esophageal
   speculum
formalin-fixed speculum
Foster-Ballenger nasal
   speculum
Fox eye speculum
Fraenkel speculum
Fraenkel speculum
Freeway speculum
Freeway-Graves speculum
Gaffee speculum
Garrigue vaginal speculum
Garrigue weighted vaginal
   speculum
Gerzog nasal speculum
Gilbert-Graves speculum
Gleason speculum
Goldbacher anoscope
   speculum
Goldstein mucosa speculum
Goldstein septal speculum
Goligher speculum
Good speculum
Graefe eye speculum
Graves bivalve speculum
Graves Britetrac vaginal
   speculum
Graves Coldlite speculum
Graves open-side vaginal
   speculum
Graves vaginal speculum
Green eye speculum

speculum (*continued*)

Gruber ear speculum
Guild-Pratt rectal speculum
Guilford-Wright bivalve
   speculum
Guist eye speculum
Guist-Black eye speculum
Guist-Bloch speculum
Gutter speculum
Guttmann vaginal speculum
Guyton-Maumenee speculum
Guyton-Park eye speculum
Guyton-Park lid speculum
Gyn-A-Lite vaginal speculum
Haglund vaginal speculum
Haglund-Stille vaginal
   speculum
Hajek-Tieck nasal speculum
Halle infant nasal speculum
Halle infant speculum
Halle nasal speculum
Halle-Tieck nasal speculum
Halle-Tieck speculum
Hardy bivalve speculum
Hardy nasal bivalve speculum
Hardy-Cushing speculum
Hardy-Duddy weighted
   vaginal speculum
Harrison speculum
Hartmann dewaxer speculum
Hartmann ear speculum
Hartmann nasal speculum
Hartmann-Dewaxer
   speculum
Hayes vaginal speculum
heavy weighted speculum
Heffernan nasal speculum
Helmholtz speculum
Helmont speculum
Henrotin vaginal speculum
Henrotin weighted vaginal
   speculum
Hertel nephrostomy
   speculum
Higbee vaginal speculum
Hinkle-James rectal speculum
Hirschman anoscope rectal
   speculum
Holinger infant esophageal
   speculum
Hood-Graves vaginal
   speculum

speculum (*continued*)

Hough-Boucheron ear speculum
House stapes speculum
Huffman infant vaginal speculum
Huffman-Graves adolescent vaginal speculum
Huffman-Graves vaginal speculum
Iliff-Park speculum
illuminated nasal speculum
illuminated speculum
Imperatori laryngeal speculum
infant eye speculum
infant vaginal speculum
Ingals nasal speculum
intranasal antral speculum
Ives rectal speculum
Jackson vaginal speculum
Jaffe eyelid speculum
Jarit-Graves vaginal speculum
Jarit-Pederson vaginal speculum
Jonas-Graves vaginal speculum
Kahn-Graves vaginal speculum
Kaiser speculum
Kalinowski ear speculum
Kalinowski-Verner ear speculum
Katena speculum
Keeler-Pierse eye speculum
Keizer-Lancaster eye speculum
Kelly rectal speculum
Kelman speculum
Killian nasal speculum
Killian rectal speculum
Killian septal speculum
Killian-Halle nasal speculum
Klaff septal speculum
KleenSpec disposable speculum
KleenSpec disposable vaginal speculum
KleenSpec vaginal speculum
Knapp eye speculum
Knapp-Culler speculum
Knolle lens speculum

speculum (*continued*)

Kogan endocervical speculum
Kogan urethra speculum
Kramer bivalve ear speculum
Kramer ear speculum
Kratz aspirating speculum
Kratz-Barraquer wire lid speculum
Kristeller vaginal speculum
Kyle nasal speculum
Lancaster eye speculum
Lancaster lid speculum
Lancaster-O'Connor speculum
Landau speculum
Landolt pituitary speculum
Lang eye speculum
Lange speculum
laryngeal speculum
Lawford speculum
LeFort urethral speculum
Lempert-Beckman-Colver endaural speculum
Lempert-Colver endaural speculum
Lester-Burch eye speculum
lid speculum
LidFix speculum
Lieberman aspirating speculum
Lieberman K-Wire speculum
lighted speculum
Lillie nasal speculum
Lindstrom-Chu aspirating speculum
Lister-Burch eye speculum
Lofberg vaginal speculum
Lucae ear speculum
Luer eye speculum
Machat adjustable aspirating wire speculum
Macon Hospital speculum
Mahoney intranasal antral speculum
Manche LASIK speculum
Martin rectal speculum
Martin vaginal speculum
Martin-Davy rectal speculum
Mason-Auvard weighted vaginal speculum
Mathews rectal speculum
Matzenauer vaginal speculum
Maumenee-Park eye speculum

speculum (*continued*)
  Maumenee-Park lid speculum
  Mayer vaginal speculum
  McBratney aspirating
    speculum
  McHugh oval speculum
  McKee speculum
  McKinney eye speculum
  McLaughlin speculum
  McPherson eye speculum
  Meller speculum
  Mellinger eye speculum
  Mellinger fenestrated blades
    speculum
  Mellinger-Axenfeld eye
    speculum
  Merz-Vienna nasal speculum
  Metcher eye speculum
  Miller vaginal speculum
  Milligan speculum
  Monosmith nasal speculum
  Montgomery vaginal
    speculum
  Montgomery-Bernstine
    speculum
  Moria one-piece speculum
  Mosher nasal speculum
  Mosher urethral speculum
  Moynihan speculum
  Moynihan-Navratil speculum
  mucosa speculum
  Mueller eye speculum
  Muir rectal speculum
  Murdock eye speculum
  Murdock-Wiener eye
    speculum
  Murdoon eye speculum
  Myles nasal speculum
  Myles-Ray speculum
  nasal bivalve speculum
  nasal speculum
  Nasa-Spec nasal speculum
  nasopharyngeal speculum
  National ear speculum
  National Graves vaginal
    speculum
  nephrostomy speculum
  New York speculum
  Nichol speculum
  Nott vaginal speculum
  Nott-Guttmann vaginal
    speculum

speculum (*continued*)
  Noyes speculum
  Omni-Park eyelid speculum
  one-hand speculum
  open-side vaginal speculum
  O'Sullivan-O'Connor vaginal
    speculum
  oval speculum
  Pannu-Kratz-Barraquer
    speculum
  Park eye speculum
  Park-Guyton eye speculum
  Park-Guyton-Callahan eye
    speculum
  Park-Guyton-Maumenee
    speculum
  Park-Maumanee eye speculum
  Park-Maumanee lid speculum
  Parks anal speculum
  Patton nasal speculum
  Patton septal speculum
  Pearce eye speculum
  Peck-Vienna nasal speculum
  Pederson vaginal speculum
  pediatric lid speculum
  pediatric speculum
  Pennington rectal speculum
  pharyngeal speculum
  Picot vaginal speculum
  Picot weighted speculum
  Pierse eye speculum
  Pilling-Hartmann speculum
  plain wire speculum
  Politzer ear speculum
  Portmann speculum
  post-urethroplasty review
    speculum
  Pratt bivalve speculum
  Pratt rectal speculum
  Pratt sigmoid speculum
  Preefer eye speculum
  Prima Series LEEP speculum
  Pritchard speculum
  proctoscopic speculum
  Prospec disposable speculum
  Proud infant turbinate
    speculum
  Pruitt rectal speculum
  Pynchon nasal speculum
  Rappazzo speculum
  Ray nasal speculum
  rectal speculum

speculum (*continued*)
Redi-Spec disposable vaginal speculum
Reipen speculum
Relat vaginal speculum
reversible lid speculum
Rica ear speculum
Rica nasal septal speculum
Rica vaginal speculum
Richard Gruber speculum
Richnau-Holmgren ear speculum
Roberts esophageal speculum
Roberts oval speculum
Rosenthal urethral speculum
round speculum
Sani-Spec vaginal speculum
Sato speculum
Sauer eye speculum
Sauer infant eye speculum
Saunders eye speculum
Sawyer rectal speculum
Scherback speculum
Scherback-Porges vaginal speculum
Schuknecht speculum
Schweizer speculum
Scott ear speculum
self-retaining speculum
Selkin speculum
Semb vaginal speculum
Senn speculum
Senturia pharyngeal speculum
septal speculum
Serdarevic speculum
Seyfert vaginal speculum
Shea speculum
shoehorn speculum
Siegle ear speculum
sigmoid speculum
Simcoe eye speculum
Simcoe wire speculum
Simcoe-Barraquer eye speculum
Simmonds vaginal speculum
Simon vaginal speculum
Simrock speculum
Sims double-ended speculum
Sims double-ended vaginal speculum
Sims rectal speculum
Sims vaginal speculum

speculum (*continued*)
Sisson-Cottle septal speculum
Sisson-Vienna nasal speculum
slotted speculum
Sluder sphenoidal speculum
SMIC ear speculum
SMIC nasal septal speculum
SMIC nasal speculum
Smirmaul eyelid speculum
Smith anal speculum
Smith eye speculum
Smith-Buie rectal speculum
SMR speculum
Sonnenschein nasal speculum
speculum anoscope
speculum forceps
speculum holder
speculum illuminator
speculum transilluminator
SRT vaginal speculum
stapes speculum
Stearns speculum
Steiner-Auvard vaginal speculum
Stevenson eye speculum
stop eye speculum
Storz ear speculum
Storz nasal speculum
Storz septal speculum
Storz-Vienna nasal speculum
Subramanian valve speculum
Sutherland-Grieshaber speculum
Sweeney posterior vaginal speculum
Swiss-pattern speculum
Swolin self-retaining vaginal speculum
Tauber speculum
Taylor vaginal speculum
Terson speculum
Thornton open-wire lid speculum
Thudichum nasal speculum
Tieck nasal speculum
Tieck-Halle infant nasal speculum
Torchia eye speculum
Toynbee ear speculum
Toynbee speculum
transsphenoidal speculum
Trelat vaginal speculum

speculum (*continued*)
Troeltsch ear speculum
tubular vaginal speculum
Turner-Warwick post-urethroplasty review speculum
Ullrich vaginal speculum
Universal speculum
urethral speculum
vaginal speculum
Vaginard metal speculum
Vauban speculum
Verner speculum
Verner-Kalinowski speculum
Vernon-David rectal speculum
Vienna Britetrac nasal speculum
Vienna nasal speculum
Vienna Britetrac nasal speculum
Vilbiss-Miller speculum
Voltolini nasal speculum
Voltolini septum speculum
Vu-Max vaginal speculum
Walton speculum
Walton-Pederson speculum
Walton-Vienna speculum
Watson speculum
Weeks eye speculum
weighted obstetrical speculum
weighted speculum
weighted vaginal speculum
Weiner speculum
Weisman-Graves open-sided vaginal speculum
Weisman-Graves vaginal speculum
Weiss speculum
Weissbarth vaginal speculum
Welch Allyn illuminated speculum
Welch Allyn KleenSpec vaginal speculum
Wellington Hospital vaginal speculum
Wiener eye speculum
Wilde ear speculum
Williams eye speculum
Wilson-Kirbe speculum
winged speculum

speculum (*continued*)
wire bivalve obstetrical speculum
wire bivalve vaginal speculum
wire eye speculum
wire lid speculum
wire speculum
wire-winged lid speculum
Worcester City Hospital vaginal speculum
Yankauer nasopharyngeal speculum
Yankauer pharyngeal speculum
Ziegler eye speculum
Zower speculum
Zylik-Michaels speculum
speculum anoscope
speculum examination
speculum forceps
speculum holder
speculum illuminator
speculum illuminator transilluminator
speculum transilluminator
Speed arthroplasty
Speed brace
Speed hand splint
speed lock clamp
Speed Lok soft stent
Speed open reduction
Speed operation
Speed osteotomy
Speed osteotomy and bone graft
Speed osteotomy graft
Speed prosthesis
Speed radial cap prosthesis
Speed radial head fracture classification
Speed sternoclavicular procedure
Speed sternoclavicular repair
Speedband ligature
Speedband multiple band ligator
Speed-Boyd fracture reduction
Speed-Boyd open reduction
Speed-Boyd radial-ulnar technique
Speed-Boyd reduction technique
Speedi Pak sinus pack
SpeedPass suture passer
SpeedReducer instrument
Speed-Sprague knife

Speedy balloon catheter
Speedy-1 Auto refractometer
Speer periosteotome
Speer suture hook
Spemann induction
Spembly cryoprobe
Spence cranioplastic roller
Spence forceps
Spence gel flotation
Spence gel mattress pad
Spence intervertebral disk
   rongeur
Spence procedure
Spence rongeur forceps
Spence urethral meatotomy
Spence-Adson clip-introducing
   forceps
Spence-Allen hypospadias repair
Spencer biopsy forceps
Spencer cannula
Spencer chalazion forceps
Spencer eye suture scissors
Spencer incontinence device
Spencer labyrinth exploration
   probe
Spencer oval punch
Spencer oval tip
Spencer plication forceps
Spencer probe
Spencer probe depth electrode
Spencer punch
Spencer rongeur forceps
Spencer stitch scissors
Spencer triangular adenoid
   punch
Spencer triangular tip
Spencer Universal adenoid
   punch tip
Spencer-Watson operation
Spencer-Watson Z-plasty
Spencer-Wells arterial forceps
Spencer-Wells chalazion forceps
Spencer-Wells hemostatic
   forceps
Spenco arch support
Spenco boot
Spenco external breast form
Spenco neoprene foam rubber
Spenco orthotic device
sperm aspiration
sperm microaspiration retrieval
   technique

Sperma-Tex preshaped mesh
spermatic artery
spermatic calculus
spermatic cord
spermatic duct
spermatic fascia
spermatic fistula
spermatic nerve
spermatic vein ligation
spermatic veins
spermatic vesicle
spermatic vessel
spermatocele implant
spermatocelectomy
spermatocystectomy
spermatocystotomy
spermatogenic cells
spermatozoon (*pl.*
   spermatozoa)
spermectomy
Spero meibomian expressor
   forceps
Spero meibomian forceps
Spetzler anterior transoral
   approach
Spetzler catheter
Spetzler clip applier
Spetzler dissector
Spetzler forceps
Spetzler lumbar-peritoneal shunt
Spetzler lumboperitoneal shunt
Spetzler MacroVac surgical
   suction device
Spetzler MicroVac suction tube
Spetzler needle holder
Spetzler scissors
Spetzler shunt
Spetzler subarachnoid catheter
Spetzler technique for shunt
   placement
Spetzler titanium aneurysm clip
Spetzler-Martin classification
SpF spinal fusion stimulator
SpF-XL stimulator
sphacelation
sphacelism
sphaceloderma
sphacelous
sphacelus
sphenocephaly
sphenoiditis
sphenoethmoidal recess

sphenoethmoidal suture
sphenoethmoidectomy
sphenofrontal suture
sphenofrontal suture line
sphenoid
  greater wing of sphenoid
  lesser wing of sphenoid
  rostrum of sphenoid
sphenoid angle
sphenoid bone
sphenoid dysplasia
sphenoid emissary foramen
sphenoid process
sphenoid sinus aperture
sphenoid sinus metastasis
sphenoid sinusotomy
sphenoidal angle
sphenoidal bone punch
sphenoidal border
sphenoidal bur
sphenoidal cannula
sphenoidal concha
sphenoidal crest
sphenoidal cyst
sphenoidal fissure
sphenoidal fontanelle
sphenoidal herniation
sphenoidal knife
sphenoidal nasal conchae
sphenoidal ostium
sphenoidal paranasal sinus
sphenoidal probe
sphenoidal process
sphenoidal punch
sphenoidal punch forceps
sphenoidal ridge
sphenoidal rostrum
sphenoidal sinus
sphenoidal sinus septum
sphenoidal sinusitis
sphenoidal spine
sphenoidal turbinate
sphenoidal turbinate bones
sphenoidal wing
sphenoidal yoke
sphenoidectomy
sphenoidostomy
sphenoidotomy
  transethmoidal
    sphenoidotomy
  transnasal sphenoidotomy
sphenomalar suture

sphenomandibular ligament
sphenomaxillary fissure
sphenomaxillary fossa
sphenomaxillary ganglion
sphenomaxillary space
sphenomaxillary suture
spheno-occipital encephalocele
spheno-occipital joint
spheno-occipital suture
spheno-occipital synchondrosis
spheno-orbital suture
sphenopalatine artery
sphenopalatine branch of
    internal maxillary artery
sphenopalatine canal
sphenopalatine fissure
sphenopalatine foramen
sphenopalatine ganglion
sphenopalatine ganglion needle
sphenopalatine ganglionectomy
sphenopalatine needle
sphenopalatine nerves
sphenopalatine notch of
    palatine bone
sphenopalatine space
sphenoparietal sinus
sphenoparietal suture
sphenoparietal suture line
sphenopetroclival region
sphenopetrosal fissure
sphenopetrosal suture
sphenopetrosal synchondrosis
sphenopharyngeal canal
sphenosquamous suture
sphenotemporal suture
sphenotic foramen
sphenovomerine suture
sphenozygomatic suture
sphere
  Carter introducer sphere
  Doherty eye sphere
  gold sphere
  Heyer-Schulte silicone sphere
  introducer for spheres
  Morgagni sphere
  Silastic sphere
  Wheeler eye sphere
sphere eye implant
sphere implant
sphere introducer (*see*
  introducer)
sphere prosthesis

spherical bur
spherical contracture
spherical eye implant
spherical form of occlusion
spherical implant
spherical lens aberration
spherical mass
spherical reamer
spherical shape
spherical 3-dimensional curve
spherical-shaped form
Sphero Flex implant
spherocentric knee prosthesis
spherocylindrical lens
spheroid articulation
spheroid joint
spheroidal cell carcinoma
sphincter
  AMS artificial urethral
    sphincter
  AMSI artificial urinary
    sphincter
  anal ileostomy with
    preservation of sphincter
  anal sphincter
  anatomical sphincter
  annular sphincter
  anorectal sphincter
  artificial sphincter
  biliary sphincter
  Boyden sphincter
  cardiac sphincter
  cardioesophageal sphincter
  choledochal sphincter
  cricopharyngeal sphincter
  double-cuff urinary sphincter
  esophageal sphincter
  external rectal sphincter
  external sphincter
  external urethral sphincter
  extrinsic sphincter
  eyelid sphincter
  functional sphincter
  gastroesophageal sphincter
  Giordano sphincter
  Henle sphincter
  hypertensive lower
    esophageal sphincter
  hypertonic sphincter
  Hyrtl sphincter
  incompetent esophageal
    sphincter

sphincter (*continued*)
  incompetent sphincter
  inguinal sphincter
  internal anal sphincter
  internal rectal sphincter
  internal sphincter
  internal urethral sphincter
  lower esophageal sphincter
    (LES)
  Lutkens sphincter
  myovascular sphincter
  Nelaton sphincter
  O'Beirne sphincter
  Oddi sphincter
  ostial sphincter
  palatopharyngeal sphincter
  pancreaticobiliary sphincter
  pharyngoesophageal
    sphincter
  precapillary sphincters
  prepyloric sphincter
  pyloric sphincter
  rectal sphincter
  upper esophageal sphincter
    (UES)
  urinary sphincter
sphincter ani
sphincter atony
sphincter contraction ring
sphincter dilator
sphincter injury
sphincter iridis
sphincter muscle
sphincter oculi
sphincter of eye
sphincter of Oddi
sphincter of Oddi dysfunction
sphincter of pupil
sphincter pharyngoplasty
sphincter reconstruction
sphincter repair
sphincter tone
sphincter vaginae
sphincter vesicae
sphincteral achalasia
sphincteralgia
sphincterectomy
sphincteric construction
sphincterismus
sphincterolysis
sphincteroplasty
sphincterorrhaphy

sphincteroscope
sphincteroscopy
sphincterotome
  Bitome bipolar
    sphincterotome
  Cotton sphincterotome
  Cremer-Ikeda sphincterotome
  Demling-Classen
    sphincterotome
  Doubilet sphincterotome
  double-channel
    sphincterotome
  ERCP sphincterotome
  Erlangen endoscopic
    sphincterotome
  Fluorotome double-lumen
    sphincterotome
  Frimberger-Karpiel 12 o'clock
    sphincterotome
  Howell rotatable
    sphincterotome
  Huibregtse-Katon
    sphincterotome
  Koch-Julian sphincterotome
  long-nosed sphincterotome
  needle-knife sphincterotome
  needle-tipped
    sphincterotome
  Olympus sphincterotome
  open sphincterotome
  precut sphincterotome
  reverse sphincterotome
  rotating sphincterotome
  shark fin sphincterotome
  single-channel wire-guided
    sphincterotome
  Ultratome double-lumen
    sphincterotome
  Ultratome triple-lumen
    sphincterotome
  Wilson-Cook double-channel
    sphincterotome
  Wilson-Cook wire-guided
    sphincterotome
  wire-guided sphincterotome
  Zimmon sphincterotome
sphincterotomy
  anal sphincterotomy
  choledochal sphincterotomy
  Doubilet sphincterotomy
  endoscopic pancreatic duct
    sphincterotomy

sphincterotomy (*continued*)
  endoscopic retrograde
    sphincterotomy (ERS)
  endoscopic sphincterotomy
    (ES)
  internal sphincterotomy
  Mulholland sphincterotomy
  Parks partial sphincterotomy
  transduodenal
    sphincterotomy
sphincterotomy basket
sphincter-saving operation
sphincter-saving procedure
sphincter-saving surgery
sphincter-saving technique
sphincter-sparing procedure
sphincter-sparing resection
sphincter-sparing technique
sphygmograph
sphygmomanometer
sphygmomanometer cuffs
sphygmometry
sphygmoscope
sphygmoscopy
SPI-Argent II peritoneal dialysis
    catheter
spica bandage
spica cast
spica cast immobilization
spica dressing
spica splint
spica table
Spicel skin graft material
spiculated calcification
spiculated lesion
spicule forceps
spiculum (*pl.* spicula)
SPIDER (steady-state projection
    imaging with dynamic
    echo-train readout)
spider angioma
spider angiomata
spider cell
spider finger
spider hemangioma
spider mole
spider nevus
spider projection
spider telangiectasia
spider telangiectasis
spider varicosity
spider vein

spider-burst
spider-web clot
Spiegel lobe
Spieghel line
Spiegler-Fendt pseudolymphoma
Spiegler-Fendt sarcoid
Spielberg dilator
Spielberg sinus cannula
Spies ethmoidal punch
Spiesman fistula probe
Spiessel internal screw fixation
Spiessel lag screw
Spiessel position screw
spigelian hernia
spigelian lobe
Spigelius hernia
Spigelius line
Spigelius lobe
Spigelman baseball finger splint
spike discharges
spike focus
spike pattern
spike retractor
spike rhythm
spike staple
spike waves
spike-and-dome complex
spike-and-sharp waves
spike-and-slow wave
spike-and-wave
spikelike emanation
spikelike formation
spikey activity
spilled teacup sign
Spiller-Frazier technique
spin technique
spina (*pl.* spinae)
spinal accessory nerve
spinal accessory nerve-facial
    nerve anastomosis
spinal analgesia
spinal analgesic
spinal anesthesia (SA)
spinal anesthetic
spinal anesthetic technique
spinal arachnoid
spinal artery
spinal arthroscope
spinal block
spinal canal
spinal catheter
spinal column stabilization

spinal compression fracture
spinal cord abscess
spinal cord circulation
spinal cord compression
spinal cord injury
spinal cord retractor
spinal cord stimulator
spinal cordotomy
spinal coronal plane deformity
spinal curet
spinal decompression
spinal dural arteriovenous fistula
spinal elevator
spinal epidural abscess (SEA)
spinal epidural space
spinal fixation
spinal fluid drainage
spinal fluid tap
spinal fracture
spinal fusion chisel
spinal fusion curet
spinal fusion elevator
spinal fusion gouge
spinal fusion instrument set
spinal fusion osteotome
spinal fusion plate
spinal fusion position
spinal fusion technique
spinal ganglion
spinal ganglion spinal gouge
spinal gouge
spinal graft tamp
spinal hematoma
spinal impactor
spinal infection biopsy
spinal inflammation
spinal injury operative
    stabilization
spinal lesion
spinal manipulation
spinal manometer
spinal marrow
spinal meningitis
spinal metastasis
spinal mobilization technique
spinal muscle
spinal needle
spinal nerves
spinal neurectomy
spinal osteotomy stabilization
spinal paralysis
spinal perforating forceps

spinal point
spinal puncture
spinal reflex
spinal retractor
spinal retractor blade
spinal rod
spinal rongeur forceps
spinal saw
spinal stenosis
spinal subarachnoid block
spinal surgery
spinal sympathetic chain
spinal tap
Spinal Technology bivalve TLSO
  brace
spinal thrust
spinal trephine
spinal turning frame
spinal vascular malformation
spinal veins
spinal-locking procedure
SpinaLogic bone growth
  stimulator
SpinalPak fusion stimulator
spinal-perforating forceps
Spinal-Stim bone growth
  stimulator
spindle
  His spindle
  Krukenberg spindle
  muscle spindle
spindle cataract
spindle cell cancer
spindle cell carcinoma
spindle cell
  hemangioendothelioma
spindle cell lipoma
spindle cell tumor
spindle colonic groove
spindle-shaped cataract
spindle-shaped incision
spindling patterns
spine
  alar spine
  angular spine
  anterior-inferior iliac spine
  anterior nasal spine (ANS)
  anterior-superior iliac spine
    (ASIS)
  anterosuperior iliac spine
    (ASIS)
  bamboo spine

spine (*continued*)
  basilar spine
  cervical spine
  Civinni spine
  cleft spine
  compensatory curvature of
    spine
  concavity of spine
  convexity of spine
  Dens view of cervical spine
  dorsal plaster spine
  dorsal spine
  erect spine
  greater tympanic spine
  Henle spine
  Hibbs onlay graft fusion of
    lumbar spine
  horny spine
  iliac spine
  ischial spines
  Knodt rod fusion of spine
  lateral curvature of spine
  lumbar spine
  lumbosacral spine
  mandibular spine
  meatal spine
  mental spine
  nasal spine
  palatine spine
  pharyngeal spine
  poker spine
  posterior nasal spine
  posterosuperior iliac spine
  rugger jersey spine
  sacral spine
  sphenoidal spine
  Spix spine
  superior iliac spine
  superior spine
  suprameatal spine
  syndesmophytes of spine
  thoracic spine
  tibial spine
  vertebral spine
spine deformity
spine fracture
spine of helix
spine of Henle
spine of maxilla
spine of sphenoid bone
SpineCATH intradiscal catheter
spin-echo image

spin-echo magnetic resonance
   imaging
spin-echo MRI
spin-echo scanning technique
Spinelli biopsy needle
Spinelli operation
Spinhaler inhaler
spinning disk nebulizer
spinning probe
spinning-top deformity
spinolamellar line
spinolaminar line
spinoneural artery
spinothalamic cordotomy
spinothalamic tract cauterized
spinous aspect
spinous interlaminar line
spinous plane
spinous process fracture
spinous process of vertebra
spinous process spreader
spinous process wire
spiny projection
Spira procedure
spiradenoma
SpiraFlo prostate stent
spiral artery
spiral arterioles
spiral band of Gossett
spiral bandage
spiral coil stent
spiral computed tomography
spiral computed tomography
   angiography
spiral CT scanner
spiral CT technique
spiral dissection
spiral drill
spiral electrode
spiral elevator
spiral endosseous implant
spiral endosteal implant
spiral flap
spiral fluted tungsten carbide
   bur
spiral fold
spiral forceps
spiral fracture
spiral ganglion
spiral groove
spiral incision
spiral joint

spiral ligament
spiral line
spiral membrane
spiral oblique fracture
spiral probe
spiral reamer
spiral reverse bandage
spiral stone dislodger
spiral suture technique
spiral sutures
spiral trochanteric reamer
spiral valve
spiral vein of modiolus
spiral vein stripper
spiral wound
spiral XCT scanner
SpiralGold oxygenator
spiral-tipped bougie
spiral-tipped catheter
spiral-wound endotracheal tube
SpiraStent stent
SpiraStent ureteral stent
Spirec drill
SpiroFlo bioabsorbable prostate
   stent
Spir-O-Flow peak flow monitor
spirogram
spirometer
   Benedict-Roth spirometer
   Bennett monitoring
      spirometer
   Calculair spirometer
   Collis spirometer
   DeVilbiss spirometer
   Eagle spirometer
   Tri-flow incentive spirometer
   Venturi spirometer
spirometry
   incentive spirometry
   Tri-flow incentive spirometry
spit cyst
Spittle biceps muscle cineplasty
Spittler procedure
Spitz nevus
Spitz-Holter flushing device
Spitz-Holter VA shunt
Spitz-Holter valve
Spitz-Holter valve implant
   material
Spivack cystostomy
Spivack gastrostomy
Spivack gastrotomy technique

Spivack operation
Spivack valve
Spivack valve technique
Spivey iris retractor
Spix spine
Spizziri cannula knife
Spizziri-Simcoe cannula
SPK transplant
splanchnic anesthesia
splanchnic AV fistula
splanchnic block
splanchnic circulation
splanchnic ganglion
splanchnic hypoperfusion
splanchnic nerve
splanchnic neurectomy
splanchnic perfusion
splanchnic retractor
splanchnicectomy
splanchnicotomy
splanchnocranium
splanchnoscopy
splanchnotribe
S-plasty
SPLATT transfer procedure
splayed alar cartilage
splayed arteries
splayed tip
splayfoot deformity
splaytooth forceps
spleen
    accessory spleen
    capsule of spleen
    colic surface of spleen
    ectopic spleen
    ellipsoid of spleen
    floating spleen
    gastric surface of spleen
    liver, kidneys, and spleen
        (LKS)
    pedicle of spleen
    phrenic surface of spleen
    ruptured spleen
spleen-preserving pancreatic
    resection
splenectomize
splenectomy
    abdominal splenectomy
    Carter splenectomy
    Federov splenectomy
    Henry splenectomy
    laparoscopic splenectomy

splenectomy (*continued*)
    Rives splenectomy
    subscapular splenectomy
    thoracicoabdominal
        splenectomy
splenectopia
splenic abscess
splenic artery
splenic AV fistula
splenic capsule
splenic cyst
splenic dullness
splenic flexure carcinoma
splenic flexure colonoscopy
splenic flexure of colon
splenic fossa
splenic hilum
splenic injury
splenic laceration
splenic lesion
splenic portogram
splenic portography
splenic pulp
splenic puncture
splenic recess of omental bursa
splenic rupture
splenic sequestration syndrome
splenic shadow
splenic souffle
splenic system angiogram
splenic tissue
splenic vein deformity
splenic vein thrombosis
splenic venogram
splenic-renal angle
splenius muscle
splenization
splenoadrenal anastomosis
splenobronchial fistula
splenocele
splenocleisis
splenocolic ligament
splenogastric omentum
splenogonadal fusion
splenogram
splenography
splenolaparatomy
splenolymph glands
splenolysis
splenomegaly
    congestive splenomegaly
    Gaucher splenomegaly

splenomegaly (*continued*)
  hemolytic splenomegaly
  hypercholesterolemic
    splenomegaly
  Niemann splenomegaly
splenoncus
splenopexy
splenoplasty
splenoportal venography
splenoportogram
splenoportography
splenoptosis
splenorenal anastomosis
splenorenal angle
splenorenal bypass shunt
splenorenal ligament
splenorenal shunt
splenorenal venous anastomosis
splenorenal venous operation
splenorrhagia
splenorrhaphy
splenosis
splenotomy
spline
  os pubis spline
  plaster spline
  stapes spline
Spline Twist microtextured
    titanium implant
splint
  4-prong finger splint
  abduction finger splint
  abduction splint
  abduction thumb splint
  acrylic cap splint
  acrylic ear splint
  acrylic splint
  acrylic surgical splint
  acrylic wafer TMJ splint
  Adam and Eve rib belt splint
  adhesive aluminum splint
  adjustable cross splint
  adjustable splint
  Adjusta-Wrist splint
  aeroplane splint
  Agnew splint
  Ainslie acrylic splint
  air splint
  AirFlex carpal tunnel splint
  airfoam splint
  airplane splint
  AliMed diabetic night splint

splint (*continued*)
  Alumafoam nasal splint
  aluminum bridge splint
  aluminum fence splint
  aluminum finger cot splint
  aluminum foam splint
  anchor splint
  Anderson splint
  Angle splint
  ankle-foot orthotic splint
  anterior acute-flexion elbow
    splint
  anterior splint
  any-angle splint
  application of splint
  Aquaplast nasal splint
  arm splint
  Asch nasal splint
  Ashhurst splint
  A-splint dental splint
  Atkins nasal splint
  bail-lock splint
  Balkan femoral splint
  ball-peen splint
  banana finger extension splint
  banjo traction splint
  baseball finger splint
  basswood splint
  Bavarian splint
  Baylor adjustable cross splint
  Baylor metatarsal splint
  Beatty aluminum finger splint
  Bend-A-Boot foot splint
  Bilson fixable-removable cross
    arch bar splint
  birdcage splint
  bite splint
  Blount splint
  board splint
  body prop positioning splint
  Boehler wire splint
  Boehler-Braun splint
  Bond arm splint
  boutonniere splint
  Bowlby arm splint
  bracketed splint
  Brady suspension splint
  Brant aluminum splint
  Breathe-Easy nasal splint
  Bremmer-Breeze splint
  bridge splint
  Bridgemaster nasal splint

splint (*continued*)

Brooke Army Hospital splint
Browne splint
Buck extension splint
Buck traction splint
buddy splint
Budin hammertoe splint
Budin toe splint
Bunnell active hand splint
Bunnell finger extension splint
Bunnell finger splint
Bunnell gutter splint
Bunnell knuckle-bender splint
Bunnell modified safety-pin splint
Bunnell outrigger splint
Bunnell reverse knuckle-bender splint
Bunnell safety pin splint
Bunny Boot foot splint
Burget nasal splint
Cabot leg splint
calibrated clubfoot splint
Camo disposable dental splint
Campbell airplane splint
Campbell traction splint
canine-to-canine lingual splint
Cannon Bio-Flek nasal splint
cap splint
Capener coil splint
Capener finger splint
Capner boutonniere splint
cardboard splint
Carl P. Jones traction splint
Carpal Lock cock-up wrist splint
Carter intranasal splint
cartilage elastic pullover kneecap splint
cast cap splint
cast lingual splint
Cawood nasal splint
Chandler felt collar splint
Chatfield-Girdlestone splint
clavicle splint
clavicular cross splint
Clayton splint
clean acrylic template splint
clubfoot splint
coaptation splint
cock-up arm splint

splint (*continued*)

cock-up hand splint
Colles splint
Comfy elbow splint
composite spring elastic splint
compression sleeve shin splint
compression splint
compressive plastic splint
Comprifix ankle splint
Cone splint
contact splint
Converse splint
copper band-acrylic splint
Cordon Colles fracture splint
Cosmolon closure for splint
counterrotational splint
countertraction splint
Craig abduction splint
Cramer wire splint
crib splint
CTS Gripfit splint
Cullen abduction splint
Culley ulna splint
Curry walking splint
Darco medical-surgical shoe and toe alignment splint
Darco toe alignment splint
Davis metacarpal splint
Delbet splint
Denis Browne clubfoot splint
Denis Browne hip splint
Denis Browne talipes hobble splint
dental splint
denture splint
Denver nasal splint
DePuy open-thimble splint
DePuy rocking-leg splint
DePuy-Potts splint
DeRoyal LMB finger splint
Digit Aid splint
digit splint
DonJoy knee splint
Dorsiwedge night splint
double-J silicone splint
double-occlusal splint
Doyle bi-valved airway splint
Doyle nasal airway splint
Doyle intranasal airway splint
Doyle nasal splint

splint (*continued*)

Doyle Shark nasal splint
drop-foot splint
DuPuy aeroplane splint
DuPuy any-angle splint
DuPuy coaptation splint
DuPuy rolled Colles splint
DuPuy-Pott splint
Dupuytren splint
Duran-Houser wire splint
dynamic splint
Early Fit night splint
Easton cock-up splint
Easy Access foot splint
Eggers contact splint
elastic plastic splint
elbow extension splint
elbow flexion splint
elephant-ear clavicle splint
EnduraSplint splint
Engelmann thigh splint
Engen palmar wrist splint
Epitrain elbow splint
Erich maxillary splint
Erich nasal splint
Essig wire acrylic splint
Essig-type splint
Extend-It finger splint
extension splint
external nasal splint
external splint
Ezeform splint
Fasplint splint
felt-collar splint
femoral splint
fence splint
Ferciot splint
Fillauer night splint
finger extension clockspring
  splint
finger flexion splint
finger splint
finger-cot splint
Finger-Hugger splint
Flexisplint
folded aluminum ear splint
fold-over finger splint
foot drop night splint
fore-and-aft splint
forearm and metacarpal splint
forearm splint
Formatray mandibular splint

splint (*continued*)

Forrester head splint
Fosler splint
Fox clavicle splint
Fox clavicular splint
FracSure splint
Fractomed splint
fracture splint
Framer splint
Freedom neutral position
  splint
Freedom Omni Progressive
  splint
Freedom Progressive Resting
  splint
Frejka pillow splint
frog splint
frog-leg splint
Froimson splint
Fruehevald splint
full occlusal splint
full-hand splint
functional resting position
  splint
functional splint
Funsten supination splint
Futura splint
Futuro splint
gait lock splint
Gallows splint
Galveston splint
Ganley splint
gauntlet splint
Gibson splint
Gilmer dental splint
Gilmer tooth splint
Glisson sling splint
gnathological splint
Gooch splint
Goode Magne-Splint magnetic
  nasal splint
Goode nasal splint
Goode-Magne nasal airway
  splint
Gordon arm splint
Granberry splint
greenstick fracture splint
Greidman splint
Guerrant-Cochran splint
Gunning jaw splint
gutter finger splint
gutter splint

splint (*continued*)

half-ring leg splint
half-ring Thomas splint
Hammond orthodontic splint
hand cock-up splint
hand splint
Hanna splint
Hare compact traction splint
Hare traction splint
Hart extension finger splint
Haynes-Griffin mandible splint
Haynes-Griffin mandibular
  splint
HealWell Cub plantar fasciitis
  night splint
Heel Free splint
Hexcelite sheet splint
Hilgenreiner splint
hinged Thomas splint
Hirschtick utility shoulder
  splint
Hodgen hip splint
Hodgen leg splint
humerus splint
HV NightSplint splint
HV SoftSplint splint
Ilfeld splint
Ilfeld-Gustafson splint
implant surgical splint
indexed splint
infant abduction splint
inflatable elbow splint
inflatable splint
Innoboot night splint
INRO surgical nail splint
interdental splint
intermediate splint
intranasal bivalve splint
intranasal splint
Isoprene plastic splint
Jacoby heel splint
jaw splint
Jelenko splint
Jet-Air splint
Jobe-Patt splint
Johnson splint
joint spring splint
Joint-Jack finger splint
Jonell countertraction finger
  splint
Jonell countertraction
  metacarpal splint

splint (*continued*)

Jonell finger splint
Jonell thumb splint
Jones arm splint
Jones forearm splint
Jones metacarpal splint
Jones nasal splint
Jones traction splint
Joseph nasal splint
Joseph septal splint
Kanavel cock-up splint
Kazanjian nasal splint
Keller-Blake half-ring leg splint
Keller-Blake leg splint
Kenny-Howard splint
Kerr abduction splint
Keystone splint
kidney internal splint
Kingsley splint
Kinney-Brown AC splint
Kirschner wire splint
Kleinert dynamic traction
  splint
Kleinert rubber-band splint
Kleinert volar pedicle splint
Klenzak double-upright splint
knee brace splint
knee immobilizer splint
knee splint
knuckle-binder splint
labial splint
labiolingual splint
Lambrinudi splint
leaf splint
leg extension splint
leg splint
Levis arm splint
Lewin baseball finger splint
Lewin-Stern finger splint
Lewin-Stern thumb splint
Liberty One splint
limb splint
lingual splint
Link boutonnière finger splint
Link stack split splint
Link toe splint
Liston splint
live splint
Lively splint
long arm splint
long leg posterior molded
  splint

splint (*continued*)
- long leg splint
- Love nasal splint
- lumiform splint
- Lynch septal splint
- Lytle metacarpal splint
- Lytle splint
- MacKay nasal splint
- magnet splint
- Magnuson abduction humeral splint
- Magnuson abduction humerus splint
- malleable metal finger splint
- Malmo hip splint
- mandible splint
- mandibular splint
- Mason splint
- Mason-Allen hand splint
- Mason-Allen Universal hand splint
- Mayer nasal splint
- McGee splint
- McIntire splint
- McKibbin splint
- McLeod padded clavicular splint
- memory splint
- metacarpal splint
- metal splint
- metatarsal splint
- Middledorpf splint
- MindSet toe splint
- modified Oppenheimer splint
- Mohr finger splint
- molded splint
- Morris splint
- Murphy splint
- Murray-Jones arm splint
- Murray-Thomas arm splint
- nasal splint
- Neiman nasal splint
- neoprene splint
- Neubeiser adjustable forearm splint
- neutral position splint
- night splint
- nose guard splint
- occlusal splint
- OCL volar splint
- O'Donaghue knee splint
- O'Donaghue stirrup splint

splint (*continued*)
- OEC forearm splint
- OEC wrist splint
- Olliger splint
- O'Malley jaw fracture splint
- Omnivac splint
- onlay splint
- open thimble splint
- Oppenheimer knuckle-bender splint
- Oppenheimer spring wire splint
- opponens splint
- Orfit splint
- Ortho Tech cock-up wrist splint
- Ortho-last splint
- Orthomedics Stretch and Heel splint
- Ortho-Mold splint
- orthopedic strap clavicle splint
- Orthoplast isoprene splint
- outrigger splint
- outrigger wrist splint
- Oval-8 finger splint
- oyster splint
- padded aluminum splint
- padded board splint
- padded plywood splint
- padded splint
- Pallab finger splint
- palmar splint
- pan splint
- Parke-Davis splint
- Pavlik harness splint
- Peabody splint
- Pearson attachment to Thomas splint
- Pearson clavicle attachment splint
- Pehr abduction splint
- pelvic splint
- PF night splint
- Phelps splint
- Phemister splint
- Phoenix outrigger splint
- Pier abduction splint
- pillow splint
- Pil-O-Splint wrist splint
- plantar fasciitis night splint
- Plastalume bulb-ended splint

splint (*continued*)

Plastalume straight splint
plaster splint
plaster-of-Paris splint
plastic splint
Plexiglas splint
pneumatic splint
Polyform splint
Polymed splint
polymethyl methacrylate ear
    splint
polyvinyl alcohol splint
Pond splint
Ponseti splint
poroplastic splint
Porzett splint
posterior splint
Pott splint
Pro-glide splint
Protecto splint
Pucci splint
Puth abduction splint
Putti splint
QualCraft splint
QuickCast splint
Quik splint
radial nerve splint
radiolucent splint
Radstat wrist splint
Rancho Los Amigos splint
Rauchfuss sling splint
Redi-Around finger splint
replant splint
resting pan splint
reverse Kingsley splint
reverse knuckle-bender splint
Robert Jones splint
rocking-leg splint
Roger Anderson well-leg
    splint
rolled Colles splint
Rolyan Gel Shell splint
Rooter splint
Rosen splint
Royalite splint
Roylan Gel Shell spica splint
Rumel aluminum bridge splint
Russell splint
safety pin splint
Safian nasal splint
sandwich-type splint
Saturn splint

splint (*continued*)

Savlon splint
Sayre splint
Scott humeral splint
Scott humerus splint
Scottish Rite splint
septal splint
Shah nasal splint
Sheffield splint
short arm plaster splint
short arm posterior molded
    splint
short leg splint
Simpson sugar-tong splint
skin splint
Slattery-McGrouther dynamic
    flexion splint
Slocum splint
Smart Splint
Sof-Gel palm shield splint
Softies wrist and forearm
    splint
Softsplint foot splint
special Colles splint
Speed hand splint
spica splint
Spigelman baseball finger
    splint
spreading hand splint
spring cock-up splint
spring-wire safety-pin splint
Stack splint
Stader splint
static splint
Stax fingertip splint
stirrup splint
Stock finger splint
Strampelli eye splint
strap clavicle splint
Stretch and Heel splint
Stromeyer splint
Stuart Gordon hand splint
Stulberg HIPciser abduction
    splint
sugar-tong plaster splint
sugar-tong splint
supination splint
Supramead nose splint
surgical splint
swan-neck splint
Swanson dynamic toe splint
Swanson hand splint

splint (*continued*)

- synergistic wrist motion splint
- Synergy splint
- talipes hobble splint
- Taylor splint
- Teare arm sling splint
- Teare arm splint
- Teflon splint
- template splint
- tennis elbow splint
- tenodesis splint
- T-finger splint
- therapeutic splint
- thermoplastic extension pan splint
- thermoplastic splint
- thigh splint
- Thomas full-ring leg splint
- Thomas full-ring splint
- Thomas hinged splint
- Thomas knee splint
- Thomas leg splint
- Thomas posterior splint
- Thomas suspension splint
- Thompson modification of Denis Browne splint
- thumb splint
- Thumz Up functional thumb splint
- Ticonium splint
- Titus forearm splint
- Titus wrist splint
- Toad finger splint
- Tobruk splint
- tong splint
- Toronto splint
- torsion bar splint
- turnbuckle elbow splint
- turnbuckle functional position splint
- ulnar splint
- Ultraflex ankle dorsiflexion dynamic splint
- Universal gutter splint
- Universal support splint
- Urias pressure splint
- utility shoulder splint
- Valentine splint
- Valpo splint
- Van Rosen splint
- Velcro extenders splint

splint (*continued*)

- Versi-Splint
- volar splint
- Volkmann splint
- von Rosen hip splint
- Wamarline wrist splint
- Warm N Form splint
- Weil splint
- well-leg splint
- Wertheim splint
- Wilson splint
- Winter splint
- wire splint
- Wirefoam splint
- wraparound splint
- Xomed Doyle nasal airway splint
- Xomed Silastic splint
- Yucca wood splint
- Zimfoam finger splint
- Zimmer airplane splint
- Zimmer clavicular cross splint
- Zim-Trac traction splint
- Zim-Zip rib belt splint
- Zollinger splint
- Zucker splint
- splint liner
- splint padding
- splinter forceps
- splinter hemorrhage
- splintered fracture
- splintered to pieces
- splinting material
- splinting of abdomen
- splinting tube
- Splintline acrylic
- Splintrex instrument
- SplintsRite stabilization device
- split anterior tibial tendon procedure
- split calvarial graft
- split cast mount
- split cuff nipple technique
- split drape
- split fixation
- split fracture
- split graft
- split hand
- split hand/split foot malformation
- split ileostomy
- split incision

split papule
split plate appliance
split Russell skeletal traction
split skin graft
split uvula
split-and-roll technique
split-bone technique
split-cord malformation
split-course technique
split-course treatment
split-finger hook
split-hand deformity
split-heel approach
split-heel fracture
split-heel incision
split-liver transplant
split-liver transplantation
split-lung ventilation
split-nail deformity
split-patellar approach
split-sheath catheter
split-sheath introducer
split-thickness flap
split-thickness graft
split-thickness implant
split-thickness periodontal flap
split-thickness prosthesis
split-thickness skin graft
splitting chisel
splitting forceps
splitting fracture
splitting lacrimal papilla
    operation
splitting of heart sounds
SpO_2-5001 oximeter
SPOA (subperiosteal orbital
    abscess)
spoiled gradient-echo imaging
spondylitic bar
spondylitic deformity
spondylitis
    ankylosing spondylitis
    Bekhterev spondylitis
    posttraumatic spondylitis
    psoriatic spondylitis
    Shober index for spondylitis
spondylolisthesis reduction
spondylolysis
spondylopathy
spondylophyte annular dissector
    perforator
spondylophyte impactor

spondylosis
spondylosyndesis
sponge
    2 × 2 strung sponge
    absorbable gelatin sponge
    absorbable sponge
    Accu-Sorb gauze sponge
    Actifoam collagen sponge
    Actifoam hemostat sponge
    Alcon sponge
    appendectomy sponge
    Bernay sponge
    Bicol collagen sponge
    Boston gauze sponge
    bronchoscopic sponge
    bronchoscopy sponge
    buffing sponge
    Bulkee super fluff sponge
    cellulose surgical sponge
    cherry sponge
    Codman Bicol sponge
    collagen sponge
    Collostat hemostatic sponge
    cotton ball sponge
    Curity cover sponge
    Curity disposable laparotomy
        sponge
    Curity gauze sponge
    Custodis sponge
    cylindrical sponge
    DeRoyal laparotomy sponge
    EndoZime sponge
    Excilon drain sponge
    Excilon dressing sponge
    Expandacell sponge
    fibrin sponge
    Fluftex gauze rolls and sponge
    free sponge
    Fuller silicone sponge
    Gardlok neurosurgical sponge
    gauze dissector sponge
    gauze rosebud sponge
    gauze sponge
    gelatin sponge
    gelatinous sponge
    Gelfoam sponge
    Graham Clark silicone sponge
    grooved silicone sponge
    Helistat absorbable collagen
        sponge
    Helistat absorbable collagen
        hemostatic sponge

sponge (*continued*)
- hemostatic sponge
- Heros chiropody sponge
- Hibbs sponge
- implant sponge
- Incert bioabsorbable implantable sponge
- InstruWipes surgical sponge
- Ivalon embolic sponge
- Johnson & Johnson gauze sponge
- K dissector sponge
- Kenwood laparotomy sponge
- Kerlix laparotomy sponge
- Kerlix packing sponge
- Kerlix super sponge
- King fluff rolls and sponge
- Kitner sponge
- Kling sponge
- K-sponge
- K-Sponge hydrocellulose sponge
- Kurkenberg sponge
- laminectomy wedge sponge
- lap sponge
- laparotomy sponge
- Lapwall laparotomy sponge
- Lincoff lens sponge
- Lincoff Silastic sponge
- lint-free sponge
- LISCO sponge
- Marlex sponge
- Masciuli silicone sponge
- Mediskin hemostatic sponge
- Medistat hemostatic sponge
- Medline gauze sponge
- Merocel sponge
- Microsponge Teardrop sponge
- Mikulicz sponge
- Miragel sponge
- Mirasorb sponge
- nasal tampon sponge
- nasopharyngeal sponge
- Naso-Tamp nasal packing sponge
- neurological sponge
- nonwoven sponge
- Nu Gauze sponge
- Nu-Brede packing and debridement sponge
- ophthalmic sponge
- Optipore scrub sponge

sponge (*continued*)
- Optipore wound-cleaning sponge
- Oto-Wick ear sponge
- Packer tunnel silicone sponge
- peanut sponge
- Pedic sponge
- pledget sponge
- polyvinyl alcohol sponge
- polyvinyl sponge
- Porolon sponge
- Pro-Ophtha absorbent stick sponge
- Prosthex sponge
- Protectaid contraceptive sponge
- radial sponge
- Ray-Tec surgical sponges
- Ray-Tec x-ray detectable surgical sponge
- Reston sponge
- Roschke dropper sponge
- rubber sponge
- saline-moistened sponge
- Sector tonsillar sponge
- Silastic sponge
- silicone sponge
- Snowflake laparotomy sponge
- Soft N Dry Merocel sponge
- soft silicone sponge
- Sof-Wick sponge
- stainless sponge
- stick sponge
- strip and point sponge
- surgical sponge
- Surgtex x-ray detectable sponge
- Taka microneurosurgical sponge
- tonsillar sponges
- Topper dressing sponges
- tracheotomy sponge
- vaginal sponge
- Vaiser eye sponge
- Venture sponge
- Versalon all purpose sponge
- Visi-Spear eye sponge
- Vistec x-ray detectable sponge
- vitrectomy sponge
- Weck sponge
- Weck-cel surgical spear sponge

sponge (*continued*)
  Weck-sorb airwick sponge
  wet lap sponge
  Wextran sponge
  x-ray detectable laparotomy
    sponge
sponge and lap count
sponge and needle count
sponge biopsy
sponge carrier (*see* carrier)
sponge clamp
sponge count
sponge dissection
sponge dissector
sponge ear curet
sponge forceps
sponge graft
sponge implant
sponge kidney
sponge patties
sponge ring
sponge silicone implant
    material
sponge stick
sponge test
sponge-and-dressing forceps
sponge-holding forceps
sponging forceps
spongiosa bone graft
spongiosa graft
spongiosa screw
spongiosa shunt
spongiosaplasty
spongiosis
spongiotic lesion
Spongostan hemostat
spongy body
spongy bone
spongy spot
spongy tissue
Sponsel osteotomy
spontaneous abortion (SAB)
spontaneous adenocarcinoma
spontaneous amputation
spontaneous breech delivery
spontaneous breech extraction
spontaneous coronary artery
    dissection
spontaneous delivery
spontaneous fracture
spontaneous gangrene of
    newborn

spontaneous hyperemic
    dislocation
spontaneous intermittent
    mandatory ventilation
    (SIMV)
spontaneous labor
spontaneous lateral ventricle
    hernia
spontaneous lesion
spontaneous miscarriage
spontaneous pneumothorax
spontaneous pseudoscar
spontaneous renal hemorrhage
spontaneous respiration
spontaneous rupture
spontaneous vaginal delivery
spontaneous ventilation
spontaneous ventilation
    anesthetic technique
spontaneous ventrolateral
    hernia
spontaneous version
spontaneous voiding
spoon
  appendectomy spoon
  Ballance mastoid spoon
  brain spatula spoon
  brain spoon
  Bunge exenteration spoon
  Castroviejo spoon
  cataract spoon
  Culler lens spoon
  Cushing brain spatula spoon
  Cushing pituitary spoon
  Cushing spatula spoon
  Daviel lens spoon
  ear spoon
  Elschnig eye spoon
  Elschnig lens spoon
  enucleation spoon
spoon
  evisceration spoon
  exenteration spoon
  eye evisceration spoon
  eye spoon
  Falk appendectomy spoon
  Fisher spoon
  gall duct spoon
  gallbladder spoon
  graft carrier spoon
  Gross ear spoon
  Hardy pituitary spoon

spoon (*continued*)
   Hatt spoon
   Hess lens spoon
   Hiebert esophageal suture spoon
   Hoke spoon
   Hoke-Roberts spoon
   intracapsular lens spoon
   Kalt eye spoon
   Kirby intracapsular lens spoon
   Kirby lens spoon
   Knapp spoon
   Kocher brain spoon
   lens spoon
   Lindner cyclodialysis spoon
   marrow spoon
   Mayo common duct spoon
   Moore gallbladder spoon
   needle spoon
   obstetrical spoon
   Ray brain spoon
   Royal spoon
   sharp spoon
   Skene uterine spoon
   spatula and spoon
   spatula spoon
   Troutman lens spoon
   uterine spoon
   Volkmann pancreatic calculus spoon
   Weber-Elschnig lens spoon
   Wells enucleation spoon
   Wells eye spoon
   Wills eye spatula and spoon
   Woodson spoon
spoon anastomosis clamp
spoon and spatula
spoon clamp
spoon curet
spoon forceps
spoon needle
spoon retractor
spoon spatula
spoon-shaped forceps
spoon-shaped hand
sporadic Burkitt lymphoma
sporadic multigland disease
sporadic multigland hyperplasia
sporadic multiple gland parathyroid hyperplasia
sporadic pituitary adenoma
sporadic renal cell carcinoma
sporadically occurring
Sportape tape
Sportelli system collimator mounted contact shield
Sports-Caster I, II knee brace
SportsFit thumb orthosis
Sport-Stirrup orthosis
SporTX pulsed direct current stimulator
SporTX stimulation device
spot cautery
spot compression
spot dermabrasion
spot face reamer
spot film
spot necrosis
spot retinoscope
spot view
SpotCheck+ handheld pulse oximeter
spot-compression paddle
spot-film roentgenography
Spot-quartz light
S-pouch reconstruction
SPR.Plus II mattress
Sprague arthroscopic technique
Sprague ear curet
Sprague-Rappaport stethoscope
sprain
   1st-degree sprain
   2nd-degree sprain
   3rd-degree sprain
   cervical sprain
   fibular collateral ankle sprain
   inversion sprain
   lumbosacral sprain
   rider's sprain
   stable sprain
   temporomandibular joint sprain
sprain fracture
sprain of joint
sprain of ligament
Spratt bone curet
Spratt ear curet
Spratt mastoid curet
Spratt nasofrontal rasp
Spratt raspatory
Spray Band dressing
spray bandage

spread (*continued*)
  infection spread
  lamina spread
  lymphatic spread
  metastatic spread
  regional spread
  venous spread
spread pattern
spread-and-cut technique
spreader (*see also* rib spreader)
  Assistant Free calibrated
    femoral-tibial spreader
  Athens suture spreader
  baby Inge bone spreader
  baby Inge laminar spreader
  Bailey rib spreader
  Beeson cast spreader
  Beeson plaster spreader
  Benson pylorus spreader
  bladder neck spreader
  Blanco valve spreader
  Blount bone spreader
  Blount laminar spreader
  Bobechko spreader
  Bores incision spreader
  Burford rib spreader
  Burford-Finochietto infant rib
    spreader
  Burford-Finochietto rib
    spreader
  Caspar disk space spreader
  Caspar vertebral body
    spreader
  cast spreader
  chest spreader
  child's rib spreader
  Cloward vertebral spreader
  conjunctival spreader
  Costenbader incision spreader
  Cox metatarsal spreader
  Davis modified Finochietto
    rib spreader
  Davis rib spreader
  DeBakey infant and child rib
    spreader
  DeBakey rib spreader
  Doyen rib spreader
  ductus spreader
  Endotec spreader
  Favaloro-Morse rib spreader
  Favaloro-Morse sternal
    spreader

spreader (*continued*)
  Finochietto rib spreader
  Finochietto-Burford rib
    spreader
  Finochietto-Stille rib spreader
  Gerbode modified Burford rib
    spreader
  Gerbode rib spreader
  Gill incision spreader
  Gross ductus spreader
  Haglund spreader
  Haglund-Stille plaster spreader
  Haight pediatric rib spreader
  Haight rib spreader
  Haight-Finochietto rib
    spreader
  Harken rib spreader
  Harrington spreader
  Henning cast spreader
  Henning plaster spreader
  Hertzler baby rib spreader
  Hertzler rib spreader
  incision spreader
  infant rib spreader
  Inge lamina spreader
  intervertebral spreader
  Jarit three-prong cast spreader
  jaw spreader
  Kimpton vein spreader
  Kirschner wire spreader
  Kwitko conjunctival spreader
  lamina spreader
  Landolt spreader
  Lefferts rib spreader
  Leksell sternal spreader
  Lemmon rib spreader
  Lemmon sternal spreader
  Lilienthal rib spreader
  Lilienthal-Sauerbruch rib
    spreader
  Matson rib spreader
  McGuire rib spreader
  Medicon spreader
  Millin bladder neck spreader
  Millin-Bacon bladder neck
    spreader
  Miltex rib spreader
  mitral valve spreader
  Mity spreader
  Morris mitral valve spreader
  Morse sternal spreader
  M-Pact cast spreader

spreader (*continued*)
- Nelson rib spreader
- Nissen rib spreader
- Overholt rib spreader
- Overholt-Finochietto rib spreader
- Park rectal spreader
- plaster spreader
- Quervain rib spreader
- Rehbein rib spreader
- rib spreader
- Ridlon spreader
- Rienhoff rib spreader
- Rienhoff-Finochietto rib spreader
- root-canal spreader
- Sauerbruch-Lilienthal rib spreader
- Saurex spreader
- Sheldon spreader
- spinous process spreader
- sternal spreader
- Stille plaster spreader
- Stille-Quervain spreader
- Struck spreader
- Suarez spreader
- Sweet rib spreader
- Sweet-Burford rib spreader
- Sweet-Finochietto rib spreader
- Tessier spreader
- Texas Scottish Rite Hospital eyebolt spreader
- Theis infant rib spreader
- Theis rib spreader
- toe spreader
- tonsillar spreader
- Tudor-Edwards rib spreader
- Tuffier rib spreader
- Turek spinous process spreader
- Turner-Warwick bladder neck spreader
- USA plaster spreader
- Ventura spreader
- vertebral spreader
- Wolfe-Bohler plaster cast spreader
- Wakai spreader
- Weinberg pediatric rib spreader
- Weinberg rib spreader

spreader (*continued*)
- Wilder band spreader
- Wilson rib spreader
- Wiltberger spinous process spreader

spreader bar
spreader grafts
spreading fistulation
spreading forceps
spreading hand splint
spreading hypoperfusion
Sprengel anomaly
Sprengel deformity
Spring catheter
spring clip
spring cock-up splint
spring finger
spring fixation
spring holder
spring hook
spring iris scissors
spring lancet
spring ligament
spring loaded biopsy instrument
spring mechanism
spring pin
spring plate
spring retractor
spring scissors
spring swivel thumb
spring wire loop
spring-assisted syringe
spring-eye needle
spring-handled forceps
spring-handled needle holder
spring-handled scissors
spring-holder instrument tray
spring-hook wire needle
Springlite lower limb prosthesis
spring-loaded biopsy gun
spring-loaded nail
spring-loaded self-retaining retractor
spring-loaded vascular stent
spring-wire retractor
spring-wire safety-pin splint
Sprint catheter
Sprint catheter with Pro/Pel coating
sprinter's fracture
Sprong sutures
Sprotte epidural needle

Sprotte spinal needle
SPT technique (station pull-
    through technique)
SPTL vascular lesion laser
SPTU stapler
spud
    Alvis spud
    Bahn spud
    Bennett foreign body spud
    Corbett foreign body spud
    curved needle eye spud
    curved needle spud
    Davis foreign body spud
    Dix foreign body spud
    Ellis foreign body spud
    eye spud
    Fisher spud
    flat eye spud
    foreign body eye spud
    foreign body spud
    Francis knife spud
    golf-club eye spud
    golf-club spud
    gouge spud
    Gross ear spud
    Hosford foreign body spud
    knife spud
    LaForce knife spud
    Levine foreign body spud
    needle spud
    O'Brien foreign body spud
    Plange spud
    Storz folding-handle eye spud
    Walter corneal spud
    Walton round gouge spud
    Whittle spud
spud dissection
spud dissector
spud gouge
spud needle
spur
    bone spur
    bony spur
    calcaneal spur
    heel spur
    hypertrophic spur
    lumbar spur
    nasal spur
    occipital spur
    olecranon spur
    plantar calcaneal spur
    scleral spur

spur (*continued*)
    septum spur
    vascular spur
    vomerine spur
spur crusher (*see* crusher)
spur formation
spur-crushing clamp
spurious aneurysm
spurious ankylosis
spurious aperture of facial canal
spurious hermaphroditism
spurious pregnancy
Spurling forceps
Spurling intervertebral disk
    forceps
Spurling intervertebral disk
    rongeur
Spurling disk forceps
Spurling laminectomy rongeur
Spurling maneuver
Spurling periosteal elevator
Spurling pituitary rongeur
Spurling retractor
Spurling rongeur forceps
Spurling sign
Spurling tissue forceps
Spurling-Kerrison down-biting
    rongeur
Spurling-Kerrison forceps
Spurling-Kerrison laminectomy
    punch
Spurling-Kerrison laminectomy
    rongeur
Spurling-Kerrison punch
Spurling-Kerrison rongeur
    forceps
Spurling-Kerrison up-biting
    rongeur
Spurling-Love-Gruenwald-
    Cushing rongeur
Sputnik Russian razor blade
Sputnik-Federov lens
sputum collection
sputum culture
sputum induction
sputum production
sputum studies
sputum tube
Spyglass angiography catheter
Spyrogel hydrogel wound
    dressing
SQ (subcuticular)

squama (*pl.* squamae)
  frontal bone squama
  mental squama
  occipital squama
  perpendicular squama
  temporal squama
squama alveolaris
squamocolumnar junction
squamofrontal
squamomastoid suture
squamoparietal suture
squamosal suture
squamosomastoid suture
squamosoparietal suture
squamososphenoid suture
squamosphenoid suture
squamotemporal
squamotympanic fissure
squamous bone
squamous border
squamous cell carcinoma (SCC)
squamous cell carcinoma of
  head and neck (SCCHN)
squamous cell carcinoma-
  inhibitory factor (SSCIF)
squamous cell papilloma
squamous cell
  pseudoepithelioma
squamous epithelial ingrowth
squamous epithelium
squamous hyperplasia
squamous ingrowth
squamous intraepithelial lesion
squamous margin
squamous odontogenic tumor
squamous papilloma
squamous suture
squamous suture lines
squamous suture of cranium
square muscle of upper lip
square prism
square punch
square specimen forceps
square wire
square-end pliers
square-ended distraction rod
square-ended hook
square-hole broach
square-off sign of shoulder
squares of dressing
square-shaped occluder
square-shouldered lesion

square-tipped arterial dissector
square-tipped artery dissector
squeeze sign
squeeze-handle forceps
Squeeze-Mark surgical marker
Squibb catheter
Squibb Sur-Fit ostomy pouch
Squibb urostomy pouch
squint hook
squinting eye
squinting patella
Squire catheter
SRH (stigmata of recent
  hemorrhage)
SR-Isosit dental restorative
  material
SR-Ivocap denture material
SR-Ivolen impression material
SR-Ivoseal impression material
S-ROM acetabular cup
S-ROM femoral stem prosthesis
S-ROM gripper
S-ROM hip prosthesis
S-ROM system prosthesis
SRP (synchronized
  retroperfusion)
SRS injectable cement
SRT vaginal speculum
SRVG (silicone elastomer ring
  vertical gastroplasty)
SS (stainless steel)
SS bobbin drain tube
SS bobbin myringotomy tube
SS staple
SS sutures
Ssabanejew-Frank gastrostomy
Ssabanejew-Frank operation
SSCIF (squamous cell
  carcinoma-inhibitory factor)
S-shaped anal anastomosis
S-shaped body
S-shaped brain retractor
S-shaped brain spatula
S-shaped deformity
S-shaped ileal pouch
S-shaped ileal pouch-anal
  anastomosis
S-shaped incision
S-shaped peripheral vascular
  clamp
S-shaped pouch
S-shaped reservoir

S-shaped retractor
S-shaped scar
S-shaped scoliosis
SSI (surgical site infection)
SSI brace (shoulder subluxation
    inhibitor brace)
SSL (subtotal supraglottic
    laryngectomy)
SSO (sagittal split osteotomy)
SSRI discontinuation syndrome
SSRO (sagittal split ramus
    osteotomy)
SST deformity
SSW forceps
ST Lalonde hook forceps
ST segment elevation
St. Bartholomew barium
    catheter
St. Clair forceps
St. Clair-Thompson abscess
    forceps
St. Clair-Thompson adenoidal
    curet
St. Clair-Thompson adenoidal
    forceps
St. Clair-Thompson adenotome
St. Clair-Thompson peritonsillar
    abscess forceps
St. George total elbow
    prosthesis
St. George total hip prosthesis
St. George total knee prosthesis
St. Jude annuloplasty ring
St. Jude bileaflet prosthetic
    valve
St. Jude cardiac device
St. Jude composite valve graft
St. Jude aortic valve prosthesis
St. Jude bileaflet heart valve
St. Jude prosthesis
St. Jude prosthetic heart valve
St. Jude valve prosthesis
St. Jude mitral valve prosthesis
St. Jude valve
St. Jude valve prosthesis
St. Luke retractor
St. Luke rongeur
St. Mark clamp
St. Mark excision
St. Mark hemorrhoidectomy
St. Mark incision
St. Mark pudendal electrode

St. Mark lipped retractor
St. Mark pelvis retractor
St. Martin eye forceps
St. Martin suturing forceps
St. Martin-Franceschetti
    secondary cataract hook
St. Urban Berlin hip joint surface
    replacement
St. Vincent tube clamp
St. Vincent tube-clamping
    forceps
St. Vincent tube-occluding
    forceps
Staar foldable intraocular lens
Staar implantable contact lens
Starr Toric implantable contact
    lens
Staar Toric lens
stab drain
stab electrode
stab form
stab incision
stab needle
stab wound
stabilization
    anterior internal stabilization
    anterior shaft-segment
        stabilization
    atlantoaxial stabilization
    atlanto-occipital stabilization
    cervical spine stabilization
    cervicothoracic junction
        stabilization
    chest wall stabilization
    columellar stabilization
    columellar subluxation
        stabilization
    coronoradicular stabilization
    definitive stabilization
    distal radioulnar joint
        stabilization
    dynamic lumbar stabilization
    flexion compression spine
        injury stabilization
    fracture stabilization
    Gruca stabilization
    iliac crest bone graft
        stabilization
    jaw stabilization
    lower cervical spine posterior
        stabilization
    lumbar spine stabilization

stabilization (*continued*)
   myoplastic muscle
     stabilization
   occipitocervical stabilization
   prophylactic operative
     stabilization
   provisional stabilization
   retentive stabilization
   rhythmic stabilization
   sacral spine stabilization
   screw stabilization
   skeletal stabilization
   spinal column stabilization
   spinal injury operative
     stabilization
   spinal osteotomy stabilization
   subluxation stabilization
   suture brow stabilization
   thoracolumbar spine
     stabilization
   TSRH crosslink stabilization
   wire stabilization
stabilization approach
stabilization of joint
stabilization plate
stabilization training
stabilized baseplate
stabilized condition
stabilized course
stabilizing bar
stabilizing fulcrum line
stabilizing guide pin
stabilocondylar knee prosthesis
Stabilor alloy
stab-in epicardial electrode
stable access cannula
stable burst fracture
stable fracture
stable reduction
stable sprain
Stableflex lens
Stableloc Colles fracture
   external fixator
Stable-Lok nut
stab-wound drain
stab-wound incision
Stack autoperfusion balloon
Stack perfusion coronary
   dilatation catheter
Stack retractor
Stack shoulder procedure
Stack splint

Stacke chisel guard
Stacke gouge
Stacke mastoidectomy
Stacke operation
Stacke probe
Staden pin guide
Stader connecting rod
Stader pin
Stader wrench
Stadie-Riggs microtome
stadium-type of ureteral orifice
Stadler splint
Staecker nerve protector
Sta-Fix tape
Stafne bone cyst
Stafne idiopathic bone cavity
stage
   desmolytic stage
   disease stage
   implant stage
   input stage
   lamina-bud stage
   maturative stage
   morphogenic stage
   patch stage
   secondary stage
   successive stages
Stage IV mattress replacement
stage of labor
staged abdominal repair (STAR)
staged breast reconstruction
staged genioplasty
staged muscle transfer
staged procedure
staged reconstruction
staghorn calculus
staghorn stone
staging
   ACJJ staging
   Breslow staging
   Enneking staging
   evaluative staging
   imaging staging
   intraoperative tumor staging
   laparoscopic staging
   Papineau bone graft staging
     (stages I-III)
   pathology and staging
   surgical evaluative staging
   surgical staging
   TNM tumor staging
staging laparotomy

staging lymphadenectomy
staging operation
staging process and imaging
staging systems in radiation
    therapy
stagnant loop syndrome
Stagnara gouge
Stagnara procedure
Staheli shelf operation
Staheli shelf procedure
Staheli technique
Stahl calipers
Stahl calipers block
Stahl calipers plate
Stahl ear
Stahl lens gauge
Stahl nucleus expressor
Stahl ophthalmic calipers
Stahli line
Stahli pigment line
Stahr gland
staining
    blood staining
    corneal staining
    extrinsic environmental
        staining
stainless irrigator
stainless spatula
stainless sponge
stainless steel
stainless steel AO plate
stainless steel balloon
    expandable stent
stainless steel blade
stainless steel bobbin
stainless steel clamp
stainless steel crown
stainless steel cup
stainless steel flexible ruler
stainless steel graft
stainless steel guidewire
stainless steel implant
stainless steel mesh
stainless steel mesh prosthesis
stainless steel mesh stent
stainless steel piston
stainless steel prosthesis
stainless steel screw
stainless steel strut
stainless steel stud
stainless steel sutures
stainless steel wire

stainless steel wire prosthesis
stainless steel wire sutures
stainless steel with molybdenum
staircase technique for lip
    reconstruction
StairClimber assist device
stairstep deformity
stairstep fracture
stairstep transcolumellar
    incision
stalagmometer
stalk
    body stalk
    connective tissue stalk
    defatting the umbilical stalk
    pituitary stalk
    polyp stalk
    rectal stalks
    umbilical stalk
stalk of polyp
stalked hydatid
Stallard blunt dissector
Stallard dissector
Stallard eyelid operation
Stallard flap operation
Stallard head clamp
Stallard operation
Stallard scleral hook
Stallard sutures
Stallard-Liegard operation
Stallard-Liegard sutures
Stallerpointe needle
Stallworthy placenta
StaLock Universal Plus suture-
    free anchor
Stalzner rectal scissors
STA-MCA (superficial temporary
    artery-middle cerebral
    artery)
STA-MCA anastomosis
STA-MCA bypass procedure
Stamey bladder neck suspension
Stamey dorsal vein apical
    retractor
Stamey Malecot catheter
Stamey modification of Pereyra
    procedure
Stamey needle
Stamey needle suspension
Stamey open-tip ureteral
    catheter
Stamey operation

Stamey paraurethral suspension
Stamey procedure
Stamey ureteral catheter
Stamey urethropexy
Stamey-Malecot catheter
Stamey-Martius procedure
Stamey-Pereyra bladder neck
   suspension
Stamey-Pereyra urethropexy
Stamler side-port fixation hook
Stamm arthrodesis
Stamm bone-cutting forceps
Stamm bunionectomy
Stamm gastroplasty
Stamm gastrostomy
Stamm gastrostomy tube
Stamm hip fusion
Stamm operation
Stamm osteotomy
Stamm procedure for
   intraarticular hip fusion
Stamm tube
Stammberger antral punch
Stammberger side-biting punch
   forceps
stammering bladder
Stamm-Kader gastrotomy
   technique
Stamm-Kader operation
Stamm-Senn gastroscopy
standard 6-lumen perfused
   catheter
standard above-elbow cast
standard arterial forceps
standard arthroscope
standard biopsy technique
standard bronchoscope
standard care sterile urethral
   catheter
standard clavicular incision
standard colonoscope
standard gastrectomy
standard duodenoscope
standard earmold
standard endoscopy
   polypectomy snare
standard ERCP catheter
standard formalin fixation
standard full-lumen
   esophagoscope
standard gastric resection
standard head halter

standard hook electrosurgical
   probe
standard Jackson laryngoscope
standard Kocher incision
standard laryngoscope
standard Lehman catheter
standard midline laparotomy
standard neck exploration
standard needle
standard open approach
standard radical neck dissection
standard retroperitoneal flank
   incision
standard right hemicolectomy
standard single port cannula
standard stripping procedure
standard surgical procedure
standard trocar
standard wire gauge
standardized curative radical
   total gastrectomy
standardized hepatectomy
standard-pattern hammer
standard-pattern mallet
standby Baumanometer
standby pacemaker
standing frame orthosis
Stanford bioptome
Stanford end-hole pigtail
   catheter
Stanford aortic dissection
Stanford-Caves bioptome
Stanford-type aortic dissection
Stange laryngoscope
Stangel fallopian tube cannula
Stangel fallopian tube miniclip
Stangel modified Barraquer
   microsurgical needle holder
Stanicor Gamma pacemaker
Stanicor Lambda demand
   pacemaker
Stanicor pacemaker
Stanischeff operation
Stankiewicz iris clip intraocular
   lens
Stanley Way procedure
Stanley-Kent bundle
Stanmore shoulder arthroplasty
Stanmore shoulder prosthesis
Stanmore total hip
Stanmore total knee
Stansel procedure

Stanton cautery clamp
Stanton cautery with mousetrap
   clamp
Stanzel needle holder
Staodyn Insight point locator
stapedectomy footplate pick
stapedectomy forceps
stapedectomy knife
stapedectomy prosthesis
stapedial artery
stapedial crus
stapedial fold
stapedial footplate auger
stapedial nerve
stapedial tendon
stapedial tendon cut
stapediolysis
stapediotenotomy
stapedius muscle
stapedius tendon
stapedius tendon knife
stapedotomy
STA-peg implant
STA-peg procedure
stapes
   base of stapes
   capitulum of stapes
   crus of stapes
   fixator muscle of base of
     stapes
   monopodal ankylotic stapes
stapes bone
stapes chisel
stapes curet
stapes dilator
stapes elevator
stapes excavator
stapes footplate
stapes forceps
stapes hoe
stapes hook
stapes mobilization
stapes needle
stapes pick
stapes piston
stapes prosthesis
stapes speculum
stapes spline
stapes superstructure
stapes tapping hammer
stapes wire guide
staphylectomy

staphylodialysis
staphyloma
staphyloncus
staphylopharyngorrhaphy
staphyloplasty
staphyloplegia
staphyloptosis
staphylorrhaphy elevator
staphylorrhaphy needle
staphyloschisis
staphylotome
staphylotomy
staple
   5-pin staple
   7-pin staple
   30-V staples
   barb staple
   barbed Richards staple
   Bio-Absorbable staple
   Blount epiphyseal staple
   Blount fracture staple
   Blount knee staple
   Bostick staple
   Coventry staple
   DePalma staple
   duToit shoulder staple
   Dwyer staple
   Ellison fixation staple
   Ethicon staple
   Fastlok implantable staple
   GIA staple
   Hernandez-Ros bone staple
   Krackow blade staple
   Lactomer absorbable
     subcuticular skin staple
   Mario-Stone staple
   meniscal staple
   metallic staple
   Nakayama staple
   orthopedic staple
   Oswestry staples
   Polysorb absorbable staple
   Proplast staples
   Proximate skin staples
   Richards fixation staple
   SGIA staples
   SinStat preformed skin staple
   skin staples
   Smith & Nephew medium
     barbed staple
   Smith and Nephew small
     barbed staple

staple (*continued*)

spike staple
SS staple
step staples
Stone staple
TA metallic staple
TA Premium-series staple
tie-over dressing with skin
   staples
titanium mandibular staple
titanium staple
von Petz staple
Wiberg fracture staple
Zimaloy epiphyseal staple
staple bone plate
staple capsulorrhaphy
staple fixation
staple forceps
staple gun (*see* stapler)
staple line dehiscence
staple procedure
staple sutures
stapled blind end
stapled coloanal anastomosis
stapled hemorrhoidectomy
stapled ileoanal anastomosis
stapled lung reduction
stapled reconstruction
stapled reconstruction
   procedure
stapled reconstruction
   technique
stapler

American vascular stapler
Appose disposable skin
   stapler
arcuate skin stapler
Auto Suture Multifire Endo
   GIA 30 stapler
Auto Suture Premium CEEA
   stapler
Auto-Suture GIA stapler
barbed stapler
Barstow stapler
CDH stapler
CEEA stapler (curved end-
   to-end anastomosis
   stapler)
circular intraluminal stapler
circular mechanical stapler
circular stapler
Cobe gun stapler

stapler (*continued*)

Concorde disposable skin
   stapler
copolymer stapler
Coventry stapler
Cricket disposable skin
   stapler
curved end-to-end
   anastomosis stapler (CEEA
   stapler)
curved intraluminal stapler
Davis-Geck surgical stapler
Day stapler
disposable intraluminal
   stapler
double-headed stapler
Downing stapler
duToit stapler
Dwyer spinal mechanical
   stapler
EEA Auto-Suture stapler
EEA circular stapler
EEA stapler
end-end stapler
Endo Babcock stapler
Endo GIA stapler
Endo hernia stapler
Endo-GIA suture stapler
Endopath hernia stapler
Endopath endoscopic
   articulation stapler
Endopath endoscopic stapler
Endopath Stealth stapler
Ethicon endosurgery circular
   stapler
gastroplasty stapler
GIA circular stapler
GIA stapler
Graftac skin stapler
Graftac-S skin stapler
Hall double-hole spinal stapler
hernia stapler
ILA stapler
Imagyn surgical stapler
Inokucki vascular stapler
intraluminal stapler
Lactomer copolymer
   absorbable stapler
LDA stapler
LDF stapler
LDS stapler
ligating and dividing stapler

stapler (*continued*)
  linear stapler
  Multifire Endo GIA stapler
  Multifire GIA stapler
  Multifire GIA-series stapler
  Multifire TA-series stapler
  Multifire VersaTack stapler
  Nakayama microvascular
    stapler
  Ni-Ti Shape Memory alloy
    compression stapler
  One-Time disposable skin
    stapler
  Oswestry-O'Brien spinal
    stapler
  PC EEA stapler
  PI disposable stapler
  PI surgical stapler
  PolyGIA stapler
  Polysorb stapler
  Precise disposable skin stapler
  Premium CEEA circular
    stapler
  Premium Plus CEEA
    disposable stapler
  Premium Poly stapler
  Proximate disposable skin
    stapler
  Proximate flexible linear
    stapler
  Proximate intraluminal stapler
  Proximate linear cutter
    stapler
  Proximate linear stapler
  Proximate-ILS curved
    intraluminal stapler
  Reflex skin stapler
  Roticulator clamp stapler
  Royal disposable skin stapler
  SDsorb meniscal stapler
  SGIA 50 disposable stapler
  SGIA stapler
  Signet disposable skin stapler
  Soviet mechanical bronchial
    stapler
  SPTU Soviet stapler
  Staplizer powered
    metaphyseal stapler
  STI-1 needle-shaped tissue
    stapler
  Surgeon's Choice stapler
  Surgiport stapler

stapler (*continued*)
  TA-30 stapler
  TA-50 stapler
  TA-55 stapler
  TA-60 stapler
  TA-90 stapler
  TA-90-BN stapler
  TL-90 stapler
  UG-70 stapler
  Uhlrich stapler
  United States Surgical circular
    stapler
  UPO-16 stapler
  Versatack stapler
  Vista disposable skin stapler
  Vital skin stapler
  Vogelfanger blood vessel
    stapler
  Vogelfanger-Beattie stapler
  Watt skin closure stapler
  Weck stapler
  Wiberg fracture stapler
  Yamagishi stapler
Staples elbow arthrodesis
Staples esophagojejunostomy
Staples osteotomy nail
Staples repair
Staples technique
stapling device (*see* stapler)
stapling instruments
stapling procedure
stapling technique
Staplizer powered metaphyseal
    stapler
  macular star
STAR (staged abdominal repair)
Star ventilator
Star X CO_2 laser
STAR LOCK multi-purpose
    threaded implant
STAR LOCK Press-Fit cylinder
    implant
Star/Vent 1-stage dental screw
    implant
Starcam camera
starch bandage
starch-based copolymer dressing
Starck cardiodilator
Starck dilator
Stark graft
Stark vulsellum forceps
Starling reflex

Starlinger uterine dilator
Starlite endodontic implant
    starter kit
Starlite Omni-AT bur
Starlite point
StarMed video otoscope
Starr ball heart prosthesis
Starr ball heart valve
Starr fixation forceps
Starr forceps
Starr polyimide loop intraocular
    lens
Starr Toric intraocular lens
Starr-Bloodwell low-profile valve
Starr-Edwards aortic valve
    prosthesis
Starr-Edwards ball valve
    prosthesis
Starr-Edwards heart valve
Starr-Edwards hermetically
    sealed pacemaker
Starr-Edwards mitral prosthesis
Starr-Edwards prosthetic aortic
    valve
Starr-Edwards prosthetic ball
    valve
Starr-Edwards prosthetic mitral
    valve
Starr-Edwards prosthetic valve
Starr-Edwards Silastic valve
Starr-Edwards silicone rubber
    ball valve
Starr-Edwards valve prosthesis
STARRT (selective tubal
    assessment to refine
    reproductive therapy)
Star-shaped omphaloplasty
    technique
Startanius blade implant
starter awl
starter broach
stasis (*pl.* stases)
    bile stasis
    duodenal stasis
    ileal stasis
    intestinal stasis
    urinary stasis
    venous stasis
stasis changes
stasis dermatitis
stasis eczema
stasis edema

stasis gallbladder
stasis syndrome
stasis ulcer
stasis vascular ulcer
stat (immediately)
Stat 2 Pumpette disposable IV
    pump
Stat aspirating instrument
Stat aspirator
Stat cutting instrument
Stat Scrub handwasher machine
Statak soft tissue attachment
    device
Statak suture anchor
State colorectal anastomosis
State end-to-end anastomosis
Statham cautery
Statham electromagnetic flow
    meter
Statham external transducer
Statham pressure transducer
Statham strain gauge
Statham transducer
Statham transensor
static air mattress
static compression
static dilation technique
static fixation
Sta-Tic impression material
static instability of wrist
static sling
static splint
static tendon transfer
static topical occlusive
    hemostatic pressure device
station pull-through esophageal
    manometry technique
station pull-through operation
station pull-through technique
    (SPT technique)
stationary angle guide
stationary bridge
stationary cataract
Sta-tite 2 ply elastic roll gauze
Sta-Tite gauze dressing
StatLock-Foley catheter
statoconic membrane
Stat-Padz defibrillator patch
Stat-Temp II liquid crystal
    temperature monitor
Stat-Temp II temperature device
Stat-Trace electrode

Status-X machine
Staude tenaculum forceps
Staude uterine tenaculum
Staude uterine tenaculum
    forceps
Staude-Jackson tenaculum
    forceps
Staude-Jackson uterine
    tenaculum
Staude-Moore forceps
Staude-Moore tenaculum
Staude-Moore uterine tenaculum
Staude-Moore uterine tenaculum
    forceps
Stauffer modification
Stauffer syndrome
Staunig position
Staunton sphygmomanometer
staurion
Stax fingertip splint
stay knot
stay suture retractor
stay suture technique
stay sutures
Stayce adjustable clamp
Stayoden 9000F TENS unit
Stay-Rite clamp
StaySharp Super-Cut face-lift
    scissors
STC 900-series travel chair
STD+ titanium total hip
    prosthesis
STE (subperiosteal tissue
    expander)
Steady Strider ankle-foot
    orthosis
steady-state gradient-echo
    imaging
steal procedure
Stealth angioplasty balloon
    catheter
Stealth catheter balloon
Stealth free-hand diamond knife
Stealth frame
steam cautery
Stearns speculum
steatogenous
Stecher arachnoid knife
Stecher microruler
Stecher position
Stedman aspirator
Stedman awl

Stedman continuous suction
    tube
Stedman saw
Stedman suction pump
Stedman suction pump aspirator
Stedman suction tube
steel embolization coil
steel ligature
steel mallet
steel mesh
steel mesh sutures
steel plate
steel ruler
steel sutures
steel wire prosthesis
Steele articulator
Steele bronchial dilator
Steele classification of intra-
    articular fractions (types
    I-III)
Steele dilator
Steele filling instrument
Steele osteotomy
Steele periosteal elevator
Steele-Stewart operation
Steelquist amputation
steel-winged butterfly needle
steep Trendelenburg position
steeple flap
steerable angioplastic guidewire
steerable catheter
steerable cystoscopy
steerable decapolar electrode
    catheter
steerable guidewire
steerable guidewire catheter
steerable wire
steering catheter
steering-wheel injury
Steerocath catheter
Steffee instrumentation
    technique
Steffee pedicle plate
Steffee plate
Steffee prosthesis
Steffee screw
Steffee screw plate
Steffee spinal instrumentation
Steffee thumb arthroplasty
Steichen neurovascular free flap
Steichen technique
Steide fracture of femur

Steiger joint
Stein cheiloplasty
Steinhauser internal screw
    fixation
Stein intraocular implant lens
Stein membrane perforator
Stein operation
Stein-Abbe lip flap
Steinach operation
Steinbach mallet
Steinberg infiltration block
Steinberg thumb sign
Steinbrocker classification
Steindler arthrodesis
Steindler flexorplasty
Steindler matricectomy
Steindler operation
Steindler procedure
Steindler stripping
Steindler technique
Steiner electromechanical
    morcellator
Steiner-Auvard vaginal retractor
Steiner-Auvard vaginal speculum
Steinert disease
Steinert laser-assisted
    intrastromal keratomileusis
    set
Steinert-Deacon incision gauge
Steinhauser bone clamp
Steinhauser electromucotome
Steinhauser internal screw
    fixation
Steinhauser lag screw
Steinhauser plate
Steinhauser position screw
Steinhauser-Castroviejo
    electromucotome
Stein-Kazanjian lower lip flap
Stein-Leventhal syndrome
Steinmann calibrated pin
Steinmann calibration pin
Steinmann extension
Steinmann extension nail
Steinmann fixation pin
Steinmann holder
Steinmann intestinal forceps
Steinmann intestinal grasping
    forceps
Steinmann pin chuck
Steinmann pin fixation
Steinmann pin with ball bearing

Steinmann pin with Crowe pilot
    point
Steinmann tendon forceps
Steinmann traction
Steinmann traction bow
Steinmann traction tractor
Steinmann tractor
Steis bone marrow transplant
    needle
Stela electrode lead
Steldent alloy
Stelid pacing lead
Stelix pacing lead
stellatae renis, venulae
stellate abscess
stellate block
stellate block anesthesia
stellate border breast lesion
stellate cataract
stellate fracture
stellate ganglion
stellate ganglion block
stellate ganglion block
    anesthesia
stellate ganglion block
    anesthetic technique
stellate ganglion blockade
stellate incision
stellate laceration
stellate pattern
stellate pseudoscar
stellate skull fracture
stellate veins of kidney
Stellbring synovectomy rongeur
Stellbrink fixation device
stellectomy
Stellite ring material of
    prosthetic valve
stem cell concentrator
stem cell gene therapy
stem extractor
stem pessary
stem prosthesis
stem rasp
stem removal
stem spoon separator
stem-cell marrow harvesting
stemmed tibial prosthesis
Stemp clamp
Stemp compound
stencil wire
Stener lesion

Stener-Gunterberg sacrum
   resection
Stengstrom nerve cutter
stenopeic disk
stenopeic iridectomy
stenosed aortic valve
stenosing tendinitis
stenosing tenosynovitis
stenosis (*pl.* stenoses)
   acquired nasopharyngeal
      stenosis
   ampullary stenosis
   anal stenosis
   anorectal stenosis
   antral stenosis
   benign papillary stenosis
   buttonhole mitral stenosis
   capillary stenosis
   carotid artery stenosis
   cervical stenosis
   choanal stenosis
   choledochoduodenal
      junctional stenosis
   cicatricial stenosis
   esophageal stenosis
   fish-mouth mitral stenosis
   Getty technique for spinal
      stenosis
   glottic stenosis
   granulation stenosis
   high-flow arterial stenosis
   hypertrophic pyloric stenosis
   hypopharyngeal stenosis
   iatrogenic nasal stenosis
   idiopathic hypertrophic
      subaortic stenosis (IHSS)
   ileostomy stenosis
   laryngeal stenosis
   laryngotracheal stenosis
   meatal stenosis
   nasal stenosis
   nasopharyngeal stenosis
   papillary stenosis
   piriform aperture stenosis
   postischemic stenosis
   preventricular stenosis
   pulmonic stenosis
   pyloric stenosis
   rectal stenosis
   spinal stenosis
   stomal stenosis
   subaortic stenosis

stenosis (*continued*)
   subglottic stenosis
   subvalvular aortic stenosis
   supraglottic stenosis
   supravalvular aortic stenosis
   tracheal stenosis
   tricuspid stenosis
   valvular stenosis
stenosis clamp
stenostenosis
stenostomia
stenotic cleft
stenotic disease
stenotic esophagogastric
      anastomosis
stenotic femoral artery
stenotic lesion
stenotic segment
stenotic valve
Stensen canal
Stensen duct
Stensen duct caruncle
Stensen foramen
Stensen plexus
Stensen veins
Stenstrom alar cartilage
      technique
Stenstrom foot flap
Stenstrom nerve holder
Stenstrom otoplasty
Stenstrom rasp
Stenstrom raspatory
Stenstrom technique in
      otoplasty
stent
   Aboulker stent
   absorbable stent
   Acculink self-expanding stent
   ACS Multi-Link Duet coronary
      stent
   ACS Multi-Link Tristar
      coronary stent
   ACS OTW HP coronary
   ACS Rx Multi-Link coronary
      stent
   activated balloon expandable
      intravascular stent
   active MRI stent (AMRIS)
   ACT-one coronary stent
   adherent stent
   adjustable vaginal stent
   American Heyer-Schulte stent

stent (*continued*)

AMS urethral stent
Amsterdam biliary stent
Anastaflo stent
AneuRx aortic aneurysm stent-graft
AngioStent cardiovascular stent
antegrade internal stent
antegrade ureteral stent
antibiotic-coated stent
antihemorrhagic stent
Atkinson tube stent
AVE GFX coronary stent
AVE Micro stent
bailout stent
balloon expandable intravascular stent
balloon expandable stent
balloon expandable flexible coil stent
balloon expandable metallic stent
Bard coil stent
Bard colorectal stent
Bard soft double-pigtail stent
Bard XT coronary stent
Bardex stent
Beamer stent
beStent 2 coronary stent
beStent balloon-expandable stent
beStent 2 laser-cut stent
biliary stent
bioabsorbable double-spiral stent
biodegradable stent
BioDivYsio stent
BioSorb resorbable urology stent
BlackBeauty ureteral stent
Braun stent
Bx Velocity coronary artery stent
Bx Velocity sirolimus-coated stent
Carcon stent
CardioCoil self-expanding coronary stent
Carey-Coons soft stent
carotid stent
CarotidCoil stent

stent (*continued*)

Carpentier stent
Carson internal/external endopyelotomy stent
cell-seeded stent
C-Flex Amsterdam stent
C-Flex ureteral stent
Champion stent
coil vascular stent
composite polymer stent
Conley tracheal stent
conventional stent
Cook FlexStent stent
Cook intracoronary stent
Cook ureteral stent
Cook Urosoft stent
Cordis Crossflex stent
Cordis radiopaque tantalum stent
core mold stent
Corinthian stent
Corvita stent
Cotton-Huibregtse biliary stent
Cotton-Leung biliary stent
covered Gianturco stent
Cragg stent
CrossFlex coil stent
CrossFlex LC coronary artery stent
Crown stent
Cypher sirolimus-eluting stent
Cysto Flex stent
Dacron stent
Dacron-covered stent
Dart coronary stent
Devon-Pura stent
DISA S-flex coronary stent
diversion stent
Dobbhoff biliary stent
double-J dangle stent
double-J indwelling catheter stent
double-J silicone internal ureteral catheter stent
double-J stent catheter stent
double-J ureteral stent
double-pigtail stent
Doyle silicone stent
drug-coated stent
drug-eluting stent
Dua stent
Duet coronary stent

stent (*continued*)

Dumon silicone stent
Dumon tracheobronchial stent
Dynalink biliary self-expanding stent
Dynamic Y stent
Elastalloy esophageal stent
Elastalloy Ultraflex Strecker nitinol stent
Eliminator biliary stent
Eliminator pancreatic stent
eluting stent
endobiliary stent
Endocare Horizon prostatic stent
Endocare nitinol stent
EndoCoil biliary stent
EndoCoil esophageal stent
endoesophageal stent
endoluminal stent
endovascular stent
Enforcer SDS coronary stent
Entract stent
EsophaCoil biliary stent
EsophaCoil self-expanding esophageal stent
esophageal stent
esophageal Strecker stent
esophageal Z-stent stent
expandable esophageal stent
expandable intrahepatic portacaval shunt stent
expandable metallic stent
Express stent
expulsion stent
Fader Tip ureteral stent
fibrin film stent
flat wire coil stent
Flexima biliary stent
FlexStent stent
foam rubber stent
foam rubber vaginal stent
FocalSeal-R neurosurgical stent
Focustent coronary stent
Freedom stent
free-standing stent
Freitag stent
French stent
gauze stent
Geenan pancreatic stent

stent (*continued*)

gelatin-covered mesh stent
gfx coronary stent
Gianturco expandable metallic biliary stent
Gianturco expanding metallic stent
Gianturco metal urethral stent
Gianturco zigzag stent
Gianturco-Rosch self-expandable biliary Z-stent
Gianturco-Roubin flexible coil stent
Gianturco-Roubin FlexStent coronary stent
Gibbon indwelling ureteral stent
Gibbon ureteral stent
Global Therapeutics Freedom stent
Global Therapeutics V-Flex stent
Guidant Multi-Link Tetra coronary stent
hand-crimped stent
hand-mounted stent
Harrell Y stent
Harrison fetal bladder stent
heat-expandable stent
helical coil stent
helical-ridged ureteral stent
Hepamed-coated Wiktor stent
heparin-coated Palmaz-Schatz stent
Hood stoma stent
Hood-Westaby T-Y stent
Horizon stent
Huibregtse biliary stent
Hydromer coated polyurethane stent
HydroPlus stent
iliac artery stent
indwelling ureteral stent
InStent CarotidCoil stent
interdigitating coil stent
IntraCoil nitinol stent
intracoronary stent
intraoral stent
Intra-prostatic stent
IntraStent DoubleStrut biliary endoprosthesis
intravascular stent

stent (*continued*)

INX stainless steel stent
iridium-192 loaded stent
IRIS coronary stent
Jasin Frontal Ostent stent
JJIS stent
J-Maxx stent
Johnson & Johnson biliary
stent
Johnson & Johnson coronary
stent
Jomed stent
JoStent coronary stent
Kaminsky stent
keel stent
kidney internal stent
kissing stent
Koken nasal stents
labial stent
lacrimal stent
laryngeal stent
lighted stent
Lubri-Flex ureteral stent
Lubri-Flex urologic stent
luminal stent
Luminexx biliary stent
Magic Wallstent
magnetic internal ureteral
stent
main pancreatic duct stent
Mardis soft stent
maxillary stent
Medinol NIRside slotted stent
Medinvent vascular stent
Meditronic coronary stent
Medivent self-expanding
coronary stent
Medivent vascular stent
Medtronic beStent stent
Medtronic interventional
vascular stent
Medtronic coronary stent
MegaLink biliary stent
Memotherm colorectal stent
Memotherm endoscopic
biliary stent
Memotherm Flexx biliary
stent
Memotherm nitanol stent
Mentor biliary stent
MeroGel nasal stent
MeroGel sinus stent

stent (*continued*)

mesh stent
metal Z stent
metal-augmented polymer
stent
metal-coated stent
metallic stent
methyl methacrylate ear stent
Microvasive stent
Mini Crown stent
mini-Monoka canalicular stent
Monoka canalicular stent
Montgomery laryngeal stent
MPD stent
multicellular stent
Multi-Flex stent
Multilink Duet stent
Multilink Pixel stent
Navius stent
Neville stent
NexStent carotid stent
NIR Elite over-the-wire stent
NIR ON Ranger balloon
expandable stent
NIR ON Ranger premounted
stent
NIR paclitaxel-coated
coronary stent
NIR Primo balloon
expandable stent
NIR Primo Monorail stent
NIR with SOX coronary stent
NIR with SOX over-the-wire
coronary stent
Niroyal Advance balloon
expandable stent
Niroyal Elite Monorail
coronary stent
NIRstent stent
nitinol mesh stent
nitinol self-expanding coil
stent
nitinol subglottic stenosis
stent
nitinol thermal memory stent
Novastent stent
occlusal stent
OmniLink biliary stent
OmniStent stent
Orlowski stent
Ossof-Sisson surgical stent
ostiomeatal stent

stent (*continued*)

paclitaxel-coated coronary stent
Palmaz arterial stent
Palmaz balloon expandable iliac stent
Palmaz biliary stent
Palmaz Corinthian transhepatic biliary stent
Palmaz vascular stent
Palmaz-Schatz balloon expandable stent
Palmaz-Schatz biliary stent
Palmaz-Schatz coronary stent
Palmaz-Schatz Crown balloon expandable stent
Palmaz-Schatz Mini Crown stent
pancreatic duct stent
Paragon Champion stent
Paragon coronary stent
Paragon nitinol stent
Passager stent
patent stent
Percuflex Amsterdam stent
Percuflex biliary stent
Percuflex endopyelotomy stent
Percuflex flexible biliary stent
Percuflex Plus ureteral stent
percutaneous stent
percutaneous ureteral stent
Perflex stainless steel stent
piano-style guidewire stent
pigtail biliary stent
pigtail stent
plastic stent
polyethylene stent
polymer-coated, drug-eluting stent
polymeric endoluminal paving stent
polytetraflouroethylene-covered stent
polyurethane stent
porous metallic stent
PowerGrip stent
premounted stent
ProstaCoil self-expanding stent
Prostakath urethral stent
prostatic stent

stent (*continued*)

PTFE-covered Palmaz stent
Pura-Vario stent
Quadracoil ureteral stent
radioactive stent
radioisotope stent
radiopaque nitinol stent
radiopaque tantalum stent
Radius self-expanding stent
Rains stent
Reliance urinary control stent
renovascular stent
Retromax endopyelotomy stent
ring biliary stent
rolled Instat stent
Roubin-Gianturco flexible coil stent
Rusch stent
RX Herculink Plus biliary stent
SMART bile duct stent
SMART biliary stent
Salman FES stent
SAXX renal stent
Schatz-Palmaz tubular mesh stent
Schneider stent
Schneider Wallstent
self-expandable metallic stent
self-expanding coil stent
self-expanding metallic stent
self-expanding stainless steel stent
self-retaining coil stent
shape memory alloy stent
Shikani middle meatal antrostomy stent
Siegel stent
Silastic indwelling ureteral stent
Silastic stent
silicone-coated, metallic self-expanding stent
Silitek ureteral stent
Silitek Uropass stent
silver-coated stent
single pigtail stent
single-J urinary diversion stent
SinuSpacer turbinate stent
slotted tube articulated stent

stent (*continued*)

- SoloPass Percuflex biliary stent
- Song stent
- Speed Lok soft stent
- SpiraFlo prostate stent
- spiral coil stent
- SpiraStent ureteral stent
- SpiroFlo bioabsorbable prostate stent
- spring-loaded vascular stent
- stainless steel balloon expandable stent
- stainless steel mesh stent
- straight stent
- Strecker balloon expandable stent
- Strecker coronary stent
- Strecker esophageal stent
- Strecker tantalum stent
- Stryker stent
- Supra G coronary stent
- Supramid occluding stent
- Surgitek Double-J closed-tip ureteral stent
- Surgitek double-J ureteral stent
- Surgitek Quadra-Coil ureteral stent
- Surgitek Tractfinder ureteral stent
- Surgitek Uropass stent
- Symphony stent
- synthetic stent
- Talent LPS endoluminal stent
- tandem stent
- Tannenbaum stent
- tantalum balloon expandable stent
- tantalum wire stent
- Tenax coronary stent
- Tensum coronary stent
- thermal memory stent
- thermoexpandable stent
- thermoplastic stent
- Titan stent
- titanium urethral stent
- Tower stent
- transhepatic biliary stent
- transpapillary cystopancreatic stent
- Trimble suture stent

stent (*continued*)

- trismus stent
- Tristar coronary stent
- T-tube stent
- tubular slotted stent
- T-Y stent
- Ultraflex Microvasive stent
- Ultraflex nitinol expandable esophageal stent
- Ultraflex self-expanding stent
- uncoated mesh stent
- Universal stent
- ureteral stent
- UroCoil self-expanding stent
- Uro-Guide stent
- Urolume urethral stent
- Urosoft stent
- U-tube stent
- vaginal stent
- Vantec urinary stent
- VascuCoil peripheral vascular stent
- vein graft stenting stent
- vein-coated stent
- Velocity stent
- Vistaflex balloon expandable, platinum alloy biliary stent
- Wallstent expanding metallic stent
- Wallstent spring-loaded stent
- Westaby stent
- whistle stent
- Wiktor balloon expandable coronary stent
- Wiktor GX coronary stent
- Wilson-Cook French stent
- wire-mesh self-expandable stent
- XT radiopaque coronary stent
- Z stent
- zigzag stent
- Zimmon biliary stent

stent construction
stent cutter
stent dressing
stent evaluation
stent expansion
stent funnel
stent graft
stent implantation
stent introducer
stent jail

stent mass
stent placement
stent plugging
stent sandwich
stent skin graft
stent strut
stent tube with pigtail curl
stent-induced intimal
    hyperplasia
stenting catheter
stenting technique
stentless porcine aortic valve
    prosthesis
stent-through-wire mesh
    technique
Stenver position
Stenver x-ray view
Stenzel fracture rod
Stenzel rod prosthesis
step deformity
Step device
step drill
step graft
step graft operation
Step laparoscopic trocar
step screw
step staples
Step trocar
step-by-step technique
step-cut lengthening
step-cut osteotomy
step-cut reamer
step-down cannula
step-down drill
step-down osteotomy
stepdown therapy
step-down transformer
Stephee joint replacement
Stephens soft IOL-inserting forceps
Stephenson corneal trephine
Stephenson needle holder
Stephenson-Donovan transfer
Stepita meatal clamp
stepladder incision
stepladder incision technique
stepladder sign
stepladder technique for lip
    reconstruction
step-off fracture
step-osteotomy
stepped-down cautery
Stepty P hemostasis bandage

step-up transformer
stepwise sutures
stercoraceous
stercoral abscess
stercoral appendicitis
stercoral fistula
stercoral ulcer
stereo x-ray views
stereoarthrolysis
stereoencephalotome
stereoencephalotomy
StereoGuide breast biopsy
    equipment
StereoGuide collimator
StereoGuide needle
StereoGuide stereotactic needle
    core biopsy
stereo-identical point
stereolithography cage
stereoroentgenography
stereoscopic microscope
stereotactic aspiration biopsy
stereotactic automated technique
stereotactic brain biopsy
stereotactic breast biopsy
    needle
stereotactic catheter drainage
stereotactic cordotomy
stereotactic core biopsy
    technique
stereotactic core breast biopsy
stereotactic craniotomy
stereotactic device
stereotactic frame
stereotactic guidance
stereotactic head frame
stereotactic instrumentation
stereotactic laser
stereotactic lesion
stereotactic localization frame
stereotactic needle core biopsy
stereotactic needle core biopsy
    procedure
stereotactic operation
stereotactic percutaneous
    needle biopsy
stereotactic radiation therapy
stereotactic retractor
stereotactic surgery
stereotactic surgical ablation
stereotactic vacuum-assisted
    biopsy device (SVAB)

stereotactic-assisted radiation
  therapy
stereotactic-assisted radiation
  therapy kit
stereotactic-focused radiation
  therapy
stereotactic-guided biopsy
stereotaxic device
stereotaxic hypophysectomy
stereotaxic instrument
stereotaxic laser
stereotaxic neuroradiography
stereotaxic neurosurgery
stereotaxic procedure
stereotaxic surgery
stereotaxic technique
stereotaxy
Steri-Band bandage
SteriCam endoscopic camera
Stericare copolymer absorbent
  dressing
Stericare hydrogel gauze
  dressing
Steri-Cath catheter
Steri-Cuff disposable tourniquet
  cuff
Steri-Drape
Steriflex-Braun bacterial filter
sterile abscess
sterile absorbent gauze
sterile adhesive bubble dressing
sterile adhesive plaster
sterile adhesive tape
sterile bone wax
sterile compression dressing
sterile connecting tube
sterile drape
sterile dressing
sterile dry dressing
sterile electrodermatome blade
sterile examination
sterile field
sterile field barrier
sterile fluffs
sterile fluid
sterile forceps holder
sterile isolation bag
sterile matrix
sterile procedure
sterile pustule
sterile saline
sterile site

sterile specimen
sterile tape
sterile technique
sterile towels
sterile transverse rod
sterile vacuum collection tube
sterile vaginal examination
sterilely draped
sterilely prepped and draped
sterilization
  Bleier clip for tubal
    sterilization
  defined sterilization
  eugenic sterilization
  Falope-ring tubal sterilization
  fractional sterilization
  gas sterilization
  irradiation sterilization
  laparoscopic sterilization
  laparoscopic tubal
    sterilization
  Madlener sterilization
  Pomeroy sterilization
  postpartum sterilization
  puerperal sterilization
  steam sterilization
  tubal sterilization
sterilized fibrillar bovine
    collagen
sterilizer forceps
sterilizing basket
Steri-Oss dental implant device
Steri-Oss endosteal dental
    implant
Steri-pads gauze pad
Steri-Pads
Steriseal disposable cannula
Steri-Sleeve sleeve
Steri-Strip skin closure
Steri-Stripped incision
Steri-Strips
Steritapes closure
Steritek ICP mini monitor
Sterivac drain
Sterling iris spatula
Sterling-Spring orthodontic
    wire
Sterling-Sylva irrigator
Stern dental attachment
Stern position
Sterna-Band self-locking sutures
sternal angle

sternal approximator (*see* approximator)
sternal biopsy
sternal blade
sternal border
sternal cartilage
sternal cleft
sternal clip
sternal depression
sternal fissure
sternal fragment
sternal infection
sternal instruments
sternal joint
sternal knife
sternal lead
sternal line
sternal muscle
sternal needle
sternal needle holder
sternal notch distance
sternal perforating awl
sternal plane
sternal position
sternal punch
sternal punch forceps
sternal puncture by aspiration
sternal puncture by curettage
sternal puncture medullogram
sternal puncture needle
sternal retractor
sternal retractor blade
sternal saw
sternal shears
sternal spreader
sternal trephine
sternal wire sutures
sternal-occipital-mandibular immobilizer (SOMI)
sternal-occipital-mandibular immobilization
sternal-splitting incision
Sternberg sign
Sternberger antibody sandwich technique
Stern-Castroviejo locking forceps
Stern-Castroviejo suturing forceps
sternectomy
Stern-McCarthy electrode
Stern-McCarthy electrotome

Stern-McCarthy electrotome resectoscope
Stern-McCarthy knife
Stern-McCarthy panendoscope
Stern-McCarthy resectoscope
sternoclavicular angle
sternoclavicular articulation
sternoclavicular disk
sternoclavicular joint
sternoclavicular joint dislocation
sternoclavicular joint reconstruction
sternoclavicular joint reduction
sternoclavicular junction
sternoclavicular ligament
sternoclavicular notch
sternoclavicularis muscle
sternocleidomastoid (SCM)
sternocleidomastoid (SCM) tumor of infancy
sternocleidomastoid artery
sternocleidomastoid fascia
sternocleidomastoid flap
sternocleidomastoid hemorrhage
sternocleidomastoid muscle
sternocleidomastoid musculocutaneous flap
sternocleidomastoid myocutaneous flap
sternocleidomastoid region
sternocleidomastoid vein
sternocleidomastoideus muscle
sternocostal articulation
sternocostal joint
sternocostal ligament
sternocostal muscle
sternocostal surface of heart
sternohyoid muscle
sternohyoideus muscle
sternomanubrial junction
sternomastoid muscle
sterno-occipital-mandibular immobilization orthosis
sterno-occipital-mandibular immobilizer brace (SOMI brace)
sterno-occipitomanubrial immobilizer
sternoschisis
sternothyroid muscle

sternothyroid muscle flap laryngoplasty
sternothyroideus muscle
sternotomy
  horizontal sternotomy
  McNeill-Chamberlain sternotomy
  median sternotomy
  vertical sternotomy
sternotomy dehiscence
sternotomy incision
sternotomy retractor
sternotomy saw
sternotomy wound
sternotracheal
sternotrypesis
sternoxiphoid plane
sternum
  clavicular incisure of sternum
  clavicular notch of sternum
  costal incisures of sternum
  costal notch of sternum
  jugular notch of sternum
  reflection of sternum
sternum cartilage
sternum depressed
sternum saw
sternum turnover procedure
sternum-perforating awl
sternum-splitting approach
sternum-splitting procedure
Ster-O₂-Mist ultrasonic cup
steroid concentration
steroid eluting electrode
steroid injection
steroid ulcer
Stertzer brachial guiding catheter
Stertzer-Myler extension wire
stethoscope
  Albion-Ford stethoscope
  Allen fetal stethoscope
  binaural stethoscope
  Bowles stethoscope
  Cammann stethoscope
  combination stethoscope
  DeLee-Hillis obstetrical head stethoscope
  DeLee-Hillis obstetrical stethoscope
  DeLee-Hillis stethoscope
  diaphragm stethoscope

stethoscope (continued)
  Doppler fetal stethoscope
  Doppler stethoscope
  Doppler ultrasound stethoscope
  Doptone fetal stethoscope
  Duo-Sonic stethoscope
  electronic stethoscope
  esophageal stethoscope
  fetal stethoscope
  Ford stethoscope
  Gordon stethoscope
  Howell tunable diaphragm stethoscope
  Leff stethoscope
  Littman Class II pediatric stethoscope
  micromembranous stethoscope
  Pilling stethoscope
  Rieger stethoscope
  Scanmate stethoscope
  Sprague-Rappaport stethoscope
  Tiemann stethoscope
  tunable diaphragm stethoscope
  ultrasound stethoscope
  Wechsler obstetrical stethoscope
Stetten colostomy crusher
Stetten intestinal clamp
Stetten spur crusher
Stevens elevator
Stevens eye knife
Stevens eye scissors
Stevens fixation forceps
Stevens hook
Stevens iris forceps
Stevens lacrimal retractor
Stevens muscle hook
Stevens muscle hook retractor
Stevens needle holder
Stevens stitch scissors
Stevens tenotomy hook
Stevens tenotomy scissors
Stevens tissue knife
Stevens traction hook
Stevens-Charles sleeve
Stevens-Johnson syndrome
Stevenson alligator forceps
Stevenson alligator scissors

Stevenson capsule punch
Stevenson clamp
Stevenson cupped-jaw forceps
Stevenson eye speculum
Stevenson grasping forceps
Stevenson lacrimal retractor
Stevenson lacrimal sac retractor
Stevenson-LaForce adenotome
Stevenson microsurgical forceps
Stevenson needle holder
Stevenson operation
Stevenson punch
Stevenson refractor
Stevenson retractor
Stevenson scissors
Stevens-Street elbow prosthesis
Stewart cartilage knife
Stewart cruciate ligament guide
Stewart crypt hook
Stewart distal clavicular excision
Stewart guide
Stewart hook
Stewart incision
Stewart knife
Stewart lenticular nuclear snare
Stewart ligament guide
Stewart rectal hook
Stewart sutures
Stewart technique
Stewart-Hamilton cardiac output
    technique
Stewart-Harley ankle procedure
Stewart-Treves syndrome
Steytler-Van Der Walt procedure
STH total hip prosthesis
STI-1 needle-shaped tissue
    stapler
Stichs wound clip
stick-and-carrol appliance
stick sponge
stick ties
Stickler disease
Stickler syndrome
stick-on electrode
stick-tie suture technique
stick-tie sutures
Stieda disease
Stieda fracture
Stieglitz unipolar nasal snare
Stieglitz splinter forceps
Stiegmann-Goff endoscopic
    ligator

Stiegmann-Goff technique
Stierlen lens loop
Stifcore aspiration needle
Stifcore transbronchial
    aspiration needle
stiff abdomen
stiff neck
stiff pupil
stiff ray
stiffening of joint
stiffening wire
stiff-heart syndrome
stifle joint
Stifneck immobilizing collar
stigma (*pl.* stigmas, stigmata)
stigmata of recent hemorrhage
    (SRH)
Stiles-Bunnell transfer
Stiles-Bunnell transfer technique
stilet, stilette (*see* stylet)
stiletto knife
Stilith implantable cardiac pulse
    generator
still radiography technique
stillbirth
stillborn infant
Stille bone chisel
Stille bone drill
Stille bone drill set
Stille bone gouge
Stille bone rongeur
Stille brace
Stille bur
Stille cast cutter
Stille cheek retractor
Stille chisel
Stille clamp
Stille coarctation hook
Stille conchotome
Stille cranial drill
Stille dissecting scissors
Stille drill
Stille flat pliers
Stille forceps
Stille gallstone forceps
Stille Gigli saw
Stille Gigli-saw guide
Stille Gigli-saw wire
Stille gouge
Stille hand drill
Stille heart retractor
Stille insufflator

Stille kidney clamp
Stille kidney forceps
Stille laryngeal applicator
Stille mallet
Stille osteotome
Stille periosteal elevator
Stille plaster shears
Stille plaster spreader
Stille rib shears
Stille rongeur
Stille rongeur forceps
Stille saw
Stille scissors
Stille shears
Stille Super Cut scissors
Stille tissue forceps
Stille trephine
Stille uterine dilator
Stille vessel clamp
Stille-Adson forceps
Stille-Aesculap plaster shears
Stille-Babcock forceps
Stille-Bailey-Senning rib
    contractor
Stille-Barraya intestinal forceps
Stille-Barraya intestinal-grasping
    forceps
Stille-Barraya vascular forceps
Stille-Beyer rongeur
Stille-Bjork forceps
Stille-Björk (see Bjork)
Stille-Bjork (also Björk)
Stille-Broback knee retractor
Stille-Crafoord forceps
Stille-Crafoord raspatory
Stille-Crafoord clamp
Stille-Crafoord coarctation clamp
Stille-Crile forceps
Stille-Doyen rasp
Stille-Doyen raspatory
Stille-Edwards rasp
Stille-Edwards raspatory
Stille-Ericksson rib shears
Stille-French cardiovascular
    needle holder
Stille-Giertz rib shears
Stille-Gigli wire saw
Stille-Halsted forceps
Stille-Horsley bone-cutting
    forceps
Stille-Horsley rib forceps
Stille-Horsley rib shears

Stille-Horsley rongeur
Stille-Joseph saw
Stille-Langenbeck elevator
Stille-Lauer bone rongeur
Stille-Leksell rongeur
Stille-Liston bone forceps
Stille-Liston bone-cutting forceps
Stille-Liston double-action
    rongeur
Stille-Liston rib-cutting forceps
Stille-Liston rongeur
Stille-Luer angular duckbill
    rongeur
Stille-Luer bone rongeur
Stille-Luer forceps
Stille-Luer multiple-action rongeur
Stille-Luer rongeur forceps
Stille-Luer-Echlin bone rongeur
Stille-Mathieu needle holder
Stille-Mayo dissecting scissors
Stille-Mayo-Hegar needle
Stille-Metzenbaum needle holder
Stillenberg raspatory
Stille-pattern bone chisel
Stille-pattern bone drill
Stille-pattern bone gouge
Stille-pattern osteotome
Stille-pattern rib shears
Stille-pattern trephine and bone
    drill set
Stille-Quervain spreader
Stiller sign
Stille-Ruskin rongeur
Stille-Russian forceps
Stille-Seldinger needle
Stille-Sherman bone drill
Stille-Stiwer osteotome
Stille-Stiwer plaster shears
Stille-Waugh forceps
Stille-Zaufal-Jansen rongeur
Stille knife
Stillman cleft
Stillman technique
Stimitrode electrode
Stimoceiver implant material
Stimprene electrotherapy brace
Stimprene wrap
Stimson anterior shoulder
    reduction technique
Stimson dressing
Stimson maneuver
Stimson pedicle clamp

stimulated gracilis neosphincter
 technique
stimulated graciloplasty
stimulating catheter
stimulating effect
stimulating electrode
stimulating skin retraction
stimulation
 bladder stimulation
 bone growth stimulation
 carotid sinus stimulation
 cerebellar stimulation
 cochlear electrical stimulation
 deep brain stimulation
 dorsal column stimulation
 double simultaneous
  stimulation (DSS)
 double-burst stimulation
 electric nerve stimulation
 electric stimulation
 electrogalvanic stimulation
 electronic stimulation
 faradic stimulation
 flash stimulation
 galvanic stimulation
 intraoperative cavernous
  nerve stimulation
 lateral electrical spine
  stimulation (LESS)
 mechanical stimulation
 muscle stimulation
 nerve stimulation
 peripheral nerve stimulation
 photic stimulation
 phrenic nerve stimulation
 reflex stimulation
 tactile stimulation
 transcutaneous electrical
  nerve stimulation (TENS)
stimulation of peripheral nerves
Stimulite honeycomb seating
 pad
stimulus response
Stimuplex block needle
Stimuplex-S nerve stimulator
STING (subureteric Teflon
 injection)
stipple cell
stippled epiphysis
stippled tongue
stippling
STIR technique

stirrups
 ankle air stirrup
 Finochietto stirrup
 Lloyd-Davis stirrups
 low stirrups
 Navratil stirrups
 obstetrical stirrups
stirrup anastomosis
stirrup bone
stirrup brace
stirrup splint
stirrup-loop curet
stitch
 alar suspension stitch
 Allgower stitch
 baseball stitch
 basting stitch
 bow-tie stitch
 Bunnell stitch
 Connell stitch
 crown stitch
 cuticular stitch
 dermoepidermal Gillies stitch
 extramucosal stitch
 figure-8 stitch
 Fothergill stitch
 Frost stitch
 funnel stitch
 Gambee stitch
 imbricating stitch
 intracuticular stitch
 Kessler stitch
 key stitch
 lock stitch
 locking stitch
 market stitch
 mattress stitch
 McCall stitch
 Parker-Kerr basting stitch
 Prolene stitch
 quilting stitch
 roll stitch
 running-locked stitch
 self-locking stitch
 seromuscular stitch
 shoelace stitch
 skin stitch
 subcuticular stitch
 subperiosteal pulling stitch
 tagging stitch
 Tamai stitch
 tilt stitch

stitch (*continued*)
  tracheal safety stitch
  triple-throw square knot
    stitch
stitch abscess
stitch scissors
stitch-removing knife
Stitt catheter
Stiwer biopsy forceps
Stiwer bone-holding forceps
Stiwer curet
Stiwer dressing forceps
Stiwer finger-ring saw
Stiwer furuncle knife
Stiwer grooved director
Stiwer hand drill
Stiwer laryngeal mirror
Stiwer retractor
Stiwer scalpel handle
Stiwer scissors
Stiwer sponge forceps
Stiwer tendon dissector
Stiwer tissue forceps
Stiwer towel clamp
Stiwer trocar
Stock eye trephine
Stock finger splint
stock implant
Stock operation
Stocker cyclodiathermy
    puncture needle
Stocker line
Stocker needle
Stocker operation
Stockert cardiac pacing
    electrode
Stockfisch appliance
Stockholm technique for radium
    therapy
stockinette
  Bel-Air orthopedic stockinette
  bias stockinette
  bias-cut stockinette
  Delta-Net stockinette
  double stockinette
  surgical stockinette
  tube stockinette
stockinette amputation bandage
stockinette bandage
stockinette cap
stockinette dressing
stocking anesthesia

stocking nevus
stocking-and-glove-type
    hypesthesia
stocking-glove anesthesia
stocking-glove distribution
stockings
  adjustable thigh antiembolism
    stockings (ATS)
  antiembolism stockings
  Camp-Sigraris stockings
  CircAid elastic stockings
  compression stockings
  elastic compression stockings
  Fast-Fit vascular stockings
  Jobst elastic stockings
  Jobst stockings
  Jobst VPGS stockings
  Jobst-Stride support stockings
  Jobst-Stridette support
    stockings
  Juzo stockings
  Linton stockings
  Medi vascular stockings
  Medi-Strumpf elastic stockings
  pneumatic compression
    stockings
  Sigvaris compression
    stockings
  Sigvaris compression
    stockings
  Sigvaris support stockings
  support stockings
  TED stockings
  thigh-high embolic stockings
  thromboembolic disease
    stockings
  True Form support stockings
  Vairox high compression
    vascular stockings
  Vairox vascular stockings
  VenES antiembolism
    stockings
  VenES II Medical stockings
  VenES vascular stockings
  venous pressure gradient
    support stockings (VPGSS)
  Zimmer antiembolism
    support stockings
stocking-seam incision
Stockman meatal clamp
Stockman penile clamp
Stoerck loop

Stoerk blennorrhea
Stoesser stripper
Stoffel operation
Stokes amputation
Stokes lens
Stokes operation
Stokes sign
Stokes-Adams seizures
Stokes-Adams syndrome
Stokes-Gritti amputation
Stoll dilution egg count
    technique
Stolte capsulorrhexis forceps
Stolte dissector
Stolte tonsillar dissector
Stolte-Stille elevator
Stoltz laparoscope
Stoltz pubiotomy
stoma (*pl.* stomas, stomata)
    abdominal stoma
    antral stoma
    artificial stoma
    bowel stoma
    colonoscopy per stoma
    diverting stoma
    dusky stoma
    end stoma
    end-loop stoma
    fibromuscular stoma
    flush with skin stoma
    gastric stoma
    gastroenterostomy stoma
    gastrointestinal stoma
    ileal loop stoma
    ileostomy stoma
    loop stoma
    nippled stoma
    permanent stoma
    prolapsed stoma
    retracted stoma
    rosebud stoma
    Silastic collar-reinforced
        stoma
    tracheostomy stoma
stoma button
stoma cap microporous
    adhesive
stoma closure
stoma hernia
stoma irrigator drain
stoma site
stoma-centering guide

stomach
    anastomosis of bile duct to
        stomach
    cardia of stomach
    cascade stomach
    cup-and-spill stomach
    dumping stomach
    fold of stomach
    greater curvature of stomach
    Holzknecht stomach
    hourglass stomach
    insufflation of stomach
    intrathoracic stomach
    lavage of stomach
    leather bottle stomach
    lesser curvature of stomach
    mucous lake of stomach
    pylorus of stomach
    reflux from stomach
    rugae of stomach
    rugal pattern of stomach
    suction stomach
    Sugiura devascularization of
        esophagus and stomach
stomach acid
stomach adenocarcinoma
stomach brush
stomach bubble
stomach calculus
stomach cancer
stomach cancer metastasis
stomach capacity
stomach cardiomyotomy
stomach clamp
stomach contents
stomach distention
stomach irrigation tube
stomach lining
stomach magnet
stomach rugae
stomach spasms
stomach stapling
stomach tube
stomach ulcer
stomach wall
Stomahesive
stomal bag
stomal colonoscopy
stomal complication
stomal intussusception
stomal invagination
stomal stenosis

stomal ulcer
stoma-measuring device
Stomate decompression tube
Stomate extension tube
Stomate low-profile gastrostomy
 kit
stomatitis
 angular stomatitis
 aphthous stomatitis
 fusospirochetal stomatitis
 gangrenous stomatitis
 membranous stomatitis
 mercurial stomatitis
 mycotic stomatitis
 necrotizing ulcerative
  stomatitis
 ulcerative stomatitis
 vesicular stomatitis
 Vincent stomatitis
 viral vesicular stomatitis
stomatitis medicamentosa
stomatitis papulosa
stomatitis traumatica
stomatodynia
stomatodysodia
stomatoglossitis
stomatognathic
stomatomalacia
stomatonecrosis
stomatonoma
stomatoplasty
stomatorrhagia
stomatorrhaphy
stomatoschisis
stomatoscopy
stomoschisis
stone
 apatite urine tract stones
 autochthonous stone
 bile duct stone
 biliary tract stone
 bilirubinate stone
 black faceted stone
 bladder stone
 calcium bilirubinate stone
 caliceal stone
 CBD (common bile duct)
 CBD stone
 cholesterol stone
 common bile duct stone
 common duct stone
 cystine urinary tract stones

stone (*continued*)
 disintegrating stones
 dissolution of stone
 dissolving kidney stone
 duct stone
 endoscopic extraction
  pancreatic duct stone
 extraction of bile duct stone
 extraction of kidney stone
 extraction of ureteral stone
 extraction of pancreatic stone
 faceted stone
 gallbladder stone
 impacted stone
 intraglandular stone
 intrahepatic stone
 intraluminal stone
 Jackstone-type urinary
  bladder stone
 kidney stone
 metabolic stone
 noncalcified stone
 passage of stone
 puncta calcific stone
 radiolucent stone
 radiononopaque stone
 residual stone
 salivary stone
 skin stones
 staghorn stone
 struvite urinary tract stones
 transduodenal excision of
  common duct stone
 ureteral stone
 urinary stone
stone basket (*see* basket)
stone basket screw mounted
 handle
Stone bunionectomy
Stone clamp
Stone clamp-applying forceps
Stone clamp-locking device
stone cutter's phthisis
stone dislodger (*see* dislodger)
stone dislodger filiform
stone extraction
stone extractor
Stone eye implant
stone fragmentation
stone granuloma formation
Stone hip arthrodesis
stone impaction

Stone implant
Stone intestinal clamp
Stone intestinal forceps
Stone lens nucleus prolapser
stone locking device
stone placenta
Stone procedure for hallux
   rigidus
stone removal
stone retriever
stone staple
Stone stomach clamp
stone surgery
Stone tissue forceps
stone-age scalpel
stone-crushing forceps
stone-extraction forceps
stone-grasping forceps
Stone-Holcombe anastomosis
   clamp
Stone-Holcombe intestinal
   clamp
stone-holding basket
Stoneman forceps
stone-retrieval balloon
stone-retrieval basket
StoneRisk diagnostic monitoring
   kit
Stonetome stone removal device
stony hard
Stookey cranial rongeur
Stookey reflex
Stookey rongeur
Stookey-Scarff operation
stool
   abdominal stool
   bloody stool
   impacted stool
   incontinent of stool
   melenic stool
   mucous stool
   pathologic stool
   pencil-shaped stools
   residual stool
   retained stool
   ribbon stools
   ribbon-shaped stools
   scybalous stool
   solid stool
stool collector
stool evacuation
stool impaction

stop collar telescope
stop eye speculum
stop needle
stopcock
Stopko irrigator
Stop-Leak gel flotation cushion
Stop-Leak gel flotation mattress
Stoppa hernia repair
Stoppa procedure
Stoppa laparoscopy repair
stop-valve airway obstruction
Storer thoracoabdominal
   retractor
Storey clamp
Storey gall duct forceps
Storey thoracic forceps
Storey-Hillar dissecting forceps
Stork arthroscope
Stormer viscosimeter
Storn Von Leeuwen chamber
Storq guidewire
Story orbital elevator
Storz adjustable headrest
Storz adjustable magnifier
Storz anterior commissure
   laryngoscope
Storz antrum punch
Storz applicator
Storz arthroscope
Storz arthroscopy operating
   instruments
Storz aspiration biopsy needle
Storz atraumatic distending
   obturator
Storz attachment
Storz band
Storz binocular loupe
Storz binocular prism
Storz binocular prism loupe
Storz biopsy forceps
Storz biopsy thoracoscope
Storz bladder evacuator
Storz bougie-urethrotome
Storz bronchial catheter
Storz bronchoscope
Storz bronchoscopic forceps
Storz bronchoscopic specimen
   collector
Storz bronchoscopic suction
   tube
Storz bronchoscopic telescope
Storz cable

Storz camera
Storz capsular forceps
Storz Capsulor intraocular lens
Storz cataract knife
Storz catheter adapter
Storz catheter connector
Storz chalazion trephine
Storz cholangiograsper
Storz choledochoscope
Storz ciliary forceps
Storz cold-light fountain
Storz cold-punch resectoscope
Storz conductor
Storz continuous irrigation-
    suction resectoscope
Storz corneal bur
Storz corneal forceps
Storz corneal trephine
Storz corneoscleral punch
Storz cotton carrier
Storz curved forceps
Storz cystoscope
Storz cystoscope tip
Storz cystoscope-urethroscope
Storz cystoscopic electrode
Storz cystoscopic forceps
Storz cystoscopic rongeur
Storz cystoscopic scissors
Storz deflecting obturator
Storz delicate iris scissors
Storz diagnostic laparoscope
Storz DiaPhine trephine
Storz direct-vision cystoscope
Storz disposable blade
Storz disposable cannula
Storz disposable fiberoptic light
    pipe
Storz disposable trephine
Storz disposable trocar
Storz duckbill rongeur
Storz ear knife handle
Storz ear knife set
Storz ear speculum
Storz Easy shield
Storz emergency ventilation
    bronchoscope
Storz endocamera
Storz endomagnifier
Storz esophageal conductor
Storz esophagoscope
Storz esophagoscopic forceps
Storz evacuator

Storz examination insert tube
Storz examining arthroscope
Storz eyepiece
Storz eyepiece attachment
Storz face shield
Storz face-shield headband
Storz fiberoptic cable
Storz fiberoptic cable adapter
Storz fiberoptic light cable
Storz fiberoptic light source
Storz flexible biopsy
    instruments
Storz flexible esophageal
    conductor
Storz flexible injection needle
Storz folding emergency
    ventilation bronchoscope
Storz folding-handle ear knife
Storz folding-handle eye spud
Storz forceps
Storz grasping biopsy forceps
Storz guillotine
Storz gynecological instruments
Storz hair transplant trephine
Storz handpiece
Storz head holder
Storz headlight
Storz high-frequency cord
Storz hysteroscope
Storz infant bronchoscope
Storz infection ventilation
    laryngoscope
Storz Injectimed
Storz insert tube
Storz inserter
Storz intranasal antral punch
Storz intraocular scissors
Storz intratracheal tube
Storz iris hook
Storz iris scissors
Storz keratome
Storz keratometer
Storz kidney stone forceps
Storz knife
Storz Laparoflator insufflator
Storz laparoscope
Storz laryngopharyngoscope
Storz laser
Storz magnet
Storz meatal clamp
Storz meniscotome
Storz microcalipers

Storz microscope
Storz microserrefine
Storz microsurgical bipolar
    coagulator
Storz Microsystems plate cutter
Storz Microsystems plate-
    holding forceps
Storz miniature forceps
Storz miniplate
Storz Monolith lithotripter
Storz Monolith lithotriptor
Storz nasal speculum
Storz nasopharyngeal biopsy
    forceps
Storz needle cannula
Storz needle holder
Storz nephroscope
Storz operating esophagoscope
Storz operating laparoscope
Storz optical biopsy forceps
Storz optical esophagoscope
Storz otolaryngological
    instruments
Storz panendoscope
Storz pediatric esophagoscope
Storz peritoneoscope
Storz pigtail probe
Storz plate
Storz Premiere Microvit
    vitrector
Storz proctoscopic instruments
Storz punch
Storz radial incision marker
Storz resectoscope
Storz resectoscope cable
Storz resectoscope curet
Storz resectoscope electrode
Storz retractor
Storz rhinomanometer
Storz rongeur
Storz safety-sterility disk
Storz scleral buckling balloon
    catheter
Storz scope
Storz septal speculum
Storz sheath
Storz sheath-handle ear knife
Storz Sine-U-View endoscope
Storz sinus biopsy forceps
Storz snare
Storz speculum
Storz stitch scissors

Storz stone dislodger
Storz stone-crushing forceps
Storz stone-extraction forceps
Storz suction tube
Storz suprapubic cystoscope
Storz syringe
Storz teaching attachment
Storz Teflon forceps guard
Storz telescope
Storz tonometer
Storz tube
Storz twist hook
Storz twisted snare wire
Storz Universal lens loop
Storz urological instruments
Storz vent tube introducer
Storz wire-cutting scissors
Storz-Atlas eye magnet
Storz-Beck tonsillar snare
Storz-Beck-Schenck snare
Storz-Bell erysiphake
Storz-Bonn suturing forceps
Storz-Bowman lacrimal probe
Storz-Bruening anastigmatic
    aural magnifier
Storz-Bruening diagnostic head
Storz-Bruening ear magnifier
Storz-Castroviejo needle holder
Storz-DeKock 2-way bronchial
    catheter
Storz-Denecke headlight
Storz-Doesel-Huzly
    bronchoscope tube
Storz-Duredge cataract knife
Storz-Duredge keratome
Storz-Duredge steel cataract
    knife
Storz-Ellik evacuator
Storz-Hopkins laryngoscope
Storz-Hopkins telescope
Storz-Iglesias resectoscope
Storz-Kirkheim urethrotome
Storz-LaForce adenotome
Storz-LaForce-Stevenson
    adenotome
Storz-Moltz tonometer
Storz-Moltz tonsillectome
Storz-Riecker laryngoscope
Storz-Schitz tonometer
Storz-Ultrata forceps
Storz-Urban surgical microscope
Storz-Utrata forceps

Storz-Vienna nasal speculum
Storz-Walker retinal detachment
    unit
Storz-Westcott conjunctival
    scissors
Stough punch
Stout continuous loop wire
Stout continuous wiring
stout-neck curet
Straatsma intraocular implant
    lens
strabismus
    convergent strabismus
    divergent strabismus
    muscular strabismus
strabismus correction
strabismus forceps
strabismus hook
strabismus needle
strabismus operation
strabismus scissors
strabismus surgery
strabismus tucker
straddle fracture
straddling aorta
straddling embolus
straight-ahead bronchoscopic
    telescope
straight aneurysm clip
straight AP pelvic injection
straight arterioles of kidney
straight blade
straight catheter
straight catheter guide
straight cautery
straight chest tube
straight clamp
straight coagulating forceps
straight connector
straight Crile clamp
straight cutting knife
straight dural hook
straight elevator
straight fissure bur
straight flush percutaneous
    catheter
straight forceps
straight graft
straight guidewire
straight hemostat
straight incision
straight inclined plane elevator

straight knot-tying forceps
straight lacrimal cannula
straight laryngeal mirror
straight line bayonet forceps
straight magnifying mirror
straight Maryland forceps
straight microbipolar forceps
straight micromonopolar
    forceps
straight microscissors
straight monopolar
    electrosurgical dissector
straight mosquito clamp
straight mosquito hemostat
straight needle
straight nerve hook
straight osteotome
straight periosteal elevator
straight rasp
straight reamer
straight retinal probe
straight retractor
straight ring curet
straight rongeur
straight scissors
straight shank bur
straight single tenaculum
    forceps
straight sinus
straight stem femoral
    component
straight stent
straight stylet
straight suture needle
straight suturing needle
straight tenaculum
straight tenotomy scissors
straight tube stylet
straight tubular graft
straight tying forceps
straight tympanoplasty knife
straight walker brace
straight-blade electrode
straight-blade laryngoscope
straight-end cup forceps
straightener
    Asch septal straightener
    Asch straightener
    Cottle-Walsham septal
      straightener
    septal straightener
    Walsham straightener

straightening maneuver
Straight-In male sling
straight-needle electrode
straight-on radiograph
straight-pin teeth
straight-point electrode
straight-point needle
StraightShot arterial cannula
straight-stem prosthesis
straight-tip bipolar forceps
straight-tip electrode
straight-tip jeweler's bipolar
    forceps
straight-tipped catheter
straight-wire electrode
strain fracture
strain gauge
strain pattern
strain x-rays
strain/counterstrain technique
strain-gauge manometer
strain-gauge transducer
Straith chin implant
Straith eyelid operation
Straith nasal implant
Straith nasal splint kit
Straith operation
Straith otoplasty
Straith profilometer
Straith Z-plasty
Strampelli eye splint
Strampelli implant
Strampelli implant cataract
    lens
Strampelli-Valvo operation
Strandell retractor
Strandell-Stille retractor
Strandell-Stille tendon hook
stranding
    fascial stranding
    mesenteric stranding
    soft tissue stranding
strandy infiltrate
strangulated bowel
strangulated bowel obstruction
strangulated hemorrhoid
strangulated incisional hernia
strangulated inguinal hernia
strangulated paraesophageal
    hernia
strangulated viscus
strangulation obstruction

strap
    API universal foam chin strap
    breast strap
    buddy strap
    Campbell rest strap
    catheter leg strap
    chin strap
    Circumpress chin strap
    lingual strap
    Montgomery straps
    palatal strap
    Press Lift chin strap
    safety strap
    Silastic strap
    supinator strap
    tourniquet strap
strap clavicle splint
Strap Lok ankle brace
strap muscles
Strap operation
strap sling
strap-on pump
Strasbourg-Fairfax in vitro
    fertilization needle
Strassburger tissue forceps
Strassman metroplasty
Strassman operation
Strassman technique
Strassman-Jones-Tompkins
    metroplasty
Strassmann uterine forceps
Strassmann uterine-elevating
    forceps
strata (*sing.* stratum)
Stratasis urethral sling
StrataSorb composite wound
    dressing
stratification
stratified clot
stratified squamous epithelium
Stratos orthotic
Stratte clamp
Stratte forceps
Stratte kidney clamp
Stratte needle holder
stratum (*pl.* strata)
stratum corneum
stratum corneum epidermidis
stratum disjunctum
stratum functionale
stratum germinativum
    epidermidis

stratum granulosum
stratum granulosum epidermidis
stratum intermedium
stratum lucidum epidermidis
stratum malpighii
stratum spinosum epidermidis
stratum subcutaneum
Stratus instrument
Straub technique
Straus curved retrobulbar needle
Strauss cannula
Strauss dental attachment
Strauss meatal clamp
Strauss metal clamp
Strauss needle
Strauss penile clamp
Strauss proctoscope
Strauss sigmoidoscope
Strauss sign
Strauss syndrome
Strauss-Valentine penile clamp
strawberry angioma
strawberry birthmark
strawberry cervix
strawberry gallbladder
strawberry hemangioma
strawberry mark
strawberry tongue
strawberry tumor
straw-colored ascites
straw-colored fluid
straw-colored urine
Strayer meniscal knife
Strayer operation to lengthen
    heel cord
Strayer procedure
Strayer tendon technique
streak retinoscope
streaked ovaries
Streamline peripheral catheter
Streatfield operation
Streatfield-Fox operation
Streatfield-Snellen operation
streblodactyly
streblomicrodactyly
Strecker balloon-expandable
    stent
Strecker coronary stent
Strecker esophageal stent
Strecker tantalum stent
Street diamond-shaped nail
Street medullary pin

Street rod
Street tonsillar syringe
Street-Stevens humeral
    replacement
Strelinger catheter-introducing
    forceps
Strelinger colon clamp
Strelinger right-angle colon
    clamp
Strempel dermatome
strength
    compressive strength
    edge strength
    extremity strength
    extrinsic muscle strength
    graft strength
    grasp strength
    grip strength
    tensile strength
    triple strength
    wet strength
    wound tensile strength
strength and mobility
streptococcal septicemia
streptomicrodactyly
Stress Cath catheter
Stress echo bed
stress fracture
stress incontinence
stress lesion
stress on cannula
stress on needle
stress roentgenogram
stress rupture
stress skin lines
stress test
stress ulcer
stress ulcer hemorrhage
stress ulceration
stress-bearing area
Stress-Ray varus-valgus device
stress-strain curve
Stretch and Heel splint
Stretch balloon
Stretch cardiac device
Stretch gauze roll
stretch injury
stretch marks
Stretch Net wound dressing
stretch reflex
stretch stricture
stretch-and-spray technique

stretching of iris
stretching of muscle
stretching of nerve
Stretta operation
Stretta procedure
Stretzer bent-tip USCI catheter
striae of abdomen
striae of breasts
striae of pregnancy
striae of thighs
striate atrophy of skin
striate body
striate vein
striated duct
striated muscle
striated muscle innervation
striated reticulum
striation
Strickland modification
Strickland technique
Strickland tendon repair
stricture
    Abbe operation for
        esophageal stricture
    anal stricture
    annular stricture
    antral stricture
    Bates operation for urethral
        stricture
    benign biliary stricture
    bile duct stricture
    bridle stricture
    cicatricial stricture
    contractile stricture
    dilated stricture
    ductal stricture
    esophageal stricture
    false stricture
    fracturing the stricture
    functional stricture
    impassable stricture
    impermeable stricture
    irritable stricture
    juncture stricture
    longitudinal esophageal
        stricture
    organic stricture
    peptic stricture
    permanent stricture
    pyloric stricture
    rectal stricture
    recurrent stricture

stricture (*continued*)
    spasmodic stricture
    spastic stricture
    stretch stricture
    temporary stricture
    UPJ stricture (ureteropelvic
        junction stricture)
    ureteropelvic junction
        stricture
    urethral stricture
    Wickwitz esophageal stricture
stricture formation
stricture scope
stricturoplasty
stricturotome
stricturotomy
Stride cardiac pacemaker
stridor
    congenital laryngeal stridor
    inspiratory stridor
    laryngeal stridor
strike-through drainage
string bladder
string carcinoma
string cell carcinoma
string test for peptic ulcer
Stringer catheter-introducing
        forceps
Stringer newborn throat forceps
Stringer tracheal catheter
string-of-beads appearance
stringy infiltration
stringy opacification
stringy vitreous floaters
strip
    abrasive strip
    adhesive tape strips
    autogenous strip
    bacitracin strips
    cardiac monitor strip
    circumferential strip
    collodion strip
    Cottonoid strips
    Cover-Strip wound closure
        strips
    demineralized flexible laminar
        bone strip
    EKG monitor strip
    fascia lata strip
    fascial strip
    felt strip
    flexible laminar bone strip

strip (*continued*)
   fluorescein strip
   gauze strip
   Gelfoam strip
   gold strip
   Gore-Tex strips
   lead strip
   Mylar strip
   Pacific Coast flexible laminar
      bone strip
   packing strip
   rayon strip
   rhythm strip
   Silverlon wound packing strips
   skin closure strips
   Suture Strip
   Suture Strip Plus wound
      closure strip
   tear strips
   Ultimatic flexible laminar
      bone strip
strip and point sponge
strip biopsy
strip biopsy resection technique
strip craniectomy
strip of gauze
strip perforation
strip procedure
strip resection
striped muscle
stripped and ligated
stripper
   Alexander rib stripper
   Babcock jointed vein stripper
   Babcock vein stripper
   Bartlett fascia stripper
   Brand tendon stripper
   Bunnell tendon stripper
   Bunt tendon stripper
   Callahan zonule lens stripper
   Cannon vein stripper
   Carroll forearm tendon
      stripper
   cartilage stripper
   chest tube stripper
   Clark vein stripper
   clot stripper
   Codman vein stripper
   Cole polyethylene vein
      stripper
   Cole vein stripper
   Crawford fascial stripper

stripper (*continued*)
   Crile stripper
   Crile vagotomy stripper
   DeBakey intraluminal stripper
   disposable stripper
   Dorian rib stripper
   Doyen rib stripper
   Doyle vein stripper
   Dunlop thrombus stripper
   elevator and stripper
   Emerson vein stripper
   endarterectomy stripper
   endonerve stripper
   Endostat fiber stripper
   endotracheal stripper
   external vein stripper
   extraluminal stripper
   fascia lata stripper
   fascia stripper
   Fischer tendon stripper
   Friedman olive-tip vein stripper
   Friedman vein stripper
   Furlong tendon stripper
   Grierson tendon stripper
   Hall-Chevalier stripper
   Holley vascular stripper
   hydraulic vein stripper
   IM tendon stripper
   improved Webb stripper
   interchangeable vein stripper
   internal vein stripper
   intraluminal stripper
   jointed vein stripper
   Joplin tendon stripper
   Keeley vein stripper
   Kurten vein stripper
   LaVeen helical stripper
   Leigh zonule lens stripper
   Lempka vein stripper
   Levy-Okun stripper
   Linton vein stripper
   Martin endarterectomy
      stripper
   Masson fascial stripper
   Matson rib stripper
   Matson-Alexander rib stripper
   Matson-Mead periosteal
      stripper
   Mayo external vein stripper
   Mayo vein stripper
   Mayo-Myers external vein
      stripper

stripper (*continued*)
  Meyer olive-tipped vein
    stripper
  Meyer spiral vein stripper
  Myers intraluminal stripper
  Myers vein stripper
  Nabatoff vein stripper
  Nelson rib stripper
  Nelson-Roberts stripper
  New Orleans endarterectomy
    stripper
  Obwegeser stripper
  olive-tipped stripper
  orthopedic surgical stripper
  periosteum stripper
  Phelan vein stripper
  pigtail tendon stripper
  polyethylene vein stripper
  Price-Thomas rib stripper
  ramus stripper
  reusable vein stripper
  rib elevator and stripper
  rib stripper
  rib-edge stripper
  ring stripper
  Roberts-Nelson rib stripper
  Samuels vein stripper
  Shaw carotid artery clot
    stripper
  Shaw carotid clot stripper
  slotted tendon stripper
  Smith cartilage stripper
  Smith posterior cartilage
    stripper
  spiral vein stripper
  Stoesser stripper
  Stukey stripper
  surgical stripper
  tendon stripper
  thrombus stripper
  Trace hydraulic vein stripper
  Trace vein stripper
  vagotomy stripper
  vein stripper
  Verner stripper
  Webb interchangeable
    stripper
  Webb vein stripper
  Wilson vein stripper
  Wurth vein stripper
  Wylie endarterectomy
    stripper

stripper (*continued*)
  Zollinger-Gilmore intraluminal
    vein stripper
  Zollinger-Gilmore vein
    stripper
  zonule stripper
stripper and elevator
stripper with bullet end
stripping
  cord stripping
  dissection and stripping
  greater saphenous vein
    ligation and stripping
  internal vein stripping
  ligation and stripping
  Linton vein stripping
  periosteal stripping
  saphenous vein ligation and
    stripping
  segmental stripping
  Steindler stripping
  vein stripping
stripping and dissection
stripping and ligation
stripping of membrane
stripping of cord
stripping of kidney capsule
stripping of vocal cord
Stripseal catheter
Strobex Mark II electrosurgical
  unit
stroboscopic microscope
Stroembeck (*see* Strömbeck)
stroke ejection rate
stroke index
stroke risk
stroke victim
stroma (*pl.* stromata)
  fibrovascular stroma
  myxochondroid stroma
  myxoid stroma
  ovarian stroma
  portio and stroma
stroma of thyroid gland
stromal desmoplasia
stromal hyperplasia
stromal line
stromal tissue
Strömbeck (*see* Strombeck)
Strombeck (*also* Strömbeck,
  Stroembeck)
Strombeck breast reduction

Strombeck incision
Strombeck mammaplasty
Strombeck mammaplasty
   incision
Strombeck operation
Strombeck technique for
   reduction mammaplasty
Strömbeck template
Stromeyer cephalhematocele
Stromeyer splint
Stromeyer-Little operation
Stromgren ankle brace
strontium-90 ophthalmic beta
   ray applicator
Strubel lid everter
Struck spreader
structural abnormality
structural anomaly
structural blepharoptosis
structural lesion
structural pathology
structural surgery
structure
   abdominal structure
   accessory structure
   adnexal structures
   bipenniform structure
   cardiovascular structures
   coiled bony structure
   collecting structures
   congested vascular structures
   deep structure
   delicate structure
   demineralized bony structure
   dense bony structure
   elbow structure
   genetic structures
   graft structure
   hilar structure
   implant structure
   intact bone structure
   islet structures
   ligamentous structure
   midline structures
   muscular structure
   musculocartilaginous
      structure
   musculofascial structures
   neck of organ or structure
   open-pore structure
   osseous structures
   removal of fetal structure

structure (*continued*)
   rodlike structure
   skeletal structure
   subcortical structures
   subintimal structure
   subtentorial structures
   superficial structures
   supporting structures
   supraglottic structures
   surrounding structures
   underlying structures
   valve structure
   vascular structure
Struempel (*also* Strümpel)
Struempel ear alligator forceps
Struempel ear punch
Struempel ear punch forceps
Struempel forceps
Struempel rongeur
Struempel-Voss ethmoidal
      forceps
Struempel-Voss ethmoidal
      forceps
Struempel-Voss nasal forceps
Strully cardiovascular scissors
Strully curet
Strully dissecting scissors
Strully dressing forceps
Strully dural scissors
Strully dural twist hook
Strully Gigli-saw handle
Strully hook
Strully hook scissors
Strully nerve root retractor
Strully neurological scissors
Strully neurosurgical scissors
Strully retractor
Strully ruptured disk curet
Strully scissors
Strully tissue forceps
Strully-Kerrison rongeur
struma
      cast iron struma
      Hashimoto struma
      ligneous struma
      Riedel struma
      substernal struma
struma aberranta
struma lymphomatosa
struma maligna
struma nodosa
strumectomy

Strümpel (*see* Struempel)
Strunksy sign
strut
   Adkins strut
   Anderson nasal strut
   calipers strut
   columellar strut
   dorsal strut
   Harrington strut
   House calipers strut
   implant substructure strut
   Judet strut
   Magnuson strut
   miniplate strut
   Nalebuff-Goldman strut
   nasal strut
   pinch nose strut
   piston strut
   Plasti-Pore strut
   polyethylene strut
   Rehbein internal steel strut
   Robinson strut
   slipped strut
   stainless steel strut
   stent strut
   Stribs strut
   substernal metallic strut
   sutured-in-place columellar
      strut
   Teflon strut
   TORP strut
   tricuspid valve strut
   valve outflow strut
   wire-loop strut
   wire-lop strut
strut bar
strut bar hook
strut calipers
strut forceps
strut fracture
strut fusion technique
strut graft
strut guide
strut hook
strut measuring instrument
strut pick
strut plate fixation
strut rhinoplasty
Struthers ligament
strut-type pin
struvite calculus
struvite crystal formation

struvite urinary tract stones
Struyken angular punch tip
Struyken conchotome
Struyken ear forceps
Struyken nasal forceps
Struyken nasal-cutting forceps
Struyken punch
Struyken turbinate forceps
StrykeFlow electrocautery
   probe
StrykeFlow suction irrigator
Stryker arthroscope
Stryker autopsy saw
Stryker blade
Stryker bur
Stryker cartilage knife
Stryker cast cutter
Stryker chip camera
Stryker chondrotome
Stryker CircOlectric bed
Stryker CircOlectric fracture
   frame
Stryker Dacron prosthetic
   ligament
Stryker dermabrader
Stryker dermatome
Stryker drain
Stryker drill
Stryker equipment
Stryker fracture frame
Stryker fracture table
Stryker frame
Stryker illuminated retractor
Stryker impact osteotome
Stryker knee arthrometer
Stryker lag screw
Stryker microdebrider
Stryker microirrigator
Stryker MixEvac
Stryker oscillating saw
Stryker perforator
Stryker resector
Stryker Rolo-dermatome
Stryker saw
Stryker saw trephine
Stryker screw
Stryker screwdriver
Stryker stent
Stryker suction irrigator
Stryker Surgilav machine
Stryker turning fracture frame
Stryker wedge suture anchor

Stryker-School meniscal knife
STSG (split-thickness skin graft)
STT (scaphoid-trapezium-
   trapezoid)
STT joint
Stuart articulator
Stuart Gordon hand splint
Stubbs adenoidal curet
Stubbs curet
Stuck laminectomy self-retaining
   retractor
Stuck self-retaining laminectomy
   retractor
Stucker bile duct dilator
Stuckrad magnifying
   laryngopharyngoscope
Studer pouch
Studer pouch procedure
Studer reservoir urinary
   diversion
study
   angioaortic arch study
   Bucky studies
   baseline study
   cardiac study
   choledochogram study
   cinephonation study
   conduction nerve study
   cystometric study
   diagnostic study
   Doppler study
   double-contrast study
   dual-contract study
   echocardiographic study
   electrocorticogram study
   electrophysiologic study
   endoscopic study
   followup studies
   fluoroscopic study
   function study
   isotope scanning studies
   isotope studies
   imaging study
   immunohistochemical study
   injection study
   iodized oil study
   Imatron C-100 system for
     heart studies
   lung function studies
   Iotrol study
   localization study
   marker transit studies

study (*continued*)
   oblique study
   pelvimetry study
   perfusion study
   phonocardiogram study
   posteroanterior study
   pyelographic study
   preliminary studies
   pulmonary function studies
   radiographic studies
   radiologic studies
   radioencephalogram study
   radiologic magnification study
   randomized study
   renogram study
   repeat study
   retrococcygeal air study
   retrospective study
   scintigraphic study
   single-contrast study
   skiagram study
   selective studies
   serial studies
   sputum studies
   sonoencephalographic study
   tachography study
   tomographic study
   tracer study
   uptake studies
   unenhanced study
   uroflow study
   Vabra endometrial study
   vibrocardiography study
   x-ray study
Stuhler-Heise fixator
Stukey stripper
Stulberg hip positioner
Stulberg HIPciser abduction
   splint
Stulberg Mark II leg positioner
Stumer perforating bur
stump
   amputation stump
   appendiceal stump
   Baylor stump
   blind stump
   bronchial stump
   burying of appendiceal stump
   cardiac stump
   cervical stump
   cone-shaped amputation
     stump

stump (*continued*)
  conical stump
  duodenal stump
  forklike stump
  gastric stump
  invaginated stump
  inverting appendiceal stump
  mature stump
  pedicle stump
  rectal stump
  revision of amputation stump
  tracheal stump
  umbilical stump
stump dehiscence
stump embolization syndrome
stump hallucination
stump invagination
stump inverted
stump leak
stump ligation
stump of appendix
stump of bronchus
stump of esophagus
stump of pedicle
stump pressure
stump shrinker
stump shrinking
stump sock
Sturge-Weber syndrome
Sturgis tenaculum
Sturmdorf amputation of cervix
Sturmdorf cervical needle
Sturmdorf cervical reamer
Sturmdorf colporrhaphy
Sturmdorf obstetrical sutures
Sturmdorf operation
Sturmdorf pedicle needle
Sturmdorf reamer
Sturmdorf suture technique
Sturmdorf sutures
Stutsman nasal snare
stuttering urinary stream
STx Saunders lumbar disk
    device
stye
Styles forceps
stylet
  Bing stylet
  bipolar irrigating stylet
  Bruening forceps stylet
  cardiovascular stylet
  catheter stylet

stylet (*continued*)
  catheter wire stylet
  Cook locking stylet
  Cooper endotracheal stylet
  Frazier stylet
  Frigitronics disposable
    cryosurgical stylet
  Hockey Stick articulating stylet
  illuminating stylet
  Inrad HiLiter ultrasound-
    enhanced stylet
  Jelco intravenous stylet
  jet stylet
  K-stylet
  Katz-Berci optical stylet
  L-stylet
  lighted stylet
  locking stylet
  Malis irrigating forceps stylet
  malleable stylet
  optical stylet
  retractable stylet
  Rumel ratchet tourniquet
    eyed stylet
  S-stylet
  straight stylet
  straight tube stylet
  surgical stylet
  tourniquet-eyed ratchet stylet
  Trachlight lighted intubating
    stylet
  transmyocardial pacing stylet
  transseptal stylet
  transthoracic pacing stylet
  Tubestat lighted stylet
  Universal curved-tube stylet
  Universal straight-tube stylet
  ureteral stylet
  wire stylet
stylet-scope endoscope
styletted catheter
styletted tracheobronchial
    catheter
Stylex syringe
styloglossus, muscle
stylohyoid branch
stylohyoid ligament
stylohyoid muscle
stylohyoid nerve
stylohyoid process syndrome
stylohyoid syndrome
styloid bone

styloid diaphragm
styloid process
styloid syndrome
styloiditis
stylomandibular artery
stylomandibular ligament
stylomandibular membrane
stylomandibular tunnel
stylomastoid artery
stylomastoid foramen
stylomastoid vein
stylomastoideum
   foramen stylomastoideum
stylomaxillary
stylopharyngeal muscle
stylopharyngeal nerve
stylopharyngeus muscle
styloradial reflex
stylostaphyline
Stylus cardiovascular sutures
Stylus suture needle
S-type dental implant
styptic cotton
styptic wool
Styrofoam dressing
Suarez retractor
Suarez spreader
Suarz continence ring
Suave-Kapandji arthroplasty
Sub-4 Platinum Plus wire kit
subacromial bursa
subacromial space
subacute condition
subacute inflammation
subanesthetic concentration
subannular mattress sutures
subantral augmentation
subaortic stenosis
subapical osteotomy
subaponeurotic abscess
subaponeurotic fascial cleft
subaponeurotic space
subarachnoid anesthesia
subarachnoid bleeding
subarachnoid block
subarachnoid block anesthesia
   (SAB anesthesia)
subarachnoid cavity
subarachnoid cisterna
subarachnoid hemorrhage
subarachnoid injection
subarachnoid pathways

subarachnoid sac
subarachnoid screw
subarachnoid septum
subarachnoid shunt
subarachnoid space
subarachnoid ureterostomy
subarachnoidal cisterns
subarachnoidal sinus
subarcuate fossa
subareolar region
subastragalar amputation
subastragalar dislocation
subaurale
subauricular region
subcallosal gyrus
subcapital fracture
subcapsular cataract
subcapsular cortex
subcapsular flap
subcapsular hemorrhage
subcapsular nephrectomy
subcapsular opacity
subcapsular renal hematoma
subcardinal veins
subcarinal angle
subcarinal lymphadenopathy
subcecal fossa
subchondral bone
subchondral bony resorption
subchondral cyst
subchorial hemorrhage
subchorial space
subchorionic hematoma
subchorionic hemorrhage
subchoroidal approach
subcilial blepharoplasty malar
   implant insertion
subciliary approach
subciliary incision
subclavian aortic anastomosis
subclavian apheresis catheter
subclavian arteriogram
subclavian arteriovenous fistula
subclavian artery aneurysm
subclavian artery occlusion
subclavian cannula
subclavian catheter
subclavian central venous
   catheter insertion
subclavian dialysis catheter
subclavian duct
subclavian endarterectomy

subclavian flap technique
subclavian groove
subclavian hemodialysis catheter
subclavian injury
subclavian introducer
subclavian line
subclavian loop
subclavian nerve
subclavian peel-away sheath
subclavian perivascular block
subclavian steal syndrome
subclavian sulcus of lung
subclavian Tegaderm dressing
subclavian triangle
subclavian vein access catheter
subclavian vein catheterization
subclavian vein patch
    angioplasty
subclavian vessel exposure
subclavian-carotid bypass
subclavian-subclavian bypass
subclavicular approach
subclavicular murmur
subclavius muscle
subcollateral gyrus
subcomplete resection
subcondylar deformity
subcondylar fracture of the
    mandible
subcondylar greenstick fracture
    of the mandible
subcondylar osteotomy
subconjunctival hemorrhage
subconjunctival injection
subconjunctival needle
subcoracoid dislocation
subcoracoid shoulder
    dislocation
subcoracoid space
subcortical encephalopathy
subcortical hemorrhage
subcortical structures
subcostal area
subcostal artery
subcostal flank incision
subcostal groove
subcostal incision
subcostal line
subcostal muscles
subcostal nerve
subcostal plane
subcostal position

subcostal retractions
subcostal transperitoneal incision
subcostal trocar
subcostal vein
subcostalis muscle
subcrepitant rales
subcutaneous (sc, SQ, subcu)
subcutaneous adipose tissue
subcutaneous augmentation
    material (SAM)
subcutaneous anastomosis
subcutaneous angiolipoma
subcutaneous bleeders
subcutaneous calcification
subcutaneous connective tissues
subcutaneous fascia
subcutaneous fasciotomy
subcutaneous fat
subcutaneous fat lines
subcutaneous fat necrosis
subcutaneous flap
subcutaneous fracture
subcutaneous hemangioma
subcutaneous hematoma
subcutaneous implantation
subcutaneous injection
subcutaneous intraocular node
subcutaneous laterodigital
    reverse flap
subcutaneous leash
subcutaneous lipoma
subcutaneous mass
subcutaneous mastectomy
subcutaneous metastasis
subcutaneous morphine pump
subcutaneous necrotizing
    infection
subcutaneous nodule
subcutaneous operation
subcutaneous patch electrode
subcutaneous pedicled flap
subcutaneous perineal mass
subcutaneous peritoneal
    administration device
subcutaneous plane
subcutaneous rhytidectomy
subcutaneous saw
subcutaneous suture
subcutaneous swelling
subcutaneous temporal nerves
subcutaneous temporofacial
    facelift

subcutaneous
    temporomandibular facelift
subcutaneous tenotomy
subcutaneous tissue expander
subcutaneous tumor
subcutaneous tunneling device
subcutaneous tunnels
subcutaneous turnover flap
subcutaneous veins of abdomen
subcutaneous venous arch at
    root of fingers
subcutaneous wound
subcutaneously
subcuticular
subcuticular level
subcuticular pull-out skin
    sutures
subcuticular pull-out sutures
subcuticular stitch
subcuticular suture technique
subcuticular sutures
subcuticular wire
subdeltoid bursa
subdeltoid fat plane obliteration
subdermal accordion
subdermal graft
subdermal implant
subdermal layer
subdermal nasal tissue
subdermal plexus of vessels
subdermal prosthesis
subdiaphragmatic abscess
subdiaphragmatic fields
subdiaphragmatic hernia
subdiaphragmatic involvement
subdiaphragmatic radiation
    therapy
subdiaphragmatic space
subdiaphragmatic
    sympathectomy
subdigastric lymph nodes
subdural abscess
subdural block
subdural cavity
subdural fluid
subdural grid electrode
subdural grid implantation
subdural hematoma
subdural hemorrhage
subdural hygroma
subdural puncture
subdural space

subdural strip electrode
subduroperitoneal shunt
subendocardial infarction
subendocardial injury
subendocardial ischemia
subendocardial myocardial
    infarction (SEMI)
subependymal extension
subependymal hemorrhage
subepicardial fat
subepicardial injury
subepicranial space
subepidermal abscess
subepidermal collagen
subepidermal nodular fibrosis
subepidermal vesiculation
subepithelial connective tissue
    graft
subepithelial hemorrhage
subepithelial membrane
subepithelial nerve plexus
subepithelial plexus
subeschar infection
subfalcial herniation
subfascial carpal tunnel
    decompression
subfascial hematoma
subfascial lane
subfascial palmar space
subfascial web space
subfrontal approach
subfrontal-transbasal approach
subgaleal abscess
subgaleal dissection
subgaleal drain
subgaleal elevation
subgaleal fascia
subgaleal flap
subgaleal hematoma
subgaleal hemorrhage
subgaleal plane
subgaleal space
subgingival curettage
subgingival space
subglandular capsular
    contracture
subglenoid dislocation
subglenoid shoulder dislocation
subglottic area
subglottic cavity
subglottic edema
subglottic forceps

subglottic hemangioma
subglottic squamous cell
   carcinoma
subglottic stenosis
subgluteal hematoma
subhepatic abscess
subhepatic space
subhuman primary donor
subhyaloid hemorrhage
subhyoid laryngotomy
subhyoid region
subimplant membrane
subinguinal fossa
subinguinal incision
subintimal hemorrhage
subintimal structure
subinvolution of uterus
subjacent tissue
sublabial adhesion
sublabial approach
sublabial incision
sublabial midline rhinoseptal
   approach
sublabial perforation
sublabial transsphenoidal
   approach
sublaminar fixation
sublaminar wire
sublethal x-ray damage repair
subligamentous dissection
Sublimaze anesthesia
sublimis sling
sublimis tendon
sublingual artery
sublingual caruncle
sublingual crescent
sublingual cyst
sublingual ducts
sublingual fibrogranuloma
sublingual fold
sublingual fossa
sublingual fovea
sublingual ganglion
sublingual glands
sublingual hematoma
sublingual mucosa
sublingual nerve
sublingual obstruction
sublingual papilla
sublingual ridge
sublingual saliva
sublingual salivary gland

sublingual space
sublingual space abscess
sublingual sulcus
sublingual tablet
sublingual ulcer
sublingual vein
sublobular veins
subluxated
subluxation
   facet subluxation
   forward subluxation
   radioulnar subluxation
   rotary subluxation
   temporomandibular joint
     subluxation
   unilateral facet subluxation
   Volkmann subluxation
subluxation stabilization
subluxed radial head
subluxed shoulder
submalar deficiency
submalar hollowing
submammary abscess
submammary crease
submammary dissector
submammary incision
submammary line
submandibular augmentation
submandibular chronic
   sclerosing sialadenitis
submandibular duct
submandibular fossa
submandibular fovea
submandibular ganglion
submandibular gland
submandibular lymph nodes
submandibular obstruction
submandibular saliva
submandibular salivary gland
submandibular space
submandibular space abscess
submandibular triangle
submandibular trigone
submandibulectomy
submasseteric space
submasseteric space abscess
submaxilla
submaxillary caruncle
submaxillary cellulitis
submaxillary duct
submaxillary fossa
submaxillary ganglion

submaxillary gland
submaxillary nerves
submaxillary region
submaxillary saliva
submaxillary salivary gland
submaxillary space
submaxillary triangle
submedial
submembranous placental
    hematoma
submental access
submental approach
submental artery
submental artery flap
submental fat pad
submental fistula
submental glands
submental hematoma
submental incision
submental island flap
submental laxity
submental liposuction
submental lymph nodes
submental region
submental space
submental space abscess
submental triangle
submental tuck approach
submental vein
submental vertex roentgenogram
submental-submandibular
    liposculpture
submentocervical view
submentonian dermo-fatty flap
submentoplasty
submentovertical axial
    projection
submerged tonsil
submerged tooth
submicroinfusion catheter
submillimetric accuracy
submitral area
submitral calcification
submitted for biopsy
submitted for frozen section
submitted for microsection
submitted to pathologist
submucosa
submucosal cleft palate
submucosal connective tissue
submucosal dissection
submucosal gastric hemorrhage

submucosal gland hypertrophy
submucosal hemorrhage
submucosal implant
submucosal invasion
submucosal resection
submucosal space
submucosal urethral
    augmentation
submucosal vascular dilation
submucosal vascular pattern
submucosal venous plexus
submucosal vessels
submucous chisel
submucous cleft
submucous cleft palate
submucous curet
submucous dissection
submucous dissector
submucous elevator
submucous fibrosis
submucous knife
submucous layer
submucous leiomyoma
submucous membrane
submucous myomata
submucous resection (SMR)
submucous resection and
    rhinoplasty
submucous retractor
submuscular breast
    augmentation
submuscular implant
submuscular implantation
submuscular pocket
subnasal
subnasion
suboccipital approach
suboccipital craniectomy
suboccipital decompression
suboccipital dural defect
suboccipital incision
suboccipital nerve
suboccipital Ommaya reservoir
suboccipital plexus
suboccipital puncture
suboccipital triangle
suboccipital trigeminal
    rhizotomy
suboccipital-subtemporal
    approach
suboccipital-transmeatal
    approach

suboccipitobregmatic diameter
suboccluding ligature
suboptimal examination
suboptimal surgery
suborbicularis oculi fat (SOOF)
suborbicularis skin
suborbital mimetic muscle
    elevation (SOMME)
subpapillary zone
subpectoral augmentation
subpectoral implant
subpectoral implantation
subpectoral implantation
    technique
subpectoral plane
subpectoral reconstruction
subpectoral-subserratus muscle
    implantation
subperichondrial dissection
subperichondrial excision
subperiosteal abscess
subperiosteal abscess of frontal
    sinus
subperiosteal amputation
subperiosteal approach
subperiosteal bone
subperiosteal brow lift
subperiosteal calcification
subperiosteal dissection
subperiosteal elevation
subperiosteal exposure
subperiosteal facelift
subperiosteal fracture
subperiosteal glass beadinserter
subperiosteal hematoma
subperiosteal hemorrhage
subperiosteal implant
subperiosteal malar cheek lift
subperiosteal mid-face lift
subperiosteal minimally invasive
    facelift
subperiosteal minimally invasive
    laser endoscopic facelift
    (SMILE facelift)
subperiosteal minimally invasive
    laser endoscopic
    rhytidectomy (SMILE
    rhytidectomy)
subperiosteal orbital abscess
    (SPOA)
subperiosteal pulling stitch
subperiosteal resection

subperiosteal tissue expander
    (STE)
subperiosteal vomerine-
    ethmoidal plane
subperiosteally resected
subperitoneal abscess
subperitoneal appendicitis
subperitoneal Baldy-Webster
    hysteropexy
subperitoneal space
subpharyngeal
subphrenic abscess
subphrenic collection
subphrenic space
subplatysmal facelift
subplatysmal facelift technique
subplatysmal fat
subplatysmal plane
subpleural mass
subpleural mediastinal plexus
subpontic hyperostosis
subpubic angle
subpubic hernia
subpulmonic pleural space
subpyramidal fossa
Sub-Q-Set subcutaneous
    continuous infusion device
Subramanian aortic clamp
Subramanian clamp
Subramanian classic miniature
    aortic clamp
Subramanian miniature aortic
    clamp
Subramanian sidewinder aortic
    clamp
Subramanian valve speculum
subretinal damage
subretinal fluid
subretinal fluid cannula
subretinal hemorrhage
subretinal neovascular
    membrane
subretinal space
subretinal surgery
Subrini penile prosthesis
subscaphocephaly
subscapular angle
subscapular artery
subscapular bursa
subscapular flap
subscapular fossa
subscapular muscle

subscapular nerves
subscapular splenectomy
subscapular system free flap
subscapularis tendon
subsegmental area
subsegmental hepatectomy
subsegmental resection
subselective embolization
subserosa
subserous fascia
subsigmoid fossa
sub-SMAS rhytidectomy
    (superficial
    musculoaponeurotic
    system)
sub-SMAS plane
subspinous dislocation
substance concentration
substantia (*pl.* substantiae)
substernal angle
substernal gland
substernal goiter
substernal metallic strut
substernal struma
substernal thyroid
substitute
  AlloMatrix injectable putty
    bone graft substitute
  Biobrane skin substitute
  bone graft substitute
  Dardik vein substitute
  EZ-Derm temporary skin
    substitute
  Mediform dural substitute
  Oxycyte perfluorocarbon-
    based blood substitute
  skin substitute
  unilaminar skin substitute
substitution transfusion
substitutional cardiac surgery
substrate phase of wound
    healing
substructure
subsuperficial
    musculoaponeurotic system
    rhytidectomy (sub-SMAS)
    rhytidectomy)
subsynaptic web
subtalar arthrodesis
subtalar articulation
subtalar dislocation
subtalar joint

subtalar motion
subtarsal
subtemporal decompression
subtemporal dissection
subtemporal-intradural approach
subtend
subtendinous bursa
sub-Tenon anesthesia cannula
subtentorial lesion
subtentorial structures
subtentorial tumor
subthalamus
subtotal cataract extraction
subtotal cleft palate
subtotal colectomy
subtotal cystectomy
subtotal esophagectomy
subtotal esophagoplasty
subtotal excision
subtotal gastrectomy
subtotal gastric exclusion
subtotal gastric resection
subtotal glossectomy
subtotal hepatectomy
subtotal hysterectomy
subtotal laminectomy
subtotal laryngectomy
subtotal orbital exenteration
subtotal pancreatectomy
subtotal removal of tumor
subtotal resection
subtotal supraglottic
    laryngectomy (SSL)
subtotal thyroidectomy
subtraction films
subtraction scintigraphy
subtraction technique
subtrigonal spheroids
subtrochanteric femoral
    fracture
subtrochanteric fracture
subtrochanteric incision
subtrochanteric osteotomy
subumbilical incision
subumbilical space
subungual abscess
subungual exostosis
subungual hematoma
subungual hyperkeratosis
subungual keratoacanthoma
    (SUKA)
subungual melanoma

subungual squamous cell
  carcinoma
subunit
suburethral melanoma
suburethral rectus fascial sling
  procedure
suburethral sling procedure
subvalvular aortic stenosis
subvertebral muscles
subvesical duct
subvesical fascia
subvolution
subxiphoid
subzonal insemination
succedaneous teeth
succenturiate lobe
succenturiate placenta
successful passage of instrument
successional teeth
successive approximation
successive responses
successive stages
succinate dehydrogenase
succinic dehydrogenase
succinylcholine anesthetic agent
succinylcholine drip
succulent nodes
succus
succussion
succussion sounds
succussion splash
sucker
sucker tip
sucking pad
sucking wound
Sucquet anastomosis
Sucquet canals
Sucquet-Hoyer anastomosis
Sucquet-Hoyer canals
suction
  Adson suction
  airway suction
  Barton suction
  bellows suction
  Bowen suction
  bulb suction
  closed-box suction
  continuous nasogastric
    suction
  continuous NG suction
  continuous suction
  Cooley cardiovascular suction

suction (*continued*)
  C-P suction
  DeLee suction
  Dia suction
  ear forceps with suction
  Emerson suction
  Ferguson suction
  flexible dental suction
  Frazier suction
  gastric suction
  Gomco suction
  Hamrick suction
  Harris tube suction
  Hemovac suction
  Humphrey coronary sinus
    suction
  intubation and suction
  lavage and suction
  low intermittent suction
  Melco suction
  nasogastric suction
  Ortholav suction
  perilimbal suction
  Pleur-Evac suction
  Printz suction
  Robinson tonsillar suction
  Rosen suction
  SureTran suction
  syringe suction
  Tis-U-Trap endometrial
    suction
  Turner-Warwick suction
  underwater suction
  Vactro perilimbal suction
  Wangensteen suction
  wound incision and suction
  Yankauer suction
suction abortion
suction adapter
suction airway
suction and intubation
suction aspiration
suction aspirator
suction assisted
suction biopsy
suction biopsy needle
suction biter
suction bulb
Suction Buster catheter
suction cannula
suction catheter
suction cautery

suction connector
suction cup
suction curet
suction curettage
suction cutter
suction cylinder
suction D&C
suction device
suction dilatation and curettage
suction dissection
suction dissector
suction drain
suction drainage
suction elevator
suction evacuator
suction extraction
suction forceps
suction hemostatic agent
suction injury
suction irrigator
suction knife
suction lipectomy
suction machine
suction magnet
suction ophthalmodynamometer
suction plate
suction pressure pump
suction probe
suction pump
suction pump aspirator
suction punch
suction reservoir
suction ring
suction stomach
suction suspension
suction tip (*see* tip)
suction tip curet
suction tonsillar dissector
suction tube
suction tube (*see* tube)
suction tube clip
suction tube obturator
suction unit
suction-assisted lipectomy
    (SAL)
suction-assisted lipocontouring
suction-assisted lipolysis
suction-coagulation tube
suction-coagulator
suction-electrocoagulator
suctioning
suction-irrigation technique

suction-irrigator (*see also*
    irrigator)
  House-Radpour suction-
    irrigator
  House-Stevenson suction-
    irrigator
  Kurze suction-irrigator
  Nezhat suction-irrigator
suctorial pad
Suda papilla classification
Sudan needle
Sudarsky cryoprobe
sudden infant death syndrome
    (SIDS)
Sudeck critical point
sudomotor nerves
sudoriferous cyst
sudoriferous duct
sudoriferous glands
sudorific centers
sudoriparous glands
Suetens-Gybels-Vandermeulen
    angiographic localizer
suffocative goiter
Sugar aneurysm clip
Sugar clip
Sugarbaker operation
Sugarbaker retrocolic clamp
sugar-tong cast
sugar-tong plaster splint
sugar-tong splint
Suggs catheter
Sugioki osteotomy of hip
Sugita aneurysm clip
Sugita catheter
Sugita cross-legged clip
Sugita fork
Sugita head clamp
Sugita head holder
Sugita jaws clip applier
Sugita microsurgical table
Sugita multipurpose head
    frame
Sugita retractor
Sugita side-curved bayonet clip
Sugita temporary straight clip
Sugita-Ikakogyo clip
Sugiura abdominal pull-through
    operation
Sugiura devascularization of
    esophagus and stomach
Sugiura esophageal varices

Sugiura procedure for
  esophageal varices
Suh ventilation tube
suitable beam film localization
suitcase kidney
SUKA (subungual
  keratoacanthoma)
Suker cyclodialysis spatula
Suker iris forceps
Suker spatula knife
Sukhtian-Hughes fixation
  device
sulcal epithelium
sulcated tongue
sulci (*sing.* sulcus)
sulci cutis
sulci in brain
sulciform
sulciolar gastric mucosa
sulcular epithelium
sulcus (*pl.* sulci)
  alveolabial sulcus
  alveolingual sulcus
  alveolobuccal sulcus
  anterolateral sulcus
  aortic sulcus
  auriculocephalic sulcus
  blunting of sulcus
  buccal sulcus
  calcaneal sulcus
  calcarine sulcus
  cardiohepatic sulcus
  carotid sulcus
  central cerebral sulcus
  cingulate sulcus
  coronal sulcus
  coronary sulcus
  costophrenic sulcus
  gingival sulcus
  gingivobuccal sulcus
  gingivolabial sulcus
  gingivolingual sulcus
  Harrison sulcus
  implant gingival sulcus
  infraorbital sulcus
  infrapalpebral sulcus
  intergluteal sulcus
  internal spiral sulcus
  interparietal sulcus
  intraparietal sulcus
  labial sulcus
  labial-buccal sulcus

sulcus (*continued*)
  labiodental sulcus
  labiomarginal sulcus
  lateral cerebral sulcus
  lateral sulcus
  lingual sulcus
  lip sulcus
  longitudinal sulcus
  mandibular sulcus
  medial bicipital sulcus
  median lingual sulcus
  median sulcus
  mentolabial sulcus
  Monro sulcus
  mylohyoid sulcus
  nasolabial sulcus
  occlusal sulcus
  oculomotor sulcus
  palatine sulcus
  palatovaginal sulcus
  palpebral-malar sulcus (tear
    trough)
  paraglenoid sulcus
  paralingual sulcus
  paramedial sulcus
  periconchal sulcus
  peroneal sulcus
  petrosal sulcus
  postauricular sulcus
  posterior median sulcus
  posterior sulcus
  posterointermediate sulcus
  posterolateral sulcus
  preauricular sulcus
  prejowl anterior mandibular
    sulcus
  prejowl sulcus
  retroauricular sulcus
  retrocentral sulcus
  retroglandular sulcus
  sigmoid sulcus
  sublingual sulcus
  superior temporal sulcus
  supratarsal sulcus
  temporal sulcus
  terminal sulcus
  tonsillolingual sulcus
  transverse occipital sulcus
  Turner intraparietal sulcus
  tympanic sulcus
  vomeral sulcus
  vomerovaginal sulcus

sulcus (*continued*)
  V-Z advancement in buccal
    sulcus
  Waldeyer sulcus
sulcus angle
sulcus anthelicis transversus
sulcus auriculae posterior
sulcus auriculae anterior
sulcus blunting
sulcus cruris helicis
sulcus ethmoidalis
sulcus fixated position
sulcus fixation
sulcus for greater palatine nerve
sulcus gluteus
sulcus hamuli pterygoidei
sulcus matricis unguis
sulcus of heart
sulcus of lung
sulcus of mandibular neck
sulcus of mastoid canaliculus
sulcus of nasal process of
    maxilla
sulcus of pterygoid hamulus
sulcus of subclavian artery
sulcus of wrist
sulcus olfactorius nasi
sulcus pterygopalatinus
sulcus spinosus
sulcus tumor
Sulfix-6 cement
sulfur colloid liver scan
sulfur colloid nuclear medicine
sulfur colloid scan
Sullivan bubble cushion
Sullivan gum scissors
Sullivan III nasal continuous
    positive air pressure device
Sullivan nasal variable positive
    airway pressure unit
Sullivan raspatory
Sullivan sinus rasp
Sullivan variable stiffness cable
Sully shoulder stabilizer brace
SULP II balloon catheter
SULP II catheter
Sultrin impregnated vaginal
    pack
Sulzer prosthesis
Summerskill operation
Summit alloy
Summit excimer laser

Summit Krumeich-Barraquer
    microkeratome
Summit LoDose collimator
summit of nose
Summit Omnimed excimer laser
Summit Apex laser
Summit Excimed laser
Sumner clamp
Sumner elevator
Sumner sign
sump
  Argyle silicone Salem sump
  Salem sump
  Saratoga sump
  van Sonnenberg sump
sump catheter
sump drain
sump drainage
sump nasogastric tube
sump Penrose drain
sump pump
sump pump catheter
sump suction tube
sump syndrome
sump tube
SUNCT syndrome
Sunday elevator
Sunday staphylorrhaphy elevator
Sunderland classification for
    nerve injuries (grades I-IV)
Sunderland nerve injury
    classification
Sundt aneurysm clip-applier
Sundt booster clip
Sundt carotid endarterectomy
    shunt
Sundt encircling clip
Sundt straddling clip
Sundt-Kees aneurysmal clip
Sundt-Kees booster clip
Sundt-Kees encircling patch clip
Sundt-Kees graft clip
sunflower cataract
sunken acetabulum
sunken-eye appearance
sunken-face appearances
sunken-in face
sunrise projection
sunrise view of patella on x-ray
sunset view of patella on x-ray
Super Arrow-Flex catheterization
    sheath

Super Cut laminectomy rongeur
Super Dopplex SDI vascular test unit
Super Eidersoft bed pad
Super Epitron high-frequency epilator
Super Field slit lamp lens
Super Grip sleeve
Super Pak posterior nasal pack
Super PEG tube
Super punctum plug
Super Stimm stimulator
Super Torque Plus catheter
super wet technique
super wrap
Super-9 guiding cardiac device
Super-9 guiding catheter
super-absorptive polymer dressing
Superblade blade
SuperCat self-tapping implant
Supercath intravenous catheter
superciliary arch
superciliary depressor muscle
superconducting magnet
superconducting quantum interference device
SuperCup acetabular cup prosthesis
Super-Dent orthodontic cement
SuperEBA cement
superficial abdominal fascia
superficial abrasion
superficial angioma
superficial basal cell carcinoma
superficial basal cell epithelioma
superficial bleeders
superficial blood vessels
superficial brachial artery
superficial brachial flap
superficial bullae
superficial burn
superficial circumflex iliac artery
superficial circumflex iliac vein
superficial dermis
superficial destruction
superficial dorsal veins
superficial epigastric artery
superficial epigastric vein
superficial erosion
superficial excision

superficial facial fascia
superficial fascia
superficial fascial system (SFS)
superficial fat
superficial femoral arch
superficial fibular nerve
superficial flexor muscle
superficial frostbite
superficial granulomatous pyoderma
superficial hemangioma
superficial implant
superficial implantation
superficial infection
superficial inguinal ring
superficial keratectomy
superficial laceration
superficial lamellar keratoplasty
superficial layers
superficial liposculpture
superficial malignant melanoma
superficial middle cerebral vein
superficial middle petrosal nerve
superficial musculoaponeurotic system (SMAS)
superficial nerve
superficial nodes
superficial palmar arch
superficial palmar artery
superficial palmar branch of radial artery
superficial parotidectomy
superficial perineal artery
superficial perineal fascia
superficial perineal space
superficial peroneal nerve
superficial petrosal artery
superficial plane rhytidectomy
superficial plantar arch
superficial radial nerve
superficial reflex
superficial renal cortical perfusion (SRCP)
superficial rhytids
superficial sclera
superficial SMAS rhytidectomy
superficial spreading melanoma
superficial structures
superficial suture technique
superficial sutures
superficial temporal artery

superficial temporal artery-to-MCA bypass
superficial temporal branch of external carotid artery
superficial temporal crest
superficial temporal fascia
superficial temporal vein
superficial transverse fibers
superficial transverse muscle of perineum
superficial ulceration
superficial upper lateral shave
superficial valvular insufficiency
superficial varicosities
superficial vein
superficial venous markings
superficial vertebral veins
superficial wound
superficialis tendon
superficially explored
superfine fiberscope
Superflex elastic dressing
Superflow Judkins catheter
Superflow guiding catheter
Superform Contours orthotic
SuperGlide needle
Superglue adhesive
Superglue tissue adhesive
superimposed bowel gas
superimposed depression
superimposition
superinfection
superior alveolar artery
superior alveolar nerve
superior ampullar nerve
superior anastomotic vein
superior angle
superior annulus
superior arcuate bundle
superior articular facet
superior articulating process
superior aspect
superior astragalonavicular ligament
superior auricular artery
superior auricular muscle
superior azygos vein
superior border
superior border of petrous portion of temporal bone
superior bulb of internal jugular vein

superior cantholysis
superior cardiac cervical nerve
superior carotid ganglion
superior carotid triangle
superior cerebellar artery
superior cerebellar peduncle
superior cerebellar vein
superior cerebral veins
superior cervical cardiac nerve
superior cervical chain
superior cervical ganglion
superior cervical ganglionectomy
superior clunial nerves
superior colliculus
superior commissure
superior constrictor muscle
superior constrictor pharngeal muscle
superior corner
superior costal facet
superior crus
superior crus of antihelix
superior cul-de-sac
superior dermal pedicle
superior dislocation
superior duodenal fold
superior duodenal fossa
superior duodenal recess
superior edge
superior epigastric artery
superior epigastric veins
superior fascia of urogenital diaphragm
superior flap
superior flexure of duodenum
superior fornix
superior fovea
superior frontal gyrus
superior ganglion
superior ganglion of glossopharyngeal nerve
superior gemellus muscle
superior gluteal artery
superior gluteal flap
superior gluteal nerve
superior gluteal neurovascular bundle
superior gluteal veins
superior hemorrhoidal artery
superior hemorrhoidal branch of inferior mesenteric artery

superior hemorrhoidal vein
superior iliac spine
superior incudal ligament
superior intercostal vein
superior iridotomy
superior joint space
superior labial artery
superior labial region
superior labial veins
superior lacrimal duct
superior lacrimal gland
superior laryngeal artery
superior laryngeal cavity
superior laryngeal nerve
superior laryngeal vein
superior laryngotomy
superior lateral cutaneous nerve
    of arm
superior ligament of incus
superior lip
superior lobe
superior longitidunal muscle of
    tongue
superior longitudinal sinus
superior lumbar hernia
superior mallear ligament
superior malposition
superior margin
superior marginotomy
superior maxilla
superior maxillary bone
superior maxillary foramen
superior maxillary retrognathia
superior meatus
superior mediastinum
superior mesenteric angiogram
superior mesenteric artery
superior mesenteric ganglion
superior mesenteric lymph
    nodes
superior mesenteric vein
superior mesenteric-caval
    anastomosis
superior mesenterorenal bypass
    technique
superior muscle
superior nasal concha
superior nasal venule of retina
superior oblique muscle
superior oblique tendon
superior occipital gyrus
superior omental recess

superior ophthalmic vein
superior orbital fissure
superior orbital fissure
    syndrome (SOFS)
superior orbital rim
superior ossicular chain
superior palpebral arch
superior palpebral region
superior palpebral vein
superior pancreaticoduodenal
    artery
superior parathyroid gland
superior parietal lobe
superior parietal lobule
superior pelvic aperture
superior pelvic strait
superior perihilar mass
superior petrosal ridge
superior petrosal sinus
superior pharyngeal artery
superior pharyngeal constrictor
superior phrenic vein
superior pole of calyx
superior pole of thyroid
superior pole traction rippling
superior portion of
    mesencephalon
superior posterior serratus
    muscle
superior pulmonary vein
superior radial tenotomy scissors
superior ramus
superior rectal artery
superior rectal fold
superior rectal veins
superior rectus
superior rectus bridle sutures
superior rectus forceps
superior rectus muscle
superior rectus traction sutures
superior root ansa cervicalis
superior sagittal sinus
superior sagittal sinus
    thrombosis (SSS)
superior sector iridectomy
superior segment of lung
superior semilunar lobule
superior spine
superior stratum
Superior suction catheter
superior superficial epigastric
    artery

superior suprarenal artery
superior surface of horizontal
    plate of palatine bone
superior tarsal muscle
superior temporal fissure
superior temporal gyrus
superior temporal sulcus
superior temporal venule of
    retina
superior thoracic aperture
superior thoracic pedicle screw
superior thyroid artery
superior thyroid gland
superior thyroid notch
superior thyroid vein
superior tibial articulation
superior tracheobronchial
    lymph nodes
superior tracheotomy
superior turbinal crest of
    maxilla
superior turbinal crest of
    palatine bone
superior turbinate
superior turbinate bone
superior tympanic artery
superior ulnar collateral artery
superior vagal ganglion
superior vena cava
superior vena cava syndrome
superior vena cavography
superior venula nasalis retinae
superior vesical artery
superior-intradural approach
superiorly based
superiorly milked
superjacent
superlag screw
supernatant
supernumerary auricles
supernumerary bone
supernumerary digits
supernumerary gland
supernumerary limb
supernumerary organ
supernumerary tendon
superoinferior projection
superoinferior tangential
    projection
superolateral aspect
superolateral surface of maxilla
superomedial

superovulation induction
Super-Plus Trimshield pad
SuperQuad assistive device
supersede
superselective microcoil
    embolization
SuperSkin thin film dressing
Superstat hemostatic wound
    pad
superstructure
supervascularization
superwet preoperative
    subcutaneous infiltration
supinated oblique view on x-ray
supination deformity
supination injury
supination reflex
supination splint
supination, external rotation
    fracture (SER fracture, SEX
    fracture)
supination-adduction fracture
supination-eversion fracture
supination-eversion injury
supination-external rotation
    injury
supination-external rotation
    fracture
supination-inversion rotation
    injury
supination-plantar flexion injury
supinator crest
supinator longus reflex
supinator muscle
supinator strap
supine C-Trax traction
supine film
supine hypotensive syndrome
supine mediolateral view
supine position
supine-oblique approach
Supolene sutures
Suppan procedure for nail
    deformity
supple neck
supplemental lobe
supplementary analgesia
supplementary marginotomy
support measures
support ridge
support stockings
support suture technique

support sutures
supported angioplasty
supporting area
supporting bone
supporting cell
supporting stitches
supporting structures
supporting tissue
supporting vessel
supportive halo cast
supportive intervention
supportive measures
supportive therapy
supportive tissue
supportive treatment
suppository
   prostaglandin suppository
   rectal suppository
   vaginal suppository
suppressant
suppurate chronic inflammation
suppuration
suppurative acute inflammation
suppurative appendicitis
suppurative exudate
suppurative granulomatous
   inflammation
suppurative infection
suppurative inflammation
suppurative labyrinthitis
suppurative osteomyelitis
suppurative otitis media (SOM)
suppurative sialadenitis
suppurative tenosynovitis
suppurative tonsillitis
Supra G coronary stent
supra-acetabular groove
supra-alar pinching
supra-annular mitral valve
   replacement
supra-annular suture ring
supra-aortic angiography
supra-areolar area
supra-arytenoid cartilage
supra-auricular point
suprabasal clefting
suprabuccal
supracallosal gyrus
supracardiac silhouette
supracardinal veins
supracerebellar approach
supracervical amputation

supracervical hysterectomy
supracervical incision
suprachoroid lamina
suprachoroid layer
suprachoroidal hemorrhage
supraciliary canal
supraclavicular adenopathy
supracondylar
supracricoid laryngectomy
supracricoid partial
   laryngectomy
supracristal plane
supradiaphragmatic
   diverticulum
supradiaphragmatic
   sympathectomy
supraduction
suprahyoid
suprahyoid epiglottitis
suprahyoid gland
suprahyoid muscles
suprahyoid neck dissection
suprahyoid space
supralaryngeal tension
Supralen cradle orthotic
Supralen Schaefer orthotic
supralevator abscess
supralevator anorectal space
supralevator pelvic
   exenteration
supralevator perirectal abscess
supralevator space
supramalleolar
supramalleolar flap
supramalleolar orthosis
supramammary
supramandibular
supramarginal gyrus
supramarginalis
   gyrus supramarginalis
supramastoid crest
supramastoid fossa
supramaxilla
supramaxillary
Supramead nose splint
suprameatal spine
supramediastinal mantle
supramental
supramental mandibular
   alveolus
supramesocolic surgical
   procedure

Supramid bridle collagen
   sutures
Supramid Extra sutures
Supramid eye muscle sleeve
Supramid graft
Supramid implant
Supramid lens
Supramid lens implant sutures
Supramid mesh implant
Supramid occluding stent
Supramid polyamide mesh
Supramid prosthesis
Supramid ptosis sleeve
Supramid ptosis sling
Supramid snare
Supramid suction tube
Supramid sutures
Supramid-Allen implant
supramohyoid neck dissection
supranasal
supranormal hemodynamic
   therapy
supranuclear lesion
supraocclusion
supraomental space
supraomohyoid neck dissection
supraoptic anastomosis
supraoptic canal
supraoptic commissure
supraoptico-hypophyseal axis
supraorbital air cell
supraorbital arch
supraorbital arch of frontal bone
supraorbital area
supraorbital artery
supraorbital bandeau
supraorbital bar
supraorbital canal
supraorbital ethmoid
supraorbital foramen
supraorbital fracture
supraorbital margin
supraorbital nerve
supraorbital notch
supraorbital pericranial flap
supraorbital plate
supraorbital point
supraorbital reflex
supraorbital region
supraorbital remodeling
supraorbital ridge
supraorbital rim

supraorbital rim of frontal bone
supraorbital vein
supraorbital-pterional approach
suprapapillary Roux-en-Y
   duodenojejunostomy
suprapatellar effusion
suprapatellar plica
suprapatellar pouch
suprapatellar reflex
supraperichondrial dissection
supraperiosteal flap
supraperiosteal implant
supraphysiologic fluid
   technique
suprapiriform foramen
suprapleural membrane
suprapubic appendectomy
   incision
suprapubic aspiration
suprapubic bag
suprapubic cannula
suprapubic catheter
suprapubic cystoscope
suprapubic cystostomy
suprapubic cystotomy
suprapubic drain
suprapubic excision of prostate
suprapubic hemostatic bag
suprapubic hernia
suprapubic incision
suprapubic lithotomy
suprapubic needle aspiration
suprapubic Pfannenstiel incision
suprapubic prostatectomy
suprapubic rami
suprapubic reflex
suprapubic region
suprapubic retractor
suprapubic self-retaining
   retractor
suprapubic sinus
suprapubic suction drain
suprapubic tenderness
suprapubic transvesical
   prostatectomy
suprapubic trocar
suprapubic tube
suprapubic urethroplasty
suprapubic urethrovesical
   suspension operation
suprarenal area
suprarenal arteries

suprarenal body
suprarenal capsule
suprarenal epithelioma
suprarenal filter placement
suprarenal ganglion
suprarenal glands
suprarenal Greenfield filter
suprarenal impression
suprarenal medulla
suprarenal plexus
suprarenal vein
suprascapular artery
suprascapular nerve
suprascapular nerve
    compression
suprascapular nerve
    entrapment
suprascapular notch
suprascapular vein
suprasellar aneurysm
suprasellar cisterna
suprasellar low-density lesion
suprasellar tumor
suprasphincteric fistula
supraspinatus fossa
supraspinatus tendon
supraspinous fossa
supraspinous muscle
suprasternal examination
suprasternal fascia
suprasternal fossa
suprasternal notch
suprasternal notch-to nipple
    distance (SN-N)
suprasternal plane
suprasternal pulsation
suprasternal region
suprasternal retraction
suprasternal space
supratarsal sulcus
supratentorial approach
supratentorial arteriovenous
    malformation
supratentorial craniotomy
supratentorial lesion
supratentorial space
supratip deformity
supratip fullness
supratonsillar fossa
supratrochlear artery
supratrochlear depression
supratrochlear nerve

supratrochlear nerve block
supratrochlear veins
supraumbilical incision
supraumbilical raphe
supraumbilical reflex
supravaginal hysterectomy
supravaginal septum
supravalvular aortic stenosis
supravalvular aortogram
supraventricular crest
supravesical fossa
supravesical hernia
supreme cardiac nerves
Supreme electrophysiology
    catheter
supreme nasal concha
supreme turbinate bone
Suraci elevator hook
Suraci zygoma hook elevator
sural arteries
sural artery flap
sural island flap for foot and
    ankle reconstruction
sural nerve biopsy
sural nerve cable graft
sural nerve entrapment
Sur-Catch paired-wire stone
    basket
surcingle
Sure Seal Golden Drain catheter
Sure Sport pad
Sure Step brace
SureBite biopsy forceps
SureCath port access catheter
Sure-Closure
Sure-Closure device
Sure-Cut biopsy needle
Surefit anterior chamber
    intraocular lens
Surefit intraocular lens
SureFlex prosthetic foot
SureFlex nickel-titanium file
Sureflow catheter
SureGrip breathing bag
SureGrip manual resuscitator
Surelite blood lancet
SurePress absorbent padding
SurePress compression dressing
SurePress compression wrap
SurePress high-compression
    bandage
SureScan scanning handpiece

SureSeal cellulose sponge
  bandage
SureSeal pressure bandage
SureSharp blood collecting
  needle
SureSharp dental needle
SureSite transparent adhesive
  film dressing
Suretac bioabsorbable shoulder
  fixation device
Suretac drill
Suretac guidewire
Surevue contact lens
Surewing winged infusion set
Surfacaine anesthetic agent
surface
  articular surface
  bosselated surface
  concave anterior surface
  concave posterior surface
  conjunctivotarsal surface
  corneal surface
  cortical surface
  cut surface
  debrided bone surface
  diaphragmatic surface
  distal surface
  dorsal condylar surface
  dorsal surface
  dorsolateral surface
  epicardial surface
  implant-bearing surface
  inferior surface
  inner surface
  internal surface
  joint surface
  labial surface
  lateral surface
  lingual surface
  masticating surface
  maxillary surface
  medial surface
  mesial surface
  occlusal surface
  oral surface
  outer surface
  palatine surface
  peritoneal surface
  plantar surface
  plateau joint surface
  pleural surface
  raw surface

surface (*continued*)
  reconstruction occlusal
    surface (RecOS)
  serosal surface
  severed surface
  skin surface
  sloping surface
  thenar surface
  ventral surface
  vertebral surface
  visceral surface
  volar surface
  working occlusal surface
  zero variance of articular
    surfaces
surface analgesia
surface anatomy
surface anesthesia
surface antibody
surface area
surface biopsy
surface cell layer
surface coil
surface cooling hypothermia
surface cooling technique
surface electrode
surface eye implant
surface implant
surface irradiation
surface membrane
surface replacement hip
    arthroplasty
surface tension
surface trauma
surface vessels
surface wrinkling retinopathy
surface-coil MRI
surface-projection rendering
    image
surfactant
surfactant test
Surfasoft dressing
Sur-Fast needle
surfer's nodules
Surfidac sutures
Surfit adhesive
Sur-Fit colostomy bag
Sur-Fit colostomy irrigation
    sleeve
Sur-Fit disposable insert
Sur-Fit flexible and drainable
    pouch

Sur-Fit irrigation sleeve tail closure
Sur-Fit mini pouch
Sur-Fit Natura pouch
Sur-Fit night drainage container set
Sur-Fit urinary drainage bag
Sur-Fit urostomy pouch
Sur-Fit drainable pouch
Surflo catheter
Surflo winged infusion set
Surgair bur
Surgairtome air drill
Surgaloy metallic sutures
Surgaloy sutures
Surgaloy wire
Surgamid polyamide sutures
SurgAssist stapler
surgeon-dependent technique failure
Surgeon's Choice stapler
Surgeon's Choice surgical stapler
surgeon's footstool
surgeon's headlight
surgeon's knot
surgeon's knot sutures
surgeon's regular needle
surgery (*see also* operation, procedure technique)
  1st ray surgery
  abdominal surgery
  ablative cardiac surgery
  access flap in osseous surgery
  adjustable-suture strabismus surgery
  adult cardiovascular surgery
  adult scoliosis surgery
  aesthetic surgery
  ambulatory surgery
  anorectal surgery
  anterior cervical spine surgery
  anterior cervicothoracic junction surgery
  anterior lower cervical spine surgery
  antiglaucoma surgery
  antireflux surgery
  antiseptic surgery
  aortic reconstructive surgery
  apically repositioned flap in mucogingival surgery
  arterial reconstructive surgery

surgery (*continued*)
  arthroscopic laser surgery
  arthroscopic surgery
  aseptic surgery
  asymmetric surgery
  augmentation surgery
  bariatric surgery
  Barr-Record clubfoot surgery
  bat ear surgery
  beating-heart bypass surgery
  bench surgery
  Bio-Pump for bypass surgery
  body-contour surgery
  Bosker TMI surgery
  breast surgery
  breast-conserving surgery
  Brent pressure earrings for keloid surgery
  Broomhead ankle surgery
  bypass surgery
  cardiac surgery
  cardiothoracic surgery
  cardiovascular surgery
  carotid surgery
  cataract surgery
  cervical decompression surgery
  cervical disk surgery
  cervicothoracic junction surgery
  Chaves scapula surgery
  Chaves-Rapp scapula surgery
  ciliodestructive surgery
  cineplastic surgery
  clean contaminated surgery
  clinical surgery
  closed heart surgery
  closed surgery
  collimated beam handpiece for laser surgery
  colon and rectal surgery
  colorectal surgery
  combination surgery
  computer-assisted stereotactic surgery
  conchal surgery
  concomitant antireflux surgery
  conservation surgery
  conservative surgery
  contraindication to surgery
  conventional surgery

surgery (*continued*)
  corneal surgery
  coronary artery bypass
    surgery (CABS)
  coronary bypass surgery
  cosmetic surgery
  cranial base surgery
  craniofacial reconstructive
    surgery
  craniofacial surgery
  craniomaxillofacial surgery
  cranio-orbital surgery
  cryogenic eye surgery
  cryogenic surgery
  curative surgery
  curative-intent surgery
  cystoreductive surgery
  cytoreductive surgery
  debulking surgery
  decompressive surgery
  definitive surgery
  dental restorative surgery
  dental surgery
  dentofacial surgery
  diagnostic surgery
  dialysis access surgery
  dirty surgery
  double jaw surgery
  DREZ surgery
  ear surgery
  ECA-PCA bypass surgery
  ectopic parts surgery
  elective cosmetic surgery
    (ECS)
  elective surgery
  emergency surgery
  emergent surgery
  endocrine surgery
  endoscopic cardiac surgery
  endoscopic sinus surgery
  endoscopic surgery
  endoscopic video-assisted
    surgery
  endovascular surgery
  enhancement surgery
  epilepsy surgery
  esthetic surgery
  ex situ bench surgery
  ExciMed ultraviolet laser
    surgery
  excisional cardiac surgery
  experimental surgery

surgery (*continued*)
  exploratory surgery
  extracorporeal surgery
  eye muscle surgery
  eyelid surgery
  failed surgery
  featural surgery
  femorodistal reconstructive
    surgery
  fetal surgery
  filtration surgery
  fistulizing surgery
  flexible endoscopic surgery
  functional endoscopic sinus
    surgery (FESS)
  gastric bypass surgery
  gastric reduction surgery
  gastrointestinal surgery
  general surgery
  general thoracic surgery
  glaucoma surgery
  gynecological surgery
  hand surgery
  hand-assisted laparoscopic
    surgery (HALS)
  hazard of surgery
  heart surgery
  helical surgery
  hepatic resectional surgery
  hepatobiliary surgery
  hip replacement surgery
  hypotensive surgery
  hypothermic surgery
  hysteroscopic surgery
  ileal pouch surgery
  ileus following abdominal
    surgery
  image-guided surgery (IGS)
  implant surgery
  in utero murine craniofacial
    surgery
  inadequate surgery
  inpatient surgery
  intestinal surgery
  intra-abdominal surgery
  intradural tumor surgery
  intralacrimal surgery
  intranasal sinus surgery
  intraorbital surgery
  intrusive surgery
  ionic surgery
  irradiation and surgery

surgery (*continued*)
　jejunoileal bypass surgery
　Kelikian knee surgery
　keyhole surgery
　knee replacement surgery
　labyrinthine surgery
　lacrimal surgery
　laparoscopic bariatric surgery
　laparoscopic colorectal
　　cancer surgery
　laparoscopically assisted
　　surgery
　laparoscopic-assisted aortic
　　reconstructive surgery
　laryngeal framework surgery
　laser surgery
　laser-filtering surgery
　levator aponeurosis surgery
　Lich-Gregoire repair in kidney
　　transplant surgery
　lid surgery
　limb-salvage surgery
　limb-sparing surgery
　limitation of surgery
　local surgery
　lower extremity surgery
　lung volume reduction
　　surgery
　major abdominal surgery
　major nonvascular abdominal
　　surgery
　major surgery
　mandibular surgery
　map-guided endocardial
　　resection surgery
　Marzola hair restoration
　　surgery
　maxillary surgery
　maxillofacial surgery
　microlaryngeal surgery
　microscopically controlled
　　surgery
　microvascular surgery
　midface suspension face-lift
　　surgery
　minimal access general
　　surgery
　minimally invasive robotic
　　heart valve surgery
　minor surgery
　Mohs micrographic surgery
　　(MMS)

surgery (*continued*)
　mucogingival surgery
　nasal endoscopic surgery
　navigated brain tumor surgery
　navigational surgery
　nephron-sparing surgery
　neurologic surgery
　neurological surgery
　neuroma relocation surgery
　nonbench surgery
　noncardiac surgery
　nonvascular abdominal
　　surgery
　oblique flap in mucogingival
　　surgery
　obstetrical surgery
　oculoplastic surgery
　oncoplastic surgery
　open anti-reflux surgery
　open disk surgery
　open heart surgery
　operative surgery
　oral and maxillofacial surgery
　　(OMS)
　oral restorative surgery
　oral surgery
　orbital surgery
　orthognathic surgery
　orthopedic surgery
　osseous surgery
　out-of-body surgery
　palliative surgery
　pancreatic surgery
　parathyroid surgery
　parenchymal sparing surgery
　pediatric cardiovascular
　　surgery
　pediatric ophthalmic surgery
　pediatric surgery
　pelvic colonic surgery
　penile venous ligation surgery
　periapical surgery
　peripheral vascular surgery
　plastic and reconstructive
　　surgery
　plastic surgery
　port-access technique for
　　coronary bypass surgery
　portal decompression surgery
　portal-systemic shunt surgery
　posterior lower cervical spine
　　surgery

surgery (*continued*)

  posterior lumbar interbody
    fusion surgery
  posterior lumbar spine and
    sacrum surgery
  posterior upper cervical spine
    surgery
  preprosthetic surgery
  pretransplant surgery
  primary perineal hypospadias
    surgery
  prophylactic surgery
  ptosis surgery
  pulmonary surgery
  Pulvertaft interweaving
    method for hand surgery
  pure refractive surgery
  pylorus-preserving surgery
  radiation surgery
  radical curative surgery
  radical surgery
  radioimmunoguided surgery
  reconstructive preprosthetic
    surgery
  reconstructive surgery
  rectal surgery
  rectovaginal surgery
  refractive surgery
  rejuvenation surgery
  remedial surgery
  renal sparing surgery
  reoperative aesthetic surgery
  reoperative bariatric surgery
  reoperative carotid surgery
  reoperative pelvic surgery
  reparative cardiac surgery
  replacement surgery
  resective surgery
  retinal surgery
  retrograde intrarenal surgery
  reversal jejunoileal bypass
    surgery
  right ventricle-pulmonary
    artery conduit surgery
  rigid endoscopic surgery
  robotic surgery
  salvage surgery
  same-day surgery
  scoliosis surgery
  secondary surgery
  second-look surgery
  segmental surgery

surgery (*continued*)

  sex reassignment surgery
  sham surgery
  shunt surgery
  silicone gel-filled mammary
    implant explanation
    surgery
  sinus surgery
  site-specific surgery
  small bowel surgery
  sonic surgery
  spare parts surgery
  sphincter-saving surgery
  spinal surgery
  stereotactic surgery
  stereotaxic surgery
  stone surgery
  strabismus surgery
  structural surgery
  suboptimal surgery
  subretinal surgery
  substitutional cardiac surgery
  suspension microlaryngeal
    surgery
  symmetric surgery
  targeted surgery
  tattoo surgery
  telepresence surgery
  telerobotic-assisted
    laparoscopic surgery
  thoracic surgery
  thyroglossal cyst surgery
  total hip replacement surgery
  total knee replacement
    surgery
  transperitoneal hand-assisted
    laparoscopic surgery
  transplantation surgery
  transsexual surgery
  transsphenoidal surgery
  transsphincteric surgery
  trauma surgery
  triple bypass heart surgery
  Tronzo hip surgery
  tubal reconstruction surgery
  tumor surgery
  Unilink system for hand
    surgery
  upper gastrointestinal tract
    surgery
  urogenital surgery
  urologic surgery

surgery (*continued*)
  vaginal surgery
  valvular heart surgery
  vascular abdominal surgery
  video-assisted thoracoscopic
    surgery (VATS)
  video-assisted thorascopic
    surgery (VATS)
  videoscopic hernia surgery
  Visco surgery
  vitreoretinal surgery
  vitreous surgery
  volume reduction surgery
    (VRS)
  weight reduction surgery
surgery complication
Surg-E-Trol instruments
SurgiAssist surgical leg holder
Surgiblade
Surgibone
Surgi-Bra breast support
Surgica K6 laser
surgical abdomen
surgical ablation
surgical abscess
surgical absence of (breast, limb,
    uterus, etc.)
surgical amputation
surgical anastomosis
surgical anatomy
surgical anesthesia
surgical ankylosis
surgical appliance
surgical appliance adhesive
surgical approach
surgical aspirator
surgical assistant
surgical biopsy
surgical blade
surgical bone impression
surgical bur
surgical cannula
surgical cholecystectomy
surgical cholecystostomy
surgical chromic sutures
surgical classification of
    gynecomastia (grades 1, 2A,
    2B, 3)
surgical clip
surgical clip applier
surgical closure
surgical complications

surgical compression garment
surgical consultation
surgical contraception
surgical contractor
surgical correction
surgical corset
surgical course
surgical curet
surgical current
surgical cutter
surgical cystgastrostomy
surgical debridement
surgical debulking
surgical decompression
surgical defect
surgical diagnosis
surgical diathermy
surgical disease
surgical dome
surgical drain
surgical drapes
surgical dressing
surgical electrode
surgical emergency
surgical emphysema
surgical endarterectomy
surgical engine
surgical enucleation
surgical enucleation procedure
surgical enucleation technique
surgical estrogen ablation
surgical evaluative staging
surgical excision
surgical excision biopsy
surgical exploration
surgical exposure
surgical extirpation
surgical failure
surgical field
surgical file
surgical film
surgical fixation
surgical flap
surgical gauze
surgical general rasp
surgical gouge
surgical grade stainless steel
    wire
surgical gut sutures
surgical hammer
surgical hand scrubs
surgical handle

surgical hazard
surgical history
surgical immobilization of joint
surgical implantation
surgical incision
surgical infection
surgical instrument guide
surgical intervention
surgical iridectomy
surgical isolator
surgical keratometer
surgical keratometry
surgical knife handle
surgical knot
surgical laser
surgical lesion
surgical ligation
surgical limbus
surgical linen sutures
surgical loupe
surgical maggot therapy
surgical mallet
surgical management
surgical maneuver
surgical margin
surgical marking pen
surgical mask
surgical menopause
surgical metallic mesh
surgical microscope
surgical neck
surgical neck fracture
surgical neck of humerus
surgical neck of tooth
surgical needle
surgical nerve stimulator
surgical neurangiographic
    technique
Surgical no-Bounce mallet
Surgical Nu-Knit
Surgical Nu-Knit absorbable
    hemostatic material
surgical option
surgical orthodontics
surgical otoscope
surgical pancreatic disease
surgical pathogens
surgical pathology
surgical patient arm shield
surgical permit
surgical pharmacology
surgical pin driver

surgical placement
surgical portal decompression
surgical power magnet
surgical prep
surgical procedure
surgical prosthesis
surgical pulp exposure
surgical recovery
surgical reduction
surgical removal (of organ,
    tissue, etc.)
surgical repair
surgical resection
surgical retractor
surgical risk
surgical saw
surgical saw blade
surgical scar
surgical scissors
surgical shock
surgical shoe
surgical silk sutures
Surgical Simplex cement
Surgical Simplex P radiopaque
    adhesive
Surgical Simplex P radiopaque
    bone cement
surgical site
surgical skin graft expander
surgical snare
surgical soft diet
surgical spatula
surgical splint
surgical sponge
surgical staging
surgical stapling biopsy gun
surgical steel gauze
surgical steel sutures
surgical stockinette
surgical stripper
surgical stylet
surgical suction pump
surgical suite
surgical supplies
surgical suture technique
surgical sutures
surgical swelling
surgical sympathectomy
surgical technique
surgical technology
surgical telescope
surgical template

surgical therapy
surgical trauma
surgical treatment
surgical triangle
surgical urachus
surgical vagolysis
surgical vagotomy
surgical wound
surgical wound classification
surgical wound infection
surgical wound surveillance
surgical-assist leg holder
surgical-assisted rapid palatal
    expansion (SA-RPE)
surgically absent
surgically denervated area
surgically implanted
    hemodialysis catheter
surgically implanted pump
surgically implanted tube
surgically severed limb
surgical-orthopedic drill
Surgicel dressing
Surgicel fibrillator absorbable
    hemostat
Surgicel gauze
Surgicel gauze dressing
Surgicel hemostatic material
Surgicel implant
Surgicel implant placement
Surgicel implantation
Surgicel Nu-Knit absorbable
    hemostat
Surgicel Nu-Knit dressing
Surgiclip
Surgicraft Copeland fetal scalp
    electrode
Surgicraft pacemaker electrode
Surgicraft sutures
Surgicraft suture needle
Surgicutt incision device
Surgidac braided polyester
    sutures
Surgidac sutures
Surgidev intraocular lens
Surgidev iris clip
Surgidev anterior chamber
    intraocular lens
Surgidev lens
Surgidev sutures
SurgiFish visceral retainer
Surgifix dressing

Surgifix outer expandable netting
Surgiflex bandage
Surgiflex dressing
Surgiflex WAVE suction-
    irrigation device
Surgiflex WAVE
    suction/irrigation probe
Surgifoam absorbable gelatin
    sponge
Surgiguide template
Surgigut sutures
Surgikos disposable drape
Surgilar sutures
Surgilase high-powered CO_2
    laser
Surgilase laser
Surgilase smoke evacuator
Surgilase Nd:YAG laser
Surgilast tubular elastic dressing
Surgilav drain
Surgilav machine
Surgilene blue monofilament
    polypropylene sutures
Surgilene sutures
Surgilift
SurgiLight OptiVision YAG laser
Surgilon braided nylon sutures
Surgilon sutures
Surg-I-Loop silicone loop
Surgiloope sutures
Surgimed clamp
SurgiMed sutures
Surgimedics cholangiography
    catheter
Surgimedics TMP air aspirator
    needle
Surgimedics TMP multiperfusion
    set
Surgin hemorrhage occluder pin
Surgineedle pneumoperitoneum
    needle
Surgipad combined dressing
SurgiPeace analgesia pump
Surgiport disposable trocar
Surgiport stapler
Surgiport trocar and sleeve
Surgiprep
SurgiPro hernia mesh
SurgiPro Prolene mesh
Surgipro sutures
Surgipulse CO_2 laser
Surgiset sutures

SurgiSis mesh
SurgiSis sling
Surgisite drape
Surgistar corneal trephine
Surgistar ophthalmic blade
Surgi Stim
Surgitable hand surgery table
Surgitek button
Surgitek catheter
Surgitek double-J closed-tip
     ureteral stent
Surgitek double ureteral catheter
Surgitek double-J ureteral stent
Surgitek expander
Surgitek Flexi-Flate penile
     implant
Surgitek Flexi-Flate penile
     prosthesis
Surgitek Flexi-rod penile
     prosthesis
Surgitek graduated cystoscope
Surgitek handpiece
Surgitek implant
Surgitek inflatable penile
     prosthesis
Surgitek mammary implant
Surgitek mammary prosthesis
Surgitek percutaneous
     endoscopic gastrostomy
Surgitek penile prosthesis
Surgitek ureteral stent
Surgitek T-Span tissue expander
Surgitome bur
Surgitool prosthetic valve
Surgitube dressing
Surgitube tubular gauze
Surgivac drain
Surgivac drainage
Surgiview laparoscope
Surgiwand suction/irrigation
     device
Surgiwip suture ligature
Surgiwip sutures
Surgtech gloves
Surgtex x-ray detectable sponge
Surital anesthesia
Surpass catheter
Surpass guidewire
surrogate host
surrounding graft material
surrounding structures
surrounding tissues

surveillance
  graft surveillance
  ongoing surveillance
  surgical wound surveillance
surveillance endoscopy
surveillance procedure
surveillance technique
Surveyor monitor
suspected transfusion reaction
Suspend sling
suspended in saline solution
suspended operating illuminator
suspended-pedicle approach
suspension
  Abell uterine suspension
  Abell-Gilliam suspension
  Aldridge-Studdefort urethral
     suspension
  Alexander-Adams uterine
     suspension
  balanced suspension
  Baldy-Webster uterine
     suspension
  barium suspension
  bladder neck suspension
  bladder suspension
  Burch bladder suspension
  Burch iliopectineal ligament
     urethrovesical suspension
  Cobb-Ragde bladder neck
     suspension
  Coffey uterine suspension
  corporeal sacrospinous
     suspension
  corset suspension
  cuff suspension
  cystourethral suspension
  Davis uterine suspension
  Doleris uterine suspension
  endoscopic bladder neck
     suspension
  extraperitoneal laparoscopic
     bladder neck suspension
  fascial suspension
  fingertrap suspension
  flexible hinge suspension
  Frangenheim-Goebell-Stoeckel
     fascia lata suspension
  frontalis suspension
  Gilliam uterine suspension
  Gilliam-Doleris uterine
     suspension

suspension (*continued*)
  Gittes-Loughlin bladder neck
    suspension
  interposition uterine
    suspension
  Lynch suspension
  Manchester uterine
    suspension
  Marshall-Marchetti-Krantz
    uterine suspension
  Milton-Adams suspension
  minimal-incision pubovaginal
    suspension
  nasal valve suspension
  Olshausen suspension
  paraurethral suspension
  Pereyra bladder neck
    suspension
  Pereyra bladder suspension
  Pereyra needle suspension
  Pereyra paraurethral
    suspension
  Pereyra vesicourethral
    suspension
  Raz bladder neck suspension
  Raz 4-quadrant suspension
  Raz needle suspension
  Raz urethral suspension
  retropubic Lapides-Ball
    bladder neck suspension
  sacrospinous ligament
    suspension
  Silesian belt suspension
  Stamey bladder neck
    suspension
  Stamey needle suspension
  Stamey paraurethral
    suspension
  Stamey-Pereyra bladder neck
    suspension
  suction suspension
  supracondylar suspension
  urethral suspension
  uterine suspension
  vesicourethral suspension
suspension anastomosis
suspension feeder
suspension laryngoscope
suspension laryngoscopy
suspension microlaryngeal
  surgery
suspension microlaryngoscopy

suspension of kidney
suspension of uterus
suspension sling
suspension traction
suspension vector
suspension-type socket
suspensory bandage
suspensory dressing
suspensory ligament
suspensory muscle
suspensory sling operation
suspicious abnormality
suspicious area
suspicious lesion
Sussman 4-mirror gonioscope
Sustagen nasogastric tube
Sustain HA-coated screw
  implant
Sustain hydroxyapatite
  biointegrated dental
  implant
sustained pressure technique
sustentacular tissue
Sutcliffe laser shield and
  retracting instrument
Sutherland eye scissors
Sutherland hamstring transfer
Sutherland hip procedure
Sutherland lens
Sutherland rotatable
  microsurgery instrument
Sutherland scissors
Sutherland thigh procedure
Sutherland vitreous forceps
Sutherland-Greenfield osteotomy
Sutherland-Grieshaber forceps
Sutherland-Grieshaber scissors
Sutherland-Grieshaber speculum
Sutherland-Rowe incision
Sutro procedure
Sutter double-stem silicone
  implant prosthesis
Sutter MCP finger joint
  prosthesis
Sutter-CPM knee device
Sutter-Smeloff heart valve
  prosthesis
Sutton biopsy needle
Sutton disease
Sutton needle
Sutton ulcer
Sutupak sutures

sutura (*pl.* suturae)
sutural bones
sutural cataract
sutural ligament
Suturamid sutures
suturation
sutures (*see also* ligature, stitch)
  20-day gut sutures
  absorbable sutures
  Acier stainless steel sutures
  Acufex bioabsorbable Suretac
    sutures
  Acutrol sutures
  adjustable external sutures
  alar cinch sutures
  Albert sutures
  Alcon sutures
  Allison sutures
  already-threaded sutures
  alternating sutures
  aluminum wire sutures
  aluminum-bronze wire sutures
  American silk sutures
  Ancap braided-silk sutures
  Ancap silk sutures
  anchor sutures
  anchoring sutures
  angiocatheter with looped
    polypropylene sutures
  angle sutures
  anterior palatine sutures
  Appolito sutures
  apposition sutures
  approximation sutures
  arcuate sutures
  Argyll Robertson sutures
  Arlt sutures
  Arruga encircling sutures
  arterial silk sutures
  Atraloc sutures
  Atraloc-Ethilon sutures
  atraumatic braided silk
    sutures
  atraumatic chromic sutures
  atraumatic sutures
  Aureomycin sutures
  Auto Sutures (AS)
  Axenfeld sutures
  B&S gauge sutures (Brown-
    Sharp)
  Babcock wire sutures
  back-and-forth sutures

sutures (*continued*)
  Barraquer silk sutures
  Barraquer sutures
  barrel knot sutures
  baseball sutures
  basilar sutures
  bastard sutures
  basting sutures
  Bauer-Black sutures
  Bell sutures
  Bertrandi sutures
  Bigelow sutures
  bilateral coronal suture
  BioSorb sutures
  Biosyn sutures
  biparietal suture
  black braided nylon sutures
  black braided silk sutures
  black braided sutures
  black silk sutures
  black twisted sutures
  Blalock sutures
  blanket sutures
  blue cotton sutures
  blue twisted cotton sutures
  blue-black monofilament
    sutures
  bolster sutures
  Bondek absorbable sutures
  bone step-off at ZF suture
  bone step-off at
    zygomaticofrontal sutures
  bone wax sutures
  Bonney sutures
  bony sutures
  Bozeman sutures
  braided Ethibond sutures
  braided Mersilene sutures
  braided Nurolon sutures
  braided nylon sutures
  braided polyamide sutures
  braided polyester sutures
  braided silk sutures
  braided sutures
  braided Vicryl sutures
  braided wire sutures
  Bralon sutures
  bregmamastoid sutures
  bregmatomastoid sutures
  bridle sutures
  bronchial sutures
  bronze sutures

sutures (*continued*)

bronze wire sutures
Brown & Sharpe suture gauge
  (B&S suture gauge)
Buckston sutures
bulb sutures
bunching sutures
Bunnell sutures
Bunnell wire pull-out sutures
buried sutures
button sutures
Beclard sutures
cable wire sutures
Callaghan sutures
capitonnage sutures
Caprolactam sutures
cardinal sutures
Cardioflon sutures
Cardionyl sutures
cardiovascular Prolene sutures
cardiovascular silk sutures
cardiovascular sutures
Cargile sutures
Carrel sutures
catgut sutures (CGS)
celluloid linen sutures
celluloid sutures
cervical sutures
chain sutures
Champion sutures
Cherney sutures
Chinese fingertrap sutures
Chinese twisted silk sutures
chloramine catgut sutures
chromated catgut sutures
chromic blue dyed sutures
chromic catgut mattress
  sutures
chromic catgut sutures
chromic collagen sutures
chromic gut sutures
chromic sutures
chromicized catgut sutures
cinch sutures
circular sutures
circumcisional sutures
clavate clove-hitch sutures
clavate sutures
clove-hitch sutures
Cloward stitch sutures
Coakley sutures
coaptation sutures

sutures (*continued*)

coated polyester sutures
coated sutures
coated Vicryl Rapide sutures
coated Vicryl sutures
cobbler's sutures
cocoon thread sutures
collagen absorbable sutures
collagen sutures
compound sutures
concha-mastoid sutures
conchomastoidal sutures
conchoscaphal sutures
Connell inverting sutures
Connell sutures
continuous catgut sutures
continuous circular inverting
  sutures
continuous cuticular sutures
continuous hemostatic
  sutures
continuous interlocking
  sutures
continuous inverting sutures
continuous key pattern
  sutures
continuous Lembert sutures
continuous locked sutures
continuous mattress sutures
continuous over-and-over
  sutures
continuous running locked
  sutures
continuous running sutures
continuous silk sutures
continuous sutures
continuous U-shaped sutures
corneal sutures
corneoscleral sutures
corneoscleroconjunctival
  sutures
coronal suture
cotton Deknatel sutures
cotton nonabsorbable sutures
cotton sutures
Cottony Dacron hollow
  sutures
Cottony Dacron sutures
cranial sutures
cranial vault sutures
crown sutures
CTI sutures

sutures (*continued*)
  Cushing sutures
  cushioning sutures
  Custodis sutures
  cutaneous sutures
  cuticular sutures
  Czerny sutures
  Czerny-Lembert sutures
  D&G sutures
  Dacron bolstered sutures
  Dacron sutures
  Dacron traction sutures
  Dafilon sutures
  Dagrofil sutures
  Daily sutures
  Davis-Geck eye sutures
  Davis-Geck sutures
  deep suspension sutures
  defect closed with sutures
  Degnon sutures
  dekalon sutures
  Deklene polypropylene sutures
  Deklene sutures
  Deknatel silk sutures
  Deknatel sutures
  delayed sutures
  DeMartel sutures
  dentate sutures
  dermal sutures
  dermal tension nonabsorbing
    sutures
  Dermalene polyethylene
    sutures
  Dermalene sutures
  Dermalon cuticular sutures
  Dermalon sutures
  Dexon absorbable synthetic
    polyglycolic acid sutures
  Dexon II sutures
  Dexon Plus sutures
  Dexon subcuticular sutures
  Dexon sutures
  DG Softgut sutures
  direct radial sutures
  Docktor sutures
  domal creation sutures
  dome-binding sutures
  Donnati sutures
  double right-angle sutures
  double-armed mattress sutures
  double-armed retention
    sutures

sutures (*continued*)
  double-armed sutures
  double-button sutures
  doubled black silk sutures
  doubled chromic catgut
    sutures
  doubled pursestring sutures
  doubled sutures
  double-running penetrating
    keratoplasty sutures
  double-stop sutures
  doubly armed sutures
  doubly ligated sutures
  Douglas sutures
  Drews sutures
  Dulox sutures
  Dupuytren sutures
  dural tenting sutures
  Duvergier sutures
  echelon sutures
  edge-to-edge sutures
  Edinburgh sutures
  EEA Auto sutures
  elastic sutures
  Emmet sutures
  Endo Knot sutures
  Endoloop sutures
  end-on mattress sutures
  end-over-end running sutures
  EPTFE vascular sutures
    (expanded
    polytetrafluoroethylene
    vascular sutures)
  Equisetene sutures
  Ethibond polybutilate-coated
    polyester sutures
  Ethibond polyester sutures
  Ethibond sutures
  Ethicon micropoint sutures
  Ethicon Sabreloc sutures
  Ethicon silk sutures
  Ethicon sutures
  Ethicon-Atraloc sutures
  Ethiflex retention sutures
  Ethiflex sutures
  Ethilon nylon sutures
  Ethilon sutures
  Ethi-pack sutures
  ethmoidomaxillary sutures
  everting interrupted sutures
  everting mattress sutures
  everting sutures

sutures (*continued*)

  expanded polytetrafluoroethylene (EPTFE) suture

  expanded polytetrafluoroethylene vascular sutures (EPTFE)

  extrachromic sutures

  eye sutures

  eyelid crease sutures

  Faden sutures

  false sutures

  far sutures

  far-and-near sutures

  far-near sutures

  FiberWire sutures

  figure-of-8 sutures

  filament sutures

  fine chromic sutures

  fine silk sutures

  fine sutures

  fingertrap sutures

  Finsterer sutures

  fish-mouth sutures

  fixation sutures

  flat sutures

  Flaxedil sutures

  Flexitone sutures

  Flexon steel sutures

  Flexon sutures

  formaldehyde catgut sutures

  Foster sutures

  Fothergill sutures

  Frater sutures

  free ligature sutures

  free-tie sutures

  French sutures

  Friedman sutures

  frontal sutures

  frontoethmoidal suture

  frontolacrimal suture

  frontomalar sutures

  frontomaxillary sutures

  frontonasal sutures

  frontoparietal sutures

  frontosphenoid sutures

  frontozygomatic sutures

  Frost sutures

  funicular sutures

  Furniss sutures

  furrier's sutures

  Gaillard-Arlt sutures

sutures (*continued*)

  Gambee sutures

  gastrointestinal surgical gut sutures

  gastrointestinal surgical linen sutures

  gastrointestinal surgical silk sutures

  Gely sutures

  general closure sutures

  general eye surgery sutures

  GI pop-off silk sutures

  GI silk sutures

  Giampapa sutures

  Gianturco sutures

  Gibson sutures

  Gillies horizontal dermal sutures

  glover's sutures

  glue-in sutures

  Gore-Tex sutures

  gossamer silk sutures

  Gould sutures

  granny knot sutures

  green braided sutures

  green Mersilene sutures

  green monofilament polyglyconate sutures

  Gregory stay sutures

  groove sutures

  Gudebrod sutures

  guide sutures

  Gussenbauer sutures

  gut chromic sutures

  gut plain sutures

  gut sutures

  guy steadying sutures

  guy sutures

  guy-steading sutures

  Guyton sutures

  Guyton-Friedenwald sutures

  half-hitch sutures

  Halsted interrupted mattress sutures

  Halsted mattress sutures

  Halsted sutures

  Hamis sutures

  harelip sutures

  harmonic suture

  Harrington sutures

  Harris sutures

  Heaney sutures

sutures (*continued*)

heavy monofilament sutures
heavy retention sutures
heavy silk retention sutures
heavy silk sutures
heavy wire sutures
helical sutures
hemostatic sutures
Herculon sutures
Hill sutures
horizontal mattress sutures
horizontal sutures
horsehair sutures
horseshoe sutures
Horsley sutures
Hu-Friedy PermaSharp sutures
IKI catgut sutures
imbricated sutures
imbricating sutures
implanted sutures
incisive sutures
India rubber sutures
infraorbital sutures
intact skin sutures
interdermal buried sutures
interdomal sutures
interendognathic sutures
interlocking sutures
intermaxillary sutures
intermediate sutures
intermittent sutures
internasal sutures
interpalpebral sutures
interparietal sutures
interplate cranial sutures
interrupted black silk sutures
interrupted chromic catgut
    sutures
interrupted chromic sutures
interrupted cotton sutures
interrupted far-near sutures
interrupted fine silk sutures
interrupted Lembert sutures
interrupted mattress sutures
interrupted near-far sutures
interrupted plain catgut
    sutures
interrupted pledgeted sutures
interrupted silk sutures
interrupted sutures
interrupted vertical mattress
    sutures

sutures (*continued*)

intestinal sutures
intracuticular nylon sutures
intracuticular running sutures
intracuticular sutures
intradermal mattress sutures
intradermal polyglactic acid
    sutures
intradermal sutures
intradermic sutures
intrafascicular sutures
intraluminal sutures
inverted knot sutures
inverted sutures
inverting sutures
Investa sutures
iodine catgut sutures
iodized surgical gut sutures
iodochromic catgut sutures
Ivalon sutures
Jobert de Lamballe sutures
Jobert sutures
Jones sutures
jugal sutures
Kal-Dermic sutures
Kalt sutures
kangaroo tendon sutures
Keisley sutures
Kelly plication sutures
Kelly sutures
Kelly-Kennedy sutures
Kessler sutures
Kessler-Kleinert sutures
Kirby sutures
Kirschner sutures
Kleinert sutures
Krackow sutures
Krause transverse sutures
Kustner sutures
Kypher sutures
lace sutures
lacidem sutures
lacrimoconchal sutures
lacrimoethmoidal sutures
lacrimomaxillary sutures
lacrimoturbinal sutures
Lahey sutures
lambdoid sutures
lambdoidal sutures
lancet sutures
Lang sutures
Lapra-Ty suture clip

sutures (*continued*)

large-caliber nonabsorbable sutures
LaRoque sutures
lateral crural spanning sutures
lateral trap sutures
lead sutures
lead-shot tie sutures
LeDentu sutures
LeDran sutures
LeFort sutures
Lembert sutures
Lempert sutures
Lespinasse sutures
Ligapak sutures
ligation sutures
ligature sutures
limbal sutures
limbic sutures
Linatrix sutures
Lindner corneoscleral sutures
linear polyethylene sutures
linen sutures
linen thread sutures
Linvatec meniscal anchor sutures
lip sutures
Littre sutures
living sutures
lock sutures
locked sutures
locking running sutures
locking sutures
lock-stitch sutures
Loeffler sutures
longitudinal sutures
Look sutures
loop sutures
Lukens catgut sutures
lumbar sutures
Lytle sutures
malar periosteum SMAS flap fixation sutures
malomaxillary sutures
mamillary sutures
Mannis sutures
Marlex sutures
Marshall V-sutures
mastoid sutures
mastoid-conchal sutures
mattress sutures
Maunsell sutures

sutures (*continued*)

Maxam sutures
Maxon absorbable sutures
Maxon sutures
Mayo linen sutures
Mayo sutures
McCannel sutures
McGraw sutures
McKissock sutures
McLean corneoscleral sutures
McLean sutures
Measuroll sutures
median palatine suture
medium chromic sutures
Medrafil sutures
Medrafil wire sutures
Meigs sutures
Mers sutures
Mersilene braided nonabsorbable sutures
Mersilene sutures
Mersilk sutures
mesh sutures
metal band sutures
metallic sutures
metopic sutures
Micrins microsurgical sutures
Micro-Glide corneal sutures
MicroMite anchor sutures
micropoint sutures
middle palatine sutures
mild chromic sutures
Millipore sutures
Miralene sutures
modified Frost sutures
Monocryl poliglecaprone sutures
Monocryl sutures
monofilament absorbable sutures
monofilament clear sutures
monofilament green sutures
monofilament nylon sutures
monofilament polypropylene sutures
monofilament skin sutures
monofilament steel sutures
monofilament sutures
monofilament wire sutures
Monosof sutures
multifilament steel sutures
multifilament sutures

sutures (*continued*)
multistrand sutures
Mustarde sutures
nasal sutures
nasofrontal sutures
nasomaxillary sutures
natural sutures
near-and-far sutures
near-far sutures
Needle-Less sutures
nerve sutures
Nesta stitch sutures
neurocentral sutures
neurological sutures
neurosurgical sutures
Nissen sutures
nonabsorbable surgical
   sutures
nonabsorbable sutures
noneverting sutures
noose sutures
Novofil sutures
Nurulon sutures
nylon monofilament sutures
nylon retention sutures
nylon sutures
obstetrical double-armed
   sutures
occipital sutures
occipitomastoid sutures
occipitoparietal sutures
occipitosphenoidal sutures
O'Connell sutures
Oertli sutures
oiled silk sutures
on-edge mattress sutures
opaque wire sutures
Ophthalon sutures
outer interrupted silk sutures
over-and-over sutures
over-and-over whip sutures
overlapping sutures
Owen sutures
Oyloidin sutures
Pagenstecher linen thread
   sutures
Pagenstecher sutures
Palatine suture
palatoethmoid sutures
palatoethmoidal sutures
palatomaxillary sutures
Palfyn sutures

sutures (*continued*)
Panacryl absorbable sutures
Panacryl sutures
Panalok absorbable sutures
Pancoast sutures
pants-over-vest sutures
Paré sutures
parietal sutures
parietomastoid sutures
parieto-occipital sutures
Parker-Kerr basting sutures
Parker-Kerr sutures
patch-reinforced mattress
   sutures
PDS Endoloop sutures
PDS sutures (polydioxanone
   sutures)
PDS Vicryl sutures
Pearsall Chinese twisted
   sutures
Pearsall silk sutures
pericostal sutures
perinatal support sutures
perineal support sutures
perineurial sutures
Perlon sutures
Perma-Hand braided silk
   sutures
Perma-Hand silk sutures
Perma-Hand sutures
PermaSharp PGA sutures
Petit sutures
petrobasilar sutures
petroclival sutures
petrosphenobasilar sutures
petrosquamous sutures
petrotympanic suture
pickup spatula sutures
Pilling sutures
pin sutures
pink twisted cotton sutures
plain catgut sutures
plain collagen sutures
plain gut sutures
plain interrupted sutures
plain sutures
plane sutures
plastic sutures
pledget sutures
pledgeted Ethibond sutures
pledgeted mattress sutures
pledgeted sutures

sutures (*continued*)

plicating sutures
plication sutures
poliglecaprone 25 sutures
polyamide sutures
polybutester sutures
Polydek sutures
polydioxanone sutures (PDS)
polyester fiber sutures
polyester sutures
polyethylene sutures
polyfilament sutures
polygalactic acid sutures
polyglactic acid sutures
polyglactin 910 sutures
polyglecaprone 25 sutures
polyglycolate sutures
polyglycolic acid sutures
polyglycolic sutures
polyglyconate sutures
polypropylene button sutures
polypropylene sutures
Polysorb sutures
pop-off sutures
posterior palatine sutures
postplaced sutures
Potts tie sutures
precut sutures
premaxillary sutures
preplaced sutures
presection sutures
presphenoethmoid sutures
primary sutures
Prolene polypropylene sutures
Prolene sutures
Pronova sutures
Proxi-Strip sutures
pulley sutures
pull-out sutures
pull-out wire sutures
Pulvertaft sutures
Purlon sutures
pursestring sutures
PVB sutures
pyoktanin catgut sutures
pyoktanin sutures
pyroglycolic acid sutures
Quickert sutures
quilt sutures
quilted sutures
radial sutures
Ramdohr sutures

sutures (*continued*)

Ramsey County pyoktanin
  catgut sutures
Rankin sutures
Rapide wound sutures
RB1 sutures
reabsorbable sutures
reconstructive sutures
rectus traction sutures
reef knot sutures
reinforcing sutures
relaxation sutures
removal of sutures
retained sutures
retention sutures
reverse-cutting sutures
rhabdoid suture
ribbon gut sutures
Richardson angle sutures
Richardson sutures
Richter sutures
Rigal sutures
right-angle mattress sutures
rip-cord sutures
Ritisch sutures
rost sutures
round block sutures
row of sutures
rubber sutures
running chromic sutures
running continuous sutures
running imbricating sutures
running nylon penetrating
  keratoplasty sutures
running subcuticular sutures
running sutures
running-locked sutures
Sabreloc sutures
Saenger sutures
safety-bolt sutures
Safil synthetic absorbable
  surgical sutures
sagittal suture
Sani-dril sutures
Sarot bold sutures
scalp sutures
scapha-concha mattress
  sutures
secondary sutures
seminal sutures
seromuscular sutures
seromuscular-to-edge sutures

sutures (*continued*)

seroserosal silk sutures
seroserosal sutures
serrated sutures
seton sutures
sewing-machine stitch sutures
SH popoff sutures
Sharpoint ophthalmic
  microsurgical sutures
Shirodkar sutures
Shoch sutures
shoelace sutures
shotted sutures
Siemens PTCA open-heart
  sutures
silicone-treated surgical silk
  sutures
silicone-treated sutures
silk braided sutures
silk interrupted mattress
  sutures
silk Mersilene sutures
silk nonabsorbable sutures
silk pop-off sutures
silk stay sutures
silk sutures
silk traction sutures
silk-braided sutures
silkworm gut sutures
silkworm gut sutures
silky Polydek sutures
silver sutures
silverized catgut sutures
Simon sutures
simple running sutures
simple sutures
Sims sutures
single-armed sutures
single-handed knot sutures
single-running sutures
skin sutures
skull base sutures
sleeper sutures
sling sutures
slotted sutures
Smead-Jones sutures
Snellen sutures
Sofsilk coated and braided
  sutures
Sofsilk nonabsorbable silk
  sutures
Softgut chromic sutures

sutures (*continued*)

Softgut surgical chromic
  catgut sutures
Softgut sutures
solid-state silk sutures
Spanish blue virgin silk
  sutures
spatula needle sutures
sphenoethmoidal sutures
sphenofrontal sutures
sphenomalar sutures
sphenomaxillary sutures
spheno-occipital sutures
spheno-orbital sutures
sphenoparietal sutures
sphenopetrosal sutures
sphenosquamous sutures
sphenotemporal sutures
sphenovomerine sutures
sphenozygomatic sutures
spiral sutures
Sprong sutures
squamomastoid sutures
squamoparietal sutures
squamosal sutures
squamosomastoid sutures
squamosoparietal sutures
squamososphenoid sutures
squamosphenoid sutures
squamous sutures
SS sutures
stainless steel sutures
stainless steel wire sutures
Stallard sutures
Stallard-Liegard sutures
staple sutures
stay sutures
steel mesh sutures
steel sutures
stepwise sutures
Sterna-Band self-locking
  sutures
sternal wire sutures
Stewart sutures
stick-tie sutures
Sturmdorf obstetrical sutures
Sturmdorf sutures
Stylus cardiovascular sutures
subannular mattress sutures
subcutaneous sutures
subcuticular pull-out skin
  sutures

sutures (*continued*)

subcuticular pull-out sutures
subcuticular sutures
superficial sutures
superior rectus bridle sutures
superior rectus traction
  sutures
Supolene sutures
support sutures
Supramid bridle collagen
  sutures
Supramid Extra sutures
Supramid lens implant sutures
Supramid sutures
Surfidac sutures
Surgaloy metallic sutures
Surgaloy sutures
surgeon's knot sutures
surgical chromic sutures
surgical gut sutures
surgical linen sutures
surgical silk sutures
surgical steel sutures
surgical sutures
Surgicraft sutures
Surgidac sutures
Surgidev sutures
Surgigut sutures
Surgilar sutures
Surgilene blue monofilament
  polypropylene suture
Surgilene sutures
Surgiloid sutures
Surgilon braided nylon
  sutures
Surgilon monofilament
  polypropylene sutures
Surgilon sutures
Surgilone monofilament
  polypropylene sutures
Surgilone sutures
Surgilope sutures
SurgiMed sutures
Surgipro sutures
Surgiset sutures
Sutupak sutures
Suturamid sutures
Sutureloop colposuspension
  sutures
swaged sutures
swaged-on sutures
Swedgeon sutures

sutures (*continued*)

Swiss blue virgin silk sutures
synthetic absorbable sutures
Synthofil sutures
tacking sutures
Tagima sutures
tantalum wire monofilament
  sutures
tantalum wire sutures
tantalum wire tension sutures
Tapercut sutures
Taylor sutures
Teflon-coated Dacron sutures
Teflon-pledgeted sutures
temporal sutures
temporomalar sutures
temporozygomatic sutures
tendon sutures
tension sutures
tension-requiring sutures
tentalum wire tension sutures
tenting sutures
Tevdek pledgeted sutures
Tevdek sutures
Thermo-Flex sutures
Thiersch sutures
thoracic sutures
thread sutures
through-and-through
  continuous sutures
through-and-through
  reabsorbable sutures
through-and-through sutures
through-the-wall mattress
  sutures
Ti-Cron sutures (*also* Tyrcron)
tie sutures
tied down over cotton sutures
tiger gut sutures
Tinel sutures
Tom Jones sutures
tongue sutures
tongue-in-groove sutures
tonsillar sutures
track sutures
traction sutures
transcutaneous-
  transconjunctival sutures
transfixation sutures
transfixing sutures
transfixion sutures
transition sutures

sutures (*continued*)

transosseous sutures
transscleral sutures
transverse palatine sutures
transverse row of sutures
traumatic sutures
true sutures
Trumbull sutures
twisted cotton sutures
twisted dermal sutures
twisted linen sutures
twisted silk sutures
twisted sutures
twisted virgin silk sutures
Tycron sutures (*also* Ti-Cron)
tympanomastoid sutures
Tyrrell-Gray sutures
U-double-barrel sutures
UltraFix MicroMite anchor
   sutures
umbilical tape sutures
unabsorbable sutures
undyed sutures
unilateral coronal sutures
uninterrupted sutures
U-shaped continuous sutures
uteroparietal sutures
Van Hillman sutures
vascular silk sutures
Verhoeff sutures
vertical mattress sutures
vertical sutures
VEST traction sutures
Vicryl pop-off sutures
Vicryl Rapide absorbable
   sutures
Vicryl Rapide sutures
Vicryl SH sutures
Vicryl sutures
Vienna wire sutures
virgin silk sutures
Viro-Tec sutures
visceroparietal sutures
von Pirquet sutures
Werner sutures
whipstitch sutures
white braided silk sutures
white braided sutures
white nylon sutures
white silk sutures
white sutures
white twisted sutures

sutures (*continued*)

wing sutures
wire sutures
wire Zytor sutures
Wölfler sutures
Woodbridge sutures
Worst Medallion sutures
Wysler sutures
ZF sutures
zygomaticofrontal sutures
zygomaticomaxillary sutures
zygomaticosphenoidal sutures
zygomaticotemporal sutures
Zytor sutures
suture anastomosis
suture anchor
suture anchor technique
suture and tying forceps
suture brow stabilization
suture button
suture carrier
suture clip
suture clip applier
suture clip forceps
suture closure
suture closure technique
suture cushion
suture cutter
suture failure
suture fixation
suture forceps
suture guide
suture holder
suture hole drill
suture hook
suture joint
suture lancet
suture ligated
suture ligation
suture ligature
suture line
suture line cancer
suture line of skull
Suture Lok device
suture material
suture needle
suture needle holder
suture passer
suture pickup hook
suture pickup spatula
suture plication
suture pusher

suture repair
suture ring
suture scissors
suture shape shifter
suture sizes (1-0, 2-0, 3-0, 4-0 [or 0, 00, 000, 0000], 5-0, etc.)
suture sizing
suture spacer
Suture Strip
Suture Strip Plus
Suture Strip Plus wound closure strip
suture tag forceps
suture wire
suture wire-cutting scissors
suture-carrying forceps
sutured in place
sutured parallel with wound edges
sutured plaque electrode
suture-holding forceps
sutureless bowel anastomosis
sutureless colostomy closure
sutureless laparoscopic extraperitoneal inguinal herniorrhaphy
sutureless pacemaker electrode
sutureless valve prosthesis
suture-line dehiscence
Sutureloop colposuspension sutures
SutureMate needle rest
suture-pulling forceps
suture-release needle
suture-removing scissors
sutures attached to arterial wall
sutures tied down over cotton
sutures tied over rubber shoes
SutureStrip Plus wound closure
suture-tying forceps
suture-tying platform forceps
suturing forceps
suturing instruments
suturing needle
suturing of cyst inside out
suturing silks
sutural diastasis
SVBG (saphenous vein bypass grafting)
Sven Johansson driver
Sven Johansson extender

Sven Johansson femoral neck nail
SVR (surgical ventricular restoration)
swab stick
swaged arthroscopic needles
swaged needle
swaged sutures
swaged-on needle
swaged-on sutures
swaging graft
swallowing center
swallowing mechanism
swamp carcinoma
Swan aortic clamp
Swan corneoscleral punch
Swan discission knife
Swan eye needle holder
Swan gouge
Swan incision
Swan knife-needle
Swan lancet
Swan needle
Swan operation
Swan punch
Swan spade-type needle knife
Swan-Brown arterial forceps
Swan-Ganz balloon flotation catheter
Swan-Ganz bipolar pacing catheter
Swan-Ganz catheterization
Swan-Ganz flow-directed catheter
Swan-Ganz guidewire catheter
Swan-Ganz pacing catheter
Swan-Ganz pulmonary artery catheter
Swan-Ganz pulmonary catheterization
Swan-Ganz thermodilution catheter
Swan-Ganz tube
Swan-Jacob goniotomy pliers
Swank high-flow arterial blood filter
swan-neck clamp
swan-neck deformity
swan-neck deformity reduction
swan-neck finger deformity
swan-neck gouge
swan-neck Missouri catheter

swan-neck pediatric Coil-Cath
catheter
swan-neck splint
Swann-Morton surgical blade
Swann-Sheldon needle
Swanson arthroplasty
Swanson carpal lunate implant
Swanson carpal scaphoid
implant
Swanson classification of
congenital skeletal limb
deficiency
Swanson condylar arthroplasty
Swanson dynamic toe splint
Swanson elevator
Swanson finger joint implant
Swanson finger joint prosthesis
Swanson flexible hallux valgus
prosthesis
Swanson great toe implant
Swanson great toe prosthesis
Swanson hand splint
Swanson hemi-implant
Swanson implant
Swanson intramedullary broach
Swanson knife
Swanson mallet
Swanson metacarpal prosthesis
Swanson metacarpophalangeal
implant
Swanson metatarsal broach
Swanson metatarsal prosthesis
Swanson operation
Swanson osteotome
Swanson prosthesis
Swanson radial head implant
Swanson radial head implant
arthroplasty
Swanson radiocarpal implant
Swanson reamer
Swanson reconstruction
Swanson scaphoid awl
Swanson Silastic elbow
prosthesis
Swanson Silastic implant
Swanson Silastic prosthesis
Swanson silicone wrist
arthroplasty
Swanson small joint implant
Swanson technique
Swanson trapezium implant
Swanson ulnar head implant

Swanson wrist joint implant
Swanson wrist prosthesis
Swartz Series Fast-Cath
introducer
swayback deformity
swayback nose
swaying of body
Sweeper curet
sweat duct
sweat gland carcinoma
sweat gland adenocarcinoma
sweat gland adenoma
Swede O Universal brace
Swede O Universal orthosis
Swede-Vent self-tapping external
hex implant
Swedgeon already-threaded
needle
Swedish approach
Swedish Helparm device
Swedish knee cage
Swedish-pattern chisel
Sween-A-Peel wound dressing
Sweeney posterior vaginal
retractor
Sweeney posterior vaginal
speculum
Sweet amputation retractor
Sweet antral trocar
Sweet clip-applying forceps
Sweet delicate pituitary
scissors
Sweet dissecting forceps
Sweet electric magnet
Sweet esophageal scissors
Sweet eye magnet
Sweet ligature forceps
Sweet magnet
Sweet method
Sweet original magnet
Sweet punch
Sweet locator
Sweet
Sweet retractor
Sweet rib spreader
Sweet scissors
Sweet sternal punch
Sweet trocar
Sweet-Burford rib spreader
Sweet-Finochietto rib spreader
sweetheart retractor
Sweet Tip bipolar lead

swelling
    boggy swelling
    corneal swelling
    diffuse swelling
    eyelid swelling
    fugitive swelling
    fusiform swelling
    genital swelling
    giant swelling
    glassy swelling
    induration and swelling
    inflammation and swelling
    joint swelling
    knee swelling
    labial swelling
    labioscrotal swelling
    periarticular soft tissue
        swelling
    periorbital swelling
    rhomboid swelling
    scrotal swelling
    subcutaneous swelling
    surgical swelling
    testicular swelling
Swenko bag
Swenson abdominal pull-
    through procedure
Swenson cholangiography tube
Swenson operation
Swenson papillotome
Swenson pull-through
    procedure
Swenson ring-jawed holding
    clamp
Swenson wire-guided
    papillotome/sphincterotome
Swets goniotomy cannula
Swets goniotomy knife
Swiderski nasal chisel
swift-cut phaco incision knife
SwiftLase scanner
swimmer's ear
swimmer's knee
swimmer's view of cervical
    spine on x-ray
swimmer's x-ray view
swimming pool granuloma
swine xenograft
Swing Phase Lock knee lock
Swinger car bed
Swiss Balance orthotic
Swiss ball

Swiss blade
Swiss blade breaker
Swiss blade holder
Swiss blue virgin silk sutures
Swiss bulldog clamp
Swiss Kiss intrastent balloon
    inflation device
Swiss Lithoclast pneumatic
    lithotripsy probe
Swiss MP joint implants
Swiss roll embedding technique
Swiss-cheese endometrium
Swiss-cheese hyperplasia
Swiss-pattern osteotome
Swiss-pattern speculum
Swissray scanner
switch flap
switch operation
switch procedure
switched B-gradient technique
Switzerland dilatation catheter
swivel adapter
swivel connector tubing
swivel dislocation
swivel hook
swivel joint suture holder
swivel knife
swivel tracheostomy tube
Swivel-Strap ankle brace
Swivel-Strap brace
SWMF (Semmes-Weinstein nylon
    monofilament)
Swolin self-retaining vaginal
    speculum
Sydenham mouth gag
Sydney crease
Sydney line
Sydney gastritis classification
Syed radium applicator
Syed template
Syed template flange
Syed template implant
Syed-Neblett implant
Syed-Neblett template
Sylva anterior chamber irrigator
Sylva eye irrigator
Sylva I&A unit
Sylva irrigating cannula
Sylva irrigator
sylvian approach
sylvian aqueduct
sylvian area

sylvian artery
sylvian dissection
sylvian fissure
sylvian fistula
sylvian fossa
sylvian hematoma
sylvian line
sylvian point
sylvian waves
Symbion artificial heart
Symbion cardiac device
Symbion Jarvik-7 artificial heart
Symbion pneumatic assist
    device
Symbion total artificial heart
Symbios dual-chamber
    pacemaker
Symbios pacemaker
symbiosis
symblepharon
    anterior symblepharon
    posterior symblepharon
    total symblepharon
symblepharon ring
symblepharopterygium
symbrachydactyly
Syme amputation at ankle
Syme amputation of foot
Syme amputation prosthesis
Syme ankle disarticulation
    amputation
Syme Dycor prosthetic foot
Syme external urethrotomy
Syme foot prosthesis
Syme operation
Syme procedure
Syme prosthesis
Syme urethrotomy
Symington anococcygeal body
symmastia
symmelia
symmetric gangrene
symmetric surgery
symmetric syndactyly
symmetric thumb duplication
symmetric vertebral fusion
symmetrical bilateral cleft
symmetrical in contour
symmetrical nest
symmetrical sacral plate
symmetrical thoracic vertebral
    plate

symmetry
    breast symmetry
    detailed evaluation of facial
        symmetry (DEFS)
    facial symmetry
    inverse symmetry
    philtral symmetry
Symmetry endobipolar
    generator
symmetry operation
symmetry plane
Symmonds enterocele repair
Symmonds hysterectomy
    retractor
Symmonds needle
Symmonds vaginal prolapse
    repair
sympathectomy
    cervical sympathectomy
    chemical sympathectomy
    Ionescu sympathectomy
    lumbar sympathectomy
    periarterial sympathectomy
    Smithwick sympathectomy
    subdiaphragmatic
        sympathectomy
    supradiaphragmatic
        sympathectomy
    surgical sympathectomy
    thoracic sympathectomy
    transdiaphragmatic
        sympathectomy
sympathectomy hook
sympathectomy retractor
sympathectomy scissors
sympathetic block
sympathetic block anesthesia
sympathetic blockade
sympathetic blockade anesthetic
    technique
sympathetic carotid plexus
sympathetic chain
sympathetic ganglia
sympathetic ganglion
sympathetic ganglion block
    anesthetic technique
sympathetic nerve
sympathetic nerve block
sympathetic nerve fibers
sympathetic raspatory
sympathetic reaction
sympathetic saliva

sympathetic trunk
sympathetically independent
    pain syndrome (SIPS)
sympathicectomy
sympathicodiaphtheresis
sympathicotripsy
sympathoexcitation reflex
sympatholysis
symphalangism
    syndromic symphalangism
    true symphalangism
Symphony stent
symphyseal fracture
symphysial height of mandible
symphysion
symphysiorrhaphy
symphysiotomy
symphysis (*pl.* symphyses)
    amphiarthrotic pubic
        symphysis
    mandibular symphysis
    pleural symphysis
    pubic symphysis
symphysis mandibulae
symphysis menti
symphysis pubis
symphysis to umbilicus
symphysodactyly
symplastic tissue
symptom formation
symptom magnification
        syndrome
symptomatic gallstone
symptomatic laryngocele
symptomatic traumatic
        dissection
symptomatology
Syms traction
Syms tractor
synapse
synaptic blocking agents
synaptic transmission
synarthrodial joint
Synatomic knee prosthesis
Synatomic total knee prosthesis
Synatomic total knee system
    with Porocoat
synchondrectomy
synchondrodial joint
synchondroseotomy
synchondroses of cranium
synchondroses of skull

synchondrosis (*pl.*
    synchrondroses)
anterior intraoccipital
    synchondrosis
carpal synchondrosis
congenital carpal
    synchondrosis
congenital synchondrosis
intercarpal joint
    synchondrosis
intersphenoidal
    synchondrosis
occipitosphenoidal
    synchondrosis
petro-occipital synchondrosis
posterior intraoccipital
    synchondrosis
spheno-occipital
    synchondrosis
sphenopetrosal synchondrosis
synchondrosis arycorniculata
synchondrosteotomy
synchondrotomy
Synchro neurovascular
    guidewire
synchrocyclotron operation
SynchroMed drug administration
    device
SynchroMed implantable pump
SynchroMed programmable
    pump
synchronized fibrillation
synchronized intermittent
    mandatory ventilation
    (SIMV)
synchronized intermittent
    mechanical ventilation
synchronized retroperfusion
    (SRP)
synchronizing cords
synchronous amputation
synchronous bilateral breast
    cancer
synchronous bladder
    reconstruction
synchronous burst pacemaker
synchronous hepatic metastasis
synchronous hermaphroditism
synchronous intermittent
    mandatory ventilation
synchronous lesion
synchronous metastasis

synchronous mode pacemaker
synchronous pacemaker
synchronous resection
synchronous with heart beat
synchrony
Synchrony pacemaker
Synchrosonic stimulator
synchrotron-based transvenous
  angiography
synchysis of vitreous
synclitism
syncope
  Adams-Stokes syncope
  cardiac syncope
  carotid sinus syncope
  carotid syncope
  laryngeal syncope
syncytial cell
syncytial knots
syncytiovascular membrane
syndactylism
syndactylism release
syndactylization
syndactyly
  complete syndactyly
  complicated syndactyly
  double syndactyly
  incomplete syndactyly
  partial syndactyly
  reduction syndactyly
  simple syndactyly
  single syndactyly
  symmetric syndactyly
  triple syndactyly
syndactyly release
syndactyly repair
syndectomy
syndesmectomy
syndesmochorial placenta
syndesmodial joint
syndesmo-odontoid
syndesmopexy
syndesmophytes of spine
syndesmoplasty
syndesmorrhaphy
syndesmosis screw
syndesmotic screw
syndesmotomy
synchondrosis
syndrome
  3rd and 4th pharyngeal
    pouch syndrome

syndrome (*continued*)
  abdominal compartment
    syndrome
  abdominal muscle deficiency
    syndrome
  acquired immunodeficiency
    syndrome (AIDS)
  acrofacial syndrome
  acute coronary syndrome
  acute disconnection
    syndrome
  acute radiation syndrome
  acute respiratory distress
    syndrome (ARDS)
  adherence syndrome
  adhesive syndrome
  adrenal feminization
    syndrome
  adult respiratory distress
    syndrome (ARDS)
  afferent loop syndrome
  aglossia-adactylia syndrome
  amniotic infection syndrome
  androgen insensitivity
    syndrome
  angio-osteohypertrophy
    syndrome
  ankyloglossia superior
    syndrome
  anomalous innominate artery
    compression syndrome
  anterior cavernous syndrome
  anterior chest wall syndrome
  anterior spinal artery
    syndrome
  auriculotemporal nerve
    syndrome
  basal cell nevus syndrome
  bent-nail syndrome
  bile-plug syndrome
  billowing mitral valve
    syndrome
  black patch syndrome
  blind loop syndrome
  blind pouch syndrome
  blue rubber bleb nevus
    syndrome
  blue toe syndrome
  body cast syndrome
  bowel bypass syndrome
  brady-tachy syndrome
  brittle nail syndrome

syndrome (*continued*)

burner syndrome
burning feet syndrome
calcaneal spur syndrome
callosal disconnection
  syndrome
camptomelic syndrome
cancer susceptibility syndrome
capsular exfoliation syndrome
caput ulnae syndrome
carotid sinus syndrome
carotid steal syndrome
carpal tunnel syndrome
cast syndrome
cat cry syndrome
cauda equina syndrome
cavernous sinus syndrome
celiac artery compression
  syndrome (CCS)
celiac band syndrome
central anticholinergic
  syndrome
central cord syndrome
central heel pad syndrome
cephalopolysyndactyly
  syndrome
cerebellomedullary
  malformation syndrome
cerebellopontine angle
  syndrome
cerebrocostomandibular
  syndrome (CCMS)
cervical acceleration-
  deceleration syndrome
cervical compression
  syndrome
cervical fusion syndrome
cervical rib syndrome
cheilitis-glossitis-gingivitis
  syndrome
chronic hyperventilation
  syndrome
chronic pain syndrome
classic multiple organ failure
  syndrome
cleft palate and lateral
  synechia syndrome (CPLS)
click-murmur syndrome
clinical syndrome
clivus syndrome
cloverleaf skull syndrome
cluster tic syndrome

syndrome (*continued*)

coarctation syndrome
common peroneal nerve
  syndrome
compartment compression
  syndrome
compartment syndrome
compensatory
  antiinflammatory response
  syndrome (CARS)
complex regional pain
  syndromes (CRPS)
compression syndrome
congenital alveolar synechia
  syndrome
congenital central
  hypoventilation syndrome
congenital ring syndrome
constriction ring syndrome
cord traction syndrome
coronary syndrome
craniofacial syndromes
cri du chat syndrome
crush syndrome
cubital tunnel syndrome
cutaneomucouveal syndrome
D chromosome ring
  syndrome
deafferentation pain
  syndrome
dentopulmonary syndrome
dialysis disequilibrium
  syndrome
dialysis encephalopathy
  syndrome
disconnection syndrome
DISH syndrome
dorsal wrist syndrome (DWS)
double-crush syndrome
dry eye syndrome
dumping syndrome
dural shunt syndrome
ectopic ACTH syndrome
embryonic fixation syndrome
empty sella syndrome
entrapment syndrome
euthyroid sick syndrome
excited skin syndrome
exertional anterior
  compartment syndrome
exertional deep posterior
  compartment syndrome

syndrome (*continued*)

exfoliation syndrome
exploding head syndrome
extra-articular pain syndrome
extrapyramidal syndrome
failed back surgery syndrome
familial aortic ectasia
syndrome
familial atypical multiple mole
melanoma syndrome
(FAMMM)
familial cardiac myxoma
syndrome
familial cholestasis syndrome
familial polyposis syndrome
female urethral syndrome
feminization syndrome
fetal alcohol syndrome
fetal aspiration syndrome
fetal face syndrome
fetal hydantoin syndrome
fetal valproate syndrome
fibrofascial compartment
syndrome
fibular tunnel syndrome
first arch syndrome
flapping valve syndrome
flexor origin syndrome
floppy valve syndrome
functional prepubertal
castration syndrome
gastrocardiac syndrome
gastrojejunal loop obstruction
syndrome
glomangiomatous osseous
malformation syndrome
glucagonoma syndrome
head-bobbing doll syndrome
heart and hand syndrome
hemangioma-
thrombocytopenia
syndrome
hemispheric disconnection
syndrome
hemolytic uremic syndrome
hepatorenal syndrome
hereditary cancer syndrome
hereditary flat adenoma
syndrome
hyaline membrane syndrome
hymenal syndrome
hyoid syndrome

syndrome (*continued*)

hypersensitive xiphoid
syndrome
hyperventilation syndrome
hypoglossia-hypodactylia
syndrome
hypoglossia-hypodactyly
syndrome
hypoplastic left heart
syndrome
hypothenar hammer
syndrome
immotile cilia syndrome
impaired regeneration
syndrome
impingement syndrome
infantile choriocarcinoma
syndrome
inflammatory bowel
syndrome (IBS)
inherited cancer syndrome
innominate artery
compression syndrome
intersection syndrome
iridocorneal endothelial
syndrome
iridocorneal epithelial
syndrome
irritable bowel syndrome
jugular foramen syndrome
kissing spine syndrome
lactic acidosis and stroke-like
syndrome
levator ani syndrome
levator scapulae syndrome
loculation syndrome
long-face syndromes
lower nephron syndrome
malignant external otitis
syndrome
mandibulofacial dysostosis
syndrome
mangled extremity syndrome
man-in-the-barrel syndrome
massive bowel resection
syndrome
maternal deprivation
syndrome
meconium aspiration
syndrome
meconium plug syndrome
median cleft face syndrome

syndrome (*continued*)

  megacystis-megaureter
    syndrome
  megacystis-microcolon-
    intestinal hypoperistalsis
    syndrome
  middle fossa syndrome
  milkman's syndrome
  minimal brain dysfunction
    syndrome
  minimal change nephrotic
    syndrome
  minimal lesion nephrotic
    syndrome
  mitral valve prolapse syndrome
  muellerian duct derivation
    syndrome
  mole melanoma syndrome
  monofixation syndrome
  mucocutaneous lymph node
    syndrome
  mucosal neuroma syndrome
  mucous plug syndrome
  multiple endocrine neoplasia
    syndrome
  multiple hamartoma
    syndrome
  multiple mucosal neuroma
    syndrome
  multiple organ dysfunction
    syndrome (MODS)
  multiple organ failure
    syndrome
  multiple pterygium syndrome
  myofascial pain syndrome
    (MPS)
  myofascial pain-dysfunction
    syndrome
  nail-patella syndrome
  nail-patella-elbow syndrome
  naviculocapitate fracture
    syndrome
  nephritic syndrome
  nephrotic syndrome
  nerve compression-
    degeneration syndrome
  neurocutaneous syndrome
  neuroleptic malignant
    syndrome (NMS)
  neurological syndrome
  neurovascular compression
    syndrome

syndrome (*continued*)

  nevoid basal cell carcinoma
    syndrome
  nonocclusive mesenteric
    ischemia syndrome
  nutcracker's syndrome
  obesity-hypoventilation
    syndrome
  occipital condyle syndrome
  ocular mucous membrane
    syndrome
  oculobuccogenital syndrome
  oculomandibulofacial
    syndrome
  oculopharyngeal syndrome
  oculovertebral syndrome
  optic tract syndrome
  orbital apex syndrome
  orbital compartment
    syndrome
  organic short bowel
    syndrome
  orofacial dysfunction
    syndrome
  orofaciodigital syndrome
  osteogenesis imperfecta
    congenita syndrome
  osteomyelofibrotic syndrome
  osteopathia striata syndrome
  osteoporosis pseudoglioma
    syndrome
  otomandibular syndrome
  ovarian hyperstimulation
    syndrome
  ovarian overstimulation
    syndrome
  ovarian vein syndrome
  pacemaker syndrome
  pain syndrome
  parasellar syndrome
  paratrigeminal syndrome
  pericardiotomy syndrome
  pericolic membrane
    syndrome
  peritubal syndrome
  peroneal compartment
    syndrome
  persistent muellerian duct
    syndrome
  petrosphenoidal syndrome
  pharyngeal pouch syndrome
  piriformis syndrome

syndrome (*continued*)

placental hemangioma syndrome

polar bear syndrome

popliteal web syndrome

postadrenalectomy syndrome

postcardiotomy syndrome

postcholecystectomy syndrome

postcolonoscopy distention syndrome

postcommissurotomy syndrome

postembolization syndrome

posterior interosseous nerve compression syndrome

postfundoplication syndrome

postgastrectomy syndrome

postirradiation syndrome

postlaminectomy syndrome

postperfusion syndrome

postpericardiotomy syndrome

postphlebitic syndrome

postpolypectomy coagulation syndrome

post-tubal ligation syndrome

postvagotomy syndrome

pre-excitation syndrome

prolapsed mitral valve syndrome

pronator syndrome

pronator teres syndrome

proximal loop syndrome

prune belly syndrome

pseudo-blind loop syndrome

pseudoexfoliation syndrome

pseudolymphoma syndrome

pseudoxanthoma elasticum syndrome

pterygopalatine fossa syndrome

pulmonary acid aspiration syndrome

pulmonary sulcus syndrome

quadriga syndrome

quadrilateral space syndrome

radial tunnel syndrome

rapid tumor lysis syndrome

recurrent abdominal pain syndrome (RAPS)

red ear syndrome

red-eyed shunt syndrome

syndrome (*continued*)

renal crush syndrome

respiratory distress syndrome

retinoblastoma-mental retardation syndrome

retrosphenoidal syndrome

rib tip syndrome

scalded-skin syndrome

scalenus anterior syndrome

scalenus anticus syndrome

scaphocapitate syndrome

scapuloperoneal syndrome

scimitar syndrome

sepsis syndrome

short face syndrome

short gut syndrome

short bowel syndrome

shoulder impingement syndrome

sick sinus syndrome

sinus tarsi syndrome

slipped rib cartilage syndrome

slipping rib syndrome

slit ventricle syndrome

solitary rectal ulcer syndrome

somatostatinoma syndrome

splenic sequestration syndrome

stagnant loop syndrome

staphylococcal scalded skin syndrome

stasis syndrome

stiff-heart syndrome

stump embolization syndrome

stylohyoid process syndrome

stylohyoid syndrome

styloid syndrome

subclavian steal syndrome

sudden infant death syndrome (SIDS)

sump syndrome

superior orbital fissure syndrome (SOFS)

superior vena cava syndrome

supine hypotensive syndrome

sympathetically independent pain syndrome (SIPS)

symptom magnification syndrome

systemic inflammatory response syndrome (SIRS)

tarsal tunnel syndrome

syndrome (*continued*)
 temporomandibular joint
  pain-dysfunction syndrome
 terminal reservoir syndrome
 testicular feminization
  syndrome
 tethered-cord syndrome
 thoracic compression
  syndrome
 thoracic endometriosis
  syndrome
 thoracic outlet syndrome
 TMJ syndrome
 tooth-and-nail syndrome
 transient compartment
  syndrome
 transplant lung syndrome
 transurethral resection
  syndrome
 triad syndrome
 trichorhinophalangeal
  syndrome
 trisomy 8 syndrome
 trisomy C syndrome
 tumor lysis syndrome
 twin-twin transfusion
  syndrome (TTTS)
 ulnar carpal abutment
  syndrome
 ulnar impaction syndrome
 ulnar tunnel syndrome
 urethral syndrome
 uterine hernia syndrome
 uveoencephalitic syndrome
 uveomeningeal syndrome
 valgus extension overload
  syndrome
 van der Hoeve syndrome
 vanished testis syndrome
 vascular ring syndrome
 VATER association syndrome
 VATER syndrome
 velocardiofacial syndrome
 vertebral subluxation
  syndrome
 vibration syndrome
 vibrator hand syndrome
 visual deprivation syndrome
 vitreoretinal traction
  syndrome
 whistling face syndrome
 yellow nail syndrome

syndrome of crocodile tears
syndromic craniosynostosis
syndromic symphalangism
syndromic synostosis
synechia (*pl.* synechiae)
synechia formation
synechia spatula
synechialysis
synechotomy
synechtenterotomy
synergic muscles
synergism
synergist
Synergist Erection penile
  prosthesis
Synergist vacuum erection
  device
synergistic muscle
synergistic necrotizing cellulitis
synergistic pressor effect
synergistic wrist motion splint
Synergy splint
Synergy ultrasound
Synergyst pacemaker
syngeneic graft
syngeneic transplantation
syngenesioplastic transplant
syngenesioplastic
  transplantation
syngraft
synkinesis
synkinetic
synmastia
SynMesh mesh
Syn-optics camera
synoptoscopy
synosteotomy
synostosis (*pl.* synostoses)
 bicoronal synostosis
 bilateral coronal synostosis
 compensatory synostosis
 coronal synostosis
 cranial suture synostosis
 cranial synostosis
 Crouzon syndromic synostosis
 metopic synostosis
 multiple-suture synostosis
 plagiocephaly without
  synostosis
 radioulnar synostosis
 sagittal suture synostosis
 sagittal synostosis

synostosis (*continued*)
  single-suture synostosis
  syndromic synostosis
  tarsal synostosis
  tribasilar synostosis
  unicoronal synostosis
  unilambdoid synostosis
  unilateral coronal synostosis
synostotic frontal plagiocephaly
  (SFP)
Synovator arthroscopic blade
synovectomy
synovectomy blade
synovectomy rongeur
synovia (*sing.* synovium)
synovial biopsy
synovial capsule
synovial cavity
synovial chondroma
synovial cyst
synovial dissector
synovial fistula
synovial flap
synovial fluid
synovial fluid examination
synovial fold
synovial ganglion
synovial gland
synovial hemangioma
synovial hernia
synovial herniation
synovial joint
synovial membrane
synovial osteochondromatosis
synovial plica
synovial proliferation
synovial sac
synovial sarcoma
synovial separator
synovial sheath
synovial villi
synoviochondromatosis
synovitis
synovium (*sing.* synovia)
synovium biopsy forceps
synpolydactyly
Syntel embolectomy catheter
Syntex screw
Synthaderm dressing
Synthaderm occlusive wound
  dressing
Synthes AO reconstruction plate

Synthes compression hip screw
Synthes dorsal distal plate
Synthes dorsal distal radius plate
Synthes external fixator
Synthes facial curet
Synthes facial drill
Synthes guide pin
Synthes maxillofacial locking
  reconstruction plate
Synthes maxillofacial titanium
  plate
Synthes metallic plate
Synthes Microsystem plate cutter
Synthes mini-depth gauge
Synthes screw
Synthes stainless steel
  minifragment plate
Synthes titanium elastic nail
Synthes titanium minifragment
  plate
Synthes transbuccal trocar
synthesis
synthetic absorbable sutures
synthetic augmentation
synthetic barrier dressing
synthetic bone
synthetic bone graft
synthetic graft
synthetic human growth
  hormone
synthetic hygroscopic cervical
  dilator
synthetic implant
synthetic mesh
synthetic sapphire tip
synthetic stent
synthetic suture material
synthetic wool
Synthofil sutures
synulosis
synulotic
Syrex syringe
syringe
  2-way syringe
  Accuguide syringe
  air syringe
  Alcock bladder syringe
  Alexander syringe
  Alexander-Reiner ear syringe
  Allegist syringe
  all-metal ear syringe
  Anel lacrimal syringe

syringe (*continued*)

Anel syringe
antral syringe
Arnold-Bruening syringe
Arrow Raulerson introducer
　syringe
Asepto aspirating syringe
Asepto bulb syringe
Asepto irrigation syringe
aspirating syringe
aspiration syringe
Autoblock safety syringe
BD Luer syringe
BD Luer-Lok syringe
BD Multifit control syringe
BD Yale syringe
bladder syringe
Boehm drop syringe
Bruening pressure syringe
bulb syringe
bulbous-tip ear syringe
Canyons irrigation syringe
Carpule syringe
catheter-tip syringe
Centrix syringe
chip syringe
Cibacalcin double-chambered
　syringe
colonoscope syringe
Concord line draw syringe
control syringe
CR resin syringe
D-syringe
Davidson syringe
dental syringe
DeVilbiss irrigating syringe
displacement syringe
disposable syringe
Duval irrigating syringe
Dynacor ear syringe
Dynacor ulcer syringe
ear syringe
Eccentric syringe
electric syringe
ENSI syringe
ExtraSafe syringe
E-Z syringe
Fink-Weinstein 2-way
　syringe
Fischer syringe
Fluorescite syringe
FNA-21 syringe

syringe (*continued*)

Fortuna syringe
fountain syringe
Fragmatome flute syringe
Fuchs 2-way eye syringe
Fuchs retinal detachment
　syringe
Gabriel syringe
Gas-Lyte ABG syringe
GC syringe
Gemini syringe
glycerin syringe
Goldstein anterior chamber
　syringe
Goldstein eye syringe
Goldstein lacrimal syringe
Green-Armytage syringe
Heath anterior chamber
　syringe
Higginson irrigation syringe
hypodermic syringe
Ilopan disposable syringe
impression material syringe
Infuset GP syringe
intraligamentary syringe
IPAS syringe
irrigation syringe
Irrigo syringe
Irrivac syringe
Isaacs aspiration syringe
Isosal syringe
Kaufman syringe
Kramer syringe
lacrimal syringe
laryngeal syringe
LaVeen inflation syringe
Lehman syringe
Lewy Teflon glycerin-mixture
　syringe
Ligmajet syringe
Luer tip syringe
Luer-Lok B-D syringe
Luer-Lok syringe
Max-I-Probe endodontic
　irrigation syringe
metal syringe
MPL aspirating syringe
Multi-Fit Luer-Lok control
　tonsillar syringe
Namic angiographic syringe
Neisser syringe
Nourse bladder syringe

syringe (*continued*)
Osciflator balloon inflation syringe
OutBound syringe
Pallin spring-assisted syringe
Parker-Heath anterior chamber syringe
Parker-Heath eye syringe
PDL intraligamentary syringe
PermaRidge delivery syringe
Pierce syringe
Pitkin syringe
plastic syringe
Politzer air syringe
Pomeroy ear syringe
Pravay syringe
Pritchard syringe
Proetz displacement syringe
Pulsator anaerobic syringe
Raulerson introducer syringe
record syringe
Reiner ear syringe
Reiner-Alexander ear syringe
Reiner-Alexander syringe
retinal detachment syringe
Riches bladder syringe
Robb syringe
Rochester syringe
Roughton-Scholander syringe
rubber-bulb syringe
Rudolph calibrated super syringe
Sana-Lok syringe
Schein syringe
sinus suction syringe
spring-assisted syringe
Storz syringe
Street tonsillar syringe
Stylex syringe
Syrex syringe
tapered-tip ear syringe
Teflon glycerin-mixture syringe
Terumo insulin syringe
Thompson syringe
Tobald syringe
tonsillar syringe
Toomey syringe
tuberculin syringe
Tubex metal syringe
Ultraject contrast media syringe

syringe (*continued*)
Ultraject prefilled syringe
van Buren cervix syringe
VanishPoint syringe
Vim Gabriel aspirating syringe
Vim tonsil syringe
Visitec syringe
Yale Luer-Lok syringe
syringe cap
syringe extension
syringe infusion pump
syringe liposculpture
syringe pump
syringe push
syringe suction
syringe-assisted liposuction
syringectomy
syringe-type infusion pump
syringing
syringohydromyelic cavity
syringomyelia
syringomyelic hemorrhage
syringotome
syringotomy
syrinx shunt
SysStim muscle stimulator
systematic anatomy
systematic approach
systematic sextant biopsy
systemic adjuvant therapy
systemic anticoagulation
systemic antifungal therapy
systemic arteriovenous fistula
systemic blood flow
systemic cancer
systemic chemotherapy
systemic chondromalacia
systemic circulation
systemic condition
systemic corticosteroid
systemic disease
systemic dissection
systemic examination
systemic hypoperfusion
systemic inflammatory response syndrome (SIRS)
systemic lesion
systemic mycosis
systemic oxygen extraction
systemic perfusion
systemic pressure

systemic radioimmunoglobulin
  therapy
systemic reaction
systemic scleroderma
systemic sepsis
systemic shock
systemic treatment
systemic venous circulation
systemic-pulmonary artery shunt
systemic-to-pulmonary artery
  anastomosis
systolic ejection rate
systolic murmur
systolic pressure
SyvekPatch
Szabo-Berci endoscopic needle
  driver set
Szabo-Berci needle

Szabo-Berci needle driver
Szilagyi approach
Sztehlo umbilical clamp
Szulc bone cutter
Szulc eye magnet
Szulc grommet
Szulc orbital implant material
Szulc vascular dilator
Szuler eustachian bougie
Szuler vascular forceps
Szultz corneal forceps
Szymanowski operation
Szymanowski-Kuhnt operation
Sedillot elevator-raspatory
Sedillot operation
Sedillot periosteal elevator
Sedillot raspatory
Sezary erythroderma

T
...

20-day gut sutures
2-1/2 gland parathyroidectomy
24-hour ambulatory gastric pH
   monitor
24-hour esophageal probe
25 Gold portable CO_2 laser
270-degree laparoscopic
   posterior fundoplasty
2-angled polypropylene loop
2-arm goniometer
2-bladed dilator
2-bottle drainage
2-buttress defect
2-clamp anastomosis
2D Doppler
2D echo (2-dimensional echo)
2-dimensional echocardiogram
2-dimensional
   echocardiography
2-dimensional Fourier transform
   gradient-echo imaging
2-dimensional Fourier
   transformation imaging
2-dimensional monitoring
2-field dissection
2-flap palatoplasty repair
2-flap palatoplasty technique
2-hole miniplate
2-hole plate
2-holed miniplate
2-hydroxyethyl methacrylate
   (HEMA)
2-joule erbium laser
2-layer anastomosis
2-layer enteroenterostomy
2-layer latex closure
2-layer open technique
2-loop ileal J-pouch
2-microphone acoustical
   rhinometer
2-needle technique
2-Optifit toric lens
2-part fracture

2-paste polysulfide rubber
   impression material
2-patch technique
2-piece implant
2-piece ostomy pouch
2-pin technique
2-plan deformity
2-plane fluoroscopy
2-plane occlusion
2-point discrimination test
2-point nerve block
2-portal technique
2-poster orthosis
2-pour technique
2-prong dural hook
2-prong rake retractor
2-pronged dural hook
2-pronged retractor
2-pronged stem finger prosthesis
2-quadrant hemorrhoidectomy
2-ridge philtrum
2-sleeve technique
2-stage hip fusion
2-stage operation
2-stage pancreatoduodenectomy
2-stage procedure
2-stage repair
2-stage Sarns cannula
2-stage Syme amputation
2-stage tendon graft
   reconstruction
2-stage tendon grafting
   technique
2-step corneal section
2-step grafting
2-step procedure
2-step technique
2-stream irrigating forceps
2-team dissection
2-toothed forceps
2-trocar laparoscopic
   cholecystectomy
2-turn epicardial lead

2-way adapter for K-Temp thermometer
2-way bag
2-way cataract-aspirating cannula
2-way catheter
2-way hemostatic bag
2-way syringe
2-way towel clip
2-wing drain
2-wing Malecot drain
3 major leads
3 zones of a burn wound
30-30 papillotome
30-V staples
3-1/2 gland
3-armed basket forceps
3-armed stellate incision
3-axis gradient coil
3-bladed clamp
3-bottle drainage
3-bottle tidal suction tube
3-buttress defect
3-chambered heart
3-clamp technique
3-cornered therapy
3D Accuscan facial implant
3-D CEMRA (contrast-enhanced MR angiography)
3-D computer reconstruction
3D CT (3-dimensional computed tomography)
3D IVUS (intravascular ultrasound)
3D PTB walker
3D short-leg walker
3D surface digitizer scanner
3D-flat Lactosorb plate
3DFT gradient-echo MR imaging
3-dimensional computed tomography (3D CT)
3-dimensional computed tomography scans
3-dimensional conformal radiation therapy
3-dimensional CT
3-dimensional fast spin-echo magnetic resonance imaging
3-dimensional Fourier transform gradient-echo imaging
3-dimensional hyaluron-based scaffold (Hyalograft C)

3-dimensional image
3-dimensional interlocking hip (TDI hip)
3-dimensional projection reconstruction imaging
3-dimensional reconstruction
3-dimensional sonic digitizer
3Dscope laparoscope
3-field dissection
3-field lymphadenectomy
3-finger spica cast
3-flanged nail
3-flanged spike
3-footed intraocular lens
3-head camera
3-hole aspiration cannula
3-hole plate
3i implant
3-in-one block
3-legged cage heart valve
3-loop ileal pouch
3-loop technique
3-lumen thrombectomy catheter
3M bone mill
3M Clean Seals waterproof bandage
3M Coban LF self-adherent wrap
3M drape
3M dressing
3M filling instrument
3M implant
3M intraocular lens
3M limb isolation bag
3M mammary implant
3M matrix tape
3M Microdon dressing
3M Micropore surgical tape
3M No Sting barrier film
3M Reston self-adhering foam pad and roll
3M scanner
3M small aperture Steri-Drape drape
3M SoftCloth adhesive wound dressing
3M syndrome
3M Tegaderm HP high MVTR transparent dressing
3M Tegaderm transparent dressing with absorbent pad
3M Tegapore wound contact material

3M Tegasorb hydrocolloid
  dressing
3M Vi-Drape
3-mirror contact lens
3-mirror intraocular lens
3-paddle tensor fasciae latae free
  flap
3-part fracture
3-piece acrylic intraocular lens
3-piece modified J-loop
  intraocular lens
3-piece silicone intraocular lens
3-pillow orthopnea
3-plane deformity
3-point chuck
3-point fixation intraocular lens
3-point head holder
3-point pinch
3-point spreader bag
3-portal technique
3-prong fork
3-prong grasping forceps
3-prong rake blade retractor
3-pronged forceps
3-pronged grasper
3-pronged grasping forceps
3-pronged polyp retriever
3-pronged rake blade
3-pronged retractor
3-quadrant hemorrhoidectomy
3rd and 4th pharyngeal pouch
  syndrome
3rd branchial anomaly
3rd cartilaginous ring
3rd cranial nerve oculomotor
3rd generation lithotriptor
3rd intention wound closure
3rd molar
3rd nerve
3rd occipital nerve
3rd parallel pelvic plane
3rd peroneal muscle
3rd trimester
3rd ventricle of brain
3rd-degree burn
3rd-degree hemorrhoid
3rd-degree radiation injury
3rd-degree sprain
3rd-grade fusion
3rd-spacing
3-snip punctum operation
3-square flap

3-stage procedure
3-step tenotomy
3-trocar technique
  cholecystectomy
3-turn epicardial lead
3-vein graft
3-vessel umbilical cord
3-wall orbital decompression
3-way bridge
3-way catheter
3-way Foley catheter
3-way irrigating catheter
3-way stopcock
10th cranial nerve (Vagus)
12th cranial nerve (hypoglossal)
T band
T bar
T clamp
T fracture
T rotating joint
T self-retaining drainage tube
T&A (tonsillectomy and
  adenoidectomy)
T&A suction tip
T&C (type and crossmatch)
T1-weighted spin-echo image
T-28 hip prosthesis
T2-weighted spin-echo image
TA II loading unit
TA metallic staple
TA Premium-series staple
Ta-182 (tantalum-182)
TA-30 stapler
TA-50 stapler
TA-55 stapler
TA-60 stapler
TA-90 stapler
TA-90-BN stapler
Taarnhoj operation
TAB (therapeutic abortion)
Tabb crural nipper
Tabb double-ended flap knife
Tabb ear curet
Tabb ear elevator
Tabb ear knife
Tabb knife pick
Tabb myringoplasty knife
Tabb pick knife
Tabb ruler
tabes dorsalis
tabescent
tabetic foot

table bones of skull
table of skull
table-fixed retractor
Tab-Strap knee immobilizer
TAC (total abdominal
    colectomy)
TAC atherectomy catheter
TAC2 atrial caval cannula
Tachdjian classification
Tachdjian hamstring technique
Tachdjian procedure
Tach-EZ dental attachment
tachography study
tachyarrhythmia
tachycardia
tachycardia-terminating
    pacemaker
Tachylog pacemaker
tachypacing
tachypnea
tachysystole
Tacit threaded anchor
tack
    ACE bone screw tack
    ArthroRivet soft tissue tack
    biodegradable surgical tack
    Caspari soft tissue tack
    Cody sacculotomy tack
    Cody tack
    Effler tack
    Graftac absorbable skin tack
    inserter tack
    titanium tack
tack hammer
tack inserter
tack operation
tack-and-pin forceps
tacking sutures
tackler's arm
Tacoma sacral plate
TACT (tuned aperture computed
    tomography)
Tacticon peripheral neuropathy
    kit
Tacticon peripheral neuropathy
    screening device
Tactilaze angioplasty
Tactilaze angioplasty laser
Tactilaze angioplasty laser
    catheter
tactile anesthesia
tactile corpuscles

tactile disk
tactile fremitus
tactile papilla
tactile probe
tactile sensation
tactile stimulation
tactile tension
Tactyl 1 glove
Tactylon synthetic surgical glove
TAD guidewire
T-adapter
    Universal T-adapter
TAF (tumor angiogenic factor)
tag
    anal tags
    auricular tag
    cutaneous tag
    external skin tag
    fibrous anal tags
    hemorrhoidal skin tags
    hemorrhoidal tags
    perianal skin tag
    perineal skin tag
    peritonsillar tags
    question tag
    radioactive tag
    rectal skin tag
    rectal tags
    sentinel tag
    skin tag
    toe tag
    tonsillar tag
TAG instrumentation
TAG suture anchor
Tagarno cine projector for
    angiogram
tagged muscles
tagging stitch
Tagima sutures
tagliacotian operation
tagliacotian rhinoplasty
Tagliacozzi flap
Tagliacozzi nasal reconstruction
TAH (total abdominal
    hysterectomy)
Tahoe ligature
tail fold
tail of breast
tail of helix
tail of pancreas
tail of Spence
tail sign

tailbone
tailgut cyst
Taillefer valve
tailor bunionectomy
tailoring of flap
tailor's ankle
tailor's bunion
tailor-tacking
Tait flap
Tait graft
Tait perineoplasty
Tajima suture technique
Taka microneurosurgical sponge
Takagi arthroscope
Takahashi cutting forceps
Takahashi elevator
Takahashi ethmoid forceps
Takahashi ethmoid punch
Takahashi iris retractor forceps
Takahashi nasal forceps
Takahashi nasal punch
Takahashi neurosurgical forceps
Takahashi punch
Takahashi rongeur
Takaro clip
Takata laser
Takayasu disease
Takayasu syndrome
Take-apart forceps
Take-apart instrument
Take-apart scissors
takedown abdominal approach
takedown of adhesions
takedown of anastomosis
takedown procedure
takeoff of vessel
Take-Out extractor
taking down of adhesions
Takumi PTCA catheter
TAL (tendon Achilles lengthening)
TAL (total autogenous
    latissimus)
TAL breast reconstruction
Talairach stereotactic frame
talar accessory test
talar avulsion fracture
talar component
talar dislocation
talar neck fracture
talar osteochondral fracture
talar tendon
talar tilt test

talc insufflation
talc operation
talc plaque
talc poudrage
Talent endoluminal stent-graft
Talent stent graft
tali (*sing.* talus)
talipes calcaneovalgus
talipes calcaneovarus
talipes calcaneus
talipes cavovalgus
talipes cavus
talipes correction
talipes equinovalgus
talipes equinovarus
talipes equinus
talipes hobble splint
talipes planovalgus
talipes valgus
talipes varus
talipomanus
talking tracheostomy tube
Talley pump
Talma operation
talocalcaneal angle
talocalcaneal articulation
talocalcaneal fusion
talocalcaneal ligament
talocalcaneonavicular articulation
talocalcaneonavicular ligament
talocrural joint
talofibular ligament
Talon balloon dilatation catheter
Talon cranial fixation device
talonavicular articulation
talonavicular fusion
talonavicular joint
talonavicular ligament
talus (*pl.* tali)
talus foot deformity
talus head
Tamai clamp approximator
Tamai stitch
Tamai technique
tamp
  bone tamp
  graft tamp
  interbody graft tamp
  Kiene bone tamp
  KyphX Inflatable Xpander
    bone tamp
  spinal graft tamp

tamper
tampon applicator
tampon forceps
tampon injury
tampon tube
tamponade
　balloon tamponade
　cardiac tamponade
　esophageal tamponade
　esophagogastric tamponade
　ferromagnetic tamponade
　finger tamponade
　nasal tamponade
　nontraumatic cardiac
　　tamponade
　postnasal balloon tamponade
　Rose tamponade
tamponade action
tamponage
tamponing
tamponment
Tamsco curet
Tamsco forceps
Tamsco wire-cutting scissors
Tan otoplasty
Tan spatula
Tanagho bladder neck
　reconstruction
Tanagho modification of Burch
　procedure
tandem applicator
Tandem cardiac device
tandem clipping technique
tandem colonoscopy
tandem connector
tandem construction
tandem insertion
tandem lesion
tandem scanning confocal
　microscope
tandem stent
Tandem thin-shaft
　transureteroscopic balloon
　dilatation catheter
Tandem triple-lumen ERCP
　cannula
TandemHeart PTVA
　(percutaneous transseptal
　ventricular assist)
TandemHeart ventricular assist
　device
Tang retractor

tangent screen examination
tangential beam
tangential biopsy
tangential clamp
tangential colonic submucosal
　injection
tangential cut
tangential excision
tangential field
tangential forceps
tangential incision
tangential occlusion clamp
tangential pediatric clamp
tangential plane
tangential port
tangential projection
tangential section
tangential view on x-ray
tangential wound
Tanne corneal cutting block
Tanne corneal patch
Tanne corneal punch
Tannenbaum stent
Tanner herniorrhaphy
Tanner mesh graft dermacarrier
Tanner mesher
Tanner operation
Tanner esophagogastrojejunstomy
Tanner anti-bile reflux operation
Tanner-Vandeput graft
Tanner-Vandeput mesh
　dermatome
Tano device
Tano double-mirror peripheral
　vitrectomy lens
Tano eraser
Tano ring
Tansini breast amputation
Tansini gastric resection
Tansini operation
Tansini removal of liver cyst
Tansini sign
Tansley operation
tantalum O ring
tantalum balloon-expandable
　stent
tantalum balloon-expandable
　stent with helical coil
tantalum bronchogram
tantalum clip
tantalum cranioplasty
tantalum eye implant

tantalum fixation
tantalum gauze
tantalum graft
tantalum hemostasis clip
tantalum implant
tantalum material
tantalum mesh
tantalum mesh eye implant
tantalum mesh graft
tantalum mesh implant
tantalum mesh prosthesis
tantalum plate
tantalum prosthesis
tantalum ring
tantalum sheet
tantalum stapes prosthesis
tantalum wire
tantalum wire fixation
tantalum wire monofilament
 sutures
tantalum wire sutures
tantalum wire tension sutures
tantalum-178 generator
tantalum-182 (Ta-182)
tantalum-ball marker
tantalum-wire stent
Tanzer auricle reconstruction
Tanzer operation
tap
 abdominal tap
 belly tap
 bloody tap
 bone marrow tap
 cisternal tap
 diagnostic spinal tap
 peritoneal tap
 screw tap
 spinal fluid tap
 spinal tap
 ventricular tap
tap drill
tap-water wet dressing
Tapcath esophageal electrode
tape
 3M matrix tape
 3M Micropore surgical tape
 adhesive tape
 appendix tapes
 appy tape
 Aquasorb Border dressing
 Blenderm tape
 Broselow tape

tape (*continued*)
 brow tape
 buddy tape
 CaraGlass fiberglass casting
  tape
 casting tape
 Cath-Secure tape
 C-Casting tape
 circling silicone tape
 circular tape
 CollaTape tape
 color-coding tape
 colored tape
 ColorZone tape
 compression tape
 Cordran tape
 Covaderm tape
 Cutter cast tape
 Dacron retraction tape
 Deknatel wound closure tape
 Delta-lite casting tape
 Dermicare hypoallergenic
  paper tape
 Dermicel hypoallergenic cloth
  tape
 Dermicel hypoallergenic
  knitted tape
 Dermiclear tape
 Dermiform hypoallergenic
  knitted tape
 Dermilite tape
 Dermiview hypoallergenic
  transparent tape
 Durapore hypoallergenic
  tape
 Elastikon elastic tape
 fiberglass casting tape
 foam tape
 Haelan tape
 Hypafix retention tape
 Hy-Tape latex-free surgical
  tape
 Hy-Tape surgical tape
 instrument coding tape
 Johnson & Johnson
  waterproof tape
 lap tapes
 Leukofix surgical tape
 Leukoflex surgical tape
 Leukopor surgical tape
 Leukosilk surgical tape
 Leukotape P sports tape

tape (*continued*)
  MaxCast fiberglass casting
    tape
  Medipore H soft cloth surgical
    tape
  Medipore H surgical tape
  Meditape tape
  Mefix adhesive tape
  Mersilene tape
  Microfoam surgical tape
  Micropore hypoallergenic tape
  Micropore tape
  microprobe surgical tape
  moist tape
  moistened tape
  Montgomery tape
  OCL flexible casting tape
  paper tape
  Polyderm border with
    Covaderm tape
  polyester-reinforced Dacron
    tape
  polyethylene retractor tape
  Powerflex tape
  restraining tape
  Scanpor surgical tape
  Scanpore hypoallergenic tape
  Scotchcast casting tape
  Scotchflex casting tape
  secured with tape
  Shur-Strip wound closure tape
  Silastic tape
  Sportape tape
  Sta-Fix tape
  sterile adhesive tape
  sterile tape
  Sure-Closure wound closure
    tape
  Teflon tape
  Transpore eye tape
  Transpore surgical tape
  TSH-01 transdermal tape
  umbilical tape
  Vascor sterile retraction tape
  vascular tape
  Velcro tapes
  Xtra Gentle surgical tape
  Zonas porous tape
tape ligature
tape marker
Taper guidewire
taper hand file

taper needle
Tapercut needle
Tapercut sutures
tapered blade
tapered bougie
tapered brain spatula
tapered catheter
tapered fissure bar
tapered Micro-Vent implant
tapered needle
tapered pin
tapered reamer
tapered rubber bougie
tapered torque guidewire
tapered-shaft punctum plug
tapered-spring needle holder
tapered-tip ear syringe
tapered-tip hydrophilic-coated
    push catheter
taper-jaw forceps
taper-jaw rongeur
Taperloc femoral component
Taperloc femoral prosthesis
Taper-Lock external hex implant
taper-point needle holder
taper-point suture needle
TaperSeal hemostatic device
tapetum (*pl.* tapeta)
tapetum alveoli
Tapia syndrome
tapinocephaly
tapping hammer
tapping of chest for fluid
Tapsul pill electrode
Taq extender
TARA (total articular
    replacement arthroplasty)
TARA prosthesis
TARA retropubic retractor
TARA total hip prosthesis
Tardy osteotome
tardy palsy
Tardy's triad
target cell
target gland
target lesion
target plasma concentration (TPC)
target sign
target tissue
target volume
target-controlled infusion (TCO)
targeted brain biopsy

targeted cryoablation device
targeted surgery
targeting drill guide
target-to-nontarget ratio
Tarin space
Tarlov cyst
Tarlov nerve elevator
Tarnier axis-traction forceps
Tarnier cranioclast
Tarnier obstetrical forceps
Tarrant position
tarsal amputation
tarsal arch
tarsal arteries
tarsal asthenopia
tarsal bar
tarsal bone
tarsal bone fracture
tarsal canal
tarsal coalition
tarsal cyst
tarsal dislocation
tarsal fold
tarsal gland
tarsal joint
tarsal laceration
tarsal membrane
tarsal muscle
tarsal plate
tarsal sinus
tarsal strip canthoplasty
tarsal strip procedure
tarsal synostosis
tarsal tunnel
tarsal ulcer
tarsal wedge osteotomy
tarsectomy
   Kuhnt tarsectomy
   Mikulicz tarsectomy
   Vladimiroff tarsectomy
tarsitis
tarsocheiloplasty
tarsoclasis
tarsoconjunctival composite graft
tarsoconjunctival flap
tarsoconjunctival glands
tarsodermal fixation technique
tarsoepiphyseal aclasis
tarsomalacia
tarsometatarsal amputation
tarsometatarsal articulations
tarsometatarsal dislocation

tarsometatarsal fracture-
   dislocation
tarsometatarsal ligament
tarsometatarsal truncated-wedge
   arthrodesis
tarso-orbital
tarsophalangeal reflex
tarsophyma
tarsoplasia
tarsoplasty
tarsorrhaphy
tarsotibial amputation
tarsotomy
tarsus (*pl.* tarsi)
tarsus inferior palpebrae
tarsus orbital septum
tarsus osseus
tarsus superior palpebrae
Tascon prosthetic valve
Tashiro repair
Tasia operation
Tasserit shoulder attachment
Tassett vaginal cup bag
Tatagiba line
Tate flap
tattoo injury
tattoo removal
tattoo surgery
tattooing instrument
tattooing needle
Tatum clamp
Tatum meatal clamp
Tatum Tee intrauterine device
Tatum ureteral transilluminator
Tauber catheter
Tauber hook
Tauber ligature carrier
Tauber ligature hook
Tauber male urethrographic
   catheter
Tauber needle
Tauber speculum
Tauber vaginal spatula
Taucher tunneler
Taufic cholangiography clamp
Taussig operation
Taussig-Bing anomaly
Taussig-Bing malformation
Taussig-Bing syndrome
Taussig-Morton node dissection
Taussig-Morton operation
Taut capillary drain

Taut cholangiographic catheter
Taut cystic duct catheter
Taut percutaneous introducer
Taveras injector
Tavernetti-Tennant-Cutter knee
Tawara node
Tay choroiditis
Tay spot
Taylor approach
Taylor aspirator
Taylor back brace
Taylor blade
Taylor brace
Taylor brain scissors
Taylor Britetrac retractor
Taylor catheter holder
Taylor clavicle support
Taylor craniotomy scissors
Taylor curet
Taylor dissecting forceps
Taylor dural scissors
Taylor fiberoptic retractor
Taylor forceps
Taylor gastric balloon
Taylor gastroscope
Taylor halter device
Taylor knife
Taylor laminectomy blade
Taylor Merocel ear wick
Taylor neurosurgical scissors
Taylor percussion hammer
Taylor pinwheel
Taylor position
Taylor procedure
Taylor pulmonary dilator
Taylor reflex hammer
Taylor retractor
Taylor scissors
Taylor speculum
Taylor spinal frame
Taylor spinal retractor
Taylor spinal retractor blade
Taylor spine brace
Taylor splint
Taylor suture technique
Taylor sutures
Taylor technique
Taylor thoracolumbosacral
    orthosis
Taylor tissue forceps
Taylor vaginal speculum
Taylor-Cushing dressing forceps

Taylor-Daniel-Weiland technique
Taylor-Knight brace
Taylor-Townsend-Corlett iliac
    crest bone graft
Tay-Sachs disease
T-band matrix
T-bandage dressing
T-bar elevator
T-bar of Kazanjian
T-bar retractor
T-binder pressure dressing
T-breast reduction
TBSA (total body surface area)
T-buttress plate
TC CO_2 monitor
TC IV total knee
TC needle holder
TC pin cutter
TC ring-handle pin and wire
    extractor
Tc-99m phosphate bone
    imaging
TCA (trichloroacetic acid)
TCA peel
TCB (transconjunctival
    blepharoplasty)
TCCK unconstrained knee
    prosthesis
T-cell depleted bone marrow
    transplantation
T-cell line
TcHIDA scan
T-clamp
TCN (terminal capillary
    network)
TCNS (transcutaneous nerve
    stimulator)
T-condylar fracture
T-contact lens
TCS knee immobilizer
TDD (thoracic duct drainage)
TDI hip (3-dimensional
    interlocking hip)
TDMAC heparin shunt
T-drain
TE fistula (tracheoesophageal
    fistula)
TE MOO mode beam laser
TEA (thromboendarterectomy)
teacup fracture
Teale amputation
Teale director

Teale gorget
Teale gorget lithotrite
Teale lithotomy gorget guide
Teale operation
Teale tenaculum
Teale tenaculum forceps
Teale uterine forceps
Teale uterine vulsellum forceps
Teale vulsellum forceps
Teale-Knapp operation
tear
  Boerhaave tear
  bucket-handle tear
  cartilage tear
  crocodile tears
  cruciate ligament tear
  degenerative tear
  esophageal tear
  flap meniscal tear
  gastric tear
  horseshoe tear
  Lachman tear
  lunotriquetral ligament tear
  lunotriquetral tear
  Mallory-Weiss mucosal tear
  meniscal tear
  mop-end tear
  mucosal tear
  parrot-beak meniscus tear
  perineal tear
  rectal tear
  retinal tear
  rotator cuff tear
  skier's tear
  syndrome of crocodile tears
  TFCC meniscus tear
  traumatic tear
  triquetral impingement
    ligament tear (TILT)
tear at 1 (2, 3, etc.) o'clock
tear clearance rate
tear duct tube
tear of capsule
tear of ligament
tear of meniscus
tear of mucosa
tear of muscle
tear sac
tear strips
tear trough style implant
tearaway introducer sheath
tearaway sheath

teardrop dissector
teardrop foramen
teardrop fracture
teardrop line
Teardrop microsponge
teardrop vertebral outgrowth
teardrop-shaped breast implant
teardrop-shaped nipple-areola
    complex
Teare arm sling
Teare arm sling splint
Teare arm splint
Teare snare
TearSaver punctum plug
Teaser device
Tebbets rhinoplasty set
Tebbets ribbon retractor
Tebbetts ribbon retractor
TEC (transluminal extraction
    catheter)
TEC positioning laser
TEC atherectomy device
TEC extraction catheter
TEC liner
TECA-TD20 EMG machine
TechMate 500 automatic
    immunostaining device
Techmedica implant
Techmedica prosthesis
Techmedica total hip
Techmedica total pelvis
technetium (Tc)
technetium bone scan
technetium pertechnetate
    scan
technetium pyrophosphate
technetium scintigram
technetium-99m scan
Technicare camera
Technicare scanner
Techni-Care wound cleanser
technique
  1st-pass technique
  1st rib resection via
    subclavicular approach
    technique
  1-line screening technique
  1-lung ventilation anesthetic
    technique
  1-phase subperiosteal implant
    technique
  1-pour technique

technique (*continued*)

133Xe intravenous injection
technique
2-flap palatoplasty technique
2-layer open technique
2-needle technique
2-patch technique
2-pin technique
2-portal technique
2-pour technique
2-sleeve technique
2-stage tendon grafting
technique
2-step technique
3-clamp technique
3-loop technique
3-portal technique
4-flap Webster-Bernard
technique
4-maximal breath
preoxygenation technique
4-port technique
4-portal technique
abdominal pressure technique
abduction traction technique
ablative technique
Ace-Colles frame technique
acid etch bonding technique
acupuncture technique
adduction traction technique
afterloading technique
agglutination technique
airbrasive technique
air-gap technique
airway occlusion technique
Albee technique
Albert suture technique
Alexander technique
Allison technique
alternating suture technique
American laryngectomy
technique
Amplatz technique
amputation technique
Amspacher-Messenbaugh
technique
Anderson-Hutchings
technique
Andrews technique
anesthetic technique
angiographic road-mapping
technique

technique (*continued*)

angle bisection technique
angle suture technique
antegrade double balloon-
double wire technique
antegrade/retrograde
cardioplegia technique
anterior quadriceps
musculocutaneous flap
technique
anterior sandwich patch
closure technique
anterograde transseptal
technique
antireflux ureteral
implantation technique
AO technique
APOLT technique
Appolito suture technique
apposition suture technique
approximation suture
technique
Araki-Sako technique
arcuate suture technique
Argyll-Robertson suture
technique
Arlt suture technique
Armaly-Drance technique
Armistead technique
Aronson-Prager technique
arrester-heart
revascularization technique
arterial cannulation anesthetic
technique
arthrographic capsular
distention and rupture
technique
ascending technique
aseptic technique
ASIF screw fixation technique
Asnis technique
assay technique
assisted reproductive
technique
Atasoy V-Y technique
Atkinson technique
atraumatic suture technique
atrial-well technique
autologous fat-injection
techniques
autologous fat-transplanting
techniques

technique (*continued*)
  autoradiographic technique
  Auto-Suture technique
  Avila technique
  avulsion technique
  Axenfeld suture technique
  Axer technique
  axillary block anesthetic
    technique
  axillary perivascular technique
  Ayre spatula-Zelsmyr
    cytobrush technique
  Babcock suture technique
  back-and-forth suture
    technique
  Badgley technique
  Baek musculocutaneous
    pedicle technique
  bag-of-bones technique
  Bailey-Badgley technique
  Bailey-Dubow technique
  Baker technique
  Balacescu technique
  Balacescu-Golden technique
  balanced anesthetic technique
  balanced force
    instrumentation technique
  balloon catheter technique
  balloon tamponade technique
  balloon-catheter and basket-
    retrieval technique
  Bandi technique
  Banks-Laufman technique
  Barcat technique
  bare scleral technique
  Barkan technique
  Baron technique
  Barraquer suture technique
  barrier technique
  Barron hemorrhoidal banding
    technique
  Barsky technique
  baseball suture technique
  basic technique
  basilar suture technique
  basket extraction technique
  basket fragmentation
    technique
  basketing technique
  Bass technique
  Bassini technique
  bastard suture technique

technique (*continued*)
  Batchelor technique
  Batch-Spittler-McFaddin
    technique
  Bauer technique
  Bauer-Tondra-Trusler
    technique
  Baumgard and Schwartz
    technique
  Baumgard-Schwartz tennis
    elbow technique
  Beall-Webel-Bailey technique
  Beckenbaugh technique
  Becker technique
  Beclard suture technique
  Becton technique
  Begg light wire differential
    force technique
  behavioral technique
  Bell-Tawse open reduction
    technique
  Belsey fundoplication
    technique
  Belt technique
  bench surgical technique
  Bentall composite graft
    technique
  Bentall inclusion technique
  Berke-Leahy technique
  Berman-Gartland technique
  Bernard-Burow technique
  Bertrandi suture technique
  Beverly-Douglas lip-tongue
    adhesion technique
  bilateral inguinal hernia repair
    technique
  Billroth I technique
  Billroth II technique
  bilobed skin flap technique
  biohazard operating
    technique
  bioprogressive technique
  biopsy technique
  biparietal suture technique
  Bircher-Weber technique
  bisecting angle technique
  bisecting-the-angle technique
  bitewing technique
  Black technique
  Black-Brostrom staple
    technique
  Blackburn technique

technique (*continued*)
  bladder neck preserving
    technique
  Blair technique
  Blair-Byars hypospadias
    technique
  Blair-Morris technique
  Blair-Omer technique
  blanket suture technique
  Blaskovics eyelid shortening
    technique
  Bleck recession technique
  Blenderm patch technique
  blind nasal intubation
    anesthetic technique
  blind nasotracheal intubation
    anesthetic technique
  blind-spot projection
    technique
  block technique
  Bloom-Raney modification of
    Smith-Robinson
    technique
  Blount tracing technique
  Blundell-Jones technique
  blunt dissection and snare
    technique
  body scanning technique
  Bohlman cervical fusion
    technique
  Bohlman triple-wire
    technique
  bolster suture technique
  bolus chase technique
  bolus intravenous anesthetic
    technique
  bone graft harvesting
    technique
  bone technique
  Bonfiglio modification of
    Phemister technique
  Bonola technique
  boost technique
  bootstrap two-vessel
    technique
  Bora technique
  bougienage technique
  Bowers technique
  Bowles technique
  Box technique
  Boyd-Anderson technique
  Boyden chamber technique

technique (*continued*)
  Boyd-McLeod tennis elbow
    technique
  Boyes brachioradialis transfer
    technique
  Bozeman suture technique
  Braasch bulb technique
  brachial plexus block
    anesthetic technique
  Brackett technique
  Brackett-Osgood-Putti-Abbott
    technique
  Brackin technique
  Brady-Jewett technique
  Brand tendon transfer
    technique
  Brannon-Wickstrom
    technique
  Braun pinch graft technique
  Braun-Jaboulay technique
  breast-conserving technique
  Brecher new methylene blue
    technique
  Brecher-Cronkite technique
  bregmatomastoid suture
    technique
  Brenner gastrojejunostomy
    technique
  Brett technique
  bridle suture technique
  Brockenbrough technique
  Brockhurst technique
  Brockman technique
  bronchoscopy anesthetic
    technique
  Brooks technique
  Brooks-Jenkins atlantoaxial
    fusion technique
  Brooks-Seddon transfer
    technique
  Brostrom ligament repair
  Brown technique
  Brown-Beard technique
  Brown-Brenn technique
  Brown-Wickham technique
  Bruhat technique
  Bruser technique
  Bryan technique
  Bryan-Morrey technique
  Buck-Gramcko technique
  Bucky technique
  Buerhenne technique

technique (*continued*)

Bugg-Boyd technique
Buie technique
bulk pack technique
bunching suture technique
Buncke technique
Bunnell atraumatic technique
Bunnell suture technique
Bunnell tendon transfer
    technique
Buratto technique
Burch bladder suspension
    technique
Burgess technique
buried mass far-and-near
    suture technique
Burkhalter modification of
    Stiles-Bunnell technique
Burkhalter transfer technique
Burman technique
Burow technique
Burrows technique
Butler technique
button suture technique
button technique
buttonhole suture technique
Buxton bolus suture
    technique
bypass technique
cable wire suture technique
Callahan fusion technique
Camino catheter technique
Camitz technique
Campbell technique
canal wall-up technique
Canale technique
cap technique
Cape Town technique
Capello technique
Capener technique
capitonnage suture technique
capping technique
capsule flap technique
capsule forceps technique
cardioplegic technique
cardiovascular imaging
    technique
Carey Ranvier technique
Carnesale technique
carotid preservation
    technique
Carrel suture technique

technique (*continued*)

Carrell fibular substitution
    technique
Carroll technique
cartilage case-grafting
    technique
cartilage-breaking technique
cartilage-molding technique
cartilage-weakening technique
catheterization technique
catheter-securing technique
caudal epidural anesthetic
    technique
cavernosal alpha blockade
    technique
Cave-Rowe shoulder
    dislocation technique
celiac plexus block anesthetic
    technique
cell separation technique
cement technique
cementless technique
central anesthetic technique
central slip sparing technique
central venous cannulation
    anesthetic technique
cephalotrigonal technique
cervical plexus block
    anesthetic technique
cervical screw insertion
    technique
cervical spondylotic
    myelopathy fusion
    technique
chain suture technique
Chakirgil technique
Chambers technique
Chandler technique
channel shoulder pin
    technique
Chapchal technique
Charters technique
Chaves-Rapp muscle transfer
    technique
Cherney suture technique
chevron marking technique
chevron technique
chew-in technique
Chiari technique
Childress ankle fixation
    technique
chloramine-T technique

technique (*continued*)

Cho technique
Cho tendon technique
cholangiographic technique
Chow technique
Chrisman-Snook ankle technique
Cierny-Mader technique
Cincinnati technique
circular suture technique
circulatory arrest anesthetic technique
circumcision suture technique
clamp-and-sew technique
clamshell technique
Clancy ligament technique
Clark transfer technique
Clark-Axer technique
classic DSRS technique
classical technique
Clayton-Fowler technique
clearance technique
Cleveland-Bosworth-Thompson technique
clip technique
closed technique
closed tubule fixation technique
closed-circuit anesthetic technique
closed-gloving technique
Cloward technique
Coakley suture technique
coaptation suture technique
cobalt-60 moving strip technique
Cobb scoliosis measuring technique
Cobb technique
cobbler's suture technique
Codivilla tendon lengthening technique
Coffey technique (I, II, III)
Coffey-Witzel jejunostomy technique
Cofield technique
Cohen cross-trigonal technique
cold resurfacing technique
cold saline-induced paresthesia technique

technique (*continued*)

Cole technique
Coleman flatfoot technique
Coleman-Noonan technique
Coleman-Stelling-Jarrett technique
Collis broken femoral stem technique
Collis-Nissen fundoplication technique
Coltart fracture technique
combination of isotonics technique
combined spinal-epidural anesthetic technique
compensation technique
composite addition technique
composite pelvic resection technique
compound suture technique
compression technique
computer-assisted continuous infusion anesthetic technique
computer-controlled drug administration anesthetic technique
computer-controlled infusion anesthetic technique
conization technique
Conn technique
Connell suture technique
Connolly technique
continuous gum technique
continuous infusion anesthetic technique
continuous pull-through technique
continuous spinal anesthetic technique
continuous suture technique
continuous-wave technique
contoured anterior spinal plate technique
contraceptive technique
contract-relax technique
controlled release anesthetic technique
controlled water-added technique
conventional technique
Converse technique

technique (*continued*)

- Conway technique
- Conyers technique
- Coonse-Adams technique
- Cope technique
- Copeland technique
- coracoclavicular technique
- Corbin technique
- coronal arc technique
- coronary flow reserve technique
- Cortel technique
- costotransversectomy technique
- Cotrel cast technique
- cough CPR technique
- Counsellor-Flor modification of McIndoe technique
- Cox technique
- Cozen-Brockway technique
- crash technique
- Crawford graft inclusion technique
- Crawford-Marxen-Osterfeld technique
- Creech technique
- Crego tendon transfer technique
- cricoid pressure anesthetic technique
- Crobin technique
- cross-facial technique
- cross-section technique
- Crown suture technique
- cruciform suture technique
- crush vasectomy technique
- crushing technique
- Crutchfield reduction technique
- cryosurgical technique
- Cubbins shoulder dislocation technique
- Culcher-Sussman technique
- culturing technique
- cup-patch technique
- Cupper suture technique
- cupula technique
- Curtin technique
- Curtis technique
- Curtis-Fisher knee technique
- Cushing suture technique
- cushioning suture technique

technique (*continued*)

- cut-and-sew technique
- cutaneous suture technique
- cut-as-you-go technique
- cutdown technique
- cuticular suture technique
- Cutler-Beard technique
- Cyriax technique
- Czerny suture technique
- Czerny-Lembert suture technique
- Daivd technique
- Darrach technique
- Darrach-McLaughlin shoulder technique
- Davey-Rorabeck-Fowler decompression technique
- David technique
- Davis drainage technique
- de Andrade-MacNab technique
- de novo needle-knife technique
- Debeyre-Patte-Elmelik rotator cuff technique
- debridement technique
- decompression technique
- decortication technique
- defibrillation technique
- DEFT technique
- degloving technique
- delayed primary suture technique
- delayed skin flap technique
- Delerm-Elbaz technique
- deliberate hypotension anesthetic technique
- demand-adapted administration anesthetic technique
- Denis Browne urethroplasty technique
- Dennis technique
- DePalma modified patellar technique
- depth pulse technique
- dermal brassiere technique
- dermal orbicular pennant technique
- dermal pedicle technique
- dermal suture technique
- dermofat technique

technique (*continued*)
  descending technique
  Desting prostatic dilatation
    technique
  destructive interference
    technique
  Devonshire technique
  Dewar posterior cervical
    fusion technique
  Dewar-Barrington clavicular
    dislocation technique
  Dewar-Harris shoulder
    technique
  Deyerle femoral fracture
    technique
  diagnostic technique
  Diamond-Gould technique
  Dias-Gingerich technique
  Dickinson calcaneal bursitis
    technique
  Dickson transplant technique
  Dickson-Willien technique
  Dieffenbach-Duplay
    hypospadias technique
  differential force technique
  differential spinal block
    anesthetic technique
  digital subtraction technique
  dilator-and-sheath technique
  dilution-filtration technique
  Dimon-Hughston technique
  Diprivan technique
  direct insertion technique
  direct/indirect technique
  display technique
  distal pedicle flap technique
  distal tunnel technique
  distraction technique
  Dixon technique
  Dolenc technique
  Doll trochanteric
    reattachment technique
  Doppler auto-correlation
    technique
  Dor fundoplication technique
  dot-blot technique
  dotter technique
  Dotter-Judkins technique
  double contrast technique
  double pedicle technique
  double stapling technique
    (DST)

technique (*continued*)
  double-armed suture technique
  double-balloon technique
  double-button suture
    technique
  double-dummy technique
  double-emulsion-solvent-
    extraction technique
  double-folded cup-patch
    technique
  double-freeze technique
  double-looped
    semitendinosus technique
  double-rod technique
  double-sealant technique
  double-staple technique
  double-stapled ileoanal
    reservoir technique
  double-stapled technique
  double-stick technique
  double-tube technique
  double-wire technique
  Douglas bag technique
  dowel technique
  doweling spondylolisthesis
    technique
  Drake tandem clipping
    technique
  DREZ modification of
    Eriksson technique
  drilling technique
  driven equilibrium Fourier
    transform technique
  Drummond spinous wiring
    technique
  Drummond wire technique
  dry field technique
  dual impression technique
  dual-plane techniques
  Duckworth-Smith technique
  duct-to-mucosa technique
  Dufourmental technique
  dunking technique
  Dunn technique
  Dunn-Brittain foot
    stabilization technique
  Duplay I technique
  Duplay II technique
  Dupuytren suture technique
  DuVries deltoid ligament
    reconstruction technique
  Dyban technique

technique (*continued*)

dye dilution technique

dynamic bolus tracking
technique

Eames technique

Eastwood technique

Eaton-Littler technique

Eaton-Malerich fracture-
dislocation technique

Eberle contracture release
technique

ECG signal-averaging
technique

Ecker-Lotke-Glazer tendon
reconstruction technique

Eden technique

edge-to-edge suture technique

Eftekhar broken femoral stem
technique

Eggers tendon transfer
technique

Eisenberger technique

Eklund technique

elliptical excision technique

Ellis skin traction technique

Ellis-Jones peroneal tendon
technique

Ellison technique

Elmslie-Trillat technique

Elsahy technique

Emmet suture technique

en bloc, no touch technique

Ender femoral fracture
technique

endobronchial intubation
anesthetic technique

endodontic technique

endofluoroscopic technique

EndoForehead operative
techniques

endorectal ileoanal pull-
through technique

endoscope-assisted
technique

endoscopic mucosal resection
technique

endoscopic mucosal
technique

endoscopic technique

endoscopic-assisted
microsurgical technique

endoscopic-assisted technique

technique (*continued*)

endovascular stenting
technique

end-to-end reconstruction
technique

end-to-side
vasoepididymostomy
technique

entangling technique

enucleation technique

epiaortic imaging technique

epidural blood patch
anesthetic technique

epineural suture technique

epithelialization technique

Erickson-Leider-Brown
technique

Eriksson brachial block
technique

Eriksson ligament technique

erysiphake technique

esophageal banding technique

ESP face-lift technique

Essex-Lopresti axial fixation
technique

Essex-Lopresti calcaneal
fracture technique

Essex-Lopresti reduction
technique

Euchidia technique

Evans ankle reconstruction
technique

eversion technique

everting interrupted suture
technique

evoked potential technique

ex situ-in situ technique

ex vivo technique

exchange technique

excisional biopsy technique

excision-curettage technique

extended mesh technique

extended-incision technique

extra-anatomic bypass
technique

extra-anatomical renal
revascularization technique

extra-articular technique

extracorporeal technique

extraction balloon technique

extradural anesthetic
technique

technique (*continued*)

extrastimulus technique

extravesical ureteral reimplantation technique

extremity mobilization technique

extubation anesthetic technique

FA technique

facet excision technique

Fahey technique

Fahey-O'Brien technique

Fairbanks technique

Falk vesicovaginal fistula technique

fanning-out technique

far-and-near suture technique

Farmer technique

fascial anchoring technique

fast exposure technique

fat-suppression technique

feathering technique

feeder-frond technique

femoral 3-in-1 technique

Fericot technique

Ferguson technique

Ferkel torticollis technique

ferning technique

fiberoptic bronchoscopy anesthetic technique

fiberoptic endoscopy anesthetic technique

fiberoptic tracheal intubation anesthetic technique

Fick technique

Ficoll-Hypaque technique

Fielding modification of Gallie technique

figure-of-8 suture technique

filing first technique

finger fracture technique

Finochietto-Billroth I gastrectomy technique

Fischer curet technique

Fish cuneiform osteotomy technique

fixation suture technique

fixation technique

FLAK technique

Flamm technique

flap technique

Flatt technique

technique (*continued*)

flicker-fusion frequency technique

Flick-Gould technique

flip-flap technique

floppy Nissen fundoplication technique

flow detection technique

flow interruption technique

flow mapping technique

fluid loading anesthetic technique

fluorescent antibody staining technique (FAST)

fluorometric technique

fluoroscopic pushing technique

flush-and-bathe technique

flushing technique

Flynn technique

Flynn-Richards-Saltzman technique

Fones technique

Forbes graft technique

Forbes modification of Phemister graft technique

Ford triangulation technique

fore-and-aft suture technique

Forest-Hastings technique

forward triangle technique

Fourier-acquired steady-state technique (FAST)

Fowler technique

Fowles dislocation technique

Fowles technique

Franke technique

Fraunfelder no-touch technique

free ligature suture technique

Freebody-Bendall-Taylor fusion technique

freehand suturing technique

Freeman resurfacing technique

free-root insertion technique

French fracture technique

Fried clubfoot technique

Fried-Hendel tendon technique

Froimson technique

frontalis sling technique

Frost suture technique

technique (*continued*)
   functional technique
   furrier's suture technique
   fusion technique
   Gaenslen split-heel technique
   galeal scoring technique
   Gallie atlantoaxial fusion
      technique
   Gallie wiring technique
   Galveston technique
   Gambee suture technique
   Ganley technique
   Garceau tendon technique
   gaseous laparoscopy
      technique
   gasless laparoscopy technique
   gastric valve tightening
      technique
   gated technique
   Gaur balloon distention
      technique
   G-banding technique
   general anesthetic technique
   George Lewis technique
   George Winter elevator torque
      technique
   Ger technique
   Getty decompression
      technique
   Giampapa suturing technique
   Giannestras modification of
      Lapidus technique
   Gibson suture technique
   gift wrap suture technique
   Gilbert-Tamai-Weiland
      technique
   Gill sliding graft technique
   Gillies-Millard cocked-hat
      technique
   Gills technique
   Gil-Vernet technique
   Gittes technique
   Gledhill technique
   Glen Anderson technique
   gliding-hole-first technique
   gloved-fist technique
   Glover suture technique
   gloving technique
   Glynn-Neibauer technique
   Goebel-Frangenheim-Stoeckel
      technique
   gold plate technique

technique (*continued*)
   gold seed implantation
      technique
   Goldberg technique
   Goldmann kinetic technique
   Goldmann static technique
   Goldner-Clippinger technique
   Goldstein spinal fusion
      technique
   Gomco technique
   Goodwin technique
   Goodwin-Hohenfellner
      technique
   Goodwin-Scott technique
   Gordon joint injection
      technique
   Gordon-Bronstrom technique
   Gordon-Taylor technique
   Gould suture technique
   gowning technique
   grabbing technique
   gracilis flap technique
   grasping technique
   Graves technique
   gravimetric technique
   Green-Banks technique
   Gregory Pell sectioning
      technique
   Greulich-Pyle technique
   Grice-Green technique
   Grimelius technique
   Gritti-Stokes knee amputation
      technique
   groove suture technique
   Grosse-Kempf tibial technique
   Groves-Goldner technique
   Gruber suture technique
   Gruentzig PTCA technique
   Guhl technique
   guidewire and mini-snare
      technique
   guidewire exchange
      technique
   Guilford stapedectomy
      technique
   guillotine technique
   Gussenbauer suture
      technique
   Guttmann technique
   guy suture technique
   Guyon ankle amputation
      technique

technique (*continued*)

Guyton-Friedenwald suture technique
Hackethal stacked nailing technique
Hakme's technique
half-mouth technique
Hall technique
Halsted suture technique
Hamas technique
Hamou technique
hanging-drop technique
Hardinge technique
harelip suture technique
Hark technique
Harman technique
Harman-Fahey technique
Harmon transfer technique
Harriluque technique
Harris suture technique
Harris-Beath technique
Hartel technique
Hartmann reconstruction technique
Hass technique
Hassmann-Brunn-Neer elbow technique
Hasson technique
Hauri technique
Hauser patellar realignment technique
Hawkins inside-out nephrostomy technique
Hawkins single-stick technique
head turn technique
Heaney technique
Heifitz technique
helical suture technique
hemostat technique
hemostatic suture technique
Henderson technique
Hendler unitunnel technique
Henning inside-to-outside technique
Henry acromioclavicular technique
hepatic vascular isolation technique
Hermodsson internal rotation technique
Herold-Torok technique

technique (*continued*)

Hey-Groves fascia lata technique
Hey-Groves ligament reconstruction technique
Hey-Groves-Kirk technique
Heyman-Herndon-Strong technique
Hibbs technique
Higgings technique
high-amplitude sucking technique
high-heat casting technique
high-kV technique
high-tension suturing technique
Hill cluster harvest technique
Hill-Nahai-Vasconez-Mathes technique
Hitchcock tendon technique
Hodgson technique
Hofmeister technique
Hohl-Moore technique
Hoke technique
Hoke-Kite technique
hold-relax technique
hole-in-one technique
Hood technique
Hoppenfeld-Deboer technique
Hori technique
horizontal mattress suture technique
hot biopsy technique
Hotchkiss-McManus PAS technique
hot-dog technique
Houghton-Akroyd fracture technique
House technique
Hovanian transfer technique
Howard technique
Howard-Schatz laser technique
Huber technique
Hughes modification of Burch technique
Hughston technique
Hughston-Jacobson technique
Hungerford technique
Hunt-Early technique
Huntington technique
Huntington tibial technique

technique (*continued*)
- Hyams conization technique
- hybridization-subtraction technique
- hybridoma technique
- hydroflow technique
- hydrogen inhalation technique
- hygroscopic technique
- hypogastric plexus block anesthesia technique
- hypothermia anesthetic technique
- hypothermic technique
- Hakanson technique
- Ilizarov bone-lengthening technique
- Ilizarov bone-straightening technique
- Ilizarov limb-lengthening technique
- Illouz liposuction technique
- Illouz original liposuction technique
- image-related screening technique
- imaging technique
- imbricated suture technique
- immediate extension technique
- immersion technique
- immunohistochemical technique
- implantation technique
- implanted suture technique
- impression technique
- incision-halving technique
- indicator-dilution technique
- indirect technique
- indocyanine green indicator dilution technique
- induced hypotension anesthetic technique
- induction anesthetic technique
- infiltration anesthetic technique
- infusion technique
- Inglis-Cooper technique
- Inglis-Ranawat-Straub technique
- Ingram technique

technique (*continued*)
- inhalation anesthetic technique
- injection technique
- inotrope resuscitation technique
- Insall ligament reconstruction technique
- insemination swim-up technique
- insertion technique
- inside-out technique
- inside-to-outside technique
- insufflation anesthetic technique
- intact canal wall technique
- intercostal nerve block anesthetic technique
- interference screw technique
- interlocking suture technique
- internal jugular vein cannulation anesthetic technique
- internal jugular vein catheterization anesthetic technique
- internal jugular vein puncture anesthetic technique
- internal jugular vein puncture technique
- interpleural anesthetic technique
- interrupted suture technique
- interscalene block anesthetic technique
- interspinous segmental spinal instrumentation technique
- interventional technique
- intra-articular anesthetic technique
- intracorporeal knotting technique
- intradermal mattress suture technique
- intradermal tattooing technique
- intramuscular preanesthetic medication anesthetic technique
- intraoperative computer-assisted spinal orientation technique

technique (*continued*)

intraperitoneal technique
intrathecal cannulation anesthetic technique
intrathecal morphine anesthetic technique
intravenous cannulation anesthetic technique
intravenous oxygen-15 water bolus technique
intubation anesthetic technique
invaginating suture technique
invagination technique
invasive technique
inverting knot technique
irrigation techniques
Irwin technique
ischemic-tourniquet technique
isocentric technique
isolation technique
isometric technique
Ivalon suture technique
J loop technique
Jaboulay-Doyen-Winkleman technique
Jacobs locking-hook spinal rod technique
Jacobson technique
Jakob technique
Janecki-Nelson technique
Jansey technique
Jeffrey technique
jejunoileal bypass reversal technique
Jerne technique
jet ventilation anesthetic technique
J-loop technique
Jobert suture technique
Johnson pelvic fracture technique
Johnson staple technique
Johnston pursestring suture technique
Jones-Jones wedge technique
Jones technique
Jones-Barnett technique
Jones-Brackett technique
Jones-Politano technique
Joplin technique

technique (*continued*)

Jorgensen technique
Judd pyloroplasty technique
Judkins cardiac catheterization technique
Judkins femoral catheterization technique
Judkins-Sones technique
jugular technique
Kader-Senn gastrotomy technique
Kalt suture technique
kangaroo tendon suture technique
Kapandji technique
Kapel elbow dislocation technique
Kapel technique
Kaplan technique
Karapandzic technique
Kashiwagi technique
Kates-Kessel-Kay technique
Kato thick smear technique
Kaufer tendon technique
Kaufmann technique
Kawamoto technique
Kazanjian vestibuloplasty technique
Kehr technique
Kelikian-Clayton-Loseff technique
Kelikian-Riashi-Gleason technique
Kellogg-Speed fusion technique
Kelly suture technique
Kendrick technique
Kendrick-Sharma-Hassler-Herndon technique
Kennedy ligament technique
Kern technique
Kerrison technique
Kesselring curet technique
Kessler suture technique
Kety-Schmidt inert gas saturation technique
keyhole tenodesis technique
Keystone technique
Kidde cannula technique
Kidner technique
King technique

technique (*continued*)
  King-Richards dislocation technique
  King-Steelquist technique
  Kirby sliding technique
  Kirk thigh amputation technique
  Kirschner suture technique
  kissing balloon technique
  Kjolbe technique
  Klein technique
  Kleinert technique
  Kleinschmidt technique
  Klisic-Jankovic technique
  Knoll refraction technique
  Knott technique
  Koch technique
  Koenig technique
  Kronig technique
  Krawkow-Cohn technique
  Krawkow-Thomas-Jones technique
  Krempen-Craig-Sotelo tibial nonunion technique
  Kristeller technique
  Kuettner technique
  Kuhnt-Szymanowski technique
  Kumar spica cast technique
  Kumar-Cowell-Ramsey technique
  Kutler finger amputation technique
  Kyoto-Barrett-Boyes perfusion technique
  Loeffler suture technique
  Labbe gastrotomy technique
  labiolingual technique
  lace suture technique
  lag technique
  Lamaze childbirth technique
  Lamaze technique
  Lamb-Marks-Bayne technique
  Lambrinudi technique
  Langenskiold technique
  laparoscopic colposuspension technique
  laparoscopic lymph node dissection technique
  laparoscopic Nissen fundoplication technique

technique (*continued*)
  laparoscopic para-aortic lymph node sampling technique
  laparoscopic stripping technique
  Lapidus hammertoe technique
  large-core technique
  Larson technique
  laryngeal mask insertion anesthetic technique
  laryngoscopy anesthetic technique
  laser dissection technique
  laser welding technique
  Lash technique
  Lassus technique
  lateral bending technique
  lateral window technique
  Laurell technique
  layer technique
  Lazarus-Nelson technique
  LCVP-aided technique
  LDN technique
  Le Dran suture technique
  Le Fort suture technique
  Leach technique
  Leadbetter modification technique
  Leboyer delivery technique
  LeDentu suture technique
  LeDuc technique
  Lee technique
  Lefevre gastrectomy technique
  Lehman technique
  Leibolt technique
  Lejour technique
  Leksell technique
  Lembert suture technique
  Lenart-Kullman technique
  lens suture technique
  lesser sac technique
  letterbox technique
  Lewit stretch technique
  Lich extravesical technique
  Lich-Gregoir technique
  Lichtman technique
  lid-loading technique
  lid-sharing technique
  Liebolt radioulnar technique

technique (*continued*)
  ligate-divide-staple technique
  ligation suture technique
  light-around-wire technique
  Limberg technique
  limb-saving technique
  Lindholm technique
  lingual split-bone technique
  lipo layering technique
  lipoinjection technique
  liposuction technique
  Lipscomb technique
  Lipscomb-Henderson-Elkins
    technique
  Lister technique
  Littler technique
  Littler-Cooley technique
  Lloyd-Roberts fracture
    technique
  Lloyd-Roberts-Lettin
    technique
  local standby anesthesia
    technique
  localization technique
  locking suture technique
  lock-stitch suture technique
  long cone technique
  loop gastric bypass technique
  loop-on mucosa suture
    technique
  Losee modification of
    MacIntosh technique
  Losee sling and reef
    technique
  loss-of-resistance technique
  lost wax pattern technique
  Lottes reduction technique
  LowDye taping technique
  low-flow anesthetic technique
  Lown technique
  Ludloff technique
  lumbar accessory movement
    technique
  lumbar anesthetic technique
  Luque instrumentation
    concave technique
  Luque instrumentation
    convex technique
  Luque sublaminar wiring
    technique
  LUS scanning technique
  Lyden technique

technique (*continued*)
  Lyden-Lehman technique
  Lynn technique
  MacIntosh technique
  macroelectrode recording
    technique
  Madden technique
  Magerl translaminar facet
    screw fixation technique
  Magilligan measuring
    technique
  Magnuson reduction
    technique
  MAGPI technique
  Ma-Griffith technique
  Maitland technique
  Majestro-Ruda-Frost tendon
    technique
  Malawer excision technique
  Mallory technique
  mammaplasty reduction
    technique
  Mancini technique
  mandibular swing technique
  mandibular-sparing technique
  Mankin technique
  Mann technique
  Mann-DuVries technique
  manometric technique
  Manske technique
  mantle technique
  manual push-pull technique
  Maquet technique
  Marbach-Weil technique
  March technique
  Marcus-Balourdas-Heiple ankle
    fusion technique
  Marks-Bayne technique
  Marlex plug technique
  Marshall ligament repair
    technique
  Marshall-McIntosh technique
  marsupialization technique
  Martin reduction technique
  masking technique
  masquerade technique
  massive dose technique
  MAST technique
  Mathieu technique
  Matti-Russe technique
  maxillary sinus Foley catheter
    balloon placement technique

technique (*continued*)
Mazet technique
McCauley technique
McConnell knee technique
McConnell medial glide
patellar taping technique
McCraw technique
McElfresh-Dobyns-O'Brien
technique
McElvenny technique
McFarland-Osborne technique
McFarlane technique
McGoon technique
McIndoe technique
McKeever-Buck elbow
technique
McKissock pedicle flap
technique
McLaughlin-Hay technique
McLean technique
McMaster technique
McReynolds open reduction
technique
McSpadden endodontic
technique
McVay technique
Meares-Stamey technique
mechanical ventilation
anesthetic technique
Mehn-Quigley technique
Meigs suture technique
membrane catheter technique
Menghini biopsy technique
Mensor-Scheck technique
Merendino technique
Merrill Supramid suturing
technique
Messerklinger technique
Meyerding-Van Demark
technique
Michal II technique
microelectrode recording
technique
microelectrode technique
microetching technique
micrograft punctiform
technique
microinvasive technique
micromanipulation technique
microsurgery technique
microsurgical technique
microtransducer technique

technique (*continued*)
microtubulotomy technique
microvascular technique
midface degloving technique
Milch cuff resection of ulna
technique
Milch elbow technique
Milford mallet finger
technique
Millard forked flap technique
Millard rotation-advancement
technique
Millen technique
Miller technique
Millesi modified technique
minilaparotomy technique
minimal leak technique
minimal-access technique
minimally invasive surgical
technique
Mital elbow release technique
miter technique
Mitrofanoff continent urinary
diversion technique
Mizuno technique
Mizuno-Hirohata-Kashiwagi
technique
modified anterior scoring
technique
modified Belsey
fundoplication technique
modified Bernard-Burow
technique
modified brachial technique
modified Cantwell technique
modified Child technique
modified Hassan open
technique
modified piggyback
technique
modified Pomeroy technique
modified Sacks-Vine push-pull
technique
modified Seldinger technique
modified Skoog technique
modified technique
modified Toupe technique
modified V-Y advancement
technique
Moe scoliosis technique
Mohs fresh tissue
chemosurgery technique

technique (*continued*)

Mohs micrographic surgery
  by fixed-tissue technique
molecular technique
monitored anesthesia care
  anesthetic technique
monitoring technique
monorail technique
Monticelli-Spinelli distraction
  technique
Moore technique
morcellation technique
Morgan-Casscells meniscus
  suturing technique
Morrison technique
Mose technique
motor point block anesthetic
  technique
moving strip x-ray technique
M-plasty technique
Mubarak-Hargens
  decompression technique
mucoperiosteal flap
  technique
mucosal relaxing incision
  technique
Mueller technique
Mullins blade technique
multiplanar endoscopic facial
  rejuvenation technique
multiplanar upper facial
  rejuvenation technique
multiple inert gas elimination
  technique (MIGET)
multiple-port incision
  technique
muscle advancement
  technique
muscle energy technique
muscle-splitting technique
Mustarde technique
Muti technique
Nalebuff-Millender lateral band
  mobilization technique
nasotracheal intubation
  anesthetic technique
nasovesicular catheter
  technique
Nealon technique
near-and-far suture technique
needle thoracentesis
  technique

technique (*continued*)

needle-knife technique
needle-through-needle single
  interspace technique
nerve stimulator anesthetic
  technique
nerve suture technique
neural archresection
  technique
neuroablative technique
neuroleptanalgesia anesthetic
  technique
Neviaser acromioclavicular
  technique
Neviaser-Wilson-Gardner
  technique
Nicholas 5-in-1 reconstruction
  technique
Nicholas ligament technique
Nickel-Perry technique
Niebauer-King technique
Nikaidoh-Bex technique
Nirschl technique
Nissen fundoplication
  technique
Nissen-Rosseti fundoplication
  technique
nitrous oxide-opioid-
  barbiturate anesthetic
  technique
no-leak technique
nonsterile technique
noose suture technique
Norfolk technique
Northern blot technique
no-touch surgical technique
no-touch technique
Oakley-Fulthorpe technique
Ober tendon technique
Ober-Barr transfer technique
O'Brien akinesia technique
Obtura injectable technique
Ockerblad ureter technique
off-center isoperistaltic
  technique
Ogata technique
Ogura technique
Okamura technique
Ollier technique
Omer technique
Omer-Capen technique
onlay technique

technique (*continued*)

onlay-tube-onlay urethroplasty technique
open drop technique
open flap technique
open harvesting technique
open Hasson technique
open laparoscopic technique
open palm technique
open technique
open-gloving technique
open-patch technique
open-sky technique
operative technique
O'Phelan technique
optimal technique
oral anesthetic technique
Orandi technique
orbital exenteration gastroscopic access technique
Orr technique
Orticochea scalping technique
Osborne-Cotterill elbow technique
Osgood modified technique
Osmond-Clarke technique
Ostrup harvesting technique
Otlinger technique
Ouchterlony gel diffusion technique
outside-to-outside arthroscopy technique
over-and-over suture technique
Overhauser technique
overlapping suture technique
over-the-wire technique
Oxford technique
Pacey technique
pacing technique
Pack technique
Pagenstecher suture technique
Palfyn suture technique
palliative technique
Palmer technique
Palmer-Widen shoulder technique
Palomo technique

technique (*continued*)

Panas ptosis correction technique
Pancoast suture technique
Pang technique
pants-over-vest technique
Papineau technique
Paquin technique
paradoxical technique
parallel technique
paralleling technique
paresthesia anesthetic technique
Parker-Kerr suture technique
Parrish-Mann hammertoe technique
Parvin gravity technique
Pare suture technique
PAS technique
passive gliding technique
patch technique
Paterson technique
patient-controlled analgesia anesthetic technique
Paulos ligament technique
Pauwels technique
Peacock transposing technique
peg-and-socket technique
Pelosi technique
pelviscopic clip ligation technique
Perclose technique
Percoll technique
percutaneous insertion technique
percutaneous interventional technique
percutaneous Judkins technique
percutaneous transfemoral technique
perfusion hypothermia technique
perfusion measurement technique
perfusion technique
periareolar technique
peribulbar anesthetic technique
pericostal suture technique

technique (*continued*)
peripheral nerve block
    anesthetic technique
Perry technique
Perry-Nickel technique
Perry-O'Brien-Hodgson
    technique
Perry-Robinson cervical
    technique
Petit suture technique
Pheasant elbow technique
Phemister onlay bone graft
    technique
Phemister-Bonfiglio technique
phrenic nerve block
    anesthetic technique
Pichlmayer technique
Pierrot-Murphy tendon
    technique
pin suture technique
pinch-grasp injection
    technique
plaque technique
plastic matrix technique
plastic suture technique
plicating suture technique
Polya technique
Ponka anesthetic technique
Ponka local anesthesia
    technique
Ponsky pull or guidewire
    insertion technique
porcelain cervical ditching
    technique
Porstmann technique
Porter-Richardson-Vainio
    technique
Positran technique
posterior flap technique
posterolateral
    costotransversectomy
    technique
postresection filling
    technique
Pratt technique
premuscular mesh technique
presaturation technique
preservation technique
pressure half-time technique
primary suture technique
Pringle vascular control
    technique

technique (*continued*)
Proetz displacement
    technique
prograde technique
projection-reconstruction
    technique
projective technique
pseudobiopsy technique
Puddu tendon technique
pulley suture technique
pull-out wire suture
    technique
pull-through technique
pulmonary artery
    catheterization anesthetic
    technique
Pulvertaft weave technique
puppet technique
pursestring suture technique
push plus refraction
    technique
push-back technique
push-pull T technique
Putti technique
quadrant sampling technique
Quartey technique
quick angulation technique
Quickert 3-suture technique
quilt suture technique
Quenu nail plate removal
    technique
radiographic technique
radioguided technique
radiologic technique
radionuclide technique
Radley-Liebig-Brown
    technique
Rainville technique
Ralston-Thompson
    pseudoarthrosis technique
Ranawat-DeFiore-Straub
    technique
rapid pull-through esophageal
    manometry technique
rapid scan technique
rapid-sequence induction
    anesthetic technique
Rapp technique
Rashkind balloon technique
Ray-Clancy-Lemon technique
Rayhack technique
reattribution technique

technique (*continued*)

rebreathing technique
Rebuck skin window technique
recanalization technique
recombinant DNA technique
reconstruction technique
reconstructive technique
recovery technique
rectal anesthetic technique
reducing technique
reduction technique
refractive operative technique
regional anesthetic technique
Reichel-Polya technique
Reichenheim technique
relaxation technique
Renard technique
rescue technique
resectional technique
restorative proctocolectomy technique
retained papilla technique
retention suture technique
retrobulbar anesthetic technique
retrograde tracheal intubation anesthetic technique
retromuscular prosthetic technique
reverse wedge technique
revival techniques
Reynolds-Horton alar cartilage technique
rhythmic initiation technique
ribbon arch technique
Richardson suture technique
Richards-Saltzman-Flynn technique
Richter suture technique
Ricketts-Abrams technique
Rideau technique
right-angle technique
Riordan tendon transfer technique
Risser technique
Ritter-Oleson technique
Roberts technique
Robicsek technique
Robinson-Southwick fusion technique
Rockwood-Green technique

technique (*continued*)

Rogers cervical fusion technique
rollerball technique
roll-tube technique
Rood technique
Rosalki technique
Ross technique
rotation skin flap technique
Roveda technique
Royle-Thompson transfer technique
RPT technique
Rumel technique
running continuous suture technique
running technique
running vascular technique
running W-plasty technique
Russe technique
Russell technique
Ryerson technique
sacral bar technique
Saeed technique
Saenger suture technique
safety technique
Sage technique
Sage-Clark technique
Saha transfer technique
Sakellarides-DeWeese technique
saline technique
Salter technique
Saltzman-Flynn-Richards technique
salvage technique
Sammarco-DiRaimondo modification of Elmslie technique
Sarmiento trochanteric fracture technique
Scaglietti closed reduction technique
scanning technique
scapular island flap technique
Schatz laser technique
Schauwecker patellar wiring technique
Scheie technique
Schepens technique
Schepsis-Leach technique
Schiller D&C technique

technique (*continued*)
Schlatter gastrectomy
 technique
Schneider technique
Schnute wedge resection
 technique
Schober technique
Schonander technique
Schoonmaker-King single-
 catheter technique
Schrudde curet technique
Schwartz-Baumgard technique
scleral search coil technique
Scott glenoplasty technique
screw insertion technique
Scudder technique
Scuderi technique
sealed envelope technique
Sealy-Laragh technique
secondary suture technique
section freeze substitution
 technique
sectional technique
Seddon technique
segment-oriented technique
Seldinger percutaneous
 technique
Seldinger retrograde wire
 intubation technique
Seldinger-Desilet technique
selective bronchial
 catheterization anesthetic
 technique
Sell-Frank-Johnson extensor
 shift technique
Semb nephrectomy technique
semitendinosus technique
Semm Z technique
sensorineural acuity level
 technique
Serafin technique
seromuscular suture
 technique
seroserous suture technique
Sever modification of
 Fairbank technique
Sewall technique
sextant technique
Shaberg-Harper-Allen
 technique
Shambaugh technique
sharp dissection technique

technique (*continued*)
Sharrard transfer technique
shave excision technique
Sheehan-Dodge technique
Sherk-Probst technique
Shirodkar suture technique
shish-kebab technique
shoelace technique
short lever accessory
 movement technique
short-scar technique
short-cone technique
shorthand vertical mattress
 stitch suture technique
Siegel technique
Silber technique
Silfverskiold lengthening
 technique
silver dollar technique
Simmons technique
Simon suture technique
Simonton technique
simple suture technique
Sims suture technique
Singer-Blom endoscopic
 tracheoesophageal
 puncture technique
single proximal portal
 technique
single space technique
single-armed suture technique
single-port technique
single-pour technique
single-shot imaging technique
skewer technique
skin expansion technique
skin flap rotation technique
skin window technique
skin-only periareolar-approach
 mastopexy technique
skin-surfacing technique
Skoog technique
sleeve technique
sliding fat pad technique
sliding skin flap technique
sliding technique
sling and blanket technique
sling and reef technique
sling suture technique
sling/wrapping technique
slit catheter technique
Slocum amputation technique

technique (*continued*)
- Slocum fusion technique
- slot-blot technique
- SMAS face-lift technique
- smiley-face knotting technique
- Smith Indian technique
- Smith technique
- Smith-Petersen technique
- Smith-Robinson technique
- snapshot GRASS technique
- snare technique
- Snellen suture technique
- Sofield femoral deficiency technique
- soluble gas technique
- Somerville technique
- Sones brachial cutdown technique
- Sones cineangiography technique
- sonication technique
- Soto-Hall bone graft technique
- Southern blot technique
- spaghetti fat grafting technique
- Sparks mandrel technique
- Speed-Boyd radial-ulnar technique
- Speed-Boyd reduction technique
- sperm microaspiration retrieval technique
- sphincter-saving technique
- sphincter-sparing technique
- Spiller-Frazier technique
- spin technique
- spinal anesthetic technique
- spinal fusion technique
- spinal mobilization technique
- spin-echo scanning technique
- spiral CT technique
- spiral suture technique
- Spivack gastrotomy technique
- Spivack valve technique
- split cuff nipple technique
- split-and-roll technique
- split-bone technique
- split-course technique
- spontaneous ventilation anesthetic technique
- Sprague arthroscopic technique

technique (*continued*)
- spread-and-cut technique
- SPT technique (station pull-through technique)
- Staheli technique
- Stamm-Kader gastrotomy technique
- standard biopsy technique
- standard technique
- Stanisavljevc technique
- stapled reconstruction technique
- Staples technique
- stapling technique
- STAR technique
- Stark-Moore-Ashworth-Boyes technique
- star-shaped omphaloplasty technique
- startle technique
- Starzl technique
- static dilation technique
- station pull-through esophageal manometry technique
- station pull-through technique (SPT technique)
- stay suture technique
- Steffee instrumentation technique
- Steichen technique
- Steindler technique
- stellate ganglion block anesthetic technique
- Stenstrom alar cartilage technique
- Stent skin graft technique
- stenting technique
- stent-through-wire mesh technique
- step-by-step technique
- stepladder incision technique
- stereotactic automated technique
- stereotactic core biopsy technique
- stereotaxic technique
- sterile technique
- Sternberger antibody sandwich technique
- Stewart technique

technique (*continued*)

Stewart-Hamilton cardiac output technique
stick-tie suture technique
Stiegmann-Goff technique
Stiles-Bunnell transfer technique
still radiography technique
Stillman technique
Stimson anterior shoulder reduction technique
stimulated gracilis neosphincter technique
strain/counterstrain technique
Strassman technique
Straub technique
Strayer tendon technique
stretch-and-spray technique
Strickland technique
strip biopsy resection technique
strut fusion technique
Studebaker technique
Sturmdorf suture technique
subclavian flap technique
subcuticular suture technique
subpectoral implantation technique
subperiosteal implant one-phase technique
subplatysmal face-lift technique
subtraction technique
suction-irrigation technique
superwet technique
superficial suture technique
superior mesenterorenal bypass technique
support suture technique
supraphysiologic fluid technique
surface cooling technique
surgical enucleation technique
surgical neurangiographic technique
surgical suture technique
surgical technique
surveillance technique
sustained pressure technique
suture anchor technique
suture closure technique
Swanson technique

technique (*continued*)

Swiss roll embedding technique
switched B-gradient technique
sympathetic blockade anesthetic technique
sympathetic ganglion block anesthetic technique
Tachdjian hamstring technique
Tajima suture technique
Tamai technique
tandem clipping technique
tarsodermal fixation technique
Taylor suture technique
Taylor-Daniel-Weiland technique
Teimourian-Adhan technique
Teimourian curet technique
telemetric technique
telescoping suture technique
tendon suture technique
tension band wiring technique
tension suture technique
Terzis technique
test dose anesthetic technique
Teuffer technique
Thal fundoplication technique
thermal dilution technique
thermal expansion technique
thermocatalytic technique
thermodilution technique
Thiersch suture technique
thiopental-sufentanil-desflurane-nitrous oxide anesthetic technique
Thomas technique
Thomas-Thompson-Straub transfer technique
Thompson reduction technique
Thompson-Henry technique
Thompson-Loomer technique
thoracic epidural anesthetic technique
thoracolumbar spondylosis surgical technique
threaded-hole-first technique
through-and-through suture technique

technique (*continued*)
thyroid surgical technique
thyroidectomy technique
Tillman resurfacing technique
tissue-expansion technique
tissue-sparing technique
titration technique
Todd-Evans stepladder tracheal
dilatation technique
Tohen tendon technique
Tom Jones suture technique
Tompkins median bivalving
technique
tongue-and-groove suture
technique
tongue-in-groove technique
topical anesthetic technique
Torg technique
Torgerson-Leach modified
technique
total etch technique
total fundoplication
technique
total intravenous anesthetic
technique
Toupe technique
tracheal extubation anesthetic
technique
tracheal intubation anesthetic
technique
tracheal suction anesthetic
technique
traction suture technique
transanal stapling technique
transarterial anesthetic
technique
transcranial electrical
stimulation anesthetic
technique
transdermal anesthetic
technique
transfixing suture technique
transiliac bar technique
translaryngeal guided
intubation anesthetic
technique
transmucosal drug
administration anesthetic
technique
transperitoneal technique
transtracheal jet ventilation
anesthetic technique

technique (*continued*)
trapezius stimulation
anesthetic technique
Trethowan-Stamm-Simmonds-
Menelaus-Haddad technique
triangulation technique
triple-wire technique
trocar technique
trocar-cannula technique
Trueta technique
Trusler aortic valve technique
T-tube technique
tubal ligation band technique
tube-shift technique
tube-within-tube technique
Tuffier morcellement
technique
Tullos technique
tumbling technique
tumescent technique
Turco clubfoot release
technique
turn-and-suction biopsy
technique
Turnbull technique
twisted suture technique
twist-off technique
Uchida technique
ultrasonographic technique
ultrasound anesthetic
technique
uncut Collis-Nissen
fundoplication technique
underlay fascia technique
unilateral inguinal hernia
repair technique
uninterrupted suture
technique
unitunnel technique
unlocking spiral technique
upgated technique
Urbaniak technique
Ussing chamber technique
Van Beek-Zook technique
Van Lint modified technique
Van Millingen eyelid repair
technique
vascular isolation technique
Vastamaki technique
Veleanu-Rosianu-Ionescu
technique
velocity catheter technique

technique (*continued*)
- venous access technique
- ventral bending technique
- Verdan technique
- Verhoeff suture technique
- vertical mattress suture technique
- vertical-cut technique
- Vest technique
- vest-over-pants technique
- Vidal-Ardrey fracture technique
- video transurethral resection technique
- video-assisted technique
- videofluoroscopic technique
- Vim-Silverman technique
- Visnevskyh anesthetic technique
- Velpius-Compere tendon technique
- volumetric technique
- Volz-Turner reattachment technique
- von Haberer-Finey gastrectomy technique
- V-Y advancement technique
- Wolfler suture technique
- Wadsworth technique
- Wagner limb-lengthening technique
- Wagner open reduction technique
- Wagner resurfacing technique
- Wagner-Baldwin technique
- Wagoner cervical technique
- Waldhausen subclavian flap technique
- Wallace technique
- Wanger reduction technique
- Wardill technique
- Warner-Farber ankle fixation technique
- Warwick and Ashken technique
- wash technique
- washed-field technique
- water-suppression technique
- Watkins fusion technique
- Watson technique
- Watson-Cheyne technique

technique (*continued*)
- wax pattern thermal expansion technique
- wax-matrix technique
- Weaver-Dunn acromioclavicular technique
- Weber-Brunner-Freuler-Boitzy technique
- Weber-Vasey traction-absorption wiring technique
- Weckesser technique
- Weine technique
- Weinstein-Ponseti technique
- Weir pattern skin flap technique
- Weir-pattern skin flap technique
- Welch technique
- Wertheim-Bohlman technique
- West-Soto-Hall patellar technique
- wet technique
- whipstitch suture technique
- Whitesides technique
- Whitesides-Kelly cervical technique
- Whitman technique
- whole blood lysis technique
- Wickham technique
- Willi glass crown technique
- Williams-Haddad technique
- Wilson technique
- Wilson-Jacobs tibial fracture fixation technique
- Wilson-McKeever shoulder technique
- window technique
- Windson-Insall-Vince grafting technique
- Winograd technique
- Winter elevation torque technique
- Winter spondylolisthesis technique
- wire removal technique
- Wirth-Jager tendon technique
- Woodward technique
- xenon-133 technique
- xenon-washout technique
- Yankauer suction technique

technique (*continued*)
  Yasargil technique
  Young technique
  Young-Dees technique
  Y-suture technique
  Zancolli rerouting technique
  Zarins-Rowe ligament
    technique
  Zavala technique
  Zazepen-Gamidov technique
  Zeier transfer technique
  Zielde technique
  Zocchi ultrasound-assisted
    lipoplasty technique
  Z-plasty technique
  Z-suture technique
  Zuker and Manketlow
    technique
Technomed Sonolith lithotriptor
Techstar percutaneous closure
  device
Techstar suturing closure device
Tecnol ankle support
Tecnol back support
Tecnol elbow support
Tecnol knee support
Tecnol wrist support
tectocephaly
tectonic keratoplasty
Tectonic magnet
tectorial membrane
tectospinal decussation
tectum of brain stem
tectum of midbrain
TED (thromboembolic disease)
TED hose
TED pneumatic compression
  boots
TED socks
TED stockings
Tedlar bag
TEE (transesophageal
  echocardiography)
Teebi hypertelorism syndrome
Teebi-Shalout syndrome
teeth
  acrylic resin teeth
  barred teeth
  bicuspid teeth
  canine teeth
  carious teeth
  connate teeth

teeth (*continued*)
  cross-pin teeth
  cuspid teeth
  decayed teeth
  deciduous teeth
  erupted teeth
  extraction of teeth
  false teeth
  Fournier teeth
  fused teeth
  geminate teeth
  Huschke auditory teeth
  impacted teeth
  inferior teeth
  labial teeth
  lower teeth
  malacotic teeth
  mandibular teeth
  maxillary teeth
  morsal teeth
  multicuspid teeth
  natural teeth
  premolar teeth
  rake teeth
  screwdriver teeth
  straight-pin teeth
  succedaneous teeth
  successional teeth
  tissue forceps with teeth
  tissue forceps without teeth
teeth ligation
teeth malocclusion
teeth malposition
Teevan lithotrite
Tefcat intrauterine insemination
  catheter
Teflo-Kapton freezing bag
Teflon Bardic plug
Teflon block
Teflon bolster
Teflon button
Teflon cannula
Teflon catheter
Teflon clip
Teflon coating
Teflon collar button
Teflon endolymphatic shunt tube
Teflon ERCP cannula
Teflon ERCP catheter
Teflon felt bolster
Teflon felt patch
Teflon felt pledget

Teflon glycerin-mixture
   injection needle
Teflon glycerin-mixture syringe
Teflon graft
Teflon guiding catheter
Teflon implant
Teflon injection catheter
Teflon injector
Teflon intracardiac patch
Teflon intracardiac patch
   prosthesis
Teflon iris retractor
Teflon liner
Teflon material
Teflon mesh implant
Teflon mesh prosthesis
Teflon mold
Teflon nasobiliary drain
Teflon needle
Teflon needle catheter
Teflon orbital floor implant
Teflon paste injection for
   incontinence
Teflon patch
Teflon piston
Teflon plate
Teflon pledget
Teflon pledget suture buttress
Teflon plug
Teflon probe
Teflon prosthesis
Teflon sheath
Teflon sheeting prosthesis
Teflon shunt tube
Teflon Silastic loop
Teflon sling rectopexy
Teflon sling repair
Teflon splint
Teflon strut
Teflon strut-cutting block
Teflon tape
Teflon tip
Teflon trileaflet prosthesis
Teflon tube
Teflon wire piston prosthesis
Teflon woven prosthesis
Teflon-coated Dacron sutures
Teflon-coated driver
Teflon-coated guidewire
Teflon-coated hollow-bore
   needle
Teflon-covered needle

Teflon-Delrin cutting block
Teflon-pledgeted sutures
Teflon-tipped catheter
Teflon-wire piston
Tef-wire prosthesis
Tegaderm occlusive dressing
Tegaderm semipermeable
   dressing
Tegaderm semipermeable
   occlusive dressing
Tegaderm transparent dressing
Tegagel hydrogel dressing
Tegagen alginate wound
   dressing
Tegapore contact-layer wound
   dressing
Tegasorb occlusive dressing
Tegasorb ulcer dressing
tegmen (*pl.* tegmina)
tegmen cellulae
tegmen cranii
tegmen mastoideum
tegmental cells
tegmental region
tegmental wall
tegmentum (*pl.* tegmenta)
tegmentum of midbrain
TEGwire balloon
TEGwire balloon dilatation
   catheter
TEGwire guide
Tehl clamp
Teimourian-Adhan technique
Teimourian aspirator lipoplasty
Teimourian curet technique
Tek tube
Tekno coagulator
Tekno forceps
Tek-Pro needle
Tekscan in-shoe monitoring
   device
Tektronix digital oscilloscope
telangiectases
telangiectasia macularis eruptiva
   perstans (TMEP)
telangiectasia verrucosa
telangiectasis (*pl.*
   telangiectases)
telangiectatic angioma
telangiectatic cancer
telangiectatic erythema
telangiectatic facial birthmark

telangiectatic fibroma
telangiectatic glioma
telangiectatic osteogenic
  sarcoma
telangiectatic wart
telangiectaticum
telangiitis
telangioma
telangiosis
telecanthus
telecentric fundus camera
telecobalt therapy
Telectronics Guardian ATP 4210
  device
Telectronics lithium pacer
Telectronics pacemaker
telecurietherapy
telemetric monitoring
telemetric pressure sensor
telemetric technique
telemetry monitor
telemonitoring
telencephalic malformation
telephone probe
telepresence surgery
teleradiography
teleradiology
Telerobotic-assisted laparoscopy
teleroentgenogram
telescope
  ACMI microlens Foroblique
    telescope
  ACMI microlens telescope
  angled telescope
  Atkins esophagoscopic
    telescope
  Best direct forward-vision
    telescope
  biopsy telescope
  bioptic telescope
  Bridge telescope
  bronchoscopic telescope
  Broyles telescope
  Burns bridge telescope
  catheterizing Foroblique
    telescope
  clamp-on telescope
  convertible telescope
  direct forward-vision
    telescope
  direct-vision telescope
  double-catheterizing telescope

telescope (*continued*)
  endoscopic telescope
  examining telescope
  fiberoptic right-angle
    telescope
  Foroblique bronchoscopic
    telescope
  high-vision surgical telescope
  Holinger bronchoscopic
    telescope
  Hopkins direct-vision
    telescope
  Hopkins endoscopy telescope
  Hopkins forward-oblique
    telescope
  Hopkins lateral telescope
  Hopkins nasal endoscopy
    telescope
  Hopkins pediatric telescope
  Hopkins retrospective
    telescope
  Hopkins rigid telescope
  Hopkins rod lens telescope
  infant telescope
  Keeler panoramic surgical
    telescope
  Kramer direct-vision
    telescope
  laryngeal-bronchial telescope
  lateral microlens telescope
  LUMINA-operating telescope
  LUMINA-SL telescope
  Luxtec illuminated surgical
    telescope
  Luxtec surgical telescope
  McCarthy Foroblique
    operating telescope
  McCarthy miniature telescope
  Microlens direct-vision
    telescope
  Microlens Foroblique
    telescope
  Mueller telescope
  nasal endoscopic telescope
  Negus telescope
  operating telescope
  pediatric telescope
  retrospective bronchoscopic
    telescope
  right-angle examining
    telescope
  right-angle telescope

telescope (*continued*)
  Selsi sport telescope
  solid-rod rigid telescope
  stop collar telescope
  Storz bronchoscopic
    telescope
  Storz-Hopkins telescope
  straight ahead bronchoscopic
    telescope
  surgical telescope
  Surgi-Spec telescope
  transilluminating telescope
  Tucker direct-vision telescope
  Vest direct forward-vision
    telescope
  Walden telescope
  Zeiss binocular prism
    telescope
telescope adapting bridge
telescope bridge
telescope catheter
telescope of cystocope
telescoped navel
telescopic view guide
telescoping brace
telescoping crossbite
telescoping guide
telescoping medullary rod
telescoping plugged catheter
telescoping rod
telescoping septal fracture
telescoping suture technique
teletherapy
Teletrast gauze
Telfa 4 x 4 bandage
Telfa adhesive pads
Telfa bolster
Telfa Clear nonadherent wound
  dressing
Telfa gauze
Telfa gauze dressing
Telfa island dressing
Telfa pad
Telfa plastic film dressing
Telfa Plus barrier island dressing
Telfa sterile adhesive pad
Telfa Xtra absorbent island
  dressing
Telfamax ultra absorbent
  dressing
TelGen-FD guided tissue
  regeneration membrane

TelGen-FD plastic membrane
TeliCam intraoral camera
TeLinde hysterectomy
TeLinde operation
TeLinde-Everett operation
telorbitism
telorism
Telos fracture table
Telos radiographic stress device
Telson hinged walking heel
Temarack flexure joint
Temens curet
TEMNO biopsy needle
temperature and galvanic skin
    response biofeedback device
temperature gradient
temperature probe
temperature-dependent
    dermatosis
temperature-sensing pacemaker
Temperlite saw blade
temperoparietal facial flap
    interposition
template
  acetabular cup template
  flange of Syed template
  implant template
  McKissock keyhole areolar
    template
  Moore template
  rod template
  Strombeck template
  surgical template
  Surgiguide template
  Syed template
  Syed-Neblett template
  Thompson template
  tissue expander template
  tissue sizer template
  total toe template
  wire template
  x-ray template
template markings
template splint
Temple procedure
Temple University nail
Temple University plate
Temple-Fay laminectomy retractor
Templeton-Zim carpal tunnel
    projection
Tempo denture liner
temporal aponeurosis

temporal arcade
temporal area
temporal arteries
temporal arteriole of retina
temporal arteritis
temporal artery biopsy
temporal bone anomaly
temporal bone bank
temporal bone fracture
temporal bone holder
temporal canal
temporal canthus
temporal diameter
temporal diploic vein
temporal electrode
temporal facial nerve
temporal fascia
temporal fascial flap
temporal field
temporal fossa abscess
temporal giant cell arteritis
temporal gyrus
temporal horn of lateral
    ventricle
temporal incision
temporal island pedicle scalp flap
temporal line
temporal lobe
temporal lobectomy
temporal margin
temporal muscle
temporal muscle and fascia flap
temporal nerves
temporal plane
temporal process of mandible
temporal process of zygomatic
    bone
temporal region
temporal retina
temporal space
temporal squama
temporal sulcus
temporal surface of frontal bone
temporal surface of great wing
temporal surface of zygomatic
    bone
temporal suture
temporal trephine
temporal vein
temporal venule
temporal-cerebral arterial
    anastomosis

temporalis fascia graft
temporalis fascia flap
temporalis flap
temporalis muscle
temporalis muscle flap
temporalis muscle transposition
temporalis muscle-fascia transfer
temporalis sling
temporalis superficialis fascia
temporalis transfer clamp
temporal-pterygomaxillary fossa
temporary aortic shunt
    subclavian-subclavian bypass
temporary base
temporary callus
temporary cartilage
temporary clip
temporary diverting colostomy
temporary end colostomy
temporary endodontic
    restorative material (TERM)
temporary fecal diversion
temporary lip augmentation
temporary loop ileostomy
temporary magnet
temporary material
temporary nerve blockade
temporary pacemaker
temporary pacing catheter
temporary pacing wire
temporary percutaneous SCS
    electrode
temporary pervenous lead
temporary prosthesis
temporary skin replacement
temporary stricture
temporary transvenous
    pacemaker
temporary vascular clip
temporary vessel clip
temporoauricular
temporofacial graft
temporofrontal
temporohyoid
temporomalar suture
temporomandibular arthralgia
temporomandibular arthrosis
temporomandibular articular
    disk
temporomandibular articulation
temporomandibular dysfunction
    (TMD)

temporomandibular endoscopic
　lift
temporomandibular joint
temporomandibular joint (TMJ)
temporomandibular joint
　ankylosis
temporomandibular joint
　articular eminence
temporomandibular joint
　articulation
temporomandibular joint capsule
temporomandibular joint click
temporomandibular joint
　dislocation
temporomandibular joint
　dysfunction (TMD, TMJ)
temporomandibular joint fossa
temporomandibular joint
　hypermobility
temporomandibular joint
　osteoarthritis (TMJ-OA)
temporomandibular joint pain-
　dysfunction syndrome
temporomandibular joint
　radiograph
temporomandibular joint
　remodeling
temporomandibular joint sprain
temporomandibular joint
　subluxation
temporomandibular joint
　synovial fluid
temporomandibular ligament
temporomandibular luxation
temporomandibular pain-
　dysfunction (TMPD)
temporomandibular pain-
　dysfunction disorder (TMPD)
temporomaxillary articulation
temporomaxillary joint
temporo-occipital
temporoparietal fascia
temporoparietal fascial flap (TPFF)
temporoparietal muscle
temporoparieto-occipital flap
temporoparieto-occipital
　rotation flap
temporosphenoid
temporozygomatic suture
TempTrac temperature monitor
Tempur-Med hospital
　replacement mattress

Tempur-Med lumbar pad
Tempur-Med pillow
Tempur-Med stretch pad
Tempur-Med wheelchair
　cushion
Tempur-Pedic pressure relieving
　Swedish mattress
Tempur-Pedic pressure relieving
　Swedish pillow
Tempur-Plus mattress
Temrex dental cement
Ten balloon
Ten system balloon catheter
Tena pouch
tenacious adhesion
tenacious mucoid secretion
tenaculum
　Abel-Aesculap-Pratt tenaculum
　Adair breast tenaculum
　Adair uterine tenaculum
　Adair-Allis tenaculum
　Aesculap-Pratt tenaculum
　atraumatic tenaculum
　Barrett uterine tenaculum
　Bierer tenaculum
　Braun uterine tenaculum
　Braun-Schroeder single-tooth
　　tenaculum
　breast tenaculum
　Brophy tenaculum
　bullet tenaculum
　cervical tenaculum
　cleft palate tenaculum
　Coakley tenaculum
　Collen-Pozzi tenaculum
　Corey tenaculum
　Cottle sharp tenaculum
　Cottle single-prong tenaculum
　Crossen puncturing
　　tenaculum
　DeLee tenaculum
　double-hook skin tenaculum
　double-tooth tenaculum
　Dudley tenaculum
　Duplay uterine tenaculum
　Emmet uterine tenaculum
　Emmet cervical tenaculum
　Ferguson tenaculum
　Gaylor tenaculum
　goiter tenaculum
　Hulka uterine tenaculum
　Jackson tracheal tenaculum

tenaculum (*continued*)
  Jacob uterine tenaculum
  Jacobs uterine tenaculum
  Jarcho uterine tenaculum
  Joseph tenaculum
  Kahn traction tenaculum
  Kahn trigger tenaculum
  Kelly uterine tenaculum
  Kennett tenaculum
  Kustner tenaculum
  Lahey goiter tenaculum
  Lahey thyroid tenaculum
  Lillie-White tenaculum
  lion-jaw tenaculum
  Marlex atraumatic obstetrical
    tenaculum
  Marlex atraumatic tenaculum
  Museux tenaculum
  nasal tenaculum
  New tenaculum
  Newman uterine tenaculum
  Potts tenaculum
  Potts-Smith tenaculum
  Pozzi tenaculum
  Pratt tenaculum
  Revots vulsellum tenaculum
  ring-toothed tenaculum
  Ritchie cleft palate tenaculum
  Sargis uterine tenaculum
  Schroeder forceps tenaculum
  Schroeder uterine tenaculum
  Schwartz tenaculum
  screw tenaculum
  sharp-toothed tenaculum
  Sims tenaculum
  single-tooth tenaculum
  Skene uterine tenaculum
  Staude uterine tenaculum
  Staude-Jackson uterine
    tenaculum
  Staude-Moore uterine
    tenaculum
  straight tenaculum
  Sturgis tenaculum
  Teale tenaculum
  Tensor tenaculum
  Thoms tenaculum
  thyroid tenaculum
  tonsillar screw tenaculum
  tonsillar tenaculum
  toothed tenaculum
  tracheal tenaculum

tenaculum (*continued*)
  traction tenaculum
  uterine tenaculum
  Watts tenaculum
  Weisman tenaculum
  White tenaculum
  Wylie uterine tenaculum
tenaculum forceps
tenaculum holder
tenaculum hook
tenaculum hook loop
tenaculum traction
tenaculum-reducing forceps
Tenador male pouch
Tenax coronary stent
Tenckhoff 2-cuff catheter
Tenckhoff peritoneal catheter
Tenckhoff peritoneal dialysis
    catheter
Tenckhoff renal dialysis catheter
tender line
tender mass
tender point
Tender subcutaneous infusion
    set
Tender Touch extractor
Tender Touch vacuum birthing
    cup
tender trigger points (TrPs)
TenderCloud pressure pad
Tenderfoot incision-making device
Tenderlett device
tenderness
  abdominal tenderness
  deep abdominal tenderness
  epigastric regionepigastric
    tenderness
  exquisite tenderness
  flank tenderness
  focal tenderness
  generalized tenderness
  intercostal tenderness
  joint tenderness
  localized tenderness
  point tenderness
  rebound tenderness
  suprapubic tenderness
tenderness on palpation
tenderness on pressure
tenderness on rebound
tenderness to percussion
tenderness to touch

Tendersorb ABD pad
tendines (*sing.* tendo)
tendineus
  arcus tendineus
tendinitis
  bicipital tendinitis
  calcific tendinitis
  rotator cuff tendinitis
  stenosing tendinitis
tendinitis ossificans traumatica
tendinomyoplastic amputation
tendinoplasty
tendinosutures
tendinotrochanteric ligament
tendinous
tendinous arch
tendinous arch of levator ani
tendinous center
tendinous chiasm
tendinous chiasm of flexor
    digitorum sublimis muscle
tendinous galea
tendinous insertion
tendinous intersection
tendinous ring
tendinous sheath
tendinous spot
tendinous xanthoma
tendo (*pl.* tendines)
tendo cricoesophageus
tendo oculi
tendo palpebrarum
tendocalcaneus
tendolysis
tendon
  Achilles tendon
  advancement of tendon
  anterior tibial tendon
  attenuation of tendon
  attrition rupture of extensor
    tendon
  calcaneal tendon
  central tendon
  common tendon
  communis tendon
  conjoined tendon
  coronary tendon
  cricoesophageal tendon
  divided tendon
  ECRL tendon
  ECU tendon
  EIP tendon

tendon (*continued*)
  EPL tendon
  extensor digiti minimi tendon
  extensor digitorum communis
    tendon
  extensor tendon
  FDP tendon
  FDS tendon
  flexor carpi radialis tendon
  flexor carpi ulnaris tendon
  flexor tendon
  FPL tendon
  graft of tendon
  hamstring tendon
  heel tendon
  inferior crus of lateral canthal
    tendon
  infraspinatus tendon
  intermediate tendon
  kangaroo tendon
  keeper tendon
  Kessler suture repair of
    tendon
  lacerated tendon
  lengthening of tendon
  Lockwood tendon
  long abductor tendon
  Magnuson transplantation of
    subscapularis tendon
  masseter tendon
  medial canthal tendon
  oblique tendon
  ocular tendon
  palmaris longus tendon
  patellar tendon
  peroneal tendon
  plantaris tendon
  posterior tibial tendon
  profundus tendon
  proprius tendon
  pulled tendon
  pulley tendon
  quadriceps tendon
  recessing of tendon
  rider's tendon
  ruptured flexor tendon
  severed tendon
  shortening of tendon
  snapping tendon
  stapedial tendon
  stapedius tendon
  sublimis tendon

tendon (*continued*)
  subscapularis tendon
  superficialis tendon
  superior oblique tendon
  supernumerary tendon
  supraspinatus tendon
  talar tendon
  tenotomy of ocular tendon
  transfer of tendon
  transplantation of tendon
  transposition of tendon
  trefoil tendon
  Tsuge technique to
    reconstruct hand tendons
  Yergason sign for subluxation
    of biceps tendon
  Zinn tendon
tendon Achilles lengthening (TAL)
tendon adhesions
tendon advancement
tendon aspiration and injection
tendon blockage
tendon calcaneus
tendon carrier
tendon cartilage
tendon centralization
tendon corpuscles
tendon dislocation
tendon excursion
tendon forceps
tendon gouge
tendon graft
tendon hook
tendon implant
tendon injury
tendon insertion
tendon intact
tendon interposition arthroplasty
tendon knife
tendon laceration
tendon lengthening
tendon necrosis
tendon needle
tendon passer (*see* passer)
tendon plate
tendon prosthesis
tendon rebalancing
tendon release
tendon repair
tendon rupture
tendon severed
tendon sheath

tendon sheath irrigation
tendon shortening
tendon
tendon suture technique
tendon sutures
tendon transfer
tendon transplant
tendon transplantation
tendon tucker (*see* tucker)
tendon-holding forceps
tendon-passing forceps
tendon-pulling forceps
tendon-retrieving forceps
tendon-seizing forceps
tendon-tucking instruments
tendon-tunneling forceps
tendoplastic amputation
tendoplasty
tendoscopy
tendosynovial tissue sarcoma
tendosynovitis (*variant of*
  tenosynovitis)
tendotome
tendotomy
tendovaginitis
Tendril DX implantable pacing
  lead
tenectomy
tenesmus
tenia of thalamus
teniamyotomy
Tennant anchor lens-insertion
  hook
Tennant Anchorflex anterior
  chamber intraocular lens
Tennant Anchorflex lens implant
Tennant eye needle holder
Tennant eye spatula
Tennant intraocular implant lens
Tennant intraocular lens forceps
Tennant iris hook
Tennant lens
Tennant lens forceps
Tennant needle holder
Tennant nuclear ball rotator
Tennant spatula
Tennant thumb-ring needle
  holder
Tennant titanium suturing forceps
Tennant tying forceps
Tennant-Colibri corneal forceps
Tennant-Maumenee forceps

Tennant-Troutman superior
   rectus forceps
Tenner eye cannula
Tenner lacrimal cannula
Tennessee capsular polisher
tennis elbow
tennis elbow splint
tennis leg
Tennis Racquet angiographic
   catheter
Tennis Racquet catheter
tennis thumb
tennis toe
Tennison cheiloplasty
Tennison operation
Tennison Z-plasty
Tennison-Randall cleft lip repair
Tennison-Randall operation
Tennison-Randall triangular flap
   repair
tennis-racket incision
tenodesis
   Andrews tenodesis
   ECU tenodesis
   Jones tenodesis
tenodesis splint
tenography
tenolysis
   de Quervain tenolysis
   Quervain tenolysis
tenomyoplasty
tenomyotomy
tenon capsule
tenon fascia
tenon membrane
tenon space
tenonectomy
tenonometer
tenontomyoplasty
tenontomyotomy
tenontoplasty
tenontotomy
tenophyte
tenoplastic reconstruction
tenoplasty
tenorrhaphy
tenostosis
tenosuspension
tenosutures
tenosynovectomy
tenosynovial
   chondrometaplasia

tenosynovitis
   adhesive tenosynovitis
   coccidioidomycosis
      tenosynovitis
   de Quervain tenosynovitis
   flexor tenosynovitis
   gonococcal flexor
      tenosynovitis
   granulomatous
      tenosynovitis
   localized nodular
      tenosynovitis
   stenosing tenosynovitis
   suppurative tenosynovitis
   villonodular pigmented
      tenosynovitis
   villous tenosynovitis
tenosynovitis crepitans
tenosynovitis hypertrophica
tenosynovitis serosa chronica
tenosynovitis stenosans
tenotome
tenotomies
tenotomy
   three-step tenotomy
   adductor tenotomy
   Arruga tenotomy
   curb tenotomy
   Dolfin extensor tenotomy
   free tenotomy
   graduated tenotomy
   subcutaneous tenotomy
   Z-marginal tenotomy
tenotomy hook
tenotomy knife
tenotomy of ocular tendon
tenotomy operation
tenotomy scissors
tenovaginitis
TENS (transcutaneous electrical/
      electrode nerve
      stimulation/stimulator)
TENS machine
TENS pad
TENS unit
tense abdomen
tense ascites
tensegrity
tensile strength
Tensilon anesthetic agent
Tensilon implant
tensiometer

tension
  continuous tension
  extraocular tension
  eyeball under tension
  interfacial surface tension
  intraocular tension
  intravenous tension
  laryngeal tension
  muscle tension
  muscular tension
  ocular tension
  reduce tension
  supralaryngeal tension
  surface tension
  tactile tension
  wound tension
tension band fixation
tension band wiring technique
tension clamp
tension fracture
tension isometer
tension nose
tension planes
tension repair
tension skin lines
tension suture technique
tension sutures
tension-control suture technique
    in open rhinoplasty
tension-free anastomosis
tension-free closure
tension-free hernioplasty
tension-free hiatoplasty
tension-free mesh implantation
tension-free mesh repair
tension-free prosthetic mesh
    repair
tension-free repair
tension-free scalp fixation
tensionless anastomosis
tension-requiring sutures
tension-stress effect of
    mechanical force
tension-type headaches (TTH)
Tensoplast elastic adhesive
    dressing
Tensor elastic bandage roll
Tensor elastic dressing
tensor fascia femoris flap
tensor fascia lata
tensor fascia lata muscle flap
tensor fasciae latae

tensor fasciae latae flap
tensor fasciae latae muscle
tensor insertion
tensor muscle
tensor tenaculum
tensor tympani muscle
tensor veli palatini
tensor veli palatini muscle
Tensum coronary stent
tentalum wire tension suture
tented
tenting of diaphragm
tenting of hemidiaphragm
tenting sign
tenting sutures
tentorial herniation
tentorial laceration
tentorial line
tentorial nerve
tentorial notch
tentorium cerebelli
tentorium cyst
tentorium of cerebellum
tentorium of hypophysis
Tenzel bipolar forceps
Tenzel calipers
Tenzel double-end periosteal
    elevator
Tenzel periosteal elevator
Tenzel rotational cheek flap
Tenzel semicircular flap
TEP repair
Tepas retractor
tepee incision
tepid water
Teq-Trode electrode
teras (pl. terata)
teratic implantation
teratocarcinoma
teratogenic potential
teratogenicity
teratogen-induced malformation
teratoid tumor
teratologic dislocation
teratomata (pl. teratomata)
  adult teratoma
  benign cystic teratoma
  cystic teratoma
  immature ovarian teratoma
  mature teratoma
Terblanche decompression of
    common bile duct

terebration
teres knife
teres major muscle
teres major skin island
teres minor
teres minor muscle
teres muscle
Terino anatomical chin implant
Terino facial implant retractor
Terino malar shell
Terlux cement
TERM (temporary endodontic restorative material)
term delivery
term pregnancy
terminal adapter electrode
terminal aorta
terminal artery
terminal bile duct
terminal cancer
terminal carcinoma
terminal care
terminal colostomy
terminal condition
terminal crest
terminal device
terminal disease
terminal duct carcinoma
terminal electrode adapter
terminal electrode nerve stimulator (TENS)
terminal extensor mechanism
terminal ganglion
terminal hinge position
terminal ileal loop
terminal ileal pouch
terminal ileal resection
terminal ileal segment
terminal ileostomy
terminal ileum intubation
terminal jaw relation record
terminal ligature
terminal line
terminal nerves
terminal occlusion
terminal phalanx
terminal plane
terminal reservoir syndrome
terminal sigmoid colostomy
terminal state
terminal sulcus
terminal Syme procedure

terminal tuft fracture
terminal vein
terminal ventricle
terminal web
termination of labor
termination of pregnancy
termination of procedure
terminoterminal anastomosis
Ter-Pogossian applicator
Ter-Pogossian cervical radium applicator
Terrien degeneration
Terrillon operation
Terry fingernail sign
Terry keratometer
Terry keratotomy
Terry line
Terry nail sign
Terry silicone capsular polisher
Terry skin lines
Terry-Mayo needle
Terry-Thomas sign
Terson capsular forceps
Terson extracapsular forceps
Terson operation
Terson speculum
tertiary amputation
tertiary carina
tertiary contractions
tertiary dehiscence
tertiary peristaltic activity
tertiary radicle
tertiary sequestrum
tertiary transmission
tertiary vitreous
tertiary wound closure
Terumo AV fistula needle
Terumo dental needle
Terumo dialyzer
Terumo Doppler fetal heart rate monitor
Terumo Glidewire
Terumo guidewire
Terumo hydrophilic guidewire
Terumo hypodermic needle
Terumo insulin syringe
Terumo coaxial catheter
Terumo hydrophilic-polymer-coated microcatheter
Terumo intravenous catheter
Terumo transducer protector
Terumo Meditech guidewire

Terumo-Clirans dialyzer
Terumo-Radiofocus hydrophilic polymer-coated guidewire
Terwilliger amputation
Terwilliger excision
Terzis technique
Tes Tape dressing
Tesa hand-held electronic digital calipers
Tesberg esophagoscope
TESE (testicular sperm extraction)
Tesio catheter
Tesla magnet
Tesla measurement
Tesla Signa magnetic resonance imager
tessellated fundus
Tessier bone bender
Tessier classification of craniofacial clefts (Tessier numbers 0-14)
Tessier cleft axis
Tessier craniofacial cleft
Tessier craniofacial instrument
Tessier craniofacial operation
Tessier disimpaction device forceps
Tessier disimpaction elevator
Tessier dislodger
Tessier elevator
Tessier facial dysostosis operation
Tessier operation
Tessier osteomicrotome
Tessier osteotome
Tessier osteotomy
Tessier rib morcellizer
Tessier spreader
Tessier type of frontal bone advancement
test dose anesthetic technique
test injection
testectomy
testes (*sing.* testis)
testes in scrotum
testicle transplant
testicular abscess
testicular appendage
testicular artery
testicular atrophy
testicular biopsy

testicular cancer
testicular carcinoma
testicular choriocarcinoma
testicular duct
testicular ectopia
testicular feminization syndrome
testicular implant
testicular lymphoma
testicular metastasis
testicular plexus
testicular prosthesis
testicular rupture
testicular shock
testicular swelling
testicular torsion
testicular tubules
testicular vein
testing drum knife
testis (*pl.* testes)
    bellclapper deformity of testis
    ectopic testis
    inverted testis
    obstructed testis
    parenchyma testis
    pulpy testis
    rete testis
    undescended testis
testis fracture
testis tumor
Testoderm patch
tethered spinal cord
tethered-bowel sign
tethered-cord syndrome
tetracaine hydrochloride anesthetic agent
tetracycline hydrochloride sclerotherapy
tetralogy of Fallot
tetrapolar esophageal catheter
Teufel cervical brace
Teuffer technique
Teuffer tendocalcaneus repair
Teurlings wrist brace
Tevdek graft
Tevdek implant
Tevdek pledgeted sutures
Tevdek prosthesis
Tew cranial retractor
Tew needle
Tew spinal retractor
Texal-Muller chest binder
Texas cannula

Texas cannula tip
Texas catheter
Texas condom catheter
Texas Goodstein sharp tip
Texas Scottish Rite Hospital (TSRH) instrumentation
Texas Scottish Rite Hospital corkscrew device
Texas Scottish Rite Hospital eyebolt spreader
Texas Scottish Rite Hospital hook holder
Texas Scottish Rite Hospital hook inserter
Texas Scottish Rite Hospital mini-corkscrew device
Texas Scottish Rite Hospital pedicle screw
Texas Scottish Rite Hospital trial hook
T-excision abdominoplasty
Textor operation
Textor vasectomy clamp
textured saline breast implant
T-fastener gastropexy
TFCC (triangular fibrocartilage complex)
TFCC meniscus tear
TFCC tear
TFE-coated wire guide
T-finger splint
T-Foam bed pad
T-Foam cushion
T-Foam mattress
T-Foam pillow
TFT cervix (tight fingertip dilated)
TG Osseotite single-stage procedure implant
TG140 needle
TGA (transposition of great arteries)
TGAR (total graft area rejected)
T-Gel cushion
TGF (transforming growth factor)
T-grommet ventilation tube
TGV (transposition of great vessels)
Thackray dental forceps
Thackray hip prosthesis

Thackray mouth gag
Thackston retropubic bag
Thal esophageal stricture repair
Thal esophagogastroscopy
Thal esophagogastrostomy
Thal fundic patch operation
Thal fundoplasty
Thal fundoplication procedure
Thal fundoplication technique
Thal gastric patch
Thal hiatal hernia repair
thalamectomy
thalamic circulation
thalamic plane
thalamic tumor
thalamic-subthalamic hemorrhage
thalamocaudate arteriovenous malformation
thalamomammillary bundle
thalamotomy
    anterior thalamotomy
    dorsomedial thalamotomy
    parafascicular thalamotomy (PFT)
thalamus
Thal-Mantel obturator
Thal-Nissen fundoplasty
Thal-Quick chest tube
Tham flap
T-handle bone awl
T-handle elevator
T-handle Jacob chuck
T-handle reamer
T-handle wrench
T-handle Zimmer chuck
T-handled awl
T-handled cup curet
THARIES (total hip articular replacement by internal eccentric shells)
Tharies femoral resurfacing component
Tharies hip arthroplasty
Tharies hip component
Tharies hip replacement prosthesis
Tharies surface hip replacement
Thatcher nail
Thatcher screw

THC (transhepatic cholangiogram)
Asta-Cath female catheter guide
Beachcomber prosthetic foot
Closer arterial closure device
Corner cushion
Dale tracheostomy tube holder
edge-coated blade
Heeler inflatable heel protector
Hockey Stick articulating stylet
MMG Golden drain
Richie brace
Rope stretch and traction device
Rope stretching device
Sensar foldable acrylic posterior chamber intraocular lens
Shark disposable biopsy forceps
Side Rester cushion
Treaser surgical instrument
Unloader brace
thebesian circulation
thebesian valve
thebesian vein
theca (*pl.* thecae)
theca cordis
theca folliculi
theca lutein cells
theca vertebralis
thecal cell tumor
thecal puncture
thecal sac compression
thecal whitlow
theca-lutein cyst
thecoperitoneal Pudenz-Schulte shunt
thecostegnosis
Theden bandage
Theile glands
Theirsch-Duplay repair
Theis infant rib spreader
Theis rib spreader
Theis self-retaining retractor
Theis self-retaining rib retractor
Theis vein retractor
thelarche
theleplasty
thelerethism
thelorrhagia
thenar atrophy
thenar cleft
thenar compartment
thenar eminence
thenar fascia
thenar flap
thenar muscle
thenar muscle hypoplasia
thenar space
thenar space abscess
thenar surface
thenar web space
Theobald lacrimal dilator
Theobald sinus probe
TheraBeads microwaveable moist heat pack
Therabite mobilizer
Thera-Boot bandage
Thera-Boot compression dressing
Thera-Boot compression wrap
Theracloud pillow
Thera-Med cold pack
Theramini electrotherapy stimulator
therapeutic abortion (TAB)
therapeutic anesthesia
therapeutic angiogenesis
therapeutic approach
therapeutic colonoscopy
therapeutic D&C
therapeutic dermabrasion
therapeutic dissection
therapeutic effect
therapeutic endoscopy
therapeutic insemination
therapeutic intervention
therapeutic iridectomy
therapeutic irradiation
therapeutic laparoscopy
therapeutic lymph node dissection (TLND)
therapeutic measures
therapeutic nerve block
therapeutic side-viewing duodenoscope
therapeutic splint
therapeutic support
therapeutic treatment

therapeutic upper endoscopy
Therapeutica sleeping pillow
Thera-Pos elbow orthosis
Thera-Pos knee orthosis
TheraPulse pulsating air
    suspension bed
Thera-Putty therapy device
TherArc pillow
TheraRest mattress
TheraSeed implant
TheraSkin wound dressing
Therasleep cervical pillow
TheraSnore device
TheraSnore oral appliance
Thera-Soft hand-wrist orthosis
Therasonics lithotriptor
Therasound transducer
Thera-SR pacemaker
Therastream microcatheter
Theratotic firm foot orthosis
Theratotic soft foot orthosis
Theratouch stimulator
Therma Jaw hot urologic
    forceps
ThermaChoice catheter
ThermaChoice thermal balloon
    ablation
ThermaChoice uterine balloon
Thermaderm epilator
Thermafil plastic carrier
Thermafil Plus obturator
thermal ablation
thermal agents
thermal anesthesia
thermal burn
thermal coefficient expansion
thermal conductivity detector
thermal death point
thermal dilution technique
thermal dose
thermal effect
thermal expansion technique
thermal imaging
thermal injury
thermal keratoplasty
thermal knife
thermal memory stent
thermal plastic wrap
thermal quenching
thermal relaxation times
Thermal responsive non-latex
    nitrile surgical glove

thermal therapy
thermal perfusion balloon
    angioplasty
Thermalator heating unit
thermally-altered epidermis
Thermapad pad
ThermaStim muscle stimulator
ThermaStim muscle warming
    device
Thermedics cardiac device
Thermedics HeartMate 1001P
    left anterior assist device
Thermedics left ventricular
    assist device
Thermex-II transurethral
    prostate heating device
thermic anesthesia
thermistor needle
thermistor probe
thermistor thermodilution
    catheter
Thermo Cardiosystems left
    ventricular assist device
Thermo orthotic
thermocatalytic technique
thermocauterectomy
thermocautery
thermocoagulation
thermocouple
thermodilution
thermodilution balloon catheter
thermodilution catheter
    introducer kit
thermodilution pacing catheter
thermodilution Swan-Ganz
    catheter
thermodilution technique
thermoexpandable stent
thermoflex sutures
ThermoFlex thermotherapy unit
ThermoFX mesh
Thermograph temperature
    monitor
thermographic examination
thermographic scanner
thermography
thermoluminescent dosimeter
thermoluminescent dosimeter
    rod
thermophore
Thermophore bandage
Thermophore hot pack

Thermophore moist heat pad
thermoplastic extension pan
    splint
thermoplastic impression
    material
thermoplastic orthosis
thermoplastic polymer
thermoplastic splint
thermoplastic stent
thermopore
Therm-O-Rite blanket
Thermos pacemaker
thermosetting polymer
Thermoskin arthritic knee wrap
Thermoskin back wrap
Thermoskin brace
Thermoskin brand
Thermoskin heat retainer
thermotherapy
thermotic pump
Thero-Skin gel padding
TherOx infusion guidewire
Theurig sterilizer forceps
THI needle
thialbarbitone anesthetic agent
thiamylal sodium anesthetic
    agent
thick adhesions
thick elastic tissue
thick visceral peel
thickened bone
thickened folds
thickened musculature
thickened pleura
thickened scar
thickened skin
thickened synovial membrane
thickening
    cortical thickening
    intimal thickening
    leaflet thickening
    mediastinal thickening
    parametrial thickening
    periosteal thickening
    pleural thickening
    sclerodermalike skin
        thickening
    sclerotic thickening
thick-layer autoradiography
thick-split graft
thick-walled Dacron-backed
    implant

thick-walled gallbladder
Thiersch anal incontinence
    operation
Thiersch canaliculi
Thiersch cerclage
Thiersch graft
Thiersch graft operation
Thiersch implant
Thiersch knife
Thiersch medium-split free graft
Thiersch operation
Thiersch procedure for rectal
    prolapse
Thiersch prosthesis
Thiersch repair of rectal
    procidentia
Thiersch ring
Thiersch skin graft
Thiersch skin graft knife
Thiersch suture technique
Thiersch sutures
Thiersch thin-split free graft
Thiersch wire
Thiersch-Duplay proximal tube
    procedure
Thiersch-Duplay tube graft
Thiersch-Duplay urethral
    construction
Thiersch-Duplay urethroplasty
thigh balloon
thigh bone
thigh flap
thigh graft arteriovenous fistula
thigh joint
thigh lift
thigh splint
thigh tourniquet
thigh-high embolic stockings
thighplasty
Thillaye bandage
Thillaye dressing
thin acupuncture needle
thin adhesions
thin basement membrane
thin disk
thin disposable cannula
thin film dressing
thin osteotomy
thin plastic membrane
ThinLine bipolar cardiac pacing
    lead
Thinline uncovered orthotic

Thinlith pacemaker
thin-needle biopsy
thin-needle percutaneous
 cholangiogram
ThinPrep procedure
ThinPrep processor
thin-section axial image
thin-shaft nasal scissors
THINSite topical wound
 dressing
THINSite with Biofilm hydrogel
 topical wound dressing
thin-skin paddle
thin-split graft
thin-wall introducer catheter
thin-walled needle
thin-wire Ilizarov fixation
thiol augmentation
thiol modification
thiopental sodium anesthetic
 agent
thiopental-sufentanil-desflurane-
 nitrous oxide anesthetic
 technique
Thiry fistula
Thiry-Vella fistula
Thole goniometer
Thole pelvimeter
Thom flap laryngeal
 reconstruction
Thoma clamp
Thoma tissue retractor
Thomas Allis forceps
Thomas Allis tissue forceps
Thomas brace
Thomas bur
Thomas calipers
Thomas cervical collar brace
Thomas classification
Thomas collar
Thomas collar cervical orthosis
Thomas cryoextractor
Thomas cryoprobe
Thomas cryoptor
Thomas curet
Thomas extrapolated bar graft
Thomas femoral shunt
Thomas fixation forceps
Thomas fixator
Thomas fracture frame
Thomas full-ring leg splint
Thomas full-ring splint

Thomas heel
Thomas heel orthosis
Thomas hinged splint
Thomas hyperextension frame
Thomas I&A cannula
Thomas keratome
Thomas knee splint
Thomas knife
Thomas leg splint
Thomas leg splint with Pearson
 attachment
Thomas long-term endotracheal
 tube holder
Thomas magnet
Thomas needle
Thomas operation
Thomas pelvimeter
Thomas pessary
Thomas posterior splint
Thomas procedure
Thomas retractor
Thomas ring
Thomas scissors
Thomas shot compression
 forceps
Thomas shunt
Thomas spatula
Thomas splint
Thomas splint with Pearson
 attachment
Thomas suspension splint
Thomas technique
Thomas uterine curet
Thomas uterine tissue-grasping
 forceps
Thomas vascular access shunt
Thomas Waldon wrench
Thomas walking brace
Thomas walking calipers brace
Thomas-Thompson-Straub
 gluteus medius procedure
Thomas-Thompson-Straub
 transfer
Thomas-Thompson-Straub
 transfer technique
Thomas-Warren incision
Thomayer sign
Thombostat
Thompson adenoid curet
Thompson adenoid punch
Thompson anterolateral
 approach

Thompson anteromedial
   approach
Thompson antral rasp
Thompson bronchial catheter
Thompson carotid artery clamp
Thompson carotid vascular clamp
Thompson chin support
Thompson curet
Thompson direct full-vision
   resectoscope
Thompson dowel
Thompson drape
Thompson endoprosthesis
Thompson evacuator
Thompson excision
Thompson femoral head
Thompson femoral head
   prosthesis
Thompson femoral neck
   prosthesis
Thompson fracture frame
Thompson frontal sinus
   raspatory
Thompson hemiarthroplasty hip
   prosthesis
Thompson hip prosthesis
   forceps
Thompson hyperextension
   fracture frame
Thompson line
Thompson lithotrite
Thompson modification of
   Denis Browne splint
Thompson operation
Thompson posterior radial
   approach
Thompson procedure
Thompson prosthesis
Thompson punch
Thompson rasp
Thompson raspatory
Thompson reduction technique
Thompson resection
Thompson resectoscope
Thompson retractor
Thompson rib shears
Thompson root extractor
Thompson sinus rasp
Thompson squeeze test of
   Achilles
Thompson squeeze test of
   gastrocnemius

Thompson stem rasp
Thompson syndrome
Thompson syringe
Thompson technique
Thompson telescoping V-
   osteotomy
Thompson template
Thompson-Compere hip
   arthrodesis
Thompson-Epstein classification
   of hip dislocations
Thompson-Epstein femoral
   fracture classification
Thompson-Henry approach
Thompson-Henry technique
Thompson-Loomer technique
Thompson-Terwilliger
   procedure
Thompson-Walker scissors
Thoms cervical collar brace
Thoms pelvimeter
Thoms tenaculum
Thoms tissue forceps
Thoms tissue-grasping forceps
Thoms-Allis intestinal forceps
Thoms-Allis tissue forceps
Thomsen rib shears
Thoms-Gaylor biopsy forceps
Thoms-Gaylor biopsy punch
Thoms-Gaylor uterine forceps
Thomson adenoidal punch
Thomson lung clamp
Thomson operation
ThoraCath catheter
thoracectomy
thoracentesis needle
thoracic anesthesia
thoracic aneurysm
thoracic aorta
thoracic aortic aneurysm repair
thoracic aortic disease
thoracic aortic dissection
thoracic aortography
thoracic approach
thoracic arch aortogram
thoracic artery forceps
thoracic axis
thoracic cage curvature
thoracic cardiac nerve
thoracic catheter
thoracic cavity
thoracic clamp

thoracic compression syndrome
thoracic disk herniation
thoracic diskectomy
thoracic drain
thoracic drainage tube
thoracic duct drainage (TDD)
thoracic duct fistula
thoracic empyema
thoracic endometriosis
    syndrome
thoracic epidural analgesia
thoracic epidural anesthetic
    technique
thoracic epidural catheterization
thoracic esophagogastrostomy
thoracic esophagus
thoracic facet fusion
thoracic fascia
thoracic ganglia
thoracic ganglion
thoracic hemostatic forceps
thoracic inferior vena cava
thoracic inlet
thoracic inlet vascular injury
thoracic kidney
thoracic laminectomy
thoracic lesion
thoracic nerve block
thoracic outlet compression
thoracic outlet syndrome
thoracic plane
thoracic region
thoracic roentgenogram
thoracic scissors
thoracic short
    esophagomyotomy
thoracic spinal cord
thoracic spinal fusion
thoracic spine biopsy
thoracic spine fracture
thoracic spine kyphotic
    deformity
thoracic spine scoliotic deformity
thoracic surgery
thoracic sutures
thoracic sympathectomy
thoracic tissue forceps
thoracic trocar
thoracic vein
thoracic vertebrae
thoracic vertebral body
thoracic viscera

thoracic wall
thoracicoabdominal incision
thoracicoabdominal
    splenectomy
thoracicolumbar division
thoracoabdominal
    esophagogastrectomy
thoracoabdominal (TA)
thoracoabdominal stapler
thoracoabdominal aneurysm
thoracoabdominal aortic
    aneurysm repair
thoracoabdominal
    esophagectomy
thoracoabdominal
    esophagogastrectomy
thoracoabdominal extrapleural
    approach
thoracoabdominal incision
thoracoabdominal injury
thoracoabdominal
    retroperitoneal
    lymphadenectomy
thoracoacromial artery
thoracoacromial flap
thoracoacromial pedicle
thoracoacromial vein
thoracobronchotomy
thoracoceloschisis
thoracocentesis
thoracocyllosis
thoracocyrtosis
thoracodidymus
thoracodorsal artery
thoracodorsal fascia flap
thoracodorsal nerve
thoracoepigastric flap
thoracoepigastric veins
thoracogastroschisis
thoracolaparotomy
thoracolumbar aponeurosis
thoracolumbar burst fracture
thoracolumbar division
thoracolumbar fascia
thoracolumbar junction surgical
    exposure
thoracolumbar nerve block
thoracolumbar pedicle screw
thoracolumbar retroperitoneal
    approach
thoracolumbar spinal
    orthosis

Thorlakson multipurpose
retractor
Thorlakson upper occlusive
clamp
Thorn maneuver
Thorn syndrome
Thornell microlaryngoscopy
Thornell operation
Thornton arcuate blade
Thornton corneal marker
Thornton corneal press-on ruler
Thornton double corneal ruler
Thornton episcleral forceps
Thornton fixating ring
Thornton fixation forceps
Thornton intraocular forceps
Thornton iris retractor
Thornton 360-degree arcuate
marker
Thornton low-profile marker
Thornton malleable spatula
Thornton nail
Thornton needle
Thornton open-wire lid
speculum
Thornton plate
Thornton screw
Thornton side plate
Thornton T-incision diamond
knife
Thornton tri-square blade
Thornton-Fine ring
Thornwald antral drill
Thornwald antral irrigator
Thornwald antral perforator
Thornwald antral trephine
Thornwald irrigator
Thornwald perforator
Thornwald trephine
THORP (titanium hollow-screw
osseointegrating
reconstruction plate)
Thorpe calipers
Thorpe conjunctival forceps
Thorpe corneal forceps
Thorpe corneoscleral forceps
Thorpe curet
Thorpe fixation forceps
Thorpe foreign body forceps
Thorpe foreign body knife
Thorpe 4-mirror goniolaser
Thorpe 4-mirror goniolaser lens

Thorpe 4-mirror goniolens
Thorpe 4-mirror vitreous fundus
laser line
Thorpe gonioprism lens
Thorpe plastic lens
Thorpe pupillary membrane
scissors
Thorpe slit lamp
Thorpe surgical gonioscope
Thorpe-Castroviejo calipers
Thorpe-Castroviejo cataract
scissors
Thorpe-Castroviejo corneal
forceps
Thorpe-Castroviejo fixation
forceps
Thorpe-Castroviejo goniolens
Thorpe-Castroviejo scissors
Thorpe-Castroviejo vitreous
foreign body forceps
Thorpe-Westcott cataract
scissors
THORP-type mandibular
reconstruction plate
Thow gastrostomy tube
THR (total hip replacement)
Thrasher intraocular forceps
Thrasher lens implant forceps
thread sutures
threaded cortical dowel
threaded eye needle
threaded guide pin
threaded interbody fusion cage
threaded portion of nail
threaded rod
threaded titanium acetabular
prosthesis (TTAP)
threaded-hole-first technique
threader
    Allen wire threader
    Borchard wire threader
    cannulated wire threader
    Frackelton wire threader
    wire threader
threader rod holder pliers
ThreadLoc driver mount screw
ThreadLoc implant
ThreadLoc retaining screw
thread-locking device
thready pulse
threatened abortion
threatened labor

threatened miscarriage
threatened premature delivery
threatened transplant rejection
three color concept of wound
   classification
threshold
  absolute threshold
  bone threshold
  displacement threshold
  double-point threshold
  fibrillation threshold
  low threshold
  ventilation threshold
Threshold inspiratory muscle
   trainer device
throat anesthesia
throat forceps
throat irrigation tube
throat mucosa
throat scissors
throat smear
throat swab
throat washings
Throat-E-Vac suction device
throbbing aorta
throbbing pain
Throckmorton reflex
thrombectomy
thrombectomy catheter
thrombi (*sing.* thrombus)
thrombin clotting time
thrombin time
thromboangiitis obliterans
thrombocytopenic
   hemangiomatosis
thromboembolic complication
thromboembolic disease (TED)
thromboembolic disease hose
thromboembolic disease socks
thromboembolic disease
   stockings
thromboembolic event
thromboembolic fistula
thromboembolism
thromboendarterectomy (TEA)
Thrombogen absorbable
   hemostat
thrombogenic disorder
thrombogenic foreign body
thrombolysis
thrombolysis in myocardial
   infarction classification

thrombolytic therapy
thrombopenia
thrombophlebitis
thromboplastin
thrombosed graft
thrombosed hemorrhoid
thrombosed internal and
   external hemorrhoid
thrombosed veins
thrombosis
   (*pl.* thromboses)
  agonal thrombosis
  arterial thrombosis
  bland thrombosis
  cerebral thrombosis
  cerebral venous sinus
   thrombosis (CVST)
  coronary thrombosis
  creeping thrombosis
  deep venous thrombosis
   (DVT)
  embolic thrombosis
  graft thrombosis
  ileofemoral deep vein
   thrombosis
  incomplete thrombosis
  inferior dental thrombosis
  mesenteric thrombosis
  microvascular thrombosis
  nonocclusive mesenteric
   thrombosis
  portal vein thrombosis
  recanalizing thrombosis
  sinus thrombosis
  splenic vein thrombosis
  superior sagittal sinus
   thrombosis (SSS)
  venous thrombosis
Thrombostat
thrombosuction catheter
thrombotic complication
thrombotic disease
thrombotic gangrene
thrombotic occlusion
thrombus (*pl.* thrombi)
  agonal thrombus
  ball-valve thrombus
  currant jelly thrombus
  organizing thrombus
thrombus extension
thrombus formation
thrombus stripper

through-and-through avulsion injury
through-and-through buttonhole fashion excision
through-and-through continuous sutures
through-and-through defect
through-and-through fracture
through-and-through laceration
through-and-through reabsorbable sutures
through-and-through suture technique
through-and-through sutures
through-cutting forceps tip
through-knee amputation
through-the-scope balloon
through-the-scope balloon dilation
through-the-scope balloon removal
through-the-scope bougie
through-the-scope catheter probe
through-the-scope dilator (TTS dilator)
through-the-scope injection needle
through-the-wall mattress sutures
throw-away manual dermatome blade
thrower's fracture
thrower's elbow
Thruflex balloon
Thruflex PTCA balloon catheter
Thrust femoral prosthesis
thrust manipulation
Thudichum nasal speculum
thulium:YAG laser angioplasty
thulium-holmium:YAG laser
thulium-holmium-chromium:yttrium-aluminum-garnet (THC:YAG) laser
thumb abduction
thumb cushion
thumb deformity
thumb duplication correction
thumb finger
thumb forceps
thumb fracture

thumb fusion
thumb hypoplasia
thumb metacarpophalangeal joint approach
thumb pad
thumb polydactyly
thumb reconstruction
thumb reflex
thumb retractor
thumb sign
thumb spica bandage
thumb spica cast
thumb splint
thumb tissue forceps
thumb-dressing forceps
thumb-index contracture
thumb-index web space
thumb-in-palm deformity
Thumb-Saver introducer clamp
Thumper device
ThumZ'Up functional thumb splint
Thunberg restrictor
Thunberg tube
Thurmond iris retractor
Thurmond nucleus-irrigating cannula
Thurmond retractor
Thurston-Holland fragment forceps
Thymapad stimulus electrode
thymectomize
thymectomy
thymic aplasia
thymic carcinoma
thymic cyst
thymic duct
thymic nodule
thymic tumor
thymic vein
thymopexy
thymus gland
thymus gland excision
thymus retractor
thymusectomy
thyrocervical trunk
thyrochondrotomy
thyrocricoidectomy
thyrocricotomy
thyroepiglottic muscle
thyroepliglottic ligament
thyrofissure

thyroglossal cyst
thyroglossal duct cystectomy
thyroglossal fistula
thyroglossal sinus
thyrohyal space
thyrohyoid fold
thyrohyoid laryngotomy
thyrohyoid ligament
thyrohyoid membrane
thyrohyoid muscle
thyroid
   aberrant thyroid
   accessory thyroid
   desiccated thyroid
   inferior pole of thyroid
   intrathoracic thyroid
   lingual thyroid
   lobectomy of thyroid
   nodular thyroid
   pyramid of thyroid
   pyramidal lobe of thyroid
   retrosternal thyroid
   substernal thyroid
   superior pole of thyroid
thyroid abscess
thyroid acropachy
thyroid adenoma
thyroid ala
thyroid artery
thyroid axis
thyroid body
thyroid bruit
thyroid cancer
thyroid capsule
thyroid carcinoma
thyroid cartilage
thyroid collar
thyroid drain
thyroid eminence
thyroid endocrine disorder
thyroid foramen
thyroid forceps
thyroid ganglion
thyroid gland
thyroid hormone serum
   concentration
thyroid hyperplasia
thyroid ima artery
thyroid ima vein
thyroid imaging
thyroid isthmectomy
thyroid isthmus

thyroid lamina
thyroid lobe
thyroid lobectomy
thyroid loop
thyroid malignoma
thyroid needle biopsy
thyroid nodule ablation
thyroid notch
thyroid operation
thyroid plexus
thyroid region
thyroid resection
thyroid retractor
thyroid scan
thyroid sheet
thyroid storm
thyroid surgical technique
thyroid tenaculum
thyroid tissue
thyroid traction forceps
thyroid tray
thyroid tumor
thyroid uptake
thyroid vein
thyroidal hernia
thyroidea accessoria
thyroidectomize
thyroidectomy
   complete thyroidectomy
   gasless endoscopic
     thyroidectomy
   subtotal thyroidectomy
   transsternal thyroidectomy
thyroidectomy technique
thyroiditis
thyroidorrhaphy
thyroidotomy
thyrolaryngeal fascia
thyrolingual duct
thyrolingual trunk
thyromegaly
thyroparathyroidectomy
thyropharyngeal muscle
thyroplasty
thyrotome
thyrotomy
thyrotoxic complement-fixation
   factor
thyrotoxic goiter
thyrotoxic myopathy
thyrotoxicosis
thyroxine

Ti (titanium)
Ti alloy screw
TI measurement (transischial measurement)
Ti rotor
Ti/CoCr hip prosthesis
Ti-28 total hip replacement
TIA (transient ischemic attack)
Ti-BAC acetabular component
Ti-BAC acetabular cup
Ti-BAC hip prosthesis
Tibbs arterial cannula
Tibbs semiautomatic suturing device
tibia
    medial plateau of tibia
    Paterson pseudarthrosis of tibia
    proximal tibia
    saber tibia
    Sofield pseudarthrosis of tibia
tibia valga
tibia vara
tibial aligner
tibial artery
tibial augmentation block
tibial bending fracture
tibial bolt
tibial broach
tibial calipers
tibial collateral ligament
tibial compartment
tibial condyle fracture
tibial crest
tibial cutter guide
tibial cutting block
tibial diaphysial fracture
tibial driver
tibial endoprosthesis
tibial fixation plate
tibial fracture
tibial fracture brace proximal support
tibial guide pin
tibial impactor
tibial insertion
tibial lymph node
tibial muscle
tibial nerve
tibial open fracture
tibial peg holes
tibial perforator

tibial pin
tibial plafond fracture
tibial plate
tibial plateau fracture
tibial plateau fracture-dislocation
tibial plateau prosthesis
tibial prosthesis
tibial pulse
tibial relocation plate
tibial resection guide
tibial resection jig
tibial retractor
tibial shaft fracture
tibial sign
tibial spine
tibial stress reaction
tibial torsion
tibial tray
tibial triplane fracture
tibial tubercle
tibial tuberosity
tibial tuberosity fracture
tibial vein
tibialis anterior (anticus) flap
tibialis anterior muscle
tibialis posterior dislocation
tibialis posterior muscle
tibialis sign
tibioadductor reflex
tibiocalcaneal arthrodesis
tibiocollateral ligament
tibiofemoral articulation
tibiofemoral fossa
tibiofemoral prosthesis
tibiofibular articulation
tibiofibular clear space
tibiofibular diastasis
tibiofibular fusion
tibiofibular joint
tibiofibular joint dislocation
tibiofibular ligament
tibiofibular line
tibiofibular mortise
tibiofibular syndesmosis
tibioperoneal trunk
tibioperoneal trunk angioplasty
tibioperoneal vessel angioplasty
tibioscaphoid
tibiotalar fusion
tibiotalar joint
tibiotalocalcaneal arthrodesis
tibiotalocalcaneal fusion

tibiotarsal articulation
Tibone posterior
    capsulorrhaphy
Tickner tissue forceps
Ticonium splint
Ti-Cron sutures (*See also* Tyrcron)
tics and fasciculations
Ticsay transpubic needle
tic-tac-toe classification for
    mutilating injuries of the
    hand (types I-VII; subtypes
    A-C; vascular status 0-1)
tidal air
tidal drainage
tidal volume
tidal wave
tie (*see* also sutures)
  cable tie
  catgut plain ties
  free tie
  gauze neck tie
  Jensen ties
  plain tie
  Quickert grooved director
    and tongue tie
  secured with ties
  silk ties
  slip-knot ties
  stick ties
  table tie
tie sutures
Tieck nasal speculum
Tieck-Halle infant nasal
    speculum
tied down over cotton sutures
tied over rubber shoes
Tiedemann nerve
Tiedmann rongeur
Tielle absorptive dressing
Tielle hydropolymer dressing
Tiemann bullet forceps
Tiemann coude catheter
Tiemann Foley catheter
Tiemann Meals tenolysis knife
Tiemann nail
Tiemann Neoflex catheter
Tiemann stethoscope
Tiemann-Meals tenolysis knife
tie-on needle
tie-over bolster
tie-over dressing
tie-over dressing with skin staples

tie-over Sellotape dressing
tier
  Addix tier
  Adson knot tier
  Jacobson knot tier
  knot tier
tiered-therapy antiarrhythmic
    device
ties (*see* sutures)
ties-over-stent
Tiger blade
Tiger blade resector
tiger gut sutures
Tiger Shark forceps
tight adhesions
tight contracture
tight fingertip dilated cervix
    (TFT cervix)
tight Nissen repair
tight seal
tightener (*see also* wire
    tightener)
  Kirschner wire tightener
  Nordt knot tightener
  wire tightener
tightening wrench
Tikhoff-Linberg operation
Tikhoff-Linberg procedure
Tikhoff-Linberg shoulder girdle
    resection
Tiko pliable iris retractor
Tiko rake retractor
Tilastan femoral components
Tilastin hip prosthesis
Tilderquist eye needle holder
Tilderquist needle holder
tile plate facet replacement
Tile-Pennal classification of
    pelvic ring fractures
Tillary double-ended retractor
Tillaux fracture of ankle
Tillaux-Chaput fracture
Tillaux-Kleiger fracture
Tillaux-Phocas syndrome
Tillett operation
Tilley dressing forceps
Tilley-Henckel forceps
Tilley-Lichwitz trocar
Tillman resurfacing technique
Tillyer bifocal lens
TILT (triquetral impingement
    ligament tear)

Tilt and Turn Paragon bed
tilt stitch
tilt table
tilt test
tilting-disk aortic valve
    prosthesis
tilting-disk heart valve
tilting-disk valve
Timberlake catheter
Timberlake electrode
Timberlake evacuator
Timberlake irrigating tip
Timberlake obturator
Timberlake resectoscope
Timbrall-Fisher incision
time
   acquisition time
   aeration time
   anesthesia time
   anesthetic time
   aortic crossclamp time
   bleeding time
   capillary refill time
   circulation time
   concentration times
   conduction time
   contraction time
   crossclamp time
   door-to-balloon times
   Duke bleeding time
   echo time
   ejection time
   electrode response time
   emptying time
   fixing time
   forced expiratory time
   image acquisition time
   inversion time
   ischemic time
   Ivy bleeding time
   lag time
   lysis time
   mean circulation time
   nondialysis time
   pre-ejection time
   procedure time
   prothrombin time
   scalar time
   thermal relaxation times
   thrombin clotting time
   thrombin time
   transit time

time-cycled ventilation
timed contractions
timed-sequential therapy
time-of-flight positron emission
    tomographic camera
TiMesh cranial mesh
TiMesh emergency screw
TiMesh hardware
TiMesh orbital mesh
TiMesh orthognathic strap plate
TiMesh patient-configured
    titanium craniomaxillofacial
    implant
TiMesh screw
TiMesh titanium mesh
TiMesh titanium tray
TIMI classification
TINA monitor
tin-bullet probe
T-incision marker
Tindall scissors
tined lead
tined lead pacemaker
tined ventricular electrode
Tinel sign
Tinel sutures
Tinel tapered reamer
Tinel tourniquet
tingling of fingertips
tingling sensation
tinkling bowel sounds
Tinnant gauge
tinnitus masker
Tiny Tytan ventilation tube
Tiny-Tef ventilation tube
TiOblast dental implant
tip (*see also* suction tip)
   accelerator tip
   ACMI cystoscopic tip
   Adson brain suction tip
   aerosol-barrier pipette tip
   Air-Shield-Vickers syringe tip
   Andrews suction tip
   aortographic suction tip
   Artus cutting tip
   aspirating tip
   Bard cystoscope tip
   Batt tip
   B-D irrigating tip
   Becker dissector tip
   Becker flat dissector tip
   Becker twist dissector tip

tip (*continued*)
 Binkhorst tip
 bipolar diathermy forceps tip
 Bishop-Harman tip
 Blasucci tip
 Blue rectal suction tip
 Bovie coagulation tip
 brain suction tip
 Brawley nasal suction tip
 Brawley suction tip
 broad, boxy or ball tips (the three Bs of tip surgery)
 Bruening biting tip
 buccal fat extractor tip
 Buie rectal suction tip
 bulbosity of nasal tip
 bulbous nasal tip
 cannula tip
 catheter tip
 Clerf aspirating tip
 Cobra cannula tip
 Cobra K cannula tip
 Cobra cannula tip
 Colorado electrocautery tip
 coned heparin tip
 conical inserter tip
 Cordes punch forceps tip
 Corometrics Spiral electrode tip
 coronary perfusion tip
 CUSA laparoscopic tip
 custom tip
 cystoscope tip
 diamond-dusted tip
 diathermy tip
 disposable cannula tip
 disposable ear tip
 disposable otoscopic ear tips
 double-articulated forceps tip
 double-articulated laryngeal forceps tip
 droopy nasal tip
 Ducor tip
 eel cobra tip
 electrosurgical resectoscope tip
 epsilon tip
 exploratory suction tip
 Extended Wear self-adhering urinary external catheter with removable tip
 eye-irrigating tip

tip (*continued*)
 E-Z Clean cautery tip
 Fell sucker tip
 flap tip
 flared ABS tip
 Flexoreamer Batt tip
 forceps tip
 Fournier tip
 Fragmatome tip
 Frazier nasal suction tip
 Gasparotti bevel tip
 Gess cannula tip
 Girard irrigating tip
 glass nasal suction tip
 grasping forceps tip
 Grieshaber vitrectomy tip
 Grossan nasal irrigator tip
 guillotine cutting tip
 Hanafee catheter tip
 Henke punch forceps tip
 Hetter pyramid tip
 Hildreth tip
 House oiler tip
 House-Urban tip
 Hydro-Dissection tip
 Illouz modified tip
 Illouz standard tip
 Implantech SE-100 smoke aspiration tip
 infraguide tip
 interchangeable forceps tips
 interchangeable laryngeal forceps tips
 irrigating tip
 irrigating-aspirating tip
 Jackson square punch tip
 Japanese suction tip
 Kahler double-action tip
 Keel tip
 Keeler lancet tip
 Keeler micro spear tip
 Keeler puncture tip
 Keeler razor tip
 Keeler round tip
 Keeler triple-facet tip
 Kelman irrigation-aspiration tip
 K-Flexofile Batt tip
 Killian cutting forceps tip
 Killian double-articulated forceps tip
 KleenSpec otoscope tip
 Klein 1-hole infiltrator tip

tip (*continued*)

Klein cannula tip
Klein multihole infiltrator tip
Knolle irrigating loop with I&A tip
Krause forceps tip
Krause oval punch tip
Krause punch forceps tip
Krause square-basket tip
Krause through-cutting forceps tip
laryngeal forceps tip
laser tip
leaflet tip
Leasure round punch tip
Leon cobra tip
Marlow Primus tip
mastoid tip
Mayo coronary perfusion tip
Medtronic tip
MegaDyne E-Z clean cautery tip
Mercedes tip
metal irrigating tip
Micro-Probe tip
MicroTip phaco tip
mitral valve leaflet tip
modified submental retractor, flared tip
Myerson biting tip
nasal suction tip
nasal tip
nasal-cutting tip
Nu-Tip disposable scissor tip
oiler tip
olive tip
Omni laser tip
overprojecting nasal tip
parenthesis tip
petrous tips
Pinocchio tip
Pinto dissector tip
plastic suction tip
plumbeous zirconate titanate tip
Polaris Mansfield/Webster deflectable tip
Poole suction tip
punch forceps tip
punch tip
pyramid Toomey tip
Quad cutting tip

tip (*continued*)

Radovan tissue expander tip
Ritter double-orifice tip
Ritter single-orifice tip
Roane bullet tip
Rosenberg dissector tip
rotary cutting tip
rubber acorn tip
rubber tip
Savary-Gilliard tip
Saverburger irrigation/aspiration tip
Scheinmann biting tip
Schuknecht suction tip
SE-100 smoke aspiration tip
Seiffert tip
serrated grasping tip
Simcoe cannula tip
Simcoe interchangeable tip
Sims suction tip
SITE guillotine cutting tip
Skimmer laryngeal blade tip
Slip-Coat tip
soft palate tip
Sondermann suction tip
spatula cannula tip
Spencer oval tip
Spencer triangular tip
Spencer Universal adenoid punch tip
splayed tip
Storz cystoscope tip
Struyken angular punch tip
sucker tip
suction tip
Surgi-Fine reusable cannula tip
synthetic sapphire tip
T&A suction tip
Teflon tip
Texas cannula tip
Texas Goodstein sharp tip
through-cutting forceps tip
Timberlake irrigating tip
Tischler-Morgan tip
Toledo dissector tip
Toledo flap dissector tip
Toledo standard dissector tip
Toledo V-dissector tip
tonsil suction tip
Toomey pyramid tip

tip (*continued*)
  Tracer Hybrid wire guide
    with Slip-Coat tip
  Trevisani cannula tip
  Tricut laryngeal blade tip
  TriEye tip
  triport tip
  tulip tip
  tungsten tip
  TurboSonic tip
  Ultrafyn cautery tip
  ultrasonic tip
  Unitri tip
  Universal adenoid punch tip
  Universal handle for punch
    tips
  Universal handle with nasal-
    cutting tips
  Universal Kerrison set and
    tips
  uvula tip
  V. Mueller cystoscopy tip
  valve tip
  vitrectomy tip
  vitrector tip
  Wagener punch tip
  Watson-Williams punch tip
  weighted tip
  Woolner tip
  Yankauer antral-punch tip
  Yankauer multi-orifice tip
  Yankauer single-orifice tip
  Yankauer suction tip
  Yankauer tonsil suction tip
tip angle
tip bifidity
tip bossing
tip graft
tip guard
tip projection
tip ptosis
tip rhinoplasty
tip rotation
tip-deflecting catheter
tip-deflecting guidewire
tipping movement
tip-plasty
TIPS shunt procedure
TIPS (transjugular intrahepatic
    portosystemic shunt)
Tip-Trol handle
tire eye implant

tire implant
tire-grooved silicone
tire-iron maneuver
Tischler cervical biopsy forceps
Tischler cervical biopsy punch
Tischler cervical biopsy punch
    forceps
Tischler cervical forceps
Tischler punch
Tischler-Morgan biopsy punch
Tischler-Morgan tip
Tischler-Morgan uterine biopsy
    forceps
Ti-Screw suture anchor
Tisseel biologic fibrogen
    adhesive
Tisseel fibrin glue
Tisseel fibrin sealant
Tisseel surgical glue
Tissell VH kit
tissue
  abdominal adipose tissue
  aberrant breast tissue
  aberrant tissue
  accessory mammary tissue
  acinar tissue
  adipose tissue
  adjacent tissue
  adventitial tissue
  analogous tissue
  aneurysm tissue
  aortic aneurysm tissue
  appendiceal tissue
  areolar tissue
  autodigestion of pancreatic
    tissue
  autogenous composite tissue
  avascular tissue
  axillary breast tissue
  basement tissue
  border tissue
  breast tissue
  brown adipose tissue
  bruised tissue
  calcified tissue
  cancellous tissue
  cancerous tissue
  cartilaginous tissue
  caseated tissue
  caudal condensation of the
    transverse fascial tissues
  chordal tissue

tissue (*continued*)
chorionic tissue
cicatricial tissue
compact tissue
connective tissue
cribriform tissue
cryostat tissue
dartoid tissue
debrided necrotic tissue
debridement of bruised tissue
debridement of necrotic
    tissue
decidual tissue
deciduous tissue
degenerated tissue
degenerating decidual tissue
denuded tissue
dermal tissue
dermoadipose tissue
devitalized soft tissue
devitalized tissue
diseased tissue
donor organs and tissues
drainage of tissues
earlobe adipose tissue
ectopic endometrial tissue
ectopic tissue
elastic tissue
elastotic tissue
embedded tissue
endometrial tissue
endoscopically harvested
    tissue
endothelial tissue
envelope of tissue
episcleral tissue
epithelial tissue
epivaginal connective tissue
erectile tissue
ethanol-treated freeze-dried
    bone tissue
excision of tissue
exposed tissue
extraperitoneal tissue
fatty tissue
fetal tissue
fibrinous tissue
fibroadipose tissue
fibroblastic tissue
fibrofatty subcutaneous tissue
fibrofatty tissue
fibroglandular tissue

tissue (*continued*)
fibrohyaline tissue
fibrolipomatous tissue
fibromyxomatous connective
    tissue
fibrous connective tissue
fibrous tissue
firm tissue
friable tissue
frozen tissue
Gamgee tissue
gelatinous tissue
glandular tissue
granulation tissue
granulomatous tissue
grayish tissue
gut-associated lymphoid tissue
    (GALT)
hard tissue
harvest tissue
healthy tissue
heart tissue
hemangiomatous tissue
hematopoietic tissue
heterologous tissue
heterotopic tissue
hyperplastic tissue
hypertrophic granulation
    tissue
impassable scar tissue
incision into organ or tissue
incision of organ or tissue
incorporated tissue
inflammation of tissue
inflammatory tissue
injured tissue
intact tissues
interstitial tissues
intertubular tissue
intervening tissues
intravesical prostatic tissue
isodense with surrounding
    tissues
junctional tissue
keratinized tissue
kidney tissue
Kuhnt intermediary tissue
lardaceous tissue
layer of tissue
lesion of tissue
lipomatous-like tissue
loose connective tissue

tissue (*continued*)
lung tissue
lymph node-bearing tissue
lymphadenoid tissue
lymphatic tissue
lymphoid tissue
membranous tissue
mesenchymal tissue
mineralized tissue
mucous tissue
muscle tissue
muscular tissues
musculoskeletal tissue
myeloid tissue
myxomatous tissue
nasion soft tissue
necrotic tissue
nephrogenic tissue
nerve tissue
nervous tissues
nodal tissue
nonmalignant tissue
nonviable tissue
oral tissues
osseous tissue
osteogenic tissue
oxygen-starved tissue
pancreatic tissue
parasternal tissue
parenchymal tissue
parenchymatous tissue
passage of tissue
periarticular soft tissues
perichondrial-periosteal tissue
perineal tissue
periorbital soft tissue
perirenal tissues
periurethral tissues
placental tissue
polypoid tissue
postnecrotic tissue
prostatic tissue
pursestring effect of the
    tissue
radionecrotic tissue
reconnected tissue
redundant tissue
residual tissue
rest tissue
reticulated tissue
rubber tissue
scar tissue

tissue (*continued*)
sclerous tissues
skeletal tissue
skin-equivalent tissue
SMAS tissue
soft tissue
splenic tissue
spongy tissue
stromal tissue
subcutaneous adipose tissue
subcutaneous connective
    tissues
subcutaneous tissue
subdermal nasal tissue
subjacent tissue
submucosal connective tissue
supporting tissue
supportive tissue
surrounding tissues
sustentacular tissue
symplastic tissue
target tissue
thick elastic tissue
thyroid tissue
tonsillar tissue
transplantation tissue
underlying tissue
uterine tissue
vaginal tissue
vaporizing diseased tissue
vascular tissue
vascularized soft tissue
vascularized tissue
wedge of tissue
weight-bearing tissue
tissue ablation
tissue anchor guide (TAG)
tissue approximation
tissue attenuation
tissue band
tissue bank
tissue bed
tissue biopsy
tissue burn
tissue coagulation
tissue compartments
tissue compression
tissue culture
tissue damage
tissue desiccation needle
tissue desiccation needle
    electrode

tissue dissection
tissue Doppler imaging
tissue drain
tissue dressing forceps
tissue engineering
tissue equivalent material
tissue expander
tissue expander template
tissue expansion
tissue fluid
tissue forceps with teeth
tissue forceps without teeth
tissue fusion
tissue glue
tissue gouge
tissue graft
tissue graft press
tissue harvest
tissue homogeneity
tissue hyperplasia
tissue interposition
tissue macrophage
tissue mandrel implant material
tissue mass
tissue molding
tissue morcellator
tissue occlusion clamp
tissue perfusion
tissue pH monitoring
tissue plane
tissue plane dissector
tissue press
tissue process
tissue protector
tissue reactivity
tissue reflectance oximeter
tissue regeneration
tissue rejection
tissue remodeling
tissue repair
tissue retractor
tissue samples
tissue scissors
tissue sizer template
tissue spaces
Tissue Tek-II cryostat
tissue texture abnormality
tissue transplant
tissue transplantation
tissue turgor
tissue typing
tissue wedge

tissue welding by laser
tissue-bearing area
tissue-borne macrophage
tissue-cultured skin
tissue-engineered cartilage
tissue-expansion technique
tissue-graft engineering
tissue-grasping forceps
Tissue-Guard bovine pericardial
    patch
tissue-holding forceps
TissueLink monopolar floating
    ball
TissueLink technology
tissue-sparing technique
tissue-specific antigen
tissue-spreading forceps
Tis-U-Trap endometrial suction
Tis-U-Trap endometrial suction
    catheter
Tital balloon catheter
Titan Apollo elastic flexion table
Titan endoprosthesis
Titan femoral component
Titan hip cup
Titan Mega PTCA dilatation
    catheter
Titan Meridian Intersegmental
    Traction table
Titan Nova manual flexion-
    extension multi-flex table
Titan slow-speed handpiece
Titan stent
titanium (Ti)
titanium alloy implant
titanium alloy needle
titanium aneurysm clip
titanium ball heart valve
titanium ball prosthesis
titanium cable
titanium cage heart valve
titanium elastic nail
titanium fixation device
titanium foil
titanium half pin
titanium hollow-screw
    osseointegrating
    reconstruction plate
    (THORP)
titanium implant material
titanium mandibular staple
titanium mesh

titanium mesh screw
titanium mesh tray
titanium microconnector
titanium microsurgical bipolar
    forceps
titanium mini bur hole covering
titanium miniplate
titanium needle
titanium optimized design plate
    (TOD plate)
titanium plasma sprayed dental
    implant
titanium prosthesis
titanium rigid fixation
titanium ring
titanium screw
titanium staple
titanium tack
titanium urethral stent
titanium wire
titanium wound retractor
titanium-sprayed implant
Titan-Mega catheter
titration technique
Titus decompressor
Titus forearm splint
Titus tongue depressor
Titus venoclysis needle
Titus wrist splint
Tivanium hip prosthesis
Tivnen tonsillar forceps
Tivnen tonsil-seizing forceps
TJF Olympus endoscope
TK Optimizer knee prosthesis
TKR (total knee replacement)
TKS laser
TL-90 stapler
TLC Baxter balloon catheter
T-lens therapeutic contact lens
TLG (tumescent liposuction
    garment)
T-loop
TLP (total
    laryngopharyngectomy)
TLS suction drain
TLS surgical drain
TLS surgical marker
TLSO brace (thoracolumbar
    standing orthosis brace)
TMA (transmetatarsal
    amputation)
T-malleable retractor

TMD (temporomandibular
    dysfunction)
TMI (transmandibular implant)
TMI implant
TMJ (temporomandibular joint)
TMJ acrylic
TMJ ankylosis
TMJ fossa-eminence prosthesis
TMJ halter
TMJ head positioner
TMJ syndrome
TMJ-OA (temporomandibular
    joint osteoarthritis)
T-model endaural retractor
TMP (transmembrane pressure)
TMPD (temporomandibular
    pain-dysfunction disorder)
TNB (Tru-Cut needle biopsy)
TNM (tumor, nodes, metastases)
TNM carcinoma classification
TNM classification of malignant
    tumors
TNM tumor staging
TNS (transcutaneous nerve
    stimulator)
Toad finger splint
to-and-fro anesthesia
to-and-fro friction sounds
to-and-fro murmur
Tobald syringe
Tobey ear forceps
Tobey ear rongeur
Tobey-Ayer maneuver
Tobin anatomical malar
    prosthetic implant
toboggan-shaped septal cartilage
    columella-tip graft
Tobold knife
Tobold laryngeal forceps
Tobold laryngeal knife
Tobold tongue depressor
Tobold-Fauvel grasping
    forceps
Tobolsky elevator
tobramycin-impregnated PMMA
    implant
Tobruk splint
Tocantins bone marrow biopsy
    needle
tocolysis
tocolytic agent
tocolytic therapy

TOD plate (titanium optimized design plate)
Todd bodies
Todd bur hole button
Todd button
Todd cautery
Todd electrocautery
Todd eye cautery needle
Todd foreign body gouge
Todd gouge
Todd needle
Todd stereotaxic guide
Todd-Evans stepladder tracheal dilatation technique
Todd-Heyer cannula guide
toddler fracture
Todd-Wells guide
Todd-Wells stereotactic frame
Todd-Wells stereotaxic guide
Todd-Wells stereotaxic instrument
Todd-Wells stereotaxic unit
toe
    claw toe
    contracted toe
    curly toes
    downgoing toes
    fanning of toes
    Girdlestone-Taylor operation for claw toes
    great toe
    hammertoe
    Hoffmann claw toe
    Jones repair of first toe
    little toe
    mallet toe
    Morton toe
    pigeon toe
    Ruiz-Mora operation for claw toe
    sausage toe
    second toe
    tennis toe
    transplanted toe
    turf toe
    upgoing toes
    webbed toes
toe bones
toe fillet flap
toe fillet flap procedure
toe flexed
toe loop
toe plate

toe prosthesis
toe pulp neurosensory flap
toe sign
toe spica cast
toe spreader
toe tag
toe-block anesthesia
toedrop brace
toeing in
toeing out
toenail
Toennis anastomosis scissors
Toennis director
Toennis dissecting scissors
Toennis dissector
Toennis dural hook
Toennis ES stand-alone constant-current electrical stimulator
Toennis needle holder
Toennis retractor
Toennis scissors
Toennis tumor-grasping forceps
Toennis-Adson dissector
Toennis-Adson dural scissors
Toennis-Adson scissors
Toennis-Adson utility scissors
toe-phalanx transplantation
toe-spread sign for Morton neuroma
toe-to-hand transfer
toe-to-thumb flap
toe-to-thumb microvascular transplant
toe-to-thumb prosthesis
toe-to-thumb transfer
Tofflemire matrix band
Tofflemire retainer
Tohen tendon technique
Tohen transfer
toilet mastectomy
Toitu cardiovascular monitor
Tolantins bone marrow infusion catheter
Toldt ligament
Toldt line
Toldt membrane
Toledo dissector
Toledo dissector tip
Toledo flap dissector tip
Toledo roller
Toledo standard dissector tip
Toledo V-dissector cannula

Toledo V-dissector tip
Tolentino cutter
Tolentino prism lens
Tolentino ring
Tolentino vitrectomy lens
Tolentino vitreoretinal cutter
Tolentino vitreous cutter
Tolman micrometer
Tolman tonometer
Tolosa-Hunt syndrome
toluidine blue
Tom Jones hysterectomy closure
Tom Jones suture technique
Tom Jones sutures
Tomac catheter
Tomac clip
Tomac foam rubber traction
    dressing
Tomac forceps
Tomac goniometer
Tomac knitted rubber elastic
    dressing
Tomac sphygmomanometer
Tomac vest-style holder
Tomac-Nelaton catheter
Tomas iris hook
Tomas suture hook
Tomasini brace
Tomasini split
TomCat PTCA guidewire
Tomenius gastroscope
Tomey trabeculectomy punch
Tomkins anesthesia unit
Tommy hip bar
Tommy trapeze bar
tomogram
tomograph
tomographic cut
tomographic examination
tomographic images
tomographic study
tomography
    3-dimensional computed
        tomography (3D CT)
    automated computerized axial
        tomography (ACAT)
    computed axial tomography
        (CAT)
    computed tomography (CT)
    computer tomography
    computerized axial
        tomography (CAT)

tomography (*continued*)
    computerized cranial
        tomography (CCT)
    computerized tomography
        (CT)
    CTI positron emission
        tomography (PET) scanner
    dynamic computed
        tomography
    emission computerized
        tomography (ECT)
    plesiosectional tomography
    polycycloidal tomography
    positron computed
        tomography
    positron emission
        tomography (PET)
    quantitative computed
        tomography (QCT)
    spiral computed tomography
    transaxial tomography
    transversal tomography
    transverse tomography
    xenon-enhanced computed
        tomography (XECT)
Tomomatic brain scanner
Tompkins aspirator
Tompkins median bivalving
        technique
Tompkins operation
TomTec echo platform
tone
    anal sphincter tone
    anal tone
    bowel tones
    cheek tone
    fetal heart tones (FHT)
    flexor tone
    heart tones
    hypoactive bowel tones
    muscle tone
    muscular tone
    normoactive bowel tones
    postural tone
    sphincter tone
    Williams tracheal tone
tone and elasticity
tone burst
tone contraction
tone decay
tone-reducing ankle-foot
        orthosis

tong splint
tongs (*see also* traction tongs)
   Ace Universal tongs
   adjustable skull traction tongs
   Barton tongs
   Barton-Cone tongs
   biopsy tongs
   Boehler tongs
   cervical traction tongs
   Cherry traction tongs
   Cohen-Eder tongs
   Crutchfield skull tongs
   Crutchfield traction tongs
   Crutchfield-Raney traction
     tongs
   Eder tongs
   Gardner tongs
   Gardner-Wells skull tongs
   Gardner-Wells traction tongs
   Heifitz traction tongs
   Raney-Crutchfield skull
     traction tongs
   Reynolds tongs
   skull tongs
   traction tongs
   Trippi-Wells tongs
   Vinke tongs
   Wells-Gardner tongs
tongue
   adherent tongue
   amyloid tongue
   apex of tongue
   arcuate papillae of tongue
   bald tongue
   base of tongue (BOT)
   beefy tongue
   bifid tongue
   body of tongue
   cecal foramen of tongue
   cerebriform tongue
   cleft tongue
   coated tongue
   cobblestone tongue
   conoid papillae of tongue
   corolliform papillae of tongue
   crenation of tongue
   crocodile tongue
   Crombie tongue
   deep artery of tongue
   dorsal veins of tongue
   dorsum of tongue
   encrusted tongue

tongue (*continued*)
   extrinsic muscle of tongue
   filmy tongue
   fissured tongue
   forked tongue
   frenulum of tongue
   frenum of tongue
   furrowed tongue
   geographic tongue
   glandular foramen of tongue
   inferior longitudinal muscle of
     tongue
   inferior surface of tongue
   intramuscular glands of
     tongue
   intrinsic muscle of tongue
   lobulated tongue
   longitudinal muscle of tongue
   longitudinal raphe of tongue
   lymphatic follicle of tongue
   magenta tongue
   mappy tongue
   margin of tongue
   median groove of tongue
   motor nerve of tongue
   mucoepidermoid carcinoma
     of the tongue
   mucous membrane of tongue
   plicated tongue
   raspberry tongue
   root of tongue
   scrotal tongue
   septum of tongue
   smoker's tongue
   stippled tongue
   strawberry tongue
   sulcated tongue
   superior longitudinal muscle
     of tongue
   transverse muscle of tongue
   vertical muscle of tongue
   villous papillae of tongue
   white hairy tongue
   wrinkled tongue
tongue biting
tongue blade
tongue depressor (*see* depressor)
   Andrews tongue depressor
   Andrews-Pynchon tongue
     depressor
   Balmer tongue depressor
   Beatty tongue depressor

tongue depressor (*continued*)
  Blakesley tongue depressor
  Boebinger tongue depressor
  Bosworth tongue depressor
  Bruening tongue depressor
  Buchwald tongue depressor
  Chamberlain tongue
    depressor
  Colver-Dawson tongue
    depressor
  Dorsey tongue depressor
  Dunn tongue depressor
  Farlow tongue depressor
  Granberry tongue depressor
  Hamilton tongue depressor
  Israel tongue depressor
  Jobson-Pynchon tongue
    depressor
  Kellogg tongue depressor
  Layman tongue depressor
  Lewis tongue depressor
  metal tongue depressor
  Mulling tongue depressor
  oral screw tongue depressor
  Pirquet tongue depressor
  Proetz tongue depressor
  Pynchon tongue depressor
  Pynchon-Lillie tongue depressor
  Titus tongue depressor
  Tobold tongue depressor
  tongue depressor
  Weder tongue depressor
  wood tongue depressor
tongue flap
tongue forceps
tongue fracture
tongue plate
tongue plate electrode
tongue plication
tongue retractor
tongue retractor blade
tongue sutures
tongue thrust classification
tongue thrust therapy
tongue traction
tongue-and-groove suture
    technique
tongue-in-groove advancement
tongue-in-groove arrangement
tongue-in-groove operation
tongue-in-groove sutures
tongue-in-groove technique

tongue-jaw-neck dissection
tongue-retaining device
tongue-seizing forceps
tongue-shaped villi
tongue-tie operation
tonic contraction
tonicity
Tonkaflo pump
Tonnis clip
Tonnis dura hook
Tonnis dura knife
Tonnis-Adson neurodissector
tonoclonic spasm
tonography
Tonomat applanation tonometer
tonometer (*see also*
    microtonometer)
  air-puff tonometer
  Alcon tonometer
  Allen-Schiotz tonometer
  Allen-Schiotz plunger
    retractor tonometer
  applanation tonometer
  Bailliart tonometer
  Ballenger-Sluder tonometer
  Barraquer applanation
    tonometer
  Barraquer operating room
    tonometer
  Bell tonometer
  Berens tonometer
  biprism applanation
    tonometer
  calibration tonometer
  Carl Zeiss tonometer
  Challenger digital applanation
    tonometer
  Coburn tonometer
  CT-10 computerized
    tonometer
  Daniels tonometer
  Draeger tonometer
  electronic tonometer
  Gartner tonometer
  Goldmann applanation
    tonometer
  Gradle tonometer
  Harrington tonometer
  hemostatic tonometer
  hollow visceral tonometer
  impression tonometer
  indentation tonometer

tonometer (*continued*)
  Intermedics intraocular
    tonometer
  Jena-Schiotz tonometer
  Keeler Pulsair noncontact
    tonometer
  Krakau tonometer
  LaForce tonometer
  Lombart tonometer
  Mack tonometer
  MacKay-Marg tonometer
  Maklakoff tonometer
  McLean tonometer
  Meding tonsil enucleator
    tonometer
  Mueller electronic tonometer
  Musken tonometer
  non-contact tonometer
  Nuvistor electronic tonometer
  Pach-Pen tonometer
  Perkins applanation
    tonometer
  pneumatic tonometer
  pressure phosphene
    tonometer
  ProTon portable tonometer
  Pulsair tonometer
  Recklinghausen tonometer
  Reichert noncontact
    tonometer
  Rosner tonometer
  Roush tonometer
  Ruedemann tonometer
  Sauer tonometer
  Sauer-Storz tonometer
  Schiotz tonometer
  Sklar tonometer
  Sklar-Schiotz jewel tonometer
  Sluder tonometer
  Sluder-Demarest tonometer
  Sluder-Sauer tonometer
  Storz tonometer
  Storz-Moltz tonometer
  Storz-Schitz tonometer
  Tolman tonometer
  Tonomat applanation
    tonometer
  Tono-Pen tonometer
tonometry
  applanation tonometry
  digital tonometry
  Schiotz tonometry

Tono-Pen tonometer
tonsil
  buried tonsil
  cerebellar tonsil
  cryptic tonsil
  crypts of palatine tonsil
  crypts of pharyngeal tonsil
  crypts of tonsils
  eustachian tonsil
  faucial tonsil
  Gerlach tonsil
  intact tonsils
  lingual tonsils
  Luschka tonsil
  palatine tonsil
  pharyngeal tonsil
  resected tonsil
  submerged tonsil
tonsil clamp
tonsil dissector
tonsil forceps
tonsil guillotine
tonsil position
tonsil sponge
tonsil suction dissector
tonsil suction tip
tonsil suction tube
tonsil-dissecting scissors
tonsil-holding forceps
tonsillar abscess
tonsillar abscess forceps
tonsillar artery
tonsillar artery forceps
tonsillar calculus
tonsillar calipers
tonsillar clamp
tonsillar compressor
tonsillar crypts
tonsillar curet
tonsillar dissector
tonsillar electrode
tonsillar elevator
tonsillar enucleator
tonsillar expressor
tonsillar exudate
tonsillar fold
tonsillar fossa
tonsillar guillotine
tonsillar hemostat
tonsillar hemostatic forceps
tonsillar hernia
tonsillar herniation

tonsillar hook
tonsillar knife
tonsillar loop
tonsillar needle
tonsillar needle holder
tonsillar needle holder forceps
tonsillar nerves
tonsillar pillar grasping forceps
tonsillar pillar retractor
tonsillar punch
tonsillar punch forceps
tonsillar retractor
tonsillar scissors
tonsillar screw
tonsillar screw tenaculum
tonsillar separator
tonsillar slitter
tonsillar snare
tonsillar snare wire
tonsillar sponges
tonsillar spreader
tonsillar suction tube
tonsillar suture hook
tonsillar suture needle
tonsillar sutures
tonsillar syringe
tonsillar syringe extension
tonsillar tag
tonsillar tampon
tonsillar tenaculum
tonsillar tissue
tonsillectome
    Ballenger-Sluder tonsillectome
    Beck tonsillectome
    Beck-Mueller tonsillectome
    Beck-Schenck tonsillectome
    Brown tonsillectome
    Daniels hemostatic
        tonsillectome
    hemostatic tonsillectome
    LaForce hemostatic
        tonsillectome
    lingual tonsillectome
    Mack lingual tonsillar
        tonsillectome
    Meding tonsil enucleator
        tonsillectome
    Molt-Storz tonsillectome
    Myles guillotine tonsillectome
    Sauer hemostatic
        tonsillectome
    Sauer-Sluder tonsillectome

tonsillectome (*continued*)
    Sauer-Storz tonsillectome
    Searcy tonsillectome
    Seiffert tonsillectome
    Sluder tonsillar tonsillectome
    Sluder-Ballenger tonsillectome
    Sluder-Demarest tonsillectome
    Sluder-Sauer tonsillectome
    Storz-Moltz tonsillectome
    Tydings tonsillectome
    Van Osdel tonsillar enucleator
        tonsillectome
    Whiting tonsillectome
tonsillectome loop
tonsillectomy
    Cheever tonsillectomy
    faucial and lingual
        tonsillectomy
    faucial tonsillectomy
    LaForce tonsillectomy
    lingual tonsillectomy
    quinsy tonsillectomy
    Sluder tonsillectomy
    snare tonsillectomy
tonsillectomy and
    adenoidectomy (T&A)
tonsillectomy with operating
    microscope
tonsil-ligating forceps
tonsillitis
tonsilloadenoidectomy
tonsillolingual sulcus
tonsilloscope
tonsillotome
tonsillotomy
tonsils
tonsil-seizing forceps
tonsil-suturing forceps
tonsil-suturing instrument
tonus fracture
Tooke angled corneal knife
Tooke blade
Tooke corneal forceps
Tooke iris knife
Tooke spatula
Tooke-Johnson corneal knife
Toomey adaptor
Toomey angled cannula
Toomey bladder evacuator
Toomey evacuator
Toomey forceps
Toomey pyramid tip

Toomey standard cannula
Toomey suction tube
Toomey surgical steel
   instrument set
Toomey syringe
Toomey syringe kit
tooth
   cheek tooth
   extraction of tooth
   incisal surface of tooth
   lingual surface of tooth
   malpositioned tooth
   maxillary anterior tooth
   maxillary posterior tooth
   migrated tooth
   migration of tooth
   missing tooth
   multirooted tooth
   pulpless tooth
   snaggle tooth
   submerged tooth
   surgical neck of tooth
   Turner tooth
   wisdom tooth
tooth band
tooth bud
tooth cement
tooth elevator
tooth extraction
tooth fracture
tooth guard
tooth hemisection
tooth immobilization
tooth ligation
tooth migration
tooth perforation
tooth plane
tooth position
tooth socket
tooth transplantation
tooth-and-nail syndrome
tooth-borne distraction device
toothed forceps
toothed pickup
toothed retractor
toothed tenaculum
toothed thumb forceps
toothed tissue forceps
tooth-extracting forceps
toothless forceps
tooth-like calcification
tooth-to-tooth position

TOP ejector punch
Topaz CO_2 laser
Topaz flexion table
Topaz pacemaker
Topcon aspheric lens
Topcon camera
Topcon chart projector
Topcon keratometer
Topcon digital lensometer
Topcon refractor
Topcon auto refractometer
Topcon camera
Topcon series slit lamp
Topcon non-contact specular
   microscope
Topcon fundus camera
Topcon retinal camera
Topcon stereoscopic fundus
   camera
Topel knot
top-entry (open body) hook
tophaceous
Top-Hat supra-annular aortic
   valve
tophus (*pl.* tophi)
   dental tophus
   gouty tophus
topical anesthesia
topical anesthetic
topical anesthetic spray
topical anesthetic technique
topical application
topical cocaine anesthetic
   agent
topical corticosteroid
topical cream
topical oropharyngeal
   anesthesia
topical therapy
TopiFoam gel-backed self-
   adhering foam pad
Topinard facial angle
topographic
   scanning/indocyanine
   green angiography
   combination instrument
topography
toposcopic catheter
Topper cannula
Topper dressing sponges
Topper nonadherent gauze
Topper sponge

TopSS scanning laser ophthalmoscope
top-valve airway obstruction
Torbot cement
Torbot plastic pouch
Torbot rubber pouch
Torchia capsular forceps
Torchia capsular polisher
Torchia conjunctival scissors
Torchia corneal knife
Torchia eye speculum
Torchia lens hook
Torchia lens implantation forceps
Torchia microbipolar forceps
Torchia microcorneal scissors
Torchia nucleus-aspirating cannula
Torchia tissue forceps
Torchia tying forceps
Torchia vectis loop
Torchia-Colibri forceps
Torchia-Kuglen hook
Torchia-Vannas micro-iris scissors
Torcon angiographic catheter
Torcon selective angiographic catheter
torcular tourniquet
Torek esophagectomy
Torek operation
Torek orchiopexy
Torek resection of thoracic esophagus
Torek-Bevan operation
Torg classification
Torg knee reconstruction
Torg technique
Torgerson-Leach modified technique
toric ablation
toric intraocular lens
Torkildsen operation
Torkildsen shunt
Torkildsen shunt procedure
Torkildsen shunt ventriculocisternostomy
Torkildsen tube
Torkildsen ventriculocisternostomy
Torktherm torque control catheter

torlone fixation pin
torn cartilage
torn knee cartilage
torn lateral meniscus
torn ligament
torn medial meniscus
torn muscle
Tornwaldt abscess
Tornwaldt bursa
Tornwaldt cyst
Torode-Zieg classification
Toronto orthosis
Toronto parapodium orthosis
Toronto pelvic fracture classification
Toronto splint
Toronto 2-stage mammaplasty
Toronto-Western catheter
TORP (total ossicular reconstructive/replacement prosthesis)
    Brackmann TORP
    Cervital TORP (total ossicular replacement prosthesis)
    Plasti-Pore TORP (Plasti-Pore total ossicular replacement prosthesis)
TORP ossicular prosthesis
TORP strut
Torpedo eye patch
Torpin automatic uterine gauze packer
Torpin cul-de-sac resection
Torpin obstetrical lever
Torpin operation
Torpin vectis blade
Torpin vectis extractor
torque guide
torque heel
torque ratchet wrench
torque wrench
torque-control balloon catheter
torque-type prosthesis
torr units of pressure
Torrence steel hook
torrential hemorrhage
Torres cross-action forceps
Torres needle holder
Torrington French spring needle
torsion bar splint
torsion forceps
torsion fracture

torsional fracture
torsional rigidity
torso crease
torso injury
torso phased-array coil
torso presentation
torticollis
tortuosity of glands
tortuosity of vessel
tortuous aorta
tortuous esophagus
tortuous root canal
tortuous telangiectasis
tortuous varicosities
tortuous vessels
torus (*pl.* tori)
torus crush
torus fracture
torus frontalis
torus levatorius
torus mandibularis
torus occipitalis
torus palatinus
To-San tissue expander
Toshiba helical CT scanner
Toshiba biplane transesophageal transducer
Toshiba brain scanner
Toshiba echocardiograph machine
Toshiba electrocardiography machine
Toshiba helical CT scanner
Toshiba microendoprobe
Toshiba microendoscope
Toshiba MR scanner
Toshiba ultrasound
Toshiba colonoscope
Toshiba video endoscope
Toshiba helical CT scanner
total abdominal colectomy (TAC)
total abdominal evisceration
total abdominal hysterectomy (TAH)
total alloplastic TMJ reconstruction prosthesis
total anesthesia
total ankle arthroplasty
total anodontia
total articular replacement arthroplasty (TARA)

total articular resurfacing arthroplasty
total artificial heart
total autogenous latissimus (TAL)
total autogenous latissimus breast reconstruction
total axial node irradiation
total biopsy
total bladder resection
total blood loss
total blood volume
total body
total body irradiation
total body surface area (TBSA)
total breech delivery
total breech extraction
total capsulectomy
total cardiopulmonary bypass
total cataract
total cataract extraction
total cleft palate
total colectomy (TC)
total colonoscopy
total condylar knee prosthesis
total contact bivalve ankle-foot orthosis
total contact cast
total cystectomy
total dehiscence
total ear obliteration
total elbow arthroplasty
total endoscopic esophagectomy
total enteral nutrition (TEN)
total etch technique
total ethmoidectomy
total excisional operation
total extraperitoneal repair
total fundoplication
total fundoplication procedure
total fundoplication technique
total gastrectomy
total gastric wrap
total glossectomy
total graft area rejected (TGAR)
total hip arthroplasty
total hip prosthesis
total hip replacement (THR)
total hip replacement surgery
total hypophysectomy
total hysterectomy

total intravenous anesthesia (TIVA)
total intravenous anesthetic technique
total ipsilateral lobectomy
total joint arthroplasty
total joint replacement
total keratoplasty
Total Knee prosthetic knee
total knee arthroscopy (TKA)
total knee prosthesis
total knee replacement (TKR)
total knee replacement surgery
total laparoscopic esophagectomy
total laryngectomy
total laryngectomy with radical neck dissection
total laryngopharyngectomy (TLP)
total L-chain concentration
total left hepatectomy
total lobectomy
total lymphoid irradiation
total mastectomy
total meniscectomy
total mesorectal excision (TME)
total midface osteotomy
total nodal irradiation
total obstruction
total ossicular prosthesis
total ossicular reconstruction/replacement prosthesis (TORP)
total pancreatectomy
total parenteral alimentation
total parenteral nutrition (TPN)
total parotidectomy
total patellofemoral joint arthroplasty
total pelvic exenteration
total penile reconstruction
total perineal rupture
total placenta previa
total pneumonectomy
total protein concentration
total push therapy
total retrocolic end-to-side gastrojejunostomy
total shoulder arthroplasty
total spinal anesthesia
total surgical removal

total symblepharon
total thoracic esophagectomy
total time to intubation (TTI)
total toe template
total top implant
total unilateral vestibular deafferentation
total upper lip resection
total vascular exclusion
total wrist arthroplasty
totally extraperitoneal inguinal herniorrhaphy
totally implantable catheter
Totco Autoclip
Totco clip
Toti operation
Toti procedure
Toti trephine
Toti trephine drill
Toti-Mosher operation
Tott ring remover
Touchlite zoom lens
touch-up peels
touch-up procedure
Touhy-Borst connector
Touhy-Borst side-arm introducer
Touma dissector
Touma T-type grommet ventilation tube
Toupe procedure
Toupe technique
Toupet fundoplasty
Toupet fundoplication
Toupet hemifundoplication
Toupet wrap for severe GERD
Tourguide guiding catheter
Tournikwik tourniquet
tourniquet
    Adams modification of Bethune tourniquet
    Adams tourniquet
    automatic rotating tourniquet
    automatic tourniquet
    Bethune lobectomy tourniquet
    Bethune lung tourniquet
    Bodenstab tourniquet
    Campbell-Boyd tourniquet
    cardiovascular tourniquet
    Carr lobectomy tourniquet
    caval tourniquet
    Conn pneumatic tourniquet

tourniquet (*continued*)
Conn Universal tourniquet
cotton-covered tourniquet
Davol tourniquet
deflated tourniquet
Digikit finger tourniquet
Disposiquet disposable
   tourniquet
double loop tourniquet
Drake tourniquet
Dupuytren tourniquet
Esmarch tourniquet
Field tourniquet
flexible tourniquet
forearm tourniquet
Fouli tourniquet
garrote tourniquet
Gaylord pneumatic tourniquet
Gill renal tourniquet
Grafco tourniquet
Holcome gastric tourniquet
horseshoe tourniquet
Ideal automatic tourniquet
inflated tourniquet
inflation of tourniquet
Johnson & Johnson
   tourniquet
Kidde tourniquet
Kidde-Robbins tourniquet
Linton tourniquet
lobectomy tourniquet
lung tourniquet
Medi-quet surgical tourniquet
Momberg tourniquet
nonpneumatic tourniquet
Pac-Kit Army-type tourniquet
Penrose tourniquet
Petit tourniquet
pneumatic ankle tourniquet
pneumatic tourniquet
Profex arthroscopic
   tourniquet
Quicket tourniquet
ratchet tourniquet
Robbins automatic tourniquet
Roberts-Nelson lobectomy
   tourniquet
Roper-Rumel tourniquet
rotating tourniquet
Rumel cardiac tourniquet
Rumel cardiovascular
   tourniquet

tourniquet (*continued*)
Rumel myocardial tourniquet
Rumel ratchet tourniquet
Rumel-Belmont tourniquet
Rumpuffet vessel tourniquet
Samway tourniquet
Satinsky tourniquet
scalp tourniquet
Sebra arm tourniquet
Shenstone tourniquet
Signorini tourniquet
single-loop tourniquet
SMIC auricular tourniquet
Spanish tourniquet
Sure-Snare tourniquet
Surgikit Velcro tourniquet
thigh tourniquet
Tinel tourniquet
torcular tourniquet
Tournikwik tourniquet
Trussdale tourniquet
U.S. Army tourniquet
Uniquet disposable
   intravenous tourniquet
Universal tourniquet
Velcro tourniquet
Velket-Velcro tourniquet
Weiner tourniquet
Wright pneumatic tourniquet
tourniquet band
tourniquet control
tourniquet cuff
tourniquet inflation unit
tourniquet occlusion
tourniquet strap
tourniquet tightened
tourniquet-eyed obturator
tourniquet-eyed ratchet stylet
Tourtual canal
Tourtual membrane
Tovell tube
towel clamp
towel clip
towel clip forceps
towel drape
Tower forceps
Tower fracture table
Tower interchangeable retractor
Tower muscle forceps
Tower prong
Tower rib retractor
Tower spinal retractor

Tower stent
Tower table
Towne position
Towne projection
  roentgenogram
Towne view of skull on x-ray
Towne x-ray view
Townley anatomic instruments
Townley anatomic knee
  replacement
Townley bone graft screw
Townley calipers
Townley femur calipers
Townley forceps
Townley implant
Townley inside-outside femur
  calipers
Townley knee prosthesis
Townley screw
Townley TARA prosthesis
Townley tissue forceps
Townley total knee prosthesis
Townley-Paton operation
Townsend biopsy punch
Townsend endocervical biopsy
  curet
Townsend knee brace
Townsend-Gilfillan plate
Townsend-Gilfillan screw
toxemia curet
toxic goiter
toxic granulation
toxic megacolon
toxicity
Toxoplasma lymphadenitis
Toynbee curet
Toynbee diagnostic tube
Toynbee ear speculum
Toynbee maneuver
Toynbee otoscope
Toynbee speculum
TPE ankle-foot orthosis
TPE biomechanical foot orthosis
TPFF (temporoparietal fascia
  flap)
T-piece
T-pin handle
T-plate
TPN (total parenteral nutrition)
TPN catheter
TPN line
TPS-coated cylinder

TPS-coated screw
Tröltsch (see Troeltsch)
Tromner reflex
Trömner (see Tromner)
Troemner (see Tromner)
Tromner (also Trömner,
  Troemner)
TR-28 hip prosthesis
trabecula (pl. trabeculae)
trabecular bone
trabecular bone fracture
trabecular carcinoma
trabecular degeneration
trabecular membrane
trabecular meshwork
trabecular region
trabecular vein
trabeculated bladder
trabeculated bone lesion
trabeculation
  coarse trabeculation
  mild trabeculation
  muscular trabeculation
trabeculectomy
trabeculodialysis
trabeculoplasty
trabeculotome
trabeculotomy
trabeculotomy probe
Trabucco double balloon
  catheter
Trac Plus catheter
trace anesthetic
Trace hydraulic vein stripper
Trace vein stripper
TraceHybrid wire guide
Tracer Blood Glucose monitor
tracer catheter
Tracer hybrid wire guide
Tracer Hybrid wire guide with
  Slip-Coat tip
Tracer over-the-wire
  intravascular mapping
  catheter
Tracer ST wire
TrachCare multi-access catheter
trachea
tracheal adenoma
tracheal agenesis
tracheal aspiration
tracheal atresia
tracheal bifurcation angle

tracheal biopsy
tracheal bistoury
tracheal block
tracheal bougie
tracheal bronchial knife
tracheal bronchus
tracheal button
tracheal calcification
tracheal cannula
tracheal cartilage
tracheal catheter
tracheal catheterization
tracheal compression
tracheal deviation
tracheal dilator
tracheal extubation anesthetic
    technique
tracheal fenestration
tracheal fistula
tracheal forceps
tracheal fracture
tracheal gland
tracheal hemostat
tracheal hemostatic forceps
tracheal hook
tracheal incision
tracheal intubation
tracheal intubation anesthetic
    technique
tracheal knife
tracheal lavage
tracheal ligation
tracheal mucosa
tracheal muscle
tracheal obstruction
tracheal papilloma
tracheal reconstruction
tracheal reflex
tracheal repair
tracheal retractor
tracheal rings
tracheal safety stitch
tracheal scalpel
tracheal scissors
tracheal secretions
tracheal stenosis
tracheal stump
tracheal suction anesthetic
    technique
tracheal suction tube
tracheal tampon
tracheal tenaculum

tracheal topical analgesia
tracheal tree
tracheal tube
tracheal tube brush
tracheal tube cuff
tracheal tube with obturator
tracheal tug
tracheal ulceration
tracheal vein
tracheal wall
tracheal web
trachealis muscle
trachelectomy
trachelomastoid muscle
trachelopexy
tracheloplasty
trachelorrhaphy
trachelotome
trachelotomy
tracheobiliary fistula
tracheobronchial anomaly
tracheobronchial foreign body
tracheobronchial suction tube
tracheobronchial tree
tracheobronchoesophageal
    fistula
tracheobronchoesophagoscope
tracheocele
tracheocricotomy
tracheocutaneous fistula
tracheoesophageal (TE)
tracheoesophageal dilator
tracheoesophageal fistula
tracheoesophageal fistula
    closure
tracheoesophageal junction
tracheoesophageal puncture
    dilator
tracheoesophageal shunt
tracheofissure
tracheogram
tracheography
tracheolaryngotomy
tracheopharyngeal shunt
tracheoplasty
tracheopulmonary secretions
tracheorrhaphy
tracheoscope
    Haslinger tracheoscope
    Jackson tracheoscope
tracheoscopy
TracheoSoft tracheostomy tube

tracheostomy
  Bjork flap tracheostomy
  cricothyroidotomy and
    tracheostomy
  elective dilatational
    tracheostomy
  emergency tracheostomy
  flap tracheostomy
  Great Ormand Street
    tracheostomy
  Portex tracheostomy
tracheostomy button
tracheostomy cannula
tracheostomy hook
tracheostomy scissors
tracheostomy stoma
tracheostomy tray
tracheostomy trocar
tracheostomy tube
tracheotome
tracheotomic bistoury
tracheotomize
tracheotomy
  Bose tracheotomy
  inferior tracheotomy
  laryngofissure with
    tracheotomy
  low tracheotomy
  superior tracheotomy
tracheotomy cannula
tracheotomy hook
tracheotomy set
tracheotomy site
tracheotomy sponge
tracheotomy tube
Trachlight lighted intubating
    stylet
trachoma forceps
trachoma gland
Trach-Talk device
track sutures
track valve
Tracker infusion catheter
Tracker knee brace
Tracker microcatheter
Tracker Soft Stream side-hole
    microinfusion catheter
Tracker-18 catheter
tracker-assisted laser
Tracheoflex tracheostomy tube
tract
  aberrant AV bypass tract

tract (*continued*)
  alimentary tract
  atriofascicular bypass tract
  atrio-His tract
  atrio-Hisian bypass tract
  atrionodal bypass tract
  Bertrand tract
  biliary tract
  black box of upper GI tract
  Breckenmacher tract
  Burdach tract
  bypass tract
  corticobulbar tract
  corticospinal tract
  digestive tract
  fasciculoventricular bypass
    tract
  fistulous tract
  flow tract
  Foville tract
  gastrointestinal tract
  geniculocalcarine tract
  genitourinary tract
  Goll tract
  Gowers tract
  Gudden tract
  Helweg tract
  hepatic outflow tract
  horizontal tract
  ileal inflow tract
  iliotibial tract
  inflammatory sinus tract
  inflow tract
  intact motor tract
  internodal tract
  intestinal tract
  intramural fistulous tract
  James accessory tract
  James atrionodal bypass tract
  James intranodal tract
  left ventricular inflow tract
  left ventricular outflow tract
  Lissauer tract
  long tract
  Meynet tract
  nodoventricular bypass tract
  olfactory tract
  olivocerebellar tract
  optic tract
  osteomeatal sinus tract
  outflow tract
  pancreaticobiliary tract

tract (*continued*)
    pin tract
    pulmonary conduit outflow
        tract
    pulmonary outflow tract
    pyramidal tract
    respiratory tract
    right ventricular inflow tract
    right ventricular outflow tract
    sensory tract
    sinonasal tract
    sinus tract
    spinothalamic tract
    transection of nerve tracts
    upper respiratory tract
    urinary tract
    urogenital tract
    ventricular flow tract
    ventricular outflow tract
    vertical tract
tract dilation
traction
    Ace Trippi-Wells tong cervical
        traction
    Ace Universal tong cervical
        traction
    Agnew traction
    AOA-CHICK halo traction
    Apley traction
    axis traction
    balanced traction
    bellows traction
    Bremer halo cervical traction
    Bremer halo crown traction
    Bremmer halo traction
    Bryant traction
    Buck extension traction
    Carrie Tracheoflex
    cervical AOA halo traction
    cervical traction
    C-Flex supine cervical traction
    Cotrel traction
    Crego bow traction
    Crego wire traction
    Crile head traction
    Crutchfield skeletal traction
    Crutchfield tongs traction
    Dale traction
    device for transverse traction
    direct transverse traction
        (DTT)
    Dunlop elbow traction

traction (*continued*)
    elastic traction
    extension traction
    external traction
    Freiberg traction
    Frejka traction
    gentle traction
    Georgiade intraoral traction
    Georgiade visor cervical
        traction
    Goodley cervical traction
    halo traction
    halo-femoral traction
    halo-pelvic traction
    halo-to-bale traction
    halter traction
    handle traction
    Handy-Buck traction
    head halter cervical traction
    head halter traction
    Hoke-Martin traction
    Holter traction
    Homestretch lumbar traction
    Houston halo cervical traction
    Houston halo traction
    intermaxillary traction
    intermittent traction
    internal traction
    Jones suspension traction
    Kestler ambulatory head
        traction
    Keys-Kirschner traction
    King traction
    Kirschner skeletal traction
    Kirschner wire traction
    Kuhlman cervical traction
    Lowsley prostatic traction
    lumbosacral support pelvic
        traction
    Lyman Smith traction
    manual traction
    maxillomandibular traction
    McBride tripod-pin traction
    Miami collar cervical traction
    moleskin traction
    Neufeld rolling traction
    pelvic traction
    Perkins traction
    Philadelphia collar cervical
        traction
    Pierson traction
    placed in traction

traction (*continued*)

- pounds of traction
- Russell pin traction
- Russell skeletal cervical traction
- Saunders cervical HomeTrac traction
- Sayre suspension traction
- skeletal traction
- skin traction
- skull traction
- split Russell skeletal traction
- Steinmann traction
- supine C-Trax traction
- suspension traction
- Syms traction
- tenaculum traction
- tongue traction
- transfer traction
- tripod pin traction
- Vinke tong skull traction
- Watson-Jones traction
- well-leg traction
- Zimfoam head halter traction

traction anchor
traction aneurysm
traction bar
traction belt
traction bow
traction detachment
traction device
traction diverticulum
traction forceps
traction fracture
traction halter collar
traction handle (*see* handle)
traction legging
traction spur from disk degeneration
traction suture technique
traction sutures
traction table
traction tenaculum
traction tongs (*see* tongs)
traction tongs screw
traction wrinkling
tractor

- Anderson tractor
- axial tractor
- banjo tractor
- Blackburn skull traction tractor

tractor (*continued*)

- Boehler tractor
- Bryant tractor
- Buck tractor
- Conco tractor
- curved tractor
- Dunlop tractor
- Exo-Bed tractor
- Exo-Static overhead tractor
- extension tractor
- Fisk tractor
- Freiberg tractor
- halo tractor
- Hamilton pelvic traction screw tractor
- Handy-Buck extension tractor
- Hoke-Martin tractor
- Kestler ambulatory head tractor
- Kirschner wire tractor
- Lowsley prostatic tractor
- Lowsley suprapubic tractor
- Lyman-Smith tractor
- Muirhead-Little pelvic rest tractor
- Naugh os calcis apparatus tractor
- Neufeld tractor
- Orr-Buck extension tractor
- Perkins split-weight tractor
- prostatic tractor
- Pugh tractor
- Rankin prostatic tractor
- Russell tractor
- skull tractor
- Steinmann traction tractor
- Syms tractor
- Trimline mobile tractor
- Tupper tractor
- Vinke skull tractor
- Watson-Jones tractor
- Wells tractor
- Young prostatic tractor
- Zimcode traction frames tractor
- Zim-Trac traction splint tractor

tractotomy
Tradition brace
traditional lipoplasty
TRAFO orthosis
tragal border

tragal cartilage
tragus (*pl.* tragi)
tragus House hook
tragus muscle
Trailblazer screw guide
Trailblazer wire
trailer gauze
Trainor operation
Trainor-Nida operation
trajector
Trake-Fit endotracheal tube
Trake-Fit tracheal tube holder
Trakstar balloon catheter
TRAM (transverse rectus
     abdominis
     musculocutaneous)
TRAM flap
TRAM flap breast reconstruction
TRAM flap hernia
TRAM flap procedure
TRAM procedure
TRAMP (transversus and rectus
     abdominis
     musculoperitoneal)
trampoline fracture
transabdominal approach
transabdominal cholangiography
transabdominal colonoscopy
transabdominal laparoscopic
     herniorrhaphy
transabdominal preperitoneal
     hernioplasty
transabdominal preperitoneal
     repair
transabdominal repair
transabdominal transducer
transacromial approach
transacromial incision
transanal approach
transanal endoscopic
     microsurgery
transanal endoscopic
     microsurgical resection
transanal excision
transanal mucosectomy with
     handsewn anastomosis
transanal pouch advancement
transanal puncture
transanal stapling technique
transannular patch
transantral approach
transantral ethmoidal approach

transantral ethmoidectomy
transantral orbital
     decompression
transaortic valve gradient
transareolar mastectomy
transareolar mastocele
transarterial anesthetic
     technique
transarticular screw
transarticular wire fixation
transaxial scan plane
transaxial tomography
transaxillary approach
transaxillary breast
     augmentation (TBA)
transaxillary incision
transaxillary needle
transaxillary subpectoral
     augmentation
transbasal
transblepharoplasty approach
transblepharoplasty forehead lift
transblepharoplasty procedure
transblepharoplasty
     subperiosteal midface
     elevation
transbrachial arch aortogram
transbrachioradialis approach
transbronchial lung biopsy
transbronchial needle aspiration
transbuccal trocar
transcallosal transventricular
     approach
transcalvarial suture fixation
transcanine approach
transcapillary hydrostatic
     pressure gradient
transcapitate fracture
transcapitate fracture-dislocation
transcapitellar wire fixation
transcarpal amputation
transcatheter ablation
transcatheter arterial
     embolization therapy
transcatheter closure
transcatheter closure of atrial
     septal defect
transcatheter device
transcatheter umbrella implant
     material
transcavernous transpetrous
     apex approach

transcellular fluid
Transcend Acetabular System
transcerebellar hemispheric
    approach
transcervical approach
transcervical femoral fracture
transcervical fracture
transcervical resection
transcervical tubal access catheter
transchondral fracture
transclavicular approach
transcoccygeal approach
transcochlear approach
transcolonic endoscopy
transcondylar fracture
transconjunctival approach
transconjunctival blepharoplasty
    (TCB)
transconjunctival endoscopic
    orbital decompression
transconjunctival lower lid
    blepharoplasty
transconjunctival retractor
transcorneal transillumination
transcoronal eyebrow lift
transcortical transventricular
    approach
transcranial Doppler probe
transcranial electrical
    stimulation anesthetic
    technique
transcranial facial bipartition
transcranial frontal-temporal-
    orbital approach
transcranial monobloc
    frontofacial advancement
transcranial projection
transcranial roentgenogram
transcranial temporomandibular
    joint radiograph
transcranial-supraorbital
    approach
transcubital approach
transcutaneous biopsy
transcutaneous broadband
    sector transducer
transcutaneous carbon dioxide
    monitor
transcutaneous cranial electrical
    stimulator
transcutaneous electrical nerve
    stimulation (TENS)

transcutaneous electrical nerve
    stimulator (TENS)
transcutaneous electrical
    neuromuscular stimulator
    (TENS)
transcutaneous extraction
    catheter
transcutaneous nerve stimulator
    (TCNS, TNS)
transcutaneous neuromuscular
    electrical stimulator
transcutaneous oxygen monitor
transcutaneous oxygen
    monitoring
transcutaneous pacemaker
transcutaneous stimulator
transcutaneous-transconjunctival
    suture
transcylindrical cholecystectomy
transcystic approach
transcystic drainage
transcystoscopically
Transcyte skin substitute graft
transdermal administration
transdermal analgesic
transdermal anesthesia
transdermal anesthetic
    technique
transdermal fentanyl device
transdiaphragmatic
    sympathectomy
transducer-tipped catheter
transduction
transduodenal approach
transduodenal
    choledocholithotomy
transduodenal endoscopic
    decompression
transduodenal excision of
    common duct stone
transduodenal fiberscopic duct
    injection
transduodenal sphincterotomy
transdural approach
Transeal transparent adhesive
    film dressing
Transeal transparent wound
    dressing
transected vertical gastric
    bypass
transection incision
transection of artery

transection of nerve roots
transection of nerve tracts
transection of tube
transection of vein
transection plane
Transelast surgical drape
transelectrical nerve stimulator
transendoscopic
    electrocoagulation
transendoscopic procedure
transendoscopic ultrasound
transensor
transepiglottic laryngotomy
transepiphyseal fracture
transesophageal echocardiography
transesophageal
    echocardiography probe
transesophageal endoscopy
transesophageal ligation of
    varices
transesophageal probe
transesophageal varix ligation
transethmoidal hypophysectomy
transethmoidal sphenoidotomy
transfemoral balloon occlusion
transfemoral endoaortic
    occlusion catheter
transfemoral liver biopsy
transfemoral venous
    catheterization
transfer
    Bateman tendon transfer
    Brand tendon transfer
    Brooks-Seddon transfer
    Bunnell tendon transfer
    buried free forearm flap transfer
    composite free tissue transfer
    dermal fat free tissue transfer
    double paddle peroneal tissue
        transfer
    Eggers tendon transfer
    facial paralysis reconstruction
        with free muscle transfer
    facial paralysis reconstruction
        with gracilis free muscle
        transfer
    facial paralysis reconstruction
        with pectoralis minor
        muscle transfer
    facial paralysis reconstruction
        with rectus abdominis
        muscle transfer

transfer (*continued*)
    free muscle transfer
    free omental flap transfer
    free tissue transfer (FTT)
    free toe transfer
    gamete intrafallopian transfer
        (GIFT)
    gracilis free muscle transfer
    Green-Grice transfer
    hypoglossal-to-facial nerve
        transfer
    ilium microvascular transfer
    island frontalis muscle
        transfer
    key-slot patella tendon
        transfer
    Lamb transfer
    Linscheid tendon transfer
    Mantelow transfer
    masseter muscle transfer
    Mayer trapezius transfer
    microvascular bone transfer
    microvascular free flap
        transfer
    microvascular free gracilis
        transfer
    microvascular free tissue
        transfer
    microvascular toe transfer
    muscle transfer
    Mustard iliopsoas transfer
    Ober-Barr brachioradialis
        transfer
    Peabody tibialis tendon
        transfer
    pectoralis minor muscle
        transfer
    rectus abdominis muscle
        transfer
    regional muscle transfer
    Roux-Goldthwait patellar
        tendon transfer
    Royal Moore opponens
        pollicis transfer
    Royle-Thompson transfer
    scapular flap transfer
    segmental microvascular
        transfers
    Sharrard iliopsoas transfer
    Slocum pes transfer
    staged muscle transfer
    static tendon transfer

transfer (*continued*)
  Stephenson-Donovan transfer
  Stiles-Bunnell transfer
  Sutherland hamstring transfer
  temporalis muscle-fascia
    transfer
  tendon transfer
  Thomas-Thompson-Straub
    transfer
  toe-to-hand transfer
  toe-to-thumb transfer
  Tohen transfer
  Trillat patellar tendon transfer
  vascularized whole joint
    transfer
  Velpeau tendon transfer
  Zancolli lasso tendon transfer
  zygote intrafallopian tube
    transfer (ZIFT)
transfer forceps
transfer of tendon
transfer traction
transference of muscle
transfibular approach
transfibular arthrodesis
transfixation incision
transfixing suture technique
transfixing sutures
transfixion bolt
transfixion screw
transfixion sutures
transformation
transformer
  cautery transformer
  current transformer
  filament transformer
  step-down transformer
  step-up transformer
transforming growth factor
  (TGF)
transfrontal approach
transfusion
  autologous transfusion
  blood transfusion
  coagulation factor transfusion
  donor transfusion
  donor-specific transfusion (DST)
  double-volume exchange
    transfusion
  exchange transfusion
  exsanguination transfusion
  immediate transfusion

transfusion (*continued*)
  incompatible blood
    transfusion
  intraperitoneal transfusion
  intrauterine transfusion
  intravenous transfusion
  IV transfusion
  massive transfusions
  placental transfusion
  plasma transfusion
  reciprocal transfusion
  replacement transfusion
  serum transfusion
  substitution transfusion
transfusion therapy
transfusion-related acute lung
    injury (TRALD)
transfusion-related air embolism
transgastric fine-needle
    aspiration biopsy
transgastric ligation
transgastric plication
transgastrostomic enteroscopy
transgenic therapy
transglottic squamous cell
    carcinoma
transgluteal approach
transhamate fracture
transhamate fracture-dislocation
transhepatic antegrade biliary
    drainage procedure
transhepatic approach
transhepatic biliary stent
transhepatic catheterization
transhepatic cholangiogram
    (THC)
transhepatic cholangiography
transhepatic embolization
transhepatic portacaval shunt
transhepatic portography
transhiatal approach
transhiatal blunt esophagectomy
transhiatal esophagectomy
    (THE)
transhiatal esophagojejunostomy
transient anesthesia
transient compartment
    syndrome
transient edema
transient hiatal hernia
transient lesion
transient osteoporosis of hip

TransiGel hydrogel-impregnated gauze
TransiGel woven gauze dressing
transiliac amputation
transiliac bar technique
transiliac fracture
transiliac rod fixation
transilluminating telescope
transillumination
transilluminator (*see also* illuminator)
  all-purpose transilluminator
  Briggs transilluminator
  Coldlite transilluminator
  Finnoff transilluminator
  hooded transilluminator
  Lancaster transilluminator
  National transilluminator
  rotating transilluminator
  Shunn gun transilluminator
  speculum illuminator transilluminator
  speculum transilluminator
  Tatum ureteral transilluminator
  Welch Allyn transilluminator
  Whitelite transilluminator
  Widner transilluminator
transischial measurement (TI measurement)
transition sutures
transitional cell carcinoma
transitional development
transitional lumbosacral joint
transitional lumbosacral vertebra
transitional tumor
transitional vertebra
transitional zone biopsy
transit-time flowmeter
transjugular hepatic biopsy
transjugular insertion
transjugular intrahepatic portal systemic shunt
transjugular liver biopsy
transjunctional lipectomy
translabial access
translabyrinthine and suboccipital approach
translaryngeal guided intubation anesthetic technique
translaryngeal tracheal intubation

translateral films
translation injury
translational fracture
translational position
translatory movement
translocation Down syndrome
translocation needle
translucent drain tube
translucent myringotomy tube
translumbar aortogram
translumbar inferior vena cava catheter
transluminal angioplasty
transluminal angioplasty catheter
transluminal balloon
transluminal balloon angioplasty
transluminal coronary angioplasty
transluminal coronary angioplasty guidewire
transluminal coronary artery angioplasty
transluminal endarterectomy catheter
transluminal extraction atherectomy
transluminal extraction catheter (TEC)
transmandibular approach
transmandibular implant (TMI)
transmandibular reconstruction
transmandibular-glossopharyngeal approach
transmastoid approach
transmaxillary approach
transmeatal approach
transmeatal atticotomy
transmeatal incision
transmeatal labyrinthotomy
transmeatal tympanoplasty incision
transmediastinal posterior esophagoplasty
transmembrane pressure (TMP)
transmesenteric hernia
transmesenteric plication
transmetacarpal replantation
transmetatarsal amputation (TMA)
transmission electron microscope (TEM)

transmission electron
    microscopy (TEM)
transmission image
transmit-receive coil
transmitter
transmucosal drug
    administration anesthetic
    technique
transmural antitachycardia
    pacemaker
transmural approach
transmural closure
transmural electrical stimulator
transmural hydrostatic pressure
    gradient
transmural inflammation
transmural resection
transmyocardial pacing stylet
transnasal administration
transnasal bile duct
    catheterization
transnasal biopsy
transnasal drain
transnasal endoscopy
transnasal intraduodenal feeding
    catheter
transnasal ligation of internal
    maxillary artery
transnasal pancreaticobiliary
    drain
transnasal sphenoidotomy
transolecranon approach
transomental posterior
    gastroenterostomy
Transonic flow probe
Transonic flowmeter
Transonic laser Doppler
    perfusion monitor
transoral approach
transoral catheter
transoral endoscopy
transoral odontoid resection
transoral projection
transoral retractor
Transorb wound dressing
Transorbent multilayer dressing
Transorbent topical wound
    dressing
transorbital leukotomy
transorbital lobotomy
transosseous holes
transosseous implant

transosseous suture
transosteal implant
transpalatal approach
transpalatal bar
transpalpebral approach
transpalpebral corrugator
    muscle
transpapillary approach
transpapillary biopsy
transpapillary cannulation
transpapillary catheterization
transpapillary cystopancreatic
    stent
transpapillary drain
transpapillary endoscope
transpapillary endoscopic
    cholecystotomy
transpapillary endoscopic
    endoprosthesis
transparent adhesive film
    dressing
transparent drape
transparent dressing
transparent elastic band ligating
    device
transpedicular approach
transpedicular screw
transpedicular screw-rod
    fixation
transpedicular segmental
    fixation
transpedicularly implanted
    anterior spinal support
    device
transpelvic amputation
transpericardial pacemaker
transperitoneal approach
transperitoneal cesarean section
transperitoneal exposure
transperitoneal hand-assisted
    laparoscopic surgery
transperitoneal laparoscopic
    adrenalectomy
transperitoneal nephrectomy
transperitoneal technique
Transpire wrist orthosis
transplacental hemorrhage
transplant
    acute rejection of liver
        transplant
    adult-to-adult living related
        donor living transplant

transplant (*continued*)
  alloplastic transplant
  autogenous transplant
  autologous bone marrow
    transplant
  auxiliary transplant
  Baffle transplant
  Berens corneal transplant
  Berens corneoscleral
    transplant
  Berens pterygium transplant
  bone marrow transplant
  cadaveric hand transplant
  cadaveric transplant
  cadaveric whole organ
    transplant
  cardiac transplant
  corneal transplant
  domino transplant
  donor transplant
  Elmslie-Trillat patellar tendon
    transplant
  fat transplant
  fetal tissue transplant
  free groin transplant
  Gallie transplant
  great toe transplant
  hair transplant
  Hauser transplant
  heart transplant
  heart-lung transplant
  hepatic transplant
  heterotopic transplant
  homogenous transplant
  Hughston patellar transplant
  kidney transplant
  lamellar corneal transplant
  laser hair transplant
  liver transplant
  living-related small bowel
    transplant
  Lower-Shumway cardiac
    transplant
  McReynolds pterygium
    transplant
  organ transplant
  orthotopic cardiac transplant
  orthotopic liver transplant
    (OLT)
  orthotopic transplant
  pancreas transplant (PTX)
  penetrating corneal transplant

transplant (*continued*)
  piggyback heart transplant
  placental tissue transplant
  primarily vascularized organ
    transplant
  pterygium transplant
  recipient of organ transplant
  reduced liver transplant (RLT)
  reduced-size transplant
  rejected transplant
  rejection cardiomyopathy
    transplant
  rejection of transplant
  renal transplant
  small bowel transplant
  SPK transplant
  split-liver transplant
  syngenesioplastic transplant
  tendon transplant
  testicle transplant
  tissue transplant
  toe-to-thumb microvascular
    transplant
transplant lung syndrome
transplant nephrectomy
transplant rejection
transplant spatula
transplant trephine
transplantation
  adrenal medulla
    transplantation
  allogeneic transplantation
  allograft tissue
    transplantation
  allograft transplantation
  anhepatic stage of liver
    transplantation
  autogenous tooth
    transplantation
  autologous blood stem cell
    transplantation
  autologous bone marrow
    transplantation (ABMT)
  autologous fat transplantation
  auxiliary partial orthotopic
    liver transplantation
    (APOLT)
bone marrow transplantation
Bosworth femoroischial
    transplantation
brain transplantation
bridge organ transplantation

transplantation (*continued*)
  cadaveric donor
    transplantation
  cardiac transplantation
  clinical intestinal
    transplantation
  composite tissue
    transplantation
  corneal transplantation
  Cowen-Loftus toe-phalanx
    transplantation
  cryopreserved extrapelvic
    ovarian transplantation
  double toe transplantation
  femoroischial transplantation
  fetal liver transplantation
  fetal thymus transplantation
  fresh extrapelvic ovarian
    transplantation
  hair transplantation
  heart transplantation
  heart-lung transplantation
  hepatic transplantation
  hepatocyte transplantation
  heterotopic transplantation
  homogenous tooth
    transplantation
  homotopic transplantation
  intestinal transplantation
  kidney transplantation
  laser hair transplantation
  liver transplantation
  living-related donor
    transplantation
  living-related liver
    transplantation (LRLT)
  lung transplantation
  Malt technique in liver
    transplantation
  muscle-tendon
    transplantation
  neonatal pulmonary
    transplantation
  organ transplantation
  orthotopic heart
    transplantation
  orthotopic liver
    transplantation
  orthotopic transplantation
  osteoarticular allograft
    transplantation
  pancreas transplantation

transplantation (*continued*)
  pancreas-kidney
    transplantation
  pancreatic transplantation
  pancreaticoduodenal
    transplantation
  piggyback liver
    transplantation
  pigment cell transplantation
  pituitary gland transplantation
  pulmonary transplantation
  renal transplantation
  segmental gracilis muscle
    transplantation
  simultaneous kidney-pancreas
    transplantation
  simultaneous pancreas-kidney
    transplantation
  SPK transplantation
  split-liver transplantation
  syngeneic transplantation
  syngenesioplastic
    transplantation
  T-cell depleted bone marrow
    transplantation
  tendon transplantation
  tissue transplantation
  toe-phalanx transplantation
  tooth transplantation
  valve transplantation
  xenograft transplantation
transplantation metastasis
transplantation of cornea
transplantation of kidney
transplantation of muscle
transplantation of ocular muscle
transplantation of tendon
transplantation surgery
transplantation tissue
transplanted fat cells
transplanted organ
transplanted stamp graft
transplanted toe
transplant-grafting forceps
transpleural approach
Transpore eye tape
Transpore surgical tape
Transpore surgical tape dressing
Transport catheter
transport tube
transporter
transposed omentum

transposition
  bilateral advancement
    transposition (BAT)
  bilateral gluteus maximus
    transposition
  carotid-subclavian
    transposition
  Dellon ulnar nerve
    transposition
  gracilis muscle transposition
  muscle transposition
  nipple transposition
  omental transposition
  parotid duct transposition
  portacaval transposition
  valve transposition
  Z-plasty transposition
transposition flap
transposition of colon
transposition of graft
transposition of great arteries
  (TGA)
transposition of great vessels
  (TGV)
transposition of pulmonary
  veins
transposition of tendon
transposition operation
transpubic incision
transpubic needle
transpupillary laser
transpyloric feeding tube
transpyloric plane
transpyloric tube
transradial approach
transrectal approach
transrectal multiplane
  3-dimensional transducer
transrectal perineal needle biopsy
transrectal probe
transrectal transphincteric
  approach
transrectal ultrasonography
  (TRUS)
transrectal ultrasound-guided
  sextant biopsy
transrectus incision
transsacral anesthesia
transsacral block
transsacral fracture
Trans-Scan 2100 noninvasive
  physiological monitor

transscaphoid dislocation
  fracture
transscaphoid fracture
transscaphoid perilunate
  dislocation
transscleral suture
transscrotal orchiopexy
transseptal approach
transseptal cannula
transseptal catheter
transseptal left heart
  catheterization
transseptal ligament
transseptal sheath
transseptal stylet
transsexual surgery
transsinus approach
transsphenoidal approach
transsphenoidal bipolar forceps
transsphenoidal curet
transsphenoidal dissector
transsphenoidal enucleator
transsphenoidal evacuation
transsphenoidal
  hypophysectomy
transsphenoidal microsurgical
  resection
transsphenoidal operation
transsphenoidal pituitary
  resection (TPR)
transsphenoidal removal
transsphenoidal resection
transsphenoidal speculum
transsphenoidal surgery
transsphincteric anal fistula
transsphincteric surgery
transsternal approach
transsternal thyroidectomy
transsylvian approach
transsyndesmotic screw
transtelephonic exercise
  monitor
transtentorial approach
transtentorial herniation
transthoracic approach
transthoracic biopsy
transthoracic catheter
transthoracic diameter
transthoracic diskectomy
transthoracic dissection
transthoracic esophagectomy
transthoracic hepatotomy

transthoracic needle aspiration
transthoracic needle aspiration
　biopsy
transthoracic Nissen
　fundoplication
transthoracic pacemaker
transthoracic pacing stylet
transthoracic percutaneous fine-
　needle aspiration biopsy
transthoracic ultrasound
transthoracic vertebral body
　resection
transthoracotomy
transtorcular approach
transtracheal anesthesia
transtracheal aspiration
transtracheal jet ventilation
　anesthetic technique
transtracheal oxygen catheter
transtriquetral fracture
transtriquetral fracture-
　dislocation
transtrochanteric approach
transtrochanteric osteotomy
transtubercular plane
transudate
transudation of fluid
transudative ascites
transudative inflammation
transfusion-related lung injury
　(TRLI)
transumbilical breast
　augmentation (TUBA)
transureteroureteral anastomosis
transureteroureterostomy
transurethral balloon dilatation
transurethral balloon dilation
transurethral biopsy
transurethral catheter
transurethral collagen injection
　therapy
transurethral laser incision
transurethral needle ablation
transurethral needle ablation of
　the prostate
transurethral perineal biopsy
transurethral prostatectomy
transurethral resection (TUR)
transurethral resection of
　bladder tumor (TURBT)
transurethral resection of
　prostate (TURP)

transurethral resection
　syndrome
transurethral thermo-ablation
　therapy
transvaginal approach
transvaginal Burch procedure
transvaginal cone
transvaginal fallopian tube
　catheterization
transvaginal puncture
transvaginal tubal catheterization
transvaginal ultrasonographic
　examination
transvaginal ultrasound
Transvene tripolar electrode
Transvene-RV lead
transvenous approach
transvenous catheter pacemaker
transvenous defibrillator lead
transvenous digital subtraction
　angiogram
transvenous electrodes
transvenous implantation of
　pacemaker leads
transvenous liver biopsy
transvenous pacemaker
transvenous pacemaker catheter
transvenous pacer
transvenous packing
transvenous therapy
transvenous ventricular demand
　pacemaker
transventricular closed
　valvotomy
transventricular dilator
transventricular mitral valve
　commissurotomy
transventricular valvotomy
transversal tomography
transversalis fascia
transversalis, fascia
transverse abdominal incision
transverse abdominal island flap
transverse acetabular ligament
transverse amputation
transverse and rectus abdominis
　musculoperitoneal
　(TRAMP) composite flap
transverse anthelicine groove
transverse aponeurotic arch
transverse appendectomy
　incision

transverse approach
transverse arch
transverse arteriotomy
transverse artery of face
transverse artery of neck
transverse artery of scapula
transverse arytenoid muscle
transverse axis
transverse bipolar montage
transverse bundles of palmar
    aponeurosis
transverse carpal ligament
transverse cervical artery
transverse cervical nerve
transverse cervical veins
transverse cesarean section
transverse circumflex vessels
transverse colectomy
transverse colon
transverse colostomy
transverse comminuted fracture
transverse commissure
transverse connector
transverse costal facet
transverse diameter
transverse diameter of inlet
transverse diameter of pelvic
    outlet
transverse discrepancy
transverse disk
transverse facial artery
transverse facial cleft
transverse facial fracture
transverse facial vein
transverse fascia
transverse fibers
transverse fixation
transverse folds of rectum
transverse foramen
transverse fracture
transverse furrow
transverse gradient coil
transverse head
transverse hermaphroditism
transverse horizontal axis
transverse humeral ligament
transverse incision
transverse lie presentation
transverse ligament
transverse ligament of
    Landsmeer
transverse mastectomy incision

transverse maxillary fracture
transverse mesocolon
transverse metacarpal ligament
transverse metatarsal ligament
transverse mucosal rugae
transverse muscle
transverse muscle of tongue
transverse myocutaneous flap
transverse nasal groove
transverse nerve
transverse occipital
    protuberance
transverse occipital sulcus
transverse orientation
transverse osteotomy
transverse palatal suture
transverse palatine folds
transverse palatine ridge
transverse palatine suture
transverse pelvic inlet
transverse perineal muscle
transverse plane
transverse presentation
transverse process
transverse projection
transverse rectal folds
transverse rectus abdominis
    muscle flap
transverse rectus abdominis
    muscle flap procedure
transverse rectus abdominis
    musculocutaneous (TRAM)
    flap
transverse rectus abdominis
    musculocutaneous flap
    breast reconstruction
transverse rectus abdominis
    myocutaneous (TRAM) flap
transverse rectus abdominis
    myocutaneous procedure
    (TRAM procedure)
transverse relaxation rate
transverse resection
transverse rhytids
transverse row of sutures
transverse saw
transverse scapular ligament
transverse section
transverse section imaging
transverse sheet
transverse sinus
transverse skin incision

transverse sulcus of heart
transverse suture
transverse suture of Krause
transverse tarsal articulation
transverse tarsal joint
transverse temporal gyri
transverse tomography
transverse vein
transverse vesical fold
transverse wave
transverse widening of
    cribriform plate
transversectomy
transverse-loop rod colostomy
transversely oriented endplate
    compression fracture
transversospinal muscle
transversosostomy
transversotomy
transversus abdominis
    aponeurosis
transversus abdominis muscle
transversus linguae muscle
transversus perinei profundus
    muscle
transversus situs
transversus thoracis muscle
transvesical prostatectomy
transxiphoid approach
Trantas operation
TranZgraft
trap
    DeLee tracheal trap
    disposable specimen trap
    EndoDynamics suction polyp
        trap
    Juhn trap
    Juhn tympanocentesis trap
    Lukens trap
trap incision
trapdoor approach
trapdoor fragment
trapdoor incision
trapdoor scleral buckle
    operation
trapdoor technique for retinal
    detachment
TrapEase filter
trapeze bar
trapezial fracture
trapeziectomy
trapeziometacarpal fusion

trapeziometacarpal joint
    replacement prosthesis
trapezium bone
trapezium fracture
trapezium implant
trapezius flap
trapezius muscle
trapezius muscle/myocutaneous
    flap
trapezius ridge sign
trapezius stimulation anesthetic
    technique
trapezoid body
trapezoid bone
trapezoid ligament
trapezoid line
trapezoidal incision
trapezoidal keratotomy
Trapezoidal-28 total hip
    prosthesis
Trapper catheter exchange
    device
Traquair periosteal elevator
transverse process fracture
Trattner urethrographic catheter
Traube murmur
Traube neurological hammer
Traube semilunar space
Traube sign
Traube space
trauma
    auricular trauma
    autoerotic rectal trauma
    birth trauma
    blunt abdominal trauma
    cerebral trauma
    cranial trauma
    foreign body trauma
    head trauma
    iatrogenic trauma
    joint trauma
    laryngotracheal trauma
    major trauma
    midface trauma
    multiple trauma
    multisystem trauma
    neurological trauma
    occlusal trauma
    occult trauma
    oral trauma
    penetrating abdominal trauma
    penetrating trauma

trauma (*continued*)
  rectal trauma
  sudden trauma
  surface trauma
  surgical trauma
trauma from occlusion
trauma induced saddle bag
trauma surgery
trauma-related death
TraumaSeal topical wound
  closure device
traumatherapy
traumatic abscess
traumatic alopecia
traumatic amputation
traumatic anesthesia
traumatic atlantooccipital
  dislocation
traumatic avulsion
traumatic blepharoptosis
traumatic brain death
traumatic brain injury (TBI)
traumatic capsule
traumatic cataract
traumatic cervical disk
  herniation
traumatic crescent
traumatic diaphragmatic hernia
traumatic dislocation
traumatic false aneurysm
traumatic fever
traumatic fibroma
traumatic fistula
traumatic fracture
traumatic gangrene
traumatic grasping forceps
traumatic hemorrhage
traumatic inflammation
traumatic injury
traumatic internal carotid artery
  dissection
traumatic intracranial hematoma
traumatic lacerations
traumatic laryngitis
traumatic lesion
traumatic lipodystrophy
traumatic luxation
traumatic occlusion
traumatic pain
traumatic perforation
traumatic progressive
  encephalopathy

traumatic rupture
traumatic shock
traumatic sutures
traumatic tattoo
traumatic tear
traumatic ulcer
traumatic wound
traumatogenic occlusion
traumatogenic pulpal occlusion
traumatopnea
traumatopneic wound
traumatosis
traumatotherapy
Trauner operation
Trautman Locktite hook
Trautman Locktite prosthesis
Trautmann angle
Trautmann triangle
Trautmann triangular space
Travel jejunostomy
Travel operation
Travenol bag
Travenol biopsy needle
Travenol dialyzer
Travenol heart bag
Travenol infuser
Travenol infusion pump
Travenol infusor device
Travenol needle
Travenol twin coil for
  hemodialysis
Travert needle
Treace drill
Treace microdrill
Treace stapes drill
Treace Tytan ventilation tube
Treacher Collins deformity
Treacher Collins syndrome
treadmill electrocardiogram
treadmill exercise stress test
treatment
  Abdopatch Gel Z self-adhesive
    scar treatment
  acupuncture treatment
  anoplasty treatment
  Bier combined treatment
  Brandt treatment
  burn scar treatment
  Carrel treatment
  Carrel-Dakin treatment
  cholecystectomy treatment
  compression rod treatment

treatment (*continued*)
  conservative surgical treatment
  conservative treatment
  continuous medical treatment
  conventional treatment
  cyclic treatment
  definitive treatment
  Elliot treatment
  embolization treatment
  endoscopic treatment
  endourologic treatment
  esophageal dilation treatment
  experimental treatment
  Fowler-Murphy treatment
  graft treatment
  hemodialysis treatment
  Imre treatment
  initial treatment
  intensive treatment
  Keating-Hart treatment
  laparoscopic treatment
  laser treatment
  long-term treatment
  Mammopatch gel self-adhesive scar treatment
  mantle radiation treatment
  Marx protocol for ORN treatment
  Murphy treatment
  Ochsner treatment
  Orr treatment
  Pad Medipatch Gel Z self-adhesive scar treatment
  proposed treatment
  protracted treatment
  radiation treatment
  Retan treatment
  rib field treatment
  split-course treatment
  subsequent treatment
  supportive treatment
  surgical treatment
  systemic treatment
  therapeutic treatment
  Trueta treatment
  Ultroid device for hemorrhoid treatment
  Zircate treatment
treatment and observation
treatment port
treatment sequelae
treatment table
treatment-resistant
tree
  biliary tree
  bronchial tree
  cannulation of the biliary tree
  endobronchial tree
  pinch tree
  pipe tree
  tracheal tree
  tracheobronchial tree
trefoil balloon catheter
trefoil deformity
trefoil Schneider balloon
trefoil tendon
Treitz arch
Treitz fossa
Treitz hernia
Treitz ligament
Treitz muscle
Trelat palate raspatory
Trelat raspatory
Trelat speculum
Trelat vaginal speculum
Trelex mesh
Trelex natural mesh
Trelles metal scleral shield
trellis formation
Tremble sphenoid cannula
tremor
  coarse tremor
  fibrillary tremor
  fibrillatory tremors
  fine tremor
  flapping tremor
  muscular tremors
  ocular tremor
  passive tremor
  striocerebellar tremor
trench foot
trench hand
trench mouth
Trendelenburg cannula
Trendelenburg operation
Trendelenburg position
Trendelenburg pulmonary embolectomy
Trendelenburg synchondroseotomy
Trendelenburg tampon
Trendelenburg vein ligation

Trendelenburg-Crafoord
    coarctation clamp
Trendelenburg-position
    lithotomy
Trenkle screwdriver
Trent eye pick
Trent eye retractor
trephination
trephine
    antral trephine
    Arroyo trephine
    Arruga eye trephine
    Arruga lacrimal trephine
    automated trephine
    automatic corneal trephine
    Bard-Parker trephine
    Barraquer corneal trephine
    Barron disposable trephine
    Barron epikeratophakia
        trephine
    Barron radial vacuum
        trephine
    Barron-Hessburg corneal
        trephine
    Becker skull trephine
    Blackburn trephine
    Blakesley lacrimal trephine
    Boiler septal trephine
    Bonaccolto trephine
    Boston model trephine
    Brown-Pusey corneal trephine
    cam-guided trephine
    Cardona corneal prosthesis
        trephine
    Castroviejo corneal transplant
        trephine
    Castroviejo corneal trephine
    Castroviejo transplant
        trephine
    chalazion trephine
    Cloward trephine
    corneal prosthesis trephine
    corneal trephine
    cranial trephine
    Cross scleral trephine
    dacryocystorhinostomy
        trephine
    Damshek sternal trephine
    Davis trephine
    DeMartel trephine
    D'Errico skull trephine
    DeVilbiss trephine

trephine (*continued*)
    DiaPhine trephine
    Dimitry chalazion trephine
    Dimitry
        dacryocystorhinostomy
        trephine
    disposable trephine
    electric trephine
    Elliot corneal trephine
    Elliot eye trephine
    Elschnig trephine
    exploratory trephine
    Franceschetti corneal
        trephine
    Galt skull trephine
    Gradle corneal trephine
    Green automatic corneal
        trephine
    Greenwood spinal trephine
    Grieshaber calibrated corneal
        trephine
    Grieshaber corneal trephine
    Guyton corneal transplant
        trephine
    hand trephine
    hand-held trephine
    Hanna trephine
    Harris trephine
    Hessburg vacuum trephine
    Hessburg-Barron vacuum
        trephine
    Hippel trephine
    Horsley trephine
    Iliff lacrimal trephine
    Jentzer trephine
    Katena trephine
    Katena-Barron trephine
    Katzin trephine
    Keyes cutaneous trephine
    King corneal trephine
    lacrimal trephine
    Lahey Clinic skull trephine
    Lahey trephine
    Leksell trephine
    Lichtenberg corneal trephine
    Lichtwicz antral trephine
    Londermann corneal trephine
    Lorie antral trephine
    Martinez disposable corneal
        trephine
    Maumenee trephine
    M-brace corneal trephine

trephine (*continued*)
  Michele trephine
  mini trephine
  Moria trephine
  Mueller electric corneal
    trephine
  Mueller electric trephine
  nasal trephine
  Paton corneal trephine
  Paton see-through corneal
    trephine
  pattern trephine
  Paufique corneal trephine
  Pharmacia corneal trephine
  Phemister biopsy trephine
  Polley-Bickel trephine
  punch trephine
  razor-blade trephine
  Robertson corneal trephine
  Rochester bone trephine
  Schanz trephine
  Scheie trephine
  Schuknecht temporal
    trephine
  Schwartz trephine
  scleral trephine
  sclerectomy with trephine
  Scoville skull trephine
  Searcy chalazion trephine
  septal trephine
  Sidney Stephenson corneal
    trephine
  sinus trephine
  Sisler lacrimal trephine
  skull trephine
  spinal trephine
  Stephenson corneal trephine
  sternal trephine
  Stille trephine
  Stock eye trephine
  Storz chalazion trephine
  Storz corneal trephine
  Storz disposable trephine
  Storz hair transplant trephine
  Stryker saw trephine
  Surgistar corneal trephine
  temporal trephine
  Thornwald antral trephine
  Toti trephine
  transplant trephine
  Troutman tenotomy trephine
  Turkel trephine

trephine (*continued*)
  Von Hippel mechanical
    trephine
  Walker corneal trephine
  Weck trephine
  Wilder trephine
  Wilkins trephine
trephine blade
trephine cutout
trephine drill
trephine marker
trephine needle biopsy
trephinement
trephiner
trephining
Treponema pallidum
    immobilization
Trestle prostatic bridge
Trethowan bunionectomy
Trethowan-Stamm-Simmonds-
    Menelaus-Haddad
    technique
Treves fold
Treves intestinal clamp
Treves operation
Trevisani cannula
Trevisani cannula tip
Tri W-G table
triad
  Andersen triad
  Beck triad
  Bezold triad
  Charcot triad
  Dieulafoy triad
  Falta triad
  Franke triad
  Grancher triad
  hepatic triad
  Kartagener triad
  O'Donoghue triad
  Osler triad
  portal triad
  Saint triad
  Whipple triad
Triad hydrophilic wound dressing
triad knee repair
triad of symptoms
Triad PET balloon
Triad prosthesis
triad syndrome
triaditis
TriaDyne bed

trial acetabular cups
trial basis
trial component
trial cup
trial driver
trial fracture frame
trial frame
trial implant
trial of conservative therapy
trial of labor
trial point
trial prosthesis
trial reduction
trial results
trial visit
triamcinolone
triangle
  Assezat triangle
  auscultatory triangle
  badger's triangle
  Béclard triangle
  Bermuda Triangle
  Bonwill triangle
  Burger triangle
  Burow triangle
  Calot triangle
  cardiohepatic triangle
  carotid triangle
  cephalic triangle
  clavipectoral triangle
  Codman triangle
  cystohepatic triangle
  digastric triangle
  Einthoven triangle
  facet of the soft triangle
  facial triangle
  femoral triangle
  Gerhardt triangle
  Grynfelt triangle
  Henke triangle
  Hesselbach triangle
  iliofemoral triangle
  inferior carotid triangle
  infraclavicular triangle
  inguinal triangle
  Kager triangle
  Kiesselbach triangle
  Labbe triangle
  Lesgaft triangle
  Livingston triangle
  lumbocostoabdominal triangle
  Macewen triangle

triangle (*continued*)
  mesenteric triangle
  occipital triangle
  omoclavicular triangle
  Pawlik triangle
  retromandibular triangle
  retromolar triangle
  scalenovertebral triangle
  Scarpa triangle
  Semon triangle
  subclavian triangle
  submandibular triangle
  submaxillary triangle
  submental triangle
  suboccipital triangle
  superior carotid triangle
  supraclavicular triangle
  surgical triangle
  Trautmann triangle
  Ward triangle
triangle of Calot
triangle of Farabeuf
triangle of Langenbeck
triangle of lingual artery
triangle of Livingston
triangle of Trautmann
triangle of Ward
triangle Secto dissector
Tri-angle shoulder abduction brace
triangular advancement flap
triangular ankle fusion frame
triangular aponeurosis
triangular bandage
triangular bipolar montage
triangular bone
triangular capsulotomy
triangular cartilage
triangular crest
triangular defect
triangular dressing
triangular eminence
triangular encompassing clip
triangular fibrocartilage
  complex (TFCC)
triangular fibrocartilage
  complex debridement
triangular fibrocartilage complex
  meniscus tear
triangular fibrocartilage
  complex tear
triangular fibrocartilage
  compound

triangular fibrocartilage
    meniscus
triangular fold
triangular fontanelle
triangular fossa
triangular island flap
triangular ligament
triangular muscle
triangular punch forceps
triangular rasp
triangular resection of leaflet
triangular space
triangular vaginal patch sling
triangulated pedicle screw
triangulation technique
triatrial heart
triaxial elbow prosthesis
triaxial hinge
triaxial semiconstrained elbow
    prosthesis
triaxial total elbow arthroplasty
tribasilar synostosis
tributaries and perforators
triceps flap
triceps muscle
triceps reflex
triceps surae jerk
triceps surae reflex
tricepsplasty
trichiasis operation
trichiasis repair
trichloroacetic acid (TCA)
trichloroacetic acid peel
trichloroethylene anesthetic agent
trichorhinophalangeal syndrome
trick knee
Tricodur compression support
    bandage
Tricodur Epi (elbow)
    compression support
    bandage
Tricodur Omos (shoulder)
    compression support
    bandage
Tricodur Talus (ankle)
    compression support
    bandage
tricompartmental knee
    replacement
Tri-Con component
Tricon-M cruciate-sparing
    prosthesis

Tricon-M patellar prosthesis
Tricon-M total knee prosthesis
Tricon-P tibial component with
    Flex-Lok pegs
Tri-Core cervical support pillow
tricorrectional bunionectomy
tricrotic pulse
tricrotic wave
tricuspid annuloplasty
tricuspid aortic valve
tricuspid atresia
tricuspid commissurotomy
tricuspid orifice
tricuspid position
tricuspid stenosis
tricuspid valve
tricuspid valve annuloplasty
tricuspid valve disease
tricuspid valve repair
tricuspid valve strut
tricuspid valvotomy
tricuspid valvulotomy
Tricut blade
Tricut laryngeal blade tip
trident hand
Trident Omega blade
Trident resection ablator
tridodecylmethylammonium
    chloride graft coating
    material (TDMAC)
Tri-Ex radiopaque triple-lumen
    extraction balloon
TriEye cannula
TriEye tip
trifacet knife
tri-fin chisel
triflange intramedullary nail
triflange nail
Tri-Float pressure reduction
    mattress
Tri-flow incentive spirometer
Tri-flow incentive spirometry
triflow oxygen
trifurcate incision
trifurcation injury
trifurcation involvement
trigeminal artery
trigeminal cavity
trigeminal decompression
trigeminal electrode
trigeminal ganglion
trigeminal gland

trigeminal impression
trigeminal knife
trigeminal nerve (cranial nerve 5)
trigeminal nerve artifact
trigeminal nerve compression
trigeminal nerve paralysis
trigeminal nerve sign
trigeminal neuralgia
trigeminal pulse
trigeminal retractor
trigeminal rhizotomy
trigeminal scissors
trigeminal self-retaining
    retractor
trigeminal-facial nerve reflex
trigeminofacial reflex
trigeminus cannula
trigeminus reflex
trigeminus scissors
trigeminy
trigger area
trigger cannula
trigger digit
trigger finger
trigger finger release
trigger point
trigger point injection
trigger reaction
trigger thumb
triggered ventilation
TriggerWheel device
trigone
    retromolar trigone
    submandibular trigone
    urogenital trigone
trigonectomy
trigonocephaly
Triguide catheter
trilaminate cushion
trileaflet aortic prosthesis
trileaflet aortic valve
trileaflet prosthesis
Trilene anesthetic agent
Trilicon external breast
    prosthesis
Trillat patellar tendon transfer
Trillat procedure
Trillaux fracture
trilobar hyperplasia
trilobate placenta
trilobed cloverleaf skull
trilobed skull

Tri-Lock acetabular cup
Tri-Lock total hip prosthesis
    with Porocoat
Tri-lock total hip system with
    Porocoat
trilocular heart
Trilogy acetabular cup
Trilogy pulse generator
Trilogy pacemaker
Trilogy low-profile balloon
    dilatation catheter
trilogy of Fallot
Trilogy single-chamber
    pacemaker
Trilucent breast implant
trimalar fracture
trimalleolar ankle fracture
trimalleolar fracture
Trimar anesthetic agent
Trimble suture stent
Trimedyne holmium laser
Trimedyne Optilase 1000 device
Tri-Met apnea monitor
Trimline knee immobilizer
Trimline mobile tractor
trimmer
    Dyonics meniscal trimmer
    margin trimmer
    model trimmer
    Septotome septum trimmer
trimodality therapy
Trinkle bone drill
Trinkle brace
Trinkle chuck
Trinkle chuck adapter
Trinkle power drill
Trinkle twist drill
trinocular microscope
Trionix camera
Trionix scanner
Trios M pacemaker
trip
    House-Urban oiler trip
tripanel, convoluted 4-strap
    (TCS) knee immobilizer
tripartite patella
tripartite placenta
triphalangeal thumb
triphalangeal thumb deformity
trip-hammer pulse
Triphasix generator
Tripier amputation

Tripier operation
Tripier operation throw square
     knot
triplane arthrodesis
triplane fracture
triplane tibial fracture
triplant implant
triple amputation
triple anastomosis
triple arthrodesis
triple bypass heart surgery
triple hemisection
triple hook
triple innominate osteotomy
triple intrathecal therapy
triple ligamentous repair
triple lobe hepatectomy
triple lumen implant
triple point
triple strength
triple syndactyly
triple thermistor coronary sinus
     catheter
triple vessel disease
triple voiding cystogram
triple-A repair (AAA; abdominal
     aortic aneurysm)
triple-angle
triple-edge diamond-blade knife
triple-lumen Arrow catheter
triple-lumen balloon flotation
     thermistor catheter
triple-lumen biliary manometry
     catheter
triple-lumen central catheter
triple-lumen central venous
     catheter
triple-lumen infusion
triple-lumen manometric
     catheter
triple-lumen manometry
     catheter
triple-lumen needle
triple-lumen perfusion to
     measure jejunal absorption
triple-lumen Sengstaken-
     Blakemore tube
triple-lumen sump drain
triple-throw square knot stitch
triple-wire procedure
triple-wire technique
triplication of ureter

tripod cane
tripod fracture
tripod grasper
tripod grasping forceps
tripod intraocular lens
tripod pin traction
tri-point K-wire sleeve
tripolar catheter
tripolar Damato curve catheter
tripolar defibrillation coil
     electrode
tripolar electrode catheter
tripolar lead
tripolar with Damato curve
     catheter
Tri-Port hemostasis introducer
     sheath kit
Tri-Port sub-Tenon anesthesia
     cannula
triport tip
Trippi-Wells tongs
tripronged loop
triquetral bone
triquetral fracture
triquetral impingement ligament
     tear (TILT)
triquetrolunate dislocation
triquetropisiform articulation
triquetrous cartilage
triradial resector blade
triradiate acetabular extensile
     approach
triradiate cartilage
triradiate line
triradiate transtrochanteric
     approach
triradiate transtrochanteric
     unilateral approach
triscaphe fusion
triscaphe joint
Triseptin surgical scrub
trismus stent
trisomy 8 syndrome
trisomy C syndrome
Tristar coronary stent
TriStar trocar
TriStim TENS unit
triticeal cartilage
triturator
Triumph VR pacemaker
trivalve
trivascular umbilical cord

TriVex procedure
Trizol RNA extractor
TroCam endoscope
TroCam endoscopic camera
Trocan disposable CO_2 trocar
Trocan disposable CO_2 trocar
  and cannula
trocar
  abdominal trocar
  Abelson cricothyrotomy
    trocar
  accessory trocar
  Allen cecostomy trocar
  American Heyer-Schulte-
    Robertson suprapubic
    trocar
  amniotic trocar
  AMS disposable trocar
  anasarca trocar
  antral trocar
  Apple trocar
  Arbuckle-Shea trocar
  Argyle trocar
  aspirating trocar
  Axiom thoracic trocar
  Babcock empyema trocar
  Babcock trocar
  Barnes internal
    decompression trocar
  B-D Potain thoracic trocar
  Beardsley cecostomy trocar
  Bernay hydrocele trocar
  Billroth ovarian trocar
  Birch trocar
  Bishop antrum trocar
  bladder trocar
  blunt trocar
  Bluntport disposable trocar
  Boettcher antral trocar
  bore trocar
  brain trocar
  brain-exploring trocar
  Bulau trocar
  Bueleau empyema trocar
  Cabot trocar
  Campbell suprapubic trocar
  Castens ascites trocar
  Castens hydrocele trocar
  cecostomy trocar
  Charlton antral trocar
  Circon ACMI trocar
  Coakley antral trocar

trocar (*continued*)
  conical trocar
  Cook urological trocar
  Corb biopsy trocar
  Core Dynamics disposable
    trocar
  core trocar
  cricothyroid trocar
  cricothyrotomy trocar
  Cross needle trocar
  Curschmann trocar
  Davidson thoracic trocar
  Dean antral trocar
  Dean trocar
  decompressive trocar
  Denker trocar
  Dexide laparoscopic trocar
  Diamond-Flex trocar
  Diederich empyema trocar
  Douglas antral trocar
  Douglas nasal trocar
  Doyen trocar
  Duchenne trocar
  Duke trocar
  Durham tracheotomy trocar
  Emmet ovarian trocar
  empyema trocar
  Endo Tip Storz trocar
  Endopatch disposable surgical
    trocar
  Endopath laparoscopic trocar
  ensheathing trocar
  Entree trocar
  Entree Plus trocar
  Ethicon disposable trocar
  Faulkner trocar
  Fein antral trocar
  Fein antrum trocar
  fiberglass sleeve trocar
  Fleurant bladder trocar
  Frazier brain-exploring trocar
  Frazier trocar
  Gallagher trocar
  gallbladder trocar
  Haeggstrom antral trocar
  Hargin antral trocar
  Hargin antrum trocar
  Hasson laparoscopic trocar
  Havlicek trocar
  Hunt angiographic trocar
  Hurwitz thoracic trocar
  hydrocele trocar

trocar (*continued*)

Ingram trocar
InnerDyne trocar
intercostal trocar
internal decompression trocar
intestinal decompression
   trocar
intestinal trocar
Jako laser trocar
Jarit disposable trocar
Johannson-Stille cystotomy
   trocar
Judd trocar
Kemp trocar
Kidd trocar
Kido suprapubic trocar
Klima-Rosegger trocar
Kolb trocar
Krause antral trocar
Kreutzmann trocar
Landau pelvic access trocar
Laparosac trocar
laparoscopic trocar
laryngeal trocar
Lichtwicz abdominal trocar
Lichtwicz antral trocar
Lillie antral trocar
Livermore trocar
Lovelace gallbladder trocar
Lower trocar
Marlow disposable trocar
Mayo-Ochsner trocar
Monoscopy locking trocar
Morson trocar
Myerson antral trocar
Myerson antrum trocar
Nagashima antroscope trocar
Neal catheter trocar
Nelson empyema trocar
Nelson thoracic trocar
Nelson-Patterson empyema
   trocar
nested trocar
Ochsner gallbladder trocar
Ochsner thoracic trocar
Olympus disposable trocar
Optiview trocar
Origin trocar
ovarian trocar
Patterson empyema trocar
Patterson-Nelson empyema
   trocar

trocar (*continued*)

Penn trocar
Pierce antral trocar
Pierce-Kyle trocar
piloting trocar
plain vesical trocar
Poole trocar
Potain aspirating trocar
prostatic trocar
pyramidal tip trocar
rectal trocar
Reddick-Saye trocar
Reuter-Wolfe trocar
Rica Universal trocar
Richard Wolf laparoscopic
   trocar
Roberts abdominal trocar
Robertson suprapubic trocar
Robinson-Brauer trocar
Ruskin antral trocar
Schwartz trocar
Sewall antral trocar
sharp trocar
Singleton empyema trocar
sinoscopy trocar
Snyder Urevac trocar
Solos disposable trocar
Southey anasarca trocar
Southey-Leech trocar
standard trocar
Step laparoscopic trocar
Stiwer trocar
Storz disposable trocar
subcostal trocar
suprapubic trocar
Surgiport disposable trocar
Sweet antral trocar
Synthes transbuccal trocar
thoracic trocar
Thoracoport trocar
Tilley-Lichwitz trocar
tracheostomy trocar
transbuccal trocar
TriStar trocar
Ueckermann cricothyroid
   trocar
Ueckermann-Denker trocar
Uni-Shunt split trocar
Universal abdominal trocar
Van Alyea antral trocar
Veirs trocar
Veress trocar

trocar (*continued*)
  Visiport optical trocar
  Walther aspirating bladder
    trocar
  Wangensteen internal
    decompression trocar
  Weck disposable trocar
  Wiener-Pierce antral trocar
  Wilson amniotic trocar
  Wilson-Baylor amniotic trocar
  Wisap disposable trocar
  Wolf needle trocar
  Wolf-Cottle trocar
  Wright-Harloe empyema
    trocar
  Ximed disposable trocar
  Yankauer antral trocar
trocar cystostomy
trocar gas leak
trocar injury
trocar needle
trocar sheath
trocar site hernia
trocar technique
trocar tunneling instrument
trocar wound bleed
trocar wound site complication
trocar-cannula technique
trocar-point Kirschner wire
trocar-related injury
Trocath peritoneal dialysis
    catheter
trochanter
  greater trochanter
  lesser trochanter
trochanter holder
trochanter-holding clamp
trochanteric awl
trochanteric bolt
trochanteric bursae of gluteus
    maximus
trochanteric crest
trochanteric depression
trochanteric pin
trochanteric plate
trochanteric rasp
trochanteric reamer
trochanteric router
trochanteric wire
trochanterplasty
trochlea
trochlear fossa

trochlear nerve (cranial nerve 4)
trochlear nerve sign
trochlear notch
trochlear process
trochlear ridge
trochoid articulation
trochoid joint
trochoidal articulation
Troeltsch (*also* Tröltsch)
Troeltsch dressing forceps
Troeltsch ear forceps
Troeltsch ear speculum
Troeltsch eustachian catheter
Troeltsch speculum
Troilius capsulotomy knife
Troisier ganglion
Troisier node
Trokel lens
Trokel-Peyman laser lens
Tröltsch (*see* Troeltsch)
Trombotect tube
Tromner percussion hammer
Tromner reflex
Trömner (see Tromner)
Tromner (also Trömner,
    Troemner)
Troemner (see Tromner)
Troncoso gonioscope
Troncoso gonioscopic lens
    implant
Troncoso implant
Troncoso tubular lens
Tronothane hydrochloride
    anesthetic agent
Tronzo approach to hip
Tronzo classification of
    trochanteric fractures
Tronzo elevator
Tronzo hip surgery
Tronzo intertrochanteric
    fracture classification
Tronzo lateral approach to hip
Tronzo prosthesis
Tronzo screw
Tronzo total hip
trophectoderm biopsy
trophic cicatrix
trophic fracture
trophic lesion
trophic nerve
trophic ulcer
trophoblastic tumor

trophoneurosis
  lingual trophoneurosis
  Romberg trophoneurosis
tropism
Trotter forceps
Trotter syndrome
trough
  deep tear troughs
  gingival trough
  infraorbital tear trough
  vestibular trough
trough and peak levels
trough gouge
trough level
trough line
trousers
  military antishock trousers
    (MAST)
  pneumatic antishock trousers
Trousseau dilating forceps
Trousseau dilator
Trousseau esophageal bougie
Trousseau mouth gag
Trousseau point
Trousseau spot
Trousseau tracheal dilator
Trousseau-Jackson esophageal
    dilator
Trousseau-Jackson tracheal
    dilator
Troutman alpha-chymotrypsin
    cannula
Troutman blade
Troutman bladebreaker
Troutman cannula
Troutman cataract extractor
Troutman chisel
Troutman conjunctival scissors
Troutman corneal dissector
Troutman corneal forceps
Troutman corneal knife
Troutman corneal punch
Troutman corneal scissors
Troutman corneal section
    scissors
Troutman eye dissector
Troutman eye implant
Troutman gouge
Troutman implant
Troutman iris spatula
Troutman lens loupe
Troutman lens spatula

Troutman lens spoon
Troutman magnetic implant
Troutman mastoid chisel
Troutman mastoid gouge
Troutman microsurgery forceps
Troutman microsurgical scissors
Troutman needle
Troutman needle holder
Troutman nonincisional lamellar
    dissector
Troutman operation
Troutman punch
Troutman rectal forceps
Troutman scissors
Troutman superior rectus
    forceps
Troutman suture scissors
Troutman tenotomy trephine
Troutman tying forceps
Troutman wave-edge corneal
    dissector
Troutman-Barraquer corneal
    fixation forceps
Troutman-Barraquer corneal
    forceps
Troutman-Barraquer iris forceps
Troutman-Barraquer iris spatula
Troutman-Barraquer
    minibladebreaker
Troutman-Barraquer-Colibri
    forceps
Troutman-Barraquer needle
    holder
Troutman-Castroviejo corneal
    section scissors
Troutman-Castroviejo scissors
Troutman-Katzin corneal
    transplant scissors
Troutman-Llobera fixation
    forceps
Troutman-Llobera Flieringa
    forceps
Troutman-Llobera-Flieringa
    forceps
Troutman-Tooke corneal knife
Trowbridge triple-speed drill
Trowbridge-Campau bone drill
Trowbridge-Campau eye magnet
Tru Taper Ethalloy needle
Truarc blood vessel ring
Truarc trachea tube
Truarc wire

Tru-Area Determination wound
measuring device
Truc flap
Truc operation
Tru-Chrome band material
Tru-Clip
Tru-Cut biopsy needle
Tru-Cut biopsy needle holder
Tru-Cut liver biopsy needle
Tru-Cut needle
Tru-Cut needle biopsy (TCNB,
TNB)
true aneurysm
true apex (TA)
true collateral ligament
true cords
true dermatochalasis
true exfoliation
True Form support stockings
true generalized microdontia
true hernia
true knot
true labor
true lateral x-ray view
true pelvis
true ribs
True separator
True sheathless catheter
true sutures
true symphalangism
true vocal cords
True/Flex intramedullary nail
trueFISP MRI (true fast imaging
with steady state
precession MRI)
Trueta technique
Trueta treatment
TrueTorque wire guide
TrueVision transvaginal probe
Trulife silicone breast form
Truline forceps
Trumble arthrodesis
Trumble hip arthrodesis
Trumbull sutures
trumpet cannula
trumpet needle guide
trumpeting on x-ray
truncal abrasions
truncal lesion
truncal vagotomy
truncal vagotomy and
gastroenterostomy

truncated cone
truncated NMR probe
truncated osteotomy
truncated tarsometatarsal wedge
arthrodesis
truncated-wedge arthrodesis
truncus arteriosus
truncus brachiocephalicus
truncus celiacus
truncus clamp
truncus costocervicalis
truncus pulmonalis
truncus thyrocervicalis
trunk
anterior vagal trunk
bicarotid trunk
brachiocephalic trunk
celiac trunk
costocervical trunk
jugular trunk
linguofacial trunk
lumbosacral trunk
lymphatic trunk
posterior vagal trunk
pulmonary trunk
sympathetic trunk
thyrocervical trunk
thyrolingual trunk
tibioperoneal trunk
vagal trunk
trunk duplication
trunk movement
trunk muscles
trunk valves
trunnion-bearing hip prosthesis
Trupower aspherical lens
Trupp ventricular needle
TruPro lacrimal cannula
TruPulse CO_2 laser
Tru-Pulse CO_2 skin resurfacing
laser
Trurell sigmoidoscope
TRUS (transrectal
ultrasonography)
Trush grasping forceps
trusion
mandibular trusion
maxillary trusion
Trusler aortic valve technique
Trusler clamp
Trusler infant vascular clamp
Trusler-Dean scissors

Trussdale tourniquet
TruStep foot prosthesis
Tru-Support bandage
Truszkowski dural dissector
Tru-Trac high-pressure PTA
    balloon
Truvision Omni lens
TruWave pressure transducer
TruZone peak flow meter
Trylon hemostatic forceps
Trelat raspatory
Trelat speculum
Trelat vaginal speculum
T-Scan 2000
Tscherne classification
Tscherne-Gotzen tibial fracture
    classification
TSH (thyroid stimulating
    hormone)
TSH-01 transdermal tape
T-shaped AO plate
T-shaped capsulotomy
T-shaped Edwards-Barbaro
    syringeal shunt
T-shaped forceps
T-shaped fracture
T-shaped graft
T-shaped incision
T-shaped scar
T-Span tissue expander
T-spatula
T-spica bandage
T-spine
T-splint
TSRH buttressed laminar hook
TSRH circular laminar hook
TSRH crosslink stabilization
TSRH double-rod construct
TSRH pedicle hook
TSRH rod fixation
TSTI (tumor-specific
    transplantation immunity)
Tsuge technique to reconstruct
    hand tendons
Tsuge tendon repair
Tsuji laminaplasty
TT-3 needle
T-TAC catheter
T-tack gastropexy
TTAP (threaded titanium
    acetabular prosthesis)
TTC (T-tube cholangiogram)

TTS (through the scope)
TTS Aire-Cuf tracheostomy tube
TTS balloon dilation
TTS catheter
TTS dilator
T-tube (see also tube)
    American Heyer-Schulte
        T-tube
    bar T-tube
    Cattell forked-type T-tube
    cul-de-sac irrigation T-tube
    Deaver T-tube
    forked T-tube
    Goode T-tube
    Hyst T-tube
    insertion of T-tube
    Kehr T-tube
    Montgomery T-tube
    Whelan-Moss T-tube
T-tube catheter
T-tube cholangiogram (TTC)
T-tube cholangiography
T-tube drain
T-tube drainage
T-tube incision
T-tube placement
T-tube round suction tube
T-tube stent
T-tube technique
T-tube tract
    choledochofiberoscopy
T-tube tract choledochoscopy
T-type dental
T-type ileocystoplasty
T-type matrix band
T-type myringotomy tube
tubal abortion
tubal block
tubal hook
tubal implantation into uterus
tubal inflation
tubal insufflation
tubal insufflation cannula
tubal insufflator
tubal ligation
tubal ligation band technique
tubal obstruction
tubal occlusion
tubal patency
tubal pregnancy
tubal reconstruction surgery
tubal ring

tubal scissors
tubal sterilization
Tubbs aortic dilator
Tubbs dilator
Tubbs mitral valve dilator
Tubbs 2-bladed dilator
Tubbs valvulotome
Tubby knife
Tubby tenotomy knife
Tubby-Steindler operation
tube (*see also* suction tube)
   3-bottle tidal suction tube
   Abbott tube
   Abbott-Miller tube
   Abbott-Rawson double-lumen
     gastrointestinal tube
   Abbott-Rawson
     gastrointestinal double-
     lumen tube
   Abramson tube
   AccuMark calibrated infant
     feeding tube
   ACMI Valentine tube
   Activent ear tube
   Adson aspirating tube
   Adson brain suction tube
   Adson neurosurgical suction
     tube
   Adson straight suction tube
   Adson suction tube
   AF tube (antifog tube)
   air inflatable tube
   air tube
   Aire-Cuf endotracheal tube
   Aire-Cuf tracheostomy tube
   Air-Lon laryngectomy tube
   Air-Lon tracheal tube
   Alesen tube
   American circle nephrostomy
     tube
   American Heyer-Schulte
     T-tube
   American tracheotomy
     tube
   Amersham tube
   Amsterdam tube
   Amstrong beveled grommet
     drain tube
   Amstrong beveled grommet
     myringotomy tube
   Amstrong ventilation tube
   anaerobic culture tube

tube (*continued*)
   Andersen mercury-weighted
     tube
   Anderson flexible suction
     tube
   Anderson suction tube
   Andrews suction tube
   Andrews-Pynchon suction
     tube
   Andrews-Yankauer suction
     tube
   anesthesia tube
   anesthetic tube
   angled pleural tube
   angled suction tube
   anode tube
   Anthony aspirating tube
   Anthony mastoid suction tube
   Anthony mastoid tube
   Anthony suction tube
   Anthony tube
   antifog tube
   antral drainage tube
   antral wash tube
   antrum-irrigating tube
   aortic sump tube
   Argyle chest tube
   Argyle endotracheal tube
   Argyle tube
   Argyle-Dennis tube
   Argyle-Salem sump tube
   Armour endotracheal tube
   Armstrong beveled grommet
     drain tube
   Armstrong beveled grommet
     myringotomy tube
   Armstrong ventilation tube
   Armstrong V-vent tube
   Arrow tube
   ascites drainage tube
   ascites suction tube
   Asepto suction tube
   aspirating tube
   Aspisafe nasogastric tube
   Atkins-Cannard tracheotomy
     tube
   Atkinson silicone rubber tube
   auditory tube
   Ayre tube
   Babcock tube
   Baerveldt glaucoma implant
     tube

tube (*continued*)

Baerveldt shunt tube
Baker intestinal decompression tube
Baker jejunostomy tube
Baker self-sumping tube
Baldwin butterfly ventilation tube
Bard gastrostomy feeding tube
Bard PEG tube
Bardic tube
Barnes nasal suction tube
Barnes suction tube
Baron ear tube
Baron suction tube
Baron-Frazier suction tube
Bavrona tube
Baylor cardiovascular sump tube
Baylor intracardiac sump tube
Baylor sump tube
Beall-Feldman-Cooley sump tube
Beardsley empyema tube
bedside suction tube
Bellini tube
Bellocq tube
Bellucci nasal suction tube
Bellucci suction tube
Bel-O-Pak suction tube
Benjamin tube
Ben-Jet tube
Bettman empyema tube
bicanalicular silicone tube
Bilboa-Dotter nasogastric tube
Billroth tube
binocular tube
Biolite ventilation tube
Biosystems feeding tube
bivalved tube
Bivona Fome-Cuf tube
Bivona customized tracheostomy tube
Bivona sleep apnea tracheostomy tube
Bivona tracheostomy tube
bladder flap tube
bladder tube
Blake esophageal tube
Blakemore esophageal tube
Blakemore nasogastric tube
Blakemore-Sengstaken tube

tube (*continued*)

Blue Line cuffed endotracheal tube
blue Shepard grommet tube
blunt suction tube
bobbin myringotomy tube
Bonina-Jacobson tube
Bonnano tube
Bonney uterine tube
Bouchut laryngeal tube
Bourdon tube
Bower PEG tube
Bowman tube
Boyce tube
brain suction tube
Brawley nasal suction tube
breathing tube
Bron suction tube
bronchial tube
bronchitis suction tube
Broncho-Cath double-lumen endotracheal tube
Broncho-Cath endotracheal tube
bronchoscopic aspirating tube
bronchoscopic suction tube
bronchoscopy disposable suction tube
Broyles tube
Bruecke tube
buccal tube
Bucy suction tube
Bucy-Frazier suction tube
Buie rectal suction tube
Buie suction tube
Butler tonsil suction tube
Butler tonsillar suction tube
Buyes air-vent suction tube
bypass tube
calibrated grasping tube
calix tube
Caluso PEG gastrostomy tube
Camel tube
Cantor intestinal tube
capillary tube
Carabelli endobronchial tube
Carden bronchoscopy tube
Carden double-lumen endotracheal tube
Carden laryngoscopy tube
Carl Zeiss myringotomy tube

tube (*continued*)

Carlens double-lumen
  endotracheal tube
Carmalt tube
Carman rectal tube
Carrel tube
cartilaginous tube
Casselberry sphenoid tube
Casselberry sphenoid washing
  tube
Castelli tube
Castelli-Paparella collar-button
  tube
Castelli-Paparella
  myringotomy tube
catheterization of eustachian
  tube
cathode ray tube (CRT)
Cattell forked-type T- tube
Cattell gallbladder tube
Causse-Shea tube
Celestin endoesophageal tube
Celestin esophageal tube
Celestin latex rubber tube
cerebromedullary tube
cesium tube
Chaffin suction tube
Chaffin sump tube
Chaffin-Pratt suction tube
Chaoul voltage x-ray tube
Charnley drain tube
Chassin tube
Chauffin-Pratt tube
Chaussier tube
chest tube
Chevalier Jackson tracheal
  tube
cholangiography tube
Christopher-Williams
  overtube
Christopher-Williams tube
Cilastin tube
circle nephrostomy tube
ClearCut II with smoke eater
  tube
Clerf laryngectomy tube
Clerk laryngectomy tube
closed drainage tube
closed suction drainage tube
closed suction tube
closed water-seal suction tube
closed-suction tube

tube (*continued*)

coagulation suction tube
coagulation-aspiration tube
coagulation-aspirator tube
Coakley wash tube
Cole endotracheal tube
Cole orotracheal tube
Cole pediatric tube
Cole uncuffed endotracheal
  tube
collar-button tube
collecting tube
collection tube
Collin tube
colostomy tube
Colton empyema tube
Combitube endotracheal tube
Comfit endotracheal tube
Compat surgical feeding tube
Cone suction tube
Cone tube
Cone-Bucy suction tube
conical centrifuge tube
Connell breathing tube
Connell ether vapor tube
Contigen tube
continuous suction tube
Cook County Hospital
  tracheal suction tube
Cook County suction tube
Cook County tracheal suction
  tube
Cooley aortic sump tube
Cooley cardiovascular suction
  tube
Cooley graft suction tube
Cooley intracardiac suction
  tube
Cooley suction tube
Cooley sump suction tube
Cooley sump tube
Cooley vascular suction tube
Cooley-Anthony suction tube
Coolidge tube
Cope loop nephrostomy
  tube
Cope nephrostomy tube
corneal tube
cornual resection of fallopian
  tube
coronary sinus suction tube
Corpak feeding tube

tube (*continued*)

Corpak weighted-tip, self-
lubricating tube
Costen suction tube
Cottle suction tube
Coupland nasal suction
tube
Coupland suction tube
C-P suction tube
Crawford tube
cricothyrotomy trocar tube
Crookes tube
Crookes-Hittorf tube
cuffed endotracheal tube
cuffed tracheostomy tube
cuffed tube
cuffless tube
CUI myringotomy tube
culture tubes
Cummings tube
cystostomy tube
Dakin tube
Dandy suction tube
David pharyngolaryngectomy
tube
Davol colon tube
Davol suction tube
Dawson-Yuhl suction tube
Deane tube
Deaver tube
DeBakey suction tube
DeBakey-Adson suction tube
Debove tube
decompressive tube
DeLee tube
Denker tube
Dennis intestinal tube
Depaul tube
Devers gallbladder tube
DeVilbiss suction tube
Devine tube
Devine-Millard-Frazier
fiberoptic suction tube
Devine-Millard-Frazier suction
tube
diagnostic ear tube
diagnostic tube
Diamond tube
DIC tracheostomy tube
digestive tube
digit tube
discharge tube

tube (*continued*)

disposable Yankauer
aspirating tube
disposable Yankauer suction
tube
Dobbhoff feeding tube
Dobbhoff gastrectomy feeding
tube
Dobbhoff gastric
decompression tube
Dobbhoff nasogastric feeding
tube
Dobbhoff PEG tube
Doesel-Huzly bronchoscopic
tube
Dominici tube
Donaldson drain tube
Donaldson eustachian tube
Donaldson myringotomy tube
Donaldson Silastic ear tube
Donaldson Teflon tube
Donaldson ventilation tube
double setup endotracheal
tube
double-cannula tracheostomy
tube
double-cuffed tube
double-focus tube
double-lumen endobronchial
tube
double-lumen suction
irrigation tube
double-lumen tube
doughnut tip suction tube
drain tube
drainage tube
drain-to-wall suction tube
Dreiling tube
dressed tube
Dryden-Quickert tube
dual-lumen sump nasogastric
tube
Duke tube
Dumon-Gilliard prosthesis
pushing tube
Dumon-Harrell tracheal tube
Dundas-Grant tube
duodenal tube
Duplay tube
Duralite tube
Durham tracheostomy tube
Dynamic digit extensor tube

tube (*continued*)

E. Benson Hood Laboratories esophageal tube
E. Benson Hood Laboratories salivary bypass tube
ear suction tube
Eastman suction tube
Edlich gastric lavage tube
Edlich lavage tube
EDTA-Vacutainer tube
Einhorn tube
electron multiplier tube
embryonic neural tube
Emerson suction tube
empyema tube
encircling silicone tube
encircling tube
end tube
endobrachial double-lumen tube
endobronchial tube
endoesophageal tube
endolymphatic shunt tube
endolymphatic tube
endoscopic tube
Endosoft reinforced cuffed tube
endotracheal tube
Endotrol endotracheal tube
Endotrol tracheal tube
Endo-Tube nasal jejunal feeding tube
EnteraFlo feeding tube
enteroclysis tube
enterolysis tube
EntriFlex small-bowel feeding tube
EntriStar feeding tube
EntriStar percutaneous endoscopic gastrostomy (PEG) tube
Eppendorf tube
ESKA-Buess esophageal tube
Esmarch tube
esophageal tube
esophagonasogastric tube
esophagoscopic tube
ET tube
Ethox lavage tube
Ethox rectal tube
eustachian tube
Ewald stomach tube

tube (*continued*)

examination insert tube
extension tube
fallopian tubes
Faucher stomach tube
Fay suction tube
Fazio-Montgomery tube
feeding gastrostomy tube
feeding tube
fenestrated tracheostomy tube
fenestrated tube
Ferguson brain suction tube
Ferguson-Frazier suction tube
fermentation tube
Feuerstein drainage tube
Feuerstein ear tube
Feuerstein myringotomy drain tube
Feuerstein split ventilation tube
fiberoptic lighted suction tube
fiberoptic suction tube
fiberoptic tube
field emission tube
fil D'Arion silicone tube
Finsterer myringotomy split tube
Finsterer suction tube
Fitzpatrick suction tube
flanged Teflon tube
flash tube
flexible rubber endoscopic tube
flexible rubber tube
flexible suction tube
Flexiflo enteral feeding tube
Flexiflo Inverta-PEG tube
Flexiflo Sacks-Vine tube
Flexiflo Stomate low-profile gastrostomy tube
Flexiflo suction feeding tube
Flexiflo tap-fill enteral tube
Flexiflo Taptainer tube
Flexiflo tungsten-weighted feeding tube
Flexiflo Versa-PEG tube
flow regulated suction tube
fluffy-cuffed tube
flush tube
fold of uterine tube
Fome-Cuf endotracheal tube

tube (*continued*)

Fome-Cuf pediatric tracheostomy tube
Foregger tube
four-lumen tube
Franco triflange ventilation tube
Frazier aspirating tube
Frazier brain suction tube
Frazier Britetrac nasal suction tube
Frazier fiberoptic suction tube
Frazier insulated suction tube
Frazier modified suction tube
Frazier nasal suction tube
Frazier straight suction tube
Frazier suction tube
Frazier tube
Frazier-Ferguson aspirating tube
Frazier-Ferguson ear suction tube
Frazier-Paparella mastoid suction tube
Frazier-Paparella mastoid tube
Frazier-Paparella suction tube
Frazier-Paparella tube
Frederick-Miller tube
French chest tube
Friend aspirating tube
frontal sinus wash tube
Fuller bivalve trach tube
Fuller tube
fusion tube
Gabriel Tucker tube
gallbladder tube
gas tube
gastric aspiration tube
gastric lavage tube
gastric tube
gastroduodenal tube
gastroenterostomy tube
gastrointestinal tube
gastrojejunostomy tube
Gastro-Port II feeding tube
gastrostomy feeding tube
gastrostomy tube
gavage tube
Geiger-Müller tube
Geissler tube
Geissler-Pluecker tube
Gillquist suction tube

tube (*continued*)

Gillquist-Stille arthroplasty suction tube
Gilman-Abrams gastric tube
Gilman-Abrams tube
Glasser gastrostomy tube
Glover suction tube
glutaraldehyde-tanned bovine collagen tube
Gomco suction tube
Goode Trim tube
Goode T-tube
Goode T-tube ventilating tube
Goode tube
Goodhill-Pynchon tonsillar suction tube
Goodhill-Pynchon tube
Gore-Tex tube
Gott tube
Gowen decompression tube
Grafco Martin laryngectomy tube
graft suction tube
granulation tube
Great Ormond Street tube
Great Ormond Street pediatric tracheostomy tube
Greiling gastroduodenal tube
Greiling tube
grommet drain tube
grommet myringotomy tube
grommet tube
grommet ventilating tube
Guibor canalicular tube
Guibor eye tube
Guibor Silastic tube
Guilford-Wright suction tube
Guisez tube
Gwathmey suction tube
Haering tube
Hagan surface suction tube
Hakim tube
Haldane tube
Haldane-Priestly tube
Hardy suction tube
Har-el pharyngeal tube
Harris tube
Heimlich tube
Heimlich-Gavrilu gastric tube
Helsper tracheostomy vent tube

tube (*continued*)

Hemagard collection tube
hemodialysis tube
Hemovac suction tube
heparin-bonded Bott-type
    tube
heparin-bonded tube
Herring tube
Hilger tracheal tube
Hi-Lo Jet tracheal tube
Hi-Lo tracheal tube
Hittorf tube
Hodge intestinal
    decompression tube
Holinger aspirating tube
Holinger open-end aspirating
    tube
Hollister tube
Holter tube
Honore-Smathers tube
horizontal tube
Hossli suction tube
hot cathode tube
hot cathode x-ray tube
Hotchkiss ear suction tube
Hough-Cadogan suction tube
House endolymphatic shunt
    tube
House shunt tube
House suction tube
House suction-irrigator tube
House-Baron suction tube
House-Radpour suction tube
House-Stevenson suction tube
House-Urban tube
Hubbard airplane vent tube
Hugly aspirating tube
Humphrey coronary sinus-
    sucker suction tube
Humphrey coronary sinus
    suction tube
Hunsaker jet ventilation tube
Hurwitz gastrostomy tube
Hymlek portable chest tube
Hyperflex tracheostomy
    tube
image Orthicon tube
Immergut suction tube
Immergut suction-coagulation
    tube
implanted tube
infant feeding tube

tube (*continued*)

infundibulum of fallopian
    tube
infundibulum of uterine tube
infusion tube
ingress tube
insert tube
insertion of tube
insufflation of fallopian tubes
insulated suction tube
intercostal tube
intestinal tube
intracardiac suction tube
intracardiac sump tube
intraluminal tube
intranasal tube
intratracheal tube
intubation tube
irrigating tube
irrigator-suction tube
Isolator lysis-centrifugation
    tube
Israel suction tube
isthmus of fallopian tube
Jackson aspirating tube
Jackson cane-shaped tracheal
    tube
Jackson cane-shaped tube
Jackson laryngectomy tube
Jackson open-end aspirating
    tube
Jackson silver tracheostomy
    tube
Jackson tracheal tube
Jackson velvet-eye aspirating
    tube
Jackson warning stop tube
Jackson-Pratt suction tube
Jackson-Rees endotracheal
    tube
Jacques gastric tube
Jacques stomach tube
Jako laryngeal suction tube
Jako laser aspirating tube
Jako suction tube
Jarit-Poole abdominal suction
    tube
Jarit-Yankauer suction tube
Javid bypass tube
jejunal feeding tube
jejunostomy tube
Jergesen tube

tube (*continued*)
Jesberg aspirating tube
Jiffy tube
Joel-Baker tube
Johns Hopkins tube
Johnson coagulation suction
  tube
Johnson intestinal tube
Jones Pyrex tube
Jones tear duct tube
J-shaped tube
Jutte tube
Kangaroo silicone
  gastrostomy feeding tube
Kaslow gastrointestinal tube
Kaslow intestinal tube
Kaslow irrigation tube
Kaslow stomach tube
Kay-Cross suction tip suction
  tube
Kehr gallbladder tube
Keidel tube
Kelly tube
Keofeed feeding tube
Keyes-Ultzmann syringe tube
KeyMed esophageal tube
Kidd tube
Kidd U-tube
Killian suction tube
Killian washing tube
Kimpton-Brown tube
Kistner plastic tracheostomy
  tube
Kistner plastic tube
Kistner tracheostomy tube
Klein ventilation tube
Knoche tube
knuckle of tube
Kobelt tube
Kos ear suction tube
Kozlowski tube
K-Tube
Kuhn endotracheal tube
Kurze suction tube
Kurze suction-irrigator tube
Lacor tube
lacrimal tube
Lahey tube
Lahey Y-tube
Lanz low-pressure cuff
  endotracheal tube
Lanz tracheostomy tube

tube (*continued*)
Lapides tube
Lar-A-Jext laryngectomy tube
large-bore gastric lavage tube
LaRocca lacrimal tube
LaRocca nasolacrimal tube
laryngeal tube
laryngectomy tube
Laryngoflex reinforced
  endotracheal tube
Laser-Trach wrapped
  endotracheal tube
Laser-Shield wrapped
  endotracheal tube
Laser-Trach endotracheal tube
Lasertubus tracheal tube
latex tube
Leiter tube
Lell tracheal tube
Lenard ray tube
Lennarson suction tube
Lentz tracheotomy tube
Leonard tube
Lepley-Ernst tracheal tube
Lester Jones tube
Levin duodenal tube
Levin-Davol tube
Lewis laryngectomy tube
Lezius suction tube
life-saving suction tube
life-saving tube
Lindeman-Silverstein Arrow
  tube
Lindeman-Silverstein
  ventilation tube
Lindholm anatomical tracheal
  tube
Lindholm tracheal tube
Linton esophageal tube
Linton-Nachlas tube
Lloyd tube
Loening stomach tube
long intestinal tube
Lonnecken tube
Lo-Pro tracheal tube
Lord-Blakemore tube
Lore suction tube
Lore-Lawrence tracheotomy
  tube
Lorenz tube
Luer speaking tube
Luer tracheal tube

tube (*continued*)

Lukens collecting tube
Lukens suction tube
Lyon tube
Lyster tube
M-A tube (Miller-Abbott tube)
MacKenty antral tube
MacKenty laryngectomy tube
Mackler esophageal tube
Mackler intraluminal tube
Mackray short-cuffed endobronchial tube
Madoff suction tube
Magill endotracheal tube
Maingot gallbladder tube
Malecot gastrostomy tube
Malecot nephrostomy tube
Malis-Frazier suction tube
malleable multipore suction tube
Mallinckrodt endotracheal tube
Mark IV nasogastric tube
Martin drainage tube
Martin laryngectomy tube
Martin tracheostomy tube
Mason suction tube
Massie sliding nail tube
mastoid suction tube
Matzner tube
McCollum tube
McGowan-Keeley tube
McIver nephrostomy tube
McKesson mouth tube
McMurtry-Schlesinger shunt tube
Mead Johnson tube
mediastinal tube
Medina ileostomy catheter tube
Medoc-Celestin pulsion tube
medullary tube
membranous tube
mercury-weighted tube
mesh myringotomy tube
metal-weighted Silastic feeding tube
Methodist suction tube
Methodist vascular suction tube
Mett tube
MIC bolus gastrostomy tube

tube (*continued*)

MIC gastroenteric tube
MIC jejunal tube
MIC jejunostomy tube
MIC-Key gastrostomy tube
microbore Tygon tube
Microfuge tube
Microgel surface-enhanced ventilation tube
microlaryngeal endotracheal tube
Micron bobbin ventilation tube
Miescher tube
Miller endotracheal tube
Miller-Abbott double-channel intestinal tube
Miller-Abbott double-lumen intestinal tube
Miller-Abbott intestinal tube
Miller-Abbott tube (M-A tube)
Millin suction tube
Mill-Rose tube
Milroy-Piper suction tube
Minnesota 4-lumen tube
Mixter tube
MLT tube
modified suction tube
Molteno shunt tube
molybdenum rotating-anode x-ray tube
molybdenum target tube
Momberg tube
Monoject suction tube
Monoka tube
monomer suction biopsy tube
Montando tube
Montefiore tracheal tube
Montgomery esophageal tube
Montgomery salivary bypass tube
Montgomery T-piece tube
Montgomery tracheal tube
Montgomery T-tube
Moore tube
Morch swivel tracheostomy tube
Morch tracheostomy tube
Moretz Tiny Tytan ventilation tube
Moretz Tytan ventilation tube
Morsch-Retec respirator tube

tube (*continued*)

  Morse suction tube
  Morse-Andrews suction tube
  Morse-Ferguson suction tube
  Mosher esophagoscope tube
  Mosher intubation tube
  Mosher lifesaver tube
  Mosher life-saving tracheal
    suction tube
  Mosher lifesaving tube
  Mosher suction tube
  Moss balloon triple-lumen
    gastrostomy tube
  Moss feeding tube
  Moss gastric decompression
    tube
  Moss gastrostomy tube
  Moss Mark IV gastrostomy
    tube
  Moss Mark IV nasal tube
  Moss Mark IV tube
  Moss nasal tube
  Moss Suction Buster tube
  Moteno shunt tube
  Moulton lacrimal duct tube
  Mousseau-Barbin esophageal
    tube
  Mousseau-Barbin prosthetic
    tube
  Mueller suction tube
  Mueller-Frazier suction tube
  Mueller-Poole suction tube
  Mueller-Pynchon suction tube
  Mueller-Yankauer suction
    tube
  Muldoon tube
  multiholed tube
  multiple-lumen tube
  Murphy drip tube
  Murphy endotracheal tube
  muscular tube
  Myerson wash tube
  myringotomy drain tube
  myringotomy tube
  Nachlas gastrointestinal tube
  Nachlas-Linton tube
  nasal suction tube
  nasal tube
  nasobiliary tube
  nasocystic drainage tube
  nasoduodenal feeding tube
  nasoendotracheal tube

tube (*continued*)

  nasoenteric feeding tube
  nasoesophageal feeding tube
  nasogastric feeding tube
  nasogastric tube
  nasoileal tube
  nasojejunal feeding tube
  nasojejunal tube
  nasolacrimal tube
  nasopharyngeal tube
  nasotracheal tube
  Natelson tube
  NCC Hi-Lo Jet endotracheal
    tube
  nephrostomy tube
  Neuber bone tube
  Neuber drainage tube
  neural tube
  New Luer-type speaking tube
  New speaking tube
  New York glass suction tube
  New York Hospital suction
    tube
  Newvicon camera tube
  Newvicon vacuum chamber
    pickup tube
  Newvicon vacuum tube
  NG feeding tube
  NG tube
  Nilsson suction tube
  Nilsson-Stille abortion suction
    tube
  Nishizaki-Wakabayashi suction
    tube
  Norton endotracheal tube
  Nunez ventricular ventilation
    tube
  Nuport PEG tube
  Nutraflex Poole tube
  Nyhus-Nelson gastric
    decompression tube
  Nyhus-Nelson jejunal feeding
    tube
  Nystroem abdominal suction
    tube
  O'Beirne sphincter tube
  obstructed shunt tube
  obstructed tube
  Ochsner gallbladder tube
  O'Dwyer intubation tube
  O'Hanlon-Poole suction tube
  Olshevsky tube

tube (*continued*)

Olympus gastrostomy tube
Ommaya ventricular tube
opaque myringotomy tube
open-end aspirating tube
oral endotracheal tube
oral esophageal tube
oroendotracheal tube
orogastric Ewald tube
orogastric tube
orotracheal tube
Ossoff-Karlan laser suction
   tube
otopharyngeal tube
ovarian tube
overcouch tube
Oxford nonkinking cuffed
   tube
Panda gastrostomy tube
Panda nasoenteric feeding
   tube
Panje tube
Paparella myringotomy tube
Paparella polyethylene tube
Paparella ventilation tube
Paparella-Frazier suction
tube
parasol tube
Parker tube
patent fallopian tube
patent tube
Paul drainage tube
Paul intestinal drainage tube
Paul-Mixter tube
PE tube (polyethylene tube;
   pressure equalization
   tube)
pear-shaped extension tube
Pedia-Trake tube
pediatric feeding tube
pediatric nasogastric tube
PEG tube (percutaneous
   endoscopic gastrostomy
   tube)
Penrose tube
percutaneous nephrostomy
   tube
Per-Lee equalizing tube
Per-Lee middle ear tubes
Per-Lee myringotomy tube
Per-Lee ventilating tubes
Per-Lee ventilation tube

tube (*continued*)

Perspex tube
Pertrach percutaneous
   tracheostomy tube
Pezzar tube
Pfluger tube
pharyngeal tube
pharyngotympanic tube
photoelectric multiplier tube
photomultiplier tube
pickup tube
Pierce antral wash tube
Pierce washing tube
pigtail nephrostomy tube
Pilling duralite tracheal tube
Pilling duralite tube
Pilling tracheostomy tube
Pitot tube
Pitt talking tracheostomy tube
Pitt tracheostomy tube
plastic tube
plastic-cuffed tracheostomy
   tube
pleural suction tube
pleural tube
Pleur-Evac suction tube
plugged tube
Plumicon camera tube
Polisar-Lyons adapted tracheal
   tube
Polisar-Lyons tracheal tube
polyethylene drainage tube
polyethylene tube
polyvinyl chloride
   endotracheal tube
polyvinyl tube
Ponsky PEG tube
Ponsky-Gauderer PEG tube
Poole abdominal suction tube
Poole suction tube
Poppen suction tube
Portex Blue Line
   tracheostomy tube
Portex Per-Fit tracheostomy
   tube
Portex preformed blue line
   tracheal tube
Portex speaking tube
Portex tracheostomy tube
Porto-vac suction tube
postnasal tube
postpyloric feeding tube

tube (*continued*)

precipitin tube
preformed polyvinyl chloride endotracheal tube
pressure equalization tube
pressure equalizing tube
Pribram suction tube
primordial catheter tube
Procter-Livingston tube
Proctor suction tube
Pudenz tube
Puestow-Olander gastrointestinal tube
Puestow-Olander GI tube
pus tube
Pynchon suction tube
pyramidal tube
Pyrex tube
Questek laser tube
Quickert tube
Quickert-Dryden tube
Quincke tube
Quinton tube
radiopaque intestinal tube
Radius enteral feeding tube
Radpour-House suction tube
RAE endotracheal tube
RAE Flex tracheal tube
Raimondi tube
Ramirez straight Silastic tube
Rand-House suction tube
Rand-Radpour suction tube
Raney tube
Ray tube
rectal tube
rectifier tube
red rubber endotracheal tube
Redivac suction tube
red-top tube
Rehfuss duodenal tube
Rehfuss stomach tube
Reinecke-Carroll lacrimal tube
reinforced tracheostomy tube
Replogle tube
respiratory tube
retractable fiberoptic tube
Reuter bobbin stainless steel drain tube
Reuter bobbin tube
Reuter bobbin ventilation tube
Reynolds tube

tube (*continued*)

Rhoton-Merz suction tube
Rica mastoid suction tube
right-angle chest tube
Ring-McLean sump tube
Ritter suprapubic suction tube
Robertshaw double-lumen endotracheal tube
Robinson equalizing tube
Rochester suction tube
Rochester tracheal tube
roll tube
Roller pump suction tube
Rosen suction tube
rotating anode tube
rubber endoscopic tube
rubber tube
Rubin Brandborg biopsy tube
Rubin hydraulic biopsy tube
Rubin-Quinton small-bowel biopsy tube
Rusch laryngectomy tube
Rusch red rubber rectal tube
Ruschelit polyvinyl chloride endotracheal tube
Russell suction tube
Ruysch tube
Ruysch-Armor tube
Ryle duodenal tube
Sachs brain suction tube
Sachs suction tube
Sachs-Vine PEG tube (percutaneous endoscopic gastrostomy tube)
Safar tube
Safety Clear Plus endotracheal tube
safety tube
Salem duodenal sump tube
Salem nasogastric tube
Salem sump action nasogastric tube
Salem sump tube
salivary bypass tube
salivary tube
salvarsan throat irrigation tube
salvarsan tube
Samco tube
Samson-Davis infant suction tube

tube (*continued*)

Sandoz balloon replacement tube
Sandoz Caluso PEG gastrostomy tube
Sandoz feeding/suction tube
Sandoz nasogastric feeding tube
Sandoz suction tube
Sandoz suction/feeding tube
Sapporo shunt tube
Sarns intracardiac suction tube
Saticon vacuum chamber pickup tube
Saticon vacuum tube
S-B tube (Sengstaken-Blakemore tube)
scavenging tube
Schachowa tube
Schall laryngectomy tube
Schmiedt tube
Schuknecht suction tube
Schuler aspiration/irrigation tube
Scott nasal suction tube
Scott suction tube
Scott-Harden tube
Securat suction tube
semicanal of auditory tube
Sengstaken nasogastric tube
Sengstaken-Blakemore esophagogastric tamponade tube
Senning suction tube
Sensiv endotracheal tube
separator tube
Seroma-Cath drainage tube
Seroma-Cath feeding tube
seton tube
Shah myringotomy tube
Shah permanent ventilation tube
Shaldon tube
Sharley tracheostomy tube
Shaw tube
Shea polyethylene drainage tube
Shea-type parasol myringotomy tube
Sheehy collar-button tube
Sheehy collar-button ventilating tube

tube (*continued*)

Sheehy collar-button ventilation tube
Sheehy Tytan ventilation tube
Sheldon-Pudenz tube
Shepard drain tube
Shepard grommet tube
Shepard grommet ventilation tube
Shepard Teflon tube
Shepard ventilation tube
Sheridan tube
Sherman suction tube
Shiley cuffless fenestrated tube
Shiley cuffless tracheostomy tube
Shiley disposable cannula low pressure cuffed tracheostomy tube
Shiley endotracheal tube
Shiley extra-length single cannula tracheostomy tube
Shiley fenestrated low pressure cuffed tracheostomy tube
Shiley French sump tube
Shiley laryngectomy tube
Shiley low-pressure cuffed tracheostomy tube
Shiley neonatal tracheostomy tube
Shiley pediatric tracheostomy tube
Shiley single cannula cuffed tracheostomy tube
Shiley sump tube
Shiley tracheostomy tube
Shiley-Bjork tube
Shiner tube
short-length tracheal tube
shunt tube
sigmoidoscope insulated suction tube
sigmoidoscope suction tube
Silastic eustachian tube
Silastic intestinal tube
Silastic sucker suction tube
Silastic tracheostomy tube
silicone tube
silicone-lubricated endotracheal tube

tube (*continued*)
Silverstein permanent
  aeration tube
Silverstein tube
Singer-Blom tube
sinus wash tube
siphon suction tube
small-bowel tube
SMIC mastoid suction tube
Smith tube
smoke evacuator suction tube
smoke removal tube
Smokeeter tube
Snyder Hemovac suction tube
Snyder Surgivac suction tube
Snyder Urevac suction tube
Softech endotracheal tube
SoftForm tube
Soileau Tytan ventilation tube
solid-phase extraction tube
Southey capillary drainage
  tube
Southey-Leech tube
Souttar tube
speaking tube
Spetzler MicroVac suction
  tube
spiral-wound endotracheal
  tube
splinting tube
sputum tube
SS bobbin drain tube
SS bobbin myringotomy tube
Stamm gastrostomy tube
Stedman continuous suction
  tube
Stedman suction tube
stent tube
sterile connecting tube
sterile vacuum collection tube
stomach irrigation tube
stomach tube
Stomate decompression tube
Stomate extension tube
Storz anti-fog tube
Storz bronchoscopic suction
  tube
Storz examination insert tube
Storz flash tube
Storz insert tube
Storz intratracheal tube
Storz suction tube

tube (*continued*)
Storz-Doesel-Huzly
  bronchoscope tube
straight chest tube
Stroud-Baron ear suction tube
suction tube
suction-coagulation tube
Suh ventilation tube
sump nasogastric tube
sump suction tube
sump tube
Super PEG tube
Supramid suction tube
suprapubic tube
surgically implanted tube
Sustagen nasogastric tube
Swan-Ganz tube
Swenson cholangiography
  tube
swivel tracheostomy tube
T self-retaining drainage tube
talking tracheostomy tube
tampon tube
tear duct tube
Teflon endolymphatic shunt
  tube
Teflon shunt tube
Tek tube
test tube
T-grommet ventilation tube
Thal-Quick chest tube
thoracic drainage tube
thoracostomy tube
thoracotomy tube
Thora-Klex chest tube
Thow gastrostomy tube
throat irrigation tube
Thunberg tube
tight-to-shaft Aire-Cuf
  tracheostomy tube
Tiny Tytan ventilation tube
Tiny-Tef ventilation tube
tonsil suction tube
tonsillar suction tube
Toomey suction tube
Torkildsen tube
Touma T-type grommet
  ventilation tube
Tovell tube
Toynbee diagnostic tube
tracheal suction tube
tracheal tube

tube (*continued*)

tracheobronchial suction tube
TracheoSoft tracheostomy
  tube
tracheostomy tube
tracheotomy tube
Tracheoflex tracheostomy
  tube
Trake-Fit endotracheal tube
transection of tube
translucent drain tube
translucent myringotomy tube
transport tube
transpyloric feeding tube
transpyloric tube
triple-lumen Sengstaken-
  Blakemore tube
Trombotect tube
Tru-Arc trachea tube
TTS Aire-Cuf endotracheal
  tube
TTS Aire-Cuf tracheostomy
  tube
T-tube round suction tube
T-type myringotomy tube
tube attachment device
tube changer
tube dressing
tube foam
tube graft
Tucker aspirating tube
Tucker flexible-tip tube
Tucker suction tube
Tucker tracheal tube
Tufts suction tube
Turkel tube
Turner-Warwick fiberoptic
  suction tube
Turner-Warwick illuminating
  suction tube
twist-in drain tube
twist-in myringotomy tube
Tygon tube
tympanoscopy ventilation
  tube
tympanostomy tube
Tytan grommet ventilation
  tube
Tytan ventilation tube
underwater-seal suction tube
underwater-seal tube
Univent endotracheal tube

tube (*continued*)

urinary drainage tube
uterine tube
U-tube tube
V. Mueller-Frazier suction tube
V. Mueller-Poole suction tube
Vacutainer vacuum tube
vacuum tube
Valentine irrigation tube
valve tube
Van Alyea antral wash tube
vascular suction tube
Veillon tube
velvet-eye aspirating tube
velvet-eye tube
ventilation tube
ventricular ventilation tube
Ventrol Levin tube
Venturi bobbin myringotomy
  tube
Venturi collar-button
  myringotomy tube
Venturi grommet
  myringotomy tube
Venturi pediatric
  myringotomy tube
Vernon antral tube
Vernon antral wash tube
Versatome laser fiber tube
vertical tube
Vidicon camera tube
Vidicon vacuum chamber
  pickup tube
Vidicon vacuum tube
Vinyon-N cloth tube
Vivonex gastrostomy tube
Vivonex Moss tube
Voltolini ear tube
Von Eichen antral tube
Von Eichen antral wash tube
Vortex tracheostomy tube
Vortex tracheotomy tube
Walter-Poole suction tube
Walter-Yankauer suction tube
Wangensteen duodenal tube
Wangensteen suction tube
Wannagat suction tube
Waring tonsil suction tube
warning stop tube
wash tube
washing tube
water-seal chest tube

tube (*continued*)
  Watkins suction tube
  Watzke tube
  Webster infusion tube
  Weck coagulating suction
    tube
  Weck suction tube
  Welch Allyn suction tube
  Wendl tube
  Wepsic suction tube
  Wesolowski Dacron tube
  West tube
  Williams esophageal tube
  Wilson-Cook nasobiliary tube
  Wilson-Cook feeding tube
  Winsburg-White bladder tube
  wire-wound endotracheal
    tube
  Witzel tube
  Wolf suction tube
  Woodbridge tube
  Wookey skin tube
  woven Dacron tube
  Wullstein microsuction tube
  Xomed endotracheal tube
  Xomed straight-shank tube
  Xomed Treace ventilation tube
  Xomed Tytan ventilation tube
  x-ray tube
  Yankauer aspirating tube
  Yankauer suction tube
  Yankauer washing tube
  Yasargil microsuction tube
  Yasargil suction tube
  Yeder suction tube
  Ygon tube
  Zeiss binocular tube
  Zollner suction tube
  Z-wave tube
  Zyler tube
tube attachment device
tube carrier
tube cecostomy
tube changer
tube decompression
tube dressing
tube extrusion
tube feeding
tube flap
tube flap graft
tube foam
tube gastrostomy

tube gauze
tube graft
tube inflation
tube inserted
tube insufflator
tube introducer
tube intubation
tube leakage
tube obstruction
tube pedicle graft
tube placement
tube prosthesis
tube removal
tube replacement
tube stockinette
tubed free skin graft
tubed groin flap
tubed pedicle flap
tubed-pedicle delayed groin flap
Tubegauz elastic net
Tubegauz seamless tubular
    knitted cotton bandage
tubeless cystostomy
tubeless lithotriptor
Tube-Lok tracheotomy dressing
tube-occluding clamp
tube-occluding forceps
Tuber syringe
tubercle
  adductor tubercle
  articular tubercle
  auricular tubercle
  Burlar tubercle
  Chassaignac tubercle
  corniculate tubercle
  cuneiform tubercle
  Darwin tubercle
  darwinian tubercle
  dissection tubercle
  Farre tubercles
  genial tubercle
  Gerdy knee tubercle
  Gerdy tubercle
  Ghon tubercle
  greater tubercle
  labial tubercle
  lesser tubercle
  Lister tubercle
  marginal tubercle
  maxillary tubercles
  mental tubercle
  Montgomery tubercles

tubercle (*continued*)
  peroneal tubercle
  pharyngeal tubercle
  philtral tubercle
  pubic tubercle
  Santorini tubercle
  scaphoid tubercle
  supraglenoid tubercle
  tibial tubercle
  Wrisberg tubercle
  zygomatic tubercle
tubercle of upper lip
tuberculous abscess
tuberculous caseation
tuberculous infiltration
tuberculous lesion
tuberculous otitis media
tuberosity
  calcaneal tuberosity
  ischial tuberosity
  malar tuberosity
  maxillary tuberosity
  radial tuberosity
  reduction tuberosity
  sacral tuberosity
  tibial tuberosity
tuberosity fragment
tuberosity reduction
tuberous carcinoma
tuberous sclerosis complex
tuberous sclerosis-associated
    renal cell carcinoma
tuberous xanthoma
tube-shift technique
Tubestat lighted stylet
tube-within-tube technique
Tubex gauze dressing
Tubex injector
Tubex metal syringe
Tubifast bandage
Tubigrip dressing
Tubigrip elastic support
    bandage
Tubi-Grip elastic support
    bandages
tubing
  Catalano tubing
  connector tubing
  Dakin tubing
  evacuator tubing
  Extendex tubing
  flexible tubing

tubing (*continued*)
  foam tubing
  Holter tubing
  hyperalimentation tubing
  Intramedic tubing
  polyvinyl tubing
  shunt tubing
  swivel connector tubing
  Tygon surgical tubing
  Tygon tubing
tubing adapter
tubing clamp
tubing clamp forceps
tubing compressor
tubing forceps
tubing hand roller
tubing introducer forceps
Tubinger gall stone forceps
Tubinger self-retaining retractor
Tubipad bandage
Tubiton tubular bandage
tubo-insufflation
tuboligation
tubo-ovarian
tubo-ovarian abscess
tubo-ovarian cyst
tubo-ovarian pregnancy
tubo-ovarian varicocele
tuboplasty
  balloon tuboplasty
tuboplasty surgical kit
tubouterine implantation
tubouterine pregnancy
tubular adenoma
tubular aneurysm
tubular basement membrane
tubular blade
tubular breasts
tubular cancer
tubular carcinoma
tubular colonic duplication
tubular defect
tubular dressing
tubular ectasia
tubular forceps
tubular gland
tubular Gore SAM material
tubular gouge
tubular graft
tubular magnet
tubular necrosis
tubular plate

tubular polyp
tubular reconstruction
tubular slotted stent
tubular vaginal speculum
tubular vertical gastroplasty
tubularized bladder neck
   reconstruction
tubularized cecal flap
tubule
  Bellini tubules
  collecting tubule
  convoluted seminiferous
    tubules
  Miescher tubule
  mucous tubule
  renal tubule
  seminiferous tubules
  testicular tubules
Tubulitec cavity liner
tubulization
tubulovillar lesion
tubulovillous adenoma
tubulovillous polyp
tuck position
tuck procedure
tucker (*see also* tendon tucker)
  Bishop tendon tucker
  Bishop-Black tendon tucker
  Bishop-DeWitt tendon tucker
  Bishop-Peter tendon tucker
  Burch-Greenwood tendon
    tucker
  Cooley cardiac tucker
  Crafoord-Cooley tucker
  DeBakey tucker
  Fink tendon tucker
  Green tucker
  Harrison tucker
  Kelly combined packer and
    tucker
  ligature tucker
  Ruedemann-Todd tendon
    tucker
  Smith-Petersen tucker
  Smuckler tucker
  strabismus tucker
  tendon tucker
Tucker anterior commissure
   laryngoscope
Tucker appendix clamp
Tucker aspirating tube
Tucker bead forceps

Tucker bougie
Tucker bronchoscope
Tucker cardiospasm dilator
Tucker dilator
Tucker direct-vision telescope
Tucker esophagoscope
Tucker flexible-tip tube
Tucker hallux forceps
Tucker hemorrhoidal ligator
Tucker laryngoscope
Tucker mediastinoscope
Tucker mid-lighted optic slide
   laryngoscope
Tucker reach-and-pin forceps
Tucker retrograde bougie
Tucker slotted laryngoscope
Tucker staple forceps
Tucker suction tube
Tucker tack and pin forceps
Tucker telescope
Tucker tracheal tube
Tucker tube
Tucker vertebrated guide
Tucker vertebrated lumen finder
Tucker-Holinger laryngoscope
Tucker-Jako laryngoscope
Tucker-Levine vocal cord
   retractor
Tucker-Luikart blade
Tucker-McLane axis-traction
   forceps
Tucker-McLane obstetrical
   forceps
Tucker-McLane-Luikart forceps
Tudor operation
Tudor-Edwards bone-cutting
   forceps
Tudor-Edwards costotome
Tudor-Edwards rib shears
Tudor-Edwards rib spreader
Tudor-Edwards spreader
Tudor-Thomas graft
Tudor-Thomas operation
Tufcote epilation probe
Tuffier abdominal retractor
Tuffier abdominal spatula
Tuffier arterial forceps
Tuffier bone bender
Tuffier forceps
Tuffier morcellement
   technique
Tuffier operation

Tuffier retractor
Tuffier rib retractor
Tuffier rib spreader
Tuffier spreader
Tuffier-Raney laminectomy
    retractor
Tuffnell bandage
tuft fracture
tuft of bone
tufted angioma
Tufts suction tube
Tuke bone saw
Tukey post-hoc correction
Tulevech lacrimal cannula
Tuli heel cup
Tulip cannula
Tulip harvesting system for
    suction lipectomy
tulip pedicle screw
tulip probe
tulip sheath
tulip tip
tulle gras dressing
Tullos technique
tumble flap
tumble-flap hypospadias
    repair
tumbler flap
tumbler graft
tumbler skin flap
tumbling E cube
tumbling fashion
tumbling procedure
tumbling technique
tumbling technique operation
tumbling-technique cataract
    extraction
tumefaction
tumescent
tumescent absorbent bandage
    dressing
tumescent anesthesia
tumescent infiltrator cannula
tumescent liposuction
tumescent liposuction garment
    (TLG)
tumescent technique
tumescent technique breast
    reduction
Tum-E-Vac gastric lavage kit
tummy tuck flap
tumofactive asymmetry

tumor
    abdominal tumor
    Abrikosov tumor
    acinic cell tumor
    adenopapillary tumor
    adnexal skin tumor
    anterior pillar tumor
    aortic body tumor
    atypical carcinoid tumor
    basaloid tumor
    Bednar tumor
    benign mesenchymal tumor
    benign mixed tumor
    benign tumor
    bleeding tumor
    body tumor
    Brigham brain tumor
    Brooke tumor
    brown tumor
    calcifying epithelial
        odontogenic tumor
    canine transmissible tumor
    capsule tumor
    carcinoid tumor
    cardiac tumor
    carotid body tumor
    cartilaginous tumor
    central giant cell tumor
    cerebellopontine angle tumor
    cerebral tumor
    ceruminous gland tumor
    common duct tumor
    conjunctival tumor
    cord tumor
    corticoadrenal tumor
    craniopharyngeal duct tumor
    Cruveilhier tumor
    Cushing tumor
    cystic tumor
    de novo tumor
    debulking of tumor
    deep tumor
    deep-lobe parotid tumor
    dermal analogue tumor
    dermoid tumor
    doubling time for tumor
    duct tumor
    ectodermal tumor
    EIC-negative breast tumor
    embryonal tumor
    encapsulated tumor
    endocardial tumor

tumor (*continued*)
- endotracheal tumor
- epidermoid tumor
- esophageal tumor
- Ewing tumor
- excavated tumor
- excavation of tumor
- excision of tumor
- extra-axial brain tumor
- fatty tumor
- fibrofatty tumor
- focal tumor
- fungating tumor
- gastric tumor
- gastrin-secreting non-beta islet cell tumor
- giant cell tumor
- glomus jugulare tumor
- glomus tumor
- Godwin tumor
- granular cell tumor
- granulosa-theca cell tumor
- Grawitz tumor
- gritty tumor
- gross tumor
- growing tumor
- hepatic tumor
- Hurthle cell tumor
- Hürthle (*see* Hurthle)
- Huerthle (*see* Hurthle)
- Hurthle (*also* Hürthle, Huerthle)
- hyperplastic tumor
- impinging on tumor
- infantile vascular tumor
- innocuous tumor
- inoperable tumor
- intra-axial brain tumor
- intracranial tumor
- intraparotid mesenchymal tumor
- invasive tumor
- islet cell tumor
- isolated metastatic tumor
- keloid tumor
- keratinizing epithelial odontogenic tumor
- Klatskin tumor
- Krukenberg tumor
- lip tumor
- lipogenic tumor
- liver tumor

tumor (*continued*)
- malignant mesenchymal tumor
- malignant odontogenic tumor
- malignant tumor
- massive tumor
- mediastinal tumor
- melanotic neuroectodermal tumor
- mesenchymal mixed tumor
- mesenchymal tumor
- mesodermal tumor
- metachronous tumor
- metastatic tumor
- midline tumor
- mixed tumor
- mucinous tumor
- mucoepidermoid tumor
- muellerian tumor
- multicentric glomus tumor
- muscle tumor
- myocardial tumors
- nerve tumor
- neuroectodermal tumor
- nodular tumor
- nonepithelial tumor
- odontogenic tumor
- ophthalmic tumor
- ovarian tumor
- Pancoast tumor
- pancreatic islet cell tumor
- papillary tumor
- parapharyngeal tumor
- parotid tumor
- periampullary tumor
- pericardial tumor
- pituitary tumor
- pontine tumor
- Pott puffy tumor
- primary brain tumor
- primary intra-axial brain tumor
- puffy tumor
- radiocurable tumor
- radioresistant tumor
- Rathke tumor
- recurrent tumor
- reduce size of tumor
- renal tumor
- resectable tumor
- residual tumor
- retroperitoneal tumor

tumor (*continued*)
  Rokitansky tumor
  ropy tumor
  salivary gland tumor
  Schwann tumor
  serous tumor
  skin tumor
  small-cell tumor
  soft tissue tumor
  solid tumor
  spindle cell tumor
  squamous odontogenic tumor
  strawberry tumor
  subcutaneous tumor
  subtentorial tumor
  subtotal removal of tumor
  sulcus tumor
  suprasellar tumor
  teratoid tumor
  testis tumor
  thalamic tumor
  thecal cell tumor
  thymic tumor
  thyroid tumor
  TNM classification of
    malignant tumors
  transitional tumor
  transurethral resection of
    bladder tumor (TURBT)
  trophoblastic tumor
  ulcerogenic tumor
  unresectable tumor
  urothelial tumor
  vascular tumor
  vasoformative tumor
  villous tumor
  Warthin tumor
  warty cicatricial tumor
  Wilms tumor
  Zollinger-Ellison tumor
tumor ablation
tumor angiogenic factor (TAF)
tumor blush
tumor capsule
tumor defect
tumor embolism
tumor encapsulation
tumor forceps
tumor imaging
tumor infiltration
tumor invasion
tumor lysis factor

tumor lysis syndrome
tumor marker
tumor necrosis factor
tumor of infancy
tumor plop
tumor probe
tumor removal
tumor resection
tumor screw
tumor surgery
tumor therapy
tumor, node, metastasis (TNM)
tumor, node, metastasis
    carcinoma classification
tumor-bearing kidney
tumor-free margin
tumor-grasping forceps
tumor-like bone condition
tumorlike necrosis
tumorous portion
tumor-related death
tumor-replacement
    endoprosthesis
tumor-specific transplantation
    immunity (TSTI)
tumor-to-tumor metastasis
tunable diaphragm stethoscope
tunable dye laser
tunable dye laser lithotripsy
tunable dye laser with Hexascan
tunable flashlamp-excited
    pulsed dye laser
tunable notch filter
tunable tinnitus masker
tungsten arc lamp
tungsten carbide bur
tungsten eye shield
tungsten microdissection needle
tungsten microelectrode
tungsten tip
tungsten-halogen slit lamp
tunica (*pl.* tunicae)
tunica abdominalis
tunica adventitia
tunica conjunctiva
tunica dartos
tunica fibrosa hepatis
tunica fibrosa lienis
tunica intima
tunica media
tunica mucosa ventriculi
tunica mucosa vesicae felleae

tunica muscularis coli
tunica muscularis intestini
    tenuis
tunica muscularis recti
tunica muscularis ventriculi
tunica propria
tunica serosa coli
tunica serosa hepatis
tunica serosa intestini tenuis
tunica serosa lienis
tunica serosa peritonei
tunica serosa ventriculi
tunica serosa vesicae felleae
tunica vaginalis
tunicary hernia
Tun-L-Cath epidural catheter
tunnel
    aortic-left ventricular tunnel
    aortopulmonary tunnel
    carpal tunnel
    crossing tunnels
    cubital tunnel
    double tunnel
    extramucosal tunnels
    fibro-osseous tunnel
    Phalen sign for carpal tunnel
    pullys in fibro-osseous tunnel
    radial tunnel
    release of carpal tunnel
    Shipps cholangiographic tunnel
    stylomandibular tunnel
    subcutaneous tunnels
    tarsal tunnel
    ulnar tunnel
    Whitzel tunnel
tunnel and sling fixation
tunnel creation
tunnel drill guide
tunnel flap
tunnel graft
tunnel projection
tunnel view
tunnel view on x-ray
tunnel x-ray view
tunnelable ventricular ICP
    catheter
tunneled bougie
tunneled eye implant
tunneled implant
tunneled supraclavicular island
    flap for head and neck
    reconstruction

tunneler
    Crafoord-Cooley tunneler
    DeBakey tunneler
    Eidemiller tunneler
    Favaloro tunneler
    Oregon tunneler
    Taucher tunneler
tunneling instrument
tunnelization
TunneLoc interference screw
tunnel-type implant material
Tunstal connector
Tuohy aortography needle
Tuohy catheter
Tuohy lumbar aortography
    needle
Tuohy needle
Tuohy spinal needle
Tuohy-Borst adapter
Tuohy-Borst side-arm
    introducer
Tuohy-Borst micropuncture
    introducer
Tupman osteotomy plate
Tupper arthroplasty
Tupper hand-holder and
    retractor
Tupper retractor
Tupper tractor
TUR (transurethral resection)
turbid fluid
turbid milky fluid
turbid peritoneal fluid
turbidity
turbinate
    bulbous turbinates
    inferior turbinate
    infracted turbinate
    infraction of turbinate
    middle turbinate
    nasal turbinate
    neck of middle turbinate
    sphenoidal turbinate
    superior turbinate
turbinate bone
turbinate electrode
turbinate forceps
turbinate knife
turbinate scissors
turbine pneumotach
turbinectomy
turbinectomy scissors

Turbinger gastric reconstruction
turbo-bit craniotome
Turbo-Jet dental bur
TurboSonic tip
TurboStaltic pump
turbo-tip of phacoemulsification unit
TURBT (transurethral resection of bladder tumor)
Turbuhaler inhaler
Turchik instrument holder
Turck bundle
Turck (*also* Türck, Tuerck)
Türck (*see* Turck)
Tuerck (*see* Turck)
Turco clubfoot release
Turco clubfoot release technique
Turco operation for talipes equinovarus
Turco-Spinella tendo calcaneus repair
Turcot syndrome
Turek spinous process spreader
turf toe
turgescence
turgescent vessel
turgid
turgor
Turk line
Turkel bone biopsy trephine set
Turkel liver biopsy needle
Turkel prostatic punch
Turkel trephine
Turkel tube
turkey gobbler neck
Turkey sternal needle
turkey-claw clamp
turn-and-suction biopsy technique
turnbuckle ankle brace
turnbuckle cast
turnbuckle distractor
turnbuckle elbow splint
turnbuckle functional position splint
turnbuckle knee brace
turnbuckle wrist orthosis
Turnbull adhesion forceps
Turnbull applicator
Turnbull cannula

Turnbull colostomy
Turnbull end-loop ileostomy
Turnbull forceps
Turnbull multiple ostomy
Turnbull multiple ostomy operation
Turnbull nail nipper
Turnbull nipper
Turnbull technique
turned-down tendon flap
turned-up pulp deformity
Turner biopsy needle
Turner cord elevator
Turner cystoscopic fulgurating electrode
Turner dilator
Turner elevator
Turner gouge
Turner hip pin
Turner intraparietal sulcus
Turner operation
Turner periosteal elevator
Turner pin
Turner prosthesis
Turner sign
Turner spinal gouge
Turner tooth
Turner-Babcock tissue forceps
Turner-Doyen retractor
Turner-Warwick adult retractor ring
Turner-Warwick bladder neck spreader
Turner-Warwick blade
Turner-Warwick diathermy scissors
Turner-Warwick fiberoptic suction tube
Turner-Warwick illuminating suction tube
Turner-Warwick incision
Turner-Warwick needle
Turner-Warwick needle holder
Turner-Warwick pediatric perineal retractor ring
Turner-Warwick posterior urethral retractor
Turner-Warwick post-urethroplasty review speculum
Turner-Warwick prostate retractor
Turner-Warwick stone forceps

Turner-Warwick suction
Turner-Warwick urethroplasty
Turner-Warwick urethroplasty
    needle
Turner-Warwick-Adson forceps
turning fracture frame
turnover flap
turnover skin flap
TURP (transurethral resection of
    prostate)
Turrell angular rotating punch
Turrell biopsy forceps
Turrell biopsy punch
Turrell proctoscope
Turrell rectal biopsy forceps
Turrell sigmoidoscope
Turrell specimen forceps
Turrell-Wittner rectal biopsy
    forceps
Turrell-Wittner rectal forceps
turret exostosis
turricephaly twig
Turvy internal screw fixation
Tusge technique to reconstruct
    hand tendons
Tutofix cortical pin
Tutofix pin
Tutoplast processed allograft
Tuttle dressing forceps
Tuttle obstetrical forceps
Tuttle proctoscope
Tuttle sigmoidoscope
Tuttle test
Tuttle thoracic forceps
Tuttle thumb forceps
Tuttle tissue forceps
Tuttle-Singley thoracic forceps
Tuwave galvanic stimulator/
    TENS unit
Twardon grommet
T-wave
Tweed analysis
Tweedy canaliculus knife
tweezers
    Dumont tweezers
    Laser Tweezers
twilight anesthesia
twill dressing
Twin Flash scanner
twin formation
Twin Jet nebulizer
twin knife

twin-barreled fibular graft
twin-coil dialyzer
Twining line
Twining position
twin-pattern chisel
twin-twin transfusion syndrome
    (TTTS)
Twisk forceps
Twisk microscissors
Twisk needle holder
Twisk scissors
twist drill
twist drill catheter
twist fixation hook
Twist MTX implant
Twist Ti implant
twisted cotton nonabsorbable
    surgical sutures
twisted cotton sutures
twisted dermal sutures
twisted fundoplication
twisted linen sutures
twisted silk sutures
twisted suture technique
twisted sutures
twisted virgin silk sutures
twisted wire loop
twisted wire snare loop
twister
    Baumgarten Vital wire twister
    Cone wire twister
    orthotic coiled spring twister
    wire twister
twist-in drain tube
twist-in drain tube inserter
twist-in myringotomy tube
twisting injury
Twist-Lock drill guard
Twist-Mate ligator
twist-off technique
twitch depression
twitching
    fibrillar twitching
    muscular twitching
Twombly operation
Twombly-Ulfelder operation
Tworek bone marrow-aspirating
    needle
Tworek screw guide
Tworek transorbital leukotome
Tworek Universal gouge
T-Y stent

Tycos gauge
Tycos manometer
Tycos pressure infusion line
Tycos sphygmomanometer
Tycron sutures (*see also* Ti-
    Cron)
Tydings automatic ratchet snare
Tydings forceps
Tydings knife
Tydings snare
Tydings tonsillar clamp
Tydings tonsillar forceps
Tydings tonsillar knife
Tydings tonsillar snare
Tydings tonsillectome
Tydings-Lakeside forceps
Tydings-Lakeside tonsillar
    forceps
Tydings-Lakeside tonsil-seizing
    forceps
Tygon catheter
Tygon esophageal prosthesis
Tygon surgical tubing
Tygon tube
tying forceps
tylectomy
Tyler Gigli saw
Tyler spiral Gigli saw
tylosis
tympanectomy
tympani
    canaliculus chordae tympani
    canaliculus of chorda
        tympani
    cavum tympani
    membrana tympani
    semicanal for tensor tympani
tympanic annulus
tympanic antrum
tympanic artery
tympanic bone
tympanic cavity
tympanic ganglion
tympanic membrane
tympanic muscle
tympanic nerve
tympanic notch
tympanic orifice
tympanic plexus
tympanic sinus
tympanic sulcus
tympanic vein

tympanicus
    annulus tympanicus
    anulus tympanicus
    canaliculus tympanicus
tympanites
tympanitic abdomen
tympanitis
tympanogram
tympanography
tympanomandibular cartilage
tympanomastoid abnormality
tympanomastoid abscess
tympanomastoid cavity
tympanomastoid fissure
tympanomastoid suture
tympanomastoidectomy
tympanomeatal
tympanomeatal flap
tympanometry
tympanoplastic knife
tympanoplasty
    Austin-Shea tympanoplasty
    columellar type II
        tympanoplasty
    Lempert incision for radical
        tympanoplasty
    type I tympanoplasty
    type II tympanoplasty
    type III tympanoplasty
    type IV tympanoplasty
    Wullstein tympanoplasty
tympanoplasty (type I, II, II,
    IV, V)
tympanoplasty forceps
tympanoplasty knife
tympanoplasty mastoidectomy
tympanoscope
Tympan-O-Scope
tympanoscopy ventilation tube
tympanosquamous fissure
tympanostomy tube
tympanosympathectomy
tympanotomy flap
tympanum
tympanum perforator
tympanum perforator handle
tympany
Tym-tap ear aspirator
Tyndall light
type
    collagen type
    dysplastic type

type (*continued*)
 Fitzpatrick classification of
  sun-reactive skin types
  (types I-IV)
 scapulohumeral type
 undifferentiated type
type and crossmatch (T&C)
type B-1, -2 lesion
type C pelvic ring fracture
type I acrocephalosyndactyly
type I imperforate anus
type I tympanoplasty
type I, II, III, IIIA, IIIB, IIIC open
 fracture
type II acrocephalosyndactyly
type II earlobe cleft
type II imperforate anus
type II tympanoplasty
type III imperforate anus
type IV imperforate anus
type IV tympanoplasty
type V tympanoplasty
typhlectomy
typhlopexy
typhlorrhaphy

typhlostomy
typhlotomy
typhloureterostomy
Typhoon cutter blade
Typhoon microdebrider blade
typical coloboma
typical skin lesion
Tyrer nerve root retractor
Tyrrell clamp
Tyrrell foreign body forceps
Tyrrell hook retractor
Tyrrell iris hook
Tyrrell skin hook
Tyrrell tympanic membrane
 hook
Tyrrell-Gray sutures
Tyshak balloon
Tyshak balloon valvuloplasty
 catheter
Tyson glands
Tytan grommet ventilation
 tube
Tytan tube inserter
Tytan ventilation tube
Tzanck operation

U.S. Army double-ended retractor
U.S. Army bone chisel
U.S. Army gauze scissors
U.S. Army gouge
U.S. Army osteotome
U.S. Army retractor
U.S. Army tourniquet
U.S. Army umbilical scissors
U.S. Army-pattern gauze scissors
U.S. Army-pattern knife
U.S. Army-pattern osteotome
U.S. Army-pattern retractor
UAC catheter (umbilical artery catheter)
UAL (ultrasound-assisted lipectomy)
UBC brace (University of British Columbia brace)
UC strip catheter tubing fastener
UCAC diagnostic catheter
UCB orthosis (University of California Berkeley orthosis)
UCBL prosthesis
Uchida fimbriectomy
Uchida incision
Uchida operation
Uchida technique
Uchida tubal banding
Uchida tubal ligation
UCI knee prosthesis
UCI total knee replacement
UCI-Barnard aortic valve
Uckermann cotton applicator
UCLA (unilateral cleft lip/alveolus)
UCLA functional long-leg brace
UCLA ureterosigmoidostomy
U-clip
UCOheal orthotic
UCOlite orthotic
U-connector
U-crimper

U-double-barrel sutures
Uebe applicator
Ueckermann cricothyroid trocar
Ueckermann-Denker trocar
Uematsu shoulder arthrodesis
UES (upper esophageal sphincter)
UF (ultrafiltrate, ultrafiltration)
U-flap
UGI (upper gastrointestinal tract)
UGI endoscope
UGI endoscopy
UHI hip prosthesis
Uhl anomaly
Uhl malformation
Uhlrich stapler
UHMWP (ultra-high-molecular-weight polyethylene)
UICC tumor classification
Ulanday double cannula
ulatrophy
Ulbrich wart curet
ulcer
   acid peptic ulcer
   active duodenal ulcer
   Allingham ulcer
   amputating ulcer
   anastomotic ulcer
   angry-looking ulcer
   anterior wall antral ulcer
   antral ulcer
   aphthoid ulcer
   aphthous ulcer
   arterial ulcer
   atonic ulcer
   Bairnsdale ulcer
   Barrett ulcer
   bear claw ulcer
   benign ulcer
   bulbar peptic ulcer
   Cameron ulcer
   channel ulcer

ulcer (*continued*)

cold ulcer
collar button-like ulcer
corneal ulcer
Cruveilhier ulcer
Curling stress ulcer
Cushing stress ulcer
cystoscopic ulcer
decubitus ulcer
dendritic ulcer
diabetic foot ulcer
Dieulafoy ulcer
duodenal ulcer
esophageal ulcer
focal colonic mucosal ulcer
follicular ulcer
gastric ulcer
gastroduodenal ulcer
gastrointestinal ulcer
gastrojejunal ulcer
Graham closure of ulcer
gravitational ulcer
greater curvature ulcer
hard ulcer
herpetic ulcer
hindfoot ulcer
Hunner ulcer
incisural ulcer
indolent radiation-induced
  rectal ulcer
indolent ulcer
inflamed ulcer
intractable ulcer
Jacob ulcer
jejunal ulcer
juxtapyloric ulcer
kissing ulcer
Kocher dilatation ulcer
lesser curvature ulcer
linear ulcer
malignant ulcer
Mann-Williamson ulcer
marginal ulcer
Marjolin ulcer
Martorell ulcer
Meleney ulcer
metatarsal ulcer
minute bleeding mucosal
  ulcer
moorean ulcer
necrotic ulcer
oropharyngeal ulcer

ulcer (*continued*)

penetrating ulcer
peptic ulcer
perambulating ulcer
perforated acid peptic ulcer
perforated ulcer
perforating ulcer
phagedenic ulcer
phlegmonous ulcer
plantar forefoot ulcer
postbulbar duodenal ulcer
postbulbar ulcer
postsurgical recurrent ulcer
prepyloric gastric ulcer
punched-out ulcer
punctate ulcer
pyloric channel ulcer
rake ulcer
recalcitrant ulcer
recurrent aphthous ulcer
recurrent ulcer
ring ulcer
rodent ulcer
Rokitansky-Cushing ulcer
rose-thorn ulcer
round ulcer
Saemisch ulcer
sea anemone ulcer
serpiginous ulcer
sickle cell ulcer
sloughing ulcer
soft ulcer
stasis ulcer
stasis vascular ulcer
stercoral ulcer
steroid ulcer
stomach ulcer
stomal ulcer
stress ulcer
string test for peptic ulcer
sublingual ulcer
Sutton ulcer
tarsal ulcer
traumatic ulcer
trophic ulcer
undermining ulcer
varicose ulcers
vascular ulcer
venous stasis ulcer
venous ulcer
V-shaped ulcer
warty ulcer

ulcer bed
ulcer disease
ulcer dressing
ulcerated area
ulcerated granuloma
ulcerated lesion
ulcerated nodule
ulcerated wound
ulcerating adenocarcinoma
ulcerating area
ulcerating granuloma
ulcerating lesion
ulceration
  agranulocytic ulceration
  anastomotic ulceration
  collar-button ulceration
  corneal ulceration
  deep ulceration
  duodenal ulceration
  esophageal ulceration
  gastric ulceration
  necrotic ulceration
  patchy ulceration
  radiation-induced ulceration
  serpiginous ulceration
  stress ulceration
  superficial ulceration
  tracheal ulceration
  varicose ulceration
  venous leg ulceration
ulcerative inflammation
ulcerative lesion
ulcerative stomatitis
ulcerogenic fistula
ulcerogenic tumor
ulceromembranous
Uldall subclavian hemodialysis
    cannula
Uldall subclavian hemodialysis
    catheter
ulectomy
Ullman line
Ulloa operation
Ullrich bone-holding forceps
Ullrich dressing forceps
Ullrich drill guard
Ullrich fistula knife
Ullrich laminectomy retractor
Ullrich self-retaining
    laminectomy retractor
Ullrich self-retaining retractor
Ullrich tubing clamp

Ullrich uterine knife
Ullrich vaginal speculum
Ullrich-Aesculap forceps
Ullrich-St. Gallen forceps
Ullrich-St. Gallen self-retaining
    retractor
ulna
ulnar artery
ulnar aspect
ulnar bursa
ulnar carpal abutment syndrome
ulnar claw hand
ulnar club hand
ulnar collateral ligament
ulnar deviation deformity
ulnar drift deformity
ulnar extensor muscle
ulnar flexor muscle
ulnar fracture
ulnar groove
ulnar head excision
ulnar hemiresection
    interposition arthroplasty
ulnar impaction syndrome
ulnar ligament
ulnar nerve
ulnar nerve block
ulnar nerve palsy
ulnar notch
ulnar rasp
ulnar recurrent artery
ulnar reflex
ulnar resection
ulnar ruler
ulnar shaft
ulnar splint
ulnar styloid bone
ulnar thumb
ulnar tunnel syndrome
ulnar variance
ulnar veins
ulnar wrist pain
ulnar-minus variance
ulnar-plus variance
ulnar-plus neutral variance
ulnar-positive variance
ulnarward
ulnocarpal joint
ulnocarpal ligament
ulnoradial
ulotomy
ULP (ultra low profile)

Ulta-Cut Cobb curet
Ultec hydrocolloid dressing
Ultec Pro alginate hydrocolloid
   dressing
Ultex bifocal lens
Ultex implant
Ultex lens
Ultex hydrocolloid dressing
Ultima Bloc bite block
Ultima femoral component
Ultimate knee
ultimobranchial body
Ultra balloon catheter
Ultra COM monitor
Ultra Dream Ride car bed
Ultra Duet Colostomy irrigating
   sleeve
ultra low profile (ULP)
ultra low resistance voice
   prosthesis
Ultra mag lens
Ultra pacemaker
Ultra Stim silver electrode
Ultra ultrasonic aspirator
Ultra view slit lamp lens
ultra x-ray
Ultrabrace orthosis
ultrabrachycephalic
Ultra-Care heel/elbow protector
Ultracast alloy
UltraCision harmonic
   laparoscopic cutting shears
UltraCision ultrasonic knife
UltraCon rigid gas permeable
   contact lens
Ultracor prosthetic valve
Ultra-Core biopsy needle
Ultra-Cut blade resector
Ultra-Cut Cobb curet
Ultra-Cut Cobb spinal gouge
Ultra-Cut Cobb spinal
   instrument
Ultra-Cut Hibbs gouge
Ultra-Cut Hoke osteotome
Ultra-Cut Smith-Petersen
   osteotome
Ultra-Cut surgical instruments
ultradelicate split-thickness
   scalp skin (UDSTS)
UltraEase ultrasound pad
UltraEdge keratome blade
ultrafast CT scanner

ultrafast magnetic resonance
   imaging
Ultrafera wound dressing
ultrafiltrate (UF)
ultrafiltration
UltraFine erbium laser
UltraFix anchor
UltraFix anchor suture
Ultraflex ankle dorsiflexion
   dynamic splint
Ultraflex esophageal prosthesis
Ultraflex stent
Ultraflex nitinol expandable
   esophageal stent
Ultraflex self-adhering male
   external catheter
Ultraflex self-expanding stent
Ultraflex stent
ultraflow
UltraFoam seating cushion
UltraForm therapeutic mattress
UltraFuse catheter
Ultrafyn cautery tip
UltraGait walker boot
ultra-high-frequency ventilation
ultra-high-magnification
   endoscopy
ultra-high-molecular-weight
   polyethylene (UHMWP)
Ultra-Image A-scan scanner
Ultraject contrast media syringe
Ultraject prefilled syringe
UltraKlenz wound cleanser
UltraLine laser
UltraLine Nd:YAG laser fiber
UltraLite flow-directed
   microcatheter
ultralow anterior resection
Ultramark ultrasound
Ultramark transducer
Ultramark echocardiograph
Ultramark scanner
Ultramatic refractor
Ultramer catheter
ultramicroscope
Ultra-Neb nebulizer
UltraPower bur guard
ultraprognathous skull
UltraPulse CO_2 laserbrasion
UltraPulse CO_2 laser
UltraPulse surgical laser
ultrapulsed laser

Ultrascope obstetrical
    Doppler
Ultra-Select guide wire
Ultra-Select nitinol PTCA guide
    wire
UltraShaper keratome
Ultra-Sil cannula
UltraSling sling
ultrasmall-shafted balloon
ultrasonic aspirating device
ultrasonic aspiration
ultrasonic attenuation
ultrasonic bone-cutting
    instrument
ultrasonic cannula
ultrasonic cataract removal
    lancet
ultrasonic cleaner
ultrasonic cleaner basket
ultrasonic diathermy
ultrasonic diathermy
    electrosurgical unit
ultrasonic dissection
ultrasonic dissector
ultrasonic electrode
ultrasonic flow director
ultrasonic fragmentation
ultrasonic fragmentation of
    urinary calculi
ultrasonic harmonic scalpel
ultrasonic lancet
ultrasonic liposculpturing
ultrasonic liposuction
ultrasonic lithotresis
ultrasonic lithotripsy
ultrasonic lithotriptor
ultrasonic micrometer
ultrasonic microscope
ultrasonic nebulizer
ultrasonic probe
ultrasonic scalpel
ultrasonic stone crusher
ultrasonic surgical aspirator
ultrasonic therapy
ultrasonic tip
ultrasonic wand
ultrasonically activated
    scalpel
ultrasonogram
ultrasonographic technique
ultrasonographically-guided
    injection

ultrasonography
    B-mode ultrasonography
    Doppler duplex
        ultrasonography
    Doppler ultrasonography
    endoscopic color Doppler
        ultrasonography
    endoscopic Doppler
        ultrasonography
    endoscopic ultrasonography
    gray-scale ultrasonography
    intraoperative
        ultrasonography (IOUS)
    intrarectal ultrasonography
    laparoscopic intracorporeal
        ultrasonography (LICU)
    laparoscopic ultrasonography
        (LUS)
    obstetrical ultrasonography
    ophthalmic ultrasonography
    real-time ultrasonography
    transrectal ultrasonography
        (TRUS)
    urologic ultrasonography
ultrasonography-guided fine-
        needle aspiration
        biopsy
UltraSorb suture anchor
ultrasound
    abdominal ultrasound
    Acuson ultrasound
    ADR Ultramark ultrasound
    Advantage ultrasound
    Alcon ultrasound
    Aloka linear ultrasound
    Aloka OB/GYN ultrasound
    Aloka sector ultrasound
    Ansaldo ultrasound
    A-scan ultrasound
    Aspen digital ultrasound
    ATL real-time ultrasound
    ATL Ultramark-series
        ultrasound
    Axisonic ultrasound
    BladderManager ultrasound
    BladderScan ultrasound
    B-mode ultrasound
    Bruel-Kjaer ultrasound
    B-scan ultrasound
    cardiac ultrasound
    catheter probe ultrasound
    color Doppler ultrasound

ultrasound (*continued*)
  colorvascular Doppler
    ultrasound
  continuous-wave ultrasound
  CooperVision ultrasound
  diagnostic ultrasound
  Diasonics ultrasound
  Doppler pulsed ultrasound
  Doppler ultrasound
  duplex ultrasound
  Dynatron ultrasound
  Eccocee ultrasound
  EchoEye ultrasound
  echo-guided ultrasound
  Elscint ultrasound
  endoanal ultrasound
  endorectal ultrasound (ERU)
  EndoSound endoscopic
    ultrasound
  General Electric ultrasound
  gray-scale ultrasound
  HDI ultrasound
  Hewlett-Packard ultrasound
  Hitachi ultrasound
  Interspec XL ultrasound
  Intertherapy intravascular
    ultrasound
  intraductal ultrasound
  intraluminal ultrasound
  intraoperative ultrasound
    (IOUS)
  Intrascan ultrasound
  Irex Exemplar ultrasound
  laparoscopic ultrasound
  LeFort urethral ultrasound
  Netra intravascular ultrasound
  NeuroSectOR ultrasound
  Olympus endoscopic
    ultrasound
  pelvic ultrasound
  Performa ultrasound
  Pie Medical ultrasound
  power Doppler ultrasound
  PowerVision ultrasound
  pulsed Doppler ultrasound
  pulsed-wave ultrasound
  real-time ultrasound
  renal ultrasound
  Rich-Mar external ultrasound
  RT Advantage ultrasound
  Shimadzu cardiac
    ultrasound

ultrasound (*continued*)
  Siemens Sonoline Elegra
    ultrasound
  Siemens Sonoline Prima
    ultrasound
  Siemens ultrasound
  SieScape ultrasound
  Sonicator portable ultrasound
  Sonoline Prima ultrasound
  Sonos cardiovascular
    ultrasound
  Spectra-Diasonics ultrasound
  Synergy ultrasound
  Toshiba Sonolayer ultrasound
  transendoscopic ultrasound
  transthoracic ultrasound
  transvaginal ultrasound
  Ultramark ultrasound
  vaginal probe ultrasound
  Vingmed ultrasound
ultrasound anesthetic technique
ultrasound bone analyzer
ultrasound cardiogram
ultrasound catheter probe
ultrasound examination
ultrasound guidance
ultrasound image
ultrasound inhaler
ultrasound liposuction
ultrasound monitor
ultrasound pad
ultrasound scan
ultrasound spatula
ultrasound stethoscope
ultrasound therapy
ultrasound transducer
ultrasound-assisted CAST
    liposuction
ultrasound-assisted lipectomy
    (UAL)
ultrasound-assisted lipoplasty
    (UAL)
ultrasound-assisted liposuction
ultrasound-assisted
    percutaneous endoscopic
    gastrostomy
ultrasound-guided anterior
    subcostal liver biopsy
ultrasound-guided automated
    large-core breast
    biopsy
ultrasound-guided biopsy

ultrasound-guided compression repair (UGCR)

ultrasound-guided core breast biopsy

ultrasound-guided core-needle biopsy (US-CNB)

ultrasound-guided echo biopsy

ultrasound-guided fine-needle aspiration

ultrasound-guided fine-needle aspiration biopsy (US-FNAB)

ultrasound-guided shock wave therapy

ultrasound-guided stereotactic biopsy

ultrastiff wire

Ultrastop anti-fogging solution

Ultrata capsulorrhexis forceps

UltraTag RBC kit

Ultra-Thin balloon

ultra-thin surgical blade

Ultratome double-lumen sphincterotome

Ultratome triple-lumen sphincterotome

Ultratone electrical transcutaneous neuromuscular stimulator

ultraviolet blood irradiation

ultraviolet detector

ultraviolet light

ultraviolet microscope

ultraviolet-blocking intraocular lens

Ultra-vue amniocentesis needle

Ultrex cylinder

Ultrex Plus penile prosthesis

Ultroid coagulator

Ultroid device for hemorrhoid treatment

Ultroid for nonsurgical hemorrhoidal management

umbilectomy

umbilical areola

umbilical artery

umbilical artery catheter (UAC)

umbilical artery catheterization

umbilical catheter

umbilical circulation

umbilical clamp

umbilical clip

umbilical cord anomaly

umbilical cord clamp

umbilical cord hematoma

umbilical fissure

umbilical fistula

umbilical fold

umbilical fossa

umbilical graft

umbilical hernia

umbilical hernia repair with omphalectomy

umbilical hernia repair with umbilectomy

umbilical herniorrhaphy

umbilical ligament

umbilical notch

umbilical plane

umbilical region

umbilical ring

umbilical scissors

umbilical skin-knife incision

umbilical stalk

umbilical stump

umbilical tape

umbilical tape drain

umbilical tape sutures

umbilical vein catheter

umbilical vein catheterization

umbilical vein graft

umbilical venous catheter

umbilicated mass

umbiliclamp

umbiliclip

umbilicoplasty

umbilicus

Umbilicutter clamp

umbrella closure

umbrella dissector

umbrella filter

umbrella graft

umbrella punctum plug

umbrella retractor

umbrella-type prosthesis

UMI amniocentesis kit

UMI catheter

UMI Cath-Seal sheath

UMI needle

UMI transseptal Cath-Seal catheter introducer

unabsorbable sutures

unanticipated hepatic disease

unassisted delivery

unassisted respiration
unattended laboratory operation
unavoidable hemorrhage
unbanded gastroplasty
unbridling
unbuckled flat position
uncal herniation
unciform bone
uncinate bone
uncinate groove
uncinate gyrus
uncinate procedure
uncinate process
uncinate process fracture
uncoated mesh stent
uncommitted metaphysial lesion
uncomplicated birth
uncomplicated delivery
uncomplicated postoperative
    course
unconditioned
unconscious
unconsciousness
unconstrained knee prosthesis
unconstrained prosthesis
unconstrained shoulder
    arthroplasty
uncontaminated
uncontrollable bleeding
uncontrollable pain
uncotomy
uncovertebral joint
uncut Collis-Nissen
    fundoplication
uncut Collis-Nissen
    fundoplication procedure
underarm orthosis
undercut
underfill rippling
underfill wrinkling
underhung bite
underlay fascia technique
underlay fascial graft
underlayer cantilever bone graft
underlying chest muscles
underlying fascia
underlying skin
underlying structures
underlying tissue
undermineralized bone graft
undermining resorption
undermining ulcer

underrunning
undersensing malfunction of
    pacemaker
undersized prosthesis
underwater Bovie
underwater diathermy
underwater drainage
underwater electrode
underwater seal
underwater suction
underwater-seal drainage
underwater-seal suction tube
underwater-seal tube
undescended testicle
undescended testis
undetermined cause
undetermined etiology
undifferentiated
    adenocarcinoma
undifferentiated carcinoma
undifferentiated connective
    tissue disease
undifferentiated lesion
undifferentiated lymphoma
undifferentiated squamous cell
    carcinoma
undifferentiated type
undisplaced fracture
Undritz anomaly
undulating membrane
undyed sutures
unenhanced helical CT
unenhanced study
unesthetic contour deformity
uneven contour
unfractionated heparin therapy
unfurling of antihelix
Unger adenoid pressure roller
ungual process
ungual tuft
unguis (pl. ungues)
UNI reservoir
UNI shunt catheter
UNI2 wrist implant
uniarticular
uniaxial joint
uniaxial strain gauge
unibevel chisel
unicaliceal kidney
unicameral bone cyst
Unicare breast pump
Unicat knife

Unicath all-purpose catheter
unicommissural aortic valve
unicompartmental knee
    arthroplasty
unicompartmental knee implant
unicompartmental knee
    replacement
unicondylar fracture
unicondylar prosthesis
unicoronal synostosis
unicystic ameloblastoma
Uni-Flate penile prosthesis
Uniflex calibrated step drill
Uniflex distal targeting awl
Uniflex dressing
Uniflex intramedullary nail
unifocal optic nerve lesion
unifocal PVCs
Uni-Gard piggyback connector
Unigraft bone graft material
Unigraft knife
Unilab Surgibone
Unilab Surgibone implant
unilambdoid synostosis
unilaminar membrane
unilaminar skin substitute
Unilase CO_2 laser
unilateral adductor paralysis
unilateral anesthesia
unilateral aortofemoral graft
unilateral approach
unilateral bar
unilateral calcaneal brace
unilateral cleft
unilateral cleft lip nose
unilateral cleft lip nose
    deformity
unilateral cleft of lip and palate
unilateral condylar fracture
unilateral coronal suture
unilateral coronal synostosis
unilateral diaphragmatic
    elevation
unilateral facet subluxation
unilateral facial atrophy
unilateral facial hypertrophy
unilateral fracture
unilateral hemidysplasia
    cornification disorder
unilateral hemilaminectomy
unilateral hermaphroditism
unilateral hernia

unilateral hypertrophy
unilateral hypophysectomy
unilateral inguinal hernia repair
unilateral inguinal hernia repair
    procedure
unilateral inguinal hernia repair
    technique
unilateral interfacetal dislocation
unilateral lobectomy
unilateral macroglossia
unilateral mesioclusion
unilateral Millard repair
unilateral neck exploration
unilateral nevoid telangiectasia
unilateral pedicle cannulation
unilateral plagiocephaly
unilateral procedure
unilateral resection
unilateral sacroiliac approach
unilateral salpingo-
    oophorectomy
unilateral subcostal incision
unilateral vocal cord paralysis
    (UVCP)
Unilink anastomotic device
Unilink system for hand surgery
Unilith pacemaker
unilobar disease
unilocular cyst
unilocular cystic lesion
unilocular joint
unimalleolar fracture
Unimar J-needle
Unimar Pipelle curet
UniMax laser micromanipulator
unimpaired function
uninhibited neurogenic
    bladder
uninterrupted suture
technique
uninterrupted sutures
union broach retention drill
union broach retention pin
unipedicled flap
unipennate muscle
uniplanar intraocular lens
unipolar atrial pacemaker
unipolar atrioventricular
    pacemaker
unipolar cautery
unipolar cutting loop
unipolar electrode

unipolar hand-switching needle-point electrocautery forceps
unipolar J-tined passive-fixation lead
unipolar lead
unipolar limb leads
unipolar pacemaker
unipolar pacemaker lead
unipolar sequential pacemaker
UniPort hemostasis introducer sheath kit
UniPuls electrostimulation instrument
unique noncolorectal liver metastasis
Uniquet disposable intravenous tourniquet
UniShaper single-use keratome
Uni-Shunt abdominal slip clip
Uni-Shunt catheter passer
Uni-Shunt cranial anchoring clip
Uni-Shunt hydrocephalus shunt
Uni-Shunt right-angle clip
Uni-Shunt split trocar
Uni-Shunt with elliptical reservoir
Uni-Shunt with reservoir introducer
Uni-sump drain
unit membrane
unit spinal rod
Unitech instruments
Unitech Toomey cannula
United Max-E pouch
U.S. Surgical circular stapler
Unitek appliance
Unitek I decubitus mattress
uniting cartilage
uniting duct
uni-tip deformity
Unitome knife
Unitrax modular endoprosthesis
Unitri cannula
Unitri tip
unitunnel technique
Unity pacemaker
Unity-C cardiac pacemaker
Univalve cast
Univent endotracheal tube
Universal condenser
Universal wrist implant

Universal abdominal trocar
Universal adenoid punch tip
Universal antral punch
Universal appliance
Universal aspirator
Universal bone plate
Universal cannula
Universal catheter access port
Universal chuck handle
Universal clip remover
Universal condenser
Universal conformer
Universal connector
Universal curved-tube stylet
Universal cystoscope
Universal drainage catheter
Universal drill
Universal drill point
Universal electron microscope
Universal esophagoscope
Universal eye shield
Universal femoral head prosthesis
Universal fixation screw
Universal forceps
Universal gastroscope
Universal goniometer
Universal gutter splint
Universal hand drill with chuck key
Universal handle
Universal handle for punch tips
Universal handle with nasal-cutting tips
Universal head holder
Universal joint cervix
Universal joint device
Universal Kerrison rongeur
Universal Kerrison set and tips
Universal laminectomy set
Universal lamp
Universal malleable valvulotome
Universal mirror handle
Universal nasal instrument handle
Universal nasal saw
Universal nasal saw blade
Universal nerve hook
Universal prosthesis
Universal proximal femur prosthesis (UPF prosthesis)
Universal punch

Universal radial component
universal recipient
Universal retractor
Universal saw
Universal sheath
Universal slit lamp
Universal speculum
Universal speculum holder
Universal splint
Universal stent
Universal straight-tube stylet
universal subperiosteal implant
Universal support splint
Universal T-adapter
Universal tourniquet
Universal trocar
Universal 2-speed hand drill
Universal vaginal probe
Universal valve prosthesis
    sewing ring
Universal wire clamp
Universal wire scissors
University forceps
University of Akron artificial
    heart
University of British Columbia
    brace (UBC brace)
University of California
    Biomechanics Laboratory
    heel cup
University of California Berkeley
    orthosis (UCB orthosis)
University of Illinois biopsy
    needle
University of Illinois marrow
    needle
University of Illinois sternal
    puncture needle
University of Iowa cotton
    applicator
University of Kansas corneal
    forceps
University of Kansas eye spatula
University of Kansas forceps
University of Kansas hook
University of Kansas spatula
University of Michigan Mixter
    thoracic forceps
Univision low-vision
    microscopic lens
Uniweave catheter
Unloader brace

unlocking spiral technique
unmeshed split-thickness skin
    graft
unmonitored local anesthesia
unmyelinated nerve fibers
Unna boot
Unna boot bandage
Unna boot cast
Unna boot dressing
Unna comedo extractor
Unna disease
Unna extractor
Unna paste
Unna paste boot
Unna wrap
Unna-Flex compression dressing
Unna-Flex compression wrap
Unna-Flex paste bandage
Unna-Pak compression dressing
unossified cartilage
unpedicled flap
unreamed femoral nail
unreduced dislocation
unrepositioned flap
unresectable extrahepatic
    disease
unresectable lesion
unresectable metastasis
unresectable periampullary
    cancer
unresectable squamous cell
    carcinoma
unresectable tumor
unripe cataract
unroof
unroofing
unruptured ectopic pregnancy
unruptured vascular anomalies
Unschuld sign
unsegmented bar
unstable bladder
unstable fracture
unstable fracture-dislocation
unstable joint
unstable zygomatic complex
    fracture
unstimulated graciloplasty
unstrained jaw relation
unstriated muscle
untethering procedure
ununited fracture
unwounded dermis

up-and-down flap
up-and-down staircases
    procedure
up-angle hook
up-angled curet
upbiting biopsy forceps
upbiting cup forceps
upbiting punch
upbiting rongeur
upcupped forceps
upcurved basket forceps
Updegraff cleft palate needle
Updegraff hook
Updegraff needle
Updegraff staphylorrhaphy
    needle
updraft nebulizer
updrawn pupil
UPF prosthesis (Universal
    proximal femur prosthesis)
upgated technique
upgoing toes
UPJ (ureteropelvic junction)
UPJ stricture (ureteropelvic
    junction stricture)
U-pouch construction
UPP (urethral pressure profile)
upper abdomen
upper abdominal evisceration
upper abdominal midline
    incision
upper abdominal organs
upper adenoma
upper airway obstruction
upper alimentary endoscopy
upper arch
upper blepharoplasty
upper body dressing
upper bound
upper cervical region
upper cervical spine anterior
    exposure
upper cervical spine fusion
upper cervical spine procedure
upper endoscopy and
    colonoscopy
upper esophageal sphincter (UES)
upper esophagoscope
upper esophagus
upper extremity
upper extremity myoelectric
    prosthesis

upper extremity nerve block
upper eyelid
upper face rejuvenation
upper ganglion
upper gastrointestinal (UGI)
    tract
upper gastrointestinal bleeding
upper gastrointestinal
    endoscopy
upper gastrointestinal tract
    surgery
upper GI hemorrhage
upper GI series
upper GI tract foreign body
Upper Hands self-retaining
    retractor
upper intestinal endoscopy
upper jaw
upper jaw bone
upper lateral nasal cartilage
upper lateral scissors
upper lid
upper limb
upper lip
upper lip length
upper lobe of lung
upper mantle field
upper midline incision
upper occlusive clamp
upper panendoscopy
upper respiratory tract
upper respiratory tract infection
upper reticular dermal peel
upper reticular dermal
    penetration
upper thorax aperture
upper tooth to upper lip
    relationship
upper tract disease
upper trapezius flap
upper universal forceps
upper-lateral exposing retractor
UPPP
    (uvulopalatopharyngoplasty)
Uppsala gall duct forceps
upright film
upright position
upright-Y incision
uptake
    fluorescein uptake
    I-131 uptake
    radioactive uptake

uptake (*continued*)
  resin uptake
  thyroid uptake
uptake studies
upturned forceps
upward bent forceps
upward masking
upward movement
upward-cutting triangular knife
upward-gaze incision
urachal carcinoma
urachal cyst
urachal fistula
urachal fold
urachal fossa
urachal sinus of bladder
urachus (*pl.* urachi)
uraniscochasma
uraniscoplasty
uraniscorrhaphy
uranoplastic
uranoplasty
uranorrhaphy
uranoschisis
uranoschism
uranostaphyloplasty
uranostaphylorrhaphy
uranostaphyloschisis
uranosteoplasty
urate-associated inflammation
Urban mastectomy
Urban microscope
Urban microsurgery camera
Urban operation
Urban retractor
Urbaniak neurovascular free flap
Urbaniak scapular flap
Urbaniak technique
Urbanski strut guide
Urbantschitsch eustachian
    bougie
Urbantschitsch nasal forceps
urea hydrolysis
urea-impermeable membrane
Ureflex ureteral catheter
uremic gastrointestinal
    lesion
uremic inflammation
Uresil biliary catheter
Uresil embolectomy
    thrombectomy catheter
Uresil irrigation catheter

Uresil occlusion balloon
    catheter
Uresil radiopaque silicone-band
    vessel loops
Uresil carotid shunt
ureter
  angulation of ureter
  bifurcation of ureter
  circumcaval ureter
  double ureter
  ectopic ureter
  kinking of ureter
  postcaval ureter
  proximal ureter
  reimplantation of ureter
  retrocaval ureter
  retroiliac ureter
  triplication of ureter
ureter implantation
ureteral basket stone dislodger
ureteral biopsy
ureteral bladder augmentation
ureteral bougie
ureteral brush biopsy kit
ureteral carcinoma
ureteral catheter
ureteral catheter forceps
ureteral catheter obturator
ureteral catheterization
ureteral clamp
ureteral dilatation catheter
ureteral dilation
ureteral dilator
ureteral duplication
ureteral ectopia
ureteral fistula
ureteral illuminator
ureteral implant
ureteral injury
ureteral isolation forceps
ureteral meatotome
ureteral meatotomy
ureteral meatotomy electrode
ureteral occlusion catheter
ureteral orifice
ureteral patch procedure
ureteral perforation
ureteral reflux
ureteral stent placement
ureteral stoma removal
ureteral stone
ureteral stone basket

ureteral stone dilator
ureteral stone dislodger
ureteral stone extractor
ureteral stone forceps
ureteral stone retriever
ureteral stylet
ureteral visualization instrument
ureterectasis
ureterectomy
ureteric fold
ureteric opening
ureteric plexus
ureteric retrieval net
ureteric ridge
ureteritis
ureterocecostomy
ureterocele
ureterocelectomy
ureterocentesis
ureterocolectomy
ureterocolic fistula
ureterocolonic anastomosis
ureterocolostomy
ureterocutaneostomy
ureterocutaneous fistula
ureterocystanastomosis
ureterocystoneostomy
ureterocystoscope
ureterocystostomy
ureteroduodenal fistula
ureteroenteroanastomosis
ureteroenterostomy
ureterogram
ureteroileal anastomosis
ureteroileal loop
ureteroileobladder anastomosis
ureteroileocutaneous
    anastomosis
ureteroileostomy
ureterointestinal anastomosis
ureterolithiasis
ureterolithotomy
ureterolysis
ureteromeatotomy
ureteroneocystostomy
ureteroneocystostomy
    herniation
ureteroneocystotomy
ureteroneopyelostomy
ureteronephrectomy
ureteropelvic junction (UPJ)
ureteropelvic junction stricture

ureteropelvic obstruction
ureteropelvioneostomy
ureteropelvioplasty
    DeWeerd ureteropelvioplasty
    Foley ureteropelvioplasty
    Foley Y-type
        ureteropelvioplasty
    Prince ureteropelvioplasty
    Scardino ureteropelvioplasty
    Y-type ureteropelvioplasty
    Y-V ureteropelvioplasty
ureteroperitoneal
    fistula
ureteropexy
ureteroplasty
ureteroplication
ureteroproctostomy
ureteropyelogram
ureteropyelography
ureteropyeloneostomy
ureteropyelonephrostomy
ureteropyeloplasty
ureteropyelostomy
ureterorectoneostomy
ureterorenofiberscope
ureterorenoscope
ureterorenoscope procedure
    sheath
ureterorenoscopy
ureterorrhaphy
ureteroscopy
ureterosigmoid anastomosis
ureterosigmoidostomy
ureterostomy
    cutaneous ureterostomy
    Sober ureterostomy
    subarachnoid ureterostomy
ureterotomy
ureterotrigonoenterostomy
ureterotrigonosigmoidostomy
ureterotubal anastomosis
ureteroureteral anastomosis
ureteroureterostomy
    van Hook
        ureteroureterostomy
ureterouterine fistula
ureterovaginal fistula
ureterovesical implantation
ureterovesical junction (UVJ)
ureterovesical obstruction
ureterovesicoplasty
ureterovesicostomy

urethra
  bulbous urethra
  cavernous portion of urethra
  cavernous urethra
  dilatation of urethra
  double urethra
  hypoplastic urethra
  membranous urethra
  navicular fossa of male urethra
  pendulous urethra
  prostatic urethra
urethral artery
urethral barrier device
urethral bougie
urethral bougienage
urethral calculus
urethral candle
urethral carcinoma
urethral catheter
urethral catheterization
urethral chill
urethral coaptation
urethral crest
urethral crest of male
urethral dilatation
urethral dilation
urethral dilator
urethral diverticulectomy
urethral epithelium
urethral female dilator
urethral filiforms
urethral forceps
urethral gland
urethral groove
urethral incompetence
urethral instillation cannula
urethral instrumentation
urethral intermittent catheter
    and tray
urethral male dilator
urethral meatotomy
urethral meatus
urethral meatus dilator
urethral opening
urethral orifice
urethral plate
urethral pressure profile (UPP)
urethral reconstruction
urethral sound
urethral speculum
urethral stricture
urethral suspension

urethral syndrome
urethral vesicle suspension
    procedure
urethral wall
urethral whip bougie
urethrascope
urethrectomy
urethreurynter
urethroblennorrhea
urethrocavernous fistula
urethrocecal anastomosis
urethrocele
urethrocutaneous fistula
urethrocystogram
urethrocystography
urethrocystopexy
urethrocystoscope
urethrogram
urethrographic cannula
urethrographic cannula clamp
urethrographic catheter
urethrographic clamp
urethrography
urethrohymenal fusion
urethrolithotomy
urethrometer
urethrometry
urethroperineal fistula
urethroperineoscrotal
urethropexy
  Aldridge urethropexy
  anterior urethropexy
  Burch retropubic urethropexy
  Raz urethropexy
  Stamey urethropexy
  Stamey-Pereyra urethropexy
urethrophyma
urethroplasty
  Badenoch urethroplasty
  Blandy urethroplasty
  Cecil-Culp urethroplasty
  Cohen urethroplasty
  Fischmann urethroplasty
  Johanson urethroplasty
  mesh graft urethroplasty
  suprapubic urethroplasty
  Thiersch-Duplay urethroplasty
  Turner-Warwick urethroplasty
  Waterhouse urethroplasty
  Wehrbein urethroplasty
urethroplasty needle
urethrorectal fistula

urethrorrhaphy
urethroscope
  ACMI urethroscope
  Albarran urethroscope
  Ballenger urethroscope
  female urethroscope
  Guiteras urethroscope
  Lowsley urethroscope
  obturator urethroscope
  posterior urethroscope
urethroscopic examination
urethroscopy
urethrostomy
urethrotome
  bougie urethrotome
  Hertel urethrotome
  Huffman-Huber infant
    urethrotome
  infant urethrotome
  Keitzer infant urethrotome
  Kirkheim-Storz urethrotome
  Maisonneuve urethrotome
  Otis urethrotome
  Riba urethrotome
  Sachs urethrotome
  Storz-Kirkheim urethrotome
urethrotome blade
urethrotomy
  Cock urethrotomy
  direct-vision internal
    urethrotomy (DVIU)
  endoscopic optical
    urethrotomy
  external urethrotomy
  internal urethrotomy
  Syme external urethrotomy
urethrovaginal fistula
urethrovaginal space
urethrovesical angle
urethrovesicular differential reflux
Urias pressure splint
Uribe orbital implant
uric acid
Uridome catheter
Uri-Drain leg bag
Uri-Drain male incontinence
    device
Uridrop catheter
Urihesive expandable adhesive
urinary bladder
urinary bladder hernia
urinary blockage

urinary calculus
urinary catheter
urinary catheterization
urinary control urethral insert
urinary diversion
urinary diversion procedure
urinary drainage
urinary drainage tube
urinary fistula
urinary hesitancy
urinary incontinence
urinary incontinence clamp
urinary incontinence prosthesis
urinary infection
urinary leg bag
urinary meatus
urinary opening
urinary output
urinary reflux
urinary reservoir
urinary retention
urinary sphincter
urinary stasis
urinary stone
urinary stream
urinary stress incontinence (USI)
urinary symptoms
urinary tract abnormality
urinary tract anomaly
urinary tract disease
urinary tract disorder
urinary tract infection
urinary tract injury
urinary tract obstruction
urinary tract reconstruction
urinary urgency
urinary volume
urinary washings
urinary-umbilical fistula
urinary-vaginal fistula
urine
  clear urine
  cloudy urine
  effluxed clear urine
  extravasation of urine
  hazy urine
  incontinent of urine
  milky urine
  residual urine
  retained urine
  straw-colored urine
  stream of urine

urine collection device
urine culture
urine specimen collection
Urist-Matchett-Brown total hip
Uro-Bond silicone adhesive
Urocam video camera
Urocare Foley catheter
Urocare latex reusable leg bag
Uro-Cath molded latex male external catheter
UroCoil self-expanding stent
Uro-Con Texas style male external catheter
UroCystom unit
urodynamic catheter
Uroflo cystometer
uroflometer
uroflow study
uroflowmeter
uroflowmetry
Urofoam adhesive foam strip for male external catheter
urogenital anomaly
urogenital diaphragm
urogenital fistula
urogenital fold
urogenital membrane
urogenital region
urogenital surgery
urogenital tract
urogenital trigone
urogenital vestibule
UroGold laser
urogram
  ascending urogram
  descending urogram
  excretion urogram
  excretory urogram
  intravenous urogram
  oral urogram
  retrograde urogram
urography
  antegrade urography
  ascending urography
  cystoscopic urography
  descending urography
  excretion urography
  excretory urography
  intravenous urography
  IV urography

urography (*continued*)
  oral urography
  percutaneous antegrade urography
Uro-Guide stent
Urolase CO_2 laser
Urolase fiber laser
Urolase neodymium:YAG laser fiber
urologic anesthesia
urologic catheter
urologic complication
urologic laparoscopic surgical procedure
urologic operation
urologic surgery
urologic surgery instrument set
urologic surgical procedure
urologic system cancer
urologic ultrasonography
urological catheter
urological evaluation
Uroloop electrode
Uroloop instrument
Urolume endourethral Wallstent prosthesis
Urolume urethral stent
Uromat dilation
UroMax high-pressure balloon catheter
uroplastique material
UroQuest On-Command catheter
urorectal membrane
Uro-Safe vinyl disposable leg bag
UroSan Plus external catheter
Urosheath incontinence device
UroSnare cystoscopic tumor snare
Urosoft stent
urostomy pouch
urothelial basement membrane
urothelial carcinoma
urothelial tumor
urothelioma
urothelium
Urovac bladder evacuator
Urquhart periosteal elevator
Urrets-Zavalia depressor
Urrets-Zavalia localizer
Urrets-Zavalia probe

Urrets-Zavalia retinal surgical lens
Urschel first rib rongeur
Urschel-Leksell rongeur
urticarial vasculitis
US 1005 uroflow meter
USA plaster spreader
USA retractor
USA laparoscope
USCI angioplasty guiding sheath
USCI Bard catheter
USCI bifurcated Vasculour prosthesis
USCI cannula
USCI catheter
USCI Finesse guiding catheter
USCI Goetz bipolar electrode
USCI guidewire
USCI guiding catheter
USCI Hyperflex guidewire
USCI introducer
USCI Mini-Profile balloon dilatation catheter
USCI bipolar electrode
USCI pacing electrode
USCI PET balloon
USCI Positrol coronary catheter
USCI probe
USCI Sauvage Bionit bifurcated vascular prosthesis
USCI Sauvage side-limb prosthesis
USCI Sauvage graft
USCI shunt
USCI Vario permanent pacemaker
U-shaped arch
U-shaped cannula
U-shaped continuous sutures
U-shaped curve
U-shaped forceps
U-shaped incision
U-shaped interdigitated muscle flap
U-shaped retractor
U-shaped scalp flap
U-shaped scar
U-shaped skin excision
Usher Marlex mesh dressing
Usher Marlex mesh graft
Usher Marlex mesh implant

Usher Marlex mesh implant material
Usher Marlex mesh prosthesis
Usher-Bellis hernia repair
USI (urinary stress incontinence)
Uskow pillars
U-splint
Ussing chamber
Ussing chamber technique
U-stitch
usual anatomic position
U-sutures
Utah arm electronic prosthesis
Utah artificial arm
Utah total artificial heart
UTAS 2000 electroretinography instrument
uteri
    adnexa uteri
    cavum uteri
    cervix uteri
    corpus uteri
    descensus uteri
    discission of cervix uteri
    fibromyomata uteri
    leiomyomata uteri
    membrane of cervix uteri
    myomata uteri
    os uteri
uterine adenocarcinoma
uterine anomaly
uterine appendage
uterine artery forceps
uterine aspiration
uterine aspirator
uterine atony
uterine biopsy curet
uterine biopsy forceps
uterine biopsy punch
uterine biopsy punch forceps
uterine bleeding
uterine canal
uterine cannula
uterine cavity
uterine cervix
uterine clamp
uterine compression
uterine configuration
uterine cornual access catheter
uterine corpus
uterine cramping

uterine cuff
uterine curet
uterine curettage
uterine curettement
uterine curettings
uterine cycle
uterine descensus
uterine didelphys
uterine dilatation
uterine dilator
uterine elevator
uterine enlargement
uterine evacuation
uterine evacuator
uterine evaluation
Uterine Explora Curette
    endometrial sampling
    device
uterine fibroid
uterine fibroidectomy
uterine fibroma
uterine forceps
uterine fundus
uterine gland
uterine hemorrhage
uterine hernia
uterine hernia syndrome
uterine incision
uterine injector
uterine irrigating curet
uterine knife
uterine leiomyosarcoma
uterine lining
uterine manipulating forceps
uterine manipulator
uterine mucus
uterine muscle
uterine myoma
uterine myomata
uterine myomectomy
uterine needle
uterine nerve
uterine orifice
uterine ostial access catheter
uterine papillary serous
    carcinoma
uterine perforation
uterine placenta
uterine plexus
uterine polyp forceps
uterine pregnancy
uterine probe

uterine procidentia
uterine prolapse repair
uterine radium insertion
uterine reflection
uterine sarcoma
uterine scissors
uterine scrapings
uterine secundines
uterine segment
uterine self-retaining cannula
uterine shadow
uterine sound
uterine specimen forceps
uterine spoon
uterine suction curet
uterine suspension
uterine suspension operation
uterine tenaculum
uterine tenaculum forceps
uterine tenaculum hook
uterine tissue
uterine trigger cannula
uterine tube
uterine tube fimbria
uterine vacuum aspirating curet
uterine vacuum cannula
uterine veins
uterine vessels
uterine vulsellum forceps
uterine wall
uterine-dressing forceps
uterine-elevating forceps
uterine-grasping forceps
uterine-holding forceps
uterine-irrigating curet
uterine-manipulating forceps
uterine-packing forceps
uteroabdominal pregnancy
Uterobrush endometrial sample
    collector
uterocentesis
uterofixation
uterolysis
utero-ovarian pregnancy
uteroparietal suture
uteropelvic ligaments
uteroperitoneal fistula
uteropexy
uteroplacental apoplexy
uteroplacental circulation
uteroplacental insufficiency
uteroplasty

uterorectal fistula
uterosacral block
uterosacral fold
uterosacral ligament
uterosalpingography
uterotubal pregnancy
uterovaginal fistula
uterovaginal plexus
uterovesical fold
uterovesical junction (UVJ)
uterus
  anteflexed uterus
  anterior uterus
  atony of uterus
  Baldy-Webster operation for
    retrodisplacement of uterus
  bicollis uterus
  bicornis uterus
  bicornuate uterus
  bilocularis uterus
  bipartitus uterus
  boggy uterus
  bosselated uterus
  broad ligament of uterus
  cochleate uterus
  contracted uterus
  contraction of uterus
  cordiformis uterus
  cornual portion of uterus
  corpus of uterus
  Coulevaire uterus
  dehiscence of uterus
  didelphic uterus
  double uterus
  effleurage of uterus
  enlarged uterus
  fibroid of uterus
  fibroid tumor of uterus
  fibroid uterus
  firm uterus
  freely mobile uterus
  freely movable uterus
  fundal portion of uterus
  Gilliam suspension of uterus
  gravid uterus
  horn of uterus
  insufflation of uterus
  interposition of uterus
  inverted uterus
  involution of uterus
  isthmus of uterus
  lateral version of uterus

uterus (*continued*)
  lyre of uterus
  mobilized uterus
  procidentia of uterus
  pubescent uterus
  rent in uterus
  retroflexed uterus
  retroverted uterus
  round ligament of uterus
  rudimentary uterus
  ruptured uterus
  septate uterus
  small uterus
  smooth-walled uterus
  subinvolution of uterus
  suspension of uterus
  tubal implantation into uterus
  ventrofixation of uterus
  ventrosuspension of uterus
uterus arcuatus
uterus didelphys
uterus massaged
uterus mobilized
uterus normal in length
uterus normal in size and shape
uterus packed with gauze
uterus septus
uterus simplex
uterus sounded
uterus unicornis
utility arch
utility bandage scissors
utility forceps
utility glove
utility scissors
utility shears
utility shoulder splint
utility-type incision
Utrata capsulorrhexis
    forceps
Utrata foldable lens cutter
utricle
utricular duct
utricular nerve
utriculoampullar nerve
utriculosaccular duct
utriculosaccularis
U-tube drain
U-tube stent
U-tube tube
U-turn maneuver
U-type dental implant

UVCP (unilateral vocal cord
  paralysis)
uvea-fixated intraocular lens
uveal melanoma
uveal metastasis
uveal staphyloma
uvea-supported intraocular
  lens
uveitis
uveoencephalitic syndrome
uveomeningeal syndrome
uveoparotid fever
UV-Flash ultraviolet germicidal
  exchange device
UVJ (ureterovesical junction)
UVR-absorbing intraocular
  lens
uvula
  bifid uvula
  cleft uvula
  elongated uvula
  forked uvula
  palatine uvula

uvula (*continued*)
  pendulous uvula
  split uvula
uvula muscle
uvula palatina
uvula retractor
uvula tip
uvula vesicae
uvular muscle
uvular retractor
uvulatome
uvulectomy
uvulitis
uvulopalatine musculature
uvulopalatopharyngoplasty
uvulopalatoplasty (UPP)
uvulopalatoplasty procedure
uvulopharyngeal
uvuloptosis
uvulotome
uvulotomy
U wave
Uyemura operation

V-flap
V-line
V-umbilicoplasty
V. Mueller amputating saw
V. Mueller aortic clamp
V. Mueller auricular appendage
    clamp
V. Mueller biopsy forceps
V. Mueller blunt hook
V. Mueller bone-cutting forceps
V. Mueller bulldog clamp
V. Mueller cross-action bulldog
    clamp
V. Mueller curved operating
    scissors
V. Mueller cystoscopy tip
V. Mueller diamond rasp
V. Mueller embolectomy
    catheter
V. Mueller fiberoptic retractor
V. Mueller lasar Rhoton
    microforceps
V. Mueller laser Backhaus towel
    forceps
V. Mueller laser Crile micro-
    arterial forceps
V. Mueller laser Heaney needle
    holder
V. Mueller laser Julian needle
    holder
V. Mueller laser micro-Allis
    forceps
V. Mueller laser Rhoton
    microneedle holder
V. Mueller laser Rhoton
    microscissors
V. Mueller laser Rhoton
    microtying forceps
V. Mueller laser Singley tissue
    forceps
V. Mueller laser tubal scissors
V. Mueller mastoid curet
V. Mueller myringotomy blade

V. Mueller nonperforating towel
    forceps
V. Mueller operating scissors
V. Mueller paracervical nerve
    block needle
V. Mueller pudendal nerve block
    needle
V. Mueller ruler
V. Mueller ruler calipers
V. Mueller TUR drape
V. Mueller tying forceps
V. Mueller Universal handle
V. Mueller vascular loop
V. Mueller vena cava clamp
V. Mueller Balfour abdominal
    retractor
V. Mueller Frazier suction tube
V. Mueller Gigli saw
V. Mueller LaForce adenotome
V. Mueller Poole suction tube
V. Mueller Vital laser Babcock
    forceps
V. Mueller Vital laser Mayo
    dissecting scissors
V. Mueller Vital laser Potts-Smith
    forceps
V. Mueller Tip-Trol handle
V.M. & Co. (*see* V. Mueller)
V/Q lung scan (ventilation-
    perfusion lung scan)
V1 halo ring
V1, V2, V3, V4, V5, V6 EKG leads
V33W high-density endocavity
    probe
VA (visual acuity)
VA magnetic implant
VA magnetic orbital implant
Vabra aspirator
Vabra assembly
Vabra cannula
Vabra catheter
Vabra cervical aspirator
Vabra curettage

Vabra endometrial biopsy
Vabra endometrial study
Vabra suction curet
Vabra uterine aspiration
   curettage
VAC (vacuum assisted closure)
Vacher self-retaining retractor
Vac-Lok immobilization cushion
Vac-Pac positioner
Vac-Pak pad
VACTERL anomaly
Vactro perilimbal suction
Vacuconstrictor erection device
Vacurette catheter
Vacurette suction curet
Vacutainer drain
Vacutainer holder
Vacutainer needle
Vacutainer tube
Vacutainer vacuum tube
Vacutome knife
Vacutron suction regulator
vacuum abortion
vacuum aspiration
vacuum aspiration catheter
vacuum aspirator
vacuum assisted closure (VAC)
vacuum assisted closure
   dressing
vacuum constriction device
vacuum curet
vacuum curettage
vacuum drain
vacuum drainage
vacuum entrapment device
vacuum erection device (VED)
vacuum extraction
vacuum extraction device
vacuum extraction operation
vacuum fixation ring
vacuum hand pump
vacuum intrauterine cannula
vacuum intrauterine probe
vacuum pillow
vacuum retractor
vacuum sinusitis
vacuum thoracic drainage
vacuum tube
vacuum tumescence-constrictor
   device
vacuum tumescence-
   enhancement therapy

vacuum uterine cannula
vacuum vaginal delivery
vacuum-assisted closure device
vacuuming needle
vacuum-operated viscous
   restraint
VAD (ventricular assist device;
   vascular/venous access
   device)
vagal accessory nerve
vagal apnea
vagal body
vagal dilator
vagal ganglion
vagal nerve
vagal trunk
vagina
   cul-de-sac of vagina
   double vagina
   lyre of vagina
   rudimentary vagina
   rugae of vagina
   vestibule of vagina
   Wharton construction of
      artificial vagina
vagina bulbi
vaginal adenocarcinoma
vaginal agenesis
vaginal aluminum electrode
vaginal anomaly
vaginal artery
vaginal atrophy
vaginal bag
vaginal birth
vaginal birth after cesarean
   section (VBAC)
vaginal bleeding
vaginal candle
vaginal carcinoma
vaginal celiotomy
vaginal cervix
vaginal cesarean section
vaginal cone biopsy
vaginal construction
vaginal contraceptive film
vaginal cuff
vaginal cuff clamp
vaginal cylinder
vaginal cystourethropexy
vaginal delivery
vaginal dilator
vaginal dimple

vaginal epithelialization
vaginal examination
vaginal fistula
vaginal flow
vaginal folds
vaginal foreign body
vaginal fornix
vaginal gland
vaginal graft
vaginal hernia
vaginal hysterectomy
vaginal hysterectomy forceps
vaginal inflammation
vaginal laceration
vaginal laser measuring rod
vaginal ligaments
vaginal lithotomy
vaginal lubrication
vaginal lumen
vaginal malformation
vaginal mucosa
vaginal muscles
vaginal needle suspension
    procedure
vaginal nerves
vaginal orifice
vaginal outlet
vaginal pack
vaginal packing
vaginal pad
vaginal plexus
vaginal probe ultrasound
vaginal process of sphenoid
    bone
vaginal prolapse prosthesis
vaginal radium insertion
vaginal reconstruction
vaginal repair
vaginal retractor
vaginal spatula
vaginal speculum
vaginal speculum loop
vaginal sponge
vaginal stent
vaginal suppository
vaginal surgery
vaginal suspension procedure
vaginal swab
vaginal tampon
vaginal tissue
vaginal varicose vein
vaginal vault repair

vaginal vertex delivery
vaginal wall approach
vaginal wall repair
vaginal wall sling procedure
vaginal, cervical, endocervical
    smears (VCE smears)
vaginalectomy
vaginalis
    phimosis vaginalis
    processus vaginalis
    tunica vaginalis
vaginectomy
vaginismus
vaginitis
vaginocutaneous fistula
vaginofixation
vaginolabial hernia
vaginoperineal fistula
vaginoperineal reconstruction
vaginoperineoplasty
vaginoperineotomy
vaginoplasty
    colon interposition
        vaginoplasty
    free flap vaginoplasty
    intestinal vaginoplasty
    penile skin inversion
        vaginoplasty
vaginoplasty procedure
vaginorectal examination
vaginorrhaphy
vaginoscope
    Huffman infant vaginoscope
    Huffman vaginoscope
    Huffman-Huber infant
        vaginoscope
    Huffman-Huber vaginoscope
    infant vaginoscope
vaginoscopy
vaginotomy
vagolysis
    highly selective vagolysis
    selective vagolysis
    surgical vagolysis
vagotomy
    abdominal vagotomy
    highly selective vagotomy
    laparoscopic vagotomy
    laser laparoscopic vagotomy
    selective vagotomy
    surgical vagotomy
    truncal vagotomy

vagotomy and antrectomy with gastroduodenostomy
vagotomy and pyloroplasty
vagotomy retractor
vagotomy stripper
vagovagal reflex
Vag-Pack
vagus nerve (cranial nerve 10)
Vail lid everter
Vail lid retractor
Vail syndrome
Vainio arthroplasty
Vairox high compression vascular stockings
Vaiser eye sponge
Vaiser-Cibis muscle retractor
Vakutage curet
Valdoni clamp
Valentine irrigation tube
Valentine irrigator
Valentine position
Valentine splint
Valentine tube
valgus
    abductio valgus
    Coleman operation for talipes valgus
    cubitus valgus
    Devonshire operation for talipes valgus
    forefoot valgus
    genu valgus
    Grice procedures for talipes valgus
    Grice-Green procedure for talipes valgus
    hallux valgus
    Hark operation for talipes valgus
    Harris-Beath operation for talipes valgus
    Herndon-Heyman operation for talipes valgus
    Hoke operation for talipes valgus
    Ingram operation for talipes valgus
    Lowsman operation for talipes valgus
    Miller operation for talipes valgus
    pes valgus

valgus (*continued*)
    talipes valgus
    Young operation for talipes valgus
valgus bar
valgus deformity
valgus extension overload syndrome
valgus-external rotation injury
Valin forceps
Valin hemilaminectomy self-retaining retractor
valise handle graft
vallate papilla
Valle hysteroscope
vallecula (*pl.* valleculae)
vallecula epiglottica
vallecula for petrosal ganglion
vallecular pouch
Valleix point
Valleix uterine probe
Valleylab cautery
Valleylab ball electrode
Valleylab electrocautery
Valleylab electrosurgical instruments
Valleylab laparoscope
Valleylab loop electrode
Valleylab pencil
Vallis instrument for hair transplant
Valls needle biopsy
Valls prosthesis
Valls-Ottolenghim-Schajowicz needle biopsy
Valpo splint
Valsalva antrum
Valsalva ligaments
Valsalva maneuver
Valsalva muscle
Valsalva sinus
Valtchev uterine manipulator
Valtchev uterine mobilizer
Valtrac absorbable biofragmentable anastomosis ring
Valtrac anastomosis device
Valtrac anastomosis ring
valvanocautery
valve (*see also* graft, implant, prosthesis)
    3-legged cage heart valve

valve (*continued*)
    4A Magovern heart valve
    4-legged cage heart valve
    Abrams-Lucas flap heart valve
    absent pulmonary valve
    Accu-Flo pressure valve
    ACMI irrigating valve
    Ahmed glaucoma artificial
        valve
    Ambu-E valve
    Angell-Shiley bioprosthetic
        heart valve
    Angell-Shiley xenograft
        prosthetic valve
    Angiocor prosthetic valve
    annuloplasty valve
    anterior nasal valve
    antisiphon valve
    aortic bioprosthetic valve
    aortic valve
    apicoaortic conduit heart valve
    apicoaortic shunt heart valve
    Arenberg-Denver valve
    Argyle anti-reflux valve
    Argyle-Salem sump anti-reflux
        valve
    artificial valve
    atrioventricular valve
    auriculoventricular valve
    auscultation sites of heart
        valves
    Bacstop check valve
    ball heart valve
    ball valve
    ball-and-cage prosthetic valve
    ball-cage valve
    ball-occluder valve
    ball-type valve
    Bard-Apter valve
    Bauer air valve
    Bauhin valve
    Baxter mechanical valve
    Beall disk heart valve
    Beall heart valve
    Beall mitral valve
    Beall prosthetic valve
    Beall-Surgitool ball-cage
        prosthetic valve
    Beall-Surgitool disk prosthetic
        valve
    Benchekroun ileal valve
    Bennett valve

valve (*continued*)
    Beraud valve
    Beverly referential valve
    Bianchi valve
    Bicer-val mitral heart valve
    Bicer-val prosthetic valve
    bicuspid aortic valve
    bicuspid valve
    bileaflet heart valve
    bileaflet tilting-disk prosthetic
        valve
    Biocor heart valve
    Biocor porcine stented aortic
        valve
    Biocor porcine stented mitral
        valve
    Biocor prosthetic valve
    Biocor stentless porcine
        aortic valve
    biological tissue valve
    bioprosthetic heart valve
    bioprosthetic valve
    Bio-Vascular prosthetic valve
    Bjork (*also* Björk)
    Björk (*see* Bjork)
    Bjork-Shiley heart valve
    Bjork-Shiley mitral valve
    Bjork-Shiley Monostrut valve
    Bjork-Shiley prosthetic aortic
        valve
    Bjork-Shiley prosthetic mitral
        valve
    bladder irrigating valve
    Blom-Singer postlaryngectomy
        valve
    Blom-Singer voice valve
    blunting of valve
    Bochdalek valve
    bovine heart valve
    bovine pericardial valve
    Braunwald heart valve
    Braunwald-Cutter ball
        prosthetic valve
    Braunwald-Cutter caged-ball
        heart valve
    Braunwald-Cutter prosthetic
        valve
    breast implant valve
    bulb and thumb screw valve
    butterfly heart valve
    caged-ball heart valve
    caged-disk heart valve

valve (*continued*)

Capetown aortic prosthetic valve
CarboMedics bileaflet prosthetic heart valve
CarboMedics Top-Hat supra-annular valve
cardiac valve
Carpentier pericardial valve
Carpentier ring heart valve
Carpentier-Edwards bioprosthetic valve
Carpentier-Edwards mitral annuloplasty valve
Carpentier-Edwards pericardial valve
Carpentier-Edwards porcine prosthetic valve
Carpentier-Edwards porcine supra-annular valve
caval valve
cleft mitral valve
Codman Hakim programmable valve
Codman-Medos programmable valve
colic valve
commissural pulmonary valve
competent ileocecal valve
competent valve
convexoconcave disk prosthetic valve
convexoconcave heart valve
Cooley-Bloodwell low profile valve
Cooley-Bloodwell-Cutter valve
Cooley-Cutter disk prosthetic valve
Coratomic prosthetic valve
Cordis-Hakin valve
Cross-Jones disk prosthetic valve
Cross-Jones mitral valve
CRx valve
CryoLife-O'Brien stentless porcine heart valve
cryopreserved homograft valve
CryoValve-SG valve
CSF flushing valve
Cutter mitral valve
Cutter-Smeloff disk valve

valve (*continued*)

Cutter-Smeloff heart valve
Cutter-Smeloff mitral valve
DeBakey heart valve
DeBakey prosthetic valve
DeBakey-Surgitool prosthetic valve
Delrin disk heart valve
Delta valve
Denver valve
Denver-Krupin valve
Diamond valve
diastolic fluttering aortic valve
disk valve
doming of valve
double spring ball valve
double-angled valve
Dua antireflux valve
dual-chamber flushing valve
Duostat rotating hemostatic valve
Duraflow heart valve
Duromedics bileaflet mitral valve
dysfunctional nasal valve
dysplastic valve
early opening of valve
eccentric monocuspid tilting-disk prosthetic valve
echo-dense valve
ectatic aortic valve
Edmark mitral valve
Edwards heart valve
Edwards Prima Plus valve
Edwards seamless heart valve
Edwards-Carpentier aortic valve
Edwards-Duromedics bileaflet heart valve
Edwards-Duromedics prosthetic valve
Elgiloy frame of prosthetic valve
Emiks heart valve
esophagogastric flap valve
eustachian valve
expiratory valve
failed nipple valve
fascia lata heart valve
fenestrated valve
fibrotic mitral valve

valve (*continued*)
Fink valve
flail mitral valve
flexible cardiac valve
floating disk heart valve
floppy mitral valve
flushing valve
Foltz valve
free-hand allograft valve
Freestyle valve
Frumin valve
GateWay Y-adapter rotating
   hemostatic valve
Georgia valve
glutaraldehyde-tanned bovine
   heart valve
glutaraldehyde-tanned porcine
   heart valve
Gott butterfly heart valve
Hakim high-pressure valve
Hakim precision valve
Hall prosthetic heart valve
Hall prosthetic valve
Hall-Kaster disk prosthetic
   valve
Hall-Kaster heart valve
Hammersmith heart valve
hammocking of valve
Hancock aortic prosthetic
   valve
Hancock bioprosthetic heart
   valve
Hancock bioprosthetic valve
Hancock heterograft heart
   valve
Hancock modified orifice
   valve
Hancock pericardial
   prosthetic valve
Hancock porcine heterograft
   heart valve
Hancock porcine heterograft
   valve
Hancock porcine valve
Hans Rudolph 3-way valve
Harken ball heart valve
Harken prosthetic valve
Harken-Starr valve
Hasner valve
heart valve
Heidbrink expiratory spill
   valve

valve (*continued*)
Heimlich chest drainage valve
Heimlich heart valve
Heister valve
Hemex prosthetic valve
heterograft valve
Heyer valve
Heyer-Pudenz valve
Heyer-Schulte valve
hinged-leaflet aortic valve
hockey-stick tricuspid valve
hollow Silastic disk heart
   valve
Holter elliptical valve
Holter high-pressure valve
Holter medium-pressure valve
Holter mini-elliptical valve
Holter straight valve
Holter-Hausner valve
homograft valve
Houston valve
Hufnagel caged-ball heart
   valve
Hufnagel disk heart valve
Hufnagel prosthetic valve
Hufnagel-Kay heart valve
Huschke valve
hypoplastic valve
ileocecal valve
incompetent aortic valve
incompetent atrioventricular
   valve
incompetent ileocecal valve
incompetent mitral valve
incompetent pulmonic valve
incompetent tricuspid valve
incompetent valve
Intact xenograft prosthetic
   valve
Intramed angioscopic valve
Ionescu tri-leaflet valve
Ionescu-Shiley artificial
   cardiac valve
Ionescu-Shiley bioprosthetic
   valve
Ionescu-Shiley bovine
   pericardial valve
Ionescu-Shiley heart valve
Ionescu-Shiley low-profile
   prosthetic valve
Ionescu-Shiley pericardial
   valve

valve (*continued*)
  Ionescu-Shiley porcine
    heterograft heart valve
  Ionescu-Shiley standard
    pericardial prosthetic valve
  irrigating valve
  Jatene arterial switch valve
  Jatene-Macchi prosthetic valve
  Kay-Shiley disk prosthetic
    valve
  Kay-Shiley heart valve
  Kay-Shiley mitral valve
  Kay-Suzuki heart valve
  Kerckring valve
  Krause valve
  Krupin glaucoma valve
  Krupin-Denver eye valve
  Lanz pressure regulating valve
  leaky valve
  Leather antegrade valve
  Leather retrograde valve
  lens mitral heart valve
  LeVeen valve
  Lewis-Leigh positive-pressure
    nonrebreathing valve
  Lifemed heterologous heart
    valve
  Liks disk rotation heart valve
  Lillehei-Kaster pivoting-disk
    prosthetic valve
  Liotta-BioImplant prosthetic
    valve
  Lopez enteral valve
  low-profile mitral heart valve
  Magnuson valve
  Magovern heart valve
  Magovern-Cromie ball-cage
    prosthetic valve
  Malteno glaucoma artificial
    valve
  Medos valve
  Medos-Hakim valve
  Medtronic Hancock valve
  Medtronic Intact porcine
    bioprosthesis valve
  Medtronic prosthetic valve
  Medtronic-Hall heart valve
  Medtronic-Hall monocuspid
    tilting-disk valve
  midsystolic closure of aortic
    valve
  Mischler valve

valve (*continued*)
  mitral valve
  Mitroflow pericardial
    prosthetic valve
  monocuspid tilting disk heart
    valve
  Monostrut Bjork-Shiley valve
  Monostrut heart valve
  Monostrut valve
  Montgomery speaking valve
  Morse valve
  Mosaic heart
  multipurpose valve
  narrowed valve
  nasal valve
  native valve
  nipple valve
  nonrebreathing valve
  notching of pulmonic valve
  Omnicarbon prosthetic valve
  Omniscience heart valve
  Omniscience prosthetic valve
  Omniscience tilting-disk valve
  Orbis-Sigma cerebrospinal
    fluid valve
  Panje voice valve
  parachute mitral valve
  parachute valve
  Passy-Muir tracheostomy and
    ventilator speaking valves
  Pelco prosthetic valve
  Pemco prosthetic valve
  peristaltic valve
  pivotal disk heart valve
  poppet valve
  porcine heart valve
  porcine valve
  premature closure of valve
  prolapsed valve
  prosthetic ball valve
  prosthetic heart valve
  prosthetic valve
  Pudenz valve
  Pudenz-Heyer-Schulte valve
  Puig-Massana-Shiley
    annuloplasty valve
  pulmonary valve
  pulmonic valve
  Pyrolite heart valve
  quadricuspid pulmonary
    valve
  Quattro mitral valve

valve (*continued*)

Raimondi spring peritoneal valve
rectal valve
reducing valve
retrograde valve
rheumatic mitral valve
Rosenmüeller valve
Ross pulmonary porcine valve
Samuels valve
Sanders valve
SCDK-Cutter valve
Schulte valve
semilunar valve
Sheldon-Pudenz valve
Shiley heart valve
Silastic disk heart valve
silicone ball heart valve
Singer-Blom valve
Smeloff prosthetic valve
Smeloff-Cutter ball-cage prosthetic valve
Smokevac trumpet valve
Sophy pressure valve
Sorin cardiac prosthetic valve
Sorin prosthetic valve
spiral valve
Spitz-Holter valve
Spivack valve
St. Jude Medical bileaflet heart valve
St. Jude Medical bileaflet prosthetic valve
St. Jude Medical prosthetic heart valve
Starr ball heart valve
Starr-Bloodwell low-profile valve
Starr-Edwards heart valve
Starr-Edwards prosthetic aortic valve
Starr-Edwards prosthetic ball valve
Starr-Edwards prosthetic mitral valve
Starr-Edwards prosthetic valve
Starr-Edwards Silastic valve
Starr-Edwards silicone rubber ball valve
Stellite ring material of prosthetic valve
stenosed aortic valve

valve (*continued*)

stenotic valve
Surgitool prosthetic valve
Taillefer valve
Tascon prosthetic valve
thebesian valve
tilting-disk heart valve
tilting-disk valve
titanium ball heart valve
titanium cage heart valve
Top-Hat supra-annular aortic valve
track valve
tricuspid aortic valve
tricuspid valve
trileaflet aortic valve
trunk valves
UCI-Barnard aortic valve
Ultracor prosthetic valve
unicommissural aortic valve
Vascor porcine prosthetic valve
velopharyngeal valve
VentEasy isolation valve
ventricular valve
Wada monocuspid tilting-disk heart valve
Wada-Cutter disk prosthetic valve
Wessex prosthetic valve
xenograft heart valve
Xenomedica prosthetic valve
Xenotech prosthetic valve
valve ablation
valve bladder
valve dilator
valve formation
valve holder
valve hook
valve leaflet excision scissors
valve of Bauhin
valve of Heister
valve of Houston
valve of Kerckring
valve outflow strut
valve prosthesis
valve replacement
valve ring
valve scissors
valve structure
valve tip
valve transplantation

valve transposition
valve tube
valved conduit anastomosis
valved graft
valved voice prosthesis
valve-ended catheter
valvotome
valvotomy
  aortic valvotomy
  balloon valvotomy
  bicuspid valvotomy
  Brock valvotomy
  closed valvotomy
  double-balloon valvotomy
  mitral valvotomy
  percutaneous mitral balloon
    valvotomy
  percutaneous mitral valvotomy
  pulmonary valvotomy
  single-balloon valvotomy
  transventricular closed
    valvotomy
  transventricular valvotomy
  tricuspid valvotomy
valvotomy knife
valvula (*pl.* valvulae)
valvula ileocolica
valvula pylori
valvular aortic disease
valvular defect
valvular disease
valvular heart disease
valvular heart surgery
valvular incompetence
valvular insufficiency
valvular sclerosis
valvular stenosis
valvulectomy
valvuloplasty
  aortic valvuloplasty
  bailout valvuloplasty
  balloon aortic valvuloplasty
  balloon mitral valvuloplasty
  balloon pulmonary
    valvuloplasty
  balloon valvuloplasty
  Carpentier tricuspid
    valvuloplasty
  catheter balloon valvuloplasty
    (CBV)
  double-balloon valvuloplasty
  Kay tricuspid valvuloplasty

valvuloplasty (*continued*)
  percutaneous aortic
    valvuloplasty (PAV)
  percutaneous balloon aortic
    valvuloplasty
  percutaneous balloon
    valvuloplasty
  percutaneous mitral balloon
    valvuloplasty
  pulmonary balloon
    valvuloplasty
  pulmonary valvuloplasty
  retrograde valvuloplasty
  single-balloon valvuloplasty
valvuloplasty balloon catheter
valvulotome
  Bailey-Glover-O'Neill
    valvulotome
  Bakst valvulotome
  bread-knife valvulotome
  Brock valvulotome
  Carmody valvulotome
  curved valvulotome
  Derra valvulotome
  Dogliotti valvulotome
  expansile valvulotome
  Gerbode mitral valvulotome
  Gohrbrand valvulotome
  Harken valvulotome
  Himmelstein pulmonary
    valvulotome
  Leather venous valvulotome
  LeMaitre valvulotome
  Longmire valvulotome
  Longmire-Mueller curved
    valvulotome
  Malm-Himmelstein pulmonary
    valvulotome
  Mills valvulotome
  Niedner valvulotome
  Potts expansile valvulotome
  Potts-Riker valvulotome
  pulmonary valvulotome
  Sellor valvulotome
  Tubbs valvulotome
  Universal malleable
    valvulotome
valvulotomy
  aortic valvulotomy
  bicuspid valvulotomy
  mitral valvulotomy
  open valvulotomy

valvulotomy (*continued*)
  pulmonary valvulotomy
  tricuspid valvulotomy
valvulotomy procedure
Van Alyea antral cannula
Van Alyea antral trocar
Van Alyea antral wash tube
Van Alyea frontal sinus cannula
Van Alyea sphenoid cannula
Van Alyea trocar
Van Alyea tube
Van Aman pigtail catheter
Van Buchem disease
Van Buchem syndrome
Van Buren bone-holding forceps
Van Buren canvas roll sound
Van Buren catheter
Van Buren catheter guide
Van Buren cervix syringe
Van Buren dilating sound
Van Buren dilator
Van Buren disease
Van Buren operation
Van Buren sequestrum forceps
Van Buren urethral sound
Van de Graaf generator
Van de Kramer fecal fat
  procedure
Van der Hoeve syndrome
Van der Pas hysteroscope
Van der Woude syndrome
Van Doren uterine biopsy punch
  forceps
Van Doren uterine forceps
Van Gorder approach
Van Gorder arthrodesis
Van Gorder operation
Van Herick modification
Van Hillman suture
Van Hook operation
van Hoorn maneuver
Van Hove bag
Van Lint akinesia
Van Lint anesthesia
Van Lint block
Van Lint conjunctival flap
Van Lint injection
Van Lint lid block
Van Lint modified technique
Van Lint-Atkinson akinesia
Van Lint-Atkinson lid akinetic
  block

Van Lint-O'Brien akinesia
Van Mandach capsule fragment
  and clot forceps
Van Millingen eyelid repair
  technique
Van Millingen graft
Van Millingen operation
Van Nes rotationplasty
Van Osdel antral wash bottle
Van Osdel guillotine
Van Osdel irrigating cannula
Van Osdel tonsillar enucleator
Van Osdel tonsillar knife
Van Osdel tonsillectome
Van Rosen splint
Van Ruben forceps
Van Slyke analysis
Van Sonnenberg gallbladder
  catheter
van Sonnenberg sump
van Sonnenberg sump catheter
van Sonnenberg sump drain
van Sonnenberg-Wittich
  catheter
Van Struyken nasal forceps
Van Struyken nasal punch
Van Struyken punch
Van Tassel angled pigtail
  catheter
Van Tassel pigtail catheter
Vancaillie uterine cannula
Vance percutaneous Malecot
  nephrostomy catheter
Vance prostatic aspiration
  cannula
Vanderpool forceps
Vanderbilt arterial forceps
Vanderbilt clamp
Vanderbilt deep-vessel forceps
Vanderbilt forceps
Vanderbilt University hemostatic
  forceps
Vanderbilt University vessel
  clamp
Vanderbilt University vessel
  forceps
Vanderbilt vessel clamp
Vanghetti cineplasty
Vanghetti limb prosthesis
Vanguard endovascular aortic
  graft
vanished testis syndrome

vanishing bone disease
VanishPoint syringe
Vannas abscess knife
Vannas capsulotomy
Vannas capsulotomy scissors
Vannas corneal scissors
Vannas fixation forceps
Vannas iridocapsulotomy scissors
Vannas knife
Vannas microcapsulotomy
    scissors
Vantage Performance monitor
Vantage tube-occluding forceps
Vantec dilator
Vantec grasping forceps
Vantec loop retriever
Vantec occlusion balloon catheter
Vantec stone basket
Vantec ureteral balloon
    dilatation catheter
Vantec urinary stent
Vantos vacuum
Vantos vacuum extraction
Vantos vacuum extractor
VAPC dorsiflexion assist orthosis
vaporization
vaporizing diseased tissue
vapor-permeable dressing
Vaportome resection electrode
Vaportome roller electrode
Vaportrode roller electrode
VAPR coagulation and cautery
    device
Varco dissecting clamp
Varco gallbladder clamp
Varco gallbladder forceps
Varco thoracic forceps
Vari bladebreaker
Vari/Moist wound dressing
variable axis knee
variable flow insufflator
variable rate pacemaker
variable screw placement
variable stiffness endoscope
variable-dose patient-controlled
    anesthesia (VDPCA)
variable-release compression
Varian CT scanner
variance
    ulnar variance
    ulnar-minus variance
    ulnar-plus variance

variance (*continued*)
    ulnar-plus/neutral variance
    ulnar-positive variance
    zero variance
Vari-Angle clip
Vari-angle clip applier
Vari-Angle McFadden clip
    applier
Vari-Angle temporary clip
    approximator
variceal band ligation
variceal bleed
variceal decompression
variceal hemorrhage
variceal wall
varicella gangrenosa
varicelliform lesion
varicelliform rash
varices (*sing.* varix)
    actively bleeding varices
    alcoholic varices
    anastomotic varices
    aneurysmal varices
    aneurysmoid varices
    bleeding esophageal varices
    Child esophageal varices
    colonic varices
    downhill esophageal varices
    ectopic varices
    esophageal varices
    esophagogastric varices
    fundal varices
    gastric varices
    ileal varices
    injection of varices
    papillary varices
    paraesophageal varices
    Sugiura esophageal varices
    Sugiura procedure for
        esophageal varices
    transesophageal ligation of
        varices
Varick elastic dressing
varicoblepharon
varicocele
    Davat operation for varicocele
    tubo-ovarian varicocele
    Vidal operation for varicocele
varicocele ligation
varicocelectomy
varicophlebitis
varicose aneurysm

varicose ulceration
varicose ulcers
varicose vein stripping and
    ligation
varicose veins
varicosis
varicosities
varicotomy
Vari-Duct hip and knee orthosis
Varidyne drain
variegated lesions
Variflex catheter
VariFlex prosthetic foot
Varigray implant
Varigray lens
Varigray lens implant
Variject needle
VariLift spinal cage
Varilus lens
Varilux implant
Varilux lens implant
Varioligator kit
VariSoft steerable guidewire
Vari-Stim hand-held nerve
    stimulator
Vari-Stim unit
Varivas loop graft
Varivas R vein graft
varix (*pl.* varices)
varix ligation
varus
    abductio varus
    cubitus varus
    forefoot varus
    hallux varus
    metatarsus primus varus
    pes varus
    talipes varus
varus hindfoot deformity
varus knee
varus osteotomy
varus-valgus plane
vas (*pl.* vasa)
vas aberrans
vas clamp
vas deferens (*pl.* vasa
    deferentia)
vas efferens
vas hook
vas isolation forceps
vasa (*sing.* vas)
vasa brevia

vasa deferentia
vasa nervorum
Vasamedics implantable prism
    laser probe
Vas-Cath catheter
Vas-Cath peripheral angioplasty
    catheter
Vasceze vascular access flush
    device
Vasclip alternative to vasectomy
Vasconcelos amputation
Vasconcelos-Barretto clamp
Vasconez tensor fascia lata flap
Vasconez tensor fasciae latae
    flap
Vasco-Posada orbital retractor
Vascor porcine prosthetic valve
Vascor sterile retraction tape
VascuClamp minibulldog vessel
    clamp
VascuClamp vascular clamp
VascuCoil peripheral vascular
    stent
Vascufil sutures
Vascu-Guard bovine pericardial
    surgical patch
Vascu-Guard peripheral vascular
    patch
vascular abdominal surgery
vascular abnormality
vascular access catheter
vascular access device (VAD)
vascular access flush device
vascular anastomosis
vascular anatomy
vascular angiography
vascular anomaly
vascular bed
vascular birthmark
vascular bulldog
vascular bundle implant
vascular bundle implantation
    into bone
vascular cannulation
vascular catheter
vascular channel
vascular circle of optic nerve
vascular clamp
vascular clip
vascular clip applier
vascular collapse
vascular complication

vascular compression
vascular compromise
vascular congestion
vascular control
vascular decompensation
vascular dilator
vascular disease
vascular dissector
vascular ectasia
vascular endothelial growth
   factor (VEGF)
vascular endothelium
vascular engorgement
vascular epiploic arch
vascular exclusion
vascular extravasation
vascular fold
vascular forceps
vascular graft
vascular graft clamp
vascular hemostatic device
vascular hypotension
vascular injury
vascular invasion
vascular isolation technique
vascular laceration
vascular laceration repair
vascular lesion therapy
vascular loop
vascular malformation
vascular malformation birthmark
vascular mass
vascular metastasis
vascular needle holder
vascular nerve
vascular nevus
vascular obstruction
vascular occlusion
vascular occlusive disease
vascular pattern
vascular pedicle
vascular perforation
vascular pericyte of Zimmerman
vascular permeability
vascular procedure
vascular proliferation
vascular prosthesis
vascular reaction
vascular reconstruction
vascular redistribution
vascular reflex
vascular resistance

vascular retractor
vascular ring
vascular ring syndrome
vascular scissors
vascular sealing device
vascular sheath
vascular silk sutures
vascular space
vascular spasm
vascular spider
vascular spring retractor
vascular spur
vascular structure
vascular suction tube
vascular tape
vascular tissue
vascular tissue forceps
vascular tumor
vascular tunic
vascular ulcer
vascular/venous assist device
   (VAD)
vascularity flap
vascularized bone graft (VBG)
vascularized calvarial flap
vascularized fascial patch
vascularized free flap
vascularized graft
vascularized island bone flap
vascularized metaphyseal bone
   graft
vascularized scapular bone graft
vascularized sensate neoclitoris
vascularized soft tissue
vascularized tendon graft
vascularized tibial bone flap
vascularized tissue
vascularized whole joint transfer
vasculature
VascuLink vascular access graft
VascuLink vascular access
   guidewire
vasculitic lesion
vasculitis
   Churg-Strauss vasculitis
   cutaneous vasculitis
   granulomatous vasculitis
   large vessel vasculitis
   livedo vasculitis
   necrotizing vasculitis
   nodular granulomatous
     vasculitis

vasculitis (*continued*)
  nodular vasculitis
  rheumatoid vasculitis
  segmental hyalinizing
    vasculitis
  small vessel vasculitis
  urticarial vasculitis
vasculo-Behçet disease
vasculogenesis
vasculopathy
Vasculour DeBakey graft
vascula (*pl.* vasculum)
VascuPatch
Vascu-Sheath catheter
Vascushunt carotid balloon
    shunt
Vascutech circular blade
Vascutek gelseal vascular graft
Vascutek knitted vascular
    graft
Vascutek vascular prosthesis
Vascutek woven vascular graft
vasectomized
vasectomy
  Burdizzo clamp vasectomy
  Burdizzo vasectomy
  crossover vasectomy
  intra-abdominal vasectomy
  percutaneous vasectomy
  Vasclip alternative to
    vasectomy
  Young vasectomy
vasectomy forceps
vasectomy reversal
Vaseline gauze
Vaseline gauze dressing
Vaseline petrolatum gauze
    dressing
Vaseline petrolatum packing
Vaseline wick dressing
Vaseline-coated gauze
vaselinized nasal tamponage
vasoactive agglutinate
VasoCath catheter
vasoconstriction
vasoconstrictive agent
vasoconstrictor nerve
vasocutaneous fistula
vasodepression
vasodepressor material
vasodilatation
vasodilating agent

vasodilation
  active vasodilation
  local vasodilation
  passive vasodilation
  regional vasodilation
vasodilator
vasodilator administration
vasodilator infusion
vasoepididymectomy
vasoepididymostomy
vasoformative tumor
vasogram
vasography
vasoligation
vasomotor activity
vasomotor center
vasomotor reaction
vasomotor rhinitis
vasomotor spasm
vaso-orchidostomy
vasopressor
vasopressor agent
vasopressor reflex
vasopuncture
vasoresection
vasorrhaphy
VasoSeal hemostatic device
VasoSeal vascular hemostatic
    device
vasosection
vasosensory nerve
vasospasm
vasospastic angina
vasostomy
vasotomy
vasotribe
vasotripsy
vasovagal attack
vasovasostomy
vasovasostomy clamp
vasovesiculectomy
VasPort access port
VasTack needle
Vastamaki hand surgery
vastus lateralis flap
vastus lateralis muscle
vastus medialis muscle
vastus medialis obliquus muscle
vastus medialis obliquus,
    musculus (VMO)
VAT pacemaker
Vater ampulla

Vater corpuscles
Vater fold
Vater papilla
VATER syndrome
Vater-Pacini corpuscles
VATS procedure
VATS wedge resection
Vaughan periosteotome
Vaughan-Jackson lesion
Vaughn sterilizer forceps
vault
    bony vault
    cartilaginous vault
    cecal vault
    cranial vault
    middle nasal vault
    nasal vault
    pharyngeal vault
    vaginal vault
Vaumgartner Vital needle holder
Vaxcel catheter
VAX-D therapy table
VBAC (vaginal birth after
    cesarean section)
V-banded gastroplasty
Vbeam pulsed dye laser
VBG (vascularized bone graft)
VBG (vertical-banded
    gastroplasty)
VBH head holder
V-blade plate
VC2 atrial caval cannula
VCE smears (vaginal, cervical,
    endocervical smears)
VCUG (voiding
    cystourethrogram;
    vesicoureterogram)
VDD pacemaker
Veau classification
Veau cleft lip repair
Veau elevator
Veau operation
Veau palatoplasty
Veau straight-line closure
Veau-Axhausen operation
Veau-Wardill palatal push-back
Veau-Wardill palatoplasty
Veau-Wardill-Kilner cleft palate
    repair
Veau-Wardill-Kilner palatoplasty
Veau-Wardill-Kilner pushback
    operation

Veau-Wardill-Kilner repair
Vecchietti operation
vectis
    cul-de-sac irrigating vectis
    irrigating vectis
    Sheets irrigating vectis
    Snellen vectis
    Wess vectis
vectis blade
vectis cesarean section forceps
vectis loop
vector guide to knee system
    from Dyonics
Vector intertrochanteric nail
Vector large-lumen catheter
Vector large-lumen guiding
    catheter
vector loop
vector lunate joint
vector of aging
vector of skin pull
vectorcardiogram
vectorcardiography
Vectra vascular access
Vectra vascular access graft
VED (vacuum erection device)
Veeder tip sling
Veeder tip snare
Veeneklaas syndrome
Veenema retropubic retractor
Veenema retropubic self-
    retaining retractor
Veenema-Gusberg needle
Veenema-Gusberg prostatic
    biopsy cut
Veenema-Gusberg prostatic
    biopsy needle
Veenema-Gusberg prostatic
    biopsy punch
Veenema-Gusberg prostatic
    punch
vegetations
vegetative bacteria
vegetative lesions
VEGF (vascular endothelial
    growth factor)
Vehe carver
Vehmehren costotome
Veidenheimer resection
    clamp
veiling of the alar rim
Veillon tube

vein
- accessory cephalic vein
- accessory hemiazygos vein
- accessory saphenous vein
- adrenal veins
- afferent veins
- anastomotic vein
- angular facial vein
- angular vein
- antebrachial vein
- anterior auricular vein
- anterior cardiac veins
- anterior cerebral vein
- anterior condylar vein
- anterior facial vein
- anterior intercostal veins
- anterior jugular vein
- anterior labial vein
- anterior scrotal veins
- anterior temporal diploic vein
- anterior tibial vein
- appendicular vein
- aqueduct of vestibule vein
- arcuate veins
- ascending lumbar vein
- auditory veins
- auricular veins
- autogenous vein
- axillary vein
- azygos vein
- basal vein
- basilic vein
- basivertebral veins
- beveled vein
- brachial veins
- brachiocephalic veins
- Breschet veins
- bronchial veins
- Browning vein
- bulb of inferior jugular vein
- Burow vein
- canaliculus vein
- cannulation of femoral artery and vein
- cardiac veins
- cardinal vein
- carotid vein
- cephalic vein
- cerebellar veins
- cerebral vein
- cervical vein
- choroid vein

vein (*continued*)
- ciliary veins
- cilioretinal vein
- circumflex femoral veins
- circumflex iliac vein
- colic vein
- collapsed jugular vein
- common anterior facial vein
- common facial vein
- common iliac vein
- component thin-walled veins
- condylar emissary vein
- conjunctival veins
- coronary veins
- costoaxillary vein
- cubital vein
- cutaneous vein
- cystic vein
- decannulation of femoral artery and vein
- deep cervical vein
- deep circumflex iliac vein
- deep dorsal vein
- deep facial vein
- deep femoral vein
- deep inferior epigastric vein
- deep lingual vein
- deep temporal vein
- deep vein
- digital vein
- diploic vein
- dorsal digital veins
- dorsal lingual veins
- dorsal metacarpal veins
- dorsal metatarsal veins
- dorsal vein
- dorsispinal vein
- duodenal vein
- emissary vein
- emulgent vein
- epigastric inferior vein
- epigastric vein
- episcleral vein
- erasing of vein
- esophageal vein
- ethmoidal veins
- external carotid vein
- external iliac vein
- external jugular vein
- external mammary vein
- external nasal veins
- external palatine vein

vein (*continued*)

- external pterygoid vein
- external pudendal vein
- external radial vein
- facial vein
- femoral vein
- femoropopliteal vein
- fibular veins
- frontal diploic vein
- frontal vein
- Galen vein
- gastric veins
- gastroepiploic vein
- genicular veins
- gluteal veins
- gonadal veins
- great cardiac vein
- great cerebral vein
- great saphenous vein
- greater saphenous vein
- hemiazygos vein
- hemorrhoidal veins
- hepatic veins
- highest intercostal vein
- hypogastric vein
- ileal veins
- ileocolic vein
- iliac vein
- ilioinguinal vein
- iliolumbar vein
- incompetent vein
- inferior alveolar vein
- inferior cerebellar veins
- inferior cerebral veins
- inferior gluteal veins
- inferior labial veins
- inferior laryngeal vein
- inferior ophthalmic vein
- inferior palpebral vein
- inferior phrenic vein
- inferior rectal vein
- inferior thyroid vein
- inferior vein
- innominate veins
- intercapital veins
- intercostal vein
- interlobar veins
- internal auditory vein
- internal cerebral veins
- internal iliac vein
- internal jugular vein
- internal maxillary vein

vein (*continued*)

- internal pudendal vein
- internal thoracic vein
- interosseous veins
- interventricular vein
- intervertebral vein
- intrarenal vein
- jejunal and ileal veins
- jejunal veins
- jugular vein
- Kohlrausch veins
- Krukenberg veins
- Kuhnt postcentral vein
- Labbé vein (*also* Labbe)
- labial veins
- labyrinthine veins
- lacrimal veins
- laryngeal vein
- Latarjet vein
- lateral sacral veins
- lateral thoracic vein
- left colic vein
- left gastric vein
- left gastroepiploic vein
- left inferior pulmonary vein
- left superior pulmonary vein
- left suprarenal vein
- left testicular vein
- left umbilical vein
- lesser ovarian vein
- lienal vein
- ligation of vein
- lingual vein
- lumbar veins
- lumen of vein
- main renal vein
- mammary vein
- Marshall oblique vein
- masseteric vein
- mastoid emissary vein
- maxillary veins
- Mayo pyloric vein
- median antebrachial vein
- median basilic vein
- median cephalic vein
- median cubital vein
- median vein
- mediastinal veins
- meningeal veins
- mesenteric superior vein
- mesenteric vein
- metacarpal veins

vein (*continued*)

metatarsal veins
middle cardiac vein
middle colic vein
middle meningeal vein
middle rectal vein
middle temporal vein
middle thyroid vein
muscular veins
musculocutaneous vein
musculophrenic veins
nasal vein
nasofrontal vein
neck veins
oblique vein
obturator veins
occipital diploic vein
occipital emissary vein
occipital vein
omphalomesenteric veins
ophthalmic vein
ophthalmomeningeal vein
ovarian vein
palatine vein
palmar digital veins
palmar metacarpal veins
palpebral veins
pampiniform vein
pancreatic veins
pancreaticoduodenal veins
paraumbilical veins
paraventricular veins
parietal emissary vein
parotid veins
patency of veins
perforating vein
pericallosal veins
pericardiac veins
pericardiacophrenic veins
peroneal veins
pharyngeal veins
phrenic veins
plantar digital veins
plantar metatarsal vein
popliteal vein
portal vein
postcardinal veins
postcentral vein
posterior auricular vein
posterior facial vein
posterior intercostal veins
posterior labial veins

vein (*continued*)

posterior scrotal veins
posterior temporal diploic
   vein
posterior tibial vein
precardinal veins
prepyloric vein
pudendal vein
pulmonary vein
pyloric vein
radial veins
ranine vein
rectal vein
renal veins
retinal vein
retroauricular vein
retromandibular vein
Retzius veins
right colic vein
right gastric vein
right gastroepiploic vein
right inferior pulmonary vein
right ovarian vein
right superior pulmonary vein
right suprarenal vein
right testicular vein
Rosenthal ascending vein
Ruysch veins
sacral veins
salvatella vein
Santorini parietal vein
saphenous vein
Sappey vein
sausaging of vein
scrotal veins
short gastric veins
sigmoid veins
small cardiac vein
small saphenous vein
smallest cardiac veins
Soemmering arterial vein
Soemmering external radial
   vein
spermatic veins
spinal veins
spiral vein
splenic vein
stellate veins
Stensen veins
sternocleidomastoid vein
striate vein
stylomastoid vein

vein (*continued*)

subcardinal veins
subclavian vein
subcostal vein
sublingual vein
sublobular veins
submental vein
superficial circumflex iliac vein
superficial dorsal veins
superficial epigastric vein
superficial middle cerebral vein
superficial temporal vein
superficial vein
superficial vertebral veins
superior anastomotic vein
superior azygos vein
superior bulb of internal jugular vein
superior cerebellar vein
superior cerebral veins
superior epigastric veins
superior gluteal veins
superior hemorrhoidal vein
superior intercostal vein
superior labial veins
superior laryngeal vein
superior mesenteric vein
superior ophthalmic vein
superior palpebral vein
superior phrenic vein
superior pulmonary vein
superior rectal veins
superior thyroid vein
supracardinal veins
supraorbital vein
suprarenal vein
suprascapular vein
supratrochlear veins
temporal diploic vein
temporal vein
terminal vein
testicular vein
thebesian vein
thoracic vein
thoracoacromial vein
thoracoepigastric veins
thrombosed veins
thymic vein
thyroid ima vein
thyroid vein

vein (*continued*)

tibial vein
trabecular vein
tracheal vein
transection of vein
transposition of pulmonary veins
transverse cervical veins
transverse facial vein
transverse vein
tympanic vein
ulnar veins
umbilical vein
uterine veins
vaginal varicose vein
varicose veins
vertebral vein
vesalian vein
Vesalius vein
vestibular veins
vidian vein
Vieussens veins
vitelline vein
vortex vein
wormy veins
vein decompression
vein dilator
vein graft
vein graft cannula
vein graft ring marker
vein graft stenting stent
vein hook retractor
vein obstruction
vein occlusion
vein of Galen
vein of Galen malformation
vein of Labbe
vein of Thebesius
vein patch
vein patch angioplasty
vein patch graft
vein retractor
vein sign
vein stripper (*see* stripper)
vein stripping
vein-coated stent
Veingard dressing
Veinlase captured-pulse laser
Veirs canaliculus repair
Veirs canaliculus rod
Veirs cannula
Veirs dacryocystorhinostomy set

Veirs malleable rod
Veirs needle
Veirs operation
Veirs rod
Veirs trocar
velamenta cerebri
velamentous insertion
velamentum (*pl.* velamenta)
velar area
velar assimilation
velar insufficiency
velar tail
Velcro belt
Velcro binder
Velcro crackles
Velcro dressing
Velcro extenders splint
Velcro fastener dressing
Velcro rales in lungs
Velcro splint
Velcro tapes
Velcro tourniquet
Veleanu-Rosianu-Ionescu
    procedure
Veleanu-Rosianu-Ionescu
    technique
Velex woven Dacron vascular
    graft
Veley head holder
Veley headrest
Velket-Velcro tourniquet
Vella fistula
velocardiofacial syndrome
velocimeter
velocimetry
Velocity stent
velolaryngeal endoscope
velopharyngeal closure
velopharyngeal competence
    (VPC)
velopharyngeal function
velopharyngeal incompetence
    (VPI)
velopharyngeal insufficiency (VPI)
velopharyngeal isthmus
velopharyngeal portal
velopharyngeal seal
velopharyngeal valve
velopharynx
veloplasty
velosynthesis
velour collar graft

velour graft
velour patch
Velpeau axillary view
Velpeau bandage
Velpeau cast
Velpeau deformity
Velpeau dressing
Velpeau fossa
Velpeau hernia
Velpeau shoulder immobilizer
Velpeau sling
Velpeau sling-dressing
Velpeau snare
Velpeau stockinette dressing
Velpeau tendon transfer
Velpeau wrap
Velroc dressing
velum (*pl.* vela)
    anterior medullary velum
    aponeurosis of velum
    artificial velum
    Baker velum
    nursing velum
    palatine velum
velvet-eye aspirating tube
velvet-eye tube
vena azygos
vena cava clamp
vena cava clip
vena cava forceps
vena cava to pulmonary artery
    shunt
vena cava-gallbladder line
vena caval cannula
vena caval clamp
vena caval clip
vena caval forceps
vena caval obstruction
vena caval scissors
vena caval umbrella
vena caval umbrella filter
vena comitans of hypoglossal
    nerve
Vena Tech dual vena cava filter
Venable bone plate
Venable hip screw
Venable screw
Venable-Stuck fracture pin
Venable-Stuck nail
venacavogram
venacavography
VenaFlo needle

VenaFlow vascular graft
Venaport catheter
Venaport coronary sinus guiding
  catheter
venectomy
VenES antiembolism stocking
VenES vascular stocking
venesection
venesuture
Venflon cannula
Venflon needle
Veni-Gard stabilization dressing
venipuncture needle
venipuncture side
venisection
venisutures
Vennes pancreatic dilation set
Venn-Watson classification
venobiliary fistula
venocapillary congestion
Venocath catheter
venoclysis cannula
venoconstriction
Venodyne boot
Venodyne pneumatic
  compressive device
Venodyne pneumatic inflation
  device
Venoflow PTFE graft
venogram
venography
  intraosseous venography
  jugular venography
  magnetic resonance
    venography (MRV)
  percutaneous splenoportal
    venography
  portal venography
  renal venography
  splenic venography
  splenoportal venography
venolysis
veno-occlusive disease
venoperitoneostomy
venorrhaphy
venoscope
venotomy
venotripsy
venous access
venous access device (VAD)
venous access port
venous access technique

venous air embolism (VAE)
venous anastomosis
venous aneurysm
venous angiocardiography
venous angle
venous anomaly
venous aortography
venous bifurcation
venous bleeding
venous cannula
venous cannulation
venous capacitance bed
venous catheter
venous circulation
venous claudication
venous compression
venous congestion
venous cutdown
venous distention
venous drainage
venous embolism
venous embolization
venous engorgement
venous flap
venous flow
venous foramen
venous gangrene
venous graft
venous groove
venous hemodynamics
venous hemorrhage
venous hypertension
venous injury
venous insufficiency
venous interposition graft
venous intravasation
venous invasion
venous irrigation catheter
venous lakes
venous leg ulceration
venous line
venous loop
venous malformation
venous needle
venous obstruction
venous occlusion
venous plethysmograph
venous plexus
venous pressure
venous pressure gradient
  support stockings (VPGSS)
venous pulse

venous puncture
venous reflux
venous return
venous sclerosis
venous sheath
venous sheath patch
venous shunt
venous sinus flow void
venous sinus of dura mater
venous spread
venous stasis
venous stasis disease
venous stasis ulcer
venous thrombectomy catheter
venous thromboembolism
venous thrombosis
venous ulcer
venous valvular competence
venous varicosity
venous vertebral plexus
venous wave
venous web
venous web disease
venous Y connector
venous Y adapter
venous-related complication
venous-to-venous anastomosis
venovenostomy
venovenous bypass (VVB)
venovenous extracorporeal
    bypass
vent implant
Ventak
    automatic implantable
      cardioverter-defibrillator
      (AICD)
Ventak AICD pacemaker
Ventak Mini II automatic
    implantable cardioverter-
    defibrillator (AICD)
Ventak Mini III implantable
    defibrillator
Ventak automatic implantable
    cardioverter-defibrillator
    (AICD)
Ventak pacemaker
Ventak Prizm dual chamber
    implantable defibrillator
Ventak Prizm implantable
    defibrillator
Ventana automated
    immunostainer

Ventana Immuno-automated
    machine
VentCheck monitor
VentEasy II isolation valve
vented earmold
Ventex dressing
Ventfoam traction dressing
venti-mask
Ventifoam traction dressing
ventilated mask
ventilation
    airway pressure release
      ventilation (APRV)
    alveolar ventilation
    artificial ventilation
    assist-control mode ventilation
    assisted ventilation
    bag-and-mask ventilation
    bagged mask ventilation
    bag-valve-mask-assisted
      ventilation
    continuous mandatory
      ventilation (CMV)
    continuous positive pressure
      ventilation (CPPV)
    continuous-flow ventilation
      (CFV)
    control of ventilation
    controlled mechanical
      ventilation (CMV)
    controlled ventilation
    control-mode ventilation
    cuirass ventilation
    difficult ventilation
    emergency ventilation
    extended mandatory minute
      ventilation (EMMV)
    forced mandatory intermittent
      ventilation
    forced ventilation
    hand ventilation
    heart synchronized ventilation
    HFJ ventilation
    high-frequency jet ventilation
      (HFJV)
    high-frequency oscillatory
      ventilation (HFOV)
    high-frequency positive-
      pressure ventilation (HFPPV)
    high-frequency ventilation
      (HFV)
    inspired ventilation (IV)

ventilation (*continued*)
  intermittent demand
    ventilation
  intermittent mandatory
    ventilation (IMV)
  intermittent mechanical
    ventilation
  intermittent positive pressure
    ventilation (IPPV)
  inverse-ratio ventilation
  jet ventilation
  local exhaust ventilation
  low-frequency jet ventilation
  manual ventilation
  maximal voluntary
    ventilation
  maximum voluntary
    ventilation (MVV)
  mechanical ventilation
  mouth-to-mouth ventilation
  neonate ventilation
  noninvasive positive-pressure
    ventilation (NPPV)
  one-lung ventilation (OLV)
  oscillatory ventilation
  partial liquid ventilation
  percutaneous transtracheal
    ventilation (PTV)
  positive-pressure ventilation
    (PPV)
  postoperative ventilation
  pressure control inverse ratio
    ventilation (PCIRV)
  pressure control ventilation
    (PCV)
  pressure support ventilation
    (PSV)
  pressure-controlled inverse
    ratio ventilation (PCIRV)
  pressure-regulated volume
    control ventilation
  prolonged postoperative
    ventilation
  proportional assist
    ventilation
  pulmonary ventilation
  single lung ventilation
  split-lung ventilation
  spontaneous intermittent
    mandatory ventilation
    (SIMV)
  spontaneous ventilation

ventilation (*continued*)
  synchronized intermittent
    mandatory ventilation
    (SIMV)
  synchronized intermittent
    mechanical ventilation
  synchronous intermittent
    mandatory ventilation
    (SIMV)
  time-cycled ventilation
  transtracheal jet ventilation
  triggered ventilation
  ultra-high-frequency
    ventilation
  volume-cycled decelerating-
    flow ventilation
ventilation adapter
ventilation agent
ventilation bronchoscope
ventilation circuit
ventilation collateralization
ventilation defect
ventilation equivalent
ventilation index (VI)
ventilation inserter
ventilation lung scan
ventilation peak pressure
ventilation perfusion scan
ventilation threshold
ventilation tube
ventilation-perfusion abnormality
ventilation-perfusion imaging
ventilation-exchange bougie
ventilation-perfusion defect
ventilation-perfusion lung scan
    (V/Q lung scan)
ventilator (*see also* respirator)
  Aequitron ventilator
  Amadeus ventilator
  Amsterdam ventilator
  Babybird ventilator
  Babyflex ventilator
  Bear adult-volume ventilator
  Bear Cub infant ventilator
  Bennett pressure-cycled
    ventilator
  Bio-Med pediatric ventilator
  Bird ventilator
  Bird pressure-cycled ventilator
  blow-by ventilator
  Bourns infant ventilator
  Bourns-Bear ventilator

ventilator (*continued*)
  Breeze infant ventilator
  Carass ventilator
  CPAP ventilator
  critical care ventilator
  cuirass ventilator
  Drager ventilator
  Emerson postoperative
    ventilator
  Hamilton ventilator
  Healthdyne ventilator
  high frequency oscillatory
    ventilator
  high-frequency jet ventilator
  high-frequency oscillation
    ventilator
  Infant Star high-frequency
    ventilator
  Infrasonics ventilator
  IVAC ventilator
  Lifecare ventilator
  Max ventilator
  mechanical ventilator
  MicroVent ventilator
  Monaghan ventilator
  Morch ventilator
  MVV ventilator
  nebulization ventilator
  Newport ventilator
  Ohio critical care ventilator
  Peep ventilator
  Pneumotron ventilator
  PneuPak ventilator
  Porta-Lung noninvasive
    extrathoracic ventilator
  pressure ventilator
  pressure-cycled ventilator
  pressure-preset ventilator
  Pulmo-Aide ventilator
  Puritan-Bennett ventilator
  Searle volume ventilator
  Sechrist infant ventilator
  Sechrist neonatal ventilator
  Servo ventilator
  Siemens Servo ventilator
  Siemens-Elema Servo ventilator
  Smart Trigger Bear ventilator
  Star ventilator
  TBird ventilator
  Venturi ventilator
  Veolar ventilator
  Vickers Neovent ventilator

ventilator (*continued*)
  VIP Bird neonatal ventilator
  Vix infant ventilator
  volume-limited ventilator
  Wave ventilator
  wean off ventilator
  Yung percutaneous mastoid
    ventilator
ventilator pressure manometer
ventilator-induced lung injury
    (VILI)
ventilatory assistance
ventilatory capacity
ventilatory depression
ventilatory equivalent
venting catheter
venting percutaneous
    gastrostomy
Vent-O-Vac aspirator
vent-plate implant
Ventra catheter
ventral aorta
ventral aspect
ventral bending technique
ventral celiotomy
ventral cleft of thyroid cartilage
ventral column
ventral hernia repair
ventral herniorrhaphy
ventral nerve root
ventral nerve root rhizotomy
ventral root
ventral sacrococcygeal muscle
ventral septal defect
ventral surface
ventral tegmental decussation
Ventric ICP catheter
ventricle
  4th ventricle
  bulb of occipital horn of
    lateral ventricle
  cerebral ventricles
  decannulation of ventricle
  double-outlet right ventricle
  Galen ventricle
  horn of lateral ventricle
  Krause ventricle
  laryngeal ventricle
  lateral ventricle
  left ventricle
  Morgagni ventricle
  posterior vein of left ventricle

ventricle (*continued*)
  right ventricle
  temporal horn of lateral
    ventricle
  terminal ventricle
  Vieussens ventricle
Ventricor pacemaker
ventricular aberration
ventricular aneurysm
ventricular angiogram
ventricular aqueduct
ventricular arrhythmia monitor
ventricular assist device (VAD)
ventricular asynchronous
    pacemaker
ventricular band
ventricular bigeminy
ventricular block
ventricular cannula
ventricular capture
ventricular catheter
ventricular catheter introducer
ventricular contraction
ventricular defect
ventricular demand pacemaker
ventricular demand pulse
    generator
ventricular demand-inhibited
    pacemaker
ventricular demand-triggered
    pacemaker
ventricular depolarization
    abnormality
ventricular dilation
ventricular ejection
ventricular end-diastolic pressure
ventricular endomyocardial
    biopsy
ventricular enlargement
ventricular exclusion
ventricular failure
ventricular fibrillation (V-fib)
ventricular flow tract
ventricular fluid
ventricular flutter
ventricular fold
ventricular ganglion
ventricular heart failure
ventricular hypertrophy
ventricular inflow anomaly
ventricular inflow tract
    obstruction

ventricular laryngocele
ventricular lead
ventricular ligament
ventricular loop
ventricular needle
ventricular outflow tract
ventricular outflow tract
    obstruction
ventricular pacemaker
ventricular perforation
ventricular pressure
ventricular puncture
ventricular rate
ventricular response
ventricular sacculation
ventricular septal defect (VSD)
ventricular septal defect closure
ventricular septal wound defect
ventricular tachycardia
ventricular tap
ventricular trigeminy
ventricular valve
ventricular ventilation tube
ventricular wall
ventricular-suppressed
    pacemaker
ventricular-triggered pacemaker
ventriculoarterial graft
ventriculoatrial shunt
ventriculoatriostomy
ventriculocaval shunt
ventriculocholecystostomy
ventriculocisternal shunt
ventriculocisternostomy
ventriculocordectomy
ventriculogram
ventriculogram retractor
ventriculography
  bubble ventriculography
  cardiac ventriculography
  cerebral ventriculography
ventriculography catheter
ventriculomyocardiotomy
ventriculomyotomy
ventriculoperitoneal shunt (VP
    shunt)
ventriculoperitoneal shunt
    placement
ventriculoperitoneal shunting
    procedure
ventriculoperitoneostomy
ventriculoplasty

ventriculopuncture
ventriculorrhaphy
ventriculoscope
ventriculoscopy
ventriculoseptal defect
ventriculoseptopexy
ventriculoseptoplasty
ventriculostomy
ventriculotomy
ventriculovenostomy
ventriculus (*pl.* ventriculi)
ventrigulography
Ventritex Angstrom implantable
    cardioverter-defibrillator
Ventritex Cadence device
Ventritex generator
Ventrix True Tech ICP catheter
ventrocystorrhaphy
ventrofixation of uterus
ventrohysteropexy
Ventrol Levin tube
ventrolateral hernia
ventrolateral mass
ventroposterolateral (VPL)
ventroposterolateral thalamic
    electrode (VPL thalamic
    electrode)
ventrorostral
ventroscopy
ventrosuspension of uterus
ventrotomy
ventrum penis flap
Ventura spreader
Ventureyra ventricular catheter
Venturi aspiration vitrectomy
    device
Venturi bobbin myringotomy
    tube
Venturi collar-button
    myringotomy tube
Venturi grommet myringotomy
    tube
Venturi insufflator
Venturi mask
Venturi meter
Venturi pediatric myringotomy
    tube
Venturi spirometer
Venturi tube
Venturi ventilation adapter
Venturi ventilator
venular lesion

venule
    high endothelial venule
    main venule (MV)
    nasal venule
    pericytic venules
    postcapillary venules
    temporal venule
venule engorgement
Veolar ventilator
VEP (visual evoked potential)
VER (visual evoked response)
Veraguth fold
Veratex cotton roll
Verbatim balloon catheter
Verbrugge bone clamp
Verbrugge bone-holding clamp
Verbrugge bone-holding forceps
Verbrugge forceps
Verbrugge needle
Verbrugge retractor
Verbrugge-Mueller bone lever
Verbrugge-Souttar craniotome
Verdan graft
Verdan hand procedure
Verdan osteoplastic thumb
    reconstruction
Verdan technique
Verdan tendon repair
Verdi scissors
Veress laparoscopic cannula
Veress needle
Veress peritoneum cannula
Veress pneumoperitoneum
    needle
Veress spring-loaded
    laparoscopy needle
Veress trocar
Veress-Frangenheim needle
Verga lacrimal groove
verge
    anal verge
    nasal verge
    rectal verge
Verhoeff advancement
Verhoeff capsular forceps
Verhoeff cataract forceps
Verhoeff dissecting scissors
Verhoeff expressor
Verhoeff lens expressor
Verhoeff operation
Verhoeff scissors
Verhoeff sclerotomy

Verhoeff suture technique
Verhoeff sutures
Verhoeff-Chandler capsulotomy
Verhoeff-Chandler operation
Veridian umbilical clamp
VeriFlex guidewire
Verifuse ambulatory infusion
   pump
Veripath peripheral guiding
   catheter
Veri-Soft graft
Verlow brace
Vermale amputation
Vermale operation
Verman needle biopsy
vermian fossa
vermicular appendage
vermiculation
vermiculous
vermiform appendage
vermiform appendix
vermiform body
vermiform process
vermifugal
vermilion
   central vermilion
   dry vermilion
   lip vermilion
   wet vermilion
vermilion Abbe flap
vermilion border of lip
vermilion enhancement
vermilion laceration
vermilion margin
vermilion surface of lip
vermilion transitional zone
vermilion zone
vermilionectomy
vermilion-free margin
vermilion-skin junction
vermilion-skin junction tattoo
vermilion-white line
   malalignment
verminous aneurysm
vermis incision
vermis of cerebellum
Vermont spinal fixator
Vermont spinal fixator
   articulation
Verner operation for talipes
   equinovarus
Verner speculum

Verner stripper
Verner-Joel cutter
Verner-Joseph scissors
Verner-Kalinowski speculum
Verner-Smith monitor
Vernet syndrome
Verneuil operation
Vernier calipers
vernix membrane
Vernon antral wash tube
Vernon scissors
Vernon wire cutter
Vernon wire-cutting scissors
Vernon-David operation
Vernon-David proctoscope
Vernon-David rectal speculum
Verocay bodies
VerreScope microlaparoscope
verruca (*pl.* verrucae)
   plantar verruca
   recalcitrant verruca
   seborrheic verruca
verruca acuminata
verruca digitata
verruca filiformis
verruca plana
verruca plana juvenilis
verruca plana senilis
verruca plantaris
verruca senilis
verruca simplex
verruca vulgaris
verrucae (*sing.* verruca)
verruciform leukoplakia
verruciform xanthoma
verruciformis
verrucosa
verrucose
verrucous angiokeratoma
verrucous carcinoma
verrucous hemangioma
verrucous hyperplasia
verrucous lesion
verrucous leukoplakia
verrucous scrofuloderma
verrucous xanthoma
verrucuous carcinoma
Versabond bone cement
VersaClimber exercise machine
Versadopp Doppler probe
Versafil tissue expander
Versaflex steerable catheter

Versaflow pump
Versa-Fx femoral device
Versalok low-back fixation
   device
Versalon all purpose sponge
Versa-PEG gastrostomy kit
Versaport trocar
VersaPulse holmium laser
VersaPulse Select laser
Versatack stapler
VersaTack stapling device
Versatome laser fiber
Versatome laser fiber tube
Versatrac lumbar retractor
Versatrax cardiac pacemaker
Versed anesthesia
Verse-Webster clamp
version
   abdominal version
   bimanual version
   bipolar version
   Braxton Hicks version
   cephalic version
   combined internal and
      external version
   combined version
   Denman spontaneous version
   ductions and versions
   external version
   Hicks version
   internal version
   pelvic version
   podalic version
   postural version
   Potter version
   spontaneous version
   Wigand version
   Wright version
Versi-Splint
Versi-Splint carry bag
vertebra (*pl.* vertebrae)
vertebrae
   Bell-Dally dislocation of first
      cervical vertebra
   cervical vertebrae
   coccygeal vertebrae
   codfish appearance of
      vertebrae
   dorsal vertebrae
   dorsal vertebra
   endplate of vertebrae
   fish vertebrae

vertebrae (*continued*)
   fused vertebrae
   lumbar vertebrae
   olisthetic vertebra
   radix arcus vertebrae
   sacral vertebrae
   scalloping of vertebrae
   spinous process of vertebra
   thoracic vertebrae
   transitional lumbosacral
      vertebra
   transitional vertebra
   wedging of olisthetic vertebra
   wedging of vertebra
vertebra plana fracture
vertebrae cervicales
vertebrae coccygeae
vertebrae lumbales
vertebrae sacrales
vertebrae thoracicae
vertebral angiography
vertebral arch
vertebral arch fusion defect
vertebral arteriogram
vertebral arteriography
vertebral artery
vertebral artery disease
vertebral artery reconstruction
vertebral body biopsy instruments
vertebral body corpectomy
vertebral body decompression
vertebral body fracture
vertebral body impactor
vertebral canal
vertebral column
vertebral compression
vertebral disk
vertebral dissection
vertebral endplate
vertebral epidural space
vertebral epiphysitis
vertebral exposure
vertebral foramen
vertebral fusion
vertebral ganglion
vertebral groove
vertebral interspace
vertebral nerve
vertebral notch
vertebral osteosynthesis fusion
   rate
vertebral outgrowth

vertebral plexus
vertebral prominence
vertebral region
vertebral resection
vertebral ribs
vertebral spine
vertebral spreader
vertebral stable burst fracture
vertebral subluxation complex
vertebral subluxation syndrome
vertebral surface
vertebral vein
vertebral wedge compression
   fracture
vertebral, anus,
      tracheoesophageal, radial,
      and renal anomaly
vertebral body corpectomy
vertebrated catheter
vertebrated probe
vertebrectomy
vertebroarterial foramen
vertebrocostal
vertebrocostal ribs
vertebromammary diameter
vertebrosacral
vertebrosternal ribs
vertex (*pl.* vertices)
vertex of bony cranium
vertex position
vertex presentation
vertical angulation
vertical axis
vertical axis of eye
vertical bipedicle flap
vertical bone loss
vertical bone self-retaining
   retractor
vertical bony height
vertical bur-hole incision
vertical compression
vertical corrugator line
vertical divergence position
vertical dysplasia
vertical elliptical incision
vertical face-lift
vertical facial height
vertical flap
vertical flap pyeloplasty
vertical forceps
vertical fracture
vertical gastric bypass

vertical glabellar crease
vertical glabellar frown lines
vertical groove
vertical incision
vertical lateral glabellar rhytids
vertical lateral parapatellar
   incision
vertical lip biopsy
vertical mammaplasty
vertical mandibular opening
vertical mattress suture technique
vertical mattress sutures
vertical maxillary excess (VME)
vertical midline approach
vertical midline incision
vertical muscle
vertical muscle of tongue
vertical nipple asymmetry
vertical oblique pattern fracture
vertical osteotomy
vertical osteotomy of ramus of
   mandible
vertical overbite
vertical overlap
vertical partial laryngectomy
vertical pedicle technique breast
   reduction
vertical plane
vertical plate of palatine
vertical ramus mandibular
   osteotomy
vertical raphe
vertical rectus plication
vertical resorption
vertical retractor
vertical rhomboid
   deepithelialization
vertical ring curet
vertical ring gastroplasty (VRG)
vertical scar
vertical self-retaining bone
   retractor
vertical shear fracture
vertical Silastic ring gastroplasty
vertical skin excision
vertical sternotomy
vertical suspension reflex
vertical sutures
vertical talus
vertical tooth fracture
vertical tract
vertical tube

vertical uterine incision
vertical-banded gastroplasty
     (VBG)
vertical-cut technique
verticalis linguae muscle
verticality
verticomental
verticosubmental projection
VertiGraft
VertiGraft textured allograft
     bone guidewire
verumontanum
Verwey eyelid operation
vesalian bone
vesalian foramen
vesalian vein
Vesalius bone
Vesalius foramen
Vesalius vein
Vesely nail
Vesely-Street nail
Vesica percutaneous bladder
     neck suspension kit
Vesica Sling Kit
vesical artery
vesical calculus
vesical diverticulectomy
vesical fascia
vesical fistula
vesical gland
vesical hernia
vesical lithotomy
vesical orifice
vesical retinaculum
vesical retractor
Vesicant
vesicle
   Baer vesicle
   chorionic vesicle
   graafian vesicle
   Malpighi vesicles
   matrix vesicles
   membrane-bound electron
      lucent cytoplasmic vesicles
   Naboth vesicles
   ocular vesicle
   olfactory vesicle
   ophthalmic vesicle
   optic vesicle
   prostatic vesicle
   pulmonary vesicles
   seminal vesicles

vesicle (*continued*)
   simple vesicle
   spermatic vesicle
vesicle hernia
vesicoabdominal fistula
vesicoacetabular fistula
vesicoamniotic shunt
vesicobullous lesion
vesicocervical fistula
vesicocervical space
vesicoclysis
vesicocolic fistula
vesicocutaneous fistula
vesicoenteric fistula
vesicofixation
vesicointestinal fistula
vesicointestinal reflex
vesicolithotomy
vesico-ovarian fistula
vesicoperineal fistula
vesicoprostatic calculus
vesicoprostatic plexus
vesicopustular eruption
vesicorectal fistula
vesicosalpingovaginal fistula
vesicosigmoidostomy
vesicospinal center
vesicostomy
vesicotomy
vesicoureteral fistula
vesicoureteral reflux
vesicoureterogram (VCUG)
vesicourethral anastomosis
vesicourethral orifice
vesicourethral suspension
vesicourethroplasty
vesicouterine deflection
vesicouterine excavation
vesicouterine fistula
vesicouterine ligament
vesicouterine peritoneum
vesicouterine pouch
vesicovaginal fascia
vesicovaginal fistula
vesicovaginal lithotomy
vesicovaginal repair
vesicovaginorectal fistula
vesicula (*pl.* vesiculae)
vesicular acute inflammation
vesicular appendage
vesicular dermatitis
vesicular eruption

vesicular granulomatous
   inflammation
vesicular stomatitis
vesiculated
vesiculation
  creeping vesiculation
  intraepidermal vesiculation
  subepidermal vesiculation
vesiculectomy
vesiculiform
vesiculobullous lesion
vesiculography
vesiculopapular
vesiculopustular
vesiculotomy
Vess chair
vessel
  aberrant vessel
  absorbent vessels
  accessory blood vessels
  anastomosis of retinal and
    choroidal vessels
  anastomotic vessel
  angioneurotic edema of vessels
  bifurcation of vessels
  bleeding vessel
  blood vessels
  capillary vessel
  cardinal vessel
  carotid vessel
  choke vessel
  choroidal vessels
  ciliary vessels
  circumflex vessel
  collateral vessel
  constricted blood vessels
  deep epigastric vessels
  dilated vessel
  ectatic vessel
  efferent vessel
  external iliac vessel
  external pudic vessel
  fasciocutaneous vessel
  feeding vessels
  friable vessel
  gastroepiploic vessels
  ghost vessels
  gluteal vessels
  great vessels
  hemorrhoidal vessels
  hyaloid vessel
  hypogastric vessel

vessel (*continued*)
  iliac vessels
  inferior vessels
  intercostal vessels
  interlacing blood vessels
  internal spermatic vessels
  intraepithelial vessels
  ligation of vessels
  lymph vessel
  lymphatic vessels
  mammary vessels
  meningeal vessels
  minor vessel
  mucosal blood vessel
  Mustard transposition of great
    vessels
  narrowed blood vessel
  nutrient vessel
  occluded blood vessel
  occluded intracranial vessel
  omphalomesenteric vessels
  opticociliary vessels
  palatine vessel
  perforator vessel
  periosteal vessel
  peripheral blood vessels
  peroneal vessels
  pudendal vessels
  pudic vessel
  pulmonary vessels
  recipient vessel
  Senning correction of
    transposition of great vessels
  small blood vessel
  spermatic vessel
  subdermal plexus of vessels
  submucosal vessels
  superficial blood vessels
  supporting vessel
  surface vessels
  takeoff of vessel
  tortuosity of vessel
  tortuous vessels
  transposition of great vessels
    (TGV)
  transverse circumflex vessels
  turgescent vessel
  uterine vessels
vessel band
vessel caliber mismatch
vessel clamp
vessel clip

vessel clip-applying forceps
vessel dilator
vessel distention
vessel exposure
vessel forceps
vessel knife
vessel ligation
vessel loop
vessel pediatric forceps
vessel peripheral clamp
vessel peripheral forceps
vessel prosthesis
vessel punch
vessel retractor
vessel-occluding clamp
vessel-sizing catheter
VEST ambulatory ventricular
    function monitor
Vest direct forward-vision
    telescope
Vest lens
vest restraint
Vest technique
Vest telescope
Vest traction sutures
VestaBlate system balloon device
vestibular abscess
vestibular canal
vestibular clamp
vestibular crest
vestibular cyst
vestibular deafferentation
vestibular depth
vestibular disease
vestibular dysfunction
vestibular epithelium
vestibular fissure
vestibular fold
vestibular function
vestibular ganglion
vestibular gland
vestibular labyrinth
vestibular lamina
vestibular ligament
vestibular membrane
vestibular mucosa
vestibular nerve
vestibular oral plate
vestibular osteotomy
vestibular papilla
vestibular region
vestibular saccule

vestibular trough
vestibular veins
vestibular web
vestibular window
vestibule
    buccal vestibule
    bulb of vestibule
    cochlear recess of vestibule
    Gibson vestibule
    labial vestibule
    laryngeal vestibule
    mandibular vestibule
    nasal vestibule
    pyloric vestibule
    Sibson vestibule
    urogenital vestibule
vestibule of cheek
vestibule of inner ear
vestibule of mouth
vestibule of pharynx
vestibule of vagina
vestibulitis
vestibulocochlear artery
vestibulocochlear nerve (cranial
    nerve 8)
vestibulo-infraglottic duct
vestibulo-ocular reflex
vestibuloplasty
vestibulotomy
vestibulum (*pl.* vestibula)
vestibulum glottidis
vestibulum laryngis
vestibulum nasi
vestibulum oris
vestibulum vaginae
vestigial muscle
vestigial nodule
vest-over-pants hernia repair
vest-over-pants herniorrhaphy
vest-over-pants inguinal
    herniorrhaphy
vest-over-pants technique
Vezien abdominal scissors
V-fib (ventricular fibrillation)
VG slit lamp
VIA arterial blood gas and
    chemistry monitor
VIABIL biliary endoprosthesis
viability
    fetal viability
    flap viability
    organ viability

Viadrape drape
Viamonte-Hobbs dye injector
Viamonte-Hobbs electrosurgical
    unit
Viamonte-Hobbs injector
    hydrotherapy
Viamonte-Jutzy electrosurgical
    unit
Viasorb occlusive film dressing
Viasorb wound dressing
Viboch graft retractor
Viboch iliac graft retractor
vibrating line
vibrating scissors
vibration amplification of sound
    energy at resonance
    (VASER) study
vibration disease
vibration syndrome
vibrational angioplasty
vibrator hand syndrome
vibratory hammer
vibratory massage
vibrocardiography
Vibrodilator
Vibrodilator probe
Vicat needle
vice-grip pliers
vicious cicatrix
Vick-Blanchard hemorrhoidal
    forceps
Vickers isolator
Vickers microdensitometer
Vickers microsurgical
    instrument
Vickers needle holder
Vickers ventilator
Vickers ring-tip forceps
Vickers Venti-mask
Vicor pacemaker
Vicq d'Azyr bundle
Vicq d'Azyr operation of larynx
Vicryl mesh
Vicryl pop-off sutures
Vicryl Rapide absorbable
    sutures
Vicryl SH sutures
Vicryl sutures
Victor blood lancet knife
Victor-Bonney forceps
Victoreen digital densitometer
Victoreen dosimeter

Victor-Gomel microsurgical
    tubal reconstruction
Victoria's Secret short incision
    abdominoplasty
Victorian collar dressing
Victorian collar-type dressing
Victory alloy
Vidal device
Vidal operation for varicocele
Vidal-Ardrey fracture technique
Vidal-Ardrey modified Hoffman
    device
Vidal-Hoffman fixator frame
Vidaurri cannula
Vidaurri irrigator
video densitometer
video duodenoscope
video endoscope
video endoscopy
video esophagoscopy
video fluoroscopy
video image colonoscope
video image gastrointestinal scope
video monitor
video otoscope
video processor
video push enteroscope
video small-bowel enteroscopy
video specular microscope
video thoracoscopic drainage
video transurethral resection
    technique
video-assisted excisional biopsy
video-assisted gastrectomy
video-assisted technique
video-assisted thoracic surgical
    procedure
video-assisted thoracoscopic
    surgery (VATS)
video-assisted thorascopic
    surgery (VATS)
video-assisted transsternal
    radical esophagectomy
videoendoscope
    double-channel
        videoendoscope
    fiberoptic videoendoscope
videofluoroscopic technique
videolaparoscopic
    cardiomyotomy
videolaparoscopic guidance
videolaseroscopy

video-rate 2-photon laser
    scanning microscope
videoscopic evaluation
videoscopic fundoplication
videoscopic hernia surgery
videoscopic repair
videostroboscopy
videourodynamic evaluation
vidian artery
vidian canal
vidian nerve
vidian vein
vidianectomy
Vidicon camera tube
Vidicon vacuum chamber
    pickup tube
Vidicon vacuum tube
Vi-Drape bowel bag
Vi-Drape drape
Vi-Drape dressing
Vi-Drape surgical film
Vienna Britetrac nasal speculum
Vienna nasal speculum
Vienna wire sutures
Viers erysiphake
Viers operation
Viers rod
Vieth-Mueller horopter
Vieussens annulus
Vieussens ganglion
Vieussens loop
Vieussens veins
Vieussens ventricle
view
    abdominal view
    anterior view
    anteroposterior x-ray view
    apical lordotic x-ray view
    Arcelin view
    baseline view
    biplane view
    bird's eye view
    Breuerton x-ray view
    buccal view
    Caldwell view
    Carter-Rowe view
    caudocranial hemiaxial view
    caudocranial view
    Chausse view
    chin-nose view
    comparison views
    coned-down view

view (*continued*)
    cone-down view
    craniocaudad views
    craniocaudal views
    cross-sectional view
    dorsal view
    frog-leg view
    frontal view
    gently brought into view
    Granger x-ray view
    Harris-Beath x-ray view
    Hughston view
    incisal quadrant view
    inlet views
    intaglio view
    Judet hip x-ray view
    Judet x-ray view
    jughandle view
    Low-Beer view
    laparoscopic transhiatal view
    laryngoscopic view
    lateral oblique transcranial view
    lateral views
    lateral x-ray view
    long axis view
    lordotic view
    mandibular occlusal view
    maxillary occlusal view
    Mayer view
    mediolateral view
    mortise x-ray view
    oblique spot view
    oblique view
    occipitomeatal view
    occlusal quadrant view
    Owen view
    PA view (posteroanterior view)
    panoramic view
    Panorex view
    pantomographic view
    plain view
    plantar view
    posterior view
    posteroanterior view
    retromammary view
    roentgenographic view
    side view
    skyline view
    spot view
    Stenver view
    stereo views
    submentocervical view

view (*continued*)
  sunrise view
  sunset view
  supine mediolateral view
  swimmer's x-ray view
  tangential view
  Towne x-ray view
  true lateral x-ray view
  tunnel view
  Velpeau axillary view
  von Rosen view
  Waters view
  worm's eye view
  x-ray view
ViewSite video monitor
VigiFoam dressing
vigilance monitoring
Vigilon drain
Vigilon gel dressing
Vigilon primary wound dressing
Vigilon semipermeable
    nonocclusive dressing
Vigilon synthetic occlusive
    dressing
Vigor pacemaker
Viking cannula
Viking II nerve monitoring device
Vilbiss-Miller speculum
Vilex cannulated screw
Vilex plastic surgery instrument
Villalta retractor
Villaret syndrome
Villasensor-Navarro fixation ring
Villasensor ultrasonic pachymeter
villi (*sing.* villus)
  chorionic villi
  duodenal villi
  finger-like villi
  intestinal villi
  jejunal villi
  leaflike villi
  lingual villi
  placental villi
  pleural villi
  ridged-convoluted villi
  synovial villi
  tongue-shaped villi
villoglandular polyp
villoma
villonodular pigmented
    tenosynovitis
villonodular synovitis

villous adenoma
villous duct cancer
villous fold
villous papillae of tongue
villous papilloma
villous polyp
villous tenosynovitis
villous tumor
villus (*pl.* villi)
villusectomy
Vim needle
Vim tonsil syringe
vimentin filament
Vim-Silverman biopsy needle
Vim-Silverman technique for
    liver biopsy
Vimule pessary
VIN (vulvar intraepithelial
    neoplasia)
Vincent angina
Vincent disease
Vincent infection
Vincent stomatitis
Vincent white mycetoma
Vineberg cardiac
    revascularization
Vineberg operation
Vineberg procedure
Vinethene and ether
Vingmed ultrasound
Vinke skull tractor
Vinke tong skull traction
Vinke tong traction
Vinke tongs
vinyl ether anesthetic agent
vinyl ethyl ether anesthetic agent
vinyl ethyl methacrylate
vinyl palatal appliance
vinyl polysiloxane impression
    material
Vioform gauze dressing
violaceous lesion
violin-string adhesions
Viomedex surgical marking pen
VIP Bird neonatal ventilator
VIP chemotherapy pump
Viper PTA catheter
Virag injector
Virag operation
viral arthritis
viral envelope
viral hepatitis

viral infection
viral labyrinthitis
viral sialadenitis
viral vesicular stomatitis
viral wart
ViraType probe
Virchow angle
Virchow brain knife
Virchow cartilage knife
Virchow cells
Virchow chisel
Virchow corpuscles
Virchow crystals
Virchow disease
Virchow law
Virchow metastasis
Virchow node
Virchow sentinel node
Virchow skin graft knife
Virchow space
Virchow-Holder angle
Virchow-Robin space
    dilatation
Virchow-Troisier node
Virden rectal catheter
Virgin hip screw
virgin silk sutures
virginal abdomen
virginal hypertrophy
virginal introitus
virginal membrane
Virginia needle
virilization
Viro-Tec sutures
virtual cautery
virtual colonoscopy
virtual cystoscopy
virtual labor monitor
virtual point
Virtus splinter clamp
Virtus splinter forceps
virucidal agent
virulent appendix
virulent cancer
Visa PTCA catheter
VISA multi-patient monitor
Visatec cystotome
VISC (vitreous infusion suction
    cutter)
viscera (*sing.* Viscus)
    abdominal viscera
    intra-abdominal viscera

viscera (*continued*)
    pelvic viscera
    thoracic viscera
viscera retainer
viscera-holding forceps
visceral anesthesia
visceral angiography
visceral aortography
visceral arteriography
visceral cranium
visceral edema
visceral fascia
visceral forceps
visceral herniation
visceral injury
visceral lamina
visceral layer
visceral lesion
visceral muscle
visceral pain
visceral perfusion
visceral peritoneum
visceral pleura
visceral space
visceral surface
visceral traction reflex
viscerobronchial cardiovascular
    anomaly
viscerocardiac reflex
viscerocranium
visceromotor manifestations
visceromotor reflex
visceroparietal suture
visceroperitoneal
visceropleural
visceroptosis
viscerosensory reflex
viscerotrophic reflex
Vischer lumboiliac incision
viscid secretion
viscidity
Visco surgery
Viscoat
viscoelastic agents
viscoelastic deformation
viscoelastic property of skin
Viscoflow angled cannula
Viscoheel orthosis
Viscoheel prosthesis
Viscoheel SofSpot orthosis
Viscoheel SofSpot prosthesis
Viscolens lens

Viscopaste gauze dressing
viscosimeter
viscosity
Viscospot heel cushion
viscous bile
viscous secretion
viscus (*pl.* viscera)
   abdominal viscus
   abdominopelvic viscus
   hollow viscus
   intraperitoneal viscus
   perforated viscus
   strangulated viscus
viscus injury
viscus perforation
vise forceps
Vishnevskys anesthetic
   technique
VISI (volar intercalated
   segmental instability)
Visi-Black surgical needle
Visicath endoscope
Visicath viewing catheter
Visi-Drape ophthalmic drape
Visiflex drape
VISI-FLOW irrigation starter set
Visijet hydrokeratome
Visilex mesh
Visilex polypropylene mesh
vision
   central vision
   field of vision (FOV)
   finger vision
   foveal vision
   halo vision
   impaired vision
   laparoscopic vision
   monocular vision
   peripheral vision
   scotopic vision
Vision camera
Vision MRI scanner
Vision PTCA catheter
Vision Tech lens
Vision Ten V-scan scanner
Visiport optical trocar
Visiport port
Visi-Spear eye sponge
Visitec angled lens hook
Visitec anterior chamber cannula
Visitec aspiration unit
Visitec cannula

Visitec capsule polisher curet
Visitec circular knife
Visitec lens
Visitec corneal shield
Visitec corneal suture
   manipulating hook
Visitec cortex extractor
Visitec crescent knife
Visitec cystotome
Visitec double iris hook
Visitec double-cutting cystotome
Visitec EdgeAhead knife
Visitec I&A cannula
Visitec iris retractor
Visitec lens pusher
Visitec manipulator
Visitec needle
Visitec nucleus removal loop
Visitec retrobulbar needle
Visitec RK zone marker
Visitec stiletto knife
Visitec straight lens hook
Visitec syringe
Visitec vitrectomy unit
Visi-Tube catheter
Vismark skin marker
visor angle
visor flap
visor flap operation
visor osteotomy
Vista disposable skin stapler
Vista pacemaker
Vista T pacemaker generator
Vistaflex balloon expandable,
   platinum alloy biliary stent
Vistaflex biliary stent
Vistec x-ray detectable sponge
Vistnes applier bar
Vistnes rubber band
visual closure
visual endoscopically controlled
   laser
visual evoked potential (VEP)
visual evoked response (VER)
visual fixation
visual function evaluation
visual hemostatic forceps
visual inspection
visual laser ablation
visual line
visual obturator
visual plane

visual point
visualization
 direct visualization
 double-contrast visualization
 en face visualization
 endoscopic visualization
 fluoroscopic visualization
 laryngoscopic visualization
Visual-Tech machine
Visulas argon C laser
Visulas Nd:YAG laser
Visulas YAG C laser
visuscope
visuscope ophthalmoscope
VISX excimer laser
Vit Commander vitreous cutter
VitaCuff dressing
VitaCuff infection control device
VitaCuff tissue-interface barrier
Vita-Gel acrylic
Vitagraft arteriovenous shunt
Vitagraft vascular graft
vital capacity
Vital Cooley microvascular
 needle holder
Vital French-eye needle holder
Vital general tissue forceps
Vital intestinal forceps
Vital intracardiac needle holder
Vital iris scissors
vital knot
Vital lung-grasping forceps
Vital microsurgery needle
 holder
Vital microvascular needle
 holder
Vital needle holder forceps
Vital neurosurgical needle
 holder
vital organs
Vital Ryder microvascular
 needle holder
Vital scissors
Vital skin stapler
Vital tissue forceps
Vital wire-cutting scissors
Vital Adson tissue forceps
Vital Babcock tissue forceps
Vital Baumgartner needle
 holder
Vital Castroviejo eye needle
 holder

Vital Cooley French-eye needle
 holder
Vital Cooley general tissue
 holder
Vital Cooley intracardiac needle
 holder
Vital Cooley neurosurgical
 needle holder
Vital Cooley operating scissors
Vital Cooley wire-cutting
 scissors
Vitalcor cardioplegia infusion
 cannula
Vitalcor venous return catheter
Vital Cottle dorsal angled
 scissors
Vital Crile-Wood needle holder
Vital Cushing tissue forceps
Vital DeBakey cardiovascular
 needle holder
Vital Derf eye needle holder
Vital Duval intestinal forceps
Vital Evans pelvic tissue forceps
Vital Finochietto needle holder
Vital Fomon angular scissors
Vital Halsey eye-needle holder
Vital Heaney needle holder
Vital Jacobson spring-handled
 needle holder
Vital Julian needle holder
Vital Kalt eye needle holder
Vital Knapp iris scissors
Vital Knapp strabismus scissors
Vitallium alloy cobalt-chrome
 prosthesis
Vitallium cap
Vitallium clip
Vitallium cup
Vitallium device
Vitallium drill
Vitallium Elliott knee plate
Vitallium eye implant
Vitallium graft
Vitallium Hicks radius plate
Vitallium hip prosthesis
Vitallium implant
Vitallium implant material
Vitallium mesh
Vitallium miniplate
Vitallium Moore self-locking
 prosthesis
Vitallium nail

Vitallium plate
Vitallium prosthesis
Vitallium screw
Vitallium Wainwright blade plate
Vitallium Walldius mechanical
    knee plate
Vital Masson needle holder
Vital Mayo dissecting scissors
Vital Mayo-Hegar needle holder
Vital Metzenbaum dissecting
    scissors
Vital Mills vascular needle
    holder
Vital Neivert needle holder
Vital Nelson dissecting scissors
Vital New Orleans needle holder
Vitalock cluster acetabular
    component
Vitalock solid-back acetabular
    component
Vitalock talon acetabular
    component
Vital Olsen-Hegar needle holder
Vital Potts-Smith forceps
Vital Rochester needle holder
Vital Ryder needle holder
Vital Sarot needle holder
Vital Stratte needle holder
Vital Wangensteen needle holder
Vital Wangensteen tissue forceps
Vital Webster needle holder
Vita-Stat automatic device
Vitatrax II pacemaker
Vitatron catheter electrode
Vitatron Diamond pacemaker
Vitatron catheter
Vitatron Jade pacemaker
Vitatron Legacy pacemaker
Vitatron Ruby pacemaker
Vitatron Topaz pacemaker
Vitax female catheter
Vitek fibrin sealant
Vitek interpositional implant
vitelline circulation
vitelline duct anomaly
vitelline fistula
vitelline membrane
vitelline vein
vitellointestinal cyst
Vitesse laser catheter
Vitesse coronary catheter
vitiligines

vitiliginous
Vitox femoral head
Vitrasert intraocular implant
Vitrathene jacket
vitreal hemorrhage
vitreal membrane
vitrectomy
    anterior vitrectomy
    closed vitrectomy
    open-sky vitrectomy
    posterior vitrectomy
vitrectomy sponge
vitrectomy tip
vitrector
    Alcon vitrector
    catheter vitrector
    Cilco vitrector
    CooperVision vitrector
    Frigitronics vitrector
    Kaufman vitrector
    Machemer VISC vitrector
    mechanical vitrector
    Microvit vitrector
    ocutome vitrector
    O'Malley vitrector
    Peeler-Cutter vitrector
    Peyman vitrector
    Storz vitrector
vitrector probe
vitrector tip
Vitremer glass-ionomer
    restorative material
vitreolenticular
vitreophage
vitreoretinal infusion cutter
vitreoretinal surgery
vitreoretinal traction syndrome
vitreoretinopathy
vitreous abscess
vitreous aspiration
vitreous base
vitreous body
vitreous breakthrough
    hemorrhage
vitreous cavity
vitreous chamber
vitreous detachment
vitreous floater
vitreous fluff
vitreous fluid
vitreous foreign body
vitreous hemorrhage

vitreous hernia
vitreous herniation
vitreous humor
vitreous infusion suction cutter (VISC)
vitreous knife
vitreous membrane
vitreous opacity
vitreous ossification
vitreous pencil
vitreous space
vitreous strand scissors
vitreous surgery
vitreous sweep spatula
vitreous transplant needle
vitreous-aspirating cannula
vitreous-aspirating needle
vitreous-grasping forceps
Vivalith II pulse generator
Vivalith-10 pacemaker
Vivatron pacemaker
vivo
Vivonex gastrostomy tube
Vivonex jejunostomy catheter
Vivonex Moss tube
Vivosil graft
Vivosil implant
Vivosil prosthesis
Vix infant ventilator
Vladimiroff (also Wladimiroff)
Vladimiroff operation
Vladimiroff tarsectomy
Vladimiroff-Mikulicz amputation
V-lance blade
V-lance eye knife
VLAP (visual laser ablation of the prostate)
V-Lok disposable blood pressure cuff
V-medullary nail
VMO (vastus medialis obliquus)
VNO (vomeronasal organ)
VNUS catheter
vocal cord injection
vocal cord medialization
vocal cordectomy
vocal cordotomy
vocal cords
vocal dysfunction
vocal fold approximation
vocal fold fixation therapy
vocal ligament

vocal muscle
vocal process
vocalis muscle
VoCoM thyroplasty implant
Voda catheter
Vogel adenoid curet
Vogel infant adenoid curet
Vogel nephropexy
Vogel operation
Vogel otoplasty
Vogel-Bale-Hohner head holder
Vogelfanger blood vessel stapler
Vogelfanger-Beattie stapler
Vogler hysterectomy forceps
Vogt angle
Vogt cataract
Vogt cephalodactyly
Vogt forceps
Vogt operation
Vogt point
Vogt toothed capsular forceps
Vogt-Barraquer corneal needle
Vogt-Barraquer eye needle
Vogt-Hueter point
voice box
voice button
voice intensity controller
voice prosthesis
voice restoration
voiding cystogram
voiding cystourethrogram (VCUG)
voiding flow rate
volar angulation deformity
volar artery
volar aspect
volar beak ligament
volar beak of the metacarpal
volar carpal ligament
volar epineurolysis
volar finger approach
volar flap advancement
volar intercalated segmental instability (VISI)
volar interosseous fascia
volar ligament
volar midline approach
volar midline oblique incision
volar pad
volar plate arthroplasty

volar plate arthroplasty
    technique fracture-
    dislocation
volar plate deficiency
volar plate injury
volar plate repair
volar radial approach
volar radiocarpal ligament
volar regions of fingers
volar regions of hand
volar semilunar wrist dislocation
volar shelf arthroplasty
volar splint
volar surface
volar tissue flap
volar transverse incision
volar ulnar approach
volar zigzag finger incision
volarward approach
volatile anesthesia
volatile anesthetic
volition oral movement
Volk conoid implant
Volk conoid lens
Volk conoid ophthalmic lens
Volk fundal lens
Volk high-resolution aspherical
    lens
Volk Minus noncontact adapter
Volk PanRetinal lens
Volk Plus noncontact adapter
Volk retinal scale adapter
Volk aspherical lens
Volkmann bone curet
Volkmann bone hook
Volkmann canal
Volkmann cheilitis
Volkmann claw hand deformity
Volkmann contracture
Volkmann curet
Volkmann finger retractor
Volkmann fracture
Volkmann hand retractor
Volkmann ischemic contracture
Volkmann ischemic paralysis
Volkmann membrane
Volkmann operation for hydrocele
Volkmann oval curet
Volkmann pancreatic calculus
    spoon
Volkmann pocket retractor
Volkmann rake

Volkmann rake retractor
Volkmann retractor
Volkmann splint
Volkmann spoon
Volkmann subluxation
Volkmann vas hook
Voller curet
volsellum (see vulsellum)
voltage clamp
Voltolini ear tube
Voltolini nasal speculum
Voltolini septum speculum
Voltolini tube
Voltz wrist joint prosthesis
volume
    abdominal volume
    biopsy volume
    bony volume
    breast volume
    circulating blood volume
    circulation volume
    corpuscular volume
    end-diastolic volume
    end-systolic volume
    flow volume
    fluid volume
    forced expiratory volume
    gas volume
    gland volume
    injection volume
    intrathoracic gas volume
    least-wrinkled fill volume
    packed cell volume
    residual volume
    target volume
    tidal volume
    total blood volume
    urinary volume
volume expansion
volume reduction surgery (VRS)
volume-cycled decelerating-flow
    ventilation
volume-deficient face
volume-limited ventilator
volumetric fat reduction
volumetric infusion pump
volumetric pump
volumetric solution
volumetric technique
voluminous hernia
voluntary control
voluntary guarding

voluntary movement
voluntary muscle
voluntary voiding
Voluson sector transducer
volvulus
  cecal volvulus
  colonic volvulus
  gastric volvulus
  Noble procedure for volvulus
  reduction of volvulus
  sigmoid volvulus
volvulus reduction
Volz arthroplasty
Volz elbow hinge
Volz total elbow
Volz-Turner reattachment
  technique
vomer bone
vomer flap
vomer forceps
vomer mucosa
vomer osteotome
vomer septal forceps
vomeral groove
vomeral sulcus
vomerine canal
vomerine cartilage
vomerine gouge
vomerine groove
vomerine ridge
vomerine spur
vomerobasilar canal
vomeronasal cartilage
vomeronasal organ (VNO)
vomeropremaxillary crest
vomerorostral canal
vomerosphenoidal articulation
vomerovaginal canal
vomerovaginal groove
vomerovaginal sulcus
Von Ammon operation
Von Andel biliary dilation
  catheter
Von Andel dilation catheter
von Bergmann hernia
von Bergmann operation
von Bezold abscess
von Blaskovics-Doyen operation
von Brum flap
von Brunn membrane
von Brunn nests in bladder
  carcinoma

von Burow operation
von Ebner glands
von Ebner line
von Economo disease
Von Eichen antral cannula
Von Eichen antral tube
Von Eichen antral wash tube
von Gies joint
von Graefe (*see* Graefe)
von Haberer gastrectomy
von Haberer gastroenterostomy
von Haberer-Aquirre
  gastrectomy
von Haberer-Finney gastrectomy
  technique
von Haberer-Finney anastomosis
von Haberer-Finney gastrectomy
von Haberer-Finney
  gastroenterostomy
von Hackler operation
Von Hippel (*see* Hippel)
von Ihring plane
von Kraske operation
Von Lackum surcingle
Von Lackum transection shift
  jacket brace
von Langenbeck bipedicle
  mucoperiosteal flap
von Langenbeck cleft lip repair
von Langenbeck incision
von Langenbeck method repair
von Langenbeck operation
von Langenbeck palatal flap
von Langenbeck palate closure
von Langenbeck pedicle flap
von Langenbeck periosteal
  elevator
von Langenbeck periosteal
  repair
Von Mandach capsule fragment
  forceps
Von Mandach clot forceps
von Meyenburg disease
Von Noorden flap
Von Noorden incision
von Petz clip
von Petz forceps
von Petz intestinal clamp
von Petz staple
von Petz stomach clamp
von Pirquet sutures
von Recklinghausen disease

von Rosen hip splint
von Rosen view for determining
   hip dislocation
von Saal medullary pin
von Seemen rongeur
von Spee curve
von Willebrandt knee
Voorhees bag
Voorhees needle
Voris intervertebral disk rongeur
Voris IV disk rongeur
Voris-Oldberg intervertebral disk
   forceps
Voris-Oldberg IV disk rongeur
   forceps
Voris-Wester forceps
Voronoff operation
Vorse occluding clamp
Vorse tube-occluding clamp
Vorse tube-occluding forceps
Vorse-Webster forceps
Vorse-Webster tube-occluding
   clamp
Vortex Clear-Flow port
Vortex router
Vortex tracheostomy tube
Vortex tracheotomy tube
vortex vein
VortX vascular occlusion coil
Voshell bursa
Voss hanging-hip operation
Vossius lenticular ring
Vostal radial fracture
   classification
Voyager Aortic IntraClusion
   device
Vozzle Vacu-Irrigator
VP shunt (ventriculoperitoneal
   shunt)
VPC (velopharyngeal
   competence)
VPGSS (venous pressure
   gradient support stockings)
VPI (velopharyngeal
   incompetence)
VPI (velopharyngeal
   insufficiency)
VPI nonadhesive condom
   catheter
VPI nonadhesive pouch
VPI stone basket
VPI urinary leg bag

VPI-Ambrose resectoscope
   forceps
VPI-Jacobellis microhematuria
   catheter set
VPL (ventroposterolateral)
VPL thalamic electrode
   (ventroposterolateral
   thalamic electrode)
VRG (vertical ring gastroplasty)
VSD (ventricular septal defect)
V-shaped erosion
V-shaped incision
V-shaped scar
V-shaped skin excision
V-shaped ulcer
V-shaped wound
V-sign
V-slit lamp
VSP plate
V-sutures
V-tach (ventricular tachycardia)
V-to-Y fashion closure
V-type intertrochanteric plate
Vueport balloon-occlusion
   catheter
Vueport balloon-occlusion
   guiding catheter
vulcanite bur
vulcanite chisel
vulcanite dental plate
vulcanization
Vulpius operation
Vulpius procedure
Vulpius-Compere operation
Vulpius-Compere procedure for
   tight heel cords
Vulpius-Stoffel procedure
vulsella (*sing.* vulsellum)
vulsella forceps
vulsellum (*pl.* vulsella) (*see also*
   forceps)
   Bland cervical traction
      vulsellum
   Donald vulsellum
   Fenton bulldog vulsellum
   Skene uterine vulsellum
vulsellum clamp
vulsellum forceps
vulva
vulvar adenoid cystic
   adenocarcinoma
vulvar biopsy

W arch
W procedure
W. D. Johnson epicardial
    retractor
W.W. Walker appliance
Woelfe (*see* Wolfe)
Woelfler (*see* Wolfler)
Wolfe (*also* Wölfe, Woelfe)
Wölfe (*see* Wolfe)
Wolfe-Bohler cast remover
Wolfe-Bohler plaster cast
    spreader
Wolfe-Boehler cast breaker
Wolfe-Boehler cutter
Wolfler (*also* Wölfler, Woelfer)
Wölfler (*see* Wolfler)
Wolfler gastroenterostomy
Wolfler gland
Wolfler operation
Wolfler sign
Wolfler suture technique
Wolfler sutures
Wotzer (*also* Wötzer, Woetzer)
Wötzer (*see* Wotzer)
Wotzer operation
Woetzer (*see* Wotzer)
Waardenburg syndrome
Waardenburg-Klein syndrome
W-abdominoplasty
Wachendorf membrane
Wachenheim-Reder sign
Wachsberger bur
Wachtenfeldt butterfly clip
Wachtenfeldt clip-applying
    forceps
Wachtenfeldt clip-removing
    forceps
Wachtenfeldt suture clip
Wachtenfeldt wound clip
Wachtenfeldt-Stille retractor
Wackenheim clivus line
Wacker Sil-Gel silicone
    cement

Wada hingeless heart valve
    prosthesis
Wada monocuspid tilting-disk
    heart valve
Wada valve prosthesis
Wada-Cutter disk prosthetic
    valve
Wadia elevator
Wadsworth elbow approach
Wadsworth hinge
Wadsworth lid clamp
Wadsworth lid forceps
Wadsworth posterolateral
    approach
Wadsworth scissors
Wadsworth technique
Wadsworth-Todd electrocautery
Wadsworth-Todd eye cautery
Waffle seating cushion
Wagener ear hook
Wagener punch tip
Wagner advancement
Wagner antral punch
Wagner bone lever
Wagner classification
Wagner disease
Wagner external fixator
Wagner fracture reduction
Wagner hammer
Wagner hand operation
Wagner knife
Wagner laryngeal brush
Wagner leg-lengthening
    distraction device
Wagner leg-lengthening device
Wagner limb-lengthening
    technique
Wagner modification of Syme
    amputation
Wagner needle holder
Wagner open reduction
    technique
Wagner operation

Wagner procedure to correct
  leg length discrepancy
Wagner punch
Wagner reduction technique
Wagner resurface prosthesis
Wagner resurfacing technique
Wagner rongeur
Wagner skin incision
Wagner skull resection
Wagner tibial lengthening
  procedure
Wagner 2-stage Syme
  amputation
Wagner-Baldwin technique
wagon wheel fracture
Wagoner approach
Wagoner cervical technique
Wagoner operation
Wagoner osteotomy
Wagoner posterior approach
Wagstaffe fracture
Wainstock eye suturing forceps
Wainwright osteotomy plate
waisting of nerve contour
WAK (wearable artificial kidney)
Wakai spreader
Wakeling fetal heart monitor
Walb knife
Walcher position
Waldeau fixation forceps
Waldem-Marshall curved
  dissecting scissors
Walden-Aufricht nasal retractor
Waldenstrom (*also* Waldenström,
  Waldenstroem)
Waldenström (*see* Waldenstrom)
Waldenstroem (*see*
  Waldenstrom)
Waldenstrom laryngeal forceps
Waldeyer colon
Waldeyer fascia
Waldeyer fluid
Waldeyer forceps
Waldeyer fossa
Waldeyer glands
Waldeyer ring
Waldeyer ring lesion
Waldeyer well-circumscribed
  lesion
Waldeyer space
Waldeyer sulcus
Waldeyer throat ring

Waldeyer tonsillar ring
Waldhausen procedure
Waldhausen subclavian flap
  repair of coarctation of
  aorta
Waldhausen subclavian flap
  technique
Wales rectal bougie
Wales rectal dilator
Walker articulator
Walker aspirator
Walker cautery
Walker coagulating electrode
Walker coagulator
Walker corneal trephine
Walker curet
Walker dissector
Walker electrode
Walker elevator
Walker everter
Walker forceps
Walker gallbladder retractor
Walker hollow quill pin
Walker lid everter
Walker lid retractor
Walker magnet
Walker needle
Walker pin
Walker retractor
Walker ring curet
Walker ruptured-disk curet
Walker scissors
Walker scleral ruler
Walker submucous elevator
Walker suction tonsillar
  dissector
Walker tonsil dissector
Walker tonsil suction dissector
Walker tonsillar needle
Walker trephine
Walker ureteral meatotomy
  electrode
Walker-Apple corneal scissors
Walker-Atkinson corneal scissors
Walker-Lee eye knife
Walker-Lee sclerotome
Walker-Murdock wrist sign
walking calipers
walking epidural anesthetic
walking heel cast
Walkmann episiotomy
  scissors

wall
  abdominal wall
  adipose layers of anterior
    abdominal wall
  anterior abdominal wall
  anterior wall
  aortic wall
  bladder wall
  bowel wall
  burying of fimbriae in uterine
    wall
  cavity wall
  chest wall
  cyst wall
  depressed chest wall
  duct wall
  fibromuscular walls
  gallbladder wall
  hardening of artery walls
  inferior wall
  infratemporal wall
  interior chest wall
  jugular wall
  lateral wall
  mastoid wall
  medial wall
  membranous wall
  midabdominal wall
  muscular wall
  musculofascial wall
  pelvic wall
  pharyngeal wall
  posterior abdominal wall
  posterior wall
  prolapsed vaginal wall
  relaxed anterior wall
  stomach wall
  sutures attached to arterial wall
  tegmental wall
  thoracic wall
  tracheal wall
  urethral wall
  uterine wall
  vaginal wall
  variceal wall
  ventricular wall
wall push maneuver
Wallace cesarean forceps
Wallace Flexihub central venous
    pressure cannula
Wallace rule of nines
Wallace technique

Wallace-Maloney knife
Wallach colposcope
Wallach Colpostat-V6
Wallach cryosurgical pencil
Wallach Endocell device
Wallach freezer cryosurgical
    device
Wallach cryosurgical instrument
Wallach pencil
Wallach pencil cryosurgical
    device
Wallach surgical devices
Wallach ZoomScope colposcope
Wallach ZoomStar colposcope
Wallach-Papette disposable
    cervical cell collector
Walldius knee arthroplasty
Walldius knee prosthesis
Walldius total knee prosthesis
Walldius Vitallium mechanical
    knee prosthesis
Wallenberg syndrome
wallerian degeneration
Wallgraft endoprosthesis
Wallich curet
Wallner interstitial prostate
    implanter
Wallstent biliary endoprosthesis
Wallstent delivery device
Wallstent esophageal prosthesis
Wallstent expanding metallic
    stent
Wallstent iliac endoprosthesis
Wallstent carotid stent
Wallstent spring-loaded stent
Wal-Pil-O neck pillow
Walser corneoscleral punch
Walser matrix
Walsh chisel
Walsh dermal curet
Walsh footplate chisel
Walsh hook
Walsh hook-type dermal
    curet
Walsh pressure ring
Walsh procedure
Walsh tissue forceps
Walsham nasal forceps
Walsham septal forceps
Walsham septum-straightening
    forceps
Walsham straightener

Walsh-Ogura orbital
  decompression
Walter corneal spud
Walter forceps
Walter nasal retractor
Walter Reed classification for
  HIV infection
Walter Reed implant
Walter Reed operation
Walter splinter forceps
Walter spud
Walter-Deaver retractor
Walter-Poole suction tube
Walter-Yankauer suction tube
Waltham-Street bougie
Walthardt operation
Walther aspirating bladder trocar
Walther canal
Walther catheter
Walther dilator
Walther duct
Walther female catheter
Walther fracture
Walther ganglion
Walther kidney pedicle clamp
Walther pedicle clamp
Walther sound
Walther tissue forceps
Walther trocar
Walther urethral dilator
Walther urethral sound
Walther-Crenshaw meatal clamp
Walther-Crenshaw meatus clamp
Walton comedo extractor
Walton corneoscleral punch
Walton curet
Walton ear knife
Walton extractor
Walton foreign body gouge
Walton gouge
Walton knife
Walton meniscal clamp
Walton meniscal forceps
Walton meniscus clamp
Walton punch
Walton rib shears
Walton rongeur
Walton round gouge spud
Walton scissors
Walton speculum
Walton-Allis tissue forceps
Walton-Liston bone rongeur

Walton-Liston forceps
Walton-Pederson speculum
Walton-Ruskin bone rongeur
Walton-Schubert punch
Walton-Schubert uterine biopsy
  forceps
Walton-Vienna speculum
waltzed flap
waltzed skin flap
Walzl hysterectomy forceps
Wamarline wrist splint
wandering abscess
wandering atrial pacemaker
  (WAP)
wandering gallbladder
wandering heart
wandering kidney
wandering liver
wandering of disarticulated
  components
wandering ovary
wandering pacemaker
Wang applicator
Wang lens
Wang needle
Wang-Binford edge detector
Wangensteen anastomosis clamp
Wangensteen awl
Wangensteen carrier
Wangensteen clamp
Wangensteen colostomy
Wangensteen deep ligature
  carrier
Wangensteen dissector
Wangensteen drain
Wangensteen drainage
Wangensteen dressing
Wangensteen duodenal tube
Wangensteen gastric-crushing
  anastomotic clamp
Wangensteen herniorrhaphy
Wangensteen internal
  decompression trocar
Wangensteen intestinal forceps
Wangensteen intestinal needle
Wangensteen ligature carrier
Wangensteen needle
Wangensteen needle holder
Wangensteen operation
Wangensteen patent ductus
  clamp
Wangensteen retractor

Wangensteen suction
Wangensteen suction tube
Wangensteen suction unit
Wangensteen tissue forceps
Wangensteen tissue inverter
Wangensteen trocar
Wangensteen tube
Wangensteen-Vital needle holder
Wanger reduction technique
waning chest pain
Wannagat injection needle
Wannagat suction tube
WAP (wandering atrial
    pacemaker)
Wappler bridge
Wappler cold cautery
Wappler cystoscope
Wappler cystoscope with
    microlens optics
Wappler electrode
Wappler microlens
    cystourethroscope
Wappler polypectomy snare
Ward elevator
Ward French needle
Ward French-eye needle
Ward nasal chisel
Ward nasal osteotome
Ward periosteal elevator
Ward triangle on pelvic x-ray
Ward-French needle
Ward-Hendrick incision
Wardill palatoplasty
Wardill pharyngoplasty
Wardill technique
Wardill-Kilner cleft palate repair
Wardill-Kilner 4-flap uranoplasty
Wardill-Kilner operation
Wardill-Kilner procedure
Wardill-Kilner V-Y palatal repair
Wardill-Kilner-Veau operation
Ward-Lempert lens
Ward-Lempert lens loupe
Ward-Mayo operation
Ward-Mayo vaginal hysterectomy
Ware cancer cell collector
Waring tonsil suction tube
Warm Springs brace
Warne penile sheath
Warner-Farber ankle fixation
    technique
Warner-Farber operation

warning stop tube
Warren flap
Warren incision
Warren operation
Warren splenorenal shunt
Warren-Mack rotating drill
Warren-Wilder retriever
Warsaw hip prosthesis
wart
    acuminate wart
    common wart
    electrodesiccation of wart
    filiform wart
    flat wart
    Hassall-Henle wart
    intra-anal wart
    mucocutaneous wart
    penile wart
    perianal wart
    periungual wart
    plantar wart
    rectal warts
    senile wart
    soft wart
    telangiectatic wart
    venereal wart
    viral wart
Wartenberg neurological
    hammer
Wartenberg pinwheel
Wartenberg sign
Wartenberg symptom
Wartenberg syndrome
Warthin clamp
Warthin crusher
Warthin forceps
Warthin spur crusher
Warthin spur-crushing clamp
Warthin area
Warthin sign
Warthin tumor
wart-like excrescence
warty cicatricial tumor
warty dyskeratoma
warty horn
warty ulcer
Warwick-Ashken technique
Warwick James elevator
wash catheter
wash impression material
wash technique
wash tube

washed clot
washed intrauterine
    insemination
washed-field technique
washer crimper
washer holder
WasherLoc implant
washer-sterilizer
washing catheter
washing tube
washings
    bronchial washings
    gastric washings
    Gravlee washings
    lung washings
    multiple washings
    nasal washings
    pelvic washings
    segmental washings
    throat washings
    urinary washings
Washington regimen
Washio skin flap
washout cannula
washout pyelography
Wasko common duct probe
Wasmann gland
wasp-waist laryngoscope
Wassel classification of thumb
    polydactyly
Wassel thumb duplication
Wassel thumb duplication
    classification
Wassmund procedure
Watanabe arthroscope
Watanabe arthroscopy
Watanabe catheter
Watanabe discoid meniscus
    classification
Watanabe pin
Watanabe pin holder
Watanabe pin remover
watchmaker forceps
Watco knee immobilizer
Water cesarean section
water cushion lithotriptor
water cystometer
water density line
water dissection
water dressing
water fissures in lens
water gauge

Water Pik irrigator
water probe
water scalpel
water vapor monitoring
water vapor transmission rates
    (WVTRs)
waterfall deformity
Waterfield needle
water-filled balloon sheath
Waterhouse transpubic
    procedure
Waterhouse urethroplasty
water-infusion esophageal
    manometry catheter
watering-can scrotum
Waterlase Millennium laser
Waterman folding bronchoscope
Waterman rib contractor
Waterman sump drain
water-perfused catheter
Waters extraoral radiography
Waters muscle stimulator
Waters operation
Waters position
Waters view of sinuses
Waters view radiograph
Waters view roentgenogram
Waters x-ray position
water-seal chest tube
water-seal drain
water-seal drainage
water-soluble contrast
    esophagogram
Waterston extrapericardial
    anastomosis
Waterston groove
Waterston operation
Waterston pacing wire
Waterston shunt
Waterston-Cooley procedure
Waterston-Cooley shunt
water-suppression technique
Waters-Waldron position
watertight closure
watertight seal
watertight skin closure
Watkins fusion technique
Watkins operation
Watkins spinal fusion
Watkins suction tube
Watkins transposition operation
    for uterine prolapse

Watkins-Wertheim operation
Watson capsule biopsy
Watson duckbill forceps
Watson heart valve holder
Watson operation
Watson scaphoid shift test
Watson
    scaphotrapeziotrapezoidal
    fusion
Watson skin-grafting knife
Watson speculum
Watson technique
Watson tonsil-seizing forceps
Watson-Cheyne dry dissector
Watson-Cheyne technique
Watson-Cheyne wedge
    resection
Watson-Jones ankle procedure
Watson-Jones anterior approach
Watson-Jones arthrodesis
Watson-Jones bone gouge
Watson-Jones bone lever
Watson-Jones dressing
Watson-Jones elevator
Watson-Jones fracture repair
Watson-Jones frame
Watson-Jones gouge
Watson-Jones guide pin
Watson-Jones incision
Watson-Jones lateral approach
Watson-Jones ligament
    reconstruction
Watson-Jones nail
Watson-Jones operation
Watson-Jones procedure
Watson-Jones reconstruction
Watson-Jones repair of ankle
    fracture
Watson-Jones tibial fracture
    classification
Watson-Jones tibial tubercle
    avulsion fracture
    classification
Watson-Jones traction
Watson-Jones tractor
Watson-Williams conchotome
Watson-Williams ethmoidal
    punch
Watson-Williams ethmoid-biting
    forceps
Watson-Williams frontal sinus
    rasp

Watson-Williams intervertebral
    disk rongeur
Watson-Williams nasal forceps
Watson-Williams nasal polypus
Watson-Williams nasal punch
Watson-Williams needle
Watson-Williams polyp forceps
Watson-Williams punch tip
Watson-Williams rasp
Watson-Williams rongeur
Watson-Williams sinus rasp
Watson-Williams sinus raspatory
Watt skin closure stapler
wattled submental region
Watts locking clamp
Watts tenaculum
Watzke band
Watzke cuff
Watzke forceps
Watzke operation
Watzke scissors
Watzke self-holding sleeve
    operation
Watzke Silicone sleeve
Watzke tube
Waugh ankle prosthesis
Waugh dissection forceps
Waugh dressing forceps
Waugh knee prosthesis
Waugh operation
Waugh prosthesis
Waugh tissue forceps
Waugh-Brophy forceps
Waugh-Clagett
    pancreaticoduodenostomy
wave guide catheter
Wave ventilator
wave-edge knife
wave-tooth forceps
WaveWire guidewire
wax bougie
wax curet
wax expansion
wax pack
wax pattern thermal expansion
    technique
waxlike rigidity
waxlike secretion
wax-matrix technique
wax-removing spatula
wax-tipped bougie
waxy cast

waxy exudate
waxy finger
waxy kidney
Way operation
Wayfarer prosthesis
Wayne laminectomy seat
Wayne U-crimper
wearable artificial kidney
wearable cardioverter-
    defibrillator device
Weary brain spatula
Weary nerve hook
Weary nerve hook retractor
Weary nerve root retractor
Weary patch graft
Weary spatula
Weaveknit vascular graft
Weavenit implant
Weavenit patch graft
Weavenit valve prosthesis
Weavenit vascular prosthesis
Weaver chalazion clamp
Weaver chalazion curet
Weaver chalazion forceps
Weaver sinus probe
Weaver trocar introducer
Weaver-Dunn acromioclavicular
    technique
Weaver-Dunn procedure
Weaver-Dunn repair of
    acromioclavicular separation
Weaver-Dunn resection
Weaver-Dunn technique
web
    duodenal web
    esophageal web
    hepatic web
    intestinal web
    laryngeal web
    myringeal web
    postcricoid web
    subsynaptic web
    terminal web
    thenar web
    tracheal web
    venous web
    vestibular web
web creep
web formation
web ligament
Web needle holder
web of fingers

web of larynx
web space
web space deepening
web space flap
web space incision
Webb bolt
Webb bolt nail
Webb cannula
Webb interchangeable stripper
Webb pin
Webb retractor
Webb stove bolt
Webb stove nail
Webb vein stripper
Webb-Balfour abdominal
    retractor
Webb-Balfour self-retaining
    abdominal retractor
Webb-Balfour self-retaining
    retractor
webbed fingers
webbed toes
Weber aortic clamp
Weber canaliculus knife
Weber catheter
Weber classification of fractures
Weber Cockayne syndrome
Weber colonic insufflator
Weber douche
Weber eye knife
Weber gland
Weber hip implant
Weber insufflator
Weber iris knife
Weber nasal douche
Weber physical injury
    classification
Weber point
Weber procedure
Weber rectal catheter
Weber retractor
Weber sign
Weber tissue scissors
Weber winged catheter
Weber-Brunner-Freuler open
    reduction
Weber-Christian disease
Weber-Danis ankle injury
    classification
Weber-Elschnig lens
Weber-Elschnig lens loupe
Weber-Elschnig lens spoon

Weber-Fergusson incision
Weber-Fergusson procedure
Weber-Fergusson-Longmire
  incision
Weber-Vasey traction-absorption
  wiring technique
Webril bandage
Webril dressing
Webril immobilization
web-spacer
Webster abdominal retractor
Webster cheiloplasty
Webster coronary sinus catheter
Webster flap
Webster infusion cannula
Webster infusion tube
Webster knife
Webster line
Webster meniscectomy scissors
Webster modification of
  Bernard-Burow cheiloplasty
Webster needle holder
Webster operation
Webster orthogonal electrode
  catheter
Webster retractor
Webster ruler
Webster skin graft knife
Webster skin lines
Webster tube
Webster-Halsey needle holder
Webster-Kleinert needle holder
Webster-Vital needle holder
Wechsler obstetrical
  stethoscope
Weck astigmatism ruler
Weck ceiling-mount operating
  microscope
Weck clamp
Weck clip
Weck clip applier
Weck coagulating suction tube
Weck dermatome
Weck disposable cannula
Weck disposable trocar
Weck electrosurgery pencil
Weck endoscopic suture punch
Weck eye shield
Weck hemoclip
Weck hysterectomy forceps
Weck instrument holder
Weck iris scissors

Weck knife
Weck microscope
Weck microsurgical tray
Weck operating microscope
Weck rectal biopsy forceps
Weck shears
Weck sponge
Weck stapler
Weck suction tube
Weck suture scissors
Weck suture-removal scissors
Weck towel forceps
Weck trephine
Weck tube
Weck uterine biopsy forceps
Weck wire-cutting scissors
Weck-blade knife
Weck-cel dressing
Weck-cel graft
Weck-cel implant
Weck-cel microsponge
Weck-cel operating microscope
Weck-cel prosthesis
Weck-cel sponge
Weck-cel surgical spear sponge
Weck-Edna nonperforating
  towel clamp
Wecker iris spatula
Wecker silver spatula
Weckesser technique
Weck-Harms forceps
Weck-Prep blade
Weck-Prep razor
Weck-sorb airwick sponge
Weck-Spencer suture scissors
weddellite calculus
Wedelstaedt chisel
Weder dissector
Weder retractor
Weder tongue depressor
Weder-Solenberger tonsil pillar
  retractor
Weder-Solenberger tonsillar
  retractor
wedge adjustable cushioned
  heel (WACH)
wedge arteriogram
wedge biopsy
wedge catheter
wedge colon resection
wedge compression
  fracture

Wedge electrosurgical resection
   device
wedge elevator
wedge excision
wedge excisional biopsy
wedge filter
wedge fracture
wedge graft
wedge heel
wedge hepatectomy
wedge hepatic biopsy
wedge incision
wedge liver biopsy
wedge of skin
wedge of tissue
wedge ostectomy
wedge osteotomy
wedge pressure
wedge pressure balloon catheter
wedge resection
wedge resection clamp
wedge-and-groove joint
wedge-line needle
wedge-shaped sleeve
   aneurysmal resection
wedge-shaped support
wedge-shaped uncomminuted
   fragment
wedge-shaped uncomminuted
   tibial plateau fracture
wedging of olisthetic vertebra
wedging of vertebra
weekend facelift
Weeker operation
Weeks eye forceps
Weeks eye speculum
Weeks needle
Weeks operation
Weeks speculum
weeping lesion
Weerda distending operating
   laryngoscope
Weerda endoscope
Wegener granulomatosis
Wegner line
Wehbe arm holder
Wehrbein hypospadias repair
Wehrbein urethroplasty
Wehrbein-Smith hypospadias
   repair
Wehrs incus prosthesis
Weiger-Zollner forceps

weight reduction surgery
weight-activated locking knee
weightbearing
   complete weightbearing
   full weightbearing (FWB)
   gradual weightbearing
   partial weightbearing (PWB)
weightbearing brace
weight-bearing tissue
weighted glove
weighted obstetrical speculum
weighted posterior retractor
weighted radiograph
weighted retractor
weighted speculum
weighted tip
weighted vaginal speculum
weight-reduction operation
weight-relieving orthosis
Weil basal layer
Weil basal zone
Weil cannula
Weil ear forceps
Weil ethmoidal forceps
Weil implant
Weil lacrimal cannula
Weil pelvic sling
Weil pelvic snare
Weil pituitary rongeur
Weil rongeur
Weil sling
Weil splint
Weiland classification
Weiland iliac crest bone graft
Weil-Blakesley conchotome
Weil-Blakesley ethmoidal
   forceps
Weil-Blakesley intervertebral
   disk rongeur
Weil-modified Swanson implant
Weimert epistaxis packing
Weinberg blade
Weinberg Joe's hoe double-
   ended retractor
Weinberg modification of
   pyloroplasty
Weinberg operation
Weinberg pediatric rib spreader
Weinberg pyloroplasty
Weinberg retractor
Weinberg rib spreader
Weinberg spreader

Weinberg vagotomy retractor
Weine technique
Weiner cannula
Weiner operation
Weiner speculum
Weiner tourniquet
Weiner uterine biopsy forceps
Weingartner ear forceps
Weingartner rongeur
Weinstein horizontal retractor
Weinstein intestinal retractor
Weinstein-Ponseti technique
Weir appendectomy
Weir excision
Weir incision
Weir operation
Weir pattern skin flap
Weir pattern skin flap technique
Weir resection of the alar base
Weir wedge
Weir-pattern skin flap technique
Weis chalazion forceps
Weis operation
Weisbach angle
Weisenbach forceps
Weisenbach sterile forceps
   holder
Weisinger operation
Weisman cannula
Weisman ear curet
Weisman infant ear curet
Weisman tenaculum
Weisman uterine tenaculum
   forceps
Weisman-Graves open-sided
   vaginal speculum
Weisman-Graves vaginal
   speculum
Weiss eye knife
Weiss forceps
Weiss gold dilator
Weiss hook
Weiss needle
Weiss procedure
Weiss speculum
Weiss spring
Weissbarth vaginal speculum
Weissman classification
Weiss-pattern knife
Weitbrecht cartilage
Weitbrecht ligament
Weitlaner brain retractor

Weitlaner hemostat
Weitlaner hinged retractor
Weitlaner microsurgery retractor
Weitlaner self-retaining retractor
Weitter plaster knife
Welch Allyn anal biopsy forceps
Welch Allyn anoscope
Welch Allyn battery handle
Welch Allyn cord handle
Welch Allyn dual-purpose
   otoscope
Welch Allyn flexible
   sigmoidoscope
Welch Allyn forceps
Welch Allyn halogen penlight
Welch Allyn hook
Welch Allyn illuminated
   speculum
Welch Allyn instrument
Welch Allyn Kleenspec
   laryngoscope
Welch Allyn KleenSpec vaginal
   speculum
Welch Allyn laryngoscope
Welch Allyn laryngoscope blade
Welch Allyn LumiView portable
   binocular microscope
Welch Allyn operating otoscope
Welch Allyn ophthalmoscope
Welch Allyn probe
Welch Allyn proctoscope
Welch Allyn rectal probe
Welch Allyn retinoscope
Welch Allyn sigmoidoscope
Welch Allyn single fiber
   illumination headlight
Welch Allyn speculum
Welch Allyn standard
   retinoscope
Welch Allyn streak retinoscope
Welch Allyn suction tube
Welch Allyn transilluminator
Welch Allyn tube
Welch Allyn video colonoscope
Welch Allyn video endoscope
Welch technique
Welcker angle
Weldon miniature bulldog clamp
well-aerated lungs
Wellaminski antral perforator
well-circumscribed lesion
well-compensated

well-controlled
well-defined
well-demarcated margin
well-demarcated scar
well-developed
well-differentiated adenoma
well-differentiated carcinoma
well-epithelialized
Weller cartilage forceps
Weller cartilage scissors
Weller dissecting scissors
Weller meniscal forceps
Weller total hip joint prosthesis
Wellington Hospital vaginal
  retractor
Wellington Hospital vaginal
  speculum
well-leg cast
well-leg holder
well-leg raising test
well-leg splint
well-leg support
well-leg traction
well-localized adenoma
Wells cannula
Wells clamp
Wells enucleation scissors
Wells enucleation scoop
Wells enucleation spoon
Wells eye spatula
Wells eye spoon
Wells forceps
Wells irrigator
Wells Johnson cannula
Wells pedicle clamp
Wells pick
Wells posterior rectopexy
Wells rectopexy
Wells scleral suture pick
Wells scoop
Wells spoon
Wells tractor
Wells-Gardner tongs
Wellwood-Ferguson introducer
Welsh cortex extractor
Welsh cortex-stripper cannula
Welsh erysiphake
Welsh flat olive-tipped double
  cannula
Welsh iris retractor
Welsh olive-tipped needles
Welsh ophthalmic forceps

Welsh ophthalmological forceps
Welsh pupil spreader-retractor
  forceps
Welsh pupil-spreader forceps
Welsh rubber bulb erysiphake
Welsh Silastic erysiphake
Welt bronchoscopic treatment
  unit
Welt bronchoscopic unit
Wenckebach block
Wenckebach disease
Wendell Hughes operation
Wendl tube
Wenger slotted plate
Wepfer gland
Wepsic fiberoptic cautery
Wepsic suction tube
Werb operation
Werb rhinostomy scissors
Werb right-angle probe
Werdnig-Hoffmann disease
Wergeland double cannula
Wergeland double needle
Wermer syndrome
Wernekinck decussation
Werner sutures
Werner syndrome
Wernicke area of brain
Wernicke disease
Wernicke sign
Wertheim clamp
Wertheim deep-surgery scissors
Wertheim forceps
Wertheim hysterectomy
Wertheim hysterectomy forceps
Wertheim kidney pedicle clamp
Wertheim needle holder
Wertheim operation
Wertheim splint
Wertheim uterine forceps
Wertheim vaginal forceps
Wertheim-Bohlman technique
Wertheim-Cullen clamp
Wertheim-Cullen compression
  forceps
Wertheim-Cullen hysterectomy
  forceps
Wertheim-Cullen kidney pedicle
  clamp
Wertheim-Cullen kidney pedicle
  forceps
Wertheim-Cullen pedicle clamp

Wertheim-Cullen pedicle
    forceps
Wertheim-Navratil forceps
Wertheim-Navratil needle
Wertheim-Reverdin clamp
Wertheim-Reverdin pedicle
    clamp
Wertheim-Schauta operation
Wertheim-Taussig operation
Werther disease
Wescott stitch scissors
Wesenberg-Hamazaki body
Weser dental hinge
Wesley Jessen lens
Wesolowski bifurcation
    replacement
Wesolowski bypass graft
Wesolowski Dacron tube
Wesolowski prosthesis
Wesolowski Teflon graft
Wesolowski vascular graft
Wesolowski vascular prosthesis
Wesolowski Weavenit vascular
    prosthesis
Wessex prosthetic valve
Wesson mouth gag
Wesson perineal retractor
Wesson perineal self-retaining
    retractor
Wesson vaginal retractor
West blunt dissector
West blunt elevator
West bone chisel
West bone gouge
West cannula
West chisel
West gouge
West hand dissector
West lacrimal cannula
West lacrimal chisel
West lacuna skull
West nasal chisel
West nasal gouge
West nasal-dressing forceps
West operation
West osteotome
West patellectomy
West plastic dissector
West Point view of shoulder on
    x-ray
West Shur cartilage clamp
West tube

Westaby stent
West-Beck periosteotome
West-Beck spoon curet
Westberg space
Westcott biopsy needle
Westcott conjunctival scissors
Westcott double-end scissors
Westcott microscissors
Westcott spring-action scissors
Westcott stitch scissors
Westcott tenotomy scissors
Westcott utility scissors
Westcott-Scheie scissors
West-Engstler skull
Wester meniscal clamp
Wester meniscectomy scissors
Westerman-Jensen needle
Westermark uterine dressing
    forceps
Westermark-Stille forceps
western boot in open fracture
Western external urinary
    catheter
Westfield-style acromioclavicular
    immobilizer
Westin-Hall incision
Westlake bull's eye bulb
Westmacott dressing forceps
Weston rectal snare
Westphal gall duct forceps
Westphal hemostat
Westphal hemostatic forceps
Westphal sign
West-Soto-Hall knee
    procedure
West-Soto-Hall patellar
    technique
wet bandage
wet colostomy
wet compress
wet dressing
wet gangrene
wet lap sponge
wet leather sign
wet line of the lip
wet lung
wet pack
wet packing
wet reading of x-ray
wet smear
wet technique
wet technique liposuction

wet technique with liposuction
     breast reduction
wet vermilion
wet-field cautery
wet-field coagulator
wet-field electrocautery
wet-field eraser cautery
wet-sheet pack
wet-to-dry dressing
Wetzel grid
Weve electrode
Weve operation
Wexler abdominal retractor
Wexler Bantam self-retaining
     retractor
Wexler catheter
Wexler deep-spreader blade
     abdominal retractor
Wexler large-frame abdominal
     retractor
Wexler lateral side-blade
     abdominal retractor
Wexler malleable-blade
     abdominal retractor
Wexler self-retaining retractor
Wexler Universal joint
     abdominal retractor
Wexler vaginal retractor
Wexler large abdominal
     retractor
Wexler-Balfour retractor
Wexler-Bantam retractor
Wexteel scissors
Wextran sponge
Weyers syndrome
Weyers-Fulling syndrome
Weyers-Thier syndrome
whalebone eustachian bougie
whalebone eustachian probe
whalebone filiform bougie
whalebone filiform catheter
Wharton construction of
     artificial vagina
Wharton duct
Wharton operation
Wharton tumor
Wharton-Jones operation
Wharton-Jones V-Y operation
wheal-and-flare reaction
Wheaton brace
Wheaton Pavlik harness brace
Wheaton tissue homogenizer

wheel bur
wheelchair cushion
wheelchair pad
Wheeler blade
Wheeler cyclodialysis spatula
Wheeler cystoscope
Wheeler cystotome
Wheeler discission knife
Wheeler eye implant
Wheeler eye sphere
Wheeler graft
Wheeler graft material
Wheeler halving procedure
Wheeler halving repair
Wheeler implant
Wheeler incision
Wheeler iris knife
Wheeler iris spatula
Wheeler malleable-shape knife
Wheeler operation
Wheeler plaque forceps
Wheeler procedure
Wheeler prosthesis
Wheeler spatula
Wheeler sphere eye implant
Wheeler spherical eye implant
Wheeler vessel forceps
Wheeler-Reese operation
Wheelhouse operation
Whelan-Moss T-tube
W-hernia
whewellite calculus
Whip appliance
whip bougie
Whip-Mix articulator
Whipple incision
Whipple operation
Whipple pancreatectomy
Whipple
     pancreaticoduodenectomy
Whipple
     pancreaticoduodenostomy
Whipple
     pancreatoduodenectomy
Whipple procedure
Whipple resection
Whipple triad
whipstitch suture technique
whipstitch sutures
whirlybird excavator
whirlybird knife
whirlybird needle

whirlybird probe
whirlybird stapes excavator
whisk-packets dressing
Whisper guidewire
whistle bougie
whistle stent
Whistler bougie
whistle-tip catheter
whistle-tip drain
whistle-tip Foley catheter
whistle-tip ureteral catheter
whistling face syndrome
whistling rales
Whitacre operation
Whitacre spinal needle
Whitaker malar sizer
Whitcomb-Kerrison
    laminectomy punch
Whitcomb-Kerrison
    laminectomy rongeur
White bone chisel
white braided silk sutures
white braided sutures
White chisel
White clamp
White classification
white dural fold
white fat
white fibers
white fibrocartilage
white fixation
White foam pessary
White forceps
white gangrene
White glaucoma pump shunt
white graft rejection
white hairy tongue
White hammer
white lesion
white line of Toldt
White mallet
White mastoid rongeur
white matter
white nylon sutures
White operation
White Plume absorbent gauze
White posterior ankle fusion
White procedure to shorten
    femur
white roll-flare vermilion border
White scissors
White screwdriver

white silk sutures
White slide procedure
white sutures
White tenaculum
White tonsil forceps
White tonsil hemostat forceps
White tonsil-seizing forceps
white twisted sutures
white-centered hemorrhage
Whitecloud-LaRocca fibular strut
    graft
white-graft reaction
Whitehead classification
Whitehead deformity
Whitehead mouth gag
Whitehead operation
Whitehead-Jennings mouth gag
White-Lillie retractor
White-Lillie tonsil forceps
Whitelite transilluminator
White-Oslay forceps
White-Oslay prostatic forceps
White-Oslay prostatic lobe-
    holding forceps
White-Proud uvular retractor
Whiteside total hip prosthesis
Whitesides-Kelly cervical
    technique
White-Smith forceps
Whiting mastoid curet
Whiting mastoid rongeur
Whiting tonsillectome
whitlow
    herpetic whitlow
    melanotic whitlow
    thecal whitlow
Whitman arch support
Whitman arthroplasty
Whitman astragalectomy
Whitman femoral neck
    reconstruction
Whitman fracture appliance
Whitman fracture frame
Whitman frame
Whitman operation
Whitman osteotomy
Whitman plate
Whitman procedure for long
    thoracic nerve palsy
Whitman talectomy procedure
Whitman technique
Whitman-Thompson procedure

Whitmore bag
Whitmore-Jewett classification for
    staging of prostate cancer
Whitnall ligament
Whitnall sling operation
Whitnall tubercle of zygoma
Whitney single-use plastic curet
Whitney superior rectus forceps
Whittle spud
Whitver penile clamp
Whitzel tunnel
WHO (wrist-hand orthosis)
whole abdominopelvic
    irradiation
whole blood lysis technique
whole body irradiation
whole bone transplant graft
whole brain irradiation
whole lobar graft
whole pelvis radiation
whole-abdomen irradiation
whole arm fusion
whole body counter
whole body digital scanner
whole body extract
whole brain radiation therapy
whole face injection approach
whole gut irrigation
whole pelvis irradiation
Wholey balloon occlusion
    catheter
Wholey guidewire
Wholey Hi-Torque floppy
    guidewire
Wholey Hi-Torque modified
    J-guidewire
Wholey Hi-Torque standard
    guidewire
Wholey wire
Wholey-Edwards catheter
whorled cells
whorled collagen fibers
Wiberg fracture staple
Wiberg fracture stapler
Wiberg patellar classification
Wiberg raspatory
Wiberg shelf procedure
Wicherkiewicz eyelid repair
Wicherkiewicz operation
Wichman retractor
wick dressing
Wickham striae

Wickham technique
Wickham-Miller triradiate
    optical kidney stone
    grasper
Wickman uterine forceps
Wickstrom wrist arthrodesis
Wickwitz esophageal stricture
wide debridement
wide decompression
wide elliptical anastomosis
wide excision
wide field
wide local excision
wide mucosa-to-mucosa Roux-en-Y
    hepaticojejunostomy
wide plane
wide resection biopsy
wide sigmoid sinus
wide skin incision
wide-angle glaucoma
Wideband urinary catheter
wide-field eyepiece
wide-field radiation therapy
wide-field total laryngectomy
widely patent orifice
wide-mouth sac
widened retrogastric space
widening of abdominal aorta
widening of suture lines
wide-open anastomosis
wide-range radiation therapy
wide-seal diaphragm
wide-set breast cleavage
Widia needle holder
Widman flap
Wid-Med resectoscope
Widner transilluminator
Wiechel scissors
Wiechel-Stille bile duct scissors
Wieder decompressor
Wieder dental retractor
Wieder dissector
Wieder pillar retractor
Wieder tonsillar dissector
Wieder-Solenberger pillar
    retractor
Wieger ligament
Wiegerinck culdocentesis
    puncture set
Wiener antral rasp
Wiener antral raspatory
Wiener breast reduction

Wiener corneal hook
Wiener eye knife
Wiener eye needle
Wiener eye speculum
Wiener eyelid repair
Wiener gold plate
Wiener hysterectomy forceps
Wiener keratome
Wiener MRI filter
Wiener nasal rasp
Wiener operation
Wiener rasp
Wiener scleral hook
Wiener speculum
Wiener suture hook
Wiener Universal frontal sinus
    rasp
Wiener Universal frontal sinus
    raspatory
Wiener-Pierce antral rasp
Wiener-Pierce antral trocar
Wiener-Pierce trocar
Wiener-Sauer intranasal tear-sac
    operation instruments
Wies chalazion forceps
Wies entropion excision
Wies entropion incision
Wies forceps
Wies operation
Wies procedure
Wiet graft-measuring instrument
Wiet otologic cup forceps
Wiet otologic scissors
Wiet retractor
Wigand endoscopic instrument
Wigand maneuver
Wigand version
Wigby-Taylor position
Wigderson ribbon retractor
Wigmore plaster saw
Wikco ankle machine
Wikstrom (also Wiström and
    Wikstroem)
Wikström (see Wikstrom)
Wikstrom artery forceps
Wikstrom gallbladder clamp
Wikstroem (see Wikstrom)
Wikström gallbladder clamp
Wikström-Stilgust clamp
Wiktor balloon-expandable
    coronary stent
Wiktor coronary stent

Wild laser
Wild lens
Wild operating microscope
Wild surgical microscope
Wildcat wire
Wilde ear forceps
Wilde ear polyp snare
Wilde ear speculum
Wilde ethmoidal exenteration
    forceps
Wilde ethmoidal forceps
Wilde ethmoidal punch
Wilde incision
Wilde intervertebral disk
    forceps
Wilde intervertebral disk
    rongeur
Wilde laminectomy forceps
Wilde nasal punch
Wilde nasal snare
Wilde nasal-cutting forceps
Wilde nasal-dressing forceps
Wilde septal forceps
Wilde-Blakesley ethmoidal
    forceps
Wilde-Blakesley scissors
Wilde-Bruening ear snare
Wilde-Bruening nasal snare
Wilder band spreader
Wilder cystitome knife
Wilder cystoscope
Wilder cystotome
Wilder dilating forceps
Wilder dilator
Wilder eye knife
Wilder foreign body hook
Wilder lacrimal dilator
Wilder lens hook
Wilder lens loupe
Wilder lens scoop
Wilder pick
Wilder retractor
Wilder scleral depressor
Wilder scleral self-retaining
    retractor
Wilder scoop
Wilder sign
Wilder trephine
Wildermuth ear
Wildervanck syndrome
Wildervanck-Smith syndrome
Wilde-Troeltsch forceps

Wildgen-Reck localizer
Wildgen-Reck metal locator
  magnet
Wildhirt laparoscope
Wiles prosthesis
Wilhelm cystoscope
Wilkadium alloy
Wilke boot
Wilke boot brace
Wilke boot prosthesis
Wilkerson choanal bur
Wilkerson intraocular lens-
  insertion forceps
Wilkes self-retaining retractor
Wilkin classification of radial
  neck fractures
Wilkins radial fracture
  classification
Wilkins trephine
Wilkinson abdominal retractor
Wilkinson abdominal self-
  retaining retractor
Wilkinson operation
Wilkinson ring frame abdominal
  retractor
Wilkinson self-retaining
  abdominal retractor
Wilkinson-Deaver blade
  abdominal retractor
Wilkoro alloy
Willauer intrathoracic forceps
Willauer raspatory
Willauer scissors
Willauer thoracic scissors
Willauer-Allis thoracic forceps
Willauer-Allis thoracic tissue
  forceps
Willauer-Allis tissue forceps
Willauer-Deaver retractor
Willauer-Gibbon periosteal
  elevator
Willett clamp
Willett placenta previa forceps
Willett placental forceps
Willett scalp flap forceps
Willi glass crown technique
William Harvey arterial blood
  filter
William Harvey cardiotomy
  reservoir
William microlumbar disk
  excision

Williams back brace
Williams cardiac device
Williams cartilage knife
Williams clamp
Williams colpopoiesis
Williams craniotome
Williams cystoscopic needle
Williams dilator
Williams diskectomy
Williams diskectomy forceps
Williams ear perforator
Williams esophageal tube
Williams eye speculum
Williams gastrointestinal forceps
Williams interlocking Y nail
Williams internal pelvimeter
Williams intestinal forceps
Williams lacrimal dilator
Williams lacrimal probe
Williams guiding catheter
Williams lumbosacral orthosis
Williams microclip
Williams microlumbar retractor
Williams microsurgery saw
Williams operation
Williams orthosis
Williams overtube sleeve
Williams pelvimeter
Williams perforator
Williams position
Williams probe
Williams procedure
Williams rod
Williams rod self-retaining
  retractor
Williams screwdriver
Williams sign
Williams speculum
Williams splinter forceps
Williams tissue forceps
Williams tonsil electrode
Williams tonsillar electrode
Williams tracheal tone
Williams leg holder
Williams uterine forceps
Williams vessel-holding forceps
Williams vulvovaginoplasty
Williamsburg forceps
Williams-Haddad procedure
Williams-Haddad technique
Williamson biopsy needle
Williamson-Noble scissors

Williams-Richardson operation
Williams-Watson ethmoidal
    punch
Williger bone curet
Williger ear curet
Williger elevator
Williger hammer
Williger raspatory
Williger separator
Willis antrum
Willis circle
Willis pancreas
Willis pouch
Willis retractor
willow fracture
Wills eye lacrimal retractor
Wills eye spatula and spoon
Wills Hospital eye cautery
Wills Hospital ophthalmic
    forceps
Wills Hospital ophthalmology
    forceps
Wills Hospital utility forceps
Wills utility forceps
Willstein diamond bur
Willy Meyer mastectomy
    incision
Willy Meyer radical mastectomy
Wilmer chisel
Wilmer conjunctival and utility
    scissors
Wilmer conjunctival scissors
Wilmer cryosurgical iris
    retractor
Wilmer iris forceps
Wilmer iris retractor
Wilmer iris scissors
Wilmer operation
Wilmer refractor
Wilmer retractor
Wilmer wedge chisel
Wilmer-Bagley iris expressor
Wilmer-Bagley lens expressor
Wilmer-Bagley retractor
Wilmer-Converse conjunctival
    scissors
Wilms amputation
Wilms operation
Wilms tumor
Wilson amniotic perforator
Wilson amniotic trocar
Wilson ankle fusion

Wilson approach
Wilson arthrodesis
Wilson awl
Wilson Bimetric arch
Wilson bolt
Wilson bone graft
Wilson bunionectomy
Wilson chamber
Wilson clamp
Wilson fracture
Wilson fracture appliance
Wilson frame
Wilson graft
Wilson intraocular scissors
Wilson knee test
Wilson leads
Wilson muscle
Wilson operation
Wilson plate
Wilson procedure
Wilson retractor
Wilson rib spreader
Wilson right-angled awl
Wilson spinal frame
Wilson spinal fusion plate
Wilson splint
Wilson spreader
Wilson stripper
Wilson technique
Wilson trocar
Wilson vein stripper
Wilson vitreous foreign body
    forceps
Wilson wrench
Wilson-Baylor amniotic trocar
Wilson-Cook biopsy forceps
Wilson-Cook bronchoscope
    biopsy forceps
Wilson-Cook Carey capsule set
Wilson-Cook catheter
Wilson-Cook coagulation
    electrode
Wilson-Cook colonoscope
    biopsy forceps
Wilson-Cook dilating balloon
Wilson-Cook double-channel
    sphincterotome
Wilson-Cook 8-wire basket stone
    extractor
Wilson-Cook electrode
    needle
Wilson-Cook endoprosthesis

Wilson-Cook esophageal balloon prosthesis
Wilson-Cook feeding tube
Wilson-Cook feeding tube kit
Wilson-Cook fine-needle-aspiration catheter
Wilson-Cook French stent
Wilson-Cook gastric balloon
Wilson-Cook gastroscope biopsy forceps
Wilson-Cook grasping forceps
Wilson-Cook hot biopsy forceps
Wilson-Cook low-profile esophageal prosthesis set
Wilson-Cook mechanical lithotriptor
Wilson-Cook minibasket
Wilson-Cook ministent retriever
Wilson-Cook nasobiliary tube
Wilson-Cook papillotome
Wilson-Cook plastic prosthesis
Wilson-Cook polypectomy snare
Wilson-Cook Protector guidewire
Wilson-Cook retrieval forceps
Wilson-Cook standard wire guide
Wilson-Cook stone basket
Wilson-Cook Tracer guidewire
Wilson-Cook tripod retrieval forceps
Wilson-Cook wire-guided sphincterotome
Wilson-Jacobs patellar graft
Wilson-Jacobs procedure
Wilson-Jacobs tibial fracture fixation technique
Wilson-Jones patellar operation
Wilson-Jones procedure
Wilson-Kirbe speculum
Wilson-McKeever arthroplasty
Wilson-McKeever procedure
Wilson-McKeever shoulder procedure
Wilson-McKeever shoulder technique
Wiltberger anterior cervical approach
Wiltberger fusion
Wiltberger spinous process spreader
Wiltberger spreader
Wiltek papillotome

Wilton-Webster coronary sinus catheter
Wilton-Webster coronary sinus thermodilution catheter
Wilton-Webster thermodilution flow and pacing catheter
Wiltse bilateral lateral fusion
Wiltse iliac retractor
Wiltse rod
Wiltse system spinal rod
Wiltse-Bankart retractor
Wiltse-Gelpi self-retaining retractor
WinABP ambulatory blood pressure monitor
Winberger line on x-ray
Winchester syndrome
Wincor enucleation scissors
windblown deformity
windblown hand
Windmill suction evacuation unit
window
   acoustic window
   aortic pulmonary window
   aortic window
   aorticopulmonary window
   aortopulmonary window
   bone window
   Lieberman sigmoidoscope with swinging window
   nasoantral window
   oval window
   pleuropericardial window
   Rebuck window
   round window
   sigmoidoscope with swinging window
   skin window
   soft tissue window
   vestibular window
window clip
window operation
window rasp
window rasp marker
window technique
windowed esophageal balloon
windowing of cortex
windshield wiper sign
windsock deformity
Windson-Insall-Vince bone graft
Windson-Insall-Vince grafting technique

Winer catheter
wing clip
wing of scapula
wing plate
wing sutures
winged catheter
winged retractor blade
winged scapula
winged shunt
winged speculum
winged steel needle
winged V double flap
winged V-flap operation
Wingfield fracture frame
Winiwarter
  cholecystoenterostomy
Winiwarter operation
Winiwarter-Buerger disease
Winkelmann hydrocele repair
Winkelmann circumcision
  clamp
winking patella
Winkler body
Winkler disease
Winograd ingrown nail
  procedure
Winograd nail plate removal
Winograd procedure
Winograd technique
Winquist femoral shaft fracture
  classification
Winquist-Hansen femoral
  fracture classification
Winsburg-White bladder tube
Winsburg-White retractor
Winslow foramen
Winslow ligament
Winslow pancreas
Winston cervical clamp
Winston catheter
Winter anterior osteotomy
Winter arch bar
Winter classification
Winter convex fusion
Winter elevation torque
  technique
Winter elevator
Winter facial fracture appliance
Winter ovum forceps
Winter placental forceps
Winter procedure
Winter shunt

Winter splint
Winter spondylolisthesis
  technique
Winter syndrome
Winter-Eber resectoscope
Winter-Nassauer placental
  forceps
Winternitz sound
Winters shunt
wire (*see also* guidewire)
  ACS exchange wire
  ACS gold-standard wire
  ACS microglide wire
  Amplatz torque wire
  Ancrofil clasp wire
  arch wire
  atrial pacing wire
  auger wire
  Australian orthodontic wire
  Australian Special Plus wire
  Babcock stainless steel suture
    wire
  Babcock stainless suture wire
  Babcock suture wire
  Baron suction tube-cleaning
    wire
  bayonet-point wire
  beaded cerclage wire
  beaded guidewire
  Beath guidewire
  Bentson exchange straight
    guidewire
  Bentson wire
  Birtcher Hyfrecator cautery
    guidewire
  Birtcher Hyfrecator cautery
    wire
  bone fixation wire
  braided wire
  brass wire
  Brooker wire
  buddy wire
  Bunnell pull-out wire
  catheter forming wires
  central core wire
  cerclage wire
  cesium-137 wire
  Charnley trochanter wire
  circumcoronal wire
  circumdential wire
  closer wire
  Coffin transpalatal wire

wire (*continued*)

coiled spiral pusher wire
Cole pull-out wire
Commander PTCA wire
Compere fixation wire
continuous loop wire
control wire
Cope wire
Cordis Stabilizer marker wire
coronary wire
Cragg Convertible wire
Cragg infusion wire
crenulated tantalum wire
crimped wire
crimper wire
Crozat orthodontic wire
curved J-exchange wire
cut snare wire
Dall-Miles cerclage wire
delivery wire
Dentaflex wire
diathermy wire
dock wire
docking wire
double keyhole loop wire
double-woven wire
Drummond wire
ear cut snare wire
ear snare wire
Eder-Puestow wire
eel wire
endocardial wire
epicardial pacing wire
Eve-Neivert tonsillar wire
extra-stiff Amplatz wire
Fegerstra wire
flexible steerable wire
Force wire
forming wires
Geenan Endotorque wire
Gigli spiral saw wire
Gigli-saw wire
Gilmer wire
Hahnenkratt orthodontic wire
Hancock temporary cardiac
   pacing wire
high-torque wire
hinged-loop snare wire
Hi-Per Flex exchange wire
House piston wire
Ideal arch wire
insertion of wire

wire (*continued*)

interdental wire
intermaxillary wire
interosseous wire
intracoronary Doppler flow
   wire
intramedullary wire
intraoral wire
intravascular Doppler-tipped
   guidewire
Isola wire
Isotac pilot wire
Ivy wire
J exchange wire
Jagwire wire
Jarabak arch wire
J-guidewire
Johnson canaliculus wire
J-tip guidewire
J-tip wire
J-tipped wire
J-wire
K wire
Katzen infusion wire
Kazanjian wire
Killip wire
Kirschner boring wire
Kirschner wire (K-wire)
labial wire
Lassoe wire
ligature tie wire
ligature wire
lingual wire
Linx extension wire
Lunderquist coat hanger wire
Lunderquist wire
Lunderquist working wire
Lunderquist nephrostomy
   wire
Luque cerclage wire
Luque sublaminar wire
magnet wire
Markley orthodontic wire
measuring wire
Micro-Glide exchange wire
monofilament snare wire
monofilament stainless steel
   wire
Mullan wire
multifilament wire
nasal snare wire
needle-knife wire

wire (*continued*)

    Neivert-Eves tonsillar wire
    nitinol shape-memory alloy
      wire
    olive wire
    outrigger wire
    over-tying wire
    pacing electrode wire
    pacing wire
    Pathfinder exchange
      guidewire
    Pathfinder wire
    PD orthodontic wire
    piston wire
    platinum wire
    prosthesis smooth wire
    protector plus wire
    Puestow wires
    pull-out wire
    pusher wire
    Quadcat wire
    QuickSilver hydrophilic-
      coated guidewire
    RadiMedical fiberoptic
      pressure-monitoring wire
    rectal cautery wire
    rectangular wire
    Remaloy wire
    Remanium wire
    Respond wire
    Risdon wire
    Roadrunner wire
    Robicheck wire
    Rosen guidewire
    Rosen wire
    Rotablator wire
    Rotafloppy wire
    round chuck-end Kirschner
      wire
    Sadowsky hook wire
    Sage wire
    Schuknecht wire
    Scimed-Choice floppy wire
    Seeker guidewire
    Seldinger retrograde wire
    separating wire
    Shiffrin bone wire
    Shinobi wire
    silk guidewire
    silver suture wire
    Silverstein malleus clip
      wire

wire (*continued*)

    Simcoe anterior chamber
      retaining wire
    Sippy esophageal dilator
      pusher wire
    smooth transfixion wire
    snare wire
    space-age wire
    spinous process wire
    square wire
    stainless steel wire
    steerable wire
    stencil wire
    Sterling-Spring orthodontic
      wire
    sternal wire
    Stertzer-Myler extension
      wire
    stiffening wire
    Stille Gigli-saw wire
    Storz twisted snare wire
    Stout continuous loop wire
    subcuticular wire
    sublaminar wire
    Surgaloy wire
    surgical grade stainless steel
      wire
    suture wire
    TAD guidewire
    tantalum wire
    Taper guidewire
    temporary pacing wire
    Terumo-Radiofocus
      hydrophilic polymer-coated
      guidewire
    Thiersch wire
    titanium wire
    tonsillar snare wire
    torque attenuating diameter
      wire
    Tracer wire
    Trailblazer wire
    trocar-point Kirschner
      wire
    trochanteric wire
    Truarch wire
    Ultra-Select nitinol PTCA
      guidewire
    ultrastiff wire
    veneer retention wire
    Waterston pacing wire
    Wildcat wire

wire (*continued*)
  Wironit clasp wire
  Wirotom clasp wire
  Zimaloy beaded suture wire
wire appliance
wire arch
wire bivalve vaginal speculum
wire bivalve obstetrical
  speculum
wire bivalve vaginal speculum
wire carbide-jaw suture
  scissors
wire crimper
wire cutter
wire drill
wire driver
wire extrusion
wire eye speculum
wire fixation
wire fixation bolt
wire frame spectacles
wire guide
wire insertion
wire knot
wire lid speculum
wire ligature
wire localization
wire loop
wire loop dilator
wire loop fixation
wire loop stapes dilator
wire mandrin
wire mesh eye implant
wire mesh graft
wire mesh implant
wire mesh prosthesis
wire needle holder
wire osteosynthesis
wire osteotomy plane
wire pass bur
wire passer
wire probe
wire prosthesis-crimping
  forceps
wire removal technique
wire saw
wire scissors
wire side blade
wire snare
wire speculum
wire splint
wire stapes prosthesis

wire stylet
wire stylet catheter
wire stabilization
wire stapes prosthesis
wire sutures
wire threader
wire tightener
wire twister
wire template
wire Zytor sutures
wire-bending die
wire-closure forceps
wire-crimper forceps
wire-crimping forceps
wire-cutting scissors
wire-cutting suture scissors
wired jaw
wire-fat ear prosthesis
Wirefoam splint
wire-Gelfoam prosthesis
wire-guided balloon-assisted
  endoscopic biliary stent
  exchange
wire-guided breast biopsy
wire-guided hydrostatic balloon
wire-guided metal spiral
  retrieval device
wire-guided oval intracostal
  dilator
wire-guided papillotome
wire-guided placement
wire-guided polyvinyl bougie
wire-guided sphincterotome
wire-loop keratoscope
wire-loop lesion
wire-loop strut
wire-mesh self-expandable stent
wire-passing awl
wire-passing bur
wire-pulling forceps
wire-tightening clamp
wire-twister needle holder
wire-twisting forceps
wire-winged lid speculum
wire-wound cannula
wire-wound endotracheal tube
wiring
  circumferential wiring
  circummandibular wiring
  circumzygomatic wiring
  compression wiring
  continuous loop wiring

wiring (*continued*)
  copper wiring
  Coventry wiring
  craniofacial suspension wiring
  Essig wiring
  facet fracture stabilization
    wiring
  facet subluxation stabilization
    wiring
  Gilmer wiring
  interfragmentary wiring
  interosseous wiring
  Ivy loop wiring
  mandibular wiring
  multiple loop wiring
  perialveolar wiring
  piriform aperture wiring
  pyriform aperture wiring
  Stout continuous wiring
  Stout wiring
  tension band wiring
wiring of jaw
wiring retractor
Wironit clasp wire
Wirosol investment material
Wirotom clasp wire
Wirovest investment material
Wirsung dilation
Wirsung duct
Wirsung pancreatic duct
Wirth-Jager posterior cruciate
    reconstruction
Wirth-Jager tendon technique
Wirthlin splenorenal clamp
Wirthlin splenorenal shunt
    clamp
Wisap diagnostic laparoscope
Wisap disposable cannula
Wisap disposable trocar
Wisap insufflator
Wisap operating laparoscope
Wisconsin laryngoscope
Wisconsin laryngoscope blade
Wise breast incision
Wise dilator
Wise iridotomy laser lens
Wise operation
Wise orbital retractor
Wise pattern in breast reduction
Wise pattern mastopexy
Wise retractor
Wise sphincterotomy laser lens

Wiseguide catheter
Wise-type pattern
Wis-Foregger laryngoscope
Wishard tip catheter
Wishard ureteral catheter
wishbone retractor
Wis-Hipple laryngoscope
Wissinger rod
Wissinger set
Wister forceps holder
Wister nipper
Wister vascular clamp
Wister wire-and-pin cutter
witch's chin deformity
Withers tendon passer
Witkop-von Sallman syndrome
Witt dental light
Wittner biopsy punch
Wittner cervical biopsy punch
Wittner cervical punch
Wittner uterine biopsy forceps
Witzel duodenostomy
Witzel enterostomy
Witzel enterostomy catheter
Witzel gastrostomy
Witzel jejunostomy
Witzel operation
Witzel tube
Witzel tunnel for feeding
    jejunostomy
Wixson hip positioner
Wizard cardiac device
Wizard disposable inflation
    device
Wizard gamma counter
Wizard microdebrider
Wizdom guidewire
W-J classification for staging of
    prostate cancer
Wladimiroff (*see* Vladimiroff)
Woakes nasal saw
Wobig entropion repair
Woelfe (*see* Wolfe)
Woelfer (*see* Wolfler)
Woetzer (*see* Wotzer)
Wölfe (*see* Wolfe)
Wolfe (*also* Wölfe, Woelfe)
Woelfe-Boehler cast breaker
Woelfe-Boehler cutter
Wohlfart-Kugelberg-Welander
    disease
Wolf antral needle

Wolf arthroscope
Wolf biopsy forceps
Wolf biting basket forceps
Wolf cannula
Wolf cataract delivery forceps
Wolf catheter
Wolf chisel knife
Wolf curved basket forceps
Wolf curved scissors
Wolf curved-basket forceps
Wolf dermal curet
Wolf disposable cannula
Wolf drain
Wolf drainage cannula
Wolf draw knife
Wolf endoscope
Wolf eye forceps
Wolf fiberoptic cord
Wolf full-thickness free graft
Wolf graft
Wolf hemostatic bag
Wolf implant
Wolf insufflation laparoscope
Wolf laparoscope
Wolf lithotrite
Wolf meniscal knife
Wolf meniscal retractor
Wolf mouth gag
Wolf needle trocar
Wolf nephrostomy catheter
Wolf nephrostomy bag catheter
Wolf panendoscope
Wolf Piezolith 2300 lithotripsy
    device
Wolf procedure for plantar
    callosity
Wolf prosthesis
Wolf return-flow cannula
Wolf rigid panendoscope
Wolf scissors
Wolf suction tube
Wolf uterine cuff forceps
Wolf-Castroviejo needle holder
Wolf-Cottle trocar
Wolfe (also Wölfe, Woelfe)
Wolfe breast carcinoma
    classification
Wolfe breast dysplasia
Wolfe cheiloplasty
Wolfe classification of breast
    dysplasia
Wolfe eye forceps

Wolfe graft
Wolfe implant
Wolfe loop electrode
Wolfe mammographic
    parenchymal patterns
Wolfe operation
Wolfe prosthesis
Wolfe ptosis operation
Wolfe uterine cuff forceps
Wölfe (see Wolfe)
Wolfe-Boehler cast breaker
Wolfe-Boehler cutter
Wolfe-Böhler cast remover
Wolfe-Böhler plaster cast
    spreader
Wolfe-Kawamoto bone graft
Wolfe-Kawamoto iliac graft
Wolfe-Krause graft
Wolfe-Krause implant
Wolfenden position
Wolferman drill
Wolff dermal curet
Wolff drain
Wolff operation
wolffian body
wolffian cyst
wolffian drain
wolffian duct
wolffian duct carcinoma
Wolf-Henning gastroscope
Wolf-Hirschhorn syndrome
Wolf-Knittlingen gastroscope
Wölfler (see Wolfler)
Wolfler (also Wölfler, Woelfler)
Wolfler gastroenterostomy
Wolfler gland
Wolfler operation
Wolfler sign
Wolfler suture technique
Wolfler sutures
Wolfman xanthomatosis
Wolf-Post rhinoscope
Wolfring glands
Wolf-Schindler gastroscope
Wolfson clamp
Wolfson forceps
Wolfson gallbladder retractor
Wolfson intestinal clamp
Wolfson retractor
Wolfson spur crusher
Wolfson spur-crushing clamp
Wolf-Veress needle

Wolf-Yoon applicator
Wolf-Yoon ring
Wolman xanthomatosis
Wolvek approximator
Wolvek fixation device
Wolvek sternal approximation
    fixation
Wolvek sternal approximation
    fixation device
Wolvek sternal approximator
Womack procedure
Wong-Staal scissors
Wood aortography needle
Wood applicator
Wood black light
Wood bulldog clamp
Wood colonic kit
Wood lamp
Wood needle
Wood operation
Wood osteotome
Wood screw
wood tongue blade
wood tongue depressor
Woodbridge sutures
Woodbridge tube
Wood-Doig vacuum biopsy
    instrument
Woodman operation
Woodruff catheter
Woodruff nasopalatine plexus
Woodruff screw
Woodruff screwdriver
Woodruff spatula knife
Woodruff ureteropyelographic
    catheter
Woods screw maneuver
Woods tonsillar scissors
Woodson dental periosteal
    elevator
Woodson double-ended
    dissector
Woodson dural separator
Woodson dural separator and
    packer
Woodson elevator
Woodson gauze packer
Woodson plug
Woodson probe
Woodson spatula
Woodson spoon
Woodward antral raspatory

Woodward elevation of scapula
Woodward
    esophagogastroscopy
Woodward
    esophagogastrostomy
Woodward hemostat
Woodward hemostatic forceps
Woodward operation
Woodward procedure
Woodward rasp
Woodward retractor
Woodward scapula procedure
Woodward sound
Woodward technique
Woodward thoracic artery
    forceps
Woodward thoracic hemostatic
    forceps
Woodward-Potts intestinal
    forceps
Wookey neck flap
Wookey pharyngoesophageal
    reconstruction
Wookey radical neck dissection
Wookey skin tube
wool roll dressing
Wooler mitral anuloplasty
Woolley tibia punch
Wool'n Gel seating cushion
Woolner tip
Wooten eye needle
Worcester City Hospital vaginal
    speculum
Worcester instrument holder
Word Bartholin gland catheter
Word catheter
Woringer-Kolopp disease
Work-Bruening diagnostic head
Workhorse percutaneous
    transluminal angioplasty
    balloon catheter
Workhorse PTCA balloon
    catheter
working bite relation
working diagnosis
working element resectoscope
working occlusal surface
working occlusion
working radiograph
world standard Olsen bipolar
    cable
worm-eaten appearance

wormian bone
wormy veins
Worrall deep retractor
Worrall headband
Worst corneal bur
Worst double-ended pigtail
    probe
Worst gonioprism contact lens
Worst intraocular lens
Worst lobster-claw lens
Worst Medallion lens
Worst Medallion sutures
Worst needle
Worst operation
Worst pigtail probe
Worth advancement forceps
Worth chisel
Worth cystitome
Worth muscle forceps
Worth operation
Worth ptosis operation
Worth strabismus forceps
Wötzer (see Wotzer)
Wotzer (also Wötzer, Woetzer)
Wotzer operation
wound
    3 zones of a burn wound
    abdominal gunshot wound
    aseptic wound
    avulsed wound
    blowing wound
    burn wound
    chronic wound
    clean wound
    closure of wound
    collagen hemostatic material
        for wounds
    contaminated wound
    contused wound
    corneal wound
    corneoscleral wound
    debridement of wound
    deep penetrating wound
    dehiscence of wound
    delayed closure of wound
    dirty wound
    disrupted operative wound
    disruption of operative
        wound
    drainage from wound
    drainage of wound
    draining wound

wound (continued)
    dressed wound
    exit wound
    flank gunshot wound
    flank wound
    fragment wound
    full-jacketed bullet wound
    fungating wound
    gaping wound
    granulating wound
    gunshot wound
    healing wound
    incised wound
    incision and packing of
        wound
    incision and resuture of
        wound
    infected wound
    lacerated wound
    laparoscopic trocar wound
    margin of wound
    minor wound
    missile-caused wound
    Mohs wound
    neck wound
    nonpenetrating wound
    open wound
    operative wound
    penetrating wound
    perforating wound
    pressure wound
    probing of wound
    problematic wound
    punctate wound
    puncture wound
    pyelotomy wound
    radiation wound
    redressed wound
    sacral wound
    secondary closure of wound
    separate stab wound
    septic wound
    seton wound
    silicone-treated wound
    spiral wound
    stab wound
    sternotomy wound
    subcutaneous wound
    sucking wound
    superficial wound
    surgical wound
    tangential wound

wound (*continued*)
  thoracotomy wound
  traumatic wound
  traumatopneic wound
  ulcerated wound
  V-shaped wound
wound abscess
wound approximation
wound ballistics
wound bed
wound biopsy
wound botulism
wound care
wound cautery
wound cavity
wound cleaning
wound clip
wound closure
wound complication
wound contraction
wound covering
wound debridement
wound dehiscence
wound discharge
wound disruption
wound drain
wound drainage
wound drainage collector
wound drainage reservoir
wound dressing
wound edge
wound entrance
wound excision
wound failure
wound fever
wound fibroblast
wound forceps
wound healing
wound hematoma
wound hernia
wound incision and suction
wound infection
wound irrigated
wound irrigation
wound ischemia
wound isolation
wound lip
wound margins
wound matrix contraction
wound necrosis
wound packed
wound protector

wound seroma
wound tensile strength
wound tension
wound towels
wound-clip forceps
Wound-Evac kit
Woun'Dres hydrogel dressing
Woun'Dres natural collagen
    hydrogel wound dressing
Wound-Span Bridge II dressing
woven bone
woven bougie
woven catheter
woven cotton gauze
woven Dacron catheter
woven Dacron graft
woven Dacron tube
woven elastic bandage
woven Teflon
woven-loop stone dislodger
woven-silk catheter
woven-tube vascular graft
    prosthesis
woven-tube vascular prosthesis
W-plasty in scar revision
W-plasty revision
wrap hematoma
wraparound dressing
wraparound flap
wraparound inactive electrode
wraparound neurovascular free
    flap
wraparound periapical lesion
wraparound splint
wrapping of abdominal aortic
    aneurysm
wrapping of aneurysm
Wrattan eye filter
wrench
  Allen wrench
  Barton tongs wrench
  compression wrench
  Fox wrench
  Harrington flat wrench
  hexagonal wrench
  Kurlander orthopedic wrench
  orthopedic wrench
  slotted wrench
  socket wrench
  Stader wrench
  T-handle wrench
  Thomas Waldon wrench

wrench (*continued*)
   tightening wrench
   torque ratchet wrench
   torque wrench
   Wilson wrench
Wright Care-TENS device
Wright Care-TENS unit
Wright fascia needle
Wright knee plate
Wright knee prosthesis
Wright maneuver
Wright nasal snare
Wright needle
Wright operation
Wright ophthalmic needle
Wright peak flowmeter
Wright plate
Wright pneumatic tourniquet
Wright ptosis needle
Wright respirometer
Wright snare
Wright test
Wright tonsillar snare
Wright Universal brace
Wright version
Wright-Crawford needle
Wright-Giemsa evaluation
Wright-Guilford cutting block
Wright-Guilford curet
Wright-Guilford double-edged
   knife
Wright-Guilford drum elevator
Wright-Guilford elevator knife
Wright-Guilford flap knife
Wright-Guilford footplate pick
Wright-Guilford incudostapedial
   knife
Wright-Guilford middle ear
   instrument
Wright-Guilford roller knife
Wright-Guilford stapes pick
Wright-Guilford wire cutter
Wrightington radiograph
Wright-Rubin forceps
Wright-Rubin forceps guard
Wrigley forceps
wringer injury
wrinkle line
wrinkled tongue
wrinkling membrane
Wrisberg cartilage
Wrisberg ganglion

Wrisberg lesion
Wrisberg ligament
Wrisberg nerve
Wrisberg tubercle
wrist
   center of rotation of wrist
   CFV wrist
   coronal MRI of wrist
   degenerative joint of wrist
   dynamic instability of wrist
   extensor retinaculum of wrist
   Gill-Stein arthrodesis of wrist
   Hamas total wrist
   metacarpal of wrist
   midcarpal disarticulation of
      wrist
   range of motion of the wrist
   SLAC wrist
   spaghetti wrist
   static instability of wrist
   sulcus of wrist
wrist arthrodesis
wrist block
wrist bone
wrist deformity
wrist disarticulation
wrist dislocation
wrist drop
wrist excision
wrist extension
wrist flexion
wrist flexion test
wrist fusion
wrist ganglion
wrist ganglionectomy
wrist joint
wrist mechanics
wrist prosthesis
wrist radial deviation
wrist reconstruction
Wrist Restore brace
wrist restraint
wrist scar
wrist ulnar deviation
Wristaleve
Wristaleve support
wrist-driven prehension orthosis
wristdrop
wrist-hand orthosis (WHO)
W-shape forceps
W-shaped anal anastomosis
W-shaped ileal pouch

W-shaped ileal pouch-anal
   anastomosis
W-shaped incision
W-shaped pouch
W-sitting position
Wucher atrophy
Wuerzberg (see Wurzburg)
Wullen stone dislodger
Wullstein bur
Wullstein chuck adapter
Wullstein curet
Wullstein double-edged knife
Wullstein drill
Wullstein ear forceps
Wullstein ear knife
Wullstein ear scissors
Wullstein ear self-retaining
   retractor
Wullstein high-speed bur
Wullstein microsuction tube
Wullstein ototympanoscope
   otoscope
Wullstein retractor
Wullstein ring curet
Wullstein scissors
Wullstein self-retaining ear
   retractor
Wullstein transplant spatula
Wullstein tympanoplasty
Wullstein tympanoplasty forceps
Wullstein-House cup-shaped
   forceps
Wullstein-House forceps
Wullstein-Paparella forceps
Wullstein-Weitlaner self-retaining
   retractor
Wullstein-Weitlaner self-retaining
   retractor
Wullstein-Zollner operation
Wunderer modification activator
Wurd catheter
Wurmuth spatula
Wurth spur crusher
Wurth vein stripper
Wurzburg (also Würzburg,
   Wuerzburg)
Würzburg (see Wurzburg)
Wurzburg (see Wurzburg)

Wurzburg plate
Wurzburg plating set
Wurzburg-Walter Lorenz rigid
   fixation set
Wurzelheber dental elevator
Wutzer hernia
Wutzer operation
Wutzler circumcision scissors
Wutzler scissors
W-V palatal repositioning
W-Y operation
W-Y palatal repositioning
W-Y palatoplasty
Wyburn-Mason syndrome
Wyeth amputation
Wyeth operation
Wyler subdural strip electrode
Wylie J clamp
Wylie carotid artery clamp
Wylie dilator
Wylie drain
Wylie endarterectomy set
Wylie endarterectomy spatula
Wylie endarterectomy stripper
Wylie forceps
Wylie hypogastric clamp
Wylie lumbar bulldog clamp
Wylie operation
Wylie pessary
Wylie renal vein retractor
Wylie spatula
Wylie splanchnic retractor
Wylie stem pessary
Wylie stripper
Wylie tenaculum forceps
Wylie uterine dilator
Wylie uterine director
Wylie uterine forceps
Wylie uterine tenaculum
Wylie uterine tenaculum forceps
Wylie-Post rhinoscope
Wyllys-Andrews operation
Wynn cleft lip operation
Wynn cleft lip repair
Wynne-Evans tonsillar
   dissector
Wyse reduction mammaplasty
Wysler sutures

X-body
X-paralysis
X-Acto blade
X-Acto gouge
X-Acto knife
Xanar CO$_2$ laser
Xanar laser adapter
Xanar laser bronchoscope
xanthelasmatosis
xanthochromia
xanthoderma
xanthogranulomatous
xanthoma of joint
xanthomatosis of bone
Xantopren impression material
Xase complex
X-Cel dental x-ray unit
X-clamp
XECT (xenon-enhanced
    computed tomography)
Xemex pulmonary artery catheter
XenoDerm graft
xenogeneic bone
xenogeneic graft
xenograft
    bovine pericardial heart valve
        xenograft
    Carpentier-Edwards xenograft
    Hancock porcine xenograft
    Ionescu-Shiley pericardial
        xenograft
    pericardial xenograft
    porcine xenograft
    swine xenograft
xenograft heart valve
xenograft transplantation
xenograft wound covering
Xenomedica prosthetic valve
xenon arc coagulator
xenon arc photocoagulation
    cautery
xenon arc photocoagulator
xenon cold light fountain

xenon lamp
xenon lung ventilation imaging
xenon photocoagulator
xenon ventilation scan
xenon-133 technique
xenon-chloride excimer
xenon-enhanced computed
    tomography (XECT)
xenon-washout technique
Xenophor femoral prosthesis
Xenotech graft
Xenotech prosthetic
Xenotech prosthetic valve
xenotransplantation
Xeroflo dressing
Xeroform dressing
Xeroform gauze
xerogram
xerography
xeroma
xeromammogram
xeromammography
xeromycteria
xerophthalmia
xeroradiography
xerostomia
xerostomic mucositis
xerotic keratitis
Ximed disposable cannula
Ximed disposable trocar
xiphicostal
xiphisternal crunching sound
xiphisternal joint
xiphisternum
xiphoid angle
xiphoid cartilage
xiphoid process
xiphoid to os pubis incision
xiphoid to umbilicus incision
xiphoidectomy
xiphoid-to-pubis midline
    abdominal incision
xiphoid-to-umbilicus incision

xiphomanubrial junction
xiphoumbilical depression
Xi-scan fluoroscope
XL illuminator
X-long cement forceps
Xoman drill
Xomed Doyle nasal airway splint
Xomed dual-chamber balloon
Xomed endotracheal tube
Xomed intraoral artificial larynx
Xomed Kartush insulated
    retractor
Xomed Kartush tympanic
    membrane patcher
Xomed micro-oscillating saw
Xomed rectal probe
Xomed Silastic splint
Xomed sinus irrigation kit
Xomed sinus-secretion collector
Xomed straight-shank tube
Xomed Treace ventilation tube
Xomed Tytan ventilation tube
Xomed-Treace nerve integrity
    monitor
XP peritympanic hearing
    instrument
Xpanderm
Xpeedior catheter
XPS Straightshot micro tissue
    resector
x-ray
    abdominal x-ray (AXR)
    chest x-ray
    diagnostic x-ray
    foreign body seen on x-ray
    Hughston knee view on x-ray
    inversion ankle stress x-ray
    KUB x-ray
    Nulling pattern on x-ray
    Overhauser effect on x-ray
    Panorex x-ray
    plain x-ray
    plantar axial x-ray
    prior to x-ray
    refracted x-ray
    repeat chest x-ray
    rising sun appearance of
        olecranon on x-ray
    serial cephalometric x-rays
    serial chest x-rays
    signet ring sign on x-ray
    strain x-rays
    sunrise view of patella on x-ray

x-ray (*continued*)
    sunset view of patella on x-ray
    supinated oblique view on x-ray
    swimmer's view of cervical
        spine on x-ray
    tangential view on x-ray
    Towne view of skull on x-ray
    trumpeting on x-ray
    tunnel view on x-ray
    ultra x-ray
    Ward triangle on pelvic x-ray
    West Point view of shoulder
        on x-ray
    wet reading of x-ray
    Winberger line on x-ray
    Y-line on x-ray
    Y-view on x-ray
x-ray absorptiometry
x-ray absorption
x-ray beam
x-ray burn
x-ray calipers
x-ray cassette
x-ray control
x-ray dermatitis
x-ray detectable laparotomy
    sponge
x-ray dosage
x-ray findings
x-ray generator
x-ray image
x-ray microscope
x-ray pelvimetry
x-ray study
x-ray template
x-ray therapy
x-ray tomographic microscope
x-ray tube
x-ray view
XRT (x-ray therapy)
X-Sizer catheter
XT coronary stent
XT radiopaque coronary stent
Xtra Gentle surgical tape
X-Trode electrode catheter
X-Trode stent
XXL balloon dilatation catheter
Xylocaine jelly
Xylocaine with epinephrine
Xyrel pacemaker
xyster raspatory
Xyticon bipolar demand
    pacemaker

Y axis
Y B Sore cushion
Y-angle
Y-body
Y-cartilage
Y-configuration closure
Y-flap
Y-incision
Y-mesh hernia repair
Yacoub and Radley-Smith
     classification
Y adapter
Yaeger lid plate
YAG (yttrium-aluminum-garnet)
YAG laser
YAG laser capsulotomy
Yale brace
Yale Luer-Lok needle
Yale Luer-Lok syringe
Yalon intraocular lens
Yamagishi stapler
Yamanda myelotomy knife
Yang needle
Yankauer antral punch
Yankauer antral punch tip
Yankauer antral trocar
Yankauer aspirating tube
Yankauer bronchoscope
Yankauer catheter
Yankauer ear curet
Yankauer esophagoscope
Yankauer ether inhaler
Yankauer ethmoid forceps
Yankauer ethmoid-cutting
     forceps
Yankauer eustachian catheter
Yankauer eustachian
     instruments
Yankauer hook
Yankauer laryngoscope
Yankauer ligature passer
Yankauer middle meatus cannula
Yankauer multi-orifice tip

Yankauer nasopharyngeal
     speculum
Yankauer nasopharyngoscope
Yankauer needle
Yankauer operation
Yankauer periosteal elevator
Yankauer pharyngeal speculum
Yankauer probe
Yankauer punch
Yankauer salpingeal curet
Yankauer salpingeal knife
Yankauer salpingeal probe
Yankauer scissors
Yankauer septal needle
Yankauer single-orifice tip
Yankauer speculum
Yankauer suction
Yankauer suction technique
Yankauer suction tip
Yankauer suction tube
Yankauer suture needle
Yankauer tonsil suction tip
Yankauer tonsillar scissors
Yankauer trocar
Yankauer washing tube
Yankauer-Little tube forceps
Yannuzzi fundus laser lens
Yarmo morcellizer
Yarsargil bayonet needle holder
Yasargil aneurysm clip-applier
Yasargil aneurysmal clip
Yasargil angled forceps
Yasargil applying forceps
Yasargil arachnoid knife
Yasargil artery forceps
Yasargil bayonet needle holder
Yasargil bayonet scissors
Yasargil bipolar forceps
Yasargil carotid clamp
Yasargil clip
Yasargil clip applier
Yasargil clip-applying forceps
Yasargil craniotomy

Yasargil cross-legged clip
Yasargil curet
Yasargil dissector
Yasargil flat serrated ring
    forceps
Yasargil instrument
Yasargil knife
Yasargil ligature carrier
Yasargil microclip
Yasargil microdissector
Yasargil microforceps
Yasargil microinstruments
Yasargil microneedle holder
Yasargil microraspatory
Yasargil microscissors
Yasargil microscope
Yasargil microsuction tube
Yasargil microvascular bayonet
    scissors
Yasargil microvessel clip-
    applying forceps
Yasargil needle holder
Yasargil neurological instrument
Yasargil neurosurgical bipolar
    forceps
Yasargil permanent aneurysm
    clip
Yasargil pituitary rongeur
Yasargil raspatory
Yasargil retractor
Yasargil scissors
Yasargil scoop
Yasargil spring hook
Yasargil straight forceps
Yasargil suction tube
Yasargil surgical microscope
Yasargil technique
Yasargil-Aesculap instrument
Yasargil-Aesculap spring clip
Yasargil-Leyla brain retractor
Yashica Dental Eye camera
Yates correction
Yazujian cataract bur
Yazujian eye knife
Y-bandage
Y-bandage dressing
Y-bone plate
Y-connector
Y-double incision
Y-drain
Yeates drain
Yeder suction tube

Yee posterior shoulder
    approach
Yellen circumcision clamp
yellow body
yellow bone marrow
yellow cartilage
yellow fibers
yellow lesion
yellow ligament
yellow marrow
yellow nail syndrome
yellow point
Yellow Springs probe
yellow-eyed dilating bougie
yellow-ochre hemorrhage
yellow-tip aspirator
Yeoman biopsy punch
Yeoman probe
Yeoman proctoscope
Yeoman punch
Yeoman rectal biopsy forceps
Yeoman sigmoidoscope
Yeoman test
Yeoman uterine biopsy forceps
Yeoman uterine forceps
Yeoman-Wittner rectal biopsy
    forceps
Yeoman-Wittner rectal forceps
Yergason sign for subluxation of
    biceps tendon
Y-fracture
Y-glass rod
Y-graft
Y-hook
Yield nonadherent gauze dressing
Y-incision
Y-Knot device
Y-ligament
Y-line
Y-line on x-ray
Y-nailing of arm
yoke block
yoke bone
yoke of mandible
yoke of maxilla
yoke transposition procedure
yoked muscles
Yoon fallopian tube ligation ring
Yoon tubal sterilization ring
Yoon ring applicator
York-Mason incision
York-Mason procedure

York-Mason repair
Yoshida dental x-ray unit
Yoshida tonsil dissector
Y-osteotomy
Yotsuyanagi retroauricular
  chondrocutaneous flap
Youens lens manipulation
  cannula
Youlten nasal inspiratory peak
  flow meter
Young anterior prostatic
  retractor
Young approach
Young bifid retractor
Young bladder retractor
Young boomerang needle
  holder
Young bulb retractor
Young clamp
young cyst
Young cystoscope
Young cystoscopic rongeur
Young dilator
Young dissector
Young epispadias repair
Young flatfoot procedure
Young forceps
Young intestinal forceps
Young lateral prostatic retractor
Young lateral retractor
Young ligature carrier
Young lobe forceps
Young needle holder
young onset cancer
Young operation for talipes
  valgus
Young pediatric rectal dilator
Young pelvic fracture
  classification
Young procedure
Young prostatectomy
Young prostatectomy forceps
Young prostatic enucleator
Young prostatic forceps
Young prostatic retractor
Young prostatic tractor
Young rectal dilator
Young renal pedicle clamp
Young rubber dam fracture
  frame
Young rubber dam holder
Young technique

Young tongue forceps
Young tongue-seizing forceps
Young tractor
Young epispadias repair
Young urological dissector
Young uterine forceps
Young vaginal dilator
Young vasectomy
Young-Dees bladder neck
  reconstruction
Young-Dees operation
Young-Dees procedure
Young-Dees technique
Young-Dees-Leadbetter bladder
  neck reconstruction
Young-Dees-Leadbetter
  operation
Younge endometrial curet
Younge irrigator
Younge uterine biopsy curet
Younge uterine biopsy forceps
Younge uterine curet
Younge uterine forceps
Younge-Kevorkian forceps
Young-Hryntschak boomerang
  needle holder
Young-Millin boomerang needle
  holder
Yount fasciotomy
Yount operation
Yount procedure
Y-plasty
Y-plasty procedure
Y-plate
Y-port connector
Y-screw
Y-shaped fracture
Y-shaped graft
Y-shaped incision
Y-shaped scar
Y-shaped skin paddle
YSI Foley probe
YSI neonatal temperature probe
Y-suture technique
Y-sutures
Y-T fracture
Y-trough catheter
yttrium pellets
yttrium-aluminum-garnet (YAG)
yttrium-aluminum-garnet laser
  (YAG laser)
Y-tube

Z

Z-angle
Z-clamp hysterectomy forceps
Z-cleft palate repair
Z-cut osteotomy
Z-direction
Z-disk
z-epicanthoplasty
Z-excision
Z-fixation nail
Z-flap incision
Z-incision
Z-line
Z-mammaplasty
Z-marginal tenotomy
Z-Med balloon catheter
Z-plane
Z-plastic relaxing operation
Z-plasty
   4-flap Z-plasty
   Cozen-Brockway Z-plasty
   double opposing Z-plasty
   Furlow double Z-plasty
   Furlow double opposing
     Z-plasty
   Furlow double reversing Z-
     plasty
   Nahigian Z-plasty
   Spencer-Watson Z-plasty
   Straith Z-plasty
   Tennison Z-plasty
Z-plasty approach
Z-plasty closure
Z-plasty for ectropion
Z-plasty incision
Z-plasty local flap graft
Z-plasty operation
Z-plasty procedure
Z-plasty revision
Z-plasty scar
Z-plasty technique
Z-plasty transposition
Z-plate
Z-point

Z-procedure
Z-retractor
Z sampler endometrial sampling
   device
Z-Sampler endometrial suction
   curet
Z-Scissors hysterectomy
   scissors
Z-screw
Z-shaped anastomosis
Z-shaped incision
Z-shaped scar
Z-shaped suture line
Z-stent
Z-suture technique
Z-sutures
Z-technique in laparoscopy
Z-track
ZTT acetabular cup
Z-type deformity
Z-wave tube
Zachary-Cope clamp
Zachary-Cope-DeMartel clamp
Zachary-Cope-DeMartel colon
   clamp
Zachary-Cope-DeMartel triple-
   colon clamp
Zadik ingrown nail procedure
Zahn lines
Zahn ribs
Zahradnicek operation
Zaias nail biopsy
Zalkind lung retractor
Zalkind-Balfour center-blade
   retractor
Zalkind-Balfour self-retaining
   retractor
Zalkind-Balfour blade
Zamboni biopsy solution
Zamorano-Dujovny localizing
   unit
Zancolli capsulodesis
Zancolli capsuloplasty

Zancolli capsulorrhaphy of
    fingers
Zancolli clawhand deformity
Zancolli claw-hand deformity
    repair
Zancolli lasso intrinsicplasty
Zancolli lasso tendon transfer
Zancolli operation
Zancolli procedure for clawhand
    deformity
Zancolli reconstruction
Zancolli rerouting technique
Zancolli static lock procedure
Zancolli laser procedure
Zanelli position
Zang metatarsal cap implant
Zang space
Zarins-Rowe ligament technique
Zarins-Rowe procedure
Zaufel bone rongeur
Zaufel sign
Zaufel-Jansen bone rongeur
Zaufel-Jansen ear hook
Zavala lung biopsy needle
Zavala technique
Zavanelli maneuver
Zavod bronchospirometry
    catheter
Zazepen-Gamidov technique
Zebra exchange guidewire
Zeichner implant
Zeimman herniorrhaphy
Zein loop
Zeir procedure for long thoracic
    nerve palsy
Zeiss aspheric lens
Zeiss beam splitter
Zeiss binocular head magnifier
Zeiss binocular prism telescope
Zeiss binocular tube
Zeiss camera equipment
Zeiss carbon arc slit lamp
Zeiss cine adapter
Zeiss coagulator
Zeiss diploscope microscope
Zeiss drape
Zeiss electron microscope
Zeiss endoscope
Zeiss eyepiece
Zeiss fundus camera
Zeiss gonioscope
Zeiss glands

Zeiss goniolens
Zeiss hammer lamp
Zeiss instruments
Zeiss lens loupe
Zeiss light coagulation for
    retinal detachment
Zeiss microscope
Zeiss microscope eyepiece
Zeiss operating camera
Zeiss operating field loupe
Zeiss operating microscope
Zeiss ophthalmological
    instruments
Zeiss ophthalmic surgical
    microscope
Zeiss ophthalmoscope
Zeiss phase-contrast microscope
Zeiss photocoagulator
Zeiss projection lensometer
Zeiss surgical microscope
Zeiss surgical laser
Zeiss slit lamp
Zeiss small-beam splitter
Zeiss stone dislodger
Zeiss unit
Zeiss ureteral stone dislodger
Zeiss vertex refractionometer
Zeiss-Barraquer cine microscope
Zeiss-Barraquer surgical
    microscope
Zeiss-Bruening anastigmatic
    auriscope
Zeiss-Cohan-Barraquer
    microscope
Zeiss-Contraves operating
    microscope
Zeiss-Gullstrand lens
Zeiss-Gullstrand loupe
Zeiss-Jena surgical microscope
Zeiss-Nordenson fundus camera
Zeiss-Opton ophthalmoscope
Zeiss-Scheimpflug camera
Zelicof orthopedic awl
Zelsmyr Cytobrush cell collector
    for Pap smear
Zenith endovascular graft
Zenker dissecting and ligature
    forceps
Zenker diverticulum
Zenker fixation
Zenker forceps
Zenker pouch

Zenker raspatory
Zenker retractor
Zenotech graft
Zenotech graft material
Zenotech synthetic ligament
Zephyr rubber elastic dressing
Zeppelin clamp
Zeppelin obstetrical forceps
zero variance of articular
    surfaces
Zerowet splash shield irrigator
Zervas hypophysectomy kit
Zest Anchor Advanced
    Generation (ZAAG) bone
    anchor
Zest implant
Zest implant anchor
Zest subperiosteal implant
Zeta probe nylon filter
ZF (zygomaticofrontal)
ZF region
ZF suture
Zickel classification
Zickel subtrochanteric rod
Zickel intramedullary nail
Zickel nail fixation
Zickel nailing of femur
Zickel subtrochanteric fracture
    operation
Zickel supracondylar rod
Ziegler blade
Ziegler cauterization
Ziegler cautery
Ziegler cautery electrode
Ziegler cilia forceps
Ziegler dilator
Ziegler ectropion repair
Ziegler electrocautery
Ziegler eye needle-knife
Ziegler eye speculum
Ziegler forceps
Ziegler iridectomy
Ziegler iris knife
Ziegler iris knife-needle
Ziegler iris needle
Ziegler knife
Ziegler knife-needle
Ziegler lacrimal dilator
Ziegler lacrimal probe
Ziegler needle
Ziegler needle probe
Ziegler needle-knife

Ziegler operation
Ziegler probe
Ziegler puncture
Ziegler speculum
Ziegler wash bottle
Ziegler-Furniss clamp
Zielke bifid hook
Zielke curet
Zielke derotator bar
Zielke gouge
Zielke instrument for scoliosis
    spinal fusion
Zielke pedicular instrumentation
Zielke rod
Zielke scoliosis gouge
Zielke screw
Zieman hernia repair
Zieman operation
ZIFT (zygote intrafallopian tube
    transfer)
zigzag approach
zigzag bilateral cleft lip repair
zigzag compensatory deformity
zigzag finger incision
zigzag incision
zigzag repair
zigzag stent
zigzagplasty
Zim carpal tunnel projection
Zimalate twist drill
Zimalate twist drill bit
Zimaloy beaded suture wire
Zimaloy cobalt-chromium-
    molybdenum alloy
Zimaloy epiphyseal staple
Zimaloy femoral head prosthesis
Zimaloy hip prosthesis
Zimaloy knee prosthesis
Zimaloy operation
Zimaloy staple
Zimany bilobed flap
Zimberg esophageal hiatal
    retractor
Zimcode traction frame
Zimcode traction frames tractor
Zimfoam finger splint
Zimfoam head halter
Zimfoam head halter traction
Zimfoam pad
Zimfoam pad and patient
    positioner
Zimfoam padding

Zimfoam pin
Zimfoam splint
Zimmer airplane splint
Zimmer antiembolism support
   stockings
Zimmer arm sling
Zimmer arthroscope
Zimmer bolt
Zimmer bone cement
Zimmer bur
Zimmer cartilage clamp
Zimmer hip prosthesis
Zimmer clamp
Zimmer clavicular cross sling
Zimmer clavicular cross splint
Zimmer clip
Zimmer hip screw
Zimmer dermatome
Zimmer drill
Zimmer driver
Zimmer driver-extractor
Zimmer extractor
Zimmer femoral condyle blade
   plate
Zimmer fracture frame
Zimmer frame
Zimmer Gigli-saw blade
Zimmer goniometer
Zimmer gouge
Zimmer hand drill
Zimmer head halter
Zimmer hip plate
Zimmer intramedullary knee
   instrumentation
Zimmer intramedullary nail
Zimmer low viscosity cement
Zimmer low viscosity adhesive
Zimmer nail
Zimmer Orthair oscillator
Zimmer Orthair ream driver
Zimmer Orthair reciprocator
Zimmer Orthairtome
Zimmer osteotomy
Zimmer pin
Zimmer prosthesis
Zimmer protractor
Zimmer saw
Zimmer screw
Zimmer screwdriver
Zimmer shoulder prosthesis
Zimmer skin graft mesher
Zimmer sling

Zimmer snare
Zimmer splint
Zimmer Statak sutures
Zimmer suction irrigator
Zimmer telescoping nail
Zimmer Ti-BAC acetabular
   components
Zimmer tibial bolt
Zimmer tibial nail cap
Zimmer tibial prosthesis
Zimmer total hip prosthesis
Zimmer Universal drill
Zimmer Universal knee
   immobilizer with Zimfoam
   padding
Zimmer-Hoen forceps
Zimmer-Kirschner hand drill
Zimmerman
   vascular pericyte of
   Zimmerman
Zimmerman operation
Zimmer-Schlesinger forceps
Zimmon biliary stent
Zimmon catheter
Zimmon endoscopic biliary
   stent set
Zimmon endoscopic pancreatic
   stent set
Zimmon esophagogastric
   balloon tamponade set
Zimmon papillotome
Zimmon sphincterotome
Zim-Trac traction splint
Zim-Trac traction splint tractor
Zim-Zip rib belt splint
zinc ball electrode
zinc gelatin impregnated gauze
zinc oxide bandage
zinc oxide-eugenol dental
   sealant (ZOE dental sealant)
zinc oxide-eugenol impression
   material
Zinco fixed ankle walker
Zinco shoulder immobilizer
Zinco thoracolumbar brace
Zinn annulus
Zinn aponeurosis
Zinn artery
Zinn cap
Zinn circle
Zinn circlet
Zinn corona

Zinn endoillumination infusion
   cannula
Zinn ligament
Zinn membrane
Zinn tendon
Zinn zone
Zinn zonule
Zinnanti clamp
Zinnanti uterine
   manipulator/injector
Zinnanti uterine manipulator
Zinnanti Z-clamp
Zipper anti-disconnect device
Zipper hypoallergenic
   tracheostomy tube neck
   band
zipper ring
zipper scar
zippered mesh
Zipser meatal clamp
Zipser meatal dilator
Zipser penile clamp
Zipster rib guillotine
Zipzoc compression wrap
Zipzoc stocking compression
   dressing
Ziramic femoral head prosthesis
Zirconia orthopedic prosthesis
Zirconia orthopedic prosthetic
   head
zirconium silicate abrasive
Zitelli bilobed nasal flap
Zitron pacemaker
Zlotsky-Ballard
   acromioclavicular injury
   classification
ZMC (zygomatic maxillary
   complex)
Zmurkiewicz brain clip
Zmurkiewicz clip applier
Zoalite lamp
Zobec sponge dressing
Zocchi ultrasound-assisted
   lipoplasty technique
ZOE dental sealant (zinc oxide
   eugenol dental sealant)
Zoeffle soft intraocular lens
Zoellner hook
Zoellner needle
Zoellner raspatory
Zoellner scissors
Zoellner stapes hook

Zoellner-Clancy procedure
Zoladex implant
Zoll defibrillator
Zoll noninvasive pacemaker
Zoll external defibrillator
Zollinger classification
Zollinger leg holder
Zollinger multipurpose tissue
   forceps
Zollinger splint
Zollinger-Ellison syndrome
Zollinger-Ellison tumor
Zollinger-Gilmore vein stripper
Zollner line
Zöllner (*see* Zollner)
Zollner (*also* Zöllner, Zoellner)
Zoellner (*see* Zollner)
Zollner suction tube
zonal aberration
zonal anatomy
zonal approach to the midface
zonary placenta
Zonas porous adhesive tape
   dressing
Zonas porous tape
zone
   abdominal wall zones (1-4)
   barrier zone
   basement membrane zone
   basement tissue zone
   buccomandibular zone
   calcification zone
   cell-free zone
   cell-poor zone
   cell-rich zone
   cornuradicular zone
   degenerative zone
   dentofacial zone
   echo zone
   facial danger zones
   flexor zone
   grenz zone
   high pressure zone (HPZ)
   inflammatory zone
   intermediate zone
   interpalpebral zone
   Lissauer zone
   Looser zone
   Marchant zone
   marginal zone
   middle zone
   necrotic zone

zone (*continued*)
 occlusal zone
 subpapillary zone
 vermilion transitional zone
 vermilion zone
 Weil basal zone
 Zinn zone
zone of injury
zonogram
zonography
zonular cataract
zonular fibers
zonular placenta
zonular space
zonule fibers
zonule of Zinn
zonule separator
zonule stripper
zonulolysis
zonulysis
zoograft
zooplastic graft
zooplasty
Zoroc resin plaster dressing
zosteriform
Zovickian flap
Zower speculum
Zucker cardiac catheter
Zucker multipurpose bipolar
 catheter
Zucker splint
Zuckerkandls dehiscence
Zucker-Myler cardiac device
Zuelzer awl
Zuelzer hook plate
Zuelzer plate
Zuker-Manketlow technique
Zuker bipolar pacing electrode
Zuma coronary guiding
 catheter
Zuma guiding catheter
ZUMI uterine manipulator
Zurich dilatation catheter
Zurich growth centile diagram
Zwanck radium pessary
Zweifel angiotribe
Zweifel angiotribe forceps
Zweifel appendectomy clamp
Zweifel needle holder
Zweifel pressure clamp
Zweifel-DeLee cranioclast
Zweymuller hip prosthesis

Zweymuller-Alloclassic
 prosthesis
Zyclast collagen
Zyderm collagen implant
Zyderm collagen injection
Zyderm collagen
Zyderm implant
Zyderm injection
Zydone analgesic
zygapophyseal joint
zygion (*pl.* zygia)
zygodactyly
zygoma elevator
zygoma fracture
zygoma hook
zygomatic arch fracture
zygomatic arch radiograph
zygomatic body fracture
zygomatic bone
zygomatic branch
zygomatic breadth
zygomatic buttress of maxilla
zygomatic complex fracture
zygomatic crest of great wing of
 sphenoid bone
zygomatic eminence
zygomatic fissure
zygomatic foramen
zygomatic fossa
zygomatic ligament
zygomatic malar complex (ZMC)
zygomatic margin
zygomatic maxillary complex
 (ZMC)
zygomatic maxillary complex
 fracture
zygomatic muscle
zygomatic nerve
zygomatic osteocutaneous
 ligament
zygomatic osteomyelitis
zygomatic process of frontal
 bone
zygomatic process of maxilla
zygomatic process of temporal
 bone
zygomatic recess
zygomatic reflex
zygomatic region
zygomatic retaining ligament
zygomatic suture line
zygomatic tubercle

zygomatic-coronoid ankylosis
zygomaticoauricular
zygomaticofacial branch
zygomaticofacial canal
zygomaticofacial foramen
zygomaticofacial nerve
zygomaticofrontal (ZF)
zygomaticofrontal region
zygomaticofrontal suture
zygomaticofrontal suture lines
zygomaticomandibular muscle
zygomaticomaxillary buttress
zygomaticomaxillary complex
zygomaticomaxillary fracture
zygomaticomaxillary
    hypoplasia
zygomaticomaxillary osteotomy
zygomaticomaxillary region
zygomaticomaxillary suture
zygomatico-orbital artery
zygomatico-orbital foramen
zygomatico-orbital fracture
zygomaticosphenoid fissure
zygomaticosphenoidal suture
zygomaticotemporal branch
zygomaticotemporal canal
zygomaticotemporal foramen
zygomaticotemporal nerve
zygomaticotemporal space
zygomaticotemporal suture
zygomaticus major muscle
zygomaticus minor muscle
zygomaticus muscle
zygomaxillare ridge
zygomaxillary point
zygote intrafallopian tube
    transfer (ZIFT)
Zyler head halter
Zyler tube
Zylik cannula
Zylik microclip
Zylik operation for talipes
    equinovarus
Zylik ophthalmoendoscope
Zylik-Joseph hook
Zylik-Michaels retractor
Zylik-Michaels scissors
Zylik-Michaels speculum
Zyoptix laser
Zyplast implant
Zyplast injectable collagen
Zyranox femoral head
Zytor sutures
Zywiec electrode